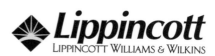

Pathophysiology
Concepts of Altered Health States

SIXTH EDITION

Pathophysiology
Concepts of Altered Health States

Carol Mattson Porth

RN, MSN, PhD (Physiology)
Professor Emeritus, School of Nursing
University of Wisconsin—Milwaukee
Milwaukee, Wisconsin

Mary Pat Kunert
RN, PhD
Consultant

With 28 Contributors

LIPPINCOTT WILLIAMS & WILKINS
A **Wolters Kluwer** Company

Philadelphia • Baltimore • New York • London
Buenos Aires • Hong Kong • Sydney • Tokyo

Acquisitions Editor: Lisa Stead
Managing Editor: Barclay Cunningham
Editorial Assistant: Karin McAndrews
Production Editor: Debra Schiff
Senior Production Manager: Helen Ewan
Art Director: Carolyn O'Brien
Interior Designer: Melissa Olson
Manufacturing Manager: William Alberti
Indexer: Maria Coughlin
Compositor: Circle Graphics
Printer: R.R. Donnelley-Willard

6th Edition

ISBN: 0-7817-2881-9

Care has been taken to confirm the accuracy of the information presented and to describe generally accepted practices. However, the authors, editors, and publisher are not responsible for errors or omissions or for any consequences from application of the information in this book and make no warranty, express or implied, with respect to the content of the publication.

The authors, editors, and publisher have exerted every effort to ensure that drug selection and dosage set forth in this text are in accordance with the current recommendations and practice at the time of publication. However, in view of ongoing research, changes in government regulations, and the constant flow of information relating to drug therapy and drug reactions, the reader is urged to check the package insert for each drug for any change in indications and dosage and for added warnings and precautions. This is particularly important when the recommended agent is a new or infrequently employed drug.

Some drugs and medical devices presented in this publication have Food and Drug Administration (FDA) clearance for limited use in restricted research settings. It is the responsibility of the health care provider to ascertain the FDA status of each drug or device planned for use in his or her clinical practice.

Learning without thought is labor lost.

—CONFUCIUS

*This book is dedicated to the students, past and present,
for whom this book was written.*

Contributors

Debra Ann Bancroft, R.N., M.S.N., F.N.P.-C.
Rheumatology Nurse Practitioner
Rheumatic Disease Center
Milwaukee, Wisconsin

Diane Book, M.D.
Assistant Professor, Neurology
Medical College of Wisconsin
Milwaukee, Wisconsin

Edward W. Carroll, M.S., Ph.D.
Clinical Assistant Professor
Department of Biomedical Sciences, College of Health Sciences
Marquette University
Milwaukee, Wisconsin

Kathryn Ann Caudell, R.N., Ph.D.
Clinical Research and Education Manager
Amgen-Oncology Professional Services
Edgewood, New Mexico

Robin Curtis, Ph.D.
Associate Professor, Retired
Department of Cellular Biology, Neurobiology, and Anatomy
The Medical College of Wisconsin
Milwaukee, Wisconsin

Sheila Curtis, R.N., M.S.
Senior Lecturer (Retired)
University of Wisconsin-Milwaukee, School of Nursing
Milwaukee, Wisconsin

Elizabeth C. Devine, R.N., Ph.D., F.A.A.N.
Professor, School of Nursing
University of Wisconsin-Milwaukee
Milwaukee, Wisconsin

Jane Dresser, R.N., M.N., M.E.D., A.P.N.
Clinical Specialist, Adult Mental Health
Medical Psychiatric Nursing Consultant Service
Milwaukee, Wisconsin

W. Michael Dunne, Jr., Ph.D. D.(A.B.M.M.)
Professor of Pathology and Immunology
Washington University School of Medicine
Medical Director, Microbiology
Barnes-Jewish Hospital
St. Louis, Missouri

Susan A. Fontana, R.N., Ph.D., C.S.-F.N.P. N.E.T.
Certified Family Nurse Practitioner
Associate Professor, School of Nursing
University of Wisconsin-Milwaukee
Milwaukee, Wisconsin

Kathryn J. Gaspard, Ph.D.
Senior Lecturer, School of Nursing
University of Wisconsin-Milwaukee
Milwaukee, Wisconsin

Clarence E. Grim, M.S., M.D., F.A.C.P., F.A.C.C.
Professor of Medicine and Epidemiology
Director, Hypertension Research Clinic
Medical College of Wisconsin
Milwaukee, Wisconsin

Carlene M. Grim, R.N., M.S.N., Sp. D.N.
President, Care Research and Education, Inc.
Milwaukee, Wisconsin

Kathleen E. Gunta, R.N., M.S.N., O.N.C.
Clinical Nurse Specialist, Orthopaedics
St. Luke's Medical Center
Milwaukee, Wisconsin

Safak Guven, M.D., F.A.C.P., F.A.C.E.
Associate Professor
Endocrinology, Diabetes, and Metabolism
American Hospital
Istanbul, Turkey

Candace L. Hennessy, R.N., Ph.D.
Patient Care Director
Froedtert Hospital
Milwaukee, Wisconsin

Georgianne H. Heymann, R.N., B.S.N.
Milwaukee, Wisconsin
Former Science Editor,
The New Book of Knowledge, Grollier Publishers

Mary Kay Jiricka, R.N., M.S.N., C.S., C.C.R.N.
Clinical Nurse Specialist
St. Luke's Medical Center
Milwaukee, Wisconsin

Julie A. Kuenzi, R.N., M.S.N., C.D.E, B.C.-A.D.M.
Diabetes Care Center Manager
Diabetes Nurse Specialist
Froedtert Hospital and Medical College of Wisconsin
Milwaukee, Wisconsin

Mary Pat Kunert, R.N., Ph.D.
Associate Professor
School of Nursing
Marquette University
Milwaukee, Wisconsin

Cyril Llamoso, M.D.
Infectious Disease Specialist
Milwaukee Health Services
Milwaukee, Wisconsin

Judy Wright Lott, R.N.C., D.S.N., N.N.P.
Associate Professor
Louise Herrington School of Nursing
Baylor University
Dallas, Texas

Glen Matfin, B.S.C., M.B. C.H.B., M.R.C.P.(UK),
    F.A.C.E, F.A.C.P.
Medical Cardiovascular and Metabolism Research
Bayer Pharmaceuticals
West Haven, Connecticut

Patricia McCowen Mehring, R.N.C., M.S.N., O.G.N.P.
Department of Obstetrics and Gynecology,
Division of Reproductive Medicine
Medical College of Wisconsin
Milwaukee, Wisconsin

Janice Smith Pigg, B.S.N., R.N., M.S.
Nurse Consultant-Rheumatology
Smith-Pigg Consultants
Cedarburg, Wisconsin

Janice Kuiper Pikna, M.S.N., R.N., C.S.
Clinical Nurse Specialist, Gerontology
Froedtert Hospital, Senior Health Program
Milwaukee, Wisconsin

Joan Pleuss, M.S., R.D., C.D.E.
Senior Research Dietitian
Clinical Research Center
Medical College of Wisconsin, Froedtert Memorial
    Lutheran Hospital
Milwaukee, Wisconsin

Gladys Simandl, R.N., Ph.D.
Associate Professor
Columbia College of Nursing
Milwaukee, Wisconsin

Cynthia V. Sommer, Ph.D., M.T.(A.S.C.P.)
Associate Professor, Department of Biological Sciences
University of Wisconsin-Milwaukee
Milwaukee, Wisconsin

Kathleen A. Sweeney, R.N., B.S.N.
Women's Outreach Coordinator
HIV Primary Care Support Network
Medical College of Wisconsin
Milwaukee, Wisconsin

Jill M. White Winters, R.N., Ph.D.
Associate Professor
School of Nursing
Marquette University
Milwaukee, Wisconsin

Reviewers

Karen S. Bailey, R.N., M.S.N., F.N.P.-C.
Assistant Professor, Department of Nursing
Marshall University
Huntington, West Virginia

Patricia M. Biteman, R.N., M.S.N.
Nursing Instructor, Department of Nursing
Humboldt State University
Arcadia, California

Thomas Buettner, M.S., Ph.D. (A.B.D.)
Missouri Baptist College and St. Louis University
St. Louis, Missouri

Jacqueline Burchum, R.N., M.S.N., C.S.
Assistant Professor and Coordinator of Nursing,
*   Extended Programs, Loewenberg School of Nursing*
University of Memphis
Jackson, Tennessee

Donald R. Colborn, Ph.D.
Associate Professor of Biology and Chemistry,
*   Natural Sciences*
Missouri Baptist College
St. Louis, Missouri

Claire B. Corbin, B.S.N., M.S.
Dean, School of Nursing
Carolinas College of Health Sciences
Charlotte, North Carolina

Andrea Cullinan, R.N., M.S., M.A., F.N.P.
Nursing Instructor, Division of Nursing
Glendale Community College
Glendale, Arizona

Deda Dolan, M.S.N., C.R.N.P.
Associate Professor, Nursing
University of Mobile
Mobile, Alabama

Kathleen Walsh Free, R.N., M.S.N., A.R.N.P.
Associate Clinical Professor, Division of Nursing
Indiana University
New Albany, Indiana

Patricia Frontczak, R.N., M.S.N.
Nursing Faculty, School of Nursing
Southwestern Michigan College
Dowagiac, Michigan

Sharon George, M.S.N., Ph.D. student
Clinical Assistant Professor, College of Nursing
The University of Alabama in Huntsville
Huntsville, Alabama

Sandra M. Grinnell, R.N., M.S.N., C.I.M.I.,
    Ph.D. student
Assistant Professor, School of Nursing
Medcenter One, College of Nursing
Bismarck, North Dakota

Jennifer G. Hensley, R.N., M.S.N., C.N.M.,
    Ed.D., L.C.C.E.
Assistant Professor, Nursing
Beth-El College of Nursing-University of Colorado
Colorado Springs, Colorado

Kerry Hull, Ph.D.
Assistant Professor, Biology Department
Bishops University
Lennoxville, Quebec City, Canada

Lori L. Kelly, M.S.N.
Assistant Professor of Nursing, Department of Nursing
Thomas More College
Crestview, Kentucky

James D. Kieffer, Ph.D.
Department of Biology
University of New Brunswick
Saint John, New Brunswick, Canada

Elizabeth M. Long, R.N., M.S.N., C.G.N.P., C.N.S.
Instructor, Department of Nursing
Gerontological Nurse Practitioner, Dr. Joseph Finley
*   and Associates*
Lamar University
Beaumont, Texas

M. Denise McHugh, R.N., M.S.N., Ph.D. student
Assistant Professor, College of Nursing
University of Wisconsin Oshkosh
Oshkosh, Wisconsin

**Mary Margaret Mooney, P.B.V.M., D.N.Sc.,
   A.R.N.P., F.A.A.N.**
Professor and Chair, Department of Nursing and Health
Clarke College
Dubuque, Iowa

Julie Moore, R.N.C., M.S.N., M.P.H., W.H.N.P.
Assistant Professor of Nursing, Division of Nursing
Hawaii Community College
Hilo, Hawaii

Meenakshi Natarajan, B.Sc.(Hons.), M.Sc.
Faculty
ICT Northumberland College
Halifax, Nova Scotia, Canada

Jan Pollock, B.S.
PTA Program Director, Department Chair, Allied Health
Davenport University
Lansing, Michigan

Catherine Reavis, R.N., Ed.D., C.S., F.N.P., C.N.O.R.
Associate Professor, School of Nursing
Texas Tech University, Health Sciences Center
Lubbock, Texas

Cathy L. Rozmus, R.N., D.S.N., F.A.C.C.E., L.C.C.E.
Vice President for Academic Affairs
Georgia Southwestern
Americus, Georgia

Sheila C. Schmuck, R.N., M.S.N.
Assistant Professor, Division of Nursing
University of Virginia's College at Wise
Wise, Virginia

Nan Smith-Blair, R.N., Ph.D.
Assistant Professor, Eleanor Mann School of Nursing
University of Arkansas
Fayetteville, Arkansas

Nancy Stephenson, R.N., C.S., Ph.D.
Assistant Professor, School of Nursing
East Carolina University School of Nursing
Greenville, North Carolina

Jill D. Steuer, R.N., C.N.S., Ph.D.
Associate Professor, School of Nursing
Capital University
Columbus, Ohio

Nancy A. Stotts, R.N., Ed.D., F.A.A.N.
Professor, Department of Physiological Nursing
School of Nursing, University of California-San Francisco
San Francisco, California

Betty Sylvesp, B.S.N., M.S.N., Ph.D student
Instructor, College of Nursing
University of Southern Mississippi
Hattiesburg, Mississippi

Margaret Terzaghi-Howe, Doctor of Science
Instructor, Natural Science and Mathematics
Mesa State College
Montrose, Colorado

Patricia A. Wessels, R.N., B.S., M.S.N.
Associate Professor of Nursing, School of Nursing
Viterbo College
La Crosse, Wisconsin

Preface

This edition marks the 20th anniversary of *Pathophysiology: Concepts of Altered Health States*. From its original edition of 650 pages, published in 1982, it has grown to over 1400 pages. The preparation of each new edition has been both challenging and humbling. Challenging to incorporate the myriad of new information; humbling to realize that despite advances in science and technology, illness and disease continue to occur and take their toll in terms of the physiologic as well as the social, psychological, and economic well-being of individuals, their families, the community, and the world at large. Nothing illustrates this realization as dramatically as the evolution of the worldwide AIDS epidemic for which science has yet to develop a vaccine or a cure.

As the others before it, the sixth edition has been carefully critiqued, reorganized, updated, and revised. The illustrations have grown from a modest 275 in the first edition to 675 in this edition. Seventy-five new illustrations have been added to this edition and another 75 have been significantly modified or replaced with new illustrations. This edition also sees the addition of three new chapters: "Concepts of Health and Disease," which introduces health and disease from a historical as well as the epidemiological viewpoint and serves as an introduction to concepts throughout the book; "Sleep and Sleep Disorders," which focuses on the physiology and developmental aspects of sleep disorders (a problem that is becoming more prevalent in a society that is increasingly faced with sleep-disturbing stresses such as those associated with long-term illnesses, family responsibilities, job schedules, and intercontinental travel); and the "Neurobiology of Thought and Mood Disorders," which focuses on anxiety and psychiatric disorders.

As a nurse-physiologist, my major emphasis with each revision has been to relate normal body functioning to the physiologic changes that participate in disease production and occur as a result of disease, as well as the body's remarkable ability to compensate for these changes. The beauty of physiology is that it integrates all of the aspects of the individual cells and organs of the human body into a total functional whole that can be used to explain both the physical and psychological aspects of altered health. Indeed, it has been my philosophy to share the beauty of the human body and to emphasize that in disease as in health, there is more "going right" in the body than is "going wrong." This book is an extension of my career and, as such, of my philosophy. It is my hope that readers will learn to appreciate the marvelous potential of the body,

incorporating it into their own philosophy and ultimately sharing it with their clients.

As with previous editions, every attempt has been made to develop a text that is current, accurate, and presented in a logical manner. The content has been arranged so that concepts build on one another. Words are defined as content is presented. Concepts from physiology, biochemistry, physics, and other sciences are reviewed as deemed appropriate. A conceptual model that integrates the developmental and preventive aspects of health has been used. Selection of content was based on common health problems, including the special needs of children and elderly persons. Although intended as a course textbook, it is also designed to serve as a reference book that students can take with them and use in their practice once the course is finished. The book was written with undergraduate students in mind, but is also appropriate for graduate students in nurse practitioner and clinical nurse specialist programs and for students in other health care disciplines.

The integration of full color into the design and illustrations has continued. This offers not only visual appeal, but enhances conceptual learning, linking text content to illustration content. This edition also retains the list of suffixes and prefixes, the table of normal laboratory values, and the glossary that was in the fifth edition. Objectives continue to appear at the beginning of each major section in a chapter and summary statements appear at the end. Two new features of the book are the key concept boxes and the inclusion of Internet addresses at the end of many of the chapters. The key concept boxes help the reader retain and utilize text information by providing a mechanism to incorporate text information into a larger conceptual unit as opposed to rotely memorizing a string of related and unrelated facts. The Internet addresses are intended not only to help the reader keep pace with the times, but to broaden the reader's perspective in terms of a more global approach to learning and practice. The Internet sites also encourage readers to investigate areas of individual interest and update knowledge in world of ever-changing information.

The writing of this book has been a meaningful endeavor for the authors. It was accomplished through an extensive review of the literature and through the use of critiques provided by students, faculty, and content specialists. As this vast amount of information was processed, inaccuracies or omissions may have occurred. Readers are encouraged to contact us about such errors. Such feedback is essential to the continual development of the book.

Acknowledgments

First and foremost, I would like to acknowledge James J. Smith, M.D., Ph.D. (1914–2001), former Chairman of the Physiology Department, Medical College of Wisconsin, who was my mentor during doctoral studies and supportive colleague and friend throughout our association. Dr. Smith's view of physiology was one of an integrated science with fundamental applications for all health professions. His steady guidance and encouragement served as an inspiration throughout the writing of the various editions of this book.

As in past editions, many persons participated in the creation of this work. The contributing authors deserve a special mention, for they worked long hours to supply essential content. To put a book of this magnitude together without their help would have been impossible. Although Marion Broome, Susan Dietz, Susan Gallagher-Lepak, Camille Kolotylo, Sylvia Eichner McDonald, Marianne Sigda, Stephanie Stewart, and Nancie Urban were not able to contribute to the sixth edition, their previous participation as contributing authors greatly facilitated its preparation. I would also like to acknowledge Mary Pat Kunert's efforts in making this edition a reality. She served as a consultant for the project and assisted in rewriting some of the pivotal chapters in the book.

Several other persons deserve special recognition. Georgianne Heymann, R.N., B.S.N., assisted in editing the manuscript. As with previous editions, she provided not only excellent editorial assistance, but also encouragement and support when the tasks associated with manuscript preparation became most frustrating. Beth Peterman and Ann Curley deserve mention for their determination and dedication while pursuing their library research tasks.

It is often said that a picture is worth a thousand words. This is particularly true in a book such as this, where illustrations form the basis for understanding difficult concepts. I would like to acknowledge Jennifer Smith for her tireless efforts in preparing the new and modified illustrations for this edition. Carole Hilmer also deserves mention. She prepared the illustrations for previous editions of the book, many of which continue to be used. I would also like to acknowledge the contributions of other authors who have shared their illustrations and photos.

I would also like to recognize the efforts of the editorial and production staff at Lippincott Williams & Wilkins that were directed by Lisa Stead, Acquisitions Editor. I particularly want to thank Barclay Cunningham, who served as Managing Editor, and Debra Schiff for her work as Production Editor.

Past and present students in my classes also deserve a special salute, for they are the inspiration upon which this book is founded. They have provided the questions, suggestions, and contact with the "real world" of patient care that have directed the organization and selection of content for the book.

And last, but not least, I would like to acknowledge my family, my friends, and my colleagues for their patience, their understanding, and their encouragement through the entire process.

Contents

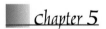

unit III

Integrative Body Functions   179

unit IV

Hematopoietic Function   249

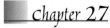

chapter 28

Alterations in Respiratory Function: Respiratory Tract Infections, Neoplasms, and Childhood Disorders   605

chapter 29

Alterations in Respiration: Alterations in Ventilation and Gas Exchange   633

Unit VIII

Renal Function and Fluid and Electrolytes   671

chapter 30

Control of Renal Function   673

chapter 31

Alterations in Fluids and Electrolytes   693

chapter 32
Alterations in Acid-Base Balance   735

chapter 33
Alterations in Renal Function   753

chapter 34
Renal Failure   777

chapter 35
Alterations in Urine Elimination   795

unit IX
Gastrointestinal Function   813

chapter 36
Control of Gastrointestinal Function   815

chapter 37

Alterations in Gastrointestinal Function   831

chapter 38

Alterations in Function of the Hepatobiliary System and Exocrine Pancreas   859

unit X

Endocrine Function   889

chapter 39

Mechanisms of Endocrine Control   891

Glenn Matfin, Safak Guven, and Julie A. Kuenzi

chapter 40

Alterations in Endocrine Control of Growth and Metabolism   903

Glenn Matfin, Safak Guven, and Julie A. Kuenzi

chapter 41
Diabetes Mellitus   925
Safak Guven, Julie A. Kuenzi, and Glenn Matfin

unit XI
Genitourinary and Reproductive Function   953

chapter 42
Structure and Function of the Male Reproductive System   955

chapter 43
Alterations in Structure and Function of the Male Genitourinary System   965

chapter 44
Structure and Function of the Female Reproductive System   983
Patricia McCowen Mehring

chapter 45
Alterations in Structure and Function of the Female Reproductive System   997
Patricia McCowen Mehring

Chapter 46

Sexually Transmitted Diseases   1029

Patricia McCowen Mehring

Unit XII

Neural Function   1041

Chapter 47

Organization and Control of Neural Function   1043

Edward W. Carroll and Robin L. Curtis

Chapter 48

Somatosensory Function and Pain   1091

Elizabeth C. Devine

chapter 49

Alterations in Motor Function   1123

Carol M. Porth and Robin L. Curtis

chapter 50

Disorders of Brain Function   1159

Diane Book

chapter 51

Sleep and Sleep Disorders   1201

chapter 52

Neurobiology of Thought, Mood, and Anxiety Disorders   1219

Mary Pat Kunert and Jane Dresser

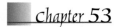

unit XIII

Special Senses   1235

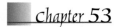

chapter 53

Control of Special Senses   1237

Edward W. Carroll, Sheila M. Curtis, and Robin L. Curtis

chapter 54

Alterations in Vision   1263

Edward W. Carroll and Sheila M. Curtis

chapter 55

Alterations in Hearing and Vestibular Function   1291

Susan A. Fontana

unit XIV

Musculoskeletal Function   1309

chapter 56

Structure and Function of the Skeletal System   1311

Concepts of Health and Disease

Early peoples were considered long-lived if they reached 30 years of age—that is, if they survived infancy. For many centuries, infant mortality was so great that large families became the tradition; many children in a family ensured that at least some would survive. Life expectancy has increased over the centuries, and today an individual in a developed country can expect to live about 71 to 79 years. Although life expectancy has increased radically since ancient times, human longevity has remained fundamentally unchanged.

The quest to solve the mystery of human longevity, which appears to be genetically programmed, began with Gregor Mendel (1822–1884), an Augustinian monk. Mendel laid the foundation of modern genetics with the pea experiments he performed in a monastery garden. Today, geneticists search for the determinant, or determinants, of the human life span. Up to this time, scientists have failed to identify an aging gene that would account for a limited life span. However, they have found that cells have a finite reproductive capacity. As they age, genes are increasingly unable to perform their functions. The cells become poorer and poorer at making the substances they need for their own special tasks or even for their own maintenance. Free radicals, mutation in a cell's DNA, and the process of programmed cell death are some of the factors that work together to affect a cell's functioning.

Chapter 1

Concepts of Health and Disease

Georgianne H. Heymann and Carol M. Porth

The concepts of what constituted health and disease at the beginning of the last century were far different from those of this century. In most of the industrialized nations of the world, people now are living longer and enjoying a healthier lifestyle. Much of this has been made possible by recent advances in science and technology. There has been an increased knowledge of immune mechanisms; the discovery of antibiotics to cure infections; and the development of vaccines to prevent disease, chemotherapy to attack cancers, and drugs to control the manifestations of mental illness.

The introduction of the birth control pill and improved prenatal care have led to decreased birth rates and declines in infant and child mortality. The benefits of science and technology also have increased the survival of infants born prematurely and of children with previously untreatable illnesses, such as immunodeficiency states and leukemia. There also has been an increase in the survival of the very seriously ill and critically injured persons of all age groups. Consequently, there has been an increase in longevity, a shift in the age distribution of the population, and an increase in age-related diseases. Coronary heart disease, stroke, and cancer have now replaced pneumonia, tuberculosis, and diarrhea and enteritis—the leading causes of death in the 1900s.

This chapter, which is intended to serve as an introduction to the book, is organized into four sections: health and society, historical perspectives on health and disease, perspectives on health and disease in individuals, and perspectives on health and disease in populations. The chapter is intended to provide the reader with the ability to view within a larger framework the historical aspects of health and disease and the relationship of health and disease to individuals and populations, and to introduce the reader to terms, such as *etiology* and *pathogenesis*, that are used throughout this text.

Health and Society

Everyone who is born holds dual citizenship in the kingdom of the well and in the kingdom of the sick. Although we all prefer to use only the good passport, sooner or later each of us is obligated, at least for a spell, to identify ourselves as citizens of that other place.[1]

After you have completed this section of the chapter, you should be able to meet the following objectives:

✦ Describe the concepts used to establish belief systems within a community and the effects on its health care practices

◆ Identify a disease believed to be generated by specific emotions and the characteristics ascribed to it

◆ Explain how mythologizing disease can be detrimental to individuals in a society

There is a long history that documents the concern of humans for their own health and well-being and that of their community. It is not always evident what particular beliefs were held by early humans concerning health and disease. Still, there is evidence that whenever humans formed social groups, some individuals have taken the role of the healer, responsible for the health of the community by preventing disease and curing the sick.

In prehistoric times, people believed that angry gods or evil spirits caused ill health and disease. To cure the sick, the gods had to be pacified or the evil spirits driven from the body. In time, this task became the job of the healers, or tribal priests. They tried to pacify the gods or drive out the evil spirits using magic charms, spells, and incantations. There also is evidence of surgical treatment. Trephining involved the use of a stone instrument to cut a hole in the skull of the sick person. It is believed that this was done to release spirits responsible for illness. Prehistoric healers probably also discovered that many plants can be used as drugs.

The community as a whole also was involved in securing the health of its members. It was the community that often functioned to take care of those considered ill or disabled. The earliest evidence of this comes from an Old Stone Age cave site, Riparo del Romio, in southern Italy. There the remains of an adolescent dwarf were found. Despite his severe condition, which must have greatly limited his ability to contribute to either hunting or gathering, the young man survived to the age of 17 years. He must have been supported throughout his life by the rest of the community, which had incorporated compassion for its members into its belief system.[2] Communities such as this probably existed throughout prehistory; separated from each other and without any formal routes of communication, they relied on herbal medicines and group activity to maintain health.

Throughout history, peoples and cultures have developed their health practices based on their belief systems. Many traditions construed sickness and health primarily in the context of an understanding of the relations of human beings to the planets, stars, mountains, rivers, spirits, and ancestors, gods and demons, the heavens and underworld. Some traditions, such as those reflected in Chinese and Indian cultures, although concerned with a cosmic scope, do not pay great attention to the supernatural.

Over time, modern Western thinking has shed its adherence to all such elements. Originating with the Greek tradition—which dismissed supernatural powers, although not environmental influences—and further shaped by the flourishing anatomic and physiologic programs of the Renaissance, the Western tradition was created based on the belief that everything that needed to be known essentially could be discovered by probing more deeply and ever more minutely into the flesh, its systems, tissues, cells, and DNA.[3] Through Western political and economic domination, these health beliefs now have powerful influence worldwide.

Every society has its own ideas and beliefs about life, death, and disease. It is these perceptions that shape the concept of health in a society. Although some customs and beliefs tend to safeguard human communities from disease, others invite and provoke disease outbreaks.

The beliefs that people have concerning health and disease can change the destiny of nations. The conquering of the Aztec empire may be one example. Historians have speculated how Hernando Cortez, starting off with fewer than 600 men, could conquer the Aztec empire, whose subjects numbered millions. Historian William H. McNeill suggests a sequence of events that may explain how a tiny handful of men could subjugate a nation of millions.

Although the Aztecs first thought the mounted, gun-powered Spaniards were gods, experience soon showed otherwise. Armed clashes revealed the limitations of horseflesh and of primitive guns, and the Aztecs were able to drive Cortez and his men from their city. Unbeknownst to the Aztecs, the Spaniards had a more devastating weapon than any firearm: smallpox. An epidemic of smallpox broke out among the Aztecs after their skirmishes with the Spaniards. Because the population lacked inherited or acquired immunity, the results were catastrophic. It is presumed that

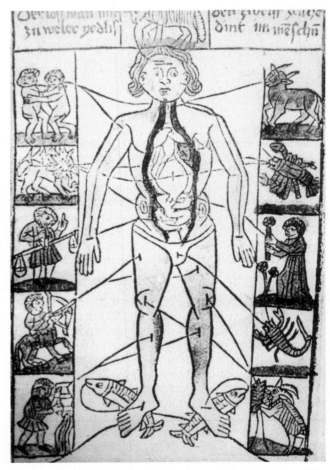

Influences of zodiac signs on the human body. (Courtesy of the National Library of Medicine)

a quarter to a third of the population died from the initial onslaught.

Even more devastating were the psychological implications of the disease: it killed only American Indians and left Spaniards unharmed. A way of life built around the old Indian gods could not survive such a demonstration of the superior power of the God the Spaniards worshipped. It is not hard to imagine then that the Indians accepted Christianity and submitted meekly to Spanish control.[4] Although we live in an age of science, science has not eliminated fantasies about health; the stigmas of sickness and the moral meanings that they carry continue. Whereas people in previous centuries wove stories around leprosy, plague, and tuberculosis to create fear and guilt, the modern age has created similar taboos and mythologies about cancer and acquired immunodeficiency syndrome (AIDS).

The myth of tuberculosis (TB) was that a person who suffered from it was of a melancholy, superior character—sensitive, creative, a being apart. Melancholy, or sadness, made one "interesting" or romantic. The general perception of TB as "romantic" was not just a literary device. It was a way of thinking that insinuated itself into the sensibilities and made it possible to ignore the social conditions, such as overcrowding and poor sanitation and nutrition, that helped breed tuberculosis.

The infusion of beliefs into public awareness often is surreptitious. Just as tuberculosis often had been regarded sentimentally, as an enhancement of identity, cancer was regarded with irrational revulsion, as a diminution of the self.[1] Current accounts of the psychological aspects of cancer often cite old authorities, starting with the Greek physician Galen, who observed that "melancholy women" are more likely to get breast cancer than "sanguine women."

Grief and anxiety were cited as causes of cancer, as well as personal losses. Public figures such as Napoleon, Ulysses S. Grant, Robert A. Taft, and Hubert Humphrey have all had their cancers diagnosed as the reaction to political defeat and the end to their political ambitions. Although distress can affect immunologic responsiveness, there is no scientific evidence to support the view that specific emotions, or emotions in general, can produce specific diseases—or that cancer is the result of a "cancer personality," described as emotionally withdrawn, lacking self-confidence, and depressive.

These disease mythologies contribute to the stigmatizing of certain illnesses and, by extension, of those who are ill. The beliefs about health and disease have the power to trap or empower people. They may inhibit people from seeking early treatment, diminish personal responsibility for practicing healthful behaviors, or encourage fear and social isolation. Conversely, they also can be the impetus for compassion to those who are ill, commitment to improving one's own health, and support for efforts to improve the health status of others.

In summary, what constitutes health and disease changes over time. Prehistoric times were marked by beliefs that angry gods or evil spirits caused ill health and disease. To cure the sick, the gods had to be pacified or the evil spirits driven from the body. Tribal healers, or priests, emerged to accomplish this task. Prehistoric healers used a myriad of treatments, including magic charms, spells, and incantations; surgical treatment; and plant medicines.

Throughout history, the concept of health in a society has been shaped by its beliefs about life, death, and disease. Some beliefs and customs, such as exhibiting compassion for disabled community members, tend to safeguard human communities and increase the quality of life for all community members. Others invite and provoke disease outbreaks, such as myths about the causes of disease.

Even though science and technology have advanced the understanding and treatment of disease, misconceptions and fantasies about disease still arise. In previous centuries, diseases such as leprosy, plague, and tuberculosis were fodder for taboos and mythologies; today it is cancer and AIDS. The psychological effects of disease mythologies can be positive or negative. At their worst, they can stigmatize and isolate those who are ill; at their best, they can educate the community and improve the health of its members.

Health and Disease: A Historical Perspective

After you have completed this section of the chapter, you should be able to meet the following objectives:

✦ Describe the contributions of the early Greek, Italian, and English scholars to the understanding of anatomy, physiology, and pathology
✦ State two important advances of the nineteenth century that helped to pave the way for prevention of disease
✦ State three significant advances of the twentieth century that have revolutionized diagnosis and treatment of disease
✦ Propose developments that will both hamper and contribute to the promotion of health and the elimination of disease in the twenty-first century

It has been said that those who do not know history are condemned to repeat it. There are many contributors to the understanding of how the body is constructed and how it works, and what disease is and how it can be treated, which in turn leads to an understanding of what health is and how can it be maintained.

Much of what we take for granted in terms of treating the diseases that afflict humankind has had its origin in the past. Although they are seemingly small contributions in terms of today's scientific advances, it is the knowledge produced by the great thinkers of the past that has made possible the many things we now take for granted.

THE INFLUENCE OF EARLY SCHOLARS

Knowledge of anatomy, physiology, and pathology as we now know it began to emerge with the ancient Greeks. They were the first to recognize the distinction between internal and external causes of illness.

To Hippocrates and his followers we owe the foundations of the clinical principles and the ethics that grew into modern medical science. Hippocrates (460–377 BC) was a blend of scientist and artist. He believed that disease occurred when the four humors—blood from the heart, yellow bile from the liver, black bile from the spleen, and phlegm from the brain—became out of balance. These humors were said to govern character as well as health, producing phlegmatic, sanguine, choleric, and melancholic personalities. This belief paralleled the even older Chinese tradition, which was founded on the complementary principles of yin (female principle) and yang (male), whose correct proportions were essential for health. Hippocrates is identified with an approach to health that dictated plenty of healthy exercise, rest in illness, and a moderate, sober diet.

It was Aristotle (384–322 BC) who, through his dissection of small animals and description of their internal anatomy, laid the foundations for the later scrutiny of the human body. For Aristotle, the heart was the most important organ. He believed it to be the center of the blood system as well as the center of the emotions. However, Aristotle's main contributions were made to science in general.

The person who took the next major step was Galen (AD 129–199), a physician to the emperors and gladiators of ancient Rome. Galen expanded on the Hippocratic doctrines and introduced experimentation into the study of

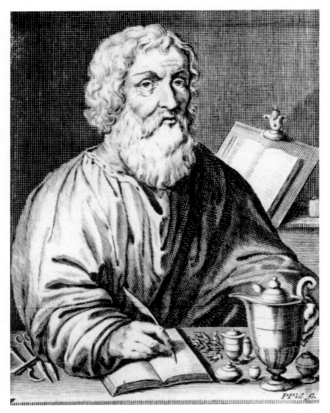

Hippocrates: A blend of scientist and scholar. (Courtesy of the National Library of Medicine)

healing. His work came to be regarded as the encyclopedia of anatomy and physiology. He demoted the heart—in his view the liver was primary for venous blood, whereas the seat of all thought was the brain. He described the arteries and veins, and even revealed the working of the nervous system by severing a pig's spinal cord at different points and demonstrating that corresponding parts of the body became paralyzed. According to Galen, the body carried three kinds of blood that contained spirits charged by various organs: the veins carried "natural spirit" from the liver; the arteries, "vital spirit" from the lungs; the nerves, "animal spirit" from the brain. The heart merely warmed the blood. After Galen's death, however, anatomic research ceased and his work was considered infallible for almost 1400 years.

As the great medical schools of universities reformed the teaching of anatomy in the early 1500s and integrated it into medical studies, it became apparent to anatomists that Galen's data—taken from dogs, pigs, and apes—often were riddled with error. It was only with the work of Andreas Vesalius (1514–1564) that Galen's ideas truly were challenged.

Vesalius, professor of anatomy and surgery at Padua, Italy, dedicated a lifetime to the study of the human body. Vesalius carried out some unprecedentedly scrupulous dissections and used the latest in artistic techniques and printing for the more than 200 woodcuts in his *De Humani Corporis Fabrica* ("On the Fabric [Structure] of the Human Body"). He not only showed just what bodily parts looked like, but how they worked. The book, published in 1543, set a new standard for the understanding of human anatomy. With this work, Vesalius became a leading figure in the revolt against Galen's teachings.

One of the most historically significant discoveries was made by William Harvey (1578–1657), an English physician and physiologist. He established that the blood circulates in a closed system impelled mechanically by a "pumplike" heart. He also measured the amount of blood in the circulatory system in any given unit of time—one of the first applications of quantitative methods in biology. Harvey's work, published in *On the Motion of the Heart and Blood in Animals* (1628), provided a foundation of physiologic principles that led to an understanding of blood pressure and set the stage for innovative techniques such as cardiac catheterization.

With the refinement of the microscope by the Dutch lens maker Anton van Leeuwenhoek (1632–1723), the stage was set for the era of cellular biology. Another early user of the microscope, English scientist Robert Hooke (1635–1703) published his *Micrographia* in 1665 in which he formally described the plant cells in cork, presented his theories of light and combustion, and his studies of insect anatomy. His book presented the great potential of the microscope for biologic investigation. In it he inaugurated the modern biologic usage of the word *cell*. A century later, German-born botanist Mathias Schleiden (1804–1881) and physiologist Theodor Schwann (1810–1882) observed that animal tissues also were composed of cells.

Although Harvey contributed greatly to the understanding of anatomy and physiology, he was not interested in the chemistry of life. It was not until French chemist

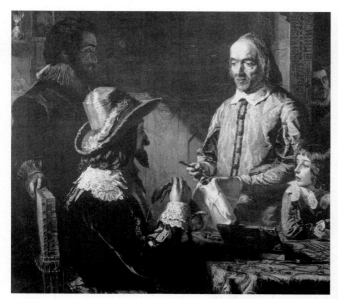

Willam Harvey's most eminent patient, King Charles I, and the future King Charles II look on as Harvey displays a dissected deer heart. (Courtesy of the National Library of Medicine)

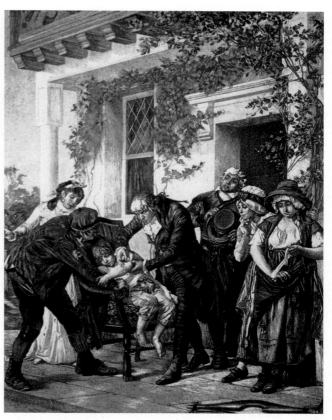

Painting by Georges-Gaston Mélingue (1894). The first vaccination. Here Dr. Jenner introduces cowpox taken from dairymaid Sarah Nelmes (right) and introduces it into two incisions on the arm of James Phipps, a healthy 8-year-old boy. The boy developed cowpox, but not smallpox, when Jenner introduced the organism into his arm 48 days later. (Courtesy of the National Library of Medicine)

Antoine Lavoisier (1743–1794), who was schooled as a lawyer but devoted to scientific pursuits, overturned 100-year-old theories of chemistry and established the basis of modern chemistry that new paths to examine body processes, such as metabolism, opened up. His restructured chemistry also gave scientists, including Louis Pasteur, the tools to develop organic chemistry.

In 1796, Edward Jenner (1749–1823) conducted the first vaccination by injecting the fluid from a dairymaid's cowpox lesion into a young boy's arm. The vaccination by this English country doctor successfully protected the child from smallpox. Jenner's discovery led to the development of vaccines to prevent many other diseases as well. Jenner's classic experiment was the first officially recorded vaccination.

THE NINETEENTH CENTURY

The nineteenth century was a time of spectacular leaps forward in the understanding of infectious diseases. For many centuries, rival epidemiologic theories associated disease and epidemics like cholera with poisonous fumes given off from dung heaps and decaying matter (poisons in the air, exuded from rotting animal and vegetable material, the soil, and standing water) or with contagion (person-to-person contact).

In 1865, English surgeon Joseph Lister (1827–1912) concluded that microbes caused wound infections. He began to use carbolic acid on wounds to kill microbes and reduce infection after surgery. However, Lister was not alone in identifying hazards in the immediate environment as detrimental to health. English nurse Florence Nightingale (1820–1910) was a leading proponent of sanitation and hygiene as weapons against disease. It was at the English

base at Scutari during the Crimean War (1854–1856) that Nightingale waged her battle. Arriving at the army hospital with a party of 38 nurses, Nightingale found nearly 2000 wounded and sick inhabiting foul, rat-infested wards. The war raged on, deluging the hospital with wounded as Nightingale not only organized the nursing care of the wounded, but provided meals, supplied bedding, and saw to the laundry. Within 6 months she had brought about a transformation and slashed the death rate from approximately 40% to 2%.[3]

From the 1860s, the rise of bacteriology, associated especially with chemist and microbiologist Louis Pasteur in France and bacteriologist Robert Koch in Germany, established the role of microorganismal pathogens. Almost for the first time in medicine, bacteriology led directly to dramatic new cures.

The technique of pasteurization is named after Louis Pasteur (1822–1895). He introduced the method in 1865 to prevent the souring of wine. Pasteur's studies of fermentation convinced him that it depended on the presence of microscopic forms of life, with each fermenting medium

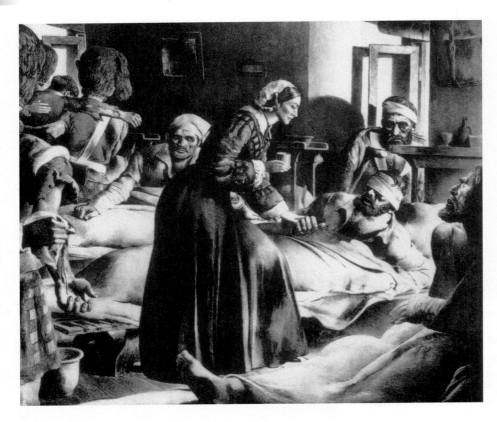

Florence Nightingale caring for wounded at Scutari, Turkey, during the Crimean War. (Courtesy of the National Library of Medicine)

serving as a unique food for a specific microorganism. He developed techniques for culturing microbes in liquid broths. Through his work, he was able to dispel the disease theory that predominated in the mid-nineteenth century attributing fevers to "miasmas," or fumes, and laid the foundation for the germ theory of disease.

The anthrax bacillus, discovered by Robert Koch (1843–1910), was the first microorganism identified as a cause of illness. Koch's trailblazing work also included identifying the organism responsible for tuberculosis and the discovery of a tuberculosis skin-testing material.

In 1895, German physicist Wilhelm Röntgen (1845–1923) discovered X rays. For the first time without a catastrophic event, the most hidden parts of a human body were revealed. Even though he understood that it was a significant discovery, Röntgen did not initially recognize the amazing diagnostic potential of the process he had discovered.

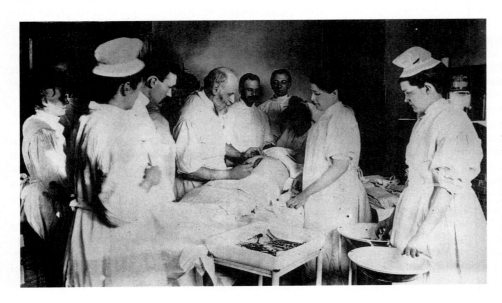

The operating room. With the advent of anesthesia, knowledge of how microbes cause disease, and availability of incandescent lighting in the operating room, surgery became an option for treating disease. Rubber gloves had not yet been invented and the surgical team worked with bare hands to perform surgery. (Hahnemann Hospital, Chicago, IL. Courtesy Bette Clemons, Phoenix, AZ)

THE TWENTIETH CENTURY

The twentieth century was a period of revolutionary industry in the science and politics of health. Concerns about the care of infants and children and the spread of infectious disease became prevailing themes in public and political arenas alike. It was during this time that private duty and public health nursing emerged as the means of delivering health care to people in their homes and in their communities. Social service agencies like the Henry Street Settlement in New York, founded by Lillian Wald, sent nurses into tenements to care for the sick.[5] The placement of nurses in schools began in New York City in 1902 at the urging of Wald, who offered to supply a Henry Street nurse for 1 month without charge.[5] Efforts to broaden the delivery of health care from the city to rural areas also were initiated during the early 1900s. The American Red Cross, which was reorganized and granted a new charter by Congress in 1905, established a nursing service for the rural poor that eventually expanded to serve the small town poor as well.[5]

Scientific discoveries and innovations abounded in the twentieth century. In the early 1900s, German bacteriologist Paul Ehrlich (1854–1915) theorized that certain substances could act as "magic bullets," attacking disease-causing microbes but leaving the rest of the body undamaged. In 1910 he introduced his discovery: using the arsenic compound Salvarsan, he had found an effective weapon against syphilis. Through his work, Ehrlich launched the science of chemotherapy.

The first antibiotic was discovered in 1928 by English bacteriologist Sir Alexander Fleming (1881–1955). As he studied the relationship between bacteria and the mold *Penicillium*, he discovered its ability to kill staphylococci. However, it was not until the 1940s that later researchers, who were searching for substances produced by one microorganism that might kill other microorganisms, produced penicillin as a clinically useful antibiotic.

By the 1930s, innovative researchers had produced a cornucopia of new drugs that could be used to treat many of the most common illnesses that left their victims either severely disabled or dead. The medical community now had at its disposal medications such as digoxin to treat heart failure; sulfa drugs, which produced near-miraculous cures for infections such as scarlet fever; and insulin to treat diabetes.

With the discovery of insulin, a once-fatal disease known from antiquity no longer carried a death sentence. Working together, Canadian physician Sir Frederick Banting (1891–1941) and physiologist Charles Best (1899–1978) isolated insulin from the pancreas of a dog in 1921. The extract, when given to diabetic dogs, restored their health. In January of 1922, they successfully treated a young boy dying of diabetes with their pancreatic extracts. Although still incurable, it became possible to live with diabetes.

One disease that remained not only incurable but untreatable through much of the twentieth century was tuberculosis. With no cure or preventive vaccine forthcoming, efforts at the turn of the century were dedicated to controlling the spread of tuberculosis. It was then that an alliance between organized medicine and the public resulted in the formation of voluntary local organizations to battle the disease. These organizations focused on education to counteract the fear of tuberculosis; at the same time, they warned against the disease. In 1904, the local organizations joined together to form a national organization, the National

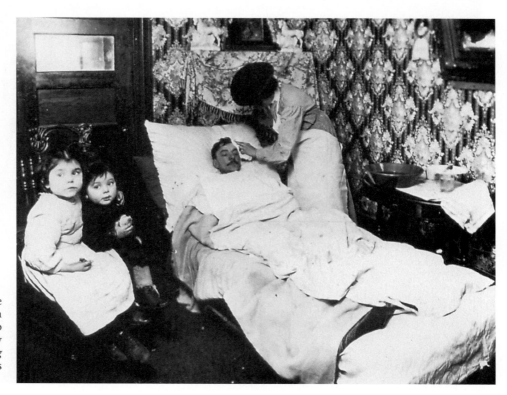

At the turn of the century, social service agencies like Henry Street Settlement in New York sent nurses into tenements to care for the sick. (Schorr T.M., Kennedy S.M. [1999]. *100 years of American nursing* [p. 12]. Philadelphia: Lippincott Williams & Wilkins)

Association for the Study and Prevention of Tuberculosis. In 1918, the name was changed to the National Tuberculosis Association, which was renamed the American Lung Association in 1973.[6]

The national and local tuberculosis associations played a vital role in educating the public by running campaigns urging people to have skin tests and chest x-rays as a means of diagnosing tuberculosis. Once tuberculosis was diagnosed, an individual was likely to be sent to a sanatorium or tuberculosis hospital. There, good nourishment, fresh air, and bed rest were prescribed in the belief that if the body's natural defenses were strengthened, they would be able to overcome the tuberculosis bacillus. For almost half a century, this would be the prevailing treatment. It was not until 1945, with the introduction of chemotherapy, that streptomycin was used to treat tuberculosis.

Outbreaks of poliomyelitis, which had increased in the early decades of the 1900s, served as the impetus for the work of American microbiologist Jonas Salk (1914–1995). At its peak, the virus was claiming 50,000 victims annually in the United States.[3] Test trials of Salk's vaccine with inactivated virus began in 1953, and it proved to prevent the development of polio. By 1955, the massive testing was complete and the vaccine was quickly put into wide use.

Surgical techniques also flourished during this time. A single technical innovation was responsible for opening up the last surgical frontier—the heart. Up to this time, the heart had been out of bounds; surgeons did not have the means to take over the function of the heart for long enough to get inside and operate.[7] American surgeon John Gibbon (1903–1973) addressed this problem when he developed the heart-lung machine. Dramatic advances followed its successful use in 1953—probably none more so than the first successful heart transplantation performed in 1967 by South African surgeon Christiaan Barnard (1922–).

For centuries, the inheritance of traits had been explained in religious or philosophical terms. Although English naturalist Charles Darwin's (1809–1882) work dispelled long-held beliefs about inherited traits, it was Austrian botanist Gregor Mendel's (1822–1884) revolutionary theories on the segregation of traits, largely ignored until 1902, that laid the groundwork for establishing the chromosome as the structural unit of heredity. Many other scientists and researchers contributed to the storehouse of genetic knowledge. With the work by American geneticist James Watson (1928–) and British biophysicists Francis Crick (1916–) and Maurice Wilkins (1916–) in the early 1950s, which established the double-helical structure of DNA, the way to investigating and understanding our genetic heritage was opened.

It is difficult, if not impossible, to single out all the landmark events of the twentieth century that contributed to the health of humankind. Among the other notable achievements are the development of kidney dialysis, oral contraceptives, transplant surgery, the computed axial tomography (CAT) scanner, and coronary angioplasty.

Not all of the important advances in modern medicine are as dramatic as open heart surgery. Often they are the

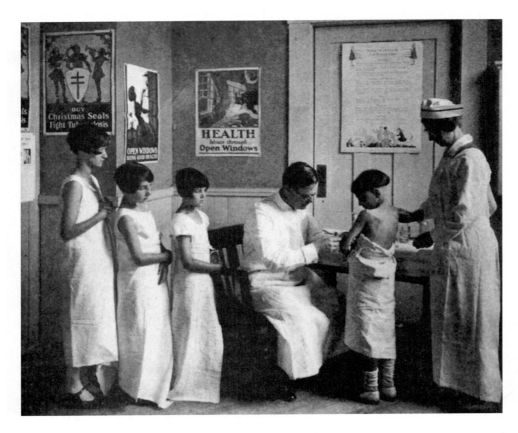

A tuberculosis skin testing clinic. (Schorr T.M., Kennedy S.M. [1999]. *100 years of American nursing* [p. 49]. Philadelphia: Lippincott Williams & Wilkins)

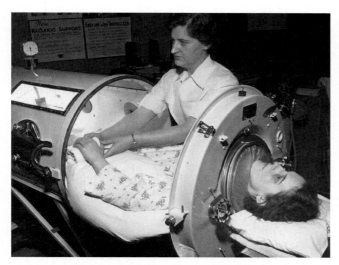

The "iron lung", which used negative pressure to draw air into the lungs, was used to provide ventilatory support for persons with "bulbar polio". (Schorr T.M., Kennedy S.M. [1999]. *100 years of American nursing* [p. 91]. Philadelphia: Lippincott Williams & Wilkins)

result of dogged work by many people and yield results only after a number of years, and then they frequently go unheralded. For example, vaccination programs, control of infectious diseases through improvements in sanitation of water and waste disposal, safer and healthier foods free from microbial contamination, identification of health risks from behaviors such as smoking, and improved prenatal care all have saved many lives in the twentieth century.

THE TWENTY-FIRST CENTURY

The twenty-first century reveals new horizons, but also new problems. In greater numbers than ever, goods and people travel the world. There is unprecedented physical mobility—travel and migration from villages to cities and country to country—and interconnectedness. However, the benefits of physical mobility and interconnectedness are accompanied by risks. Diseases such as AIDS are evidence that nothing is regional, local, or limited in its reach.

In 1976, the World Health Organization (WHO) actually succeeded in eliminating smallpox from the face of the earth. This triumph gave substance to the idea that other infections, like measles, also might disappear if sufficient efforts were directed at worldwide campaigns to isolate and cure them. However, new infectious diseases, such as Lyme disease and Legionnaire's disease, and new forms of old diseases, such as resistant strains of tuberculosis and malaria, have emerged and are readily spread worldwide. The powerful interventions used to fight these infections have had the unexpected effect of accelerating their biologic evolution and making them impervious to one after another form of chemical attack.

Pathogens also can be introduced into the food chain and travel worldwide. The discovery that beef from cattle infected with bovine spongiform encephalopathy (BSE) may be the source of Creutzfeldt-Jakob disease led many countries to ban beef products from the United Kingdom when BSE was found to be prevalent in English herds. The introduction of such pathogens can be the result of ignorance, carelessness, or greed. Tobacco is a product that serves as a pathogen. In a quest for ever-increasing profits, the tobacco industry created a demand for its product by artificially raising the nicotine content of cigarettes so as to increase their addictive potential. This was done with the knowledge of the health risks of tobacco products, thanks to experiments conducted by the tobacco companies' own medical scientists, but kept secret.

If there is a blueprint for future advances, it is in the genes. The twenty-first century is destined to be dominated by advances in genetics. With the mapping of the human genome comes hope of cure for some of the most dreaded crippling and fatal diseases. The mapping of the human genome also has posed new ethical dilemmas, for with it comes the potential to predict the future health of persons based on their genes. It soon may be possible to differentiate between persons who will develop certain debilitating diseases and those who will not.

Although advances in science and technology will continue to provide new treatments for many diseases, it has become apparent that there are more impressive rewards to be had by preventing diseases from becoming established in the first place. Ultimately, maintaining health is more resource conservative and cost effective than relying on treatment of disease. Many decades ago, we learned that even though the "magic bullets" such as antibiotics had the ability to cure what was once considered incurable, much of our freedom from communicable disease is due to clean water, efficient sanitation, and good nutrition. We have become increasingly aware of the importance of preventive measures against noninfectious conditions, especially cancer and coronary heart disease. There is no better way to prevent disease and maintain health than by leading a healthy life, and increasingly, it will be the individual who is responsible for ensuring a healthy passage through life.

In summary, Greek scholars were responsible for establishing the fundamentals of anatomy, physiology, and pathology that served as the earliest knowledge base for understanding health and disease. It was Hippocrates (460–377 BC) and his followers who laid the foundations of the clinical principles and ethics that grew into modern science. Although his belief that disease occurred when the four humors—blood, yellow and black bile, and phlegm—became out of balance was disproved, his approach to health that dictated plenty of healthy exercise, rest in illness, and a moderate, sober diet remains valid. Galen (AD 129–199) took the next major step, expanding on Hippocratic doctrines and introducing experimentation into the study of healing. His work, gleaned through his role as physician to the emperors and gladiators of Rome and animal dissections, came to be regarded as the encyclopedia of anatomy and physiology and was considered infallible for almost 1400 years.

Significant challenges to long-held beliefs began with the work of Andreas Vesalius (1514–1564), professor of anatomy and surgery at Padua, Italy. His published work *On the Fabric [Structure] of the Human Body* showing how the parts of the body looked and worked set a new standard for the understanding of human anatomy. Other significant early contributions were made by scholars such as William Harvey (1578–1657), the English physician and physiologist, who in his book *On the Motion of the Heart and Blood in Animals* provided a physiologic framework for the circulation of blood; Anton van Leeuwenhoek (1632–1723), the Dutch lens maker who refined the microscope and set the stage for the era of cellular biology; and Edward Jenner (1749–1823), the English country physician, who conducted the first successful vaccination.

The nineteenth century was a time of major discoveries that paved the way for understanding infectious diseases. Significant contributions were made by such scientists as Joseph Lister, the English surgeon who concluded that microbes caused wound infections; German bacteriologist Robert Koch, who discovered the anthrax bacillus, thus identifying for the first time a microorganism and the illness it caused; and French chemist and microbiologist Louis Pasteur, who developed the technique of pasteurization. Perhaps the most notable technical innovation of the century was the discovery of X rays by German physicist Wilhelm Röntgen.

The scientific undertakings and discoveries of the twentieth century were revolutionary. In 1910, Paul Ehrlich introduced chemotherapy, and in 1928, Sir Alexander Fleming discovered the first antibiotic as he studied the relationship between bacteria and the mold *Penicillium*. Diseases that had once been fatal or crippling were managed or prevented by new advances, such as the discovery of insulin by Sir Frederick Banting and Charles Best in 1922 and the development of the polio vaccine by Jonas Salk in 1953. Technical innovations set the stage for new surgical techniques. The creation of the heart-lung machine by American surgeon John Gibbon paved the way for coronary bypass surgery and the first successful heart transplantation in 1967, which was performed by Christiaan Barnard, a South African surgeon. Other important advances included kidney dialysis, oral contraceptives, the CAT scanner, and coronary angioplasty. Public health programs also were responsible for greatly affecting the health of populations, such as those dedicated to increasing vaccination, improving sanitation of water and waste disposal, and identifying health risks.

Knowledge about the influence of heredity on health and disease originated with Charles Darwin's (1809–1882) evolutionary theories about inherited traits and with Gregor Mendel's (1822–1884) theories on the segregation of traits, which laid the groundwork

for establishing the chromosome as the structural unit of heredity. In the early 1950s, geneticist James Watson of the United States and British biophysicists Francis Crick and Maurice Wilkins presented their findings on the double-helical structure of DNA.

The twenty-first century is predicted to be a time of great advances in the field of genetics, already evidenced by the substantial mapping of the human genome that has taken place. Scientists look to genetic research to provide advances that not only will predict who may develop disease, but will provide new treatments for those diseases. However promising future advances may appear, it is readily apparent that prevention is an equally important tool in maintaining health.

Perspectives on Health and Disease in Individuals

After you have completed this section of the chapter, you should be able to meet the following objectives:

✦ State the World Health Organization definition of health
✦ Describe the function of adaptation as it relates to health and disease
✦ State a definition of pathophysiology
✦ Characterize the disease process in terms of etiology, pathogenesis, morphology, clinical manifestations, and prognosis
✦ Explain the meaning of reliability, validity, sensitivity, specificity, and predictive value as it relates to observations and tests used in the diagnosis of disease

What constitutes health and disease often is difficult to determine because of the way different people view the topic. What is defined as health is determined by many factors, including heredity, age and sex, cultural and ethnic differences, as well as individual, group, and governmental expectations.

HEALTH

The WHO in 1948 defined health as a "state of complete physical, mental, and social well-being and not merely the absence of disease and infirmity."[8] Although ideal for many people, this was an unrealistic goal. At the World Health Assembly in 1977, representatives of the member governments of WHO agreed that their goal was to have all citizens of the world reach a level of health by the year 2000 that allows them to live a socially and economically productive life.[8] The U.S. Department of Health and Human Services in *Healthy People 2010* described the determinants of health as an interaction between an individual's biology and behavior, physical and social environments, government policies and interventions, and access to quality health care.[9]

HEALTH AND DISEASE AS STATES OF ADAPTATION

The ability of the body to adapt both physically and psychologically to the many stresses that occur in both health and disease is affected by a number of factors, including age, health status, psychosocial resources, and the rapidity with which the need to adapt occurs (see Chapter 9). Generally speaking, adaptation affects the whole person. When adapting to stresses that are threats to health, the body uses those behaviors that are the most efficient and effective. It does not use long-term mechanisms when short-term adaptation is sufficient. The increase in heart rate that accompanies a febrile illness is a temporary response designed to deliver additional oxygen to tissues during the short period that the elevated temperature increases metabolic needs. On the other hand, hypertrophy of the left ventricle is a long-term adaptive response that occurs in persons with chronic hypertension.

Adaptation is further affected by the availability of adaptive responses and the ability of the body to select the most appropriate response. The greater the number of available responses, the more effective the capacity to adapt. Adaptive capacity is decreased with extremes of age and with disease conditions that limit the availability of adaptive responses. The immaturity of the infant impairs the ability to adapt, as does the decline in functional reserve that occurs in the elderly. For example, infants have difficulty concentrating urine because of the immaturity of their renal tubular structures, and therefore are less able than an older child or adult to cope with decreased water intake or exaggerated water losses. Similarly, persons with preexisting heart disease are less able to adapt to health problems that require recruitment of cardiovascular responses. Adaptation also is less effective when changes in health status occur suddenly rather than gradually. For instance, it is possible to lose a liter of blood through chronic gastrointestinal bleeding without developing signs of shock. On the other hand, a sudden hemorrhage that causes the loss of an equal amount of blood is apt to produce hypotension and circulatory shock. Even in advanced disease states, the body retains much of its adaptive capacity and is able to maintain the internal environment within relatively normal limits.

DISEASE

The term *pathophysiology*, which is the focus of this book, may be defined as the physiology of altered health. The term combines the words *pathology* and *physiology*. Pathology (from the Greek *pathos*, meaning "disease") deals with the study of the structural and functional changes in cells, tissues, and organs of the body that cause or are caused by disease. Physiology deals with the functions of the human body. Thus, pathophysiology deals not only with the cellular and organ changes that occur with disease, but with the effects that these changes have on total body function. Pathophysiology also focuses on the mechanisms of the underlying disease and provides the background for preventive as well as therapeutic health care measures and practices.

A disease has been defined as any deviation from or interruption of the normal structure or function of a part, organ, or system of the body that is manifested by a characteristic set of symptoms or signs; the etiology, pathology, and prognosis may be known or unknown.[10] The aspects of the disease process include the etiology, pathogenesis, morphologic changes, clinical manifestations, diagnosis, and clinical course.

Etiology

The causes of disease are known as *etiologic factors*. Among the recognized etiologic agents are biologic agents (*e.g.*, bacteria, viruses), physical forces (*e.g.*, trauma, burns, radiation), chemical agents (*e.g.*, poisons, alcohol), and nutritional excesses or deficits. At the molecular level, it is important to distinguish between sick molecules and molecules that cause disease.[11] This is true of diseases such as cystic fibrosis, sickle cell anemia, and familial hypercholesterolemia, in which genetic abnormality of a single amino acid, transporter molecule, or receptor protein produces widespread effects on health.

Most disease-causing agents are nonspecific, and many different agents can cause disease of a single organ. For example, lung disease can result from trauma, infection, exposure to physical and chemical agents, or neoplasia. With severe lung involvement, each of these agents has the potential to cause respiratory failure. On the other hand, a single agent or traumatic event can lead to disease of a number of organs or systems. For example, severe circulatory shock can cause multiorgan failure.

Although a disease agent can affect more than a single organ and a number of disease agents can affect the same organ, most disease states do not have a single cause. Instead, most diseases are multifactorial in origin. This is particularly true of diseases such as cancer, heart disease, and diabetes. The multiple factors that predispose to a particular disease often are referred to as *risk factors*.

One way to view the factors that cause disease is to group them into categories according to whether they were present at birth or acquired later in life. *Congenital conditions* are defects that are present at birth, although they may not be evident until later in life. Congenital malformation may be caused by genetic influences, environmental factors (*e.g.*, viral infections in the mother, maternal drug use, irradiation, or intrauterine crowding), or a combination of genetic and environmental factors. Not all genetic disorders are evident at birth. Many genetic disorders, such as familial hypercholesterolemia and polycystic kidney disease, take years to develop. *Acquired defects* are those that are caused by events that occur after birth. These include injury, exposure to infectious agents, inadequate nutrition, lack of oxygen, inappropriate immune responses, and neoplasia. Many diseases are thought to be the result of a genetic predisposition and an environmental event or events that serves as a trigger to initiate disease development.

Pathogenesis

Pathogenesis is the sequence of cellular and tissue events that take place from the time of initial contact with an etiologic agent until the ultimate expression of a disease. Etiology describes what sets the disease process in motion, and pathogenesis, how the disease process evolves. Although the two terms often are used interchangeably, their meanings are quite different. For example, atherosclerosis often is cited as the cause or etiology of coronary heart disease. In reality, the progression from fatty streak to the occlusive vessel lesion seen in persons with coronary heart disease represents the pathogenesis of the disorder. The true etiology of atherosclerosis remains largely uncertain.

Morphology

Morphology refers to the fundamental structure or form of cells or tissues. *Morphologic changes* are concerned with both the gross anatomic and microscopic changes that are characteristic of a disease. *Histology* deals with the study of the cells and extracellular matrix of body tissues. The most common method used in the study of tissues is the preparation of histologic sections that can be studied with the aid of a microscope. Because tissues and organs usually are too thick to be examined under a microscope, they must be sectioned to obtain thin, translucent sections. Histologic sections play an important role in the diagnosis of many types of cancer. A *lesion* represents a pathologic or traumatic discontinuity of a body organ or tissue. Descriptions of lesion size and characteristics often can be obtained through the use of radiographs, ultrasonography, and other imaging methods. Lesions also may be sampled by biopsy and the tissue samples subjected to histologic study.

Clinical Manifestations

Disease can be manifest in a number of ways. Sometimes the condition produces manifestations, such as fever, that make it evident that the person is sick. Other diseases are silent at the onset and are detected during examination for other purposes or after the disease is far advanced.

Signs and *symptoms* are terms used to describe the structural and functional changes that accompany a disease. A *symptom* is a subjective complaint that is noted by the person with a disorder, whereas a *sign* is a manifestation that is noted by an observer. Pain, difficulty in breathing, and dizziness are symptoms of a disease. An elevated temperature, a swollen extremity, and changes in pupil size are objective signs that can be observed by someone other than the person with the disease. Signs and symptoms may be related to the primary disorder or they may represent the body's attempt to compensate for the altered function caused by the pathologic condition. Many pathologic states are not observed directly—one cannot see a sick heart or a failing kidney. Instead, what can be observed is the body's attempt to compensate for changes in function brought about by the disease, such as the tachycardia that accompanies blood loss or the increased respiratory rate that occurs with pneumonia.

It is important to recognize that a single sign or symptom may be associated with a number of different disease states. For example, an elevated temperature can indicate the presence of an infection, heat stroke, brain tumor, or any number of other disorders. A differential diagnosis that describes the origin of a disorder usually requires information regarding a number of signs and symptoms. For example, the presence of fever, a reddened sore throat, and positive throat culture describes a "strep throat" infection. A *syndrome* is a compilation of signs and symptoms (*e.g.*, chronic fatigue syndrome) that are characteristic of a specific disease state. *Complications* are possible adverse extensions of a disease or outcomes from treatment. *Sequelae* are lesions or impairments that follow or are caused by a disease.

Diagnosis

A *diagnosis* is the designation as to the nature or cause of a health problem (*e.g.*, bacterial pneumonia or hemorrhagic stroke). The diagnostic process usually requires a careful history and physical examination. The history is used to obtain a person's account of his or her symptoms, their progression, and the factors that contribute to a diagnosis. The physical examination is done to observe for signs of altered body structure or function.

The development of a diagnosis involves weighing competing possibilities and selecting the most likely one from among the conditions that might be responsible for the person's clinical presentation. The clinical probability of a given disease in a person of a given age, sex, race, lifestyle, and locality often is influential in arrival at a presumptive diagnosis. Laboratory tests, radiologic studies, CT scans, and other tests often are used to confirm a diagnosis.

Normality. An important factor when interpreting diagnostic test results is the determination of whether they are normal or abnormal. Is a blood count above normal, within the normal range, or below normal? Normality usually determines whether further tests are needed or if interventions are necessary. What is termed a *normal* value for a laboratory test is established statistically from test results obtained from a selected sample of people. The normal values refer to the 95% distribution (mean plus or minus two standard deviations [mean $\pm$ 2 SD]) of test results for the reference population.[12] Thus, the normal levels for serum sodium (135 to 145 mEq/L) represent the mean serum level for the reference population $\pm$ 2 SD. The normal values for some laboratory tests are adjusted for sex or age. For example, the normal hemoglobin range for women is 12.0 to 16.0 g/dL and for men, 14.0 to 17.4 g/dL.[13] Serum creatinine level often is adjusted for age in the elderly (see Chapter 30), and normal values for serum phosphate differ between adults and children.

Reliability, Validity, Sensitivity, Specificity, and Predictive Value. The quality of data on which a diagnosis is based may be judged for its reliability, validity, sensitivity, specificity, and predictive value.[14,15] *Reliability* refers to the extent to which an observation, if repeated, gives the same result. A poorly calibrated blood pressure machine may give inconsistent measurements of blood pressure, particularly of pressures in either the high or low range. Reliability also depends on the persons making the measurements. For example, blood pressure measurements may vary from one observer to another because of the technique that is used (*e.g.*, different observers may deflate the cuff at a different rate, thus obtaining different values), the way the numbers on the manometer are read, or differences in hearing acuity. *Validity* refers to the extent to which a measurement tool measures what it is intended to measure. This often is assessed by comparing a measurement method with the best possible method of measure that is available. For example, the validity of blood pressure measurements obtained by a sphygmomanometer might be compared with those obtained by intra-arterial measurements.

Measures of sensitivity and specificity are concerned with determining how well the test or observation identifies people with the disease and people without the disease. *Sensitivity* refers to the proportion of people with a disease who are positive for that disease on a given test or observation (called a *true-positive* result). *Specificity* refers to the proportion of people without the disease who are negative on a given test or observation (called a *true-negative* result). A test that is 95% specific correctly identifies 95 of 100 normal people. The other 5% are *false-positive* results. A false-positive test result, particularly for conditions such as human immunodeficiency virus (HIV) infection, can be unduly stressful for the person being tested (see Chapter 20). In the case of HIV testing, a positive result on the initial antibody test is followed up with a more sensitive test. On the other hand, *false-negative* test results in conditions such as cancer can delay diagnosis and jeopardize the outcome of treatment.

Predictive value is the extent to which an observation or test result is able to predict the presence of a given disease or condition. A *positive predictive value* refers to the proportion of true-positive results that occurs in a given population. In a group of women found to have "suspect breast nodules" in a cancer screening program, the proportion later determined to have breast cancer would constitute the positive predictive value. A *negative predictive value* refers to the true-negative observations in a population. In a screening test for breast cancer, the negative predictive value represents the proportion of women without suspect nodules who do not have breast cancer. Although predictive values rely in part on sensitivity and specificity, they depend more heavily on the prevalence of the condition in the population. Despite unchanging sensitivity and specificity, the positive predictive value of an observation rises with prevalence, whereas the negative predictive value falls.

Clinical Course

The clinical course describes the evolution of a disease. A disease can have an acute, subacute, or chronic course. An *acute disorder* is one that is relatively severe, but self-limiting. *Chronic disease* implies a continuous, long-term process. A chronic disease can run a continuous course or it can present with exacerbations (aggravation of symptoms and severity of the disease) and remissions (a period during which there is a lessening of severity and a decrease in symptoms). *Subacute disease* is intermediate or between acute and chronic: it is not as severe as an acute and not as prolonged as a chronic disease.

The spectrum of disease severity for infectious diseases such as hepatitis B can range from preclinical to persistent chronic infection. During the *preclinical stage*, the disease is not clinically evident but is destined to progress to clinical disease. As with hepatitis B, it is possible to transmit the virus during the preclinical stage. *Subclinical disease* is not clinically apparent and is not destined to become clinically apparent. It is diagnosed with antibody or culture tests. Most cases of tuberculosis are not clinically apparent and evidence of their presence is established by skin tests. *Clinical disease* is characterized by signs and symptoms. A persistent chronic infectious disease persists for years, sometimes for life. *Carrier status* refers to an individual who harbors an organism but is not infected as evidenced by antibody response or clinical manifestations. This person still can infect others. Carrier status may be of limited duration or it may be chronic, lasting for months or years.

In summary, health is determined by many factors, including genetics, age and sex, and cultural and ethnic differences. The WHO defines health as a "state of complete physical, mental, and social well-being and not merely the absence of disease and infirmity."

The ability of the body to adapt to changes that occur in both health and disease is affected by such factors as age, health status, and psychosocial resources. Adaptation is further affected by the availability and number of adaptive responses. Extreme age and disease conditions, such as when changes occur suddenly rather than gradually, also affect the capacity to adapt.

The term *pathophysiology* may be defined as the physiology of altered health. A *disease* has been defined as any deviation from or interruption of the normal structure or function of any part, organ, or system of the body that is manifested by a characteristic set of symptoms or signs and whose etiology, pathology, and prognosis may be known or unknown. The causes of disease are known as *etiologic factors*. Recognized etiologic agents include biologic agents (bacteria, viruses), physical forces (trauma, burns, radiation), chemical agents (poisons, alcohol), and nutritional excesses or deficits. *Pathogenesis* describes how the disease process evolves. *Morphology* refers to the structure or form of cells or tissues; *morphologic changes* are changes in structure or form that are characteristic of a disease.

Disease can manifest itself through signs and symptoms. A symptom is a subjective complaint, such as pain or dizziness; a sign is an observable manifestation, such as an elevated temperature or a reddened sore throat. A syndrome is a compilation of signs and symptoms that are characteristic of a specific disease state.

The clinical course of a disease describes its evolution. It can be acute (relatively severe, but self-limiting), chronic (continuous or episodic, but taking place over a long period), or subacute (not as severe as acute or as prolonged as chronic). Within the disease spectrum, a disease can be designated preclinical, or not clinically evident; subclinical, not clinically apparent and not destined to become clinically apparent; or clinical, characterized by signs and symptoms.

Perspectives on Health and Disease in Populations

After you have completed this section of the chapter, you should be able to meet the following objectives:

✦ Define the term *epidemiology*
✦ Compare the meaning of the terms *incidence* and *prevalence* as they relate to measures of disease frequency
✦ Compare the sources of information and limitations of mortality and morbidity statistics
✦ Characterize the natural history of a disease
✦ Differentiate primary, secondary, and tertiary levels of prevention

The health of individuals is closely linked to the health of the community and to the population it encompasses. The ability to traverse continents in a matter of hours has opened the world to issues of populations at a global level. Diseases that once were confined to local areas of the world now pose a threat to populations throughout the world.

As we move into the twenty-first century, we are continually reminded that the health care system and the services it delivers are targeted to particular populations. Managed care systems are focused on a population-based approach to planning, delivering, providing, and evaluating health care. The focus of health care also has begun to emerge as a partnership in which individuals are asked to assume greater responsibility for their own health.

EPIDEMIOLOGY AND PATTERNS OF DISEASE

Epidemiology is the study of disease in populations. It was initially developed to explain the spread of infectious diseases during epidemics and has emerged as a science to study risk factors for multifactorial diseases, such as heart disease and cancer. Epidemiology looks for patterns, such as age, race, dietary habits, lifestyle, or geographic location of persons affected with a particular disorder. In contrast to biomedical researchers, who seek to elucidate the mechanisms of disease production, epidemiologists are more concerned with whether something happens than how it happens.[16] For example, the epidemiologist is more concerned with whether smoking itself is related to cardiovascular disease and whether the risk of heart disease decreases when smoking ceases. On the other hand, the biomedical researcher is more concerned about the causative agent in cigarette smoke and the pathway by which it contributes to heart disease.

Much of our knowledge about disease comes from epidemiologic studies. Epidemiologic methods are used to determine how a disease is spread, how to control it, how to prevent it, and how to eliminate it. Epidemiologic methods also are used to study the natural history of disease, to evaluate new preventative and treatment strategies, to explore the impact of different patterns of health care delivery, and to predict future health care needs. As such, epidemiologic studies serve as a basis for clinical decision making, allocation of health care dollars, and development of policies related to public health issues.

Prevalence and Incidence

Measures of disease frequency are an important aspect of epidemiology. They establish a means for predicting what diseases are present in a population and provide an indication of the rate at which they are increasing or decreasing. A *disease case* can be either an existing case or the number of new episodes of a particular illness that is diagnosed within a given period. *Incidence* is the number of new cases arising in a population during a specified time. It is determined by dividing the number of new cases of a disease by the population at risk for development of the disease during the same period. *Prevalence* is the number of people in a population who have a particular disease at a given point in time or period. It is determined by dividing the existing number of cases by the population at risk for development of the disorder during the same period. Incidence and prevalence rates always are reported as proportions (*e.g.*, cases per 100 or cases per 100,000).

Morbidity and Mortality

Morbidity and mortality statistics provide information about the functional effects (morbidity) and death-producing (mortality) characteristics of a disease. These statistics are useful in terms of anticipating health care needs, planning of public education programs, directing health research efforts, and allocating health care dollars.

Mortality or death statistics provide information about the trends in the health of a population. In most countries, people are legally required to record certain facts such as age, sex, and cause of death on a death certificate. Internationally agreed classification procedures (the International Classification of Diseases by the WHO) are used for coding the cause of death and the data are expressed as death rates.[8] Crude mortality rates (*i.e.*, number of deaths in a given period) do not account for age, sex, race, socioeconomic status, and other factors. For this reason, mortality often is expressed as death rates for a specific population, such as the infant morality rate. Mortality also can be described in terms of the leading causes of death according to age, sex, race, and ethnicity. Among all persons 65 years of age and older, the five leading causes of death in the United States are heart disease, cancer, stroke, chronic obstructive lung disease, and pneumonia and influenza[9] (Fig. 1-1). In 1997, for example, diabetes was the third leading cause of death among American Indians 65 years of age and older, the fourth leading cause of death among older Hispanic and black persons, and the sixth leading cause of death among older white persons and Asian Americans.[9]

Morbidity describes the effects an illness has on a person's life. Many diseases, such as arthritis, have low death rates but have a significant impact on a person's life. Morbidity is concerned not only with the occurrence or incidence of a disease, but with persistence and the long-term consequences of the disease.

DETERMINATION OF RISK FACTORS

Conditions suspected of contributing to the development of a disease are called *risk factors*. They may be inherent to the person (high blood pressure or overweight) or external

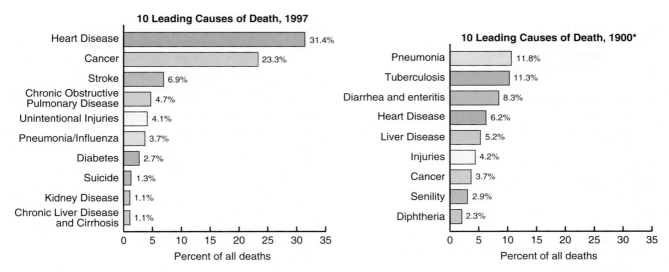

FIGURE 1-1   The 10 leading causes of death as a percentage of deaths in the United States, 1900 and 1997. (U.S. Department of Health and Human Services. [2000]. *Healthy people 2010.* Centers for Disease Control and Prevention, National Center for Health Statistics, National Vital Statistics System. [Unpublished data, 1997.] Accessible at http://web.health.gov/healthypeople/)

(smoking or drinking alcohol). There are different types of studies used to determine risk factors, including cross-sectional studies, case-control studies, and cohort studies. *Cross-sectional studies* use the simultaneous collection of information necessary for classification of exposure and outcome status. They can be used to compare the prevalence of a disease in those with the factor (or exposure) with the prevalence of a disease in those who are unexposed to the factor, such as the prevalence of coronary heart disease in smokers and nonsmokers. *Case-control studies* are designed to compare persons known to have the outcome of interest (*cases*) and those known not to have the outcome of interest (*control*). Information on exposures or characteristics of interest is then collected from persons in both groups. For example, the characteristics of maternal alcohol consumption in infants born with fetal alcohol syndrome (cases) can be compared with those in infants born without the syndrome (control). A *cohort* is a group of persons who were born at approximately the same time or share some characteristics of interest. Persons enrolled in a cohort study (also called a *longitudinal study*) are followed over a period to observe some health outcome. A cohort may consist of a single group of persons chosen because they have or have not been exposed to suspected risk factors; two groups specifically selected because one has been exposed and the other has not; or a single exposed group in which the results are compared with the general population. The Framingham Study, which examined the characteristics of people who would later experience coronary heart disease, and the Nurses' Health Study, which initially explored the relationship between oral contraceptives and breast cancer, are two well-known cohort studies.

The Framingham Study

One of the best-known examples of a cohort study is the Framingham Study, which was carried out in Framingham,

Massachusetts.[17] Framingham was selected because of the size of the population, the relative ease with which the people could be contacted, and the stability of the population in terms of moving into and out of the area. This longitudinal study, which began in 1950, was set up by the U.S. Public Health Service to study the characteristics of people who would later develop coronary heart disease. The study consisted of 5000 persons, aged 30 to 59 years, selected at random and followed for an initial period of 20 years, during which time it was predicted that 1500 of them would develop coronary heart disease. The advantage of such a study is that it can study a number of risk factors at the same time and determine the relative importance of each. Another advantage is that the risk factors can be related later to other diseases such as stroke. Chart 1-1 describes some of the significant milestones from the Framingham Study.

The Nurses' Health Study

A second well-known cohort study is the Nurses' Health Study, which was developed by Harvard University and Brigham and Women's Hospital. The study began in 1976 with a cohort of 121,700 female nurses, 30 to 55 years of age, living in the United States.[18] Initially designed to explore the relationship between oral contraceptives and breast cancer, nurses in the study have provided answers to detailed questions about their menstrual cycle, smoking habits, diet, weight and waist measurements, activity patterns, health problems, and medication use. They have collected urine and blood samples, and even provided researchers with their toenail clippings.[19] In selecting the cohort, it was reasoned that nurses would be well organized, accurate, and observant in their responses, and that physiologically they would be no different from other groups of women. It also was anticipated that their childbearing, eating, and smoking patterns would be similar to those of other working women.

CHART 1-1

Framingham Study: Significant Milestones

- 1960—Cigarette smoking found to increase risk of heart disease
- 1961—Cholesterol level, blood pressure, and electro-cardiogram abnormalities found to increase risk of heart disease
- 1967—Physical activity found to reduce risk of heart disease and obesity to increase risk of heart disease
- 1970—High blood pressure found to increase risk of stroke
- 1976—Menopause found to increase risk of heart disease
- 1977—Effects of triglycerides and low-density lipoprotein (LDL) and high-density lipoprotein (HDL) cholesterol noted
- 1978—Psychosocial factors found to affect heart disease
- 1986—First report on dementia
- 1988—High levels of HDL cholesterol found to reduce risk of death
- 1994—Enlarged left ventricle shown to increase risk of stroke
- 1996—Progression from hypertension to heart failure described
- 1997—Report of cumulative effects of smoking and high cholesterol on the risk of atherosclerosis

(Abstracted from Framingham Heart Study. [2001]. Research milestones. [On-line.] Available: http://rover.nhlbi.nih.gov/about/framingham/timeline.htm.)

The Nurses' Health Study has yielded over 250 published papers on subjects as diverse as body mass index, weight change, and risk of adult-onset asthma in women;[20] smoking cessation and time course to decreased risk of coronary heart disease in middle-aged women;[21] electric blanket use and breast cancer;[22] waist circumference, waist:hip ratio, and risk of breast cancer;[23] and aspirin and risk of colorectal cancer.[24] After 25 years, 90% of the nurses still respond promptly to the biennial questionnaire—a rate that far exceeds the average for other longitudinal studies.

NATURAL HISTORY

The *natural history* of disease refers to the progression and projected outcome of a disease without medical intervention. By studying the patterns of a disease over time in populations, epidemiologists can better understand its natural history. A knowledge of the natural history can be used to determine disease outcome, establish priorities for health care services, determine the effects of screening and early detection programs on disease outcome, and compare the results of new treatments with the expected outcome without treatment.

There are some diseases for which there are no effective treatment methods available, or the current treatment measures are effective only in certain people. In this case, the natural history of the disease can be used as a predictor of outcome. For example, the natural history of hepatitis C indicates that 80% of people who become infected with the virus fail to clear the virus and progress to chronic infection.[25] Information about the natural history of a disease and the availability of effective treatment methods provides directions for preventive measures. In the case of hepatitis C, careful screening of blood donations and education of intravenous drug abusers can be used to prevent transfer of the virus. At the same time, scientists are striving to develop a vaccine that will prevent infection in persons exposed to the virus. The development of vaccines to prevent the spread of infectious diseases such as polio and hepatitis B undoubtedly has been motivated by knowledge about the natural history of these diseases and the lack of effective intervention measures. With other diseases, such as breast cancer, early detection through use of breast self-examination and mammography increases the chances for a cure.

Prognosis refers to the probable outcome and prospect of recovery from a disease. It can be designated as chances for full recovery, possibility of complications, or anticipated survival time. Prognosis often is presented in relation to treatment options—that is, the expected outcomes or chances for survival with or without a certain type of treatment. The prognosis associated with a given type of treatment usually is presented along with the risk associated with the treatment

LEVELS OF PREVENTION

Basically, leading a healthy life contributes to the prevention of disease. There are three fundamental types of prevention: primary prevention, secondary prevention, and tertiary prevention[26] (Chart 1-2). *Primary prevention* is directed at keeping disease from occurring by removing all risk factors. Immunizations are examples of primary prevention. *Secondary prevention* detects disease early when it is still asymptomatic and treatment measures can effect a cure. The use of a Papanicolaou (Pap) smear for early detection of cervical cancer is an example of secondary prevention. *Tertiary prevention* is directed at clinical interventions that prevent further deterioration or reduce the complications of a disease once it has been diagnosed. An example is the use of β-adrenergic drugs to reduce the risk of death in persons

---

CHART 1-2

Levels of Prevention

- Primary prevention: Actions aimed at prevention of disease
- Secondary prevention: Actions aimed at early detection and prompt treatment of disease
- Tertiary prevention: Treatment and rehabilitation measures aimed at preventing further progress of the disease

who have had a heart attack. Tertiary prevention measures also include measures to limit physical impairment and social consequences of an illness.

Primary prevention often is accomplished outside the health care system. Chlorination and fluoridation of water supplies and laws that mandate seat belt use are examples of community-wide primary prevention. There are fewer community-wide efforts directed at secondary prevention, and those that are available usually do not involve the entire community. Examples include breast self-examination education programs and blood pressure screening programs. Nevertheless, many health care clinics are becoming increasingly devoted to primary and secondary prevention through such activities as prenatal and well-child care, immunizations, lifestyle counseling, and screening for early disease detection or risk factors. There are many fewer tertiary prevention efforts outside the health care system.

In summary, the health of individuals is closely linked to the health of the community and to the population it encompasses. Epidemiology is the study of disease in populations. It looks for patterns such as age, race, and dietary habits of persons who are affected with a particular disorder to determine under what circumstances the particular disorder will occur. Using epidemiologic methods, researchers determine how a disease is spread, how to control it, how to prevent it, and how to eliminate it.

Epidemiologists use measures of disease frequency to predict what diseases are present in a population and as an indication of the rate at which they are increasing or decreasing. Incidence is the number of new cases arising in a population during a specified time. Prevalence is the number of people in a population who have a particular disease at a given point in time or period.

Morbidity and mortality provide epidemiologists with information about the functional effects and death-producing characteristics of a disease. Mortality or death statistics provide information about the trends in the health of a population. Morbidity describes the effects an illness has on a person's life. It is concerned with the incidence of disease as well as its persistence and long-term consequences.

Conditions suspected of contributing to the development of a disease are called *risk factors*. They may be inherent to a person (high blood pressure) or external (smoking). Studies used to determine risk factors include cross-sectional studies, case-control studies, and cohort studies. Cross-sectional studies use the simultaneous collection of information necessary for classification of exposure and outcome status. Case-control studies are designed to compare subjects who are known to have the outcome of interest (cases) with those who are known not to have the outcome of interest (control). Cohort studies involve groups of persons who were born at approximately the time or share some characteristic of interest. The Framingham Study, which examined the characteristics of people in whom coronary heart disease would later develop, and the

Nurses' Health Study, which initially explored the relationship between oral contraceptives and breast cancer, are two well-known cohort studies.

The natural history of disease refers to the progression and projected outcome of a disease without medical intervention. It can be used to determine disease outcome, establish priorities for health care services, provide direction for prevention and early detection programs, and compare treatment methods and their outcomes with untreated outcomes. *Prognosis* is the term used to designate the probable outcome and prospect of recovery from a disease.

The three fundamental types of prevention are primary prevention, secondary prevention, and tertiary prevention. Primary prevention, such as immunizations, is directed at removing risk factors so disease does not occur. Secondary prevention, such as a Pap smear, detects disease when it still is asymptomatic and curable with treatment. Tertiary prevention, such as β-adrenergic drugs to reduce the risk of death in persons who have had a heart attack, focuses on clinical interventions that prevent further deterioration or reduce the complications of a disease.

Related Web Sites

Framingham Heart Study   www.nhlbi.nih.gov/about/framingham
ICIDH-2—International Classification of Functioning, Disability and Health   www.who.int/icidh
National Library of Medicine   www.nlm.nih/gov
Nurses' Health Study home page   www.channing.harvard.edu/nhs
U.S. News and World Report article on Nurses' Health Study, 3/22/99   www.usnews.com/usnews/issue/990322/nycu/22nur.htm
WHOSIS—World Health Organization Statistical Information System   www.who.int/whosis

References

1. Sontag S. (1990). *Illness as metaphor*. New York: Doubleday, Anchor Books.
2. James P., Thorpe N. (1995). *Ancient inventions*. New York: Random House, Inc., Ballantine Books.
3. Porter R. (1998). *The greatest benefit to mankind: A medical history of humanity*. New York: W.W. Norton & Company.
4. McNeill W.H. (1998). *Plagues and peoples*. New York: Doubleday, Anchor Books.
5. Schorr T.M., Kennedy M.S. (1999). *100 years of American nursing*. Philadelphia: Lippincott Williams & Wilkins.
6. American Lung Association. (1982, March). From Koch to today. *American Lung Association Bulletin* 68, 2–3.
7. Le Fanu J. (2000). *The rise and fall of modern medicine*. New York: Carroll & Graf.
8. World Health Organization. (2001). *About WHO: Definition of health; disease eradication/elimination goals*. [On-line.] Available: http//www.who.int/aboutwho/en/history/htm. Accessed June 21, 2001.
9. U.S. Department Health and Human Services. (2000). *Healthy people 2010*. National Health Information Center. [On-line.] Available: http://web.health.gov/healthypeople/.
10. *Dorland's illustrated medical dictionary* (29th ed., p. 511). (2000). Philadelphia: W.B. Saunders.

11. Waldenstrom J. (1989). Sick molecules and our concepts of illness. *Journal of Internal Medicine* 225, 221–227.

12. Brigden M.L., Heathcote J.C. (2000). Problems with interpreting laboratory tests. *Postgraduate Medicine* 107 (7), 145–162.

13. Fischbach F. (2000). *A manual of laboratory and diagnostic tests* (6th ed., p. 74). Philadelphia: Lippincott Williams & Wilkins.

14. Bates B. (1995). *A guide to physical assessment and history taking* (6th ed., pp. 641–642). Philadelphia: J.B. Lippincott.

15. Dawson-Saunders B., Trapp R.G. (1990). Evaluating diagnostic procedures. In Dawson-Saunders B., Trapp R.G. (Eds.), *Basic and clinical biostatistics* (pp. 229–244). Norwalk, CT: Appleton & Lange.

16. Vetter N., Mathews I. (1999). *Epidemiology and public health maintenance*. Edinburgh: Churchill Livingstone.

17. Framingham Heart Study. (2001). *Framingham Heart Study: Design, rationale, objectives, and research milestones.* [On-line.] Available: http://www.nhlbi.nih.gov/about/framingham/design.htm. Accessed June 21, 2001.

18. Brophy B. (1999, March 9). Doing it for science. *U.S. News and World Report.*

19. Garland M., Morris J.S., Stamfer M.J., Colditz G.A., Spate V.L., Baskett C.K., Rosner B., Speizer F.E., Willett W.C., Hunter D.J. (1995). Prospective study of toenail selenium levels and cancer among women. *Journal of the National Cancer Institute* 87, 497–505.

20. Carmago C.A., Weiss S.T., Zhang S., Willett W.C., Speizer F.E. (1999). Prospective study of body mass index, weight gain, and risk of adult-onset asthma in women. *Archives of Internal Medicine* 159, 2582–2588.

21. Kawachi I., Colditz G.A., Stamfer M.J., Willett W.C., Manson J.E., Rosner B., Speizer F.E., Hennekens C.H. (1994). Smoking cessation and time course of decreased risks of coronary heart disease in middle-aged women. *Archives of Internal Medicine* 154, 169–175.

22. Laden F., Neas L.M., Tolbert P.E., Holmes M.D., Hankinson S.E., Spiegelman D., Speizer F.E., Hunter D.J. (2000). Electric blanket use and breast cancer in the Nurses' Health Study. *American Journal of Epidemiology* 152, 41–49.

23. Huang Z., Willett W.C., Colditz G.A., Hunter D.J., Manson J.E., Rosner B., Speizer F.E., Hankinson S.E. (1999). Waist circumference, waist:hip ratio, and risk of breast cancer in the Nurses' Health Study. *American Journal of Epidemiology* 150, 1316–1324.

24. Giovannucci E., Egan K.M., Hunter D.J., Stampfer M.J., Colditz G.A., Willett W.C., Speizer F.E. (1995). Aspirin and the risk of colorectal cancer in women. *New England Journal of Medicine* 333, 609–614.

25. Liang J., Reherman B., Seeff L.B., Hoofnagle J.H. (2000). Pathogenesis, natural history, treatment, and prevention of hepatitis C. *Annals of Internal Medicine* 132, 296–305.

26. Stanhope M., Lancaster J. (2000). *Community and public health nursing* (5th ed., p. 43). St. Louis: Mosby.

Chapter 2

Concepts of Altered Health in Children

Judy Wright Lott

*C*hildren are not miniature adults. Physical and psychological maturation and development strongly influence not only the type of illnesses children experience, but their responses to these illnesses. Although many signs and symptoms are the same in persons of all ages, some diseases and complications are more likely to occur in the child. This chapter provides an overview of the developmental stages of childhood and their relationship to the health care needs of children. Specific diseases are presented throughout other sections of the book.

At the beginning of the 20th century, a child's chances of reaching adulthood in the United States were limited. The infant mortality rate was 200 deaths per 1000 live births.[1] Infectious diseases were rampant, and children, owing to their immature and inexperienced immune systems, as well as frequent exposure to other infected children, were especially vulnerable. With the introduction of antibiotics, infectious disease control, and nutritional and technologic advances, infant mortality decreased dramatically. Although infant mortality has declined over past decades, the record low of 7.2 infant deaths per 1000 live births in 1998 placed the United States only 26th in relation to other industrialized nations.[2,3] Also of great concern is the difference in mortality rates for white and nonwhite infants. Infant death rates among African Americans, Native Americans, Alaska Natives, and Hispanics/Latinos in 1998 were all above the national average of 7.2 deaths per 1000 live births. The greatest disparity exists for African Americans,

whose infant death rate (14.3 per 1000 in 1998) is nearly 2½ times that of white infants (6.0 per 1000 in 1996). Recent data indicate that the racial disparities between white and African-American infant mortality rates are increasing.[1-4]

One of the more perplexing causes of infant mortality is the incidence of preterm birth among women of all races and classes. Despite continued, gradual declines in the overall infant mortality rate during the latter part of the 20th century, the incidence of premature births continues as a challenge to reducing the racial disparities and in reducing the overall incidence. Prematurity and low birth weight is the leading cause of death in African-American infants. For white infants, the leading cause of death is congenital anomalies.[1-3] Sudden infant death syndrome (SIDS) is the third leading cause of overall infant mortality among all races in the United States, accounting for approximately 10% of infant deaths.[4]

Congenital anomalies (birth defects) account for the most infant mortality, causing approximately one in five infant deaths overall. Efforts to decrease mortality rates are aimed at improving access to prenatal care and understanding the underlying causes of neonatal (*i.e.*, infants younger than 28 days of age) mortality, congenital anomalies, and preterm delivery, which are still poorly understood despite continuing research. Many of the major causes of death during the postneonatal period (*i.e.*, age 28 days to 1 year)—SIDS, death from infectious diseases (*e.g.*, pneumonia, influenza), and accidents—may be preventable through health promotion efforts such as routine infant care, immunizations, and teaching of parenting skills, including the "back-to-sleep" program.

Growth and Development

After you have completed this section of the chapter, you should be able to meet the following objectives:

✦ Characterize the use of percentiles to describe growth and development during infancy and childhood

✦ Describe the major events that occur during prenatal development from fertilization to birth

✦ Define the terms *low birth weight, small for gestational age,* and *large for gestational age*

✦ Identify reasons for abnormal uterine growth

✦ Describe assessment methods for determination of gestational age

The phrase *growth and development* describes a process whereby a fertilized ovum becomes an adult person. *Physical growth* describes changes in the body as a whole or in its individual parts. *Development*, on the other hand, embraces other aspects of differentiation, such as changes in body function and psychosocial behaviors.

Physical growth occurs in a cephalocaudal direction. Relative body proportions change over the life span. In early fetal development, the head is the largest part of the body, but this changes as the individual grows (Fig. 2-1).

The average newborn weighs approximately 3000 to 4000 g and is 50 to 53 cm long. The first year is a period of rapid growth demonstrated by lengthening of the trunk and accumulation of subcutaneous fat.[5] After the first year and before entering into puberty, the legs grow more rapidly than any other part of the body.

The onset of puberty is marked by a significant alteration in body proportions because of the effects of the pubertal growth spurt. The feet and hands are the first to grow. Because the trunk grows faster than the legs, at adolescence a large portion of the increase in height is a result of trunk growth. The brain is another organ that undergoes a period of rapid growth. At birth, the brain is 25% of adult size; at 1 year, it is 50% of adult size; and at 5 years, it is 90% of adult size. The size of the head reflects brain growth.[6] Linear growth is a result of skeletal growth. After maturation of the skeleton is complete, linear growth is complete. By 2 years of age, the length is 50% of the adult height. Beginning with the third year, the growth rate is 5 to 6 cm for the next 9 years. During the adolescent period, there is a growth spurt. Males may add approximately 20 cm and females 16 cm to height during this time. Weight is rapidly increased after birth. By 6 months of age, the birth weight is doubled, and by 1 year, it is tripled. The average weight increase is 2 to 2.75 kg per year until the adolescent growth spurt begins.[7]

Growth and development encompass a complex interaction between genetic and environmental influences. The experience of each child is unique, and the patterns of growth and development may be profoundly different for individual children within the context of what is called *normal.* Because of the wide variability, these norms often can be expressed only in statistical terms.

Evaluation of growth and development requires comparison of an individual's growth and development to a standard of growth and development. Statistics are calculations derived from measurements that are used to describe the sample measured or to make predictions about the rest of the population that the sample represented. Because all individuals grow and develop at different rates, the standard for growth and development must somehow take this individual variation into account. The standard typically is derived from measurements made on a sample of individuals deemed representative of the total population. When multiple measurements of biologic variables such as height, weight, head circumference, and blood pressure are made, most values fall around the center or middle of all the values. Plotting the data on a graph yields a bell-shaped curve, which depicts the normal distribution of these continuously variable values (Fig. 2-2).

The mean and standard deviation are common statistics used in describing the characteristics of a population. The mean represents the average of the measurements. It is the sum of the values divided by the number of values. A normal bell-shaped curve is symmetric, with the mean falling in the center of the curve and with one half of the values falling on either side of the mean. The standard de-

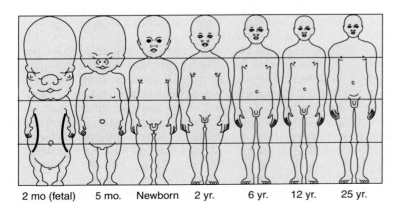

FIGURE 2-1 Changes in body proportions from the 2nd fetal month to adulthood. (Robbins W.J., Brody S., Hogan A.G., et al. [1928]. *Growth*. New Haven: Yale University Press. By permission of publisher)

2 mo (fetal)   5 mo.   Newborn   2 yr.   6 yr.   12 yr.   25 yr.

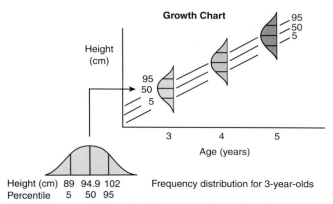

Growth Chart

Height (cm)

Age (years)

Height (cm) 89 94.9 102
Percentile   5   50   95

Frequency distribution for 3-year-olds

FIGURE 2-2 Relationship between percentile lines on the growth curve and frequency distributions of height at different ages. (Behrman R.E., Kliegman R.M., Jenson H.B. [2000]. *Nelson textbook of pediatrics* [16th ed., pp. 23–65]. Philadelphia: W.B. Saunders)

viation determines how far a value varies or deviates from the mean. The points one standard deviation above and below the mean include 68% of all values, two standard deviations 95% of all values, and three standard deviations 99.7% of all values.[5] If a child's height is within one standard deviation of the mean, he or she is as tall as 68% of children in the population. If a child's height is greater than three standard deviations, he or she is taller than 99.7% of children in the population.

The bell-shaped curve can also be marked by percentiles, which are useful for comparison of an individual's values with other values. When quantitative data are arranged in ascending and descending order, a middle value called the *median* can be described with one half (50%) of the values falling on either side. The values can be further divided into percentiles. A percentile is a number that indicates the percentage of values for the population that are equal to or below the number. Percentiles are used most often to compare an individual's value with a set of norms. They are used extensively to develop and interpret physical growth charts and measurements of ability and intelligence.

PRENATAL GROWTH AND DEVELOPMENT

Human development is considered to begin with fertilization, the union of sperm and ovum resulting in a zygote. The process begins with the intermingling of a haploid number of paternal (23, X or Y) and maternal (23, X) chromosomes in the ampulla of the oviduct that fuse to form a zygote. Within 24 hours, the unicellular organism becomes a two-cell organism and, within 72 hours, a 16-cell organism, called a *morula*. This series of mitotic divisions is called *cleavage*. During cleavage, the rapidly developing cell mass travels down the oviduct to the uterus by a series of peristaltic movements. The morula enters the uterus approximately 3 days after fertilization. On the fourth day, the morula is separated into two parts by fluid from the uterus. The outer layer gives rise to the placenta (trophoblast), and the inner layer gives rise to the embryo (embryo-

blast). The structure is now called a *blastocyst*. By the sixth day, the blastocyst attaches to the endometrium. This is the beginning of implantation, and it is completed during the second week of development.[8]

Prenatal development is divided into two main periods. The first, or embryonic, period begins during the second week and continues through the eighth week after fertilization.[6,8] During the embryonic period, the main organ systems are developed and many function at a minimal level (see Chapter 4). The second, or fetal, period begins during the ninth week. During the fetal period, the growth and differentiation of the body and organ systems occur.

Embryonic Development

Human development progresses through three phases.[6] During the first stage of embryonic development, there is growth through an increase in cell numbers and the elaboration of cell products. The second stage of development is one of morphogenesis (development of form), which includes mass cell movement. During this stage, the movement of cells allows them to interact with each other in the formation of tissues and organs. The third stage is the stage of differentiation or maturation of physiologic processes. Completion of differentiation results in organs that are capable of performing specialized functions.

With the onset of embryonic development, which begins during the second week of gestation, the trophoblast continues its rapid proliferation and differentiation, and the embryoblast evolves into a bilaminar embryonic disk. This flattened, circular plate of cells gives rise to all three germ layers of the embryo (*i.e.*, ectoderm, mesoderm, endoderm). The third week is a period of rapid development, noted for the conversion of the bilaminar embryonic disk into a trilaminar embryonic disk through a process called *gastrulation*.[6,8] The ectoderm differentiates into the epidermis and nervous system, and the endoderm gives rise to the epithelial linings of the respiratory passages, digestive

 Prenatal Development

➤ The prenatal period, which begins with implantation of the blastocyst, is divided into two periods: the embryonic period and the fetal period.

➤ The embryonic period spans the second through the eighth weeks of gestation. This period is marked by the formation of the germ layers, early tissue differentiation, and development of the major organs and systems of the body.

➤ The fetal period extends from the ninth week to birth. Development during the fetal period is largely concerned with rapid growth and differentiation of tissues, organs, and body systems.

tract, and glandular cells of organs such as the liver and pancreas. The mesoderm becomes smooth muscle tissue, connective tissue, blood vessels, blood cells, bone marrow, skeletal tissue, striated muscle tissue, and reproductive and excretory organs.

The notochord, which is the primitive axis about which the axial skeleton forms, is also formed during the third week (see Chapter 47). The neurologic system begins its development during this period. *Neurulation*, a process that involves formation of the neural plate, neural folds, and their closure, is completed by the fourth week. Disturbances during this period can result in brain and spinal defects such as spina bifida. The cardiovascular system is the first functional organ system to develop. The primitive heart, which beats and circulates blood, develops during this period (see Chapter 24).

By the fourth week, the neural tube is formed. The embryo begins to curve and fold into a characteristic "C"-shaped structure. The limb buds are visible, as are the otic pits (*i.e.*, primordia of the internal ears) and the lens placodes (primordia of the lens of the eyes). The fifth week is notable for the rapid growth of the head secondary to brain growth.

During the sixth week, the upper limbs are formed by fusion of the swellings around the branchial groove. In the seventh week, there is the beginning of the digits, and the intestines enter the umbilical cord (umbilical herniation). By the eighth week, the embryo is human-like in appearance—eyes are open, and eyelids and ear auricles are easily identified.

Fetal Development

The fetal period extends from the ninth week to birth.[6,8] During the 9th to 12th weeks, fetal head growth slows, whereas body length growth is greatly accelerated. By the 11th week, the intestines in the proximal portion of the cord have returned to the abdomen. The primary ossification centers are present in the skull and long bones, and maturation of the fetal external genitalia is established by the 12th week. During the fetal period, the liver is the major site of red blood cell formation (*i.e.*, erythropoiesis); at 12 weeks, this activity has decreased and erythropoiesis begins in the spleen. Urine begins to form during the 9th to 12th weeks and is excreted into the amniotic fluid.[8]

The 13th through 16th weeks are notable for ossification of the skeleton, scalp hair patterning, and differentiation of the ovaries in female fetuses. By the 17th through 20th week, growth has slowed. The fetal skin is covered with a fine hair called *lanugo* and a white, cheeselike material called *vernix caseosa*. Eyebrows and head hair are visible. In male fetuses, the testes begin to descend, and in female fetuses, the uterus is formed. Brown fat also forms during this period. Brown fat is a specialized type of adipose tissue that produces heat by oxidizing fatty acids. It is similar to white fat but has larger and more numerous mitochondria, which provide its brown color. Brown fat is found near the heart and blood vessels that supply the brain and kidneys and is thought to play a role in maintaining the temperature of these organs during exposure to environmental changes that occur after birth.

During the 21st through 25th weeks, there is a significant fetal weight gain. The type II alveolar cells of the lung begin to secrete surfactant (see Chapter 28). The pulmonary system becomes more mature and able to support respiration during the 26th through 29th weeks. Breathing movements are present owing to central nervous system (CNS) maturation. At this age a fetus often survives if born prematurely and given intensive care. There also is an increasing amount of subcutaneous fat, with white fat making up 3.5% of body weight.[6]

The 30th through 34th weeks are significant for an increasing amount of white fat (8% of body weight), which gives the fetal limbs an almost chubby appearance.[6] During the 35th week, grasp and the pupillary light reflex are present. If a normal-weight fetus is born during this period, it is premature by "date" as opposed to premature by "weight."[6]

Expected time of birth is 266 days, or 38 weeks after fertilization, or 40 weeks after the last menstrual period (LMP).[6] At this time, the neurologic, cardiovascular, and pulmonary systems are developed enough for the infant to make the transition to extrauterine life. The survival of the newborn depends on this adaptation after the placenta is removed.

Fetal Growth and Weight Gain. Development during the fetal period is primarily concerned with rapid growth and differentiation of tissues, organs, and systems. Fetal weight gain is linear from 20 weeks' gestation through 38 weeks' gestation. In the last half of pregnancy, the fetus gains 85% of birth weight. After 38 weeks of gestation, the rate of growth declines, probably related to the constraint of uterine size and decreased placental function. After birth, weight gain again increases similar to intrauterine rates. Birth weight can be affected by a variety of factors, including maternal nutrition, genetic factors, maternal chronic diseases, placental abnormalities, sex, socioeconomic factors, multiple births, chromosomal abnormalities, and infectious diseases.

BIRTH WEIGHT AND GESTATIONAL AGE

At birth, the average weight of the full-term newborn is 3000 to 4000 g. In the past, infants weighing less than 2500 g were classified as premature. In 1961, infants weighing less than 2500 g were classified as low birth weight (LBW). Lubchenco and Battaglia established standards for birth weight, gestational age, and intrauterine growth in the United States in the 1960s[9,10] (Fig. 2-3). With these standards, gestational age can be assessed and normal and abnormal growth can be identified. The Colorado Growth Curve places newborns into percentiles.[9] The 10th through 90th percentiles of intrauterine growth encompass 80% of births.[11] Growth is considered abnormal when a newborn falls above or below the 90th and 10th percentiles, respectively.

An infant is considered term when born between the beginning of the 38th week and completion of the 41st week. An infant is considered premature when born before the end of the 37th week and postmature when born after the end of the 41st week. The lowest mortality rates occur among newborns with weights between 3000 and 4000 g with gestational ages of 38 to 42 weeks.[12–14]

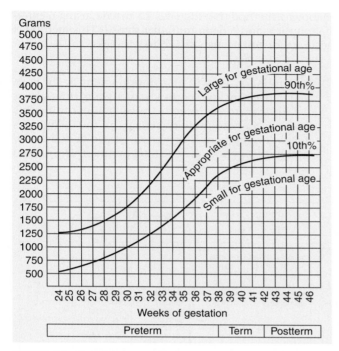

FIGURE 2-3 Classification of newborns by birth weight and gestational age. (Redrawn from Battaglia F.C., Lubchenco L.O. [1967]. A practical classification of newborn infants by weight and gestational age. *Journal of Pediatrics* 71, 159)

Abnormal Intrauterine Growth

Growth of the fetus in the uterus depends on a multitude of intrinsic and extrinsic factors. Optimal fetal growth depends on efficient placental function, adequate provision of energy and growth substrates, appropriate hormonal environment, and adequate room in the uterus. Birth weight variability in a population is primarily determined by maternal heredity, intrinsic fetal growth potential, and environmental factors. Abnormal growth, which can occur at any time during fetal development, can have immediate and long-term consequences for the infant.

Small for Gestational Age. *Small for gestational age* (SGA) is a term that denotes fetal undergrowth. SGA is defined as birth weight less than two standard deviations below the mean for gestational age, or below the 10th percentile. It often is used interchangeably with *intrauterine growth retardation* (IUGR). Worldwide, between 30% and 40% of infants born at weights less than 2500 g are SGA. Mortality rates of severely affected SGA infants are five to six times those of normally grown infants of comparable gestational age.

Fetal growth retardation can occur at any time during fetal development. Depending on the time of insult, the infant can have symmetric or proportional growth retardation or asymmetric or disproportional growth retardation. Impaired growth that occurs early in pregnancy during the hyperplastic phase of growth results in a symmetric growth retardation. Because mitosis is affected, organs and tissues are smaller owing to decreased cell number. Head circum-

ference, length, and weight usually are represented within similar percentile grids, although the head may be smaller, as in microcephaly.[15] This is irreversible postnatally. Causes of proportional IUGR include chromosomal abnormalities, congenital infections, and exposure to environmental toxins.

Impaired growth that occurs later in pregnancy during the hypertrophic phase of growth results in asymmetric growth retardation.[12–14] Infants with IUGR due to intrauterine malnutrition often have weight reduction out of proportion to length or head circumference but are spared impairment of head and brain growth.[7] Tissues and organs are small because of decreased cell size, not decreased cell numbers. Postnatally, the impairment may be partially corrected with good nutrition.

Maternal, placental, and environmental factors affect fetal growth. Because of the effects on the placenta (it also is undergrown), the risk for perinatal complications is higher. These include birth asphyxia, hyperglycemia, polycythemia, meconium (*i.e.*, dark green, mucilaginous newborn stool) aspiration, and hypothermia. The long-term effects of growth retardation depend on the timing and severity of the insult. Many of these infants have developmental disabilities on follow-up examination, especially if the growth retardation is symmetric. They may remain small, especially if the insult occurs early. If the insult occurs later because of placental insufficiency or uterine restraint, with good nutrition catch-up growth can occur and the infant may attain appropriate growth.

Large for Gestational Age. *Large for gestational age* (LGA) is a term that denotes fetal overgrowth. The definition of LGA is birth weight greater than two standard deviations above the mean for gestation, or above the 90th percentile. The excessive growth may result from a genetic predisposition or may be stimulated by abnormal conditions in utero. Infants of diabetic mothers may be LGA, especially if the diabetes was poorly controlled during pregnancy. Maternal hyperglycemia exposes the fetus to increased levels of glucose, which stimulates fetal secretion of insulin. Insulin increases fat deposition, and the result is a macrosomic (large body size) infant. Infants with macrosomia have enlarged viscera and are large and plump because of an increase in body fat. Complications when an infant is LGA include birth asphyxia and trauma due to mechanical difficulties during the birth process, hypoglycemia, and polycythemia.[12]

Assessment Methods

The methods of assessing gestation can be divided into two categories: prenatal assessment and postnatal assessment. *Prenatal assessment* of gestational age most commonly includes careful menstrual history, physical milestones during pregnancy (*e.g.*, uterine size, detection of fetal heart rate and movements), and prenatal tests for maturity (*e.g.*, ultrasound, amniotic fluid studies). Nägele's rule uses the first day of the LMP to calculate the day of labor by adding 7 days to the LMP and counting back 3 months.[12] This method often can be inaccurate if the mother is not a good historian or has a history of irregular menses, which interferes with identification of a normal cycle.

Postnatal assessment of gestational age is most commonly done by examination of external physical and neuromuscular characteristics alone or in combination. The most common methods used in nurseries today were developed by Dubowitz or Ballard. The Dubowitz method is comprehensive and includes 21 criteria using external physical (11) and neuromuscular (10) signs[16] (Fig. 2-4). The estimate of gestational age is best done within 48 hours of birth and is accurate within 2 weeks. The method is less accurate for infants born at less than 30 weeks' gestational age. The Ballard method is an abbreviated Dubowitz method that includes 12 criteria, using 6 external physical and 6 neuromuscular signs.[11] This method is accurate for gestational ages 26 to 44 weeks.

In summary, growth and development begin with union of ovum and sperm and is ongoing throughout a child's life to adulthood. Abnormalities during this process can have profound effects on the infant. Prenatal development is composed of two periods—the embryonic period and the fetal period. During these

A

Neurological sign	Score					
	0	1	2	3	4	5
Posture						
Square window (wrist)	90°	60°	45°	30°	0°	
Ankle dorsiflexion	90°	75°	45°	20°	0°	
Arm recoil	180°	90°-180°	<90°			
Leg recoil	180°	90-180°	<90°			
Popliteal angle	180°	160°	130°	110°	90°	<90°
Heel to ear						
Scarf sign						
Head lag						
Ventral suspension						

B

External sign	Score				
	0	1	2	3	4
Oedema	Obvious oedema hands and feet pitting over tibia	No obvious oedema hands and feet, pitting over tibia	No oedema		
Skin texture	Very thin, gelatinous	Thin and smooth	Smooth, medium thickness Rash or superficial peeling	Slight thickening Superficial cracking and peeling esp. hands & feet	Thick and parchment-like, superficial or deep cracking
Skin color (infant not crying)	Dark red	Uniformly pink	Pale pink variable over body	Pale. Only pink over ears, lips, palms or soles	
Skin opacity (trunk)	Numerous veins and venules clearly seen, esp over abdomen	Veins and tributaries seen	A few large vessels seen over abdomen	A few large vessels indistinctly seen over abdomen	No blood vessels seen
Lanugo (over back)	No lanugo	Abundant, long and thick over whole back	Hair thinning especially over lower back	Small amount of lanugo and bald areas	At least half of back devoid of lanugo
Plantar creases	No skin creases	Faint red marks over anterior half of sole	Definite red marks over more than anterior half, indentations over less than anterior third	Indentations over more than anterior third	Definite deep indentations over more than anterior third
Nipple formation	Nipple barely visible, no areola	Nipple well defined, areola smooth and flat, diameter <0.75 cm	Areola stippled, edge not raised, diameter <0.75 cm	Areola stippled, edge raised, diameter >0.75 cm	
Breast size	No breast tissue palpable	Breast tissue on one or both sides 0.5 cm diameter	Breast tissue both sides, one or both 0.5-1.0 cm	Breast tissue both sides, one or both >1 cm	
Ear form	Pinna flat and shapeless, little or no incurving of edge	Incurving of part of edge of pinna	Partial incurving whole of upper pinna	Well-defined incurving whole of upper pinna	
Ear firmness	Pinna soft, easily folded, no recoil	Pinna soft, easily folded, slow recoil	Cartilage to edge of pinna, but soft in places, ready recoil	Pinna firm, cartilage to edge, instant recoil	
Genitalia Males	Neither testis in scrotum	At least one testis high in scrotum	At least one testis right down		
Females (with hips half abducted)	Labia majora widely separated, labia minora protruding	Labia majora almost cover labia minora	Labia majora completely cover labia minora		

FIGURE 2-4 (A) Neurologic characteristics of the Dubowitz examination. Neurologic criteria are recorded and added to a final score as performed for the physical assessment. (**B**) External characteristics of the Dubowitz examination. Physical criteria are recorded and a final score is obtained following the addition of each category's score. (Dubowitz L., Dubowitz V. [1977]. *Gestational age of the newborn.* Reading, MA: Addison-Wesley)

periods, the zygote becomes the newborn with the organ maturity to make the adjustments necessary for extrauterine life. Infants born before this process is completed are called *premature* and can have major problems with extrauterine adjustments. Postnatal growth is rapid and ongoing and proceeds in an orderly and predictable manner.

Infancy

After you have completed this section of the chapter, you should be able to meet the following objectives:

+ Describe the use of the Apgar score in evaluating infant well-being at birth
+ List three injuries that can occur during the birth process
+ Describe physical growth and organ development during the first year of life
+ Explain how the common health care needs of the premature infant differ from the health care needs of the term newborn or infant
+ Differentiate between organic and nonorganic failure to thrive syndrome

Infancy is defined as that time from birth to approximately 18 months of age. This is a period of rapid physical growth and maturation. The infant begins life as a relatively helpless organism and, through a process of progressive development, gains the skills to interact and cope with the environment. The infant begins life with a number of primitive reflexes and little body control. By 18 months, a child is able to run, grasp and manipulate objects, feed himself or herself, play with toys, and communicate with others.

GROWTH AND DEVELOPMENT

Physical growth is rapid during infancy. After birth, there is a period of relative starvation as the infant adjusts to enteral feeding. Infants lose approximately 5% to 10% of their birth weight, but within days, they begin to gain weight, and by 2 weeks, they are back to birth weight. Average birth weight for a term newborn is 3000 to 4000 g, and this weight usually is doubled by 6 months and tripled by approximately 1 year after birth.

The median height at birth is 49.9 cm for girls and 50.5 cm for boys. During the first 6 months, height increases by 2.5 cm per month. By 1 year, the increase in length is 50% of the birth length. This increase is primarily in trunk growth. Median head circumference at birth is 34.5 cm for girls and 34.8 cm for boys. There is a rapid increase in head circumference in the first year, which is a good indicator of brain growth. Head circumference increases by 1.5 cm per month the first 6 months and 0.5 cm per month the second 6 months. Chest circumference at birth is smaller than head circumference. By 1 year, the head and chest are approximately equal in circumference. After 1 year, chest circumference exceeds head circumference.[7] After birth, most organ systems continue to grow and mature in an orderly fashion. Variations in growth and development are responsible for the differences in body proportions. For example, during the fetal period, the head is the predominant part because of the rapidly growing brain, whereas during infancy, the trunk predominates, and in childhood, the legs predominate. The patterns of growth are cephalocaudal, proximodistal, and mass (size) to specific.

Organ systems must continue to grow and mature after delivery. Many are at a minimal level of functioning at birth. This often places the infant at risk for health problems.

 Infancy

> Infancy, which is the time from birth to 18 months of age, is a period of rapid physical growth and maturation.

> From an average birth weight of 3000 to 4000 g in the full-term infant and a median height of 49.9 cm for girls and 50.5 cm for boys, the infant manages to triple its weight and increase its length by 50% at 1 year of age.

> Developmentally, the infant begins life with a number of primitive reflexes and little body control. By 18 months, a child is able to run, grasp and manipulate objects, feed self, play with toys, and communicate with others.

> Basic trust, the first of Erikson's psychosocial stages, develops as infants learn that basic needs are met regularly.

> At the age of 18 months or the end of the infancy period, the emergence of symbolic thought causes a reorganization of behaviors with implications for the many developmental domains that lie ahead as the child moves to the early childhood stage of development.

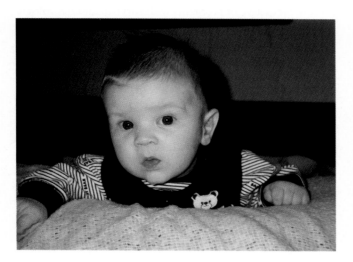

The respiratory system must make the transition from an intrauterine to an extrauterine existence. Onset of respiration must begin at birth for survival. The first breaths expand the alveoli and initiate gas exchange. The infant's respiratory rate initially is rapid and primarily abdominal, but with maturation, it gradually slows. Maturation of the respiratory system includes an increase in the number of alveoli and growth of the airways. Infants are obligatory nose breathers until 3 to 4 months of age; any upper airway obstruction may cause respiratory distress.[7] The trachea is small and close to the bronchi, and the bronchi's branching structures enable infectious agents to be easily transmitted throughout the lungs. The softness of the supporting cartilage in the trachea, along with its small diameter, place the infant at risk for airway obstruction. The auditory (eustachian) tube is short and straight and closely communicates with the ear, putting the infant at risk for middle ear infections (see Chapter 55).

Birth initiates major changes in the cardiovascular system. The fetal shunts, the foramen ovale and ductus arteriosus, begin to close, and the circulation of blood changes from a series to a parallel circuit (see Chapter 24). At birth, the size of the heart is large in relation to the chest cavity. The size and weight of the heart double the first year. Initially, the right ventricle is more muscular than the left ventricle, but this reverses in infancy. The heart rate gradually slows, and systolic blood pressure rises.

The gastrointestinal system is immature, and most digestive processes are poorly functioning until approximately 3 months of age. Solid food may pass incompletely digested and be evident in the stool. At birth, sucking may be poor and require several days to become effective. The tongue thrust reflex is present and aids in sucking, but it disappears at approximately 6 months of age. Stomach capacity increases rapidly in the first months, but because of the limited capacity and rapid emptying, infants require frequent feeding.[7] The infant's genitourinary system is functionally immature at birth. There is difficulty in concentrating urine, and the ability to adjust to a restricted fluid intake is limited. The small bladder capacity causes frequent voiding.

The nervous system undergoes rapid maturation and growth during the infancy period. In contrast to other systems that grow rapidly after birth, the nervous system grows proportionately more rapidly before birth. The most rapid period of fetal brain growth is between 15 and 20 weeks of gestation, at which time there is a significant increase in neurons. A second increase occurs between 30 weeks' gestation and 1 year of age. At birth, the average brain weighs approximately 325 g. By 1 year of age, the weight has tripled, and the brain weighs approximately 1000 g.[7] One of the best indicators of brain growth is head circumference, which increases six times as much during the first year as it does during the second year of life.

The maturation of the nervous system includes an increase in neuron size, in size and number of glial cells, and in interneural connections and branching of axons and dendrites. As this maturation progresses, the level of functioning of the infant increases from simple to complex, from primative reflexes to purposeful movement.

Cortical control of motor functions is closely associated with myelination of nerve fibers. Myelination of the various nerve tracts progresses rapidly after birth and follows a cephalocaudal and proximodistal direction sequence, beginning with the spinal cord and cranial nerves, followed by myelination of the brain stem and corticospinal tracts.[7] In general, sensory pathways become myelinated before motor pathways. The acquisition of fine and gross motor skills depends on this myelination and maturation.

The first year of life also is filled with psychosocial developmental milestones for the infant. Basic needs must be met before the infant can accomplish these developmental tasks. Erikson described the development of a sense of trust as the task of the first stage.[17] If trust is not acquired, the infant becomes mistrustful of others and frustrated with his or her inability to control the surrounding environment.

COMMON HEALTH PROBLEMS

The birth process is a critical event. Prenatal influences, birth trauma, and prematurity have an immediate impact on survival and health. The common health problems in this section have been divided into three subsections: health problems of the newborn, special needs of the premature infant, and health problems of the infant.

Health Problems of the Newborn

Distress at Birth and the Apgar Score.   The Apgar score, devised by Dr. Virginia Apgar, is a scoring system that evaluates infant well-being at birth.[15] The system addresses five categories (*i.e.*, heart rate, respiratory effort, muscle tone, reflex irritability, color), with a total score ranging from 0 to 10, depending on the degree to which these functions are presented (Table 2-1). Evaluations are performed at 1 minute and 5 minutes after delivery. A score of 0 to 3 is indicative of severe distress, 4 to 6 of moderate distress, and 7 to 10 of mild to no distress. Most infants score 6 to 7 at 1 minute and 8 to 9 at 5 minutes. If the score is 7 or less, the evaluation should be repeated every 5 minutes until a score of 7 or greater is obtained. An abnormal score at 5 minutes is more predictive of problems with survival and neurologic outcome than at 1 minute.[12]

Birth Injuries.   Injuries sustained during the birth process are responsible for a significant amount of neonatal mortality and morbidity. In 1991, birth injuries ranked as the eighth leading cause of infant death in the United States. Predisposing factors for birth injuries include macrosomia, prematurity, cephalopelvic disproportion, and dystocia (*i.e.*, abnormal labor or childbirth).[12,18]

Caput succedaneum is a localized area of scalp edema caused by sustained pressure of the presenting part against the cervix. An accumulation of serum or blood forms above the periosteum from the high pressure caused by the obstruction. The caput succedaneum may extend across suture lines and have overlying petechiae, purpura, or ecchymosis. No treatment is needed, and it usually resolves over the first week of life.[12,18]

TABLE 2-1 ◆ Apgar Score Assessment

Criterion	Score*		
	0	1	2
Heart rate	Absent	<100	>100
Respiratory effort	Absent	Weak, irregular	Crying
Muscle tone	Limp	Some flexion	Well flexed
Reflex irritability	No response	Grimace	Cry, gag
Color	Pale	Cyanotic	Pink
Total	0	5	10

* The Apgar score should be assigned at 1 minute and 5 minutes after birth, using a timer. Each criterion is assessed and assigned a 0, 1, or 2. The total score is the assigned Apgar score. If resuscitation is required beyond the 5 minutes, additional Apgar scores also may be assigned as a method to document the response of the newborn to the resuscitation.

Cephalohematoma is a subperiosteal collection of blood from ruptured blood vessels. The margins are sharply delineated and do not cross suture lines. It usually is unilateral, but it may be bilateral, and it usually occurs over the parietal area. The swelling may not be apparent for 24 to 48 hours because subperiosteal bleeding is slow. The overlying skin is not discolored. An underlying skull fracture may be present. Treatment is not needed unless the cephalohematoma is large and results in severe blood loss or significant hyperbilirubinemia. Skull fracture and intracranial hemorrhage are associated complications. An uncomplicated cephalohematoma usually resolves within 2 weeks to 3 months.[11,15]

Skull fractures are uncommon because the infant's compressible skull is able to mold to fit the contours of the birth canal. However, fractures can occur and more often follow a forceps delivery or severe contraction of the pelvis associated with prolonged, difficult labor. Skull fractures may be linear or depressed. Uncomplicated linear fractures often are asymptomatic and do not require treatment. Depressed skull fractures are observable by the palpable indentation of the infant's head. They require surgical intervention if there is compression of underlying brain tissue. A simple linear fracture usually heals within several months.[12,18]

The clavicle is the most frequently fractured bone during the birth process. It is more common in LGA infants and occurs when delivery of the shoulders is difficult in vertex (*i.e.*, head) or breech presentations. The infant may or may not demonstrate restricted motion of the upper extremity, but passive motion elicits pain. There may be discoloration or deformity and, on palpation, crepitus (*i.e.*, a crackling sound from bones rubbing together), and irregularity may be found. Treatment consists of immobilizing the affected arm and shoulder and providing pain relief.[12,18]

The brachial plexuses are situated above the clavicles in the anterolateral bases of the neck. They are composed of the ventral rami of the fifth cervical nerves through the first thoracic nerves. During vertex deliveries, excessive lateral traction of the head and neck away from the shoulders may cause a stretch injury to the brachial plexus on that side. In a breech presentation, excessive lateral traction on the trunk before delivery of the head may tear the lower roots of the cervical cord. If the breech presentation includes delivery with the arms overhead, an injury to the fifth and sixth cervical roots may result. When injury to the brachial plexus occurs, it causes paralysis of the upper extremity. The paralysis often is incomplete.[12,18,19]

Brachial plexus injuries include three types: Erb-Duchenne paralysis (*i.e.*, upper arm), Klumpke's paralysis (*i.e.*, lower arm), and paralysis of the entire arm. Risk factors include an LGA infant and a difficult, traumatic delivery. Erb-Duchenne paralysis occurs with injury to the fifth and sixth cervical roots. It is the most common type of brachial plexus injury and manifests with variable degrees of paralysis of the shoulder and arm. The position of the affected arm is adducted and internally rotated, with extension at the elbow, pronation of the forearm, and flexion of the wrist. When the infant is lifted, the affected extremity is limp. The Moro reflex is impaired or absent, but the grasp reflex is present.

Klumpke's paralysis results from injury to the seventh and eighth cervical and first thoracic nerve roots. It is rare and presents with paralysis of the hand. The infant has wrist drop, the fingers are relaxed, and the grasp reflex is absent. The Moro reflex is impaired, with the upper extremity extending and abducting normally while the wrist and fingers remain flaccid.[12,18,19]

Treatment of brachial plexus injuries includes immobilization, appropriate positioning, and an exercise program. Most infants recover in 3 to 6 months. If paralysis persists beyond this time, surgical repair (neuroplasty, end-to-end anastomosis, nerve grafting) may be done.[19]

Congenital Malformations. Congenital malformations are anatomic or structural abnormalities present at birth (see Chapter 7). They are a major cause of morbidity and mortality in children. In 1998, congenital anomalies accounted for 22% of infant deaths, including 24% of neonatal deaths and 18% of infant deaths beyond the neonatal period.[3,4] Anomalies of the cardiovascular system and CNS account for most deaths due to congenital anomalies.[3] Some stages of embryonic development are more at risk than others for development of congenital malformations after teratogen exposure. The causes of congenital malformations may be classified as genetic, environmental, or multifactorial.

Special Needs of the Premature Infant

Infants born before 37 weeks' gestation are considered premature. They often fall into the LBW category, defined as birth weight less than 2500 g. LBW and prematurity often go hand in hand. Most infants weighing less than 2500 g, and almost all weighing less than 1500 g, are premature. Mortality and morbidity are increased in the premature population and are inversely proportional to the length of gestation. The shorter the time of gestation, the greater is the risk of death or disability. This is because of the immaturity of the organ systems, which interferes with the successful transition to an extrauterine life. Immaturity predisposes this population to the complications of prematurity. Included in this group are those premature infants who have grown abnormally during their shortened gestation (*i.e.*, LGA or SGA). Abnormal growth places an added stress on their transition to extrauterine life.

Despite the advances in obstetric management since the late 1960s, the rate of premature delivery has not significantly changed. The incidence of preterm births (<37 weeks' gestation) has gradually increased since the mid-1980s from 9.5% to 11%. The cause of this increase is not known. African Americans are two to three times more likely to have a preterm delivery; almost one of every five African-American births is premature.[20] In the United States, LBW is responsible for two thirds of neonatal deaths despite an increase in the survival rate of the LBW infant. Contributing risk factors for prematurity also are associated with LBW. Risk factors associated with prematurity and LBW include maternal age (*i.e.*, younger than 16, older than 35 years), race (*i.e.*, African American more than white), socioeconomic status, marital status (*i.e.*, single more than married), smoking, substance abuse, malnutrition, poor or no prenatal care, medical risks predating pregnancy, and medical risks in current pregnancy.[12,21]

The premature infant is poorly equipped to withstand the rigors of extrauterine transition. The organ systems are immature and may not be able to sustain life. The respiratory system may not be able to support gas exchange; the skin may be thin and gelatinous and easily damaged; the immune system is compromised and may not effectively fight infection; and the lack of subcutaneous fat puts the infant at risk for temperature instability. Complications of prematurity include respiratory distress syndrome, pulmonary hemorrhage, transient tachypnea, congenital pneumonia, pulmonary air leaks, bronchopulmonary dysplasia, recurrent apnea, glucose instability, hypocalcemia, hyperbilirubinemia, anemia, intraventricular hemorrhage, necrotizing enterocolitis, circulatory instability, hypothermia, bacterial or viral infection, retinopathy of prematurity, and disseminated intravascular coagulopathies.

Respiratory Problems.   *The respiratory distress syndrome* (RDS), frequently referred to as *hyaline membrane disease*, is the most common complication of prematurity. In the United States, RDS develops in approximately 10% to 15% of newborns weighing less than 2500 g and 60% of infants born at 29 weeks' gestation. The incidence of RDS is lower in African-American than in white infants and in female than in male infants.

The primary cause of RDS is the lack of surfactant in the lungs. Surfactant is produced by type II alveolar cells in the lungs. It is a combination of several phospholipids that lowers the alveolar surface tension and facilitates lung expansion (see Chapters 27 and 28). At 24 weeks' gestation, there are small amounts of surfactant and few terminal air sacs (*i.e.*, primitive alveoli) with underdeveloped pulmonary vascularity. If an infant is born at this time, there is little chance of survival. By 26 to 28 weeks, there usually is sufficient surfactant and lung development to permit survival.

The availability of exogenous surfactant replacement therapy has improved the outcome of RDS and has been recognized as the main factor responsible for the 6.2% decrease in the infant mortality rate in the United States from 1989 to 1990. However, because the survival rate of the sickest infants has improved and because their management is more complex, the incidence of other complications has increased. These include air leak syndromes, bronchopulmonary dysplasia, and intracranial hemorrhage.[12,21]

Apnea and *periodic breathing* are other common respiratory problems in premature infants. Because the respiratory center in the medulla oblongata is underdeveloped in the premature infant, the ability for sustained ventilatory drive often is impaired. *Apnea* is defined as cessation of breathing; it is characterized by failure to breathe for 20 seconds or more and often is accompanied by bradycardia or cyanosis. Among infants weighing less than 1.5 kg, 50% require intervention for significant apneic spells.[12,21] Although apnea may be caused by an underlying disease process such as infection, this is not apnea of prematurity and should not be treated as such.

Periodic breathing commonly occurs in those infants weighing less than 1.8 kg. It is an intermittent failure to breathe for periods lasting less than 10 to 15 seconds. Management of apnea and periodic breathing includes use of medications or ventilatory support until the CNS is developed and able to sustain adequate ventilatory drive.[12,21]

Intraventricular Hemorrhage.   Intraventricular hemorrhage (IVH) is a common problem almost exclusive to premature infants. It ranks second only to RDS as a major cause of death in the premature infant. For infants born after less than 35 weeks' gestation or weighing less than 1400 g, the incidence is 40% to 50%, with the most immature at the highest risk of IVH. The hemorrhage often occurs in a subependymal germinal matrix layer. This is a periventricular structure located between the caudate nucleus and the thalamus at the level of or slightly posterior to the foramen of Monro. The germinal matrix is an early developmental structure that contains a fragile vascular area that is poorly supported by connective tissue. By term, this structure is gone.

Risk factors for IVH include pneumothorax, hypotension, acidosis, coagulopathy, transport, volume expansion, and bicarbonate infusion. The proposed mechanisms for IVH include a hypoxic-ischemic insult resulting in cerebral hyperperfusion of the germinal matrix area that causes vessel rupture. Another proposed mechanism is disruption of vascular integrity in the germinal matrix caused by hypotension. Four grades of hemorrhage have been identified.[12,18] Most hemorrhages resolve, but the more severe hemorrhages may obstruct the flow of cerebrospinal fluid, causing a progressive hydrocephalus (Table 2-2).

Necrotizing Enterocolitis.

Necrotizing enterocolitis (NEC) is an acquired gastrointestinal disease process that is a major problem in preterm infants. The incidence is 1% to 5% of admissions to the neonatal intensive care unit. Although approximately 90% of infants affected are preterm infants weighing less than 1500 g, 10% of infants affected are term infants. The mortality rate varies from 20% to 40%.

The exact cause of NEC is unknown but is thought to be multifactorial. Risk factors for NEC include birth asphyxia, umbilical artery catheterization, patent ductus arteriosus, polycythemia, enteral feeding, and medications such as indomethacin, vitamin E, and xanthines.[22] There is agreement that the process begins with diminished perfusion of the intestinal wall, which results in ischemia and hypoxia that leads to necrosis and gangrene. Although bacterial infection plays a role in the disease, it is not thought to be the initiating event. Milk feeding has been implicated. Approximately 93% of infants in whom NEC develops have been fed enterally.[23] Human milk and commercial formulas serve as substrates for bacterial growth in the gut.

The ileum is most commonly affected, followed by the ascending colon, cecum, transverse colon, and rectosigmoid. The necrosis of the intestine may be superficial, affecting only the mucosa or submucosa, or may extend through the entire intestinal wall. Perforation can occur and lead to peritonitis.[22,24] The manifestations of NEC are variable, but the usual presentation includes abdominal distention, gastric aspirates, bilious stools, lethargy, apnea, and hypoperfusion. The infant often appears septic. Laboratory examination may reveal leukocytosis or leukopenia, neutropenia, thrombocytopenia, glucose instability, electrolyte imbalance, metabolic acidosis, hypoxia, hypercapnia, and disseminated intravascular coagulation. Blood cultures are positive for only approximately 30% of these patients. Microorganisms reported in NEC include *Escherichia coli*, *Klebsiella*, *Enterobacter*, *Pseudomonas*, *Salmonella*, *Clostridium difficile*, and *Clostridium perfringens*.[22]

Clinical diagnosis is primarily radiographic. The radiographic hallmark of NEC is pneumatosis intestinalis or intramural air. Pneumoperitoneum is indicative of intestinal perforation. A large, stationary, distended loop of intestine on repeated radiographs may indicate gangrene, and a gasless abdomen may indicate peritonitis.[22]

Treatment includes cessation of feedings, stomach decompression, broad-spectrum antibiotic coverage, and supportive treatment. Intestinal perforation requires surgical intervention. Intestinal resection of dead intestine with a diverting ostomy is the procedure of choice.[22]

Health Problems of the Infant

Infants are prone to numerous health problems during the first year of life, which may become serious if not recognized and treated appropriately. Many of them may be precipitated by the relative immaturity of the organ systems. Infants are prone to nutritional disturbances, feeding difficulties, problems with food allergies, gastroesophageal reflux, and colic. Injuries, the major cause of death during infancy, are caused by events such as aspiration of foreign objects, suffocation, motor vehicle accidents, falls, poisoning, burns, and drowning. Childhood diseases may be a problem if the infant is not adequately immunized.

Issues Related to Nutrition.

Good nutrition is important during infancy because of rapid growth. Human milk or commercial infant formulas form the basis for the early nutritional needs of the newborn and young infant. The American Academy of Pediatrics recommends breast-feeding for the first 12 months of life. Human milk from a well-nourished mother is easily digested, provides sufficient nutrients and calories for normal growth and development, and has the added benefit of offering some immune protection. Fluoride is recommended for breast-fed infants and those receiving formula made with water containing less than 0.3 ppm of fluoride. Dietary or supplemental iron is added at approximately 6 months of age, when the fetal iron stores are depleted.

TABLE 2-2 ✦ Classification of Periventricular/Intraventricular Hemorrhage

Grade	Location of Hemorrhage and Radiologic Appearance
Mild (grade I)	Subependymal region, germinal matrix
Moderate (grade II)	Subependymal hemorrhage with minimal filling (10%–40%) of lateral ventricles with no or little ventricular enlargement
Severe (grade III)	Subependymal hemorrhage with significant filling of lateral ventricles (>50%) with significant ventricular enlargement
Periventricular hemorrhagic infarction	Intraparenchymal venous hemorrhage

(From Fanaroff A.A., Martin R.J. [1997]. The central nervous system: Intracranial hemorrhage. In *Neonatal-perinatal medicine: Diseases of the fetus and infant* [6th ed., pp. 891–893]. Philadelphia: W.B. Saunders and Volpe J.J. [1995]. Intracranial hemorrhage: Germinal matrix hemorrhage of the premature infant. In *Neurology of the newborn* [3rd ed., pp. 403–463]. Philadelphia: W.B. Saunders.)

Mothers who do not choose to breast-feed their child or who are unable to breast-feed may choose a commercial formula. Several companies produce infant formulas that contain the essential nutrients for infants. Although there are some minor differences, most infant formulas are similar, regardless of which company produces the formula.

Some infants may experience difficulties in consuming mother's milk or infant formulas that are based on cow's milk because of lactase deficiency. Lactase is an enzyme that breaks down lactose, the carbohydrate found in human milk and cow's milk. Some infant formulas contain carbohydrates other than lactose. These formulas are made from soybeans. Other feeding intolerances also may occur. Treatment of any milk or formula intolerance depends on identification of the specific offender and elimination of it from the diet. Newborns and infants frequently exhibit "spitting up" or regurgitation of formula, despite the absence of a formula intolerance. In general, cow's milk-based formulas are preferable to soy-based formulas, and changing to a soy-based formula should be undertaken only when there is a proven case of intolerance. It is important that all claims of formula intolerance be thoroughly investigated before an infant is changed to a soy-based formula. Education of the parents about the signs and symptoms of intolerance and reassurance that spitting up formula is normal may be all that is required. An infant who is gaining weight, appears alert and well-nourished, has adequate stools, and demonstrates normal hunger is unlikely to have a formula intolerance.

One area of infant nutrition that is still the subject of much controversy is the introduction of solid foods. There is great variation in advice regarding when to start solid foods and what solid foods to introduce. In general, human milk or iron-fortified infant formulas should supply most infant nutrition during the first year of life. However, solid foods usually are introduced beginning at 6 months. When solid foods are being introduced, they should be considered as supplemental to the total nutrition and not as the main component of nutrition. Solid foods should be introduced only by spoon-feeding. The addition of cereal to formula in a bottle or in "infant feeders" is not recommended. It has never been shown that early introduction of solid foods causes the infant to sleep longer at night.

Bland infant cereals, such as rice cereal, usually are introduced first. Slow progression to the addition of individual vegetables, fruits, and, finally, meats occurs as the infant learns to chew and swallow food. Infants also become able to drink from a cup rather than a bottle during this time. The addition of desserts is not recommended because these add calories without adding substantial nutrition.

Sometime between 9 and 12 months, the infant's intake of solid foods and formula increases, and the infant can be weaned from the breast or bottle. Much anxiety can accompany weaning, so it should be done gradually. Mothers may need reassurance that their infant is progressing normally at that time.

Irritable Infant Syndrome or Colic.

Colic is usually defined as paroxysmal abdominal pain or cramping in an infant and usually is manifested by loud crying, drawing up of the legs to the abdomen, and extreme irritability. Episodes of colic may last from several minutes to several hours a day. During this time, most efforts to soothe the infant or relieve the distress are unsuccessful. Colic is most common in infants younger than 3 months of age but can persist up to 9 months of age.

Caring for an infant with colic can be frustrating. There is no single etiologic factor that causes colic; therefore, the treatment of colic is not precise. Many nonmedical techniques and pharmacologic preparations such as antispasmodics, sedatives, and antiflatulents have been tried. Nonpharmacologic interventions should be attempted before administration of drugs. Support of the parents is probably the single most important factor in the treatment of colic. Many times the mother (or primary care provider) may be afraid to state just how frustrated she is with her inability to console the infant. An open discussion of this frustration can help the mothers or care providers recognize that their feelings of frustration are normal; frequently, this gives them the added support needed to deal with their infant.

Failure to Thrive.

Failure to thrive is a term that refers to inadequate growth of the child due to the inability to obtain or use essential nutrients. Failure to thrive may be organic or nonorganic. Organic failure to thrive is the result of a physiologic cause that prevents the infant from obtaining or using nutrients appropriately. An example of organic failure to thrive is inadequate growth of an infant with deficient energy reserve because of a congenital defect that makes sucking and feeding difficult. Nonorganic failure to thrive is the result of psychological factors that prevent adequate intake of nutrition. An example of nonorganic failure to thrive is inadequate weight gain due to inadequate intake of nutrients because of parental neglect.

Diagnosis of the type of failure to thrive depends on careful examination and history of the infant and serial follow-up evaluations. An individual infant's growth can be compared with the standards for normal growth and development. Cases of organic failure to thrive usually are easier to diagnose than cases of nonorganic failure to thrive. Diagnosis of nonorganic failure to thrive requires extensive investigation of history, family situation, relationship of the care provider to the infant, and evaluation of feeding practices. The nonorganic basis should be considered early in every case of failure to thrive.

Therapy for failure to thrive depends on the cause. Because long-term nutritional deficiencies can result in impaired physical and intellectual growth, provision of optimal nutrition is essential. Methods to increase nutritional intake by adjusting caloric density of the formula or by parenteral nutrition may be required in cases of organic failure to thrive.

Sudden Infant Death Syndrome.

Defined as the sudden death of an infant younger than 1 year of age that remains unexplained after autopsy, investigation of the death scene, and review of the history, SIDS is the third leading cause of overall infant mortality among all races in the United States, accounting for approximately 10% of infant deaths.[4] SIDS is the leading cause of infant death in the United States during the postneonatal period, between 1 and 12 months of age. Approximately 7000 infants die of SIDS each year.[23,25,26] The specific cause of SIDS is not known. Factors associated with an increased prevalence of SIDS include prone sleeping position, African-American or Native-American race, prematurity, LBW, young maternal age, lack of prenatal care or inadequate prenatal care, smoking or substance use during pregnancy, and exposure to environmental cigarette smoke.[4]

The prone sleeping position is a significant risk factor in SIDS. The frequency of SIDS is more than threefold greater when infants sleep on their stomachs compared with sleeping on their backs.[4] Population-based education programs to decrease the practice of having infants sleep on their stomachs have resulted in a substantial decrease in SIDS.

The exact cause of SIDS is unknown. Theories center on brain stem abnormality, which prevents effective cardiorespiratory control. Features of SIDS include prolonged sleep apnea, increased frequency of brief inspiratory pauses, excessive periodic breathing, and impaired response to increased carbon dioxide or decreased oxygen. A diagnosis of SIDS can be made only if an autopsy is performed to exclude other causes of death. Differentiation of child abuse from SIDS is an important consideration, and each case of SIDS must be subjected to careful examination.

Support of the family of an infant with SIDS is crucial. Parents frequently feel guilty or inadequate as parents. The fact that there must be close scrutiny to differentiate a SIDS death from a death by child abuse adds to the guilt and disappointment felt by the family. After a diagnosis of SIDS is made, it is important that the parents and other family members receive information about SIDS. Health care providers need to be fully aware of resources available to families with a SIDS death. The siblings of the child who died should not be overlooked. Children also need information and support to get through the grief process. Children may blame themselves for the death or fear that they, too, may die of SIDS. Too many times, they are not given information because the adults are trying to protect them.

Injuries. Injuries are the major cause of death in infants 6 to 12 months of age. Aspiration of foreign objects, suffocation, falls, poisonings, drowning, burns, and other bodily damage may occur because of the infant's increasing ability to investigate the environment. Childproofing the environment can be an important precaution to prevent injuries. No home or environment can be completely childproofed, but close supervision of the child by a competent care provider is essential to prevent injury.

Motor vehicle accidents are responsible for a significant number of infant deaths. After 1 year of age, motor vehicle accidents become the number one cause of accidental death. Most states require that infants be placed in an approved infant safety restraint while riding in a vehicle. The middle of the back seat is considered the safest place for the infant to ride. Many hospitals do not discharge an infant unless there is a safety restraint system in the car. If a family cannot afford a restraint system, programs are available that donate or loan the family a restraint. Health care providers must be involved in educating the public about the dangers of carrying infants in vehicles without taking proper precautions to protect them.

Infectious Diseases. One of the most dramatic improvements in infant health has been related to widespread immunization of infants and children to the major childhood communicable diseases, including diphtheria, pertussis, tetanus, polio, measles, mumps, rubella, hepatitis, and *Haemophilus influenzae* type B infection. Immunizations to these infectious diseases have greatly reduced morbidity and mortality in infants and young children. These immunizations are given at standard times as part of health promotion in infants and children. However, these immunization programs have not completely eradicated these diseases, but have only lowered their prevalence. Immunization programs are effective only if all children receive the immunizations. Although most immunizations can be received through local health departments at no or low cost, many infants or young children do not routinely receive immunizations or do not receive the full regimen of immunizations. Methods to improve compliance and access to immunizations are needed.

> In summary, infancy is defined as that period from birth to 18 months of age. During this time, growth and development are ongoing. The relative immaturity of many of the organ systems places the infant at risk for a variety of illnesses. Birth initiates many changes in the organ systems as a means of adjusting to postnatal life. The birth process is a critical event, and maladjustments and injuries during the birth process are a major cause of death or disability. Premature delivery is a significant health problem in the United States. The premature infant is at risk for numerous health problems because of the interruption of intrauterine growth and immaturity of organ systems.

Early Childhood

After you have completed this section of the chapter, you should be able to meet the following objectives:

+ Define *early childhood*
+ Describe the growth and development of early childhood
+ Discuss the common health problems of early childhood

Early childhood is considered the period of 18 months through 5 years of age. During this time, the child passes through the stages of toddler (*i.e.*, 18 months to 3 years) and preschooler (*i.e.*, 3 to 5 years). There are many changes as the child moves from infancy through the toddler and preschool years. The major achievements are the development and refinement of locomotion and language, which take place as children progress from dependence to independence.[12,21]

GROWTH AND DEVELOPMENT

Early childhood is a period of continued physical growth and maturation. Compared with infancy, physical growth is not as dramatic. Weight gain during the toddler stage is

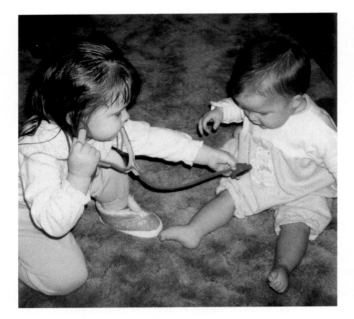

1.8 to 2.7 kg per year (an average of 2.3 kg per year). At 2 years, the average weight is 12 kg, and by 2.5 years the birth weight has quadrupled. By the preschool years, growth slows considerably. The average weight gain is approximately 2.3 kg per year, and almost all organ systems have reached full maturity. At 3 years, the average weight is 14.5 kg, and by 6 years, it has increased to 21 kg. During early childhood, height increases an average 7.5 cm per year and comes primarily through an increase in leg length. At 2 years of age, the average height is 86.6 cm, and by 6 years, it has reached 116 cm. In the first 2 years of life, head circumference increases by 2.5 cm per year. After 2 years of age, head circumference growth slows, and by 5 years, the average increase in head circumference is 1.25 cm per year.[7]

The maturation of organ systems is ongoing during early childhood. The respiratory system continues its growth and maturation, but because of the relative immaturity of the airway structures, otitis media and respiratory infections are common. The barrel-shaped chest that is characteristic of infancy has begun to change to a more adult shape. The respiratory rate of infancy has slowed and averages 20 to 30 breaths per minute. Respirations remain abdominal until 7 years of age.[7]

Neural growth remains rapid during early childhood. Growth is primarily hypertrophic. The brain is 90% of adult size by 2 years of age. The cephalocaudal, proximo-distal principle is followed as myelinization of the cortex, brain stem, and spinal cord is completed. The spinal cord is completely myelinated by 2 years of age. At that time, control of anal and urethral sphincters and the motor skills of locomotion can be achieved and mastered. The continuing maturation of the neuromuscular system is increasingly evident as complex gross and fine motor skills are acquired throughout early childhood.

Growth and maturation in the musculoskeletal system continue with ossification of the skeletal system, growth of

 Early Childhood

➤ Early childhood, which encompasses the period from 18 months through 5 years of age, is a period of continued growth and development.

➤ During this time, the child passes through the stages of toddler (*i.e.*, 18 months to 3 years) and preschooler (*i.e.*, 3 years through 5 years).

➤ The major achievements are the development and refinement of locomotion and language, which take place as children progress from dependence to independence.

➤ During early childhood, the child begins to develop independence. The toddler must acquire a sense of autonomy while overcoming a sense of doubt and shame. The preschooler must acquire a sense of initiative and develop a conscience.

➤ Learning is ongoing and progressive and includes interactions with others, appropriate social behavior, and sex role functions.

the legs, and changes in muscle and fat proportions. Legs grow faster than the trunk in early childhood; after the first year of life, approximately two thirds of the increase in height is leg growth. Muscle growth is balanced by a corresponding decrease in adipose tissue accumulation.

During early childhood, many important psychosocial tasks are mastered by the child. Independence begins to develop, and the child is on the way to becoming a social being in control of the environment. Development and refinement of gross and fine motor abilities allow involvement with a potentially infinite number of tasks and activities.

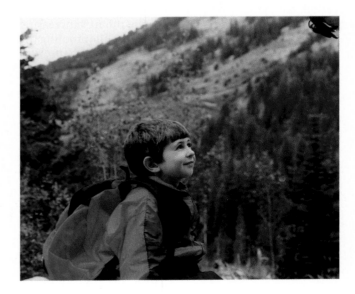

Learning is ongoing and progressive and includes interactions with others, appropriate social behavior, and sex role functions. Erikson described the tasks that must be accomplished in early childhood. The toddler must acquire a sense of autonomy while overcoming a sense of doubt and shame. The preschooler must acquire a sense of initiative and develop a conscience.[17]

COMMON HEALTH PROBLEMS

The early childhood years can pose significant health risks to the growing and maturing child. Injuries are the leading cause of death in children between the ages of 1 and 4 years; only adolescents experience more injuries. Locomotion, together with a lack of awareness of danger, places toddlers and preschoolers at special risk for injuries. Motor vehicle accidents are responsible for almost 50% of all accidental deaths in this group. Many of the injuries and deaths can be prevented by appropriate restraints in car seats and seat belts. Other major causes of injuries include drowning, burns, poisoning, falls, aspiration and suffocation, and bodily damage.[7]

Infectious diseases can be a problem for children during early childhood because of their susceptibility. This also may be the time when children first enter day care, which increases their exposure to other children and infectious diseases. The major disorders include the communicable childhood diseases (*e.g.,* common cold, influenza, varicella [chicken pox], and gastrointestinal tract infections).[6]

Child maltreatment is an increasing problem in the United States. Although the numbers vary according to the methods and definitions used, the best estimates indicate that approximately 1.4 million children in the United States undergo some form of abuse.[27] Child maltreatment includes physical and emotional neglect, physical abuse, and sexual abuse. Neglect is the most common type of maltreatment and can take the form of deprivation of basic necessities or failure to meet the child's emotional needs. It is often attributed to poor parenting skills. Physical abuse is the deliberate infliction of injury. The cause is probably multifactorial, with predisposing factors that include the parent, child, and environment. Sexual abuse is on the rise and includes a spectrum of types. The typical abuser is male. Children often do not report the abuse because they are afraid of not being believed.[7,27]

In summary, early childhood is defined as the period from 18 months to 5 years of age—the toddler and preschool years. Growth and development continue but are not as dramatic as during the prenatal and infancy periods. Early childhood is a time when most organ systems reach maturity and the child becomes an independent, mobile being. There continue to be significant health risks during this period, especially from infectious diseases and injuries. Injuries are the leading cause of death during this period. Child abuse is rapidly increasing as a major health problem.

Early School Years to Late Childhood

After you have completed this section of the chapter, you should be able to meet the following objectives:

+ Define *early school years*
+ Characterize the growth and development that occurs during the early school years
+ Discuss the common health problems of the early school years

In this text, early school years or late childhood is defined as the period in which a child begins school through the beginning of adolescence. These 6 years involve a great deal of change, but when one recollects "childhood," these are the years most often remembered. The experiences of this period have a profound effect on the physical, cognitive, and psychosocial development of the child, which influence the adult that the child will become.

GROWTH AND DEVELOPMENT

Although physical growth is steady throughout the early school years, it is slower than in the previous periods and the adolescent period to follow. During late childhood, children typically gain approximately 3 to 3.5 kg and grow an average of 6 cm per year.[5] The average 6-year-old is 116 cm tall and weighs approximately 21 kg. By 12 years of age, the same child may weigh 40 kg and be 150 cm tall. There is only a slight difference in the body sizes of boys and girls during this period, with boys being only slightly taller and heavier than girls.[7]

During late childhood, a child's legs grow longer, posture improves, and his or her center of gravity descends to

 Middle Childhood

➤ The middle childhood years (6 to 12 years) are those during which the child begins school through the beginning of adolescence.

➤ Growth during this period averages 3 to 3.5 kg and 6 cm per year, and occurs in approximately three to four bursts per year that last for approximately 8 weeks.

➤ Muscular strength, coordination, and stamina increase progressively, as does the ability to perform complex movements such as shooting basketballs, playing the piano, and dancing.

➤ During this stage, the child develops the cognitive skills that are needed to consider several factors simultaneously and to evaluate oneself and perceive others' evaluations.

a lower point. These changes make children more graceful and help them to be successful at climbing, bike riding, roller skating, and other physical activities. Body fat distribution decreases and, in combination with the lengthening skeleton, gives the child a thinner appearance. As the body fat decreases, lean muscle mass increases. By 12 years of age, boys and girls have doubled their body strength and physical capabilities. Although muscular strength increases, the muscles are still relatively immature and injury from overstrenuous activities, such as difficult sports, can occur. With the gains in length, the head circumference decreases in relation to height, waist circumference decreases in relation to height, and leg length increases in relation to height.

Facial proportions change as the face grows faster in relation to the rest of the cranium. The brain and skull grow very little during late childhood. Primary teeth are lost and replaced by permanent teeth. When the permanent teeth first appear, they may appear to be too big for the mouth and face. This is a temporary imbalance that is alleviated as the face grows. Caloric requirements usually are lower compared with previous periods and with the adolescent period to follow. Cardiac growth is slow. Heart rate and respiratory rates continue to decrease, and blood pressure gradually rises. Growth of the eye continues, and the normal farsightedness of the preschool child is gradually converted to 20/20 vision by approximately 11 to 12 years. Frequent vision assessment is recommended during late childhood as part of normal routine health screenings.[7]

Bone ossification and mineralization continues. Bones cannot resist muscle pressure and pull as well as mature bones. Precautions should be taken to prevent alterations in bone structure, such as providing properly fitting shoes and adequate desks to prevent poor posture. Children should be checked routinely and often for scoliosis (see Chapter 58) during this period.

Toward the end of late childhood, the physical differences between the two sexes become apparent. Females usually enter pubescence approximately 2 years before males, resulting in noticeable differences in height, weight, and development of secondary sex characteristics. There is much individual variation among children of the same sex. These differences can be extremely difficult for children to cope with.

Entry into the school setting has a major impact on the psychosocial development of the child at this age. The child begins to form relationships with other children, forming groups. Peers become more important as the child moves out of the security of the family and into the bigger world. Usually during this period, children begin to form closer bonds with individual "best friends." However, the best friend relationships may frequently change. The personality of the child begins to appear. Although the personality is still developing, the basic temperament and approach to life become apparent. Although changes in personality occur with maturity, the basic elements may not change. The major task of this stage, as identified by Erikson, is the development of industry or accomplishment.[17] Failure to meet this task results in a sense of inferiority or incompetence, which can impede further progress.

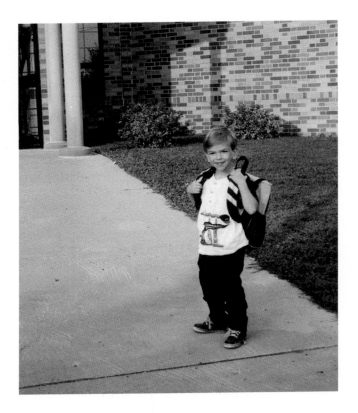

COMMON HEALTH PROBLEMS

Because of the high level of immune system competence in late childhood, these children have an immunologic advantage over earlier years. Respiratory infections are the leading cause of illness at this time, followed by gastrointestinal disorders. The chief cause of mortality is accidents, primarily motor vehicle accidents. Immunization against the major communicable diseases of childhood has greatly improved the health of children in their early childhood years.

Health promotion includes appropriate dental care. The incidence of dental caries has decreased since the addition of fluoride to most water systems in the United States. However, there is still a high incidence of dental caries during late childhood that is related to inadequate dental care and a high amount of dietary sugar. Children at the early part of this stage may not be as effective in brushing their teeth and may require adult assistance, but they may be reluctant to allow parental help.

Infections with bacterial and fungal agents are a common problem in childhood. These infections commonly occur as respiratory, gastrointestinal, or skin diseases. Infections of the skin occur more frequently in this age group than in any other age group, probably related to increased exposure to skin lesions. Other acute or chronic health problems may surface for the first time. Asthma, caused by allergic reactions, frequently manifests for the first time during the early school years. Epilepsy also may be first diagnosed during this period. Many childhood cancers also may appear. Developmental disabilities or specific learning disabilities may become apparent as the child enters school.

In summary, early school years to late childhood is defined as that period from beginning school through adolescence. During these 6 years, growth is steady but much slower than in the previous periods. Entry into school begins the formation of relationships with peers and has a major impact on psychological development. This is a wonderful period of relatively good health secondary to an immunologic advantage, but respiratory disease poses a leading cause of illness, and motor vehicle accidents are the major cause of death. Several chronic health problems such as asthma, epilepsy, and childhood cancers may surface during this time.

Adolescence

After you have completed this section of the chapter, you should be able to meet the following objectives:

✦ Define what is meant by the period known as *adolescence*
✦ Characterize the physical and psychosocial changes that occur during adolescence
✦ Cite the developmental tasks that adolescents need to fulfill
✦ Describe common concerns of parents regarding their adolescent child
✦ Discuss how the changes that occur during adolescence can influence the health care needs of the adolescent

Adolescence is a transitional period between childhood and adulthood. During adolescence, there are significant physical, social, psychological, and cognitive changes. The changes of adolescence do not occur on a strict timeline; instead, they occur at different times according to a unique internal calendar known only to the person. For definition's sake, adolescence is considered to begin with the development of secondary sex characteristics, around 11 or 12 years of age, and to end with the completion of somatic growth from approximately 18 to 20 years of age. Girls usually begin and end adolescence earlier than boys. The adolescent period is conveniently referred to as the *teenaged years*, from 13 through 19 years of age.

Several "tasks" that adolescents need to fulfill have been identified. These tasks include achieving independence from parents, adopting peer codes and making personal lifestyle choices, forming or revising individual body image and coming to terms with one's body image if it is not "perfect," and establishing sexual, ego, vocational, and moral identities.

GROWTH AND DEVELOPMENT

Adolescence is influenced by hormonal activity that is influenced by the CNS. Physical growth occurs simultaneously with sexual maturation.

Adolescents typically experience gains of 20% to 25% in linear growth. An adolescent growth spurt, which lasts approximately 24 to 36 months, accounts for most of this somatic growth. The age at onset, the duration, and the

Adolescent Period

➤ The adolescent period, which extends from 13 through 19 years of age, is a time of rapid changes in body size and shape, and physical, psychological, and social functioning.

➤ Adolescence is a time when hormones and sexual maturation interact with social structures in fostering the transition from childhood to adulthood.

➤ The development tasks of adolescence include achieving independence from parents, adopting peer codes and making personal lifestyle choices, forming or revising individual body image, and coming to terms with one's body image.

extent of the growth vary between males and females and among individuals. In females, the growth spurt usually begins around 10 to 14 years of age. It begins earlier in females than in males and ends earlier, with less dramatic changes in weight and height. Females usually gain approximately 5 to 20 cm in height and 7 to 25 kg in weight. Most females have completed their growth spurt by 16 or 17 years of age. Males begin their growth spurt later, but it usually is more pronounced, with an increase in height of 10 to 30 cm and an increase in weight of 7 to 30 kg. Males may continue to gain in height until 18 to 20 years of age. Increases in height are possible until approximately 25 years of age.[28]

The changes in physical body size are not random but have a characteristic pattern. Growth in arms, legs, hands, feet, and neck appears first, then increases in hip and chest size occur, followed in several months by increases in shoulder width and depth and in trunk length. These changes may be difficult for the adolescent and parents. Adolescents may change shoe sizes several times over several months. Although brain size is not significantly increased during adolescence, the size and shape of the skull and facial bones change. The features of the face may appear to be out of proportion until full adult growth is attained.[6,28] Muscle mass and strength also increase during adolescence. Sometimes, there may be a discrepancy between the growth of bone and muscle mass, creating a temporary dysfunction with slower or less smooth movements resulting from the mismatch of bone and muscle. Body proportions undergo typical changes during adolescence. In males, the thorax becomes broader, and the pelvis remains narrow. In females, the opposite occurs: the thorax remains narrow, and the pelvis widens.

Organ systems also undergo changes in function, and some have changes in structure. The heart increases in size as the result of increased muscle cell size. Heart rate decreases to normal adult rates, whereas blood pressure increases rapidly to adult rates. Circulating blood volume and hemoglobin concentration increase. Males demonstrate greater changes in blood volume and higher hemoglobin concentrations because of the influence of testosterone and the relatively higher muscle mass.

With adolescence, skin becomes thicker, and additional hair growth occurs in both sexes. Sebaceous and sweat gland activity increases. Plugged sebaceous glands frequently result in acne (see Chapter 61). Increased sweat gland activity results in perspiration and body odor. The eyes undergo changes that may contribute to increased myopia. Auditory acuity peaks in adolescence and begins to decline after approximately 13 years of age.

Voice changes are of significant importance during adolescence for both sexes; however, the change is more pronounced in males. The voice change results from the growth of the larynx. There is more growth of the larynx in males than in females. The paranasal sinuses reach adult proportions, which increases the resonance of the voice, adding to the adult sound of the voice.[6,28]

Changes in the endocrine system are of great importance in the initiation and continuation of the adolescent growth spurt. The hormones involved include growth hormone (GH), thyroid hormones, adrenal hormones, insulin, and the gonadotropic hormones. GH regulates growth in childhood but is essentially replaced by sex hormones as the primary impetus for growth during adolescence. The exact role of GH in the adolescent growth spurt is unclear. Thyroid hormone, a significant hormone in the regulation of metabolism during childhood, continues to be important during adolescence. The relation of thyroid hormone to the other hormones and its role in the adolescent growth spurt is unclear. The thyroid gland becomes larger during adolescence, and it is believed that production of thyroid hormones is increased during this period. Insulin is necessary for appropriate growth at all stages, including adolescence. Insulin must be present for GH to be effective. The pancreatic islets of Langerhans increase in size during adolescence.[6,28]

The anterior pituitary gland produces the gonadotropic hormones, follicle-stimulating hormone and luteinizing hormone. These hormones influence target organs to secrete sex hormones. The ovaries respond by secreting estrogens and progesterone, and the testes respond by producing androgens, resulting in the maturation of the primary sex characteristics and the appearance of secondary sex characteristics. Primary sex characteristics are those involved in reproductive function (*i.e.*, internal and external genitalia). The secondary sex characteristics are the physical signs that signal the presence of sexual maturity but are not directly involved in reproduction (*i.e.*, pubic and axillary hair). Androgens initiate the beginning of the growth spurt. Sex hormones, including androgens, also conclude height growth by causing bone maturity, epiphyseal closure of bones, and discontinuation of skeletal growth.

The dramatic and extensive physical changes that occur during the transition from child to adult are matched only by the psychosocial changes that occur during the adolescent period. It is not possible to develop one guide that ad-

equately describes and explains the tremendous changes that occur during adolescence because the experience is unique for each adolescent. There are, fortunately, some commonalities within the process that can be used to facilitate understanding of these changes. The transition from child to adult is not a smooth, continuous, or uniform process. There are frequent periods of rapid change, followed by brief plateaus. These periods can change with little or no warning, which makes living with an adolescent difficult at times.

One thing that persons who deal with adolescents must remember is that, no matter how rocky the transition from child to adult, adolescence is not a permanent disability! Eighty percent of adolescents go through adolescence with little or no lasting difficulties. Health care professionals who care for adolescents may need to offer support to worried parents that the difficulties their adolescent is experiencing and that the entire family is experiencing as a result may be normal. The adolescent also may need reassurance that his or her feelings are not abnormal.[6,28]

Common concerns identified by adolescents include conflicts with parents, conflicts with siblings, concerns about school, and concerns about peers and peer relationships. Personal identity is an overwhelming concern expressed by adolescents. Common health problems experienced by adolescents are headache, stomachache, and insomnia. These disorders may be psychosomatic in origin. Adolescents also may exhibit situational anxiety and mild depression. The health care worker may need to refer adolescents for specialized counseling or medical care if any of the health care concerns are exaggerated.

Parents of adolescents also may have concerns about their child during the adolescent period. Common concerns related to the adolescent's behavior include rebelliousness, wasting time, risk-taking behaviors, mood swings, drug experimentation, school problems, psychosomatic complaints, and sexual activity.[28] The period of adolescence is one of transition from childhood to adulthood. It is filled with conflicts as the adolescent attempts to take on an adult role. Communication between the adolescent and family can help make the transition less stressful.

COMMON HEALTH PROBLEMS

Adolescence is considered to be a relatively healthy period; however, significant morbidity and mortality do occur. Health promotion is of extreme importance during the adolescent period. There are fewer actual physical health problems during this period, but there is a greater risk of morbidity and mortality from other causes, such as accidents, homicide, or suicide.

Several factors contribute to the risk for injury during adolescence. The adolescent is unable always to recognize potentially dangerous situations, possibly because of a discrepancy between physical maturity and cognitive and emotional development. Certain behavioral and developmental characteristics of the adolescent exaggerate this problem. Adolescents may feel the need to challenge parental or other authority. They also have a strong desire to "fit in" with the peer group. Adolescents exhibit a type of magical thinking and have a need to experiment with potentially dangerous situations or behaviors.

More than 80% of deaths during adolescence are attributed to injuries. Leading causes of nonintentional injuries are automobile accidents (number 1), motorcycle accidents, and drowning (number 2). Other accidental injuries include falls, striking objects, firearm mishaps (number 3), and sports. Accidental injuries kill more adolescents every year than all other causes of death combined, with males accounting for four of five injury victims. Automobile accidents account for 50% of all deaths of adolescents from ages 16 through 19 years.[6,28] Drowning, which is more common in males than females, decreases in prevalence after 18 years of age. Most drownings occur on weekends from May through August, are associated with alcohol use, and occur in fresh water rather than in the ocean. Firearm injuries are the third leading cause of nonintentional mortality in adolescents. Firearm accidents occur much more frequently to males between the ages of 15 to 24 years than to males of any other age.[6] Many of these accidents occur in the adolescent's home while cleaning or playing with the gun.

Other nonintentional causes of death include poisoning, skateboard injuries, all-terrain vehicle accidents, and participation in sports. However, most sports injuries are not fatal. Approximately one third to one half of all injuries occur in the school. Falls are the most common cause of injury in high schools, with contusions, abrasions, swelling, sprains, strains, and dislocations being the most common injuries.[2,26] Cancer is the fourth leading cause of death in adolescents, but it is the leading cause of death from nonviolent sources. There is an increased incidence of certain types of cancer during adolescence, including lymphomas, Hodgkin's disease, and bone and genital tumors. Leukemia is the leading cause of cancer mortality in persons between the ages of 15 and 24 years.[28]

Adolescents also are subject to intentional injuries, such as homicide and suicide. Suicide rates have risen dramatically for adolescents since the 1950s, to approximately 13 to 14 per 100,000. Most of the increase can be attributed to the greater number of suicides committed by white males. It also is thought that the rate of adolescent suicide may be higher than what is reported because of underreporting on death certificates. Almost 60% of suicides involve firearms.[28]

The increasing prevalence of sexual activity among adolescents has created unique health problems. These include adolescent pregnancy, sexually transmitted diseases, and human immunodeficiency virus (HIV) transmission. Associated problems include substance abuse, such as alcohol, tobacco, inhalants, and other illicit drugs. Health care providers must not neglect discussing sexual activity with the adolescent. Nonjudgmental, open, factual communication is essential for dealing with an adolescent's sexual practices. Discussion of sexual activity frequently is difficult for the adolescent and the adolescent's family. If a rela-

tionship exists between the adolescent and the health care provider, this may provide a valuable forum for the adolescent to get accurate information about safe sex, including contraception and avoidance of high-risk behaviors for acquiring sexually transmitted diseases or acquired immunodeficiency syndrome (AIDS).[28]

Substance abuse among adolescents increased rapidly in the 1960s and 1970s but has declined since that time. However, substance abuse still is prevalent in the adolescent age group. Health care workers must be knowledgeable about the symptoms of drug abuse, the consequences of drug abuse, and the appropriate management of adolescents with substance abuse problems. Substance abuse among adolescents includes tobacco products, cigarettes and "smokeless" tobacco (*e.g.*, snuff, chewing tobacco). Other substances include alcohol, marijuana, stimulants, inhalants, cocaine, hallucinogens, tranquilizers, and sedatives. Adolescents are at high risk for succumbing to the peer pressure to participate in substance abuse. They have a strong desire to fit in and be accepted by their peer group. It is difficult for them to "just say no." Magical thinking leads adolescents to believe that they will not get "hooked" or that the bad consequences will not happen to them. Adolescents and the rest of society are constantly bombarded with the glamorous side of substance use. Television shows, movies, and magazine advertisements are filled with beautiful, healthy, successful, happy, and popular persons who are smoking cigarettes or drinking beer or other alcoholic beverages. Adolescents are trying to achieve the lifestyle depicted in those ads, and it takes tremendous willpower to resist that temptation. It is important that adolescents be provided with "the rest of the story" through education and constant communication.[6,28]

Pregnancy has become a major problem of the teen years. Approximately 1 million adolescents in the United States become pregnant annually.[2] Four of every 10 teenage females become pregnant before reaching 20 years of age. One fifth of all pregnancies occur within the first month after beginning sexual activity; one half occur within the first 6 months of sexual activity. Of the slightly more than 1 million adolescent pregnancies, 47% delivered, 40% had therapeutic abortions, and 13% had spontaneous abortions.[6]

Adolescent pregnancy carries significant risks to the mother and to the fetus or newborn. The topic of adolescent pregnancy involves issues related to physical and biologic maturity of the adolescent, growth requirements of the adolescent and fetus, and unique prenatal care requirements of the pregnant adolescent. Emotional responses and psychological issues regarding relationships of the adolescent in her family and with the father of the baby, as well as how the pregnancy will affect the adolescent's future, must be considered.

In summary, adolescence is a transitional period between childhood and adulthood. It begins with development of secondary sex characteristics (11 to 12 years) and ends with cessation of somatic growth (18 to

20 years). This is the period of the major growth spurt, which is more pronounced in males. The endocrine system is of great importance with its numerous hormonal changes and their initiation and continuation of the growth spurt. Psychosocial changes are equally dramatic during this period and often place tremendous pressure on relationships between adults and the adolescent. Adolescence is a relatively healthy period, but significant morbidity and mortality exist as a result of accidents, homicide, and suicide. The increasing prevalence of sexual activity and substance abuse places the adolescent at risk for HIV infection; alcohol, tobacco, and other drug abuse; and adolescent pregnancy.

Related Web Sites

General Children References
Children's Bureau, U.S. Department of Health and Human
  Services   www.acf.dhhs.gov/programs/cb

Child Maltreatment
National Clearinghouse on Child Abuse and Neglect
  Information   www.calib.com/nccanch
National Center for Injury Prevention and Control Fact Sheet:
  The Co-occurrence of Intimate Partner Violence Against
  Mothers and Abuse of Children   www.cdc.gov/ncipc/
  factsheets/dvcan.htm

Sudden Infant Death Syndrome
American Academy of Pediatrics—ways to help reduce the risk
  of SIDS   www.aap.org/new/sids/reduceth.htm
SIDS Alliance   www.sidsalliance.org
National SIDS & Infant Death Program Support Center—
  downloadable brochures   sids-id-psc.org/brochures.htm
Healthtouch Online—An Overview Of Sudden Infant Death
  Syndrome   www.healthtouch.com/bin/EContent_HT/
  showAllLfts.asp?lftname=SLEEP027&cid=HT

Low Birth Weight, Prematurity, Infant Mortality
The Future of Children: Low Birth Weight
  www.futureofchildren.org/LBW/index.htm
Neonatology on the Web   www.neonatology.org
Racial and Ethnic Disparities in Infant Mortality
  raceandhealth.hhs.gov/3rdpgblue/infant/red.htm

Adolescence
Microsoft Encarta Online Encyclopedia: Adolescence
  encarta.msn.com
Journal of the American Academy of Child and Adolescent Psychiatry: Suicide and violence prevention: parent education
  in the emergency department   www.findarticles.com/
  m2250/3_38/54171862/p1/article.jhtml
Children's Hospital Medical Center of Cincinnati—health
  information resources   www.cincinnatichildrens.com/
  resources/

References

1. U.S. Department of Health and Human Services. (2000). *Healthy children 2000*. Washington, DC: Author.
2. Murphy S.L. (1998). Deaths: Final data for 1998. *National Vital Statistics Reports* 48(11).
3. Centers for Disease Control and Prevention, National Center for Health Statistics. (1998). *Health, United States, 1998*.
4. Brenner R.A., Simons-Morton B.G., Bhaskar B., Mehta N., Melnick V.L., Revenis M., et al. (1998). Prevalence and predictors of the prone sleep position among inner-city infants. *JAMA* 280, 341–346.
5. Needlman R.D. (2000). Growth and development. In Behrman R.E., Kliegman R.M., Jenson H.B. (Eds.), *Nelson textbook of pediatrics* (16th ed., pp. 23–65). Philadelphia: W.B. Saunders.
6. Moore K.L., Persaud T.V.N. (1998). *The developing human* (6th ed.). Philadelphia: W.B. Saunders.
7. Whaley L.F., Wong D.L. (1995). *Nursing care of infants and children* (5th ed., pp. 2–28, 106–154, 337–363). St. Louis: Mosby–Year Book.
8. Larsen, W.J. (1997). *Human embryology* (2nd ed.). NY: Churchill Livingstone.
9. Lubchenco L.O., Hansman C., Dressler M., et al. (1963). Intrauterine growth as estimated from liveborn birthweight data at 24 to 42 weeks of gestation. *Pediatrics* 32, 793–800.
10. Battaglia F.C., Lubchenco L.O. (1967). A practical classification of newborn infants by weight and gestational age. *Journal of Pediatrics* 71, 748–758.
11. Ballard J.L., Novak K., Driver M. (1979). A simplified score on assessment of fetal maturation in newly born infants. *Journal of Pediatrics* 95, 769–774.
12. Katz K., Nishioka, E. (1998). Neonatal assessment. In Kenner C., Lott J.W., Flandermeyer A. (Eds.), *Comprehensive neonatal nursing: A physiologic perspective* (pp. 223–251). Philadelphia: W.B. Saunders.
13. Harmon J. (1998). High-risk pregnancy. In Kenner C., Lott J.W., Flandermeyer A. (Eds.), *Comprehensive neonatal nursing: A physiologic perspective* (pp. 133–143). Philadelphia: W.B. Saunders.
14. Nagey D.A., Viscardi R.M. (1993). Retarded intrauterine growth. In Jeffrey J., Pomerance C., Richardson J. (Eds.), *Neonatology for the clinician*. Norwalk, CT: Appleton & Lange.
15. Apgar V. (1953). A proposal for a new method of evaluation of the newborn infant. *Current Research in Anesthesia and Analgesia* 32, 260.
16. Dubowitz L.M., Dubowitz V., Goldberg C. (1970). Clinical assessment of gestational age in the newborn infant. *Journal of Pediatrics* 77, 1–10.
17. Erikson E. (1963). *Childhood and society*. New York: W.W. Norton.
18. Blackburn S.T. (1998). Assessment and management of neurologic dysfunction. In Kenner C., Lott J.W., Flandermeyer A. (Eds.), *Comprehensive neonatal nursing: A physiologic perspective* (pp. 564–607). Philadelphia: W.B. Saunders.
19. Stoll B.J., Kliegman R.M. (2000). The fetus and the neonatal infant. In Behrman R.E., Kliegman R.M., Jenson H.B. (Eds.), *Nelson textbook of pediatrics* (16th ed., pp. 487–492). Philadelphia: W.B. Saunders.
20. Shiono P.H., Behrman R.E. (1995). Low birth weight: Analysis and recommendations. In *Low birth weight: The future of children, 5*. The David and Lucille Packard Foundation.
21. Cifuentes J., Haywood J.L., Ross M., Carlo W. (1998). Assessment and management of respiratory dysfunction. In Kenner C., Lott J.W., Flandermeyer A. (Eds.), *Comprehensive neonatal nursing: A physiologic perspective* (pp. 252–305). Philadelphia: W.B. Saunders.
22. McCollum L., Thigpen J. (1998). Assessment and management of gastrointestinal dysfunction. In Kenner C., Lott J.W., Flandermeyer A. (Eds.), *Comprehensive neonatal nursing: A physiologic perspective* (pp. 371–408). Philadelphia: W.B. Saunders.
23. Valdes-Dopena M. (1992). The sudden infant death syndrome: Pathologic findings. *Clinical Perinatology* 19, 701–716.

24. Lefrak L., Dowling D. (1998). Nutrition: Physiologic basis of metabolism and management of enteral and parenteral nutrition. In Kenner C., Lott J.W., Flandermeyer A. (Eds.), *Comprehensive neonatal nursing: A physiologic perspective* (pp. 354–370). Philadelphia: W.B. Saunders.

25. Hunt C. (2000). Sudden infant death syndrome. In Behrman R.E., Kliegman R.M., Jenson H.B. (Eds.), *Nelson textbook of pediatrics* (16th ed., pp. 2139–2143). Philadelphia: W.B. Saunders.

26. Hoffman H.J., Hellman L.S. (1992). Epidemiology of the sudden infant death syndrome: Maternal, neonatal, and postnatal risk factors. *Clinical Perinatology* 19, 717–738.

27. Wissow L.S. (1995). Child abuse and neglect. *New England Journal of Medicine* 332, 1425–1431.

28. Neinstein L.S., Kaufman F.R. (1991). *Adolescent health care: A practical guide* (pp. 3–37, 561–575). Baltimore: Williams & Wilkins.

Chapter 3

Concepts of Altered Health in Older Adults

Janice Kuiper Pikna

For age is opportunity no less than youth, itself, though in another dress. And as the evening twilight fades away the sky is filled with stars, invisible by day.

—Henry Wadsworth Longfellow

Aging is a natural, lifelong process that brings with it unique biopsychosocial changes. These changes create special health care needs for the older adult population that merit consideration. Because the prediction for the future is a continuous increase in the older adult population, there is a need to focus on the special health care needs of this group. *Gerontology* is the discipline that studies aging and the aged from biologic, psychological, and sociologic perspectives. It explores the dynamic processes of complex physical changes, adjustments in psychological functioning, and alterations in social identities. Through a holistic approach, health care providers specializing in gerontology seek to assist older adults in maximizing their functional abilities while attempting to prevent and minimize illness and disability.

An important first distinction is that aging and disease are not synonymous. Unfortunately, a common assumption is that growing older is inevitably accompanied by illness, disability, and overall decline in function. The fact is that the aging body can accomplish most, if not all, of the functions of its youth; the difference is that they may take longer, require greater motivation, and be less precise. But as in youth, maintenance of physiologic function occurs through continued use.

The Elderly and Theories of Aging

After you have completed this section of the chapter, you should be able to meet the following objectives:

- State a definition for *young-old, middle-old,* and *old-old,* and characterize the changing trend in the elderly population
- State a philosophy of aging that incorporates the positive aspects of the aging process
- Compare the focus of programmed change and stochastic theories of aging

WHO ARE THE ELDERLY?

The older adult population is typically defined in chronologic terms and includes individuals 65 years of age and older. This age was chosen somewhat arbitrarily, and historically it is linked to the Social Security Act of 1935. With this Act, the first national pension system in the United States, which designated 65 years as the pensionable age, was developed. Since then, the expression *old age* has been understood to apply to anyone older than 65 years. Because there is considerable heterogeneity among this group, older adults often are subgrouped into young-old (65 to 74 years), middle-old (75 to 84 years), and old-old (85+ years) to reflect more accurately the changes in function that occur. Age parameters, however, are somewhat irrelevant because chronologic age is a poor predictor of biologic function. However, chronologic age does help to quantify the number of individuals in a group and allows predictions to be made for the future.

In 1998, 12.7% of the total United States population (approximately 34.4 million) was 65 years of age or older, and the proportion has increased yearly. This older adult population is expected to grow to nearly 70 million by the year 2030 (Fig. 3-1). The older adult population itself is getting older. Average life expectancy has increased as a result of overall advances in health care technology, improved nutrition, and improved sanitation. Women who are now 65 years of age can expect to live an additional 19 years (84 years of age), and men an additional 15.8 years (80.8 years old).[1]

Aging can be thought of somewhat as a women's issue because women tend to outlive men. In 1998, there was a sex ratio of 143 women for every 100 men older than 65 years in the United States. This ratio increases to as high as 241 women for every 100 men in the 85 years and older age group. Marital status also changes with advancing age. In 1998, one half of all older women living in the community were widows, and there were four times as many widows (8.4 million) as there were widowers (2 million).[1]

Although 3.7 million older adults were in the workforce in 1998 (*i.e.*, working or actively seeking work), most were retired.[1] Retirement represents a significant role change for

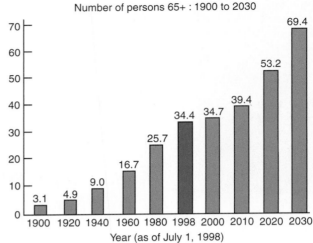

Number of persons 65+ : 1900 to 2030

FIGURE 3-1 Number of people 65 years and older, 1990 to 2030 (in millions). (Used with permission from American Association of Retired Persons. [1999]. *A profile of older Americans.* Washington, DC: AARP)

older adults. Attitudes and adjustment to retirement are influenced by preretirement lifestyles and values. Individuals with leisure pursuits during their work life seem to adjust better to retirement than those whose lives were dominated by work. For many of today's cohort of older adults, the work ethic of the Great Depression remains profoundly ingrained as the central purpose in life. When work is gone, a significant loss is felt, and something must be substituted in its place. Because leisure has not always been a highly valued activity, older adults may have difficulty learning to engage in meaningful leisure pursuits.

Loss of productive work is just one of many losses that can accompany the aging process. Loss of a spouse is a highly significant life event that commonly has negative implications for the survivor. Experts cite an increased mortality among recently bereaved older adults (especially men), an increased incidence of depression, psychological distress, and loneliness, and higher rates of chronic illness. Loss of physical health and loss of independence are other changes that can affect the psychosocial aspects of aging, as can relocation, loss of friends and relatives, and changes in the family structure.

Poverty is common among the elderly population. In 1998, approximately 3.4 million persons (10.5%) of those 65 years of age and older lived below the poverty line, with a median income of $18,166 for men and $10,054 for women. The income for African-American elderly was even lower. The main sources of income for older persons in 1996 were Social Security (91% of older persons), income from assets (63%), public and private pensions (43%), earnings (21%), and public assistance (6%).[1]

Contrary to popular belief, most older adults live in community settings. Most live in some type of family setting, with a spouse, their children, or other relatives, and

 The Elderly

➤ The older population, which is subgrouped into the young-old (65 to 74 years), the middle-old (75 to 84 years), and the old-old (85+ years), has increased dramatically during the past century and is expected to continue to grow as the result of overall advances in health care technology, improved nutrition, and improved sanitation.

➤ As the result of increased years, many older adults are confronted with retirement, changes in lifestyle, loss of significant others, and a decline in physical functioning.

➤ Although aging brings with it a unique set of biophysiologic changes, it is not synonymous with disease and disability. Most older adults can perform most or all of the activities they performed in earlier years, although they often take longer and require greater motivation.

approximately 31% live alone. Only 4.2% of all individuals 65 years of age and older reside in long-term care facilities or nursing homes. However, this number increases to 19.8% for persons 85 years of age or older.[1]

Older adults are the largest consumers of health care. In 1994 to 1995, more than half of the population (52.5%) reported having one or more disabilities. One third had at least one severe disability and approximately one sixth (14%) had difficulties with activities of daily living (ADL). Almost half of all adult hospital beds are filled with patients 65 years of age and older.[2]

THEORIES OF AGING

The lifestyle changes that occur with aging have been described in various developmental theories. Probably the most widely known is Erikson's eight stages of development. According to his theory, the first seven developmental stages span the period from childbirth through middle adulthood. The eighth stage, in older adulthood, focuses on "ego integrity versus despair." Ego integrity is the acceptance of one's life in relation to humanity and one's place in history. Lack of ego integrity leads to despair, signified by a nonacceptance of one's lifestyle and a fear of death. Despair may be manifested as apathy, depression, or decreased life satisfaction.[3,4]

The stages of physical change that occur as part of the aging process are less well articulated. Several theories attempt to explain the biology of aging through a variety of scientific observations at the molecular, cellular, organ, and system levels. No one theory explains all of the aging processes, but each holds some clues. In reality, it is reasonable to suppose that there are multiple influences that affect the aging process. The various theories of aging can be categorized as programmed change theories or stochastic theories. *Programmed change theories* propose that the changes that occur with aging are genetically programmed, whereas *stochastic theories* maintain that the changes result from an accumulation of random events or damage from environmental agents or influences. It is accepted now that the process of aging and longevity is multifaceted, with both genetics and environmental factors playing a role. In animal studies, genetics accounted for less that 35% of the effects of aging, whereas environmental influences accounted for over 65% of the effects.[5]

Programmed change theory resides with genetic influences that determine physical condition, occurrence of disease, age of death, cause of death, and other factors contributing to longevity.[6] At the cellular level, Hayflick observed more than 25 years ago that cultured human fibroblasts have a limited ability to replicate (approximately 50 population doublings) and then die.[7,8] Before achieving this maximum, they slow their rate of division and manifest identifiable and predictable morphologic changes characteristic of senescent cells. Another explanation of cellular aging resides with an enzyme called *telomerase* that is believed to govern chromosomal aging through its action on telomeres, the outermost extremities of the chromosome arms. With each cell division, a small segment of telomeric deoxyribonucleic acid (DNA) is lost, unless a cell has a constant supply of telomerase. In the absence of telomerase, the telomeres shorten, resulting in senescence-associated gene expression and inhibition of cell replication. It is thought that in certain cells, such as cancer cells, telomerase maintains telomere length, thereby enhancing cell replication. Currently, there is interest in developing telomerase therapy that could be used to initiate cell death in selected targets such as cancer cells and preventing cell senescence in other cell types, such as the chondrocytes in joints, the retinal epithelial cells in the eye, and the lymphocytes in the immune system.[9]

The function and longevity of cells in the various tissues of the body are determined by double-stranded DNA and its specific repair enzymes. DNA undergoes continuous change in response both to exogenous agents and intrinsic processes. It has been suggested that aging results from conditions that produce mutations in DNA or deficits in DNA repair mechanisms. The oxidative free radical theory is a stochastic idea in which aging is thought to result partially from oxidative metabolism and the effects of free radical damage (see Chapter 5). The major byproducts of oxidative metabolism include superoxides that react with DNA, ribonucleic acid, proteins, and lipids, leading to cellular damage and aging. Another damage theory, the wear and tear theory, proposes that accumulated damage to vital parts of the cell leads to aging and death. Cellular DNA is cited as an example. If repair to damaged DNA is incomplete or defective, as is thought to occur with aging, declines in cellular function might occur.[6]

Although these theories help to explain some of the biologic phenomena of aging, many questions remain. It seems likely that the human genome project will begin to explain some of the questions regarding the genetics of aging, but much needs to be answered regarding the effects of environmental influences on aging.

In summary, aging is a natural, lifelong process that brings with it unique biopsychosocial changes. Aging is not synonymous with disease or ill health. The aging body can accomplish most or all of the functions of its youth, although they may take longer, require greater motivation, and be less precise.

The older adult population is typically defined in chronologic terms as individuals 65 years of age and older and can be further defined as young-old (65 to 74 years), middle-old (75 to 84 years), and old-old (85+ years). The number of older persons has increased and is expected to continue to grow in the future, with an anticipated 70 million Americans older than age 65 by the year 2030.

There are two main types of theories used to explain the biologic changes that occur with aging: programmed change theories, which propose that aging changes are genetically programmed, and stochastic theories, which maintain that aging changes result from an accumulation of random events or damage from environmental hazards.

Physiologic Changes of Aging

After you have completed this section of the chapter, you should be able to meet the following objectives:

+ Describe common skin changes that occur with aging
+ Explain how muscle changes that occur with aging affect high-speed performance and endurance
+ Describe the process of bone loss that occurs with aging
+ State the common changes in blood pressure regulation that occur with aging
+ List the changes in respiratory function that occur with aging
+ Relate aging changes in neural function to the overall function of the body
+ Briefly discuss the effects of aging on vision, hearing, taste, and smell
+ Describe three changes that occur in the gastrointestinal tract with aging
+ State the significance of decreased lean body mass on interpretation of the glomerular filtration rate using serum creatinine levels

The physiologic changes seen in the elderly reflect not only the aging process, but the effects of years of exposure to environmental agents such as sunlight and cigarette smoke, and disease processes such as diabetes mellitus. Overall, there is a general decline in the structure and function of the body with advancing age. The decline results in a decreased reserve capacity of the various organ systems that consequently produces reduced homeostatic capabilities, making the older adult more vulnerable to stressors such as illness, trauma, surgery, medications, and environmental changes.

Research to identify true age-related changes as opposed to disease states is difficult. Studies using cross-sectional methodologies are the easiest to perform; however, mortality can confound the results. Although longitudinal studies tend to be more precise, they require years to perform and may not be able to account for numerous variables that enter into the aging equation, such as environment, occupation, and diet. However, it is important to differentiate, as much as possible, those changes that occur in the body as a result of aging from those that occur owing to disease. This distinction allows for more accurate diagnosis and treatment of disease conditions and helps to avoid inappropriate labeling of aging changes.

Regardless of the difficulty in defining normal aging as it relates to the various organ systems, there is a pattern of gradual loss that occurs. Many of these losses begin in early adulthood, but because of the large physiologic reserve of most organ systems, the decrement does not become functionally significant until the loss reaches a certain level. Some changes, such as those that affect the skin and posture, are more visible, whereas others, such as those affecting the kidney, may go unnoticed until the person is challenged with situations such as eliminating medications.

SKIN

Changes in the skin more obviously reflect the aging process than do changes in other organ systems (see Chapter 61). Aging can impinge on the primary functions of the skin:

protection from the environment, temperature regulation, maintenance of fluid and electrolyte balance, sensory regulation, and excretion of metabolic wastes. Exposure to sunlight and harsh weather accelerates aging of the skin.

With aging, the skin becomes wrinkled and dry and develops uneven pigmentation. The thickness of the dermis, or middle layer of skin, decreases by approximately 20%, which gives the skin an overall thin and transparent quality. This is especially true for areas exposed to sunlight. Dermal collagen fibers rearrange and degenerate, resulting in decreased skin strength and elasticity. Cellularity and vascularity of the dermis decrease with advancing age and can cause vascular fragility, leading to senile purpura (*i.e.,* skin hemorrhages) and slow skin healing. Delayed wound healing may be influenced by other factors such as poor nutrition and circulation and by changes in immune function.[10,11] The function of the sebaceous glands diminishes with age and leads to a decrease in sebum secretion. The decrease in size, number, and activity of the eccrine sweat glands causes a decrease in their capacity to produce sweat.[10,11]

Fingernails and toenails become dull, brittle, and thick, mostly as a result of decreased vascularity of the nail beds. Age-related changes in hair occur as well. Owing to a decline in melanin production by the hair follicle, approximately one half of the population older than 50 years of age has at least 50% gray hair, regardless of sex or original hair color. Changes in hair growth and distribution also are seen.[10,11] Hair on the scalp, axillae, and pubis becomes more sparse, and the hairs of the ears and nostril coarsen. Skin disorders are common among the older adult population and can include skin cancers, keratoses (*i.e.,* warty lesions), xerosis (*i.e.,* excessive dryness), dermatitis, and pruritus (*i.e.,* generalized itching).

STATURE AND MUSCULOSKELETAL FUNCTION

Aging is accompanied by a progressive decline in height, especially among older women. This decline in height is attributed mainly to compression of the spinal column. Body composition changes as well. The amount of fat increases, and lean body mass and total body water decrease with advancing age.

With aging, there is a reduction in muscle size and strength that is related to a loss of muscle fibers and a reduction in the size of the existing fibers. Although the decline in strength that occurs with aging cannot be halted, its progress can be slowed with exercise. There is a decline in high-speed performance and reaction time because of a decrease in type II muscle fibers.[12,13] Impairments in the nervous system also can cause movements to slow. However, type I muscle fibers, which offer endurance, are thought to remain consistent with age (see Chapter 12).

Numerous studies have reported a loss of bone mass with aging, regardless of sex, race, or body size. With aging, the process of bone formation (*i.e.,* renewal) is slowed in relation to bone resorption (*i.e.,* breakdown), resulting in a loss of bone mass and weakened bone structure. This is especially true for postmenopausal women. By 65 years of age, most women have lost two thirds of their skeletal mass owing to a decrease in estrogen production.[13] Skeletal bone loss is not a uniform process. At approximately 30 years of age, bone loss begins, predominantly in the trabecular bone (*i.e.*, fine network of bony struts and braces in the medullary cavity) of the heads of the femora and radii and in the vertebral bodies.[13] By 80 years of age, women have lost nearly 43% of their trabecular bone, and men have lost 27%. This process becomes pathologic (*i.e.*, osteoporosis) when it significantly increases the predisposition to fracture and associated complications (see Chapter 58).

The prevalence of joint disease is increased among the elderly. By age 65 years, 80% of the population has some articular disease. Osteoarthritis is so common among the elderly that it is often incorrectly assumed to be a normal age-related change rather than a disease. The synovial joints ultimately are affected by osteoarthritis, most commonly the joints of the hands, feet, knees, hips, and shoulders. It is characterized by cartilage loss and new bone formation, accounting for a distortion in articulation, limited range of motion, and joint instability (see Chapter 59). Age is the single greatest risk factor for development of osteoarthritis, in part because of the mechanical impact on joints over time, but it also is related to injury, altered physical condition of the articular cartilage, obesity (*e.g.*, knee), congenital deformity (*e.g.*, hip), crystal deposition in articular cartilage (*e.g.*, knee), and heredity. Pain, immobility, and joint inflammation often ensue. Treatment is aimed at minimizing risk factors, weight loss if indicated, exercise to increase muscle strength, and pain relief measures.

CARDIOVASCULAR FUNCTION

Cardiovascular disease remains the leading cause of morbidity and mortality in older adults. It often is difficult to separate true age-related changes in the cardiovascular system from disease processes. The aorta and arteries tend to become stiffer and less distensible with age, the heart becomes less responsive to the catecholamines, the maximal exercise heart rate declines, and there is a decreased rate of diastolic relaxation.[14]

Although approximately 40% of older adults have hypertension, the disorder is not considered a normal age-related process.[15] The elevation in blood pressure is more pronounced for the systolic blood pressure than for the diastolic blood pressure, probably as a result of increased aortic stiffness. In the elderly, compensatory cardiovascular mechanisms often are delayed or insufficient, so that a drop in blood pressure due to position change or consumption of a meal is common.[16,17] Orthostatic hypotension, or a significant drop in systolic blood pressure on assumption of the upright position, is more common among the elderly (see Chapter 23). Even in the absence of orthostatic hypotension, the elderly respond to postural stress with diminished changes in heart rate and diastolic pressure. This altered response to orthostatic stress is thought to result from changes in autonomic nervous system function, inadequate functioning of the circulatory system, or both.[18]

Senescent cardiac muscle typically displays a decreased response to β-adrenergic stimulation and circulating catecholamines, and there is increased diastolic stiffness of the ventricles that impedes filling, probably because of a slower rate of diastolic relaxation. Although early diastolic filling decreases by approximately 50% between 20 and 80 years of age, filling volumes are maintained, most likely as a result of an enhanced atrial contraction and its contribution to ventricular filling. The afterload (*i.e.*, opposition to left ventricular ejection) rises steadily with age as the ascending aorta becomes more rigid and the resistance in peripheral arterial vessels increases. Although the overall size of the heart does not increase, the thickness of the left ventricular wall may increase with age, in part responding to the increased afterload that develops because of blood vessel changes.[14] The resting heart rate remains unchanged or decreases only slightly with age; however, the maximum heart rate that can be achieved during maximal exercise is decreased.

Despite aging changes and cardiovascular disease, overall cardiovascular function at rest in most healthy elderly persons is considered adequate to meet the body's needs. Cardiac output is essentially maintained in healthy older adults (men more than women) during exercise despite the decreased heart rate response, apparently because of a greater stroke volume resulting from increased end-diastolic volume (*i.e.*, Frank-Starling mechanism) during exercise.[17,19]

RESPIRATORY FUNCTION

As lung function changes with age, it often is difficult to differentiate the effects of age from those of environmental and disease factors. Maximal oxygen consumption (Vo_2 max), a measure used to determine overall cardiopulmonary function, declines with age. Numerous studies have indicated that Vo_2 max can improve significantly with exercise and that the Vo_2 max of older adult master athletes can meet and exceed that of their younger counterparts.

A progressive loss of elastic recoil in the lung is caused by changes in the amount of elastin and composition of collagen fibers. Calcification of the soft tissues of the chest wall causes increased stiffness and thus increases the workload of the respiratory muscles. There is a loss of alveolar structure that decreases the surface area of gas exchange. Although the total lung capacity remains constant, the consequences of these changes result in an increased residual lung volume, and functional reserve capacity and a decline in vital capacity. There is a linear decrease in arterial oxygen tension (Po_2) of approximately 20 mm Hg from 20 to 70 years of age. This is thought to result primarily from the ventilation-perfusion mismatching of the aging lung.[20]

NEUROLOGIC FUNCTION

Changes at the structural, chemical, and functional levels of the nervous system occur with normal aging, but overall they do not interfere with day-to-day routines unless specific neurologic diseases come into play. The weight of the brain decreases with age, and there is a loss of neurons in the brain and spinal cord. Neuron loss is most pronounced in the cerebral cortex, especially in the superior temporal area. Additional changes take place in the neurons and supporting cells. Atrophy of the neuronal dendrites results in impaired synaptic connections, diminished electrochemical reactions, and neural dysfunction. Synaptic transmissions also are affected by changes in the chemical neurotransmitters dopamine, acetylcholine, and serotonin. As a result, many neural processes slow. Lipofuscin deposits (*i.e.*, yellow, insoluble intracellular material) are found in greater amounts in the aged brain.[21]

Sensorimotor changes show a decline in motor strength, slowed reaction time, diminished reflexes (especially in the ankles), and proprioception changes. These changes can cause the balance problems and slow, more deliberate movements that are frequently seen in older individuals.[22]

Even though changes in the brain are associated with aging, overall cognitive abilities remain intact. Although language skills and attention are not altered with advanced age, performance and constructional task abilities can decline, as can short-term memory and immediate recall. A change in personality or significant cognitive deficits is considered unusual with normal aging, and if either occur, evaluation is in order. Dementia and/or depression can frequently be the cause.

SPECIAL SENSES

Sensory changes with aging can greatly affect the older adult's level of functioning and quality of life. Vision and hearing impairments due to disease states, for example, can interfere with communication and may lead to social isolation and depression.

Vision

There is a general decline in visual acuity with age, and nearly all individuals older than 55 years of age require vision correction for reading or distance. The decline occurs as a result of a smaller pupil diameter, loss of refractive power of the lens, and an increase in the scattering of light. The most common visual problem among older adults is presbyopia, or difficulty focusing on near objects. It is caused mainly by decreased elasticity of the lens and atrophy of the ciliary muscle (see Chapter 54).

Glare and abrupt changes in light pose particular problems for older adults. Both are reasons why the elderly frequently give up night driving; they also increase their risk for falls and injury. Color discrimination changes also take place with aging. In particular, older adults have more difficulty identifying blues and greens. This is thought to be related to problems associated with filtering short wavelengths of light (*i.e.*, violet, blue, green) through a yellowed, opaque lens. Corneal sensitivity also may diminish with age, so that older adults may be less aware of injury or infection.[23]

Ophthalmologic diseases and disorders are common in the elderly. Cataracts, glaucoma, and macular degeneration are seen frequently and can greatly impair vision and function. Low-vision aids, such as special magnifiers and high-intensity lighting that mimics sunlight, can assist in optimizing vision in otherwise uncorrectable ophthalmologic problems.

Hearing

Hearing loss is common among older adults, and some degree of impairment is almost inevitable with advancing age. It has been reported that 25% of independent individuals 65 to 74 years of age and 40% of those 75 years of age and older have a hearing impairment, whereas as many as 70% of institutionalized older adults have difficulty hearing.[24,25]

Presbycusis, or the hearing loss of old age, is characterized by a gradual, progressive onset of bilateral and symmetric sensorineural hearing loss of high-frequency tones (see Chapter 55). The hearing deficit often has both a peripheral and a central component. Speech discrimination, or the ability to distinguish among words that are near-homonyms or distinguish words spoken by several different speakers, often is impaired.[24] Accelerated speech and shouting can increase distortion and further compound the problem. When speaking to hearing-impaired older adults, it is helpful to face them directly so they can observe lip movements and facial expressions. Speech should be slow and direct. Loudness can be irritating. Rephrasing misunderstood messages also can improve understanding of the spoken word. Hearing aids can be effective for various levels of hearing loss and may greatly improve the ability to hear and communicate. However, the usefulness of a hearing aid may be limited if the hearing deficit is multifactorial, with both a central and a peripheral component.

Cerumen (*i.e.*, ear wax) impaction in the external auditory canal also is commonly seen in older adults and can impair hearing. The cerumen glands, which are modified apocrine sweat glands, atrophy and produce drier cerumen. This may be partially responsible for more frequent cerumen impactions in the older adult population.[24,25]

Taste and Smell

Olfaction, or the sense of smell, declines with aging possibly as a result of generalized atrophy of the olfactory bulbs and a moderate loss of olfactory neurons. Smell is a protective mechanism and persons who cannot smell may be at risk for exposure to environmental hazards. For example, people who cannot smell smoke would be at particular risk if a fire broke out.

The sense of taste decreases with aging, but it is believed to be less affected than olfaction. Because taste and smell are necessary for the enjoyment of food flavor, older adults may not enjoy eating as much as in their youth. Drugs and disease also may affect taste. Alterations in taste and smell, along with other factors such as eating alone, decreased ability to purchase and prepare food, and the high cost of some foods, may account for poor nutritional intake in some older adults. Conversely, the lack of sensory feedback may lead the person to eat more and gain weight.

IMMUNE FUNCTION

An overall decline in immune system capabilities with aging can pose an increased risk for some infections (see Chapter 18). Involution of the thymus gland is complete by approximately 45 to 50 years of age, and although the total number of T cells remains unchanged, there are changes in the function of helper T cells that alter the cellular immune response of older adults. There also is evidence of an increase in various autoantibodies (*e.g.*, rheumatoid factor) as a person ages, increasing the risk of autoimmune disorders. Older adults are more susceptible to urinary tract infections, respiratory tract infections, wound infections, and nosocomial infections. The mortality rate from influenza and bronchopneumonia is increased for the older adult population. Local organ factors and coincident diseases probably play a bigger role in the acquisition of these infections than age-related changes in immunity.[26]

Early detection of infections is more difficult in older adults because the typical symptoms, such as fever and elevated white blood cell count, often are absent.[27] A change in mental status or decline in function often is the only presenting sign. It has been reported that frank delirium occurs in 50% of older adults with infections.[28] Thus, infections in the elderly may be far advanced at the time of diagnosis.

GASTROINTESTINAL FUNCTION

The gastrointestinal tract shows less age-associated change in function than many other organ systems. Although tooth loss is common and approximately 40% of the older adult population is edentulous, it is not considered part of the normal aging process. Poor dental hygiene with associated caries and periodontal disease is the main reason for the loss. *Edentia*, or toothlessness, can lead to dietary changes and can be associated with malnutrition. Use of dentures can enhance mastication; however, taste sensation is inhibited. Because of improved dental technology and the fluoridated water supply, more persons are able to keep their teeth into their later years. *Xerostomia*, or dry mouth, also is common, but it is not universal among older adults, and typically occurs as a result of decreased salivary secretions. Other causes of dry mouth can include medications, such as anticholinergics and tranquilizers, radiation therapy, and obstructive nasal diseases that induce mouth breathing.

Soergel and colleagues (1964) coined the term *presbyesophagus* to denote changes in esophageal function, such as decreased motility and inadequate relaxation of the lower esophageal sphincter, that occur with aging.[29] However, in studies that controlled for disease states such as diabetes mellitus and neuropathies, no increase in abnormal motility was observed. In general, the physiologic function of the esophagus appears to remain intact with advancing age.

Atrophy of the gastric mucosa and a decrease in gastric secretions can occur in older adults. Achlorhydria (*i.e.*, decrease in hydrochloric acid secretion) occurs, probably as a result of a loss of parietal cells. Although not universal, achlorhydria is more prevalent among older adults and can cause impaired gastric absorption of substances requiring an acid environment.

Atrophic gastritis and decreased secretion of intrinsic factor are more common with aging and result in a malabsorption of vitamin B_{12}. Because vitamin B_{12} is necessary for the maturation of red blood cells, a deficiency can lead to a type of macrocytic anemia called *pernicious anemia*. Vitamin B_{12} deficiency also can cause neurologic abnormalities such as peripheral neuropathy, ataxia, and even dementia.

Treatment consists of regular periodic vitamin B_{12} replacement therapy through injection because the oral form is not absorbed owing to a lack of intrinsic factor.[30]

The small intestine shows some age-related morphologic changes, such as mucosal atrophy; however, absorption of most nutrients and other functions appear to remain intact. Absorption of calcium, however, decreases with aging and may reflect decreased intestinal absorption along with other factors, such as reduced intake of vitamin D, decreased formation of vitamin D_3 by the skin because of reduced sun exposure, and decreased activation of vitamin D_3 by the liver and kidney.

Diverticula of the colon are common among older adults, with more than 50% of individuals older than 80 years having diverticular disease. The high incidence appears to result mainly from a low-fiber diet. Constipation, or infrequent passage of hard stool, is another frequently occurring phenomenon. It often is attributed to immobility and decreased physical activity, a low-fiber diet, decreased fluid intake, and medications; malignancies and other disease states also can be responsible. Complications of constipation can include fecal impaction or obstruction, megacolon, rectal prolapse, hemorrhoids, and laxative abuse.

RENAL FUNCTION

Although age-related anatomic and physiologic changes occur, the aging kidney remains capable of maintaining fluid and electrolyte balance remarkably well. Aging changes result in a decreased reserve capacity, which may alter the kidney's ability to maintain homeostasis in the face of illnesses or stressors. Overall, there is a general decline in kidney mass with aging, predominantly in the renal cortex. The number of functional glomeruli decreases by 30% to 50%, with an increased percentage of sclerotic or abnormal glomeruli.[31]

Numerous cross-sectional and longitudinal studies have documented a steady, age-related decline in total renal blood flow of approximately 10% per decade after 20 years of age, so that the renal blood flow of an 80-year-old person averages approximately 300 mL/minute, compared with 600 mL/minute in a younger adult. The major decline in blood flow occurs in the cortical area of the kidney, causing a progressive, age-related decrease in the glomerular filtration rate (GFR). Serum creatinine, a byproduct of muscle metabolism, often is used as a measure of GFR. The decline in GFR that occurs with aging is not accompanied by an equivalent increase in serum creatinine levels because the production of creatinine is reduced as muscle mass declines with age.[32] Serum creatinine levels often are used as an index of kidney function when prescribing and calculating drug doses for medications that are eliminated through the kidneys; this has important implications for older adults. If not carefully addressed, improper drug dosing can lead to an excess accumulation of circulating drugs and result in toxicity. A formula that adjusts for age-related changes in serum creatinine for individuals 40 through 80 years of age is available (see Chapter 34).

Renal tubular function declines with advancing age, and the ability to concentrate and dilute urine in response to fluid and electrolyte impairments is diminished. The aging kidney's ability to conserve sodium in response to sodium depletion is impaired and can result in hyponatremia. A decreased ability to concentrate urine, an age-related decrease in responsiveness to antidiuretic hormone, and an impaired thirst mechanism may account for the older adult's greater predisposition to dehydration during periods of stress and illness. Older adults also are more prone to hyperkalemia and hypokalemia when stressed than are younger individuals. An elevated serum potassium may result from a decreased GFR, lower renin and aldosterone levels, and changes in tubular function. Low potassium levels, on the other hand, are more commonly caused by gastrointestinal disorders or diuretic use. Neither is the result of aging.[32]

GENITOURINARY FUNCTION

Changes in the bladder occur with the aging process, resulting in a possible decline in function. Overall, the smooth muscle and supportive elastic tissue are replaced with fibrous connective tissue. This can cause incomplete bladder emptying and a diminished force of urine stream. Bladder capacity also decreases with age, whereas the frequency of urination increases. As elastic tissue and muscles weaken, stress incontinence becomes more prevalent.

In aging women, atrophy of perineal structures can cause the urethral meatus to recede along the vaginal wall. Atrophy of other pelvic organs occurs in the aging woman because of diminished estrogen production after menopause: vaginal secretions diminish; the vaginal lining is thinner, drier, less elastic, and more easily traumatized; and normal flora are altered. These changes can result in vaginal infections, pruritus, and painful intercourse.[33]

In aging men, benign prostatic hyperplasia (BPH) is very common. The incidence progressively increases to approximately 90% of men who are 85 years of age. The condition often is asymptomatic until approximately age 50 years. Thereafter, the incidence and severity of symptoms increase with age. BPH can cause obstructive symptoms such as urinary hesitancy, diminished force of stream, retention, and postvoid dribbling; it also can cause irritative symptoms such as frequency, nocturia, urgency, and even urge incontinence (see Chapter 43).[34]

Sexual activity remains possible into late life for men and women. In general, the duration and intensity of the sexual response cycle is diminished in both sexes. Penile erection takes longer to develop because of changes in neural innervation and vascular supply. Women take longer to experience the physiologic changes of vaginal expansion and lubrication during the excitement phase. Social factors affecting sexual behavior include the desire to remain sexually active, access to a sexually functioning partner, and availability of a conducive environment.[35,36]

In summary, there is a general decline in the structure and function of the body with advancing age, resulting in a decreased reserve capacity of the various organ systems, including the integumentary, musculoskeletal, cardiorespiratory, nervous, sensory, immune, gastrointestinal, and genitourinary systems. This results in a reduction of homeostatic capabilities, making the older adult more vulnerable to stressors such as illness, trauma, surgery, medication administration, and environmental changes.

Functional Problems of Aging

After you have completed this section of the chapter, you should be able to meet the following objectives:

+ Compare information obtained from functional assessment with that obtained from a physical examination used to arrive at a medical diagnosis
+ Cite the differences between chronic and transient urinary incontinence
+ State four risk factors for falls in older individuals
+ List five symptoms of depression in older adults
+ Name a tool that can be used for assessing cognitive function
+ State the difference between delirium and dementia

Although aging is not synonymous with disease, the aging process does lend itself to an increased incidence of illness. As chronologic age increases, so does the probability of having multiple chronic diseases. It has been estimated that 86% of older adults have at least one chronic condition, and most actually have more than one. The extent of these problems is described in Table 3-1. Older adults are more likely to experience a decline in overall health and function because of the increased incidence of chronic illness that occurs with advancing age. Because aging also brings with it a decreased ability to maintain homeostasis, illnesses often manifest in an atypical manner.

In addition to chronic illnesses, older adults suffer disproportionately from functional disabilities, or the inability to perform the necessary activities of daily living (ADL). It is most likely that the decrements in health that can accompany the aging process are responsible for these functional disabilities. Among the more common functional problems of the older adult are urinary incontinence, instability and falls, sensory impairment, depression, dementia, and delirium.

TABLE 3-1 ✦ Common Health Problems in the Elderly

Health Problems	Percentage With Problems
Arthritis	49
Hypertension	40
Heart disease	31
Hearing impairment	28
Orthopedic impairments	18
Cataracts	16
Sinusitis	15
Diabetes	13

(Data from American Association of Retired Persons. [1999]. *A profile of older Americans*. Washington, D.C.: Author.)

FUNCTIONAL ASSESSMENT

Evaluation of the older adult's functional abilities is a key component in gerontologic health care. Medical diagnoses alone are incomplete without an assessment of function. Two older adults with similar medical diagnoses of arthritis, hypertension, and osteoporosis, for example, can be at opposite ends of the spectrum of functional abilities.

Assessing functional status can be done in many different ways, using a variety of methods. Measures of function should attempt systematically and objectively to evaluate the level at which an individual is functioning in a variety of areas, including biologic, psychological, and social health.

Selection of a screening tool to measure function depends on the purpose of data collection, the individual or target population to be assessed, availability and applicability of the instruments, reliability and validity of the screening tools, and the setting or environment. An issue that arises when assessing function is the question of capability versus performance. For example, an older adult may be able to bathe without supervision; however, the long-term care facility where the person resides may discourage it for safety reasons. Among the more commonly used assessment tools are those that measure the ability to perform ADL and the patient's cognitive function.

When evaluating levels of function, determination of the older adult's ability to perform ADL and instrumental ADL (IADL) should be included. Activities of daily living are basic self-care tasks, such as bathing, dressing, grooming, ambulating, transferring (*e.g.*, from a chair to bed), feeding, and communicating. Instrumental activities of daily living are more complex tasks that are necessary to function in society, such as writing, reading, cooking, cleaning, shopping, laundering, climbing stairs, using the telephone, managing money, managing medications, and using transportation. The IADL tasks indirectly examine cognitive abilities as well because they require a certain level of cognitive skills to complete.

Several tools are available for measuring functional status. One of the more commonly used tools is the Index of Activities of Daily Living. Developed by Katz in 1963 and revised in 1970, it summarizes performance in six functions: bathing, dressing, toileting, transferring, continence, and feeding. It is used as an assessment tool to determine the need for care and the appropriateness of treatment and as a teaching aid in rehabilitation settings. Through questioning and observation, the rater forms a mental picture of the older adult's functional status as it existed during a 2-week period preceding the evaluation, using the most dependent degree of performance.[37,38] Numerous studies using the Katz Index tool show significant validity and reliability. The advantage of the tool is that it is easy to administer and provides a "snapshot" of the older adult's level of physical functioning. The disadvantage is that it does not include IADL categories that are of equal importance, especially for older adults living in the community.

URINARY INCONTINENCE

Urinary incontinence, or involuntary loss of urine, plagues over 30% of community-living individuals over age 60, 50% of hospitalized older adults, and 60% of residents in long-term care facilities. These estimates may be low because individuals often fail to report symptoms of urinary incontinence, perhaps owing to the attached social stigma. Health care professionals often neglect to elicit such information as well.

Incontinence is an expensive problem. A conservative estimate of cost for direct care of adults with incontinence is over $15 billion annually.[39] Urinary incontinence can have deleterious consequences, such as social isolation and embarrassment, depression and dependency, skin rashes and pressure sores, and financial hardship. Although urinary incontinence is a common disorder, it is not considered a normal aspect of aging. Studies reveal that 60% to 70% of community-dwelling older adults with urinary incontinence can be successfully treated and even cured.

Changes in the micturition cycle that accompany the aging process make the older adult prone to urinary incontinence. A decrease in bladder capacity, in bladder and sphincter tone, and in the ability to inhibit detrusor (*i.e.*, bladder muscle) contractions, combined with the nervous system's increased variability to interpret bladder signals, can cause incontinence (see Chapter 35). Impaired mobility and a slower reaction time also can aggravate incontinence.

The causes of incontinence can be divided into two categories: transient and chronic. Of particular importance is the role of pharmaceuticals as a cause of transient urinary incontinence. Numerous medications, such as long-acting sedatives and hypnotics, psychotropics, and diuretics, can induce incontinence. Treatment of transient urinary incontinence is aimed at ameliorating or relieving the cause on the assumption that the incontinence will resolve.

Chronic, or established, urinary incontinence occurs as a failure of the bladder to store urine or a failure to empty urine. Failure to store urine can occur as a result of detrusor muscle overactivity with inappropriate bladder contractions (*i.e.*, urge incontinence). There is an inability to delay voiding after the sensation of bladder fullness is perceived. Urge incontinence is typically characterized by large-volume leakage episodes occurring at various times of day. Urethral incompetence (*i.e.*, stress incontinence) also causes a bladder storage problem. The bladder pressure overcomes the resistance of the urethra and results in urine leakage. Stress incontinence causes an involuntary loss of small amounts of urine with activities that increase intra-abdominal pressure, such as coughing, sneezing, laughing, or exercising.[39,40]

Failure of the bladder to empty urine can occur because of detrusor instability, resulting in urine retention and overflow incontinence. Also called *neurogenic incontinence*, this type of incontinence can be seen with neurologic damage from conditions such as diabetes mellitus and spinal cord injury. Outlet obstruction, as with prostate enlargement and urethral stricture, also can cause urinary retention with overflow incontinence. Functional incontinence, or urine leakage due to toileting problems, occurs because cognitive, physical, or environmental barriers impair appropriate use of the toilet.[39,40]

After a specific diagnosis of urinary incontinence is established, treatment is aimed at correcting or ameliorating the problem. Probably the most effective interventions for older adults with incontinence are behavioral techniques. These strategies involve educating the individual and providing reinforcement for effort and progress. Techniques include bladder training, timed voiding or habit training, prompted voiding, pelvic floor muscle (*i.e.*, Kegel) exercises, and dietary modifications. Biofeedback, a training technique to teach pelvic floor muscle exercises, uses computerized instruments to relay information to individuals about their physiologic functions. Biofeedback can be helpful when used in conjunction with other behavioral treatment techniques. Use of pads or other absorbent products should be seen as a temporary help measure and not as a cure. Numerous types of products are available to meet many different consumer needs.

Pharmacologic intervention may be helpful for some individuals. Estrogen replacement therapy in postmenopausal women, for example, may help to relieve stress incontinence. Drugs with anticholinergic and bladder smooth muscle relaxant properties (*e.g.*, oxybutynin, tolterodine) may help with urge incontinence. These medications are not without side effects, however, and their use must be carefully weighed against the possible benefits.

Surgical intervention may help to relieve urinary incontinence symptoms in appropriate patients. Bladder neck suspension may assist with stress incontinence unrelieved by other interventions, and prostatectomy is appropriate for men with overflow incontinence due to enlarged prostate. However, older adults may have medical conditions that preclude surgery. Other treatments include intermittent self-catheterization for some types of overflow incontinence.

INSTABILITY AND FALLS

Unstable gait and falls are a common source of concern for the older adult population.[39,40] The literature reveals that 30% of community-dwelling individuals older than 65 years of age and 50% of nursing home residents fall each year. Most falls do not result in serious injury, but the potential for serious complications and even death is real. Accidents are the sixth leading cause of death among older adults, with falls ranking first in this category. Hip fractures are one of the most feared complications from a fall. More than 340,000 individuals fracture a hip each year; most of these are elderly women. Significant morbidity occurs as a result of a hip fracture. The literature varies, but as many as 50% of older adults who sustain a hip fracture are reported to require nursing home care for at least 1 year, and up to 20% die in the year after a hip fracture. Other bones frequently fractured by older adults who fall are the humerus, wrist, and pelvis. These bones bear the brunt of osteoporotic changes and, as a result, are more vulnerable to injury. Soft tissue injuries such as sprains and strains also can result from falls.[41–43]

An individual's activity may be restricted because of fear on the individual's or caregiver's part about possible falling. These anxieties may lead to unnecessary restrictions in independence and mobility and commonly are mentioned as a reason for institutionalization.

Although some falls have a single, obvious cause, such as a slip on a wet or icy surface, most are the result of several factors. Risk factors that predispose to falling include a combination of age-related biopsychosocial changes, chronic ill-

nesses, and situational and environmental hazards. Gait and stability require the integration of information from the special senses, the nervous system, and the musculoskeletal system. Changes in gait and posture that occur in healthy aged individuals also contribute to the problem of falls. The older person's stride shortens; the elbows, trunk, and knees become more flexed; toe and heel lift decrease while walking; and sway while standing increases. Muscle strength and postural control of balance decrease, proprioception input diminishes, and righting reflexes slow. All these factors predispose the older adult to the possibility of falling.[44]

Because the central nervous system integrates sensory input and sends signals to the effector components of the musculoskeletal system, any alteration in neural function can predispose to falls. For this reason, falls have been associated with strokes, Parkinson's disease, and normal-pressure hydrocephalus. Similarly, diseases or disabilities that affect the musculoskeletal system, such as arthritis, muscle weakness, or foot deformities, are associated with an increase in the incidence of falls. Age- and disease-related alterations in vision and hearing impair sensory input and can contribute to falls. Vestibular system alterations such as benign positional vertigo or Ménière's disease cause balance problems that can result in falls. Cognitive impairments such as dementia have been associated with an increased risk of falling, most likely because of impaired judgment and problem-solving abilities.

Input from the cardiovascular and respiratory systems influences function and ambulation. Cardiovascular diseases, especially postural hypotension, can cause recurrent falls, solely or in association with the previously mentioned factors. The dramatic drop in blood pressure on rising that is seen in postural hypotension can cause falls because of syncope and dizziness.

Medications are an important and potentially correctable cause of instability and falls. Centrally acting medications, such as sedatives and hypnotics, have been associated with an increase in the risk of falling and injury. Diuretics can cause volume depletion, electrolyte disturbances, and fatigue, predisposing to falls. Antihypertensive drugs can cause fatigue, orthostatic hypotension, and impaired alertness, contributing to the risk of falls.

Environmental hazards play a significant role in falling. More than 70% of falls occur in the home and often involve objects that are tripped over, such as cords, scatter rugs, and small items left on the floor. Poor lighting, ill-fitting shoes, surfaces with glare, and improper use of ambulatory devices such as canes or walkers also contribute to the problem.[42,43] Table 3-2 summarizes the possible causes of falls.

Preventing falls is the key to controlling the potential complications that can result. Because multiple factors usually contribute to falling, the aim of the clinical evaluation is to identify risk factors that can be modified. Assessment of sensory, neurologic, and musculoskeletal systems; direct observation of gait and balance; and a careful medication inventory can help identify possible causes. Dizziness, either transient due to a self-limiting illness or recurring, is a risk factor for falls. In one study, 24% of persons older than 72 years of age reported at least once-monthly episodes of dizziness.[45] Dizziness was associated with several conditions, including cardiovascular disorders, sensory impairment, bal-

TABLE 3-2 ✦ Risk Factors for Falls

Category of Risk Factors	Examples
Accidents and environmental hazards	Slips, trips Clutter, cords, throw rugs
Age-related functional changes	Decreased muscle strength, slowed reaction time, decreased proprioception, impaired righting reflexes, increased postural sway, altered gait, impaired visual and hearing function
Cardiovascular disorders	Aortic stenosis, cardiac dysrhythmias, autonomic nervous system dysfunction, hypovolemia, orthostatic hypotension, carotid sinus syncope, vertebrobasilar insufficiency
Gastrointestinal disorders	Diarrhea, postprandial syncope, vasovagal response
Genitourinary disorders	Urinary incontinence, urinary urgency/frequency, nocturia
Medication use	Alcohol, antihypertensives, cardiac medications, diuretics, narcotics, oral hypoglycemic agents, psychotropic medications, drug–drug interactions, polypharmacy
Metabolic disorders	Anemia, dehydration, electrolyte imbalance, hypothyroidism
Musculoskeletal disorders	Osteoarthritis, rheumatoid arthritis, myopathy
Neurologic disorders	Balance/gait disorders, cerebellar dysfunction, stroke with residual effects, cervical spondylosis, central nervous system lesions, delirium, dementia, normal-pressure hydrocephalus, peripheral neuropathy, Parkinson's disease, seizure disorder, transient ischemic attack
Prolonged bed rest	Hypovolemia, muscle weakness from disuse and deconditioning
Respiratory disorders	Hypoxia, pneumonia
Sensory impairments	Decreased visual acuity, cataract, glaucoma, macular degeneration, hearing impairment, vestibular disorders

ance disturbances, and psychological conditions. The number of medications the person took also was associated with episodes of dizziness.[45]

Preventive measures can include a variety of interventions, such as surgery for cataracts or cerumen removal for hearing impairment related to excessive ear wax accumulation. Other interventions may include podiatric care, discontinuation or alteration of the medication regimen, exercise programs, physical therapy, and appropriate adaptive devices. The home also should be assessed by an appropriate health care professional (*e.g.*, occupational therapist) and recommendations made regarding modifications to promote safety. Simple changes such as removing scatter rugs, improving the lighting, and installing grab bars in the bathtub can help prevent falling. These interventions can maximize the older adult's independence and prevent the morbidity and mortality that can occur as a result of a fall.[41–43]

SENSORY IMPAIRMENT

Although sensory impairments are not imminently life threatening, their impact on health can be substantial.[25,46,47] Hearing impairment is associated with decreased quality of life, depression, isolation, and dementia. Visual impairment is related to increased risk of falls, hip fractures, physical disability, and depression. Nursing home residents with visual impairment are more likely to require assistance with ADL and can be at risk for falls and hip fractures. Visual impairment also appears to increase mortality.[47]

Sensory impairment results not only from deficits in peripheral sensory structures but from the central processing of sensory information. The older person's difficulty in processing multisensory information is seen most strikingly when there is a rapid fluctuation in the nature of the information that is received from the environment.[24]

It has been reported that a lack of sensory information can predispose to psychological symptoms. Charles Bonnet syndrome is an organic disorder occurring in the elderly that is characterized by complex visual hallucinations. It is associated with ocular disease and, strictly speaking, is seen in older adults with preserved intellectual functions.[48] In one study, 10% of persons (mean age 75 years) with severe visual disability experienced visual hallucinations.[49] These persons retained insight into the problem and needed only reassurance that their hallucinations did not represent mental illness. Both auditory and visual impairment can have important psychological effects in association with dementia. Delusions have been associated with hearing impairment. In one study that used a case-control method, elderly persons with late-life psychosis with paranoid symptomatology were four times more likely to have hearing impairments compared with control subjects.[50]

DEPRESSION

Depression is a significant health problem that affects the older adult population. Estimates of depression in the elderly vary widely; however, there is a consensus that the size of the problem is underestimated owing to misdiagnosis and mistreatment. Approximately 15% of community-dwelling older adults are thought to have depressive symptoms. The estimate drops to approximately 3% when diagnosis is restricted to major depression. Depressive symptoms are seen in approximately 15% to 25% of nursing home residents.[51]

The term *depression* is used to describe a symptom, syndrome, or disease. As listed in the American Psychiatric Association's 1994 *Diagnostic and Statistical Manual of Mental Disorders* (DSM-IVR), the criteria for the diagnosis and treatment of a major depression include at least five of the following symptoms during the same 2-week period, with at least one of the symptoms being depressed mood or anhedonia (*i.e.*, loss of interest or pleasure): depressed or irritable mood; loss of interest or pleasure in usual activities; appetite and weight changes; sleep disturbance; psychomotor agitation or retardation; fatigue and loss of energy; feelings of worthlessness, self-reproach, or excessive guilt; diminished ability to think or concentrate; and suicidal ideation, plan, or attempt.[52]

Depressive symptomatology can be incorrectly attributed to the aging process, making recognition and diagnosis difficult. Depressed mood, the signature symptom of depression, may be less prominent in the older adult, and more somatic complaints and increased anxiety are reported, confusing the diagnosis. Symptoms of cognitive impairment can be seen in the depressed older adult. Because it can be misdiagnosed as dementia, a thorough medical evaluation is in order. Unlike true dementia, pseudodementia of depression usually improves with treatment for depression. Although they are similar in clinical presentation, there are some subtle distinctions between the two conditions (Table 3-3). Physical illnesses can complicate the diagnosis as well. Depression can be a symptom of a medical condition, such as pancreatic cancer, hypothyroidism or hyperthyroidism, pneumonia and other infections, congestive heart failure, dementia, and stroke.[51,53] Medications such as sedatives, hypnotics, steroids, antihypertensives, and analgesics also can induce a depressive state. Numerous confounding social problems, such as bereavement, loss of job or income, and loss of social support, can obscure or complicate the diagnosis.[53,54]

The course of depression in older adults is similar to that in younger persons. As many as 40% experience recurrences. Suicide rates are highest among the elderly. There is a linear increase in suicide with age, most notably among white men older than 60 years of age. Although the exact reasons are

unclear, it may be caused by the emotional alienation that can accompany the aging process, combined with complex biopsychosocial losses.[53–55]

Because diagnosis of depression can be difficult, use of a screening tool may help to measure affective functioning objectively. The *Geriatric Depression Scale*, an instrument of known reliability and validity, was developed to measure depression specifically in the noninstitutionalized older adult population. The 30-item dichotomous scale elicits information on topics relevant to symptoms of depression among older adults, such as memory loss and anxiety.[56] Many other screening tools, each with its own advantages and disadvantages, exist to evaluate the older adult's level of psychological functioning, in its entirety or as specific, separate components of function.

Treatment goals for older adults with depression are to decrease the symptoms of depression, improve the quality of life, reduce the risk of recurrences, improve health status, decrease health care costs, and decrease mortality. Pharmacotherapy (*i.e.*, use of antidepressants) is an effective treatment approach for the depressed older adult. The selection of a particular medication depends on a variety of factors, such as a prior positive or negative response, history of first-degree relatives responding to medication, concurrent nonpsychotropic medical illnesses that may interfere with medication use, concomitant use of nonpsychiatric medications that may alter the metabolism or increase the side effect profile, likelihood of adherence, patient preference, and cost.

Selective serotonin reuptake inhibitors (SSRIs), a newer class of antidepressants (*e.g.*, sertraline, paroxetine, citalopram), provide high specificity by blocking or slowing serotonin reuptake without the antagonism of neurotransmitter receptors or direct cardiac effects. Because of this, they are an attractive first choice for pharmacotherapy. Dosing is usually once per day, creating ease of administration. They also are less lethal in overdose than other types of antidepressants, such as the tricyclics, an important consideration because of the high suicide rate among older adults. The anticholinergic and cardiovascular side effects that can be problematic with tricyclic antidepressants (*e.g.*, nortriptyline, desipramine, amitriptyline) are minimal with SSRIs. Regardless of the classification, psychotropic

---

TABLE 3-3 ✦ Characteristics That Distinguish Dementia From Pseudodementia of Depression

Dementia	Pseudodementia of Depression
Insidious onset	Rapid onset
Symptoms present for long duration	Symptoms present for relatively short time
Inaccurate in answering orientation questions; attempts to cover up inaccuracies	May show lack of interest in answering questions; frequent "don't know" or "don't care" response
May try to conceal deficits	May tend to emphasize deficits; highlight disabilities
Consistently performs poorly on tasks of similar difficulty	May display marked variability in performing tasks of similar difficulty
Mood and behavior tend to be labile	Mood consistently depressed; may have superimposed agitation or anxiety
May have neurologic symptoms of dysphasia, apraxia, or agnosia	Neurologic symptoms not present

medications should be given in low doses initially and gradually titrated according to response and side effects. Response to antidepressants usually requires 4 to 6 weeks at a therapeutic dose levels. For a single episode of major depression, drug therapy usually should continue for a minimum of 6 months, and 2 to 5 years for recurrent depression, to prevent relapse.[51,53,54]

Electroconvulsive therapy (ECT) may be the treatment of choice for older adults with severe, pharmacologically resistant major depressive episodes. Studies indicate that individuals older than 60 years of age are the largest group of patients who receive ECT. Despite the negative publicity that has been associated with ECT, the evidence for its efficacy in the treatment of depression is strong. Unfortunately, relapse after ECT is common, and alternative treatment strategies, including maintenance ECT or maintenance antidepressants after ECT, are being used.[57]

"Talking therapy," such as supportive counseling or psychotherapy, is considered to be an important part of the treatment regimen, alone or in combination with pharmacotherapy or ECT. Alterations in life roles, lack of social support, and chronic medical illnesses are just a few examples of life event changes that may require psychosocial support and new coping skills. Counseling in the older adult population requires special considerations. Individuals with significant vision, hearing, or cognitive impairments may require special approaches. Many elderly persons do not see themselves as depressed and reject referrals to mental health professionals. Special efforts are needed to engage these individuals in treatment. Family therapy can be beneficial as a way to help the family understand more about depression and its complexities and as an important source of support for the older adult. Although depression can impose great risks for older adults, it is thought to be the most treatable psychiatric disorder in late life and therefore warrants aggressive case finding and intervention.

DEMENTIA

Dementia is a complex and devastating problem that is a major cause of disability in the older adult population. Although the actual prevalence of dementia is unknown, estimates range from 2.5% to 24.6% of those older than 65 years of age, with the number increasing with advanced age. In long- term care facilities, up to 70% of residents have cognitive impairments.[58]

Although there can be a decline in intellectual function with aging, dementia, sometimes called *senility*, is not a normal aging process. Dementia is a syndrome of acquired, persistent impairment in several domains of intellectual function, including memory, language, visuospatial ability, and cognition (*i.e.*, abstraction, calculation, judgment, and problem solving). Mood disturbances and changes in personality and behavior often accompany the intellectual deterioration.

Dementia can result from a wide variety of conditions, including degenerative, vascular, neoplastic, demyelinating, infectious, inflammatory, toxic, metabolic, and psychiatric disorders. Up to 70% of older adults with dementia (4 million Americans) are thought to have Alzheimer's disease, a

chronic, progressive neurologic disorder of unknown cause.[58] Multi-infarct dementia is the second most common disorder, with 10% to 20% of dementias attributed to this vascular disorder in which multiple emboli disseminate throughout the brain, causing infarctions.[52,59]

Much work is being done in the diagnosis and treatment of dementia, in particular of Alzheimer's disease.[60–62] Because there currently are no specific diagnostic tests to determine the presence of Alzheimer's disease, the diagnosis is essentially made by excluding other possible causes of the dementia symptoms.

A commonly used measure of cognitive function is the Mini-Mental State Examination (MMSE) developed by Folstein and colleagues in 1975. This tool provides a brief, objective measure of cognitive functioning and has been widely used. The MMSE, which can be administered in 5 to 10 minutes, consists of a variety of questions that cover memory, orientation, attention, and constructional abilities.[63] The test has been studied and found to fulfill its original goal of providing a brief screening tool that quantifies cognitive impairments and documents cognitive changes over time. However, it has been cautioned that this examination should not be used by itself as a diagnostic tool to identify dementia.

Currently, there is no cure for Alzheimer's disease. Medications to halt further cognitive decline, however, are available. Emphasis has been on increasing cholinergic synaptic transmission in areas of the brain that are concerned with memory and cognition. Drugs that inhibit the breakdown of acetylcholine at the synaptic cleft have been developed and have been shown to be effective in slowing the progression of the disease in some persons. At present, four drugs, tacrine, donepezil, rivastigmine, and galantamine are available in the therapeutic category of cognitive-enhancing agents. All four medications are acetylcholinesterase inhibitors whose action elevates acetylcholine concentrations in the cerebral cortex by slowing degradation of acetylcholine released by still-intact neurons. The magnitude of tacrine's cognitive-enhancing effects, the first-released drug in this category, have been modest and associated with significant side effects that preclude use. Donepezil has been shown to be a more potent, specific inhibitor of acetylcholinesterase with minimal side effects. The newer agents, rivastigmine and galantamine, are thought to be more selective in the binding and inactivation of acetylcholinesterase; however, adverse reactions, especially gastrointestinal symptoms, can impede therapeutic dosing.[64–66]

Among the neuroprotective drugs that are proposed to delay the onset or progression of Alzheimer's disease are extracts of *Ginkgo biloba*, vitamin E, nonsteroidal anti-inflammatory drugs (NSAIDs), estrogen, and calcium channel blockers. Extracts of *Ginkgo biloba*, derived from the leaf of a subtropical tree, are available in health food stores. The compounds, which supposedly have antioxidant, neurotrophic, and anti-inflammatory properties, are promoted as a remedy for memory problems in persons with Alzheimer's disease.[67] A meta-analysis of five studies that examined the efficacy of the compound on cognition concluded that *Ginkgo biloba* extract improves cognition slightly.[68] The pathology of Alzheimer's disease may involve oxidative stress and the accumulation of free radicals, leading to neuronal degeneration in the brain. Vitamin E, a fat-soluble vitamin, interacts with cell membranes, traps free radicals, and may interrupt chain reactions that damage cells.[69] In a recent meta-analysis, however, the true benefits could not be substantiated.[70] The NSAIDs are thought to decrease the inflammatory response to inflammatory mediators released from injured or degenerating nerve cells. Estrogen may have neuroprotective effects as well. In a large community study, women who used estrogen after menopause scored higher on cognitive screening tools, even after controlling for the effects of age, education, and other variables that may affect cognition.[71] Calcium channel blockers prevent calcium influx, which is proposed to cause neuronal death due to release of intracellular enzymes. There is no consensus on the use of these preventative agents, and further studies are needed before guidelines can be developed for their use in the prevention of Alzheimer's disease.

Management of older adults with Alzheimer's disease and other dementias usually involves assuming increasing responsibility for and supplying increasing care to individuals as the illness renders them incapable. Impaired judgment and cognition can prevent the older adult from making reasonable decisions and choices and eventually threatens their overall well-being. Family members often assume the monumental task of caring for older adults with dementia until the burden becomes too great, at which time many older adults may be relocated to long-term care facilities.

Some specific behavioral problems commonly are seen in older adults with dementia, including agitation, depression, hallucinations, aggressiveness, and wandering. It may be necessary to use low doses of pharmacologic agents such as neuroleptics, antidepressants, and antipsychotics. Nonpharmacologic interventions can help control behavioral problems and may preclude the need for medications. Ensuring that the individual's physical needs, such as hygiene, bowel and bladder elimination, safety, and nutrition, are met can help prevent catastrophic reactions. Providing a consistent routine in familiar surroundings also helps to alleviate stress. Matching the cognitive needs of the older adult by avoiding understimulation and overstimulation assists in preventing behavior problems.

The work of Hall has shown positive results in the care of older adults with Alzheimer's disease.[72] Hall's conceptual model, progressively lowered stress threshold (PLST), proposes that the demented individual's ability to tolerate any type of stress progressively declines as the disease advances. Interventions for the older adult with dementia therefore center on eliminating and avoiding stressors as a way to prevent dysfunctional behaviors. These stressors include fatigue, change of routine, excessive demands, overwhelming stimuli, and physical stressors. Hall's work with the PLST model has shown that individuals tend to awaken less at night, use less sedatives and hypnotics, eat better, socialize more, function at a higher level, and experience fewer episodes of anxiety, agitation, and other dysfunctional behaviors.

DELIRIUM

It is important to differentiate dementia from delirium, also referred to as *acute confusional state*. The demented older adult is far more likely to become delirious. The onset of delirium in the demented individual may be mistaken as an exacerbation of the dementia and consequently not treated.[73,74]

Delirium is an acute disorder developing over a period of hours to days and is seen frequently in hospitalized elderly patients. Prevalence rates range from 14% to 56% of hospitalized older adults and up to 90% of older adults admitted to psychiatric hospitals. Delirium is defined by the DSM-IVR as an organic mental syndrome featuring a global cognitive impairment, disturbances of attention, reduced level of consciousness, increased or decreased psychomotor activity, and a disorganized sleep-wake cycle. The severity of the symptoms tends to fluctuate unpredictably but often is more pronounced at night.[52]

Delirium can be a presenting feature of a physical illness and may be seen with disorders such as myocardial infarction, pneumonia and other infections, cancer, and hypothyroidism. Patients with drug toxicities may present with delirium. Malnutrition, use of physical restraints, and iatrogenic events also can precipitate delirium.

The exact reason that delirium occurs is unclear. It is speculated that the decreased central nervous system capacity in older adults may precipitate delirium. Other possible contributing factors include vision and hearing impairments, psychological stress, and diseases of other organ systems. Delirium has a high mortality rate, ranging between 20% and 40%. Agitation, disorientation, and fearfulness—the key symptoms of delirium—place the individual at high risk for injuries such as a fracture from a fall.[61,74]

Diagnosis of delirium involves recognition of the syndrome and identification of its causes. Management involves treatment of the underlying disease condition and symptomatic relief through supportive therapy, including good nutrition and hydration, rest, comfort measures, and emotional support. Prevention of delirium is the overall goal; avoidance of the devastating and life-threatening acute confusional state is the key to successful management and treatment.[75]

In summary, health care for older adults requires unique considerations, taking into account age-related physiologic changes and specific disease states common in this population. Although aging is not synonymous with disease, the aging process does lend itself to an increased incidence of illness. The overall goal is to assist the older adult in maximizing independence and functional capabilities and minimizing disabilities that can result from various acute and chronic illnesses.

The evaluation of the older adult's functional abilities is a key component in gerontologic health care. Medical diagnoses alone are incomplete without an assessment of function. When evaluating levels of function, determination of the older adult's ability to perform ADL and IADL should be included.

Among the functional disorders that are common in the older population are urinary incontinence, instability and falls, sensory impairment, depression, dementia, and delirium. The older adult is especially prone to urinary incontinence because of changes in the micturition cycle that accompany the aging process. Behavioral techniques can be an effective way to treat incontinence problems in the older adult population. Falls are a common source of concern for the older adult population. Although most falls do not result in serious injury, the potential for serious complications and even death is real. Most falls are the result of several risk factors, including age-related biopsychosocial changes, chronic illness, and situational and environmental hazards. Both hearing and visual impairment, which are common in the elderly, contribute to communication problems, depression, and social isolation. Depression is a significant but treatable health problem that often is misdiagnosed and mistreated in the older adult population. Dementia is a syndrome of acquired, persistent impairment in several domains of intellectual function, including memory, language, visuospatial ability, and cognition (*i.e.*, abstraction, calculation, judgment, and problem solving). Although there can be a slight decline in intellectual function with aging, dementia is not a normal aging process. Delirium is an acute confusional disorder developing over a period of hours to days and often is seen as a presenting feature of a physical illness or drug toxicity.

Drug Therapy in the Older Adult

After you have completed this section of the chapter, you should be able to meet the following objectives:

✦ Characterize drug therapy in the older adult population
✦ List five factors that contribute to adverse drug reactions in the elderly
✦ Cite cautions to be used in prescribing medications for the elderly

Drug therapy in the older adult population is a complex phenomenon influenced by numerous biopsychosocial factors. The elderly are the largest group of consumers of prescription and over-the-counter drugs. Although the older population comprises only approximately 13% of the U.S. population, they consume one third of all prescription drugs and 50% of all over-the-counter medications.[76] The incidence of adverse drug reactions in the elderly is two to three times that found in young adults. This is considered to be a conservative estimate because drug reactions are less well recognized in older adults and reactions often can mimic symptoms of specific disease states.

Errors in the administration of medications and compliance are common among the older adult population, estimated by several authorities to be between 25% and 50% for community-dwelling elderly. Reasons for this high volume of errors are numerous. Poor manual dexterity, failing eyesight, lack of understanding about the treatment regimen, attitudes and beliefs about medication use, mistrust of health care providers, and forgetfulness or confusion are but a few factors that can affect the adherence to medication regimens. The role of the health care provider also can contribute to improper medication use. There can be a tendency to treat symptoms with drugs rather than fully investigate the cause of those symptoms. To compound matters, accurate diagnosis of specific disease states can be difficult because older adults tend to underreport symptoms and because presenting symptoms are often atypical.[77,78]

Age-related physiologic changes also account for adverse effects of medications. In general, the absorption of orally ingested drugs remains essentially unchanged with age, even though the gastric pH is known to rise and gastric emptying time can be delayed. Changes in drug distribution, however, are clinically significant. Because lean body mass and total body water decrease with advancing age, water-soluble drugs such as digoxin and propranolol tend to have a smaller volume of distribution, resulting in higher plasma concentrations for a given dose and increased likelihood of a toxic reaction. Conversely, fat-soluble drugs such as diazepam are more widely distributed and accumulate in fatty tissue owing to an increase in adipose tissue with aging. This can cause a delay in elimination and accumulation of the drug over time (*i.e.*, prolonged half-life) with multiple doses of the same drug. Drug metabolism through the liver is thought to be altered owing to the decrease in hepatic blood flow seen in the older adult. Renal excretion controls the elimination of drugs from the body, and because kidney function declines with age, the rate of drug excretion decreases. This can result in an increased half-life of drugs and is why estimates of creatinine clearance are recommended to determine drug dosing.[79]

Drug use for older adults warrants a cautious approach. "Start low and go slow" is the adage governing drug prescribing in geriatric pharmacology. Older adults often can achieve therapeutic results on small doses of medications. If necessary, dosing can then be titrated slowly according to response.

Further complicating matters is the issue of polypharmacy in older adults, who often have multiple disorders that may require multiple drug therapies. Polypharmacy increases the risk of drug interactions and adverse drug reactions and decreases compliance. Drugs and disease states also can interact, causing adverse effects. For example, psychotropic drugs administered to older adults with dementia may cause a worsening of confusion; β-blocking agents administered to an individual with chronic obstructive pulmonary disease may induce bronchoconstriction; and nonsteroidal anti-inflammatory medications given to an older adult with hypertension can raise blood pressure further.

The use of certain types of medications carries a high risk for older adults and should be avoided if possible. In general, long-acting drugs or drugs with prolonged half-lives can be problematic. Many sedatives and hypnotics fit into this category, and drugs such as diazepam and flurazepam should be avoided. Other classes of drugs, such as antidepressants and anxiolytics, may provide the necessary symptomatic relief and may be more appropriate for older adults than sedatives and hypnotics. Use of these agents warrants caution, however, with consideration for the unique pharmacokinetic changes that accompany aging. Drugs that possess anticholinergic properties should also be used with caution. Anticholinergics are used for a variety of conditions; however, side effects such as dry mouth and eyes, blurred vision, and constipation are common. These drugs can also cause more serious side effects, such as confusion, urinary retention, and orthostatic hypotension. Agents that enter the central nervous system, including narcotics and alcohol, can cause a variety of problems, most notably delirium. These problems most likely occur as a result of a decreased central nervous system reserve capacity.[76,77,79]

Because of the serious implications of medication use in the elderly, strategies need to be used to enhance therapeutic effects and prevent harm. Careful evaluation of the need for the medication by the health care provider is the first step. Once decided, analysis of the individual's current medication regimen and disease states is necessary to prevent drug-drug interactions, drug-disease interactions, and adverse responses. Dosing should be at the low end, and frequency of drug administration should be kept to a minimum to simplify the routine and enhance compliance. Timing the dose to a specific activity of daily living (*e.g.*, "take with breakfast") can also improve compliance, as can special packaging devices such as pill boxes and blister packs. The cost of medications is another important factor for older adults on reduced, fixed incomes. Choosing less expensive products of equal efficacy can increase compliance. The importance of educating the individual about the medication cannot be overemphasized. Health care professionals need to provide verbal and written information on the principles of medication use and on the specific medications being used. This facilitates active, involved participation by the older adult and enhances the individual's ability to make informed decisions.[80]

In summary, drug therapy in the older adult population is a complex phenomenon influenced by numerous biopsychosocial factors. Alterations in pharmacokinetics occur with advancing age and increases the likelihood of toxic reactions. "Start low and go slow" is the adage governing geriatric pharmacology. Centrally acting drugs and drugs with long half-lives should be avoided when possible. Drug-drug interactions, drug-disease interactions, and adverse reactions increase in the elderly population. Educating the older adult about drug use is an important factor in ensuring compliance and accurate medication administration.

Related Web Sites

AHCPR Clinical Practice Guides   www.ahcpr.gov/clinic
Alzheimer's Association   www.alz.org
American Association of Retired Persons   www.aarp.org/
Gerontological Society of America   www.geron.org
National Association of Continence www.nafc.org
National Institutes of Aging   www/nih/gov/nia

NCHS Aging Activities   www.cdc.gov/nchs/agingact.htm
NursingCenter.com-clinical nursing information
   www.nursingcenter.com

References

1. American Association of Retired Persons. (1999). *A profile of older Americans*. Washington, DC: Author.
2. U.S. Department of Health and Human Services. (1996). *Profile of Medicare—30th anniversary*. Washington, DC: Health Care Financing Administration.
3. Erikson E. (1963). *Childhood and society*. New York: W.W. Norton.
4. Erikson E.H., Erikson J.M., Kivirck H.Q. (1986). *Vital involvement in old age*. New York: W.W. Norton.
5. Finch C.E., Tanzi R.E. (1997). Genetics of aging. *Science* 278, 407–412.
6. Slagboom P.E., Bastiann T.H., Beekman M., Wendendorf R.G.J., Meulenbelt I. (2000). Genetics of human aging. *Annals of the New York Academy of Science* 908, 50–61.
7. Hayflick L. (1985). Theories of biological aging. *Experimental Gerontology* 10, 145–159.
8. Hayflick L. (1979). Cell biology of aging. *Federation Proceedings* 38, 1847–1850.
9. Fossell M. (1998). Telomerase and the aging cell. *Journal of the American Medical Association* 279, 1732–1735.
10. Griffiths C.E.M. (1998). Aging of the skin. In Brocklehurst J.C., Tallis R., Fillet H. (Eds.), *Textbook of medicine and gerontology* (5th ed., pp. 1293–1298). Edinburgh: Churchill Livingstone.
11. Glogau R.G. (1997). Physiologic and structural changes associated with the aging skin. *Dermatology Clinics* 15, 555–559.
12. Taaffe D.R., Marcus R. (2000). Musculoskeletal health and the older adult. *Journal of Rehabilitation Research and Development* 37, 245–254.
13. Timiras P.S. (1994). Aging of the skeleton, joints, and muscles. In Timiras P.S. (Ed.), *Physiological basis of aging and geriatrics* (2nd ed., pp. 259–272). Boca Raton, FL: CRC Press.
14. Lakatta E.G. (1999). Cardiovascular aging research. *Journal of the American Gerontological Society* 47, 613–625.
15. Joint National Committee. (1998). *The Sixth Report of Joint National Committee on Prevention, Detection, Evaluation, and Treatment of High Blood Pressure*. NIH publication no. 98-4080. Bethesda, MD: National Institutes of Health.
16. Applegate W.B. (1998). Hypertension. In Hazzard W.R., Blass J.P., Ettinger W.H. Jr., Halter J.B., Ouslander J.G. (Eds.), *Principles of geriatric medicine and gerontology* (4th ed., pp. 713–720). New York: McGraw-Hill.
17. Lakotta E.G. (2000). Cardiovascular aging in health. *Clinical Geriatric Medicine* 16, 419–444.
18. Smith J.J., Porth C.J.M. (1990). Age and the response to orthostatic stress. In Smith J.J. (Ed.), *Circulatory response to the upright position* (pp. 121–139). Boca Raton, FL: CRC Press.
19. Fleg J.L., O'Connor F., Gerstenblith G., Becker L.C., Clulow J., Schulman S.P., et al. (1995). Impact of age on the cardiovascular response to dynamic upright exercise in healthy men and women. *Journal of Applied Physiology* 78, 890–900.
20. Timiras P.S. (1994). Aging of respiration, erythrocytes and the hematopoietic system. In Timiras P.S. (Ed.), *Physiological basis of aging and geriatrics* (2nd ed., pp. 225–233). Boca Raton, FL: CRC Press.
21. Timiras P.S. (1994). Aging of the nervous system: Structural and biochemical changes. In Timiras P.S. (Ed.), *Physiological*

basis of aging and geriatrics (2nd ed., pp. 89–102). Boca Raton, FL: CRC Press.

22. Odenheimer G.L. (1998). Geriatric neurology. *Neurology Clinics* 16, 561–567.

23. Forrester J.V. (1997). Aging and vision. *British Journal of Ophthalmology* 81, 809–810.

24. Nusbaum N.J. (1999). Aging and sensory senescence. *Southern Medical Journal* 92, 267–275.

25. Bruck. A.M. (1999). Vision, hearing problems in the elderly. *Provider* 25 (10), 101–102, 105.

26. Timiras P.S. (1994). Aging of the immune system. In Timiras P.S. (Ed.), *Physiological basis of aging and geriatrics* (2nd ed., pp. 75–87). Boca Raton, FL: CRC Press.

27. Mouton C.P., Pierce B., Espino D.V. (2001). Common infections in older adults. *American Family Practitioner* 63, 257–268.

28. Fraser D. (1997). Assessing the elderly for infection. *Journal of Gerontological Nursing* 23, 5–10.

29. Soergel K.H., Zboralske F.E., Amberg J.R. (1964). Presbyesophagus: Esophageal motility in nonagenarians. *Journal of Clinical Investigation* 43, 1472–1476.

30. Hall R.E., Wiley J.W. (1998). Age-associated change in gastrointestinal function. In Hazzard W.R., Blass J.P., Ettinger W.H. Jr., Ouslander J.G. (Eds.), *Principles of geriatric medicine and gerontology* (4th ed., pp. 835–842). New York: McGraw-Hill.

31. Lindeman R.D. (1998). Renal and electrolyte disorders. In Duthie E.H. Jr., Katz P.R. (Eds.), *Practice in geriatrics* (3rd ed., pp. 546–561). Philadelphia: W.B. Saunders.

32. Beck L.M. (1994). Aging changes in renal function. In Hazzard W.R., Blass J.P., Ettinger W.H. Jr., Ouslander J.G. (Eds.), *Principles of geriatric medicine and gerontology* (4th ed., pp. 767–776). New York: McGraw-Hill.

33. Smith M. (1998). Gynecological disorders. In Duthie E.H. Jr., Katz P.R. (Eds.), *Practice in geriatrics* (3rd ed., pp. 524–534). Philadelphia: W.B. Saunders.

34. Letran J.L., Brawer M.K. (1998). Disorders of the prostate. In Hazzard W.R., Blass J.P., Ettinger W.H. Jr., Halter J.B., Ouslander J.G. (Eds.), *Principles of geriatric medicine and gerontology* (4th ed., pp. 809–821). New York: McGraw-Hill.

35. Kaiser F.E. (1998). Sexuality. In Duthie E.H. Jr., Katz P.R., (Eds.), *Practice in geriatrics* (3rd ed., pp. 48–56). Philadelphia: W.B. Saunders.

36. Duffy L.M. (1998). Lovers, loners, and lifers: Sexuality and the older adult. *Geriatrics* 53 (Suppl. 1), S66–S69.

37. Katz S., Ford A.B., Jackson B.A., Jaffee M.W. (1963). Studies of illness in the aged: The Index of ADL. *Journal of the American Medical Association* 185, 914–919.

38. Katz S., Downs T.D., Cash H.R., Grotz R.C. (1970). Progress in development of the Index of ADL. *Gerontologist* 10, 20–30.

39. Fantl J.A., Neuman D.F., Colling J., Delancey J.B.L., Keeys C., Loughery R., et al. (1996). *Urinary incontinence in adults: Acute and chronic management.* Clinical practice guideline no. 2, 1996 update. Publication no. 96–06. Rockville, MD: Agency for Health Care Policy and Research.

40. Yee S., Phanumas D., Fields S.D. (2000). Urinary incontinence: A primary care guide to managing acute and chronic symptoms in older adults. *Geriatrics* 55 (11), 65–71.

41. Coogler C.E., Wolf S.L. (1998). Falls. In Hazzard W.R., Blass J.P., Ettinger W.H. Jr., Halter J.B., Ouslander J.G. (Eds.), *Principles of geriatric medicine and gerontology* (4th ed., pp. 1535–1546). New York: McGraw-Hill.

42. Fuller G.F. (2000). Falls in the elderly. *American Family Practitioner* 61, 2159–2168, 2173–2174.

43. Gregg E.W., Pereira M.A., Caspersen C.J. (2000). Physical activity, falls, and fractures among older adults: A review of the epidemiologic evidence. *Journal of the American Geriatric Society* 48, 883–893.

44. Hausdorff J.M., Edelberg H.K., Cudkowicz M.E., Singh M.A., Wei J.Y. (1997). The relationship between gait and falls. *Journal of the American Geriatric Society* 45, 1406.

45. Tennetti M.E., Williams C.S., Gill T.M. (2000). Dizziness among older adults: A possible geriatric syndrome. *Annals of Internal Medicine* 132, 337–344.

46. Keller B.K., Morton J.L., Thomas V.S., Potter J.F. (1999). The effect of visual and hearing impairment on functional status. *Journal of the American Gerontological Society* 47, 1319–1325.

47. Reuben D.B., Mui S., Damesyn M., Moore A.A., Greendale G.A. (1999). The prognostic value of sensory impairment in older persons. *Journal of the American Gerontological Society* 47, 930–935.

48. Mojica T.R., Baily P.P. (2000). Hallucinations in the vision-impaired elderly: The Charles Bonnet Syndrome. *Nurse Practitioner* 25 (8), 74–76.

49. Teunisse R.J., Cruysberg J.R., Hoefnagels W.H., Verbeck A.L., Zitman F.G. (1996). Visual hallucinations in psychologically normal people: Charles Bonnet's syndrome. *Lancet* 347, 794–797.

50. Almedia O.P., Howard R.J., Levy R. (1995). Psychotic states arising in late life (late paraphrenia): The role of risk factors. *British Journal of Psychiatry* 166, 215–228.

51. NIH Consensus Development Panel. (1995). Diagnosis and treatment of depression in late life. *Journal of the American Medical Association* 268, 1018–1024.

52. American Psychiatric Association. (1994). *Diagnostic and statistical manual of mental disorders* (4th ed., rev.). Washington, DC: Author.

53. Pollock B.G., Reynolds C.F. 3rd (2000). Depression late in life. *Harvard Mental Health Letter* 17 (3), 3–5.

54. Depression Guideline Panel. (1993). *Depression in primary care: Treatment of major depression* (vol. 2). Clinical practice guideline no. 5, 1993. Publication no. 93-0551. Rockville, MD: Agency for Health Care Policy and Research.

55. Bharucha A.J., Satlin A. (1997). Late life suicide: A review. *Harvard Review of Psychiatry* 5 (2), 55–65.

56. Yesavage J.A., Brink T.L., Rose T.L., Lum O., Huang V., Adey M., et al. (1983). Development and validation of a geriatric depression scale: A preliminary report. *Journal of Psychiatric Research* 17, 37–49.

57. Kelly K.G., Zisselman M. (2000). Update on electroconvulsive therapy (ECT) in older adults. *Journal of the American Geriatric Society* 48, 560–566.

58. Hendrie H.C. (1997). Epidemiology of Alzheimer's disease. *Geriatrics* 52 (Suppl. 2), S4–S8.

59. Loeb C., Meyer J.S. (2000). Criteria for diagnosis of vascular dementia. *Archives of Neurology* 67, 615–618.

60. Beck C., Cody M., Souder E., Zhang M., Small G.W. (2000). Dementia diagnostic guidelines: Methodologies, results, implementation costs. *Journal of the American Geriatric Society* 48, 1195–1203.

61. Espino D.V., Jules-Bradley A.C.A., Johnston C.L., Mouton C.P. (1998). Diagnostic approach to the confused elderly patient. *American Family Practitioner* 57, 1358–1366.

62. Bolla L.R., Filley C.M., Palmer R.M. (2000). Office diagnosis of the four major types of dementia. *Geriatrics* 55 (1), 34–48.

63. Folstein M.F., Folstein B.E., McHugh P.R. (1975). "Mini-Mental State": A practical method for grading the cognitive state of patients for the clinician. *Journal of Psychiatric Research* 12, 189–198.

64. Rogers S.L., Farlow M.R., Doody R.S., Mohs R., Friedhoff L.T. (1998). A 24-week, double-blind, placebo-controlled trial of donepezil in patients with Alzheimer's disease: American Academy of Neurology. *Neurology* 50, 136–145.

65. Spencer C.M., Noble S. (1998). Rivastigmine: A review of its use in Alzheimer's disease. *Drugs and Aging* 13, 391–411.

66. Mayeux R. (1999). Treatment of Alzheimer's disease. *New England Journal of Medicine* 341, 1670–1679.

67. LeBars P.L., Katz M.M., Berman N., Itil T.M., Freedman A.M., Schatzberg A.F. (1997). A placebo-controlled, double-blind, randomized trial of *Ginkgo biloba* for dementia. *Journal of the American Medical Association* 278, 1327–1332.

68. Oken B.S., Storzbach D.M., Kaye J.A. (1998). The efficacy of *Ginkgo biloba* on cognitive function in Alzheimer's disease. *Archives of Neurology* 55, 1409–1415.

69. Sono M., Ernesto M.S., Thomas R.G., Kaluber M.P., Schafer K., Grundman M., et al. (1997). A controlled trial of selegiline, alpha-tocopherol, or both as treatment for Alzheimer's disease. *New England Journal of Medicine* 336, 1216–1222.

70. Wolfson E., Moride V., Perrault A. (2001). Revew: Donepezil, metrifonate, rivastigmine and *Ginkgo biloba* are more effective than placebo in Alzheimer's disease. *Journal Club* 134 (1), 10.

71. Steffens D.C., Norton M.C., Plassman B.L., Tschanz J.T., Wyse B.W., Welsh-Bohmer K.A., Anthony J.C., Breitner J.C.S. (1999). Enhanced cognitive performance with estrogen use in nondemented community-dwelling older women. *Journal of the American Geriatric Society* 47, 1171–1175.

72. Hall G.R., LaBudakis D. (1999). A behavioral approach to Alzheimer's disease. The progressively lowered stress threshold model. *Advanced Nurse Practitioner* 7 (7), 39–41,81.

73. O'Keefe S.T. (1999). Delirium in the elderly. *Age and Aging* 28 (Suppl. 2): 5–8.

74. Inouye S.K., Charpentier P.A. (1996). Precipitating factors in delirium in hospitalized elderly persons. *Journal of the American Medical Association* 275, 852–857.

75. Inouye S.K., Bogarous S.T., Charpentier P.A., Leo-Summers L., Acampora D., Holford T.R., Cooney L.M. Jr. (1999). A multicomponent intervention to prevent delirium in hospitalized older patients. *New England Journal of Medicine* 340, 669–676.

76. Abrams W.B., Beers M.H., Berkow R., Fletcher A.J. (1995). *Merck manual of geriatrics* (2nd ed.). Whitehouse Station, NJ: Merck Research Laboratories.

77. Woodhouse K.W. (1994). Pharmacology of drugs in the elderly. *Journal of the Royal Society of Medicine* 87 (Suppl. 23), 2–4.

78. Aparasu R.R., Mort J.R. (2000). Inappropriate prescribing for the elderly: Beers criteria-based revew. *Annals of Pharmacology* 34, 338–346.

79. Katzung B.G. (2001). Special aspects of geriatric pharmacology. In Katzung B.G. (Ed.), *Basic and clinical pharmacology* (8th ed., pp. 1036–1044). New York: Lange Medical Books/McGraw-Hill.

80. Beyth R.J., Shorr R.J. (1998). Medication use. In Duthie E.H. Jr., Katz P.R. (Eds.), *Practice in geriatrics* (3rd ed., pp. 38–47). Philadelphia: W.B. Saunders.

Cell Function and Growth

With its elegant structure and astonishing range of functions, the living cell is an object of wonder. It is the basic unit of all living organisms. There are more than 300 trillion cells in the human body, and every second of every day, more than 10 million die and are replaced.

In 1665, these impressive structures were named. While examining a thin slice of cork, Robert Hooke (1635–1703), an English scientist and pioneer microscopist, noted that it was made up of tiny boxlike units. The units reminded him of the small enclosures in which monks lived, and he named the microscopic spaces "cells," from the Latin word cells, meaning "small enclosures."

Although Hooke, as well as other scientists, intently studied microscopic life, few guessed the significance of the cells. That would be delayed until microscopes were advanced enough to yield more detailed information. It was with the work of Anton van Leeuwenhoek (1632–1723), a Dutch biologist and microscopist, that the mysteries and importance of the cell were revealed. He ground a single lens to such perfection that he was able to produce a microscope with great resolving power—one that was capable of magnifying a specimen from approximately 50 to 300 times in diameter. Van Leeuwenhoek's work, which included constructing an aquatic microscope that he used to study red blood cells and their flow through the body, was responsible for helping scientists investigate human tissue in ways that once they only dreamed of.

Chapter 4

Cell and Tissue Characteristics

Edward W. Carroll

The *cell* is the smallest functional unit that an organism can be divided into and retain the characteristics necessary for life. Cells with similar embryonic origin or function are often organized into larger functional units called *tissues*. These tissues in turn combine to form the various body structures and organs. Although the cells of different tissues and organs vary in structure and function, certain characteristics are common to all cells. Cells are remarkably similar in their ability to exchange materials with their immediate environment, obtaining energy from organic nutrients, synthesizing complex molecules, and replicating themselves. Because most disease processes are initiated at the cellular level, an understanding of cell function is crucial to understanding the disease process. Some diseases affect the cells of a single organ, others affect the cells of a particular tissue type, and still others affect the cells of the entire organism.

This chapter discusses the structural and functional components of the cell, integration of cell function and growth, movement of molecules such as ions across the cell membrane and membrane potentials, and tissue types.

Functional Components of the Cell

After you have completed this section of the chapter, you should be able to meet the following objectives:

✦ List the major components of the cell protoplasm
✦ State why the nucleus is called the "control center" of the cell

The Functional Organization of the Cell

➤ Cells are the smallest functional unit of the body. They contain structures that are strikingly similar to those needed to maintain total body function.

➤ The nucleus is the control center for the cell. It also contains most of the hereditary material.

➤ The organelles, which are analogous to the organs of the body, are contained in the cytoplasm. They include the mitochondria, which supply the energy needs of the cell; the ribosomes, which synthesize proteins and other materials needed for cell function; and the lysosomes, which function as the cell's digestive system.

➤ The cell membrane encloses the cell and provides for intracellular and intercellular communication, transport of materials into and out of the cell, and maintenance of the electrical activities that power cell function.

✦ Explain the relationships among DNA, genes, and chromosomes
✦ Name the three types of RNA and describe their role in protein synthesis
✦ List the cellular organelles and state their functions
✦ State four functions of the cell membrane

Although diverse in their organization, all eukaryotic cells have in common structures that perform unique functions. When seen under a light microscope, three major components of the cell become evident: the nucleus, the cytoplasm, and the cell membrane (Fig. 4-1).

PROTOPLASM

The internal matrix of the cell is called *protoplasm*. Protoplasm is composed of water, proteins, lipids, carbohydrates, and electrolytes. Water makes up 70% to 85% of the cell's protoplasm. The second most abundant constituents (10% to 20%) of protoplasm are the cell proteins, which form cell structures and the enzymes necessary for cellular reactions. Proteins can also be found complexed to other compounds as nucleoproteins, glycoproteins, and lipoproteins. Lipids comprise 2% to

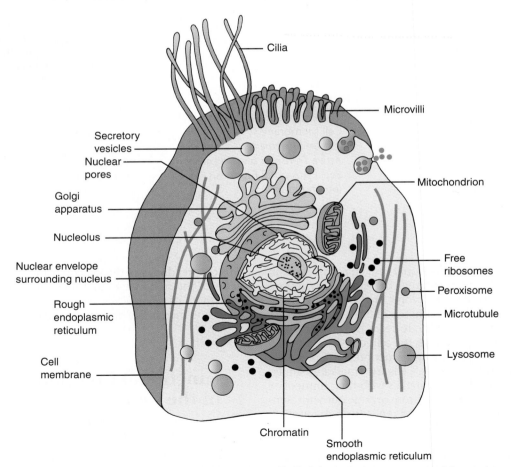

FIGURE 4-1 Composite cell designed to show in one cell all of the various components of the nucleus and cytoplasm.

3% of most cells. The most important lipids are the phospholipids and cholesterol, which are mainly insoluble in water; they combine with proteins to form the cell membrane and the membranous barriers that separate different cell compartments. Some cells also contain large quantities of triglycerides. In the fat cells, triglycerides can constitute up to 95% of the total cell mass. The fat stored in these cells represents stored energy, which can be mobilized and used wherever it is needed in the body. Few carbohydrates are found in the cell, and these are used primarily for fuel. Potassium, magnesium, phosphate, sulfate, and bicarbonate are the major intracellular electrolytes. Small quantities of sodium, chloride, and calcium ions are also present in the cell. These electrolytes facilitate the generation and transmission of electrochemical impulses in nerve and muscle cells. Intracellular electrolytes participate in reactions that are necessary for cellular metabolism. Two distinct regions of protoplasm exist in the cell: the *cytoplasm*, which lies outside the nucleus, and the *karyoplasm* or *nucleoplasm*, which lies inside the nucleus.

THE NUCLEUS

The nucleus of the cell appears as a rounded or elongated structure situated near the center of the cell (see Fig. 4-1). It is enclosed in a nuclear membrane and contains chromatin and a distinct region called the *nucleolus*. All eukaryotic cells have at least one nucleus (prokaryotic cells, such as bacteria, lack a nucleus and nuclear membrane). Some cells contain more than one nucleus; osteoclasts (a type of bone cell) typically contain 12 or more.

The nucleus is the control center for the cell. It contains deoxyribonucleic acid (DNA) that is essential to the cell because its genes contain the information necessary for the synthesis of proteins that the cell must produce to stay alive. These proteins include structural proteins and enzymes used to synthesize other substances, including carbohydrates and lipids. The genes also represent the individual units of inheritance that transmit information from one generation to another. The nucleus is also the site of ribonucleic acid (RNA) synthesis. There are three types of RNA: messenger RNA (mRNA), which copies and carries the DNA instructions for protein synthesis to the cytoplasm; ribosomal RNA (rRNA), which moves to the cytoplasm, where it becomes the site of protein synthesis; and transfer RNA (tRNA), which also moves into the cytoplasm, where it transports amino acids to the elongating protein as it is being synthesized (see Chapter 6).

The complex structure of DNA and DNA-associated proteins dispersed in the nuclear matrix is called *chromatin*. Each DNA molecule is made up of two extremely long, double-stranded helical chains containing variable sequences of four nitrogenous bases. These bases form the genetic code. Within the nucleus, each double-stranded DNA molecule is periodically coiled about basic proteins

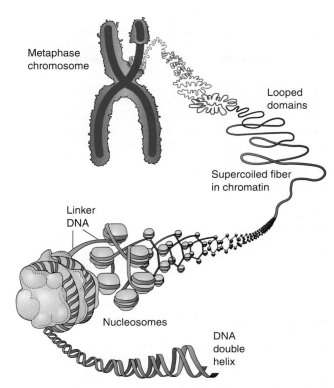

FIGURE 4-2 Increasing orders of DNA compaction in chromatin and mitotic chromosomes. (From Cormack D.H. [1993]. *Essential histology*. Philadelphia: J.B. Lippincott)

called *histones*, forming regularly spaced spherical structures called *nucleosomes* that resemble beads on a string (Fig. 4-2). The string of beads is further wound into filaments that make up the structure of chromatin. Further coiling produces structures known as *chromosomes*, which are visible during cell division.

Although each DNA molecule contains many genetic instructions, it is not made up entirely of genes. Stretches of meaningless DNA can lie between one gene and the next and sometimes reside within the gene sequence itself. The amino acid sequence of the gene that is interpreted is called an *exon*, and the interspersed meaningless portion is called an *intron*. In cells that are about to divide, the DNA must be replicated before mitosis or cell division occurs. During replication, complementary pairs of DNA are generated such that each daughter cell receives an identical set of genes.

During mitosis, the chromosomes are condensed and can be observed; at other times during the cell cycle they are not observable. In the mature or nondividing cell, chromatin may exist in a less active, condensed form called *heterochromatin* or a transcriptionally more active form called *euchromatin*. Because heterochromatic regions of the nucleus stain more intensely than regions consisting of euchromatin, nuclear staining can be used as a guide to cell activity. A more active cell, which contains greater amounts of euchromatin, does not stain or is lightly stained.

The nucleus also contains the darkly stained round body called the *nucleolus*. Although nucleoli were first described in 1781, it was not until the early 1960s that their function was identified: it was determined that rRNA is transcribed exclusively in the nucleolus.[1] Nucleoli are structures composed of regions from five different chromosomes, each with a part of the genetic code needed for the synthesis of rRNA. Cells that are actively synthesizing proteins can be recognized because their nucleoli are large and prominent and the nucleus as a whole is euchromatic.

Surrounding the nucleus is a doubled membrane called the *nuclear envelope* or *nuclear membrane*. The nuclear membrane contains many structurally complex circular pores where the two membranes fuse to form a gap filled with a thin protein diaphragm. Evidence suggests that many classes of molecules, including fluids, electrolytes, RNA, some proteins, and perhaps some hormones, can move in both directions through the nuclear pores. Nuclear pores apparently regulate which molecules pass between the cytoplasm and nucleus.

THE CYTOPLASM AND ITS ORGANELLES

The cytoplasm surrounds the nucleus, and it is in the cytoplasm that the work of the cell takes place. Cytoplasm is essentially a colloidal solution that contains water, electrolytes, suspended proteins, neutral fats, and glycogen molecules.[2] Although they do not contribute to the cell's function, pigments may also accumulate in the cytoplasm. Some pigments, such as melanin, which gives skin its color, are normal constituents of the cell. Bilirubin is a normal major pigment of bile; however, excess accumulation of bilirubin within cells is abnormal. This is evidenced clinically by a yellowish discoloration of the skin and sclera, a condition called *jaundice*.

Embedded in the cytoplasm are various *organelles*, which function as the organs of the cell. These organelles include the ribosomes, endoplasmic reticulum (ER), Golgi complex, mitochondria, lysosomes, microtubules, filaments, peroxisomes and centrioles.

Ribosomes

The ribosomes serve as sites of protein synthesis in the cell.[3] They are small particles of nucleoproteins (rRNA and proteins) that can be found attached to the wall of the ER or as free ribosomes (Fig. 4-3). Free ribosomes are scattered singly in the cytoplasm or joined by strands of mRNA to form functional units called *polyribosomes*. Free ribosomes are involved in the synthesis of proteins, mainly as intracellular enzymes.

Endoplasmic Reticulum

The ER is an extensive system of paired membranes and flat vesicles that connects various parts of the inner cell (see Fig. 4-3). The fluid-filled space, called the *matrix*, between the paired ER membrane layers is connected with the space between the two membranes of the double-layered nuclear membrane, the cell membrane, and various cytoplasmic organelles. It functions as a tubular communication system through which substances can be transported

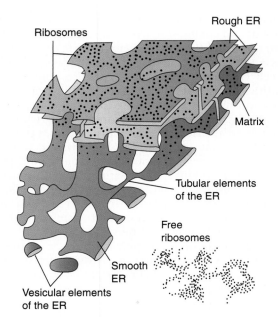

FIGURE 4-3 Three-dimensional view of the rough endoplasmic reticulum (ER) with its attached ribosomal RNA and the smooth endoplasmic reticulum.

from one part of the cell to another. A large surface area and multiple enzyme systems attached to the ER membranes also provide the machinery for a major share of the metabolic functions of the cell.

Two forms of ER exist in cells: rough and smooth. Rough ER is studded with ribosomes attached to specific binding sites on the membrane. The ribosomes, with the accompanying strand of mRNA, synthesize proteins. Proteins produced by the rough ER are usually destined for incorporation into cell membranes and lysosomal enzymes or for exportation from the cell. The rough ER segregates these proteins from other components of the cytoplasm and modifies their structure for a specific function. For example, the synthesis of digestive enzymes by the pancreatic acinar cells and the production of plasma protein by liver cells take place in the rough ER. All cells require a rough ER for the synthesis of lysosomal enzymes.

The smooth ER is free of ribosomes and is continuous with the rough ER. It does not participate in protein synthesis; instead, its enzymes are involved in the synthesis of lipid molecules, regulation of intracellular calcium, and metabolism and detoxification of certain hormones and drugs. It is the site of lipid, lipoprotein, and steroid hormone synthesis. The sarcoplasmic reticulum of skeletal and cardiac muscle cells is a form of smooth ER. Calcium ions needed for muscle contraction are stored and released from cisternae of the sarcoplasmic reticulum. Smooth ER of the liver is involved in glycogen storage and metabolism of lipid-soluble drugs.

Golgi Complex

The Golgi apparatus, sometimes called the *Golgi complex*, consists of stacks of thin, flattened vesicles or sacs. These

Golgi bodies are found near the nucleus and function in association with the ER. Substances produced in the ER are carried to the Golgi complex in small, membrane-covered transfer vesicles. Many cells synthesize proteins that are larger than the active product. Insulin, for example, is synthesized as a larger, inactive proinsulin molecule that is cut apart to produce a smaller, active insulin molecule within the Golgi complex of the beta cells of the pancreas. The Golgi complex modifies these substances and packages them into secretory granules or vesicles. Enzymes destined for export from the cell are packaged in secretory vesicles. After appropriate signals, the secretory vesicles move out of the Golgi complex into the cytoplasm and fuse to the inner side of the plasma membrane, where they release their contents into the extracellular fluid. Figure 4-4 is a diagram of the synthesis and movement of a hormone through the rough ER and Golgi complex. Besides its function in producing secretory granules, the Golgi complex is thought to produce large carbohydrate molecules that combine with proteins produced by the rough ER to form glycoproteins. The Golgi apparatus also forms the acrosomal cap on the head of the sperm.[4]

Lysosomes and Peroxisomes

The lysosomes can be viewed as the digestive system of the cell. They consist of small, membrane-enclosed sacs containing hydrolytic enzymes capable of breaking down worn-out cell parts so they can be recycled. They also break down foreign substances such as bacteria taken into the cell. All of the lysosomal enzymes are acid hydrolases, which means that they require an acid environment. The lysosomes provide this environment by maintaining a pH of approximately 5 in their interior. The pH of the cytoplasm is approximately 7.2, which protects other cellular structures from this acidity. Like many other organelles, lysosomes have a unique surrounding membrane that can be pinched off to form vesicles that are used to transport materials throughout the cytoplasm.

Lysosomal enzymes are synthesized in the rough ER and then transported to the Golgi apparatus, where they are biochemically modified and packaged as lysosomes. Unlike other organelles, the sizes and functions of lysosomes vary considerably. This diversity is determined by the type of enzyme packaged in the lysosome by the Golgi complex. Lysosomes containing hydrolytic enzymes that have not entered the digestive process are called *primary lysosomes*. *Secondary lysosomes* are those in which the hydrolytic enzymes have been activated and the chemical degradation process has begun. They form when primary lysosomes fuse with material that needs to be digested. Secondary lysosomes can be formed in one of two ways: heterophagy or autophagy (Fig. 4-5). *Heterophagocytosis* refers to the uptake of material from outside the cell. External materials are taken into the cell by an infolding of the cell membrane to form a surrounding phagocytic vesicle or *phagosome*. Primary lysosomes then fuse with phagosomes to form secondary lysosomes. Heterophagocytosis is most common in phagocytic white blood cells such as neutrophils and macrophages. *Autophagocytosis* involves the removal of damaged cellular organelles, such as mitochondria or ER, which must be removed if the cell's normal function is to continue. Autophagocytosis is most pronounced in cells undergoing atrophy.

Although enzymes in the secondary lysosomes can break down most proteins, carbohydrates, and lipids to their basic constituents, some materials remain undigested. These undigested materials may remain in the cytoplasm as *residual bodies* or be extruded from the cell. In some long-lived cells, such as neurons and heart muscle cells, large quantities of residual bodies accumulate as lipofuscin granules or age pigment. Other indigestible pigments, such as inhaled carbon particles and tattoo pigments, also accumulate and may persist in residual bodies for decades.

Lysosomes play an important role in the normal metabolism of certain substances in the body. In some inherited diseases known as *lysosomal storage diseases*, a specific

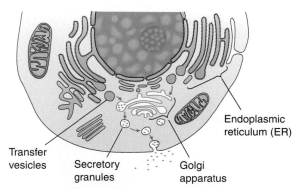

FIGURE 4-4 Hormone synthesis and secretion. In hormone secretion, the hormone is synthesized by the ribosomes attached to the rough endoplasmic reticulum. It moves from the rough ER to the Golgi complex, where it is stored in the form of secretory granules. These leave the Golgi complex and are stored within the cytoplasm until released from the cell in response to an appropriate signal.

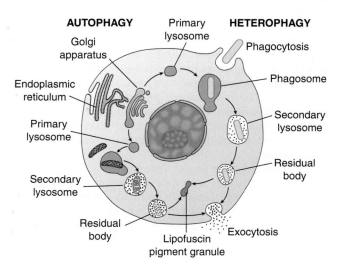

FIGURE 4-5 The process of autophagy and heterophagy, showing the primary and secondary lysosomes, residual bodies, extrusion of residual body contents from the cell, and lipofuscin-containing residual bodies.

lysosomal enzyme is absent or inactive, in which case the digestion of certain cellular substances (*e.g.*, cerebrosides, gangliosides, sphingomyelin) does not occur.[5] As a result, these substances accumulate in the cell. In Tay-Sachs disease, an autosomal recessive disorder, hexosaminidase A, which is the lysosomal enzyme needed for degrading the GM_2 ganglioside found in nerve cell membranes, is deficient. Although GM_2 ganglioside accumulates in many tissues, such as the heart, liver, and spleen, its accumulation in the nervous system and retina of the eye causes the most damage. Infants born with the disorder are normal at birth, but motor and mental deterioration and blindness soon begin to develop as GM_2 gangliosides accumulate in the nervous system. The course of the disease is rapid and relentless, and death usually occurs in the second or third year of life.

Smaller than lysosomes, spherical membrane-bound organelles called *peroxisomes* contain a special enzyme that degrades peroxides (*e.g.*, hydrogen peroxide). Peroxisomes function in the control of free radicals (see Chapter 5). Unless degraded, these highly unstable chemical compounds would otherwise damage other cytoplasmic molecules. For example, catalase degrades toxic hydrogen peroxide molecules to water. Peroxisomes also contain the enzymes needed for breaking down very–long-chain fatty acids, which are ineffectively degraded by mitochondrial enzymes. In liver cells, peroxisomal enzymes are involved in the formation of the bile acids. In a genetic disease called *adrenoleukodystrophy*, the most common disorder of peroxisomes, there is a buildup of long-chain fatty acids in the nervous system and adrenal gland.[5] The disorder, which is rapidly progressive and fatal, results in dementia and adrenal insufficiency because of the accumulation of the fatty acids.

Mitochondria

The mitochondria are literally the "power plants" of the cell because they transform organic compounds into energy that is easily accessible to the cell. Energy is not made here, but is extracted from organic compounds. Mitochondria contain the enzymes needed for capturing most of the energy in foodstuffs and converting it into cellular energy. This multistep process is generally called *cellular respiration* because it requires oxygen. Much of this energy is stored in the high-energy phosphate bonds of compounds such as adenosine triphosphate (ATP), which powers the various cellular activities. Energy that is not used or stored as ATP is dissipated as heat used to maintain body temperature.

Mitochondria are found close to the site of energy consumption in the cell (*e.g.*, near the myofibrils in muscle cells). The number of mitochondria in a given cell type is largely determined by the type of activity the cell performs and how much energy is needed to undertake this activity. For example, large increases in mitochondria have been observed in skeletal muscle that has been repeatedly stimulated to contract.

The mitochondria are composed of two membranes: an outer membrane that encloses the periphery of the mitochondrion and an inner membrane that forms shelflike projections, called *cristae* (Fig. 4-6). The outer and inner membranes form two spaces. The outer space is located between the two membranes. The inner space, which is filled with an amorphous matrix, is called the *matrix space*. The outer mitochondrial membrane is involved in lipid synthesis and fatty acid metabolism. The inner membrane contains the respiratory chain enzymes and transport proteins needed for the synthesis of ATP.[6]

Mitochondria contain their own DNA and ribosomes and are self-replicating. The DNA is found in the mitochondrial matrix and is distinct from the chromosomal DNA found in the nucleus. Mitochondrial DNA, known as the "other human genome," is a double-stranded, circular molecule that encodes the rRNA and tRNA required for intramitochrondial synthesis of proteins needed for the energy-generating function of the mitochondria. Although mitochondrial DNA directs the synthesis of 13 of the proteins required for mitochondrial function, the DNA of the nucleus encodes the structural proteins of the mitochondria and other proteins needed to carry out cellular respiration.

Mitochondrial DNA is inherited matrilineally (*i.e.*, from the mother) and provides a basis for familial lineage studies. Mutations have been found in each of the mitochondrial genes, and an understanding of the role of mitochondrial DNA in certain diseases is beginning to emerge.[7,8] Most tissues in the body depend to some extent on oxidative metabolism and can therefore be affected by mitochondrial DNA mutations.

THE CYTOSKELETON

Besides its organelles, the cytoplasm contains a network of microtubules, microfilaments, intermediate filaments, and thick filaments (Fig. 4-7). Because they control cell shape and movement, these structures are a major component of the structural elements called the *cytoskeleton*.

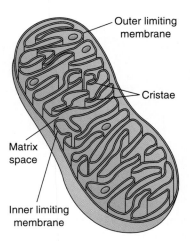

FIGURE 4-6 Mitochondrion. The inner membrane forms transverse folds called cristae, where the enzymes needed for the final step in adenosine triphosphate (ATP) production (*i.e.*, oxidative phosphorylation) are located.

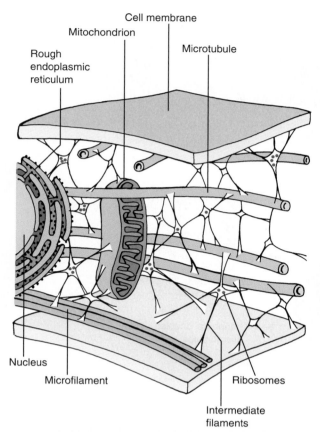

Cell membrane
Mitochondrion
Microtubule
Rough
endoplasmic
reticulum
Nucleus
Microfilament
Ribosomes
Intermediate
filaments

FIGURE 4-7 Microtubes and microfilaments of the cell. The microfilaments associate with the inner surface of the cell and aid in cell motility. The microtubules form the cytoskeleton and maintain the position of the organelles.

Microtubules

The microtubules are slender tubular structures composed of globular proteins called *tubulin*. Microtubules function in many ways, including development and maintenance of cell form; participation in intracellular transport mechanisms, including axoplasmic transport in neurons and melanin dispersion in pigment cells of the skin; and formation of the basic structure for several complex cytoplasmic organelles, including the centrioles, basal bodies, cilia, and flagella. Abnormalities of the cytoskeleton may contribute to alterations in cell mobility and function. For example, proper functioning of the microtubules is essential for various stages of leukocyte migration. In certain disease conditions, such as diabetes mellitus, alterations in leukocyte mobility and migration may interfere with the chemotaxis and phagocytosis of the inflammatory response and predispose toward the development of bacterial infection.

Microtubules can be rapidly assembled and disassembled according to the needs of the cell. The assembly of microtubules is halted by the action of the plant alkaloid colchicine. This compound stops cell mitosis by interfering with formation of the mitotic spindle and is used for cytogenetic (chromosome) studies. It is also used

as a drug for treating gout. It is thought that the drug's ability to reduce the inflammatory reaction associated with this condition stems from its ability to interfere with microtubular function of white blood cells and their migration into the area.

Cilia and Flagella. Cilia and flagella are hairlike processes extending from the cell membrane that are capable of sweeping and flailing movements, which can move surrounding fluids or move the cell through fluid media (Fig. 4-8). Both contain identically organized cores of microtubules that consist of two microtubules surrounded at the periphery by clusters of paired microtubules. Each cilium and flagellum is anchored to a basal body that is responsible for the formation of the microtubular core. Cilia are found on the apical or luminal surface of epithelial linings of various body cavities or passages such as the upper respiratory system. Removal of mucus from the respiratory passages is highly dependent on proper function of the cilia. Flagella form the tail-like structures that provide motility for sperm.

Genetic defects can result in improper microtubule formation and, as a result, the cilia may be nonfunctional. One of these disorders, the *immobile cilia syndrome*, impairs sperm motility, causing male sterility. At the same time, it immobilizes the cilia of the respiratory tract, interfering with clearance of inhaled bacteria, leading to a chronic lung disease called *bronchiectasis.*[5]

Centrioles and Basal Bodies. Centrioles and basal bodies are structurally identical organelles composed of an array of highly organized microtubules. Internally, centrioles and basal bodies have an amorphous central core surrounded by clusters formed of triplet sets of microtubules. In dividing cells, the two cylindrical centrioles form the mitotic spindle that aids in the separation and movement of the chromosomes. Basal bodies are more numerous than centrioles and are found near the cell membrane in association with cilia and flagella. They are responsible for the formation of the highly organized core of microtubules found in cilia and flagella. The internal microtubular arrangement of centrioles and basal bodies is different from that found in cilia and flagella.

Microfilaments

Microfilaments are thin, threadlike cytoplasmic structures. Three classes of microfilaments exist: thin microfilaments, which are equivalent to the thin actin filaments in muscle; intermediate filaments, which are a heterogeneous group of filaments with diameter sizes between the thick and thin filaments; and thick myosin filaments, which are present in muscle cells, but may also exist temporarily in other cells.

Muscle contraction depends on the interaction between the thin actin filaments and thick myosin filaments. Microfilaments are present in the superficial zone of the cytoplasm in most cells. Contractile activities involving the microfilaments and associated thick myosin filaments contribute to associated movement of the cytoplasm and cell membrane during endocytosis and exocytosis. Microfilaments are also present in the microvilli of the intestine. The intermediate filaments aid in supporting and maintaining the

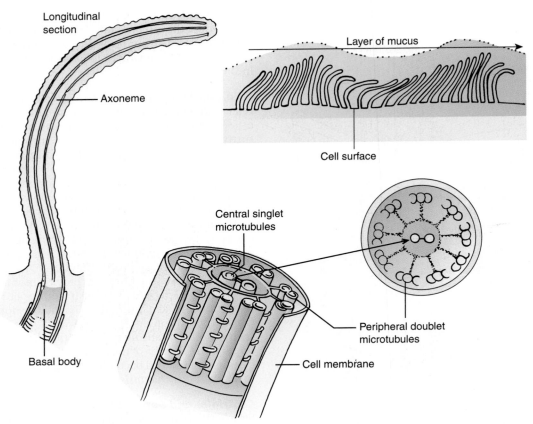

FIGURE 4-8 Structure of cilium. (Adapted from Cormack D. H. [1993]. *Essential histology* [p. 79]. Philadelphia: J.B. Lippincott)

asymmetric shape of cells. Examples of intermediate filaments are the keratin filaments that are found anchored to the cell membrane of epidermal keratinocytes of the skin and the glial filaments that are found in astrocytes and other glial cells of the nervous system. The *neurofibrillary tangle* found in the brain in Alzheimer's disease contains microtubule-associated proteins and neurofilaments, evidence of a disrupted neuronal cytoskeleton.[5]

THE CELL MEMBRANE

The cell is enclosed in a thin membrane that separates the intracellular contents from the extracellular environment. To differentiate it from the other cell membranes, such as the mitochondrial or nuclear membranes, the cell membrane is often called the *plasma membrane*. In many respects, the plasma membrane is one of the most important parts of the cell. It acts as a semipermeable structure that separates the intracellular and extracellular environments. It provides receptors for hormones and other biologically active substances, participates in the electrical events that occur in nerve and muscle cells, and aids in the regulation of cell growth and proliferation. It is also thought that the cell membrane may play an important role in the behavior of cancer cells, which is discussed in Chapter 8.

The cell membrane consists of an organized arrangement of lipids, carbohydrates, and proteins (Fig. 4-9). The main structural component of the membrane is its lipid bilayer. It is a bimolecular layer that consists primarily of phospholipids, together with glycolipids and cholesterol. The lipids form a bilayer structure that is essentially impermeable to all but lipid-soluble substances. Approximately 75% of the lipids are phospholipids, each with a hydrophilic (water-soluble) head and a hydrophobic (water-insoluble) tail. The phospholipid molecules along with the glycolipids are aligned such that their hydrophilic heads face outward on each side of the membrane and their hydrophobic tails project toward the middle of the membrane. The hydrophilic heads retain water and help cells adhere to each other. At normal body temperature, the viscosity of the lipid component of the membrane is equivalent to that of olive oil. The presence of cholesterol stiffens the membrane.

Although the basic structure of the cell membrane is provided by the lipid bilayer, most of the specific functions are carried out by proteins.[2] Some proteins, called *transmembrane proteins*, pass directly through the membrane and communicate with the intracellular and extracellular environments. Many of the transmembrane proteins are tightly bound to lipids in the bilayer and are essentially part of the membrane. These transmembrane proteins are called *integral proteins*. A second type of protein, the *peripheral proteins*, are bound to one or the other side of the membrane and do not pass into the lipid bilayer. Many of the periph-

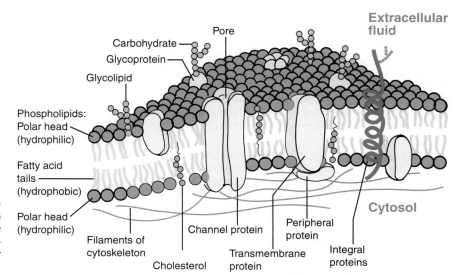

FIGURE 4-9 The structure of the cell membrane showing the hydrophilic (polar) heads and the hydrophobic (fatty acid) tails and the position of the integral and peripheral proteins in relation to the interior and exterior of the cell.

eral proteins can be removed from the membrane surface with little damage to the membrane.

The function of the membrane proteins is largely determined by the way in which they are associated with the membrane. Thus, peripheral proteins are associated with functions involving the inner or outer side of the membrane where they are located. A number of the peripheral proteins serve as receptors or are involved in intracellular signaling systems. By contrast, only the transmembrane proteins can function on both sides of the membrane or transport molecules across it.

Many of the integral transmembrane proteins form the ion channels found on the cell surface. These channel proteins have a complex morphology and are selective with respect to the substances they transmit. Mutations in these channel proteins, often referred to as *channelopathies*, are responsible for a host of genetic disorders.[9] For example, in the inherited disease called *cystic fibrosis*, the primary defect resides in an abnormal chloride channel, which results in increased sodium and water reabsorption that causes respiratory tract secretions to thicken and occlude the airways (see Chapter 29).[9] Other disorders of membrane channels, such as the potassium channel, are associated with hearing impairment, cardiac dysrhythmias, and periodic hyperkalemic paralysis.[9]

The cell surface is surrounded by a fuzzy-looking layer called the *cell coat*, or *glycocalyx*. The structure of the glycocalyx consists of long, complex carbohydrate chains attached to protein molecules that penetrate the outside portion of the membrane (*i.e.*, glycoproteins); outward-facing membrane lipids (*i.e.*, glycolipids); and carbohydrate-binding proteins called *lectins*. The cell coat participates in cell-to-cell recognition and adhesion. It contains tissue transplant antigens that label cells as self or nonself. ABO blood group antigens are contained in the cell coat of red blood cells. An intimate relationship exists between the cell membrane and the cell coat. If the cell coat is enzymatically removed, the cell remains viable and can generate a new cell coat, but damage to the cell membrane usually results in cell death.

In summary, the cell is a remarkably autonomous structure that functions in a manner strikingly similar to that of the total organism. The nucleus controls cell function and is the mastermind of the cell. It contains DNA, which provides the information necessary for the synthesis of the various proteins that the cell must produce to stay alive and to transmit information from one generation to another.

The cytoplasm contains the cell's organelles and the enzymes necessary for glycolysis. Ribosomes serve as sites for protein synthesis in the cell. The ER functions as a tubular communication system through which substances can be transported from one part of the cell to another and as the site of protein (rough ER), carbohydrate, and lipid (smooth ER) synthesis. Golgi bodies modify materials synthesized in the ER and package them into secretory granules for transport within the cell or for export from the cell. Lysosomes, which can be viewed as the digestive system of the cell, contain hydrolytic enzymes that digest worn-out cell parts and foreign materials. They are membranous structures formed in the Golgi complex from hydrolytic enzymes synthesized in the rough ER. The mitochondria serve as power plants for the cell because they transform food energy into ATP, which is used to power cell activities. Mitochondria contain their own extra-chromosomal DNA, which is used in the synthesis of mitochondrial RNAs and proteins used in oxidative metabolism. Microtubules are slender, stiff tubular structures that influence cell shape, provide a means of moving organelles through the cytoplasm, and effect movement of the cilia and of chromosomes during cell division. Several types of threadlike filaments, including actin and myosin filaments, participate in muscle contraction.

The plasma membrane is a lipid bilayer that surrounds the cell and separates it from its surrounding external environment. The cell surface is surrounded by a fuzzy-looking layer, the cell coat or glycocalyx, which contains tissue antigens and participates in cell-to-cell recognition and adhesion.

Integration of Cell Function and Replication

After you have completed this section of the chapter, you should be able to meet the following objectives:

✦ Trace the pathway for cell communication, beginning at the receptor and ending with effector response, and explain why the process is often referred to as *signal transduction*

✦ Describe the function of G proteins in signal transduction

✦ List three classifications of growth factors

✦ Relate the function of ATP to cell metabolism

✦ Differentiate anabolism and catabolism

✦ Compare the processes involved in aerobic and anaerobic metabolism

✦ Describe the five phases of the cell cycle

CELL COMMUNICATION

Cells in multicellular organisms need to communicate with one another to coordinate their function and control their growth. Cells communicate with each other by means of chemical messenger systems. In some tissues, messengers move from cell to cell through gap junctions without entering the extracellular fluid. In other tissues, cells communicate by chemical messengers secreted into the extracellular fluid. Many types of chemical messengers bind to receptors on or near the cell surface. These chemical messengers are sometimes called *first messengers* because, by one means or another, their external signal is converted into internal signals carried by a second chemical called a *second messenger*. It is the second messenger that triggers the intracellular changes that produce the desired physiologic effect. Some lipid-soluble chemical messengers move through the membrane and bind to cytoplasmic or nuclear receptors to exert their physiologic effects.

The three basic types of intercellular communication mediated by messengers in the extracellular fluid are hormonal communication, paracrine and autocrine communication, and neural communication.[10] Endocrine signaling relies on hormones carried in the bloodstream to cells throughout the body. With paracrine signaling, the chemical mediators are rapidly metabolized and act mainly on nearby cells. In autocrine signaling, a cell releases a chemical into the extracellular fluid that affects its own activity (Fig. 4-10). Synaptic signaling occurs in the nervous system, where neurotransmitters act only on adjacent nerve cells through special contact areas called *synapses*. In some parts of the body, the same chemical messenger can function as a neurotransmitter, a paracrine mediator, and a hormone secreted by neurons into the bloodstream.

Neurotransmitters, protein and peptide hormones, and other chemical messengers do not exert their effects by entering cells. Instead, their messages are conveyed across the membrane and converted (*i.e.*, transduced) by cell membrane proteins into signals within the cell, a process often called *signal transduction*. Many molecules involved in signal transduction are proteins. A unique property of proteins that allows them to function in this way is their ability to change their shape or conformation, thereby changing their function and consequently the functions of the cell. These conformational changes are often ac-

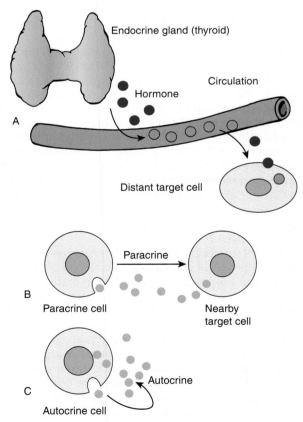

FIGURE 4-10 Examples of endocrine (**A**), paracrine (**B**), and autocrine (**C**) secretions.

 Cell Communication

➤ Cells communicate with each other and with the internal and external environments by a number of mechanisms, including electrical and chemical signaling systems that control electrical potentials, the overall function of a cell, and gene activity needed for cell division and cell replication.

➤ Chemical messengers exert their effects by binding to cell membrane proteins or receptors that convert the chemical signal into signals within the cell, in a process called *signal transduction*.

➤ Cells regulate their responses to chemical messengers by increasing or decreasing the number of active receptors on their surface.

complished through enzymes called *protein kinases* that catalyze the phosphorylation of amino acids in the protein structure.

CELL RECEPTORS

Each cell type in the body contains a distinctive set of receptor proteins that enable it to respond to a complementary set of signaling molecules in a specific, preprogrammed way. These receptors, which span the cell membrane, relay information to a series of intracellular intermediates that eventually pass the signal to its final destination. Many receptors for chemical messengers have been isolated and characterized. These proteins are not static components of the cell membrane; they increase or decrease in number according to the needs of the cell. When excess chemical messengers are present, the number of active receptors decreases in a process called *down-regulation*; when there is a deficiency of the messenger, the number of active receptors increases through *up-regulation*. There are three known classes of cell surface receptor proteins: ion channel linked, G protein linked, and enzyme linked.

Ion-Channel–Linked Receptors

Ion-channel–linked receptors are involved in the rapid synaptic signaling between electrically excitable cells. This type of signaling is mediated by a small number of neurotransmitters that transiently open or close ion channels formed by integral proteins in the cell membrane. This type of signaling is involved in the transmission of impulses in nerve and muscle cells.

G-Protein–Linked Receptors and Signal Transduction

G proteins constitute the on–off switch for signal transduction. Although there are numerous intercellular messengers, many of them rely on a class of molecules called *G proteins* to convert external signals (first messengers) into internal signals (second messengers). These internal signals induce biochemical changes in the cell that lead to the desired physiologic effects. G proteins are so named because they bind to guanine nucleotides such as guanine diphosphate (GDP) and guanine triphosphate (GTP).

Signal transduction relies on a series of orchestrated biochemical events (Fig. 4-11). All signal transduction systems have a receptor component that functions as a signal discriminator by recognizing a specific first messenger. After a first messenger binds to a receptor, conformational changes occur in the receptor, which activates the G protein. The activated G protein, in turn, acts on other membrane-bound intermediates called *effectors*. Often, the effector is an enzyme that converts an inactive precursor molecule into a second messenger, which diffuses into the cytoplasm and carries the signal beyond the cell membrane. Many members of the G-protein family have been identified. At least one subset of G proteins is present in all cells; it regulates signal transmission by the second messenger 3′,5′-cyclic adenosine monophosphate (cAMP).

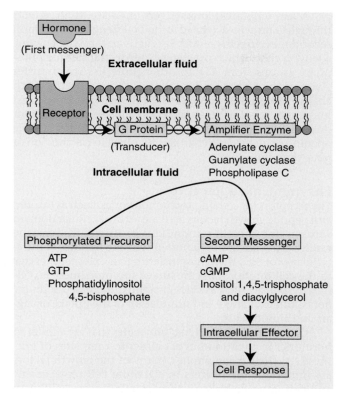

FIGURE 4-11 Signal transduction pattern common to several second messenger systems. A protein or peptide hormone is the first messenger to a membrane receptor, stimulating or inhibiting a membrane-bound enzyme by means of a G protein. The amplifier enzyme catalyzes the production of a second messenger from a phosphorylated precursor. The second messenger then activates an internal effector, which leads to the cell response. (Redrawn from Rhoades R.A., Tanner G.A. [1996]. *Medical physiology*. Boston: Little, Brown)

Although there are differences between the G proteins, all share a number of features. All are found on the cytoplasmic side of the cell membrane, and all incorporate the *GTPase cycle*, which functions as the on–off switch for G-protein activity. GTPase is an enzyme that converts GTP with its three phosphate groups to GDP with its two phosphate groups. In the inactive state, G proteins contain tightly bound GDP. When a receptor coupled to a G protein is activated, the G protein releases the GDP and binds GTP. This causes the G protein to dissociate from the receptor and activate the effector. During the process of signal transduction, GTPase converts bound GTP to GDP, thereby returning the G protein to its resting state and switching the signal off. Certain bacterial toxins can bind to the G proteins, causing inhibition or stimulation of its signal function. One such toxin, the toxin of *Vibrio cholerae*, binds and activates the stimulatory G protein linked to the cAMP system that controls the secretion of fluid into the intestine. In response to the cholera toxin, these cells overproduce fluid, leading to severe diarrhea and life-threatening depletion of extracellular fluid volume.[2]

Many chemical messengers mediate their effects through G-protein–activated second messengers. A common second messenger is cAMP. It is activated by the enzyme adenyl cyclase, which generates cAMP by transferring phosphate groups from ATP to other proteins. This transfer changes the form and function of these proteins. Such changes eventually produce the cell response to the first messenger, whether it is a secretion, muscle contraction or relaxation, or a change in metabolism. Sometimes, it is the opening of membrane channels involved in calcium ion or potassium ion influx.

Enzyme-Linked Receptors

The receptors for certain protein hormones, such as insulin, and peptide growth factors activate an intracellular domain with enzyme (protein-tyrosine kinase) activity. The enzyme catalyzes the phosphorylation of tyrosine residues of intracellular proteins, thereby transferring an external message to the cell interior. Enzyme-linked receptors mediate cellular responses such as calcium influx, increased sodium/potassium exchange, and stimulation of the uptake of sugars and amino acids.

Growth factors are signal molecules that are similar to hormones in function but act closer to their sites of synthesis. As their name implies, many of the growth factors are important messengers in signaling cell replacement and cell growth. Most of the growth factors belong to one of three groups: factors that foster the multiplication and development of various cell types (*e.g.*, growth factor and epidermal growth factor); lymphokines and cytokines, which are important in the regulation of the immune system (see Chapter 18); and colony-stimulating factors, which regulate the proliferation and maturation of white and red blood cells (see Chapter 13).

MESSENGER-MEDIATED CONTROL OF NUCLEAR FUNCTION

Some messengers, such as thyroid hormone and steroid hormones, do not bind to membrane receptors but move directly across the lipid layer of the cell membrane and are carried to the cell nucleus, where they influence DNA activity. Many of these hormones bind to a cytoplasmic receptor, and together they are carried to the nucleus. In the nucleus, the receptor–hormone complex binds to DNA, thereby increasing transcription of mRNA. The mRNAs are translated in the ribosomes, with the production of increased amounts of proteins that alter cell function.

THE CELL CYCLE AND CELL DIVISION

The life of a cell is called the *cell cycle*. It is usually divided into five phases: G_0, G_1, S, G_2, and M. Some cells may not have a G_1 phase, and others may not have a G_2 stage. However, all cells must grow, replicate their genetic material if they are to divide, and undergo the process of mitosis if they are to replicate.[11] G_0 is the stage when the cell may leave the cell cycle and either remain in a state of inactivity

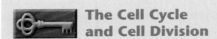

The Cell Cycle and Cell Division

> The cell cycle represents the life cycle of a cell.

> The cell cycle is divided into two main stages: mitosis, which represents the cell division stage of the cell cycle, and interphase, which represents the nondividing phase of the cell cycle.

> There are two types of cell division: mitotic cell division, which occurs in somatic cells such as liver cells, and meiosis, which occurs in the gamete-producing organs (*i.e.*, the ovaries and testes).

or reenter the cell cycle at another time. G_1 is the stage during which the cell is starting to prepare for mitosis through DNA and protein synthesis and an increase in organelle and cytoskeletal elements. The S phase is the synthesis phase, during which DNA replication occurs and the centrioles are beginning to replicate. G_2 is the premitotic phase and is similar to G_1 in terms of RNA and protein synthesis. The M phase is the phase during which cell mitosis occurs. Nondividing cells, such as mature nerve cells or cells not preparing for mitosis, are said to be in the G_0 phase of the cell cycle (Fig. 4-12).

Cell Division

Cell division, or *mitosis*, which was first described in 1875, is the process during which a parent cell divides and each

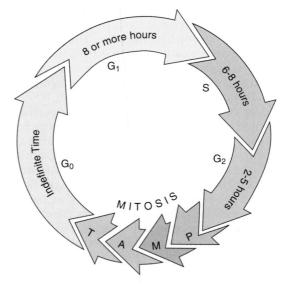

FIGURE 4-12 Cell cycle. G_0, nondividing cell; G_1, cell growth; S, DNA replication; G_2, protein synthesis; M, mitosis, which lasts for 1 to 3 hours and is followed by cytokinesis.

daughter cell receives a chromosomal karyotype identical to the parent cell.[11] Cell division provides the body with a means of replacing cells that have a limited life span such as skin and blood cells, increasing tissue mass during periods of growth, and providing for tissue repair and wound healing. Despite the early cytologic description of the four stages of mitosis, it was not until the early 1950s that the importance of the cell cycle was realized.

Mitosis, which is a dynamic and continuous process, usually lasts from 1 to 1½ hours. It is divided into four stages: prophase, metaphase, anaphase, and telophase (Fig. 4-13). The phase during which the cell is not undergoing division is called *interphase*. During *prophase*, the chromosomes become visible because of increased coiling of the DNA, the two centrioles replicate, and a pair moves to each side of the cell. Simultaneously, the microtubules of the mitotic spindle appear between the two pairs of centrioles. Later in prophase, the nuclear envelope and nucleolus disappear. *Metaphase* involves the organization of the chromosome pairs in the midline of the cell and the formation of a mitotic spindle composed of the microtubules. *Anaphase* is the period during which separation of the chromosome pairs occurs, with the microtubules pulling one member of each pair of 46 chromosomes toward the opposite cell pole. Cell division or *cytokinesis* is completed after *telophase*, the stage during which the mitotic spindle vanishes and a new nuclear membrane develops and encloses each complete set of chromosomes.

Cell division is controlled by changes in the intracellular concentrations and activity of three major groups of intracellular proteins: cyclins, cyclin-dependent kinases, and anaphase-promoting complex. These proteins complex with a protein kinase, resulting in the activation of many substrate proteins involved in DNA synthesis and mitosis. Specific cyclins are involved in the process of cell division. Cell division is also controlled by several external factors, including the presence of cytokines, various growth factors, or even adhesion factors when the cell is associated with other cells in a tissue. In addition, the cell cycle is regulated by several checkpoints that determine whether DNA replication has occurred with a high degree of fidelity. Two of the better understood are the DNA damage and the spindle formation checkpoints. If these biochemical checkpoints are not faithfully met, the cell may default to programmed cell death or apoptosis.[12]

CELL METABOLISM AND ENERGY SOURCES

Energy is the ability to do work. Cells use oxygen and the breakdown products of the foods we eat to produce the energy needed for muscle contraction, transport of ions and molecules, and the synthesis of enzymes, hormones, and other macromolecules. *Energy metabolism* refers to the processes by which fats, proteins, and carbohydrates from the foods we eat are converted into energy or complex energy sources in the cell. Catabolism and anabolism are the two phases of metabolism. *Catabolism* consists of breaking down stored nutrients and body tissues to produce energy. *Anabolism* is a constructive process in which more complex molecules are formed from simpler ones.

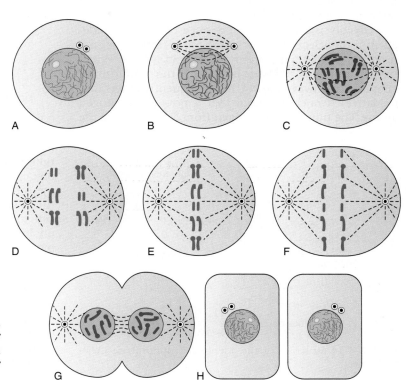

FIGURE 4-13 Cell mitosis. *A* and *H* represent the nondividing cell; *B*, *C*, and *D* represent prophase; *E* and *F* represents anaphase; and *G* represents telophase. (From Chaffee E.E., Gersheimer E.M. [1974]. *Basic physiology and anatomy* [3rd ed.]. Philadelphia: J.B. Lippincott)

The special carrier for cellular energy is ATP. ATP molecules consist of adenosine, a nitrogenous base; ribose, a five-carbon sugar; and three phosphate groups (see Fig. 4-14). The phosphate groups are attached by two high-energy bonds. Large amounts of free energy are released when ATP is hydrolyzed to form adenosine diphosphate (ADP), an adenosine molecule that contains two phosphate groups. The free energy liberated from the hydrolysis of ATP is used to drive reactions that require free energy, such as muscle contraction and active transport mechanisms. Energy from foodstuffs is used to convert ADP back to ATP. ATP is often called the *energy currency* of the cell; energy can be "saved or spent" using ATP as an exchange currency.

Two sites of energy production are present in the cell: the anaerobic (*i.e.*, without oxygen) glycolytic pathway, occurring in the cytoplasm, and the aerobic (*i.e.*, with oxygen) pathways in the mitochondria. The glycolytic pathway serves as the prelude to the aerobic pathways.

Anaerobic Metabolism

Glycolysis is the process by which energy is liberated from glucose (Fig. 4-15). It is an important energy provider for cells that lack mitochondria, the cell organelle in which aerobic metabolism occurs. This process also provides energy in situations when delivery of oxygen to the cell is delayed or impaired. Glycolysis involves a sequence of reactions that converts glucose to pyruvate, with the concomitant production of ATP from ADP. The net gain of energy from the glycolysis of one molecule of glucose is two ATP molecules.[13] Although relatively inefficient as to energy yield, the glycolytic pathway is important during periods of decreased oxygen delivery, as occurs in skeletal muscle during the first few minutes of exercise.

Glycolysis requires the presence of nicotinamide-adenine dinucleotide (NAD^+), a hydrogen carrier. The end-products of glycolysis are pyruvate and NADH. When oxygen is present, pyruvate moves into the aerobic mitochondrial pathway, and NADH subsequently enters into oxidative chemical reactions that remove the hydrogen atoms. The transfer of hydrogen from NADH during the

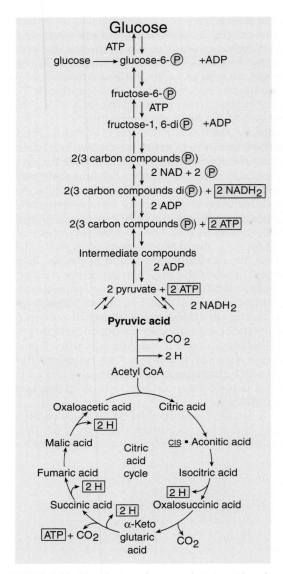

FIGURE 4-15 Glycolytic pathway and citric acid cycle.

oxidative reactions allows the glycolytic process to continue by facilitating the regeneration of NAD^+. Under anaerobic conditions, such as cardiac arrest or circulatory shock, pyruvate is converted to lactic acid, which diffuses out of the cells into the extracellular fluid. Conversion of pyruvate to lactic acid is reversible, and after the oxygen supply has been restored, lactic acid is reconverted back to pyruvate and used directly for energy or to synthesize glucose.

Much of the reconversion of lactic acid occurs in the liver, but a small amount can occur in other tissues. The liver removes lactic acid from the bloodstream and converts it to glucose in a process called *gluconeogenesis*. This glucose is released into the bloodstream to be used again by the muscles or by the central nervous system. This recycling of lactic acid is referred to as the *Cori cycle*. Heart muscle

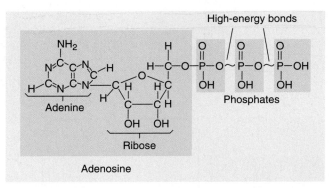

FIGURE 4-14 Structure of the adenosine triphosphate (ATP) molecule.

is also efficient in converting lactic acid to pyruvic acid and then using the pyruvic acid for fuel. Pyruvic acid is a particularly important source of fuel for the heart during heavy exercise when the skeletal muscles are producing large amounts of lactic acid and releasing it into the bloodstream.

Aerobic Metabolism

Aerobic metabolism occurs in the cell's mitochondria and involves the citric acid cycle and oxidative phosphorylation. It is here that hydrogen and carbon molecules from the fats, proteins, and carbohydrates in our diet are broken down and combined with molecular oxygen to form carbon dioxide and water as energy is released. Unlike lactic acid, which is an end-product of anaerobic metabolism, carbon dioxide and water are relatively harmless and easily eliminated from the body. In a 24-hour period, oxidative metabolism produces 300 to 500 mL of water.

The citric acid cycle, sometimes called the *tricarboxylic acid* or *Krebs cycle*, provides the final common pathway for the metabolism of nutrients (see Fig. 4-15). In the citric acid cycle, an activated two-carbon molecule of acetyl coenzyme A (acetyl-CoA) condenses with a four-carbon molecule of oxaloacetic acid and moves through a series of enzyme-mediated steps. This process produces hydrogen and carbon dioxide. As hydrogen is generated, it combines with one of two special carriers, NAD^+ or flavin adenine dinucleotide, for transfer to the electron transport system. The carbon dioxide molecule is converted to bicarbonate or carried to the lungs and exhaled. In the citric acid cycle, each of the two pyruvate molecules formed in the cytoplasm from one molecule of glucose yields another molecule of ATP along with two molecules of carbon dioxide and eight hydrogen atoms. These hydrogen atoms are transferred to the electron transport system on the inner mitochondrial membrane for oxidation. In addition to pyruvate from the glycolysis of glucose, products of amino acid and fatty acid degradation enter the citric acid cycle and contribute to the generation of ATP.[2]

Oxidative metabolism, which supplies 90% of the body's energy needs, is the process by which hydrogen generated during the citric acid cycle combines with oxygen to form ATP and water. It is accomplished by a series of enzymatically catalyzed reactions that split each hydrogen atom into a hydrogen ion and an electron. During the process of ionization, the electrons removed from the hydrogen atoms enter an electron transport system found on the inner membrane of the mitochondrion. This electron transport chain consists of electron acceptors that can be reversibly reduced or oxidized by accepting or giving up electrons. Each electron is shuttled from one acceptor to another until it reaches the end of the chain, where its final two electrons are used to reduce elemental oxygen, which combines with the hydrogen ions to form water. As the electrons move along the electron transport chain, large amounts of energy are released. This energy is used to convert ADP to ATP. Because the formation of ATP in-

volves the addition of a high-energy phosphate bond to ADP, the process is sometimes called *oxidative phosphorylation*. Cyanide poisoning kills by binding to the enzymes needed for a final step in the oxidative phosphorylation sequence.[2]

In summary, cells communicate with each other by means of chemical messenger systems. In some tissues, chemical messengers move from cell to cell through gap junctions without entering the extracellular fluid. Other types of chemical messengers bind to receptors on or near the cell surface. There are three known classes of cell surface receptor proteins: ion channel linked, G protein linked, and enzyme linked. Ion-linked signaling is mediated by neurotransmitters that transiently open or close ion channels formed by integral proteins in the cell membrane. G-protein–linked receptors rely on a class of molecules called *G proteins* that function as an on–off switch to convert external signals (first messengers) into internal signals (second messengers). Enzyme-linked receptors interact with certain peptide hormones, such as insulin and growth factors, to directly initiate the activity of the intracellular protein-tyrosine kinase enzyme. Binding of hormone or growth factor to its receptor triggers multiple cellular responses such as calcium influx, increased sodium–potassium exchange, stimulation of the uptake of sugars and amino acids, or transcription of certain key genes that control cell proliferation.

The life of a cell is called the cell cycle. It is usually divided into five phases: G_0, or the resting phase; G_1, during which the cell begins to prepare for division through DNA and protein synthesis; the S or synthetic phase, during which DNA replication occurs; G_2, which is the premitotic phase and is similar to G_1 in terms of RNA and protein synthesis; and the M phase, during which cell division occurs. Cell division, or mitosis, is the process during which a parent cell divides into two daughter cells, with each receiving an identical pair of chromosomes. The process of mitosis is dynamic and continuous and is divided into four stages: prophase, metaphase, anaphase, and telophase.

Metabolism is the process whereby the carbohydrates, fats, and proteins we eat are broken down and subsequently converted into the energy needed for cell function. Energy is converted to ATP, which serves as the energy currency for the cell. Two sites of energy conversion are present in cells: the mitochondria and the cytoplasmic matrix. The most efficient of these pathways is the aerobic citric acid pathway in the mitochondria. This pathway requires oxygen and produces carbon dioxide and water as end-products. The glycolytic pathway, which is located in the cytoplasm, involves the breakdown of glucose to form ATP. This pathway can function without oxygen by producing lactic acid.

Movement Across the Cell Membrane and Membrane Potentials

After you have completed this section of the chapter, you should be able to meet the following objectives:

✦ Discuss the mechanisms of membrane transport associated with diffusion, osmosis, endocytosis, and exocytosis and compare with active transport mechanisms
✦ Describe the function of ion channels
✦ Describe the basis for membrane potentials
✦ Explain the relationship between membrane permeability and membrane potential

The cell membrane serves as a barrier that controls which substances enter and leave the cell. This barrier function allows materials that are essential for cell function to enter the cell, while excluding those that are harmful. It is responsible for differences in the composition of intracellular and extracellular fluids.

MOVEMENT OF SUBSTANCES ACROSS THE CELL MEMBRANE

Movement through the cell membrane occurs in essentially two ways: passively, without an expenditure of energy, or actively, using energy-consuming processes. The cell membrane can also engulf a particle, forming a membrane-coated vesicle; this membrane-coated vesicle is moved into the cell by *endocytosis* or out of the cell by *exocytosis*.

Passive Movement

The passive movement of particles or ions across the cell membrane is directly influenced by chemical or electrical gradients and does not require an expenditure of energy. A difference in the number of particles on either side of the membrane creates a chemical gradient and a difference in charged particle or ions creates an electrical gradient. Chemical and electrical gradients are often linked and are called *electrochemical gradients*.

Diffusion. Diffusion refers to the process by which molecules and other particles in a solution become widely dispersed and reach a uniform concentration because of energy created by their spontaneous kinetic movements (Fig. 4-16). Electrolytes and other substances move from an area of higher to an area of lower concentration. With ions, diffusion is affected by energy supplied by their electrical charge. Lipid-soluble molecules such as oxygen, carbon dioxide, alcohol, and fatty acids become dissolved in the lipid matrix of the cell membrane and diffuse through the membrane in the same manner that diffusion occurs in water. Other substances diffuse through minute pores of the cell membrane. The rate of movement depends on how many particles are available for diffusion and the velocity of the kinetic movement of the particles. The number of openings in the cell membrane through which the particles can move also determines transfer rates. Temper-

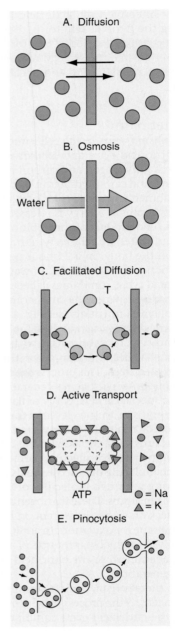

FIGURE 4-16 Mechanisms of membrane transport. (**A**) Diffusion, in which particles move to become equally distributed across the membrane. (**B**) The osmotically active particles regulate the flow of water. (**C**) Facilitated diffusion uses a carrier system. (**D**) In active transport, selected molecules are transported across the membrane using the energy-driven (ATP) pump. (**E**) The membrane forms a vesicle that engulfs the particle and transports it across the membrane, where it is released. This is called pinocytosis.

ature changes the motion of the particles; the greater the temperature, the greater is the thermal motion of the molecules. Thus, diffusion increases in proportion to the increased temperature.

Osmosis. Most cell membranes are semipermeable in that they are permeable to water but not all solute particles.

Water moves through a semipermeable membrane along a concentration gradient, moving from an area of higher to one of lower concentration (see Fig. 4-16). This process is called *osmosis*, and the pressure that water generates as it moves through the membrane is called *osmotic pressure.*

Osmosis is regulated by the concentration of non-diffusible particles on either side of a semipermeable membrane. When there is a difference in the concentration of particles, water moves from the side with the lower concentration of particles and higher concentration of water to the side with the higher concentration of particles and lower concentration of water. The movement of water continues until the concentration of particles on both sides of the membrane is equally diluted or until the hydrostatic (osmotic) pressure created by the movement of water opposes its flow.

Facilitated Diffusion. Facilitated diffusion occurs through a transport protein that is not linked to metabolic energy (see Fig. 4-16). Some substances, such as glucose, cannot pass unassisted through the cell membrane because they are not lipid soluble or are too large to pass through the membrane's pores. These substances combine with special transport proteins at the membrane's outer surface, are carried across the membrane attached to the transporter, and then released. In facilitated diffusion, a substance can move only from an area of higher concentration to one of lower concentration. The rate at which a substance moves across the membrane because of facilitated diffusion depends on the difference in concentration between the two sides of the membrane. Also important are the availability of transport proteins and the rapidity with which they can bind and release the substance being transported. It is thought that insulin, which facilitates the movement of glucose into cells, acts by increasing the availability of glucose transporters in the cell membrane.

Active Transport and Cotransport

Active transport mechanisms involve the expenditure of energy. The process of diffusion describes particle movement from an area of higher concentration to one of lower concentration, resulting in an equal distribution across the cell membrane. Sometimes, however, different concentrations of a substance are needed in the intracellular and extracellular fluids. For example, the intracellular functioning of the cell requires a much higher concentration of potassium than is present in the extracellular fluid while maintaining a much lower concentration of sodium than in the extracellular fluid. In these situations, energy is required to pump the ions "uphill" or against their concentration gradient. When cells use energy to move ions against an electrical or chemical gradient, the process is called *active transport.*

The active transport system studied in the greatest detail is the sodium–potassium pump, or Na^+/K^+ ATPase pump (see Fig. 4-16). The Na^+/K^+ ATPase pump moves sodium from inside the cell to the extracellular region, where its concentration is approximately 14 times greater than inside; the pump also returns potassium to the inside, where

its concentration is approximately 35 times greater than it is outside the cell. Energy used to pump sodium out of the cell and potassium into the cell is obtained by splitting and releasing energy from the high-energy phosphate bond in ATP by the enzyme ATPase. Were it not for the activity of the sodium–potassium pump, the osmotically active sodium particles would accumulate in the cell, causing cellular swelling because of an accompanying influx of water (see Chapter 5).

Two types of active transport systems exist: primary active transport and secondary active transport. In *primary active transport*, the source of energy (*e.g.*, ATP) is used directly in the transport of a substance. *Secondary active transport* mechanisms harness the energy derived from the primary active transport of one substance, usually sodium ions, for the cotransport of a second substance. For example, when sodium ions are actively transported out of a cell by primary active transport, a large concentration gradient develops (*i.e.*, high concentration on the outside and low on the inside). This concentration gradient represents a large storehouse of energy because sodium ions are always attempting to diffuse into the cell. Similar to facilitated diffusion, secondary transport mechanisms use membrane transport proteins. These proteins have two binding sites, one for sodium ions and the other for the substance undergoing secondary transport. Secondary transport systems are classified into two groups: *cotransport* or *symport* systems, in which the sodium ion and solute are transported in the same direction, and *countertransport* or *antiport* systems, in which sodium ions and the solute are transported in the opposite direction (Fig. 4-17). An

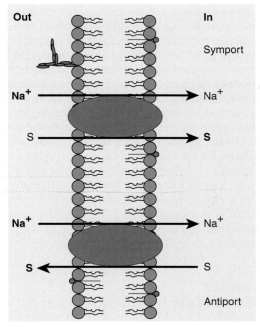

FIGURE 4-17 Secondary active transport systems. Symport or cotransport (**top**) carries the transported solute (**s**) in the same direction as the Na^+ ion. Antiport or counter-transport carries the solute and Na^+ in the opposite direction. (Rhoades R.A., Tanner G.A. [1996]. *Medical physiology.* Boston: Little, Brown)

example of cotransport occurs in the intestine, where the absorption of glucose and amino acids is coupled with sodium transport.

Endocytosis and Exocytosis

Endocytosis is the process by which cells engulf materials from their surroundings. It includes pinocytosis and phagocytosis. *Pinocytosis* involves the ingestion of small solid or fluid particles. The particles are engulfed into small, membrane-surrounded vesicles for movement into the cytoplasm. The process of pinocytosis is important in the transport of proteins and strong solutions of electrolytes (see Fig. 4-16).

Phagocytosis literally means *cell eating* and can be compared with pinocytosis, which means *cell drinking*. It involves the engulfment and subsequent killing or degradation of microorganisms and other particulate matter. During phagocytosis, a particle contacts the cell surface and is surrounded on all sides by the cell membrane, forming a phagocytic vesicle or phagosome. Once formed, the phagosome breaks away from the cell membrane and moves into the cytoplasm, where it eventually fuses with a lysosome, allowing the ingested material to be degraded by lysosomal enzymes. Certain cells, such as macrophages and polymorphonuclear leukocytes (neutrophils), are adept at engulfing and disposing of invading organisms, damaged cells, and unneeded extracellular constituents (see Chapter 18).

Receptor-mediated endocytosis involves the binding of substances such as low-density lipoproteins to a receptor on the cell surface. Binding of a ligand (*i.e.*, a substance with a high affinity for a receptor) to its receptor normally causes widely distributed receptors to accumulate in clathrin-coated pits. An aggregation of special proteins on the cytoplasmic side of the pit causes the coated pit to invaginate and pinch off, forming a clathrin-coated vesicle that carries the ligand and its receptor into the cell.

Exocytosis is the mechanism for the secretion of intracellular substances into the extracellular spaces. It is the reverse of endocytosis in that a secretory granule fuses to the inner side of the cell membrane and an opening occurs in the cell membrane. This opening allows the contents of the granule to be released into the extracellular fluid. Exocytosis is important in removing cellular debris and releasing substances, such as hormones, synthesized in the cell.

During endocytosis, portions of the cell membrane become an endocytotic vesicle. During exocytosis, the vesicular membrane is incorporated into the plasma membrane. In this way, cell membranes can be conserved and reused.

Ion Channels

The electrical charge on small ions such as Na⁺ and K⁺ makes it difficult for these ions to move across the lipid layer of the cell membrane. However, rapid movement of these ions is required for many types of cell functions, such as nerve activity. This is accomplished by facilitated diffusion through selective ion channels. Ion channels are integral proteins that span the width of the cell mem-

brane and are normally composed of several polypeptides or protein subunits that form a gating system. Specific stimuli cause the protein subunits to undergo conformational changes to form an open channel or gate through which the ions can move (Fig. 4-18). In this way, ions do not need to cross the lipid-soluble portion of the membrane but can remain in the aqueous solution that fills

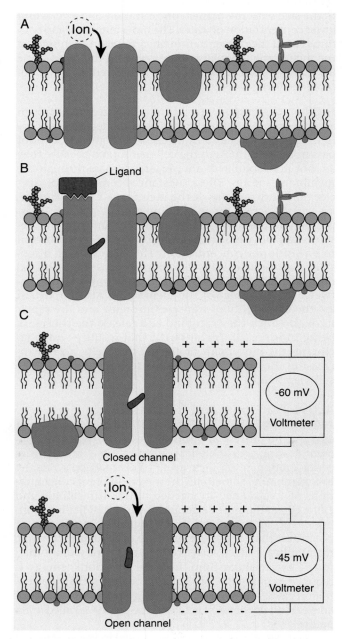

FIGURE 4-18 Ion channels. (**A**) Nongated ion channel remains open, permitting free movement of ions across the membrane. (**B**) Ligand-gated channel is controlled by ligand binding to the receptor. (**C**) Voltage-gated channel is controlled by a change in membrane potential. (Rhoades R.A., Tanner G.A. [1996]. *Medical physiology.* Boston: Little, Brown)

the ion channel. Ion channels are highly selective; some channels allow only for passage of sodium ions, and others are selective for potassium, calcium, or chloride ions. Specific interactions between the ions and the sides of the channel can produce an extremely rapid rate of ion movement. For example, ion channels can become negatively charged, promoting the rapid movement of positively charged ions.

The plasma membrane contains two basic groups of ion channels: leakage channels and gated channels. Leakage channels are open even in the unstimulated state, whereas gated channels open and close in response to specific stimuli. Three types of gated channels are present in the plasma membrane: *voltage-gated channels*, which have electrically operated gates that open when the membrane potential changes beyond a certain point; *ligand-gated channels*, which have chemically operated gates that respond to specific receptor-bound ligands, such as the neurotransmitter acetylcholine; and *mechanically gated channels*, which open or close in response to such mechanical stimulations as vibrations, tissue stretching, or pressure.[10]

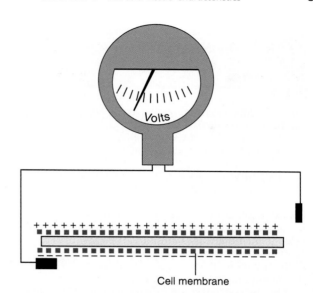

FIGURE 4-19 Alignment of charge along the cell membrane. The electrical potential is negative on the inside of the cell membrane in relation to the outside.

MEMBRANE POTENTIALS

The human body runs on a system of self-generated electricity. Electrical potentials exist across the membranes of most cells in the body. Because these potentials occur at the level of the cell membrane, they are called *membrane potentials*. In excitable tissues, such as nerve or muscle cells, changes in the membrane potential are necessary for generation and conduction of nerve impulses and muscle contraction. In other types of cells, such as glandular cells, changes in the membrane potential contribute to hormone secretion and other functions.

Electrical Potentials

Electrical potential, measured in volts (V), describes the ability of separated electrical charges of opposite polarity (+ and −) to do work. The potential difference is the difference between the separated charges. The terms *potential difference* and *voltage* are synonymous. Voltage is always measured with respect to two points in a system. For example, the voltage in a car battery (6 or 12 V) is the potential difference between the two battery terminals. Because the total amount of charge that can be separated by a biologic membrane is small, the potential differences are small and are measured in *millivolts* (1/1000 of a volt). Potential differences across the cell membrane can be measured by inserting a very fine electrode into the cell and another into the extracellular fluid surrounding the cell and connecting the two electrodes to a voltmeter (Fig. 4-19). The movement of charge between two points is called *current*. It occurs when a potential difference has been established and a connection is made such that the charged particles can move between the two points.

Extracellular and intracellular fluids are electrolyte solutions containing approximately 150 to 160 mmol/L of positively charged ions and an equal concentration of neg-

atively charged ions. These are the current-carrying ions responsible for generating and conducting membrane potentials. Usually, a small excess of positively charged ions exists at the outer surface of the cell membrane. This is represented as positive charges on the outside of the membrane and is balanced by an equal number of negative charges on the inside of the membrane. Because of the extreme thinness of the cell membrane, the accumulation of these ions at the surfaces of the membrane contributes to the establishment of a membrane potential.

Diffusion Potentials

A diffusion potential describes the voltage generated by ions that diffuse across the membrane. Two conditions are necessary for a membrane potential to occur by diffusion: the membrane must be selectively permeable, allowing a single type of ion to diffuse through membrane pores, and the concentration of the diffusible ion must be greater on one side of the membrane than on the other. In the resting or unexcited state, when the membrane is highly permeable to potassium, the concentration of potassium ions inside the cell is approximately 35 times greater than outside. Because of the large concentration gradient existing across the cell membrane, potassium ions tend to diffuse outward. As they do so, they carry their positive charges with them, and the inside becomes negative in relation to the outside. This new potential difference repels further outward movement of the positively charged potassium ions. The same phenomenon occurs during an action potential, when the membrane is highly permeable to sodium. Sodium ions move inside the cell, creating a membrane potential of the opposite polarity. An *equilibrium potential* is one in which no net movement of ions occurs because the diffusion and electrical forces are exactly balanced. An *equilibrium potential* for an ion can

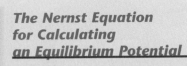

The Nernst Equation for Calculating an Equilibrium Potential

The following equation, known as the *Nernst equation*, can be used to calculate the equilibrium potential (electromotive force [EMF] in millivolts [mV] of a univalent ion at body temperature of 37°C).

$$EMF \text{ (mV)} = -61 \times \log_{10} \text{ (ion concentration inside/ion concentration outside)}$$

For example, if the concentration of an ion inside the membrane is 100 mmol/L and the concentration outside the membrane is 10 mmol/L, the EMF (mV) for that ion would be $-61 \times \log_{10}$ (100/10 [$\log_{10}$ of 10 is 1]). Therefore, it would take 61 mV of charge inside the membrane to balance the diffusion potential created by the concentration difference across the membrane for the ion.

The EMF for potassium ions using a normal estimated intracellular concentration of 140 mmol/L and a normal extracellular concentration of 4 mmol/L is −94 mV:

$$-94 \text{ mV} = -61 \times \log_{10} \text{ (140 mmol inside/4 mmol outside)}$$

This value assumes the membrane is permeable only to potassium. This value approximates the −70 to −90 mV resting membrane potential for nerve fibers measured in laboratory studies.

The EMF for sodium using a normal estimated intracellular concentration of 14 mmol/L and a normal extracellular concentration of 140 mmol/L is +61 mV:

$$+61 \text{ mV} = -61 \times \log_{10} \text{ (14 mmol/L/140 mmol/L)}$$

The equilibrium potential for sodium normally occurs at the peak of an action potential when the membrane is much more permeable to the sodium ion than to the potassium ion. When a membrane is permeable to several different ions, the diffusion potential reflects the sum of the equilibrium potentials for each of the ions.

be calculated using the *Nernst equation* (see accompanying box).

Variations in Membrane Potentials

The membrane potential can be altered by changes in membrane permeability. For example, calcium ions decrease membrane permeability to sodium ions, and vice versa. If insufficient calcium ions are available, as in severe hypocalcemia, the permeability to sodium increases. As a result, membrane excitability increases—sometimes causing spontaneous muscle movements (tetany) to occur. Local anesthetic agents (*e.g.*, procaine, cocaine) act directly on neural membranes to decrease their permeability to sodium.

In summary, movement of materials across the cell's membrane is essential for survival of the cell. Diffusion is a process by which substances such as ions move from areas of greater concentration to areas of lesser concentration in an attempt to reach a uniform distribution. Osmosis refers to the diffusion of water molecules through a semipermeable membrane along a concentration gradient. In facilitated diffusion, molecules that cannot normally pass through the cell's membranes can do so with the assistance of a carrier molecule. Diffusion of water molecules by osmosis or ions by facilitated diffusion does not require an expenditure of energy by the cell and is therefore passive in nature. Another type of transport, called *active transport*, requires the cell to expend energy in moving ions against a concentration gradient. Two types of active transport exist, primary and secondary; both require carrier proteins. The Na^+/K^+ ATPase pump is the best-known type of active transport. It is estimated that up to one third of the energy expenditure of the cell is used to maintain the Na^+/K^+ ATPase pump.

Endocytosis is a process by which cells engulf materials from the surrounding medium. Small particles are ingested by a process called *pinocytosis*; larger particles are engulfed by a process called *phagocytosis*. Some particles require bonding with a ligand, and the process is called *receptor-mediated endocytosis*. Exocytosis involves the removal of large particles from the cell and is essentially the reverse of endocytosis.

Ion channels are integral transmembrane proteins that span the width of the cell membrane and are normally composed of polypeptide or protein subunits that form a gating system. Many ions can diffuse through the cell membrane only if conformational changes occur in the membrane proteins that comprise the ion channel. Two basic groups of ion channels exist: leakage channels and gated channels.

Electrical potentials (negative on the inside and positive on the outside) exist across the membranes of most cells in the body. These electrical potentials result from the selective permeability of the cell membrane to Na^+ and K^+; the presence of nondiffusible anions inside the cell membrane; and the activity of the sodium–potassium membrane pump, which extrudes Na^+ from inside the membrane and returns K^+ to the inside. An equilibrium or diffusion potential is one in which no net movement of ions occurs because the diffusion and electrical forces are exactly balanced.

Body Tissues

After you have completed this section of the chapter, you should be able to meet the following objectives:

✦ Explain the process of cell differentiation in terms of development of organ systems in the embryo and the continued regeneration of tissues in postnatal life
✦ Explain the function of stem cells

◆ Describe the characteristics of the four different tissue types

◆ Explain the function of intercellular adhesions and junctions

◆ Characterize the composition and functions of the extracellular matrix

In the preceding sections, we discussed the individual cell, its metabolic processes, and mechanisms of communication and replication. Although cells are similar, their structure and function vary according to the special needs of the body. For example, muscle cells perform different functions from skin cells or nerve cells. Groups of cells that are closely associated in structure and have common or similar functions are called *tissues*. Four categories of tissue exist: epithelium, connective (supportive) tissue, muscle, and nerve. These tissues do not exist in isolated units, but in association with each other and in variable proportions, forming different structures and organs. This section provides a brief overview of the cells in each of these four tissue types, the structures that hold these cells together, and the extracellular matrix in which they live.

Organization of Cells Into Tissues

➤ Cells with a similar embryonic origin or function are often organized into larger functional units called *tissues*, and these tissues in turn associate with other, dissimilar tissues to form the various organs of the body.

➤ Connective tissue is the most abundant tissue of the body. It is found in a variety of forms, ranging from solid bone to blood cells that circulate in the vascular system.

➤ Epithelial tissue forms sheets that cover the body's outer surface, lines internal surfaces, and forms glandular tissue. It is supported by a basement membrane, is avascular, and must receive nourishment from capillaries in supporting connective tissues.

➤ Muscle tissue contains actin and myosin filaments that allow it to contract and provide locomotion and movement of skeletal structures (skeletal muscle), pumping of blood through the heart (cardiac muscle), and contraction of blood vessels and visceral organs (smooth muscle).

➤ Nervous tissue provides the means for controlling body function and for sensing and moving about in the external environment. It consists of two major types of cells: the neurons, which function in communication, and the neuroglial cells, which support the neurons.

CELL DIFFERENTIATION

After conception, the fertilized ovum undergoes a series of divisions, ultimately forming approximately 200 different cell types.[14] The formation of different types of cells and the disposition of these cells into tissue types is called *cell differentiation*, a process controlled by a system that switches genes on and off. Embryonic cells must become different to develop into all of the various organ systems, and they must remain different after the signal that initiated cell diversification has disappeared. The process of cell differentiation is controlled by cell memory, which is maintained through regulatory proteins contained in the individual members of a particular cell type. Cell differentiation also involves the sequential activation of multiple genes and their protein products. This means that after differentiation has occurred, the tissue type does not revert to an earlier stage of differentiation. The process of cell differentiation normally moves forward, producing cells that are more specialized than their predecessors. Usually, highly differentiated cell types, such as skeletal muscle and nervous tissue, lose their ability to undergo cell division.

Although most cells differentiate into specialized cell types, many tissues contain a few *stem cells* that apparently are only partially differentiated. These stem cells are still capable of cell division and serve as a reserve source for specialized cells throughout the life of the organism.[14] They are the major source of cells that make regeneration possible in some tissues. Stem cells have varying abilities to differentiate. Some tissues, such as skeletal muscle tissue, lack sufficient numbers of undifferentiated cells and have limited regenerative capacity. Stem cells of the hematopoietic (blood) system have the greatest potential for differentiation. These cells can potentially reconstitute the entire blood-producing and immune systems. They are the major ingredient in bone marrow transplants. Other stem cells, such as those that replenish the mucosal surface of the gastrointestinal tract, are less general but can still differentiate. Cancer cells are thought to originate from undifferentiated stem cells (see Chapter 8).

EMBRYONIC ORIGIN OF TISSUE TYPES

All of the approximately 200 different types of body cells can be classified into four basic or primary tissue types: epithelial, connective, muscle, and nervous (Table 4-1). These basic tissue types are often described by their embryonic origin. The embryo is essentially a three-layered tubular structure (Fig. 4-20). The outer layer of the tube is called the *ectoderm*; the middle layer, the *mesoderm*; and the inner layer, the *endoderm*. All of the adult body tissues originate from these three cellular layers. Epithelium has its origin in all three embryonic layers, connective tissue and muscle develop mainly from the mesoderm, and nervous tissue develops from the ectoderm.

EPITHELIAL TISSUE

Origin and Characteristics

Epithelial tissue forms sheets that cover the body's outer surface, line the internal surfaces, and form the glandular

TABLE 4-1 ✦ Classification of Tissue Types

Tissue Type	Location
Epithelial Tissue	
Covering and lining of body surfaces	
Simple epithelium	
Squamous	Lining of blood vessels, body cavities, alveoli of lungs
Cuboidal	Collecting tubules of kidney; covering of ovaries
Columnar	Lining of intestine and gallbladder
Stratified epithelium	
Squamous keratinized	Skin
Squamous nonkeratinized	Mucous membranes of mouth, esophagus, and vagina
Cuboidal	Ducts of sweat glands
Columnar	Large ducts of salivary and mammary glands; also found in conjunctiva
Transitional	Bladder, ureters, renal pelvis
Pseudostratified	Tracheal and respiratory passages
Glandular	
Endocrine	Pituitary gland, thyroid gland, adrenal, and other glands
Exocrine	Sweat glands and glands in gastrointestinal tract
Neuroepithelium	Olfactory mucosa, retina, tongue
Reproductive epithelium	Seminiferous tubules of testis; cortical portion of ovary
Connective Tissue	
Embryonic connective tissue	
Mesenchymal	Embryonic mesoderm
Mucous	Umbilical cord (Wharton's jelly)
Adult connective tissue	
Loose or areolar	Subcutaneous areas
Dense regular	Tendons and ligaments
Dense irregular	Dermis of skin
Adipose	Fat pads, subcutaneous layers
Reticular	Framework of lymphoid organs, bone marrow, liver
Specialized connective tissue	
Bone	Long bones, flat bones
Cartilage	Tracheal rings, external ear, articular surfaces
Hematopoietic	Blood cells, myeloid tissue (bone marrow)
Muscle Tissue	
Skeletal	Skeletal muscles
Cardiac	Heart muscles
Smooth	Gastrointestinal tract, blood vessels, bronchi, bladder, and others
Nervous Tissue	
Neurons	Central and peripheral neurons and nerve fibers
Supporting cells	Glial and ependymal cells in central nervous system; Schwann and satellite cells in peripheral nervous system

tissue. Underneath all types of epithelial tissue is an extracellular matrix, called the *basement membrane.* A basement membrane consists of the basal lamina and an underlying reticular layer. The terms *basal lamina* and *basement membrane* are often used interchangeably. Epithelial cells have strong intracellular protein filaments (*i.e.,* cytoskeleton) that are important in transmitting mechanical stresses from one cell to another. The cells of epithelial tissue are tightly bound together by specialized junctions. These specialized junctions enable these cells to form barriers to the movement of water, solutes, and cells from one body compartment to the next. Epithelial tissue is avascular (*i.e.,* without blood vessels) and must therefore receive oxygen and nutrients from the capillaries of the connective tissue on which the epithelial tissue rests (Fig. 4-21). Epithelial tissue contains a number of neural receptors (*i.e.,* pressure, thermal, and pain) that serve to sample the internal and external environments. To survive, epithelial tissue must be kept moist. Even the seemingly dry skin epithelium is kept moist by a nonvitalized, waterproof layer of superficial skin cells called *keratin,* which prevents evaporation of moisture from the deeper living cells.

Epithelia are derived from all three embryonic layers. Most epithelia of the skin, mouth, nose, and anus are derived from the ectoderm. Linings of the respiratory tract, the gastrointestinal tract, and the glands of the digestive tract are of endodermal origin. The endothelial lining of

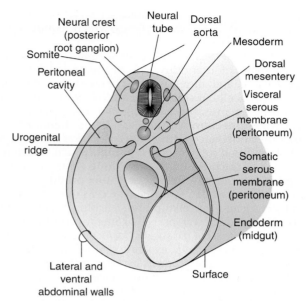

FIGURE 4-20 Cross section of a human embryo illustrating the development of the somatic and visceral structures.

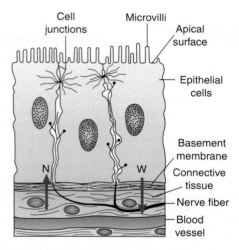

FIGURE 4-21 Typical arrangement of epithelial cells in relation to underlying tissues and blood supply. Epithelial tissue has no blood supply of its own but relies on the blood vessels in the underlying connective tissue for nutrition (**N**) and elimination of wastes (**W**).

blood vessels originates from the mesoderm. Many types of epithelial tissue retain the ability to differentiate and undergo rapid proliferation for replacing injured tissue.

Types of Epithelial Cells

Epithelial tissues are classified according to the shape of the cells and the number of layers that are present: *simple, stratified,* and *pseudostratified.* The terms *squamous* (thin and flat), *cuboidal* (cube shaped), and *columnar* (resembling a column) refer to the cells' shape (Fig. 4-22).

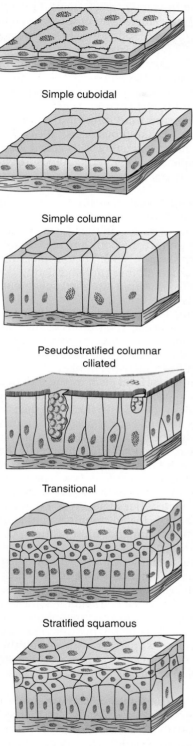

FIGURE 4-22 Representation of the various epithelial tissue types.

Simple Epithelium. *Simple epithelium* contains a single layer of cells, all of which rest on the basement membrane.

Simple squamous epithelium is adapted for filtration; it is found lining the blood vessels, lymph nodes, and alveoli of the lungs. The single layer of squamous epithelium lining the heart and blood vessels is known as the *endothelium*. A similar type of layer, called the *mesothelium*, forms the serous membranes that line the pleural, pericardial, and peritoneal cavities and cover the organs of these cavities. A *simple cuboidal epithelium* is found on the surface of the ovary and in the thyroid. *Simple columnar epithelium* lines the intestine. One form of a simple columnar epithelium has hairlike projections called *cilia*, often with specialized mucus-secreting cells called *goblet cells*. This form of simple columnar epithelium lines the airways of the respiratory tract.

Stratified and Pseudostratified Epithelium.
Stratified epithelium contains more than one layer of cells, with only the deepest layer resting on the basement membrane. It is designed to protect the body surface. *Stratified squamous keratinized* epithelium makes up the epidermis of the skin. *Keratin* is a tough, fibrous protein existing as filaments in the outer cells of skin. A stratified squamous keratinized epithelium is made up of many layers. The layers closest to the underlying tissues are cuboidal or columnar. The cells become more irregular and thinner as they move closer to the surface. Surface cells become totally filled with keratin and die, are sloughed off, and then replaced by the deeper cells. A stratified squamous nonkeratinized epithelium is found on moist surfaces such as the mouth and tongue. Stratified cuboidal and columnar epithelia are found in the ducts of salivary glands and the larger ducts of the mammary glands. In smokers, the normal columnar ciliated epithelial cells of the trachea and bronchi are often replaced with stratified squamous epithelium cells that are better able to withstand the irritating effects of cigarette smoke.

Pseudostratified epithelium is a type of epithelium in which all of the cells are in contact with the underlying intercellular matrix, but some do not extend to the surface. A pseudostratified ciliated columnar epithelium with goblet cells forms the lining of most of the upper respiratory tract. All of the tall cells reaching the surface of this type of epithelium are either ciliated cells or mucus-producing goblet cells. The basal cells that do not reach the surface serve as stem cells for ciliated and goblet cells. *Transitional epithelium* is a stratified epithelium characterized by cells that can change shape and become thinner when the tissue is stretched. Such tissue can be stretched without pulling the superficial cells apart. Transitional epithelium is well adapted for the lining of organs that are constantly changing their volume, such as the urinary bladder.

Glandular Epithelium.
Glandular epithelial tissue is formed by cells specialized to produce a fluid secretion. This process is usually accompanied by the intracellular synthesis of macromolecules. The chemical nature of these macromolecules is variable. The macromolecules typically are stored in the cells in small, membrane-bound vesicles called *secretory granules*. For example, glandular epithelia can synthesize, store, and secrete proteins (*e.g.*, insulin), lipids (*e.g.*, adrenocortical hormones, secretions of the sebaceous glands), and complexes of carbohydrates and proteins (*e.g.*, saliva). Less common are secretions such as those produced by the sweat glands, which require minimal synthetic activity.

All glandular cells arise from surface epithelia by means of cell proliferation and invasion of the underlying connective tissue, and all release their contents or secretions into the extracellular compartment. *Exocrine glands*, such as the sweat glands and lactating mammary glands, retain their connection with the surface epithelium from which they originated. This connection takes the form of epithelium-lined tubular ducts through which the secretions pass to reach the surface. Exocrine glands are often classified according to the way secretory products are released by their cells. In *holocrine* type cells (*e.g.*, sebaceous glands), the glandular cell ruptures, releasing its entire contents into the duct system. New generations of cells are replaced by mitosis of basal cells. *Merocrine* or *eccrine* type glands (*e.g.*, salivary glands, exocrine glands of the pancreas) release their glandular products by exocytosis. In apocrine secretions (*e.g.*, mammary glands, certain sweat glands), the apical portion of the cell, along with small portions of the cytoplasm, is pinched off the glandular cells. *Endocrine glands* are epithelial structures that have had their connection with the surface obliterated during development. These glands are ductless and produce secretions (*i.e.*, hormones) that move directly into the bloodstream.

CONNECTIVE OR SUPPORTIVE TISSUE

Origin and Characteristics
Connective tissue (or supportive tissue) is the most abundant tissue in the body. As its name suggests, it connects and binds or supports the various tissues. The capsules that surround organs of the body are composed of connective tissue. Bone, adipose tissue, and cartilage are specialized types of connective tissue that function to support the soft tissues of the body and store fat. Connective tissue is unique in that its cells produce the extracellular matrix that supports and holds tissues together. Connective tissue has a role in tissue nutrition. The close proximity of the extracellular matrix to blood vessels allows it to function as an exchange medium through which nutrients and metabolic wastes pass.

Most connective tissue is derived from the embryonic mesoderm, but some is derived from the neural crest, a derivative of the ectoderm. During embryonic development, mesodermal cells migrate from their site of origin and then surround and penetrate the developing organ. These cells are called *mesenchymal cells*, and the tissue they form is called *mesenchyme*. Tissues derived from embryonic mesenchymal cells include bone, cartilage, and adipose (fat) cells. Besides providing the source or origin of most connective tissues, mesenchyme develops into other structures such as blood cells and blood vessels. Connective tissue cells include fibroblasts, chondroblasts, osteoblasts, hematopoietic stem cells, blood cells, macrophages, mast cells, and adipocytes. The matrix of the umbilical cord is composed of a second type of embryonic mesoderm called *mucous connective tissue* or *Wharton's jelly*.

Adult connective tissue proper can be divided into four types: loose or areolar, reticular, adipose, and dense connective tissue. Dense connective tissue is further subdivided into irregular and regular connective tissue. Specialized connective tissues, such as blood and blood-forming tissues, are discussed in Chapter 13; cartilage and bone are discussed in Chapter 56.

Loose Connective Tissue

Loose connective tissue, also known as *areolar tissue*, is soft and pliable. Although it is more cellular than dense connective tissue, it contains large amounts of intercellular substance (Fig. 4-23). It fills spaces between muscle sheaths and forms a layer that encases blood and lymphatic vessels. Areolar connective tissue supports the epithelial tissues and provides the means by which these tissues are nourished. In an organ containing functioning epithelial tissue and supporting connective tissue, the term *parenchymal tissue* is used to describe the functioning epithelium as opposed to the connective tissue framework or stroma.

Cells of loose connective tissue include fibroblasts, mast cells, adipose or fat cells, macrophages, plasma cells, and leukocytes. Loose connective tissue cells secrete substances that form the extracellular matrix that supports and connects body cells. Fibroblasts are the most abundant of these cells. They are responsible for the synthesis of the fibrous and gel-like substance that fills the intercellular spaces of the body and for the production of collagen, elastic, and reticular fibers.

The *basal lamina* is a special type of intercellular matrix that is present where connective tissue contacts the tissue it supports. It is visible only with an electron microscope and is produced by the epithelial cells. In many locations, reticular fibers, produced by the connective tissue cells, are associated with the basal lamina. Together the basal lamina and the reticular layer form the basement membrane seen by light microscopy. A basement membrane is found along the interface between connective tissue and muscle fibers, on Schwann cells of the peripheral nervous system, on the basal surface of endothelial cells, and on fat cells. These basement membranes bond cells to the underlying or surrounding connective tissues, serve as selective filters for particles that pass between connective tissue and other cells, and contribute to cell regeneration and repair.

Adipose tissue is a special form of connective tissue in which adipocytes predominate. Adipocytes do not generate an extracellular matrix but maintain a large intracellular space. These cells store large quantities of triglycerides and are the largest repository of energy in the body. Adipose tissue helps fill spaces between tissues and helps to keep organs in place. Subcutaneous layers of fat help to shape the body. Because fat is a poor conductor of heat, adipose tissue serves as thermal insulation for the body. Adipose tissue exists in two forms. Unilocular (white) adipose tissue is composed of cells in which the fat is contained in a single, large droplet in the cytoplasm. Multilocular (brown) adipose tissue is composed of cells that contain multiple droplets of fat

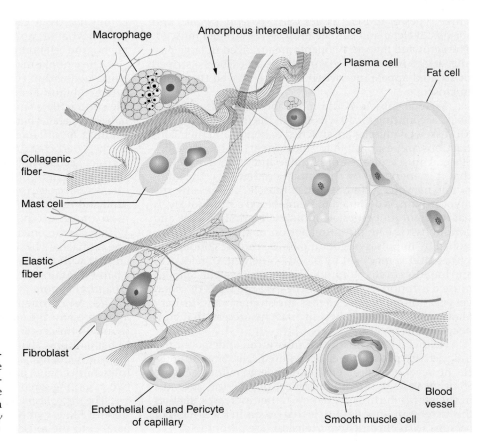

FIGURE 4-23 Diagrammatic representation of cells that may be seen in loose connective tissue. The cells lie in an intercellular matrix that is bathed in tissue fluid that originates in capillaries. (From Cormack D.H. [1987]. *Ham's histology* [9th ed.]. Philadelphia: J.B. Lippincott)

and numerous mitochondria. These two types of fat are discussed in Chapter 11.

Reticular tissue is characterized by a network of reticular fibers associated with reticular cells. These reticular cells are believed to retain multipotential capabilities similar to undifferentiated mesenchymal cells. Reticular tissues comprise the framework of the liver, bone marrow, and lymphoid tissues such as the spleen.

Dense Connective Tissue

Dense connective tissue exists in two forms: dense irregular and dense regular. Dense irregular connective tissue consists of the same components found in loose connective tissue, but there is a predominance of collagen fibers and fewer cells. This type of tissue can be found in the dermis of the skin (*i.e.*, reticular layer), the fibrous capsules of many organs, and the fibrous sheaths of cartilage (*i.e.*, perichondrium) and bone (*i.e.*, periosteum). It also forms the fascia that invests muscles and organs. Dense regular connective tissues are rich in collagen fibers and form the tendons and aponeuroses that join muscles to bone or other muscles and the ligaments that join bones to bone. Tendons and ligaments are white fibers because of an abundance of collagen. Ligaments such as the ligamenta flava of the vertebral column and the true vocal folds are called *yellow fibers* because of the abundance of elastic fibers.

MUSCLE TISSUE

Three types of muscle tissues exist: *skeletal, cardiac*, and *smooth*. Skeletal and cardiac muscles are striated muscles. The actin and myosin filaments are arranged in large parallel arrays in bundles, giving the muscle fibers a striped or striated appearance when they are viewed through a microscope.

Skeletal muscle is the most abundant tissue in the body, accounting for 40% to 45% of the total body weight. Most skeletal muscles are attached to bones, and their contractions are responsible for movements of the skeleton. Skeletal muscle differs from cardiac and smooth muscle in that it is enervated by the somatic rather than the autonomic nervous system. Cardiac muscle, comprising the myocardium, is designed to pump blood continuously. It has inherent properties of automaticity, rhythmicity, and conductivity. The pumping action of the heart is controlled by impulses originating in the cardiac conduction system and is modified by blood-borne neural mediators and impulses from the autonomic nervous system. Smooth muscle is found in the iris of the eye, the walls of blood vessels, hollow organs such as the stomach and urinary bladder, and hollow tubes, such as the ureters, that connect internal organs.

Neither skeletal nor cardiac muscle can undergo the mitotic activity needed to replace injured cells. Smooth muscle, however, may proliferate and undergo mitotic activity. Some increases in smooth muscle are physiologic, as occurs in the uterus during pregnancy. Other increases, such as the increase in smooth muscle that occurs in the arteries of persons with chronic hypertension, are pathologic.

Although the three types of muscle tissue differ significantly in structure, contractile properties, and control mechanisms, they have many similarities. In the following section, the structural properties of skeletal muscle are presented as the prototype of striated muscle tissue. Smooth muscle and the ways in which it differs from skeletal muscle are also discussed. Cardiac muscle is described in Chapter 24.

Skeletal Muscle

Skeletal muscle tissue is packaged into skeletal muscles that attach to and cover the body skeleton. Each skeletal muscle is a discrete organ made up of hundreds or thousands of muscle fibers. At the periphery of skeletal muscle fibers, randomly scattered satellite cells are found. They represent a source of undifferentiated myoblast cells that may be involved in the limited regeneration capabilities of skeletal muscle.[14,15] Even though muscle fibers predominate, substantial amounts of connective tissue, blood vessels, and nerve fibers are also present.

Organization and Structure. In an intact muscle, the individual muscle fibers are held together by several different layers of connective tissue. Skeletal muscles such as the biceps brachii are surrounded by a dense, irregular connective tissue covering called the *epimysium* (Fig. 4-24). Each muscle is subdivided into smaller bundles called *fascicles*, which are surrounded by a connective tissue covering called the *perimysium*. The number of fascicles and their size vary among muscles. Fascicles consist of many elongated structures called *muscle fibers*, each of which is surrounded by connective tissue called the *endomysium*. Skeletal muscles are syncytial or multinucleated structures, meaning there are no true cell boundaries within a skeletal muscle fiber.

The cytoplasm of the muscle fiber (*i.e.*, sarcoplasm) is contained within the sarcolemma, which represents the cell membrane. Embedded throughout the sarcoplasm are the contractile elements actin and myosin, which are arranged in parallel bundles (*i.e.*, myofibrils). The thin, lighter-staining myofilaments are composed of actin, and the thicker, darker-staining myofilaments are composed of myosin. Each myofibril consists of regularly repeating units along the length of the myofibril; each of these units is called a *sarcomere* (see Fig. 4-24). Sarcomeres are the structural and functional units of cardiac and skeletal muscle. A sarcomere extends from one Z line to another Z line. Within the sarcomere are alternating light and dark bands. The central dark band (A band) contains mainly myosin filaments, with some overlap with actin filaments. The lighter I band contains only actin filaments and straddles the Z band; therefore, it takes two sarcomeres to complete an I band. An H zone is found in the middle of the A band and represents the region where only myosin filaments are found. In the center of the H zone is a thin, dark band, the M band or line, that is produced by linkages between the myosin filaments. Z bands consist of short elements that interconnect and provide the thin actin filaments from two adjoining sarcomeres with an anchoring point.

The *sarcoplasmic reticulum*, which is comparable to the smooth ER, is composed of longitudinal tubules that run parallel to the muscle fiber and surround each myofibril.

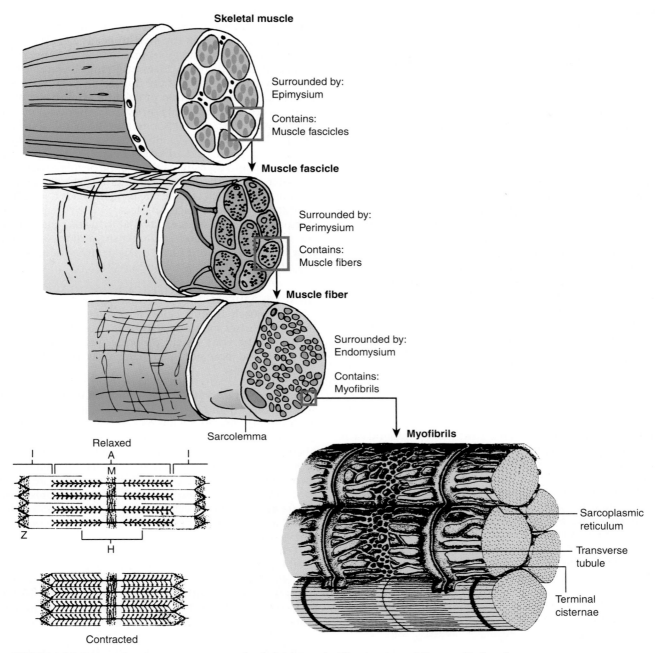

FIGURE 4-24 Connective tissue components of a skeletal muscle. The structure of the myofibril and the relationship between actin and myosin myofilaments are also shown.

This network ends in enlarged, saclike regions called the *lateral sacs* or *terminal cisternae*. These sacs store calcium to be released during muscle contraction. A binding protein called *calsequestrin* found in the terminal cisternae enables a high concentration of calcium ions to be sequestered in the cisternae. The concentration of calcium ions in the cisternae is 10,000 times higher than in the sarcoplasm.[10,15]

A second system of tubules consists of the *transverse* or *T tubules*, which are extensions of the plasma membrane and run perpendicular to the muscle fiber. The hollow portion or lumen of the transverse tubule is continuous with the extracellular fluid compartment. Action potentials, which are rapidly conducted over the surface of the muscle fiber, are in turn propagated by the T tubules and into the sarcoplasmic reticulum. As the action potential moves through the lateral sacs, the sacs release calcium, initiating muscle contraction. The membrane of the sarcoplasmic reticulum also has an active transport mechanism for pumping calcium ions back into the reticulum. This prevents interactions between calcium ions and the actin and myosin myofilaments after cessation of a muscle contraction.

Skeletal Muscle Contraction. During muscle contraction, the thick myosin and thin actin filaments slide over each other, causing shortening of the muscle fiber, although the length of the individual thick and thin filaments remains unchanged. The structures that produce the sliding of the filaments are the myosin heads that form cross-bridges with the thin actin filaments (Fig. 4-25). When activated by ATP, the cross-bridges swivel in a fixed arc, much like the oars of a boat, as they become attached to the actin filament. During contraction, each cross-bridge undergoes its own cycle of movement, forming a bridge attachment and releasing it, and moving to another site where the same sequence of movement occurs. This pulls the thin and thick filaments past each other.

Myosin is the chief constituent of the thick filament. It consists of a thin tail, which provides the structural backbone for the filament, and a globular head. Each globular head contains a binding site able to bind to a complementary site on the actin molecule. In addition to the binding site for actin, each myosin head has a separate active site that catalyzes the breakdown of ATP to provide the energy needed to activate the myosin head so it can form a cross-bridge with actin. After contraction, myosin also binds ATP, thus breaking the linkage between actin and myosin.

Myosin molecules are bundled together side by side in the thick filaments such that one half have their heads toward one end of the filament and their tails toward the other end; the other half are arranged in the opposite manner. The thin filaments are composed mainly of actin, a globular protein lined up in two rows that coil around each other to form a long helical strand. Associated with each actin filament are two regulatory proteins, tropomyosin and troponin (see Fig. 4-25). *Tropomyosin*, which lies in grooves of the actin strand, provides the site for attachment of the globular heads of the myosin filament. In the non-contracted state, *troponin* covers the tropomyosin binding sites and prevents formation of cross-bridges between the actin and myosin. During an action potential, calcium ions released from the sarcoplasmic reticulum diffuse to the adjacent myofibrils, where they bind to troponin. The binding of calcium to troponin uncovers the tropomyosin binding sites such that the myosin heads can attach and form cross-bridges. Energy from ATP is used to break the actin and myosin cross-bridges, stopping the muscle contraction. After breaking of the linkage between actin and myosin, the concentration of calcium around the myofibrils decreases as calcium is actively transported into the sarcoplasmic reticulum by a membrane pump that uses energy derived from ATP.

The basis of rigor mortis can be explained by the binding of actin and myosin. As the muscle begins to degenerate after death, the sarcoplasmic cisternae release their calcium ions, which enables the myosin heads to combine with their sites on the actin molecule. As ATP supplies diminish, no energy source is available to start the normal interaction between actin and myosin, and the muscle is in a state of rigor until further degeneration destroys the cross-bridges between actin and myosin.

Smooth Muscle

Smooth muscle is often called *involuntary muscle* because its activity arises spontaneously or through activity of the autonomic nervous system. Smooth muscle contractions are slower and more sustained than skeletal or cardiac muscle contractions.

Organization and Structure. Smooth muscle cells are spindle shaped and smaller than skeletal muscle fibers. Each smooth muscle cell has one centrally positioned nucleus. Z bands or M lines are not present in smooth muscle fibers, and the cross-striations are absent because the bundles of filaments are not parallel but crisscross obliquely through the cell. Instead, the actin filaments are attached to structures called *dense bodies*. Some of the dense bodies are attached to the cell membrane, and others are dispersed in the cell and linked together by structural proteins (Fig. 4-26).

The lack of Z lines and regular overlapping of the contractile elements provides a greater range of tension development. This is important in hollow organs that undergo changes in volume, with consequent changes in the length of the smooth muscle fibers in their walls. Even with the distention of a hollow organ, the smooth muscle fiber retains some ability to develop tension, whereas such distention would stretch skeletal muscle beyond the area where the thick and thin filaments overlap.

Smooth muscle usually is arranged in sheets or bundles. In hollow organs, such as the intestines, the bundles are organized into the two-layered muscularis externa consisting of an outer, longitudinal layer and an inner, circular layer. A thinner muscularis mucosae often lies between the muscularis externa and the endothelium. In blood vessels, the bundles are arranged circularly or helically around the vessel wall.

Smooth Muscle Contraction. As with cardiac and skeletal muscle, smooth muscle contraction is initiated by an increase in intracellular calcium. However, smooth muscle differs from skeletal muscle in the way its cross-bridges are

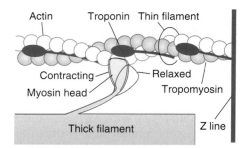

FIGURE 4-25 Molecular structure of the thin actin filament and the thicker myosin filament of striated muscle. The thin filament is a double-stranded helix of actin molecules with tropomyosin and troponin molecules lying along the grooves of the actin strands. During muscle contraction, the ATP-activated heads of the thick myosin filament swivel into position, much like the oars on a boat, form a cross-bridge with a reactive site on tropomyosin, and then pull the actin filament forward. During muscle relaxation, the troponin molecules cover the reactive sites on tropomyosin.

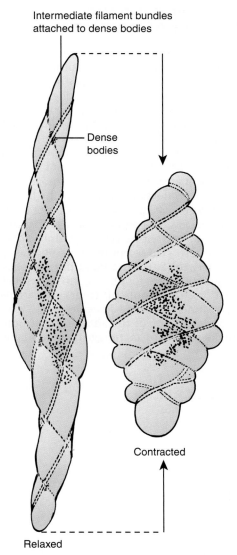

Intermediate filament bundles
attached to dense bodies

Dense
bodies

Contracted

Relaxed

FIGURE 4-26 Structure of smooth muscle showing the dense bodies. In smooth muscle, the force of contraction is transmitted to the cell membrane by bundles of intermediate fibers. (Cormack D.H. [1993]. *Essential histology* [p. 229]. Philadelphia: J.B. Lippincott)

Types of Smooth Muscle. Smooth muscle may be divided into two broad categories according to the mode of activation: multiunit and single-unit smooth muscle. In *multiunit* smooth muscle, each unit operates almost independently of the others and is often enervated by a single nerve, such as occurs in skeletal muscle. It has little or no inherent activity and depends on the autonomic nervous system for its activation. Smooth muscle of this type is found in the iris, in the walls of the vas deferens, and attached to hairs in the skin. The fibers in *single-unit* smooth muscle are in close contact with each other and can contract spontaneously without nerve or hormonal stimulation. Normally, most muscle fibers contract synchronously, hence the term *single-unit* smooth muscle. Some single-unit smooth muscle, such as that found in the gastrointestinal tract, is self-excitable. This is usually associated with a basic slow-wave rhythm transmitted from cell to cell by nexuses (*i.e.,* gap junctions) formed by the fusion of adjacent cell membranes. The cause of this slow wave is unknown. The intensity of contraction increases with the frequency of the action potential. Certain hormones, other agents, and local factors can modify smooth muscle activity by depolarizing or hyperpolarizing the membrane. The smooth muscle of the uterus and small-diameter blood vessels is also single-unit smooth muscle.

NERVE TISSUE

Nerve tissue is distributed throughout the body as an integrated communication system. Anatomically, the nervous system is divided into the central nervous system (CNS), which consists of the brain and spinal cord, and the peripheral nervous system (PNS), composed of nerve fibers and ganglia that exist outside the CNS. Nerve cells develop from the embryonic ectoderm. Nerve cells are highly differentiated and therefore incapable of regeneration in postnatal life. Embryonic development of the nervous system and the structure and function of the nervous system are discussed more fully in Chapter 47.

Structurally, nerve tissue consists of two cell types: nerve cells or neurons and glial or supporting cells. Most nerve cells consist of three parts: the soma or cell body, dendrites, and axon. The cytoplasm-filled dendrites, which are multiple, elongated processes, receive and carry stimuli from the environment, from sensory epithelial cells, and from other neurons to the cell. The axon, which is a single cytoplasm-filled process, is specialized for generating and conducting nerve impulses away from the cell body to other nerve cells, muscle cells, and glandular cells.

Neurons can be classified as afferent and efferent neurons according to their function. Afferent or sensory neurons carry information toward the CNS; they are involved in the reception of sensory information from the external environment and from within the body. Efferent or motor neurons carry information away from the CNS; they are needed for control of muscle fibers and endocrine and exocrine glands.

Communication between neurons and effector organs, such as muscle cells, occurs at specialized structures called

formed. The sarcoplasmic reticulum of smooth muscle is less developed than in skeletal muscle, and no transverse tubules are present. Smooth muscle relies on the entrance of extracellular calcium and its release from the sarcoplasmic reticulum for muscle contraction. This dependence on movement of extracellular calcium across the cell membrane during muscle contraction is the basis for the action of calcium-blocking drugs used in treatment of cardiovascular disease.

Smooth muscle also lacks the calcium-binding regulatory protein, troponin, which is found in skeletal and cardiac muscle. Instead, it relies on another cytoplasmic protein called *calmodulin*. The calcium–calmodulin complex binds to and activates the myosin-containing thick filaments, which interact with actin.

synapses. At the synapse, chemical messengers (*i.e.*, neurotransmitters) alter the membrane potential to conduct impulses from one nerve to another or from a neuron to an effector cell. In addition, electrical synapses exist in which nerve cells are linked through gap junctions that permit the passage of ions from one cell to another.

The neuroglia (*glia* means "glue") are cells that support neurons, form myelin, and have trophic and phagocytic functions. Four types of neuroglia are found in the CNS: astrocytes, oligodendrocytes, microglia, and ependymal cells. Astrocytes are the most abundant of the neuroglia. They have many long processes that surround blood vessels in the CNS. They provide structural support for the neurons, and their extensions form a sealed barrier that protects the CNS. The oligodendrocytes provide myelination of neuronal processes in the CNS. The microglia are phagocytic cells that represent the mononuclear phagocytic system in the nervous system. Ependymal cells line the cavities of the brain and spinal cord and are in contact with the cerebrospinal fluid. In the PNS, supporting cells consist of the Schwann and satellite cells. The Schwann cells provide myelination of the axons and dendrites, and the satellite cells enclose and protect the dorsal root ganglia and autonomic ganglion cells.

CELL JUNCTIONS AND CELL-TO-CELL ADHESION

Cell junctions occur at many points in cell-to-cell contact, but they are particularly plentiful and important in epithelial tissue. Three basic types of intercellular junctions are observed: tight junctions, adhering junctions, and gap junctions (Fig. 4-27). Often, the cells in epithelial tissue are joined by all three types of junctions. *Continuous tight* or occluding junctions (*i.e.*, zona occludens), which are found only in epithelial tissue, seal the surface membranes of adjacent cells together. This type of intercellular junction prevents materials such as macromolecules present in the intestinal contents from entering the intercellular space.

Adhering junctions represent a site of strong adhesion between cells. The primary role of adhering junctions may be that of preventing cell separation. Adhering junctions are not restricted to epithelial tissue; they provide adherence between adjacent cardiac muscle cells as well. Adhering junctions are found as continuous, beltlike adhesive junctions (*i.e.*, zonula adherens), or scattered, spotlike adhesive junctions called *desmosomes* (*i.e.*, macula adherens). A special feature of the adhesion belt junction is that it provides a site for anchorage of microfilaments to the cell

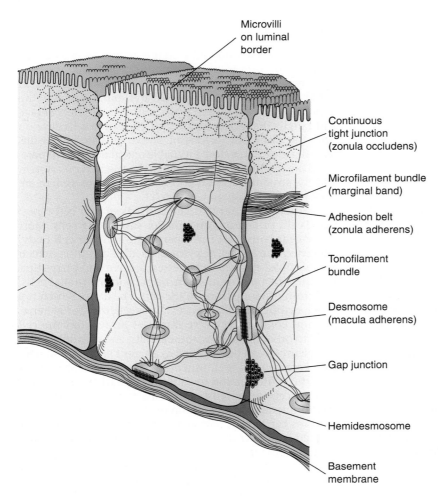

Microvilli on luminal border

Continuous tight junction (zonula occludens)

Microfilament bundle (marginal band)

Adhesion belt (zonula adherens)

Tonofilament bundle

Desmosome (macula adherens)

Gap junction

Hemidesmosome

Basement membrane

FIGURE 4-27 The chief types of intercellular junctions found in epithelial tissue. (From Cormack D.H. [1993]. *Essential histology*. Philadelphia: J.B. Lippincott)

membrane. In epithelial desmosomes, bundles of keratin-containing intermediate filaments (*i.e.*, tonofilaments) are anchored to the junction on the cytoplasmic area of the cell membrane. A primary disease of desmosomes is pemphigus. This disease is caused by a buildup of antibodies to the proteins of the desmosomes. Persons affected have skin and mucous membrane blistering.[5]

Gap junctions, or *nexus junctions*, involve the close adherence of adjoining cell membranes with the formation of channels that link the cytoplasm of the two cells. Gap junctions are not unique to epithelial tissue; they play an essential role in many types of cell-to-cell communication. Because they are low-resistance channels, gap junctions are important in cell-to-cell conduction of electrical signals (*e.g.*, between cells in sheets of smooth muscle or between adjacent cardiac muscle cells, where they function as electrical synapses). These multiple communication channels also enable ions and small molecules to pass directly from one cell to another. Gap junctions are associated with a variety of diseases, among which are inner ear deafness, cardiac arrhythmias, and Charcot-Marie-Tooth disease (the most common inherited peripheral neuropathy).[9]

Hemidesmosomes are another type of junction. They are found at the base of epithelial cells and help attach the epithelial cell to the underlying connective tissue. They resemble half a desmosome, hence their name.

EXTRACELLULAR MATRIX

Tissues are not made up solely of cells. A large part of their volume is made up of an extracellular matrix. This matrix is composed of a variety of proteins and polysaccharides (*i.e.*, a molecule made up of many sugars). These proteins and polysaccharides are secreted locally and are organized into a supporting meshwork in close association with the cells that produced them. The amount and composition of the matrix vary with the different tissues and their function. In bone, for example, the matrix is more plentiful than the cells that surround it; in the brain, the cells are much more abundant and the matrix is only a minor constituent.

Two main classes of extracellular macromolecules make up the extracellular matrix. The first is composed of polysaccharide chains of a class called *glycosaminoglycans* (GAGs), which are usually found linked to protein as proteoglycans. The second type consists of the fibrous proteins (*i.e.*, collagen and elastin) and the fibrous adhesive proteins (*i.e.*, fibronectin and laminin) that are found in the basement membrane. The members of each of these two classes of extracellular macromolecules come in a variety of shapes and sizes.

The proteoglycan and GAG molecules in connective tissue form a highly hydrated, gel-like substance, or tissue gel, in which the fibrous proteins are embedded. The polysaccharide gel resists compressive forces, the collagen fibers strengthen and help organize the matrix, the rubber-like elastin adds resilience, and the adhesive proteins help cells attach to the appropriate part of the matrix. Polysaccharides in the tissue gel are highly hydrophilic, and they form gels even at low concentrations. They also accumulate a negative charge that attracts cations such as sodium, which are osmotically active, causing large amounts of water to be sucked into the matrix. This creates a swelling pressure, or turgor, that enables the matrix to withstand extensive compressive forces. This is in contrast to collagen, which resists stretching forces. For example, the cartilage matrix that lines the knee joint can support pressures of hundreds of atmospheres by this mechanism.

Glycosaminoglycan and proteoglycan molecules in connective tissue usually constitute less than 10% by weight of fibrous tissue. Because they form a hydrated gel, the molecules fill most of the extracellular space, providing mechanical support to the tissues while ensuring rapid diffusion of water and electrolytes and the migration of cells. One GAG, hyaluronan or hyaluronic acid, is thought to play an important role as a space filler during embryonic development. It creates a cell-free space into which cells subsequently migrate. When cell migration and organ development are complete, the excess hyaluronan is degraded by the enzyme hyaluronidase. Hyaluronan is also important in directing the cell replacement that occurs during wound repair.

Three types of fibers are found in the extracellular space: collagen, elastin, and reticular fibers. *Collagen* is the most common protein in the body. It is a tough, nonliving, white fiber that serves as the structural framework for skin, ligaments, tendons, and many other structures. *Elastin* acts like a rubber band; it can be stretched and then returns to its original form. Elastin fibers are abundant in structures subjected to frequent stretching, such as the aorta and some ligaments. *Reticular fibers* are extremely thin fibers that create a flexible network in organs subjected to changes in form or volume, such as the spleen, liver, uterus, or intestinal muscle layer.

Integrins

An important class of extracellular macromolecules is the adhesion molecules. These molecules include the integrins, which are a diverse group of glycoproteins. They usually help in attaching epithelial cells to the underlying basement membrane. They can also attach to specific ligands on adjacent cells. The binding is calcium dependent and may involve actin filaments that are not associated with cell junctions.

Integrins associated with binding cells to the intracellular matrix are both magnesium and calcium dependent. One group of these integrins is associated with hemidesmosomes, whereas others are associated with the surface of white blood cells, macrophages, and platelets. Integrins usually have a relatively weak affinity for their ligands except where they are associated with cellular focal contacts and hemidesmosomes. This allows some movement between cells except where a firm attachment is required to attach the epithelial cells to the underlying connective tissue.

Certain integrins play an important role in allowing white blood cells to pass through the vessel wall, a process called *transmigration*. Persons affected with leukocyte adhesion deficiency are unable to synthesize appropriate integrin molecules. As a result, they experience repeated bacterial infections because their white blood cells are not able to transmigrate through vessel walls.

In summary, body cells are organized into four basic tissue types: epithelial, connective, muscle, and nervous. The epithelium covers and lines the body surfaces and forms the functional components of glandular structures. Epithelial tissue is classified into three types according to the shape of the cells and the number of layers that are present: simple, stratified, and pseudostratified. The cells in epithelial tissue are held together by three types of intercellular junctions: tight, adhering, and gap. They are attached to the underlying tissue by hemidesmosomes. Connective tissue supports and connects body structures; it forms the bones and skeletal system, the joint structures, the blood cells, and the intercellular substances. Adult connective tissue can be divided into four types: loose or areolar, reticular, adipose, and dense (regular and irregular).

Muscle tissue is a specialized tissue designed for contractility. Three types of muscle tissue exist: skeletal, cardiac, and smooth. Actin and myosin filaments interact to produce muscle shortening, a process activated by the presence of calcium. In skeletal muscle, calcium is released from the sarcoplasmic reticulum in response to an action potential. Smooth muscle is often called *involuntary muscle* because it contracts spontaneously or through activity of the autonomic nervous system. It differs from skeletal muscle in that its sarcoplasmic reticulum is less defined and it depends on the entry of extracellular calcium ions for muscle contraction.

Nervous tissue is designed for communication purposes and includes the neurons, the supporting neural structures, and the ependymal cells that line the ventricles of the brain and the spinal canal.

The extracellular matrix is made up of a variety of proteins and polysaccharides. These proteins and polysaccharides are secreted locally and are organized into a supporting meshwork in close association with the cells that produced them. The amount and composition of matrix vary with the different tissues and their function. Extracellular fibers include collagen fibers, which comprise tendons and ligaments; elastic fibers, found in large arteries and some ligaments; and thin reticular fibers, which are plentiful in organs that are subject to a change in volume (*e.g.*, spleen and liver).

References

1. Thiry M., Goessens G. (1996). Historical overview. In *Molecular biology intelligence unit: The nucleolus during the cell cycle.* (pp. 1–11). Georgetown, TX: R.G. Landes Co.
2. Alberts B., Bray D., Lewis J., Raff M., Roberts K., Watson J.D. (1994). *Molecular biology of the cell* (3rd ed., pp. 335–399, 485–488, 679, 738). New York and London: Garland Publishing.
3. Joachim F. (1998). How the ribosome works. *American Scientist* 86(5), 428–439.
4. Moore K.L., Persaud T.V.N. (1998). *The developing human: Clinically oriented embryology* (6th ed., pp. 17–46). Philadelphia: W. B. Saunders.
5. Cotran R.S., Kumar V., Collins T. (Eds.). (1999). *Robbins' pathologic basis of disease* (6th ed., pp. 153–156, 716, 1130, 1202, 1340). Philadelphia: W.B. Saunders.
6. Nelson D.L., Cox M.M. (2000). *Lehninger's principles of biochemistry* (3rd ed., pp. 567–597). New York: Worth Publishers.
7. The United Mitochondrial Disease Foundation. (2001). *Mitochondrial disease: Basis of disease.* [Online]. Available at http://www.umdf.org/mitodisease. Accessed June 20, 2001.
8. Wallace D.C. (1997). Mitochondrial DNA in aging and disease. *Scientific American* 277 (2), 40–47.
9. Ashcroft F.M. (2000). *Ion channels and disease* (pp. 67–96, 95–133, 211–229). San Diego: Academic Press.
10. Tortora G.J., Grabowski S. R. (2000). *Principles of anatomy and physiology* (9th ed., pp. 60–103, 268–301, 378–411). New York: John Wiley & Sons.
11. Baserga R. (1999). Introduction to the cell cycle. In Stein G.S., Baserga R., Giordano A., Denhardt D.T. (Eds.). *The molecular basis of cell cycle and growth control* (pp. 1–14) New York: Wiley-Liss.
12. J. Kimball Biology Pages. (2000, May 21). The cell cycle. [On-line]. Available at: http://www.ultranet.com/~jkimball/BiologyPages/C/CellCycle.html. Accessed July 24, 2000.
13. Mathews C.K., van Holde K.E., Ahern K.G. (2000). *Biochemistry* (3rd ed., pp. 446–482). San Francisco: Benjamin/Cummings.
14. Kerr J.B. (1999). *Atlas of functional histology* (pp. 1–24, 25–37, 81–106). London: Mosby.
15. Guyton A.C., Hall J.E. (2000). *Textbook of medical physiology* (10th ed., p. 85), Philadelphia: W.B Saunders.

Chapter 5

Cellular Adaptation, Injury, and Death and Wound Healing

When confronted with stresses that endanger its normal structure and function, the cell undergoes adaptive changes that permit survival and maintenance of function. It is only when the stress is overwhelming or adaptation is ineffective that cell injury and death occur. This chapter focuses on cellular adaptation, cell injury and death, and wound healing.

Cellular Adaptation

After you have completed this section of the chapter, you should be able to meet the following objectives:

✦ Cite the general purpose of changes in cell structure and function that occur as the result of normal adaptive processes

✦ Describe cell changes that occur with atrophy, hypertrophy, hyperplasia, metaplasia, and dysplasia and state general conditions under which the changes occur

✦ Cite three sources of intracellular accumulations

Cells adapt to changes in the internal environment, just as the total organism adapts to changes in the external environment. Cells may adapt by undergoing changes in size, number, and type. These changes, occurring singly or in combination, may lead to atrophy, hypertrophy, hyperplasia, metaplasia, and dysplasia (Fig. 5-1). Adaptive cellular responses also include intracellular accumulations and storage of products in abnormal amounts.[1,2]

There are numerous molecular mechanisms mediating cellular adaptation, including factors produced by other cells or by the cells themselves. These mechanisms depend largely on signals transmitted by chemical messengers that exert their effects by altering gene function. In general, the genes expressed in all cells fall into two categories: "housekeeping" genes that are necessary for normal function of a cell, and genes that determine the differentiating characteristics of a particular cell type. In many adaptive cellular responses, the expression of the differentiation genes is altered, whereas that of the housekeeping genes remains unaffected.[1] Thus, a cell is able to change size or form without compromising its housekeeping function. Once the stimulus for adaptation is removed, the effect on expression of the differentiating genes is removed and the cell resumes

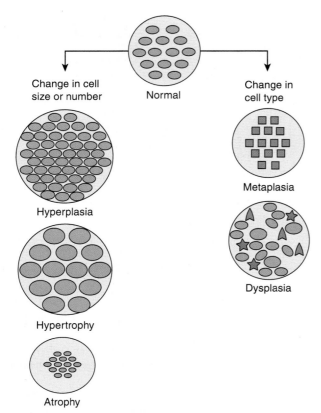

FIGURE 5-1 Adaptive cell responses involving a change in number (hyperplasia), cell size (hypertrophy and atrophy), cell type (metaplasia), or size, shape, and organization (dysplasia).

its previous state of specialized function. Whether adaptive cellular changes are normal or abnormal depends on whether the response was mediated by an appropriate stimulus. Normal adaptive responses occur in response to need and an appropriate stimulus. After the need has been removed, the adaptive response ceases.

ATROPHY

When confronted with a decrease in work demands or adverse environmental conditions, most cells are able to revert

 Cellular Adaptations

➤ Cells are able to adapt to increased work demands or threats to survival by changing their size (atrophy and hypertrophy), number (hyperplasia), and form (metaplasia).

➤ Normal cellular adaptation occurs in response to an appropriate stimulus and ceases once the need for adaptation has ceased.

to a smaller size and a lower and more efficient level of functioning that is compatible with survival. This decrease in cell size is called *atrophy*. Cell size, particularly in muscle tissue, is related to workload. As the workload of a cell diminishes, oxygen consumption and protein synthesis decrease. Cells that are atrophied reduce their oxygen consumption and other cellular functions by decreasing the number and size of their organelles and other structures. There are fewer mitochondria, myofilaments, and endoplasmic reticulum structures. When a sufficient number of cells are involved, the entire tissue or muscle atrophies.

The general causes of atrophy can be grouped into five categories: disuse, denervation, loss of endocrine stimulation, inadequate nutrition, and ischemia or a decrease in blood flow. Disuse atrophy occurs when there is a reduction in skeletal muscle use. An extreme example of disuse atrophy is seen in the muscles of extremities that have been encased in plaster casts. Because atrophy is adaptive and reversible, muscle size is restored after the cast is removed and muscle use is resumed. Denervation atrophy is a form of disuse atrophy that occurs in the muscles of paralyzed limbs. Lack of endocrine stimulation produces a form of disuse atrophy. In women, the loss of estrogen stimulation during menopause results in atrophic changes in the reproductive organs. With malnutrition and decreased blood flow, cells decrease their size and energy requirements as a means of survival.

HYPERTROPHY

Hypertrophy represents an increase in cell size and with it an increase in the amount of functioning tissue mass. It results from an increased workload imposed on an organ or body part and is commonly seen in cardiac and skeletal muscle tissue, which cannot adapt to an increase in workload through mitotic division and formation of more cells. Hypertrophy involves an increase in the functional components of the cell that allows it to achieve equilibrium between demand and functional capacity. For example, as muscle cells hypertrophy, additional actin and myosin filaments, cell enzymes, and adenosine triphosphate (ATP) are synthesized.

Hypertrophy may occur as the result of normal physiologic or abnormal pathologic conditions. The increase in muscle mass associated with exercise is an example of physiologic hypertrophy. Pathologic hypertrophy occurs as the result of disease conditions and may be adaptive or compensatory. Examples of adaptive hypertrophy are the thickening of the urinary bladder from long-continued obstruction of urinary outflow and the myocardial hypertrophy that results from valvular heart disease or hypertension. Compensatory hypertrophy is the enlargement of a remaining organ or tissue after a portion has been surgically removed or rendered inactive. For instance, if one kidney is removed, the remaining kidney enlarges to compensate for the loss.

The precise signal for hypertrophy is unknown. It may be related to ATP depletion, mechanical forces such as stretching of the muscle fibers, activation of cell degradation products, or hormonal factors.[1] Whatever the mechanism, a limit is eventually reached beyond which further enlargement of the tissue mass is no longer able to compensate for the increased work demands. The limiting factors for continued hypertrophy might be related to limitations in blood flow. In hypertension, for example, the increased workload required to pump blood against an elevated arterial pressure results in a progressive increase in left ventricular muscle mass (Fig. 5-2).

There has been recent interest in the signaling pathways that control the arrangement of contractile elements in myocardial hypertrophy. Research suggests that certain signal molecules can alter gene expression controlling the size and assembly of the contractile proteins in hypertrophied myocardial cells. For example, the hypertrophied myocardial cells of well-trained athletes have proportional increases in width and length. This is in contrast to the hypertrophy that develops in dilated cardiomyopathy, in which the hypertrophied cells have a relatively greater increase in length than width. In pressure overload, as occurs with hypertension, the hypertrophied cells have greater width than length.[3] It is anticipated that further elucidation of the signal pathways that determine the adaptive and nonadaptive features of cardiac hypertrophy will lead to new targets for treatment.

HYPERPLASIA

Hyperplasia refers to an increase in the number of cells in an organ or tissue. It occurs in tissues with cells that are capable of mitotic division, such as the epidermis, intestinal epithelium, and glandular tissue. Nerve cells and skeletal and cardiac muscle do not divide and therefore have no capacity for hyperplastic growth. There is evidence that hyperplasia involves activation of genes controlling cell proliferation and the presence of intracellular messengers that control cell replication and growth. As with other normal adaptive cellular responses, hyperplasia is a controlled process that occurs in response to an appropriate stimulus and ceases after the stimulus has been removed.

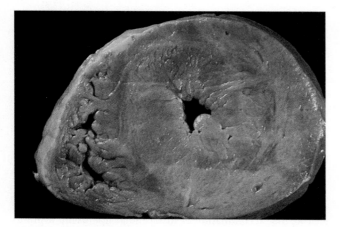

FIGURE 5-2 Myocardial hypertrophy. Cross-section of the heart in a patient with long-standing hypertension. (From Rubin E., Farber J.L. [1999]. *Pathology* [3rd ed., p. 9]. Philadelphia: Lippincott Williams & Wilkins)

The stimuli that induce hyperplasia may be physiologic or nonphysiologic. There are two common types of physiologic hyperplasia: hormonal and compensatory. Breast and uterine enlargement during pregnancy are examples of a physiologic hyperplasia that results from estrogen stimulation. The regeneration of the liver that occurs after partial hepatectomy (*i.e.*, partial removal of the liver) is an example of compensatory hyperplasia. Hyperplasia is also an important response of connective tissue in wound healing, during which proliferating fibroblasts and blood vessels contribute to wound repair. Although hypertrophy and hyperplasia are two distinct processes, they may occur together and are often triggered by the same mechanism.[1] For example, the pregnant uterus undergoes both hypertrophy and hyperplasia as the result of estrogen stimulation.

Most forms of nonphysiologic hyperplasia are due to excessive hormonal stimulation or the effects of growth factors on target tissues.[2] Excessive estrogen production can cause endometrial hyperplasia and abnormal menstrual bleeding (see Chapter 45). Benign prostatic hyperplasia, which is a common disorder of men older than 50 years of age, is thought to be related to the action of androgens (see Chapter 43). Skin warts are an example of hyperplasia caused by growth factors produced by certain viruses, such as papillomaviruses.

METAPLASIA

Metaplasia represents a reversible change in which one adult cell type (epithelial or mesenchymal) is replaced by another adult cell type. Metaplasia is thought to involve the reprogramming of undifferentiated stem cells that are present in the tissue undergoing the metaplastic changes.

Metaplasia usually occurs in response to chronic irritation and inflammation and allows for substitution of cells that are better able to survive under circumstances in which a more fragile cell type might succumb. However, the conversion of cell types never oversteps the boundaries of the primary groups of tissue (*e.g.*, one type of epithelial cell may be converted to another type of epithelial cell, but not to a connective tissue cell). An example of metaplasia is the adaptive substitution of stratified squamous epithelial cells for the ciliated columnar epithelial cells in the trachea and large airways of a habitual cigarette smoker. A vitamin A deficiency also induces squamous metaplasia of the respiratory tract. Although the squamous epithelium is better able to survive in these situations, the protective function that the ciliated epithelium provides for the respiratory tract is lost. Also, continued exposure to the influences that cause metaplasia may predispose to cancerous transformation of the metaplastic epithelium.

DYSPLASIA

Dysplasia is characterized by deranged cell growth of a specific tissue that results in cells that vary in size, shape, and appearance. Minor degrees of dysplasia are associated with chronic irritation or inflammation. The pattern is most frequently encountered in metaplastic squamous epithelium of the respiratory tract and uterine cervix. Although dysplasia is abnormal, it is adaptive in that it is potentially reversible after the irritating cause has been removed. Dysplasia is strongly implicated as a precursor of cancer. In cancers of the respiratory tract and the uterine cervix, dysplastic changes have been found adjacent to the foci of cancerous transformation. Through the use of the Papanicolaou (Pap) smear, it has been documented that cancer of the uterine cervix develops in a series of incremental epithelial changes ranging from severe dysplasia to invasive cancer. However, dysplasia is an adaptive process and as such does not necessarily lead to cancer. In many cases, the dysplastic cells revert to their former structure and function.

INTRACELLULAR ACCUMULATIONS

Intracellular accumulations represent buildup of substances that cells cannot immediately use or dispose of. The substances may accumulate in the cytoplasm (frequently in the lysosomes) or in the nucleus. In some cases the accumulation may be an abnormal substance that the cell has produced, and in other cases the cell may be storing exogenous materials or products of pathologic processes occurring elsewhere in the body. These substances can be grouped into three categories: (1) normal body substances, such as lipids, proteins, carbohydrates, melanin, and bilirubin, that are present in abnormally large amounts; (2) abnormal endogenous products, such as those resulting from inborn errors of metabolism; and (3) exogenous products, such as environmental agents and pigments that cannot be broken down by the cell.[2] These substances may accumulate transiently or permanently, and they may be harmless or in some cases may be toxic.

The accumulation of normal cellular constituents occurs when a substance is produced at a rate that exceeds its metabolism or removal. An example of this type of process is fatty changes in the liver due to intracellular accumulation of triglycerides. Liver cells normally contain some fat, which is either oxidized and used for energy or converted to triglycerides. This fat is derived from free fatty acids released from adipose tissue. Abnormal accumulation occurs when the delivery of free fatty acids to the liver is increased, as in starvation and diabetes mellitus, or when the intrahepatic metabolism of lipids is disturbed, as in alcoholism.

Intracellular accumulation can result from genetic disorders that disrupt the metabolism of selected substances. A normal enzyme may be replaced with an abnormal one, resulting in the formation of a substance that cannot be used or eliminated from the cell, or an enzyme may be missing, so that an intermediate product accumulates in the cell. For example, there are at least 10 genetic disorders that affect glycogen metabolism, most of which lead to the accumulation of intracellular glycogen stores. In the most common form of this disorder, von Gierke's disease, large amounts of glycogen accumulate in the liver and kidneys because of a deficiency of the enzyme glucose-6-phosphatase. Without this enzyme, glycogen cannot be broken down to form glucose. The disorder leads not only to an accumulation of glycogen but to a reduction in blood glucose levels. In Tay-Sachs disease, another genetic disorder, abnormal lipids accumulate in the brain and other tissues, causing motor and mental deterioration beginning at approximately 6 months of age, followed by death at 2 to 3 years of age. In a similar manner, other enzyme defects lead to the accumulation of other substances.

Pigments are colored substances that may accumulate in cells. They can be endogenous (*i.e.*, arising from within the body) or exogenous (*i.e.*, arising from outside the body). Icterus, also called *jaundice*, is a yellow discoloration of tissue caused by the retention of bilirubin, an endogenous bile pigment. This condition may result from increased bilirubin production from red blood cell destruction, obstruction of bile passage into the intestine, or toxic diseases that affect the liver's ability to remove bilirubin from the blood. Lipofuscin is a yellow-brown pigment that results from the accumulation of the indigestible residues produced during normal turnover of cell structures (Fig. 5-3). The accumulation of lipofuscin increases with age and is sometimes referred to as the *wear-and-tear pigment*. It is more common in heart, nerve, and liver cells than other tissues and is seen more often in conditions associated with atrophy of an organ.

One of the most common exogenous pigments is carbon in the form of coal dust. In coal miners or persons exposed to heavily polluted environments, the accumulation of carbon dust blackens the lung tissue and may cause serious lung disease. The formation of a blue lead line along the margins of the gum is one of the diagnostic features of lead poisoning. Tattoos are the result of insoluble pigments introduced into the skin, where they are engulfed by macrophages and persist for a lifetime.

The significance of intracellular accumulations depends on the cause and severity of the condition. Many accumulations, such as lipofuscin and mild fatty change, have no effect on cell function. Some conditions, such as the hyperbilirubinemia that causes jaundice, are reversible. Other disorders, such as glycogen storage diseases, produce accumulations that result in organ dysfunction and other alterations in physiologic function.

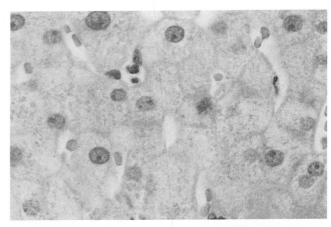

FIGURE 5-3 Accumulation of intracellular lipofuscin. A photomicrograph of the liver of an 80-year-old man shows golden cytoplasmic granules, which represent lysosomal storage of lipofuscin. (From Rubin E., Farber J.L. [1999]. *Pathology* [3rd ed., p. 13]. Philadelphia: Lippincott Williams & Wilkins)

In summary, cells adapt to changes in their environment and in their work demands by changing their size, number, and characteristics. These adaptive changes are consistent with the needs of the cell and occur in response to an appropriate stimulus. The changes are usually reversed after the stimulus has been withdrawn.

When confronted with a decrease in work demands or adverse environmental conditions, cells atrophy or reduce their size and revert to a lower and more efficient level of functioning. Hypertrophy results from an increase in work demands and is characterized by an increase in tissue size brought about by an increase in cell size and functional components in the cell. An increase in the number of cells in an organ or tissue that is still capable of mitotic division is called *hyperplasia*. Metaplasia occurs in response to chronic irritation and represents the substitution of cells of a type that are better able to survive under circumstances in which a more fragile cell type might succumb. Dysplasia is characterized by deranged cell growth of a specific tissue that results in cells that vary in size, shape, and appearance. It is a precursor of cancer.

Under some circumstances, cells may accumulate abnormal amounts of various substances. If the accumulation reflects a correctable systemic disorder, such as the hyperbilirubinemia that causes jaundice, the accumulation is reversible. If the disorder cannot be corrected, as often occurs in many inborn errors of metabolism, the cells become overloaded, causing cell injury and death.

Cell Injury and Death

After you have completed this section of the chapter, you should be able to meet the following objectives:

- ✦ Describe the mechanisms whereby physical agents such as blunt trauma, electrical forces, and extremes of temperature produce cell injury
- ✦ Differentiate between the effects of ionizing and non-ionizing radiation in terms of their ability to cause cell injury
- ✦ Explain how the injurious effects of biologic agents differ from those produced by physical and chemical agents
- ✦ State the mechanisms and manifestations of cell injury associated with lead poisoning
- ✦ State how nutritional imbalances contribute to cell injury
- ✦ Describe three types of reversible cell changes that can occur with cell injury
- ✦ Define *free radical* and relate free radical formation to cell injury and death
- ✦ Describe cell changes that occur with ischemic and hypoxic cell injury
- ✦ Relate the effects of impaired calcium homeostasis to cell injury and death
- ✦ Differentiate cell death associated with necrosis and apoptosis
- ✦ Cite the reasons for the changes that occur with the wet and dry forms of gangrene

Cells can be injured in many ways. The extent to which any injurious agent can cause cell injury and death depends in large measure on the intensity and duration of the injury and the type of cell that is involved. Cell injury is usually reversible up to a certain point, after which irreversible cell injury and death occur. Whether a specific stress causes irreversible or reversible cell injury depends on the severity of the insult and on variables such as blood supply, nutritional status, and regenerative capacity. Cell injury and death are ongoing processes, and in the healthy state, they are balanced by cell renewal.

CAUSES OF CELL INJURY

Cell damage can occur in many ways. For purposes of discussion, the ways by which cells are injured have been grouped into five categories: (1) injury from physical agents, (2) radiation injury, (3) chemical injury, (4) injury from biologic agents, and (5) injury from nutritional imbalances.

Injury From Physical Agents

Physical agents responsible for cell and tissue injury include mechanical forces, extremes of temperature, and electrical forces. They are common causes of injuries due to environmental exposure, occupational and transportation accidents, and physical violence and assault.

Mechanical Forces.   Injury or trauma due to mechanical forces occurs as the result of body impact with another object. The body or the mass can be in motion or, as sometimes happens, both can be in motion at the time of impact. These types of injuries split and tear tissue, fracture bones, injure blood vessels, and disrupt blood flow.

 Cell Injury

- ➤ Cells can be damaged in a number of ways, including physical trauma, extremes of temperature, electrical injury, exposure to damaging chemicals, radiation damage, injury from biologic agents, and nutritional factors.

- ➤ Most injurious agents exert their damaging effects through uncontrolled free radical production, impaired oxygen delivery or utilization, or the destructive effects of uncontrolled intracellular calcium release.

- ➤ Cell injury can be reversible, allowing the cell to recover, or it can be irreversible, causing cell death and necrosis.

- ➤ In contrast to necrosis, which results from tissue injury, apoptosis is a normal physiologic process designed to remove injured or worn-out cells.

Extremes of Temperature. Extremes of heat and cold cause damage to the cell, its organelles, and its enzyme systems. Exposure to low-intensity heat (43° to 46°C), such as occurs with partial-thickness burns and severe heat stroke, causes cell injury by inducing vascular injury, accelerating cell metabolism, inactivating temperature-sensitive enzymes, and disrupting the cell membrane. With more intense heat, coagulation of blood vessels and tissue proteins occurs. Exposure to cold increases blood viscosity and induces vasoconstriction by direct action on blood vessels and through reflex activity of the sympathetic nervous system. The resultant decrease in blood flow may lead to hypoxic tissue injury, depending on the degree and duration of cold exposure. Injury from freezing probably results from a combination of ice crystal formation and vasoconstriction. The decreased blood flow leads to capillary stasis and arteriolar and capillary thrombosis. Edema results from increased capillary permeability.

Electrical Injuries. Electrical injuries can affect the body through extensive tissue injury and disruption of neural and cardiac impulses. The effect of electricity on the body is mainly determined by its voltage, the type of current (*i.e.,* direct or alternating), its amperage, the resistance of the intervening tissue, the pathway of the current, and the duration of exposure.[2,4]

Lightning and high-voltage wires that carry several thousand volts produce the most severe damage.[2] Alternating current (AC) is usually more dangerous than direct current (DC) because it causes violent muscle contractions, preventing the person from releasing the electrical source and sometimes resulting in fractures and dislocations. In electrical injuries, the body acts as a conductor of the electrical current. The current enters the body from an electrical source, such as an exposed wire, and passes through the body and exits to another conductor, such as the moisture on the ground or a piece of metal the person is holding. The pathway that a current takes is critical because the electrical energy disrupts impulses in excitable tissues. Current flow through the brain may interrupt impulses from respiratory centers in the brain stem, and current flow through the chest may cause fatal cardiac arrhythmias.

The resistance to the flow of current in electrical circuits transforms electrical energy into heat. This is why the elements in electrical heating devices are made of highly resistive metals. Much of the tissue damage produced by electrical injuries is caused by heat production in tissues that have the highest electrical resistance. Resistance to electrical current varies from the greatest to the least in bone, fat, tendons, skin, muscles, blood, and nerves. The most severe tissue injury usually occurs at the skin sites where the current enters and leaves the body. After electricity has penetrated the skin, it passes rapidly through the body along the lines of least resistance—through body fluids and nerves. Degeneration of vessel walls may occur, and thrombi may form as current flows along the blood vessels. This can cause extensive muscle and deep tissue injury. Thick, dry skin is more resistant to the flow of electricity than thin, wet skin. It is generally believed that the greater the skin resistance, the greater is the amount of local skin burn, and the less the resistance, the greater are the deep and systemic effects.

Radiation Injury

Electromagnetic radiation comprises a wide spectrum of wave-propagated energy, ranging from ionizing gamma rays to radiofrequency waves (Fig. 5-4). A photon is a particle of radiation energy. Radiation energy above the ultraviolet (UV) range is called *ionizing radiation* because the photons have enough energy to knock electrons off atoms and molecules. *Nonionizing radiation* refers to radiation energy at frequencies below that of visible light. *UV radiation* represents the portion of the spectrum of electromagnetic radiation just above the visible range. It contains increasingly energetic rays that are powerful enough to disrupt intracellular bonds and cause sunburn.

Ionizing Radiation. Ionizing radiation affects cells by causing ionization of molecules and atoms in the cell, by directly hitting the target molecules in the cell, or by producing free radicals that interact with critical cell components.[1,2,5] It can immediately kill cells, interrupt cell replication, or cause a variety of genetic mutations, which may or may not be lethal. Most radiation injury is caused by localized irradiation that is used in treatment of cancer (see Chapter 8). Except for unusual circumstances such as the use of high-dose irradiation that precedes bone marrow transplantation, exposure to whole-body irradiation is rare.

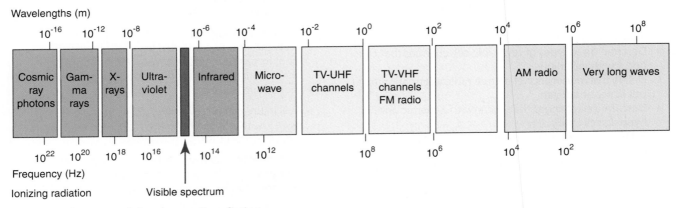

FIGURE 5-4 Spectrum of electromagnetic radiation.

The injurious effects of ionizing radiation vary with the dose, dose rate (a single dose can cause greater injury than divided or fractionated doses), and the differential sensitivity of the exposed tissue to radiation injury. Because of the effect on deoxyribonucleic acid (DNA) synthesis and interference with mitosis, rapidly dividing cells of the bone marrow and intestine are much more vulnerable to radiation injury than tissues such as bone and skeletal muscle. Over time, occupational and accidental exposure to ionizing radiation can result in increased risk for the development of various types of cancers, including skin cancers, leukemia, osteogenic sarcomas, and lung cancer.

Many of the clinical manifestations of radiation injury result from acute cell injury, dose-dependent changes in the blood vessels that supply the irradiated tissues, and fibrotic tissue replacement. The cell's initial response to radiation injury involves swelling, disruption of the mitochondria and other organelles, alterations in the cell membrane, and marked changes in the nucleus. The endothelial cells in blood vessels are particularly sensitive to irradiation. During the immediate postirradiation period, only vessel dilatation takes place (*e.g.*, the initial erythema of the skin after radiation therapy). Later or with higher levels of radiation, destructive changes occur in small blood vessels such as the capillaries and venules. Acute reversible necrosis is represented by such disorders as radiation cystitis, dermatitis, and diarrhea from enteritis. More persistent damage can be attributed to acute necrosis of tissue cells that are not capable of regeneration and chronic ischemia. Chronic effects of radiation damage are characterized by fibrosis and scarring of tissues and organs in the irradiated area (*e.g.*, interstitial fibrosis of the heart and lungs after irradiation of the chest). Because the radiation delivered in radiation therapy inevitably travels through the skin, radiation dermatitis is common. There may be necrosis of the skin, impaired wound healing, and chronic radiation dermatitis.

Ultraviolet Radiation.   Ultraviolet radiation causes sunburn and increases the risk of skin cancers (see Chapter 61). The degree of risk depends on the type of UV rays, the intensity of exposure, and the amount of protective melanin pigment in the skin. Skin damage induced by UV radiation is believed to be caused by reactive oxygen species and by damage to melanin-producing processes in the skin. UV radiation also damages DNA, resulting in the formation of pyrimidine dimers (*i.e.*, the insertion of two identical pyrimidine bases into replicating DNA instead of one). Other forms of DNA damage include the production of single-stranded breaks and formation of DNA–protein cross-links. Normally, errors that occur during DNA replication are repaired by enzymes that remove the faulty section of DNA and repair the damage. The importance of the DNA repair in protecting against UV radiation injury is evidenced by the vulnerability of persons who lack the enzymes needed to repair UV-induced DNA damage. In a genetic disorder called *xeroderma pigmentosum*, an enzyme needed to repair sunlight-induced DNA damage is lacking. This autosomal recessive disorder is characterized by extreme photosensitivity and a 2000-fold increased risk of skin cancer in sun-exposed skin.[2]

Nonionizing Radiation.   Nonionizing radiation includes infrared light, ultrasound, microwaves, and laser energy. Unlike ionizing radiation, which can directly break chemical bonds, nonionizing radiation exerts its effects by causing vibration and rotation of atoms and molecules. All of this vibrational and rotational energy is eventually converted to thermal energy. Low-frequency nonionizing radiation is used widely in radar, television, industrial operations (*e.g.*, heating, welding, melting of metals, processing of wood and plastic), household appliances (*e.g.*, microwave ovens), and medical applications (*e.g.*, diathermy). Isolated cases of skin burns and thermal injury to deeper tissues have occurred in industrial settings and from improperly used household microwave ovens. Injury from these sources is mainly thermal and, because of the deep penetration of the infrared or microwave rays, tends to involve dermal and subcutaneous tissue injury.

Chemical Injury

Chemicals capable of damaging cells are everywhere around us. Air and water pollution contains chemicals capable of tissue injury, as does tobacco smoke and some processed or preserved foods. Some of the most damaging chemicals exist in our environment, including gases such as carbon monoxide, insecticides, and trace metals such as lead.

Chemical agents can injure the cell membrane and other cell structures, block enzymatic pathways, coagulate cell proteins, and disrupt the osmotic and ionic balance of the cell. Corrosive substances such as strong acids and bases destroy cells as the substances come into contact with the body. Other chemicals may injure cells in the process of metabolism or elimination. Carbon tetrachloride (CCl_4), for example, causes little damage until it is metabolized by liver enzymes to a highly reactive free radical ($CCl_3^\bullet$). Carbon tetrachloride is extremely toxic to liver cells.

Drugs.   Many drugs—alcohol, prescription drugs, over-the-counter drugs, and street drugs—are capable of directly or indirectly damaging tissues. Ethyl alcohol can harm the gastric mucosa, liver (see Chapter 38), developing fetus (see Chapter 7), and other organs. Antineoplastic (anticancer) and immunosuppressant drugs can directly injure cells. Other drugs produce metabolic end-products that are toxic to cells. Acetaminophen, a commonly used analgesic drug, is detoxified in the liver, where small amounts of the drug are converted to a highly toxic metabolite. This metabolite is detoxified by a metabolic pathway that uses a substance (*i.e.*, glutathione) normally present in the liver. When large amounts of the drug are ingested, this pathway becomes overwhelmed and toxic metabolites accumulate, causing massive liver necrosis.

Lead Toxicity.   Lead is a particularly toxic metal. Small amounts accumulate to reach toxic levels. There are innumerable sources of lead in the environment, including flaking paint, lead-contaminated dust and soil, lead-contaminated root vegetables, lead water pipes or soldered joints, pottery glazes, and newsprint. Adults often encounter lead through occupational exposure. Lead and other metal smelter workers, miners, welders, storage battery workers, and pottery makers are particularly at risk.[1,6] Children are exposed to lead through ingestion of peeling lead paint, by breathing dust from lead paint (*e.g.*, during remodeling), or from playing in contaminated soil. There has been a substantial decline in blood lead levels of the entire population since the removal of lead from gasoline and from soldered food cans.[7] However, high lead blood levels continue to be a problem, particularly among children. In the Third National Health and Nutrition Examination Survey (NHANES III, 1988 to 1991), blood lead levels were highest in 1- to 2-year-old children and lowest in 12- to 19-year-olds.[7] The prevalence of elevated blood lead levels is higher for children living in more urbanized areas. By race or ethnicity, non-Hispanic black children residing in central cities with a population of 1 million or more have the highest proportion of elevated blood lead levels. A high percentage of Mexican-American children living in the most urbanized areas also had elevated lead levels.[8]

Lead is absorbed through the gastrointestinal tract or the lungs into the blood. A deficiency in calcium, iron, or zinc increases lead absorption. In children, most lead is absorbed through the lungs. Although children may have the same or a lower intake of lead, the absorption in infants and children is greater; thus, they are more vulnerable to lead toxicity.[2] Lead crosses the placenta, exposing the fetus to levels of lead that are comparable with those of the mother. Lead is stored in bone and eliminated by the kidneys. Approximately 85% of absorbed lead is stored in bone (and teeth of young children), 5% to 10% remains in the blood, and the remainder accumulates in soft tissue deposits. Although the half-life of lead is hours to days, bone deposits serve as a repository from which blood levels are maintained. In a sense, bone protects other tissues, but the slow turnover maintains blood levels for months to years.

The toxicity of lead is related to its multiple biochemical effects.[2] It has the ability to inactivate enzymes, compete with calcium for incorporation into bone, and interfere with nerve transmission and brain development. The major targets of lead toxicity are the red blood cells, the gastrointestinal tract, the kidneys, and the nervous system.

Anemia is a cardinal sign of lead toxicity. Lead competes with the enzymes required for hemoglobin synthesis and with the membrane-associated enzymes that prevent hemolysis of red blood cells. The resulting red cells are microscopic and hypochromic, resembling those seen in iron-deficiency anemia. The life span of the red cell is also decreased. The gastrointestinal tract is the main source of symptoms in the adult. This is characterized by "lead colic," a severe and poorly localized form of acute abdominal pain. A lead line formed by precipitated lead sulfite may appear along the gingival margins. The lead line is seldom seen in children. The kidneys are the major route for excretion of lead. Lead can cause diffuse kidney damage, eventually leading to renal failure. Even without overt signs of kidney damage, lead toxicity leads to hypertension.

In the nervous system, lead toxicity is characterized by demyelination of cerebral and cerebellar white matter and death of cortical cells. When this occurs in early childhood, it can affect neurobehavioral development and re-

sult in lower IQ levels and poorer classroom performance.[9] Peripheral demyelinating neuropathy may occur in adults. The most serious manifestation of lead poisoning is acute encephalopathy. It is manifested by persistent vomiting, ataxia, seizures, papilledema, impaired consciousness, and coma. Acute encephalopathy may manifest suddenly, or it may be preceded by other signs of lead toxicity such as behavioral changes or abdominal complaints.

Because of the long-term neurobehavioral and cognitive deficits that occur in children with even moderately elevated lead levels, the Centers for Disease Control and Prevention and the American Academy of Pediatrics have issued recommendations for childhood lead screening.[10–12] A safe blood level of lead is still uncertain. At one time, 25 $\mu g/dL$ was considered safe. Surveys have shown abnormally low IQs in children with levels as low as 10 to 15 $\mu g/dL$; in 1991, the safe level was lowered to 10 $\mu g/dL$.[13]

Screening for lead toxicity involves use of capillary blood obtained from a finger stick to measure free erythrocyte protoporphyrin (EP). Elevated levels of EP result from the inhibition by lead of the enzymes required for heme synthesis in red blood cells. The EP test is useful in detecting high lead levels but usually does not detect levels below 20 to 25 $\mu g/dL$. Thus, capillary screening test values greater than 10 $\mu g/dL$ should be confirmed with those from a venous blood sample. This test also reflects the effects of iron deficiency, a condition that increases lead absorption.[13]

Because the symptoms of lead toxicity usually are vague, diagnosis is often delayed. Anemia may provide the first clues to the disorder. Laboratory tests are necessary to establish a diagnosis. Measurement of lead levels in venous blood is usually used. Treatment involves removal of the lead source and, in cases of severe toxicity, administration of a chelating agent. Asymptomatic children with blood levels of 45 to 69 $\mu g/dL$ usually are treated. A public health team should evaluate the source of lead because meticulous removal is needed.

Injury From Biologic Agents

Biologic agents differ from other injurious agents in that they are able to replicate and can continue to produce their injurious effects. These agents range from submicroscopic viruses to the larger parasites. Biologic agents injure cells by diverse mechanisms. Viruses enter the cell and become incorporated into its DNA synthetic machinery. Certain bacteria elaborate exotoxins that interfere with cellular production of ATP. Other bacteria, such as the gram-negative bacilli, release endotoxins that cause cell injury and increased capillary permeability.

Injury From Nutritional Imbalances

Nutritional excesses and nutritional deficiencies predispose cells to injury. Obesity and diets high in saturated fats are thought to predispose persons to atherosclerosis. The body requires more than 60 organic and inorganic substances in amounts ranging from micrograms to grams. These nutrients include minerals, vitamins, certain fatty acids, and specific amino acids. Dietary deficiencies can occur in the form of starvation, in which there is a deficiency of all nutrients and vitamins, or because of a selective deficiency of a single nutrient or vitamin. Iron-deficiency anemia, scurvy, beriberi, and pellagra are examples of injury caused by the lack of specific vitamins or minerals. The protein and calorie deficiencies that occur with starvation cause widespread tissue damage.

MECHANISMS OF CELL INJURY

The mechanisms by which injurious agents cause cell injury and death are complex. Some agents, such as heat, produce direct cell injury; other factors, such as genetic derangements, produce their effects indirectly through metabolic disturbances and altered immune responses. There seem to be at least three major mechanisms whereby most injurious agents exert their effects: free radical formation, hypoxia and ATP depletion, and disruption of intracellular calcium homeostasis.

Free Radical Injury

Many injurious agents exert their damaging effects through a reactive chemical species called a *free radical*.[2,14–16] Free radical injury is rapidly emerging as a final common pathway for tissue damage by many injurious agents.

In most atoms, the outer electron orbits are filled with paired electrons moving in opposite directions to balance their spins. A free radical is a highly reactive chemical species arising from an atom that has a single unpaired electron in an outer orbit (Fig. 5-5). In this state, the radical is highly unstable and can enter into reactions with cellular constituents, particularly key molecules in cell membranes and nucleic acids. Moreover, free radicals can establish chain reactions, sometimes thousands of events long, as the molecules they react with in turn form free radicals. Chain reactions may branch, causing even greater damage. Uncontrolled free radical production causes damage to cell membranes, cross-linking of cell proteins, inactivation of enzyme systems, or damage to the nucleic acids that make up DNA.

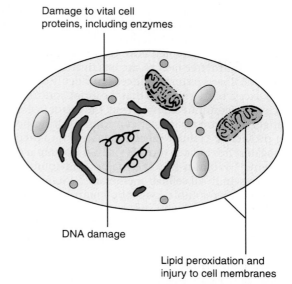

FIGURE 5-6 Mechanisms of free radical cell damage.

Free radical formation is a byproduct of many normal cellular reactions in the body, including energy generation, breakdown of lipids and proteins, and inflammatory processes. For example, free radical generation is the main mechanism for killing microbes in phagocytic white blood cells. Molecular oxygen (O_2), with its two unpaired outer electrons, is the most frequent source of free radicals. During the course of normal cell metabolism, cells process energy-producing oxygen into water; in some reactions, a superoxide radical is formed. Lipid oxidation (*i.e.*, peroxidation) is another source of free radicals. Exogenous sources of free radicals include tobacco smoke, certain pollutants and organic solvents, hyperoxic environments, pesticides, and radiation. Some of these compounds and certain medications are metabolized to free radical intermediates that cause oxidative damage to target tissues.

Although the effects of these reactive free radicals are wide-ranging, three types of effects are particularly important in cell injury: lipid peroxidation, oxidative modification of proteins, and DNA effects (Fig. 5-6). Destruction of the phospholipids in cell membranes, including the outer plasma membrane and those of the intracellular organelles, results in loss of membrane integrity. Free radical attack on cell proteins, particularly those of critical enzymes, can interrupt vital processes throughout the cell. DNA is an important target of the hydroxyl free radical. Damage can involve single-stranded breaks in DNA, modification of base pairs, and cross-links between strands. In most cases, various DNA repair pathways can repair the damage. However, if the damage is extensive, the cell dies. The effects of free radical–mediated DNA changes have also been implicated in aging and malignant transformation of cells.

Under normal conditions, most cells have chemical mechanisms that protect them from the injurious effects of free radicals. These mechanisms commonly break down when the cell is deprived of oxygen or exposed to certain

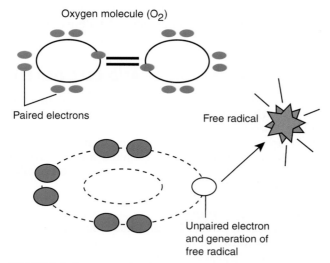

FIGURE 5-5 Oxygen molecule and generation of free radical.

chemical agents, radiation, or other injurious agents. Free radical formation is a particular threat to tissues in which the blood flow has been interrupted and then restored. During the period of interrupted flow, the intracellular mechanisms that control free radicals are inactivated or damaged. When blood flow is restored, the cell is suddenly confronted with an excess of free radicals that it cannot control.

Scientists continue to investigate the use of free radical scavengers to protect against cell injury during periods when protective cellular mechanisms are impaired. Defenses against free radicals include vitamin E, vitamin C, and β-carotene.[17] Vitamin E is the major lipid-soluble antioxidant present in all cellular membranes. Vitamin C is an important water-soluble cytosolic chain-breaking antioxidant; it acts directly with superoxide and singlet oxygen radicals. β-carotene, a pigment found in most plants, reacts with singlet oxygen and can also function as an antioxidant.

Hypoxic Cell Injury

Hypoxia deprives the cell of oxygen and interrupts oxidative metabolism and the generation of ATP. The actual time necessary to produce irreversible cell damage depends on the degree of oxygen deprivation and the metabolic needs of the cell. Well-differentiated cells, such as those in the heart, brain, and kidneys, require large amounts of oxygen to provide energy for their special functions. Brain cells, for example, begin to undergo permanent damage after 4 to 6 minutes of oxygen deprivation. A thin margin can exist between the time involved in reversible and irreversible cell damage. One study found that the epithelial cells of the proximal tubule of the kidney in the rat could survive 20 but not 30 minutes of ischemia.[18]

Hypoxia can result from an inadequate amount of oxygen in the air, respiratory disease, ischemia (*i.e.*, decreased blood flow due to circulatory disorders), anemia, edema, or inability of the cells to use oxygen. Ischemia is characterized by impaired oxygen delivery and impaired removal of metabolic end-products such as lactic acid. In contrast to pure hypoxia, which affects the oxygen content of the blood and affects all of the cells in the body, ischemia commonly affects blood flow through small numbers of blood vessels and produces local tissue injury. In cases of edema, the distance for diffusion of oxygen may become a limiting factor. In hypermetabolic states, the cells may require more oxygen than can be supplied by normal respiratory function and oxygen transport. Hypoxia also serves as the ultimate cause of cell death in other injuries. For example, toxins from certain microorganisms can interfere with cellular use of oxygen, and a physical agent such as cold can cause severe vasoconstriction and impair blood flow.

Hypoxia literally causes a power failure in the cell, with widespread effects on the cell's functional and structural components. As oxygen tension in the cell falls, oxidative metabolism ceases, and the cell reverts to anaerobic metabolism, using its limited glycogen stores in an attempt to maintain vital cell functions. Cellular pH falls as lactic acid accumulates in the cell. This reduction in pH can have profound effects on intracellular structures. The nuclear chromatin clumps and myelin figures, which derive from

destructive changes in cell membranes and intracellular structures, are seen in the cytoplasm and extracellular spaces.

One of the earliest effects of reduced ATP is acute cellular swelling caused by failure of the energy-dependent sodium/potassium (Na^+/K^+) ATPase membrane pump, which extrudes sodium from and returns potassium to the cell. With impaired function of this pump, intracellular potassium levels decrease, and sodium and water accumulate in the cell. The movement of fluid and ions into the cell is associated with dilatation of the endoplasmic reticulum, increased membrane permeability, and decreased mitochondrial function.[2] To this point, the cellular changes due to ischemia are reversible if oxygenation is restored. If the oxygen supply is not restored, however, there is a continued loss of essential enzymes, proteins, and ribonucleic acid through the hyperpermeable membrane of the cell. Injury to the lysosomal membranes results in leakage of destructive lysosomal enzymes into the cytoplasm and enzymatic digestion of cell components. Leakage of intracellular enzymes through the permeable cell membrane into the extracellular fluid is used as an important clinical indicator of cell injury and death. These enzymes enter the blood and can be measured by laboratory tests.

Impaired Calcium Homeostasis

Calcium functions as a messenger for the release of many intracellular enzymes. Normally, intracellular calcium levels are kept extremely low compared with extracellular levels. These low intracellular levels are maintained by energy-dependent membrane-associated calcium/magnesium (Ca^{2+}/Mg^{2+}) ATPase exchange systems.[2] Ischemia and certain toxins lead to an increase in cytosolic calcium because of increased influx across the cell membrane and the release of calcium stored in the mitochondria and endoplasmic reticulum. The increased calcium level activates a number of enzymes with potentially damaging effects. The enzymes include the phospholipases responsible for damaging the cell membrane, proteases that damage the cytoskeleton and membrane proteins, ATPases that break down ATP and hasten its depletion, and endonucleases that fragment chromatin. Although it is known that injured cells accumulate calcium, it is unknown whether this is the ultimate cause of irreversible cell injury.

REVERSIBLE CELL INJURY AND CELL DEATH

The mechanisms of cell injury can produce sublethal and reversible cellular damage or lead to irreversible injury with cell destruction or death (Fig. 5-7). Cell destruction and removal can involve one of two mechanisms: apoptosis, which is designed to remove injured or worn-out cells, or cell death and necrosis, which occurs in irreversibly damaged cells.

Reversible Cell Injury

Reversible cell injury, although impairing cell function, does not result in cell death. Two patterns of reversible cell injury can be observed under the microscope: cellular

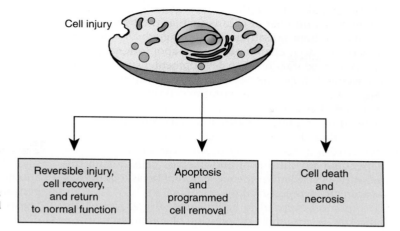

FIGURE 5-7 Outcomes of cell injury: reversible cell injury, apoptosis and programmed cell removal, cell death and necrosis.

swelling and fatty change. Cellular swelling occurs with impairment of the energy-dependent Na^+/K^+ ATPase membrane pump, usually as the result of hypoxic cell injury.

Fatty changes are linked to intracellular accumulation of fat. When fatty changes occur, small vacuoles of fat disperse throughout the cytoplasm. The process is usually more ominous than cellular swelling, and although it is reversible, it usually indicates severe injury. These fatty changes may occur because normal cells are presented with an increased fat load or because injured cells are unable to metabolize the fat properly. In obese persons, fatty infiltrates often occur within and between the cells of the liver and heart because of an increased fat load. Pathways for fat metabolism may be impaired during cell injury, and fat may accumulate in the cell as production exceeds use and export. The liver, where most fats are synthesized and metabolized, is particularly susceptible to fatty change, but fatty changes may also occur in the kidney, the heart, and other organs.

Cell Death

In each cell line, the control of cell number is regulated by a balance of cell proliferation and cell death. Cell death can involve apoptosis or necrosis. Apoptotic cell death involves controlled cell destruction and is involved in normal cell deletion and renewal. For example, blood cells that undergo constant renewal from progenitor cells in the bone marrow are removed by apoptotic cell death. Necrotic cell death is a pathologic form of cell death resulting from cell injury. It is characterized by cell swelling, rupture of the cell membrane, and inflammation.

Apoptosis. *Apoptosis*, from Greek *apo* for "apart" and *ptosis* for "fallen," means *fallen apart*. Apoptotic cell death, which is equated with cell suicide, eliminates cells that are worn out, have been produced in excess, have developed improperly, or have genetic damage. In normal cell turnover, this process provides the space needed for cell replacement. The process, which was first described in 1972, has become one of the most vigorously investigated processes in biology.[19] Apoptosis is thought to be involved in several physiologic and pathologic processes. Current research is focusing on the genetic control mechanisms of apoptosis in

an attempt to understand the pathogenesis of many disease states such as cancer and autoimmune disease.

Apoptotic cell death is characterized by controlled autodigestion of cell components. Cells appear to initiate their own death through the activation of endogenous enzymes. This results in cell shrinkage brought about by disruption of the cytoskeleton, condensation of the cytoplasmic organelles, disruption and clumping of nuclear DNA, and a distinctive wrinkling of the cell membrane.[2] As the cell shrinks, the nucleus breaks into spheres, and the cell eventually divides into membrane-covered fragments. During the process, membrane changes occur, signaling surrounding phagocytic cells to engulf the apoptotic cell and complete the degradation process (Fig. 5-8).

Apoptosis is thought to be responsible for several normal physiologic processes, including programmed destruction of cells during embryonic development, hormone-dependent involution of tissues, death of immune cells, cell death by cytotoxic T cells, and cell death in proliferat-

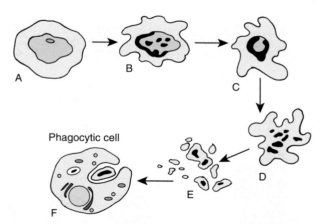

FIGURE 5-8 Apoptotic cell removal: (**A**) shrinking of the cell structures, (**B** and **C**) condensation and fragmentation of the nuclear chromatin, (**D** and **E**) separation of nuclear fragments and cytoplasmic organelles into apoptotic bodies, and (**F**) engulfment of apoptotic fragments by phagocytic cell.

ing cell populations. During embryogenesis, in the development of a number of organs such as the heart, which begins as a single pulsating tube and is gradually modified to become a four-chambered pump, apoptotic cell death allows the next stage of organ development. It also separates the webbed fingers and toes of the developing embryo (Fig. 5-9). The control of immune cell numbers and destruction of autoreactive T cells in the thymus have been credited to apoptosis. Cytotoxic T cells and natural killer cells are thought to destroy target cells by inducing apoptotic cell death. Apoptotic cell death occurs in the hormone-dependent involution of endometrial cells during the menstrual cycle and in the regression of breast tissue after weaning from breast-feeding.

Apoptosis appears to be linked to several pathologic processes. For example, suppression of apoptosis may be a determinant in the growth of cancers. Apoptosis is also thought to be involved in the cell death associated with certain viral infections, such as hepatitis B and C, and in cell death caused by a variety of injurious agents, such as mild thermal injury and radiation injury. Apoptosis may also be involved in neurodegenerative disorders such as Alzheimer's disease, Parkinson's disease, and amyotrophic lateral sclerosis (ALS). The loss of cells in these disorders does not induce inflammation; although the initiating event is unknown, apoptosis appears to be the mechanism of cell death.[20]

Several mechanisms appear to be involved in initiating cell death by apoptosis. As in the case of endometrial changes that occur during the menstrual cycle, the process can be triggered by the addition or withdrawal of hormones. In hepatitis B and C, the virus seems to sensitize the hepatocytes to apoptosis.[21] Certain oncogenes and suppressor genes involved in the development of cancer seem to play an active role in stimulation or suppression of apoptosis. Injured cells may induce apoptotic cell death through increased cytoplasmic calcium, which leads to activation of nuclear enzymes that break down DNA. In some instances, gene transcription and protein synthesis, the events that produce new cells, may be the initiating factors. In other cases, cell surface signaling or receptor activation appears to be the influencing force.

Necrosis. Necrosis refers to cell death in an organ or tissue that is still part of a living person. Necrosis differs from apoptosis in that it involves unregulated enzymatic digestion of cell components, loss of cell membrane integrity with uncontrolled release of the products of cell death into the intracellular space, and initiation of the inflammatory response. In contrast to apoptosis, which functions in removing cells so they can be replaced by new cells, necrosis often interferes with cell replacement and tissue regeneration.

With necrotic cell death, there are marked changes in the appearance of the cytoplasmic contents and the nucleus. These changes often are not visible, even under the microscope, for hours after cell death. The dissolution of the necrotic cell or tissue can follow several paths. The cell can undergo liquefaction (*i.e.*, liquefaction necrosis); it can be transformed to a gray, firm mass (*i.e.*, coagulation necrosis); or it can be converted to a cheesy material by infiltration of fatlike substances (*i.e.*, caseous necrosis). *Liquefaction necrosis* occurs when some of the cells die but their catalytic enzymes are not destroyed. An example of liquefaction necrosis is the softening of the center of an abscess with discharge of its contents. During *coagulation necrosis*, acido-

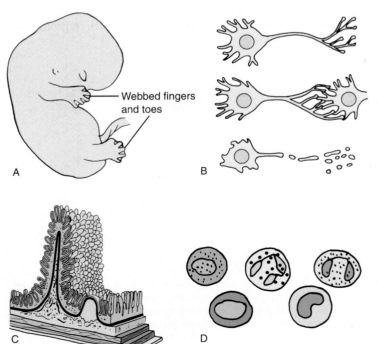

A

B

Webbed fingers and toes

C

D

FIGURE 5-9 Examples of apoptosis: (**A**) separation of webbed fingers and toes in embryo, (**B**) development of neural connections, (**C**) removal of cells from intestinal villa, and (**D**) removal of senescent blood cells. (**C** from Chaffee E.E., Lytle I.M. [1980]. *Basic physiology and anatomy* [4th ed.]. Philadelphia: J.B. Lippincott)

sis develops and denatures the enzymatic and structural proteins of the cell. This type of necrosis is characteristic of hypoxic injury and is seen in infarcted areas. *Infarction* (*i.e.*, tissue death) occurs when an artery supplying an organ or part of the body becomes occluded and no other source of blood supply exists. As a rule, the infarct's shape is conical and corresponds to the distribution of the artery and its branches. An artery may be occluded by an embolus, a thrombus, disease of the arterial wall, or pressure from outside the vessel. *Caseous necrosis* (*i.e.*, soft, cheeselike center) is a distinctive form of coagulation necrosis. It is most commonly associated with tubercular lesions and is thought to result from immune mechanisms.

Gangrene

The term *gangrene* is applied when a considerable mass of tissue undergoes necrosis. Gangrene may be classified as dry or moist. In dry gangrene, the part becomes dry and shrinks, the skin wrinkles, and its color changes to dark brown or black. The spread of dry gangrene is slow, and its symptoms are not as marked as those of wet gangrene. The irritation caused by the dead tissue produces a line of inflammatory reaction (*i.e.*, line of demarcation) between the dead tissue of the gangrenous area and the healthy tissue (Fig. 5-10). Dry gangrene usually results from interference with arterial blood supply to a part without interference with venous return and is a form of coagulation necrosis.

In moist or wet gangrene, the area is cold, swollen, and pulseless. The skin is moist, black, and under tension. Blebs form on the surface, liquefaction occurs, and a foul odor is caused by bacterial action. There is no line of demarcation between the normal and diseased tissues, and the spread of tissue damage is rapid. Systemic symptoms are usually severe, and death may occur unless the condition can be arrested. Moist or wet gangrene primarily results from interference with venous return from the part. Bacterial invasion plays an important role in the development of wet gangrene and is responsible for many of its prominent symptoms. Dry gangrene is confined almost ex-

clusively to the extremities, but moist gangrene may affect the internal organs or the extremities. If bacteria invade the necrotic tissue, dry gangrene may be converted to wet gangrene.

Gas gangrene is a special type of gangrene that results from infection of devitalized tissues by one of several *Clostridium* bacteria. These anaerobic and spore-forming organisms are widespread in nature, particularly in soil; gas gangrene is prone to occur in trauma and compound fractures in which dirt and debris are embedded. Some species have been isolated in the stomach, gallbladder, intestine, vagina, and skin of healthy persons. The bacteria produce toxins that dissolve the cell membranes, causing death of muscle cells, massive spreading edema, hemolysis of red blood cells, hemolytic anemia, hemoglobinuria, and renal toxicity.[22] Characteristic of this disorder are the bubbles of hydrogen sulfide gas that form in the muscle. Gas gangrene is a serious and potentially fatal disease. Because the organism is anaerobic, oxygen is sometimes administered in a hyperbaric chamber.

In summary, cell injury can be caused by a number of agents, including physical agents, chemicals, biologic agents, and nutritional factors. Among the physical agents that generate cell injury are mechanical forces that produce tissue trauma, extremes of temperature, electricity, radiation, and nutritional disorders. Chemical agents can cause cell injury through several mechanisms: they can block enzymatic pathways, cause coagulation of tissues, or disrupt the osmotic or ionic balance of the cell. Biologic agents differ from other injurious agents in that they are able to replicate and continue to produce injury. Among the nutritional factors that contribute to cell injury are excesses and deficiencies of nutrients, vitamins, and minerals.

Injurious agents exert their effects largely through generation of free radicals, production of cell hypoxia, or unregulated intracellular calcium levels. Partially reduced oxygen species called *free radicals* are important mediators of cell injury in many pathologic conditions. They are an important cause of cell injury in hypoxia and after exposure to radiation and certain chemical agents. Lack of oxygen underlies the pathogenesis of cell injury in hypoxia and ischemia. Hypoxia can result from inadequate oxygen in the air, cardiorespiratory disease, anemia, or the inability of the cells to use oxygen. Increased intracellular calcium activates a number of enzymes with potentially damaging effects.

Injurious agents may produce sublethal and reversible cellular damage or may lead to irreversible cell injury and death. Cell death can involve two mechanisms: apoptosis or necrosis. Apoptosis involves controlled cell destruction and is the means by which the body removes and replaces cells that have been produced in excess, developed improperly, have genetic damage, or are worn out. Necrosis refers to cell death that is characterized by cell swelling, rupture of the cell membrane, and inflammation.

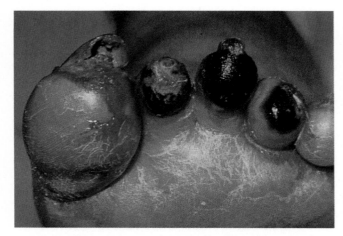

FIGURE 5-10 Gangrenous toes. (Biomedical Communications Group, Southern Illinois University School of Medicine, Springfield, IL)

Tissue Repair and Wound Healing

After you have completed this section of the chapter, you should be able to meet the following objectives:

✦ Define the terms *parenchymal* and *stromal* as they relate to the tissues of an organ

✦ Compare labile, stable, and permanent cell types in terms of their capacity for regeneration

✦ Describe healing by primary and secondary intention

✦ Trace the wound-healing process through the inflammatory, proliferative, and remodeling phases

✦ Explain the effect of malnutrition; ischemia and oxygen deprivation; impaired immune and inflammatory responses; and infection, wound separation, and foreign bodies on wound healing

✦ Discuss the effect of age on wound healing

Body organs and structures contain two types of tissues: parenchymal and stromal. The parenchymal (*i.e.*, from the Greek for "anything poured in") tissues contain the functioning cells of an organ or body part (*e.g.*, hepatocytes, renal tubular cells). The stromal tissues (*i.e.*, from the Greek for "something laid out to lie on") consist of the supporting connective tissues, blood vessels, and nerve fibers.

Injured tissues are repaired by regeneration of parenchymal cells or by connective tissue repair in which scar tissue is substituted for the parenchymal cells of the injured tissue. The primary objective of the healing process is to fill the gap created by tissue destruction and to restore the structural continuity of the injured part. When regeneration cannot occur, healing by replacement with a connective scar tissue provides the means for maintaining this continuity. Although scar tissue fills the gap created by tissue death, it does not repair the structure with functioning parenchymal cells. Because the regenerative capabilities of most tissues are limited, wound healing usually involves some connective tissue repair.

Considerable research has contributed to the understanding of chemical mediators and growth factors that orchestrate the healing process.[1,2] These chemical mediators and growth factors are released in an orderly manner from many of the cells that participate in the healing process. Some growth factors act as chemoattractants, enhancing the migration of white blood cells and fibroblasts to the wound site, and others act as mitogens, causing increased proliferation of cells that participate in the healing process.[23] For example, platelet-derived growth factor, which is released from activated platelets, attracts white blood cells and acts as a growth factor for blood vessels and fibroblasts. Many of the cytokines discussed in Chapter 18 are growth factors.

REGENERATION

Regeneration involves replacement of the injured tissue with cells of the same parenchymal type, leaving little or no evidence of the previous injury. The ability to regenerate varies with the tissue and cell type. Body cells are divided

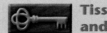

Tissue Repair and Wound Healing

➤ Injured tissues can be repaired by regeneration of the injured tissue cells with cells of the same tissue or parenchymal type, or by connective repair processes in which scar tissue is used to effect healing.

➤ Regeneration is limited to tissues with cells that are able to undergo mitosis.

➤ Connective tissue repair occurs by primary or secondary intention and involves the inflammatory phase, the proliferative phase, and the remodeling phase.

➤ Wound healing is impaired by conditions that diminish blood flow and oxygen delivery, restrict nutrients and other materials needed for healing, and depress the inflammatory and immune responses; and by infection, wound separation, and presence of foreign bodies.

into three types according to their ability to undergo regeneration: labile, stable, or permanent cells.[1]

Labile cells are those that continue to divide and replicate throughout life, replacing cells that are continually being destroyed. Labile cells can be found in tissues that have a daily turnover of cells. They include the surface epithelial cells of the skin, the oral cavity, vagina, and cervix; the columnar epithelium of the gastrointestinal tract, uterus, and fallopian tubes; the transitional epithelium of the urinary tract; and bone marrow cells.

Stable cells are those that normally stop dividing when growth ceases. These cells are capable, however, of undergoing regeneration when confronted with an appropriate stimulus. For stable cells to regenerate and restore tissues to their original state, the supporting stromal framework must be present. When this framework has been destroyed, the replacement of tissues is haphazard. The hepatocytes of the liver are one form of stable cell, and the importance of the supporting framework to regeneration is evidenced by two forms of liver disease. In some types of viral hepatitis, for example, there is selective destruction of the parenchymal liver cells, while the cells of the supporting tissue remain unharmed. After the disease has subsided, the injured cells regenerate, and liver function returns to normal. In cirrhosis of the liver, fibrous bands of tissue form and replace the normal supporting tissues of the liver, causing disordered replacement of liver cells and disturbance of hepatic blood flow and liver function.

Permanent or *fixed cells* cannot undergo mitotic division. The fixed cells include nerve cells, skeletal cells, and cardiac muscle cells. These cells cannot regenerate; once destroyed, they are replaced with fibrous scar tissue that lacks the functional characteristics of the destroyed tissue.

For example, the scar tissue that develops in the heart after a heart attack cannot conduct impulses or contract to pump blood.

CONNECTIVE TISSUE REPAIR

Connective tissue replacement is an important process in the repair of tissue. It allows replacement of nonregenerated parenchymal cells by a connective tissue scar. Depending on the extent of tissue loss, wound closure and healing occur by *primary* or *secondary* intention. A sutured surgical incision is an example of healing by primary intention. Larger wounds (*e.g.*, burns and large surface wounds) that have a greater loss of tissue and contamination, heal by secondary intention. Healing by secondary intention is slower than healing by primary intention and results in the formation of larger amounts of scar tissue. A wound that might otherwise have healed by primary intention may become infected and heal by secondary intention.

Wound healing is commonly divided into three phases: the inflammatory phase, the proliferative phase, and the maturational or remodeling phase.[24,25] In wounds healing by primary intention, the duration of the phases is fairly predictable. In wounds healing by secondary intention, the process depends on the extent of injury and the healing environment.

Inflammatory Phase

The inflammatory phase of wound healing begins at the time of injury and is a critical period because it prepares the wound environment for healing. It includes hemostasis (Chapter 14) and the vascular and cellular phases of inflammation (Chapter 18). Hemostatic processes are activated immediately at the time of injury. There is constriction of injured blood vessel and initiation of blood clotting by way of platelet activation and aggregation. After a brief period of constriction, these same vessels dilate and capillaries increase their permeability, allowing plasma and blood components to leak into the injured area. In small surface wounds, the clot loses fluid and becomes a hard, desiccated scab that protects the area.

The cellular phase of inflammation follows and is evidenced by the migration of phagocytic white blood cells that digest and remove invading organisms, fibrin, extracellular debris, and other foreign matter. The neutrophils or polymorphonuclear cells (PMNs) are the first cells to arrive and are usually gone by day 3 or 4. They ingest bacteria and cellular debris. Approximately 24 hours after the arrival of the PMNs, a larger and less specific phagocytic cell, called a *macrophage*, enters the wound area and remains for an extended period. This cell, arising from blood monocytes, is an essential cell in the healing process. Its functions include phagocytosis and release of growth factors that stimulate epithelial cell growth, angiogenesis (*i.e.*, growth of new blood vessels), and attraction of fibroblasts. When a large defect occurs in deeper tissues, PMNs and macrophages are required to remove the debris and facilitate wound closure. Although a wound may heal in the absence of PMNs, it cannot heal in the absence of macrophages.

Proliferative Phase

The proliferative phase of healing usually begins within 2 to 3 days of injury and may last as long as 3 weeks in wounds healing by primary intention. The primary processes during this time focus on the building of new tissue to fill the wound space. The key cell during this phase is the *fibroblast*. The fibroblast is a connective tissue cell that synthesizes and secretes collagen and other intercellular elements needed for wound healing. Fibroblasts also produce a family of growth factors that induce angiogenesis and endothelial cell proliferation and migration.

As early as 24 to 48 hours after injury, fibroblasts and vascular endothelial cells begin proliferating to form a specialized type of soft, pink granular tissue, called *granulation tissue*, that serves as the foundation for scar tissue development (Fig. 5-11). This tissue is fragile and bleeds easily because of the numerous, newly developed capillary buds. Wounds that heal by secondary intention have more necrotic debris and exudate that must be removed, and they involve larger amounts of granulation tissue. The newly formed blood vessels are leaky and allow plasma proteins and white blood cells to leak into the tissues. At approximately the same time, epithelial cells at the margin of the wound begin to regenerate and move toward the center of the wound, forming a new surface layer that is similar to that destroyed by the injury. In wounds that heal by primary intention, these epidermal cells proliferate and seal the wound within 24 to 48 hours.[26] When a scab has formed on the wound, the epithelial cells migrate between it and the underlying viable tissue; when a significant portion of the wound has been covered with epithelial tissue, the scab lifts off. At times, excessive granulation tissue, sometimes referred to as *proud flesh*, may form and extend above the edges of wound, preventing reepithelialization from taking place. Surgical removal or chemical cauterization of the defect allows healing to proceed.

As the proliferative phase progresses, there is continued accumulation of collagen and proliferation of fibroblasts. Collagen synthesis reaches a peak within 5 to 7 days and continues for several weeks, depending on wound size. By the second week, the white blood cells have largely left the area, the edema has diminished, and the wound begins to blanch as the small blood vessels become thrombosed and degenerate.

Remodeling Phase

The third phase of wound healing, the remodeling process, begins approximately 3 weeks after injury and can continue for 6 months or longer, depending on the extent of the wound. As the term implies, there is continued remodeling of scar tissue by simultaneous synthesis of collagen by fibroblasts and lysis by collagenase enzymes. As a result of these two processes, the architecture of the scar becomes reoriented to increase the tensile strength of the wound.

Most wounds do not regain the full tensile strength of unwounded skin after healing is completed. Carefully sutured wounds immediately after surgery have approximately 70% of the strength of unwounded skin, largely because of the placement of the sutures. This allows persons to move about freely after surgery without fear of wound separation.

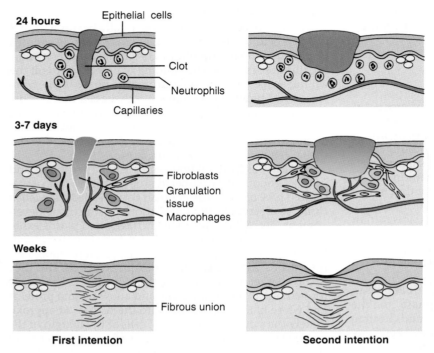

FIGURE 5-11 Healing of a skin wound by primary and secondary intention. First 24 hours: formation of a blood clot and migration of neutrophils. 3–7 days: angiogenesis, migration of macrophages and fibroblasts, and development of granulation tissue. Weeks following injury: development of the fibrous scar, disappearance of increased vascularity, and exit of inflammatory cells.

When the sutures are removed, usually at the end of the first week, wound strength is approximately 10%. It increases rapidly over the next 4 weeks and then slows, reaching a plateau of approximately 70% to 80% of the tensile strength of unwounded skin at the end of 3 months.[2] An injury that heals by secondary intention undergoes wound contraction during the proliferative and remodeling phases. As a result, the scar that forms is considerably smaller than the original wound. Cosmetically, this may be desirable because it reduces the size of the visible defect. However, contraction of scar tissue over joints and other body structures tends to limit movement and cause deformities. As a result of loss of elasticity, scar tissue that is stretched fails to return to its original length.

An abnormality in healing by scar tissue repair is *keloid* formation. Keloids are tumorlike masses caused by excess production of scar tissue. The tendency toward development of keloids is more common in African Americans and seems to have a genetic basis.

FACTORS THAT AFFECT WOUND HEALING

Many local and systemic factors influence wound healing. Although there are many factors that impair healing, science has found a few ways to hasten the normal process of wound repair. Among the causes of impaired wound healing are malnutrition; impaired blood flow and oxygen delivery; impaired inflammatory and immune responses; infection, wound separation, and foreign bodies; and age effects.

Malnutrition
Successful wound healing depends in part on adequate stores of proteins, carbohydrates, fats, vitamins, and minerals. It is well recognized that malnutrition slows the heal-

ing process, causing wounds to heal inadequately or incompletely.[27] Protein deficiencies prolong the inflammatory phase of healing and impair fibroblast proliferation, collagen, and protein matrix synthesis, angiogenesis, and wound remodeling. Carbohydrates are needed as an energy source for white blood cells. Carbohydrates also have a protein-sparing effect and help to prevent the use of amino acids for fuel when they are needed for the healing process. Fats are essential constituents of cell membranes and are needed for the synthesis of new cells.

Although most vitamins are essential cofactors for the daily functions of the body, vitamins A and C play an essential role in the healing process. Vitamin C is needed for collagen synthesis. In vitamin C deficiency, improper sequencing of amino acids occurs, proper linking of amino acids does not take place, the byproducts of collagen synthesis are not removed from the cell, new wounds do not heal properly, and old wounds may fall apart. Administration of vitamin C rapidly restores the healing process to normal. Vitamin A functions in stimulating and supporting epithelialization, capillary formation, and collagen synthesis. Vitamin A also has been shown to counteract the anti-inflammatory effects of corticosteroid drugs and can be used to reverse these effects in persons who are on chronic steroid therapy. The B vitamins are important cofactors in enzymatic reactions that contribute to the wound-healing process. All are water soluble, and with the exception of vitamin B_{12}, which is stored in the liver, almost all must be replaced daily. Vitamin K plays an indirect role in wound healing by preventing bleeding disorders that contribute to hematoma formation and subsequent infection.

The role of minerals in wound healing is less clearly defined. The macrominerals, including sodium, potassium, calcium, and phosphorus, as well as the microminerals such as copper and zinc, must be present for normal cell function. Zinc is a cofactor in a variety of enzyme systems responsible for cell proliferation. In animal studies, zinc has been found to aid in reepithelialization.

Blood Flow and Oxygen Delivery

For healing to occur, wounds must have adequate blood flow to supply the necessary nutrients and to remove the resulting waste, local toxins, bacteria, and other debris. Impaired wound healing due to poor blood flow may occur as a result of wound conditions (*e.g.*, swelling) or preexisting health problems. Arterial disease and venous pathology are well-documented causes of impaired wound healing. In situations of trauma, a decrease in blood volume may cause a reduction in blood flow to injured tissues.

Molecular oxygen is required for collagen synthesis. It has been shown that even a temporary lack of oxygen can result in the formation of less stable collagen.[28,29] Wounds in ischemic tissue become infected more frequently than wounds in well-vascularized tissue. PMNs and macrophages require oxygen for destruction of microorganisms that have invaded the area. Although these cells can accomplish phagocytosis in a relatively anoxic environment, they cannot digest bacteria.

Impaired Inflammatory and Immune Responses

Inflammatory and immune mechanisms function in wound healing. Inflammation is essential to the first phase of wound healing, and immune mechanisms prevent infections that impair wound healing. Among the conditions that impair inflammation and immune function are disorders of phagocytic function, diabetes mellitus, and therapeutic administration of corticosteroid drugs.

Phagocytic disorders may be divided into extrinsic and intrinsic defects. Extrinsic disorders are those that impair attraction of phagocytic cells to the wound site, prevent engulfment of bacteria and foreign agents by the phagocytic cells (*i.e.*, opsonization), or cause suppression of the total number of phagocytic cells (*e.g.*, immunosuppressive agents). Intrinsic phagocytic disorders are the result of enzymatic deficiencies in the metabolic pathway for destroying the ingested bacteria by the phagocytic cell. The intrinsic phagocytic disorders include chronic granulomatous disease (see Chapter 19), an X-linked inherited disease in which there is a deficiency of myeloperoxidase and nicotinamide-adenine dinucleotide peroxidase (NADPH)-dependent oxidase enzyme. Deficiencies of these compounds prevent generation of hydrogen superoxide and hydrogen peroxide needed for killing bacteria.

Wound healing is a problem in persons with diabetes mellitus, particularly those who have poorly controlled blood glucose levels. Studies have shown delayed wound healing, poor collagen formation, and poor tensile strength in diabetic animals. Of particular importance is the effect of hyperglycemia on phagocytic function. Neutrophils, for example, have diminished chemotactic and phagocytic function, including engulfment and intracellular killing of bacteria, when exposed to altered glucose levels. Small blood vessel disease is also common among persons with diabetes, impairing the delivery of inflammatory cells, oxygen, and nutrients to the wound site.

The therapeutic administration of corticosteroid drugs decreases the inflammatory process and may delay the healing process. These hormones decrease capillary permeability during the early stages of inflammation, impair the phagocytic property of the leukocytes, and inhibit fibroblast proliferation and function.

Infection, Wound Separation, and Foreign Bodies

Wound contamination, wound separation, and foreign bodies delay wound healing. Infection impairs all dimensions of wound healing. It prolongs the inflammatory phase, impairs the formation of granulation tissue, and inhibits proliferation of fibroblasts and deposition of collagen fibers. All wounds are contaminated at the time of injury. Although body defenses can handle the invasion of microorganisms at the time of wounding, badly contaminated wounds can overwhelm host defenses. Trauma and existing impairment of host defenses also can contribute to the development of wound infections.

Approximation of the wound edges (*i.e.*, suturing of an incision type of wound) greatly enhances healing and prevents infection. Epithelialization of a wound with closely approximated edges occurs within 1 to 2 days. Large, gaping wounds tend to heal more slowly because it is often impossible to effect wound closure with this type of wound. Foreign bodies tend to invite bacterial contamination and delay healing. Fragments of wood, steel, glass, and other compounds may have entered the wound at the site of injury and can be difficult to locate when the wound is treated. Sutures are also foreign bodies, and although needed for the closure of surgical wounds, they are an impediment to healing. This is why sutures are removed as soon as possible after surgery. Wound infections are of special concern in persons with implantation of foreign bodies such as orthopedic devices (*e.g.*, pins, stabilization devices), cardiac pacemakers, and shunt catheters. These infections are difficult to treat and may require removal of the device.

Bite Wounds. Animal and human bites are particularly troublesome in terms of infection.[30,31] The animal inflicting the bite, the location of the bite, and the type of injury are all important determinants of whether the wound becomes infected. Approximately 28% to 80% of all cat bites become infected. Dog bites, for unclear reasons, become infected only approximately 3% to 18% of the time. Bites inflicted by children are usually superficial and seldom become infected, whereas bites inflicted by adults have a much higher rate of infection. Puncture wounds are more likely to become infected than lacerations, probably because lacerations are easier to irrigate and debride.

Treatment of bite wounds involves vigorous irrigation and cleansing as well as debridement or removal of necrotic tissue. Whether bite wounds are closed with sutures to promote healing by primary intention depends on the location of the bite and whether the wound is already infected. Wounds that are not infected and require closure for mechanical or cosmetic reasons may be sutured. Wounds of the hand are not usually sutured because closed-space infection of the hand can produce loss of function. Antibiotics are usually administered prophylactically to persons with high-risk bites (*e.g.*, cat bites in any location and human or animal bites to the hand). All persons with bites should be evaluated to determine if tetanus or rabies prophylaxis is needed.

Effect of Age

The effects of immaturity and aging affect healing. The rate of skin replacement slows with aging.

Wound Healing in Neonates and Children. Wound healing in the pediatric population follows a course similar to that in the adult population.[32] The child has a greater capacity for repair than the adult but may lack the reserves needed to ensure proper healing. Such lack is evidenced by an easily upset electrolyte balance, sudden elevation or lowering of temperature, and rapid spread of infection. The neonate and small child may have an immature immune system with no antigenic experience with organisms that contaminate wounds. The younger the child, the more likely is the development of immune depression.

Successful wound healing also depends on adequate nutrition. Children need sufficient calories to maintain growth and wound healing. The premature infant is often born with immature organ systems and minimal energy stores but high metabolic requirements—a condition that predisposes to impaired wound healing.

Wound Healing in Aged Persons. The rate of cell replacement is slowed in normal aging skin and in the reepithelialization of open wounds.[33] The skin is more fragile and easily wounded. There is a gradual decline in immune function in the elderly. Multiple illnesses, circulatory problems, and nutritional deficits compound the wound-healing process. The elderly are more vulnerable to chronic wounds than younger persons and these wounds heal more slowly.

In summary, the ability of tissues to repair damage due to injury depends on the body's ability to replace the parenchymal cells and to organize them as they were originally. Regeneration describes the process by which tissue is replaced with cells of a similar type and function. Healing by regeneration is limited to tissue with cells that are able to divide and replace the injured cells. Body cells are divided into types according to their ability to regenerate: labile cells, such as the epithelial cells of the skin and gastrointestinal tract, which continue to regenerate throughout life; stable cells, such as those in the liver, which normally do not divide but are capable of regeneration when confronted with an appropriate stimulus; and permanent or fixed cells, such as nerve cells, which are unable to regenerate. Scar tissue repair involves the substitution of fibrous connective tissue for injured tissue that cannot be repaired by regeneration.

Wound healing occurs by primary and secondary intention and is commonly divided into three phases:

the inflammatory phase, the proliferative phase, and the maturational or remodeling phase. In wounds healing by primary intention, the duration of the phases is fairly predictable. In wounds healing by secondary intention, the process depends on the extent of injury and the healing environment. Wound healing can be impaired or complicated by factors such as malnutrition; restricted blood flow and oxygen delivery; diminished inflammatory and immune responses; and infection, wound separation, and the presence of foreign bodies.

References

1. Rubin E., Farber J.L. (Eds.). (1999). *Pathology* (3rd ed., pp. 6–13, 87–103, 329–330, 338–341). Philadelphia: Lippincott Williams & Wilkins.
2. Cotran R.S., Kumar V., Collins T. (Eds.). (1999). *Robbins pathologic basis of disease* (6th ed., pp. 6–8, 12–14, 31–43, 102–111, 310, 420, 421, 424–428). Philadelphia: W.B. Saunders.
3. Hunter J.J., Chien K.R. (1999). Signaling pathways in cardiac hypertrophy and failure. *New England Journal of Medicine* 341(17), 1276–1283.
4. Goodwin C.W. (1996). Electrical injury. In Bennett J.C., Plum F. (Eds.). *Cecil textbook of medicine* (20th ed., pp. 64–67). Philadelphia: W.B. Saunders.
5. Upton A.C. (1996). Radiation injury. In Bennett J.C., Plum F. (Eds.). *Cecil textbook of medicine* (20th ed., pp. 59–64). Philadelphia: W.B. Saunders.
6. Landrigan P.J., Todd A. C. (1994). Lead poisoning. *Western Journal of Medicine* 161, 153–156.
7. Brody D.J., Pirkle J.L, Kramer R.A. (1994). Blood lead levels in the US population: Phase I of the Third National Health and Nutrition Examination Survey (NHANES III, 1988–1991). *Journal of the American Medical Association* 272(4), 277–283.
8. Pirkle J.L., Brody D.J., Gunter E.W. (1994). The decline in blood lead levels in the United States: The National Health and Nutrition Examination Surveys (NHANES). *Journal of the American Medical Association* 272(4), 284–291.
9. Piomelli S. (1996). Lead poisoning. In Behrman R.E., Kliegman R.M., Arvin A.M. (Eds.). *Nelson textbook of pediatrics* (15th ed., pp. 2010–2013). Philadelphia: W.B. Saunders.
10. Ellis M.R., Kane K.Y. (2000). Lightening the lead load in children. *American Family Physician* 62, 545–554, 559–560.
11. Centers for Disease Control and Prevention. (1997). *Screening young children for lead poisoning: Guidance for state and local health officials.* Atlanta: Centers for Disease Control and Prevention, National Center for Environmental Health, U.S. Department of Health and Human Services, Public Health Service.
12. American Academy of Pediatrics Committee on Environmental Health. (1998). Screening for elevated blood levels. *Pediatrics* 101, 1072–1078.
13. Centers for Disease Control. (1991). *Preventing lead poisoning in young children: A statement by the Centers for Disease Control.* Atlanta: U.S. Department of Health and Human Services, Public Health Service.
14. McCord J.M. (2000). The evolution of free radicals and oxidative stress. *American Journal of Medicine* 108, 652–659.
15. Kerr M.E., Bender C.M., Monti E.J. (1996). An introduction to oxygen free radicals. *Heart and Lung* 25, 200–209.
16. Betteridge D.J. (2000). What is oxidative stress? *Metabolism* 49 (2), 3–8.

17. Machlin L.J., Bendich A. (1987). Free radical tissue damage: Protective role of antioxidant nutrients. *FASEB Journal* 1(6), 441–445.

18. Vogt M.T., Farber E. (1968). On the molecular pathology of ischemic renal cell death: Reversible and irreversible cellular and mitochondrial metabolic alterations. *American Journal of Pathology* 53, 1–26.

19. Skikumar P., Dong Z., Mikhailov V., Denton M., Weinberg J.M., Venkatachalam M.A. (1999). Apoptosis: Definitions, mechanisms, and relevance to disease. *American Journal of Medicine* 107, 490–505.

20. Thompson C.B. (1995). Apoptosis in the pathogenesis and treatment of disease. *Science* 267, 1456–1462.

21. Rust C., Gores G.J. (2000). Apoptosis and liver disease. *American Journal of Medicine* 108, 568–575.

22. Corry M., Montoya L. (1990). Gas gangrene: Certain diagnosis or certain death. *Critical Care Nursing* 9 (10), 30–38.

23. Pessa M.E., Bland K.I., Copeland E.M. III. (1987). Growth factors and determinants of wound repair. *Journal of Surgical Research* 42, 207–217.

24. Waldorf H., Fewkes J. (1995). Wound healing. *Advances in Dermatology* 10, 77–95.

25. Flynn M.B. (1996). Wound healing and critical illness. *Critical Care Clinics of North America* 8, 115–124.

26. Orgill D., Deming H.R. (1988). Current concepts and approaches to healing. *Critical Care Medicine* 16, 899–908.

27. Albina J.E. (1995). Nutrition and wound healing. *Journal of Parenteral and Enteral Nutrition* 18, 367–376.

28. Whitney J.D. (1989). Physiologic effects of tissue oxygenation on wound healing. *Heart and Lung* 18, 466–474.

29. Whitney J.D. (1990). The influence of tissue oxygenation and perfusion on wound healing. *Clinical Issues in Critical Care Nursing* 1, 578–584.

30. Fleisher G.R. (1999). The management of bite wounds. *New England Journal of Medicine* 340, 138–140.

31. Talan D.A., Citron D.M., Abrahamian F.M., Moran G.J., Goldstein E.J.C. (1999). Bacteriologic analysis of infected dog and cat bites. *New England Journal of Medicine* 340, 85–92.

32. Garvin G. (1990). Wound healing in pediatrics. *Nursing Clinics of North America* 25, 181–191.

33. Boynton P.R., Jaworski D., Paustian C. (1999). Meeting the challenges of healing chronic wounds in older adults. *Nursing Clinics of North America* 34(4), 921–932.

Chapter 6

Genetic Control of Cell Function and Inheritance

Edward W. Carroll

Genetic information is stored in the structure of *deoxy-ribonucleic acid* (DNA). DNA is an extremely stable macro-molecule found in the nucleus of each cell. Because of the stable structure of DNA, the genetic information can sur-vive the many processes of reduction division, in which the gametes (*i.e.*, ovum and sperm) are formed, and the fertilization process. This stability is also maintained throughout the many mitotic cell divisions involved in the formation of a new organism from the single-celled fertil-ized ovum called the *zygote*. The term *gene* is used to describe a part of the DNA molecule that contains the information needed to code for the types of proteins and enzymes needed for the day-to-day function of the cells in the body. In addition, a gene is the unit of heredity passed from generation to generation. For example, genes control the type and quantity of hormones that a cell pro-duces, the antigens and receptors that are present on the cell membrane, and the synthesis of enzymes needed for metabolism. Of the estimated 35,000 to 140,000 genes that humans possess, more than 5000 have been identified and more than 2300 have been localized to a particular chromosome. With few exceptions, each gene provides the instructions for the synthesis of a single protein. This chap-ter includes discussions of genetic regulation of cell func-tion, chromosomal structure, patterns of inheritance, and gene technology.

Genetic Control of Cell Function

After you have completed this section of the chapter, you should be able to meet the following objectives:

- ◆ Describe the structure of a gene
- ◆ Explain the mechanisms by which genes control cell function and another generation
- ◆ Describe the concepts of induction and repression as they apply to gene function
- ◆ Define *gene locus* and *allele*
- ◆ Describe the pathogenesis of gene mutation
- ◆ Explain how gene expressivity and penetrance deter-mine the effects of a mutant gene that codes for the production of an essential enzyme

The genetic information needed for protein synthesis is encoded in the DNA contained in the cell nucleus. A sec-ond type of nucleic acid, *ribonucleic acid* (RNA), is involved in the actual synthesis of cellular enzymes and proteins. Cells contain several types of RNA: messenger RNA, trans-fer RNA, and ribosomal RNA. *Messenger RNA* (mRNA) con-tains the transcribed instructions for protein synthesis obtained from the DNA molecule and carries them into the cytoplasm. Transcription is followed by translation, the synthesis of proteins according to the instructions carried by mRNA. *Ribosomal RNA* (rRNA) provides the machinery needed for protein synthesis. *Transfer RNA* (tRNA) reads the instructions and delivers the appropriate amino acids to the ribosome, where they are incorporated into the protein being synthesized.

The mechanism for genetic control of cell function is illustrated in Figure 6-1. The nuclei of all the cells in an organism contain the same accumulation of genes derived from the gametes of the two parents. This means that liver cells contain the same genetic information as skin and muscle cells. For this to be true, the molecular code must be duplicated before each succeeding cell division, or mitosis. In theory, although this has not yet been achieved in humans, any of the highly differentiated cells of an organism could be used to produce a complete, genetically identical organism, or *clone*. Each particular cell type in a tissue uses only part of the information stored in the genetic code. Although information required for the development and differentiation of the other cell types is still present, it is repressed.

Besides nuclear DNA, part of the DNA of a cell resides in the mitochondria. Mitochondrial DNA is inherited from the mother by her offspring (*i.e.*, matrilineal inheritance). Several genetic disorders are attributed to defects in mitochondrial DNA. Leber's hereditary optic neuropathy was the first human disease attributed to mutation in mitochondrial DNA.

GENE STRUCTURE

The structure that stores the genetic information in the nucleus is a long, double-stranded, helical molecule of DNA. DNA is composed of *nucleotides*, which consist of phos-

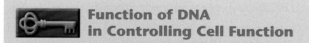

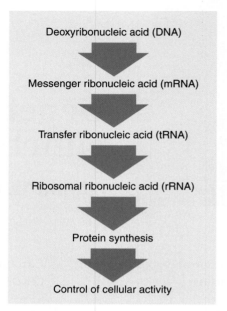

FIGURE 6-1 DNA-directed control of cellular activity through synthesis of cellular proteins. Messenger RNA carries the transcribed message, which directs protein synthesis, from the nucleus to the cytoplasm. Transfer RNA selects the appropriate amino acids and carries them to ribosomal RNA where assembly of the proteins takes place.

phoric acid, a five-carbon sugar called *deoxyribose*, and one of four nitrogenous bases. These nitrogenous bases carry the genetic information and are divided into two groups: the *purine bases*, adenine and guanine, which have two nitrogen ring structures, and the *pyrimidine bases*, thymine and cytosine, which have one ring. The backbone of DNA consists of alternating groups of sugar and phosphoric acid; the paired bases project inward from the sides of the sugar molecule. DNA resembles a spiral staircase, with the paired bases representing the steps (Fig. 6-2). A precise complementary pairing of purine and pyrimidine bases occurs in the double-stranded DNA molecule. Adenine is paired with thymine, and guanine is paired with cytosine. Each nucleotide in a pair is on one strand of the DNA molecule, with the bases on opposite DNA strands bound together by hydrogen bonds that are extremely stable under normal conditions. Enzymes called *DNA helicases* separate the two strands so that the genetic information can be duplicated or transcribed.

Several hundred to almost one million base pairs can represent a gene; the size is proportional to the protein product it encodes. Of the two DNA strands, only one is used in transcribing the information for the cell's polypeptide-building machinery. The genetic information of one strand is meaningful and is used as a template for transcription; the complementary code of the other strand does not make sense and is ignored. Both strands, however, are involved in DNA duplication. Before cell division, the two strands of the helix separate and a complementary molecule is duplicated next to each original strand. Two strands become four strands. During cell division, the newly duplicated

> ### Function of DNA in Controlling Cell Function
>
> ➤ The information needed for the control of cell structure and function is embedded in the genetic information encoded in the stable DNA molecule.
>
> ➤ Although every cell in the body contains the same genetic information, each cell type uses only a portion of the information, depending on its structure and function.
>
> ➤ The production of the proteins that control cell function is accomplished by (1) the transcription of the DNA code for assembly of the protein onto messenger RNA, (2) the translation of the code from messenger RNA and assembly of the protein by ribosomal RNA in the cytoplasm, and (3) the delivery of the amino acids needed for protein synthesis to ribosomal RNA by transfer RNA.

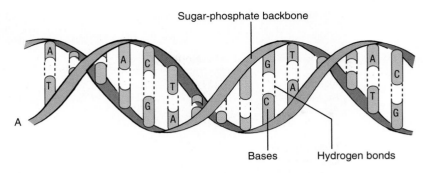

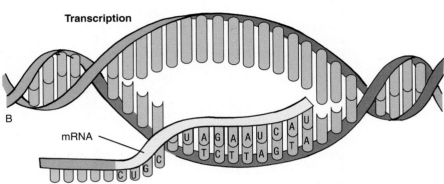

FIGURE 6-2 The DNA double helix and transcription of messenger RNA (mRNA). The top panel (**A**) shows the sequence of four bases (adenine [A], cytosine [C], guanine [G], and thymine [T]), which determines the specificity of genetic information. The bases face inward from the sugar-phosphate backbone and form pairs (*dashed lines*) with complementary bases on the opposing strand. In the bottom panel (**B**), transcription creates a complementary mRNA copy from one of the DNA strands in the double helix.

double-stranded molecules are separated and placed in each daughter cell by the mechanics of mitosis. As a result, each of the daughter cells again contains the meaningful strand and the complementary strand joined in the form of a double helix. In 1958, Meselson and Stahl characterized this replication of DNA as *semiconservative* as opposed to conservative (Fig. 6-3).

The DNA molecule is combined with several types of protein and small amounts of RNA into a complex known as *chromatin*. Chromatin is the readily stainable portion of the cell nucleus. Some DNA proteins form binding sites for repressor molecules and hormones that regulate genetic transcription; others may block genetic transcription by preventing access of nucleotides to the surface of the DNA molecule. A specific group of proteins called *histones* are thought to control the folding of the DNA strands.

GENETIC CODE

The four bases—guanine, adenine, cytosine, and thymine (uracil is substituted for thymine in RNA)—make up the alphabet of the genetic code. A sequence of three of these bases forms the fundamental triplet code used in transmitting the genetic information needed for protein synthesis. This triplet code is called a *codon* (Table 6-1). An example is the nucleotide sequence GCU (guanine, cytosine, and uracil), which is the triplet RNA code for the amino acid alanine. The genetic code is a universal language used by most living cells (*i.e.*, the code for the amino acid tryptophan is the same in a bacterium, a plant, and a human being). *Stop codes*, which signal the end of a protein molecule, are also present. Mathematically, the four bases can

be arranged in 64 different combinations. Sixty-one of the triplets correspond to particular amino acids, and three are stop signals. Only 20 amino acids are used in protein synthesis in humans. Several triplets code for the same amino

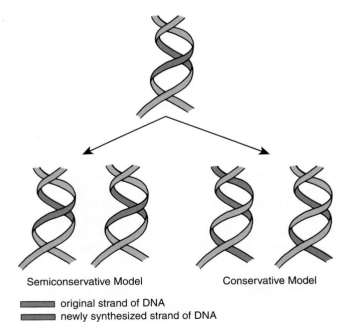

Semiconservative Model   **Conservative Model**

▭ original strand of DNA
▬ newly synthesized strand of DNA

FIGURE 6-3 Semiconservative vs conservative models of DNA replication as proposed by Meselson and Stahl in 1958. In semiconservative DNA replication, the two original strands of DNA unwind and a complementary strand is formed along each original strand.

TABLE 6-1 ✦ Triplet Codes for Amino Acids

Amino Acid	RNA Codons					
Alanine	GCU	GCC	GCA	GCG		
Arginine	CGU	CGC	CGA	CGG	AGA	AGG
Asparagine	AAU	AAC				
Aspartic acid	GAU	GAC				
Cysteine	UGU	UGC				
Glutamic acid	GAA	GAG				
Glutamine	CAA	CAG				
Glycine	GGU	GGC	GGA	GGG		
Histidine	CAU	CAC				
Isoleucine	AUU	AUC	AUA			
Leucine	CUU	CUC	CUA	CUG	UUA	UUG
Lysine	AAA	AAG				
Methionine	AUG					
Phenylalanine	UUU	UUC				
Proline	CCU	CCC	CCA	CCG		
Serine	UCU	UCC	UCA	UCG	AGC	AGU
Threonine	ACU	ACC	ACA	ACG		
Tryptophan	UGG					
Tyrosine	UAU	UAC				
Valine	GUU	GUC	GUA	GUG		
Start (CI)	AUG					
Stop (CT)	UAA	UAG	UGA			

(Guyton A. [2000]. *Textbook of medical physiology* [10th ed., p. 28]. Philadelphia: W.B. Saunders)

acid; therefore, the genetic code is said to be *redundant* or *degenerate*. For example, AUG is a part of the initiation or start signal and the codon for the amino acid methionine. Codons that specify the same amino acid are called *synonyms*. Synonyms usually have the same first two bases but differ in the third base.

PROTEIN SYNTHESIS

Although DNA determines the type of biochemical product that the cell synthesizes, the transmission and decoding of information needed for protein synthesis are carried out by RNA, the formation of which is directed by DNA. The general structure of RNA differs from DNA in three respects: RNA is a single-stranded rather than a double-stranded molecule; the sugar in each nucleotide of RNA is ribose instead of deoxyribose; and the pyrimidine base thymine in DNA is replaced by uracil in RNA. Three types of RNA are known: mRNA, tRNA, and rRNA. All three types are synthesized in the nucleus by RNA polymerase enzymes that take directions from DNA. Because the ribose sugars found in RNA are more susceptible to degradation than the sugars in DNA, the types of RNA molecules in the cytoplasm can be altered rapidly in response to extracellular signals.

Messenger RNA
Messenger RNA is the template for protein synthesis. It is a long molecule containing several hundred to several thousand nucleotides. Each group of three nucleotides forms a codon that is exactly complementary to the triplet of nucleotides of the DNA molecule. Messenger RNA is formed by a process called *transcription*, in which the weak hydrogen bonds of the DNA are broken so that free RNA nucleotides can pair with their exposed DNA counterparts on the meaningful strand of the DNA molecule (see Fig. 6-2). As with the base pairing of the DNA strands, complementary RNA bases pair with the DNA bases. In RNA, uracil replaces thymine and pairs with adenine.

During transcription, a specialized nuclear enzyme, called *RNA polymerase*, recognizes the beginning or start sequence of a gene. The RNA polymerase attaches to the double-stranded DNA and proceeds to copy the meaningful strand into a single strand of RNA as it travels along the length of the gene. On reaching the stop signal, the enzyme leaves the gene and releases the RNA strand. The RNA strand then is processed. Processing involves the addition of certain nucleic acids at the ends of the RNA strand and cutting and splicing of certain internal sequences. Splicing often involves the removal of stretches of RNA. Because of the splicing process, the final mRNA sequence is different from the original DNA template. RNA sequences that are retained are called *exons*, and those excised are called *introns*. The functions of the introns are unknown. They are thought to be involved in the activation or deactivation of genes during various stages of development.

Splicing permits a cell to produce a variety of mRNA molecules from a single gene. By varying the splicing segments of the initial mRNA, different mRNA molecules are formed. For example, in a muscle cell, the original tropomyosin mRNA is spliced in as many as 10 different ways, yielding distinctly different protein products. This permits different proteins to be expressed from a single gene and reduces how much DNA must be contained in the genome.

Transfer RNA

The clover-shaped tRNA molecule contains only 80 nucleotides, making it the smallest RNA molecule. Its function is to deliver the activated form of amino acids to protein molecules in the ribosomes (Fig. 6-4). At least 20 different types of tRNA are known, each of which recognizes and binds to only one type of amino acid. Each tRNA molecule has two recognition sites: the first is complementary for the mRNA codon and the second is for the amino acid itself. Each type of tRNA carries its own specific amino acid to the ribosomes, where protein synthesis is taking place; there it recognizes the appropriate codon on the mRNA and delivers the amino acid to the newly forming protein molecule.

Ribosomal RNA

The ribosome is the physical structure in the cytoplasm where protein synthesis takes place. Ribosomal RNA forms 60% of the ribosome, with the remainder of the ribosome composed of the structural proteins and enzymes needed for protein synthesis. As with the other types of RNA, rRNA is synthesized in the nucleus. Unlike other RNAs, ribosomal RNA is produced in a specialized nuclear structure called the *nucleolus*. The formed rRNA combines with ribosomal proteins in the nucleus to produce the ribosome, which is then transported into the cytoplasm. On reaching the cytoplasm, most ribosomes become attached to the endoplasmic reticulum and begin the task of protein synthesis.

Proteins are made from a standard set of amino acids, which are joined end-to-end to form the long polypeptide chains of protein molecules. Each polypeptide chain may have as many as 100 to more than 300 amino acids in it. The process of protein synthesis is called *translation*, because the genetic code is translated into the production language needed for protein assembly. Besides rRNA, translation requires the coordinated actions of mRNA and tRNA. Each

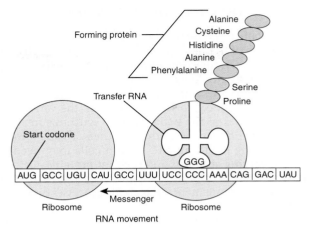

FIGURE 6-4 Messenger RNA strand is moving through two ribosomes. As each "codon" passes through, an amino acid is added to the growing protein chain, which is shown in the right-hand ribosome. The transfer RNA molecule determines which of the 20 amino acids will be added at each stage of protein formation. (Guyton A.C., Hall J.E. [2000]. *Textbook of medical physiology* [10th ed., p. 28]. Philadelphia: W.B. Saunders)

of the 20 different tRNA molecules transports its specific amino acid to the ribosome for incorporation into the developing protein molecule. Messenger RNA provides the information needed for placing the amino acids in their proper order for each specific type of protein. During protein synthesis, mRNA contacts and passes through the ribosome, which "reads" the directions for protein synthesis in much the same way that a tape is read as it passes through a tape player (Fig. 6-5). As mRNA passes through the ribosome, tRNA delivers the appropriate amino acids for attachment to the growing polypeptide chain. The long mRNA molecule usually travels through and directs protein synthesis in more than one ribosome at a time. After the first part of the mRNA is read by the first ribosome, it moves onto a second and a third. As a result, ribosomes that are actively involved in protein synthesis are often found in clusters called *polyribosomes*.

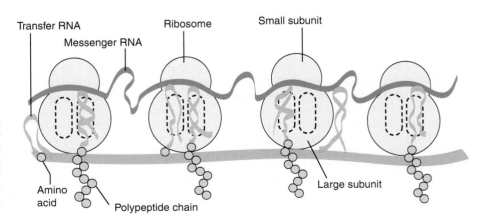

FIGURE 6-5 Structure of the ribosomes as well as their functional relation to messenger RNA, transfer RNA, and the endoplasmic reticulum during the formation of protein molecules. (Redrawn from Bloom W., Fawcett D.W. [1975]. *A textbook of histology.* [10th ed., p. 113]. Philadelphia: W.B. Saunders)

REGULATION OF GENE EXPRESSION

Although all cells contain the same genes, not all genes are active all of the time, nor are the same genes active in all cell types. On the contrary, only a small, select group of genes is active in directing protein synthesis in the cell, and this group varies from one cell type to another. For the differentiation process of cells to occur in the various organs and tissues of the body, protein synthesis in some cells must be different from that in others. To adapt to an ever-changing environment, certain cells may need to produce varying amounts and types of proteins. Certain enzymes, such as carbonic anhydrase, are synthesized by all cells for the fundamental metabolic processes on which life depends.

The degree to which a gene or particular group of genes is active is called *gene expression*. A phenomenon termed *induction* is an important process by which gene expression is increased. Except in early embryonic development, induction is promoted by some external influence. *Gene repression* is a process whereby a regulatory gene acts to reduce or prevent gene expression. Some genes are normally dormant but can be activated by inducer substances; other genes are naturally active and can be inhibited by repressor substances. Genetic mechanisms for the control of protein synthesis are better understood in microorganisms than in humans. It can be assumed, however, that the same general principles apply.

The mechanism that has been most extensively studied is the one by which the synthesis of particular proteins can be turned on and off. For example, in the bacterium *Escherichia coli* grown in a nutrient medium containing the disaccharide lactose, the enzyme galactosidase can be isolated. The galactosidase catalyzes the splitting of lactose into a molecule of glucose and a molecule of galactose. This is necessary if lactose is to be metabolized by *E. coli*. However, if the *E. coli* is grown in a medium that does not contain lactose, very little of the enzyme is produced. From these and other studies, it is theorized that the synthesis of a particular protein, such as galactosidase, requires a series of reactions, each of which is catalyzed by a specific enzyme.

At least two types of genes control protein synthesis: *structural genes* that specify the amino acid sequence of a polypeptide chain and *regulator genes* that serve a regulatory function without stipulating the structure of protein molecules. The regulation of protein synthesis is controlled by a sequence of genes, called an *operon*, on adjacent sites on the same chromosome (Fig. 6-6). An operon consists of a set of structural genes that code for enzymes used in the synthesis of a particular product and a promoter site that binds RNA polymerase and initiates transcription of the structural genes. The function of the operon is further regulated by activator and repressor operators, which induce or repress the function of the promoter. The activator and repressor sites commonly monitor levels of the synthesized product and regulate the activity of the operon through a negative feedback mechanism. Whenever product levels decrease, the function of the operon is activated, and when levels increase, its function is repressed. Regulatory genes found elsewhere in the genetic

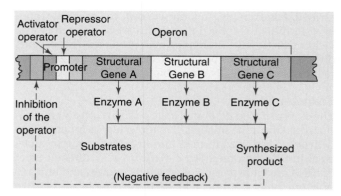

FIGURE 6-6 Function of the operon to control biosynthesis. The synthesized product exerts negative feedback to inhibit function of the operon, in this way automatically controlling the concentration of the product itself. (Guyton A., Hall J.E. [2000]. *Textbook of medical physiology* [10th ed., p. 31]. Philadelphia: W.B. Saunders)

complex can exert control over an operon through activator or repressor substances. Not all genes are subject to induction and repression.

GENE MUTATIONS

Rarely, accidental errors in duplication of DNA occur. These errors are called *mutations*. Mutations result from the substitution of one base pair for another, the loss or addition of one or more base pairs, or rearrangements of base pairs. Many of these mutations occur spontaneously; others occur because of environmental agents, chemicals, and radiation. Mutations may arise in somatic cells or in germ cells. Only those DNA changes that occur in germ cells can be inherited. A somatic mutation affects a cell line that differentiates into one or more of the many tissues of the body and is not transmissible to the next generation. Somatic mutations that do not have an impact on the health or functioning of a person are called *polymorphisms*. Occasionally, a person is born with one brown eye and one blue eye because of a somatic mutation. The change or loss of gene information is just as likely to affect the fundamental processes of cell function or organ differentiation. Such somatic mutations in the early embryonic period can result in embryonic death or congenital malformations. Somatic mutations are important causes of cancer and other tumors in which cell differentiation and growth get out of control. Each year, hundreds of thousands of random changes occur in the DNA molecule because of environmental events or metabolic accidents. Fortunately, fewer than 1 in 1000 base pair changes result in serious mutations. Most of these defects are corrected by DNA repair mechanisms. Several mechanisms exist, and each depends on specific enzymes such as DNA repair nucleases. Fishermen, farmers, and others who are excessively exposed to the ultraviolet radiation of sunlight have an increased risk for development of skin cancer as a result of potential radiation damage to the genetic structure of the skin-forming cells.

In summary, genes are the fundamental unit of information storage in the cell. They determine the types of proteins and enzymes made by the cell and therefore control inheritance and day-to-day cell function. Genes store information in a stable macromolecule called *DNA*. Genes transmit information contained in the DNA molecule as a triplet code. The arrangement of the nitrogenous bases of the four nucleotides (*i.e.*, adenine, guanine, thymine [or uracil in RNA], and cytosine) forms the code. The transfer of stored information into production of cell products is accomplished through a second type of macromolecule called *RNA*. Messenger RNA transcribes the instructions for product synthesis from the DNA molecule and carries it into the cell's cytoplasm, where ribosomal RNA uses the information to direct product synthesis. Transfer RNA acts as a carrier system for delivering the appropriate amino acids to the ribosomes, where the synthesis of cell products occurs. Although all cells contain the same genes, only a small, select group of genes is active in a given cell type. In all cells, some genetic information is repressed, whereas other information is expressed. Gene mutations represent accidental errors in duplication, rearrangement, or deletion of parts of the genetic code. Fortunately, most mutations are corrected by DNA repair mechanisms in the cell.

Chromosomes

After you have completed this section of the chapter, you should be able to meet the following objectives:

✦ Define the terms *autosomes*, *chromatin*, *meiosis*, and *mitosis*

✦ List the steps in constructing a karyotype using cytogenetic studies

✦ Explain the significance of the Barr body

Most genetic information of a cell is organized, stored, and retrieved in small intracellular structures called *chromosomes*. Although the chromosomes are visible only in dividing cells, they retain their integrity between cell divisions. The chromosomes are arranged in pairs; one member of the pair is inherited from the father, the other from the mother. Each species has a characteristic number of chromosomes. In the human, 46 single or 23 pairs of chromosomes are present. Of the 23 pairs of human chromosomes, there are 22 pairs called *autosomes* that are alike in males and females. Each of the 22 pairs of autosomes has the same appearance in all individuals, and each has been given a numeric designation for classification purposes (Fig. 6-7).

The sex chromosomes make up the 23rd pair of chromosomes. Two sex chromosomes determine the sex of a person. All males have an X and Y chromosome (*i.e.*, an X chromosome from the mother and a Y chromosome from the father); all females have two X chromosomes (*i.e.*, one from each parent). Only one X chromosome in the

Chromosome Structure

➤ The DNA that stores genetic material is organized into 23 pairs of chromosomes. There are 22 pairs of autosomes, which are alike for males and females, and one pair of sex chromosomes, with XX pairing in females and XY pairing in males.

➤ Cell division involves the duplication of the chromosomes. Duplication of chromosomes in somatic cell lines involves mitosis, in which each daughter cell receives a pair of 23 chromosomes. Meiosis is limited to replicating germ cells and results in formation of a single set of 23 chromosomes.

female is active in controlling the expression of genetic traits; however, both X chromosomes are activated during gametogenesis. In the female, the active X chromosome is invisible, but the inactive X chromosome can be demonstrated with appropriate nuclear staining. The method of inactivation is thought to involve the addition of a methyl group to the X chromosome. This inactive chromatin mass is seen as the *Barr body* in epithelial cells or as the drumstick body in the chromatin of neutrophils. The genetic sex of a child can be determined by microscopic study of cell or tissue samples. The total number of X chromosomes is equal to the number of Barr bodies plus one (*i.e.*, an inactive plus an active X chromosome). For example, the cells of a normal female have one Barr body and therefore a total of two X chromosomes. A normal male has no Barr bodies. Males with Klinefelter's syndrome (one Y, an inactive X, plus an active X chromosome) exhibit one Barr body. In the female, whether the X chromosome derived from the mother or that derived from the father is active is determined within a few days after conception; the selection is random for each postmitotic cell line. This is called the *Lyon principle*, after Mary Lyon, the British geneticist who described it.

CELL DIVISION

There are two types of cell division: mitosis (see Chapter 4) and meiosis. *Meiosis* is limited to replicating germ cells and takes place only once in a cell line. It results in the formation of gametes or reproductive cells (*i.e.*, ovum and sperm), each of which has only a single set of 23 chromosomes. Meiosis is typically divided into two distinct phases, meiotic divisions I and II. Similar to mitosis, cells about to undergo the first meiotic division replicate their DNA during interphase. During metaphase I, homologous chromosomes pair up, forming a synapsis or tetrad (two chromatids per chromosome). They are sometimes called *bivalents*. The X and Y chromosomes are not homologs and do not form bivalents. While in metaphase I, an interchange

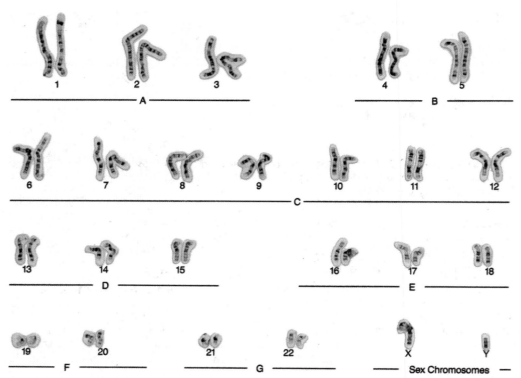

FIGURE 6-7 Karyotype of normal human boy. (Courtesy of the Prenatal Diagnostic and Imaging Center, Sacramento, CA. Frederick W. Hansen, MD, Medical Director)

of chromatid segments can occur. This process is called *crossing over* (Fig. 6-8). Crossing over allows for new combinations of genes, increasing genetic variability. After telophase I, each of the two daughter cells contains one member of each homologous pair of chromosomes and a sex chromosome (23 double-stranded chromosomes). No DNA synthesis occurs before meiotic division II. During anaphase II, the 23 double-stranded chromosomes (two chromatids) of each of the two daughter cells from meiosis I divide at their centromeres. Each subsequent daughter cell receives 23 single-stranded chromatids. Thus, a total of four daughter cells are formed by a meiotic division of one cell (Fig. 6-9).

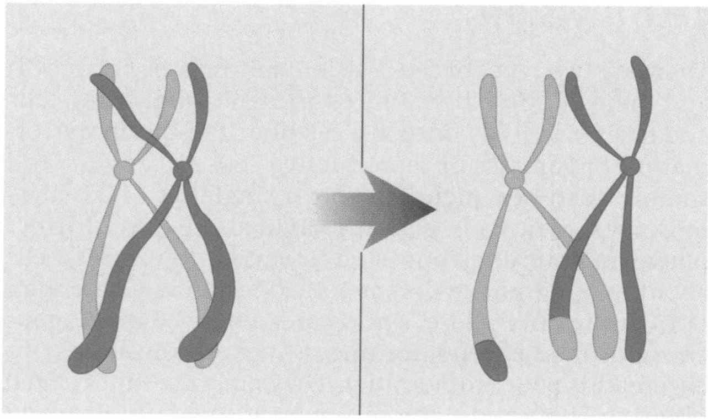

Meiosis, which only occurs in the gamete-producing cells found in either testes or ovaries, has a different outcome in males and females. In males, meiosis (spermatogenesis) results in four viable daughter cells called *spermatids* that differentiate into sperm cells. In females, gamete formation or oogenesis is quite different. After the first meiotic division of a primary oocyte, a secondary oocyte and another structure called a *polar body* are formed. This small polar body contains little cytoplasm, but it may undergo a second meiotic division, resulting in two polar bodies (Fig. 6-10). The secondary oocyte undergoes its second meiotic division, producing one mature oocyte and another polar body. Four viable sperm cells are produced during spermatogenesis, but only one ovum from oogenesis.

CHROMOSOME STRUCTURE

Cytogenetics is the study of the structure and numeric characteristics of the cell's chromosomes. Chromosome studies can be done on any tissue or cell that grows and divides in culture. Lymphocytes from venous blood are frequently used for this purpose. After the cells have been cultured, a drug called *colchicine* is used to arrest mitosis in metaphase. A chromosome spread is prepared by fixing and spreading the chromosomes on a slide. Subsequently, appropriate staining techniques show the chromosomal banding patterns so they can be identified. The chromosomes are photographed, and the photomicrograph of each chromosome is cut out and arranged in pairs according to a standard

FIGURE 6-8 Crossing over of DNA at the time of meiosis.

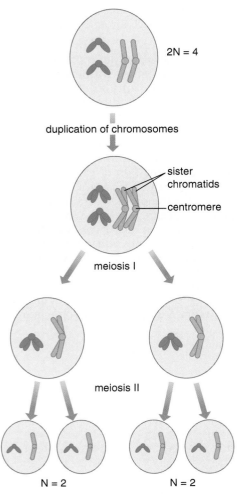

FIGURE 6-9 Separation of chromosomes at the time of meiosis.

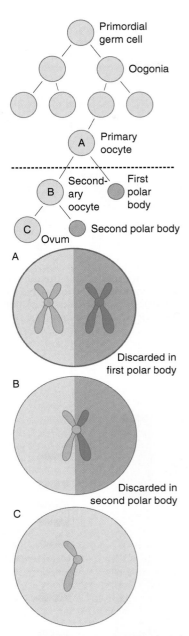

FIGURE 6-10 Essential stages of meiosis in a female, with discarding of the first and second polar bodies and formation of the ovum with the haploid number of chromosomes. The *dotted line* indicates reduction division. (Adapted from Cormack D.H. [1993]. *Essential histology*. Philadelphia: J.B. Lippincott)

classification system. The completed picture is called a *karyotype*, and the procedure for preparing the picture is called *karyotyping*. A uniform system of chromosome classification was originally formulated at the 1971 Paris Chromosome Conference and was later revised to describe the chromosomes as seen in more elongated prophase and prometaphase preparations.

In the metaphase spread, each chromosome takes the form of chromatids to form an "X" or "wishbone" pattern. Human chromosomes are divided into three types according to the position of the centromere (*i.e.*, central constriction; Fig. 6-11). If the centromere is in the center and the arms are of approximately the same length, the chromosome is said to be *metacentric*; if it is off center and the arms are of clearly different lengths, it is *submetacentric*; and if it is near one end, it is *acrocentric*. The short arm of the chromosome is designated as "p" for "petite," and the long arm is designated as "q" for no other reason than it is the next letter of the alphabet. Arms of the chromosome are indicated by the chromosome number followed by the p or q designation. Chromosomes 13, 14, 15, 21, and 22 have small masses of chromatin called *satellites* attached to their short

arms by narrow stalks. At the ends of each chromosome are special DNA sequences called *telomeres*. Telomeres allow the end of the DNA molecule to be replicated completely.

The banding patterns of a chromosome are used in describing the position of a gene. Regions on the chromosomes are numbered from the centromere outward. The regions are further divided into bands and subbands, which are also numbered (Fig. 6-12). These numbers are used in designating the position of a gene on a chromosome. For

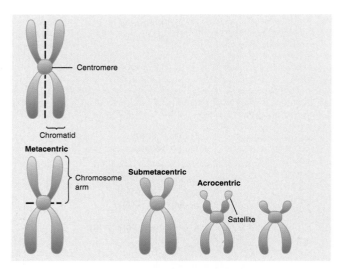

FIGURE 6-11 Three basic shapes and the component parts of human metaphase chromosomes. The relative size of the satellite on the acrocentric is exaggerated for visibility. (Adapted from Cormack D.H. [1993]. *Essential histology*. Philadelphia: J.B. Lippincott)

example, Xp22.2 refers to subband 2, band 2, region 2 of the short arm (p) of the X chromosome.

In summary, the genetic information in a cell is organized, stored, and retrieved as small cellular structures called *chromosomes*. Forty-six chromosomes arranged in 23 pairs are present in the human being. Twenty-two of these pairs are autosomes. The 23rd pair is the sex chromosomes, which determine the sex of a person. Two types of cell division occur, meiosis and mitosis. Meiosis is limited to replicating germ cells and results in the formation of gametes or reproductive cells (ovum and sperm), each of which has only a single set of 23 chromosomes. Mitotic division occurs in somatic cells and results in the formation of 23 pairs of chromosomes. A karyotype is a photograph of a person's chromosomes. It is prepared by special laboratory techniques in which body cells are cultured, fixed, and then stained to demonstrate identifiable banding patterns. A photomicrograph is then made. Often the individual chromosomes are cut out and regrouped according to chromosome number.

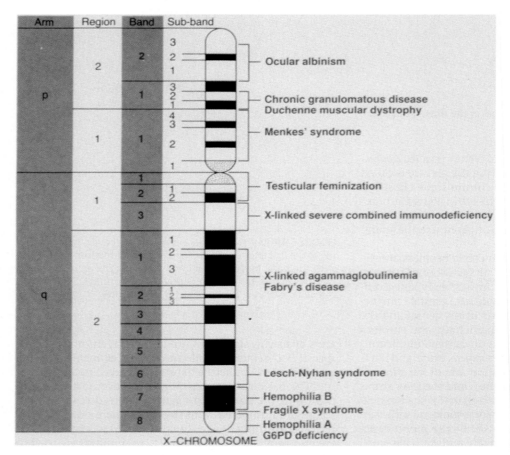

FIGURE 6-12 Details of a banded karyotype of the X chromosome. Notice the nomenclature of arms, regions, bands, and subbands. On the right side, the approximate locations of some errors that cause disease are indicated. (Cotran R.S., Kumar V., Collins T. [1999]. *Robbins pathologic basis of disease* [6th ed., p. 167]. Philadelphia: W.B. Saunders)

Patterns of Inheritance

After you have completed this section of the chapter, you should be able to meet the following objectives:

✦ Construct a hypothetical pedigree for a recessive and dominant trait according to Mendel's law
✦ Contrast genotype and phenotype
✦ Define the terms *allele, locus, expressivity,* and *penetrance*

The characteristics inherited from a person's parents are inscribed in gene pairs located along the length of the chromosomes. Alternate forms of the same gene are possible (*i.e.,* one inherited from the mother and the other from the father), and each may produce a different aspect of a trait.

DEFINITIONS

Genetics has its own set of definitions. The *genotype* of a person is the genetic information stored in the base sequence triplet code. The *phenotype* refers to the recognizable traits, physical or biochemical, associated with a specific genotype. Often, the genotype is not evident by available detection methods. More than one genotype may have the same phenotype. Some brown-eyed persons are carriers of the code for blue eyes, and other brown-eyed persons are not. Phenotypically, these two types of brown-eyed persons are the same, but genotypically they are different.

When it comes to a genetic disorder, not all persons with a mutant gene are affected to the same extent. *Expressivity* refers to the manner in which the gene is expressed in the phenotype, which can range from mild to severe. *Penetrance* represents the ability of a gene to express its function. Seventy-five percent penetrance means 75% of persons of a particular genotype demonstrate a recognizable phenotype. Syndactyly and blue sclera are genetic mutations that often do not exhibit 100% penetrance.

The position of a gene on a chromosome is called its *locus,* and alternate forms of a gene at the same locus are called *alleles.* When only one pair of genes is involved in the transmission of information, the term *single-gene trait* is used. Single-gene traits follow the Mendelian laws of inheritance.

Polygenic inheritance involves multiple genes at different loci, with each gene exerting a small additive effect in determining a trait. Most human traits are determined by multiple pairs of genes, many with alternate codes, accounting for some of the dissimilar forms that occur with certain genetic disorders. Polygenic traits are predictable, but less so than single-gene traits. *Multifactorial* inheritance is similar to polygenic inheritance in that multiple alleles at different loci affect the outcome; the difference is that multifactorial inheritance includes environmental effects on the genes.

Many other gene–gene interactions are known. These include *epistasis,* in which one gene masks the phenotypic effects of another nonallelic gene; *multiple alleles,* in which

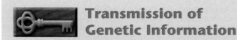

Transmission of Genetic Information

➤ The transmission of information from one generation to the next is vested in genetic material transferred from each parent at the time of conception.

➤ Alleles are the alternate forms of a gene (one from each parent), and the locus is the position that they occupy on the chromosome.

➤ The genotype of a person represents the sum total of the genetic information in the cells and the phenotype the physical manifestations of that information.

➤ Penetrance is the percentage in a population with a particular genotype in which that genotype is phenotypically manifested, whereas expressivity is the manner in which the gene is expressed.

➤ Mendelian, or single-gene, patterns of inheritance include autosomal dominant and recessive traits that are transmitted from parents to their offspring in a predictable manner. Polygenic inheritance, which involves multiple genes, and multifactorial inheritance, which involves multiple genes as well as environmental factors, are less predictable.

more than one allele affects the same trait (*e.g.,* ABO blood types); *complementary genes,* in which each gene is mutually dependent on the other; and *collaborative genes,* in which two different genes influencing the same trait interact to produce a phenotype neither gene alone could produce.

GENETIC IMPRINTING

Besides autosomal and sex-linked genes and mitochondrial inheritance, it was found that certain genes exhibited a "parent of origin" type of transmission in which the parental genomes do not always contribute equally in the development of an individual (Fig. 6-13). The transmission of this phenomenon was given the name *genomic imprinting* by Helen Crouse in 1960. Although rare, it is estimated that approximately 100 genes exhibit genomic, or genetic, imprinting. Evidence suggests there is a genetic conflict over the developing embryo: the male genome attempts to establish larger offspring, whereas the female prefers smaller offspring to conserve her energy for the current and subsequent pregnancies.

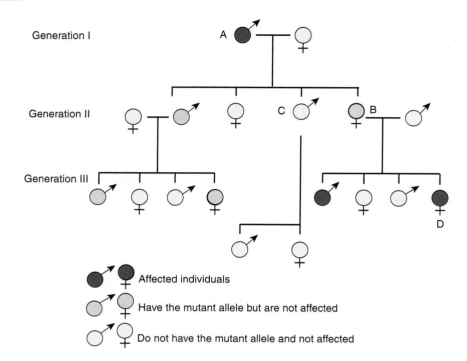

FIGURE 6-13 Pedigree of genetic imprinting. In generation I, male **A** has inherited a mutant allele from his affected mother (not shown); the gene is "turned off" during spermatogenesis, and therefore none of his offspring (generation II) will express the mutant allele, regardless if they are carriers. However, the gene will be "turned on" again during oogenesis in any of his daughters (**B**) who inherit the allele. All offspring (generation III) who inherit the mutant allele will be affected. All offspring of normal children (**C**) will produce normal offspring. Children of female **D** will all express the mutation if they inherit the allele.

It was the pathologic analysis of ovarian teratomas (tumors made up of various cell types derived from an undifferentiated germ cell) and hydatidiform moles (gestational tumors made up of trophoblastic tissue) that yielded the first evidence of genetic imprinting. All ovarian teratomas were found to have a 46,XX karyotype. The results of detailed chromosomal polymorphism analysis confirmed that these tumors developed without the paternally derived genome. Conversely, analysis of hydatidiform moles suggested that they were tumors of paternal origin.

A well-known example of genomic imprinting is the transmission of the mutations in Prader-Willi and Angelman's syndromes. Both syndromes exhibit mental retardation as a common feature. It was also found that both disorders had the same deletion in chromosome 15. When the deletion is inherited from the mother, the infant presents with Angelman's ("happy puppet") syndrome; when the same deletion is inherited from the father, Prader-Willi syndrome results.

A related chromosomal disorder is *uniparental disomy.* This occurs when two chromosomes of the same number are inherited from one parent. Normally, this is not a problem except in cases where a chromosome has been imprinted by a parent. If an allele is inactivated by imprinting, the offspring will have only one working copy of the chromosome, resulting in possible problems.

MENDEL'S LAWS

The main feature of inheritance is predictability: given certain conditions, the likelihood of the occurrence or recurrence of a specific trait is remarkably predictable. The units of inheritance are the genes, and the pattern of single-gene expression can often be predicted using Mendel's laws of genetic transmission. Techniques and discoveries since Gregor Mendel's original work was published in 1865 have led to some modification of his original laws.

Mendel discovered the basic pattern of inheritance by conducting carefully planned experiments with simple garden peas. Experimenting with several phenotypic traits in peas, Mendel proposed that inherited traits are transmitted from parents to offspring by means of independently inherited factors—now known as genes—and that these factors are transmitted as recessive and dominant traits. Mendel labeled dominant factors (his round peas) "A" and recessive factors (his wrinkled peas) "a." Geneticists continue to use capital letters to designate dominant traits and lowercase letters to identify recessive traits. The possible combinations that can occur with transmission of single-gene dominant and recessive traits can be described by constructing a figure called a *Punnet square* using capital and lowercase letters (Fig. 6-14).

The observable traits of single-gene inheritance are inherited by the offspring from the parents. During maturation, the primordial germ cells (*i.e.,* sperm and ovum) of both parents undergo meiosis, or reduction division, in which the number of chromosomes is divided in half (from 46 to 23). At this time, the two alleles from a gene locus separate so that each germ cell receives only one allele from each pair (*i.e.,* Mendel's first law). According to Mendel's second law, the alleles from the different gene loci segregate independently and recombine randomly in the zygote. Persons in whom the two alleles of a given pair are the same (AA or aa) are called *homozygotes. Heterozygotes* have different alleles (Aa) at a gene locus. A *recessive trait* is one expressed only in a homozygous pairing; a *dominant trait* is one expressed in either a homozygous or a heterozygous pairing. All persons with a dominant allele

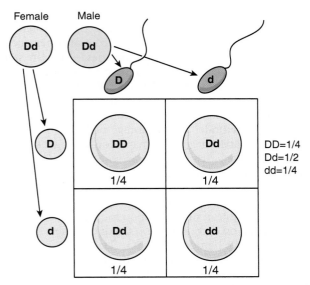

Female   Male

DD=1/4
Dd=1/2
dd=1/4

FIGURE 6-14 The Punnett square showing all possible combinations for transmission of a single gene trait (dimpled cheeks). The example shown is when both parents are heterozygous (dD) for the trait. The alleles carried by the mother are on the left and those carried by the father are on the top. The D allele is dominant and the d allele is recessive. The DD and Dd offspring have dimples and the dd offspring does not.

(depending on the penetrance of the genes) manifest that trait. A *carrier* is a person who is heterozygous for a recessive trait and does not manifest the trait. For example, the genes for blond hair are recessive and those for brown hair are dominant. Therefore, only persons with a genotype having two alleles for blond hair would be blond; persons with either one or two brown alleles would have dark hair.

PEDIGREE

A pedigree is a graphic method for portraying a family history of an inherited trait. It is constructed from a carefully obtained family history and is useful for tracing the pattern of inheritance for a particular trait.

In summary, inheritance represents the likelihood of the occurrence or recurrence of a specific genetic trait. The genotype refers to information stored in the genetic code of a person, whereas the phenotype represents the recognizable traits, physical and biochemical, associated with the genotype. Expressivity refers to the expression of a gene in the phenotype, and penetrance is the ability of a gene to express its function. The point on the DNA molecule that controls the inheritance of a particular trait is called a *gene locus*. Alternate forms of a gene at one gene locus are called *alleles*. The alleles at a gene locus may carry recessive or dominant traits. A recessive trait is one expressed only when there are two copies (homozygous) of the recessive alleles. Dominant traits are expressed with either homozygous or

heterozygous pairing of the alleles. A pedigree is a graphic method for portraying a family history of an inherited trait.

Gene Technology

After you have completed this section of the chapter, you should be able to meet the following objectives:

✦ Define genomic mapping
✦ Briefly describe the methods used in linkage studies, dosage studies, and hybridization studies

GENOMIC MAPPING

The genome is the gene complement of an organism. Genomic mapping is the assignment of genes to specific chromosomes or parts of the chromosome. The Human Genome Project, which started in 1990, is an international project to identify and localize the estimated 35,000 to 140,000 genes in the human genome. This is a phenomenal undertaking because there are approximately 3.2 billion base pairs in the human genome. The national effort toward genomic mapping is jointly coordinated by the National Institutes of Health and the Department of Energy. Organizers of the U.S. Human Genome Project hope to have the completed map by the year 2005. It is also anticipated that the project will reveal the chemical basis for as many as 4000 genetic diseases. It is expected to provide tests for screening and diagnosing genetic disorders and the basis for new treatments. To date, chromosomes 21 and 22 have been completely mapped.

Although the human genome project has received most of the publicity, genome sequencing also is underway in a variety of animals, such as the mouse and fruit fly, and other organisms, from bacteria to plants. These and other endeavors will be of benefit in animal husbandry and agriculture and the study of genetic similarities among various species. The human genome project has created an anticipation of future benefits from its undertakings as well as ethical concerns that must be dealt with by both scientists and the public.

Two types of genomic maps exist: genetic maps and physical maps. Genetic maps are like highway maps. They use linkage studies (*e.g.*, dosage, hybridization) to estimate the distances between chromosomal landmarks (*i.e.*, gene markers). Physical maps are similar to a surveyor's map. They measure the actual physical distance between chromosomal elements in biochemical units, the smallest being the nucleotide base.

Genetic maps and physical maps have been refined over the decades. The earliest mapping efforts localized genes on the X chromosome. The initial assignment of a gene to a particular chromosome was made in 1911 for the color blindness gene inherited from the mother (*i.e.*, following the X-linked pattern of inheritance). In 1968, the specific location of the Duffy blood group on the long arm of chromosome 1 was determined. The locations of more than 2300 expressed human genes have been mapped to a

Gene Mapping

> - The Human Genome Project is an attempt to map all the genes in the human genome.

> - Linked genes are found on the same chromosome; the degree of linkage of two genes is based on their physical distance from each other on the chromosome.

> - Somatic cell hybridization allows geneticists to study which chromosomes contain the coding for various enzymes.

> - In situ hybridization uses specific sequences of DNA or RNA to locate genes that do not express themselves in cell culture.

specific chromosome and most of them to a specific region on the chromosome. However, genetic mapping is continuing so rapidly that these numbers are constantly being updated. Documentation of gene assignments to specific human chromosomes is updated almost daily in the *Online Mendelian Inheritance in Man* (http://www.ncbi.nlm.nih.gov/Omim), an encyclopedia of expressed gene loci. Another source is the Genome Data Base, which is the central database for mapped genes and an international repository for most mapping information. Many methods have been used for developing genetic maps. The most important ones are family linkage studies, gene dosage methods, and hybridization studies. Often, the specific assignment of a gene is made using information from several mapping techniques.

Most of the genome mapping has been accomplished by a method called *transcript mapping*. The two-part process begins with isolating mRNAs immediately after they are transcribed. Next, the complementary DNA molecule is prepared. Although transcript mapping may provide knowledge of the gene sequence, it does not automatically mean that the function of the genetic material has been determined.

Linkage Studies

Mendel's laws were often insufficient to explain the transmission of several well-known traits such as color blindness and hemophilia A. In some families it was noted that these two conditions were transmitted together. In 1937, Bell and Haldane concluded that somehow the two mutations were coupled or "linked." Detailed analyses of other familial conditions have concluded that there are several exceptions to Mendel's laws.

Linkage studies assume that genes occur in a linear array along the chromosomes. During meiosis, the paired chromosomes of the diploid germ cell exchange genetic material because of the crossing-over phenomenon (see Fig. 6-8). This exchange usually involves more than one gene; large blocks of genes (representing large portions of the chromosome) usually are exchanged. Although the point at which the block separates from another occurs randomly, the closer together two genes are on the same chromosome, the greater the chance is that they will be passed on together to the offspring. When two inherited traits occur together at a rate significantly greater than would occur by chance, they are said to be *linked*.

Several methods take advantage of the crossing over and recombination of genes to map a particular gene. In one method, any gene that is already assigned to a chromosome can be used as a marker to assign other linked genes. For example, it was found that an extra long chromosome 1 and the Duffy blood group were inherited as a dominant trait, placing the position of the blood group gene close to the extra material on chromosome 1. Color blindness has been linked to classic hemophilia A (*i.e.*, lack of factor VIII) in some pedigrees; hemophilia A has been linked to glucose-6-phosphate dehydrogenase deficiency in others; and color blindness has been linked to glucose-6-phosphate dehydrogenase deficiency in still others. Because the gene for color blindness is found on the X chromosome, all three genes must be located in a small section of the X chromosome. Linkage analysis can be used clinically to identify affected persons in a family with a known genetic defect. Males, because they have one X and one Y chromosome, are said to be *hemizygous* for sex-linked traits. Females can be homozygous (normal or mutant) or heterozygous for sex-linked traits. Heterozygous females are known as *carriers* for X-linked defects.

One autosomal recessive disorder that has been successfully diagnosed prenatally by linkage studies using amniocentesis is congenital adrenal hyperplasia (due to 21-hydroxylase deficiency), which is linked to an immune response gene (human leukocyte antigen [HLA] type). Postnatally, linkage studies have been used in diagnosing hemochromatosis, which is closely linked to another HLA type. Persons with this disorder are unable to metabolize iron, and it accumulates in the liver and other organs. It cannot be diagnosed by conventional means until irreversible damage has been done. Given a family history of the disorder, HLA typing can determine if the gene is present, and if it is present, dietary restriction of iron intake may be used to prevent organ damage.

Dosage Studies

Dosage studies involve measuring enzyme activity. Autosomal genes are normally arranged in pairs, and normally both are expressed. If both alleles are present and both are expressed, the activity of the enzyme should be 100%. If one member of the gene pair is missing, only 50% of the enzyme activity is present, reflecting the activity of the remaining normal allele.

Hybridization Studies

A recent biologic discovery revealed that two somatic cells from different species, when grown together in the same culture, occasionally fuse to form a new hybrid cell. Two types of hybridization methods are used in genomic studies: somatic cell hybridization and in situ hybridization.

Somatic cell hybridization involves the fusion of human somatic cells with those of a different species (typically, the mouse) to yield a cell containing the chromosomes of both species. Because these hybrid cells are unstable, they begin to lose chromosomes of both species during subsequent cell divisions. This makes it possible to obtain cells with different partial combinations of human chromosomes. By studying the enzymes that these cells produce, it is possible to determine that an enzyme is produced only when a certain chromosome is present; the coding for that enzyme must be located on that chromosome.

In situ hybridization involves the use of a specific sequence of DNA or RNA to locate genes that do not express themselves in cell culture. DNA and RNA can be chemically tagged with radioactive or fluorescent markers. These chemically tagged DNA or RNA sequences are used as probes to determine gene location. The probe is added to a chromosome spread after the DNA strands have been separated. If the probe matches the complementary DNA of a chromosome segment, it hybridizes and remains at the precise location (hence the term *in situ*) on a chromosome. Radioactive or fluorescent markers are used to determine the location of the probe.

RECOMBINANT DNA TECHNOLOGY

During the past several decades, genetic engineering has provided the methods for manipulating nucleic acids and recombining genes (recombinant DNA) into hybrid molecules that can be inserted into unicellular organisms and reproduced many times over. Each hybrid molecule produces a genetically identical population, called a *clone*, that reflects its common ancestor.

The techniques of gene isolation and cloning rely on the fact that the genes of all organisms, from bacteria through mammals, are based on similar molecular organization. Gene cloning requires cutting a DNA molecule apart, modifying and reassembling its fragments, and producing copies of the modified DNA, its mRNA, and its gene product. The DNA molecule is cut apart by using a bacterial enzyme, called a *restriction enzyme*, that binds to DNA wherever a particular short sequence of base pairs is found and cleaves the molecule at a specific nucleotide site. In this way, a long DNA molecule can be broken down into smaller, discrete fragments with the intent that one fragment contains the gene of interest. More than 100 restriction enzymes are commercially available that cut DNA at different recognition sites.

The selected gene fragment is replicated through insertion into a unicellular organism, such as a bacterium. To do this, a cloning vector such as a bacterial virus or a small DNA circle that is found in most bacteria, called a *plasmid*, is used. Viral and plasmid vectors replicate autonomously in the host bacterial cell. During gene cloning, a bacterial vector and the DNA fragment are mixed and joined by a special enzyme called a *DNA ligase*. The re-

combinant vectors formed are then introduced into a suitable culture of bacteria, and the bacteria are allowed to replicate and express the recombinant vector gene. Sometimes, mRNA taken from a tissue that expresses a high level of the gene is used to produce a complementary DNA molecule that can be used in the cloning process. Because the fragments of the entire DNA molecule are used in the cloning process, additional steps are taken to identify and separate the clone that contains the gene of interest.

In terms of biologic research and technology, cloning makes it possible to identify the DNA sequence in a gene and produce the protein product encoded by a gene. The specific nucleotide sequence of a cloned DNA fragment can often be identified by analyzing the amino acid sequence and mRNA codons of its protein product. Short sequences of base pairs can be synthesized, radioactively labeled, and subsequently used to identify their complementary sequence. In this way, identifying normal and abnormal gene structures is possible. Proteins that formerly were available only in small amounts can now be made in large quantities once their respective genes have been isolated. For example, genes encoding for insulin and growth hormone have been cloned to produce these hormones for pharmacologic use.

GENE THERAPY

Although quite different from inserting genetic material into a unicellular organism such as bacteria, techniques are available for inserting genes into the genome of intact multicellular plants and animals. Promising delivery vehicles for these genes are the adenoviruses. These viruses are ideal vehicles because their DNA does not become integrated into the host genome; however, repeated inoculations are often needed because the body's immune system usually targets cells expressing adenovirus proteins. Sterically stable liposomes also show promise as DNA delivery mechanisms. This type of therapy is one of the more promising methods for the treatment of genetic disorders, certain cancers, cystic fibrosis, and many infectious diseases.

Two main approaches are used in gene therapy: transferred genes either replace defective genes or selectively inhibit deleterious genes. Cloned DNA sequences or ribosomes usually are the compounds used in gene therapy. However, the introduction of the cloned gene into the multicellular organism can influence only the few cells that get the gene. An answer to this problem would be the insertion of the gene into a sperm or ovum; after fertilization, the gene would be replicated in all of the differentiating cell types. Even so, techniques for cell insertion are limited. Not only are moral and ethical issues involved, but these techniques cannot direct the inserted DNA to attach to a particular chromosome or supplant an existing gene by knocking it out of its place.

DNA FINGERPRINTING

The technique of DNA fingerprinting is based in part on those techniques used in recombinant DNA technology and those originally used in medical genetics to detect slight variations in the genomes of different individuals. Using restrictive endonucleases, DNA is cleaved at specific regions. The DNA fragments are separated according to size by electrophoresis (*i.e.*, Southern blot) and transferred to a nylon membrane. The fragments are then broken apart and subsequently annealed with a series of radioactive probes specific for regions in each fragment. An autoradiograph reveals the DNA fragments on the membrane. When used in forensic pathology, this procedure is undertaken on specimens from the suspect and the forensic specimen. Banding patterns are then analyzed to see if they match. With conventional methods of analysis of blood and serum enzymes, a 1 in 100 to 1000 chance exists that the two specimens match because of chance. With DNA fingerprinting, these odds are 1 in 100,000 to 1 million.

In summary, the genome is the gene complement of an organism. Genomic mapping is a method used to assign genes to particular chromosomes or parts of a chromosome. The most important ones used are family linkage studies, gene dosage methods, and hybridization studies. Often the specific assignment of a gene is determined by using information from several mapping techniques. Linkage studies assign a chromosome location to genes based on their close association with other genes of known location. Recombinant DNA studies involve the extraction of specific types of messenger RNA used in synthesis of complementary DNA strands. The complementary DNA strands, labeled with a radioisotope, bind with the genes for which they are complementary and are used as gene probes. Now underway is an international project to identify and localize all 50,000 to 120,000 genes in the human genome. Genetic engineering has provided the methods for manipulating nucleic acids and recombining genes (recombinant DNA) into hybrid molecules that can be inserted into unicellular organisms and reproduced many times over. As a result, proteins that formerly were available only in small amounts can now be made in large quantities once their respective genes have been isolated. DNA fingerprinting, which relies on recombinant DNA technologies and those of genetic mapping, is often used in forensic investigations.

Bibliography

Alberts B., Bray D., Lewis J., Raff M., Roberts K., Watson J.D. (1994). *Molecular biology of the cell* (3rd ed., pp. 242–251, 379–380). New York: Garland Publishing.

Aparicio S.A.J.R. (2000). How to count . . . human genes. *Nature Genetics* 25 (2), 129–130. [On-line]. Available: http://www.nature.com. Accessed July 13, 2000.

Carlson B.M. (1999). *Human embryology and developmental biology* (2nd ed., pp. 2–23, 128–145). St. Louis: Mosby.

Ewing B., Green P. (2000). Analysis of expressed sequence tags indicates 35,000 human genes. *Nature Genetics* 25 (2)
232–234. [On-line]. Available: http://www.nature.com. Accessed July 13, 2000.

Gelehter T.D., Collins F.S. (1990). *Principles of medical genetics.* Baltimore: Williams & Wilkins.

Guyton A.C., Hall J.E. (2000). *Textbook of medical physiology* (10th ed., pp. 24–37). Philadelphia: W.B. Saunders.

Hattori M., Fujyama A., Taylor H., Watanabe H., Yada T., Park H.S., et al. (2000). The DNA sequence of human chromosome 21. *Nature* 405, 311–319. [On-line]. Available: http://www.nature.com. Accessed July 13, 2000.

Hawley R.S., Mori C.A. (1999). *The human genome: A user's guide.* San Diego: Harcourt Academic Press.

Human Genome Project. (2000). *Columbia encyclopedia* (6th ed.). [On-line]. Available: http://www.bartleby.com/65/hu/HumanG.html. Accessed October 22, 2000.

The International RH Mapping Consortium. (2000). *A new gene map of the human genome.* [On-line]. Available: http://www.ncbi.nlm.nih.gov/genemap99. Accessed July 13, 2000.

Jain H.K. (1999). *Genetics: Principles, concepts and implications.* Enfield, NH: Science Publishers.

Johns D.R. (1995). Mitochondrial DNA and disease. *New England Journal of Medicine* 333, 638–644.

Karf B. (1995). Molecular diagnosis (part I). *New England Journal of Medicine* 332, 1218–1220.

Lamb B.C. (2000). *The applied genetics of plants, animals, humans and fungi* (pp. 23–42). London: Imperial College Press.

Liang F., Holt I., Pertea G., Karamycheva S., Salzberg S.L., Quakenbush J. (2000). Gene index analysis of the human genome estimates approximately 120,000 genes. *Nature Genetics* 25 (2) 239–240. [On-line]. Available: http://www.nature.com. Accessed July 13, 2000.

Marieb E.N. (2001). *Human anatomy and physiology.* (5th ed., pp. 1159–1160). San Francisco: Addison Wesley.

Moore K.L., Persaud T.V.N. (1998). *The developing human: Clinically orientated embryology* (6th ed., pp. 17–46). Philadelphia: W.B. Saunders.

Online Mendelian Inheritance in Man. (2000). Angelman syndrome. [On-line]. Available: http://www.ncbi.nlm.nih.gov/htbin-post/Omim/dispmim?105830. Accessed October 3, 2000.

Online Mendelian Inheritance in Man. (2000). Prader-Willi syndrome. [On-line]. Available: http://www.ncbi.nlm.nih.gov/htbin-post/Omim/dispmim?176270. Accessed 10/03/00.

Ostrer H. (1998). *Non-Mendelian genetics in humans.* New York: Oxford University Press.

Rosenthal N. (1994). DNA and the genetic code. *New England Journal of Medicine* 331, 39–41.

Sadler R.W. (2000). *Langman's medical embryology* (8th ed., pp. 3–30, 112–135).

Sapienza C. (1990). Parenteral imprinting of genes. *Scientific American* 263 (4), 52–60.

Shapiro L.J. (2000). Molecular basis of genetic disorders. In Behrman R.E., Kliegman R.M., Nelson W., Jenson H.B. (Eds.), *Nelson textbook of pediatrics* (16th ed., pp. 313–325). Philadelphia: W.B. Saunders.

Snustad D.P., Simmons J.M. (Eds.). (2000). *Principles of genetics* (2nd ed., pp. 3–21, 52–71, 91–115, 665–669). New York: John Wiley & Sons.

Vogel F., Motulsky A.G. (1997). *Human genetics: Problems and approaches* (3rd ed., pp. 83–193, 360–430). New York: Springer-Verlag.

White R., Lalouel J. (1988). Chromosomal mapping with DNA markers. *Scientific American* 258 (2), 40–49.

Chapter 7

Genetic and Congenital Disorders

Genetic and Chromosomal Disorders

Single-Gene Disorders
Autosomal Dominant Disorders
Autosomal Recessive Disorders
X-Linked Disorders
Multifactorial Inheritance
Disorders
Chromosomal Disorders
*Alterations in Chromosome
Duplication*

Alterations in Chromosome Number
Alterations in Chromosome Structure

**Disorders Due to Environmental
Influences**

Period of Vulnerability
Teratogenic Agents
Radiation
Chemicals and Drugs
Infectious Agents

Diagnosis and Counseling

Genetic Assessment
Prenatal Diagnosis
Maternal Serum Markers
Ultrasound
Amniocentesis
Chorionic Villus Sampling
*Percutaneous Umbilical Blood
Sampling*
Fetal Biopsy
*Cytogenetic and Biochemical
Analyses*

Genetic and congenital defects are important at all levels of health care because they affect all age groups and can involve almost any of the body tissues and organs. Congenital defects, sometimes called *birth defects*, develop during prenatal life and usually are apparent at birth or shortly thereafter. Spina bifida and cleft lip, for example, are apparent at birth, but other malformations, such as kidney and heart defects, may be present at birth but may not become apparent until they begin to produce symptoms. Not all genetic disorders are congenital, and many are not apparent until later in life.

Birth defects, which affect more than 150,000 infants each year, are the leading cause of infant death.[1] Birth defects may be caused by genetic factors (*i.e.*, single-gene or multifactorial inheritance or chromosomal aberrations), or they may be caused by environmental factors that occurred during embryonic or fetal development (*i.e.*, maternal disease, infections, or drugs taken during pregnancy). In rare cases, congenital defects may be the result of intrauterine factors such as fetal crowding, positioning, or entanglement of fetal parts with the amnion. This chapter provides an overview of genetic and congenital disorders and is divided into three parts: (1) genetic and chromosomal disorders, (2) disorders caused by environmental agents, and (3) diagnosis and counseling.

Genetic and Chromosomal Disorders

After you have completed this section of the chapter, you should be able to meet the following objectives:

✦ Define *congenital defect*
✦ Describe three types of single-gene disorders
✦ Contrast disorders due to multifactorial inheritance with those caused by single-gene inheritance
✦ Describe two chromosomal abnormalities that demonstrate aneuploidy
✦ Describe three patterns of chromosomal breakage and rearrangement
✦ Relate maternal age and occurrence of Down syndrome

Genetic disorders involve a permanent change (or mutation) in the genome. A genetic disorder can involve a single-gene trait, multifactorial inheritance, or a chromosome disorder.

SINGLE-GENE DISORDERS

Single-gene disorders are caused by a single defective or mutant gene. The defective gene may be present on an autosome or the X chromosome and it may affect only one

131

Genetic and Chromosomal Disorders

➤ Genetic disorders are inherited as autosomal dominant disorders, in which each child has a 50% chance of inheriting the disorder, and as autosomal recessive disorders, in which each child has a 25% chance of being affected, a 50% chance of being a carrier, and a 25% chance of being unaffected.

➤ Sex-linked disorders almost always are associated with the X chromosome and are predominantly recessive.

➤ Chromosomal disorders reflect events that occur at the time of meiosis and result from defective movement of an entire chromosome or from breakage of a chromosome with loss or translocation of genetic material.

member of an autosomal gene pair (matched with a normal gene) or both members of the pair. Single-gene defects follow the mendelian patterns of inheritance (see Chapter 6) and are often called *mendelian disorders*. At last count, there were more than 6000 single-gene disorders, many of which have been mapped to a specific chromosome.[2]

The genes on each chromosome are arranged in pairs and in strict order, with each gene occupying a specific location or locus. The two members of a gene pair, one inherited from the mother and the other from the father, are called *alleles*. If the members of a gene pair are identical (*i.e.*, code the exact same gene product), the person is *homozygous*, and if the two members are different, the person is *heterozygous*. The genetic composition of a person is called a *genotype*, whereas the *phenotype* is the observable expression of a genotype in terms of morphologic, biochemical, or molecular traits. If the trait is expressed in the heterozygote (one member of the gene pair codes for the trait), it is said to be *dominant*; if it is expressed only in the homozygote (both members of the gene pair code for the trait), it is *recessive*.

Although gene expression usually follows a dominant or recessive pattern, it is possible for both alleles (members) of a gene pair to be fully expressed in the heterozygote, a condition called *codominance*. Many genes have only one normal version, called a *wild-type* allele. Other genes have more than one normal allele (alternate forms) at the same locus. This is called *polymorphism*. Blood group inheritance (*e.g.*, AO, BO, AB) is an example of codominance and polymorphism.

A single mutant gene may be expressed in many different parts of the body. Marfan's syndrome is a defect in connective tissue that has widespread effects involving skeletal, eye, and cardiovascular structures. In other single-gene disorders, the same defect can be caused by mutations at several different loci. Childhood deafness can result from 16 different types of autosomal recessive mutations.

Single-gene disorders are characterized by their patterns of transmission, which usually are obtained through a family genetic history. The patterns of inheritance depend on whether the phenotype is dominant or recessive, and whether the gene is located on an autosomal or sex chromosome (see Chapter 6). Disorders of autosomal inheritance include autosomal dominant and autosomal recessive traits. Among the approximate 6000 single-gene disorders, more than half are autosomal dominant. Autosomal recessive phenotypes are less common, accounting for approximately one third of single-gene disorders.[3] Currently, all sex-linked genetic disorders are thought to be X-linked and most are recessive. The only mutations affecting the Y-linked genes are involved in spermatogenesis and male fertility and hence are not transmitted. A few additional genes with homologs on the X chromosome have been mapped to the Y chromosome, but to date, no disorders resulting from mutations in these genes have been described.

Virtually all single-gene disorders lead to formation of an abnormal protein or decreased production of a gene product. The defect can result in defective or decreased amounts of an enzyme, defects in receptor proteins and their function, alterations in nonenzyme proteins, or mutations resulting in unusual reactions to drugs. Table 7-1 lists some of the common single-gene disorders and their manifestations.

Autosomal Dominant Disorders

In autosomal dominant disorders, a single mutant allele from an affected parent is transmitted to an offspring regardless of sex. The affected parent has a 50% chance of transmitting the disorder to each offspring (Fig. 7-1). The unaffected relatives of the parent or unaffected siblings of the offspring do not transmit the disorder. In many conditions, the age of onset is delayed, and the signs and symptoms of the disorder do not appear until later in life, as in Huntington's chorea (see Chapter 50).

Autosomal dominant disorders also may manifest as a new mutation. Whether the mutation is passed on to the next generation depends on the affected person's reproductive capacity. Many new autosomal dominant mutations are accompanied by reduced reproductive capacity; therefore, the defect is not perpetuated in future generations. If an autosomal defect is accompanied by a total inability to reproduce, essentially all new cases of the disorder will be due to new mutations. If the defect does not affect reproductive capacity, it is more likely to be inherited.

Although there is a 50% chance of inheriting a dominant genetic disorder from an affected parent, there can be wide variation in gene penetration and expression. When a person inherits a dominant mutant gene but fails to express it, the trait is described as having *reduced penetrance*. Penetrance is expressed in mathematical terms; a 50% penetrance indicates that a person who inherits the defective gene has a 50% chance of expressing the disorder. The person who has a mutant gene but does not express it is an important exception to the rule that unaffected persons do not transmit an autosomal dominant trait. These persons

TABLE 7-1 ♦ Some Disorders of Mendelian or Single-Gene Inheritance and Their Significance

Disorder	Significance
Autosomal Dominant	
Achondroplasia	Short-limb dwarfism
Adult polycystic kidney disease	Kidney failure
Huntington's chorea	Neurodegenerative disorder
Familial hypercholesterolemia	Premature atherosclerosis
Marfan's syndrome	Connective tissue disorder with abnormalities in skeletal, ocular, cardiovascular systems
Neurofibromatosis (NF)	Neurogenic tumors: fibromatous skin tumors, pigmented skin lesions, and ocular nodules in NF-1; bilateral acoustic neuromas in NF-2
Osteogenesis imperfecta	Molecular defects of collagen
Spherocytosis	Disorder of red blood cells
von Willebrand's disease	Bleeding disorder
Autosomal Recessive	
Color blindness	Color blindness
Cystic fibrosis	Disorder of membrane transport of ions in exocrine glands causing lung and pancreatic disease
Glycogen storage diseases	Excess accumulation of glycogen in the liver and hypoglycemia (von Gierke's disease); glycogen accumulation in striated muscle in myopathic forms
Oculocutaneous albinism	Hypopigmentation of skin, hair, eyes as result of inability to synthesize melanin
Phenylketonuria (PKU)	Lack of phenylalanine hydroxylase with hyperphenylalaninemia and impaired brain development
Sickle cell disease	Red blood cell defect
Tay-Sachs disease	Deficiency of hexosaminidase A; severe mental and physical deterioration beginning in infancy
X-Linked Recessive	
Bruton-type hypogammaglobulinemia	Immunodeficiency
Hemophilia A	Bleeding disorder
Duchenne dystrophy	Muscular dystrophy
Fragile X syndrome	Mental retardation

can transmit the gene to their descendants and so produce a skipped generation. Autosomal dominant disorders also can display *variable expressivity*, meaning that they can be expressed differently among individuals. Polydactyly or supernumerary digits, for example, may be expressed in the fingers or the toes.

The gene products of autosomal dominant disorders usually are regulatory proteins involved in rate-limiting components of complex metabolic pathways or key com-

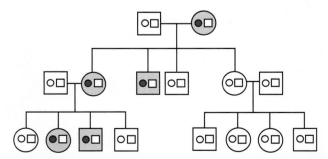

FIGURE 7-1 Simple pedigree for inheritance of an autosomal dominant trait. The small, colored circle represents the mutant gene. An affected parent with an autosomal dominant trait has a 50% chance of passing the mutant gene on to each child regardless of sex.

ponents of structural proteins such as collagen.[4,5] Two disorders of autosomal inheritance, Marfan's syndrome and neurofibromatosis (NF), are described in this chapter.

Marfan's Syndrome. Marfan's syndrome is a connective tissue disorder that is manifested by changes in the skeleton, eyes, and cardiovascular system. There is a wide range of variation in expression of the disorder. Persons may have abnormalities of one or all three systems. The skeletal deformities, which are the most obvious features of the disorder, include a long, thin body with exceptionally long extremities and long, tapering fingers, sometimes called *arachnodactyly* or *spider fingers* (Fig. 7-2), hyperextensible joints, and a variety of spinal deformities including kyphoscoliosis. Chest deformity, pectus excavatum (*i.e.,* deeply depressed sternum), or pigeon chest deformity, often is present. The most common eye disorder is bilateral dislocation of the lens due to weakness of the suspensory ligaments. Myopia and predisposition to retinal detachment also are common, the result of increased optic globe length due to altered connective tissue support of ocular structures. However, the most life-threatening aspects of the disorder are the cardiovascular defects, which include mitral valve prolapse, progressive dilation of the aortic valve ring, and weakness of the aorta and other arteries. Dissection and rupture of

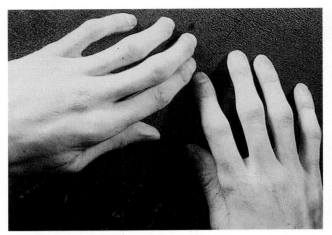

FIGURE 7-2 Long, slender fingers (arachnodactyly) in a patient with Marfan's syndrome. (Rubin E., Farber J.L. [1999]. *Pathology* [3rd ed., p. 242]. Philadelphia: Lippincott Williams & Wilkins)

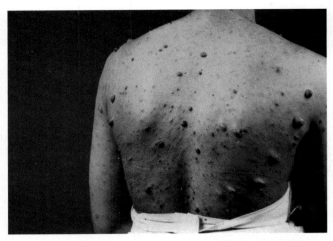

FIGURE 7-3 Neurofibromatosis on the back. (Reed and Carnick Pharmaceuticals) (Sauer G.C., Hall J.C. [1996]. *Manual of skin diseases.* Philadelphia: Lippincott-Raven)

the aorta often lead to premature death. The average age of death in persons with Marfan's syndrome is 30 to 40 years.[4]

Neurofibromatosis.   Neurofibromatosis is a condition involving neurogenic tumors that arise from Schwann cells and other elements of the peripheral nervous system.[4,5] There are at least two genetically and clinically distinct forms of the disorder: type 1 NF (NF-1), also known as *von Recklinghausen's disease,* and type 2 bilateral acoustic NF (NF-2). Both of these disorders result from a genetic defect in a protein that regulates cell growth. The gene for NF-1 has been mapped to chromosome 17, and the gene for NF-2 has been mapped to chromosome 22.

NF-1 is a relatively common disorder with a frequency of 1 in 3000.[5] Approximately 50% of cases have a family history of autosomal dominant transmission, and the remaining 50% appear to represent a new mutation. In more than 90% of persons with NF-1, cutaneous and subcutaneous neurofibromas develop in late childhood or adolescence. The cutaneous neurofibromas, which vary in number from a few to many hundreds, manifest as soft, pedunculated lesions that project from the skin. They are the most common type of lesion, often are not apparent until puberty, and are present in greatest density over the trunk (Fig. 7-3). The subcutaneous lesions grow just below the skin; they are firm and round, and may be painful. Plexiform neurofibromas involve the larger peripheral nerves. They tend to form large tumors that cause severe disfigurement of the face or an extremity. Pigmented nodules of the iris (Lisch nodules), which are specific for NF-1, usually are present after 6 years of age. They do not present any clinical problem but are useful in establishing a diagnosis.

A second major component of NF-1 is the presence of large (usually ≥15 mm in diameter), flat cutaneous pigmentations, known as *café-au-lait spots.* They are usually a uniform light brown in whites and darker brown in African Americans, with sharply demarcated edges (Fig. 7-4). Although small single lesions may be found in normal children, larger lesions or six or more spots larger than 1.5 cm

in diameter suggest NF-1. The skin pigmentations become more evident with age as the melanosomes in the epidermal cells accumulate melanin.

In addition to neurofibromatoses, persons with NF-1 have a variety of other associated lesions, the most common being skeletal lesions such as scoliosis and erosive bone defects. Persons with NF-1 also are at increased risk for development of other nervous system tumors such as meningiomas, optic gliomas, and pheochromocytomas.

NF-2 is characterized by tumors of the acoustic nerve. Most often, the disorder is asymptomatic through the first 15 years of life. The most frequent symptoms are headaches, hearing loss, and tinnitus (*i.e.,* ringing in the ears). There may be associated intracranial and spinal meningiomas. The condition is made worse by pregnancy, and oral contraceptives may increase the growth and symptoms of tumors. Persons with the disorder should be warned that severe dis-

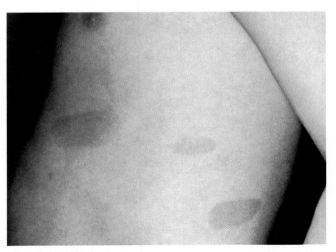

FIGURE 7-4 Neurofibromatosis with early café-au-lait spots in a 5-year-old child. (Owen Laboratories, Inc.) (Sauer G.C., Hall J.C. [1996]. *Manual of skin diseases.* Philadelphia: Lippincott-Raven)

orientation may occur during diving or swimming underwater, and drowning may result. Surgery may be indicated for debulking or removal of the tumors.

Autosomal Recessive Disorders

Autosomal recessive disorders are manifested only when both members of the gene pair are affected. In this case, both parents may be unaffected but are carriers of the defective gene. Autosomal recessive disorders affect both sexes. The occurrence risk in each pregnancy is one in four for an affected child, two in four for a carrier child, and one in four for a normal (noncarrier, unaffected) homozygous child (Fig. 7-5).

With autosomal recessive disorders, the age of onset is frequently early in life; the symptomatology tends to be more uniform than with autosomal dominant disorders; and the disorders are characteristically caused by deficiencies in enzymes rather than abnormalities in structural proteins. In the case of a heterozygous carrier, the presence of a mutant gene usually does not produce symptoms because equal amounts of normal and defective enzymes are synthesized. The "margin of safety" ensures that cells with half their usual amount of enzyme function normally. By contrast, the inactivation of both alleles in a homozygote results in complete loss of enzyme activity. Autosomal recessive disorders include almost all inborn errors of metabolism. Enzyme disorders that impair catabolic pathways result in an accumulation of dietary substances (*e.g*, phenylketonuria [PKU]) or cellular constituents (*e.g.*, lysosomal storage diseases). Other disorders result from a defect in the enzyme-mediated synthesis of an essential protein (*e.g.*, the cystic fibrosis transmembrane conductance regulator in cystic fibrosis). Two examples of autosomal recessive disorders that are not covered elsewhere in this book are PKU and Tay-Sachs disease.

Phenylketonuria. Phenylketonuria is a genetically inherited enzyme defect. It is characterized by a deficiency of phenylalanine hydroxylase, the enzyme needed for conversion of phenylalanine to tyrosine. As a result of this deficiency, toxic levels of phenylalanine accumulate in the blood. Like other inborn errors of metabolism, PKU is inherited as a recessive trait and is manifested only in the homozygote. Untreated, PKU results in severe mental retardation.

PKU occurs once in approximately 10,000 births, and damage to the developing brain almost always results when high concentrations of phenylalanine and other metabolites persist in the blood.[4] Because the symptoms of untreated PKU develop gradually and would often go undetected until irreversible mental retardation had occurred, newborn infants are routinely screened for abnormal levels of serum phenylalanine. It is important that blood samples for PKU screening be obtained at least 12 hours after birth to ensure accuracy.[6] It also is possible to identify carriers of the trait by subjecting them to a phenylalanine test, in which a large dose of phenylalanine is administered orally and the rate at which it disappears from the bloodstream is measured.

Infants with the disorder are treated with a special diet that restricts phenylalanine intake. Dietary treatment must be started early in neonatal life to prevent brain damage. The results of dietary therapy of children with PKU have been impressive. The diet can prevent mental retardation as well as other neurodegenerative effects of untreated PKU.

Tay-Sachs disease. Tay-Sachs disease is a variant of a class of lysosomal storage diseases, known as *gangliosidoses,* in which substances (gangliosides) found in membranes of nervous tissue are deposited in neurons of the central nervous system and retina because of a failure of lysosomal degradation.[4,5] The disease is particularly prevalent among eastern European (Ashkenazi) Jews. Infants with Tay-Sachs disease appear normal at birth but begin to manifest progressive weakness, muscle flaccidity, and decreased attentiveness at approximately 6 to 10 months of age. This is followed by rapid deterioration of motor and mental function, often with development of generalized seizures. Retinal involvement leads to visual impairment and eventual blindness. Death usually occurs before 4 years of age. Although there is no cure for the disease, analysis of the blood serum for a deficiency of the lysosomal enzyme, hexosaminidase A, which is deficient in Tay-Sachs disease, allows for accurate identification of the genetic carriers for the disease.

X-Linked Disorders

Sex-linked disorders are almost always associated with the X, or female, chromosome, and the inheritance pattern is predominantly recessive. Because of a normal paired gene, female heterozygotes rarely experience the effects of a defective gene. The common pattern of inheritance is one in which an unaffected mother carries one normal and one mutant allele on the X chromosome. This means that she has a 50% chance of transmitting the defective gene to her sons, and her daughters have a 50% chance of being carriers of the mutant gene. When the affected son procreates, he transmits the defective gene to all of his daughters, who become carriers of the mutant gene. Because the genes of the Y chromosome are unaffected, the affected male does not transmit the defect to any of his sons, and they will not be carriers or transmit the disorder to their children.

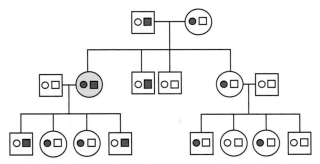

FIGURE 7-5 Simple pedigree for inheritance of an autosomal recessive trait. The small, colored circle and square represent a mutant gene. When both parents are carriers of a mutant gene, there is a 25% chance of having an affected child, a 50% chance of a carrier child, and a 25% chance of a nonaffected or noncarrier child, regardless of sex. All children (100%) of an affected parent are carriers.

X-linked recessive disorders include the fragile X syndrome, glucose-6-phosphate dehydrogenase deficiency (see Chapter 15), hemophilia A (see Chapter 14), and X-linked agammaglobulinemia (see Chapter 19).

Fragile X Syndrome. Fragile X syndrome is an X-linked disorder associated with a fragile site on the X chromosome where the chromatin fails to condense during mitosis. As with other X-linked disorders, fragile X syndrome affects males more often than females. The disorder, which affects approximately 1 in 1000 male infants, is the second most common cause of mental retardation, after Down syndrome.[7]

Affected males are mentally retarded and share a common physical phenotype that includes a long face with large mandible; large, everted ears; and large testicles (macro-orchidism). Hyperextensible joints, a high-arched palate, and mitral valve prolapse, which is observed in some cases, mimic a connective tissue disorder. Some physical abnormalities may be subtle or absent. The most distinctive feature, which is present in 90% of prepubertal males, is macro-orchidism.[5,8]

In 1991, the fragile X syndrome was mapped to a small area on the X chromosome (Xq27), now designated FMR-1 (fragile X, mental retardation 1) site.[7] The mechanism by which the normal FMR-1 gene is converted to an altered, or mutant, gene capable of producing disease symptoms involves an increase in the length of the gene. A small region of the gene that contains the CCG triplet code undergoes repeated duplication, resulting in a longer gene. The longer gene is susceptible to methylation, a chemical process that results in inactivation of the gene. When the number of repeats is small (<200), the person often has few or no manifestations of the disorder, compared with those evidenced in persons with a larger number of repeats.

In fragile X families, the probability of being affected with the disorder is related to the position in the pedigree. Later generations are more likely to be affected than earlier generations. For example, brothers of transmitting males are at a 9% risk of having mental retardation, whereas grandsons of transmitting males are at a 40% risk.[5] Approximately 20% of males who have been shown to carry the fragile X mutation are clinically and cytogenetically normal. Because male carriers transmit the trait through all their daughters (who are phenotypically normal) to affected grandchildren, they are called *transmitting males*. Approximately 50% of female carriers are affected (mentally retarded), a proportion that is higher than with other X-linked disorders.[5]

MULTIFACTORIAL INHERITANCE DISORDERS

Multifactorial inheritance disorders are caused by multiple genes and, in many cases, environmental factors. The exact number of genes contributing to multifactorial traits is not known, and these traits do not follow a clear-cut pattern of inheritance as do single-gene disorders. Multifactorial inheritance has been described as a threshold phenomenon in which the factors contributing to the trait might be compared with water filling a glass.[9] Using this analogy, one might say that expression of the disorder occurs when the glass overflows. Disorders of multifactorial inheritance can be expressed during fetal life and be present at birth, or they may be expressed later in life. Congenital disorders that are thought to arise through multifactorial inheritance include cleft lip or palate, clubfoot, congenital dislocation of the hip, congenital heart disease, pyloric stenosis, and urinary tract malformation. Environmental factors are thought to play a greater role in disorders of multifactorial inheritance that develop in adult life, such as coronary artery disease, diabetes mellitus, hypertension, cancer, and common psychiatric disorders such as manic-depressive psychoses and schizophrenia.

Although multifactorial traits cannot be predicted with the same degree of accuracy as the mendelian single-gene mutations, characteristic patterns exist. First, multifactorial congenital malformations tend to involve a single organ or tissue derived from the same embryonic developmental field. Second, the risk of recurrence in future pregnancies is for the same or a similar defect. This means that parents of a child with a cleft palate defect have an increased risk of having another child with a cleft palate, but not with spina bifida. Third, the increased risk (compared with the general population) among first-degree relatives of the affected person is 2% to 7%, and among second-degree relatives, it is approximately one-half that amount.[5] The risk increases with increasing incidence of the defect among relatives. This means that the risk is greatly increased when a second child with the defect is born to a couple. The risk also increases with severity of the disorder and when the defect occurs in the sex not usually affected by the disorder.

CHROMOSOMAL DISORDERS

Chromosomal disorders form a major category of genetic disease, accounting for a large proportion of reproductive wastage (early gestational abortions), congenital malformations, and mental retardation. Specific chromosomal abnormalities can be linked to more than 60 identifiable syndromes that are present in 0.7% of all live births, 2% of all pregnancies in women older than 35 years of age, and 50% of all first-term abortions.[3]

During cell division (*i.e.,* mitosis) in nongerm cells, the chromosomes replicate so that each cell receives a full diploid number. In germ cells, a different form of division (*i.e.,* meiosis) takes place. During meiosis, the double sets of 22 autosomes and the 2 sex chromosomes (normal diploid number) are reduced to single sets (haploid number) in each gamete. At the time of conception, the haploid number in the ovum and that in the sperm join and restore the diploid number of chromosomes. Chromosomal defects usually develop because of defective movement during meiosis or because of breakage of a chromosome with loss or translocation of genetic material.

Chromosome abnormalities are commonly described according to the shorthand description of the karyotype. In this system, the total number of chromosomes is given first, followed by the sex chromosome complement, and then the description of any abnormality. For example, a male with trisomy 21 is designated 47,XY,+21.

Alterations in Chromosome Duplication

Mosaicism is the presence in one individual of two or more cell lines characterized by distinctive karyotypes. This defect results from an accident during chromosomal duplication. Sometimes, mosaicism consists of an abnormal karyotype and a normal one, in which case the physical deformities caused by the abnormal cell line usually are less severe.

Alterations in Chromosome Number

A change in chromosome number is called *aneuploidy*. Among the causes of aneuploidy is failure of the chromosomes to separate during oogenesis or spermatogenesis. This can occur in the autosomes or the sex chromosomes and is called *nondisjunction*. Nondisjunction gives rise to germ cells that have an even number of chromosomes (22 or 24). The products of conception formed from this even number of chromosomes have an uneven number of chromosomes, 45 or 47. *Monosomy* refers to the presence of only one member of a chromosome pair. The defects associated with monosomy of the autosomes are severe and usually cause abortion. Monosomy of the X chromosome (45,X/O), or Turner's syndrome, causes less severe defects. *Polysomy*, or the presence of more than two chromosomes to a set, occurs when a germ cell containing more than 23 chromosomes is involved in conception. This defect has been described for the autosomes and the sex chromosomes. Trisomies of chromosomes 8, 13, 18, and 21 are the more common forms of polysomy of the autosomes. There are several forms of polysomy of the sex chromosomes in which extra X or Y chromosomes are present.

Trisomy 21. First described in 1866 by John Langon Down, trisomy 21, or Down syndrome, causes a combination of birth defects including some degree of mental retardation, characteristic facial features, and other health problems. According to the National Down Syndrome Association, it is the most common chromosomal disorder, occurring approximately once in every 800 to 1000 births. Currently, there are approximately 350,000 people in the United States with Down syndrome.[10]

Approximately 95% of cases of Down syndrome are caused by nondisjunction or an error in cell division during meiosis, resulting in a trisomy of chromosome 21. Most of the remaining cases are due to a translocation in which part of chromosome 21 breaks off and attaches to another chromosome (usually chromosome 14). Although there still are only 46 chromosomes in the cell, the presence of the extra part of chromosome 21 causes the features of Down syndrome (to be discussed).

The risk of having a child with Down syndrome increases with maternal age—it is 1/1300 at 25 years of age, 1/365 at 35 years, and 1/30 at 45 years of age.[11] The reason for the correlation between maternal age and nondisjunction is unknown, but is thought to reflect some aspect of aging of the oocyte. Although males continue to produce sperm throughout their reproductive life, females are born with all the oocytes they ever will have. These oocytes may change as a result of the aging process. With increasing age, there is a greater chance of a woman having been exposed to damaging environmental agents such as drugs, chemicals, and radiation. Unlike trisomy 21, Down syndrome due to a chromosome (21; 14) translocation shows no relation to maternal age but has a relatively high recurrence risk in families when a parent, particularly the mother, is a carrier.

The physical features of a child with Down syndrome are distinctive, and therefore the condition usually is apparent at birth. These features include a small and rather square head. There is upward slanting of the eyes; small, low-set, and malformed ears; a fat pad at the back of the neck; an open mouth; and a large, protruding tongue (Fig. 7-6). The child's hands usually are short and stubby, with fingers that curl inward, and there usually is only a single palmar (*i.e.*, simian) crease. Hypotonia and joint laxity also are present in infants and young children. There often are accompanying congenital heart defects and an increased risk of gastrointestinal malformations. Approximately 1% of persons with trisomy 21 Down syndrome have mosaicism (*i.e.*, cell populations with the normal chromosome number and trisomy 21); these persons may be less severely affected. Of particular concern is the much greater risk of development of acute leukemia among children with Down syndrome—10 to 20 times greater than that of other children.[5] With increased life expectancy due to improved health care, it has been found that there is an increased risk of Alzheimer's disease among older persons with Down syndrome.

There are several prenatal screening tests that can be done to determine the risk of having a child with Down syndrome. The most commonly used test is the triple screen—α-fetoprotein (AFP), human chorionic gonadotropin (HCG), and unconjugated estriol. The results of these tests, which usually are done between 15 and 20 weeks of gestation, together with the woman's age often are used to determine the probability of a pregnant woman having a child with Down syndrome. These tests are able to accurately detect only approximately 60% of fetuses with Down syndrome.

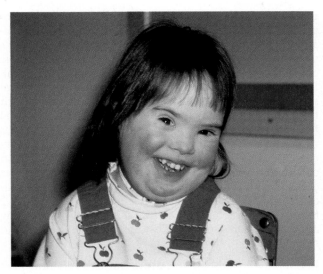

FIGURE 7-6 A child with Down syndrome. (Courtesy of March of Dimes Birth Defects Foundation, White Plains, NY)

Some women are given false-positive readings and some are given false-negative readings. In 1992, fetal nuchal (back of neck) translucency, as measured by ultrasonography in the first trimester, was proposed as another screening measure; the nucha was found to be thicker in fetuses with Down syndrome.[12] This test, which must be done by a highly trained professional, continues to be investigated as a screening method. The only way to accurately determine the presence of Down syndrome in the fetus is through chromosome analysis using chorionic villus sampling, amniocentesis, or percutaneous umbilical blood sampling.

Monosomy X. Monosomy X, or Turner's syndrome, describes a monosomy of the X chromosome (45,X/0) with gonadal agenesis, or absence of the ovaries. This disorder affects approximately 1 of every 2500 live births, and it has been estimated that over 99% of fetuses with the 45,X/0 karyotype are spontaneously aborted in the first trimester.[13] There are variations in the syndrome, with abnormalities ranging from essentially none to webbing of the neck with redundant skin folds, nonpitting lymphedema of the hands and feet, and congenital heart defects, particularly coarctation of the aorta. There also may be abnormalities in kidney development (*i.e.,* abnormal location, abnormal vascular supply, or double collecting system). There may be other abnormalities such as changes in nail growth, high-arched palate, short fourth metacarpal, and strabismus.

Characteristically, the female with Turner's syndrome is short in stature, but her body proportions are normal. She does not menstruate and shows no signs of secondary sex characteristics. When a mosaic cell line (*i.e.,* 45,X/0 and 46,X/X or 45,X/0 and 46,X/Y) is present, the manifestations associated with the chromosomal defect tend to be less severe.

Administration of female sex hormones (*i.e.,* estrogens) is used to promote development of secondary sexual characteristics and produce additional skeletal growth in women with Turner's syndrome. Growth hormone also may be used to increase skeletal growth.[14]

The diagnosis of Turner's syndrome often is delayed until late childhood or early adolescence in girls who do not present with the classic features of the syndrome.[15] Early diagnosis is an important aspect of treatment for Turner's syndrome. It allows for counseling about the phenotypic characteristics of the disorder; screening for cardiac, renal, thyroid, and other abnormalities; provision of emotional support for the girl and her family; and planning for growth hormone therapy, if appropriate.[13] Because of the potential for delay in diagnosis, it has been recommended that girls with unexplained short stature (height below the fifth percentile), webbed neck, peripheral lymphedema, coarctation of the aorta, or delayed puberty have chromosome studies done. In addition, chromosome analysis should be considered for girls who remain above the fifth percentile but have two or more features of Turner's syndrome, including high palate, nail deformities, short fourth metacarpal, and strabismus.[15]

Polysomy X. Polysomy X, or Klinefelter's syndrome, is a condition of testicular dysgenesis accompanied by the presence of one or more extra X chromosomes in excess of the normal male XY complement. Most males with Klinefelter's syndrome have one extra X chromosome (XXY). In rare cases, there may be more than one extra X chromosome (XXXY). The syndrome is characterized by enlarged breasts, sparse facial and body hair, small testes, and the inability to produce sperm.[15] Regardless of the number of X chromosomes present, the male phenotype is retained. Based on studies conducted in the 1970s, including one sponsored by the National Institutes of Health and Human Development that checked the chromosomes of more than 40,000 infants, it has been estimated that the XXY syndrome is one of the most common genetic abnormalities known, occurring as frequently as 1 in 500 to 1 in 1000 male births.[16] Although the presence of the extra chromosome is fairly common, the syndrome with its accompanying signs and symptoms that may result from the extra chromosome is uncommon. Many men live their lives without being aware that they have an additional chromosome. For this reason, it has been suggested that the term *Klinefelter's syndrome* be replaced with *XXY male.*

The condition often goes undetected at birth. The infant usually has normal male genitalia, with a small penis and small, firm testicles. At puberty, the intrinsically abnormal testes do not respond to stimulation from the gonadotropins and undergo degeneration. This leads to a tall stature with abnormal body proportions in which the lower part of the body is longer than the upper part. Later in life, the body build may become heavy, with a female distribution of subcutaneous fat and variable degrees of breast enlargement. There may be deficient secondary male sex characteristics, such as a voice that remains feminine in pitch and sparse beard and pubic hair. There may be sexual dysfunction along with the complete infertility that occurs owing to the inability to produce sperm. Regular administration of testosterone, beginning at puberty, can promote more normal growth and development of secondary sexual characteristics. Although the intellect usually is normal, most XXY males have some degree of language impairment. They often learn to talk later than do other children and often have trouble with learning to read and write.

The presence of the extra X chromosome in the XXY male results from nondisjunction during meiotic division in one of the parents. The additional X chromosome (or chromosomes) is of maternal origin in approximately two thirds of cases and of paternal origin in the remaining one third.[4] The cause of the nondisjunction is unknown. Advanced maternal age increases the risk, but only slightly.

Alterations in Chromosome Structure

Aberrations in chromosome structure occur when there is a break in one or more of the chromosomes followed by rearrangement or deletion of the chromosome parts. Among the factors believed to cause chromosome breakage are exposure to radiation sources, such as x-rays; influence of certain chemicals; extreme changes in the cellular environment; and viral infections.

Several patterns of chromosome breakage and rearrangement can occur (Fig. 7-7). There can be a *deletion* of the broken portion of the chromosome. When one chromosome is involved, the broken parts may be *inverted. Iso-*

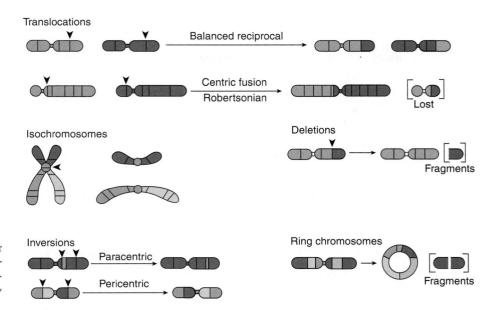

FIGURE 7-7 Rearrangement after breaks in chromosome structures. (Cotran R.S., Kumar V., Collins T. [1999]. *Pathologic basis of disease.* [6th ed., p. 169]. Philadelphia: W.B. Saunders)

chromosome formation occurs when the centromere, or central portion, of the chromosome separates horizontally instead of vertically. *Ring formation* results when deletion is followed by uniting of the chromatids to form a ring. *Translocation* occurs when there are simultaneous breaks in two chromosomes from different pairs, with exchange of chromosome parts. With a balanced reciprocal translocation, no genetic information is lost; therefore, persons with translocations usually are normal. However, these persons are translocation carriers and may have normal and abnormal children.

A special form of translocation called a *centric fusion* or *Robertsonian translocation* involves two acrocentric chromosomes in which the centromere is near the end. Typically, the break occurs near the centromere affecting the short arm in one chromosome and the long arm in the other. Transfer of the chromosome fragments leads to one long and one extremely short chromosome. The short fragments commonly are lost. In this case, the person has only 45 chromosomes, but the amount of genetic material that is lost is so small that it often goes unnoticed. Difficulty, however, arises during meiosis; the result is gametes with an unbalanced number of chromosomes.

A rare form of Down syndrome can occur in the offspring of persons in whom there has been a translocation involving the long arm of chromosome 21q and the long arm of one of the acrocentric chromosomes (most often 14 or 22). The translocation adds to the normal long arm of chromosome 21; therefore, the person with this type of Down syndrome has 46 chromosomes, but essentially a trisomy of 21q.[3]

The manifestations of aberrations in chromosome structure depend to a great extent on the amount of genetic material that is lost. Many cells sustaining unrestored breaks are eliminated within the next few mitoses because of deficiencies that may in themselves be fatal. This is beneficial because it prevents the damaged cells from becoming a permanent part of the organism or, if it occurs in the gametes, from giving rise to grossly defective zygotes. Some altered chromosomes, such as those that occur with translocations, are passed on to the next generation.

In summary, genetic disorders can affect a single gene (mendelian inheritance) or several genes (polygenic inheritance). Single-gene disorders may be present on an autosome or on the X chromosome and they may be expressed as a dominant or recessive trait. In autosomal dominant disorders, a single mutant allele from an affected parent is transmitted to an offspring regardless of sex. The affected parent has a 50% chance of transmitting the disorder to each offspring. Autosomal recessive disorders are manifested only when both members of the gene pair are affected. Usually, both parents are unaffected but are carriers of the defective gene. Their chances of having an affected child are one in four; of having a carrier child, two in four; and of having a noncarrier unaffected child, one in four. Sex-linked disorders, which are associated with the X chromosome, are those in which an unaffected mother carries one normal and one mutant allele on the X chromosome. She has a 50% chance of transmitting the defective gene to her sons, and her daughters have a 50% chance of being carriers of the mutant gene. Because of a normal paired gene, female heterozygotes rarely experience the effects of a defective gene. Multifactorial inheritance disorders are caused by multiple genes and, in many cases, environmental factors.

Chromosomal disorders result from a change in chromosome number or structure. A change in chromosome number is called *aneuploidy*. *Monosomy* involves the presence of only one member of a chromosome pair; it is seen in Turner's syndrome, in which there is monosomy of the X chromosome. *Polysomy* refers to the presence of more than two chromosomes in a set. Klinefelter's syndrome involves polysomy of the X chromosome. Trisomy 21 (*i.e.*, Down syndrome) is the most common form of chromosome disorder. Alterations in chromosome structure involve deletion or addition of genetic material, which may involve a translocation of genetic material from one chromosome pair to another.

Disorders Due to Environmental Influences

After you have completed this section of the chapter, you should be able to meet the following objectives:

+ Cite the most susceptible period of intrauterine life for development of defects due to environmental agents
+ State the cautions that should be observed when considering use of drugs during pregnancy
+ Describe the effects of alcohol and cocaine abuse on fetal development and birth outcomes
+ List four infectious agents that cause congenital defects

The developing embryo is subject to many nongenetic influences. After conception, development is influenced by the environmental factors that the embryo shares with the mother. The physiologic status of the mother—her hormone balance, her general state of health, her nutritional status, and the drugs she takes—undoubtedly influences the development of the unborn child. For example, diabetes mellitus is associated with increased risk of congenital anomalies. Smoking is associated with lower than normal neonatal weight. Alcohol, in the context of chronic alcoholism, is known to cause fetal abnormalities. Some agents cause early abortion. Measles and other infectious agents cause congenital malformations. Other agents, such as radiation, can cause chromosomal and genetic defects and produce developmental disorders.

PERIOD OF VULNERABILITY

The embryo's development is most easily disturbed during the period when differentiation and development of the organs are taking place. This time interval, which is often referred to as the period of *organogenesis*, extends from day 15 to day 60 after conception. Environmental influences during the first 2 weeks after fertilization may interfere with implantation and result in abortion or early resorption of the products of conception. Each organ has a critical period during which it is highly susceptible to environmental derangements (Fig. 7-8). Often, the effect is expressed at the biochemical level just before the organ begins to develop. The same agent may affect different organ systems that are developing at the same time.

TERATOGENIC AGENTS

A teratogenic agent is an environmental agent that produces abnormalities during embryonic or fetal development. It is important to remember that, in this case, the environment is that of the embryo and fetus. Maternal disease or altered metabolic state also can affect the environment of the embryo or fetus. For discussion purposes, teratogenic agents have been divided into three groups: radiation, drugs and chemical substances, and infectious agents. Chart 7-1 lists commonly identified agents in each of these groups. Theoretically, environmental agents can cause birth defects in three ways: by direct exposure of the pregnant woman and the embryo or fetus to the agent; through exposure of the soon-to-be-pregnant woman with an agent that has a slow clearance rate such that a teratogenic dose is retained during early pregnancy; or as a result of mutagenic effects of an environmental agent that occur before pregnancy, causing permanent damage to a woman's (or a man's) reproductive cells.

Radiation

Heavy doses of ionizing radiation have been shown to cause microcephaly, skeletal malformations, and mental retardation. There is no evidence that diagnostic levels of radiation cause congenital abnormalities. Because the question of safety remains, however, many agencies require that the day of a woman's last menstrual period be noted on all radiologic requisitions. Other institutions may require a pregnancy test before any extensive diagnostic x-ray studies are performed. Radiation is teratogenic and mutagenic, and there is the possibility of effecting inheritable changes in genetic materials. Administration of therapeutic doses of radioactive iodine (^{131}I) during the 13th week of gestation, the time when the fetal thyroid is beginning to concentrate iodine, has been shown to interfere with thyroid development.

Chemicals and Drugs

Environmental chemicals and drugs can cross the placenta and cause damage to the developing embryo and fetus. It has been estimated that only 2% to 3% of developmental defects have a known drug or environmental origin. Some of the best-documented environmental teratogens are the organic mercurials, which cause neurologic deficits and blindness. Sources of exposure to mercury include contaminated food (fish) and water.[17] The precise mechanism by which chemicals and drugs exert their teratogenic effects is largely unknown. They may produce cytotoxic (cell-killing), antimetabolic, or growth-inhibiting properties. Often their effects depend on the time of exposure (in terms of embryonic and fetal development) and extent of exposure (dosage).

Drugs top the list of chemical teratogens, probably because they are regularly used at elevated doses. Most drugs can cross the placenta and expose the fetus to both the pharmacologic and teratogenic effects. Factors that affect placental drug transfer and drug effects on the fetus include the rate at which the drug crosses the placenta, the duration of exposure, and the stage of placental and fetal develop-

Weeks

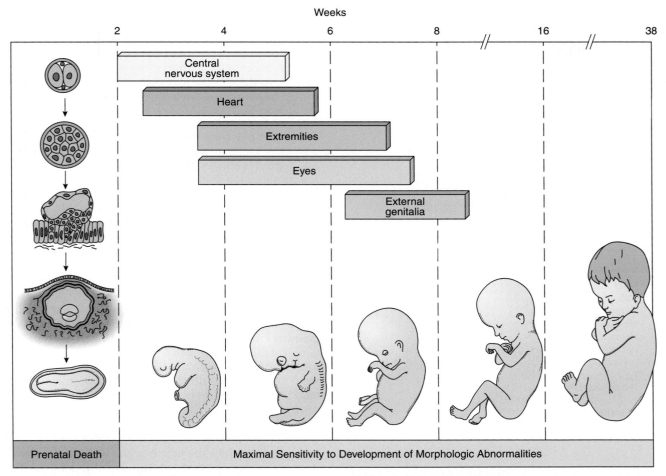

FIGURE 7-8 Sensitivity of specific organs to teratogenic agents at critical periods in embryogenesis. Exposure of adverse influences in the preimplantation and early postimplantation stages of development (*far left*) leads to prenatal death. Periods of maximal sensitivity to teratogens (*horizontal red bars*) vary for different organ systems but overall are limited to the first 8 weeks of pregnancy. (Rubin E., Farber J.L. [1999]. *Pathology* [3rd ed., p. 216]. Philadelphia: Lippincott Williams & Wilkins)

ment at the time of exposure.[18] Lipid-soluble drugs tend to cross the placenta more readily and enter the fetal circulation. The molecular weight of a drug also influences the rate of transfer and the amount of drug transferred across the placenta. Drugs with a molecular weight less than 500 can cross the placenta easily, depending on lipid solubility and degree of ionization; those with a molecular weight of 500 to 1000 cross the placenta with more difficulty; and those with molecular weights greater than 1000 cross very poorly.[18]

A number of drugs are suspected of being teratogens, but only a few have been identified with certainty.[19] Perhaps the best known of these drugs is thalidomide, which has been shown to give rise to a full range of malformations, including phocomelia (*i.e.*, short, flipper-like appendages) of all four extremities. Other drugs known to cause fetal abnormalities are the antimetabolites that are used in the treatment of cancer, the anticoagulant drug warfarin, several of the anticonvulsant drugs, ethyl alcohol, and cocaine. Some drugs affect a single developing structure; for exam-

ple, propylthiouracil can impair thyroid development and tetracycline can interfere with the mineralization phase of tooth development. More recently, vitamin A and its derivatives (the retinoids) have been targeted for concern because of their teratogenic potential. Concern over the teratogenic effects of vitamin A derivatives became evident with the introduction of the acne drug isotretinoin (Accutane). Fetal abnormalities such as cleft palate, heart defects, retinal and optic nerve abnormalities, and central nervous system malformations were observed in women ingesting therapeutic doses of the drug during the first trimester of pregnancy.[20] There also is concern about the teratogenic effects when a woman consumes high doses of vitamin A, such as those contained in some dietary supplements or vitamin pills. It is currently recommended that doses greater than 10,000 IU should be avoided.[21]

In 1983, the U.S. Food and Drug Administration established a system for classifying drugs according to probable risks to the fetus. According to this system, drugs are put into five categories: A, B, C, D, and X. Drugs in category

CHART 7-1

*Teratogenic Agents**

Radiation
Drugs and Chemical Substances
Alcohol
Anticoagulants
  Warfarin
Anticonvulsants
Cancer drugs
  Aminopterin
  Methotrexate
  6-Mercaptopurine
Isotretinoin (Accutane)
Propylthiouracil
Tetracycline
Thalidomide

Infectious Agents
Viruses
  Cytomegalovirus
  Herpes simplex virus
  Measles (rubella)
  Mumps
  Varicella-zoster virus (chickenpox)
Nonviral factors
  Syphilis
  Toxoplasmosis

* Not inclusive.

A are the least dangerous, and categories B, C, and D are increasingly more dangerous. Those in category X are contraindicated during pregnancy because of proven teratogenicity.[22] The law does not require classification of drugs that were in use before 1983.

Because many drugs are suspected of causing fetal abnormalities, and even those that were once thought to be

Teratogenic Agents

➤ Teratogenic agents such as radiation, chemicals and drugs, and infectious organisms are agents that produce abnormalities in the developing embryo.

➤ The stage of development of the embryo determines the susceptibility to teratogens. The period during which the embryo is most susceptible to teratogenic agents is the time time during which rapid differentiation and development of body organs and tissues are taking place, usually from days 15 to 60 postconception.

safe are now being viewed critically, it is recommended that women in their childbearing years avoid unnecessary use of drugs. This pertains to nonpregnant women as well as pregnant women because many developmental defects occur early in pregnancy. As happened with thalidomide, the damage to the embryo may occur before pregnancy is suspected or confirmed. Two drugs of particular importance are alcohol and cocaine.

Fetal Alcohol Syndrome.   The term *fetal alcohol syndrome* (FAS) refers to a constellation of physical, behavioral, and cognitive abnormalities resulting from maternal alcohol consumption. It has been reported that 1 in 1000 infants born in the United States manifests some characteristics of the syndrome.[23] Alcohol, which is lipid soluble and has a molecular weight between 600 and 1000, passes freely across the placental barrier; concentrations of alcohol in the fetus are at least as high as in the mother. Unlike other teratogens, the harmful effects of alcohol are not restricted to the sensitive period of early gestation, but extend throughout pregnancy.

Alcohol has widely variable effects on fetal development, ranging from minor abnormalities to FAS. Criteria for defining FAS were standardized by the Fetal Alcohol Study Group of the Research Society on Alcoholism in 1980,[24] and modifications were proposed in 1989 by Sokol and Clarren.[25] The proposed criteria are prenatal or postnatal growth retardation (*i.e.,* weight or length below the 10th percentile); central nervous system involvement, including neurologic abnormalities, developmental delays, behavioral dysfunction, intellectual impairment, and skull and brain malformation; and a characteristic face with short palpebral fissures (*i.e.,* eye openings), a thin upper lip, and an elongated, flattened midface and philtrum (*i.e.,* the groove in the middle of the upper lip). The facial features of FAS may not be as apparent in the newborn but become more prominent as the infant develops (Fig. 7-9). As the children grow into adulthood, the facial features become more subtle, making diagnosis of FAS in older individuals more difficult.[26] Each of these defects can vary in severity, probably reflecting the timing of alcohol consumption in terms of the period of fetal development, amount of alcohol consumed, and hereditary and environmental influences. Because of problems with terminology and the diagnostic criteria, the Institute of Medicine in 1996 proposed the terms *alcohol-related neurodevelopmental disorder* (ARND) and *alcohol-related birth defects* (ARBD) to describe conditions in which there is a history of maternal alcohol consumption.[27] This new terminology uses pathophysiologic diagnostic categories to describe the conditions resulting from confirmed alcohol exposure. For example, facial abnormalities, growth retardation, and central nervous system abnormalities would be classified as FAS; central nervous system and cognitive abnormalities would be classified as ARND; and birth defects as ARBD.[28]

The mechanisms whereby alcohol exerts its teratogenic effects are unclear. Evidence suggests that the effects of alcohol observed in children with FAS are related to the timing of alcohol consumption and peak alcohol dose.

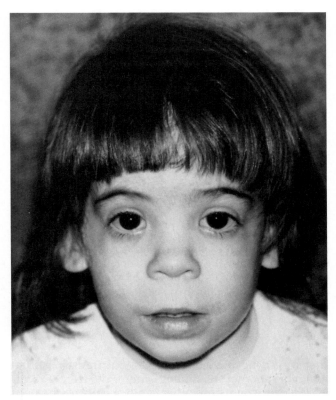

FIGURE 7-9 Child with fetal alcohol syndrome. (Clarren S.K., Smith D.W. [1978]. The fetal alcohol syndrome. *New England Journal of Medicine* 298, 1065)

The amount of alcohol that can be safely consumed during pregnancy also is unknown. Animal studies suggest that the fetotoxic effects of alcohol are dose dependent rather than threshold dependent. Studies suggest that even three drinks per day may be associated with a lower IQ at 4 years of age.[29] However, it may be that the time during which alcohol is consumed is equally important. Even small amounts of alcohol consumed during critical periods of fetal development may be teratogenic. For example, if alcohol is consumed during the period of organogenesis, a variety of skeletal and organ defects may result. When alcohol is consumed later in gestation, when the brain is undergoing rapid development, there may be behavioral and cognitive disorders in the absence of physical abnormalities. Chronic alcohol consumption throughout pregnancy may result in a variety of effects, ranging from physical abnormalities to growth retardation and compromised central nervous system functioning. Evidence suggests that short-lived high concentrations of alcohol such as those that occur with binge drinking may be particularly significant, with abnormalities being unique to the period of exposure. The recommendation of the U.S. Surgeon General is that women abstain completely from alcohol during pregnancy.[30]

Cocaine Babies. Of concern is the increasing use of cocaine by pregnant women. In 1992, approximately 45,000 women in this country used cocaine during their pregnancy.[31] Determining exposure of infants to maternal cocaine use often is difficult. In utero exposure often is ascertained by testing maternal urine for cocaine and its metabolites and by interviewing the mother. Urine testing provides evidence only of recent cocaine use, and information from an interview may be inaccurate. Urine testing of infants provides evidence only of recent exposure to cocaine.

Among the effects of cocaine use during pregnancy is a decrease in uteroplacental blood flow, maternal hypertension, stimulation of uterine contractions, and fetal vasoconstriction. The decrease in uteroplacental blood flow is associated with an increase in preterm births, intrauterine growth retardation, microcephaly, and neurologic abnormalities.[32,33] Furthermore, there appears to be a dose-related relationship between increasing levels of chronic cocaine abuse and impaired fetal growth and neurologic function.[33] Maternal hypertension may increase the risk of abruptio placentae, particularly if it is accompanied by a decrease in uteroplacental blood flow.[31] Fetal vasoconstriction has been suggested as the cause of fetal anomalies, particularly limb reduction defects and urogenital tract defects such as hydronephrosis, hypospadias, and undescended testicles, as well as ambiguous genitalia.[34,35] Exposure of the fetus to cocaine also may lead to destructive lesions of the brain, including cerebral infarction and intracranial hemorrhage. Sudden infant death syndrome (SIDS) also has been more common in infants of mothers who have used cocaine during their pregnancy.[36]

Although the immediate effects of maternal cocaine use on infant behavior are being reported, the long-term effects are largely unknown. Unfortunately, cocaine addiction often affects the behavior of the pregnant woman to the extent that the need to procure larger amounts of the drug overwhelms all other considerations of maternal and fetal well-being; other factors such as malnutrition, use of other drugs and teratogens, and lack of prenatal care also may contribute to fetal disorders.

Folic Acid Deficiency. Although most birth defect are related to exposure to a teratogenic agent, deficiencies of nutrients and vitamins also may be a factor. Folic acid deficiency has been implicated in the development of neural tube defects (*e.g.,* anencephaly, spina bifida, encephalocele). Studies have shown a reduction in neural tube defects when folic acid was taken before conception and continued during the first trimester of pregnancy.[37,38] The Public Health Service recommends that all women of childbearing age should take 400 micrograms (μg) of folic acid daily. It has been suggested that this recommendation may help to prevent as many as 50% of neural tube defects.[39] The Institute of Medicine Panel for Folate and Other B Vitamins and Choline has recently revised the Recommended Dietary Allowance for pregnant women to 600 μg.[40] These recommendations are particularly important for women who have previously had an affected pregnancy, for couples with a close relative with the disorder, and for women with diabetes mellitus and those on anticonvulsant drugs who are at increased risk for having infants with birth defects.

Since 1998, all enriched cereal grain products in the United States have been fortified with folic acid. To achieve an adequate intake of folic acid, pregnant women should couple a diet that contains folate-rich foods (*e.g.*, orange juice, dark, leafy green vegetables, and legumes) with sources of synthetic folic acid, such as fortified food products.[40]

Infectious Agents

Many microorganisms cross the placenta and enter the fetal circulation, often producing multiple malformations. The acronym TORCH stands for *t*oxoplasmosis, *o*ther, *r*ubella (*i.e.*, German measles), *c*ytomegalovirus, and *h*erpes, which are the agents most frequently implicated in fetal anomalies.[3] Other infections include varicella-zoster virus infection, listeriosis, leptospirosis, Epstein-Barr virus infection, tuberculosis, and syphilis. The TORCH screening test examines the infant's serum for the presence of antibodies to these agents. These infections tend to cause similar clinical manifestations, including microcephaly, hydrocephalus, defects of the eye, and hearing problems.

Toxoplasmosis is a protozoal infection that can be contracted by eating raw or poorly cooked meat. The domestic cat also seems to carry the organism, excreting the protozoa in its stools. It has been suggested that pregnant women should avoid contact with excrement from the family cat. The introduction of the rubella vaccine in the United States has virtually eliminated congenital rubella. The epidemiology of cytomegalovirus infection is largely unknown. Some infants are severely affected at birth, and others, although having evidence of the infection, have no symptoms. In some symptom-free infants, brain damage becomes evident over a span of several years. There also is evidence that some infants contract the infection during the first year of life, and in some of them the infection leads to retardation a year or two later. Herpes simplex type 2 infection is considered to be a genital infection and usually is transmitted through sexual contact. The infant acquires this infection in utero or in passage through the birth canal.

In summary, a teratogenic agent is one that produces abnormalities during embryonic or fetal life. It is during the early part of pregnancy (15 to 60 days after conception) that environmental agents are most apt to produce their deleterious effects on the developing embryo. A number of environmental agents can be damaging to the unborn child, including radiation, drugs and chemicals, and infectious agents. FAS is a risk for infants of women who regularly consume alcohol during pregnancy. Of recent concern is the use of cocaine by pregnant women. Because many drugs have the potential for causing fetal abnormalities, often at an early stage of pregnancy, it is recommended that women of childbearing age avoid unnecessary use of drugs. It also has been shown that folic acid deficiency can contribute to neural tube defects. The acronym TORCH stands for *t*oxoplasmosis, *o*ther, *r*ubella, *c*ytomegalovirus, and *h*erpes, which are the infectious agents most frequently implicated in fetal anomalies.

Diagnosis and Counseling

After you have completed this section of the chapter, you should be able to meet the following objectives:

✦ Describe the process of genetic assessment
✦ Cite the rationale for prenatal diagnosis
✦ Describe methods used in arriving at a prenatal diagnosis, including ultrasonography, amniocentesis, chorionic villus sampling, percutaneous umbilical fetal blood sampling, and laboratory methods to determine the biochemical and genetic makeup of the fetus

The birth of a defective child is a traumatic event in any parent's life. Usually two issues must be resolved. The first deals with the immediate and future care of the affected child, and the second with the possibility of future children in the family having a similar defect. Genetic assessment and counseling can help to determine whether the defect was inherited and the risk of recurrence. Prenatal diagnosis provides a means of determining whether the unborn child has certain types of abnormalities.

GENETIC ASSESSMENT

Effective genetic counseling involves accurate diagnosis and communication of the findings and of the risks of recurrence to the parents and other family members who need such information. Counseling may be provided after the birth of an affected child, or it may be offered to persons at risk for having defective children (*i.e.*, siblings of persons with birth defects). A team of trained counselors can help the family to understand the problem and can support their decisions about having more children.

Assessment of genetic risk and prognosis usually is directed by a clinical geneticist, often with the aid of laboratory and clinical specialists. A detailed family history (*i.e.*, pedigree), a pregnancy history, and detailed accounts of the birth process and postnatal health and development are included. A careful physical examination of the affected child and often of the parents and siblings usually is needed. Laboratory tests, including chromosomal analysis and biochemical studies, often precedes a definitive diagnosis.

The creases and dermal ridges on the palms and soles are examined in a genetic study called dermatoglyphic analysis. This is of value because the dermal ridges are formed by 16 weeks of gestation and any abnormalities document the time during which the developmental defect occurred. Dermatoglyphic analysis includes examination of the patterns of the arches on the fingertips, the flexion creases of the fifth finger, and the arch pattern of the base of the great toe.

PRENATAL DIAGNOSIS

Prenatal diagnosis should begin with measures to identify pregnancies in which there is a recognizable risk of diagnosable fetal disorder.[41] The use of a questionnaire to elicit genetic information is recommended by the American

College of Obstetricians and Gynecologists before prenatal diagnosis is undertaken.[42]

The purpose of prenatal diagnosis is not just to detect fetal abnormalities. Rather, it has the following objectives: to provide parents with information needed to make an informed choice about having a child with an abnormality; to provide reassurance and reduce anxiety among high-risk groups; and to allow parents at risk for having a child with a specific defect, who might otherwise forgo having a child, to begin pregnancy with the assurance that knowledge about the presence or absence of the disorder in the fetus can be confirmed by testing.

Among the methods used for fetal diagnosis are maternal blood screening, ultrasonography, amniocentesis, chorionic villus sampling, and percutaneous umbilical fetal blood sampling. Termination of pregnancy is indicated only in a small number of cases; in the rest, the fetus is normal and the procedure provides reassurance for the parents. Prenatal diagnosis can also provide the information needed for prescribing prenatal treatment for the fetus. For example, if congenital adrenal hyperplasia is diagnosed, the mother can be treated with adrenal cortical hormones to prevent masculinization of a female fetus.

Maternal Serum Markers

Maternal blood testing began in the early 1980s with the test for AFP. AFP is a major fetal plasma protein and has a structure similar to the albumin that is found in postnatal life. AFP is made initially by the yolk sac and later by the liver. It peaks at approximately 12 to 14 weeks in the fetus and falls thereafter. AFP is found in the amniotic fluid at approximately 1/100 the concentration found in fetal serum. AFP reaches the maternal bloodstream and can be measured by laboratory methods. The normal maternal serum AFP level rises from 13 weeks and peaks at 32 weeks of gestation. In pregnancies where the fetus has a neural tube defect (*i.e.*, anencephaly and open spina bifida) or certain other malformations such as an anterior abdominal wall defect, maternal and amniotic levels of AFP are elevated because open neural tube and ventral wall defects are associated with exposed fetal membrane and blood vessel surfaces that increase the AFP in the amniotic fluid and maternal blood. Screening of maternal blood samples usually is done between weeks 16 and 18 of gestation.[33]

Although neural tube defects have been associated with elevated levels of AFP, decreased levels have been associated with Down syndrome. The single maternal serum marker that yields the highest detection rate for Down syndrome is an elevated level of HCG. The combined use of three maternal serum markers, decreased AFP and unconjugated estriol and elevated HCG, between 16 and 20 weeks of pregnancy has been shown to detect as many as 60% of Down syndrome pregnancies.[41] The use of ultrasound to verify fetal age can reduce the number of false-positive tests with this screening method.

Ultrasound

Ultrasound is a noninvasive diagnostic method that uses reflections of high-frequency sound waves to visualize soft tissue structures. Since its introduction in 1958, it has been used during pregnancy to determine number of fetuses, fetal size, fetal position, amount of amniotic fluid that is present, and placental location. It also is possible to assess fetal movement, breathing movements, and heart pattern. Improved resolution and real-time units have enhanced the ability of ultrasound scanners to detect congenital anomalies. With this more sophisticated equipment, it is possible to obtain information such as measurements of hourly urine output in a high-risk fetus. Ultrasound makes possible the in utero diagnosis of hydrocephalus, spina bifida, facial defects, congenital heart defects, congenital diaphragmatic hernias, disorders of the gastrointestinal tract, and skeletal anomalies. Cardiovascular abnormalities are the most commonly missed malformation. A four-chamber view of the fetal heart improves the detection of cardiac malformations. Intrauterine diagnosis of congenital abnormalities permits planning of surgical correction shortly after birth, preterm delivery for early correction, selection of cesarean section to reduce fetal injury, and, in some cases, intrauterine therapy. When a congenital abnormality is suspected, a diagnosis made using ultrasound usually can be obtained by weeks 16 to 18 of gestation.

Amniocentesis

Amniocentesis involves the withdrawal of a sample of amniotic fluid from the pregnant uterus by means of a needle inserted through the abdominal wall (Fig. 7-10). The procedure is useful in women older than 35 years of age, who have an increased risk of giving birth to an infant with Down syndrome; in parents who have another child with chromosomal abnormalities; and in situations in which a parent is known to be a carrier of an inherited disease. Ultrasound is used to gain additional information and to guide the placement of the amniocentesis needle. The amniotic fluid and cells that have been shed by the fetus are studied. Usually, a determination of fetal status can be made by the 16th to 17th week of pregnancy. For chromosomal analysis, the fetal cells are grown in culture and the result is available in 10 to 14 days. The amniotic fluid also can be tested using various biochemical tests.

Early amniocentesis (before 15 weeks) can be done. However, its safety has not been established. The volume of fluid removed in relation to total amniotic fluid is greater, which may produce fetal loss or have an effect on fetal lung function.

Chorionic Villus Sampling

Sampling of the chorionic villi usually is done after 10 weeks of gestation.[43] Doing the test before that time is not recommended because of the danger of limb reduction defects in the fetus. The chorionic villi are the site of exchange of nutrients between the maternal blood and the embryo—the chorionic sac encloses the early amniotic sac and fetus, and the villi are the primitive blood vessels that develop into the placenta. The sampling procedure usually is performed using a transabdominal approach. The tissue that is obtained can be used for fetal chromosome studies, DNA analysis, and biochemical studies. The fetal tissue does not

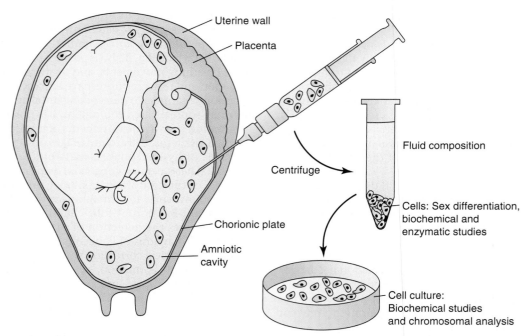

FIGURE 7-10 Amniocentesis. A needle is inserted into the uterus through the abdominal wall, and a sample of amniotic fluid is withdrawn for chromosomal and biochemical studies. (Department of Health, Education and Welfare. [1977]. *What are the facts about genetic disease?* Washington, DC: DHEW)

have to be cultured, and fetal chromosome analysis can be made available in 24 hours. DNA analysis and biochemical tests can be completed in 1 to 2 weeks.[42]

Percutaneous Umbilical Blood Sampling

Percutaneous fetal blood sampling involves the transcutaneous insertion of a needle through the uterine wall and into the umbilical artery. It is performed under ultrasound guidance and can be done any time after 16 weeks of gestation. It is used for prenatal diagnosis of hemoglobinopathies, coagulation disorders, metabolic and cytogenic disorders, and immunodeficiencies. Fetal infections such as rubella and toxoplasmosis can be detected through measurement of immunoglobulin M antibodies or direct blood cultures. Results from cytogenic studies usually are available within 48 to 72 hours. Because the procedure carries a greater risk of pregnancy loss than amniocentesis, it usually is reserved for situations in which rapid cytogenic analysis is needed or in which diagnostic information cannot be obtained by other methods.

Fetal Biopsy

Fetal biopsy is done with a fetoscope under ultrasound guidance. It is used to detect certain genetic skin defects that cannot be diagnosed with DNA analysis. It also may be done to obtain muscle tissue for use in diagnosis of Duchenne muscular dystrophy.

Cytogenic and Biochemical Analyses

Amniocentesis and chorionic villus sampling yield cells that can be used for cytogenetic and DNA analyses. Biochemical analyses can be used to detect abnormal levels of AFP and abnormal biochemical products in the maternal blood and in specimens of amniotic fluid and fetal blood.

Cytogenetic studies are used for fetal karyotyping to determine the chromosomal makeup of the fetus. They are done to detect abnormalities of chromosome number and structure. Karyotyping also reveals the sex of the fetus. This may be useful when an inherited defect is known to affect only one sex.

Analysis of DNA is done on cells extracted from the amniotic fluid or obtained by chorionic villus sampling, to detect genetic defects such as inborn errors of metabolism. The defect may be established through direct demonstration of the molecular defect or through methods that break the DNA into fragments so that the fragments may be studied to determine the presence of an abnormal gene. Direct demonstration of the molecular defect is done by growing the amniotic fluid cells in culture and measuring the enzymes that the cultured cells produce. Many of the enzymes are expressed in the chorionic villi; this permits earlier prenatal diagnosis because the cells do not need to be subjected to prior culture. DNA studies are used to detect genetic defects that cause inborn errors of metabolism such as Tay-Sachs disease, glycogen storage diseases, and familial hypercholesterolemia. Prenatal diagnoses are possible for more than 70 inborn errors of metabolism.

In summary, genetic and prenatal diagnosis and counseling are done in an effort to determine the risk of having a child with a genetic or chromosomal disorder. They often involve a detailed family history (*i.e.*, pedigree), examination of any affected and other family members, and laboratory studies including chromosomal analysis and biochemical studies. They usually are done by a genetic counselor and a specially prepared team of health care professionals. Ultrasound and amniocentesis can be used to screen for congenital defects. Ultrasound is used for determination of fetal size and position and for the presence of structural anomalies. Amniocentesis and chorionic villus sampling are used to obtain specimens for cytogenetic and biochemical studies. They are used in the prenatal diagnosis of more than 70 genetic disorders.

Related Web Sites

Centers for Disease Control and Prevention search for information on birth defects   wonder.cdc.gov/#about
March of Dimes—Birth Defect Information   www.modimes.org
Maternal Child Health Bureau
     www.mchb.hrsa.gov/index.html
Online Mendelian Inheritance of Man   www.ncbi.nlm.nih.gov/Omim

References

1. March of Dimes Birth Defects Foundation. (1999). Birth defects information. [On-line]. Available: http://www.modimes.org.
2. Online Mendelian Inheritance in Man (OMIN™). (2000). Baltimore, MD: McKusick-Nathans Institute of Genetic Medicine, John Hopkins University; and Bethesda, MD: National Center for Biotechnology Information, National Library of Medicine. [On-line]. Available: http://www.ncbi.nlm.nih.gov/omim.
3. Thompson M.W., McInnes R.R., Willard H.F. (1991). *Thompson and Thompson genetics in medicine* (5th ed., pp. 59–66, 201, 411–425). Philadelphia: W.B. Saunders.
4. Rubin E., Farber J.E. (Eds.). (1999). *Pathology* (3rd ed., pp. 221–223, 236, 241–242, 252, 257–259). Philadelphia: Lippincott Williams & Wilkins.
5. Cotran R.S., Kumar V., Collins T. (Eds.). (1999). *Robbins pathologic basis of disease* (6th ed., pp. 144–149, 155–156, 162–165, 170–171, 177–178). Philadelphia: W.B. Saunders.
6. Koch R.K. (1999). Issues in newborn screening for phenylketonuria. *American Family Physician* 60, 1462–1466.
7. National Institute of Child Health and Human Development. (2000). Facts about fragile X syndrome. [On-line]. Available: http://www.nichd.nih.gov/publications/pubs/Fragilex.htm.
8. Warren S.T. (1997). Trinucleotide repetition and fragile X syndrome. *Hospital Practice* 31 (4), 73–85, 90–98.
9. Riccardi V.M. (1977). *The genetic approach to human disease* (p. 92). New York: Oxford University Press.
10. March of Dimes. (2000). Down syndrome. [On-line]. Available: http://www.modimes.org/HealthLibrary2/FactSheets/Down_syndrome.htm.
11. Newberger D.S. (2000). Down syndrome: Prenatal risk assessment and diagnosis. *American Family Physician* 62, 825–832, 837–838.
12. Wald N.J., Watt H.C., Hacshaw A.K. (1999). Integrated screening for Down's syndrome based on tests performed during the first and second trimester. *New England Journal of Medicine* 341, 461–467.
13. Rosenfeld R.G. (2000). Turner's syndrome: A growing concern. *Pediatrics* 137, 443–444.
14. Saenger P. (1996). Turner's syndrome. *New England Journal of Medicine* 335, 1749–1754.
15. Savendahl L., Davenport M. (2000). Delayed diagnoses of Turner's syndrome: Proposed guidelines for change. *Journal of Pediatrics* 137, 455–459.
16. National Institute of Child Health and Human Development. (2000). A guide for XXY males and their family. [On-line]. Available: http://www.nichd.nih.gov/publications/pubs/klinefelter.htm.
17. Steurerwald U., Weibe P., Jorgensen P.J., Bjerve K., Brock J., Heinzow B., et al. (2000). Maternal seafood diet, methylmercury exposure, and neonatal neurologic function. *Journal of Pediatrics* 136, 599–605.
18. Katzung B.D. (1998). *Basic and clinical pharmacology* (7th ed., pp. 979–988). Stamford, CT: Appleton & Lange.
19. Koren G., Pstuszak A., Ito S. (1998). Drugs in pregnancy. *New England Journal of Medicine* 338, 1128–1137.
20. Ross S.A., McCaffery P.J., Drager U.C., DeLuca L.M. (2000). Retinoids in embryonal development. *Physiological Reviews* 80, 1021–1055.
21. Oakley G.P., Erickson J.D. (1995). Vitamin A and birth defects. *New England Journal of Medicine* 333, 1414–1415.
22. U.S. Food and Drug Administration. (2000). Pregnancy categories. [On-line]. Available: http://www.fda.gov.
23. March of Dimes. (1999). Leading categories of birth defects. [On-line]. Available: http://www.modimes.org/HealthLibrary2/InfantHealthStatistics/bdtable.htm.
24. Rosett H.L. (1980). A clinical perspective of the fetal alcohol syndrome. *Alcoholism, Clinical and Experimental Research* 4, 162–164.
25. Sokol R.J., Clarren S.K. (1980). Guidelines for use of terminology describing the impact of prenatal alcohol on the offspring. *Alcoholism, Clinical and Experimental Research* 13, 587–589.
26. Lewis D.D., Woods S.E. (1994). Fetal alcohol syndrome. *American Family Physician* 50, 1025–1032.
27. Stratton K., Howe C., Battaglia F. (Eds.). (1996). *Fetal alcohol syndrome: Diagnosis, epidemiology, prevention and treatment* (pp. 4–21). Washington, DC: National Academy Press.
28. American Academy of Pediatrics (2000). Fetal alcohol syndrome and alcohol-related neurodevelopmental disorders. *Pediatrics* 106, 358–361.
29. Ernhart C.B., Bowden D.M., Astley S.J. (1987). Alcohol teratogenicity in the human: A detailed assessment of specificity, critical period, and threshold. *American Journal of Obstetrics and Gynecology* 156, 33–39.
30. Surgeon General's advisory on alcohol and pregnancy. (1981). *FDA Drug Bulletin* 2, 10.
31. March of Dimes. (2000). Cocaine use during pregnancy. [On-line]. Available: http://www.modimes.org/HealthLibrary2/FactSheets/Cocaine_use_during_pregnancy.htm.
32. Volpe J.J. (1972). Effect of cocaine use on the fetus. *New England Journal of Medicine* 327, 399–407.
33. Chiriboga C.A., Brust C.M., Bateman D., Hauser W.A. (1999). Dose-response effect of fetal cocaine exposure on newborn neurologic function. *Pediatrics* 103, 79–85.
34. MacGregor S.N., Keith L.G., Chasnoff I.J., Rosner M.A., Chisum G.M., Shaw P., Minogue J.P. (1987). Cocaine use

during pregnancy: Adverse outcome. *American Journal of Obstetrics and Gynecology* 157, 686–690.

35. Chasnoff I.J., Chisum G.M., Kaplan W.E. (1988). Maternal cocaine use and genitourinary malformations. *Teratology* 37, 201–204.

36. Riley J.B., Brodsky N.L., Porat R. (1988). Risk of SIDS in infants with in utero cocaine exposure: A prospective study [Abstract]. *Pediatric Research* 23, 454A.

37. Committee on Genetics. (1993). Folic acid for the prevention of neural tube defects. *Pediatrics* 92, 493–494.

38. Centers for Disease Control and Prevention. (1992). Recommendations for use of folic acid to reduce the number of cases of spina bifida and other neural tube defects. *Morbidity and Mortality Weekly Report* 41, 1–8.

39. Scholl T.O., Johnson W.G. (2000). Folic acid: Influence on outcome of pregnancy. *American Journal of Clinical Nutrition* 71 (Suppl.), 1295S–1303S.

40. Bailey L.B. (2000). New standard for dietary folate intake in pregnant women. *American Journal of Clinical Nutrition* 71 (Suppl.), 1304S–1307S.

41. D'Alton M.E., DeCherney A.H. (1993). Prenatal diagnosis. *New England Journal of Medicine* 328, 114–120.

42. American College of Obstetricians and Gynecologists. (1987). *Antenatal diagnosis of genetic disorders* (pp. 1–8). Technical bulletin no. 108. Washington, DC: Author.

43. Wilson R.D. (2000). Amniocentesis and chorionic villus sampling. *Current Opinion in Obstetrics and Gynecology* 12, 81–86.

Chapter 8

Alterations in Cell Differentiation: Neoplasia

Kathryn Ann Caudell

Cancer is the second leading cause of death in the United States after cardiovascular disease. The disease affects all age groups, causing more death in children 3 to 15 years of age than any other disease. The American Cancer Society has estimated that 1.2 million Americans will develop cancer in 2000, and that one in two males and one in three females will have cancer during their lifetime. It also is estimated that approximately 552,200 Americans will die in the year from neoplastic diseases.[1] As age-adjusted cancer mortality rates increase and heart disease mortality decreases, it is predicted that cancer will become the leading cause of death in a few decades.[2] Trends in cancer survival demonstrate that relative 5-year survival rates have improved since the early 1960s. It is estimated that approximately 59% of people who develop cancer each year will be alive 5 years later.

Cancer is not a single disease. The term describes almost all forms of malignant neoplasia. Cancer can originate in almost any organ, with the prostate being the most common site in men and the breast in women (Fig. 8-1). The ability of cancer to be cured varies considerably and depends on the type of cancer and the extent of the disease at diagnosis. Cancers such as acute lymphocytic leukemia, Hodgkin's disease, testicular cancer, and osteosarcoma, which only a few decades ago had poor prognoses, are today cured in many cases. However, lung cancer, which is the leading cause of death in men and women in the United States, is resistant to therapy, and although some progress has been made in its treatment, mortality rates remain high. This chapter is divided into five sections: concepts of cell growth, characteristics of benign and malignant neoplasms, carcinogenesis and causes of cancer, diagnosis and treatment, and childhood cancers. Specific types of cancer are discussed elsewhere in this book.

Concepts of Cell Growth

After you have completed this section of the chapter, you should be able to meet the following objectives:

- ✦ Define *neoplasm* and explain how neoplastic growth differs from the normal adaptive changes seen in atrophy, hypertrophy, and hyperplasia
- ✦ Distinguish between cell proliferation and differentiation
- ✦ Describe the five phases of the cell cycle
- ✦ Characterize the properties of stem cells

CANCER INCIDENCE AND DEATHS BY SITE AND SEX-2000 ESTIMATES

CANCER INCIDENCE BY SITE AND SEX		CANCER DEATHS BY SITE AND SEX	
MALES	FEMALES	MALES	FEMALES
PROSTATE 180,400	BREAST 182,800	LUNG 89,300	LUNG 67,600
LUNG 89,500	LUNG 74,600	PROSTATE 31,900	BREAST 40,800
COLON & RECTUM 63,600	COLON & RECTUM 66,600	COLON & RECTUM 27,800	COLON & RECTUM 28,500
BLADDER 38,300	UTERUS 36,100	LYMPHOMA 14,400	PANCREAS 14,500
LYMPHOMA 35,900	LYMPHOMA 26,400	PANCREAS 13,700	OVARY 14,000
ORAL AND PHARYNX 20,200	OVARY 23,100	LEUKEMIA 12,100	LYMPHOMA 13,100
MELANOMA OF THE SKIN 27,300	MELANOMA OF THE SKIN 20,400	ESOPHAGUS 9,200	LEUKEMIA 9,600
KIDNEY 18,800	BLADDER 14,900	LIVER 8,500	UTERUS 6,500
LEUKEMIA 16,900	PANCREAS 14,600	BLADDER 8,100	NERVOUS SYSTEM 5,900
PANCREAS 13,700	LEUKEMIA 13,900	STOMACH 7,600	STOMACH 5,400
STOMACH 13,400	CERVIX 12,800	KIDNEY 7,300	MULTIPLE MYELOMA 5,400
NERVOUS SYSTEM 9,500	KIDNEY 12,400	NERVOUS SYSTEM 7,100	LIVER 5,300
ALL SITES 619,700	ALL SITES 600,400	ALL SITES 284,100	ALL SITES 268,100

FIGURE 8-1 Cancer incidence and deaths (2000 estimates) by site and sex. (Greenlee R. T., Murray T., Bolden S., et al. [2000]. Cancer statistics, 2000. *CA: A Cancer Journal for Clinicians* 50 [1], 7–33)

Cancers result from a process of altered cell differentiation and growth. The resulting tissue is called *neoplasia*. The term *neoplasm* comes from a Greek word meaning *new formation*. Unlike the tissue growth that occurs with hypertrophy and hyperplasia, the growth of a neoplasm is uncoordinated and relatively autonomous in that it lacks normal regulatory controls over cell growth and division. Neoplasms tend to increase in size and continue to grow after the stimulus has ceased or the needs of the organism have been met.

Tissue renewal and repair involves cell proliferation and differentiation. *Proliferation*, or the process of cell division, is an inherent adaptive mechanism for replacing body cells when old cells die or additional cells are needed. *Differentiation* is the process of specialization whereby new cells acquire the structure and function of the cells they replace. In adult tissues, the size of a population of cells is determined by the rates of cell proliferation, differentiation, and death by apoptosis.[3] Apoptosis, which is discussed in Chapter 5, is a form of programmed cell death designed to eliminate senescent cells or unwanted cells. A balance of cellular signals that regulate cell proliferation, differentiation, and apoptosis regulates the size of cell populations.

THE CELL CYCLE

The cell cycle is the interval between each cell division. It regulates the duplication of genetic information and appropriately aligns the duplicated chromosomes to be received by the daughter cells. In addition, pauses or checkpoints in the cell cycle determine the accuracy with which deoxyribonucleic acid (DNA) is duplicated. These checkpoints allow for any defects to be edited and repaired, thereby assuring that the daughter cells receive the full complement of genetic information, identical to that of the parent cell.[3]

The cell cycle is divided into four distinct phases referred to as G_1, S, G_2, and M (Fig. 8-2). G_1 (*gap 1*), is the postmitotic phase during which DNA synthesis ceases while

Cell Proliferation and Growth

➤ Tissue growth and repair involve cell proliferation and differentiation.

➤ Cell proliferation is the process whereby tissues acquire new or replacement cells through cell division.

➤ Cell differentiation is the orderly process in which proliferating cells are transformed into different and more specialized types. It determines the microscopic characteristics of the cell, how the cell functions, and how long it will live.

➤ Cells that are fully differentiated are no longer capable of cell division.

of cellular division or mitosis. Continually dividing cells, such as the stratified squamous epithelium of the skin, continuously cycle from one mitosis to the next. Nondividing permanent cells, such as neurons, exit the cell cycle and are unable to undergo further cell division. Cells that are not actively dividing are quiescent and reside in a resting phase, the G_0 phase. These quiescent cells reenter the cell cycle in response to extracellular nutrients, growth factors, hormones, and other signals such as blood loss or tissue injury that signal for cell renewal.[4,5]

The duration of the phases of the cell cycle vary depending on the cell type, the frequency with which the cells divide, and host characteristics such as the presence of appropriate growth factors. Very rapidly dividing cells can complete the cell cycle in less than 8 hours, whereas others can take longer than 1 year. Most of this variability occurs in the G_0 and G_1 phases. The duration of the S phase (10 to 20 hours), the G_2 phase (2 to 10 hours), and the M phase (0.5 to 1 hour) appears to be relatively constant.[5]

ribonucleic acid (RNA) and protein synthesis and cell growth take place. During the *S phase*, DNA synthesis occurs, giving rise to two separate sets of chromosomes, one for each daughter cell. G_2 (*gap 2*) is the premitotic phase and is similar to G_1 in that DNA synthesis ceases while RNA and protein synthesis continues. The *M phase* is the phase

CELL PROLIFERATION

Cell proliferation is the process by which cells divide and reproduce. In normal tissue, cell proliferation is regulated so that the number of cells actively dividing is equivalent to the number dying or being shed. In humans, there are two major categories of cells: gametes and somatic cells. The *gametes* (ovum and sperm) are *haploid*, having only one set of chromosomes from one parent, and are designed specifically for sexual fusion. After fusion, a *diploid* cell containing both sets of chromosomes is formed. This cell is the *somatic cell* that goes on to form the rest of the body.

In terms of cell proliferation, the 200 or more cell types of the body can be divided into 3 large groups: the well-differentiated neurons and cells of skeletal and cardiac muscle that are unable to divide and reproduce; the parent, or progenitor cells, that continue to divide and reproduce, such as blood cells, skin cells, and liver cells; and the undifferentiated stem cells that can be triggered to enter the cell cycle and produce large numbers of progenitor cells when the need arises. The rates of reproduction of these cells vary greatly. White blood cells and cells that line the gastrointestinal tract live several days and must be replaced constantly. In most tissues, the rate of cell reproduction is greatly increased when tissue is injured or lost. Bleeding, for example, stimulates the rapid reproduction of the blood-forming cells of the bone marrow. In some types of tissue, the genetic program for cell replication normally is repressed, but can be resumed under certain conditions. The liver, for example, has extensive regenerative capabilities under certain conditions.

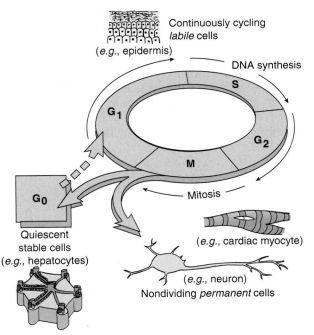

FIGURE 8-2 Cell populations and cell cycle phases. Constantly dividing labile cells continuously cycle from one mitosis to the next. Nondividing permanent cells have exited the cycle and are destined to die without further cell division. Quiescent stable cells in G_0 are neither cycling nor dying and can be induced to reenter the cell cycle at an appropriate stimulus. (Cotran R.S., Kumar V., Collins T. [1999]. *Robbins pathologic basis of disease* [6th ed., p. 90]. Philadelphia: W.B Saunders)

CELL DIFFERENTIATION

Cell differentiation is the process whereby proliferating cells are transformed into different and more specialized cell types. This process leads to a fully differentiated, adult cell that has achieved its specific set of structural, functional, and life expectancy characteristics. For example, a red blood cell is programmed to develop into a concave disk that functions as a vehicle for oxygen transport and lives approximately 120 days.

All of the different cell types of the body originate from a single cell—the fertilized ovum. As the embryonic cells increase in number, they engage in an orderly process of differentiation that is necessary for the development of all the various organs of the body. The process of differentiation is regulated by a combination of internal programming that involves the expression of specific genes and external stimuli provided by neighboring cells, exposure to substances in the maternal circulation, and a variety of growth factors, nutrients, oxygen, and ions.[6]

What makes the cells of one organ different from those of another organ is the type of gene that is expressed. Although all cells have the same complement of genes, only a small number of these genes are expressed in postnatal life. When cells, such as those of the developing embryo, differentiate and give rise to committed cells of a particular tissue type, the appropriate genes are maintained in an active state while the remainder are inactive. Normally, the rate of cell reproduction and the process of cell differentiation are precisely controlled in prenatal and postnatal life so that both of these mechanisms cease once the appropriate numbers and types of cells are formed.

The process of differentiation occurs in orderly steps; with each progressive step, increased specialization is exchanged for a loss of ability to develop different cell characteristics and different cell lines. The more highly specialized a cell becomes, the more likely it is to lose its ability to undergo mitosis. Neurons, which are the most highly specialized cells in the body, lose their ability to divide and reproduce once development of the nervous system is complete. More important, there are no reserve or parent cells to direct their replacement. However, appropriate numbers of these cell types are generated in the embryo such that loss of a certain percentage of cells does not affect the total cell population. Although these cells never divide and are not replaced if lost, they exist in sufficient numbers to carry out their specific functions. In other, less specialized tissues, such as the skin and mucosal lining, cell renewal continues throughout life.

Even in the continuously renewing cell populations, highly specialized cells are similarly unable to divide. An alternative mechanism provides for their replacement. There are progenitor cells of the same lineage that have not yet differentiated to the extent that they have lost their ability to divide. These cells are sufficiently differentiated that their daughter cells are limited to the same cell line, but they are insufficiently differentiated to preclude the potential for active proliferation. As a result, these parent or progenitor cells are able to provide large numbers of replacement cells. The progenitor cells, however, have limited capacity for self-renewal and they become restricted to producing a single type of cell.

Another type of cell, called a *stem cell*, remains incompletely differentiated throughout life. Stem cells are reserve cells that remain quiescent until there is a need for cell replenishment, in which case they divide, thereby producing

other stem cells and cells that can carry out the functions of the differentiated cell (Fig. 8-3). There are several types of stem cells, some of which include the muscle satellite cell, the epidermal stem cell, the spermatogonium, and the basal cell of the olfactory epithelium. These stem cells are unipotent in that they give rise only to one type of differentiated cell. Oligopotent stem cells can produce a small number of cells, and pluripotent stem cells, such as those involved in hematopoiesis, give rise to numerous cell types.[4] Stem cells are the primary cellular component of bone marrow transplantation, in which the stem cells in the transplanted marrow reestablish the recipient's blood production and immune system. Peripheral blood stem cell transplantation is a transplantation procedure that bypasses the need for bone marrow infusion by infusing stem cells that have been separated and removed from the donor blood.

In summary, the term *neoplasm* refers to an abnormal mass of tissue in which the growth exceeds and is uncoordinated with that of the normal tissues. Unlike normal cellular adaptive processes such as hypertrophy and hyperplasia, neoplasms do not obey the laws of normal cell growth. They serve no useful purpose, they do not occur in response to an appropriate stimulus, and they continue to grow at the expense of the host.

Cell proliferation is the process whereby cells divide and bear offspring; it normally is regulated so that the number of cells that are actively dividing is equal to the number dying or being shed.

The process of cell growth and division is called the *cell cycle*. It is divided into four phases: G_1, the postmitotic phase, during which DNA synthesis ceases while RNA and protein synthesis and cell growth take place; S, the phase during which DNA synthesis occurs, giving rise to two separate sets of chromosomes; G_2, the premitotic phase, during which RNA and protein synthesis continues; and M, the phase of cell mitosis

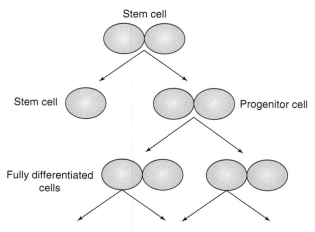

FIGURE 8-3 Mechanism of cell replacement.

or cell division. The G_0 phase is a resting or quiescent phase in which nondividing cells reside.

Cell differentiation is the process whereby cells are transformed into different and more specialized cell types as they proliferate. It determines the structure, function, and life span of a cell. There are three types of cells: well-differentiated cells that are no longer able to divide, progenitor or parent cells that continue to divide and bear offspring, and undifferentiated stem cells that can be recruited to become progenitor cells when the need arises. As a cell line becomes more differentiated, it becomes more highly specialized in its function and less able to divide.

Characteristics of Benign and Malignant Neoplasms

After you have completed this section of the chapter, you should be able to meet the following objectives:

✦ Cite the method used for naming benign and malignant neoplasms
✦ State at least six ways in which benign and malignant neoplasms differ
✦ Relate the properties of cell differentiation to the development of a cancer cell line and the behavior of the tumor
✦ Trace the pathway for hematologic spread of a metastatic cancer cell
✦ Use the concepts of growth fraction and doubling time to explain the growth of cancerous tissue
✦ Describe the general effects of cancer on body systems

Neoplasms are composed of two types of tissue: parenchymal tissue and the stroma or supporting tissue. The *parenchymal cells* represent the functional components of an organ. The *supporting tissue* consists of the connective tissue, blood vessels, and lymph structure. The parenchymal cells of a tumor determine its behavior and are the component for which a tumor is named. The supporting tissue carries the blood vessels and provides support for tumor survival and growth.

TERMINOLOGY

By definition, a *tumor* is a swelling that can be caused by a number of conditions, including inflammation and trauma. Although they are not synonymous, the terms *tumor* and *neoplasm* often are used interchangeably. Neoplasms usually are classified as benign or malignant. Neoplasms that contain well-differentiated cells that are clustered together in a single mass are considered to be *benign*. These tumors usually do not cause death unless their location or size interferes with vital functions. In contrast, malignant neoplasms are less well differentiated and have the ability to break loose, enter the circulatory or lymphatic systems, and

form secondary malignant tumors at other sites. *Malignant neoplasms* usually cause suffering and death if untreated or uncontrolled.

Tumors usually are named by adding the suffix *-oma* to the parenchymal tissue type from which the growth originated. Thus, a benign tumor of glandular epithelial tissue is called an *adenoma,* and a benign tumor of bone tissue is called an *osteoma.* The term *carcinoma* is used to designate a malignant tumor of epithelial tissue origin. In the case of a malignant adenoma, the term *adenocarcinoma* is used. Malignant tumors of mesenchymal origin are called *sarcomas* (*e.g.,* osteosarcoma). *Papillomas* are benign microscopic or macroscopic fingerlike projections that grow on any surface. A *polyp* is growth that projects from a mucosal surface, such as the intestine. Although the term usually implies a benign neoplasm, some malignant tumors also appear as polyps.[3] *Oncology* is the study of tumors and their treatment. Table 8-1 lists the names of selected benign and malignant tumors according to tissue types.

Benign and malignant neoplasms usually are differentiated by their (1) cell characteristics, (2) manner of growth, (3) rate of growth, (4) potential for metastasizing or spreading to other parts of the body, (5) ability to produce generalized effects, (6) tendency to cause tissue destruction, and (7) capacity to cause death. The characteristics of benign and malignant neoplasms are summarized in Table 8-2.

BENIGN NEOPLASMS *encapsulated*

Benign tumors are characterized by a slow, progressive rate of growth that may come to a standstill or regress, an expansive manner of growth, the presence of a well-defined fibrous capsule, and failure to metastasize to distant sites. Benign tumors are composed of well-differentiated cells that resemble the cells of the tissue of origin. For example, the cells of a uterine leiomyoma resemble uterine smooth muscle cells. For unknown reasons, benign tumors seem to have lost the ability to suppress the genetic program for cell replication but retain the program for normal cell differentiation. Benign tumors grow by expansion and are enclosed in a fibrous capsule. This is in sharp contrast to malignant neoplasms, which grow by infiltrating the surrounding tissue (Fig. 8-4). The capsule is responsible for a sharp line of demarcation between the benign tumor and the adjacent tissues, a factor that facilitates surgical removal. The formation of the capsule is thought to represent the reaction of the surrounding tissues to the tumor.[6]

Benign tumors do not undergo degenerative changes as readily as malignant tumors, and they usually do not cause death unless they interfere with vital functions because of their location. For instance, a benign tumor growing in the cranial cavity can eventually cause death by compressing brain structures. Benign tumors also can cause disturbances in the function of adjacent or distant structures by producing pressure on tissues, blood vessels, or nerves. Some benign tumors are also known for their ability to cause alterations in body function through abnormal elaboration of hormones.

TABLE 8-1 ✦ Names of Selected Benign and Malignant Tumors According to Tissue Types

Tissue Type	Benign Tumors	Malignant Tumors
Epithelial		
Surface	Papilloma	Squamous cell carcinoma
Glandular	Adenoma	Adenocarcinoma
Connective		
Fibrous	Fibroma	Fibrosarcoma
Adipose	Lipoma	Liposarcoma
Cartilage	Chondroma	Chondrosarcoma
Bone	Osteoma	Osteosarcoma
Blood vessels	Hemangioma	Hemangiosarcoma
Lymph vessels	Lymphangioma	Lymphangiosarcoma
Lymph tissue		Lymphosarcoma
Muscle		
Smooth	Leiomyoma	Leiomyosarcoma
Striated	Rhabdomyoma	Rhabdomyosarcoma
Neural Tissue		
Nerve cell	Neuroma	Neuroblastoma
Glial tissue	Glioma (benign)	Glioblastoma, astrocytoma, medullo-blastoma, oligodendroglioma
Nerve sheaths	Neurilemmoma	Neurilemmal sarcoma
Meninges	Meningioma	Meningeal sarcoma
Hematologic		
Granulocytic		Myelocytic leukemia
Erythrocytic		Erythrocytic leukemia
Plasma cells		Multiple myeloma
Lymphocytic		Lymphocytic leukemia or lymphoma
Monocytic		Monocytic leukemia
Endothelial Tissue		
Blood vessels	Hemangioma	Hemangiosarcoma
Lymph vessels	Lymphangioma	Lymphangiosarcoma
Endothelial lining		Ewing's sarcoma

MALIGNANT NEOPLASMS

Malignant neoplasms tend to grow rapidly, spread widely, and kill regardless of their original location. Because of their rapid rate of growth, malignant tumors tend to compress blood vessels and outgrow their blood supply, causing ischemia and tissue necrosis; rob normal tissues of essential nutrients; and liberate enzymes and toxins that destroy tumor tissue and normal tissue. The destructive nature of malignant tumors is related to their lack of cell differentiation, cell characteristics, rate of growth, and ability to spread and metastasize.

There are two categories of cancer—solid tumors and hematologic cancers. Solid tumors initially are confined to a specific tissue or organ. As the growth of a solid tumor progresses, cells are shed from the original tumor mass and travel through the blood and lymph system to produce metastasis in distant sites. Hematologic cancers involve the blood-forming cells that naturally migrate to the blood and lymph systems, thereby making them disseminated diseases from the beginning.

Cancer Cell Characteristics

In tissues capable of regeneration, replacement cells usually are derived from progenitor or undifferentiated stem cells. The process of cell differentiation involves changes in gene expression such that each step in the process is accomplished by expression of genes that produce more specialized cell functions. Expression of certain genes is accomplished by gene regulatory proteins that, when bound to DNA, can facilitate or inhibit transcription of adjacent genes. Combinations of these regulatory proteins generate a large number of different cells. This regulatory protein group includes proteins called *master gene-encoded regulatory proteins* that exhibit decisive coordinating effects in controlling large sets of genes. These master proteins have the ability to affect the production of many proteins in cells, thereby facilitating cellular differentiation.

TABLE 8-2 ✦ Characteristics of Benign and Malignant Neoplasms

Characteristics	Benign	Malignant
Cell characteristics	Well-differentiated cells that resemble normal cells of the tissue from which the tumor originated	Cells are undifferentiated and often bear little resemblance to the normal cells of the tissue from which they arose
Mode of growth	Tumor grows by expansion and does not infiltrate the surrounding tissues; usually encapsulated	Grows at the periphery and sends out processes that infiltrate and destroy the surrounding tissues
Rate of growth	Rate of growth usually is slow	Rate of growth is variable and depends on level of differentiation; the more anaplastic the tumor, the more rapid the rate of growth
Metastasis	Does not spread by metastasis	Gains access to the blood and lymph channels and metastasizes to other areas of the body
General effects	Usually is a localized phenomenon that does not cause generalized effects unless its location interferes with vital functions	Often causes generalized effects such as anemia, weakness, and weight loss
Tissue destruction	Usually does not cause tissue damage unless its location interferes with blood flow	Often causes extensive tissue damage as the tumor outgrows its blood supply or encroaches on blood flow to the area; also may produce substances that cause cell damage
Ability to cause death	Usually does not cause death unless its location interferes with vital functions	Usually causes death unless growth can be controlled

→ malignant

When a stem cell divides, one daughter cell retains the stem cell characteristics, and the other daughter cell becomes a progenitor daughter cell that leads to an irreversible terminal differentiation. The progeny of each progenitor cell continues along the same genetic program, with the differentiating cells undergoing multiple mitotic divisions in the process of becoming a mature cell type and with each generation of cells becoming more specialized. In this way, a single stem cell can give rise to the many cells needed for normal tissue repair or blood cell responses. When the dividing cells becomes fully differentiated, they no longer are capable of mitosis. In the immune system, for example, appropriately stimulated B lymphocytes become progressively more differentiated as they undergo successive mitotic divisions, until they become mature plasma cells that no longer can divide but are capable of releasing large amounts of membrane-bound antibody.

Cancer cells, unlike normal cells, fail to undergo normal cell proliferation and differentiation. It is thought that cancer cells develop from mutations that occur during the differentiation process (Fig. 8-5). When the mutation occurs early in the process, the resulting tumor is poorly differentiated and highly malignant; when it occurs later in the process, better differentiated and less malignant tumors result.

The term *anaplasia* is used to describe the lack of cell differentiation in cancerous tissue. Undifferentiated cancer cells are altered in appearance and nuclear size and shape from the cells in the tissue from which the cancer originated. In descending the scale of differentiation, enzymes and specialized pathways of metabolism are lost and cells undergo functional simplification.[3] Highly anaplastic cancer cells, whatever their tissue of origin, begin to resemble each other more than they do their tissue of origin. For example, when examined under the microscope, cancerous tissue that originates in the liver does not have the appearance of normal liver tissue. Some cancers display only slight anaplasia, and others display marked anaplasia.

Because cancer cells lack differentiation, they do not function properly, nor do they die in the time frame of normal cells. In some types of leukemia, for example, the lymphocytes do not follow the normal developmental process. They do not differentiate fully, acquire the ability to destroy bacteria, or die on schedule. Instead, these long-lived, defective cells continue to grow, crowding the normal developing blood cells, thereby affecting the development of other cell lineages such as the erythrocytes, platelets, and other white blood cells. This results in reduced numbers of mature, effectively functioning cells, producing white blood cells that cannot effectively fight infection, erythrocytes that cannot effectively transport oxygen to tissues, or platelets that cannot participate in the clotting system.

Alterations in cell differentiation also are accompanied by changes in cell characteristics and cell function that distinguish cancer cells from their fully differentiated normal counterparts. These changes include alterations in contact inhibition, loss of cohesiveness and adhesion, impaired cell-to-cell communication, expression of altered tissue antigens, and elaboration of degradative enzymes that participate in invasion and metastatic spread.

Contact inhibition is the cessation of growth after a cell comes in contact with another cell. Contact inhibition usually switches off cell growth by blocking the synthesis of DNA, RNA, and protein. In wound healing, contact inhibition causes fibrous tissue growth to cease at the point where

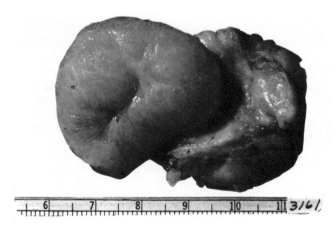

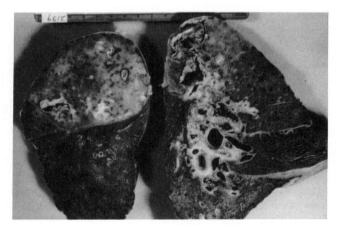

FIGURE 8-4 Photographs of a benign encapsulated fibroadenoma of the breast (**top**) and a bronchogenic carcinoma of the lung (**bottom**). The fibroadenoma has sharply defined edges, but the bronchogenic carcinoma is diffuse and infiltrates the surrounding tissues.

Benign and Malignant Neoplasms

➤ A tumor is a new growth or neoplasm.

➤ Benign neoplasms are well-differentiated tumors that resemble the tissues of origin but have lost the ability to control cell proliferation. They grow by expansion, are enclosed in a fibrous capsule, and do not cause death unless their location is such that it interrupts vital body functions.

➤ Malignant neoplasms are less well-differentiated tumors that have lost the ability to control both cell proliferation and differentiation. They grow in a crablike manner to invade surrounding tissues, have cells that break loose and travel to distant sites to form metastases, and inevitably cause suffering and death unless their growth can be controlled through treatment.

Most cancers synthesize and secrete enzymes (*i.e.*, proteases and glycosidases) that break down proteins involved in ensuring intracellular organization and cell-to-cell cohesion. The degradation of the extracellular matrix by these enzymes facilitates invasiveness of the tumor. The production of degradative enzymes, such as fibrinolysins, contributes to the breakdown of the intercellular matrix, which leads to changes in the organization of the cell's cytoskeleton and affects cell-to-cell adhesion, cellular migration, and cellular communication. Cancers of nonendocrine tissues may assume hormone synthesis to produce so-called *ectopic hormones* (discussed with paraneoplastic syndromes in the section on general effects).

the edges of the wound come together. Cancer cells, however, tend to grow rampantly without regard for other tissue. The reduced tendency of cancer cells to stick together (*i.e.*, *cohesiveness* and *adhesiveness*) permits shedding of the tumor's surface cells; these cells appear in the surrounding body fluids or secretions and often can be detected using the *Papanicolaou (Pap)* test. Impaired cell-to-cell communication may interfere with formation of intercellular connections and responsiveness to membrane-derived signals.

Cancer cells express a number of cell surface molecules or antigens that are immunologically identified as foreign. These *tissue antigens* are coded by the genes of a cell. Many transformed cancer cells revert to earlier stages of gene expression and produce antigens that are immunologically distinct from the antigens that are expressed by cells of the well-differentiated tissue from which the cancer originated. Some cancers express fetal antigens that are not produced by comparable cells in the adult. Tumor antigens may be used clinically as markers to indicate the presence or progressive growth of a cancer.

Invasion and Metastasis

Cancer spreads by direct invasion and extension, seeding of cancer cells in body cavities, and metastatic spread through the blood or lymph pathways. Unlike benign tumors, which grow by expansion and usually are surrounded by a capsule, malignant cancers grow by extensive infiltration and invasion of the surrounding tissues. The word *cancer* is derived from the Latin word meaning *crablike* because cancerous growth spreads by sending crablike projections into the surrounding tissues. The lack of a sharp line of demarcation separating them from the surrounding tissue makes the complete surgical removal of malignant tumors more difficult than removal of benign tumors. *Seeding* of cancer cells into body cavities occurs when a tumor erodes into these spaces. Most often, the peritoneal cavity is involved, but other spaces such as the pleural cavity, pericardial cavity, and joint spaces may be involved. Seeding into the peritoneal cavity is particularly common with ovarian cancers.

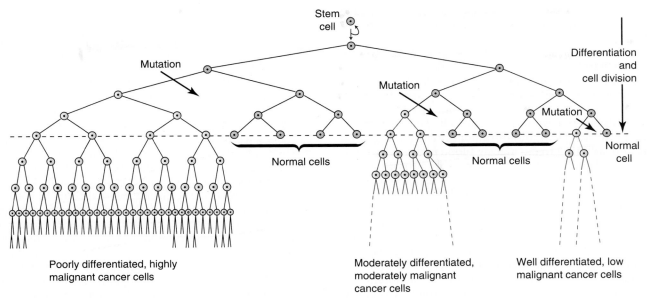

FIGURE 8-5 Mutation of a cell line. (Prescott D.M., Flexer A.S. [1986]. *Cancer, the misguided cell*. Sunderland, MA: Sinauer Associates)

The term *metastasis* is used to describe the development of a secondary tumor in a location distant from the primary tumor. Metastatic tumors retain many of the characteristics of the primary tumor from which they were derived. Because of this, it usually is possible to determine the site of the primary tumor from the cellular characteristics of the metastatic tumor. Some tumors tend to metastasize early in their developmental course, but others do not metastasize until later. Occasionally, the metastatic tumor is far advanced before the primary tumor becomes clinically detectable. Malignant tumors of the kidney, for example, may go completely undetected and be asymptomatic even when a metastatic lesion is found in the lung.

Metastasis occurs by way of the lymph channels (*i.e.,* lymphatic spread) and the blood vessels (*i.e.,* hematogenic spread).[3,7] In many types of cancer, the first evidence of disseminated disease is the presence of tumor cells in the lymph nodes that drain the tumor area. When metastasis occurs by way of the lymphatic channels, the tumor cells lodge first in the regional lymph nodes that received drainage from the tumor site. Once in the lymph node, the cells may die because of the lack of a proper environment, grow into a discernible mass, or remain dormant for unknown reasons. Because the lymphatic channels empty into the venous system, cancer cells that survive may eventually break loose and gain access to the venous system.

With hematologic spread, the blood-borne cancer cells typically follow the venous flow that drains the site of the neoplasm. Before entering the general circulation, venous blood from the gastrointestinal tract, pancreas, and spleen is routed through the portal vein to the liver. The liver is therefore a common site for metastatic spread of cancers that originate in these organs. Although the site of hematologic spread usually is related to vascular drainage of the primary tumor, some tumors metastasize to distant and un-related sites. As tumor growth progresses, malignant cells evolve and change their metastatic propensity and site preference. These metastatic cells increase their responsiveness to growth signals at distant sites by overexpressing certain growth factor receptors. They also exhibit decreased responsiveness to tissue-of-origin growth signals. Another explanation for the occurrence of metastatic site preference involves the responsiveness of metastatic cells to cytokines (*i.e.,* protein hormones synthesized and secreted from a number of cell types) released by tissue cells at the metastasis site.[8] For example, transferrin, a growth-promoting substance isolated from lung tissue, has been found to stimulate the growth of extremely malignant cells that typically metastasize to the lungs. Other organs that are preferential sites for metastasis contain their own specific sets of cytokines.

Examples of cancer cells preferentially metastasizing to distant sites include prostatic cancer spread to bone, bronchiogenic cancer spread to the adrenal glands and brain, and neuroblastoma spread to the liver and bones. Even among tumors that arise in the lung and metastasize to the brain, different tumors selectively metastasize to distinct sites in the brain. Certain organs such as the heart, skin, and skeletal muscle are rarely a site of metastasis despite ample blood flow capable of transporting metastatic cells to these tissues.

The selective nature of hematologic spread indicates that metastasis is a finely orchestrated, multistep process, and only a small, select clone of cancer cells has the right combination of gene products to perform all of the steps needed for establishment of a secondary tumor. It has been estimated that fewer than 1 in 10,000 tumor cells that leave a primary tumor survives to start a secondary tumor.[9] To metastasize, a cancer cell must be able to break loose from the primary tumor, invade the surrounding extracellular matrix, gain access to a blood vessel, survive its passage in the bloodstream, emerge from the bloodstream at a favorable location, invade the surrounding tissue, and begin to grow (Fig. 8-6).

Considerable evidence suggests that cancer cells capable of metastasis secrete enzymes that break down the surrounding extracellular matrix, allowing them to move through the degraded matrix and gain access to a blood vessel. Once in the circulation, the tumor cells are vulnerable to destruction by host immune cells. Some tumor cells gain protection from the antitumor host cells by aggregating and adhering to circulating blood components, particularly platelets, to form tumor emboli. Tumor cells that survive their travel in the circulation must be able to halt their passage by adhering to the vessel wall. Tumor cells express various cell surface attachment factors such as laminin receptors that facilitate their anchoring to laminin in the basement membranes. After attachment, the tumor cells then secrete proteolytic enzymes such as type IV collagenase that degrade the basement membrane and facilitate the migration of the tumor cells through the membrane into the interstitial area, where they subsequently establish growth of a secondary tumor.

Once in the target tissue, the process of tumor development depends on the establishment of blood vessels and specific growth factors that promote proliferation of the tumor cells. Tumor cells secrete tumor angiogenesis factor, which enables the development of new blood vessels in the tumor, a process termed *angiogenesis*.[7] The presence of stimulatory or inhibitor growth factors correlates with the site-specific pattern of metastasis. For example, a potent growth-stimulating factor has been isolated from lung tissue, and stromal cells in bone have shown to produce a factor that stimulates growth of prostatic cancer cells.[7]

The selective nature of metastasis raises the question of whether there are tumor genes that elicit or inhibit metastasis as their major function. If such genes exist, their presence could be used to predict the likelihood of cancer metastasis and provide information that could be used in designing treatment protocols. No single gene marker has been associated with metastasis of cancer cells. However, there has been interest in a tumor suppressor gene (NM23). In a series of human breast cancers, the NM23 protein levels were highest in tumors that had spread to three or fewer nodes. However, in a study investigating colon cancer metastasis, this gene was not found to suppress metastasis. These controversial findings suggest that the NM23 tumor suppressor gene may be tissue specific, suppressing breast tumors but not colon tumors.[3]

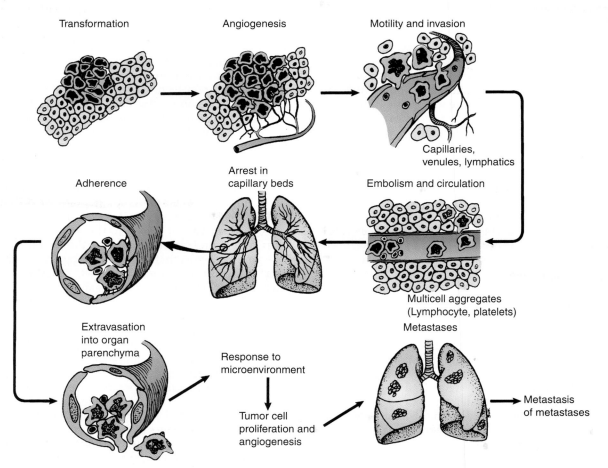

FIGURE 8-6 The pathogenesis of metastasis. (DeVita V.T. Jr., Hellman S., Rosenberg, S.A. [1997] *Cancer: Principles and practice of oncology* (5th ed., pp. 135–148). Philadelphia: Lippincott-Raven)

Tumor Growth

The rate of tissue growth in normal and cancerous tissue depends on three factors: the number of cells that are actively dividing or moving through the cell cycle, the duration of the cell cycle, and the number of cells that are being lost compared with the number of new cells being produced. One of the reasons cancerous tumors often seem to grow so rapidly relates to the size of the cell pool that is actively engaged in cycling. It has been shown that the cell cycle time of cancerous tissue cells is not necessarily shorter than that of normal cells; rather, cancer cells do not die on schedule. The growth factors that allow cells to enter the G_0 phase when they are not needed for cell replacement are lacking. A greater percentage of cells are actively engaged in cycling than occurs in normal tissue.

The ratio of dividing cells to resting cells in a tissue mass is called the *growth fraction*. The doubling time (T_D) is the length of time it takes for the total mass of cells in a tumor to double. As the growth fraction increases, the doubling time decreases. When normal tissues reach their adult size, an equilibrium between cell birth and cell death is reached. Cancer cells, however, continue to divide until limitations in blood supply and nutrients inhibit their growth. As this happens, the doubling time for cancer cells decreases. If tumor growth is plotted against time on a semilogarithmic scale, the initial growth rate is exponential and then tends to decrease or flatten out over time. This characterization of tumor growth is called the *Gompertzian model*.[5]

The rate of tumor growth is not necessarily constant and is influenced by factors such as hormones and blood supply. Menopause and pregnancy may cause a proliferation of tumor cells that previously had been static. Although it generally is thought that benign tumors grow slowly and cancerous tumors grow quickly and erratically, there are variables that can cause growth rates to vary and stray from typical growth characteristics.[3]

It also is thought that the degree of differentiation of a tumor is correlated with its growth rate. For example, undifferentiated tumors grow more rapidly than the more differentiated benign tumors. Although this is generally true, some malignant tumors apparently dormant for a number of years suddenly begin to proliferate rapidly, causing death in a short time.[3]

Experimentally, it is possible to determine the growth rate by calculating the proportion of dividing cells in the S phase and comparing this number with the total proportion of cells in that phase. Tumor growth is determined by measuring tumor volume as a function of time. Although it may seem reasonable that the T_D of tumors could be calculated by knowing the growth fraction and cell cycle phase durations, a number of cells are lost during the growth of a tumor, perhaps from necrosis, metastasis, or differentiation. For this reason, the T_D of tumors is slower than might be expected.[5]

A tumor usually is undetectable until it has doubled 30 times and contains more than 1 billion (10^9) cells. At this point, it is approximately 1 cm in size (Fig. 8-7). After 35 doublings, the mass contains more than 1 trillion (10^{12}) cells, which is a sufficient number to kill the host.

Cancer in situ is a localized preinvasive lesion. Depending on its location, this type of lesion usually can be removed surgically or treated so that the chances of recurrence are small. For example, cancer in situ of the cervix is essentially 100% curable.

General Effects

There probably is no single body function left unaffected by the presence of cancer (Table 8-3). Because tumor cells

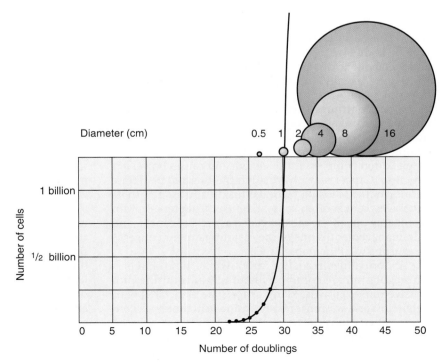

FIGURE 8-7 Growth curve of a hypothetical tumor on arithmetic coordinates. Notice the number of doubling times before the tumor reaches an appreciable size. (Adapted from Collins V.P., et al. [1956]. Observations of growth rates of human tumors. *Am J Roent Rad Ther Nuclear Med* 76, 988.)

TABLE 8-3 ◆ General Effects on Body Function Associated With Cancer Growth

Overall Effect	Related Tumor Action
Altered function of the involved tissue	Destruction and replacement of parenchymal tissue by neoplastic growth
Bleeding and hemorrhage	Compression of blood vessels, with ischemia and necrosis of tissue; or tumor may outgrow its blood supply
Ulceration, necrosis, and infection of tumor area	Ischemia associated with rapid growth, with subsequent bacterial invasion
Obstruction of hollow viscera or communication pathways	Expansive growth of tumor with compression and invasion of tissues
Effusion in serous cavities	Impaired lymph flow from the serous cavity or erosion of tumor into the cavity
Increased risk of vascular thrombosis	Abnormal production of coagulation factors by the tumor, obstruction of venous channels, and immobility
Anemia	Bleeding and depression of red blood cell production
Bone destruction	Metastatic invasion of bony structures
Hypercalcemia	Destruction of bone due to metastasis or production by the tumor of parathyroid-like hormone
Pain	Liberation of pain mediators by the tumor, compression, or ischemia of structures
Cachexia, weakness, wasting of tissues	Catabolic effect of the tumor on body metabolism along with selective trapping of nutrients by rapidly growing tumor cells
Inappropriate hormone production (*e.g.*, ADH or ACTH secretion by cancers such as bronchogenic carcinoma)	Production by the tumor of hormones or hormone-like substances that are not regulated by normal feedback mechanisms

replace normally functioning parenchymal tissue, the initial manifestations of cancer usually reflect the primary site of involvement. For example, cancer of the lung initially produces impairment of respiratory function; as the tumor grows and metastasizes, other body structures become affected.

Cancer disrupts tissue integrity. As cancers grow, they compress and erode blood vessels, causing ulceration and necrosis along with frank bleeding and sometimes hemorrhage. One of the early warning signals of colorectal cancer is blood in the stool. Cancer cells also may produce enzymes and metabolic toxins that are destructive to the surrounding tissues. Usually, tissue damaged by cancerous growth does not heal normally. Instead, the damaged area persists and often continues to grow; a sore that does not heal is another warning signal of cancer. Cancer has no regard for normal anatomic boundaries; as it grows, it invades and compresses adjacent structures. Abdominal cancer, for example, often compresses the viscera and causes bowel obstruction. Cancer may obstruct lymph flow and penetrate serous cavities, causing pleural effusion and ascites. In its late stages, cancer often causes pain (see Chapter 48). Pain is probably one of the most dreaded aspects of cancer, and pain management is one of the major treatment concerns for persons with incurable cancers.

Abnormalities in energy, carbohydrate, lipid, and protein regulation are common manifestations during progressive tumor growth. Many cancers are associated with weight loss and wasting of body fat and lean protein, a condition called *cancer cachexia*. Although anorexia, reduced food intake, and abnormalities of taste are common in peo-

ple with cancer and often are accentuated by treatment methods, the extent of weight loss and protein wasting cannot be explained in terms of diminished food intake alone. There also is a disparity between the size of the tumor and the severity of cachexia, which supports the existence of other mediators in the development of cachexia. Cachexia is thought to be the result of tumor-derived or host-derived factors that cause anorexia directly by acting on satiety centers in the hypothalamus or indirectly by injuring tissues that subsequently release anorexigenic substances.

Cachectin was the first identified cytokine associated with wasting. Cachectin was later found to be identical to tumor necrosis factor (TNF), a cytokine secreted primarily from macrophages in response to tumor cell growth or gram-negative bacterial infections.[10] TNF causes anorexia by suppressing satiety centers and by suppressing the synthesis of lipoprotein lipase, an enzyme that facilitates the release of fatty acids from lipoproteins so they can be used by tissues. TNF is an endogenous pyrogen that induces fever by its actions on cells in the hypothalamic regulatory regions of the brain. TNF also induces a number of inflammatory responses, activates the coagulation system, suppresses bone marrow stem cell division, acts on hepatocytes to increase the synthesis of specific serum proteins in response to inflammatory stimuli, and mediates endotoxic shock secondary to trauma, burns, and sepsis.[11] The role of TNF and its full impact on cancer cachexia are uncertain. It has been suggested by some that the hormone may be an endogenous antineoplastic agent. Interleukin (IL)-1, another cytokine secreted from macrophages, shares with TNF the ability to initiate cachexia.

In addition to signs and symptoms at the sites of primary and metastatic disease, cancer can produce manifestations in sites that are not directly affected by the disease. Such manifestations are collectively referred to as *paraneoplastic syndromes*. Some of these manifestations are caused by the elaboration of hormones by cancer cells, and others result from the production of circulating factors that produce nonmetastatic hematopoietic, neurologic, and dermatologic syndromes. For example, cancers may produce procoagulation factors that contribute to an increased risk of venous thrombosis. It is estimated that approximately 10% of persons with cancer are affected by these syndromes.[3] The three most common endocrine syndromes associated with cancer are the syndrome of inappropriate antidiuretic hormone secretion (see Chapter 31), Cushing's syndrome due to ectopic adrenocorticotropic hormone (now called *corticotropin*) production (see Chapter 40), and hypercalcemia (see Chapter 31). Hypercalcemia of malignancy does not appear to be related to parathyroid hormone (PTH) but to PTH-related protein, which shares several biologic actions with PTH. It also can be caused by osteolytic processes induced by cancer such as multiple myeloma or bony metastases from other cancers. The paraneoplastic syndromes may be the earliest indication that a person has cancer; they also may signal early recurrence of the disease in previously treated patients.

In summary, neoplasms may be either benign or malignant. Benign and malignant tumors differ in terms of cell characteristics, manner of growth, rate of growth, potential for metastasis, ability to produce generalized effects, tendency to cause tissue destruction, and capacity to cause death. The growth of a benign tumor is restricted to the site of origin, and the tumor usually does not cause death unless it interferes with vital functions. Cancers or malignant neoplasms, however, grow wildly and without organization, spread to distant parts of the body, and cause death unless their growth is inhibited or stopped by treatment.

There are two types of cancer: solid tumors and hematologic tumors. Solid tumors initially are confined to a specific organ or tissue, but hematologic cancers are disseminated from the onset. Cancer is a disorder of cell proliferation and differentiation. Cancer cells often are poorly differentiated compared with normal cells, and they display abnormal membrane characteristics, have abnormal antigens, produce abnormal biochemical products, and have abnormal karyotypes. All cancers result from nonlethal genetic changes that transform a normal cell into a cancer cell. The spread of cancer occurs through three pathways: direct invasion and extension, seeding of cancer cells in body cavities, and metastatic spread through vascular or lymphatic pathways. Only a proportionately small clone of cancer cells is capable of metastasis. To metastasize, a cancer cell must be able to break loose from the primary tumor, invade the surrounding extracellular matrix, gain access to a blood vessel, survive its passage in the bloodstream, emerge from the bloodstream at a favorable location, invade the surrounding tissue, and begin to grow.

Cancer disrupts tissue integrity. Cancers also produce chemical mediators called *cytokines*, such as TNF, that produce weight loss and tissue wasting. Paraneoplastic syndromes arise from the ability of neoplasms to elaborate hormones and other chemical messengers to produce nonmetastatic endocrine, hematopoietic, neurologic, and dermatologic syndromes.

Carcinogenesis and Causes of Cancer

After you have completed this section of the chapter, you should be able to meet the following objectives:

+ Describe the role of proto-oncogenes and anti-oncogenes in the transformation of a normal life line to a cancer cell line
+ Name the steps in the transformation of normal cells to cancer cells by carcinogens
+ State how lifestyle can contribute to the cancer risk through increased exposure to carcinogenic agents
+ Relate the function of the immune system to prevention of cancer

Because cancer is not a single disease, it is reasonable to assume that it does not have a single cause. More likely, cancer occurs because of interactions between multiple risk factors or repeated exposure to a single carcinogenic (cancer-producing) agent. Among the risk factors that have been linked to cancer are heredity, chemical and environmental carcinogens, cancer-causing viruses, and immunologic defects. All cancers result from nonlethal genetic changes that transform a normal cell into a cancerous cell.

ONCOGENESIS

The term *oncogenesis* refers to a genetic mechanism whereby normal cells are transformed into cancer cells. Two kinds of genes control normal cell growth and replication: growth-promoting regulatory genes called *proto-oncogenes* and growth-inhibiting regulatory genes called *anti-oncogenes*. These genes have been implicated as the principal targets of genetic damage occurring during the development of a cancer cell.[12,13] Such genetic damage may be acquired by the action of chemicals, radiation, or viruses, or it may be inherited in the germ line. Most cancers probably are multifactorial in origin, with several factors acting in concert or sequentially to produce the multiple genetic abnormalities that are characteristic of cancer cells.

Oncogenes are mutations of normal growth-regulating genes. The oncogene theory dates back to 1911, when Francis Peyton Rous discovered a virus that causes sarcomas in chickens. Over the years, various oncogenic viruses have been identified that can produce cancerous transformations in laboratory cell cultures and animals. As the research with

Oncogenesis

➤ Normal cell growth is controlled by growth-promoting proto-oncogenes and growth-suppressing anti-oncogenes. Normally, cell growth is genetically controlled so that potentially malignant cells are targeted for elimination by tumor-suppressing genes.

➤ Oncogenesis is a genetic process whereby normal cells are transformed into cancer cells. It involves mutations in the normal growth-regulating genes.

➤ The transformation of normal cells into cancer cells is multifactorial, involving the inheritance of cancer susceptibility genes and environmental factors such as chemicals, radiation, and viruses.

virus-induced cell transformation progressed, it was discovered that normal cells contain DNA sequences similar to the viral genes that cause cancerous transformation of laboratory cells. These DNA sequences, called *proto-oncogenes*, have essential roles in regulating the growth and proliferation of normal cells. Proto-oncogene products may act as growth factors, as receptors for growth factors, or as second messengers that transmit growth factor signals. The involvement of these genes in the cancer process is due to a somatic mutation that takes place in a specific target tissue, converting its proto-oncogenes into oncogenes.

Another discovery identified a different class of genes, the cancer suppressor genes or anti-oncogenes. These tumor-suppressing genes inhibit the proliferation of cells in a tumor. When this type of gene is inactivated, a genetic signal that normally inhibits proliferation is removed, thereby causing the cell to begin unregulated growth. Several human tumor suppressor genes have been identified.[3] Of particular interest in this group is the p53 gene, located on the short arm of chromosome 17. This gene, which codes for a protein that is pivotal in growth regulation and functions as a suppressor of tumor growth, has been found to be altered at some point in the development of approximately one half of human cancers.[3] Mutation of the p53 gene has been implicated in the development of lung, breast, and colon cancer—the three leading causes of cancer death.[3] The p53 gene also appears to initiate apoptosis of radiation- and chemotherapy-damaged tumor cells. Thus, tumors that retain normal p53 function are more likely to respond to such therapy than tumors that carry a defective p53 gene.[3]

Another newly discovered suppressor gene is FHIT, located in a fragile region on the short arm of chromosome 3. The fragile characteristic of its location has led researchers to suggest it may be particularly susceptible to mutation by carcinogens such as those contained in tobacco smoke. It has been found to be completely or partially absent in a number of cancers, including colon, breast, and lung.[14]

There have been numerous distinctions discovered between the proto-oncogenes and the tumor suppressor genes. The mutations that cause proto-oncogenes to change to oncogenes are thought to occur in a structural gene or a regulatory gene that results in overproduction of a normal protein product. The cell acquires a new function that often is a continuous or otherwise abnormal signal for unregulated cellular proliferation. These mutations exhibit an autosomal dominant inheritance pattern in that one defective gene and one normal allele are inherited. Fetuses that inherit this mutation usually do not survive to term. In contrast, the mutation that affects tumor suppressor genes exhibits an autosomal recessive inheritance pattern and usually occurs in both inherited genes. Individuals who inherit this type of mutation usually are at high risk for developing cancers that demonstrate a common tissue or cell type preference.[13]

Normally, proto-oncogenes are specifically turned on for only a brief period in the cell cycle. When the proto-oncogenes and their products are altered by mutation, they may operate continuously, causing unregulated cell growth. Significantly, it appears that the acquisition of a single gene mutation is not sufficient to transform normal cells into cancer cells. Instead, cancerous transformation appears to require the activation of many independently mutated genes.

The transformation of normal cells to cancer cells by carcinogenic agents is a multistep process that can be divided into three stages: initiation, promotion, and progression (Fig. 8-8). *Initiation* involves the exposure of cells to appropriate doses of a carcinogenic agent that makes them susceptible to malignant transformation. The carcinogenic agents can be chemical, physical, or biologic, and produce irreversible changes in the genome of a previously normal cell. Because the effects of initiating agents are irreversible, multiple divided doses may achieve the same effects as single exposures of the same comparable dose or small amounts of highly carcinogenic substances. The most susceptible cells for mutagenic alterations in the genome are the cells that are actively synthesizing DNA.[15]

Promotion involves the induction of unregulated accelerated growth in already initiated cells by various chemicals and growth factors. Promotion is reversible if the promoter substance is removed. Cells that have been irreversibly initiated may be promoted even after long latency periods. The latency period varies with the type of agent, the dosage, and the characteristics of the target cells. Many chemical carcinogens are called *complete carcinogens* because they can initiate and promote neoplastic transformation. *Progression* is the process whereby tumor cells acquire malignant phenotypic changes that promote invasiveness, metastatic competence, a tendency for autonomous growth, and increased karyotypic instability.[15]

Carcinogenic agents can be divided into two categories: direct-reacting agents, which do not require activation in the body to become carcinogenic, and indirect-reacting agents, called *procarcinogens*, which become active only after metabolic conversion. The carcinogenicity of some chemicals is augmented by agents that by themselves have little or no cancer-causing ability. These agents are called *promoters*. It is believed that promoters exert their effect by

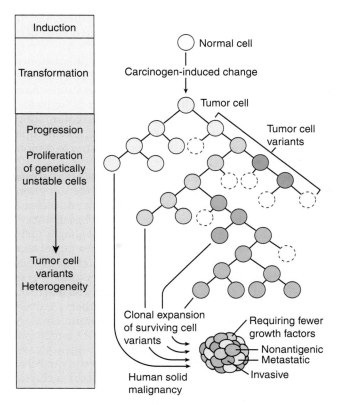

FIGURE 8-8 The process of induction, transformation, and progression and the clonal evolution of tumors. New subclones arise from descendents of the original transformed cell and with progression and the clonal evaluation of tumors. New subclones arise from the original descendants of the transformed cell with progressive growth of a tumor mass that incorporates these variants into subclones that are more aggressive and more adept at evading host defenses. (Adapted from Tannock I.F. [1983]. Biology of tumor growth. *Hospital Practice* 18, 81)

changing the expression of genetic material in a cell, increasing DNA synthesis, enhancing gene amplification (*i.e.*, number of gene copies that are made), and altering intercellular communication. Some hormones, for example, may alter the endocrine balance and act as promoters. Several carcinogenic agents may act together or with other types of carcinogenic influences, such as viruses or radiation, to produce cancer.[3]

Direct- and indirect-acting agents form highly reactive species (*i.e.*, electrophiles and free radicals) that bind with the nucleophilic residues on DNA, RNA, or cellular proteins. The action of these reactive species tends to cause cell mutation or alteration in synthesis of cell enzymes and structural proteins in a manner that alters cell replication and interferes with cell regulatory controls. Antioxidants such as vitamins A, C, and E inhibit the formation of free radicals and thus may inhibit the damaging effects of carcinogens on DNA. The direct-acting agents usually are weak carcinogens and, depending on the dose and duration of exposure, may cause cancer. Among these direct-acting agents are the alkylating drugs used in the treatment of cancer.

The indirect-acting procarcinogens require metabolic conversion to active carcinogens. Among the most potent

of the procarcinogens are the polycyclic hydrocarbons. The polycyclic hydrocarbons are of particular interest because they are produced in the combustion of tobacco and are present in cigarette smoke. They also are produced from animal fat in the process of broiling meats and are present in smoked meats and fish. Another class of procarcinogens is the aromatic amines and azo dyes. The carcinogenicity of these agents is exerted mainly in the liver, where the metabolic process that activates the procarcinogen occurs. An exception is β-naphthylamine, which is broken down in the urine and causes bladder cancer. It has been responsible for a 50-fold increase in bladder cancer in rubber industry workers and those exposed to aniline dye. Some of the azo dyes have been developed into food coloring agents, which are federally regulated in the United States. Aflatoxin B_1 is a naturally occurring carcinogen produced by some strains of *Aspergillus*, a mold that grows in improperly stored grains and nuts. It also may be found in peanuts and peanut butter. There is a high correlation between dietary levels of this food contaminant and liver cancer in some parts of Africa and the Far East. Hepatitis B also is endemic in these areas, and it has been suggested that it may contribute to the carcinogenic effects of aflatoxin B_1.[3]

Heredity

A hereditary predisposition to approximately 50 types of cancer has been observed in families. Breast cancer, for example, occurs more frequently in women whose grandmothers, mothers, aunts, and sisters also have experienced a breast malignancy. The genetic predisposition for development of cancer has been documented for a number of cancerous and precancerous lesions that follow mendelian inheritance patterns. Cancer is found in approximately 10% of persons having one affected first-degree relative, in approximately 15% of persons having two affected family members, and in 30% of persons having three affected family members. The risk increases to approximately 50% in women 65 years of age who have multiple family members with breast cancer. Two oncogenes, called *BRAC1* (breast carcinoma 1) and *BRAC2* (breast carcinoma 2), have been implicated in a genetic susceptibility to breast cancer. Li-Fraumeni syndrome, an autosomal dominant inherited disorder (*i.e.*, a mutation in the p53 tumor suppressor gene), places women at high risk for developing breast cancer in their twenties and thirties and developing other cancers, including sarcomas, leukemia, and brain tumors.[6]

Several cancers exhibit an autosomal dominant inheritance pattern. In approximately 40% of cases, retinoblastoma is inherited as an autosomal dominant trait; the remaining cases are nonhereditary. The penetrance of the genetic trait is high; in carriers of the dominant retinoblastoma gene, the penetrance for this gene is 95% for at least one tumor, and the affected person may be unilaterally or bilaterally affected.[16] Familial adenomatous polyposis of the colon also follows an autosomal dominant inheritance pattern. In people who inherit this gene, hundreds of adenomatous polyps may develop, some of which inevitably become malignant.[3] Retinoblastoma and heritable forms of cancer are discussed further in the section on childhood cancers.

Carcinogens

A carcinogen is an agent capable of causing cancer. The role of environmental agents in causation of cancer was first noted in 1775 by Sir Percivall Pott, who related the high incidence of scrotal cancer in chimneysweeps to their exposure to coal soot.[17] In 1915, a group of Japanese investigators conducted the first experiments in which a chemical agent was used to produce cancer.[17] These investigators found that a cancerous growth developed when they painted a rabbit's ear with coal tar. Coal tar has since been found to contain potent polycyclic aromatic hydrocarbons. Since then, many carcinogenic agents have been identified (Chart 8-1).

Chemical Carcinogens. More than six million chemicals have been identified. It is estimated that less than 1000 of these have been extensively examined for their carcinogenic potential.[18] Some have been found to cause cancers in animals, and others are known to cause cancers in humans. These agents include both natural (*e.g.*, aflatoxin B_1) and artificial products (*e.g.*, vinyl chloride).

Approximately 2% to 4% of cancer deaths are associated with an exposure to an occupational hazard. Those substances identified as having carcinogenic capabilities were found to be closely associated with abnormal clustering of certain cancers. For example, occupational exposure to asbestos fibers is significantly related to increased risks for developing several cancers, including lung, laryngeal, and gastrointestinal cancers, and mesothelioma. Increased incidences of leukemia are associated with benzene exposure.[6]

Herbicide exposure, particularly to the phenoxy herbicides, has been associated with an increased incidence of non-Hodgkin's lymphoma in farmers. Other studies have discovered a relationship between this class of herbicides and soft tissue sarcomas and cancers of the colon, lung, nasal passages, prostate, and ovary; leukemia; and multiple myeloma. However, definitive studies are too few to demonstrate exposure–risk relationships.

Many cancers are associated with lifestyle risk factors, such as smoking, dietary factors, and alcohol consumption. Cigarette smoke contains both procarcinogens and promoters. It is directly associated with lung and laryngeal cancer[19] and has been linked with cancers of the esophagus, pancreas, kidney, uterine cervix, and bladder. Chewing tobacco or tobacco products increases the risk of cancers of the oral cavity and esophagus. It has been estimated that 30% of current cancer deaths in the United States are related to tobacco. Not only is the smoker at risk, but others passively exposed to cigarette smoke are at risk. Environmental tobacco smoke has been classified as a "group A" carcinogen based on the U.S. Environmental Protection Agency's system of carcinogen classification. It also is estimated that between 20% and 60% of the deaths that occur each year from non–smoking-related lung cancers may be caused by environmental tobacco smoke.[20]

There is strong evidence that certain elements in the diet contribute to cancer risk. For example, benzo[*a*]pyrene and other polycyclic hydrocarbons may be produced when meat and fish are charcoal broiled or smoked or when foods are fried in fat that has been reused multiple times. Nitrosamines, which are powerful carcinogens, may be formed from nitrites that are derived from nitrates added to vegetables and foods as a preservative. Formation of these nitrosamines may be inhibited by the presence of antioxidants such as vitamin C in the stomach.

Cancer of the colon has been associated with high dietary intake of fat, protein, and beef and low intake of dietary fiber. The carcinogenic factors associated with a high-fat diet have yet to be confirmed. However, some studies have shown a relationship between high levels of fecally excreted bile acids and colon cancer. A high-fat diet increases the flow of primary bile acids. These acids are converted to secondary bile acids such as lithocholic acid and deoxycholic acid in the presence of anaerobic bacteria in the colon. These acids are thought to be tumor promoters rather than initiators.[7]

Alcohol modifies the metabolism of carcinogens in the liver and esophagus.[21] It is believed to influence the transport of carcinogens, increasing the contact between an externally induced carcinogen and the stem cells that line the upper oral cavity and esophagus. The carcinogenic effect of cigarette smoke can be enhanced by concomitant consumption of alcohol; persons who smoke and drink considerable amounts of alcohol are at increased risk for development of cancer of the oral cavity and esophagus.

CHART 8-1

Chemical and Environmental Agents Known to be Carcinogenic in Humans

Polycyclic Hydrocarbons

Soots, tars, and oils
Cigarette smoke

Industrial Agents

Aniline and azo dyes
Arsenic compounds
Asbestos
β-Naphthylamine
Benzene
Benzo[*a*]pyrene
Carbon tetrachloride
Insecticides, fungicides
Nickel and chromium compounds
Polychlorinated biphenyls
Vinyl chloride

Food and Drugs

Smoked foods
Nitrosamines
Aflatoxin B_1
Diethylstilbestrol
Anticancer drugs (*e.g.*, alkylating agents, cyclophosphamide, chlorambucil, nitrosourea)

The effects of carcinogenic agents usually are dose dependent—the larger the dose or the longer the duration of exposure, the greater the risk that cancer will develop. Some chemical carcinogens may act in concert with other carcinogenic influences, such as viruses or radiation, to induce neoplasia. There usually is a time delay ranging from 5 to 30 years from the time of chemical carcinogen exposure to the development of overt cancer. This is unfortunate because many people may have been exposed to the agent and its carcinogenic effects before the association was recognized. This occurred, for example, with the use of diethylstilbestrol, which was widely used in the United States from the mid-1940s to 1970 to prevent miscarriages. But it was not until the late 1960s that many cases of vaginal adenosis and adenocarcinoma in young women were found to be the result of their exposure in utero to diethylstilbestrol.[22]

Radiation.   The effects of *ionizing radiation* in carcinogenesis has been well documented in atomic bomb survivors, in patients diagnostically exposed, and in industrial workers, scientists, and physicians who were exposed during employment. Malignant epitheliomas of the skin and leukemia were significantly elevated in these populations.[6] Between 1950 and 1970, the death rate from leukemia alone in the most heavily exposed population groups of the atomic bomb survivors in Hiroshima and Nagasaki was 147 per 100,000 persons, 30 times the expected rate.[23]

The type of cancer that developed depended on the dose of radiation, the sex of the person, and the age at which exposure occurred. For instance, approximately 25 to 30 years after total body or trunk irradiation, there were increased incidences of leukemia and cancers of the breast, lung, stomach, thyroid, salivary gland, gastrointestinal system, and lymphoid tissues. The length of time between exposure and the onset of cancer is related to the age of the individual. For example, children exposed to ionizing radiation in utero have an increased risk for developing leukemias and childhood tumors, particularly 2 to 3 years after birth. This latency period for leukemia extends to 5 to 10 years if the child was exposed after birth and to 20 years for certain solid tumors.[6] As another example, the latency period for the development of thyroid cancer in infants and small children who received radiation to the head and neck to decrease the size of the tonsils or thymus was as long as 35 years after exposure.

The association between sunlight and the development of skin cancer has been reported for more than 100 years. William Dubreuilh, a French dermatologist, published in 1907 epidemiologic data that implicated sunlight as a cause for skin cancer. *Ultraviolet radiation* emits relatively low-energy rays that do not deeply penetrate the skin. However, the skin absorbs most of the rays, which leads to excited energy states of the nucleic acid bases, and results in photochemical reactions between DNA bases.[6] As with other carcinogens, the effects of ultraviolet radiation usually are additive, and there usually is a long delay between the time of exposure and the time that cancer can be detected.

The evidence supporting the role of ultraviolet radiation in the cause of skin cancer includes skin cancer that develops primarily on the areas of skin more frequently exposed to sunlight (*e.g.*, the head and neck, arms, hands, and legs), a higher incidence in light-complexioned individuals who lack the ultraviolet-filtering skin pigment melanin, and the fact that the intensity of ultraviolet exposure is directly related to the incidence of skin cancer, as evidenced by higher rates occurring in Australia and the American Southwest.[6] There also are studies that suggest intense, episodic exposure to sunlight, particularly during childhood, is more important in the development of melanoma than prolonged low-intensity exposure.[24]

Radon is a radioactive gas that is formed from the decay of uranium widely distributed in soil and rocks. Different geographic areas contain varying amounts. The daughter products of radon emit alpha particles that bind to the dust in the home and may be inhaled and deposited in the lungs. Studies have found that people exposed to high amounts (approaching 3000 picocuries [pCi]/L of air) of the gas, such as uranium miners, have higher incidences of bronchogenic carcinoma. Residential home monitoring began in some communities across the country in the 1980s. Although most homes in the United States have radon levels below 2 pCi/L, 4% to 5% have at least five times that amount.[17] There is concern that low-level indoor exposure (*e.g.*, in homes in areas of high radon in the soil) may contribute to lung cancer. At present, further studies are needed to determine the significance of radon as a lung cancer risk factor.[3]

Oncogenic Viruses

It has been suspected for some time that viruses play an important role in the development of certain forms of cancer, particularly leukemia and lymphoma. Ellermann in 1908 and Rous in 1911 were the first to describe the transmissibility of avian leukemia and sarcoma, respectively. Because these initial studies were carried out in birds, the interest in the findings remained isolated to avian research. Subsequent studies discovered that in rabbits, squamous cell carcinomas would develop from benign papillomas, lesions that were caused by the papillomavirus. Interest in the field of viral oncology, particularly in human populations, has burgeoned with the discovery of reverse transcriptase, the development of recombinant DNA technology, and more recently with the discovery of oncogenes and tumor suppressor genes.[19]

An oncogenic virus is one that can induce cancer. Viruses, which are small particles containing genetic (DNA or RNA) material, enter a host cell and become incorporated into its chromosomal DNA or take control of the cell's machinery for the purpose of producing viral proteins. A large number of DNA and RNA viruses (*i.e.*, retroviruses) have been shown to be oncogenic in animals. However, only a few viruses have been linked to cancer in humans.[3] Among the recognized oncogenic viruses in humans are the human T-cell leukemia virus-1 (HTLV-1), human papilloma virus (HPV), Epstein-Barr virus (EBV), and hepatitis B virus (HBV).[6] Herpes simplex type 2 also has been associated with cervical cancer, but the evidence supporting its role as a carcinogenic influence is less clear.

Although there are a number of retroviruses (RNA viruses) that cause cancer in animals, there is only one known human retrovirus that is associated with cancer. HTLV-1 is associated with a form of T-cell leukemia that is endemic in certain parts of Japan and some areas of the Caribbean and Africa, and is found sporadically elsewhere, including the United States and Europe. Like the human immunodeficiency virus, HTLV-1 is attracted to the CD4+ T cells, and this subset of T cells is therefore the major target for cancerous transformation. The virus requires transmission of infected T cells by way of sexual intercourse, infected blood, or breast milk. Adult T-cell leukemia (ATL) develops in approximately 2% to 5% of persons seropositive for HTLV-1 and is an aggressive cancer, with a median survival of 3 to 4 months from the time of diagnosis. Evidence suggests that the HTLV-1 virus has a direct effect in causing cancer because infants who are born in areas with high incidence rates but move to another part of the world exhibit the same likelihood for developing ATL. In vitro studies also have found that the virus is capable of transforming T cells contained in normal human umbilical cord blood to immortalized precancerous cells.

A second type of HTLV virus, HTLV-2, has been isolated from individuals with an unusual form of hairy cell leukemia. Hairy cell leukemia normally is the result of alterations in the B-lymphocyte lineage. However, the HTLV-2 variant involves the T-lymphocyte lineage.[3,25]

Three DNA viruses have been implicated in human cancers: HPV, EBV, and HBV. The transforming DNA viruses form stable associations with the human genome using genes that allow them to complete their replication cycle and be expressed in transformed cells. There is strong evidence to suggest that the DNA viruses act in concert with other factors to cause cancer.

There are over 60 genetically different types of HPV. Some types (*i.e.*, types 1, 2, 4, 7) have been shown to cause benign squamous papillomas (*i.e.*, warts). HPVs also have been implicated in squamous cell carcinoma of the cervix and anogenital region. HPV types 16 and 18 and, less commonly, types 31, 33, 35, and 51, have been found in approximately 85% of squamous cell carcinomas of the cervix and presumed precursors (*i.e.*, severe cervical dysplasia and carcinoma in situ).[3]

EBV is a member of the herpesvirus family. It has been implicated in the pathogenesis of four human cancers: Burkitt's lymphoma, nasopharyngeal cancer, B-cell lymphomas in immunosuppressed individuals such as those with acquired immunodeficiency syndrome (AIDS), and in some cases of Hodgkin's lymphoma. Burkitt's lymphoma, a tumor of B lymphocytes, is endemic in parts of East Africa and occurs sporadically in other areas worldwide. In persons with normal immune function, the EBV-driven B-cell proliferation is readily controlled and the person becomes asymptomatic or experiences a self-limited episode of infectious mononucleosis (see Chapter 16). In regions of the world where Burkitt's lymphoma is endemic, concurrent malaria or other infections cause impaired immune function, allowing sustained B-lymphocyte proliferation. The incidence of nasopharyngeal cancer is high in some areas of China, particularly southern China, and in the Cantonese population in Singapore. EBV genomes have been found in almost all of the nasopharyngeal tumor specimens in these areas.

HBV is the etiologic agent in the development of hepatitis B, cirrhosis, and hepatocellular carcinoma (HCC). Epidemiologic data strongly support the role of HBV in the development of human HCC. There is a significant correlation between elevated rates of HCC worldwide and the prevalence of HBV carriers. Other etiologic factors also may contribute to the development of liver cancer. Ingestion of aflatoxin and infection with hepatitis C virus have been implicated. The precise mechanism by which HBV induces HCC has not been determined, although it has been suggested that it may be the result of prolonged HBV-induced liver damage and regeneration. A number of countries endemic for HBV infection have begun widespread vaccinations against the virus. It will be interesting to observe if these vaccinations lower the incidence of HCC.[7,25]

Immunologic Defects

There is growing evidence for the immune system's participation in resistance against the progression and spread of cancer. The central concept, known as the immune surveillance hypothesis, which was first proposed by Paul Ehrlich in 1909, postulates that the immune system plays a central role in resistance against the development of tumors.[26] In addition to cancer–host interactions as a mechanism of cancer development, immunologic mechanisms provide a means for the detection, classification, and prognostic evaluation of cancers and as a potential method of treatment. *Immunotherapy* (discussed later in this chapter) is a cancer treatment modality designed to heighten the patient's general immune responses so as to increase tumor destruction.

It has been suggested that the development of cancer might be associated with impairment or decline in the surveillance capacity of the immune system. For example, increases in cancer incidence have been observed in people with immunodeficiency diseases and in those with organ transplants who are receiving immunosuppressant drugs. The incidence of cancer also is increased in the elderly, in whom there is a known decrease in immune activity. The association of Kaposi's sarcoma with AIDS further emphasizes the role of the immune system in preventing malignant cell proliferation.[17]

It has been shown that most tumor cells have molecular configurations that can be specifically recognized by immune T cells or by antibodies and hence are termed *tumor antigens*. The most relevant tumor antigens fall into two categories: unique tumor-specific antigens found only on tumor cells, and tumor-associated antigens found on tumor cells and on normal cells. Quantitative and qualitative differences permit the use of these tumor-associated antigens to distinguish cancer cells from normal cells.[27]

Virtually all of the components of the immune system have the potential for eradicating cancer cells, including T lymphocytes, B lymphocytes and antibodies, macrophages, and natural killer (NK) cells (see Chapter 18). The T-cell response is undoubtedly one of the most important host responses for controlling the growth of antigenic tumor cells; it is responsible for direct killing of tumor cells and for activation of other components of the immune system. The

T-cell immunity to cancer cells reflects the function of two subsets of T cells: the CD4+ helper T cells and CD8+ cyto-toxic T cells. The finding of tumor-reactive antibodies in the serum of people with cancer supports the role of the B cell as a member of the immune surveillance team. Anti-bodies can destroy cancer cells through complement-mediated mechanisms or through antibody-dependent cellular cytotoxicity, in which the antibody binds the can-cer cell to another effector cell, such as the NK cell, that does the actual killing of the cancer cell. NK cells do not require antigen recognition and can lyse a wide variety of target cells. The cytotoxic activity of NK cells can be aug-mented by the lymphokines, IL-2, and interferon, and NK activity can be amplified by immune T-cell re-sponses.[28] Macrophages are important in tumor immunity as antigen-presenting cells to initiate the immune re-sponse and as potential effector cells to participate in tumor cell lysis.

> In summary, because cancer is not a single disease, it is reasonable to assume that it does not have a single cause. Multiple factors probably interact at the ge-netic level to transform normal cells into cancer cells. This transformation process is called *oncogenesis*. Two kinds of genes control normal cell growth and repli-cation: growth-promoting regulatory genes (*i.e.*, proto-oncogenes) and growth-inhibiting regulatory genes (*i.e.*, anti-oncogenes). These genes are implicated as principal targets of genetic damage that occurs during the development of a cancer cell. Such genetic damage may be acquired by the action of chemicals (*i.e.*, chem-ical carcinogens), radiation, or viruses, or it may be inherited in the cell line.

Diagnosis and Treatment

After you have completed this section of the chapter, you should be able to meet the following objectives:

✦ Describe methods used in detection and diagnosis of cancer, including the Papanicolaou smear, tissue biopsy, tumor markers, and polymerase chain reaction
✦ Compare methods used in grading and staging cancers
✦ Explain the mechanism by which radiation exerts its beneficial effects in the treatment of cancer
✦ Describe the adverse effects of radiation therapy
✦ Compare the action of cell cycle–specific and cell cycle–independent chemotherapeutic drugs
✦ Describe the three mechanisms whereby biotherapy exerts its effects
✦ Describe four uses of gene therapy in the treatment of cancer

DIAGNOSTIC METHODS

The methods used in the diagnosis and staging of cancer are determined largely by the location and type of cancer suspected. A number of diagnostic procedures are used in the diagnosis of cancer, including x-ray studies, endoscopic examinations, urine and stool tests, blood tests for tumor markers, bone marrow aspirations, ultrasound imaging, magnetic resonance imaging (MRI), and computed tomog-raphy (CT) scan. Four diagnostic methods are discussed in this chapter: the Pap smear, tissue biopsy, tumor markers, and the polymerase chain reaction (PCR).

The Pap Smear

The Pap smear is an example of the type of test called *exfo-liative cytology*. It consists of a microscopic examination of a properly prepared slide by a cytotechnologist or pathol-ogist for the purpose of detecting the presence of abnor-mal cells. The usefulness of exfoliative cytology relies on the fact that the cancer cells lack the cohesive properties and intercellular junctions that are characteristic of nor-mal tissue; without these characteristics, cancer cells tend to exfoliate and become mixed with secretions surround-ing the tumor growth. The American Cancer Society rec-ommends that the test be done annually to detect cervical cancer in women who are or have been sexually active and who have reached 18 years of age. After three consecutive normal findings, the test may be performed less frequently at the discretion of the physician.[29] Exfoliative cytology also can be performed on other body secretions, includ-ing nipple drainage, pleural or peritoneal fluid, and gastric washings.

Biopsy

Tissue biopsy is the removal of a tissue specimen for micro-scopic study. Biopsies are obtained in a number of ways, in-cluding needle aspiration (*i.e.*, fine, percutaneous, or core needle); by endoscopic methods, such as bronchoscopy or cystoscopy, which involve the passage of an endoscope through an orifice and into the involved structure; or by lap-aroscopic methods. In some instances, a surgical incision is made from which biopsy specimens are obtained. Excisional biopsies are those in which all of the tumor is removed. The tumors usually are small, solid, palpable masses. If the tumor is too large to be completely removed, a wedge of tissue from the mass can be excised for examination. Tissue diagno-sis is of critical importance in designing the treatment plan should cancer cells be found.[30]

Tumor Markers

Tumor markers are antigens that are expressed on the sur-face of tumor cells or substances released from normal cells in response to the presence of tumor. Some substances, such as hormones and enzymes, are produced normally by the tissue involved but become overexpressed as a result of can-cer. Other tumor markers, such as oncofetal proteins, are produced during fetal development and are induced to re-appear later in life as a result of benign and malignant neo-plasms. Tumor markers are used for screening, diagnosis, establishing prognosis, monitoring treatment, and detecting recurrent disease.

As diagnostic tools, tumor markers have limitations. The value of a marker depends on its sensitivity, specificity, proportionality, and feasibility.[31] Sensitivity implies that the marker is apparent early in the development of the tumor and has few false-negative results. Specificity indicates that the marker is specific for the specific cancer and is not elevated in other disease conditions (*i.e.*, has few false-positive results). Proportionality means that the level of marker accurately reflects the growth of the tumor, such that higher levels reflect a larger growth. Feasibility implies that the methods are readily available, easy to use, and that the cost is not prohibitive. Nearly all markers can be elevated in benign conditions, and most are not elevated in the early stages of malignancy. Hence, tumor markers have limited value as screening tests. Extremely elevated levels of a tumor marker can indicate a poor prognosis or the need for more aggressive treatment. Perhaps the greatest value of tumor markers is in monitoring therapy in people with widespread cancer. Nearly all markers show an association with the clinical course of the disease. The levels of most markers decline with successful treatment and increase with recurrence of the tumor.

The markers that have been most useful in practice have been human chorionic gonadotropin (hCG), CA 125, prostate-specific antigen (PSA), prostatic acid phosphatase (PAP), α-fetoprotein (AFP), and carcinoembryonic antigen (CEA). HCG is a hormone normally produced by the placenta. It is used as a marker for diagnosing, prescribing treatment, and following the disease course in persons with high-risk gestational trophoblastic tumors. PSA and PAP are used as markers in prostate cancer, and CA 125 is used as a marker in ovarian cancer.

Some cancers express oncofetal antigens, which are differentiation antigens normally presented only during embryonal development.[3] The two that have proven the most useful as tumor markers are AFP and CEA. AFP is synthesized by the fetal liver, yolk sac, and gastrointestinal tract and is the major serum protein in the fetus. Elevated levels are encountered in people with primary liver cancers and have also been observed in some testicular, ovarian, pancreatic, and stomach cancers. CEA normally is produced by embryonic tissue in the gut, pancreas, and liver and is elaborated by a number of different cancers. Depending on the serum level adopted for significant elevation, CEA is elevated in approximately 60% to 90% of colorectal carcinomas, 50% to 80% of pancreatic cancers, and 25% to 50% of gastric and breast tumors.[3] As with most other tumor markers, elevated levels of CEA and AFP are found in other, noncancerous conditions, and elevated levels of both depend on tumor size so that neither is useful as an early test for cancer.

Polymerase Chain Reaction

Polymerase chain reaction is a highly sensitive in vitro technique designed to identify specific circulating tumor cells and micrometastases in leukemias, lymphomas, melanoma, neuroblastoma, and a variety of carcinomas. Tumor-specific abnormalities in the DNA of tumor cells are amplified, which allows identification of these abnormalities among cell populations containing only a few tumor cells (see Chapter 17). The PCR technique is so sensitive that one tumor cell can be identified in a million to a billion normal cells.[32]

Although PCR has been found to be superior to conventional techniques in detecting circulating tumor cells and micrometastases, several limitations are associated with this technique. Because of the extreme sensitivity of the test, there is a tendency for false-positive results to occur if certain precautions are not taken to prevent contamination of the samples. Inhibitor substances are contained in some tissues and fluids that can also decrease the sensitivity. Most tumor cells that reach the bloodstream are destroyed by mechanical or immunologic mechanisms, thereby reducing the number of cells in the peripheral circulation. The number of tumor cells identified in blood obtained from peripheral sites may not reflect the extent of circulating cells.

More research is needed to determine the extent of this technique's application to the field of oncology. Perhaps patients with low tumor burdens can be given systemic therapy at an earlier stage, when better results could be achieved. PCR also may improve preoperative staging in patients with certain epithelial cancers, which could lead to more conservative and less disfiguring surgeries.

Staging and Grading of Tumors

The two basic methods for classifying cancers are grading according to the histologic or cellular characteristics of the tumor and staging according to the clinical spread of the disease. Both methods are used to determine the course of the disease and aid in selecting an appropriate treatment or management plan. Grading of tumors involves the microscopic examination of cancer cells to determine their level of differentiation and the number of mitoses. Cancers are classified as grades I, II, III, and IV with increasing anaplasia or lack of differentiation. Staging of cancers uses methods to determine the progress and spread of the disease. Surgery may be used to determine tumor size and lymph node involvement.

The clinical staging of cancer is intended to provide a means by which information related to the progress of the disease, the methods and success of treatment modalities, and the prognosis can be communicated to others. The TNM system, which has evolved from the work of the International Union Against Cancer (IUAC) and the American Joint Committee on Cancer Staging and End Stage Reporting (AJCCS), is used by many cancer facilities. This system, which is briefly described in Chart 8-2, classifies the disease into stages using three tumor components: *T* stands for the extent of the primary tumor, *N* refers to the involvement of the regional lymph nodes, and *M* describes the extent of the metastatic involvement. The time of staging is indicated as cTNM, clinical-diagnostic staging; pTNM, postsurgical resection-pathologic staging; sTNM, surgical-evaluative staging; rTNM, retreatment staging; and aTNM, autopsy staging.[33]

CANCER TREATMENT

The goals of cancer treatment methods fall into three categories: curative, controlling, and palliative. The most common modalities are surgery, radiation, chemotherapy, hormonal therapy, and biotherapy. The treatment of cancer involves the use of a carefully planned program that combines the benefits of multiple treatment modalities and the expertise of an interdisciplinary team of specialists including medical, surgical, and radiation oncologists; clinical nurse specialists; nurse practitioners; pharmacists; and a variety of ancillary personnel.

Surgery

It is estimated that 90% of all patients with cancer will undergo a surgical procedure during the course of their management.[34] Surgery is used for diagnosis, the staging of cancer, tumor removal, and palliation (*i.e.*, relief of symptoms) when a cure cannot be achieved. The type of surgery to be used is determined by the extent of the disease, the location and structures involved, the tumor growth rate and invasiveness, the surgical risk to the patient, and the quality of life the patient will experience after the surgery. If the tumor is small and has well-defined margins, the entire tumor often can be removed. If, however, the tumor is large or involves vital tissues, surgical removal may be difficult if not impossible.

Surgical techniques consist of a number of approaches to cancer care. For example, surgery can be the primary, curative treatment for cancers that are locally or regionally contained, have not metastasized, or have not invaded major organs. It also is used as a component of adjuvant therapy when used in addition to chemotherapy or radiation therapy in other types of cancers. Surgical techniques also may be used to control oncologic emergencies such as gastrointestinal hemorrhages. Another approach includes using surgical techniques for prophylaxis in families that have a high genetically confirmed risk for developing cancer. For instance, colectomy may be suggested for families that have familial adenomatous polyposis coli. Prophylactic mastectomy also may be encouraged for women who are at very high risk for developing breast cancer.[30]

Surgical techniques have expanded to include electrosurgery, cryosurgery, chemosurgery, cytoreductive surgery, and laser surgery. Electrosurgery uses the cutting and coagulating effects of high-frequency current applied by needle, blade, or electrodes. Once considered a palliative procedure, it now is being used as an alternative treatment for certain cancers of the skin, oral cavity, and rectum. Cryosurgery involves the instillation of liquid nitrogen into the tumor through a probe. It is used in treating cancers of the oral cavity, brain, and prostate. Chemosurgery is used in skin cancers. It involves the use of a corrosive paste in combination with multiple frozen sections to ensure complete removal of the tumor. Laser surgery uses a laser beam to resect a tumor. It has been used effectively in retinal and vocal cord surgery.

Cooperative efforts among cancer centers throughout the world have helped to standardize and improve surgical procedures, determine which cancers benefit from surgical intervention, and establish in what order surgical and other treatment modalities should be used. Increased emphasis also has been placed on the development of surgical techniques, such as limb-salvage surgery, which is used in the treatment of osteogenic sarcoma to preserve functional abilities while permitting complete removal of the tumor.

Radiation Therapy

More than 50% of patients with cancer receive radiation therapy, alone or in combination with other forms of treatment. Radiation can be used alone as the primary method of treatment for Hodgkin's disease and early-stage breast, laryngeal, prostate, vaginal, and uterine cervical cancers. If radiation is used as the primary treatment for cure, the duration of treatment usually is longer and the dose is higher than in palliative treatment modalities. Radiation therapy also is used as an adjuvant treatment with surgery administered presurgically or postsurgically, with chemotherapy, or with both chemotherapy and surgery. In patients with acute lymphocytic leukemia in which the primary treatment is chemotherapy, radiation is used to treat sanctuary sites such as the central nervous system because it has been found to enhance the ability of chemotherapy to cross the blood-brain barrier. It is used as a palliative treatment to reduce symptoms in approximately 50% of patients with advanced cancers who receive radiation therapy. It is effective in reducing the pain associated with bone metastasis and, in some cases, improves mobility. Radiation also is used to treat several oncologic emergencies such as superior vena cava syndrome, spinal cord compression, bronchial obstruction, and hemorrhage.[35]

Mechanisms of Action. Ionizing radiation is radiation that is capable of ejecting one or more electrons from an atom. Ionizing radiation causes significant biologic effects with small amounts of localized energy that are powerful enough to break chemical bonds. It affects cells by direct ionization of molecules or, more commonly, by indirect ionization. Indirect ionization produced by x-rays and gamma rays causes cellular damage when these rays are absorbed into tissue and give up their energy by producing fast-moving electrons. These electrons interact with free or loosely bonded electrons of the absorber cells and subsequently produce free radicals that interact with critical cell components (see Chapter 5).[36] It can immediately kill cells,

Discovery of Ionizing Radiation

Ionizing radiation was discovered by Marie and Pierre Curie and by Wilhelm Conrad Roentgen just before the turn of the century. Development of the first cathode-ray tube followed during the 1920s, along with quantitative methods for measuring radiation dosage. The first use of radium to treat cancer occurred 1 to 2 years after development of the cathode-ray tube. During this same period, Claude Regauc (Foundation Curie in Paris) was able to demonstrate that fractionated, small, sublethal doses of radiation could permanently halt spermatogenesis, but no single lethal dose could do so without causing severe damage to the surrounding tissues. This observation linked external irradiation to the treatment of cancer. Another advance in radiation therapy was the development of radioactive cobalt. Since then, advances in technology have resulted in the sophisticated equipment that produces high-voltage x-ray and electron beams capable of delivering a therapeutic dose of radiation to the tumor with limited morbidity to surrounding tissues.

delay or halt cell cycle progression, or, at dose levels commonly used in radiation therapy, cause damage in the nucleus that results in cell death after replication. Cell damage may be sublethal, in which case a single break in the strand of DNA can repair itself if there is time before the next radiation insult. Double-stranded breaks in DNA are generally believed to be the primary damage that leads to radiation death in cells. The consequence of unrepaired DNA is that cells may continue to function until they undergo cell mitosis, at which time the genetic damage from the irradiation may result in death of the cell. The clinical significance is that the rapidly proliferating and poorly differentiated cells of a cancerous tumor are more likely to be injured by radiation therapy than are the more slowly proliferating cells of normal tissue. To some extent, however, radiation is injurious to all rapidly proliferating cells, including those of the bone marrow and the mucosal lining of the gastrointestinal tract. In addition to its lethal effects, radiation also produces sublethal injury. Recovery from sublethal doses of radiation occurs in the interval between the first dose of radiation and subsequent doses. This is why large total doses of radiation can be tolerated when they are divided into multiple, smaller fractionated doses. Normal tissue usually is able to recover from radiation damage more readily than cancerous tissue.

Radiation, Sensitivity, and Responsiveness. The term *radiosensitivity* describes the inherent properties of a tumor that determine its responsiveness to radiation. It varies widely among the different types of cancers and is thought to vary as a function of their position in the cell cycle. Fast-growing cells, for example, that have cell cycle durations of 9 or 10 hours typically are more radiosensitive in mitosis (M) or late in the G_2 phase. More slowly growing cells that have longer S phases are more radioresistant.[36] Acute lym-phocytic leukemia and lymphoma are highly radiosensitive cancers, but rhabdomyosarcomas and melanomas are much less so.

The radiation dose that is chosen for treatment of a particular cancer is determined by factors such as the radiosensitivity of the tumor type, size of the tumor, and, more important, the tolerance of the surrounding tissues. Dose-response curves, which express the extent of lethal tissue injury in relation to the dose of radiation, are determined by the number of cells that survive graded, fractional doses of radiation. With the use of fractionated doses, it is likely that the cancer cells will be dividing and in the vulnerable period of the cell cycle. This dose also allows time for normal tissues to repair the radiation damage. Studies are being conducted to find ways to increase the radiosensitivity of tumors by altering their DNA in a manner that either makes it more sensitive to radiation or less able to repair radiation damage.

Radiation responsiveness describes the manner in which a radiosensitive tumor responds to irradiation. One of the major determinants of radiation responsiveness is tumor oxygenation because oxygen is a rich source of free radicals that form and destroy essential cell components during irradiation. Many rapidly growing tumors outgrow their blood supply and become deprived of oxygen. The hypoxic cells of these tumors are more resistant to radiation than normal or well-oxygenated tumor cells. Methods of ensuring adequate oxygen delivery, such as adequate hemoglobin levels, are important. Agents that act as radiosensitizers are being investigated. These agents increase the production of free radicals during radiation in a manner similar to oxygen.

Administration. Ionizing radiation includes two distinct forms: electromagnetic waves and fast-moving, high-energy particles. Electromagnetic radiation consists of x-rays and gamma rays, both of which are similar in nature, but differ in the way they are made. X-rays are produced by electrical devices that accelerate electrons to high energy levels and abruptly stop them at a target. Gamma rays are emitted from the spontaneous decay of radioactive isotopes of elements such as cobalt and cesium. The electromagnetic radiation is energetic and extremely penetrating. Particulate radiation used in radiation therapy includes electrons, protons, alpha particles, neutrons, negative pi-mesons, and heavy ions. These particles are accelerated by electromagnetic fields in linear accelerators and cyclotrons.[36]

A number of types of equipment and beams can be used for administering radiation therapy. Large radiation therapy centers have a selection suitable for the treatment of almost any malignancy in any part of the body. Therapy can be delivered by either external beam radiation machines that have sources of radiation located some distance from the patient (sometimes called *teletherapy*) or by short-distance therapy (brachytherapy), in which a sealed radioactive source is placed close to or directly in the tumor site. Radioisotopes with a short half-life may be injected or given by mouth as a palliative or curative treatment for some forms of cancer.

External beam radiation machines deliver a penetrating radiation dose, depending on the energy or voltage rating that is used. The higher the energy, the greater the depth of penetration. The early forms of radiation therapy used x-ray machines with energy levels from 100 to 250 kV. These machines delivered low-penetrance rays that exerted their maximum tumor dose within 1 to 2 cm of the skin surface. They are now used only in superficial skin lesions or tumors located near the skin surface. The newer, megavoltage machines produce x-rays by allowing high-energy electrons to be accelerated by microwaves. These x-rays are much more penetrating and allow for treatment from a number of directions (*i.e.,* cross firing). This allows for delivery of curative doses of radiation without causing extensive damage to skin or other tissues. The megavoltage rays also spare bone structures more than lower-energy x-rays. Various beam-modifying wedges, rotational techniques, and other specific approaches are used to increase the radiation damage to the tumor site while sparing the normal surrounding tissues. Cobalt-60 machines deliver gamma rays that are comparable with megavoltage x-rays. They were once the most common type of equipment used, but because the radiation source is a radioactive isotope, it is undergoing decay and needs to be replaced every 5 to 6 years to avoid lengthy treatment times. As the name implies, linear accelerators produce megavoltage electromagnetic wave radiation by accelerating electrons in a straight line. Linear accelerators have distinct advantages, including the speed with which treatment can be given. This reduces the time the patient must spend in awkward and uncomfortable positions. Some linear accelerators also are equipped to produce particulate radiation. With particulate radiation, most of the energy is expended at a certain depth, sparing surrounding tissues.

Brachytherapy involves the insertion of sealed radioactive sources into a body cavity (intracavitary) or directly into body tissues (interstitial). Radiation sources are sealed in applicators of almost any size or shape. Most commonly they are packed into needles, beads, seeds, ribbons, or catheters, which are then implanted directly into the tumor. Removable devices make it possible to insert a radioactive material into a tumor area for a specific time (1 or 2 days to 1 week) and remove it. The radioactive sources used most commonly for this purpose are cesium-137, iridium-192, and iodine-125. Cancers of the cervix and uterus often are treated with removable cesium insertions or iridium implants. Radioactive materials with a relatively short half-life, such as gold-198, radium-226, iodine-125, or palladium-103, are commonly encapsulated and used in permanent implants. This type of treatment is used for oral, bladder, and prostate cancers.

Unsealed internal radiation sources are either injected intravenously, administered by mouth, or instilled into a body cavity. Iodine-131, which is given by mouth, is used in the treatment of thyroid cancer. Gold-198 and phosphorus-32 are instilled directly into body cavities to control effusions (*i.e.,* collections of fluid in a serous cavity).

Internal radiation sources are a source of radiation exposure as long as a sealed implant remains in the body or an unsealed implant or injected radioisotope emanates rays of radiant energy. It is essential that the type of ray that is being emitted and the half-life of the radioisotope be con-sidered when care is provided for a person receiving internal radiation. Some radioisotopes, such as phosphorus-32, produce only beta rays, which do not create a radiation hazard because of the limited range of beta radiation. Others, such as cesium implants, pose a radiation hazard because they emit gamma rays. Institutions that practice nuclear medicine must be licensed by the Atomic Energy Commission and have a radiation safety officer, who is responsible for establishing policies and maintaining radiation safety in the institution.

Adverse Effects. Radiation cannot distinguish between malignant cells and the rapidly proliferating cells of normal tissue. During radiation treatment, injury to normal cells can produce adverse effects. Radiation effects are dose and fractionation dependent. Tissues that are most frequently affected are the skin, the mucosal lining of the gastrointestinal tract, and the bone marrow. Anorexia, nausea, emesis, and diarrhea are common, depending on the site of treatment. These usually can be controlled by medication and dietary measures. Other systemic signs include fatigue, profuse perspiration, and even chills. These effects are temporary and reversible.

Radiation also causes bone marrow depression, which subsequently affects the blood count and predisposes the individual to infection and bleeding. The first cells to decrease in number are the leukocytes, then the thrombocytes (platelets), and finally the red blood cells. Frequent blood counts are used during radiation therapy to monitor bone marrow function.

External beam radiation must first penetrate the skin; depending on the total dose and type of radiation used, reactions of the skin may develop. With moderate doses of radiation to the skin, the hair falls out spontaneously or when being combed, after the 10th to the 14th day; with larger doses, erythema develops (much like a sunburn) and may turn brown; and, at higher doses, patches of dry or moist desquamation may develop. Fortunately, epithelialization takes place after the treatments have been stopped. Mucositis, desquamation of the oral and pharyngeal mucous membranes, which sometimes may be severe, may occur as a predictable side effect in people receiving head and neck irradiation. The most severe effect is dry mouth because the parotid gland is in the treatment field.

Chemotherapy

Since the early 1960s, cancer chemotherapy has evolved as a major treatment modality. More than 30 different chemotherapeutic drugs are used alone or in various combinations. Administering higher doses of multiple drugs may be used as a strategy to achieve cure or optimal palliation; however, the adverse drug interactions and side effects can be unpredictable and intense. Chemotherapeutic drugs may be the primary form of treatment, or they may be used as adjuncts to other treatments. Chemotherapy is the primary treatment for most hematologic and some solid tumors, including choriocarcinoma, testicular cancer, acute and chronic leukemia, Burkitt's lymphoma, Hodgkin's disease, and multiple myeloma.

Cancer chemotherapeutic drugs exert their effects through several mechanisms. At the cellular level, they exert their lethal action by creating adverse conditions that prevent cell growth and replication. These mechanisms include disrupting production of essential enzymes; inhibiting DNA, RNA, and protein synthesis; and preventing cell mitosis.[6,37]

For most chemotherapy drugs, the relationship between tumor cell survival and drug dose is exponential, with the number of cells surviving being proportional to drug dose, and the number of cells at risk for exposure being proportional to the destructive action of the drug. Chemotherapeutic drugs are most effective in treating tumors that have a high growth fraction because of their ability to kill rapidly dividing cells. Exponential killing implies that a proportion or percentage of tumor cells are killed, rather than an absolute number. This proportion is a constant percentage of the total number of cells. For this reason, multiple courses of treatment are needed if the tumor is to be eradicated.[5]

The anticancer drugs may be classified as either cell cycle specific or cell cycle nonspecific. Drugs are cell cycle specific if they exert their action during a specific phase of the cell cycle. For example, methotrexate, an antimetabolite, acts by interfering with DNA synthesis and thereby interrupts the S phase of the cell cycle. Drugs that are cell cycle nonspecific affect cancer cells through all the phases of the cell cycle. The alkylating agents, which are cell cycle nonspecific, act by disrupting DNA when the cells are in the resting state and when they are dividing. The site of action of various cancer drugs varies. Chemotherapeutic drugs that have similar structures and effects on cell function usually are grouped together, and these drugs usually have similar toxic and side effects. Because they differ in their mechanisms of action, combinations of cell cycle–specific and cell cycle–nonspecific agents often are used to treat cancer.

Combination chemotherapy has been found to be more effective than treatment with a single drug. With this method, several drugs with different mechanisms of action, metabolic pathways, times of onset of action and recovery, side effects, and onset of side effects are used. Drugs used in combinations are individually effective against the tumor and synergistic with each other. The regimens for combination therapy often are referred to by acronyms. Two well-known combinations are CHOP (cyclophosphamide, doxorubicin, Oncovin [vincristine], and prednisone), used in the treatment of Hodgkin's disease, and CMF (cyclophosphamide, methotrexate, and 5-fluorouracil), used in the treatment of breast cancer. The maximum possible drug doses usually are used to ensure the maximum cell killing. Routes of administration and dosage schedules are carefully designed to ensure optimal delivery of the active forms of the drugs to a tumor during the sensitive phase of the cell cycle.

Several newer chemotherapy drugs have become available. The taxanes, derived from *Taxus* (yew) plant bark, exert their effects in the M phase to inhibit mitosis. These drugs are used primarily to treat refractory ovarian and breast cancers, and are under investigation in the treatment of other solid tumors and lung cancers.[37] Liposomal therapy, in which chemotherapy drugs are encapsulated by coated liposomes, has been found to distribute more of the chemotherapy to the desired site with fewer toxic effects than the administration of the chemotherapy alone. This therapy has been approved for use to treat AIDs-related Kaposi's sarcoma and ovarian and breast cancers.[38]

Many of these drugs are administered intravenously. Venous access devices often are used for people with poor venous access and those who require frequent or continuous intravenous therapy. It can be used for home administration of chemotherapy drugs, blood sampling, and administration of blood components. These systems use an implanted venous catheter with vascular access ports. In some cases, the drugs are administered by continuous infusion using a special ambulatory infusion pump that allows the person to remain at home and maintain his or her activities.[39]

Adverse Effects. Because cancer cells are derived from normal cells, they retain many of the properties of normal cells. Chemotherapeutic drugs affect the neoplastic cells and the rapidly proliferating cells of normal tissue. The nadir (*i.e.*, lowest point) is the point of maximal toxicity for a given adverse effect of a drug and is stated in the time it takes to reach that point. The nadir for leukopenia with thiotepa, for example, occurs at 14 days after initiation of treatment. Because many toxic effects of chemotherapeutic drugs persist for some time after the drug is discontinued, the nadir times and recovery rates are useful guides in evaluating the effects of cancer therapy.

Anorexia, nausea, and vomiting are common problems associated with cancer chemotherapy. The severity of the vomiting is related to the emetic potential of the particular drug. These symptoms can occur within minutes or hours of drug administration and are thought to be due to stimulation of the chemoreceptor trigger zone (*i.e.*, vomiting center) in the medullary lateral reticular formation. The chemoreceptor trigger zone responds to levels of chemicals circulating in the blood.[40] The symptoms usually subside within 24 to 48 hours and often can be relieved by antiemetics. Newly developed antiemetics that block the serotonin 5-HT_3 receptors, such as ondansetron and granisetron, have facilitated the use of highly emetic chemotherapy drugs by more effectively reducing the nausea and vomiting induced by these drugs.[41]

Diarrhea is another problem associated with cancer chemotherapy. Chemotherapy can cause a temporary lactose intolerance or an increase in gastric motility. Pharmacologic and dietary interventions are helpful in reducing the severity of diarrhea. For example, Lomotil and Imodium are frequently prescribed, and patients should be advised to eat low-residue, small, frequent meals; avoid spicy or greasy food; drink 2 to 3 quarts of uncarbonated beverages daily; avoid extreme temperatures in foods or beverages; and use nutritional supplements when necessary.[40]

Some drugs cause stomatitis and damage to the rapidly proliferating cells of the gastrointestinal tract mucosal lining. Most chemotherapeutic drugs suppress bone marrow function and formation of blood cells, leading to anemia, leukopenia, and thrombocytopenia. With severe granulocytopenia, there is risk for developing serious infections. Fatigue is one of the most prevalent problems experienced by patients with cancer and is estimated to occur in 96% of individuals receiving chemotherapy. The cause is multifactorial and poorly understood.[42] Hair loss results from impaired proliferation of the hair follicles and is a side effect of a number of cancer drugs; it usually is temporary, and the hair tends to regrow when treatment is stopped. The rapidly proliferating structures of the reproductive system are particularly sensitive to the action of the cancer drugs. Women may experience changes in menstrual flow or have amenorrhea. Men may have a decreased sperm count (*i.e.*, oligospermia) or absence of sperm (*i.e.*, azoospermia). Many chemotherapeutic agents also may have teratogenic or mutagenic effects leading to fetal abnormalities.

Chemotherapy drugs are toxic to all cells. The mutagenic, carcinogenic, and teratogenic potential of these drugs has been strongly supported by both animal and human studies. Because of these potential risks, special care is required when handling or administering the drugs. Drugs, drug containers, and administration equipment require special disposal as hazardous waste. Several organizations, including the Occupational Safety and Health Administration (OSHA), the Oncology Nursing Society (ONS), and American Society of Hospital Pharmacists (ASHP), have developed special guidelines for the safe handling and disposal of antineoplastic drugs as well as for accidental spills and exposure.[43,44]

Epidemiologic studies have shown an increased risk of second malignancies such as acute nonlymphocytic leukemia after long-term use of alkylating agents[45,46] and semustine[47] for treatment of various forms of cancer. These second malignancies are thought to result from direct cellular changes produced by the drug or from suppression of the immune response.

Hormone Therapy

Hormone therapy consists of administration of hormones or hormone-blocking drugs. It is used for cancers that are responsive to or dependent on hormones for growth. The actions of hormones depend on the presence of specific receptors in the tumor. Among the tumors known to be responsive to hormonal manipulations are those of the breast, prostate, adrenal gland, and uterine endometrium. Hormones commonly used for cancer treatment include estrogens (*e.g.*, diethylstilbestrol, estradiol), androgens (*e.g.*, testosterone), and progestins (*e.g.*, hydroxyprogesterone). Hormone therapy also involves use of the adrenal corticosteroid hormones such as prednisone, dexamethasone, and methylprednisone. These compounds inhibit mitosis and are cytotoxic to cells of lymphocytic origin. Hormones are cell cycle nonspecific and are thought to alter the synthesis of RNA and proteins by binding to receptor sites. The side effects of hormonal treatment are directly related to the normal action of the hormones. Because dosages of these drugs usually are higher than those that normally occur in the body, the normal actions of the hormone are accentuated.[37] Hormone-blocking drugs include the antiestrogen drugs tamoxifen and leuprolide (*i.e.*, a gonadotropin-releasing hormone analog that blocks both estrogens and androgens) and the antiadrenal drug aminoglutethimide.

Biotherapy

Biotherapy involves the use of biologic response modifiers (BRMs) that change the person's own biologic response to cancer. The BRMs are products normally produced in the body that serve as regulators and messengers of normal cellular function. Although biotherapy relies heavily on immune mechanisms, it is not limited to them. Three major mechanisms by which biotherapy exerts its effects are modification of host responses, direct destruction of cancer cells by suppressing tumor growth or killing the tumor cell, and modification of tumor cell biology.

Immunotherapy techniques include active and passive immunotherapy. Active immunotherapy involves nonspecific techniques such as bacille Calmette-Guérin (BCG) and levamisole, and specific techniques such as purified or recombinant antigens. Passive immunotherapy is divided into nonspecific techniques such as lymphokine-activated killer (LAK) cells and cytokine therapy, specific techniques such as antibody therapy, and combined techniques that include LAK cells and antibodies. Active immunotherapy focuses on stimulating immune response. BCG is an attenuated strain of the bacterium that causes bovine tuberculosis. BCG acts as a nonspecific stimulant of the immune system. A second method involves the use of vaccines made from the patient's own tumor (autologous) or from pooled tumor-associated antigens (allogeneic) that have been obtained from a number of tumors. Active immunotherapy has been studied as treatment for melanoma, renal cell carcinoma, and leukemia.[27]

Adoptive immunotherapy is a technique that uses lymphokine-activated NK cells or tumor-specific T-cell immunity as a means of eradicating cancer cells. Originally, only LAK cells were used. These NK cells are grown in culture supported by IL-2. Because NK cells are nonspecific in their function, LAK cells attack both normal and tumor cells. The technique of adoptive therapy has been expanded to the production of tumor-specific T cells. These cells are derived from a person's own *tumor-infiltrating lymphocytes* (TILs) that have been expanded in the laboratory so that a large amount of cells are available for reinfusion. Because the TILs are tumor specific, they do not attack normal host cells.

Four types of biologic response modifiers are being used or investigated: interferon therapy, interleukin therapy, monoclonal antibodies, and hematopoietic growth factors. Some agents, such as the interferons, have more than one biologic action, including antiviral, immunomodulatory, and antiproliferative actions. The *interferons* are endogenous polypeptides that are synthesized by a number of cells in response to a variety of cellular or viral stimuli. The three major types of interferons are alpha (α), beta (β) and gamma (γ), each group differing in terms of their cell surface receptors. The exact physiologic roles of each of the interferons remain unclear. They appear to inhibit viral replication and also may be involved in inhibiting tumor protein synthesis and in prolonging the cell cycle and increasing the percentage of cells in the G_0 phase. Interferons stimulate NK cells and T-lymphocyte killer cells. Interferon-γ has been approved for the treatment of hairy cell leukemia, AIDS-related Kaposi's sarcoma, chronic myelogenous leukemia, and condylomata acuminata (*i.e.*, genital warts), and as adjuvant therapy for patients at high risk for recurrent melanoma.[48] Its use with other cancers, including renal cell carcinoma, colorectal cancer, cutaneous T-cell lymphoma, and multiple myeloma, is being investigated. Research is focusing on combining interferons with other forms of cancer therapy and establishing optimal doses and treatment protocols.

There are 17 identified *interleukins*, and only one, IL-2, has been approved by the U.S. Food and Drug Administration (FDA) for the treatment of metastatic renal cell carcinoma. IL-1, IL-3, IL-4, IL-6, IL-11, and IL-12 are currently under investigation in clinical trials. IL-2 has been found to reduce tumor size in a minority of patients with metastatic renal cancer and melanoma.[49]

Monoclonal antibodies (MoAbs) are highly specific antibodies derived from cloned cells or hybridomas. Scientists were able to produce large quantities of these MoAbs that were specific for tumor cells. Several MoAbs have been approved: muromonab-CD3 (OKT-3), which targets the CD3 receptor of human T cells, for the treatment of acute allograft rejection in renal transplant recipients; satumomab pendetide, used in the detection of colorectal and ovarian cancers[50]; and rituximab, an anti-CD20 MoAb used in the treatment of B-cell malignant lymphomas.[51]

Hematopoietic growth factors are growth and maturation factors that include the colony-stimulating factors (CSFs). The CSFs are factors that control the production of neutrophils and monocytes/macrophages, erythropoietin, and thrombopoietin.[52]

Bone Marrow and Peripheral Blood Stem Cell Transplantation

Bone marrow transplantation (BMT) and peripheral blood stem cell transplantation (PBSCT) are two treatment approaches for individuals with inherited disorders, immunodeficiencies, leukemias, certain solid tumors, and other cancers previously thought to be incurable. BMT techniques include *allogeneic BMT*, in which the recipient receives the bone marrow from another person who is human leukocyte antigen (HLA) matched, *syngeneic BMT*, in which the donor is an identical twin, and *autologous BMT*, in which the recipient's bone marrow is harvested and reinfused after treatment.

The first allogeneic BMT was successfully performed in 1968 to treat advanced leukemia. Since then, advances in BMT, such as supportive measures including platelet administration, graft-versus-host disease pretreatment and prophylaxis, and hematopoietic growth factors, have increased survival for a number of patients. Allogeneic transplantation is used primarily to treat all types of leukemia, but has been used in a limited fashion to treat multiple myeloma. Autologous BMT is considered when an HLA-matched donor is not available. Auto-BMTs are used for certain hematologic malignancies such as Hodgkin's and non-Hodgkin's lymphomas, and for some solid tumors such as neuroblastoma and testicular cancer. The primary goal of auto-BMT is to administer high-dose chemotherapy to achieve the maximum tumoricidal effect while providing a hematologic rescue to decrease the potentially fatal hematologic side effects.[53]

PBSCT, an alternative to BMT, uses the patient's peripheral blood stem cells to repopulate the bone marrow after extensive high-dose chemotherapy. It is a treatment option when there may be bone marrow abnormalities such as

metastases or hypocellularity. PBSCT has been found to be more advantageous than BMT for a number of reasons. Stem cells can be harvested by apheresis techniques, which are less invasive and do not require general anesthesia. PBSCT is an outpatient procedure that is easier and safer for the patient and approximately half the cost of BMT. The period of aplasia after high-dose chemotherapy is shorter, thereby reducing the risks associated with granulocytopenia, the number of transfusions the patients require, and the intensive supportive care needed during BMT. Despite the apparent advantages this technique has to offer, some disadvantages exist. Fewer pluripotent stem cells are contained in the peripheral blood; therefore, multiple leukapheresis sessions are necessary to harvest sufficient numbers of stem cells. There also may be the risk of infusing malignant cells, although this risk is less than with auto-BMT. Although there is uncertainty surrounding the number and types of cells harvested during the leukapheresis procedures and the most ideal time during the course of the disease to perform PBSCT, it represents an exciting alternative to BMT. Research is being undertaken to investigate the efficacy of PBSCT in fetal therapy, sequential PBSCTs in patients with residual disease, treatments involving combinations of PBSCT and auto-BMT, and the use of growth factors for cell mobilization to improve the quantity of cells harvested at one pheresis session.[54]

A new transplantation modality, termed *nonmyeloablative stem cell transplantation*, uses less intensive conditioning chemotherapy and the adoptive transfer of alloreactive donor lymphocytes. The less intensive chemotherapy provides sufficient immunosuppression to facilitate engraftment of the allogeneic cells. The administration of donor lymphocytes induces a graft-versus-tumor effect in which the donor lymphocytes identify and destroy the patient's remaining tumor cells. The goal of nonmyeloablative stem cell transplantation is to reduce procedure-related morbidity and mortality rates and improve the patient's long-term clinical outcomes.[55]

Gene Therapy

Gene therapy, a rapidly evolving treatment modality, is defined as the alteration of an individual's genetic material to fight or prevent disease.[56] The process by which one or more genes are inserted into a cell's genome is termed *gene transfer*. There are two major applications of gene transfer. Gene therapy involves inserting genes into the patient's genome, a technique called *somatic cell gene therapy*, to correct an error or manipulate a particular cell's biologic behavior. Gene therapy is based on Boveri's somatic mutation theory of cancer development, which proposes that malignancies result from an imbalance in the normal chromosome structure that is essential for normal growth and development. Germ-line gene therapy, which has not been approved by the FDA and the National Institutes of Health, attempts to manipulate genetically the ova and sperm to pass genetic changes to future generations.[57] *Gene marking* is the process whereby labeled genes are inserted into cells for future identification. This process will facilitate the determination of sources of relapse after auto-BMT.

Genes are transferred by chemical or physical techniques, including calcium phosphate coprecipitation, microinjection, receptor-mediated DNA transfer, and liposomal membrane fusion; or by retroviral vectors in which human genes are inserted into the genome of the virus, the virus attaches to the target cells and empties its genetic material into the cell, and, by reverse transcriptase, the new gene is inserted into the DNA of the patient's cell. Another approach involves the delivery of genes to cancer cells that destroy them or return them to normal functioning. This method involves transferring molecules into the cancer cell that increase its sensitivity to cytotoxic drugs, inserting tumor suppressor genes that stop the cancer cell's uncontrolled proliferation, and using antisense oligonucleotides and ribozymes that interfere with the transcription and translation of oncogenes.[58]

Current uses of gene therapy to correct a genetic error include the insertion of the adenosine deaminase (ADA) gene in children with severe combined immunodeficiency disease, who lack this gene, and the insertion of K-ras and p53 genes into lung cancer cells. Several techniques have been used to add a new function to cells, one of which involves inserting the multidrug resistance-1 (MDR-1) gene into bone marrow stem cells in an attempt to increase their resistance to chemotherapy. Other cancers in which gene therapy is being investigated include malignant melanoma, brain tumors such as glioblastoma and neuroblastoma, acute and chronic myelogenous leukemia, and breast cancer.[59]

In summary, the methods used in the diagnosis of cancer vary with the type of cancer and its location. Because many cancers are curable if diagnosed early, health care practices designed to promote early detection are important. These practices include breast self-examination in the female, testicular self-examination in the male, and consulting a physician when any of the early warning signals of cancer are present. Pap smears and tissue biopsies are used to detect the presence of cancer cells and in diagnosis. There are two basic methods of classifying tumors: (1) grading according to the histologic or tissue characteristics, and (2) clinical staging according to spread of the disease. Histologic studies are done in the laboratory using cells or tissue specimens. The TNM system for clinical staging of cancer uses tumor size, lymph node involvement, and presence of metastasis.

Treatment plans that use more than one type of therapy, often in combination, are providing cures for a number of cancers that a few decades ago had a poor prognosis, and are increasing the life expectancy in other types of cancer. Surgical procedures are more precise as a result of improved diagnostic equipment and new techniques such as laser surgery. Radiation equipment and radioactive sources permit greater and more controlled destruction of cancer cells while causing less damage to normal tissues. Successes with immunotherapy techniques offer hope that the body's own defenses can be used in fighting cancer. BMT and PBSCT

allow for a greater tumoricidal effect while replenishing the pluripotent stem cells. Gene therapy, although investigational, may provide a foundation for the development of more effective treatments in the future.

Childhood Cancers

After you have completed this section of the chapter, you should be able to meet the following objectives:

✦ Cite the early warning signs of cancer in children
✦ Discuss possible concerns of adult survivors of childhood cancer

In the United States, cancer is the second leading cause of death in children 1 to 14 years of age.[1] Between 1974 and 1991, children younger than 14 years of age exhibited a 1% average yearly increase in the incidence of all malignant neoplasms, with a 1.6% average increase in the incidence of acute lymphocytic leukemia and a greater than 2% increase for astroglial tumors, rhabdomyosarcomas, germ cell tumors, and osteosarcomas.[60] The spectrum of cancers that affect children differs markedly from those that affect adults. Although most adult cancers are of epithelial cell origin (*e.g.*, lung cancer, breast cancer, colorectal cancers), childhood cancers usually involve the hematopoietic system, nervous system, or connective tissue. Chart 8-3 lists the most common forms of solid childhood cancers.

As with adult cancers, there probably is no one cause of childhood cancer. However, many forms of childhood cancer repeat in families and may result from polygenic or single-gene inheritance, chromosomal aberrations (*e.g.*, translocations, deletions, insertions, inversions, duplications), exposure to mutagenic environmental agents, or a combination of these factors (see Chapter 7). If cancer develops in one child, the risk of cancer in siblings is approximately twice that of the general population, and if the disease develops in two children, the risk is even greater.

Heritable forms of cancer tend to have an earlier age of onset, a higher frequency of multifocal lesions in a single organ, and bilateral involvement of paired organs or multiple primary tumors. The two-hit hypothesis has been used as one explanation of heritable cancers.[3] The first "hit" or

---

CHART 8-3

Common Solid Tumors of Childhood

Brain and nervous system tumors
　Medulloblastoma
　Glioma
Neuroblastoma
Wilms' tumor
Rhabdomyosarcoma and embryonal sarcoma
Retinoblastoma
Osteosarcoma
Ewing's sarcoma

mutation occurs prezygotically (*i.e.*, in germ cells before conception) and is present in the genetic material of all somatic cells. Cancer subsequently develops in one or several somatic cell lines that undergo a second mutation.

Children with heritable disorders are at increased risk for developing certain forms of cancer. For example, Down syndrome is associated with increased risk of leukemia; primary immunodeficiency disorders (see Chapter 19) are associated with lymphoma, leukemia, and brain cancer; and xeroderma pigmentosum is associated with basal and squamous cell carcinoma and melanoma.

DIAGNOSIS AND TREATMENT

The early diagnosis of childhood cancers often is overlooked because the signs and symptoms often are similar to those of common childhood diseases and because cancer occurs less frequently in children than in adults.[61] Symptoms of prolonged fever, unexplained weight loss, and growing masses (especially in association with weight loss) should be viewed as warning signs of cancer in children. Diagnosis of childhood cancers involves many of the same methods that are used in adults. Accurate disease staging is especially beneficial in childhood cancers, in which the potential benefits of treatment must be carefully weighed against potential long-term effects.

The treatment of childhood cancers is complex, intensive, prolonged, and continuously evolving. Improved therapy and supportive care have led to progressive increases in survival. For children younger than 15 years of age, the 5-year survival rate between 1989 and 1995 for all cancer sites was 75%; for acute lymphocytic leukemia, 81%; for acute myeloid leukemia, 43%; for bone cancer, 67%; for neuroblastoma, 71%; for brain and central nervous system, 64%; for Wilms' tumor, 93%; for Hodgkin's disease, 93%; and for non-Hodgkin's lymphoma, 77%.[1]

ADULT SURVIVORS OF CHILDHOOD CANCER

With improvement in treatment methods, the number of children who survive childhood cancer is continuing to increase.[62] Unfortunately, therapy may produce late sequelae, such as impaired growth, neurologic dysfunction, hormonal dysfunction, cardiomyopathy, pulmonary fibrosis, and risk of second malignancies. Although cures for large numbers of children have been possible only since the 1970s, much already is known about the potential for delayed effects.

Children reaching adulthood after cancer therapy may have reduced physical stature because of the therapy they received, particularly radiation, which retards the growth of normal tissues along with cancer tissue. The younger the age and the higher the radiation dose, the greater the deviation from normal growth. There also is concern that central nervous system radiation as a prophylactic measure in childhood leukemia has an effect on cognition and learning. Children younger than 6 years of age at the time of radiation and those receiving the highest radiation doses are most likely to have subsequent cognitive difficulties.

Delayed sexual maturation in both boys and girls can result from irradiation of the gonads. Delayed sexual maturation also is related to treatment of children with alkylating agents. Cranial irradiation may result in premature menarche in girls, with subsequent early closure of the epiphysis and a reduction in final growth achieved. Data related to fertility and health of the offspring of childhood cancer survivors are just becoming available.

Vital organs such as the heart and lungs may be affected by cancer treatment. Children who received anthracyclines (*i.e.*, doxorubicin or daunorubicin) may be at risk for developing cardiomyopathy and congestive heart failure. Pulmonary irradiation may cause lung dysfunction and restrictive lung disease. Drugs such as bleomycin, methotrexate, and bisulfan also can cause lung disease.

For survivors of childhood cancers, the risk of second cancers is reported to range from 3% to 12%. There is a special risk of second cancers in children with the retinoblastoma gene. Because of this risk, children who have been treated for cancer should be followed routinely.

In summary, although most adult cancers are of epithelial cell origin, most childhood cancers usually involve the hematopoietic system, nervous system, or connective tissue. Heritable forms of cancer tend to have an earlier age of onset, a higher frequency of multifocal lesions in a single organ, and bilateral involvement of paired organs or multiple primary tumors. The early diagnosis of childhood cancers often is overlooked because the signs and symptoms often are similar to those of other childhood diseases. With improvement in treatment methods, the number of children who survive childhood cancer is continuing to increase. As these children approach adulthood, there is continued concern that the life-saving therapy they received during childhood may produce late sequelae, such as impaired growth, neurologic dysfunction, hormonal dysfunction, cardiomyopathy, pulmonary fibrosis, and risk of second malignancies.

Related Web Sites

American Bone Marrow Donor Registry   www.abmdr.org
American Cancer Society   www.cancer.org
American Prostate Society   www.ameripros.org
American Society of Clinical Oncology   www.asco.org
American Society for Therapeutic Radiology and Oncology
      www.astro.org
CA: A Cancer Journal for Clinicians   www.ca-journal.org
National Cancer Institute   www.nci.nih.gov
National Coalition for Cancer Survivorship   www.cansearch.org
National Society of Genetic Counselors   www.nsgc.org
Oncology Nursing Society   www.ons.org

References

1. Greenlee R.T., Murray T., Bolden S., Wingo P.A. (2000). Cancer statistics, 2000. *CA: A Cancer Journal for Clinicians* 50, 7–33.

2. Li, F.P. (1996). Hereditary cancer susceptibility. *Cancer 78*, 553–557.

3. Cotran R.S., Kumar V., Collins T. (1999). Neoplasia. In *Robbins pathologic basis of disease* (6th ed., pp. 90–91, 260–327). Philadelphia: W.B. Saunders.

4. Lee W.M.F., Dang C.V. (2000). Control of cell growth and differentiation. In Hoffman R., Benz E.K., Shattil S.J., Furie B., Cohen H.J., Silberstein L.E., McGlave P. (Eds.), *Hematology: Basic principles and practice* (3rd ed., pp. 57–71). New York: Churchill Livingstone.

5. Buick, R.N. (1994). Cellular basis of chemotherapy. In Dorr R.T., Von Hoff D.D. (Eds.), *Cancer chemotherapy handbook* (pp. 3–14). Norwalk, CT: Appleton & Lange.

6. Ruddon, R.W. (Ed.). (1995). *Cancer biology* (pp. 3–60, 141–276). New York and Oxford: Oxford University Press.

7. Fidler I.J. (1997). Molecular biology of cancer: Invasion and metastasis. In DeVita V.T. Jr., Hellman S., Rosenberg S.A. (Eds.), *Cancer: Principles and practice of oncology* (5th ed., pp. 135–148). Philadelphia: Lippincott-Raven.

8. Roitt I., Brostoff J., Male D. (1996). Cell cooperation in the antibody response. In *Immunology* (4th ed., pp. 8.8–8.11). London: Mosby.

9. Liotta L.A. (1992). Cancer cell invasion and metastasis. *Scientific American 266* (2), 54–63.

10. Beutler B. (1993). Cytokines and cancer cachexia. *Hospital Practice 28*(4), 45–52.

11. Oppenheim J.J., Ruscetti F.W. (1997). Cytokines. In Stites D.P., Terr A.I., Parslow T.G. (Eds.), *Medical immunology* (9th ed., pp. 147–168). Stamford, CT: Appleton & Lange.

12. Caudell K.A., Cuaron L.J., Gallucci, B.B. (1996). Cancer biology: Molecular and cellular aspects. In McCorkle R., Grant M., Frank-Stromborg M., Baird S.B. (Eds.), *Cancer nursing: A comprehensive textbook* (2nd ed., pp. 150–170), Philadelphia: W.B. Saunders.

13. Levine, A.J. (1996). Tumor suppressor genes. In Pusztai L., Lewis C.E., Yap E. (Eds.), *Cell proliferation in cancer: Regulatory mechanisms of neoplastic cell growth* (pp. 86–104), Oxford: Oxford University Press.

14. Pennisi E. (1996). New gene forges link between fragile site and many cancers. *Science 272*, 649.

15. Pusztai L., Cooper K. (1996). Introduction: Cell proliferation and carcinogenesis. In Pusztai L., Lewis C.E., Yap E. (Eds.), *Cell proliferation in cancer: Regulatory mechanisms of neoplastic cell growth* (pp. 3–24), Oxford: Oxford University Press.

16. Knudson, A.G. (1974). Heredity and human cancer. *American Journal of Pathology 77*, 77–84.

17. Rubin E., Farber J.L. (1999). *Pathology* (3rd ed., pp. 155–212, 434). Philadelphia: Lippincott Williams & Wilkins.

18. Stellman J.M., Stellman S.D. (1996). Cancer and the workplace. *CA: A Cancer Journal for Clinicians 46*, 70–92.

19. Frank-Stromborg M., Heusinkveld K.B., Rohan K. (1996). Evaluating cancer risks and preventive oncology. In McCorkle R., Grant M., Frank-Stromborg M., Baird S.B. (Eds.), *Cancer nursing: A comprehensive textbook* (2nd ed., pp. 213–264). Philadelphia: W.B. Saunders.

20. Bartecchi C.E., MacKenzie T.D., Schrier R. (1994). The human costs of tobacco use. *New England Journal of Medicine 330*, 907–912.

21. McMillan S. (1992). Carcinogenesis. *Seminars in Oncology Nursing 8*, 10–19.

22. Poskanzer D.C., Herbst A. (1977). Epidemiology of vaginal adenosis and adenocarcinoma associated with exposure to stilbestrol in utero. *Cancer 39*, 1892–1895.

23. Jablon S., Kato H. (1972). Studies of the mortality of A-bomb survivors: 5. Radiation dose and mortality, 1950–1970. *Radiation Research 50*, 649–698.

24. Marks R. (1996). Prevention and control of melanoma: The public health approach. *CA: A Cancer Journal for Clinicians 46*, 199–216.

25. Howley P.M. (1996). Viral carcinogenesis. In Pusztai L., Lewis C.E., Yap E. (Eds.), *Cell proliferation in cancer: Regulatory mechanisms of neoplastic cell growth* (pp. 38–58). Oxford: Oxford University Press.

26. Burnett F.M. (1967). Immunologic aspects of malignant disease. *Lancet 1*, 1171.

27. Beverley P. (1996). Tumor Immunology. In Roitt I., Brostoff J., Male D. (Eds.), *Immunology* (4th ed., pp. 20.1–20.8), London: Mosby.

28. Greenberg P.D. (1997). Mechanisms of tumor immunology. In Stites D.P., Terr A.I., Parslow T.G. (Eds.), *Medical immunology* (9th ed., pp. 631–639). Stamford, CT: Appleton & Lange.

29. American Cancer Society. (1993). *American Cancer Society facts and figures: 1993*. Atlanta, GA: Author.

30. Weintraub F.N., Neumark, D.E. (1996). Surgical oncology. In McCorkle R., Grant M., Frank-Stromborg M., Baird S.B. (Eds.), *Cancer nursing: A comprehensive textbook* (2nd ed., pp. 315–330), Philadelphia: W.B. Saunders.

31. Collins M.C. (1990). Tumor markers and screening tools in cancer detection. *Nursing Clinics of North America 25*, 283–290.

32. Ghossein R.A., Rosai J. (1996). Polymerase chain reaction in the detection of micrometastases and circulating tumor cells. *Cancer 78*, 10–16.

33. American Joint Committee on Cancer. (1997). *AJCC cancer staging manual/American Joint Committee on Cancer* (5th ed). Philadelphia: Lippincott-Raven.

34. Daly J.M., Wanebo J., DeCosse J.J. (1993). Principles of surgical oncology. In Calabresi P., Schein P.S. (Eds.), *Medical oncology: Basic principles and clinical management of cancer*. (2nd ed.). Philadelphia: W.B. Saunders.

35. Hilderley L.J., Dow K.H. (1996). Radiation oncology. In McCorkle R., Grant M., Frank-Stromborg M., Baird S.B. (Eds.), *Cancer nursing: A comprehensive textbook* (2nd ed., pp. 331–358). Philadelphia: W.B. Saunders.

36. Hall E.J., Cox J.D. (1994). Physical and biologic basis of radiation therapy. In Cox J.D. (Ed.), *Moss' radiation oncology: Rationale, technique, results* (7th ed., pp. 3–66), St. Louis: Mosby.

37. Guy J.L., Ingram B.A. (1996). Medical oncology: The agents. In McCorkle R., Grant M., Frank-Stromborg M., Baird S.B. (Eds.), *Cancer nursing: A comprehensive textbook* (2nd ed., pp. 359–394), Philadelphia: W.B. Saunders.

38. Bogner J.R., Kronawitter U., Rolinski B., Goebel F.D., Gillitzer R., Hofschneider P.H. (1994). Liposomal doxorubicin in the treatment of advanced AIDs-related Kaposi's sarcoma. *Journal of Acquired Immune Deficiency Syndrome 7*, 463–468.

39. Martin V.R., Walker R.E., Goodman M. (1996). Delivery of cancer chemotherapy. In McCorkle R., Grant M., Frank-Stromborg M., Baird S.B. (Eds.), *Cancer nursing: A comprehensive textbook* (2nd ed., pp. 395–433), Philadelphia: W.B. Saunders.

40. Grant M., Ropka M.E. (1996). Alterations in nutrition. In McCorkle R., Grant M., Frank-Stromborg M., Baird S.B. (Eds.), *Cancer nursing: A comprehensive textbook* (2nd ed., pp. 919–943), Philadelphia: W.B. Saunders.

41. Krakoff I.H. (1996). Systemic treatment of cancer. *CA: A Cancer Journal for Clinicians 46*, 134–141.

42. Irvine D., Vincent L., Graydon J., Bubela N., Thompson L. (1994). The prevalence and correlates of fatigue in patients

receiving treatment with chemotherapy and radiotherapy. *Cancer Nursing* 17, 367–378.

43. U.S. Department of Labor, Office of Occupational Medicine, Occupational Safety and Health Administration (OSHA). (1986). *Work practice guidelines for personnel dealing with cytotoxic (antineoplastic) drugs*. Publication no. 8-1.1. Washington, DC: Author.

44. Oncology Nursing Society. (1988). *Cancer chemotherapy guideline: Module I, II, III, IV*. Pittsburgh: Oncology Nursing Press.

45. Pederson-Bjergaard J., Larson S.O. (1982). Incidence of acute nonlymphocytic leukemia, preleukemia and acute myeloproliferative syndrome up to 10 years after treatment of Hodgkin's disease. *New England Journal of Medicine* 307, 964–971.

46. Coltman C.A., Jr., Dixon D.O. (1982). Second malignancies complicating Hodgkin's disease: A Southwest Oncology Group 10 year followup. *Cancer Treatment Reports* 66, 1023–1033.

47. Boise J.D., Greene M.H., Killen J.Y., et al. (1983). Leukemia and preleukemia after adjuvant treatment of gastrointestinal cancer with semustine. *New England Journal of Medicine* 309, 1079–1084.

48. Skalla, K. (1996). The interferons. *Seminars in Oncology Nursing* 12, 97–105.

49. Royal R.E., Steinberg S.M., Krause P.S., Heywood G., White D.E., Hwu P., et al. (1996). Correlates of response to IL-2 therapy in patients treated for metastatic renal cancer and melanoma. *The Cancer Journal* 2 (2), 91–98.

50. Farrell M.M. (1996). Biotherapy and the oncology nurse. *Seminars in Oncology Nursing* 12, 82–88.

51. McLaughlin P., Grillo-Lopez A.J., Link B.K., Levy R., Czuczman M.S., Williams M.E., et al. (1998). Rituximab chimeric anti-CD20 monoclonal antibody therapy for relapsed indolent lymphoma: Half of patients respond to a four-dose treatment program. *Journal of Clinical Oncology* 16, 2825–2833.

52. Bagby G.C., Heinrich M.C. (1999). Cytokines, growth factors and hematopoiesis. In Wingard J.R., Demetri G.D. (Eds.), *Clinical applications of cytokines and growth factors* (pp. 2–55). Norwell, MA: Kluwer Academic Publishers.

53. Whedon M.B. (1995). Bone marrow transplantation nursing: Into the twenty-first century. In Buchsel P.C., Whedon M.B. (Eds.), *Bone marrow transplantation: Administrative and clinical strategies* (pp. 1–18). Boston: Jones and Bartlett.

54. Kessinger A. (2000). Reestablishing hematopoiesis with peripheral stem cells. In Armitage J.O., Antman K.H. (Eds.), *High-dose cancer therapy: Pharmacology, hematopoietins, stem cells* (3rd ed., pp. 273–282). Philadelphia: Lippincott Williams & Wilkins.

55. Carella A.M., Champlin R., Slavin S., McSweeney P., Storb R. (2000). Mini-allografts: ongoing trials in humans. *Bone Marrow Transplantation* 25, 345–350.

56. National Cancer Institute. (1993). *Questions and answers about gene therapy. Cancer facts*. Washington, DC: National Cancer Institute.

57. Robinson K.D., Abernathy E., Conrad K.J. (1996). Gene therapy of cancer. *Seminars in Oncology Nursing* 12, 142–151.

58. Bank A. (2000). Gene therapy. In Armitage J.O., Antman K.H. (Eds.), *High-dose cancer therapy: Pharmacology, hematopoietins, stem cells* (3rd ed., pp. 167–181). Philadelphia: Lippincott Williams & Wilkins.

59. Wheeler V.S. (1995). Gene therapy: Current strategies and future applications. *Oncology Nursing Forum* 22 (2 Suppl.), 20–26.

60. Gurney J.G., Davis S., Severson P.K., Fang J.Y., Risse A., Robinson L.L. (1996). Trends in cancer incidence among children in the U.S. *Cancer* 78, 532–541.

61. Crist W.M. (2000). Neoplastic diseases and tumors. In Behrman R.E., Kliegman R.M., Jensen H.B. (Eds.), *Nelson textbook of pediatrics* (16th ed., pp. 1531–1543). Philadelphia: W.B. Saunders.

62. Ward J.D. (2001). Pediatric cancer survivors. *Nurse Practitioner* 26 (12), 18–37.

Integrative Body Functions

French physiologist Claude Bernard (1813–1878) was the first to theorize that, in a closely orchestrated process, the body strives to achieve and maintain a steady state. In the middle of the 19th century, Bernard proposed his concept of the *milieu intèrieur*, or the stable internal environment, regulated by a multitude of interacting control mechanisms geared to maintain the body's chemical and physical status. He proposed that internal secretions functioned as a part of the body's regulatory mechanism, maintaining a balance in response to a range of changing conditions imposed by the external environment.

Through his experiments, Bernard discovered a number of mechanisms that were dedicated to maintaining homeostasis. One of his discoveries was the process by which internal temperature is kept constant. He was able to show that the nervous system responds to internal cold by sending chemical messages to the blood vessels to constrict in order to conserve body heat. The product of his considerable work is the classic *Introduction to the Study of Experimental Medicine (1865)*.

Stress and Adaptation

Mary Pat Kunert

Stress has become an increasingly discussed topic in today's world. The concept is discussed extensively in the health care fields, and it is found as well in economics, political science, business, and education. At the level of the popular press, the term is exploited with messages about how stress can be prevented, managed, and even eliminated.

Whether stress is more prevalent today than it was in centuries past is uncertain. Certainly, the pressures that existed were equally challenging, although of a different type. Social psychologists Richard Lazarus and Susan Folkman related that as early as the 14th century the term was used to indicate hardship, straits, adversity, or affliction.[1] In the 17th century, *stress* and related terms appeared in the context of physical sciences: *load* was defined as an external force, *stress* as the ratio of internal force created by the load to the area over which the force acted, and *strain* was the deformation or distortion of the object.[1] These concepts are still used in engineering today.

The concepts of stress and strain survived, and throughout the 19th and early 20th centuries, stress and strain were thought to be the cause of "ill health" and "mental disease."[2] By the 20th century, stress had drawn considerable attention both as a health concern and as a research focus. In 1910, when Sir William Osler delivered his Lumleian Lectures on "Angina Pectoris," he described the relationship of stress and strain to angina pectoris.[3] Approximately 15 years later, Walter Cannon, well known for his work in

physiology, began to use the word *stress* in relation to his laboratory experiments on the "fight-or-flight" response. It seems possible that the term emerged from his work with the homeostatic features of living organisms and their tendency to "bound back" and "resist disruption" when acted on by an "external force."[4] At about the same time, Hans Selye, who became known for his research and publications on stress, began using the term *stress* in a very special way to mean an orchestrated set of bodily responses to any form of noxious stimulus.[5]

During the past 60 to 70 years, thousands of studies have sought to explain Selye's theory and the stress response. A major portion of stress research has been conducted in the sciences of nursing and medicine because of the hypothesized relationship between stress and disease.

The content in this chapter has been organized into three sections: homeostasis, the stress response and adaptation to stress, and acute and chronic effects of stress.

Homeostasis

After you have completed this section of the chapter, you should be able to meet the following objectives:

✦ Cite Cannon's four features of homeostasis
✦ Describe the components of a control system, including the function of a negative feedback system

CONSTANCY OF THE INTERNAL ENVIRONMENT

The environment in which body cells live is not the external environment that surrounds the organism, but rather the local fluid environment that surrounds each cell. Claude Bernard, a 19th century physiologist, was the first to describe clearly the central importance of a stable internal environment, which he termed the *milieu intèrieur*. Bernard recognized that body fluids surrounding the cells and the various organ systems provide the means for exchange between the external and the internal environments. It is from this internal environment that body cells receive their nourishment, and it is into this fluid that they secrete their wastes. Even the contents of the gastrointestinal tract and lungs do not become part of the internal environment until they have been absorbed into the extracellular fluid. A multicellular organism is able to survive only as long as the composition of the internal environment is compatible with the survival needs of the individual cells. For example, even a small change in the pH of the body fluids can disrupt the metabolic processes of individual cells.

The concept of a stable internal environment was supported by Walter B. Cannon. He proposed that this kind of stability, which he called *homeostasis*, was achieved through a system of carefully coordinated physiologic processes that oppose change.[6] Cannon pointed out that these processes were largely automatic and emphasized that homeostasis involves resistance to both internal and external disturbances.

In his book *Wisdom of the Body*, published in 1939, Cannon presented four tentative propositions to describe the general features of homeostasis.[6] With this set of propositions, Cannon emphasized that when a factor is known to shift homeostasis in one direction, it is reasonable to expect the existence of mechanisms that have the opposite effect. In the homeostatic regulation of blood sugar, for example, mechanisms that both raise and lower blood sugar would be expected to play a part. As long as the responding mechanism to the initiating disturbance can recover homeostasis, the integrity of the body and the status of normality are retained.

Homeostasis

➤ Homeostasis is the purposeful maintenance of a stable internal environment maintained by coordinated physiologic processes that oppose change.

➤ The physiologic control systems that oppose change operate by negative feedback mechanisms that are composed of a sensor that detects a change, an integrator/comparator that sums and compares incoming data with a set point, and an effector system that returns the sensed function to within the range of the set point.

Constancy of the Internal Environment

1. Constancy in an open system, such as our bodies represent, requires mechanisms that act to maintain this constancy. Cannon based this proposition on insights into the ways by which steady states such as glucose concentrations, body temperature, and acid-base balance were regulated.
2. Steady-state conditions require that any tendency toward change automatically meet with factors that resist change. An increase in blood sugar results in thirst as the body attempts to dilute the concentration of sugar in the extracellular fluid.
3. The regulating system that determines the homeostatic state consists of a number of cooperating mechanisms acting simultaneously or successively. Blood sugar is regulated by insulin, glucagon, and other hormones that control its release from the liver or its uptake by the tissues.
4. Homeostasis does not occur by chance, but is the result of organized self-government.

(Cannon W.B. [1932]. *The wisdom of the body* (pp. 299–300). New York: W.W. Norton)

CONTROL SYSTEMS

The ability of the body to function and maintain homeostasis under conditions of change in the internal and external environment depends on the thousands of physiologic *control systems* that regulate body function. A homeostatic control system is a collection of interconnected components that function to keep a physical or chemical parameter of the body relatively constant. The body's control systems regulate cellular function, control life processes, and integrate functions of the different organ systems.

Of recent interest have been the neuroendocrine control systems that influence behavior. Biochemical messengers that exist in our brain control nerve activity, information flow, and, ultimately, behavior.[7] These control systems function in producing the emotional reactions to stressors. In persons with mental health disorders, they can interact in the production of symptoms associated with the disorder. The field of neuropharmacology has focused on the modulation of the endogenous messengers and signaling systems that control behavior in the treatment of mental disorders such as anxiety disorders, depression, and schizophrenia.

Feedback Systems

Most control systems in the body operate by *negative feedback mechanisms*, which function in a manner similar to the thermostat on a heating system. When the monitored function or value decreases below the set point of the system, the feedback mechanism causes the function or value to increase; and when the function or value is increased above the set point, the feedback mechanism causes it to

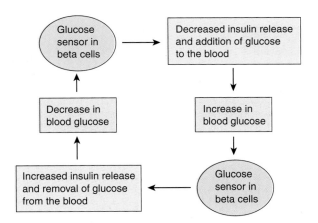

FIGURE 9-1 Illustration of negative feedback control mechanisms using blood glucose as an example.

decrease (Fig. 9-1). For example, in the negative feedback mechanism that controls blood glucose levels, an increase in blood glucose stimulates an increase in insulin, which enhances the removal of glucose from the blood. When sufficient glucose has left the bloodstream to cause blood glucose levels to fall, insulin secretion is inhibited and glucagon and other counterregulatory mechanisms stimulate the release of glucose from the liver, which causes the blood glucose to return to normal.

The reason most physiologic control systems function under negative rather than *positive feedback mechanisms* is that a positive feedback mechanism interjects instability rather than stability into a system. It produces a cycle in which the initiating stimulus produces more of the same. For example, in a positive feedback system, exposure to an increase in environmental temperature would invoke compensatory mechanisms designed to increase rather than decrease body temperature.

> In summary, physiologic and psychological adaptation involves the ability to maintain the constancy of the internal environment (homeostasis) and behavior in the face of a wide range of changes in the internal and external environments. It involves negative feedback control systems that regulate cellular function, control life's processes, regulate behavior, and integrate the function of the different body systems.

Stress

After you have completed this section of the chapter, you should be able to meet the following objectives:

- State Selye's definition of stress
- Define *stressor*
- Cite two factors that influence the nature of the stress response
- Explain the interactions among components of the nervous system in mediating the stress response

- Describe the stress responses of the autonomic nervous system, the endocrine system, the immune system, and the musculoskeletal system
- Explain the purpose of adaptation
- List at least six factors that influence a person's adaptive capacity
- Relate experience and previous learning to the process of adaptation
- Contrast anatomic and physiologic reserve
- Propose a way by which social support may serve to buffer challenges to adaptation

The increased focus on health promotion has heightened interest in the roles of stress and biobehavioral stress responses in the development of disease.[8] Stress may contribute directly to the production or exacerbation of a disease, or it may contribute to the development of behaviors such as smoking, overeating, and drug abuse that increase the risk of disease. Some of the many diseases that are being studied with this relationship in mind include depression, chronic fatigue syndrome, irritable bowel syndrome, and inflammatory diseases such as rheumatoid arthritis.[9–12]

THE STRESS RESPONSE

In the early 1930s, the world-renowned endocrinologist Hans Selye was the first to describe a group of specific anatomic changes that occurred in rats that were exposed to a variety of different experimental stimuli. He came to an understanding that these changes were manifestations of the body's attempt to adapt to stimuli. Selye described *stress* as "a state manifested by a specific syndrome of the body developed in response to any stimuli that made an intense systemic demand on it."[13] As a young medical student, Selye noticed that patients with diverse disease conditions had many signs and symptoms in common. He observed that "whether a man suffers from a loss of blood, an infectious disease, or advanced cancer, he loses his appetite, his muscular strength, and his ambition to accomplish anything; usually the patient also loses weight and even his facial expression betrays that he is ill."[14] Selye referred to this as the "syndrome of just being sick."

In his early career as an experimental scientist, Selye noted a triad of adrenal enlargement, thymic atrophy, and gastric ulcer appeared in rats he was using for his studies. These same three changes developed in response to many different or nonspecific experimental challenges. He assumed that the hypothalamic-pituitary-adrenal (HPA) axis played a pivotal role in the development of this response. To Selye, the response to stressors was a process that enabled the rats to resist the experimental challenge by using the function of the system best able to respond to it. He labeled the response the *general adaptation syndrome* (GAS): *general* because the effect was a general systemic reaction, *adaptive* because the response was in reaction to a stressor, and *syndrome* because the physical manifestations were coordinated and dependent on each other.[13]

According to Selye, the GAS involves three stages: the alarm stage, the stage of resistance, and the stage of exhaustion. The *alarm stage* is characterized by a generalized stimulation of the sympathetic nervous system and the HPA axis, resulting in the release of catecholamines and cortisol. During the *resistance stage*, the body selects the most effective and economic channels of defense. During this stage, the increased cortisol levels present during the first stage drop because they are no longer needed. If the stressor is prolonged or overwhelms the ability of the body to defend itself, the *stage of exhaustion* ensues, during which resources are depleted and signs of "wear and tear" or systemic damage appear.[15] Selye contended that many ailments, such as various emotional disturbances, mildly annoying headaches, insomnia, upset stomach, gastric and duodenal ulcers, certain types of rheumatic disorders, and cardiovascular and kidney diseases appear to be initiated or encouraged by the "body itself because of its faulty adaptive reactions to potentially injurious agents."[14]

The events or environmental agents responsible for initiating the stress response were called *stressors*. According to Selye, stressors could be endogenous, arising from within the body, or exogenous, arising from outside the body.[14] In explaining the stress response, Selye proposed that two factors determine the nature of the stress response: the properties of the stressor and the conditioning of the person being stressed. Selye indicated that not all stress was detrimental; hence, he coined the terms *eustress* and *distress*.[15] He suggested that mild, brief, and controllable periods of stress could be perceived as positive stimuli to emotional and intellectual growth and development. It is the severe, protracted, and uncontrolled situations of psychological and physical distress that are disruptive of health.[14] For example, the joy of becoming a new parent and the sorrow of losing a parent are completely different experiences, yet their stressor effect—the nonspecific demand for adjustment to a new situation—can be similar.

Stressors tend to produce different responses in different persons or in the same person at different times, indicating the influence of the adaptive capacity of the person, or what Selye called *conditioning factors*. These conditioning factors may be internal (*e.g.*, genetic predisposition, age, sex) or external (*e.g.*, exposure to environmental agents, life experiences, dietary factors, level of social support).[14] The relative risk for development of a stress-related pathologic process seems, at least in part, to depend on these factors.

Neuroendocrine-Immune Interactions

Activation and control of the stress response are mediated by the combined efforts of the nervous and endocrine systems. The neuroendocrine systems integrate signals received along neurosensory pathways and from circulating mediators that are carried in the bloodstream. In addition, the immune system both affects and is affected by the stress response.

The stress response is meant to protect the person against acute threats to homeostasis and is normally time limited. Therefore, under normal circumstances, the neural responses and the hormones that are released in the response are not around long enough to cause damage to

Stress and Adaptation

➤ Stress is a state manifested by symptoms that arise from the coordinated activation of the neuroendocrine and immune systems, which Selye called the *general adaptation syndrome*.

➤ The hormones and neurotransmitters (catecholamines and cortisol) that are released during the stress response function to alert the individual to a threat or challenge to homeostasis, to enhance cardiovascular and metabolic activity in order to manage the stressor, and to focus the energy of the body by suppressing the activity of other systems that are not immediately needed.

➤ Adaptation is the ability to respond to challenges of physical or psychological homeostasis and to return to a balanced state.

➤ There are individual differences in the ability to adapt. It is influenced by previous learning and physiologic reserve, time, genetic endowment, age, health status, nutrition, sleep-wake cycles, and psychosocial factors.

vital tissues. However, in situations in which the stress response is hyperactive or becomes habituated, the physiologic and behavioral changes (*e.g.*, immunosuppression, sympathetic system activation) induced by the response can themselves become a threat to homeostasis. If the stress response is hypoactive, with a decrease in the activity of the HPA axis, the person may be more susceptible to diseases associated with overactivity of the immune response, especially increased cytokine and autoimmune activity.[9,16]

Neuroendocrine Responses

The integration of the stress responses, which occurs at the level of the central nervous system (CNS), is complex and not completely understood. It relies on communication along neuronal pathways of the cerebral cortex, the limbic system, the thalamus, the hypothalamus, the pituitary gland, and the reticular activating system (RAS) (Fig. 9-2). The cerebral cortex is involved with vigilance, cognition, and focused attention, and the limbic system with emotional components (*e.g.*, fear, excitement, rage, anger) of the stress response. The thalamus functions as the relay center and is important in receiving, sorting out, and distributing sensory input. The hypothalamus coordinates the responses of the endocrine and autonomic nervous systems (ANS). The RAS modulates mental alertness, ANS activity, and skeletal muscle tone, using input from other neural structures. The musculoskeletal tension that occurs during the stress response reflects the increased activity of the RAS and its influence on the muscle spindles and the gamma loop (*i.e.*, descending neural pathways, gamma

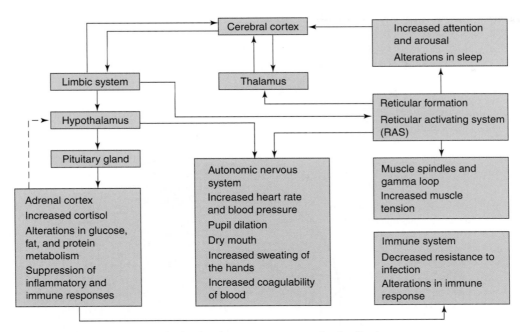

FIGURE 9-2 Stress pathways. The broken line represents negative feedback.

motor neurons, spindle muscle fibers, afferent neurons, and alpha motor neurons), which control muscle tone (see Chapter 47).

Central to the neuroendocrine component of the stress response are the locus ceruleus (LC)–norepinephrine (NE) pathway, which regulates the sympathetic nervous system component of the ANS, and corticotropin-releasing factor (CRF), which functions as the mediator of the endocrine response to stress (Fig. 9-3). The *locus ceruleus*, an area of the brain stem that is densely populated with neurons producing NE, is thought to be the central integrating site for the autonomic nervous system response to stressful stimuli. The LC-NE system has afferent pathways to the hypothalamus, the limbic system, the hippocampus, and the cerebral cortex. *Corticotropin-releasing factor* is a small peptide hormone found in both the hypothalamus and in extrahypothalamic structures, such as the limbic system and the brain stem. CRF is both an important endocrine regulator of pituitary and adrenal activity and a neurotransmitter involved in autonomic nervous system activity, metabolism, and behavior.[9,17] Receptors for CRF are distributed throughout the brain as well as many peripheral sites. CRF from the hypothalamus induces the secretion of adrenocorticotropic hormone (ACTH) from the anterior pituitary gland. ACTH, in turn, stimulates the adrenal gland to synthesize and secrete the glucocorticoid hormones (*e.g.*, cortisol).

The LC-NE system confers an adaptive advantage during a stressful situation. The sympathetic nervous system manifestation of the stress reaction has been called the *fight-or-flight response.* This is the most rapid of the stress responses and represents the basic survival response of our primitive ancestors when confronted with the perils of the wilderness and its inhabitants. The increase in sympathetic activity in the brain increases attention and arousal and thus probably intensifies memory. The heart and respiratory rates increase, the hands and feet become moist, the pupils dilate, the mouth becomes dry, and the activity of the gastrointestinal tract decreases.

The glucocorticoid hormones have a number of direct or indirect physiologic effects that mediate the stress response, enhance the action of other stress hormones, or suppress other components of the stress system. In this regard, cortisol acts both as a mediator of the stress response and an inhibitor of the stress response such that overactivation does not occur.[18] Cortisol maintains blood glucose levels by antagonizing the effects of insulin and enhances the effect of catecholamines on the cardiovascular system. It also suppresses osteoblast activity, hematopoiesis, protein and collagen synthesis, immune responses, and renal function (see Chapter 40). All of these functions are meant to protect the organism against the effects of a stressor and to focus energy on regaining balance in the face of an acute challenge to homeostasis.

The ANS and CRF responses seem to participate in a positive feedback loop in that activation of one system tends to activate the other as well, whereas the glucocorticoids inhibit the secretion of CRF and ACTH, which closes the negative feedback loop. CRF, independent of its role in the HPA axis, increases the activity of the neurons of the LC, which in turn increase the release of CRF. It has been suggested that this interaction of CRF and the LC-NE system is the mediator of the behavioral responses to stressors.[19,20]

Stress and Other Hormones. A wide variety of hormones, including growth hormones, thyroid hormone, and the reproductive hormones, also are responsive to stressful situations. Systems responsible for reproduction, growth, and immunity are directly linked to the stress system, and the

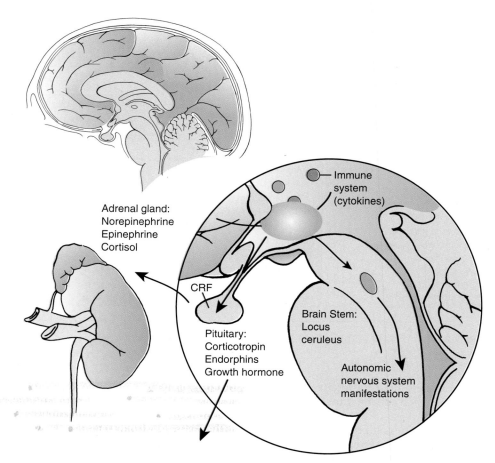

FIGURE 9-3 Neuroendocrine–immune system regulation of the stress response.

hormonal effects of the stress response profoundly influence these systems.

Although growth hormone is initially elevated at the onset of stress, the prolonged presence of cortisol leads to suppression of growth hormone, somatomedin C, and other growth factors, exerting a chronically inhibitory effect on growth. In addition, CRF directly increases somatostatin, which in turn inhibits growth hormone secretion. Although the connection is speculative, the effects of stress on growth hormone may provide one of the vital links to understanding failure to thrive in children.

Stress-induced cortisol secretion also is associated with decreased levels of thyroid-stimulating hormone and inhibition of conversion of thyroxine to the more biologically active triiodothyronine in peripheral tissues. Both changes may serve as a means to conserve energy at times of stress.

Antidiuretic hormone (ADH) also is involved in the stress response, particularly in hypotensive stress or stress due to fluid volume loss. ADH, also known as *vasopressin*, increases water retention by the kidneys, produces vasoconstriction of blood vessels, and appears to synergize CRF's capacity to increase the release of ACTH.

The reproductive hormones are inhibited by CRH at the hypophyseal level and by cortisol at the pituitary, gonadal, and target tissue level.[14] Sepsis and severe trauma can induce anovulation and amenorrhea in women and decreased spermatogenesis and decreased levels of testosterone in men.

Immune Responses

The hallmark of the stress response, as first described by Selye, is the endocrine-immune interactions (*i.e.*, increased corticosteroid production and atrophy of the thymus) that are known to suppress the immune response. In concert, these two components of the stress system, through endocrine and neurotransmitter pathways, produce the physical and behavioral changes designed to adapt to acute stress. Much of the literature regarding stress and the immune response focuses on the causal role of stress in immune-related diseases. It has been suggested that the reverse may occur; emotional and psychological manifestations of the stress response may be a reflection of alterations in the CNS resulting from the immune response. Immune cells such as monocytes and lymphocytes can penetrate the blood-brain barrier and take up residence in the brain, where they secrete cytokines and other inflammatory mediators that influence the stress response. In the case of cancer, this could mean that the subjective feelings of helplessness and hopelessness that have been repeatedly related to the onset and progression of cancers may arise secondary to the CNS effects of products released by immune cells during the early stage of the disease.[21]

The exact mechanism by which stress produces its effect on the immune response is unknown and probably varies from person to person, depending on genetic endowment and environmental factors. The most significant arguments for interactions between the neuroendocrine and immune systems derive from evidence that immune and neuroendocrine cells share common signal pathways (*i.e.*, messenger molecules and receptors), that hormones and neuropeptides can alter the function of immune cells, and that the immune system and its products (*e.g.*, cytokines) can modulate neuroendocrine function.[22] Receptors for a number of CNS-controlled hormones and neuromediators reportedly have been found on lymphocytes. Among these are receptors for glucocorticoids, insulin, testosterone, prolactin, catecholamines, estrogens, acetylcholine, and growth hormone, suggesting that these hormones influence lymphocyte function. For example, cortisol is known to suppress immune function, and pharmacologic doses of cortisol are used clinically to suppress the immune response. There is evidence that the immune system, in turn, influences neuroendocrine function.[23] It has been observed that the HPA axis is activated by cytokines such as interleukin-1, interleukin-6, and tumor necrosis factor that are released from immune cells.

A second possible route of neuroendocrine regulation of immune function is through the sympathetic nervous system and the release of catecholamines. The lymph nodes, thymus, and spleen are supplied with ANS nerve fibers. Centrally acting CRF activates the ANS through multisynaptic descending pathways, and circulating epinephrine acts synergistically with CRF and cortisol to inhibit the function of the immune system.

Not only is the quantity of immune expression changed because of stress, but the quality of the response is changed. Stress hormones differentially stimulate the proliferation of T-lymphocyte helper 2 cells (T_H2) over T_H1 cells. Because these T helper cell subtypes secrete different cytokines, they stimulate different aspects of the immune response. T_H1 cells tend to stimulate the cellular-mediated immune response, whereas T_H2 cells activate B lymphocytes and mast cells.[7]

COPING AND ADAPTATION TO STRESS

The ability to adapt to a wide range of environments and stressors is not peculiar to humans. According to René Dubos (a microbiologist noted for his study of human responses to the total environment), "adaptability is found throughout life and is perhaps the one attribute that distinguishes most clearly the world of life from the world of inanimate matter."[24] Living organisms, no matter how primitive, do not submit passively to the impact of environmental forces. They attempt to respond adaptively, each in its own unique and most suitable manner. The higher the organism on the evolutionary scale, the larger its repertoire of adaptive mechanisms and its ability to select and limit aspects of the environment to which it responds. The most fully evolved mechanisms are the social responses through which individuals or groups modify their environments, their habits, or both to achieve a way of life that is best suited to their needs.

Adaptation

Human beings, because of their highly developed nervous system and intellect, usually have alternative mechanisms for adapting and have the ability to control many aspects of their environment. Air conditioning and central heating limit the need to adapt to extreme changes in environmental temperature. The availability of antiseptic agents, immunizations, and antibiotics eliminates the need to respond to common infectious agents. At the same time, modern technology creates new challenges for adaptation and provides new sources of stress, such as increased noise, air pollution, exposure to harmful chemicals, and changes in biologic rhythms imposed by shift work and transcontinental air travel.

Of particular interest are the differences in the body's response to events that threaten the integrity of the body's physiologic environment and those that threaten the integrity of the person's psychosocial environment. Many of the body's responses to physiologic disturbances are controlled on a moment-by-moment basis by feedback mechanisms that limit their application and duration of action. For example, the baroreflex-mediated rise in heart rate that occurs when a person moves from the recumbent to the standing position is almost instantaneous and subsides within seconds. Furthermore, the response to physiologic disturbances that threaten the integrity of the internal environment is specific to the threat; the body usually does not raise the body temperature when an increase in heart rate is needed. In contrast, the response to psychological disturbances is not regulated with the same degree of specificity and feedback control; instead, the effect may be inappropriate and sustained.

Factors Affecting the Ability to Adapt

Adaptation implies that an individual has successfully created a new balance between the stressor and the ability to deal with it. The means used to attain this balance are called *coping strategies* or *coping mechanisms*. Coping mechanisms are the emotional and behavioral responses used to manage threats to our physiologic and psychological homeostasis. According to Lazarus, how we cope with stressful events depends on how we appraise the event; in other words, what does the situation mean to us?[25] Has the event caused harm or loss? Does the event pose a threat of harm or loss? And, finally, is the event a challenge rather than a threat? Previous experience and learning, physiologic reserve, time, genetic endowment and age, health status, nutrition, sleep-wake cycles, and psychosocial factors influence a person's appraisal of a stressor and the coping mechanisms used to adapt to the new situation (Fig. 9-4).

Previous Experience and Learning. Dubos cites the case of an old Chinese fisherman (the type depicted on the scrolls of the Sung dynasty) as an example of the effect that experience and learning have on adaptation[24]:

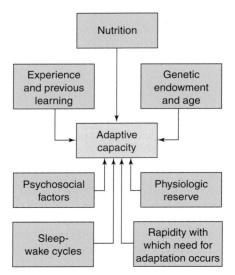

FIGURE 9-4 Factors affecting adaptation.

The fisherman appears fully at ease and relaxed in his primitive boat, floating on a misty lake, or even a polluted and crowded harbor. He has probably experienced many tribulations in the course of his years of struggle and poverty but has survived by becoming almost totally identified with his environment. He is so well adapted to it that he will probably live for many more years, without modern comfort, sanitation, or medical care, just by letting his existence be ruled by what he considers to be the unalterable laws of the seasons and nature. In the course of his life, he developed different protective mechanisms that increased his immunologic, physiologic, and psychic resistance to the physicochemical hardships, the parasites, and the social conflicts that threatened him every day. He has elected to spend the rest of his life in the environment in which he has evolved and to which he has become adapted. Robust though he appears and really is, he probably would soon become sick if he moved into an area where the parasites, physiologic stresses, and social customs differ from the ones among which he has spent his early life.

Physiologic and Anatomic Reserve. The trained athlete is able to increase cardiac output sixfold to sevenfold during exercise. The safety margin for adaptation of most body systems is considerably greater than that needed for normal activities. The red blood cells carry more oxygen than the tissues can use, the liver and fat cells store excess nutrients, and bone tissue stores calcium in excess of that needed for normal neuromuscular function. The ability of body systems to increase their function given the need to adapt is known as the *physiologic reserve.* Many of the body organs, such as the lungs, kidneys, and adrenals, are paired to provide anatomic reserve as well. Both organs are not needed to ensure the continued existence and maintenance of the internal environment. Many persons function normally with only one lung or one kidney. In kidney disease, for example, signs of renal failure do not occur until approximately 90% of the functioning nephrons have been destroyed.

Time. Adaptation is most efficient when changes occur gradually rather than suddenly. It is possible, for instance, to lose a liter or more of blood through chronic gastrointestinal bleeding over a week without manifesting signs of shock. However, a sudden hemorrhage that causes rapid loss of an equal amount of blood is likely to cause hypotension and shock.

Genetic Endowment. Adaptation is further affected by the availability of adaptive responses and flexibility in selecting the most appropriate and economical response. The greater is the number of available responses, the more effective is the capacity to adapt.

Genetic endowment can ensure that the systems that are essential to adaptation function adequately. Even a gene that has deleterious effects may prove adaptive in some environments. In Africa, the gene for sickle cell anemia persists in some populations because it provides some resistance to infection with the parasite that causes malaria.

Age. The capacity to adapt is decreased at the extremes of age. The ability to adapt is impaired by the immaturity of an infant, much as it is by the decline in functional reserve that occurs with age. For example, the infant has difficulty concentrating urine because of immature renal structures and therefore is less able than an adult to cope with decreased water intake or exaggerated water losses. A similar situation exists in the elderly owing to age-related changes in renal function.

Health Status. Physical and mental health status determines physiologic and psychological reserves and is a strong determinant of the ability to adapt. For example, persons with heart disease are less able to adjust to stresses that require the recruitment of cardiovascular responses. Severe emotional stress often produces disruption of physiologic function and limits the ability to make appropriate choices related to long-term adaptive needs. Those who have worked with acutely ill persons know that the will to live often has a profound influence on survival during life-threatening illnesses.

Nutrition. There are 50 to 60 essential nutrients, including minerals, lipids, certain fatty acids, vitamins, and specific amino acids. Deficiencies or excesses of any of these nutrients can alter a person's health status and impair the ability to adapt. The importance of nutrition to enzyme function, immune response, and wound healing is well known. On a worldwide basis, malnutrition may be one of the most common causes of immunodeficiency.

Among the problems associated with dietary excess are obesity and alcohol abuse. Obesity is a common problem. It predisposes to a number of health problems, including atherosclerosis and hypertension. Alcohol is commonly used in excess. It acutely affects brain function and, with long-term use, can seriously impair the function of the liver, brain, and other vital structures.

Sleep-Wake Cycles. Sleep is considered to be a restorative function in which energy is restored and tissues are regenerated.[26] Sleep occurs in a cyclic manner, alternating with periods of wakefulness and increased energy use. Biologic rhythms play an important role in adaptation to stress, development of illness, and response to medical treatment. Many rhythms such as rest and activity, work and leisure, and eating and drinking oscillate with a frequency similar to that of the 24-hour light-dark solar day. The term *circadian*, from the Latin *circa* ("about") and *dies* ("day"), is used to describe these 24-hour diurnal rhythms (see Chapter 51).

Sleep disorders and alterations in the sleep-wake cycle have been shown to alter immune function, the normal circadian pattern of hormone secretion, and physical and psychological functioning.[27] The two most common manifestations of an alteration in the sleep-wake cycle are insomnia and sleep deprivation or increased somnolence. In some persons, stress may produce sleep disorders, and in others, sleep disorders may lead to stress. Acute stress and environmental disturbances, loss of a loved one, recovery from surgery, and pain are common causes of transient and short-term insomnia. Air travel and jet lag constitute additional causes of altered sleep-wake cycles, as does shift work. In persons with chronic insomnia, the bed often acquires many unpleasant secondary associations and becomes a place of stress and worry rather than a place of rest.[28]

Hardiness. Studies by social psychologists have focused on individuals' emotional reactions to stressful situations and their coping mechanisms to determine those characteristics that help some people remain healthy despite being challenged by high levels of stressors. For example, the concept of *hardiness* describes a personality characteristic that includes a sense of having control over the environment, a sense of having a purpose in life, and an ability to conceptualize stressors as a challenge rather than a threat.[29] Many studies by nurses and social psychologists suggest that hardiness is correlated with positive health outcomes.[29]

Psychosocial Factors. Several studies have related social factors and life events to illness. Scientific interest in the social environment as a cause of stress has gradually broadened to include the social environment as a resource that modulates the relation between stress and health. Presumably, persons who can mobilize strong supportive resources from within their social relationships are better able to withstand the negative effects of stress on their health. Studies suggest that social support has direct and indirect positive effects on health status and serves as a buffer or modifier of the physical and psychosocial effects of stress.[30] Social networks contribute in a number of ways to a person's psychosocial and physical integrity. The configuration of significant others that constitutes this network functions to mobilize the resources of the person; these friends, colleagues, and family members share the person's tasks and provide monetary support, materials and tools, and guidance in improving problem-solving capabilities.[30] Persons with ample social networks are not as likely to experience many types of stress such as being homeless or being lonely.[9] There is also evidence that persons who have social supports or social assets may live longer and have a lower incidence of somatic illness.[31] Social support has been viewed in terms of the number of relationships a person has and the person's perception of these relationships.[32,33] Close relationships with others can involve positive effects as well as the potential for conflict and may, in some situations, leave the person less able to cope with life stressors.

In summary, the stress response is an activation of several physiologic systems (sympathetic nervous system, the HPA axis, and the immune system) that work in a coordinated fashion to protect the body against damage from the intense demands made on it. Selye called this response the *general adaptation syndrome*. The stress response is divided into three stages: the *alarm stage*, with activation of the sympathetic nervous system and the HPA axis; the *resistance stage*, during which the body selects the most effective defenses; and the *stage of exhaustion*, during which physiologic resources are depleted and signs of systemic damage appear.

The activation and control of the stress response are mediated by the combined efforts of the nervous and endocrine systems. The neuroendocrine systems integrate signals received along neurosensory pathways and from circulating mediators that are carried in the bloodstream. In addition, the immune system both affects and is affected by the stress response.

Adaptation is affected by a number of factors, including experience and previous learning, the rapidity with which the need to adapt occurs, genetic endowment and age, health status, nutrition, sleep-wake cycles, hardiness, and psychosocial factors.

Disorders of the Stress Response

After you have completed this section of the chapter, you should be able to meet the following objectives:

✦ Describe the physiologic and psychological effects of a chronic stress response
✦ Describe the three states characteristic of post-traumatic stress disorder
✦ List five nonpharmacologic methods of treating stress

For the most part, the stress response is meant to be acute and time limited. The time-limited nature of the process renders the accompanying catabolic and immunosuppressive effects advantageous. It is the chronicity of the response that is thought to be disruptive to physical and mental health.

Stressors can assume a number of patterns in relation to time. They may be classified as acute time-limited, chronic intermittent, or chronic sustained. An acute time-limited stressor is one that occurs over a short time and does not recur; a chronic intermittent stressor is one to which a person is chronically exposed. The frequency or chronicity of circumstances to which the body is asked to respond often determines the availability and efficiency of the stress responses. The response of the immune system, for example, is more rapid and efficient on second exposure to a pathogen than it is on first exposure, but chronic exposure to a stressor can fatigue the system and impair its effectiveness.

EFFECTS OF ACUTE STRESS

The reactions to acute stress are those associated with the autonomic nervous system, the fight-or-flight response. The manifestations of the stress response—a pounding headache, cold moist skin, a stiff neck—are all part of the acute stress response. Centrally, there is facilitation of neural pathways mediating arousal, alertness, vigilance, cognition, and focused attention, as well as appropriate aggression. The acute stress response can result from either psychologically or physiologically threatening events. In situations of life-threatening trauma, these acute responses may be lifesaving in that they divert blood from less essential to more essential body functions. Increased alertness and cognitive functioning enables rapid processing of information and arrival at the most appropriate solution to the threatening situation.

However, for persons with limited coping abilities, either because of physical or mental health, the acute stress response may be detrimental. This is true of persons with preexisting heart disease in whom the overwhelming sympathetic behaviors associated with the stress response can lead to dysrhythmias. For people with other chronic health problems, such as headache disorder, acute stress may precipitate a reoccurrence. In healthy individuals, the acute stress response can redirect attention from behaviors that promote health, such as attention to proper meals and getting adequate sleep. For those with health problems, it can interrupt compliance with medication regimens and exercise programs. In some situations, the acute arousal state actually can be life threatening, physically immobilizing the person when movement would avert catastrophe (*e.g.,* moving out of the way of a speeding car).

EFFECTS OF CHRONIC STRESS

The stress response is designed to be an acute self-limited response in which activation of the ANS and the HPA axis is controlled in a negative feedback manner. As with all negative feedback systems, including the stress response system, pathophysiologic changes can occur. Function can be altered in several ways, including when a component of the system fails; when the neural and hormonal connections among the components of the system are dysfunctional; and when the original stimulus for the activation of the system is prolonged or of such magnitude that it overwhelms the ability of the system to respond appropriately. In these cases, the system may become overactive or underactive.

Chronicity and excessive activation of the stress response can result from chronic illnesses as well as contribute to the development of long-term health problems. Chronic activation of the stress response is an important public health issue from both a health and a cost perspective. The National Institute for Occupational Safety and Health declared stress a hazard of the workplace.[34] It is linked to a myriad of health disorders, such as diseases of the cardiovascular, gastrointestinal, immune, and neurologic systems, as well as depression, chronic alcoholism and drug abuse, eating disorders, accidents, and suicide.

Occurrence of the oral disease acute necrotizing gingivitis, in which the normal bacterial flora of the mouth become invasive, is known by dentists to be associated with acute stress, such as final examinations.[35] Similarly, herpes simplex type 1 infection (*i.e.,* cold sores) often develops during periods of inadequate rest, fever, ultraviolet radiation, and emotional upset. The resident herpesvirus is kept in check by body defenses, probably T lymphocytes, until a stressful event occurs that causes suppression of the immune system. Psychological stress is associated in a dose-response manner with an increased risk for development of the common cold, and this risk is attributable to increased rates of infection rather than frequency of symptoms after infection.[36]

In a study in which participants were infected with the influenza virus, those persons who reported the greatest amount of premorbid stress reported the most intense influenza symptoms and had a statistically greater production of interleukin-6, a cytokine that acts as a chemotactic agent for immune cells.[37] Elderly caregivers of a spouse with dementia had a significantly higher score for emotional distress and higher salivary cortisol than matched control subjects. The higher stress was correlated with a decreased immune response to an influenza vaccine.[38] The experience of stress also has been associated with delays in wound healing.[39,40]

Post-traumatic Stress Disorder

Post-traumatic stress disorder (PTSD) is an example of chronic activation of the stress response as a result of experiencing a potentially life-threatening event. It was formerly called *battle fatigue* or *shell shock* because it was first characterized in men and women returning from combat. In general, 30% of all persons in a war zone develop PTSD. Although war is still a significant cause of PTSD, other major catastrophic events, such as major weather-related disasters, airplane crashes, terrorist bombings, and rape or child abuse, also may result in the development of the disorder. At any one time, approximately 3.6% of the adult population in the United States is affected. Although there are no studies of the prevalence of PTSD among children in the United States, there is a high prevalence of childhood exposure to life-threatening violence in the home, school, and neighborhood.[41]

PTSD is characterized by a constellation of symptoms that are experienced as states of intrusion, avoidance, and hyperarousal. *Intrusion* refers to the occurrence of "flashbacks" during waking hours or nightmares in which the past traumatic event is relived, often in vivid and frightening detail. *Avoidance* refers to the emotional numbing that accompanies this disorder and disrupts important personal relationships. Because a person with PTSD has not been able to resolve the painful feelings associated with the trauma, depression is commonly a part of the clinical picture. Survivor guilt also may be a product of traumatic situations in which the person survived the disaster but loved ones did not. *Hyperarousal* refers to the presence of increased irritability and exaggerated startle reflex. In addition, memory problems, sleep disturbances, and anxiety are commonly experienced by persons with PTSD.

Although the pathophysiology of PTSD is not completely understood, it has been suggested that its symptoms may arise from an activation of fear-related brain systems such as the amygdala and its neuronal projections to the brain stem, hypothalamus, and medulla. It has been hypothesized that the intrusive symptoms of PTSD may arise from an exaggerated sympathetic nervous system activation in response to the traumatic event. Indeed, signs of increased sympathetic activity have been demonstrated in studies of persons with PTSD.[42,43] Catecholamines also may play an important role in enhancing memory.

Persons with PTSD also demonstrate decreased cortisol levels, increased sensitivity of cortisol receptors, and an enhanced negative feedback inhibition of cortisol release with the dexamethasone suppression test. Dexamethasone is a synthetic glucocorticoid that mimics the effects of cortisol and directly inhibits the action of CRF and ACTH. This is in contrast to patients with major depression, who have a decreased sensitivity of glucocorticoid receptors, a high plasma level of cortisol, and a decreased dexamethasone suppression.[44] The hypersuppression of cortisol observed with the dexamethasone test suggests that persons with PTSD do not exhibit a classic stress response as described by Selye. Because this hypersuppression has not been described in other psychiatric disorders, it may serve as a relatively specific marker for PTSD.

Another finding in persons with PTSD is a decreased hippocampal volume.[45] One of the deleterious effects of high plasma cortisol is neuronal atrophy, particularly in the hippocampus, an area of the brain densely populated with glucocorticoid receptors and vital for cognitive skills and memory. In PTSD, the increased glucocorticoid receptor sensitivity makes the hippocampus susceptible to damage even with low cortisol levels. On the other hand, it is possible that persons who had a small hippocampal volume before a traumatic event experience the event differently from those in whom PTSD does not subsequently develop.[46]

Little is known about the risk factors that predispose people to the development of PTSD. It is important to note that less than half of all people who are exposed to a traumatic event develop PTSD. For example, only 15% to 30% of soldiers exposed to combat develop the disorder.[46] It also has been found that children exposed to violent events but who have strong family relationships rarely develop PTSD.[41] Statistics indicate there is a need for studies to determine risk factors for PTSD as a means of targeting individuals who may need intensive therapeutic measures after a life-threatening event. Research also is needed to determine the mechanisms by which the disorder develops so that it can be prevented, or if that is not possible, so that treatment methods can be created to decrease the devastating effects that this disorder has on affected individuals and their families.[42] To this end, the National Institute of Mental Health has established a mechanism (Rapid Grants) for funding studies of the acute effects of disasters.[47]

Health care professionals need to be aware that clients who present with symptoms of depression, anxiety, and alcohol or drug abuse may in fact be suffering from PTSD. The client history should include questions concerning the occurrence of violence, major loss, or traumatic events in the person's life. Debriefing, or talking about the traumatic event at the time it happens, often is an effective therapeutic tool. Crisis teams are among the first people to attend to the emotional needs of those caught in catastrophic events. Some people may need continued individual or group therapy. Often concurrent pharmacotherapy, such as antidepressants and antianxiety agents, is useful and helps the individual participate more fully in therapy.

Most important, the person with PTSD must not be made to feel responsible for the disorder or that it is evidence of a character flaw. It is not uncommon for persons with this disorder to be told to "get over it" or "just get on with it, because others have." There is ample evidence to suggest that there is a biologic basis for the individual differences in responses to traumatic events, and these differences need to be taken into account.

TREATMENT AND RESEARCH OF STRESS DISORDERS

Treatment

The treatment of stress should be directed toward helping people avoid coping behaviors that impose a risk to their health and providing them with alternative stress-reducing strategies. Purposeful priority setting and problem solving can be used by persons who are overwhelmed by the number of life stresses to which they have been exposed. Other nonpharmacologic methods used for stress reduction are relaxation techniques, guided imagery, music therapy, massage, and biofeedback.

Relaxation. Practices for evoking the relaxation response are numerous. They are found in virtually every culture and are credited with producing a generalized decrease in sympathetic system activity and musculoskeletal tension. According to Herbert Benson, a physician who worked in developing the technique, four elements are integral to the various relaxation techniques: a repetitive mental device, a passive attitude, decreased mental tonus, and a quiet environment.[48] Benson developed a noncultural method that is commonly used for achieving relaxation (see accompanying box).

Progressive muscle relaxation, originally developed by Edmund Jacobson, who did extensive research on the muscle correlates of anxiety and tension, is another method of relieving tension. He observed that tension can be defined physiologically as the inappropriate contraction of muscle fibers. His procedure, which has been modified by a number of therapists, consists of systematic contraction and relaxation of major muscle groups.[49] As the person learns to relax, the various muscle groups are combined. Eventually, the person learns to relax individual muscle groups without first contracting them.

Imagery. Guided imagery is another technique that can be used to achieve relaxation. One method is scene visualization, in which the person is asked to sit back, close the

The Relaxation Response

- Sit quietly in a comfortable position.
- Deeply relax all your muscles, beginning at your feet and progressing up to your face.
- Breathe through your nose. Become aware of your breathing. As you breathe out, say the word "one" silently to yourself. Continue for 20 minutes. When you have finished, sit quietly for several minutes, first with your eyes closed and then with them open.
- Do not worry about whether you are successful in achieving a deep level of relaxation. Maintain a positive attitude and permit the relaxation to occur at its own rate. Expect distracting thoughts, ignore them, and continue repeating "one" as you breathe out.

(Modified from Benson H. [1977]. Systemic hypertension and the relaxation response. *New England Journal of Medicine* 296, 1152)

eyes, and concentrate on a scene narrated by the therapist. Whenever possible, all five senses are involved: the person attempts to see, feel, hear, and taste aspects of the visual experience. Other types of imagery involve imagining the appearance of each of the major muscle groups and how they feel during tension and relaxation.

Music Therapy. Music therapy is used for both its physiologic and psychological effects. It involves listening to selected pieces of music as a means of ameliorating anxiety or stress, reducing pain, decreasing feelings of loneliness and isolation, buffering noise, and facilitating expression of emotion. Music is defined as having three components: rhythm, melody, and harmony.[50,51] Rhythm is the order in the movement of the music. Rhythm is the most dynamic aspect of music, and particular pieces of music often are selected because they harmonize with body rhythms such as heart rhythm, respiratory rhythm, or gait. The melody is created by the musical pitch and distance (or interval) between the musical tone. The melody contributes to the listener's emotional response to the music. The harmony results from the way pitches are blended together, with the combination of sounds described as consonant or dissonant by the listener. Music usually is selected based on a person's musical preference and past experiences with music. Depending on the setting, headphones may be used to screen out other distracting noises. Radio and television music is inappropriate for music therapy because of the inability to control the selection of pieces that are played, the interruptions that occur (*e.g.*, commercials and announcements), and the quality of the reception.

Massage Therapies. Massage is the manipulation of the soft tissues of the body to promote relaxation and relief of muscle tension. The technique that is used may involve a gentle stroking along the length of a muscle (effleurage),

application of pressure across the width of a muscle (petrissage), deep massage movements applied by a circular motion of the thumbs or fingertips (friction), squeezing across the width of a muscle (kneading), or use of light slaps or chopping actions (hacking).[52] Massage may be administered by practitioners who have received special training in its use or by less prepared persons such as parents of small children[53,54] or caregivers of confused elders.[55] It often is used as a means of physiologic relaxation and stress relief in critically ill patients.[56]

Biofeedback. Biofeedback is a technique in which an individual learns to control physiologic functioning. It involves electronic monitoring of one or more physiologic responses to stress with immediate feedback of the specific response to the person undergoing treatment. Several types of responses are used: electromyographic (EMG), electrothermal, and electrodermal (EDR).[57] The EMG response involves the measurement of electrical potentials from muscles, usually the forearm extensor or frontalis. This is used to gain control over the contraction of skeletal muscles that occurs with anxiety and tension. The electrodermal sensors monitor skin temperature in the fingers or toes. The sympathetic nervous system exerts significant control over blood flow in the distal parts of the body such as the digits of the hands and feet. Consequently, anxiety often is manifested by a decrease in skin temperature in the fingers and toes. EDR sensors measure conductivity of skin (usually the hands) in response to anxiety. Fearful and anxious people often have cold and clammy hands, which leads to a decrease in conductivity.

Research

Research in stress has focused on personal reports of the stress situation and the physiologic responses to stress. A number of interview guides and written instruments are available for measuring the personal responses to stress and coping in adults[58,59] and children.[60]

There are fewer methods available for measuring the physiologic responses to stress in humans because much of the research in the field of stress has been accomplished using animal models. There are some good reasons for this. First, the human experience of stress varies among individuals based on previous life experiences and availability of adaptive resources; therefore, it is difficult to find a stimulus that produces equivalent stress in all subjects in a study. Second, suitable methods for measuring the components of the stress response in humans are limited. Some methods require invasive procedures, many demand expensive equipment, and all require investigator competency in their use.[61] In addition, many measurement methods, such as venipuncture, can introduce additional stress to the experimental condition.

Some of the current methods for studying the physiologic manifestations of the stress response include electrocardiographic recording of heart rate, blood pressure measurement, electrodermal measurement of skin resistance associated with sweating, and biochemical analyses of hormone levels.[61] Measurements of urinary and plasma catecholamines can be used as an index of autonomic nervous system activation. Cortisol levels can be obtained from salivary samples. The effect of the stress response on the immune system can be studied through the use of blood tests to obtain immune cell (lymphocyte) counts and antibody levels.

Research that attempts to establish a link between the stress response and disease needs to be interpreted with caution owing to the influence that individual differences have in the way people respond to stress. Not everyone who experiences stressful life events develops a disease. The evidence for a link between the stress response system and the development of disease in susceptible persons is compelling but not conclusive. No study has established a direct cause-and-effect relationship between the stress response and disease occurrence. For example, depressive illness often is associated with an increase in both plasma cortisol and cerebrospinal fluid concentrations of CRF. The question that arises is whether this increased plasma cortisol is a cause or an effect of the depressive state. Although health care professionals continue to question the role of stressors and coping skills on the pathogenesis of disease states, we must resist the temptation to suggest that any disease is due to excessive stress or poor coping skills.

In summary, stress in itself is neither negative nor deleterious to health. The stress response is designed to be time limited and protective, but in situations of prolonged activation of the response because of overwhelming or chronic stressors, it could be damaging to health. PTSD is an example of chronic activation of the stress response as a result of experiencing a severe trauma. In this disorder, memory of the traumatic event seems to be enhanced. Flashbacks of the event are accompanied by intense activation of the neuroendocrine system.

Treatment of stress should be aimed at helping people avoid coping behaviors that can adversely affect their health and providing them with other ways to reduce stress. Nonpharmacologic methods used in the treatment of stress include relaxation techniques, guided imagery, music therapy, massage techniques, and biofeedback.

Research in stress has focused on personal reports of the stress situation and the physiologic responses to stress. A number of interview guides and written instruments are available for measuring the personal responses to acute and chronic stressors. Methods used for studying the physiologic manifestations of the stress response include electrocardiographic recording of heart rate, blood pressure measurement, electrodermal measurement of skin resistance associated with sweating, and biochemical analyses of hormone levels.

References

1. Lazarus R.S., Folkman S. (1984). *Stress, appraisal, and coping.* New York: Springer.
2. Hinkle L.E. (1977). The concept of "stress" in the biological and social sciences. In Lipowskin Z.J., Lipsitt D.R., Whybrow P.C. (Eds.), *Psychosomatic medicine* (pp. 27–49). New York: Oxford University Press.
3. Osler W. (1910). The Lumleian lectures in angina pectoris. *Lancet* 1, 696–700, 839–844, 974–977.
4. Cannon W.B. (1935). Stresses and strains of homeostasis. *American Journal of Medical Science* 189, 1–5.
5. Selye H. (1946). The general adaptation syndrome and diseases of adaptation. *Journal of Clinical Endocrinology* 6, 117–124.
6. Cannon W.B. (1939). *The wisdom of the body* (pp. 299–300). New York: W.W. Norton.
7. Wilcox R.E., Gonzales R.A. (1995). Introduction to neurotransmitters, receptors, signal transduction, and second messengers. In Schatzberg A.F., Nemeroff C.B. (Eds.), *Textbook of psychopharmacology* (pp. 3–29). Washington, DC: American Psychiatric Press.
8. Elenkov I.J., Webster E.L., Torpy D.J., Chrousos G.P. (1999). Stress, corticotrophin-releasing hormone, glucocorticoids, and the immune/inflammatory response: Acute and chronic effects. *Annals of the New York Academy of Sciences* 876, 1–11.
9. Chrousos G.P. (1998). Stressors, stress, and neuroendocrine integration of the adaptive response. *Annals of the New York Academy of Sciences* 851, 311–335.
10. Mitchell, A.J. (1998). The role of corticotropin releasing factor in depressive illness: A critical review. *Neuroscience and Biobehavioral Reviews* 22, 635–651.
11. Noll G., Wenzel R.R., Binggeli C., Corti C., Luscher T.F. (1998). Role of sympathetic nervous system in hypertension and effects of cardiovascular drugs. *European Heart Journal* 19 (Suppl. F), 32–38.
12. Walker J.G., Littlejohn G.O., McMurray N.E., Cutolo M. (1999). Stress system response and rheumatoid arthritis: A multilevel approach. *Rheumatology* 38, 1050–1057.
13. Selye H. (1976). *The stress of life* (rev. ed.). New York: McGraw-Hill.
14. Selye H. (1973). The evolution of the stress concept. *American Scientist* 61, 692–699.
15. Selye H. (1974). *Stress without distress* (p. 6). New York: New American Library.
16. Heim C., Ehlert U., Hellhammer D.H. (1999). The potential role of hypocortisolism in the pathophysiology of stress-related bodily disorders. *Psychoneuroendocrinology* 25, 1–35.
17. Lopez J.F., Akil H., Watson S.J. (1999). Neural circuits mediating stress. *Biological Psychiatry* 46, 1461–1471.
18. Sapolsky R.M., Romero L.M., Munck A.U. (2000). How do glucocorticoids influence stress responses? Integrating permissive, suppressive, stimulatory, and preparative actions. *Endocrine Reviews* 21, 55–89.
19. Koob G.F. (1999) Corticotropin-releasing factor, norepinephrine, and stress. *Biological Psychiatry* 46, 1167–1180.
20. Lehnert H., Schulz C., Dieterich K. (1998). Physiological and neurochemical aspects of corticotrophin-releasing factor actions in the brain: The role of the locus ceruleus. *Neurochemical Research* 23, 1039–1052.
21. Dantzer R., Kelley K.W. (1989). Stress and immunity: An integrated view of relationships between the brain and immune system. *Life Sciences* 44, 1995–2008.
22. Falaschi P., Martocchia A., Proietti A., Pastore R., D'urso R. (1994). Immune system and the hypothalamus-pituitary-adrenal axis. *Annals of the New York Academy of Sciences* 741, 223–231.
23. Woiciechowsky C., Schoning F., Lanksch W.R., Volk H.D., Docke W.D. (1999). Mechanisms of brain mediated systemic anti-inflammatory syndrome causing immunodepression. *Journal of Molecular Medicine* 77, 769–780.

24. Dubos R. (1965). *Man adapting* (pp. 256, 258, 261, 264). New Haven: Yale University Press.

25. Lazarus R. (2000). Evolution of a model of stress, coping, and discrete emotions. In Rice V.H. (Ed.), *Handbook of stress, coping, and health* (pp. 195–222). Thousand Oaks, CA: Sage Publications.

26. Adams K., Oswold I. (1983). Protein synthesis, bodily renewal and sleep-wake cycle. *Clinical Science* 65, 561–567.

27. Gillin J.C., Byerley W.F. (1990). The diagnosis and management of insomnia. *New England Journal of Medicine* 322, 239–248.

28. Moldofsky H., Lue F.A., Davidson J.R., Gorezynski R. (1989). Effects of sleep deprivation on human immune functions. *FASEB Journal* 3, 1972–1977.

29. Ford-Gilboe M., Cohen J.A. (2000). Hardiness: A model of commitment, challenge, and control. In Rice V.H. (Ed.), *Handbook of stress, coping, and health* (pp. 425–436). Thousand Oaks, CA: Sage Publications.

30. Broadhead W.E., Kaplan B.H., James S.A., et al. (1983). The epidemiologic evidence for a relationship between social support and health. *American Journal of Epidemiology* 117, 521–537.

31. Greenblatt M., Becerra R.M., Serafetinides E.A. (1982). Social networks and mental health: An overview. *American Journal of Psychiatry* 139, 977–984.

32. House J.S., Robbins C., Metzner H.L. (1982). The association of social relationships and activities with mortality: Prospective evidence from the Tecumseh Community Health Study. *American Journal of Epidemiology* 16 (1), 123–140.

33. Tilden V.P., Weinert C. (1987). Social support and the chronically ill individual. *Nursing Clinics of North America* 33, 613–620.

34. National Institute for Occupational Safety and Health. (1999). *Stress at work* (pp. 1–26). Publication no. 99-101, HE 20.7102:ST 8/4. Bethesda, MD: U.S. Department of Health and Human Services.

35. Dworkin S.F. (1969). Psychosomatic concepts and dentistry: Some perspectives. *Journal of Periodontology* 40, 647.

36. Cohen S., Tyrrell D.A.J., Smith A.P. (1991). Psychological stress and susceptibility to the common cold. *New England Journal of Medicine* 325, 606–612.

37. Cohen S., Doyle W.J., Skoner D.P. (1999). Psychological stress, cytokine production, and severity of upper respiratory illness. *Psychosomatic Medicine* 61 (2), 175–180.

38. Vedhara K., Wilcock G.K., Lightman S.L., Shanks N.M. (1999). Chronic stress in elderly carers of dementia patients and antibody response to influenza vaccination. *Lancet* 353, 627–631.

39. Rozlog L.A., Kiecolt-Glaser J.K., Marucha P.T., Sheridan J.F., Glaser, R. (1999). Stress and immunity: Implication for viral disease and wound healing. *Journal of Periodontology* 70, 786–792.

40. Cacioppo J.T., Berntson G.G., Malarkey W.B., Kiecolt-Glaser J.K., Sheridan J.F., Poehlmann K.M., Burleson M.H., Ernst J.M., Hawkley L.C. (1998). Autonomic, neuroendocrine, and immune responses to psychological stress: The reactivity hypothesis. *Annals of the New York Academy of Sciences* 840, 664–673.

41. McCloskey L.A. (2000). Posttraumatic stress in children exposed to family violence and single event trauma. *Journal of the American Academy of Child and Adolescent Psychiatry* 39, 108–115.

42. Yehuda R. (2000). Biology of posttraumatic stress disorder. *Journal of Clinical Psychiatry* 61 (Suppl. 7), 14–21.

43. Nutt D. (2000). The psychobiology of posttraumatic stress disorder. *Journal of Clinical Psychiatry* 61 (5), 24–29.

44. Yehuda, R. (1998). Psychoneuroendocrinology of posttraumatic stress disorder. *Psychiatric Clinics of North America* 21, 359–379.

45. Lombroso, P.L. (1998). Development of the cerebral cortex: XII. Stress and brain development: I. *Journal of the Academy of Child and Adolescent Psychiatry* 37, 1337–1339.

46. Sapolsky R. (1999). Stress and your shrinking brain (posttraumatic stress disorder's effect on the brain). *Discover*, 20 (3), 116.

47. National Institute of Mental Health. (2000). *Have you lived through a very scary and dangerous event? A real illness: posttraumatic stress disorder (PTSD)* (pp. 1–8). HE 20.8102:IL 6/PTSD. Bethesda, MD: National Institute of Mental Health.

48. Benson H. (1977). Systemic hypertension and the relaxation response. *New England Journal of Medicine* 296, 1152–1154.

49. Jacobson E. (1958). *Progressive relaxation*. Chicago: University of Chicago Press.

50. Chlan L., Tracy M.F. (1999). Music therapy in critical care: Indications and guidelines for intervention. *Critical Care Nurse* 19 (3), 35–41.

51. White J.M. (1999). Effects of relaxing music on cardiac autonomic balance and anxiety after acute myocardial infarction. *American Journal of Critical Care* 8, 220–230.

52. Vickers A., Zollman C. (1999). ABC of complementary therapies: Massage therapies. *British Medical Journal* 319, 1254–1257.

53. Rusy L.M., Weisman S.J. (2000). Complementary therapies for acute pediatric pain management. *Pediatric Clinics of North America* 47, 589–599.

54. Huhtala V., Lehtonen L., Heinonen R., Korvenranta H. (2000). Infant massage compared with crib vibrator in treatment of colicky infants. *Pediatrics* 105 (6), E84.

55. Rowe M., Alfred D. (1999). The effectiveness of slow-stroke massage in diffusing agitated behaviors in individuals with Alzheimer's disease. *Journal of Gerontological Nursing* 25 (6), 22–34.

56. Richards K.C. (1998). Effect of back massage and relaxation intervention on sleep in critically ill patients. *American Journal of Critical Care* 7, 288–299.

57. Fischer-Williams M., Nigl A.J., Sovine D.L. (1986). *A textbook of biological feedback*. New York: Human Sciences Press.

58. Wimbush F.B., Nelson M.L. (2000). Stress, psychosomatic illness, and health. In Rice V.H. (Ed.), *Handbook of stress, coping, and health* (pp. 143–194). Thousand Oaks, CA: Sage Publications.

59. Backer J.H., Bakas T., Bennett S.J., Pierce P.K. (2000). Coping with stress: Programs of nursing research. In Rice V.H. (Ed.), *Handbook of stress, coping, and health* (pp. 223–263). Thousand Oaks, CA: Sage Publications.

60. Ryan-Wenger N.A., Sharrer V.W., Wynd C.A. (2000). Stress, coping, and health in children. In Rice V.H. (Ed.), *Handbook of stress, coping, and health* (pp. 265–293). Thousand Oaks, CA: Sage Publications.

61. White J.M., Porth C.M. (2000). Physiological measurement of the stress response. In Rice V.H. (Ed.), *Handbook of stress, coping, and health* (pp. 69–94). Thousand Oaks, CA: Sage Publications.

Alterations in Temperature Regulation

Body heat is generated in the core tissues of the body. It is transferred to the skin surface by the blood and then released into the environment surrounding the body. Body temperature rises in fever owing to cytokine-mediated changes in the hypothalamic temperature set point and in hyperthermia due to excessive heat production, inadequate heat dissipation, or a failure of thermoregulatory mechanisms; it falls during hypothermia caused by exposure to cold. This chapter is organized into three sections: regulation of body temperature, fever and hyperthermia, and hypothermia.

Body Temperature Regulation

After you have completed this section of the chapter, you should be able to meet the following objectives:

+ Differentiate between body core temperature and skin temperature and relate the differences to methods used for measuring body temperature
+ Describe the mechanisms of heat production in the body
+ Define the terms *conduction, radiation, convection,* and *evaporation,* and relate them to the mechanisms for heat loss from the body

Virtually all biochemical processes in the body are affected by changes in temperature. Metabolic processes speed up or slow down depending on whether body temperature is rising or falling. *Core body temperature (i.e.,* intracranial, intrathoracic, and intra-abdominal) normally is maintained within a range of 36.0°C to 37.5°C (97.0°F to 99.5°F).[1,2] Within this range, there are individual differences and diurnal variations; internal core temperatures reach their highest point in late afternoon and evening and their lowest point in the early morning hours (Fig. 10-1).

Body temperature reflects the difference between heat production and heat loss and varies with exercise and extremes of environmental temperature. Properly protected, the body can function in environmental conditions that range from −50°C (−48°F) to +50°C (+122°F). Individual body cells, however, cannot tolerate such a wide range of temperatures—at −1°C (+32°F), ice crystals form, and at +45°C (+113°F), cell proteins coagulate.[3]

Most of the body's heat is produced by the deeper core tissues (*i.e.,* muscles and viscera), which are insulated from the environment and protected against heat loss by the subcutaneous tissues and skin (Fig. 10-2). Adipose tissue is a particularly good insulator, conducting heat only one third as effectively as other tissues. Heat loss occurs when the heat from the body's inner core is transferred to the skin surface by the circulating blood. If no heat were lost by the body, the temperature of the body would rise 1°C (1.8°F)

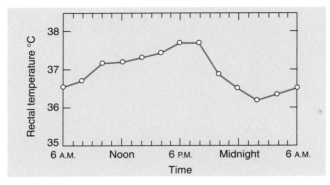

FIGURE 10-1 Normal diurnal variations in body temperature.

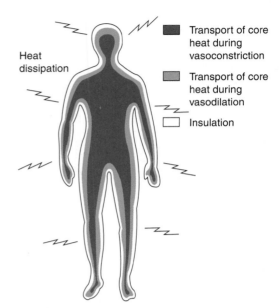

FIGURE 10-2 Control of heat loss. Body heat is produced in the deeper core tissues of the body, which is insulated by the subcutaneous tissues and skin to protect against heat loss. During vasodilatation, circulating blood transports heat to the skin surface, where it dissipates into the surrounding environment. Vasoconstriction decreases the transport of core heat to the skin surface, and vasodilatation increases transport.

per hour at rest; with light work, the temperature would rise 2°C per hour.

Temperatures differ in various parts of the body, with core temperatures being higher than those at the skin surface. In general, the rectal temperature is used as a measure of core temperature. Rectal temperatures usually range from 37.3°C (99.2°F) to 37.6°C (99.6°F).[2] Special caution must be used with this method to avoid rupturing the rectum, particularly in infants. Core temperatures may also be obtained from the esophagus using a flexible thermometer, from a pulmonary artery catheter that is used for thermodilution measurement of cardiac output, or from a urinary catheter with thermosensor that measures the temperature of urine in the bladder. Because of location, pulmonary artery and esophageal temperatures closely reflect the temperature of the heart and thoracic organs. This is the preferred measurement when body temperatures are changing rapidly and need to be followed reliably.[2] The oral temperature, taken sublingually, is usually 0.2°C (0.36°F) to 0.51°C (0.9°F) lower than the rectal temperature; however, it usually follows changes in core temperature closely. The axillary temperature also can be used as an estimate of core temperature. However, the parts of the axillary fossa must be pressed closely together for an extended period (5 to 10 minutes for a glass thermometer) because this method requires considerable heat to accumulate before the final temperature is reached. Ear-based thermometry uses an infrared sensor to measure the flow of heat from the tympanic membrane and ear canal.[2,4] The method is easy to use and has been reported to correlate well with rectal temperatures. It has become popular in the pediatric setting because of its ease and speed of measurement, acceptability to parents and children, and cost savings in personnel time required to take a child's temperature.[5] However, there continues to be debate about the accuracy of this method.[4,6] Several factors can alter the accuracy of ear-based thermometry: (1) the size of the probe cover must match the size of the ear canal; (2) the infrared reader must be directed at the tympanic membrane; and (3) the presence of any exudate (fluid or cerumen) in the ear canal or behind the tympanic membrane affects the accuracy of the reading.[6]

Core body temperature rather than the surface temperature is regulated by the *thermoregulatory center* in the hypothalamus. This center integrates input from cold and warm thermal receptors located throughout the body and generates output responses that conserve body heat or increase its dissipation. The *thermostatic set point* of the thermoregulatory center is set so that the temperature of the body core is regulated within the normal range of 36.0° to 37.5°C. When body temperature begins to rise above the normal range, heat-dissipating behaviors are initiated; when the temperature falls below the normal range, heat production

 Thermoregulation

➤ Core body temperature is a reflection of the balance between heat gain and heat loss by the body. Metabolic processes produce heat, which must be dissipated.

➤ The hypothalamus is the thermal control center—it receives information from peripheral and central thermoreceptors and compares that information with its temperature set point.

➤ Heat loss occurs through transfer of body core heat to the surface through the circulation. Heat is lost from the skin through radiation, conduction, convection, and evaporation.

➤ An increase in core temperature is effected by vasoconstriction and shivering, a decrease in temperature by vasodilation, and sweating.

is increased. Core temperatures above 41°C (105.8°F) or below 34°C (93.2°F) usually mean that the body's ability to thermoregulate is impaired (Fig. 10-3). Body responses that produce, conserve, and dissipate heat are described in Table 10-1. Spinal cord injuries that transect the cord at T6 or above can seriously impair temperature regulation because the hypothalamus can no longer control skin blood flow or sweating.

In addition to physiologic thermoregulatory mechanisms, humans engage in voluntary behaviors to help regulate body temperature. These behaviors include the selection of proper clothing and regulation of environmental temperature through heating systems and air conditioning. Body positions that hold the extremities close to the body prevent heat loss and are commonly assumed in cold weather.

MECHANISMS OF HEAT PRODUCTION

Metabolism is the body's main source of heat production. There is a 0.56°C (1°F) increase in body temperature for every 7% increase in metabolism. The sympathetic neurotransmitters, epinephrine and norepinephrine, which are released when an increase in body temperature is needed, act at the cellular level to shift metabolism so energy production is reduced and heat production is increased. This may be one of the reasons fever tends to produce feelings of weakness and fatigue. Thyroid hormone increases cellular metabolism, but this response usually requires several weeks to reach maximal effectiveness.

Fine involuntary actions such as shivering and chattering of the teeth can produce a threefold to fivefold increase in body temperature. *Shivering* is initiated by impulses from the hypothalamus. The first muscle change that occurs with

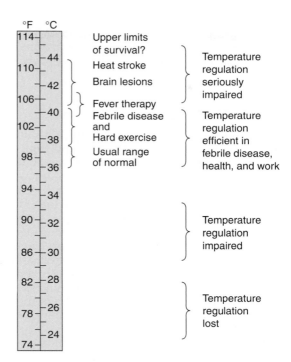

FIGURE 10-3 Body temperatures under different conditions. (Dubois, E.F. [1948]. *Fever and the regulation of body temperature.* Springfield, IL: Charles C. Thomas)

shivering is a general increase in muscle tone, followed by an oscillating rhythmic tremor involving the spinal-level reflex that controls muscle tone. Because no external work is performed, all the energy liberated by the metabolic processes from shivering is in the form of heat.[7]

TABLE 10-1 ✦ Heat Gain and Heat Loss Responses Used in Regulation of Body Temperature

Heat Gain		Heat Loss	
Body Response	*Mechanism of Action*	*Body Response*	*Mechanism of Action*
Vasoconstriction of the superficial blood vessels	Confines blood flow to the inner core of the body, with the skin and subcutaneous tissues acting as insulation to prevent loss of core heat	Dilatation of the superficial blood vessels	Delivers blood containing core heat to the periphery where it is dissipated through radiation, conduction, and convection
Contraction of the pilomotor muscles that surround the hairs on the skin	Reduces the heat loss surface of the skin	Sweating	Increases heat loss through evaporation
Assumption of the huddle position with the extremities held close to the body	Reduces the area for heat loss		
Shivering	Increases heat production by the muscles		
Increased production of epinephrine	Increases the heat production associated with metabolism		
Increased production of thyroid hormone	Is a long-term mechanism that increases metabolism and heat production		

Physical exertion increases body temperature. With strenuous exercise, more than three fourths of the increased metabolism resulting from muscle activity appears as heat within the body, and the remainder appears as external work.

MECHANISMS OF HEAT LOSS

Most of the body's heat losses occur at the skin surface as heat from the blood moves to the skin and from there into the surrounding environment. There are numerous arteriovenous (AV) shunts under the skin surface that allow blood to move directly from the arterial to the venous system. These AV shunts are much like the radiators in a heating system. When the shunts are open, body heat is freely dissipated to the skin and surrounding environment; when the shunts are closed, heat is retained in the body. The blood flow in the AV shunts is controlled almost exclusively by the sympathetic nervous system in response to changes in core temperature and environmental temperature. Contraction of the *pilomotor muscles* of the skin, which raises skin hairs and produces goose bumps, reduces the surface area available for heat loss.

Heat is lost from the body through radiation, conduction, and convection from the skin surface; through the evaporation of sweat and insensible perspiration; through the exhalation of air that has been warmed and humidified; and through heat lost in urine and feces. Of these mechanisms, only heat losses that occur at the skin surface are directly under hypothalamic control.

Conduction

Conduction is the direct transfer of heat from one molecule to another. Blood carries, or conducts, heat from the inner core of the body to the skin surface. Normally, only a small amount of body heat is lost through conduction to a cooler surface. Cooling blankets or mattresses that are used for reducing fever rely on conduction of heat from the skin to the cool surface of the mattress. Heat also can be conducted in the opposite direction—from the external environment to the body surface. For instance, body temperature may rise slightly after a hot bath.

Water has a specific heat several times greater than air, so water absorbs far greater amounts of heat than air does. The loss of body heat can be excessive and life threatening in situations of cold water immersion or cold exposure in damp or wet clothing.

The conduction of heat to the body's surface is influenced by blood volume. In hot weather, the body compensates by increasing blood volume as a means of dissipating heat. Persons who are not acclimated to a hot environment can increase their total blood volume by 10% within 2 to 4 hours of heat exposure. A mild swelling of the ankles during hot weather provides evidence of blood volume expansion. Exposure to cold produces a cold diuresis and a reduction in blood volume as a means of controlling the transfer of heat to the body's surface.

Radiation

Radiation is the transfer of heat through the air or a vacuum. Heat from the sun is carried by radiation. Heat loss by radiation varies with the temperature of the environment. Environmental temperature must be less than that of the body for heat loss to occur. Normally, approximately 60% to 70% of body heat is dissipated by radiation.

Convection

Convection refers to heat transfer through the circulation of air currents. Normally, a layer of warm air tends to remain near the body's surface; convection causes continual removal of the warm layer and replacement with air from the surrounding environment. The wind-chill factor that often is included in the weather report combines the effect of convection due to wind with the still-air temperature.

Evaporation

Evaporation involves the use of body heat to convert water on the skin to water vapor. Water that diffuses through the skin independent of sweating is called *insensible perspiration*. Insensible perspiration losses are greatest in a dry environment. Sweating occurs through the sweat glands and is controlled by the sympathetic nervous system. Unlike other sympathetically mediated functions, in which the catecholamines serve as neuromediators, sweating is mediated by acetylcholine. This means that anticholinergic drugs, such as atropine, can interfere with heat loss by interrupting sweating.

Evaporative heat losses involve insensible perspiration and sweating, with 0.58 calories being lost for each gram of water that is evaporated.[1] As long as body temperature is greater than the atmospheric temperature, heat is lost through radiation. However, when the temperature of the surrounding environment becomes greater than skin temperature, evaporation is the only way the body can rid itself of heat. Any condition that prevents evaporative heat losses causes the body temperature to rise.

In summary, body temperature is normally maintained within a range of 36.0°C to 37.4°C (97.0°F to 99.5°F). Most of the body's heat is produced by metabolic processes that occur within deeper core structures (*i.e.,* muscles and viscera) of the body. Heat loss occurs at the body's surface when heat from core structures is transported to the skin by the circulating blood. Heat is lost from the body through radiation, conduction, convection, and evaporation. The thermoregulatory center in the hypothalamus functions to modify heat production and heat losses as a means of regulating body temperature.

Increased Body Temperature

After you have completed this section of the chapter, you should be able to meet the following objectives:

◆ Characterize the mechanisms involved in body heat production and heat loss
◆ Describe the four stages of fever
◆ Explain what is meant by intermittent, remittent, sustained, and relapsing fevers

+ State the relation between body temperature and heart rate
+ Differentiate between the physiologic mechanisms involved in fever and hyperthermia
+ State the criteria for high-risk status of children 0 to 36 months of age
+ State the definition for fever in the elderly and cite possible mechanisms for altered febrile response in the elderly
+ Compare the characteristics of fevers caused by infectious agents and drug-related fevers
+ Compare the mechanisms of malignant hyperthermia and neuroleptic malignant syndrome

Both fever and hyperthermia describe conditions in which body temperature is higher than the normal range. However, true fever is due to an upward displacement of the hypothalamic set point for temperature control, whereas in hyperthermia, the set point is unchanged, but the mechanisms that control body temperature are ineffective in maintaining body temperature within a normal range during situations when heat production may be excessive (*i.e.*, strenuous exercise) or when there is exposure to high ambient temperature.

FEVER

The literature on fever dates back to the writings of Hippocrates, which contain many descriptions of febrile-course diseases, such as typhoid fever.[8] However, it was not until the development of the thermometer that measurements of body temperature became possible. One of the first studies of body temperature was reported in 1868 by the German physician Carl Wunderlich, who, during a 20-year period, studied the body temperature of 25,000 patients with observations made twice daily with a foot-long thermometer held in the axilla for 20 minutes.[9] Wunderlich observed that the thermometer was a useful instrument for providing insight into the condition of the ill person. Today, temperature is one of the most frequent physiologic responses to be monitored during illness.

Mechanisms

Fever, or *pyrexia*, describes an elevation in body temperature that is caused by a cytokine-induced upward displacement of the set point of the hypothalamic thermoregulatory center. Fever is resolved or "broken" when the factor that caused the increase in the set point is removed. Fevers that are regulated by the hypothalamus usually do not rise above 41°C (105.8°F), suggesting a built-in thermostatic safety mechanism. Temperatures above that level are usually the result of superimposed activity, such as convulsions, hyperthermic states, or direct impairment of the temperature control center.

Fever can be caused by a number of microorganisms and substances that are collectively called *exogenous pyrogens* (Fig. 10-4). Exogenous pyrogens induce host cells to produce fever-producing mediators called *endogenous pyrogens*. Research has identified at least three chemical substances that act as endogenous pyrogens: interleukin-1, interleukin-

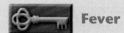

Fever

➤ Fever is an increase in body temperature (due to vasoconstriction and shivering) in response to a cytokine-induced increase in the hypothalamic set point.

➤ Fever is an adaptive response to bacterial and viral infections or to tissue injury. The growth rate of microorganisms is inhibited and immune function is enhanced.

➤ Infection or tissue injury (exogenous pyrogens) stimulates a release of endogenous pyrogens from host macrophages or endothelial cells.

➤ Endogenous pyrogens induce the production of prostaglandins in the hypothalamus, which causes an increase in temperature set point.

➤ In response to the increase in set point, the hypothalamus initiates physiologic responses to increase core temperature to match the new set point.

6, and tumor necrosis factor.[10] These chemical mediators, also known as *cytokines*, are synthesized by a number of body cell types, including endothelial cells, epithelial cells, lymphocytes, fibroblasts, and macrophages. The endogenous pyrogens increase the set point of the hypothalamic thermoregulatory center, possibly through the action of

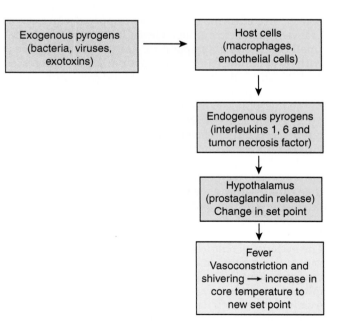

FIGURE 10-4 Mechanisms of fever production.

prostaglandin E. In response to the increase in set point, the hypothalamus neurally initiates shivering and vasoconstriction that increase the core body temperature to the new set point, and fever is established. In addition to their fever-producing actions, the endogenous pyrogens mediate a number of other responses. For example, interleukin-1 is an inflammatory mediator that produces other signs of inflammation such as leukocytosis, anorexia, and malaise (see Chapter 18).

Many noninfectious disorders, such as myocardial infarction, pulmonary emboli, and neoplasms, produce fever. In these conditions, the injured or abnormal cells incite the production of endogenous pyrogen. For example, trauma and surgery can be associated with up to 3 days of fever. Some malignant cells, such as those of leukemia and Hodgkin's disease, secrete endogenous pyrogen.

A fever that has its origin in the central nervous system is sometimes referred to as a *neurogenic fever*. It usually is caused by damage to the hypothalamus due to central nervous system trauma, intracerebral bleeding, or an increase in intracranial pressure. Neurogenic fevers are characterized by a high temperature that is resistant to antipyretic therapy and is not associated with sweating.

Purpose

The purpose of fever is not completely understood. However, from a purely practical standpoint, fever is a valuable index to health status. For many, fever signals the presence of an infection and may legitimize the need for medical treatment. In ancient times, fever was thought to "cook" the poisons that caused the illness. With the availability of antipyretic drugs in the late 19th century, the belief that fever was useful began to wane, probably because most antipyretic drugs also had analgesic effects.

There is little research to support the belief that fever is harmful unless the temperature rises above 40°C (104°F). Animal studies have demonstrated a clear survival advantage in infected members with fever compared with animals that were unable to produce a fever. It has been shown that small elevations in temperature such as those that occur with fever enhance immune function. There is increased motility and activity of the white blood cells, stimulation of interferon production, and activation of T cells.[10,11] Many of the microbial agents that cause infection grow best at normal body temperatures, and their growth is inhibited by temperatures in the fever range. For example, the rhinoviruses responsible for the common cold are cultured best at 33°C (91.4°F), which is close to the temperature in the nasopharynx; temperature-sensitive mutants of the virus that cannot grow at temperatures above 37.5°C (99.5°F) produce fewer signs and symptoms.[12]

Patterns

The patterns of temperature change in persons with fever vary and may provide information about the nature of the causative agent.[13–15] These patterns can be described as intermittent, remittent, sustained, or relapsing. An *intermittent fever* is one in which temperature returns to normal at least once every 24 hours. In a *remittent fever*, the temperature does not return to normal and varies a few degrees in either direction. In a *sustained* or *continuous fever*, the temperature remains above normal with minimal variations (usually less than 0.55°C or 1°F). A *recurrent* or *relapsing fever* is one in which there is one or more episodes of fever, each as long as several days, with one or more days of normal temperature between episodes.

Critical to the analysis of a fever pattern is the relation of heart rate to the level of temperature elevation. Normally, a 1°C rise in temperature produces a 15-bpm (beats per minute) increase in heart rate (1°F, 10 bpm).[13] Most persons respond to an increase in temperature with an appropriate increase in heart rate. The observation that a rise in temperature is not accompanied by the anticipated change in heart rate can provide useful information about the cause of the fever. For example, a heart rate that is slower than would be anticipated can occur with Legionnaires' disease and drug fever, and a heart rate that is more rapid than anticipated can be symptomatic of hyperthyroidism and pulmonary emboli.

Manifestations

The physiologic behaviors that occur during the development of fever can be divided into four successive stages: a prodrome; a chill, during which the temperature rises; a flush; and defervescence (Fig. 10-5). During the *first* or *prodromal* period, there are nonspecific complaints such as mild headache and fatigue, general malaise, and fleeting aches and pains. During the *second stage* or *chill*, there is the uncomfortable sensation of being chilled and the onset of generalized shaking, although the temperature is rising. Vasoconstriction and piloerection usually precede the onset of shivering. At this point the skin is pale and covered with goose flesh. There is a feeling of being cold and an urge to put on more clothing or covering and to curl up in a position that conserves body heat. When the shivering has caused the body temperature to reach the new set point of the temperature control center, the shivering ceases, and a sensation of warmth develops. At this point, the *third stage* or *flush* begins, during which cutaneous vasodilation occurs and the skin becomes warm and flushed. The *fourth*, or *defervescence*, stage of the febrile response is marked by the ini-

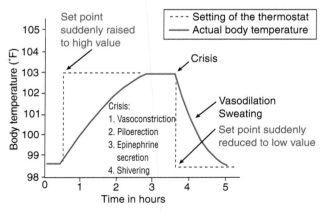

FIGURE 10-5 Effects of changing the set point of the hypothalamic temperature controller. (Guyton A.C., Hall J.E. [2000]. *Textbook of medical physiology* [10th ed., p. 831]. Philadelphia: W.B. Saunders)

tiation of sweating. Not all persons proceed through the four stages of fever development. Sweating may be absent, and fever may develop gradually with no indication of a chill or shivering.

Common manifestations of fever are anorexia, myalgia, arthralgia, and fatigue. These discomforts are worse when the temperature rises rapidly or exceeds 39.5°C (103.1°F). Respiration is increased, and the heart rate usually is elevated. Dehydration occurs because of sweating and the increased vapor losses due to the rapid respiratory rate. The occurrence of chills commonly coincides with the introduction of pyrogen into the circulation. Many of the manifestations of fever are related to the increases in the metabolic rate, increased need for oxygen, and use of body proteins as an energy source. During fever, the body switches from using glucose (an excellent medium for bacterial growth) to metabolism based on protein and fat breakdown.[16] With prolonged fever, there is increased breakdown of endogenous fat stores. If fat breakdown is rapid, metabolic acidosis may result (see Chapter 32).

Headache is a common accompaniment of fever and is thought to result from the vasodilation of cerebral vessels occurring with fever. Delirium is possible when the temperature exceeds 40°C (104°F). In the elderly, confusion and delirium may follow moderate elevations in temperature. Owing to increasingly poor oxygen uptake by the aging lung, pulmonary function may prove to be a limiting factor in the hypermetabolism that accompanies fever in older persons. Confusion, incoordination, and agitation commonly reflect cerebral hypoxemia. Febrile convulsions can occur in some children.[17] They usually occur with rapidly rising temperatures or at a threshold temperature that differs with each child.

The herpetic lesions, or fever blisters, that develop in some persons during fever are caused by a separate infection by the type 1 herpes simplex virus that established latency in the regional ganglia and is reactivated by a rise in body temperature.

Diagnosis and Treatment

Fever usually is a manifestation of a disease state, and as such, determining the cause of a fever is an important aspect of its treatment. For example, fevers from infectious diseases usually are treated with antibiotics, whereas other fevers, such as those resulting from a noninfectious inflammatory condition, may be treated symptomatically.

Sometimes it is difficult to establish the cause of a fever. A prolonged fever for which the cause is difficult to ascertain is often referred to as *fever of unknown origin* (FUO). FUO is defined as a temperature elevation of 38.3°C (101°F) or higher that is present for 3 weeks or longer.[18] Among the causes of FUO are malignancies (*i.e.*, lymphomas, metastases to the liver and central nervous system); infections such as human immunodeficiency virus or tuberculosis, or abscessed infections; and drug fever. Malignancies, particularly non-Hodgkin's lymphoma, are important causes of FUO in the elderly. Cirrhosis of the liver is another cause of FUO.

The methods of fever treatment focus on modifications of the external environment intended to increase heat transfer from the internal to the external environment, support of the hypermetabolic state that accompanies fever, protection of vulnerable body organs and systems, and treatment of the infection or condition causing the fever. Because fever is a disease symptom, its manifestation suggests the need for treatment of the primary cause.

Modification of the environment ensures that the environmental temperature facilitates heat transfer away from the body. Sponge baths with cool water or an alcohol solution can be used to increase evaporative heat losses. More profound cooling can be accomplished through the use of a cooling mattress, which facilitates the conduction of heat from the body into the coolant solution that circulates through the mattress. Care must be taken so that cooling methods do not produce vasoconstriction and shivering that decrease heat loss and increase heat production.

Adequate fluids and sufficient amounts of simple carbohydrates are needed to support the hypermetabolic state and prevent the tissue breakdown that is characteristic of fever. Additional fluids are needed for sweating and to balance the insensible water losses from the lungs that accompany an increase in respiratory rate. Fluids also are needed to maintain an adequate vascular volume for heat transport to the skin surface.

Antipyretic drugs, such as aspirin and acetaminophen, often are used to alleviate the discomforts of fever and protect vulnerable organs, such as the brain, from extreme elevations in body temperature. These drugs act by resetting the hypothalamic temperature control center to a lower level, presumably by blocking the activity of cyclo-oxygenase, an enzyme that is required for the conversion of arachidonic acid to prostaglandin E_2.[19]

Fever in Children

The mechanisms for controlling temperature are not well developed in the infant. In infants younger than 3 months, a mild elevation in temperature (*i.e.*, rectal temperature of 38°C [100.4°F]) can indicate serious infection that requires immediate medical attention.[20,21] Fever without a source occurs frequently in infants and children and is a common reason for visits to the clinic or emergency department. Approximately two thirds of children visit their health care providers with an acute febrile illness before they reach the age of 3 years.[22]

Both minor and life-threatening infections are common in the infant to 3-year age group.[20,21] The most common causes of fever in children are minor or more serious infections of the respiratory system, urinary system, gastrointestinal tract, or central nervous system. Occult bacteremia and meningitis also occur in this age group and should be ruled out. The Agency for Health Care Policy and Research Expert Panel has developed clinical guidelines for use in the treatment of infants and children 0 to 36 months of age with fever without a source.[23] The guidelines define fever in this age group as an elevation in rectal temperature of at least 38°C (100.4°F). The guidelines also point out that fever may result from overbundling or a vaccine reaction. When overbundling is suspected, it is suggested that the infant be unbundled and the temperature retaken after 15 to 30 minutes.

Fever in infants and children can be classified as low risk or high risk, depending on the probability of the infection progressing to bacteremia or meningitis. Signs of toxicity include lethargy, poor feeding, hypoventilation, poor tissue oxygenation, and cyanosis. Infants can be considered low risk if they were delivered at term and sent home with their mother without complications and have been healthy with no previous hospitalizations or previous antimicrobial therapy. A white blood cell count and urinalysis are recommended as a means of confirming low-risk status. Blood and urine cultures, chest radiographs, and lumbar puncture usually are done in high-risk infants and children to determine the cause of fever.

The mean probability of serious bacterial infection in infants younger than 3 months of age is 8.6%, and in children between 3 and 36 months, it is 4.5%.[20,23] Infants with fever who are considered to be low risk usually are managed on an outpatient basis providing the parents or caregivers are deemed reliable. Older children with fever without source also may be treated on an outpatient basis. Parents or caregivers require full instructions, preferably in writing, regarding assessment of the febrile child. They should be instructed to contact their health care provider should their child show signs suggesting sepsis. High-risk infants and infants younger than 28 days usually are hospitalized for evaluation of their fever and treatment. Parenteral antimicrobial therapy usually is initiated after samples for blood, urine, and spinal fluid cultures have been taken.

Fever in the Elderly

In the elderly, even slight elevations in temperature may indicate serious infection or disease. This is because the elderly often have a lower baseline temperature, and although they increase their temperature during an infection, it may fail to reach a level that is equated with significant fever.[24–26]

Normal body temperature and the circadian pattern of temperature variation often are altered in the elderly. Elderly persons are reported to have a lower basal temperature (36.4°C [97.6°F] in one study) than younger persons.[27] It has been recommended that the definition of fever in the elderly be expanded to include an elevation of temperature of at least 1.1°C (2°F) above baseline values.[26]

It has been suggested that 20% to 30% of elders with serious infections present with an absent or blunted febrile response.[26] When fever is present in the elderly, it usually indicates the presence of serious infection, most often caused by bacteria. The absence of fever may delay diagnosis and initiation of antimicrobial treatment. Unexplained change in functional capacity, worsening of mental status, weakness and fatigue, and weight loss are signs of infection in the elderly. They should be viewed as possible signs of infection and sepsis when fever is absent. The probable mechanisms for the blunted fever response include a disturbance in sensing of temperature by the thermoregulatory center in the hypothalamus, alterations in release of endogenous pyrogens, and the failure to elicit responses such as vasoconstriction of skin vessels, increased heat production, and shivering that increase body temperature during a febrile response.

Another factor that may delay recognition of fever in the elderly is the method of temperature measurement. Oral temperature remains the most commonly used method for measuring temperature in the elderly. It has been suggested

that rectal and tympanic membrane methods are more effective in detecting fever in the elderly. This is because conditions such as mouth breathing, tongue tremors, and agitation often make it difficult to obtain accurate oral temperatures in the elderly.

HYPERTHERMIA

Hyperthermia describes an increase in body temperature that occurs without a change in the set point of the hypothalamic thermoregulatory center. It occurs when the thermoregulatory mechanisms are overwhelmed by heat production, excessive environmental heat, or impaired dissipation of heat.[28] It includes (in order of increasing severity) heat cramps, heat syncope, heat exhaustion, and heatstroke. Malignant hyperthermia describes a rare genetic disorder of anesthetic-related hyperthermia. Fever and hyperthermia also may occur as the result of a drug reaction.

A number of factors predispose to hyperthermia. If muscle exertion is continued for long periods in warm weather, as often happens with athletes, military recruits, and laborers, excessive heat loads are generated.[28] Because adequate circulatory function is essential for heat dissipation, elderly persons and those with cardiovascular disease are at increased risk for hyperthermia. Drugs that increase muscle tone and metabolism or reduce heat loss (*e.g.*, diuretics, neuroleptics, drugs with anticholinergic action) can impair thermoregulation. Infants and small children who are left in a closed car for even short periods in hot weather are potential victims of hyperthermia. Florence Nightingale in *Notes on Nursing* observed that an excess of blankets is the most common cause of fever in the hospital.[29]

Heat Cramps

Heat cramps are slow, painful, skeletal muscle cramps and spasms, usually in the muscles that are most heavily used, that last for 1 to 3 minutes. Cramping results from salt depletion that occurs when fluid losses from heavy sweating are replaced by water alone. The muscles are tender, and the

Hyperthermia

➤ Hyperthermia is a pathologic increase in core body temperature without a change in the hypothalamic set point. The thermoregulatory center is overwhelmed by either excess heat production, impaired heat loss, or excessive environmental heat.

➤ Malignant hyperthermia is an autosomal dominant disorder in which an abnormal release of intracellular stores of calcium causes uncontrolled skeletal muscle contractions, resulting in a rapid increase in core body temperature. This usually is in response to an anesthetic.

skin usually is moist. Body temperature may be normal or slightly elevated. There almost always is a history of vigorous activity preceding the onset of symptoms.

Treatment consists of drinking an oral saline solution and resting in a cool environment. Because absorption is slow and unpredictable, salt tablets are not recommended. Salt tablets also can cause gastric irritation, vomiting, and cerebral edema. Strenuous physical activity should be avoided for several days, while dietary sodium replacement is continued.

Heat Syncope

Heat syncope is characterized by a sudden episode of unconsciousness resulting from cutaneous vasodilation and subsequent hypotension. Usually the episode follows vigorous exercise. The systolic blood pressure usually is less than 100 mm Hg, the pulse is weak, and the skin is cool and moist. The treatment consists of recumbency and rest in a cool place and administration of fluids orally or intravenously.

Heat Exhaustion

Heat exhaustion is related to a gradual loss of salt and water, usually after prolonged and heavy exertion in a hot environment. The symptoms include thirst, fatigue, nausea, oliguria, giddiness, and finally delirium. Gastrointestinal flulike symptoms are common. Hyperventilation in association with heat exhaustion may contribute to heat cramps and tetany by causing respiratory alkalosis (see Chapter 32). The skin is moist, the rectal temperature usually is higher than 37.8°C (100°F), and the heart rate is elevated, usually by more than half again the normal resting rate. Signs of heat syncope and heat cramps may accompany heat exhaustion.

Like heat cramps, heat exhaustion is treated by rest in a cool environment, the provision of adequate hydration, and salt replacement. Intravenous fluids are administered when adequate oral intake cannot be achieved.

Heatstroke

Heatstroke is a severe, life-threatening failure of thermoregulatory mechanisms resulting in an excessive rise in body temperature—a core temperature greater than 40°C (104°F), absence of sweating, and loss of consciousness. Evaporation serves as the major mechanism for heat dissipation in a warm environment, and conditions that interrupt this mechanism predispose to increased body temperature and heatstroke.

Heatstroke is seen most commonly in the elderly and disabled. An average of 1700 heatstroke-related deaths occur in the United States every year, with 80% of those deaths occurring in persons 50 years of age and older.[30] In the elderly, the problem often is one of impaired heat loss and failure of homeostatic mechanisms, such that body temperature rises with any increase in environmental temperature. Elderly persons with a decreased ability to perceive changes in environmental temperature or decreased mobility are at particular risk because they also may be unable to take appropriate measures such as removing clothing, moving to a cooler environment, and increasing fluid intake. This is particularly true of elderly persons who live alone in small and poorly ventilated housing units and who may be too confused or weak to complain or seek help at the onset of symptoms.

The symptoms of heatstroke include dizziness, weakness, emotional lability, nausea and vomiting, confusion, delirium, blurred vision, convulsions, collapse, and coma. The skin is hot and usually dry, and the pulse is typically strong initially. The blood pressure may be elevated at first, but hypotension develops as the condition progresses. As vascular collapse occurs, the skin becomes cool. Associated abnormalities include electrocardiographic changes consistent with heart damage, blood coagulation disorders, potassium and sodium depletion, and signs of liver damage.

Treatment consists of rapidly reducing the core temperature. Care must be taken that the cooling methods used do not produce vasoconstriction or shivering and thereby decrease the cooling rate or induce heat production. Two general methods of cooling are used. One method involves submersion in cold water or application of ice packs, and the other involves spraying the body with tepid water while a fan is used to enhance heat dissipation through convection. Whatever method is used, it is important that the temperature of vital structures, such as the brain, heart, and liver, be reduced rapidly, because tissue damage ensues when core temperatures rise above 43°C (109.4°F). Selective brain cooling has been achieved by fanning the face during hyperthermia.[2] Blood flows from the emissary venous pathways of the skin on the head through the bones of the skull to the brain. In hyperthermia, face fanning is thought to cool the venous blood that flows through these emissary veins and thereby produce brain cooling by enhancing heat exchange between the hot arterial blood and the surface-cooled venous blood in the intracranial venous spaces.

Drug Fever

Drug fever has been defined as fever coinciding with the administration of a drug and disappearing after the drug has been discontinued.[31–33] Drugs can induce fever by several mechanisms. They can interfere with heat dissipation; they can alter temperature regulation by the hypothalamic centers; they can act as direct pyrogens; they can injure tissues directly; or they can induce an immune response.[34]

Exogenous thyroid hormone increases metabolic rate and can increase heat production and body temperature. Peripheral heat dissipation can be impaired by atropine, antihistamines, phenothiazines, and tricyclic antidepressants, which decrease sweating, or by sympathomimetic drugs, which produce peripheral vasoconstriction. Cimetidine, a histamine type 2 (H_2)–blocking drug that decreases gastric acid production, also blocks H_2 receptors in the hypothalamus and has been known to cause fever. Bleomycin (an anticancer drug), amphotericin B (an antifungal drug), and allergic extracts and vaccines that contain bacterial and viral products all can act to induce the release of pyrogens. Intravenously administered drugs can lead to infusion-related phlebitis with production of cellular pyrogens that produce fever. Treatment with anticancer drugs can cause the release of endogenous pyrogen from the cancer cells that are destroyed.

The most common cause of drug fever is a *hypersensitivity reaction*. Hypersensitivity drug fevers develop after several weeks of exposure to the drug, cannot be explained in terms of the drug's pharmacologic action, are not related to drug dose, disappear when the drug is stopped, and reappear when the drug is readministered. The fever pattern is typically spiking in nature and exhibits a normal diurnal rhythm. Persons with drug fevers often experience other signs of hypersensitivity reactions, such as arthralgias, urticaria, myalgias, gastrointestinal discomfort, and rashes.

Temperatures of 38.8°C to 40.0°C (102°F to 104°F) are common in drug fever. The person may be unaware of the fever and appear to be well for the degree of fever that is present. The absence of an appropriate increase in heart rate for the degree of temperature elevation is an important clue to the diagnosis of drug fever. A fever often precedes other, more serious effects of a drug reaction; for this reason, the early recognition of drug fever is important. Drug fever should be suspected whenever the temperature elevation is unexpected and occurs despite improvement in the condition for which the drug was prescribed.

Malignant Hyperthermia

Malignant hyperthermia is an autosomal dominant metabolic disorder in which heat generated by uncontrolled skeletal muscle contraction can produce severe and potentially fatal hyperthermia. The muscle contraction is caused by an abnormal release of intracellular calcium from the mitochondria and sarcoplasmic reticulum (see Chapter 4).

In affected persons, an episode of malignant hyperthermia is triggered by exposure to certain stresses or general anesthetic agents. The syndrome most frequently is associated with the halogenated anesthetic agents and the depolarizing muscle relaxant succinylcholine.[35,36] There also are various nonoperative precipitating factors, including trauma, exercise, environmental heat stress, and infection. The condition is particularly dangerous in a young person who has a large muscle mass to generate heat.

During malignant hyperthermia, the body temperature can rise to as high as 43°C (109.4°F) at a rate of 1°C every 5 minutes. An initial sign of the disorder, when the condition occurs during anesthesia, is skeletal muscle rigidity. Cardiac arrhythmias and a hypermetabolic state follow in rapid sequence unless the triggering event is immediately discontinued. In addition to discontinuing the triggering agents, treatment includes measures to cool the body and the administration of dantrolene, a muscle relaxant drug that acts by blocking the release of calcium from the sarcoplasmic reticulum. There is no accurate screening test for the condition. A family history of malignant hyperthermia should be considered when general anesthesia is needed because there are anesthetic agents available that do not trigger the hyperthermic response.

Neuroleptic Malignant Syndrome

Neuroleptic malignant syndrome usually has an explosive onset and is characterized by hyperthermia, muscle rigidity, alterations in consciousness, and autonomic nervous system dysfunction. The hyperthermia is accompanied by tachy-cardia (120 to 180 bpm), cardiac dysrhythmias, labile blood pressure (70/50 to 180/130 mm Hg), postural instability, dyspnea, and tachypnea (18 to 40 breaths/minute).[37] Permanent brain damage may result, and the mortality rate is nearly 30%.[38]

The disorder is associated with neuroleptic (psychotropic) medications and may occur in as many as 1% of persons taking such drugs. Some of the most commonly implicated drugs are haloperidol, chlorpromazine, thioridazine, and thiothixene. All of these drugs block dopamine receptors in the basal ganglia and hypothalamus. Hyperthermia is thought to result from alterations in the function of the hypothalamic thermoregulatory center caused by decreased dopamine levels or from uncontrolled muscle contraction like that occurring with anesthetic-induced malignant hyperthermia. Many of the neuroleptic drugs increase muscle contraction, suggesting that this mechanism may contribute to the neuroleptic malignant syndrome.

Treatment for neuroleptic malignant syndrome includes the immediate discontinuance of the neuroleptic drug, measures to decrease body temperature, and treatment of dysrhythmias and other complications of the disorder. Bromocriptine (a dopamine agonist) and dantrolene (a muscle relaxant) may be used as part of the treatment regimen.

In summary, fever and hyperthermia refer to an increase in body temperature outside the normal range. True fever is a disorder of thermoregulation in which there is an upward displacement of the set point for temperature control. In hyperthermia, the set point is unchanged, but the challenge to temperature regulation exceeds the thermoregulatory center's ability to control body temperature. Fever can be caused by a number of factors, including microorganisms, trauma, and drugs or chemicals, all of which incite the release of endogenous pyrogens. The reactions that occur during fever consist of four stages: a prodrome, a chill, a flush, and defervescence. A fever can follow an intermittent, remittent, sustained, or recurrent pattern. The manifestations of fever are largely related to dehydration and an increased metabolic rate. Even a low-grade fever in high-risk infants or in the elderly can indicate serious infection.

The treatment of fever focuses on modifying the external environment as a means of increasing heat transfer to the external environment; supporting the hypermetabolic state that accompanies fever; protecting vulnerable body tissues; and treating the infection or condition causing the fever.

Hyperthermia includes heat syncope, heat cramps, heat exhaustion, and heatstroke. Among the factors that contribute to the development of hyperthermia are prolonged muscular exertion in a hot environment, disorders that compromise heat dissipation, and hypersensitivity drug reactions. Malignant hyperthermia is an autosomal dominant disorder that can produce a severe and potentially fatal increase in body temperature. The condition commonly is triggered by general anesthetic agents and muscle relaxants used during surgery. The neuroleptic malignant syndrome is associated with neuroleptic drug therapy and is thought to result from alterations in the function of the thermoregulatory center or from uncontrolled muscle contraction.

Decreased Body Temperature

After you have completed this section of the chapter, you should be able to meet the following objectives:

✦ Define *hypothermia*
✦ Compare the manifestations of mild, moderate, and severe hypothermia and relate them to changes in physiologic functioning that occur with decreased body temperature

HYPOTHERMIA

Hypothermia is defined as a core temperature (*i.e.*, rectal, esophageal, or tympanic) less than 35°C.[39] Core body temperatures in the range of 34°C to 35°C (93.2°F to 95°F) are considered mildly hypothermic; 30°C to 34°C (86°F to 93.2°F), moderately hypothermic; and less than 30°C (86°F), severely hypothermic.[39] In the United States from 1979 to 1995, an average of 723 deaths per year were attributable to hypothermia.[40]

Accidental hypothermia may be defined as a spontaneous decrease in core temperature, usually in a cold environment and associated with an acute problem but without a primary disorder of the temperature-regulating center. The term *submersion hypothermia* is used when cooling follows acute asphyxia, as occurs in drowning.[41] In children, the rapid cooling process, in addition to the diving reflex that triggers apnea and circulatory shunting to establish a heart–brain circulation (see Chapter 21), may account for the surprisingly high survival rate after submersion. The diving reflex is greatly diminished in adults. Children have been reported to survive 10 to 40 minutes of submersion asphyxia.[42,43] Controlled hypothermia may be used during certain types of surgeries to decrease brain metabolism.

Oral temperatures are markedly inaccurate during hypothermia because of severe vasoconstriction and sluggish blood flow. Electronic thermometers with flexible probes are available for measuring rectal, bladder, and esophageal temperatures. However, rectal and bladder temperatures often lag behind fluctuations in core temperature, and esophageal temperatures may be elevated during inhalation of heated air.[44] Most clinical thermometers measure temperature only in the range of 35°C to 42°C (95°F to 107.6°F); a special thermometer that registers as low as 25°C (77°F) or an electrical thermistor probe is needed for monitoring temperatures in persons with hypothermia.

Systemic hypothermia may result from exposure to prolonged cold (atmospheric or submersion). The condition may develop in otherwise healthy persons in the course of accidental exposure. Because water conducts heat more readily than air, body temperature drops rapidly when the body is submerged in cold water or when clothing becomes wet. In persons with altered homeostasis due to debility or disease, hypothermia may follow exposure to relatively small decreases in atmospheric temperature.

Elderly and inactive persons living in inadequately heated quarters are particularly vulnerable to hypothermia. Acute alcoholism is a common predisposing factor. Persons with cardiovascular disease, cerebrovascular disease, malnutrition, and hypothyroidism also are predisposed to hypothermia. The use of sedatives and tranquilizing drugs may be a contributing factor.[45]

Manifestations

The signs and symptoms of hypothermia include poor coordination, stumbling, slurred speech, irrationality and poor judgment, amnesia, hallucinations, blueness and puffiness of the skin, dilation of the pupils, decreased respiratory rate, weak and irregular pulse, and stupor. With mild hypothermia, intense shivering generates heat and sympathetic nervous system activity is raised to resist lowering of temperature. Vasoconstriction can be profound, heart rate is accelerated, and stroke volume is increased. Blood pressure increases slightly, and hyperventilation is common. Exposure to cold augments urinary flow (*i.e.*, cold diuresis) before there is any fall in temperature. Dehydration and increased hematocrit may develop within a few hours of even mild hypothermia, augmented by an extracellular-to-intracellular water shift.

With moderate hypothermia, shivering gradually decreases, and the muscles become rigid. Shivering usually ceases at 27°C (80.6°F). Heart rate and stroke volume are reduced, and blood pressure falls. The greatest effect of hypothermia is exerted through a decrease in the metabolic rate, which falls to 50% of normal at 28°C (82.4°F).[46] Associated with this decrease in metabolic rate is a decrease in oxygen consumption and carbon dioxide production. There is roughly a 6% decrease in oxygen consumption for every 1°C decrease in temperature. A decrease in carbon dioxide production leads to a decrease in respiratory rate. Respirations decrease as temperatures drop below 32.2°C (90°F). Decreases in mentation, the cough reflex, and respiratory tract secretions may lead to difficulty in clearing secretions and aspiration. Consciousness usually is lost at 30°C (86°F).[46]

In terms of cardiovascular function, a gradual decline in heart rate and cardiac output occurs as hypothermia

Hypothermia

➤ Hypothermia is a pathologic decrease in core body temperature without a change in the hypothalamic set point.

➤ The compensatory physiologic responses meant to produce heat (shivering) and retain heat (vasoconstriction) are overwhelmed by unprotected exposure to cold environments.

progresses. Blood pressure initially rises and then gradually falls. There is increased risk of dysrhythmia developing, probably from myocardial hypoxia and autonomic nervous system imbalance. Ventricular fibrillation is a major cause of death in hypothermia.

Carbohydrate metabolism and insulin activity are decreased, resulting in a hyperglycemia that is proportional to the level of cooling. A cold-induced loss of cell membrane integrity allows intravascular fluids to move into the skin, giving the skin a puffy appearance. Acid-base disorders occur with increased frequency at temperatures below 25°C (77°F) unless adequate ventilation is maintained. Extracellular sodium and potassium concentrations decrease, and chloride levels increase. There is a temporary loss of plasma from the circulation along with sludging of red blood cells and increased blood viscosity as the result of trapping in the small vessels and skin.

Treatment

The treatment of hypothermia consists of rewarming, support of vital functions, and the prevention and treatment of complications.[47] There are three methods of rewarming: passive rewarming, active total rewarming, and active core rewarming. *Passive rewarming* is done by removing the person from the cold environment, covering with a blanket, supplying warm fluids (oral or intravenous), and allowing rewarming to occur at the person's own pace. *Active total rewarming* involves immersing the person in warm water or placing heating pads or hot water bottles on the surface of the body, including the extremities. Active core rewarming places major emphasis on rewarming the trunk, leaving the extremities, containing the major metabolic mass, cold until the heart rewarms. *Active core rewarming* can be done by instilling warmed fluids into the gastrointestinal tract; peritoneal dialysis; by extracorporeal blood warming, in which blood is removed from the body and passed through a heat exchanger and then returned to the body; or by inhalation of an oxygen mixture warmed to 42°C to 46°C (107.6°F to 114.8°F).

Persons with mild hypothermia usually respond well to passive rewarming in a warm bed. Persons with moderate or severe hypothermia do not have the thermoregulatory shivering mechanism and require active rewarming. During rewarming, the cold acidotic blood from the peripheral tissues is returned to the heart and central circulation. If this is done too rapidly or before cardiopulmonary function has been adequately reestablished, the hypothermic heart cannot respond to the increased metabolic demands of warm peripheral tissues.

In summary, hypothermia is a potentially life-threatening disorder in which the body's core temperature drops below 35°C (95°F). Accidental hypothermia can develop in otherwise healthy persons in the course of accidental exposure and in elderly or disabled persons with impaired perception of or response to cold. Alcoholism, cardiovascular disease, malnutrition, and hypothyroidism contribute to the risk of hypothermia. The greatest effect of hypothermia is a decrease in the metabolic rate, leading to a decrease in carbon dioxide production and respiratory rate. The signs and symptoms of hypothermia include poor coordination, stumbling, slurred speech, irrationality, poor judgment, amnesia, hallucinations, blueness and puffiness of the skin, dilation of the pupils, decreased respiratory rate, weak and irregular pulse, stupor, and coma. The treatment for moderate and severe hypothermia includes active rewarming.

Related Web Sites

Agency for Healthcare Research and Quality—most recent clinical guidelines for treatment of fever   www.ahrq.gov
Centers for Disease Control and Prevention—most recent statistics on infectious diseases   www.cdc.gov
Emergency Nursing World   www.enw.org
Malignant Hyperthermia Organization of the United States   www.mhaus.org
Search and Rescue Society of British Columbia   www.sarbc.org/hypo.html

References

1. Guyton A.C., Hall J.E. (2000). *Textbook of medical physiology* (10th ed., pp. 822–833). Philadelphia: W.B. Saunders.
2. Gisolfi C.V., Mora F. (2000). *The hot brain: Survival, temperature, and the human body*. Cambridge, MA: MIT Press.
3. Vick R. (1984). *Contemporary medical physiology* (p. 886). Menlo Park, CA: Addison Wesley.
4. Erickson R.S. (1999). The continuing question of how best to measure body temperature. *Critical Care Medicine* 27, 2307–2314.
5. Beach P.S., McCormick D.P. (1991). Clinical applications of ear thermometry [Editorial]. *Clinical Pediatrics* (Suppl. 4), 3–4.
6. Knies R.B. (1998). Research applied to clinical practice: Temperature measurements in acute care. [On-line.] Available: http://www.ENW.org/Research-Thermometry.htm.
7. Jansky L. (1998). Shivering. In Blatteis C.M. (Ed.), *Physiology and pathophysiology of temperature regulation* (pp. 48–58). River Edge, NJ: World Scientific Publishing.
8. Atkins L. (1984). Fever: The old and new. *Journal of Infectious Diseases* 149, 339–348.
9. Stein M.T. (1991). Historical perspectives in fever and thermometry. *Clinical Pediatrics* (Suppl. 4), 5–7.
10. Mackowiak P.A. (1998). Concepts of fever. *Archives of Internal Medicine* 158, 1870–1881.
11. Blatteis C.M. (1998). Fever. In Blatteis C.M. (Ed.), *Physiology and pathophysiology of temperature regulation* (pp. 178–192). River Edge, NJ: World Scientific Publishing.
12. Rodbard D. (1981). The role of regional temperature in the pathogenesis of disease. *New England Journal of Medicine* 305, 808–814.
13. McGee Z.A., Gorby G.L. (1987). The diagnostic value of fever patterns. *Hospital Practice* 22(10), 103–110.
14. Cunha B.A. (1984). Implications of fever in the critical care setting. *Heart and Lung* 13, 460–465.
15. Cunha B.A. (1996). The clinical significance of fever patterns. *Infectious Disease Clinics of North America* 10, 33–43.
16. Saper C.B., Breder C.D. (1994). The neurologic basis of fever. *New England Journal of Medicine* 330, 1880–1886.
17. Champi C., Gaffney-Yocum P.A. (1999). Managing febrile seizures in children. *Nurse Practitioner* 24 (10), 28–30, 34–35.

18. Cunha B.A. (1996). Fever without source. *Infectious Disease Clinics of North America* 10, 111–127.
19. Plaisance K.I., Mackowiak P.A. (2000). Antipyretic therapy: Physiologic rationale, diagnostic implications, and clinical consequences. *Archives of Internal Medicine* 160, 449–456.
20. Baker M.D. (1999). Evaluation and management of infants with fever. *Pediatric Clinics of North America* 46, 1061–1072.
21. Park J.W. (2000). Fever without source in children. *Postgraduate Medicine* 107, 259–266.
22. Daaleman T.P. (1996). Fever without source in infants and young children. *American Family Physician* 54, 2503–2512.
23. Baraff L.J., Bass J.W., Fleisher G.R., Klein J.O., McCracken G.H. Jr., Powell K.R., Schriger D.L. (1993). Practice guidelines for the management of infants and children 0 to 36 months of age with fever without source. Agency for Health Care Policy and Research. (Erratum appears in *Ann Emerg Med.* [1993]. 22(9), 1490). *Annals of Emergency Medicine* 22(7), 1198–1210.
24. Castle S.C., Norman D.C., Yeh M., Miller D., Yoshikawa T.T. (1991). Fever response in elderly nursing home residents: Are the older truly colder? *Journal of the American Geriatric Society* 39(9), 853–857.
25. Yoshikawa T.T., Norman D.C. (1996). Approach to fever and infections in the nursing home. *Journal of the American Geriatric Society* 44, 74–82.
26. Yoshikawa T.T., Norman, D.C. (1998). Fever in the elderly. *Infectious Medicine* 15, 704–706, 708.
27. Castle S.C., Yeh M., Toledo S., et al. (1993). Lowering the temperature criterion improves detection of infections in nursing home residents. *Aging Immunology and Infectious Disease* 4, 67–76.
28. Khosla R., Guntupalli K.K. (1999). Heat-related illnesses. *Critical Care Clinics* 15, 251–263.
29. Nightingale F. (1970). *Notes on nursing* (p. 45). London: Brandon Systems Press.
30. Ballester J.M., Harchelroad F.P. (1999). Hyperthermia: How to recognize and prevent heat-related illnesses. *Geriatrics* 54 (7), 20–24.
31. Tabor P.A. (1986). Drug-induced fever. *Drug Intelligence and Clinical Pharmacy* 20, 413–420.
32. Mackowiak P.A., LeMaistre C.F. (1986). Drug fever: A critical appraisal of conventional concepts. *Annals of Internal Medicine* 106, 728–733.
33. Hofland S.L. (1985). Drug fever: Is your patient's fever drug-related? *Critical Care Nurse* 5, 29–34.
34. Johnson D.H., Cunha B.A. (1996). Drug fever. *Infectious Disease Clinics of North America* 10, 85–99.
35. Jurkat-Rott K., McCarthy T., Lehmann-Horn F. (2000). Genetics and pathogenesis of malignant hyperthermia. *Muscle and Nerve* 23, 4–17.
36. Denborough M. (1998). Malignant hyperthermia. *Lancet* 352, 1131–1136.
37. Parker W.A. (1987). Neuroleptic malignant syndrome. *Critical Care Nurse* 7, 40–46.
38. Goldwasser H.D., Hooper J.F. (1988). Neuroleptic malignant syndrome. *American Family Practice* 38 (5), 211–216.
39. Mercer J.B. (1998). Hypothermia and cold injuries in man. In Blatteis C.M. (Ed.), *Physiology and pathophysiology of temperature regulation* (pp. 246–256). River Edge, NJ: World Scientific Publishing.
40. Centers for Disease Control and Prevention. (1998). Hypothermia-related deaths, Georgia—January 1996–December 1997, and United States, 1979–1995. *Morbidity and Mortality Weekly Reports* 47, 1037.
41. Conn A.W. (1979). Near drowning and hypothermia. *Canadian Medical Association Journal* 120, 397–400.
42. Siebke H., Beivik H., Rod T. (1975). Survival after 40 minutes submersion with cerebral sequelae. *Lancet* 1, 1275–1277.
43. Moss J.F. (1988). The management of accidental severe hypothermia. *New York Journal of Medicine* 88, 411–413.
44. Danzl D.F., Pozos R.S. (1994). Accidental hypothermia. *New England Journal of Medicine* 331, 1756–1760.
45. Ballester J.M., Harchelroad F.P. (1999). Hypothermia: An easy-to-miss, dangerous disorder in winter weather. *Geriatrics* 54 (2), 51–57.
46. Wong K.C. (1983). Physiology and pharmacology of hypothermia. *Western Journal of Medicine* 138, 227–232.
47. Hanania N.A., Zimmerman J.L. (1999). Accidental hypothermia. *Critical Care Clinics* 15, 235–249.

Chapter 11

Alterations in Nutritional Status

Joan Pleuss

"You are what you eat" is a familiar maxim. To a great extent, nutrition determines how a person looks, feels, and acts. The need for adequate nutrition begins at the time of conception and continues throughout life. Nutrition provided by food or supplements in the proper proportions enables the body to maintain life, to grow physically and intellectually, to heal and repair tissue, and to maintain the stamina necessary for well-being. This chapter addresses nutritional status, overnutrition and obesity, and undernutrition.

Nutritional Status

After you have completed this section of the chapter, you should be able to meet the following objectives:

✦ Define *nutritional status*
✦ Define *calorie* and state the number of calories derived from the oxidation of 1 g of protein, fat, or carbohydrate

✦ Explain the difference between anabolism and catabolism
✦ Relate the processes of glycogenolysis and gluconeogenesis to the regulation of blood glucose by the liver
✦ Define *basal metabolic rate* and cite factors that affect it
✦ State the purpose of the Recommended Dietary Allowance of calories, proteins, fats, carbohydrates, vitamins, and minerals
✦ Describe methods used for a nutritional assessment
✦ State the factors used in determining body mass index and explain its use in evaluating body weight in terms of undernutrition and overnutrition

Nutritional status describes the condition of the body related to the availability and use of nutrients. Nutrients provide the energy and materials necessary for performing the activities of daily living; for maintaining healthy skin, muscles, and other body tissues; for replacing and healing tissues; and for the effective functioning of all body systems, including the immune and respiratory systems. Poor nutritional status can cause illness and prevent recuperation from illness.

Nutrients are derived from the digestive tract through the ingestion of foods or, in some cases, through liquid feedings that are delivered directly into the gastrointestinal tract by a synthetic tube (*i.e.*, tube feedings). The exception occurs in persons with certain illnesses in which the digestive tract is bypassed and the nutrients are infused directly into the circulatory system. Once inside the body, nutrients are used for energy or as the building blocks for tissue growth and repair. When excess nutrients are available, they frequently are stored for future use. If the required nutrients are unavailable, the body adapts by conserving and using its nutrient stores.

ENERGY METABOLISM

Energy is measured in heat units called *calories*. A calorie, spelled with a small *c* and also called a *gram calorie*, is the amount of heat or energy required to raise the temperature of 1 g of water by 1°C. A *kilocalorie* (kcal), or *large calorie*, is the amount of energy needed to raise the temperature of 1 kg of water by 1°C. Because a calorie is so small, kilocalories often are used in nutritional and physiologic studies. The oxidation of proteins provides 4 kcal/g; fats, 9 kcal/g; carbohydrates, 4 kcal/g, and alcohol, 7 kcal/g.

All body activities require energy, whether they involve an individual cell, a single organ, or the entire body. *Metabolism* is the organized process through which nutrients such as carbohydrates, fats, and proteins are broken down, transformed, or otherwise converted into cellular energy. The process of metabolism is unique in that it enables the continual release of energy, and it couples this energy with physiologic functioning. For example, the energy used for muscle contraction is derived largely from energy sources that are stored in muscle cells and then released as the muscle contracts. Because most of our energy sources come from the nutrients in the food that is eaten, the ability to store energy and control its release is important.

Adipose Tissue

More than 90% of body energy is stored in the adipose tissues of the body. Adipocytes, or fat cells, occur singly or in small groups in loose connective tissue. In many parts of the body, they cushion body organs such as the kidneys. In addition to isolated groups of fat cells, entire regions of fat tissue are committed to fat storage. Collectively, fat cells constitute a large body organ that is metabolically active in the uptake, synthesis, storage, and mobilization of lipids, which are the main source of fuel storage for the body. Some tissues, such as liver cells, are able to store small amounts of lipids, but when these lipids accumulate, they begin to interfere with cell function. Adipose tissue not only serves as a storage site for body fuels, it provides insulation for the body, fills body crevices, and protects body organs.

Studies of adipocytes in the laboratory have shown that fully differentiated cells do not divide. However, such cells have a long life span, and anyone born with large numbers of adipocytes runs the risk of becoming obese. Some im-

Energy Metabolism

➤ All body activities require energy, whether they involve a single cell, a single organ, or the entire body.

➤ Energy, which is measured in kilocalories (kcal), is obtained from foods.

➤ Fats, which are a concentrated water-free energy source, contain 9 kcal/g. They are stored in fat cells as triglycerides, which are the main storage sites for energy.

➤ Carbohydrates are hydrated fuels, which supply 4 kcal/g. They are stored in limited quantities as glycogen and can be converted to fatty acids and stored in fat cells as triglycerides.

➤ Amino acids, which supply 4 kcal/g, are used in building body proteins. Amino acids in excess of those needed for protein synthesis are converted to fatty acids, ketones, or glucose and are stored or used as metabolic fuel.

mature adipocytes capable of division are present in postnatal life; these cells respond to estrogen stimulation and are the potential source of additional fat cells during postnatal life.[1] Fat deposition results from proliferation of these existing immature adipocytes and can occur as a consequence of excessive caloric intake when a woman is breastfeeding or during estrogen stimulation around the time of puberty. An increase in fat cells also may occur during late adolescence and in middle-aged persons who already are overweight.

There are two types of adipose tissue: white fat and brown fat. White fat, which despite its name is cream colored or yellow, is the prevalent form of adipose tissue in postnatal life. It constitutes 10% to 20% of body weight in adult males and 15% to 25% in adult females. At body temperature, the lipid content of fat cells exists as an oil. It consists of triglycerides, which are three molecules of fatty acids esterified to a glycerol molecule. Triglycerides, which contain no water, have the highest caloric content of all nutrients and are an efficient form of energy storage. Fat cells synthesize triglycerides, the major fat storage form, from dietary fats and carbohydrates. Insulin is required for transport of glucose into fat cells. When calorie intake is restricted for any reason, fat cell triglycerides are broken down, and the resultant fatty acids and glycerol are released as energy sources.

Brown fat differs from white fat in terms of its thermogenic capacity or ability to produce heat. Brown fat, the site of diet-induced thermogenesis and nonshivering thermogenesis, is found primarily in early neonatal life in humans and in animals that hibernate. In humans, brown fat decreases with age but is still detectable in the sixth decade.

This small amount of brown fat has a minimal effect on energy expenditure.

Anabolism and Catabolism

There are two phases of metabolism: anabolism and catabolism. *Anabolism* is the phase of metabolic storage and synthesis of cell constituents. Anabolism does not provide energy for the body; it requires energy. *Catabolism* involves the breakdown of complex molecules into substances that can be used in the production of energy. The chemical intermediates for anabolism and catabolism are called *metabolites* (*e.g.*, lactic acid is a metabolite formed when glucose is broken down in the absence of oxygen). Both anabolism and catabolism are catalyzed by enzyme systems located in body cells. A substrate is a substance on which an enzyme acts. Enzyme systems selectively transform fuel substrates into cellular energy and facilitate the use of energy in the process of assembling molecules to form energy substrates and storage forms of energy.

Because body energy cannot be stored as heat, the cellular oxidative processes that release energy are low-temperature reactions that convert food components to chemical energy that can be stored. The body transforms carbohydrates, fats, and proteins into the intermediary compound, *adenosine triphosphate* (ATP). ATP is called the *energy currency of the cell* because almost all body cells store and use ATP as their energy source (see Chapter 4). The metabolic events involved in ATP formation allow cellular energy to be stored, used, and replenished.

Glucose Metabolism

Glucose is a six-carbon molecule; it is an efficient fuel that, when metabolized in the presence of oxygen, breaks down to form carbon dioxide and water (Fig. 11-1). Although many tissues and organ systems are able to use other forms of fuel, such as fatty acids and ketones, the brain and nervous system rely almost exclusively on glucose as a fuel source. The nervous system can neither store nor synthesize glucose; instead, it relies on the minute-by-minute extraction of glucose from the blood to meet its energy needs. In the fed and early fasting state, the nervous system requires approximately 100 to 115 g of glucose per day to meet its metabolic needs.

The liver regulates the entry of glucose into the blood. Glucose ingested in the diet is transported from the gastrointestinal tract, through the portal vein, and to the liver before it gains access to the circulatory system (Fig. 11-2). The liver stores and synthesizes glucose. When blood sugar is increased, the liver removes glucose from the blood and stores it for future use. Conversely, the liver releases its glucose stores when blood sugar drops. In this way, the liver acts as a buffer system to regulate blood sugar levels. Blood sugar levels usually reflect the difference between the amount of glucose released into the circulation by the liver and the amount of glucose removed from the blood by body cells.

Excess glucose is stored in two forms. It can be converted to fatty acids and stored in fat cells as triglycerides, or it can be stored in the liver and skeletal muscle as glycogen. Small amounts of glycogen also are stored in the skin and in some of the glandular tissues.

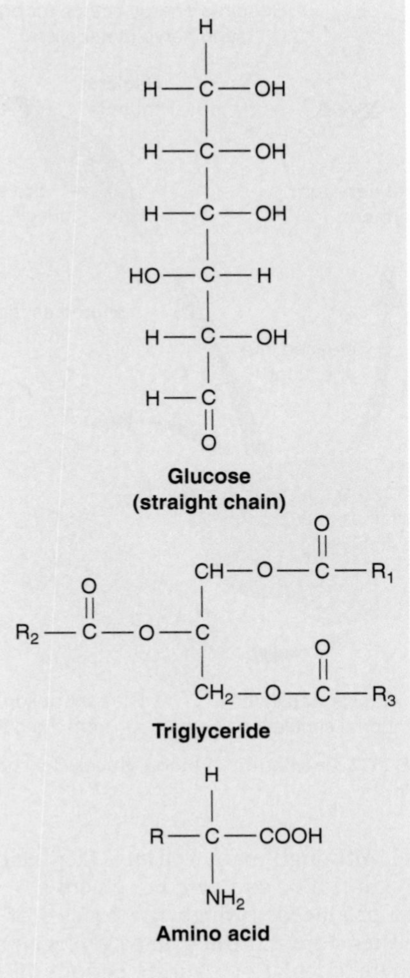

FIGURE 11-1 Glucose, triglyceride, and amino acid structure.

Glycogenolysis. Glycogenolysis, or the breakdown of glycogen, is controlled by the action of two hormones: glucagon and epinephrine. Epinephrine is more effective in stimulating glycogen breakdown in muscle, whereas the liver is more responsive to glucagon. The synthesis and degradation of glycogen are important because they help maintain blood sugar levels during periods of fasting and strenuous exercise. Only the liver is able to release its glucose stores into the blood for use by other tissues, such as the brain and nervous system. Glycogen breaks down to form a phosphorylated glucose molecule, and in this form, it is too large to pass through the cell membrane. The liver, but not skeletal muscle, has the enzyme glucose-6-phosphatase, which is needed to remove the phosphate group and allow the glucose molecule to enter the bloodstream.

Gluconeogenesis. The synthesis of glucose is referred to as *gluconeogenesis*, or the building of glucose from new sources. The process of gluconeogenesis, most of which occurs in the liver, converts amino acids, lactate, and glycerol

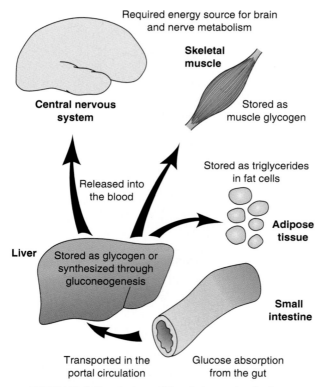

FIGURE 11-2 Regulation of blood glucose by the liver.

into glucose. Although many cells use fatty acids as a fuel source, they cannot be converted to glucose.

Glucose produced through the process of gluconeogenesis is either stored in the liver as glycogen or released into the general circulation. During periods of food deprivation or when the diet is low in carbohydrates, gluconeogenesis provides the glucose that is needed to meet the metabolic needs of the brain and other glucose-dependent tissues. Several hormones stimulate gluconeogenesis, including glucagon, glucocorticoid hormones from the adrenal cortex, and thyroid hormone.

Fat Metabolism

The average American diet provides approximately 33% of calories in the form of fats. In contrast to glucose, which yields only 4 kcal/g, each gram of fat yields 9 kcal. Another 30% to 50% of the carbohydrates consumed in the diet are converted to triglycerides for storage.

A triglyceride contains three fatty acids linked by a glycerol molecule (see Fig. 11-1). Fatty acids and triglycerides can be derived from dietary sources, they can be synthesized in the body, or they can be mobilized from fat depots. Excess carbohydrates are converted to triglycerides and transported to adipose cells for storage. One gram of anhydrous (water-free) fat stores more than six times as much energy as 1 hydrated gram of glycogen. One reason weight loss is greatest at the beginning of a fast or weight loss program is that this is when the body uses its water-containing glycogen stores. Later, when the body begins to

use energy stored as triglycerides, water losses are decreased and weight loss tends to plateau.

The mobilization of fatty acids for use in energy production is facilitated by the action of lipases (*i.e.*, enzymes) that break the triglycerides into three fatty acids and a glycerol molecule. The activation of lipases and subsequent mobilization of fatty acids is stimulated by epinephrine, glucocorticoid hormones, growth hormones, and glucagon. After triglycerides have been broken down, their fatty acids and glycerol enter the circulation and travel to the liver, where they are removed from the blood and used as a source of energy or converted to ketones.

The efficient burning of fatty acids requires a balance between carbohydrate and fat metabolism. The ratio of fatty acid and carbohydrate use is altered in situations that favor fat breakdown, such as diabetes mellitus and fasting. In these situations, the liver produces more ketones than it can use; this excess is released into the bloodstream. Ketones can be an important source of energy because even the brain adapts to the use of ketones during prolonged periods of starvation. A problem arises, however, when fat breakdown is accelerated and the production of ketones exceeds tissue use. Because ketones are organic acids, they cause ketoacidosis when they are present in excessive amounts.

Protein Metabolism

Approximately three fourths of body solids are proteins. Proteins are essential for the formation of all body structures, including genes, enzymes, contractile structures in muscle, matrix of bone, and hemoglobin of red blood cells.

Amino acids are the building blocks of proteins. Twenty amino acids are present in body proteins in significant quantities. Each amino acid has an acidic group (COOH) and an amino group (NH_2; see Fig. 11-1). Unlike glucose and fatty acids, there is only a limited facility for the storage of excess amino acids in the body. Most of the stored amino acids are contained in body proteins. Amino acids in excess of those needed for protein synthesis are converted to fatty acids, ketones, or glucose and are stored or used as metabolic fuel. Because fatty acids cannot be converted to glucose, the body must break down proteins and use the amino acids as a major source of substrate for gluconeogenesis during periods when metabolic needs exceed food intake. The liver has the enzymes and mechanisms needed to deaminate and to convert the amino groups from the amino acid to urea. The breakdown or degradation of proteins and amino acids occurs primarily in the liver, which also is the site of gluconeogenesis.

ENERGY EXPENDITURE

The expenditure of body energy results from four mechanisms of heat production (*i.e.*, thermogenesis): basal metabolic rate (BMR) or resting energy equivalent, diet-induced thermogenesis, exercise-induced thermogenesis, and thermogenesis in response to changes in environmental conditions. The amount of energy used varies with age, body size, rate of growth, and state of health.

Basal Metabolic Rate

The BMR refers to the chemical reactions occurring when the body is at rest. These reactions are necessary to provide energy for maintenance of normal body temperature, cardiovascular and respiratory function, muscle tone, and other essential activities of tissues and cells in the resting body. The resting metabolic rate constitutes 50% to 70% of body energy needs.[1] The BMR is measured using an instrument called a *metabolator* that measures the rate of oxygen use by a person. Oxygen consumption is measured under basal conditions: after a full night's sleep, after at least 12 hours without food, and while the person is awake and at rest in a warm and comfortable room. The BMR is then calculated in terms of calories per hour and normally averages approximately 60 calories per hour in young men and 53 calories per hour in young women. Women in general have a 5% to 10% lower BMR than men because of their higher percentage of adipose tissue. Factors that affect the BMR are age, sex, physical state, and pregnancy. A progressive decline in the normal BMR occurs with aging[1] (Fig. 11-3). The BMR can be used to predict the calorie needs for maintenance of nutrition.

The resting energy equivalent (REE) is used for predicting energy expenditure. Several equations that determine REE have been published. Although the Harris-Benedict equation has been the most widely used, research indicates that the World Health Organization equation has better predicting value[2] (Table 11-1). Multiplying the REE by a factor of 1.2 usually adequately predicts the caloric needs for maintenance of nutrition during health. A factor of 1.5 usually provides the needed nutrients during repletion and during illnesses such as pneumonia, long bone fractures, cancer, peritonitis, and recovery from most types of surgery.

TABLE 11-1 ✦ Equations for Predicting Resting Energy Expenditure (REE) From Body Weight Alone

Sex and Age Range (yr)	Equation to Derive REE in kcal/day*	SD†
Male		
0–3	$(60.9 \times wt) - 54$	53
3–10	$(22.7 \times wt) + 495$	62
10–18	$(17.5 \times wt) + 651$	100
18–30	$(15.3 \times wt) + 679$	151
30–60	$(11.6 \times wt) + 879$	164
>60	$(13.5 \times wt) + 487$	148
Female		
0–3	$(61.0 \times wt) - 51$	61
3–10	$(22.5 \times wt) + 499$	63
10–18	$(12.2 \times wt) + 746$	117
18–30	$(14.7 \times wt) + 496$	121
30–60	$(8.7 \times wt) + 829$	108
>60	$(10.5 \times wt) + 596$	108

*Weight (wt) of person in kilograms.
†Standard deviation (SD) of the differences between actual and computed values.
(Adapted from Food and Nutrition Board, National Research Council, NAS. [1989]. *Recommended dietary allowances* [10th ed.]. Washington, DC: National Academy Press)

Diet- and Exercise-Induced Thermogenesis

Diet-induced thermogenesis, or thermic effect of food, describes the energy used by the body for the digestion, absorption, and assimilation of food after its ingestion. It is energy expended over and above the caloric value of the food and accounts for approximately 10% of the total calories expended. When food is eaten, the metabolic rate rises and then returns to normal within a few hours. The amount of energy expended for physical activity is determined by the type of activity performed, the length of participation, and the person's weight and physical fitness. Table 11-2 describes the energy expenditures for various activities.

RECOMMENDED DIETARY ALLOWANCES AND DIETARY REFERENCE INTAKES

The *Recommended Dietary Allowances* (RDAs) define the intakes that meet the nutrient needs of almost all healthy persons in a specific age and sex group.[3] The RDAs, which are periodically updated, have been published since 1941 by the National Academy of Sciences. The RDA is used in advising persons about the level of nutrient intake they need to decrease the risk of chronic disease.

The *Dietary Reference Intake* (DRI) includes a set of at least four nutrient-based reference values, the RDA, the Adequate Intake, the Estimated Average Requirement, and the Tolerable Upper Intake Level, each of which has specific uses.[4] The *Adequate Intake* (AI) is set when there is not

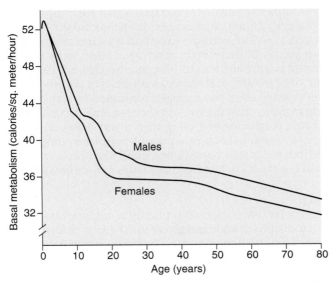

FIGURE 11-3 Normal basal metabolic rates at different ages for each sex. (Guyton A.C., Hall J.E. [1996]. *Medical physiology* [9th ed., p. 909]. Philadelphia: W.B. Saunders)

TABLE 11-2 ✦ Energy Expenditure per Hour During Different Types of Activity for a 70-kg Man

Form of Activity	Calories per Hour
Sleeping	65
Awake lying still	77
Sitting at rest	100
Standing relaxed	105
Dressing and undressing	118
Tailoring	135
Typewriting rapidly	140
"Light" exercise	170
Walking slowly (2.6 mph)	200
Carpentry, metal working, industrial painting	240
"Active" exercise	290
"Severe" exercise	450
Sawing wood	480
Swimming	500
Running (5.3 mph)	570
"Very severe" exercise	600
Walking very fast (5.3 mph)	650
Walking up stairs	1100

(Extracted from data compiled by Professor M.S. Rose. Guyton A.C., Hall J.E. [1996]. *Medical physiology* [9th ed.]. Philadelphia: W.B. Saunders)

enough scientific evidence to estimate an average requirement. The AI is derived from experimental or observational data that show a mean intake that appears to sustain a desired indicator of health. An *Estimated Average Requirement* is the intake that meets the estimated nutrient need of half of the persons in a specific group. This figure is used as the basis for developing the RDA and is expected to be used by nutrition policy makers in the evaluation of the adequacy of a nutrient for a specific group and for planning how much of the nutrient the group should consume. The *Tolerable Upper Intake Level* is the maximum intake that is judged unlikely to pose a health risk in almost all healthy persons in a specified group. It refers to the total intakes from food, fortified food, and nutrient supplements. This value is not intended to be a recommended level of intake, and there is no established benefit for persons who consume nutrients at the RDA or AI levels.

The DRIs are regularly reviewed and updated by the Food and Nutrition Board of the Institute of Medicine and the National Academy of Science. The current recommended DRIs for selected vitamins and minerals that have been released between 1997 and 2001 are listed in Table 11-3.

The *United States RDA* (USRDA) was established for the purpose of labeling foods. It takes the highest value of each nutrient for children older than 4 years of age and for adults (excluding pregnancy and lactation); therefore, the USRDA sometimes provides a margin of nutritional safety higher than the RDA.

Proteins, fats, carbohydrates, vitamins, and minerals each have their own function in providing the body with what it needs to maintain life and health. Recommended allowances have not been established for every nutrient; some are given as a safe and adequate intake, but others, such as carbohydrates and fats, are expressed as a percentage of the calorie intake.

NUTRITIONAL NEEDS

Calories

Energy requirements are greater during growth periods. Infants require approximately 115 kcal/kg at birth, 105 kcal/kg at 1 year, and 80 kcal/kg of body weight between 1 to 10 years of age. During adolescence, boys require 45 kcal/kg of body weight and girls require 38 kcal/kg of body weight. During pregnancy, a woman needs an extra 300 kcal/day above her usual requirement, and during the first 3 months of breast-feeding, she requires an additional 500 kcal.[3] Table 11-4 can be used to predict the caloric requirements of healthy adults.

Proteins

Proteins are required for growth and maintenance of body tissues, enzymes and antibody formation, fluid and electrolyte balance, and nutrient transport. Proteins are composed of amino acids, nine of which are essential to the body. These are leucine, isoleucine, methionine, phenylalanine, threonine, tryptophan, valine, lysine, and histidine. The foods that provide these essential amino acids in adequate amounts are milk, eggs, meat, fish, and poultry. Dried peas and beans, nuts, seeds, and grains contain all the essential amino acids but in less than adequate proportions. These proteins need to be combined with each other or with complete proteins to meet the amino acid requirements for protein synthesis. Diets that are inadequate in protein can result in kwashiorkor. If calories and protein are inadequate, protein-calorie malnutrition occurs.

Unlike carbohydrates and fats, which are composed of hydrogen, carbon, and oxygen, proteins contain 16% nitrogen; therefore, nitrogen excretion is an indicator of protein intake. If the amount of nitrogen taken in by way of protein is equivalent to the nitrogen excreted, the person is said to be in nitrogen balance. A person is in positive nitrogen balance when the nitrogen consumed by way of protein is greater than the amount excreted. This occurs during growth, pregnancy, or healing after surgery or injury. A negative nitrogen balance often occurs with fever, illness, infection, trauma, or burns, when more nitrogen is excreted than is consumed. It represents a state of tissue breakdown.

Fats

Dietary fats are composed primarily of triglycerides (*i.e.,* a mixture of fatty acids and glycerol). The fatty acids are saturated (*i.e.,* no double bonds), monounsaturated (*i.e.,* one double bond), or polyunsaturated (*i.e.,* two or more double bonds). The saturated fatty acids elevate blood cholesterol, whereas the monounsaturated and polyunsaturated fats lower blood cholesterol. Saturated fats usually are from animal sources and remain solid at room temperature. With the exception of coconut and palm oils (which are satu-

TABLE 11-3 ◆ Dietary Reference Intakes: Recommended Intakes for Individuals

Life Stage Group	Calcium (mg/d)	Phosphorus (mg/d)	Magnesium (mg/d)	Vitamin D (µg/d)a,b	Iron (mg/d)	Thiamin (mg/d)	Riboflavin (mg/d)	Niacin (mg/d)c	Vitamin B6 (mg/d)	Folate (µg/d)d	Vitamin B12 (µg/d)	Pantothenic Acid (mg/d)	Biotin (µg/d)	Vitamin A (µg/d)e	Vitamin C (mg/d)	Vitamin E (mg/d)f	Selenium (µg/d)
Infants																	
0–6 mo	210*	100*	30*	5*	0.27*	0.2*	0.3*	2*	0.1*	65*	0.4*	1.7*	5*	400*	40*	4*	15*
7–12 mo	270*	275*	75*	5*	11	0.3*	0.4*	4*	0.3*	80*	0.5*	1.8*	6*	500*	50*	6*	20*
Children																	
1–3 y	500*	460	80	5*	7	0.5	0.5	6	0.5	150	0.9	2*	8*	300	15	6	20
4–8 y	800*	500	130	5*	10	0.6	0.6	8	0.6	200	1.2	3*	12*	400	25	7	30
Males																	
9–13 y	1300*	1250	240	5*	8	0.9	0.9	12	1.0	300	1.8	4*	20*	600	45	11	40
14–18 y	1300*	1250	410	5*	11	1.2	1.3	16	1.3	400	2.4	5*	25*	900	75	15	55
19–30 y	1000*	700	400	5*	8	1.2	1.3	16	1.3	400	2.4	5*	30*	900	90	15	55
31–50 y	1000*	700	420	5*	8	1.2	1.3	16	1.3	400	2.4	5*	30*	900	90	15	55
51–70 y	1200*	700	420	10*	8	1.2	1.3	16	1.7	400	2.4g	5*	30*	900	90	15	55
>70 y	1200*	700	420	15*	8	1.2	1.3	16	1.7	400	2.4g	5*	30*	900	90	15	55
Females																	
9–13 y	1300*	1250	240	5*	8	0.9	0.9	12	1.0	300	1.8	4*	20*	600	45	11	40
14–18 y	1300*	1250	360	5*	15	1.0	1.0	14	1.2	400h	2.4	5*	25*	700	65	15	55
19–30 y	1000*	700	310	5*	18	1.1	1.1	14	1.3	400h	2.4	5*	30*	700	75	15	55
31–50 y	1000*	700	320	5*	18	1.1	1.1	14	1.3	400h	2.4	5*	30*	700	75	15	55
51–70 y	1200*	700	320	10*	8	1.1	1.1	14	1.5	400	2.4g	5*	30*	700	75	15	55
>70 y	1200*	700	320	15*	8	1.1	1.1	14	1.5	400	2.4g	5*	30*	700	75	15	55
Pregnancy																	
≤18 y	1300*	1250	400	5*	27	1.4	1.4	18	1.9	600i	2.6	6*	30*	750	80	15	60
19–30 y	1000*	700	350	5*	27	1.4	1.4	18	1.9	600i	2.6	6*	30*	770	85	15	60
31–50 y	1000*	700	360	5*	27	1.4	1.4	18	1.9	600i	2.6	6*	30*	770	85	15	60
Lactation																	
≤18 y	1300*	1250	360	5*	10	1.4	1.6	17	2.0	500	2.8	7*	35*	1200	115	19	70
19–30 y	1000*	700	310	5*	9	1.4	1.6	17	2.0	500	2.8	7*	35*	1300	120	19	70
31–50 y	1000*	700	320	5*	9	1.4	1.6	17	2.0	500	2.8	7*	35*	1300	120	19	70

This table presents Recommended Dietary Allowances (RDAs) in bold type and Adequate Intakes (AIs) in ordinary type followed by an asterisk (*). RDAs and AIs may both be used as goals for individual intake. RDAs are set to meet the needs of almost all (97% to 98%) individuals in a group. For healthy breast-fed infants, the AI is the mean intake. The AI for other life-stage and sex groups is believed to cover needs of all individuals in the group, but lack of data or uncertainty in the data prevent being able to specify with confidence the percentage of individuals covered by this intake.

a As cholecalciferol. 1 µg cholecalciferol = 40 IU vitamin D.

b In the absence of adequate exposure to sunlight.

c As niacin equivalents (NE). 1 mg of niacin = 60 mg of tryptophan; 0–6 mo = preformed niacin (not NE).

d As dietary folate equivalents (DFE). 1 DFE = 1 µg food folate = 0.6 µg of folic acid from fortified food or as a supplement consumed with food or as a supplement taken on an empty stomach.

e As retinol activity equivalents (RAEs). 1 RAE = 1 µg retinol, 12 µg β-carotene, 24 µg α-carotene, or 24 µg β-cryptoxanthin in foods. To calculate RAEs from REs of provitamin A carotenoids in foods, divide the REs by 2. For preformed vitamin A in foods or supplements and for provitamin A carotenoids in supplements, 1 RE = 1 RAE.

f As α-Tocopherol. α-Tocopherol includes RRR-α-tocopherol, the only form of α-tocopherol that occurs naturally in foods, and the 2R-stereoisomeric forms of α-tocopherol (RRR-, RSR-, RRS-, and RSS-α-tocopherol) that occur in fortified foods and supplements. It does not include the 2S-stereoisomeric forms of α-tocopherol (SRR-, SSR-, SRS-, and SSS-α-tocopherol), also found in fortified foods and supplements.

g Because 10% to 30% of older people may malabsorb food-bound vitamin B12, it is advisable for those older than 50 years to meet their RDA mainly by consuming foods fortified with vitamin B12 or a supplement containing vitamin B12.

h In view of evidence linking folate intake with neural tube defects in the fetus, it is recommended that all women capable of becoming pregnant consume 400 µg from supplements or fortified foods in addition to intake of food folate from a varied diet.

i It is assumed that women will continue consuming 400 µg from supplements or fortified food until their pregnancy is confirmed and they enter prenatal care, which ordinarily occurs after the end of the periconceptional period—the critical time for formation of the neural tube.

(Copyright 2001 by the National Academy of Sciences. Reprinted courtesy of the National Academy Press, Washington, DC. These reports may be accessed at www.nap.edu/books/0309071836/html.)

TABLE 11-4 ✦ Caloric Requirements Based on Body Weight and Activity Level

	Sedentary	Moderate	Active
Overweight	20–25 kcal/kg	30 kcal/kg	35 kcal/kg
Normal	30 kcal/kg	35 kcal/kg	40 kcal/kg
Underweight	30 kcal/kg	40 kcal/kg	45–50 kcal/kg

(Adapted from Goodhart R.S., Shils M.E. [1980]. *Modern nutrition in health and disease* [6th ed.]. Philadelphia: Lea and Febiger)

rated), unsaturated fats are found in plant oils and usually are liquid at room temperature.

Dietary fats provide energy, serve as carriers for the fat-soluble vitamins, are precursors of prostaglandins, and are a source of fatty acids. The polyunsaturated fatty acid linoleic acid is the only fatty acid that is required. A deficiency of linoleic acid results in dermatitis. The daily requirement is 5 g or 1% to 2% of the total daily calories. Because vegetable oils are rich sources of linoleic acid, this level can be met by including two teaspoons of oil.

Other than the requirement for linoleic acid, there is no specific requirement for dietary fat, provided there is adequate nutrition available for energy. Fat is the most concentrated source of energy. It is recommended that 30% or less of the calories in the diet should come from fats.[5]

Cholesterol is the major constituent of cell membranes and is synthesized by the body. Cholesterol metabolism and transport are discussed in Chapter 22. The daily dietary recommendation for cholesterol is less than 300 mg.

Carbohydrates

Dietary carbohydrates are composed of simple sugars, complex carbohydrates, and undigested carbohydrates (*i.e.,* fiber). Because of their vitamin, mineral, and fiber content, it is recommended that the bulk of the carbohydrate content in the diet be in the complex form rather than as simple sugars that contain few nutrients. Sucrose (*i.e.,* table sugar) is implicated in the development of dental caries.

There is no specific dietary requirement for carbohydrates. All of the energy requirements can be met by dietary fats and proteins. Although some tissues, such as the nervous system, require glucose as an energy source, this need can be met through the conversion of amino acids and the glycerol part of the triglyceride molecule to glucose. The fatty acids from triglycerides are converted to ketones and used for energy by other body tissues. A carbohydrate-deficient diet usually results in the loss of tissue proteins and the development of ketosis. Because protein and fat metabolism increases the production of osmotically active metabolic wastes that must be eliminated through the kidneys, there is danger of dehydration and electrolyte imbalances. The amount of carbohydrate needed to prevent tissue wasting and ketosis is 50 to 100 g/day. In practice, most of the daily energy requirement should be from carbohydrate. This is because protein is an expensive source of calories and because it is recommended that no more

than 30% of the calories in the diet be derived from fat. The current recommendation is that the diet should provide 50% to 60% of the calories as carbohydrates.

Vitamins

Vitamins are a group of organic compounds that act as catalysts in various chemical reactions. A compound cannot be classified as a vitamin unless it is shown that a deficiency of it causes disease. Contrary to popular belief, vitamins do not provide energy directly. As catalysts, they are part of the enzyme systems required for the release of energy from protein, fat, and carbohydrates. Vitamins also are necessary for the formation of red blood cells, hormones, genetic materials, and the nervous system. They are essential for normal growth and development.

There are two types of vitamins: fat soluble and water soluble. The four fat-soluble vitamins are vitamins A, D, E, and K. The nine required water-soluble vitamins are thiamine, riboflavin, niacin, pyridoxine (Vitamin B_6), pantothenic acid, vitamin B_{12}, folic acid, biotin, and vitamin C. Because the water-soluble vitamins are excreted in the urine, it is less likely that they may become toxic to the body, but the fat-soluble vitamins are stored in the body, and they may reach toxic levels. Table 11-5 lists sources and functions of vitamins.

Minerals

Minerals serve many functions. They are involved in acid-base balance and in the maintenance of osmotic pressure in body compartments. Minerals are components of vitamins, hormones, and enzymes. They maintain normal hemoglobin levels, play a role in nervous system function, and are involved in muscle contraction and skeletal development and maintenance. Minerals that are present in relatively large amounts in the body are called *macrominerals*. These include calcium, phosphorus, sodium, chloride, potassium, magnesium, and sulfur. The remainder are classified as *trace minerals*; they include iron, manganese, copper, iodine, zinc, cobalt, fluorine, and selenium. Table 11-6 lists mineral sources and functions.

Fiber

Fiber, the portion of food that cannot be digested by the human intestinal tract, increases stool bulk and facilitates bowel movements. Fiber decreases the incidence of digestive diseases and colorectal cancer and lowers blood sugar and cholesterol.[6] The amount of fiber believed beneficial is a daily intake of 20 to 30 g.

NUTRITIONAL ASSESSMENT

The nutritional status can be assessed by evaluating the person's dietary intake, taking anthropometric measurements, performing a physical examination, and conducting laboratory tests. The nutritional assessment can provide information regarding the adequacy of the diet, the person's body size compared with normal ranges, and the possibility of overnutrition or undernutrition.

Nutritional assessment remains more of an art than a science. A global assessment obtains information about

TABLE 11-5 ✦ Sources and Functions of Vitamins

Vitamin	Major Food Sources	Functions
Fat-Soluble Vitamins		
Vitamin A (retinol, provitamin, carotenoids)	Retinol: liver, butter, whole milk, cheese, egg yolks; provitamin A: carrots, green leafy vegetables, sweet potatoes, pumpkin, winter squash, apricots, cantaloupe, fortified margarine	Essential for normal retinal function; plays an essential role in cell growth and differentiation, particularly epithelial cells. Epidemiologic evidence suggests a role in preventing certain cancers
Vitamin D (calciferol)	Fortified dairy products, fortified margarine, fish oils, egg yolk	Increases intestinal absorption of calcium and promotes ossification of bones and teeth
Vitamin E (tocopherol)	Vegetable oil, margarine, shortening, green and leafy vegetables, wheat germ, whole-grain products, egg yolk, butter, liver	Functions as an antioxidant protecting vitamins A and C and fatty acids; prevents cell membrane injury
Water-Soluble Vitamins		
Vitamin C (ascorbic acid)	Broccoli, sweet and hot peppers, collards, brussel sprouts, kale, potatoes, spinach, tomatoes, citrus fruits, strawberries	Potent antioxidant involved in many oxidation–reduction reactions; required for synthesis of collagen; increases absorption of nonheme iron; is involved in wound healing and drug metabolism
Thiamin (vitamin B_1)	Pork, liver, meat, whole grains, fortified grain products, legumes, nuts	Coenzyme required for several important biochemical reactions in carbohydrate metabolism; thought to have an independent role in nerve conduction
Riboflavin (vitamin B_2)	Liver, milk, yogurt, cottage cheese, meat, fortified grain products	Coenzyme that participates in a variety of important oxidation–reduction reactions and an important component of a number of enzymes
Niacin (nicotinamide, nicotinic acid)	Liver, meat, poultry, fish, peanuts, fortified grain products	Essential component of the coenzymes nicotinamide adenine dinucleotide (NAD) and nicotinamide dinucleotide diphosphate (NADP), which are involved in many oxidative reduction reactions
Folacin (folic acid)	Liver, legumes, green leafy vegetables	Coenzyme in amino acid and nucleoprotein metabolism; promotes red cell formation
Vitamin B_6 (pyridoxine)	Meat, poultry, fish, shellfish, green and leafy vegetables, whole-grain products, legumes	A major coenzyme involved in the metabolism of amino acids; required for synthesis of heme
Vitamin B_{12}	Meat, poultry, fish, shellfish, eggs, dairy products	Coenzyme involved in nucleic acid synthesis; assists in development of red cells and maintenance of nerve function
Biotin	Kidney, liver, milk, egg yolks, most fresh vegetables	Coenzyme in fat synthesis, amino acid metabolism, and glycogen formation
Pantothenic acid	Liver, kidney, meats, milk, egg yolk, whole-grain products, legumes	Coenzyme involved in energy metabolism

(Data from *Vitamin facts,* National Dairy Council, and other sources)

TABLE 11-6 ◆ Sources and Functions of Minerals

Mineral	Major Sources	Functions
Calcium	Milk and milk products, fish with bones, greens	Bone formation and maintenance; tooth formation, vitamin B absorption, blood clotting, nerve and muscle function
Chloride	Table salt, meats, milk, eggs	Regulates pH of stomach, acid-base balance, osmotic pressure of extracellular fluids
Cobalt	Organ meats, meats	Aids in maturation of red blood cells (as part of B_{12} molecule)
Copper	Cereals, nuts, legumes, liver, shellfish, grapes, meats	Catalyst for hemoglobin formation, formation of elastin and collagen, energy release (cytochrome oxidase and catalase), formation of melanin, formation of phospholipids for myelin sheath of nerves
Fluoride	Fluorinated water	Strengthens bones and teeth
Iodine	Iodized salt, fish (saltwater and anadromous)	Thyroid hormone synthesis and its function in maintenance of metabolic rate
Iron	Meats, heart, liver, clams, oysters, lima beans, spinach, dates, dried nuts, enriched and whole-grain cereals	Hemoglobin synthesis, cellular energy release (cytochrome pathway), killing bacteria (myeloperoxidase)
Magnesium	Milk, green vegetables, nuts, bread, cereals	Catalyst of many intracellular nerve impulses, retention of reactions, particularly those related to intracellular enzyme reactions; low magnesium levels produce an increase in irritability of the nervous system, vasodilatation, and cardiac dysrhythmias
Phosphorus	Meats, poultry, fish, milk and cheese, cereals, legumes, nuts	Bone formation and maintenance; essential component of nucleic acids and energy exchange forms such as adenosine triphosphate (ATP)
Potassium	Oranges, dried fruits, bananas, meats, potatoes, peanut butter, coffee	Maintenance of intracellular osmolality, acid-base balance, transmission of nerve impulses, catalyst in energy metabolism, formation of proteins, formation of glycogen
Sodium	Table salt, cured meats, meats, milk, olives	Maintenance of osmotic pressure of extracellular fluids, acid-base balance, neuromuscular function; absorption of glucose
Zinc	Whole-wheat cereals, eggs, legumes	Integral part of many enzymes, including carbonic anhydrase, which facilitates combination of carbon dioxide with water in red blood cells; component of lactate dehydrogenase, which is important in cellular metabolism; component of many peptidases; important in digestion of proteins in gastrointestinal tract

many facets of nutrition, including current physical symptoms, any functional impairment, acute and chronic illnesses, a detailed physical examination, and history of dietary intake. Clinical assessment is probably one of the most valid methods of making a nutritional diagnosis and planning nutritional care.[7]

Diet Assessment

A nutritional assessment begins with an evaluation of the person's diet. This can be accomplished by recording the food consumed by actual observation or by 24-hour recall and through the administration of a questionnaire or diet history. Each technique has its own shortcomings, such as the tendency to alter behavior when it is known that the behavior is being observed or reported.

Health Assessment

Health assessment, including a health history and physical examination, reveals weight changes, muscle wasting, fat

stores, functional status, and nutritional status. Comparison of the person's current weight with previous weights identifies whether the person's weight is stable, changed drastically, or tends to fluctuate. For example, recent rapid weight loss can be a sign of cancer, a malfunctioning thyroid gland, or self-imposed starvation. A history of fluctuating weight could be associated with bulimia. Degradation of muscle, or muscle wasting, is a serious sign of malnutrition. Decreased ability to initiate or complete activities of daily living could result from a decrease in energy caused by a poor diet, a neurologic malfunction such as multiple sclerosis, or symptoms related to chronic obstructive pulmonary disease. Quality of the hair, absence of body hair, condition of gums, and skin lesions could signal poor nutritional status.

Anthropometric Measurements

Anthropometric measurements provide a means for assessing body composition, particularly fat stores and skeletal muscle mass. This is done by measuring height, weight, body circumferences, and thickness of various skinfolds. These measurements commonly are used to determine growth patterns in children and appropriateness of current weight in adults.

Body weight is the most frequently used method of assessing nutritional status; it should be used in combination with measurements of body height to establish whether a person is underweight or overweight.

Relative weight is the actual weight divided by the desirable weight and multiplied by 100. A relative weight greater than 120% is indicative of obesity. Recent changes in weight are probably a better indication of undernutrition than a low relative weight. An unintentional loss of 10% of body weight or more within the past 6 months usually is considered predictive of a poor clinical outcome, especially if weight loss is continuing.[8] The body mass index (BMI) uses height and weight to determine healthy weight (Table 11-7). It is calculated by dividing the weight in kilograms by the height in meters squared (BMI = weight [kg]/height [m²]). A BMI between 18.5 and 25 has the lowest statistical health risk.[9] A BMI of 25 to 29.9 is considered overweight; a BMI of 30 or greater as obese; and a BMI greater than 40 as very or morbidly obese.[10]

Body weight reflects both lean body mass and adipose tissue and cannot be used as a method for describing body composition or the percentage of fat tissue present. Statistically, the best percentage of body fat for men is between 12% and 20%, and for women, it is between 20% and 30%.[11] During physical training, body fat usually decreases, and lean body mass increases. Among the methods used to estimate body fat are skinfold thickness, body circumferences, hydrodensitometry, bioelectrical impedance, dual photon absorptiometry, computed tomography (CT), and magnetic resonance imaging (MRI).

Measurements of *skinfold thickness* can provide a reasonable assessment of body fat, particularly if taken at multiple sites. They can provide information about the location of the fat and can be used together with equations and tables to estimate the percentage of lean body mass and fat tissue.[12,13] However, these measurements often are difficult to perform and subject to considerable variation between observers, and do not provide information about abdominal and intramuscular fat.

The measurement of *body circumferences*, most commonly waist and hip, provides an objective measurement of body fat and supplies the information needed to calculate the waist circumference to hip circumference. The measurement of body circumference has received attention because of an interest in excess visceral or intra-abdominal fat. The waist circumference is commonly used for this purpose.[10]

Hydrodensitometry (underwater weighing) is based on the principle that fat tissue is less dense than muscle and bone.[12] It is more accurate than skinfold thickness or body circumference measurements in determining the percentage of body fat, although there are limitations. It requires access to special equipment; assumes a constant density of lean body mass, which is subject to error; and necessitates an estimation of residual gas volumes in the lungs, which often is difficult to obtain.

Another method of estimating body fat is *bioelectrical impedance*. This method is performed by attaching electrodes at the wrist and ankle that send a harmless current through the body. The flow of the current is affected by the amount of water in the body. Because fat-free tissue contains virtually all the water and the conducting electrolytes, measurements of the resistance (*i.e.*, impedance) to current flow can be used to estimate the percentage of body fat present.[12] Bioelectrical impedance is one of the most widely available techniques for assessing body fat. The method is relatively inexpensive, easy to use, and portable.

Dual photon absorptiometry also determines body fat and is replacing densitometry as the standard because of its high precision and simplicity.[12] However, it is expensive, requires exposure to a small amount of radiation, and is difficult to use in the very obese. Its advantages are that it requires minimal cooperation on the part of the person being tested and that it provides a bone mineral estimate.

TABLE 11-7 ✦ **Classification of Overweight and Obesity by BMI, Waist Circumference, and Associated Disease Risk***

| | BMI (kg/m²) | Obesity Class | Disease Risk* Relative to Normal Weight and Waist Circumference | |
			Men ≤102 cm (≤40 in) Women ≤88 cm (≤35 in)	Men >102 cm (>40 in) Women >88 cm (>35 in)
Underweight	<18.5		—	—
Normal†	18.5–24.9		—	—
Overweight	25.0–29.9		Increased	High
Obesity	30.0–34.9	I	High	Very high
	35.0–39.9	II	Very high	Very high
Extreme obesity	≥40	III	Extremely high	Extremely high

BMI, body mass index.
* Disease risk for type 2 diabetes, hypertension, and cardiovascular disease.
† Increased waist circumference also can be a marker for increased risk, even in persons of normal weight.
(Expert Panel. [1998]. Clinical guidelines on the identification, evaluation, and treatment of overweight and obesity in adults. National Institutes of Health. [On-line.] Available: http://nhlbi.nih.gov/guidelines/ob_gdlns.htm.

Computed tomography and *MRI* can be used to provide quantitative pictures from which the thickness of fat can be determined. CT scans also can be used to provide quantitative estimates of regional fat and give a ratio of intra-abdominal to extra-abdominal fat.[12] Because these methods are costly, they usually are reserved for research studies.

Laboratory Studies

Various laboratory tests can aid in evaluating nutritional status. Some of the most commonly performed tests are serum albumin to assess the protein status, total lymphocyte count and delayed hypersensitivity reaction to assess cellular immunity, and creatinine–height index to assess skeletal muscle protein. Vitamin and mineral deficiencies can be determined by measurements of their levels in blood, saliva, and other body tissues or by measuring nutrient-specific chemical reactions. All of these tests are limited by confounding factors and therefore need to be evaluated along with other clinical data.

In summary, nutritional status describes the condition of the body related to the availability and use of nutrients. Nutrients provide the energy and materials necessary for performing the activities of daily living and for the growth and repair of body tissues. Metabolism is the organized process whereby nutrients such as carbohydrates, fats, and proteins are broken down, transformed, or otherwise converted to cellular energy. Glucose, fats, and amino acids from proteins serve as fuel sources for cellular metabolism. These fuel sources are ingested during meals and stored for future use. Glucose is stored as glycogen or converted to triglycerides in fat cells for storage. Fats are stored in adipose tissue as triglycerides. Amino acids are the building blocks of proteins, and most of the stored amino acids are contained in body proteins and as fuel sources for cellular metabolism. Energy is measured in heat units called *kilocalories*.

The expenditure of body energy results from heat production (*i.e.*, thermogenesis) associated with the BMR or basal energy equivalent, diet-induced thermogenesis, exercise-induced thermogenesis, and thermogenesis in response to changes in environmental conditions.

The body requires more than 40 nutrients on a daily basis. Nutritional status reflects the continued daily intake of nutrients over time and the deposition and use of these nutrients in the body. The DRI is the Daily Recommended Intake of essential nutrients considered to be adequate to meet the known nutritional needs of healthy persons. The DRI has 22 age and sex classifications and includes recommendations for calories, protein, fat, carbohydrates, vitamins, and minerals. The nutritional status of a person can be assessed by evaluation of dietary intake, anthropometric measurements, health assessment, and laboratory tests. Health assessment includes a health history and physical examination to determine weight changes, muscle wasting, fat stores, functional status, and nutritional

status. Anthropometric measurements are used for assessing body composition; they include height and weight measurements and measurements to determine the composition of the body in relation to lean body mass and fat tissue (*e.g.*, skinfold thickness, body circumferences, hydrodensitometry, bioelectrical impedance, and CT scans).

Overnutrition and Obesity

After you have completed this section of the chapter, you should be able to meet the following objectives:

✦ Define and discuss the causes of obesity and health risks associated with obesity
✦ Differentiate upper and lower body obesity and their implications in terms of health risk
✦ Discuss the treatment of obesity in terms of diet, behavior modification, exercise, social support, and surgical methods

Obesity is defined as a condition characterized by excess body fat. Clinically, obesity and overweight have been defined in terms of the BMI. Historically, various world bodies have used different BMI cutoff points to define obesity. In 1997, the World Health Organization defined the various classifications of overweight (BMI ≥ 25) and obesity (BMI ≥ 30). This classification was subsequently adopted by the National Institutes of Health.[10] The use of a BMI cutoff of 25 as a measure of overweight raised some concern that the BMI in some men might be due to muscle rather than fat weight. However, it has been shown that a BMI cutoff of 25 can sensitively detect most overweight people and does not erroneously detect overlean people.[14]

Overweight and obesity have become national health problems, increasing the risk of hypertension, hyperlipidemia, type 2 diabetes, coronary heart disease, and other health problems. Fifty-five percent of the U.S. population is estimated to be overweight (BMI ≥ 25). Obesity is particularly prevalent among some minority groups, lower income groups, and people with less education. The prevalence of obesity (BMI ≥ 30) in the United States has increased from 12.0% in 1991 to 17.9% in 1998.[15]

CAUSES OF OBESITY

The excess body fat of obesity often significantly impairs health. This excess body fat is generated when the calories consumed exceed those expended through exercise and activity.[16] The physiologic mechanisms that lead to this imbalance are poorly understood.[17] They probably exist in different combinations among obese persons.

Although factors that lead to the development of obesity are not understood, they are thought to involve the interaction of genotype and environmental factors, which include social, behavioral, cultural, with the physiology, metabolism, and genetics of the individual.[18] Epi-

Obesity

➤ Obesity results from an imbalance between energy intake and energy consumption. Because fat is the main storage form of energy, obesity represents an excess of body fat.

➤ Overweight and obesity are determined by measurements of body mass index (BMI; weight [kg]/height [m²]) and waist circumference. A BMI of 25 to 29.9 is considered overweight; a BMI of 30 or greater as obese; and a BMI greater than 40 as very or morbidly obese.

➤ Waist circumference is used to determine the distribution of body fat. Central, or abdominal, obesity is an independent predictor of morbidity and mortality associated with obesity.

demiologic surveys indicate that the prevalence of overweight may also be related to social and economic conditions. The second (1976 through 1980) National Health and Nutrition Examination Survey (NHANES II) has shown that if American women are divided into two groups according to economic status, the prevalence of obesity is much higher among those in the poverty group.[19] In contrast, men above the poverty level had a higher prevalence of overweight than men below the poverty level.

Obesity is known to run in families, suggesting a hereditary component. The question that surrounds this observation is whether the disorder arises because of genetic endowment or environmental influences. Studies of twin and adopted children have provided evidence that heredity contributes to the disorder.[20] It is now believed that the heritability of the BMI is approximately 33%.[21]

Although genetic factors may explain some of the individual variations in terms of excess weight, environmental influences also must be taken into account. These influences include family dietary patterns, decreased level of activity because of labor-saving devices and time spent on the computer, reliance on the automobile for transportation, easy access to food, energy density of food, and supersizing of portions. The obese may be greatly influenced by the availability of food, the flavor of food, time of day, and other cues. The composition of the diet also may be a causal factor, and the percentage of dietary fat independent of total calorie intake may play a part in the development of obesity. Psychological factors include using food as a reward, comfort, or means of getting attention. Eating may be a way to cope with tension, anxiety, and mental fatigue. Some persons may overeat and use obesity as a means of avoiding emotionally threatening situations.

It has been suggested that the increased prevalence of obesity in the United States has resulted from increased caloric intake together with a sedentary lifestyle and energy-saving conveniences.[22] Even when a reasonable number of calories are consumed, fewer are expended because of inactivity. A low rate of energy expenditure may contribute to the prevalence of obesity in some families.

TYPES OF OBESITY

Two types of obesity based on distribution of fat have been described: upper body and lower body obesity. *Upper body obesity* is also referred to as *central*, *abdominal*, or *male* obesity. Lower body obesity is known as *peripheral*, *gluteal-femoral*, or *female* obesity. The obesity type is determined by dividing the waist by the hip circumference. A waist-hip ratio greater than 1.0 in men and 0.8 in women indicates upper body obesity (Fig. 11-4). Research suggests that fat distribution may be a more important factor for morbidity and mortality than overweight or obesity.

The presence of excess fat in the abdomen out of proportion to total body fat is an independent predictor of risk factors and mortality. Waist circumference is positively correlated with abdominal fat content. Waist circumference 35 inches or greater in women and 40 inches or greater in men has been associated with increased health risk[10] (see Table 11-7). Central obesity can be further differentiated into intra-abdominal, or visceral, fat and subcutaneous fat by the use of CT or MRI scans. However, intra-abdominal fat usually is synonymous with central fat distribution. One of the characteristics of abdominal fat is that fatty acids released from the viscera go directly to the liver before entering the systemic circulation, having a potentially greater impact on hepatic function. Higher levels of circulating free fatty acids in obese persons, particularly those with upper body obesity, are thought to be associated with many of the adverse effects of obesity.[16]

In general, men have more intra-abdominal fat and women more subcutaneous fat. As men age, the proportion of intra-abdominal fat to subcutaneous fat increases. After menopause, women tend to acquire more central fat distribution. Increasing weight gain, alcohol, and low levels of activity are associated with upper body obesity. These changes place persons with upper body obesity at greater

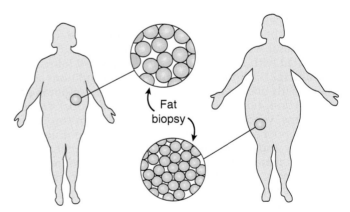

FIGURE 11-4 Distribution of body fat and size of fat cells in persons with upper and lower body obesity. (Courtesy of Ahmed Kissebah, M.D., Ph.D., Medical College of Wisconsin, Milwaukee)

risk for ischemic heart disease, stroke, and death independent of total body fat. They also tend to exhibit hypertension, elevated levels of triglycerides and decreased levels of high-density lipoproteins, hyperinsulinemia and diabetes mellitus, breast and endometrial cancer, gallbladder disease, menstrual irregularities, and infertility. Visceral fat also is associated with abnormalities of metabolic and sex hormone levels.[23]

Weight loss causes a loss of visceral fat and has resulted in improvements in metabolic and hormonal abnormalities.[24,25] Although peripheral obesity is associated with varicose veins in the legs and mechanical problems, it does not increase the risk of heart disease.[26] In terms of weight reduction, some studies have shown that persons with upper body obesity are easier to treat than those with lower body obesity. Other studies have shown no difference in terms of success with weight reduction programs between the two types of obesity.

Weight cycling (the losing and gaining of weight) has been found to have little or no effect on metabolic variables, central obesity, or cardiovascular risk factors or future amount of weight loss.[27] More research is needed to determine its effect on dietary preference for fat, psychological adjustment, disordered eating, and mortality.[28,29] It is postulated that perhaps it is the underlying obesity and not the weight fluctuation that affects life expectancy.[30]

HEALTH RISKS ASSOCIATED WITH OBESITY

Obesity affects both psychosocial and physical well-being. In the United States as well as other countries, there are many negative stereotypes associated with obesity. People, especially women, are expected to be thin, and obesity may be seen as sign of a lack of self-control. Obesity may negatively affect employment and educational opportunities as well as marital status. Obesity also may play a role in a person's treatment by health professionals.[15] Although nurses, physicians, and other health professionals are aware of the low success rate and difficulty in treating weight problems, they still may place the blame on the obese patient.[15]

In terms of health problems, obese persons are more likely to have high blood pressure, hyperlipidemia, cardiovascular disease, glucose intolerance, insulin resistance, type 2 diabetes, stroke, gallbladder disease, infertility, and cancer of the endometrium, prostate, colon, and, in postmenopausal women, the breast.[10] The increased weight associated with obesity stresses the bones and joints, increasing the likelihood of arthritis. Other conditions associated with obesity include sleep apnea and pulmonary dysfunction, nonalcoholic steatohepatitis, carpal tunnel syndrome, venous insufficiency and deep vein thrombosis, and poor wound healing.[10] Because some drugs are lipophilic and exhibit increased distribution in fat tissue, the administration of these drugs, including some anesthetic agents, can be more dangerous in obese persons. If surgery is required, the obese person heals slower than a nonobese person of the same age.

Massive obesity, because of its close association with so many health problems, can be regarded as a disease in its own right.[31] It is the second leading cause of preventable death. In men who have never smoked, the risk of death increases from 1.06 at a BMI of 24.5 to 1.67 at a BMI higher than 26.[32] The waist-hip ratio is a less reliable predictor of mortality in women than BMI.

PREVENTION OF OBESITY

Emphasis is being placed on the prevention of obesity. It has been theorized that obesity is preventable because the effect of hereditary factors is no more than moderate. A more active lifestyle together with a low-fat diet (<30% of calories) is seen as the strategy for prevention. The target audience should be young children, adolescents, and young adults.[33] Tools needed to achieve this goal include promotion of regular meals, avoidance of snacking, substituting water for calorie-containing beverages, decreased television viewing time, a low-fat diet, and increased activity. Other experts target the high-risk period from 25 to 35 years, menopause,[34] and the year after successful weight loss.

TREATMENT OF OBESITY

There are many ways to treat obesity. It is currently recommended that treatment should focus on lifestyle modification through a combination of a low-calorie diet, increased physical activity, and behavior therapy.[10] Pharmacotherapy and surgery are available as an adjunct to lifestyle changes in individuals who meet specific criteria.

Before treatment begins, an assessment should be made of the degree of overweight and the overall risk status. The patient should be assessed for the following risk factors: coronary heart disease, type 2 diabetes, sleep apnea, gynecologic abnormalities, osteoarthritis, gallstones, stress incontinence, cigarette smoking, hypertension, low-density lipoprotein cholesterol greater than 160 mg/dL, high-density lipoprotein cholesterol less than 35 mg/dL, impaired fasting glucose, family history of premature coronary heart disease, and age 45 years or older in men or 55 years or older in women. Individuals having three of these risk factors should be classified at high absolute risk. If the patient also is physically inactive and has a serum triglyceride level higher than 200 mg/dL, the absolute risk is even greater.

It also is advisable to determine the person's motivation to lose weight. Several factors can be evaluated to make this assessment. These include reasons for weight loss, previous history of weight loss attempts, social support, attitude toward physical activity, ability to participate in physical activity, time available for attempting intervention, understanding the causes of the obesity and its contribution to disease, and, finally, financial considerations.

The goals for weight loss are, at a minimum, prevention of further weight gain, reduction of current weight, and maintenance of a lowered body weight indefinitely. An algorithm has been designed for use in treating overweight and obesity. The initial goal in treatment is to lower body weight by 10% from baseline over a 6-month period. This degree of weight loss requires a calorie reduction of 300 to 500 kcal/day in individuals with a BMI of 27 to 35. For those persons with a BMI greater than 35, the calorie intake needs to be reduced by 500 to 1000 kcal/day. After 6 months, the person should be given strategies for maintaining the new weight. The person who is unable to achieve significant weight loss should be enrolled in a weight management program to prevent further weight gain.

Dietary Therapy

Dietary therapy should be individually prescribed based on the person's overweight status and risk profile. The diet should be a personalized plan that is 500 to 1000 kcal/day less than the current dietary intake. If the patient's risk status warrants it, the diet also should be decreased in saturated fat and contain 30% or less of total calories from fat. Reduction of dietary fat without a calorie deficit will not result in weight loss. Frequent contacts with a qualified dietetic professional help to achieve weight loss and then to maintain weight.

Physical Activity

Physical activity is important in the prevention of weight gain. In addition, it reduces cardiovascular and diabetes risk beyond that achieved by weight loss alone. Although physical activity is an important part of weight loss therapy, it does not lead to a significant weight loss. Exercise should be started slowly with the duration and intensity increased independent of each other. The goal should be 30 minutes or more of moderate-intensity activity on most days of the week. The activity can be performed at one time or intermittently over the day.

Behavior Therapy

Techniques for changing behavior include self-monitoring of eating habits and physical activity, stress management, stimulus control, problem solving, contingency management, cognitive restructuring, and social support.

Combined Therapy

The most successful weight loss program incorporates medical nutrition therapy, physical activity, and behavior change. Pharmacotherapy should be considered only after combined therapy has been in effect for a minimum of 6 months.

Pharmacotherapy

Drugs approved by the U.S. Food and Drug Administration can be used as an adjunct to the aforementioned regimen in some patients with a BMI of 30 or more with no other risk factors or diseases and for patients with a BMI of 27 to 29.9 with concomitant risk factors or disease. The risk factors and diseases defined as warranting pharmacotherapy are hypertension, dyslipidemia, coronary heart disease, type 2 diabetes, and sleep apnea.

Two prescription drugs are available for weight loss therapy—sibutramine and orlistat. Sibutramine inhibits the reuptake of serotonin, norepinephrine, and dopamine. The drug produces weight loss by decreasing appetite.[35] Orlistat is a lipase inhibitor that works by decreasing fat absorption in the intestine. Both sibutramine and orlistat need careful monitoring for side effects. They also are contraindicated in certain patients.

Weight Loss Surgery

This option is limited to persons with a BMI greater than 40; those with a BMI greater than 35 who have comorbid conditions and in whom efforts at medical therapy have failed; and those who have complications of extreme obesity. Vertical gastric banding and gastric bypass are two procedures that are used in subjects with acceptable operative risks. Persons who undergo surgical interventions also must continue in a program that provides guidance in nutrition and physical activity and behavioral and social support.

CHILDHOOD OBESITY

Obesity is the most prevalent nutritional disorder affecting the pediatric population in the United States. The findings from NHANES III, conducted between 1988 and 1994, showed that 14% of children and 12% of adolescents were overweight.[36] The definition for overweight for the NHANES III study was a BMI at or above the sex- and age-specific 95th percentile. A diagnosis of obesity is made when the triceps skinfold is greater than the 85th percentile and the weight for height is greater than 120% of ideal when controlled for age and sex.[37] Children who are 120% of weight expected for their height are overweight, but they are overfat only when the triceps skinfold result is greater than the 85th percentile. This distinction is important in preventing misdiagnosis of obesity and creating anxiety for the parents and the child.

The major concern of childhood obesity is that obese children will grow up to become obese adults. Even before reaching adulthood, overweight children already are experiencing mental and psychological problems because of their obesity. Pediatricians are beginning to see hypertension, dyslipidemia, and type 2 diabetes in obese children and adolescents.[38] In addition, there is a growing concern that childhood and adolescent obesity may be associated with negative psychosocial consequences such as low self-esteem and discrimination by adults and peers.[39]

Childhood obesity is determined by a combination of hereditary and environmental factors. It is associated with obese parents, higher socioeconomic status, increased parental education, small family size, and sedentary lifestyle.[40] Children with overweight parents are at highest risk; the risk for those with two overweight parents is much higher than for children in families in which neither parent is obese. One of the trends leading to childhood obesity is the increase in inactivity. Increasing perceptions that neighborhoods are unsafe has resulted in less time spent outside playing and walking and more time spent indoors engaging in sedentary activities such as television viewing. Television viewing is associated with consumption of calorie-dense snacks and decreased indoor activity. Obese children also may have a deficit in recognizing hunger sensations, stemming perhaps from parents who use food as gratification.

Because adolescent obesity is predictive of adult obesity, treatment of childhood obesity is desirable.[41,42] Weight loss without adverse health effects and maintenance of that loss are the goals. Each child should be assessed and treated individually. In young children who have mild to moderate weight problems, weight maintenance or a reduced rate of weight gain is sufficient. Studies indicate that physical activity in combination with diet therapy is more effective than diet therapy alone.[43]

When weight loss is required, a loss of 1 pound per month is reasonable together with permanent changes in food consumption and activity. The focus, however, should be on normalizing food intake, particularly fat intake, and increasing physical activity. If weight gain can be slowed or maintained during growth, lean body mass increases and some of the abnormal metabolic effects of obesity may be reversed. Family members need to be involved so they can learn to provide appropriate support and assist the child in taking responsibility for his or her own actions. Highly restrictive diets should be limited to the rare child or adolescent who has morbid complications. They should not be used for children or adolescents with renal, liver, or cardiac disease. These diets should contain a minimum of 2 g protein/kg body weight.[36] There should be close monitoring for sustained nitrogen losses, cardiac dysrhythmias, and cholelithiasis. Commercial diets are not recommended.

> In summary, obesity is defined as excess body fat resulting from consumption of calories in excess of those expended for exercise and activities. Heredity, socioeconomic, cultural, and environmental factors, psychological influences, and activity levels have been implicated as causative factors in the development of obesity. The health risks associated with obesity include hypertension and cardiovascular disease, hyperlipidemia, insulin resistance and type 2 diabetes mellitus, menstrual irregularities and infertility, cancer of the endometrium, breast, prostate, and colon, and gallbladder disease. There are two types of obesity—upper body and lower body obesity. Upper body obesity is associated with a higher incidence of complications. The treatment of obesity focuses on nutritionally adequate weight-loss diets, behavior modification, exercise, social support, and, in situations of marked obesity, surgical methods. Obesity is the most prevalent nutritional disorder affecting the pediatric population in the United States.

Undernutrition

After you have completed this section of the chapter, you should be able to meet the following objectives:

+ List the major causes of malnutrition and starvation
+ State the difference between protein-calorie starvation (*i.e.*, marasmus) and protein malnutrition (*i.e.*, kwashiorkor)
+ Explain the effect of malnutrition on muscle mass, respiratory function, acid-base balance, wound healing,

immune function, bone mineralization, the menstrual cycle, and testicular function
+ State the causes of malnutrition in the hospitalized patient
+ Compare the eating disorders and complications associated with anorexia nervosa and the binge-purge syndrome

Undernutrition ranges from the selective deficiency of a single nutrient to starvation in which there is deprivation of all ingested nutrients. Undernutrition can result from willful eating behaviors, as in anorexia nervosa and the binge-purge syndrome; lack of food availability; or health problems that impair food intake and decrease its absorption and use. Weight loss and malnutrition are common during illness, recovery from trauma, and hospitalization.

The prevalence of malnutrition in children is substantial. Globally, nearly 195 million children younger than 5 years of age are undernourished.[44] Malnutrition is most obvious in developing countries of the world, where the condition takes severe forms. Even in developed nations, malnutrition remains a problem. In 1992, it was estimated that 12 million American children consumed diets that were significantly below the recommended allowances of the National Academy of Sciences.[44]

MALNUTRITION AND STARVATION

Malnutrition and starvation are conditions in which a person does not receive or is unable to use an adequate amount of calories and nutrients for body function. Among the many causes of starvation, some are willful, such as the person with anorexia nervosa who does not consume enough food to maintain weight and health, and some are medical, such as persons with Crohn's disease who are unable to absorb their food. Most cases of food deprivation result in semistarvation with protein and calorie malnutrition.

Protein and Calorie Malnutrition

In malnutrition and starvation, the amount of food consumed and absorbed is drastically reduced. It may be primary, due to inadequate food intake, or secondary to disease conditions that produce tissue wasting. Most of the literature on malnutrition and starvation has dealt with infants and children in underdeveloped countries. Malnutrition in this population commonly is divided into two distinct conditions: marasmus and kwashiorkor.

Protein-calorie malnutrition, also referred to as *marasmus*, is characterized by loss of muscle and fat stores. Marasmus is characterized by progressive wasting from inadequate food intake that is equally deficient in calories and protein. The person appears emaciated, with sparse, dry, and dull hair and depressed heart rate, blood pressure, and body temperature. The child with marasmus has a wasted appearance, with stunted growth and loss of subcutaneous fat, but with relatively normal skin, hair, liver function, and affect.

Kwashiorkor is caused by protein deficiency. The term *kwashiorkor* comes from the African word meaning "the disease suffered by the displaced child," because the condition develops soon after a child is displaced from the breast after the arrival of a new infant and placed on a starchy gruel feeding. The child with kwashiorkor is characterized by edema, desquamating skin, discolored hair, enlarged abdomen, anorexia, and extreme apathy. The serum albumin level is less that 3.0 g/dL, and there is pitting edema of the extremities. There is less weight loss and wasting of skeletal muscles than in marasmus. Other manifestations include skin lesions, easily pluckable hair, enlarged liver and distended abdomen, cold extremities, and decreased cardiac output and tachycardia.

Marasmus-kwashiorkor is an advanced protein-calorie deficit together with increased protein requirement or loss. This results in a rapid decrease in anthropometric measurements with obvious edema and wasting and loss of organ mass.

Starvation

Starvation implies the lack of food intake. Depending on the prestarvation state, the metabolic events of starvation permit life to continue for months without caloric intake. In healthy, normally fed persons, there is fuel enough to last for more than 80 days, assuming previous use of 2000 kcal/day; approximately 85% of these calories are stored in fat tissue, 14% in body proteins, and 1% in stored carbohydrate sources.[45] Despite the limited carbohydrate stores, which are depleted within 12 to 24 hours without food, a continuing supply of glucose is essential for survival. The central nervous system uses approximately 115 g of glucose a day, and red blood cells, bone marrow, kidneys, and the peripheral nervous system use another 36 g of glucose.[45] One of the critical adaptive mechanisms in starvation is the production of new glucose (*i.e.*, gluconeogenesis). The liver uses glycerol, lactate, and amino acids in the synthesis of glucose. The glycerol skeleton, obtained from triglycerides released from fat cells, plays a significant role in glucose synthesis. Early studies established that after the first few days of starvation, free fatty acids and ketones, rather than glucose, become the predominant fuels.[46] For this reason, a state of ketosis is common during starvation.

Proteins have vital enzymatic and structural functions; the body avoids using proteins as a fuel source until the late stages of starvation. Eventually, protein wasting ensues, with substantial weight loss, the best known and most easily recognized sign of starvation. This weight loss is caused by loss of lean body tissue and fat along with diuresis. The importance of protein conservation to survival has been demonstrated in animal studies, in which a premorbid increase in nitrogen excretion due to protein use heralded the final stages of starvation.[45]

Daily weight loss can range from 1 pound to several pounds, depending on the stage of tissue wasting. Wound healing is poor, and the body is unable to fight off infection because of multiple immunologic malfunctions throughout the body. The muscles used for breathing become weakened, and respiratory function becomes compromised as muscle proteins are used as a fuel source. A reduction in respiratory function has many implications, especially for persons with burns, trauma, infection, or chronic respiratory disease and for persons who are being mechanically ventilated because of respiratory failure.

Although intellectual functioning remains intact despite the ketosis that occurs during starvation, depression and emotional lability are common. There is a diminished appetite and decreased desire for fluids because of the altered hypothalamic function that occurs with ketosis. A marked decrease in libido is observed with starvation. The female experiences anovulation and amenorrhea, and the male experiences decreased testicular function. The kidney does not go untouched by starvation. Calcium and phosphate are excreted as bone is dissolved, and uric acid is retained, which can cause gout.

Malnutrition and Wasting in Illness

Malnutrition and wasting are common in persons with trauma, sepsis, and serious illnesses such as cancer and acquired immunodeficiency syndrome. Approximately half of all persons with cancer experience tissue wasting in which the tumor induces metabolic changes leading to a loss of adipose tissue and muscle mass.[47] In healthy adults, body protein homeostasis is maintained by a cycle in which the net loss of protein in the postabsorptive state is matched by a net postprandial gain of protein.[48,49] In persons with severe injury or illness, net protein breakdown is accelerated and protein rebuilding disrupted. Consequently, these persons may lose up to 20% of body protein, much of which originates in skeletal muscle.[49] Protein mass is lost from the liver, gastrointestinal tract, kidneys, and heart. As protein is lost from the liver, hepatic synthesis of serum proteins decreases and decreased levels of serum proteins are observed. There is a decrease in immune cells and those needed for wound healing. The lungs are affected primarily by weakness and atrophy of the respiratory muscles. The gastrointestinal tract undergoes mucosal atrophy with loss of villi in the small intestine, resulting in malabsorption. The loss of protein from cardiac muscle leads to a decrease in myocardial contractility and cardiac output.

In hospitalized patients, malnutrition increases morbidity and mortality rates, incidence of complications, and length of stay. Malnutrition may present at the time of admission or develop during hospitalization. The hospitalized patient often finds eating a healthful diet difficult and commonly has restrictions on food and water intake in preparation for tests and surgery. Pain, medications, special diets, and stress can decrease appetite. Even when the patient is well enough to eat, being alone in a room where unpleasant treatments may be given is not conducive to eating. Although hospitalized patients may appear to need fewer calories because they are on bed rest, their actual need for caloric intake may be higher because of other energy expenditures. For example, more calories are expended during fever, when the metabolic rate is increased. There also may be an increased need for protein to support tissue repair after trauma or surgery.

Treatment

The treatment of severe protein-calorie malnutrition involves the use of measures to correct fluid and electrolyte abnormalities and replenish proteins, calories, and micronutrients.[50] Treatment is started with modest quantities of proteins and calories based on the person's actual weight. Concurrent administration of vitamins and minerals is needed. Either the enteral or parenteral route can be used. The treatment should be undertaken slowly to avoid complications. The administration of water and sodium with carbohydrates can overload a heart that has been weakened by malnutrition and result in congestive failure. Enteral feedings can result in malabsorptive symptoms due to abnormalities in the gastrointestinal tract. Refeeding edema is benign dependent edema that results from renal sodium reabsorption and poor skin and blood vessel integrity. It is treated by elevation of the dependent area and modest sodium restrictions. Diuretics are ineffective and may aggravate electrolyte deficiencies.

EATING DISORDERS

Eating disorders affect an estimated 5 million Americans each year.[51] These illnesses, which include anorexia nervosa, bulimia nervosa, and binge-eating disorder and their variants, incorporate serious disturbances in eating, such as restriction of intake and binging, with an excessive concern over body shape or body weight. Eating disorders typically occur in adolescent girls and young women, although 5% to 15% of cases of anorexia nervosa and 40% of cases of binge-eating disorder occur in boys and men.[51] The mortality rate from anorexia nervosa, 0.56% per year, is more than 12 times the mortality rate among young women in the general population.[51]

Eating disorders are more prevalent in industrialized societies and occur in all socioeconomic and major ethnic groups. A combination of genetic, neurochemical, developmental, and sociocultural factors is thought to contribute to the development of the disorders. The American Psychiatric Society's *Diagnostic and Statistical Manual of Mental Disorders, Text Revision* (DSM-IV-TR) has established criteria for the diagnosis of anorexia nervosa and bulimia nervosa.[52] Although these criteria allow clinicians to make a diagnosis in persons with a specific eating disorder, the symptoms often occur along a continuum between those of anorexia nervosa and bulimia nervosa. Preoccupation with weight and excessive self-evaluation of weight and shape are common to both disorders, and persons with eating disorders may demonstrate a mixture of both disorders.[52] The female athlete triad, which includes disordered eating, amenorrhea, and osteoporosis, does not meet the strict DSM-IV criteria for anorexia nervosa or bulimia nervosa, but shares many of the characteristics and therapeutic concerns of the two disorders (see Chapter 58). Persons with eating disorders may require concomitant evaluation for psychiatric illness because eating disorders often are accompanied by mood, anxiety, and personality disorders. Suicidal behavior may accompany anorexia nervosa and bulimia nervosa and should be ruled out.[51]

Anorexia Nervosa

Anorexia nervosa was first described in the scientific literature over 100 years ago by Sir William Gull.[53] The DSM-IV-

Eating Disorders

➤ Eating disorders are serious disturbances in eating, such as willful restriction of intake and binge eating, as well as excessive concern over body weight and shape.

➤ Anorexia nervosa is characterized by a refusal to maintain a minimally normal body weight (*e.g.*, at least 85% of minimal expected weight); an excessive concern over gaining weight and how the body is perceived in terms of size and shape; and amenorrhea (in girls and women after menarche).

➤ Bulimia nervosa is characterized by recurrent binge eating; inappropriate compensatory behaviors such as self-induced vomiting, fasting, or excessive exercise that follow the binge-eating episode; and extreme concern over body shape and weight.

➤ Binge eating consists of consuming unusually large quantities of food during a discrete period (*e.g.*, within any 2-hour period) along with lack of control over the binge-eating episode.

➤ Binge-eating disorders are characterized by eating behaviors such as eating rapidly, eating until becoming uncomfortably full, eating large amounts when not hungry, eating alone because of embarrassment, and disgust, depression, or guilt because of eating episodes.

TR diagnostic criteria for anorexia nervosa are (1) a refusal to maintain a minimally normal body weight for age and height (*e.g.*, at least 85% of minimal expected weight or BMI ≥ 17.5); (2) an intense fear of gaining weight or becoming fat; (3) a disturbance in the way one's body size, weight, shape is perceived; and (4) amenorrhea (in girls and women after menarche).[52] Anorexia nervosa is more prevalent among young women than men. The disorder typically begins in teenaged girls who are obese or perceive themselves as being obese. An interest in weight reduction becomes an obsession, with severely restricted caloric intake and frequently with excessive physical exercise. The term *anorexia*, meaning "loss of appetite," is a misnomer because hunger is felt, but in this case is denied.

Many organ systems are affected by the malnutrition that occurs in persons with anorexia nervosa. The severity of the abnormalities tends to be related to the degree of malnutrition and is reversed by refeeding. The most frequent complication of anorexia is amenorrhea and loss of secondary sex characteristics with decreased levels of estrogen, which can eventually lead to osteoporosis. Bone loss can occur in young women after as short a period of illness as 6 months.[51] Symptomatic compression fractures and kyphosis have been reported. Constipation, cold intolerance and failure to shiver in cold, bradycardia, hypotension, decreased heart size, electrocardiographic changes, blood and electrolyte abnormalities, and skin with lanugo (*i.e.*, increased amounts of fine hair) are common. Unexpected sudden deaths have been reported; the risk appears to increase as weight drops to less than 35% to 40% of ideal weight. It is believed that these deaths are caused by myocardial degeneration and heart failure rather than dysrhythmias.

The most exasperating aspect of the treatment of anorexia is the inability of the person with anorexia to recognize there is a problem. Because anorexia is a form of starvation, it can lead to death if left untreated. A multidisciplinary approach appears to be the most effective method of treating persons with the disorder.[54,55] The goals of treatment are eating and weight gain, resolution of issues with the family, healing of pain from the past, and efforts to work on psychological, relationship, and emotional issues.

Bulimia Nervosa and Binge Eating

Bulimia nervosa and binge eating are eating disorders that encompass an array of distinctive behaviors, feelings, and thoughts. Binge eating is characterized by the consumption of an unusually large quantity of food during a discrete time (*e.g.*, within any 2-hour period) along with lack of control over the binge-eating episode. A binge-eating/purging subtype of anorexia nervosa also exists.[52] Low body weight is the major factor that differentiates this subtype of anorexia nervosa from bulemia nervosa.

Bulimia Nervosa. Bulimia nervosa is 10 times more common in women than men; it usually begins between 13 and 20 years of age, and affects up to 3% of young women.[56] The DSM-IV-TR criteria for bulimia nervosa are (1) recurrent binge eating (at least two times per week for 3 months); (2) inappropriate compensatory behaviors such as self-induced vomiting, abuse of laxatives or diuretics, fasting, or excessive exercise that follow the binge-eating episode; (3) self-evaluation that is unduly influenced by body shape and weight; and (4) a determination that the eating disorder does not occur exclusively during episodes of anorexia nervosa.[52] The diagnostic criteria for bulimia nervosa now include subtypes to distinguish patients who compensate by purging (*e.g.*, vomiting or abuse of laxatives or diuretics) and those who use nonpurging behaviors (*e.g.*, fasting or excessive exercise). The disorder may be associated with other psychiatric disorders, such as substance abuse.[51,56]

The complications of bulimia nervosa include those resulting from overeating, self-induced vomiting, and cathartic and diuretic abuse. Among the complications of self-induced vomiting are dental disorders, parotitis, and fluid and electrolyte disorders. Dental abnormalities, such as sensitive teeth, increased dental caries, and periodontal disease, occur with frequent vomiting because the high acid content of the vomitus causes tooth enamel to dissolve. Esophagitis, dysphagia, and esophageal stricture are common. With frequent vomiting, there often is reflux of gastric contents into the lower esophagus because of re-laxation of the lower esophageal sphincter. Vomiting may lead to aspiration pneumonia, especially in intoxicated or debilitated persons. Potassium, chloride, and hydrogen are lost in the vomitus, and frequent vomiting predisposes to metabolic acidosis with hypokalemia (see Chapter 32). An unexplained physical response to vomiting is the development of benign, painless parotid gland enlargement.

The weights of persons with bulimia nervosa may fluctuate, although not to the dangerously low levels seen in anorexia nervosa. Their thoughts and feelings range from fear of not being able to stop eating to a concern about gaining too much weight. They also experience feelings of sadness, anger, guilt, shame, and low self-esteem.

Treatment strategies include psychological and pharmacologic treatments. Unlike persons with anorexia nervosa, persons with bulimia nervosa or binge eating are upset by the behaviors practiced and the thoughts and feelings experienced, and they are more willing to accept help. Pharmacotherapeutic agents include the tricyclic antidepressants (*e.g.*, desipramine, imipramine), the selective serotonin reuptake inhibitors (*e.g.*, fluoxetine), and other antidepressant medications.[56]

Binge Eating. Binge eating is characterized by recurrent episodes of binge eating at least 2 days per week for 6 months and at least three of the following: (1) eating rapidly; (2) eating until becoming uncomfortably full; (3) eating large amounts when not hungry; (4) eating alone because of embarrassment; and (5) disgust, depression, or guilt because of eating episodes.[51,54,56]

The primary goal of therapy for binge-eating disorders is to establish a regular, healthful eating pattern. Persons with binge-eating disorders who have been successfully treated for their eating disorder have reported that making meal plans, eating a balanced diet at three regular meals a day, avoiding high-sugar foods and other binge foods, recording food intake and binge-eating episodes, exercising regularly, finding alternative activities, and avoiding alcohol and drugs are helpful in maintaining their more healthful eating behaviors after treatment.

In summary, undernutrition can range from a selective deficiency of a single nutrient to starvation in which there is deprivation of all ingested nutrients. Malnutrition and starvation are among the most widespread causes of morbidity and mortality in the world. The body adapts to starvation through the use of fat stores and glucose synthesis to supply the energy needs of the central nervous system. Malnutrition is common during illness, recovery from trauma, and hospitalization. The effects of malnutrition and starvation on body function are widespread. They include loss of muscle mass, impaired wound healing, impaired immunologic function, decreased appetite, loss of calcium and phosphate from bone, anovulation and amenorrhea in women, and decreased testicular function in men.

Anorexia nervosa, bulimia nervosa, and binge eating are eating disorders that result in malnutrition. In anorexia nervosa, distorted attitudes about eating lead to serious weight loss and malnutrition. Bulimia nervosa is characterized by secretive episodes or binges of eating large quantities of easily consumed, high-caloric foods, followed by compensatory behaviors such as fasting, self-induced vomiting, or abuse of laxatives or diuretics. Binge-eating disorder is characterized by eating large quantities of food but is not accompanied by purging and other inappropriate compensatory behaviors seen in persons with bulimia nervosa.

Related Web Sites

American Dietetic Association   www.eatright.org
Food and Nutrition Information Center
   www.nal.usda.gov/fnic
National Academies of Sciences (Dietary Reference Intakes: Applications in Dietary Assessment [2001]. Available to read on-line free.)   www.nap.edu/books/0309071836/html/
National Institute of Diabetes and Digestive and Kidney Diseases—information on nutrition   www.niddk.nih.gov/health/nutrition.htm
The Diet Channel—good source for nutrition content of food   www.thedietchannel.com

References

1. Guyton A.C., Hall J.E. (1996). *Textbook of medical physiology* (9th ed., p. 909). Philadelphia: W.B. Saunders.
2. Garrel D.R., Jobin N., De Jonge L.H.M. (1996). Should we still use the Harris and Benedict equations? *Nutrition in Clinical Practice* 11, 99–103.
3. Subcommittee on the Tenth Edition of The RDAs. (1989). *Recommended dietary allowances* (10th ed.). Commission on Life Sciences-National Council. Washington, DC: National Academy Press.
4. Institute of Medicine. (2000). Introduction to dietary references intakes. In *Dietary reference intakes for vitamin C, vitamin E, selenium, and carotenoids*. Washington, DC: National Academy Press. [On-line.] Available: http://www.nap.edu/books/0309069351/html.
5. National Cholesterol Education Program Expert Panel on Detection, Evaluation, and Treatment of High Blood Cholesterol in Adults. (1993). Summary of the second report of the National Cholesterol Education Program (NCEP) Expert Panel on Detection, Evaluation, and Treatment of High Blood Cholesterol in Adults. *Journal of the American Medical Association* 269, 3015–3023.
6. Bennett W.G., Cerda J.J. (1996). Benefit of dietary fiber: Myth or medicine? *Postgraduate Medicine* 99, 153–156.
7. Hill G.L., Windsor J.A. (1995). Nutritional assessment in clinical practice. *Nutrition* 11 (2 Suppl.), 198–201.
8. Detsky A.S., Smalley P.S., Chang J. (1994). Is this patient malnourished? *Journal of the American Medical Association* 271, 54–58.
9. World Health Organization. (1989). *Measuring obesity: Classification and description of anthropometric data*. Copenhagen: World Health Organization.
10. National Cholesterol Education Program Expert Panel on Detection, Evaluation, and Treatment of High Blood Cholesterol in Adults. (1998). Clinical Guidelines on the identification, evaluation, and treatment of overweight and obesity in adults. NIH publication no. 98-4083. *Obesity Research* 6 (Suppl. 2), 51S–209S. Also available on-line: http://www.nhlbi.nih.gov/guidelines/ob_gdlns.htm.
11. Abernathy R.P., Black D.R. (1996). Healthy body weight: An alternative perspective. *American Journal of Clinical Nutrition* 63 (Suppl.), 448S–451S.
12. Willett W.C., Dietz W.H., Colditz G.A. (1999). Guidelines to healthy weight. *New England Journal of Medicine* 341, 427–434.
13. Durnin J.V., deBrun H., Feunekas G.I. (1977). A comparison of skinfold method with extent of "overweight" and various weight-height relationships in assessment of obesity. *British Journal of Nutrition* 77, 3–7.
14. Mokdad A. H., Serdula M.K., Dietz W.H., Bowman B.A., Marks J.S., Koplan, J.P. (1999). The spread of the obesity epidemic in the United States, 1991–1998. *Journal of the American Medical Association* 282, 1519–1522.
15. Allison D.B., Saunders S.E. (2000). Obesity in North America: An overview. *Medical Clinics of North America* 84, 305–328.
16. Goran M.I. (2000). Energy metabolism and obesity. *Medical Clinics of North America* 84, 347–362.
17. NIH Technology Assessment Conference Panel. (1992). Methods for voluntary weight loss and control. *Annals of Internal Medicine* 116, 942–949.
18. Hill J.O., Wyatt H.R., Melanson E.L. (2000). Genetic and environmental contributions to obesity. *Medical Clinics of North America* 84, 333–346.
19. McDowell A., Engel A., Massey J.T., Mauer K. (1981). *Plan and operation of the National Health and Nutrition Examination Survey, 1976–1980*. Vital and Health Statistics Series 1(15), 1–144. Hyattsville, MD: National Center for Health Statistics.
20. Soreneson T.J., Holst C., Stunkard A.J., Skovgaard T.J. (1992). Correlations of body mass index of adult adoptees and their biological and adoptive relatives. *International Journal of Obesity and Related Metabolic Disorders* 16, 227–236.
21. Bouchard C. (1994). *The genetics of obesity*. Boca Raton, FL: CRC Press.
22. Hill J.O., Melanson E.L. (1999). Overview of the determinants of overweight and obesity: Current evidence and research issues. *Medicine and Science in Sports and Exercise* 31 (Suppl.), S515–S521.
23. Kissebah A.H., Krakower G.R. (1994). Regional adiposity and morbidity. *Physiological Reviews* 74, 761–811.
24. Fujoka S., Matsuzawa Y., Tounaja K., Kawamoto T., Kobatake T., Keno Y., et al. (1991). Improvement of glucose and lipid metabolism associated with selective reduction of intra-abdominal fat in premenstrual women with visceral fat obesity. *International Journal of Obesity* 15, 853–859.
25. Pleuss J.A., Hoffman R.G., Sonnentag G.E., Goldstein M.D., Kissebah A.H. (1993). Effects of abdominal fat on insulin and androgen levels. *Obesity Research* 1 (Suppl. 1), 25F.
26. Ashwell M. (1994). Obesity in men and women. *International Journal of Obesity* 18 (Suppl. 1), S1–S7.
27. Jeffery R.W. (1996). Does weight cycling present a health risk? *American Journal of Clinical Nutrition* 63 (Suppl.), 452S–455S.
28. Muls E., Kempen K., Vansant G., Saris W. (1995). Is weight cycling detrimental to health? A review of the literature in humans. *International Journal of Obesity and Related Metabolic Disorders* 19 (Suppl. 3), S46–S50.
29. Williamson D.F. (1996). "Weight cycling" and mortality: How do the epidemiologists explain the role of intentional weight loss? *Journal of the American College of Nutrition* 15, 6–13.
30. Garn S.M. (1996). Fractionating healthy weight. *American Journal of Clinical Nutrition* 63 (Suppl.), 412S–414S.

31. Dwyer J. (1996). Policy and healthy weight. *American Journal of Nutrition* 63 (Suppl. 3), 415S–418S.

32. Lee I., Manson J.E., Hennekens C.H., Paffenbarger R.S. (1993). Body weight and mortality: A 27-year follow-up of middle-aged men. *Journal of the American Medical Association* 270, 2823–2828.

33. Task Force on Prevention and Treatment of Obesity. (1994). Towards prevention of obesity: Research directives. *Obesity Research* 2, 571.

34. Wing R.R. (1995). Changing diet and exercise behaviors in individuals at risk for weight gain. *Obesity Research* 3 (Suppl. 2), 277S–282S.

35. Berke E.M., Morden N.E. (2000). Medical management of obesity. *American Family Physician* 62, 419–426.

36. CDC. (1997). Update: Prevalence of overweight among children, adolescents, and adults—United States, 1988–1994. *Morbidity and Mortality Weekly Report* 46, 198–202.

37. Dietz W.H., Robinson T.N. (1993). Assessment and treatment of childhood obesity. *Pediatrics in Review* 14, 337–343.

38. Dietz W.H. (1998). Health consequences of obesity in youth: Childhood predictors of adult disease. *Pediatrics* 101 (Suppl. 3), 518–525.

39. Hill J.O., Trowbridge F.L. (1998). Childhood obesity: Future directions and research priorities. *Pediatrics* 101 (Suppl. 3), 570–574.

40. Birch L.L., Fisher J.O. (1998). Development of eating behaviors among children and adolescents. *Pediatrics* 101 (Suppl. 3), 539–554.

41. Eck L.H., Klesge R.C., Hanson C.L., Slawson D. (1992). Children at familial risk for obesity: An examination of dietary intake, physical activity and weight status. *International Journal of Obesity* 16, 71–78.

42. Schonfeld-Warden N., Warden C.H. (1997). Childhood obesity. *Pediatric Clinics of North America* 44, 339–361.

43. Sallis J.F., McKenzie T.L., Alcaraz J.E., Kolody B., Hovell M.F., Nadir P.R. (1993). Project SPARK: Effects of physical education on adiposity in children. *Annals of the New York Academy of Science* 699, 127–136.

44. Brown J.L., Pollitt E. (1996). Malnutrition, poverty, intellectual development. *Scientific American* 274(2), 38–43.

45. Sauded K., Felig P. (1976). The metabolic events of starvation. *American Journal of Medicine* 60, 117–126.

46. Cahill G.F., Jr., Herrera M.G., Morgan A.P., Soeldner J.S., Steinke J., Levy P.L., et al. (1966). Hormone–fuel interrelationships during fasting. *Journal of Clinical Investigation* 45, 1751–1769.

47. Tisdale M.J. (1999). Wasting in cancer. *Journal of Nutrition* 129 (IS Suppl), 43S–46S.

48. Chiolero R., Revelly J., Tappy L. (1999). Energy metabolism in sepsis and injury. *Journal of Nutrition* 129 (IS Suppl), 45S–51S.

49. Biolo G., Gabriele T., Ciccchi B., Situlin R., Iscara F., Gullo A., Guarnieri G. (1999). Metabolic response to injury and sepsis: Changes in protein metabolism. *Journal of Nutrition* 129 (IS Suppl), 53S–57S.

50. Baron R.B. (2001). Nutrition. In Tierney L.M., McPhee S.J., Papadakis M.A. (Eds.), *Current diagnosis and treatment* (40th ed., pp. 1232–1233). New York: Lange Medical Books/McGraw-Hill.

51. Becker A., Grinspoon S.K., Klibanski A., Herzog D.B. (1999). Eating disorders. *New England Journal of Medicine* 340, 1092–1098.

52. American Psychiatric Society. (2000). Practice guideline for treatment of patients with eating disorders (Revision). *American Journal of Psychiatry* 157, 1–38.

53. Gull W.W. (1868). Anorexia nervosa. *Transactions of the Clinical Society of London* 7, 22–27.

54. Kreipe R.E., Birndorf S.A. (2000). Eating disorders in adolescents and young adults. *Medical Clinics of North America* 84, 1027–1049.

55. Gordon A. (2001). Eating disorders: Anorexia nervosa. *Hospital Practice* 36(2), 36–38.

56. McGilley B.M., Pryor T.L. (1998). Assessment and treatment of bulimia nervosa. *American Family Physician* 57 (6), 27–43.

Chapter 12

Alterations in Activity Tolerance

Mary Kay Jiricka

Health includes both physical and psychological components; it involves the ability to work, exercise, participate in leisure activities, and perform activities of daily living. To be able to perform these activities requires that the body have sufficient physiologic and psychological energy and stamina. When the body no longer can meet these energy demands, fatigue occurs. Fatigue may be acute, as in that resulting from increased physical activity, or it may be chronic. Conditions that impair health can affect a person's activity reserve and impose certain restrictions, such as bed rest and immobility, on the ability to perform work and other activities. This chapter focuses on activity tolerance, the ability to do work, and the body's response to exercise; activity intolerance and fatigue; and the physiologic and psychosocial responses to immobility and bed rest.

Activity is defined as the process of energy expenditure for the purpose of accomplishing an effect. Human beings interact with their environment in a cyclic pattern of periods of activity and rest, both of which have physical and psychological elements. *Rest* is characterized by inactivity and requires minimal energy expenditure. Activity denotes the process of movement and requires the expenditure of energy. The form of activity known as *exercise* not only is characterized by movement and energy expenditure, but results in an overall conditioning of the body when performed on a regular basis. This section of the chapter focuses on the physiologic and psychological responses to exercise and increased workload on the body.

There is increasing interest in both the preventative and therapeutic effects of exercise. A regular program of exercise is recommended as a means of maintaining weight control and cardiovascular fitness. The athletically fit person has more reserves to call on when he or she becomes ill. Exercise also is becoming recognized as an integral part of the treatment regimen for many diseases. It is recommended as a means of lowering low-density lipoproteins and increasing high-density lipoproteins in persons with hyperlipidemia, of providing better regulation of blood glucose in persons with diabetes, and of improving activity tolerance in persons with cardiac and respiratory diseases. Regular exercise also has psychological benefits. Exercise training can improve self-esteem, remedy depressive moods, and enhance quality of life.[1]

Activity Tolerance

After you have completed this section of the chapter, you should be able to meet the following objectives:

✦ Describe the physiologic and psychological responses to exercise and work

✦ Define the term *maximal oxygen consumption* and state how it is measured

✦ Identify one physical method and two paper and pencil tools to assess work performance

ACTIVITY TOLERANCE AND WORK PERFORMANCE

There are two main types of exercise: aerobic and isometric. *Aerobic* or *endurance exercise* involves the use of oxygen for transforming substrates such as glucose, fatty acids, and amino acids into energy. It involves a change in muscle length (contraction and elongation) such as occurs when walking or running. Aerobic exercise training results in muscles that use oxygen more efficiently such that the body can do more work with less cardiac and respiratory effort. The sustained type of muscle activity used during aerobic exercise does not promote significant muscle hypertrophy, even though the exercise may go on for hours. During *isometric* or *resistance exercise*, the muscles contract against an immovable force without changing length. Isometric exercise involves activities, such as weight lifting and high-resistance exercises, that improve overall muscle strength and tone and build muscle mass. The bulging biceps and chest muscle of professional weight lifters result from high-intensity resistance exercise. Here strength, not stamina, is important. Most exercise programs use a combination of aerobic and isometric activities.

Physiologic Responses

Physical activity or exercise depends on four major components: cardiopulmonary fitness; muscle strength, flexibility, and endurance; availability of energy substrates to meet the increased energy demands imposed by increased physical activity; and motivation and mental endurance.

Cardiopulmonary Responses. The cardiopulmonary responses, which include the circulatory functions of the heart and blood vessels and the gas exchange functions of the respiratory system, work to supply oxygen and energy substrates to the working muscle groups and exchange oxygen and carbon dioxide with the atmosphere. Aerobic or cardiopulmonary exercise involves repetitive and rhythmic movements; it uses large muscle groups and results in the ability to perform vigorous exercise for an extended period. Exercise places a major stress on the cardiopulmonary system and causes various physiologic responses.[2,3]

The principal factor that determines how long and effectively a person will be able to exercise is the capacity of the heart, lungs, and circulation to deliver oxygen to the working muscles. The term *maximal oxygen consumption* ($\dot{V}O_2$ max) represents this principle. $\dot{V}O_2$ max is determined by the rate at which oxygen is delivered to the working muscles, the oxygen-carrying capacity of blood, and the amount of oxygen extracted from the blood by the working muscles. It is measured as the volume of oxygen consumed, usually in liters or milliliters, per unit of time (*i.e.*, liters/minute). The $\dot{V}O_2$ max is an important determinant of the person's capacity to perform work and can increase up to 20-fold with strenuous exercise.[4]

The cardiovascular response to increased activity and exercise includes an increase in heart rate, stroke volume (*i.e.*, amount of blood that the heart pumps with each beat), and arterial blood pressure. The increase in heart rate is mediated through neural, hormonal, and intrinsic cardiovascular mechanisms. With anticipation of exercise, the vasomotor center of the brain is stimulated to initiate sympathetic activity concomitant with inhibition of parasympathetic mechanisms. Stimulation of the sympathetic nervous system causes the release of the sympathetic neurotransmitters, norepinephrine and epinephrine. These transmitters produce an increase in heart rate and cardiac contractility. At the start of exercise, the heart rate rises immediately and continues to increase until a plateau is reached. This plateau, or steady-state heart rate, is maintained until the exercise, or activity, is terminated. Also contributing to the increased heart rate are intrinsic mechanisms in the heart. During exercise, increased blood return to the heart stimulates right atrial stretch receptors that initiate an increase in heart rate. Release of epinephrine and norepinephrine from the adrenal glands helps to sustain the increased heart rate.[2–4]

During exercise, cardiac output may increase from a resting level of 4 to 8 L/minute to as high as 15 L/minute for women and 22 L/minute for men. The increase in cardiac output is due to an increase in heart rate and stroke volume. The neurotransmitters norepinephrine and epinephrine cause the heart to beat faster and more forcefully. In addition, increased venous return stretches the myocardial fibers, which results in a more forceful contraction and a more complete emptying of the ventricles with each beat, a response called the *Frank-Starling mechanism* (see Chapter 21).[4]

With the onset of exercise, the systolic blood pressure increases because of the increase in cardiac output; however, the diastolic blood pressure changes little because of peripheral vasodilatation caused by the accumulation of metabolic waste products. The increased systolic pressure that occurs concomitant with a nearly constant diastolic blood pressure results in increases in pulse pressure and mean arterial pressure. The increase in mean arterial pressure ensures the perfusion of vital organ systems.[2–4]

The role of the respiratory system is to effect the exchange of oxygen and carbon dioxide. During exercise, the respiratory system must increase the rate of gas exchange. This takes place through a series of physiologic responses. With the increase in cardiac output, a greater volume of blood under slightly increased pressure is delivered to the pulmonary vessels in the lungs. This results in the opening of more pulmonary capillary beds, producing better alveolar perfusion and a more efficient exchange of oxygen and carbon dioxide.[3,4]

In addition to pulmonary perfusion being enhanced during exercise, pulmonary ventilation is increased. The respiratory rate and tidal volume increase, resulting in an increase in minute ventilation. This response is controlled by chemoreceptors—located in the medulla, the aorta, and the carotid arteries—that monitor blood gases and pH. During exercise, decreases in blood oxygen and pH and increases in carbon dioxide stimulate an increase in the rate and depth of respiration.[4,5]

Neuromuscular Responses. The integration of the neurologic and musculoskeletal systems is essential for body movement and participation in activity. To initiate and sustain increased activity, muscle strength, flexibility, and endurance are needed. *Muscle strength* is defined as the ability of muscle groups to produce force against resistance. *Flexibility* involves the range of movement of joints, whereas *muscle endurance* refers to the ability of the body or muscle groups to perform increased activity for an extended time.

Skeletal muscle consists of two distinct types of muscle fibers based on differences in their size, speed, and endurance: red slow-twitch (type I) and white fast-twitch (type II) muscle fibers.[4] Both heredity and activity influence the distribution of fast-twitch and slow-twitch fibers. There are hereditary differences in muscle fiber composition. Some people have considerably more fast-twitch than slow-twitch fibers, and others have more slow-twitch than fast-twitch fibers. This could determine to some extent the area of athletics for which a person is best suited.

The slow-twitch fibers, which are smaller than the fast-twitch fibers, tend to produce less overall force but are more energy efficient than fast-twitch fibers. They are better suited biochemically to perform lower-intensity work for prolonged periods of time. These fibers have a high oxidative capacity as a result of high concentrations of mitochondria and myoglobin. Slow-twitch fibers predominate in the large muscle groups such as the leg muscles and therefore play a major role in sustaining activity during prolonged exercise or endurance activities. Periods of sustained inactivity, such as prolonged immobility or bed rest, primarily affect slow-twitch fibers that quickly decondition.[4,6]

In contrast to slow-twitch fibers, fast-twitch fibers are larger and better suited for high-intensity work, but they fatigue more easily. These fibers have high myosin adenosine triphosphatase (ATPase) activity, few mitochondria, low myoglobin concentration, and high glycolytic capacity, resulting in dependence on anaerobic metabolism to supply adenosine triphosphate (ATP) for energy. Fast-twitch muscle fibers are most common in smaller muscle groups such as those found in the arms and eye. Fast-twitch fibers predominate during activities in which short bursts of intense energy are required, such as sprinting or weight lifting. Anabolic steroids enhance fast-twitch fiber activity.[4,6]

During aerobic activity, working muscles use oxygen 10 to 20 times faster than nonworking muscles. This increased oxygen demand is met by an increase in cardiac output and an increase in muscle blood flow. Skeletal muscles receive 85% to 95% of the cardiac output during aerobic activities, and 15% to 20% of the cardiac output at rest. The increased blood flow during aerobic activities is achieved through two mechanisms: dilation of blood vessels in the working muscles and constriction of blood vessels in the organs of low priority.[6]

Increased blood flow to working muscles is achieved by relaxation of the arterioles and the precapillary sphincters. Chemical changes such as decreased oxygen and pH and increased levels of potassium, adenosine, carbon dioxide, and phosphate contribute to the vasodilation during prolonged exercise and recovery from exercise.[2] Increased venous flow and, thus, increased venous return are enhanced by the alternate contraction and relaxation of working muscles.

Another mechanism that increases blood flow to the working muscles is the diversion of blood from the visceral organs. The amount of blood diverted from the visceral organs is proportional to the level of exercise, and as exercise is increased, more blood is diverted to working muscles. This redistribution of blood flow results from selective vasoconstriction in organs, such as the kidneys and gastrointestinal structures, that are less active than the working muscles.[2]

Skeletal muscles hypertrophy and undergo other anatomic changes in response to exercise training. "Trained muscles" have an increased number of capillaries surrounding each muscle fiber that facilitates the delivery of oxygen to the working muscle cells during exercise. Trained skeletal muscles are able to use oxygen more efficiently, probably because of enhanced enzymatic activity that increases oxidative capacity. Mitochondria appear to adapt by increasing the transport of oxygen and other substrates to the inner regions of the muscle fiber for more efficient use of oxygen.[2,4,7]

Metabolic and Thermal Responses. To perform physical activities, the body requires increased energy sources. Energy is obtained from creatine phosphate (a stored form of muscle energy), glucose, glycogen, and fatty acids. As the activity begins, especially aerobic activity, the body uses its energy sources in a characteristic pattern. The first sources for energy are stored ATP, creatine phosphate, and muscle glycogen. Short, intense periods of activity lasting 1 to 2 minutes exploit these energy sources through anaerobic metabolism.[8] If the activity is to be performed for a period of 3 to 40 minutes, muscle glycogen and creatine phosphate are used to meet the energy requirements through both anaerobic and aerobic metabolism. For intense, prolonged periods of activity that last more than 40 minutes, aerobic metabolism is essential. Muscle glycogen, glucose, and fatty acids are used for energy sources during prolonged activity.[4]

To supply the energy needed for increased activity, a person must consume a balanced diet and have adequate hydration. General recommendations for a balanced diet include 55% complex carbohydrate sources, 30% fat sources (mainly polyunsaturated fats), and 15% protein. Although proteins are not used for energy sources during increased activity, they have an essential role in the building and rebuilding of tissues and organs. During increased activity and exercise, it is essential that an individual maintain adequate hydration. Increased activity can result in loss of fluids from the vascular compartment. If this is allowed to progress, the person may experience severe dehydration that may lead to vascular collapse. Before and during vigorous activity, a person should replenish body fluids with water and electrolyte solutions.[4]

Under normal resting conditions, the body is able to maintain its temperature within a set range. It does this by way of two mechanisms. The first mechanism used by the body to regulate temperature is to change blood flow to the skin. When the blood vessels of the skin dilate, warm blood is shunted from the core tissues and organs to the skin surface, where heat is lost more easily to the surrounding environment. The second mechanism by which the body loses heat is through sweating, in which the evaporation of sweat from the skin surface contributes to the loss of body heat. Depending on training level and environmental conditions, the body may have difficulty regulating its temperature during vigorous exercise.[4,9] With sufficient training, the body adapts by increasing the rate of sweat production. Temperature regulation improves with training, and the trained person begins to sweat sooner, often within 1 to 2 minutes of the start of exercise. Sweat production begins even before the core temperature rises, and a cooling effect is initiated soon after the start of exercise; the sweat produced is more dilute than sweat produced by a nontrained person. Sweat normally contains large amounts of sodium chloride; production of a dilute sweat allows evaporative cooling to take place while sodium chloride is conserved.[4]

During exercise, plasma proteins are shifted from the interstitial space to the vascular space so that there is an increase in the amount of proteins in the blood. These proteins exert an osmotic force that draws fluid from the interstitial space into the vascular compartment. This contributes to an increase in vascular volume, which in turn is delivered to the working muscles and which also provides more efficient heat dissipation.[4]

Gastrointestinal Function. The gastrointestinal system is affected by intense increased physical activity. During increased physical activity, blood is shunted away from the gastrointestinal tract toward the active skeletal muscles. Gastrointestinal motility, secretory activity, and absorption are decreased. This can result in the person experiencing reflux, vomiting, bloating, and stomach pain. Other symptoms the person may experience include cramping, urge to defecate, and diarrhea.[10,11]

Hemostasis and Immune Function. Increased physical activity affects both hemostasis and the immune system. Increased epinephrine levels stimulate increased fibrinolytic activity. Thus, regular strenuous exercise can result in increased fibrinolytic activity and a slowing of coagulative activity.[4,12]

The response of the immune system to exercise is varied and depends on frequency, intensity, and duration of the exercise. Moderate-intensity exercise is associated with leukocytosis, lymphocytosis, neutrophilia, and lymphocytopenia.[13] Chronic, intense exercise may have different effects on the immune system. Recent research has focused on the relationship between chronic exercise training and the beneficial or harmful effects that may occur in the immune system. The immune system is stimulated by regular, moderate exercise, whereas it may be impaired with regular, repetitive, intense exercise. This may explain why elite athletes are susceptible to illness, especially upper respiratory tract infections.[4,14–16]

Psychological Responses

There is a mental component to the performance of increased activity and exercise. The mental aspect entails the motivation to initiate an activity, or exercise program, and

the dedication to incorporate the regimen into one's lifestyle. Positive effects of regularly performed exercise include increased energy and motivation, positive self-image and self-esteem, decreased anxiety, and better management of stress.

Assessment of Activity Tolerance

The assessment of a person's ability to tolerate exercise and perform work can be conducted in several ways. One method is to administer a paper and pencil test that enables persons to describe their normal activities, their perceived level of activity tolerance, or their level of fatigue. One example of a paper and pencil test is the Human Activity Profile (HAP).[17] The HAP originally was developed to assess the quality of life for persons participating in a rehabilitation program for chronic obstructive pulmonary disease. After investigating numerous physiologic and psychological measures, it was noted that the most important aspect of quality of life was the amount of daily activity the person was able to perform. The HAP consists of 94 items that represent common activities that require known amounts of average energy expenditure. The person marks each item based on whether he or she is still able to perform the activity or has stopped performing the activity.

Another paper and pencil test is the Fatigue Severity Scale[18] (Chart 12-1). This tool consists of nine statements that describe symptoms of fatigue. Persons are instructed to choose a number from 1 to 7 that best indicates their agreement with each statement. The tool is brief, easy to administer, and easily interpreted. Paper and pencil tests provide an objective way to assess a person's activity tolerance.

Another method for assessing activity tolerance is ergometry. Ergometry is a procedure for determining physical performance capacity. The ergometer is a specific tool that imposes a constant level of work. A specified workload,

---

CHART 12-1

Fatigue Severity Scale*

1. My motivation is lower when I am fatigued.
2. Exercise brings on my fatigue.
3. I am easily fatigued.
4. Fatigue interferes with my physical functioning.
5. Fatigue causes frequent problems for me.
6. My fatigue prevents sustained physical functioning.
7. Fatigue interferes with carrying out certain duties and responsibilities.
8. Fatigue is among my three disabling symptoms.
9. Fatigue interferes with my work, family, or social life.

*Patients are instructed to choose a number from 1 to 7 that indicates their degree of agreement with each statement; 1 indicates strongly disagree, and 7 indicates strongly agree. (Krupp L.B., LaRocca N.G., Muire-Nash J., Steinberg A.D. [1989]. The Fatigue Severity Scale: Application to patients with multiple sclerosis and systemic lupus erythematosus. *Archives of Neurology 46*, 1122)

expressed in terms of watts or joules per second, is imposed while the person performs the task. During the performance of the work, the person's physiologic status is monitored, as well as their subjective assessment of the work.[19]

Two examples of ergometers include the bicycle ergometer and the treadmill ergometer. A bicycle ergometer is a stationary bicycle that has a friction belt attached. The front wheel of the bicycle is rotated, and the braking force of the belt can be adjusted to alter the workload. A treadmill ergometer is used more frequently to assess workload performance, especially cardiac function. During treadmill testing, the person walks or runs on a moving belt. Changing the speed and incline of the treadmill alters the workload. This change usually is done in predetermined stages. During treadmill testing, the electrocardiogram is monitored continuously, and the blood pressure is checked intermittently. Usually, the person being tested continues to exercise, completing successive stages of the test, until exhaustion intervenes or a predetermined or maximal heart rate is reached.[19]

Maximal heart rate is estimated by age. Tables of maximal heart rate by age are available, but as a general rule, the predicted maximal heart rate can be estimated by subtracting age from 220 (*e.g.*, the target heart rate for a 40-year-old person would be 180 beats/minute). The person may continue to exercise until the predicted maximum heart rate is achieved, or until 85% to 90% of the predicted maximal rate is reached.

Metabolic equivalents (METs) are commonly used to express workload at various stages of work. One MET is equivalent to the energy expended in a resting position. METs are multiples of the basal metabolic rate, and as the type of activity performed (*e.g.*, walking, running) is changed, the MET requirement also changes. For example, walking at 4 miles per hour (mph), cycling at 11 mph, playing tennis (singles), or doing carpentry requires 5 to 6 METs. Running at 6 mph requires 10 METs, and running at 10 mph requires 17 METs. Physically trained persons are able to achieve workloads beyond 16 METs. Healthy sedentary persons seldom are able to exercise beyond 10 or 11 METs. In persons with coronary artery disease, workloads of 8 METs often produce angina.

During exercise stress testing, persons are asked to rate their subjective feelings of the exercise experience. A commonly used tool to measure the person's perception of the amount of work being performed is the Borg Rating of Perceived Exertion (RPE) Scale,[20] which is based on research that correlates heart rate to feelings of perceived exertion (Chart 12-2). The scale values range from 6 through 20. The numeric values on the RPE Scale increase linearly with workload, and the total scale reflects a 10-fold increase in heart rate. As the person is performing the exercise, he or she is asked to select a number that best corresponds to his or her feelings of exertion for the work being performed. The number chosen should be approximately 10 times the heart rate (*e.g.*, if the person rates the exercise experience as a 7, the heart rate should be 70 beats/minute).

A newer category of scale with ratio properties has been developed. The numbers on this scale range from 0 to 10, with 0 representing nothing; 0.5, very, very weak; and 10,

---

CHART 12-2

The 15-Grade Scale for Rating of Perceived Exertion: the RPE Scale

6
7 Very, very light
8
9 Very light
10
11 Fairly light
12
13 Somewhat hard
14
15 Hard
16
17 Very hard
18
19 Very, very hard
20

Borg G.A.V. (1973). Perceived exertion: A note on "history" and methods. *Medicine and Science in Sports* 5, 90–93.

---

very, very strong. With this method, the expressions and the numbers they represent are placed in the correct position for a ratio scale. For example, because 1 represents very weak, 0.5 represents very, very weak or half that intensity.[21]

Activity Tolerance

➤ Activity is the process of purposeful energy expenditure. Exercise, a form of activity that results in overall conditioning of the body, can be aerobic or isometric.

➤ Exercise depends on the availability of energy substrates, cardiovascular fitness, muscle strength and flexibility, and motivation.

➤ The cardiovascular response to exercise includes increased heart rate, stroke volume, and mean arterial pressure. An increased percentage of cardiac output is distributed to working muscle.

➤ Pulmonary perfusion and pulmonary ventilation increase.

➤ Psychological effects of exercise include an increase in energy and in the ability to adapt to stress.

In summary, the response of the body to increased activity and exercise assumes that a healthy, normal person is performing the increased activity. In disease states, especially diseases of the cardiovascular, pulmonary, or musculoskeletal systems, the body's response to increased activity is compromised. The normal physiologic responses cannot be elicited. When a person experiences diseases, activities of daily living and an exercise regimen must be adapted to the physiologic limitations.

The body reacts to the increased activity of exercise by a series of physiologic responses that increase its level of performance. Heart rate, cardiac output, and stroke volume increase to deliver more blood to working muscles. Minute ventilation and diffusion of oxygen and carbon dioxide increase to provide oxygen more efficiently to meet the rising metabolic demands. Local changes in the arterioles and capillaries contribute to enhanced perfusion of the working muscles. Over time and with training, temperature regulation is altered so the body is able to perform activity without increasing its core temperature. Activity tolerance is assessed by use of paper and pencil tests or with bicycle or treadmill ergometry. Persons are required to perform a prescribed amount of work. While performing this work, they are monitored for their cardiovascular response and their subjective feelings of exertion for the specified amount of working being performed.

Activity Intolerance and Fatigue

After you have completed this section of the chapter, you should be able to meet the following objectives:

✦ Differentiate acute from chronic fatigue
✦ List at least four health problems that are associated with chronic fatigue
✦ Define *chronic fatigue syndrome* and describe assessment findings, presenting symptoms, and laboratory values associated with the disorder
✦ Discuss treatment modalities for chronic fatigue syndrome

Activity intolerance can be defined as "a state in which a person has insufficient physical or psychological energy to endure or complete required or desired daily activity."[22] How frequently, how intensely, and how long people are able to carry out their activities of daily living depends on a balance between available energy (needed oxygen and nutrients) and the energy that is required to complete the desired task. Factors that influence this balance of energy include (1) overall physical condition (*e.g.,* level of fatigue, deconditioning, disease, and pain); (2) psychosocial factors (*e.g.,* depression and anxiety); and (3) lifestyle factors (*e.g.,* obesity, smoking, lack of regular exercise).[23] This section of the chapter focuses on fatigue, specifically acute fatigue and the chronic fatigue syndrome (CFS).

MECHANISMS OF FATIGUE

Fatigue is a state that is experienced by everyone at some time in his or her life. Fatigue can be a normal physical response, as in the case of extreme exercise in healthy people, or it can be a symptom that is experienced by

people with limited exercise reserve, such as people with impaired cardiorespiratory function, anemia, or malnutrition, or those on certain types of drug therapy. Fatigue also may be related to lack of sleep or mental stress. Like dyspnea and pain, fatigue is a subjective symptom. Fatigue often is described as a subjective feeling of tiredness that varies in terms of pleasantness, intensity, and duration and often is influenced by the time of day and a person's biorhythms.[24] It is different from the normal tiredness that people experience at the end of the day. Tiredness is relieved by a good night's sleep, whereas fatigue persists despite sufficient or adequate sleep. Fatigue is one of the most common symptoms reported to health care professionals, yet it is one of the least understood health care problems.

According to Piper, fatigue may be related to two major types of stressors: situational and developmental.[24,25] Situational stressors are situation specific and can be associated with five factors: (1) the environment (*e.g.,* excessive noise, temperature extremes, changes in weather); (2) drug-related incidents (*e.g.,* use of tranquilizers, alcohol, toxic chemical exposure); (3) treatment-related therapies (*e.g.,* chemotherapy, radiation therapy, surgery, anesthesia, diagnostic testing); (4) physical exertion (*e.g.,* exercise); and (5) nonphysical exertion (*e.g.,* stress, monotony). Developmental stressors are associated with two main factors: physical factors due to a disease process and emotional factors.

When fatigue is related to mental factors or emotional stress, the physiologic explanation of fatigue may be associated with the function of the reticular activating system (RAS). The RAS, which is located in the reticular formation of the pons and midbrain, is responsible for maintaining wakefulness. Stimulation of this system results in wakefulness; conversely, inhibition results in fatigue. There is a feedback system between the RAS and the cerebral cortex.[24]

Fatigue is categorized as central or peripheral. Central fatigue is fatigue that has its origin in the central nervous system (CNS). It refers to the perception of effort or impairments in the central processing of somatic or physiologic stimuli originating in the working muscles. In contrast, peripheral fatigue refers to exhaustion of muscles during exertion and occurs because of impairments in the contracting muscles or peripheral nerves. During exercise, if a person is centrally fatigued, he or she may be able to force or push themselves to complete the necessary tasks or exercise. In contrast, if someone is peripherally fatigued, that person cannot voluntarily perform the necessary activities.[26]

ACUTE PHYSICAL FATIGUE

Acute fatigue has a rapid onset, is perceived to be a normal response to the activity being performed, is relieved shortly after the activity ceases, and serves as a protective mechanism. Although acute physical fatigue can develop when insufficient oxygen or nutrients are delivered to the muscle, for the purpose of this chapter, acute fatigue is defined as muscle fatigue associated with increased activity, or exercise, that is carried out to the point of exhaustion.

Physical conditioning can influence the onset of acute fatigue. People who engage in regular exercise compared with sedentary persons are able to perform an activity for longer periods before acute fatigue develops. They probably are able to do so because their muscles use oxygen and nutrients more efficiently and their circulatory and respiratory systems are better able to deliver oxygen and nutrients to the exercising muscles.

Acute physical fatigue occurs more rapidly in deconditioned muscle. For example, acute fatigue often is seen in people who have been on bed rest because of a surgical procedure, or in people who have had their activity curtailed because of chronic illness such as heart or respiratory disease. In such cases, the acute fatigue often is out of proportion to the activity that is being performed (*e.g.,* dangling at the bedside, sitting in a chair for the first time). When resuming activity for the first time after a prolonged period of bed rest or inactivity, the person may experience tachycardia and hypotension. Unless these parameters are changed by medications such as β-adrenergic blocking drugs, heart rate and blood pressure become particularly sensitive indicators of activity tolerance or intolerance.

Another example of people who experience acute physical fatigue are those who require the use of assistive devices such as wheelchairs, walkers, or crutches. The upper arm muscles are less well adapted to prolonged exercise than the leg muscles. This is because arm muscles are primarily composed of type II muscle fibers. Type II muscle fibers, which are used when the body requires short bursts of energy, fatigue quickly. As a result, people who use wheelchairs or a pair of crutches may quickly experience fatigue until their arms become conditioned to the increased activity.

CHRONIC FATIGUE

Chronic fatigue differs from acute fatigue in terms of onset, intensity, perception, duration, and relief. In contrast to acute fatigue, chronic fatigue has an insidious onset, is typically perceived as being unusually intense relative to the amount of activity performed, lasts longer than 1 month, has a cumulative effect, and is not relieved by cessation of activity. Although acute fatigue often serves a protective function, chronic fatigue is not protective. Chronic fatigue may even lead to aversion of activity and be further accompanied by a desire to escape certain activities. Many diseases and chronic health conditions cause people to experience chronic fatigue. When it is associated with a specific disease, there often is a physiologic basis for the fatigue. When the physiologic problem is corrected, the fatigue may be relieved.[24,25] Chronic fatigue is one of the more common problems experienced by people with chronic health problems (Table 12-1). It limits the

---

TABLE 12-1 ◆ Chronic Illnesses and Causes of Chronic Fatigue

Chronic Illness	Cause of Fatigue
Acquired immunodeficiency syndrome	Impaired immune function, anorexia, muscle weakness, and psychosocial factors associated with the disease
Anemia	Decreased oxygen-carrying capacity of blood
Arthritis	Pain and joint dysfunction lead to impaired mobility, loss of sleep, and emotional factors
Cancer	Presence of chemical products and catabolic processes associated with tumor growth; anorexia and difficulty eating; effects of chemotherapy and radiation therapy; and psychosocial factors such as depression, grieving, hopelessness, and fear
Cardiac disease	
Myocardial infarction	Death of myocardial tissue results in decreased cardiac output, poor tissue perfusion, and impaired delivery of oxygen and nutrients to vital organs
Congestive heart failure	Impaired pumping ability of the heart results in poor perfusion of muscle tissue and vital organs
Neurologic disorders	
Multiple sclerosis	Demyelinating disease of CNS characterized by slowing of nerve conduction, resulting in lower extremity weakness and fatigue
Myasthenia gravis	Disorder of postsynaptic acetylcholine receptors of the myoneural junction, resulting in muscle weakness and fatigue
Chronic lung disease	Increased work of breathing and impaired gas exchange
Chronic renal failure	Accumulation of metabolic wastes; fluid, electrolyte, and acid-base disorders; decreased red blood cell count and oxygen-carrying capacity due to impaired erythropoietin production
Metabolic disorders	
Hypothyroidism	Decrease in basal metabolic rate manifested by fatigue
Diabetes mellitus	Impaired cellular use of glucose by muscle cells
Obesity	Imbalance in nutritional intake and energy expenditure; increased workload due to excess weight
Steroid myopathy	Glucocorticosteroids interfere with protein and glycogen synthesis, which leads to muscle wasting

amount of activity that a person can perform and may interfere with employment, the performance of activities of daily living, and the quality of life in general. Although fatigue often is viewed as a symptom of anxiety and depression, it is important to recognize that these psychological manifestations may be symptoms of the fatigue. For example, people with persistent fatigue due to a chronic illness may have to curtail their work schedules, decrease social activities, and limit their usual family responsibilities. These lifestyle changes may be the reasons for the depression rather than the depression being a cause of the fatigue.

Chronic fatigue is a common problem in people with cancer, particularly those who are undergoing cancer treatment (chemotherapy or radiation therapy). Studies involving patients receiving chemotherapy for a variety of cancers report incidences of fatigue ranging from 59% to 82%.[27] In all of these studies, fatigue was the most common and distressing side effect of the treatment. In people receiving radiation therapy, the incidence of fatigue ranged from 65% to 100% and was rated as the most severe effect of the treatment, especially during the last week of treatment.[27] A possible explanation for the fatigue that occurs in people with cancer involves a chemical mediator called *tumor necrosis factor* (TNF). TNF is secreted by activated macrophages, some tumor cells, and some T lymphocytes (see Chapter 18). It causes depletion of the protein stores of skeletal muscle. As a result, muscle wasting occurs, and people have to expend

---

Activity Intolerance and Fatigue

➤ Activity intolerance is the inability of a person to complete activities because of insufficient psychological or physiologic energy.

➤ Fatigue may be due to situational stressors (environment, drug, therapies, physical or mental exertion) or developmental stressors (disease or emotional factors).

➤ Acute fatigue is muscle fatigue with a rapid onset and duration limited to the duration of the exercise. The time it takes to develop acute fatigue at any level of exercise depends on conditioning.

➤ Chronic fatigue has an insidious onset, a long duration unrelated to duration of activity, and intensity not related to the intensity of activity.

➤ Chronic fatigue syndrome (CFS) is characterized by disabling fatigue and many nonspecific symptoms, including cognitive impairments, sleep disturbances, and musculoskeletal pain. The etiology of CFS is unknown, but it is associated with several chronic diseases such as fibromyalgia, depression, and irritable bowel syndrome.

---

more energy to perform simple activities such as sitting and standing.[28]

Chronic Fatigue Syndrome

Chronic fatigue syndrome is a condition of disabling fatigue of at least 6 months' duration that is typically accompanied by an array of self-reported, nonspecific symptoms such as cognitive impairments, sleep disturbances, and musculoskeletal pain. CFS probably is not a new disease. Indeed, in the 19th century the diagnosis of "neurasthenia" was a common diagnosis applied to a group of symptoms that are very similar to those found in CFS.[29] In the 20th century and now into the 21st century, CFS continues to be a relatively common diagnosis. Because of differences in who is included in the diagnostic category of CFS, the prevalence data vary among studies. In general, approximately 10% to 20% of all patients in primary practice complained of fatigue of at least 6 months' duration. In community surveys, the prevalence of CFS that is reported is considerably lower (1% to 3%); however, this does not negate the importance of CFS as a major public health issue.[30]

Definition. The etiology of CFS is unknown, there are no biologic markers for the diagnosis of CFS, and there are no definitive treatments. Furthermore, the overlap of symptoms of CFS with other syndromal disorders (*i.e.*, fibromyalgia, depression, and irritable bowel syndrome, which also are characterized by fatigue) complicates the ability to define the syndrome with any degree of certainty.[31] In fact, CFS may describe a group of similar symptoms that develop in different groups of individuals with different combinations of risk factors.[31]

In 1994, the Centers for Disease Control and Prevention (CDC), through its International Chronic Fatigue Syndrome study group, published a revised case definition of CFS.[32] To be classified as CFS, the fatigue must be clinically evaluated, cause severe mental and physical exhaustion, and result in a significant reduction in the individual's premorbid activity level. In addition, there must be evidence of the concurrent occurrence of four of the following eight symptoms: sore throat, tender cervical or axillary lymph nodes, muscle pain, multijoint pain without swelling or redness, headaches, unrefreshing sleep, and postexertional malaise lasting more than 24 hours. The fatigue and concurrent symptoms must be of 6 months' duration or longer. Chart 12-3 outlines the criteria for diagnosis of CFS.[32]

Pathophysiology. Theories of the pathogenesis of CFS include infections, a genetic predisposition, a dysfunction in the hypothalamic-pituitary-adrenal axis, or an alteration in the autonomic nervous system.[33,34] Despite much research and the development of several theories, the pathophysiology behind CFS remains unknown. The results of studies to date are intriguing, but further study is needed before conclusions are drawn. Indeed, CFS may have many causes.[35]

The fatigue experienced in CFS is similar to the fatigue associated with therapeutic doses of interferon alfa, suggesting a possible link to an underlying viral infec-

Criteria for Diagnosis of Chronic Fatigue Syndrome

Clinically evaluated fatigue
- Fatigue of ≥6 months' duration (new or definite onset)
- Not relieved by rest
- Significant reduction in premorbid occupational, educational, social, or personal activities

Concurrent experience of at least four of the following symptoms:
- Impaired memory or concentration
- Sore throat
- Tender cervical or axillary lymph nodes
- Muscle pain
- Multijoint pain
- New headaches
- Unrefreshing sleep
- Postexertional malaise

Exclusionary diagnoses
- Any active medical condition that could explain the chronic fatigue
- Any previously diagnosed but incompletely resolved medical condition that could explain the chronic fatigue
- Any past or current diagnosis of a major depressive disorder, schizophrenia, delusional disorder, dementia, or anorexia or bulimia nervosa
- Alcohol or other substance abuse within 2 years of onset of chronic fatigue symptoms

(Developed from Fukuda K., Straus S.E., Hickie I., Sharpe M.C., Dobbins J.G., Komaroff A.L. [1994]. The chronic fatigue syndrome: A comprehensive approach to its definition and study. *Annals of Internal Medicine* 121, 953–959)

tion. Infectious agents such as Epstein-Barr virus, human herpesvirus 6, enterovirus, human retrovirus, *Mycobacterium tuberculosis*, *Borrelia burgdorferi*, *Brucella*, and *Candida* have been linked to the pathogenesis of the syndrome. However, none of these agents has been conclusively linked in a cause-and-effect relationship with the development of CFS. Psychological disorders often are associated with CFS, especially anxiety and depression, but this is difficult to evaluate. Persons with CFS are more likely than the general population to have experienced a psychological disorder such as major depression or panic disorder before the development of CFS; however, it also is true that a significant proportion of those persons with CFS have not had such episodes, either before or after the development of CFS.[29] Questions arise as to whether the psychological disorders are a cause of the CFS, whether the CFS is the cause of the psychological disorders, or, finally, whether a common etiologic agent causes both CFS and psychological disorders.

Several studies suggest that CFS may be due to a primary alteration in immune function. A number of immuno-

logic abnormalities have been described in persons with CFS.[33] It is hypothesized that the immune system may overreact to an environmental agent (most likely an infectious agent) or internal stimuli and be unable to self-regulate after the infectious insult is over. Another possibility is that a viral infection may produce continued suppression of the immune system. Mononuclear cells from persons with CFS have a decreased response to antigenic stimulation and proliferate at one-half the normal rate. One of the most consistent immunologic findings is a low level of activity in natural killer cells.[36] These lymphocytes participate in the transfer of delayed hypersensitivity and the production of interleukin-2 and interferon-γ.[33,37] It has been speculated that in a situation of prolonged immune activation, natural killer cells that find their way past the blood-brain barrier may damage brain cells and cause chronic neuroendocrine abnormalities and thus CFS.[36]

Autonomic nervous system dysfunction also is thought to play a possible role in CFS. In a significant proportion of clients with CFS, there are abnormal responses to both parasympathetic and sympathetic laboratory challenges.[38] A statistically greater number of persons diagnosed with CFS have orthostatic hypotension and tachycardia with tilt table testing than do healthy control subjects.[31,38]

The role that the CNS plays in the development of CFS has been receiving increasing attention. Indeed, it has been suggested that the CNS may be the final common pathway in the development of this disorder.[31] In brain imaging studies using magnetic resonance imaging and positron emission tomography scans, white matter abnormalities and hypoperfusion of the brain stem have been found in persons with CFS.[39,40] In other studies, abnormalities of the hypothalamic-pituitary-adrenal axis, such as attenuated activity of corticotropin-releasing hormone and changes in the circadian rhythm of cortisol secretion, have been documented.

Manifestations. One of the most important findings in persons with CFS is the complaint of fatigue. Often, the symptom of fatigue is preceded by a cold or flulike illness. Frequently, the person describes the illness as recurring, with periods of exacerbations and remissions. With each subsequent episode of the illness, the fatigue increases.

Physical findings include low-grade fever. The fever is intermittent and occurs only when the illness recurs. Other findings include nonexudative pharyngitis, palpable and tender cervical lymph nodes, a mildly enlarged thyroid gland, wheezing, splenomegaly, myalgias, arthralgias, and heme-positive stool with subsequent negative sigmoidoscopies.

Psychological problems include impaired cognition, which the person describes as an inability to concentrate and perform previously mundane tasks. There are reports of mood and sleep disturbances, balance problems, visual disturbances, and various degrees of anxiety and depression.

Diagnosis and Treatment. The diagnosis of CFS is made by integration of the entire clinical picture of the client's symptoms, physical assessment findings, and the results of diagnostic tests. Usually a complete blood count; serum electrolytes, blood glucose, and total plasma proteins; Lyme disease titers; and renal, liver, and thyroid function tests, along with a urinalysis and stool guaiac analysis, are done to rule out other causes of the client's symptoms. Laboratory and other diagnostic test results often demonstrate minor abnormalities, although not of sufficient magnitude to reflect the degree of fatigue present. Common laboratory abnormalities include atypical lymphocytosis, mild anemia, elevation of the erythrocyte sedimentation rate, decreased serum phosphorus, iron deficiency, and elevated liver function test results. Chest radiographs are negative.[32] The client's symptoms must be present for at least 6 months. In some cases, the symptoms have been present for as long as 1 to 2 years before the diagnosis of CFS is made. CFS often is a diagnosis of exclusion (see Chart 12-3).

The treatment of CFS tends to be nonspecific. It centers on client education, emotional support, treatment of symptoms, and overall management of general health. Symptom management includes development of an exercise program that helps the person regain strength. Along with a structured activity program, persons should be encouraged to be as active as possible as they resume their activities of daily living.

Nutritional support also is important. A low-fat, low- to moderate-protein, high–complex-carbohydrate diet is recommended, along with a multivitamin and multimineral supplement. For overweight persons, weight loss is recommended. Alcohol should be avoided because it exacerbates the symptoms of CFS.[35]

Analgesics and nonsteroidal anti-inflammatory medications are beneficial in treating the symptoms of myalgia and arthralgia. Antidepressants may be used to treat symptoms of depression, but the medication should not be used in isolation, and appropriate supportive treatment and counseling should be provided to the person.[37]

A holistic approach to the treatment of CFS is essential. With proper treatment and support, most persons with CFS demonstrate improvement. However, relapses can occur. Persons diagnosed with CFS must continue to receive follow-up care and treatment on a regular basis. Local and national support groups are available for persons who experience CFS.

In summary, fatigue is a nonspecific, self-recognized state of physical and psychological exhaustion. It results in the person's not being able to perform routine activities and is not relieved with sleep or rest. Acute fatigue results from excessive use of the body or specific muscle groups and often is related to depletion of energy sources. Chronic fatigue often is associated with a specific disease or chronic illness and may be relieved when the effects of the disease are corrected. CFS is a complex illness that has physiologic and psychological manifestations. It is characterized by debilitating fatigue. Diagnosis often is made by a process of elimination, and treatment requires a holistic approach.

Bed Rest and Immobility

After you have completed this section of the chapter, you should be able to meet the following objectives:

+ Describe the effects of gravity on the body
+ Describe the effects of immobility and prolonged bed rest on the cardiovascular, pulmonary, renal, musculoskeletal, metabolic, and gastrointestinal body systems
+ Discuss changes in fluid and electrolyte balance associated with immobility and prolonged bed rest
+ Identify alterations in serum electrolyte and hematologic values that are related to immobility and prolonged bed rest
+ Discuss changes in sensory perception that are consequences of immobility and prolonged bed rest
+ Identify alterations in physical assessment findings that are related to the effects of immobility and prolonged bed rest
+ Describe treatment interventions that counteract the negative effects of immobility and prolonged bed rest

Immobility may be dictated by injury that requires stabilization to facilitate the healing process, or it may result from conditions that limit physical reserve. The effects of immobility can be restricted to a single extremity that is encased in a plaster cast; involve both legs, as in a person confined to a wheelchair; or involve the entire body, as in a person confined to bed rest. Bed rest and immobility are associated with various complications that include generalized weakness, orthostatic intolerance, atelectasis, pneumonia, pulmonary emboli, thrombophlebitis, muscle atrophy, osteoporosis, urinary retention, constipation, and impaired sensory perception[41-44] (Table 12-2). This section of the chapter describes the physiologic changes that occur with bed rest and immobility and the treatment interventions to counteract their effects.

Bed rest is one of the oldest and most commonly used methods of treatment for various medical conditions. Before the 1940s, bed rest was prescribed for 2 weeks after childbirth, 3 weeks after herniorrhaphy, and 4 to 6 weeks after myocardial infarction. It was believed that the complex biochemical and physical demands of physical activity diverted energy from the restorative and reparative processes of healing. Rest in bed was regarded as tantamount to optimal rest of the heart and entire body.

During World War II, the shortage of hospital beds and medical personnel forced early mobilization of many patients. As often happens with this kind of action, it soon was discovered that early mobilization lessened complications and improved patient outcome. The National Aeronautics and Space Administration (NASA) conducted research that described the damaging effects of prolonged inactivity and weightlessness. These studies indicate that weightlessness and the antigravity effects of bed rest produce similar responses.

ANTIGRAVITY EFFECTS OF BED REST

The supine position that often accompanies immobility and bed rest interferes with the effects of gravity. The force

TABLE 12-2 ✦ Complications of Bed Rest and Immobility	
System	**Complication**
Cardiovascular	Decreased cardiac output, contributing to decreased aerobic capacity; orthostatic intolerance; venous thrombophlebitis
Pulmonary	Atelectasis; relative hypoxemia; pneumonia
Musculoskeletal	Muscle atrophy and loss of strength; decreased muscle oxidative capacity contributing to decreased aerobic capacity; osteoporosis (bone loss); contractures; osteoarthritis
Gastrointestinal	Constipation
Genitourinary	Incontinence; renal calculi
Skin	Pressure ulcers
Functional	Impaired ambulation and activity tolerance
Psychological	Sensory deprivation; altered sensory perception

(Harper C.M., Lyles Y.M. [1988]. Physiology and complications of bed rest. *Journal of the American Geriatric Society 36*, 1048)

of gravity exerts beneficial effects on the body. As the body maintains a supine position, the absence of the force of gravity leads to many of the deconditioning effects associated with immobility and bed rest.

While upright, the body compensates for the effects of gravity in a variety of ways. The skeletal muscles contract and exert pressure against veins and lymph vessels. This contraction counteracts the force of gravity that would cause blood and fluid to pool in the lower extremities. Blood is kept moving through the circulatory system. Bones remain stronger because longitudinal weight bearing keeps essential minerals, such as calcium, inside the structure of the bone.

PHYSIOLOGIC RESPONSES

Cardiovascular Responses

After a period of bed rest, the cardiovascular system exhibits changes that reflect the loss of gravitational and exercise stimuli. In effect, the cardiovascular system becomes deconditioned, resulting in an exaggeration of the hemodynamic changes normally seen with standing after brief bed rest. This deconditioning is manifest in three major alterations: postural hypotension, increased cardiac workload, and venous stasis with the potential for deep venous thrombosis.

One of the most striking responses to assumption of the supine position during bed rest is the alteration of blood flow. In the supine position, approximately 500 mL of blood is redistributed from the lower extremities to the central circulation. Most of this blood is diverted to the lungs; a smaller portion is diverted to the arms and head. The increased fluid shifted to the head and thoracic cavity may result in the person experiencing headache, swelling of the nasal sinuses, nasal congestion, and puffiness of the eyelids.[45–48]

The increase in central blood volume results in an increase in stroke volume, which results in an increase in

cardiac output. In the supine position, the normal cardiac output is 7 to 8 L/minute, compared with a cardiac output of 5 to 6 L/minute for a person in the standing position. Initially, the increase in stroke volume and cardiac output is accompanied by a slight decrease in heart rate and systemic vascular resistance and the maintenance of blood

Bed Rest and Immobility

➤ The cardiovascular responses to bed rest include a redistribution of blood volume from the lower body to the central circulation, a deconditioning of the heart, and a reduction in total body water. Orthostatic intolerance may develop.

➤ Venous stasis due to bed rest encourages the development of deep vein thrombosis.

➤ Pulmonary changes due to bed rest include decreased tidal volume and functional residual capacity. Alveoli tend to collapse, resulting in areas of decreased pulmonary ventilation.

➤ Bed rest increases the risk for development of renal calculi and urinary tract infections.

➤ Muscle mass is reduced owing to disuse atrophy and bone mass is reduced because of an imbalance of activity between osteoclasts (bone resorption) and osteoblasts (bone generation).

➤ Pressure ulcers due to tissue ischemia may develop in areas in constant contact with the bed surface.

➤ Psychological effects of bed rest include anxiety and depression and decreased ability to concentrate and learn.

pressure. With extended periods of bed rest there is an increase in venous compliance, which decreases venous return to the heart and thus compromises cardiac filling, resulting in an increase in heart rate and a decrease in stroke volume. With prolonged bed rest, heart rate can increase approximately 0.5 beat/minute each day.

Bed rest also affects fluid balance. The increase in plasma volume in the central circulation stimulates baroreceptors. The stimulation of the baroreceptors results in an inhibition of antidiuretic hormone and aldosterone, with a resultant water and sodium (*i.e.*, natriuresis) diuresis. In the supine position, diuresis begins on the first day with the shift of blood from the lower extremities to the thoracic cavity. The loss of water and sodium results in an increase in hematocrit, hemoglobin, and red cell mass owing to the loss of plasma volume.[42,43,46]

After approximately 4 days of bed rest, fluid losses reach an equilibrium. A possible explanation for this is that fluid is lost from the vascular compartment with a subsequent iso-osmotic shift of fluid from the extravascular space. Extravascular hydration is sacrificed to maintain adequate isotonic vascular volume. With a decrease in the extravascular volume and the reestablishment of intravascular volume, the osmoreceptors inhibit diuresis and natriuresis. Despite the reestablishment of intravascular volume, the extravascular spaces remain dehydrated.[42,43,46,48]

Orthostatic Hypotension. During bed rest, the forces of gravity and hydrostatic pressure are removed from the cardiovascular system. After 3 to 4 days of bed rest, resumption of the upright position results in orthostatic or postural intolerance. Standing after prolonged bed rest results in a decrease in central blood volume as blood is displaced to the lower extremities and dependent parts of the body. Decreases in stroke volume and cardiac output occur along with increases in heart rate and systemic vascular resistance. The signs and symptoms of postural intolerance include tachycardia, nausea, diaphoresis, and sometimes syncope or fainting.

It has been hypothesized that the underlying pathology for the bed rest–induced orthostatic intolerance is autonomic nervous system dysfunction. The reason for this is not completely understood because catecholamine levels and adrenergic receptor sensitivity do not change significantly with bed rest. Research suggests that an additional cardiovascular response is present that may contribute to orthostatic intolerance associated with bed rest. The decrease in stroke volume also may be caused by a reduction in left ventricular size and distensibility that occurs because of an apparent physiologic cardiac atrophy in response to a decrease in the loading conditions of the heart.[49]

Cardiac Workload and Exercise Tolerance. The major cardiovascular manifestation of deconditioning associated with bed rest is an increased workload on the heart. Initially, when a person assumes the supine position, venous return to the heart increases along with an increase in stroke volume and cardiac output, which is accompanied by a slight decrease in heart rate. Over time, cardiac output and stroke volume stabilize, whereas heart rate increases. During periods of tachycardia, the time the heart spends in diastole

is decreased. With decreased time spent in diastole, the heart does not have sufficient time to fill with blood, and it has to work harder (expend more energy and use more oxygen) to perfuse vital organs and meet the metabolic demands of the body. This response is exaggerated when a person has to assume the upright position and begin activity after a prolonged period of bed rest. When a person begins submaximal exercise after prolonged bed rest, heart rate increases while stroke volume and cardiac output decrease. Between 5 and 10 weeks of reconditioning exercise is required for return of heart rate, stroke volume, and cardiac output parameters to their levels before bed rest.[45,47,50,51]

Venous Stasis. Venous stasis in the legs results from lack of skeletal muscle pump function that promotes venous return to the heart. The skeletal muscle pump function ceases after assumption of the supine position, and there is mechanical compression of veins from the position of the lower extremities against the bed. This increased pressure damages the intima of the vessel and causes platelets to adhere easily to the damaged vessel, encouraging clot formation.

The development of deep vein thrombosis (DVT) is the third major complication of bed rest. It is believed that three possible factors combine to predispose a person to thrombus formation: venous stasis, application of external pressure from the mattress against the veins, and hypercoagulability of the blood. However, most persons with DVT have other risk factors in addition to bed rest.[43] The development of DVT also predisposes to the development of pulmonary emboli. As persons begin to resume activity patterns, the risk that large thrombi may dislodge and work their way through the circulatory system and lodge in the pulmonary vessel increases.

Various theories have been advanced for the causes of the hypercoagulability and clot formation that occur with bed rest. One theory suggests that the development of dehydration with bed rest leads to an increased number of formed elements in the blood and contributes to increased blood viscosity. Increased viscosity contributes to clotting. Another theory points to the role of calcium. During bed rest, demineralization of bone occurs, and calcium and other minerals are released into the bloodstream. Calcium activates the conversion of prothrombin to thrombin, and thrombin becomes the activating enzyme that converts fibrinogen to fibrin. Fibrin then initiates the process of clot formation.[52]

Pulmonary Responses

Bed rest and assumption of the supine position produces changes in lung volumes and the mechanics of breathing. When a person is supine, the diaphragm moves upward, causing a decrease in the size of the thoracic compartment, and chest/lung expansion is limited because of the resistance of the bed. Lung expansion also is reduced by a decrease in lung compliance. In the supine position, normal tidal volume breathing is a function of the abdominal muscles, in contrast to breathing in the upright position, in which normal breathing is primarily a function of rib cage movement. Tidal volume and functional residual capacity are decreased, and the efficiency and effectiveness of ventilation are hindered. Persons must work harder to breathe, and take fewer deep breaths. Alveoli tend to collapse, resulting in areas of atelectasis and a decrease in the surface for gas exchange. These changes in function contribute to respiratory complications associated with bed rest: atelectasis, accumulation of secretions, hypoxemia, and pulmonary emboli.

Atelectasis is characterized by localized areas of lung collapse. It is caused by impaired mucociliary clearance of the airway, resulting in pooling of secretions. Also, poor fluid intake and dehydration may cause secretions to become thick and tenacious. Stasis of secretions provides an ideal medium for bacterial growth, especially pneumococcal, staphylococcal, and streptococcal organisms. To prevent the complication of pneumonia from developing, persons must perform coughing and deep-breathing exercises. However, with the combined need of overcoming resistance to chest and lung expansion and obstructed airways, more energy is required to breathe. More oxygen is used and more carbon dioxide is produced, causing the person to expend more energy to get less air.

Urinary Tract Responses

The kidneys are designed to function optimally with the body in the erect position. The anatomy of the kidney is such that urine flows from the kidney pelvis by gravity, whereas the action of peristalsis moves urine through the ureters to the bladder. Prolonged bed rest affects the renal system by altering the composition of body fluids and predisposing to the development of kidney stones. In the supine position, urine is not readily drained from the renal pelvis. Bed rest also may predispose to urinary tract infections and urinary incontinence because of positional changes and difficulty in emptying the bladder.[48,51,53]

A major complication of prolonged bed rest is the increased risk for development of kidney stones. Prolonged bed rest causes muscle atrophy, protein breakdown, decalcification of bone, hypercalcemia and hyperphosphatemia, and an increased risk for development of calcium-containing kidney stones. The urine becomes saturated with calcium salts (*i.e.*, calcium oxalate and calcium phosphate) as a result of the hypercalcemia and hyperphosphatemia, and urinary stasis resulting from the supine position favors crystallization of the stone-forming calcium salts. Moreover, urine levels of citrate, a prominent inhibitor of calcium stone formation, do not increase during bed rest.[48,51–53] Dehydration further increases the urinary concentration of stone-forming elements and risk of kidney stone formation. The pathogenesis and manifestations of kidney stones are discussed in Chapter 33.

Urinary tract infections and incontinence also may occur. The cause of incontinence is inadequate emptying of the bladder while the person is in the supine position. This position contributes to stagnation of urine in the bladder and may predispose the person to bladder and urinary tract infections.

Musculoskeletal Responses

Muscles are only as strong as they need to be to perform the work at hand. Disuse atrophy leads to loss of approximately one eighth of the muscle's strength with each week of disuse.[43,54] Weight loss occurs when normally healthy people are subjected to periods of prolonged bed rest. The weight loss occurs when people are placed on controlled diets, as well as when they are allowed to eat ad libitum.[54] The reduction in weight is associated with the loss of lean muscle mass and fat content. Immobilization also causes a reduction in force-generating capacity along with increased fatigability, primarily owing to a decrease in muscle mass and the cross-sectional area of muscle fiber.[55] The larger and the better trained the muscle, the faster the loss of muscle strength and the quicker the deconditioning occurs. For example, leg muscles lose strength and mass more quickly than muscles of the arms in persons placed on prolonged bed rest.

In addition to loss of strength, muscles atrophy, change shape and appearance, and shorten when immobilized. There also is a decrease in the oxidative capacity of the muscle mitochondria. These changes affect individual muscle fibers and total muscle mass. Atrophy of muscles is reflected as an increase in urinary nitrogen excretion and a decrease in muscle weight. Because of the decreased oxidative capacity of the mitochondria, muscles fatigue more easily.[43,56]

Along with muscle, connective tissue undergoes changes when subjected to immobility or bed rest. Periarticular connective tissue, ligaments, tendons, and articular cartilage require motion to maintain health. Changes in structure and function of connective tissue become apparent 4 to 6 days after immobilization and remain even after normal activity has been resumed. It is believed that changes in the structure of collagen fibers contribute to the connective tissue changes associated with immobility.[56]

Muscle atrophy not only contributes to wasting and weakening of muscle tissue, it plays a role in the development of *contractures*. A contracture is the abnormal shortening of muscle tissue, rendering the muscle highly resistant to stretch. Muscles weaken and shorten with disuse. Contractures occur when muscles do not have the necessary strength to maintain their integrity (*i.e.*, their proper function and full range of motion). Contractures mainly develop over joints when there is an imbalance in the muscle strength of the antagonistic muscle groups. If allowed to progress, the contracture eventually involves the muscle groups, tendons, ligaments, and joint capsule. The joint becomes limited in its full use and range of motion. Proper body alignment decreases the risk for development of contractures.[43,52]

Another consequence of prolonged immobility and bed rest for the musculoskeletal system is the loss of bone mass and the development of osteoporosis. Bone is a dynamic tissue that undergoes continual deposition and replacement of minerals in response to the dual stimuli of weight bearing and muscle pull. With immobility and bed rest, calcium loss from the bone begins almost immediately.

The maintenance of normal bone function depends on two types of cells: osteoblasts and osteoclasts. Osteoblasts function in building the osseous matrix of the bone, and osteoclasts function in the breakdown of the bone matrix. Through their opposing forces, the bone matrix is continually turned over and new bone is regenerated. Osteoblasts depend on the stress of mobility and weight bearing to perform their function. During immobility and bed rest, the process of building new bone stops, but the osteoclast cells continue to perform their function. This results in structural changes in the bone as the bone decalcifies. There also is an increase in the excretion of bone phosphorous and nitrogen. Despite the calcium loss from the bone, serum calcium remains normal because the excess calcium is excreted in the urine and feces.

Persons who experience disuse osteoporosis from prolonged immobility and bed rest develop soft, spongy bones. The bones may easily compress and become deformed. Because of lack of structural firmness, the bones may easily fracture. Persons with osteoporosis experience much pain when they begin weight-bearing activities. Despite the lack of calcium in the bone, a diet high in calcium will not enhance bone uptake of calcium. Unneeded calcium is added to the excess calcium that already is being excreted in the urine. This may precipitate the formation of calcium-containing renal stones. The best measure to prevent the occurrence of osteoporosis is to begin weight bearing as soon as possible.

Skin Responses

Except for the soles of the feet, the skin is not designed for weight bearing. However, during bed rest, the large surface area of the skin bears weight and is in constant contact with the surface of the bed. Constant pressure is transmitted to the skin, subcutaneous tissue, and muscle, especially to those tissues over bony prominences. This constant contact causes increased pressure and impairs normal capillary blood flow, which interferes with the exchange of nutrients and waste products. Tissue ischemia and necrosis may result and lead to the development of pressure ulcers. Also contributing to the development of pressure ulcers is moisture from the skin in constant contact with bed linens and the forces of friction and shear.

Metabolic and Endocrine Responses

When a person is placed on bed rest, the basal metabolic rate drops in response to decreased energy requirements of the body. Anabolic processes are slowed, and catabolic processes become accelerated. Protein breakdown occurs and leads to a protein deficiency and a negative nitrogen balance.[44] Persons in a negative nitrogen balance experience nausea and anorexia, which contribute to the catabolic state. Insulin plays a role in regulating protein metabolism and glucose use. It does this primarily by inhibiting protein breakdown.

The person on bed rest experiences an impaired responsiveness to the actions of insulin. During bed rest, it takes more insulin to maintain serum glucose. After 10 days of bed rest, there is a 100% increase in basal insulin concentration to maintain normal glucose control.[57,58] There also appears to be an induced insulin resistance that helps explain the negative nitrogen balance seen in patients who experience prolonged bed rest.

Possible reasons for the glucose unresponsiveness to hyperinsulinemia include a change in the action of insulin because of the release of a substance that acts as an insulin inhibitor (this substance is believed to act at cell membrane binding sites); a change in some aspect of the cellular membrane glucose transport system; or inhibition of the function of a second factor that has insulin-like activity. Research suggests that one or more factors are activated with physical exercise. These factors respond to the quantity of energy expenditure and are necessary for insulin, and possibly glucose, to function normally. In the absence of activity, the action of these factors may be suppressed. A final explanation for glucose unresponsiveness to hyperinsulinemia is a combination of the aforementioned causes.[57,58] Insulin sensitivity can be reduced by brief periods of hyponutrition.[59]

Persons who experience prolonged periods of bed rest have changes in the circadian release of various hormones. Normally, insulin and growth hormone peak twice a day. In people who experienced 30 days of bed rest, a single daily peak of these hormones occurred. Other hormonal changes include an afternoon peak of epinephrine rather than the normal early morning peak, and an early morning peak of aldosterone rather than the usual noonday peak that is seen in normally active persons.[60] The immune system also is subject to physiologic changes associated with bed rest or immobility. Research demonstrates that after 4 weeks of bed rest, there is an increase in interleukin-1 production, which may play a role in the bone mineral loss that occurs during bed rest. Also seen is a decrease in interleukin-2 secretion, which may play a part in the infectious diseases that often occur during periods of bed rest.[61]

Gastrointestinal Responses

Gastrointestinal responses to bed rest vary. Constipation and fecal impaction are frequent complications that occur when persons experience prolonged periods of immobility and bed rest. With inactivity, there is slowed movement of feces through the colon. The act of defecation requires the integration of the abdominal muscles, the diaphragm, and the levator ani. Muscle atrophy and loss of tone occur in the immobilized person and interfere with the normal act of defecation. Lack of privacy and the supine position may compound problems with defecation.[42,44,52,53]

Sensory Responses

Immobility reduces the quality and quantity of sensory information available from kinesthetic, visual, auditory, and tactile sensation. It also reduces the person's ability to interact with the environment. Decreased kinesthetic stimulation occurs from both immobilization and assumption of the supine or recumbent position. Responses to decreased kinesthetic stimulation include an impaired functioning of thought processes and decreased sensory perception. Prolonged immobility and bed rest have been associated with a number of impaired sensory responses. Common occurrences include both visual and auditory hallucinations, vivid dreams, inefficient thought processes, loss of contact with reality, and alteration in tactile stimulation.

In addition to sensory deprivation related to prolonged bed rest and immobility, persons may experience a sensory monotony from the hospital environment. Repetitious and meaningless sounds from cardiac monitors, respirators, and hospital personnel, along with an environment that may be void of light and a normal day-night cycle, also contribute to impaired sensory perception.

PSYCHOSOCIAL RESPONSES

Immobility often sets the stage for changes in the person's response to illness. Persons adapt to prolonged bed rest and immobility through a series of physiologic responses and through changes in affect, perception, and cognition. Affective changes include increased anxiety, fear, depression, hostility, rapid mood changes, and alterations in normal sleep patterns. These changes in mood occur with hospitalized patients who are subjected to periods of prolonged bed rest and immobility, and in persons in confinement, such as astronauts and prisoners.

Research on immobilized or isolated persons has demonstrated that the motivation to learn decreases with periods of prolonged immobility, as does the ability to learn and retain new material and transfer newly learned material to a different situation. Persons are less able and less motivated to perform problem-solving activities; they are less able to concentrate and discriminate information.[60] These studies present major implications for the timing of patient education and the preparation of education materials.

Prolonged bed rest and immobility also contribute to the social isolation of the hospitalized person. Confined to a hospital bed, the person is unable to assume certain societal roles. The roles of spouse, parent, sibling, worker, and friend are altered either temporarily or permanently while the person is hospitalized. People may respond to this isolation by exhibiting various effective and ineffective coping behaviors, including increased anxiety, depression, restlessness, fear, and rapid mood changes.

TIME COURSE OF PHYSIOLOGIC RESPONSES

The deconditioning responses to the inactivity of immobility and bed rest affect all body systems. One of the important factors to keep in mind is the rapidity with which the changes occur and the length of time required to overcome these effects. The body responds in a characteristic pattern to the effects of the supine position and bed rest (see Table 12-2). During the first 3 days of bed rest, one of the first changes to occur is a massive diuresis. Accompanying the diuresis are increases in serum osmolality, hematocrit, venous compliance, and an increase of urinary sodium and chloride excretion. Fluid losses stabilize by approximately the fourth day. By days 4 to 7, there are changes in the hemolytic system. Fibrinogen as well as fibrinolytic activity increase, and clotting time is prolonged. The cardiovascular system responds with a decrease in cardiac output and stroke volume. The basal metabolic rate decreases and glucose intolerance and a negative nitrogen balance begin to develop.

Additional effects on the hemolytic system are observed on days 8 to 14. Red blood cell number is decreased and the phagocytic ability of leukocytes is reduced. There is a decrease in lean body mass and, after 15 days of bed rest, osteoporosis and hypercalciuria occur. Aerobic power decreases, the cyclic excretion of some hormones is changed, and the person's thought patterns and sensory perception are altered[62] (Table 12-3).

TABLE 12-3 ✦ Physiologic Changes During Bed Rest

0–3 Days	4–7 Days	8–14 Days	Over 15 Days
Increases in	**Increases in**	**Increases in**	**Increases in**
Urine volume	Urine creatinine, hydroxyproline, PO_4, N, and K excretion	Urine pyrophosphate	Peak hypercalciuria
Urine Na, Cl, Ca, and osmol excretion		Sweating sensitivity	Sensitivity to thermal threshold
	Plasma globulin, phosphate and glucose levels	Exercise hyperthermia	Auditory threshold (secondary)
Plasma osmolality	Blood fibrinogen	Exercise maximal heart rate	
Hematocrit	Fibrinolytic activity and clotting time		
Venous compliance	Visual focal point		
	Hyperthermia of eye conjunctiva, dilation of retinal arteries and veins		
	Auditory threshold		
Decreases in	**Decreases in**	**Decreases in**	**Decreases in**
Total fluid intake	Near point of visual acuity	Red blood cell mass	Bone density
Extracellular and intracellular fluid	Orthostatic tolerance	Leukocyte phagocytosis	
Calf blood flow	Nitrogen balance	Tissue heat conductance	
Resting heart rate		Lean body mass	
Secretion of gastric acid			
Glucose tolerance			

(Greenleaf J.E. [1984]. Physiological responses to prolonged bed rest and fluid immersion in humans. *Journal of Applied Physiology: Respiratory, Environmental and Exercise Physiology 57*, 619–633)

INTERVENTIONS

A holistic approach should be taken when caring for persons who are immobile or require prolonged periods of bed rest. Interventions and treatment should include actions that address the person's physical and psychosocial needs. The goals of care for the immobilized person include structuring a safe environment in which the person is not at risk for nosocomial complications, providing diversional activities to offset problems with sensory deprivation, and preventing complications of bed rest by implementing an interdisciplinary plan of care.

In summary, during the last 75 years, the use of bed rest has undergone a complete reversal as a standard of treatment for a variety of medical conditions. Over time, research findings have described the deleterious consequences of inactivity. All body systems are affected by complications of immobility and prolonged bed rest.

The responses to bed rest and immobility affect all body systems. One of the important factors is the rapidity with which the changes occur and the long time required to overcome the effects of prolonged bed rest and immobility. Adverse effects of prolonged immobility and bed rest include a decreased cardiac output, orthostatic intolerance, dehydration, potential for thrombophlebitis, pneumonia, formation of renal calculi, development of pressure ulcers, sensory deprivation, and impaired thought processes.

Related Web Sites

American Association for Chronic Fatigue Syndrome (AACFS)
www.aacfs.org
Centers for Disease Control—chronic fatigue syndrome site
www.cdc.gov/ncidod/diseases/cfs/index.htm
Exercise Physiology Laboratory at NASA Johnson Space Center
www.jsc.nasa.gov/sa/sd/sd3/exl
Neuromuscular Center–Presbyterian Hospital of Dallas and the University of Texas Southwestern Medical Center at Dallas Institute for Exercise and Environmental Medicine
www.texashealth.org/nmc
Papers Presented at the Bi-Annual Research Conference of the AACFS, October 10–11, 1998   www.cfids-me.org/aacfs

References

1. Jennings G.L.R. (1995). Mechanisms for reduction of cardiovascular risk by regular exercise. *Clinical and Experimental Pharmacology and Physiology* 22, 209–211.
2. Oka R.K. (1990). Cardiovascular response to exercise. *Cardiovascular Nursing* 26 (6), 31–36.
3. Wingate S. (1991). Acute effects of exercise on the cardiovascular system. *Journal of Cardiovascular Nursing* 5 (4), 27–38.
4. Foss M.L., Keteyian, S.J. (1998). *Fox's physiological basis for exercise and sport* (6th ed.). Boston: WCB McGraw-Hill.
5. Casaburi R. (1994). Physiologic responses to training. *Clinics in Chest Medicine* 15, 215–227.
6. Crawford M.H. (1992). Physiologic consequences of systematic training. *Cardiology Clinics* 10, 209–218.
7. Simoneau J.A. (1995). Adaptation of human skeletal muscle to exercise-training. *International Journal of Obesity* 19 (Suppl. 4), S9–S13.
8. Spurway N.C. (1992). Aerobic exercise, anaerobic exercise and the lactate threshold. *British Medical Bulletin* 48, 569–591.
9. Kenney W.L., Johnson J.M. (1992). Control of skin blood flow during exercise. *Medicine and Science in Sports and Exercise* 24, 303–312.
10. Berg A., Müller H.M., Rathmann S., Deibert P. (1999). The gastrointestinal system: An essential target organ of the athlete's health and physical performance. *Exercise Immunology Review* 5, 78–95.
11. Brouns F., Beckers E. (1993). Is the gut an athletic organ? Digestion, absorption and exercise. *Sports Medicine* 15, 242–257.
12. Streiff M., Bell W.R. (1994). Exercise and hemostasis in humans. *Seminars in Hematology* 31, 155–165.
13. Nieman D.C. (1994). The effect of exercise on immune function. *Bulletin on the Rheumatic Diseases* 43 (8), 5–8.
14. Mackinnon L.T. (1997). Immunity in athletes. *International Journal of Sports Medicine* 18 (Suppl. 1), S62–S68.
15. Hughes W.T. (1998). The athlete: An immunocompromised host. *Advances in Pediatric Infectious Diseases* 13, 79–99.
16. Pyne D.B., Gleeson M. (1998). Effects of intensive exercise training on immunity in athletes. *International Journal of Sports Medicine* 19 (Suppl. 3), S183–S194.
17. Daughton D.M., Fix J.A. (1986). *Human Activity Profile (HAP) manual.* Lutz, FL: Psychological Assessment Resources, Inc.
18. Krupp L.B., LaRocca N.G., Muir-Nash J., Steinberg A.D. (1989). The Fatigue Severity Scale: Application to patients with multiple sclerosis and systemic lupus erythematosus. *Archives of Neurology* 46, 1121–1123.
19. Ulmer H.V. (1983). Work physiology: Environmental physiology. In Schmidt R.F., Thews G. (Eds.), *Human physiology* (pp. 548–564). New York: Springer-Verlag.
20. Borg G.A.V. (1973). Perceived exertion: A note on "history" and methods. *Medicine and Science in Sports* 5, 90–93.
21. Borg G.A.V. (1982). Psychophysical bases of perceived exertion. *Medicine and Science in Sports* 14, 377–381.
22. Carroll-Johnson R. (Ed.). (1989). *Classification of nursing diagnoses: Proceedings of the eighth conference* (p. 543). Philadelphia: J.B. Lippincott.
23. MacLean S. (1991). Activity intolerance. In Maas M., Buckwalter K., Hardy M.A. (Eds.), *Nursing diagnoses and interventions for the elderly* (pp. 252–262). Redwood City, CA: Addison-Wesley Nursing.
24. Piper B.F. (1986). Fatigue. In Carrieri V.K., Lindsey A.M., West C.W. (Eds.), *Pathophysiological phenomena in nursing: Human responses to illness* (pp. 219–234). Philadelphia: W.B. Saunders.
25. Piper B.F. (1989). Fatigue: Current bases for practice. In Funk S.G., Tornquist E.M., Champagne M.T., Copp L.A., Wiese R.A. (Eds.), *Key aspects of comfort: Management of pain, fatigue, and nausea* (pp. 187–198). New York: Springer-Verlag.
26. Belza B. (1994). The impact of fatigue on exercise performance. *Arthritis Care and Research* 7, 176–180.
27. Nail L.M., King K.B. (1987). Fatigue. *Seminars in Oncology Nursing* 3, 257–262.
28. St. Pierre B.A., Kasper C.E., Lindsey A.M. (1992). Fatigue mechanisms in patients with cancer: Effects of tumor necrosis factor and exercise on skeletal muscle. *Oncology Nursing Forum* 19, 419–425.
29. Evengard B., Schacterle R.S., Komaroff L. (1999). Chronic fatigue syndrome: New insights and old ignorance. *Journal of Internal Medicine* 256, 455–469.

30. Lloyd A. (1998). Chronic fatigue syndrome: Shifting boundaries and attributions. *American Journal of Medicine* 105 (3A), 7S–10S.

31. Demitrack M.A. (1998). Neuroendocrine aspects of chronic fatigue syndrome: A commentary. *American Journal of Medicine* 105 (3A), 11S–14S.

32. Fukuda K., Straus S.E., Hickie I., Sharpe M.C., Dobbins J.G., Komaroff A.L. (1994). The chronic fatigue syndrome: A comprehensive approach to its definition and study. *Annals of Internal Medicine* 121, 953–959.

33. Cho W.K., Stollerman G.H. (1992). Chronic fatigue syndrome. *Hospital Practice* 27, 221–245.

34. Demitrack M.A., Engleberg N.C. (1994). Chronic fatigue syndrome. *Current Therapy in Endocrinology and Metabolism* 5, 135–142.

35. Levine P.H. (1998). What we know about chronic fatigue syndrome and its relevance to the practicing physician. *American Journal of Medicine* 105 (3A), 100S–103S.

36. Whiteside T.L., Friberg D. (1998). Natural killer cells and natural killer cell activity in chronic fatigue syndrome. *American Journal of Medicine* 105 (3A), 27S–34S.

37. Calabrese L., Danao T., Camara E., Wilke W. (1992). Chronic fatigue syndrome. *American Family Physician* 45, 1205–1213.

38. Pagani M., Lucini D. (1999). Chronic fatigue syndrome: A hypothesis focusing on the autonomic nervous system. *Clinical Science* 96, 117–125.

39. Tirelli U., Chierichetti F., Tavio M., Simonelli D., Bianchin G., Zanco P., Ferlin G. (1998). Brain positron emission tomography (PET) in chronic fatigue syndrome: Preliminary data. *American Journal of Medicine* 105 (3A), 54S–58S.

40. Lange G., Wang S., DeLuca J., Natelson B. (1998). Neuroimaging in chronic fatigue syndrome. *American Journal of Medicine* 105 (3A), 50S–53S.

41. Harper C.M., Lyles Y.M. (1988). Physiology and complications of bed rest. *Journal of the American Geriatric Society* 36, 1047–1054.

42. Coletta E.M., Murphy J.B. (1992). The complications of immobility in the elderly stroke patient. *Journal of the American Board of Family Practice* 5, 389–397.

43. Dittmer D.K., Teasell R. (1993). Complications of immobilization and bed rest, Part 1: Musculoskeletal and cardiovascular complications. *Canadian Family Physician* 39, 1428–1437.

44. Teasell R., Dittmer D.K. (1993). Complications of immobilization and bed rest, Part 2: Other complications. *Canadian Family Physician* 39, 1440–1446.

45. Taylor H.L., Henschel A., Broek J., Keys A. (1949). Effects of bed rest on cardiovascular function and work performance. *Journal of Applied Physiology* 11, 223–239.

46. Dean E. (1993). Bedrest and deconditioning. *Neurology Report* 17(1), 6–9.

47. Convertino V.A. (1997). Cardiovascular consequences of bed rest: Effect on maximal oxygen uptake. *Medicine and Science in Sports and Exercise* 29, 191–197.

48. Faria S.H. (1998). Assessment of immobility hazards. *Home Care Provider* 3, 189–191.

49. Levine B.D., Zuckerman J.H., Pawelczyk J.A. (1997). Cardiac atrophy after bed-rest deconditioning: A nonneural mechanism for orthostatic intolerance. *Circulation* 96, 517–525.

50. Saltin B., Blomquist G., Mitchell J.H., Johnson R.L., Wildenthal K., Chapman C.B. (1968). Responses to exercise after bed rest and after training: A longitudinal study of adaptive changes in oxygen transport and body composition. *Circulation* 38 (Suppl. 7), 1–65.

51. Krasnoff J., Painter P. (1999). The physiological consequences of bed rest and inactivity. *Advances in Renal Replacement Therapy* 6, 124–132.

52. Olson E.V., Thompson L.F., McCarthy J., Johnson B.J., Edmonds R.E., Schroeder L.M., Wade M. (1967). The hazards of immobility. *American Journal of Nursing* 67, 780–797.

53. Mobily P.R., Kelley L.S. (1991). Iatrogenesis in the elderly. *Journal of Gerontological Nursing* 17 (9), 5–10.

54. Corcoran P.J. (1991). Use it or lose it: The hazards of bed rest and inactivity. *Western Journal of Medicine* 154, 536–538.

55. Ibebunjo C., Martyn J.A.J. (1999). Fiber atrophy, but not changes in acetylcholine receptor expression, contributes to the muscle dysfunction after immobilization. *Critical Care Medicine* 27, 275–285.

56. Hendricks T. (1995). The effects of immobilization on connective tissue. *Journal of Manual and Manipulative Therapy* 3 (3), 98–103.

57. Dolkas C.B., Greenleaf J.E. (1977). Insulin and glucose responses during bed rest with isotonic and isometric exercise. *Journal of Applied Physiology* 43, 1033–1038.

58. Shangraw R.E., Stuart C.A., Prince M.J., Peters E.J., Wolfe R.R. (1988). Insulin responsiveness of protein metabolism in vivo following bedrest in humans. *American Journal of Physiology* 255, E548–E558.

59. Nygren J., Thorell A., Brismar K., Karpe F., Ljungqvist O. (1997). Short-term hypocaloric nutrition but not bed rest decrease insulin sensitivity and IGF-I bioavailability in healthy subjects: The importance of glucagon. *Nutrition* 13, 945–951.

60. Rubin M. (1988). The physiology of bed rest. *American Journal of Nursing* 88, 50–58.

61. Schmitt D.A., Schaffar L., Taylor G.R., Loftin K.C., Schneider V.S., Koebel A., Abbal M., Sonnenfeld G., Lewis D.E., Reubin J.R., Ferebee R. (1996). Use of bed rest and head-down tilt to simulate spaceflight-induced immune system changes. *Journal of Interferon and Cytokine Research* 16, 151–157.

62. Greenleaf J.E., Kozlowski S. (1982). Physiological consequences of reduced physical activity during bed rest. In Terjung R.L (Ed.), *Exercise and sport sciences reviews* (pp. 84–119). Syracuse, NY: American College of Sports Medicine.

Hematopoietic Function

From ancient times, the importance of blood as a determinant of health was recognized. Its life-affecting powers are well described in the written treatises of Greek physician Galen (AD 130–200). Galen, who reigned as the foremost medical authority for nearly 1500 years, believed that an individual stayed healthy as long as four body fluids—blood, phlegm, yellow bile, and black bile—remained in the right proportion. He also believed that the four humors determined one's basic temperament. Whether an individual was sanguine, sluggish and dull, quick to anger, or melancholy was determined by the degree to which one or another of the humors predominated. The most desirable personality type was achieved when blood was thought to predominate, yielding a warm and cheerful person.

The workings of blood were traced by Galen from its creation, which he believed took place in the liver, throughout the body. He came to believe that disease manifested itself if any one of the fluids was in excess or deficient and was carried in the blood. The theory led to bloodletting—the drawing of blood from the vein of a sick person so the disease could flow out with the blood. For many centuries, bloodletting was the standard treatment for a myriad of ills.

Chapter 13

Blood Cells and the Hematopoietic System

Kathryn J. Gaspard

Blood consists of blood cells (*i.e.*, red blood cells, thrombocytes or platelets, and white blood cells) and the plasma in which the cells are suspended. Blood cells have a relatively short life span and must be continually replaced. The generation of blood cells takes place in the *hematopoietic* (from the Greek *haima* for "blood" and *poiesis* for "making") system. The hematopoietic system encompasses all of the blood cells and their precursors, the bone marrow where blood cells have their origin, and the lymphoid tissues where some blood cells circulate as they develop and mature.

Composition of Blood and Formation of Blood Cells

After you have completed this section of the chapter, you should be able to meet the following objectives:

✦ Describe the composition of plasma
✦ Name the formed elements of blood and cite their function and life span
✦ Trace the process of hematopoiesis from stem cell to mature blood cell

When blood is removed from the circulatory system, it clots. The clot contains the blood cells and fibrin strands formed from the conversion of the plasma protein fibrinogen. It is surrounded by a yellow liquid called *serum*. Blood that is kept from clotting by the addition of an anticoagulant (*e.g.*, heparin, citrate) and then centrifuged separates into layers (Fig. 13-1). The lower layer (approximately

42% to 47% of the whole-blood volume) contains the erythrocytes, or red blood cells, and is referred to as the *hematocrit*. The intermediate layer (approximately 1%) containing the leukocytes is white or gray and is called the *buffy layer*. Above the leukocytes is a thin layer of platelets that is not discernible to the naked eye. The translucent, yellowish fluid that forms on the top of the cells is the *plasma*, which comprises approximately 55% of the total volume.

PLASMA

The plasma component of blood carries the cells that transport gases, aid in body defenses, and prevent blood loss. It transports nutrients that are absorbed from the gastrointestinal tract to body cells and delivers the waste products from cellular metabolism to the kidney for elimination; it transports hormones and permits the exchange of chemical messengers; it facilitates the exchange of body heat; and it participates in electrolyte and acid-base balance and the osmotic regulation of body fluids. Plasma is 90% to 91% water by weight, 6.5% to 8% proteins by weight, and 2% other small molecular substances (Table 13-1).

PLASMA PROTEINS

The plasma proteins are the most abundant solutes in plasma. Most proteins are formed in the liver and serve a variety of functions. The major types are albumin, globulins, and fibrinogen. Albumin is the most abundant and makes up approximately 54% of the plasma proteins. It does not diffuse through the vascular endothelium and therefore

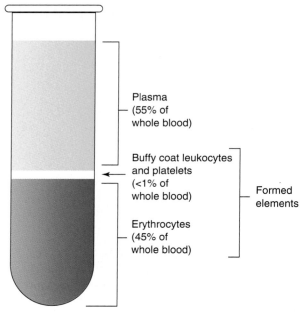

Plasma
(55% of
whole blood)

Buffy coat leukocytes
and platelets
(<1% of
whole blood)

Erythrocytes
(45% of
whole blood)

Formed
elements

FIGURE 13-1 Layering of blood components in an anticoagulated and centrifuged blood sample.

 Composition of the Blood

➤ Blood is a liquid that fills the vascular compartment and serves to transport dissolved materials and blood cells throughout the body.

➤ The most abundant of the blood cells, the erythrocytes or red blood cells, function in oxygen and carbon dioxide transport.

➤ The leukocytes, or white blood cells, serve various roles in immunity and inflammation.

➤ Platelets are small cell fragments that are involved in blood clotting.

contributes to plasma osmotic pressure and the maintenance of blood volume (see Chapter 31). Albumin also serves as a carrier for certain substances and acts as a blood buffer. The globulins comprise approximately 38% of plasma proteins. There are three types of globulins: the alpha globulins that transport bilirubin and steroids, the beta globulins that transport iron and copper, and the gamma globulins that constitute the antibodies of the immune system. Fibrinogen makes up approximately 7% of the plasma proteins and is converted to fibrin in the clotting process. The remaining 1% of circulating proteins are hormones, enzymes, complement, and carriers for lipids.

BLOOD CELLS

The blood cells include the erythrocytes or red blood cells, the leukocytes or white blood cells, and platelets (Table 13-2). The blood cells, or formed elements, are not all true cells and most survive for only a few days in the

circulation or tissues as a result of their function. They do not divide so must be continually renewed by the process of hematopoiesis in the bone marrow.

Erythrocytes

The erythrocytes, or red blood cells, are the most numerous of the formed elements. They are small, biconcave disks with a large surface area and can easily deform in small capillaries. They contain the oxygen-carrying protein, hemoglobin, that functions in the transport of oxygen. The erythrocytes are derived from the myeloid or bone marrow stem cell and live approximately 120 days in the circulation (see Chapter 15).

Leukocytes

The leukocytes, or white blood cells, constitute only 1% of the total blood volume. They originate in the bone marrow and circulate throughout the lymphoid tissues of the body. There they function in the inflammatory and immune processes. They include the granulocytes, the lymphocytes, and the monocytes (Fig. 13-2).

Granulocytes. The granulocytes are all phagocytic cells and are identifiable because of their cytoplasmic granules. These white blood cells are spherical and have distinctive multilobar nuclei. The granulocytes are divided into three

TABLE 13-1 ✦ **Plasma Components**		
Plasma	Percentage of Plasma Volume	Description
Water	90–91	
Proteins	6.5–8	
Albumin		54% Plasma proteins
Globulins		38% Plasma proteins
Fibrinogen		7% Plasma proteins
Other substances	1–2	Hormones, enzymes, carbohydrates, fats, amino acids, gases, electrolytes, excretory products

TABLE 13-2 ✦ Blood Cell Counts

Blood Cells	Number of Cells/μL	Percentage of White Blood Cells
Red blood cell count	$4.2–5.4 \times 10^6$, $3.6–5.0 \times 10^6$ *	
White blood cell count	$4.40–11.3 \times 10^3$	
Differential count		
Granulocytes		
Neutrophils		
Segs		47–63
Bands		0–4
Eosinophils		0–3
Basophils		0–2
Lymphocytes		24–40
Monocytes		4–9
Platelet count	$150–400 \times 10^3$	

* First value is for men and the second for women.

types (neutrophils, eosinophils, and basophils) according to the staining properties of the granules. Functionally, all granulocytes are phagocytes.

Neutrophils. The neutrophils, which constitute 50% to 60% of the total number of white blood cells, have granules that are neutral and hence do not stain with an acidic or a basic dye. Because these white cells have nuclei that are divided into three to five lobes, they are often called *polymorphonuclear leukocytes.*

The neutrophils are primarily responsible for maintaining normal host defenses against invading bacteria and fungi, cell remains, and a variety of foreign substances. The cytoplasm of mature neutrophils contains fine granules. These granules contain degrading enzymes that are used in destroying foreign substances and correspond to lysosomes found in other cells (see Chapter 4). Enzymes and oxidizing agents associated with these granules are capable of degrading a variety of natural and synthetic substances, including complex polysaccharides, proteins, and lipids. These enzymes are important in maintaining normal host defenses and in mediating inflammation.

The neutrophils are the first cells to arrive at the site of inflammation, usually appearing within 90 minutes of injury. They migrate to the site as a result of chemotactic factors induced by invading bacteria. Once there, they engulf the pathogen and destroy it. The neutrophil count increases greatly during the inflammatory process. When this happens, immature forms of neutrophils are released from the bone marrow. These immature cells are often called *bands* or *stabs* because of the horseshoe shape of their nuclei. They represent a storage pool of neutrophil precursors. After being released from the bone marrow, circulating neutrophils have a short life span and therefore must be constantly replaced if their numbers are to remain adequate.

The neutrophils have their origin in the myeloblasts that are found in the bone marrow (Fig. 13-3). The myeloblasts are the committed precursors of the granulocyte pathway and do not normally appear in the peripheral circulation. When they are present, it suggests a disorder of blood cell proliferation and differentiation. The myeloblasts differentiate into promyelocytes and then myelocytes. Usually, a cell is not called a *myelocyte* until it has at least 12 granules. The myelocytes mature to become metamyelocytes (Greek *meta*, for "beyond"), at which point they lose their capacity for mitosis. Subsequent development of the neutrophil involves reduction in size, with transformation from an indented to an oval to a horseshoe-shaped nucleus (*i.e.*, band cell) and then to a mature cell with a segmented nucleus. These mature neutrophils are often referred to as

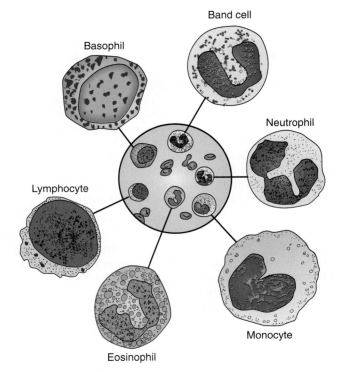

FIGURE 13-2 White blood cells.

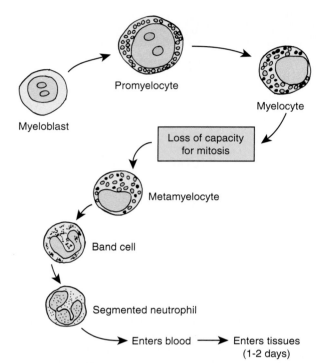

Promyelocyte

Myeloblast

Myelocyte

Loss of capacity
for mitosis

Metamyelocyte

Band cell

Segmented neutrophil

Enters blood ⟶ Enters tissues
(1-2 days)

FIGURE 13-3 Development of neutrophils. (Adapted from Cormack D.H. [1993]. *Ham's histology* [9th ed.]. Philadelphia: J.B. Lippincott)

segs because of their segmented nucleus. Development from stem cell to mature neutrophil takes approximately 2 weeks. It is at this point that the neutrophil enters the bloodstream.

After release from the marrow, the neutrophils spend only approximately 10 hours in the circulation before moving into the tissues. Their survival in the tissues lasts approximately 1 to 3 days. They die in the tissues in discharging their phagocytic function, or die of senescence. The pool of circulating neutrophils (*i.e.*, those that appear in the blood count) are in closely maintained equilibrium with a similar-sized pool of cells marginating along the walls of small blood vessels. These are the neutrophils that respond to chemotactic factors and migrate into the tissues toward the offending agent. Epinephrine, exercise, stress, and corticosteroid drug therapy can cause rapid increases in the circulating neutrophil count by shifting cells from the marginating to the circulating pool. Endotoxins or microbes have the opposite effect, producing a transient decrease in neutrophils by attracting neutrophils into the tissues.

Eosinophils. The cytoplasmic granules of the eosinophils stain red with the acidic dye eosin. These leukocytes constitute 1% to 3% of the total number of white blood cells and increase in number during allergic reactions and parasitic infections. It is thought that they release enzymes that detoxify the agents or chemical mediators associated with allergic reactions and assist in terminating the response.

Basophils. The granules of the basophils stain blue with a basic dye. These cells constitute only approximately 0.3% to 0.5% of the white blood cells. The granules in the basophils contain heparin, an anticoagulant, and histamine, a vasodilator. The basophils share properties of mast cells and are thought to be involved in allergic and stress responses.

Lymphocytes. The lymphocytes constitute 20% to 30% of the white blood cell count. They have no identifiable granules in the cytoplasm and are also called *agranulocytes*. There are two types of lymphocytes: B lymphocytes and T lymphocytes. The lymphocytes play an important role in the immune response. They move between blood and lymph tissue, where they may be stored for hours or years. Their function in the lymph nodes or spleen is to defend against microorganisms in the immune response (see Chapter 18). The B lymphocytes differentiate to form antibody-producing plasma cells and are involved in humoral-mediated immunity. The T lymphocytes are involved in cell-mediated immunity.

Monocytes and Macrophages. Monocytes are the largest of the white blood cells and constitute approximately 3% to 8% of the total leukocyte count. The life span of the circulating monocyte is approximately 1 to 3 days, three to four times longer than that of the granulocytes. These cells survive for months to years in the tissues. The monocytes, which are phagocytic cells, are often referred to as *macrophages* when they enter the tissues. The monocytes engulf larger and greater quantities of foreign material than the neutrophils. These leukocytes play an important role in chronic inflammation and are also involved in the immune response by activating lymphocytes and by presenting antigen to T cells. When the monocyte leaves the vascular system and enters the tissues, it functions as a macrophage with specific activity. The macrophages are known as *histiocytes* in loose connective tissue, *microglial cells* in the brain, and *Kupffer cells* in the liver. Some macrophages function in the alveoli.

Granulomatous inflammation is a distinctive pattern of chronic inflammation in which the macrophages form a capsule around insoluble materials that cannot be digested. Foreign body granulomas are incited by relatively inert foreign bodies, such as talc or surgical sutures. Immune granulomas are caused by insoluble particles that are capable of inciting a cell-mediated immune response. The tubercle that forms in primary tuberculosis infections is an example of an immune granuloma (see Chapter 28).

Thrombocytes

Thrombocytes, or platelets, are circulating cell fragments of the large megakaryocytes that are derived from the myeloid stem cell. They function to form a platelet plug to control bleeding after injury to a vessel wall (see Chapter 14). Their cytoplasmic granules release mediators required for hemostasis. Thrombocytes have no nucleus, cannot replicate, and, if not used, they last approximately 8 to 9 days in the circulation before they are removed by the phagocytic cells of the spleen.

HEMATOPOIESIS

The generation of blood cells begins in the endothelial cells of the developing blood vessels during the fifth week of gestation and then continues in the liver and spleen. After birth, this function is gradually taken over by the bone marrow. The marrow is a network of connective tissue containing immature blood cells. At sites where the marrow is hematopoietically active, it produces so many erythrocytes that it is red, hence the name *red bone marrow*. Fat cells are also present in bone marrow, but they are inactive in terms of blood cell generation. Marrow made up predominantly of fat cells is called *yellow bone marrow*. During active skeletal growth, red marrow is gradually replaced by yellow marrow in most of the long bones. In adults, red marrow is largely restricted to the flat bones of the pelvis, ribs, and sternum. As a person ages, the cellularity of the marrow declines. When the demand for red cell replacement increases, as in hemolytic anemia, there can be resubstitution of red marrow for yellow marrow.

Some hematopoiesis may also be generated in the spleen and the liver.

Blood Cell Precursors

The blood-forming population of bone marrow is made up of three types of cells: self-renewing stem cells, differentiated progenitor (parent) cells, and functional mature blood cells. All of the blood cell precursors of the erythrocyte (*i.e.*, red cell), myelocyte (*i.e.*, granulocyte or monocyte), lymphocyte (*i.e.*, T lymphocyte and B lymphocyte), and megakaryocyte (*i.e.*, platelet) series are derived from a small population of primitive cells called the *pluripotent stem cells* (Fig. 13-4). Their lifelong potential for proliferation and self-renewal makes them an indispensable and lifesaving source of reserve cells for the entire hematopoietic system. Several levels of differentiation lead to the development of committed unipotential cells, which are the progenitors for each of the blood cell types. These cells are referred to as *colony-forming units* or *burst-forming units*. These progenitor

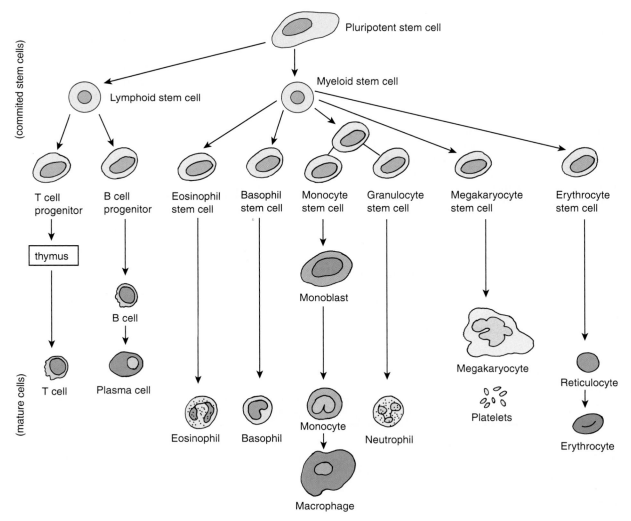

FIGURE 13-4 Major maturational stages of blood cells.

cells lose their capacity for self-renewal but retain the potential to differentiate in response to lineage-specific growth factors. They develop into the precursor cells that give rise to mature erythrocytes, myelocytes, megakaryocytes, or lymphocytes.

Disorders of hematopoietic stem cells include aplastic anemia and the leukemias. Today, potential cures for these and many other disorders require hematopoietic stem cell transplantation. Stem cell transplants correct bone marrow failure, immune deficiencies, hematologic defects and malignancies, and inherited errors of metabolism. Sources of the stem cells include bone marrow, peripheral blood, and umbilical cord blood, all of which replenish the recipient with a normal population of pluripotent stem cells. Bone marrow and peripheral blood transplants may be derived from the patient (autologous) or from a histocompatible donor (allogeneic). Autologous transplants are often used to replenish stem cells after high-dose chemotherapy or irradiation. Peripheral blood stem cells are harvested from the blood after the administration of a cytokine growth factor that increases the quantity and migration of the cells from the bone marrow. Umbilical cord blood from HLA-matched donors is a transplant option for children and carries less risk of graft-versus-host disease. Methods of collecting, propagating, and preserving stem cells are still being investigated.

Regulation of Hematopoiesis

Under normal conditions, the numbers and total mass for each type of circulating blood cell remain relatively constant. The blood cells are produced in different numbers according to needs and regulatory factors. This regulation of blood cells is thought to be at least partially controlled by hormone-like growth factors called *cytokines*. The cytokines are a family of glycoproteins that stimulate the proliferation, differentiation, and functional activation of the various blood cell precursors in bone marrow. They are produced by many blood cells and the capillary endothelium and act locally in the bone marrow by binding to cell surface receptors.

Some cytokines are colony-stimulating factors (CSFs) that were named for their ability to promote growth of blood cell colonies in culture. Lineage-specific CSFs that act on committed progenitor cells include erythropoietin (EPO), granulocyte colony-stimulating factor (G-CSF), monocyte-macrophage colony-stimulating factor (M-CSF), and thrombopoietin (TPO). There are also nonspecific cytokines that support the proliferation of the earlier hematopoietic precursors: granulocyte-monocyte colony-stimulating factor (GM-CSF) and interleukin-3, also known as multi-CSF. The CSFs act at different points in the proliferation and differentiation pathway and their functions overlap. Other cytokines, such as the many interleukins, support the development of lymphocytes and act synergistically to aid the functions of the CSFs (see Chapter 18).

The genes for most hematopoietic growth factors have been cloned and their recombinant proteins have been generated for use in a wide range of clinical problems. The clinically useful factors include EPO, TPO, G-CSF and GM-CSF. They are used to treat bone marrow failure caused by chemotherapy or aplastic anemia, the anemia of kidney failure, hematopoietic neoplasms, infectious diseases such as acquired immunodeficiency syndrome (AIDS), congenital and myeloproliferative disorders, and some solid tumors. Growth factors are used to increase peripheral stem cells for transplantation and to accelerate cell proliferation after bone marrow engraftment. Many of these uses are still investigational.

> In summary, blood is composed of plasma, plasma proteins, formed elements or blood cells, and substances such as hormones, enzymes, electrolytes, and byproducts of cellular waste. The blood cells consist of erythrocytes or red blood cells, leukocytes or white blood cells, and thrombocytes or platelets. Blood cells are generated from pluripotent stem cells located in the bone marrow. Blood cell production is regulated by chemical messengers called *cytokines* and *growth factors*.

Diagnostic Tests

After you have completed this section of the chapter, you should be able to meet the following objectives:

✦ Cite information gained from a complete blood count
✦ State the purpose of the erythrocyte sedimentation rate
✦ Describe the procedure used in bone marrow aspiration

Blood specimens can be obtained through skin puncture (capillary blood), venipuncture, arterial puncture, or bone marrow aspiration.

BLOOD COUNT

Tests of the hematologic system provide information regarding the number of blood cells and their structural and functional characteristics. A complete blood count (CBC) is a commonly performed screening test that determines the number of red blood cells, white blood cells, and platelets per unit of blood. The white cell differential count is the determination of the relative proportions (percentages) of individual white cell types. Measurement of hemoglobin, hematocrit, mean corpuscular volume (MCV), mean corpuscular hemoglobin concentration (MCHC), and mean

---

Hematopoiesis

➤ Blood cells originate from pluripotent stem cells in the bone marrow.

➤ The proliferation, differentiation, and functional abilities of the various blood cells are controlled by hormone-like growth factors called *cytokines*.

cell hemoglobin (MCH) is usually included in the CBC. Inspection of the blood smear identifies morphologic abnormalities such as a change in size, shape, or color of cells. Specific tests of red blood cell function are found in Chapter 15 and of white blood cell function in Chapter 16.

ERYTHROCYTE SEDIMENTATION RATE

The erythrocyte sedimentation rate (ESR) is a screening test for monitoring the fluctuations in the clinical course of a disease. In anticoagulated blood, red blood cells aggregate and sediment to the bottom of a tube. The rate of fall of the aggregates is accelerated in the presence of fibrinogen and other plasma proteins that are often increased in inflammatory diseases. The ESR is the distance in millimeters that a red cell column travels in 1 hour. Normal values are 1 to 13 mm/hour for men and 1 to 20 mm/hour for women.

BONE MARROW ASPIRATION AND BIOPSY

Tests of bone marrow function are done on samples obtained using bone marrow aspiration or bone marrow biopsy. Bone marrow aspiration is performed with a special needle inserted into the bone marrow cavity, and a sample of marrow is withdrawn. Usually, the posterior iliac crest is used in all persons older than 12 to 18 months of age. Other sites include the anterior iliac crest, sternum, and spinous processes T10 through L4. The sternum is not commonly used in children because the cavity is too shallow and there is danger of mediastinal and cardiac perforation. Because aspiration disturbs the marrow architecture, this technique is used primarily to determine the type of cells present and their relative numbers. Stained smears of bone marrow aspirates are usually subjected to several studies: determination of the erythroid to myeloid cell count (*i.e.*, normal ratio is 1:3); differential cell count, search for abnormal cells, evaluation of iron stores in reticulum cells, and special stains and immunochemical studies.

Bone marrow biopsy is done with a special biopsy needle inserted into the posterior iliac crest. Biopsy removes an actual sample of bone marrow tissue and allows study of the architecture of the tissue. It is used to determine the marrow-to-fat ratio and the presence of fibrosis, plasma cells, granulomas, and cancer cells. The major hazard of these procedures is the slight risk of hemorrhage. This risk is increased in persons with a reduced platelet count.

> In summary, diagnostic tests of the blood include the complete blood count, which is used to describe the number and characteristics of the erythrocytes, leukocytes, and platelets. The erythrocyte sedimentation rate is used to detect inflammation. Bone marrow aspiration is used to determine the function of the bone marrow in generating blood cells.

Bibliography

Alexander W.S. (1998). Cytokines in hematopoiesis. *International Reviews of Immunology* 16, 651–682.

Buckner C.D. (1999). Autologous bone marrow transplants to hematopoietic stem cell support with peripheral blood stem cells: A historical perspective. *Journal of Hematology* 8, 233–263.

Davoren J.B. (2000). Blood disorders. In McPhee S.J., Lingappa V.R., Ganong W.F., Lange J.D. (Eds.), *Pathophysiology of disease* (3rd ed., pp. 98–123). New York: Lange Medical Books/McGraw-Hill.

Guyton A.C., Hall J.E. (2000). *Textbook of medical physiology* (10th ed.). Philadelphia: W.B. Saunders.

Hoffman R., Benz E.J., Shattil S.J., Furie B., Cohen H.J., Silberstein L.E., McGlave P. (2000). *Hematology: Basic principles and practice* (3rd ed.). New York: Churchill Livingstone.

Kirby S.L. (1999). Bone marrow: Target for gene transfer. *Hospital Practice* 34, 59–62.

Metcalf D. (1999). Cellular hematopoiesis in the twentieth century. *Seminars in Hematology* 36 (Suppl. 7), 5–12.

Rocha V., Wagner J.E., Sobocinski K., Klein J.P., Zhang M.J., Hororwitz M.M., Gluckman E. (2000). Graft-versus-host disease in children who have received a cord-blood or bone marrow transplant from an HLA-identical sibling. *New England Journal of Medicine* 342, 1846–1854.

Rubin R.N., Leopold L. (1998). *Hematologic pathophysiology*. Madison, CT: Fence Creek Publishing.

Thomas E.D. (1999). Bone marrow transplantation: A review. *Seminars in Hematology* 36 (Suppl. 7), 95–103.

Chapter 14

Alterations in Hemostasis

Kathryn J. Gaspard

Mechanisms of Hemostasis
Vessel Spasm
Formation of the Platelet Plug
Blood Coagulation
Clot Retraction
Clot Dissolution

Hypercoagulability States
Increased Platelet Function
Increased Clotting Activity

Bleeding Disorders
Platelet Defects
Thrombocytopenia
Impaired Platelet Function

Coagulation Defects
Impaired Synthesis
of Coagulation Factors
Hereditary Disorders
Disseminated Intravascular
Coagulation
Vascular Disorders

The term *hemostasis* refers to the stoppage of blood flow. The normal process of hemostasis is regulated by a complex array of activators and inhibitors that maintain blood fluidity and prevent blood from leaving the vascular compartment. Hemostasis is normal when it seals a blood vessel to prevent blood loss and hemorrhage. It is abnormal when it causes inappropriate blood clotting or when clotting is insufficient to stop the flow of blood from the vascular compartment. Disorders of hemostasis fall into two main categories: the inappropriate formation of clots within the vascular system (*i.e.*, thrombosis) and the failure of blood to clot in response to an appropriate stimulus (*i.e.*, bleeding).

Mechanisms of Hemostasis

After you have completed this section of the chapter, you should be able to meet the following objectives:

✦ State the five stages of hemostasis
✦ Describe the formation of the platelet plug
✦ State the purpose of coagulation
✦ State the function of clot retraction
✦ Trace the process of fibrinolysis

Hemostasis is divided into five stages: vessel spasm, formation of the platelet plug, blood coagulation or de-

velopment of an insoluble fibrin clot, clot retraction, and clot dissolution (Fig. 14-1).

VESSEL SPASM

Vessel spasm is initiated by endothelial injury and caused by local and humoral mechanisms. A spasm constricts the vessel and reduces blood flow. It is a transient event that usually lasts less than 1 minute. Thromboxane A_2 (TXA_2), released from the platelets and cells, and other mediators contribute to vasoconstriction. Prostacyclin, a prostaglandin released from the vessel endothelium, produces vasodilation and inhibits platelet aggregation.

FORMATION OF THE PLATELET PLUG

The platelet plug, the second line of defense, is initiated as platelets come in contact with the vessel wall. Platelets, also called *thrombocytes*, are large fragments from the cytoplasm of bone marrow cells called *megakaryocytes*. They are enclosed in a membrane but have no nucleus and cannot reproduce. Their cytoplasmic granules release mediators for hemostasis. Although they lack a nucleus, they have many of the characteristics of a whole cell. They have mitochondria and enzyme systems capable of producing adenosine triphosphate and adenosine diphosphate (ADP) and they have the enzymes needed for synthesis of prostaglandins, which are required for their function in hemostasis. Platelets

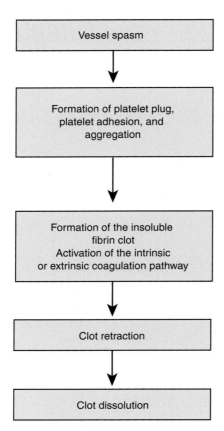

FIGURE 14-1 Steps in hemostasis.

also produce a growth factor that causes vascular endothelial cells, smooth muscle cells, and fibroblasts to proliferate and grow.

The life span of a platelet is only 8 to 9 days. Platelet production is controlled by a protein called *thrombopoietin* that causes proliferation and maturation of megakaryocytes.[1] The sources of thrombopoietin include the liver,

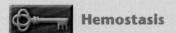

Hemostasis

➤ Hemostasis is the orderly, stepwise process for stopping bleeding that involves vasospasm, formation of a platelet plug, and the development of a fibrin clot.

➤ The blood clotting process requires the presence of platelets produced in the bone marrow, von Willebrand factor generated by the vessel endothelium, and clotting factors synthesized in the liver, using vitamin K.

➤ The final step of the process involves fibrinolysis or clot dissolution, which prevents excess clot formation.

kidney, smooth muscle, and bone marrow. Its production and release are regulated by the number of platelets in the circulation. The newly formed platelets that are released from the bone marrow spend up to 8 hours in the spleen before they are released into the blood.

Platelet plug formation involves adhesion and aggregation of platelets (Fig. 14-2A). It also requires a protein molecule called *von Willebrand factor* (vWF). This factor is produced by the endothelial cells of blood vessels and circulates in the blood as a carrier protein for coagulation factor VIII.

Platelets are attracted to a damaged vessel wall, become activated, and change from smooth disks to spiny spheres, exposing receptors on their surfaces. Adhesion to the vessel subendothelial layer occurs when the platelet receptor binds to vWF at the injury site, linking the platelet to exposed collagen fibers. The process of adhesion is controlled by local hormones and substances released by platelet granules. As the platelets adhere to the collagen fibers on the damaged vessel wall, they begin to release large amounts of ADP and TXA$_2$. Platelet aggregation and formation of a loosely organized platelet plug occurs as the ADP and TXA$_2$ cause nearby platelets to become sticky and

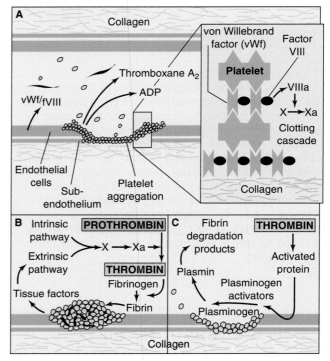

FIGURE 14-2 (**A**) The platelet plug occurs seconds after vessel injury. Von Willebrand's factor, released from the endothelial cells, binds to platelet receptors, causing *adhesion* of platelets to the exposed collagen. Platelet *aggregation* is induced by release of thromboxane A$_2$ and adenosine diphosphate. (**B**) Coagulation factors, activated on the platelet surface, lead to the formation of thrombin and fibrin, which stabilize the platelet plug. (**C**) Control of the coagulation process and clot dissolution are governed by thrombin and plasminogen activators. Thrombin activates protein C, which stimulates the release of plasminogen activators. The plasminogen activators in turn promote the formation of plasmin, which digests the fibrin strands.

adhere to the original platelets. Stabilization of the platelet plug occurs as the coagulation pathway is activated on the platelet surface and fibrinogen is converted to fibrin, thereby creating a fibrin meshwork that cements the platelets and other blood components together (see Fig. 14-2B).

Defective platelet plug formation causes bleeding in persons who are deficient in platelet receptor sites or vWF. In addition to sealing vascular breaks, platelets play an almost continuous role in maintaining normal vascular integrity. They may supply growth factors for the endothelial cells and arterial smooth muscle cells. Persons with platelet deficiency have increased capillary permeability and sustain small skin hemorrhages from the slightest trauma or change in blood pressure.

BLOOD COAGULATION

Blood coagulation is the process by which fibrin strands create a meshwork that cements blood components together (Fig. 14-3). It results from activation of the intrinsic or the extrinsic coagulation pathways (Fig. 14-4). The intrinsic pathway, which is a relatively slow process, begins in the blood itself. The extrinsic pathway, which is a much faster process, begins with trauma to the blood vessel or surrounding tissues. The terminal steps in both pathways are the same: the activation of factor X and thrombin-induced formation of fibrin, the material that stabilizes a clot. Both pathways are needed for normal hemostasis, and many interrelations exist between them. Each system is activated when blood passes out of the vascular system. The

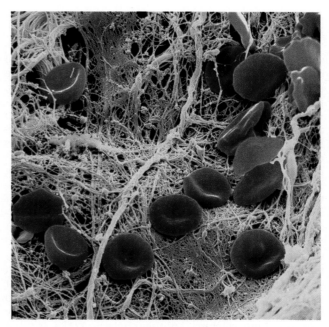

FIGURE 14-3 Scanning electron micrograph of a blood clot (×3600). The fibrous bridges that form a meshwork between red blood cells are fibrin fibers. (© Oliver Meckes, Science Source/Photo Researchers)

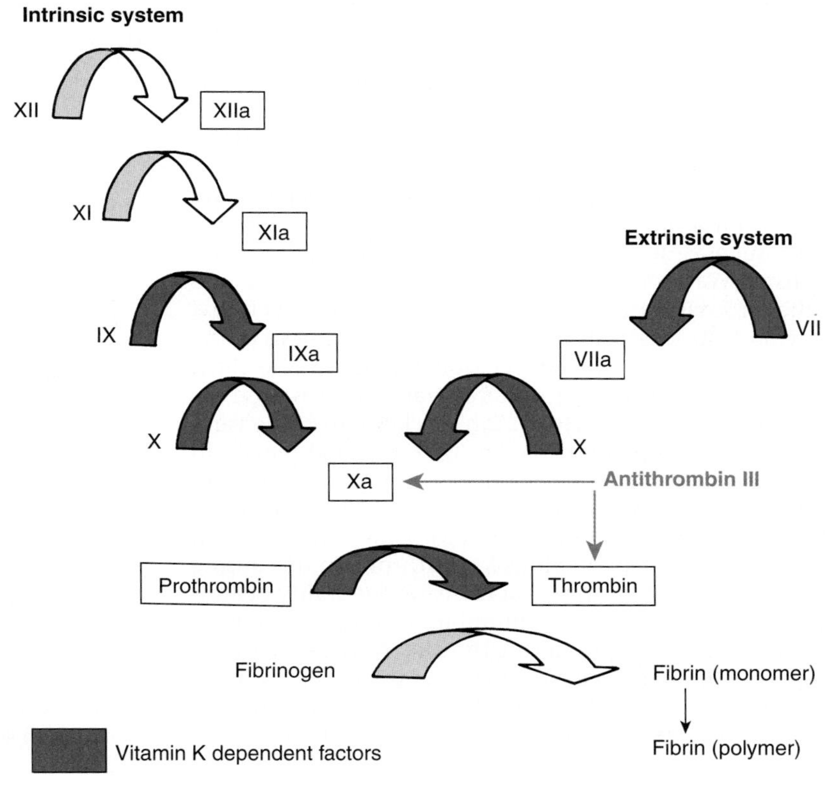

intrinsic system is activated as blood comes in contact with collagen in the injured vessel wall; the extrinsic system is activated when blood is exposed to tissue extracts. Bleeding, when it occurs because of defects in the extrinsic system,

FIGURE 14-4 Intrinsic and extrinsic coagulation pathways. The terminal steps in both pathways are the same. Calcium, factors X and V, and platelet phospholipids combine to form prothrombin activator, which then converts prothrombin to thrombin. This interaction causes conversion of fibrinogen into the fibrin strands that create the insoluble blood clot. (Adapted from Lehne, R. [1998]. *Pharmacology for nursing care* [3rd ed., p. 534]. Philadelphia: W.B. Saunders)

Intrinsic system

XII → XIIa

XI → XIa

IX → IXa

X → Xa

Extrinsic system

VII → VIIa

X → Xa

Antithrombin III

Prothrombin → Thrombin

Fibrinogen → Fibrin (monomer) → Fibrin (polymer)

■ Vitamin K dependent factors

usually is not as severe as that which results from defects in the intrinsic pathway.

The coagulation process is controlled by many substances that promote clotting (*i.e.*, procoagulation factors) or inhibit it (*i.e.*, anticoagulation factors). Each of the procoagulation factors, identified by Roman numerals, performs a specific step in the coagulation process. The action of one coagulation factor or proenzyme is designed to activate the next factor in the sequence (*i.e.*, cascade effect). Because most of the inactive procoagulation factors are present in the blood at all times, the multistep process ensures that a massive episode of intravascular clotting does not occur by chance. It also means that abnormalities of the clotting process occur when one or more of the factors are deficient or when conditions lead to inappropriate activation of any of the steps.

Calcium (factor IV) is required in all but the first two steps of the clotting process. The body usually has sufficient amounts of calcium for these reactions. Inactivation of the calcium ion prevents blood from clotting when it is removed from the body. The addition of citrate to blood stored for transfusion purposes prevents clotting by chelating ionic calcium. Another chelator, EDTA, is often added to blood samples used for analysis in the clinical laboratory.

Coagulation is regulated by several natural anticoagulants. Antithrombin III inactivates coagulation factors and neutralizes thrombin, the last enzyme in the pathway for the conversion of fibrinogen to fibrin. When antithrombin III is complexed with naturally occurring heparin, its action is accelerated and provides protection against uncontrolled thrombus formation on the endothelial surface. Protein C, a plasma protein, acts as an anticoagulant by inactivating factors V and VIII. Protein S, another plasma protein, accelerates the action of protein C. Plasmin breaks down fibrin into fibrin degradation products that act as anticoagulants. It has been suggested that some of these natural anticoagulants may play a role in the bleeding that occurs with disseminated intravascular coagulation (DIC; discussed later).

The anticoagulant drugs warfarin and heparin are used to prevent venous thrombi and thromboembolic disease, such as deep vein thrombosis and pulmonary embolism. Warfarin acts by decreasing prothrombin and other procoagulation factors. It alters vitamin K such that it reduces its availability to participate in synthesis of the vitamin K–dependent coagulation factors in the liver. Warfarin is readily absorbed after oral administration. Its maximum effect takes 36 to 72 hours because of the varying half-lives of preformed clotting factors that remain in the circulation. Heparin is naturally formed in large quantities in mast cells and in the basophilic cells of the blood. Pharmacologic preparations of heparin are extracted from animal tissues. Heparin binds to antithrombin III, causing a conformational change that increases the ability of antithrombin III to inactivate thrombin, factor Xa, and other clotting factors. By promoting the inactivation of clotting factors, heparin ultimately suppresses the formation of fibrin. Heparin is unable to cross the membranes of the gastrointestinal tract and must be given by injection.

CLOT RETRACTION

After the clot has formed, clot retraction, which requires large numbers of platelets, contributes to hemostasis by squeezing serum from the clot and joining the edges of the broken vessel.

CLOT DISSOLUTION

The dissolution of a blood clot begins shortly after its formation; this allows blood flow to be reestablished and permanent tissue repair to take place (see Fig. 14-2C). The process by which a blood clot dissolves is called *fibrinolysis*. As with clot formation, clot dissolution requires a sequence of steps controlled by activators and inhibitors (Fig. 14-5). Plasminogen, the proenzyme for the fibrinolytic process, normally is present in the blood in its inactive form. It is converted to its active form, plasmin, by plasminogen activators formed in the vascular endothelium, liver, and kidneys. The plasmin formed from plasminogen digests the fibrin strands of the clot and certain clotting factors, such as fibrinogen, factor V, factor VIII, prothrombin, and factor XII. Circulating plasmin is rapidly inactivated by α_2-plasmin inhibitor, which limits fibrinolysis to the local clot and prevents it from occurring in the entire circulation.

Two naturally occurring plasminogen activators are tissue-type plasminogen activator and urokinase-type plasminogen activator. The liver, plasma, and vascular endothelium are the major sources of physiologic activators. These activators are released in response to a number of stimuli, including vasoactive drugs, venous occlusion, elevated body temperature, and exercise. The activators are unstable and rapidly inactivated by inhibitors synthesized by the endothelium and the liver. For this reason,

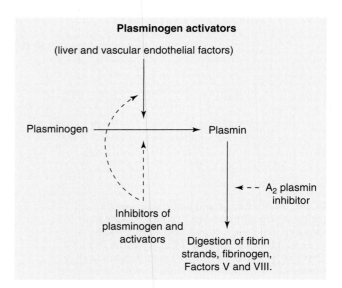

FIGURE 14-5 Fibrinolytic system and its modifiers. The *solid lines* indicate activation, and the *broken lines* indicate inactivation.

chronic liver disease may cause altered fibrinolytic activity. A major inhibitor, plasminogen activator inhibitor-1, in high concentrations has been associated with deep vein thrombosis, coronary artery disease, and myocardial infarction.[2]

> In summary, hemostasis is designed to maintain the integrity of the vascular compartment. The process is divided into five phases: vessel spasm, which constricts the size of the vessel and reduces blood flow; platelet adherence and formation of the platelet plug; formation of the fibrin clot, which cements the platelet plug together; clot retraction, which pulls the edges of the injured vessel together; and clot dissolution, which involves the action of plasmin that dissolves the clot and allows blood flow to be reestablished and tissue healing to take place. Blood coagulation requires the stepwise activation of coagulation factors, carefully controlled by activators and inhibitors.

CHART 14-1

Conditions Associated With Hypercoagulability States

Increased Platelet Function
Atherosclerosis
Diabetes mellitus
Smoking
Elevated blood lipid and cholesterol levels
Increased platelet levels

Accelerated Activity of the Clotting System
Pregnancy and the puerperium
Use of oral contraceptives
Postsurgical state
Immobility
Congestive heart failure
Malignant diseases

Hypercoagulability States

After you have completed this section of the chapter, you should be able to meet the following objectives:

✦ Compare normal and abnormal clotting
✦ State the causes and effects of increased platelet function
✦ State two conditions that contribute to increased clotting activity

There are two general forms of hypercoagulability states: conditions that create increased platelet function and conditions that cause accelerated activity of the coagulation system. Hypercoagulability represents hemostasis in an exaggerated form and predisposes to thrombosis. Arterial thrombi due to turbulence are composed of platelet aggregates, and venous thrombi due to stasis are largely composed of platelet aggregates and fibrin complexes that result from excess coagulation. Chart 14-1 summarizes conditions commonly associated with hypercoagulability states.

INCREASED PLATELET FUNCTION

The causes of increased platelet function are disturbances in flow, endothelial damage, and increased sensitivity of platelets to factors that cause adhesiveness and aggregation. Atherosclerotic plaques disturb flow, cause endothelial damage, and promote platelet adherence. Platelets that adhere to the vessel wall release growth factors that cause proliferation of smooth muscle and thereby contribute to the development of atherosclerosis. Smoking, elevated levels of blood lipids and cholesterol, hemodynamic stress, diabetes mellitus, and immune mechanisms may cause vessel damage, platelet adherence, and,

eventually, thrombosis. Cancer and some diseases are associated with high platelet counts and the potential for thrombosis. The term *thrombocytosis* is used to describe elevations in the platelet count above 1,000,000/mm³. This occurs in some malignancies and inflammatory states and after splenectomy. Myeloproliferative disorders produce excess platelets that may predispose to thrombosis or, paradoxically, bleeding when the rapidly produced platelets are defective.

INCREASED CLOTTING ACTIVITY

Factors that increase the activation of the coagulation system are stasis of blood flow and alterations in the coagulation components of the blood (*i.e.*, an increase in procoagulation factors or a decrease in anticoagulation factors).

 Hypercoagulability States

➤ Hypercoagulability states increase the risk of clot or thrombus formation in either the arterial or venous circulations.

➤ Arterial thrombi are associated with conditions that produce turbulent blood flow and platelet adherence.

➤ Venous thrombi are associated with conditions that cause stasis of blood flow with increased concentrations of coagulation factors.

Stasis causes the accumulation of activated clotting factors and platelets and prevents their interactions with inhibitors. Slow and disturbed flow is a common cause of venous thrombosis in the immobilized or postsurgical patient. Heart failure also contributes to venous congestion and thrombosis. Elevated levels of estrogen increase coagulation factors. The incidence of stroke, thromboemboli, and myocardial infarction is greater in women who use oral contraceptives, particularly after age 35, and in heavy smokers.[3] Clotting factors are also increased during normal pregnancy. These changes, along with limited activity during the puerperium (immediate postpartum period), predispose to venous thrombosis. Hypercoagulability is common in cancer and sepsis. Many tumor cells are thought to release tissue factor molecules that, along with the increased immobility and sepsis seen in patients with malignant disease, contribute to thrombosis in these patients. A reduction in anticoagulants such as antithrombin III, protein C, and protein S predisposes to venous thrombosis.[4] Deficiencies of these inhibitor proteins are uncommon inherited defects. It has been suggested that high circulating levels of homocysteine also predispose to venous and arterial thrombosis by activating platelets and altering antithrombotic mechanisms.[5]

Another cause of increased venous and arterial clotting is a condition known as the *antiphospholipid syndrome*. The syndrome is caused by the development of antiphospholipid antibodies and recurrent thrombosis of vessels of any size. Women with the disorder have a history of recurrent pregnancy losses due to ischemia and thrombosis of placental vessels. Diagnosis is based on two positive test results for lupus anticoagulant or high immunoglobulin G (IgG) or IgM anticardiolipin antibodies in tests at least 12 weeks apart. Persons with the disorder have a history of having one or more of the following: deep venous thrombosis; arterial thrombosis, including stroke, myocardial infarction, or gangrene; recurrent fetal loss; or thrombocytopenia.[6] Exactly how antiphospholipid antibodies relate to thrombosis is unclear. One suggested mechanism is that the antibodies inhibit prostacyclin production by endothelial cells, with a consequent increase in platelet aggregation. Another is that the antibodies inhibit the activation of protein C. Because protein C counteracts clotting, inhibition of its activation favors thrombosis. Treatment focuses on removal or reduction in factors that predispose to thrombosis, including advice to stop smoking and counseling against use of estrogen-containing oral contraceptives by women. Prolonged prophylactic therapy to reduce thrombus formation and immune suppression is recommended. Some studies suggest that daily aspirin is as effective as oral anticoagulants.[6]

In summary, hypercoagulability causes excessive clotting and contributes to thrombus formation. It results from conditions that create increased platelet function or that cause accelerated activity of the coagulation system. Increased platelet function usually results from disorders such as atherosclerosis that damage the vessel endothelium and disturb blood flow or from conditions such as smoking that cause increased sensitivity of platelets to factors that promote adhesiveness and aggregation. Factors that cause accelerated activity of the coagulation system include blood flow stasis, resulting in an accumulation of coagulation factors, and alterations in the components of the coagulation system (*i.e.*, an increase in procoagulation factors or a decrease in anticoagulation factors).

Bleeding Disorders

After you have completed this section of the chapter, you should be able to meet the following objectives:

✦ State the mechanisms of drug-induced thrombocytopenia and idiopathic thrombocytopenia and the differing features in terms of onset and resolution of the disorders
✦ Describe the manifestations of thrombocytopenia
✦ Describe the role of vitamin K in coagulation
✦ State three common defects of coagulation factors and the causes of each
✦ Differentiate between the mechanisms of bleeding in hemophilia A and von Willebrand disease
✦ Describe the physiologic basis of acute disseminated intravascular coagulation
✦ Describe the effect of vascular disorders on hemostasis

Bleeding disorders or impairment of blood coagulation can result from defects in any of the factors that contribute to hemostasis. Defects are associated with platelets, coagulation factors, and vascular integrity.

 Bleeding Disorders

➤ Bleeding disorders are caused by defects associated with platelets, coagulation factors, and vessel integrity.

➤ Disorders of platelet plug formation include a decrease in platelet numbers due to inadequate platelet production (bone marrow dysfunction), excess platelet destruction (thrombocytopenia), abnormal platelet function (thrombocytopathia), or defects in von Willebrand factor.

➤ Impairment of the coagulation stage of hemostasis is caused by a deficiency in one or more of the clotting factors.

➤ Disorders of blood vessel integrity result from structurally weak vessels or vessel damage due to inflammation and immune mechanisms.

PLATELET DEFECTS

Bleeding can occur as a result of a decrease in the number of circulating platelets or impaired platelet function. The depletion of platelets must be relatively severe (10,000 to 20,000/mL, compared with the normal values of 150,000 to 400,000/mL) before hemorrhagic tendencies or spontaneous bleeding become evident. Bleeding that results from platelet deficiency commonly occurs in small vessels and is characterized by petechiae (*i.e.*, pinpoint purplish-red spots) and purpura (*i.e.*, purple areas of bruising) on the arms and thighs. Bleeding from mucous membranes of the nose, mouth, gastrointestinal tract, and vagina is characteristic. Bleeding of the intracranial vessels is a rare danger with severe platelet depletion.

Thrombocytopenia

Platelets are produced by cells in the bone marrow and then stored in the spleen before being released into the circulation. Consequently, a decrease in the number of circulating platelets, a condition called *thrombocytopenia*, can result from a decrease in platelet production by the bone marrow, an increased pooling of platelets in the spleen, or decreased platelet survival due to immune destruction or nonimmune mechanisms.

Loss of bone marrow function in aplastic anemia (see Chapter 15) or replacement of bone marrow by malignant cells, such as occurs in leukemia, results in decreased production of platelets. Infection with human immunodeficiency virus (HIV) suppresses the production of megakaryocytes. Radiation therapy and drugs such as those used in the treatment of cancer may depress bone marrow function and reduce platelet production.

There may be normal production of platelets but excessive pooling of platelets in the spleen. The spleen normally sequesters approximately 30% to 40% of the platelets. When the spleen is enlarged (*i.e.*, splenomegaly), however, as many as 80% of the platelets can be sequestered in the spleen. Splenomegaly occurs in cirrhosis with portal hypertension and in lymphomas.

Premature destruction of platelets occurs by a variety of immune mechanisms (*e.g.*, antibodies produced against the platelet). In acute DIC or thrombotic thrombocytopenic purpura (TTP), excessive platelet consumption leads to a deficiency.

Drug-Induced Thrombocytopenia.

Some drugs, such as quinine, quinidine, and certain sulfa-containing antibiotics, may induce thrombocytopenia. These drugs act as a hapten (see Chapter 18) and induce antigen–antibody response and formation of immune complexes that cause platelet destruction by complement-mediated lysis. In persons with drug-associated thrombocytopenia, there is a rapid fall in platelet count within 2 to 3 days of resuming a drug or 7 or more days (*i.e.*, the time needed to mount an immune response) after starting a drug for the first time. The platelet count rises rapidly after the drug is discontinued. The anticoagulant drug heparin has been increasingly implicated in thrombocytopenia and, paradoxically, in thrombosis. The complications typically occur 5 days after the start of therapy and result from heparin-dependent antiplatelet antibodies that cause aggregation of platelets and their removal from the circulation. The antibodies often bind to vessel walls, causing injury and thrombosis. The newer, low–molecular-weight heparin has been shown to be effective in reducing the incidence of heparin-induced complications compared with the older, high–molecular-weight form of the drug.[7]

Idiopathic Thrombocytopenic Purpura.

Idiopathic thrombocytopenic purpura, an autoimmune disorder, results in platelet antibody formation and excess destruction of platelets. The IgG antibody binds to two identified membrane glycoproteins while in the circulation. The platelets, which are made more susceptible to phagocytosis because of the antibody, are destroyed in the spleen.

Acute idiopathic thrombocytopenic purpura is more common in children and usually follows a viral infection. It is characterized by sudden onset of petechiae and purpura and is a self-limited disorder with no treatment. In contrast, the chronic form is usually seen in adults and seldom follows an infection. It is a disease of young people, with a peak incidence between the ages of 20 and 50 years, and is seen twice as often in women as in men. It may be associated with other immune disorders such as acquired immunodeficiency syndrome (AIDS) or systemic lupus erythematosus. The condition occasionally presents precipitously with signs of bleeding, often into the skin (*i.e.*, purpura and petechiae) or oral mucosa. There is commonly a history of bruising, bleeding from gums, epistaxis (*i.e.*, nosebleeds), and abnormal menstrual bleeding. Because the spleen is the site of platelet destruction, splenic enlargement may occur.

Diagnosis usually is based on severe thrombocytopenia (platelet counts <20,000/mL), and exclusion of other causes. Tests for the platelet antibody are available but lack specificity (*e.g.*, they react with platelet antibodies from other sources). Treatment includes the initial use of corticosteroid drugs, often followed by splenectomy and the use of immunosuppressive agents. Use of high-dose dexamethasone, given in cycles over 1 month, has proven to be effective in persons who experience a relapse.[8]

Thrombotic Thrombocytopenic Purpura.

Thrombotic thrombocytopenic purpura is a combination of thrombocytopenia, hemolytic anemia, signs of vascular occlusion, fever, and neurologic abnormalities. The onset is abrupt and the outcome may be fatal. Widespread vascular occlusions consist of thrombi in arterioles and capillaries of many organs, including the heart, brain, and kidneys. Erythrocytes become fragmented as they circulate through the partly occluded vessels and cause the hemolytic anemia. The clinical manifestations include purpura and petechiae and neurologic symptoms ranging from headache to seizures and altered consciousness. TTP is probably caused by widespread endothelial damage that releases mediators resulting in platelet aggregation. The disorder is similar to DIC but does not involve the clotting system. Treatment for TTP includes *plasmapheresis*, a procedure that involves removal of plasma from withdrawn blood and replacement with fresh-frozen plasma. The treatment is continued until remission occurs. With plasmapheresis treatment, there is a complete recovery in 80% to 90% of cases.

Impaired Platelet Function

Impaired platelet function (also called *thrombocytopathia*) may result from inherited disorders of adhesion (*e.g.*, von Willebrand disease) or acquired defects caused by drugs, disease, or extracorporeal circulation. Chart 14-2 lists other drugs that impair platelet function. Defective platelet function is also common in uremia, presumably because of unexcreted waste products. Cardiopulmonary bypass also causes platelet defects and destruction.

Use of aspirin and other nonsteroidal anti-inflammatory drugs (NSAIDs) is the most common cause of impaired platelet function. These drugs inhibit platelet cyclooxygenase activity and consequently the synthesis of the prostaglandin TXA_2, which is required for platelet aggregation. The effect of aspirin on platelet aggregation lasts for the life of the platelet—usually approximately 8 to 9 days. In contrast to the effects of aspirin, which produce irreversible inhibition of cyclooxygenase and last for the life of the platelet, the inhibition of cyclooxygenase by other NSAIDs is reversible and lasts only for the duration of drug action.[9] Aspirin commonly is used to prevent formation of arterial thrombi. It is used in prevention of both heart attack and stroke. A 1989 report indicated a 44% reduction in risk of myocardial infarction in persons older than 50 years of age who had taken low doses of aspirin.[10]

COAGULATION DEFECTS

Impairment of blood coagulation can result from deficiencies of one or more of the known clotting factors. Deficiencies can arise because of defective synthesis, inherited disease, or increased consumption of the clotting factors. Bleeding that results from clotting factor deficiency typically occurs after injury or trauma. Large bruises, hematomas, or prolonged bleeding into the gastrointestinal or urinary tracts or joints are common.

Impaired Synthesis of Coagulation Factors

Coagulation factors V, VII, IX, X, XI, and XII; prothrombin; and fibrinogen are synthesized in the liver. In liver disease, synthesis of these clotting factors is reduced, and bleeding may result. Of the coagulation factors synthesized in the liver, factors VII, IX, and X and prothrombin require the presence of vitamin K for normal activity. In vitamin K deficiency, the liver produces the clotting factor, but in an inactive form. Vitamin K is a fat-soluble vitamin that is continuously being synthesized by intestinal bacteria. This means that a deficiency in vitamin K is not likely to occur unless intestinal synthesis is interrupted or absorption of the vitamin is impaired. Vitamin K deficiency can occur in the newborn infant before the establishment of the intestinal flora; it can also occur as a result of treatment with broad-spectrum antibiotics that destroy intestinal flora. Because vitamin K is a fat-soluble vitamin, its absorption requires bile salts. Vitamin K deficiency may result from impaired fat absorption caused by liver or gallbladder disease.

Hereditary Disorders

Hereditary defects have been reported for each of the clotting factors, but most are rare diseases. The most common bleeding disorders involve the factor VIII–vWF complex. The disorders are hemophilia A, which affects 1 in 10,000 males, and von Willebrand disease, which occurs in 1% of the population.[11] Factor IX deficiency (*i.e.*, hemophilia B) occurs in approximately 1 in 50,000 persons and is genetically and clinically similar to hemophilia A.

Hemophilia A. Circulating factor VIII is part of a complex molecule, bound to vWF. Factor VIII coagulant protein is the functional portion produced by the liver and endothelial cells. vWF, synthesized by the endothelium and megakaryocytes, binds and stabilizes factor VIII in the circulation by preventing proteolysis. It is also required for platelet adhesion to the subendothelial layer.

Hemophilia A, which is caused by a deficiency in factor VIII, is an X-linked recessive disorder that primarily affects males. Although it is a hereditary disorder, there is no family history of the disorder in approximately one third of newly diagnosed cases, suggesting that it has arisen as

---

> ### CHART 14-2
>
> #### *Drugs That May Predispose to Bleeding*
>
> **Interference With Platelet Production or Function**
> Acetazolamide
> Alcohol
> Antimetabolite and anticancer drugs
> Antibiotics such as penicillin and the cephalosporins
> Aspirin and salicylates
> Carbamazepine
> Clofibrate
> Colchicine
> Dextran
> Dipyridamole
> Thiazide diuretics
> Gold salts
> Heparin
> Nonsteroidal anti-inflammatory drugs
> Quinine derivatives (quinidine and hydroxychloroquine)
> Sulfinpyrazone
> Sulfonamides
>
> **Interference With Coagulation Factors**
> Amiodarone
> Anabolic steroids
> Warfarin
> Heparin
>
> **Decrease in Vitamin K Levels**
> Antibiotics
> Clofibrate

a new mutation in the factor VIII gene.[11] Approximately 90% of persons with hemophilia produce insufficient quantities of the factor, and 10% produce a defective form. The percentage of normal factor VIII activity in the circulation depends on the genetic defect and determines the severity of hemophilia (*i.e.*, 5% to 25% in mild hemophilia, 1% to 4% in moderate hemophilia, and 1% or less in severe forms of hemophilia). In mild or moderate forms of the disease, bleeding usually does not occur unless there is a local lesion or trauma such as surgery or dental procedures. The mild disorder may not be detected in childhood. In severe hemophilia, bleeding usually occurs in childhood (*e.g.*, it may be noticed at the time of circumcision) and is spontaneous and severe. Characteristically, bleeding occurs in soft tissues, the gastrointestinal tract, and the hip, knee, elbow, and ankle joints. Joint bleeding usually begins when a child begins to walk. Often, a target joint is prone to repeated bleeding. The bleeding causes inflammation of the synovium, with acute pain and swelling. Without proper treatment, chronic bleeding and inflammation causes joint fibrosis and contractures, resulting in major disability. There is also the potential for life-threatening intracranial hemorrhage.

Factor VIII replacement therapy is initiated when bleeding occurs or as prophylaxis with repeated bleeding episodes. The purpose is to limit the extent of tissue damage. *Cryoprecipitate*, prepared from fresh-frozen plasma, contains factor VIII. Its use is no longer recommended unless it is prepared from the father of the child with hemophilia. Highly purified factor VIII and factor IX concentrates prepared from human plasma are the usual replacement products for persons with severe hemophilia. Before blood was tested for infectious diseases, these products were prepared from multiple donor samples and carried a high risk of exposure to viruses for hepatitis and AIDS. Donor screening and the development of effective virus-inactivation procedures have effectively reduced the transmission of hepatitis viruses and HIV through clotting concentrates. However, an important clinical complication of treatment with clotting factor concentrates prior to the implementation of these procedures was the development of hepatitis B or C infection and the increased risk for chronic complications. Persons who received clotting factor concentrates before 1990 may be at risk for infection with hepatitis B and/or C and should be tested.[12]

As the quality and safety of clotting factors have risen, so has the cost, which sometimes restricts their use. Factor VIII produced by recombinant deoxyribonucleic acid (DNA) technology is now available and does not have the potential for transmitting viral disease. Although there are many advantages of recombinant factor VIII, the cost may be prohibitive. There is also the question of whether the recombinant product will incite a higher incidence of antibodies to factor VIII than plasma-derived concentrates.[13] The newer recombinant products and continuous-infusion pumps may allow prevention rather than therapy for hemorrhage.

The cloning of the factor VIII gene and progress in gene delivery systems have led to hope that hemophilia A may be cured by gene therapy. Carrier detection and prenatal diagnosis can now be done by analysis of direct gene mutation or DNA linkage studies. Prenatal amniocentesis or chorionic villus sampling is used to predict complications and determine therapy. It may eventually be used to select patients for gene addition.

Von Willebrand Disease. Von Willebrand disease, which typically is diagnosed in adulthood, is the most common hereditary bleeding disorder. Transmitted as an autosomal trait, it is caused by a deficiency of or defect in vWF. This deficiency results in reduced platelet adhesion. There are many variants of the disease, and manifestations range from mild to severe. Because vWF carries factor VIII, its deficiency may also be accompanied by reduced levels of factor VIII and results in defective clot formation. Symptoms include bruising, excessive menstrual flow, and bleeding from the nose, mouth, and gastrointestinal tract. Many persons with the disorder are diagnosed when surgery or dental extraction results in prolonged bleeding. Most cases are mild and untreated.

In severe cases, factor VIII products that contain vWF are infused to replace the deficient clotting factors. The disorder also responds to desmopressin acetate (DDAVP), a synthetic analog of the hormone vasopressin, which stimulates the endothelial cells to release vWF and plasminogen activator. DDAVP can also be used to treat mild hemophilia A and platelet dysfunction caused by uremia, heart bypass, and the effects of aspirin.[14]

DISSEMINATED INTRAVASCULAR COAGULATION

Disseminated intravascular coagulation is a paradox in the hemostatic sequence and is characterized by widespread coagulation and bleeding in the vascular compartment. It is not a primary disease but occurs as a complication of a wide variety of conditions. DIC begins with massive activation of the coagulation sequence as a result of unregulated generation of thrombin, resulting in systemic formation of fibrin. In addition, levels of all the major anticoagulants are reduced (Fig. 14-6). The microthrombi that result cause vessel occlusion and tissue ischemia. Multiple organ failure may ensue. Clot formation consumes all available coagulation proteins and platelets, and severe hemorrhage results.

The disorder can be initiated by activation of the intrinsic or extrinsic pathways. Activation through the extrinsic pathway occurs with liberation of tissue factors, as in trauma and cancers. The intrinsic pathway may be activated through extensive endothelial damage caused by viruses, infections, immune mechanisms, or stasis of blood. Obstetric disorders that involve necrotic placental or fetal tissue commonly are associated with DIC. Other inciting clinical conditions include massive trauma, burns, sepsis, shock, meningococcemia, and malignant disease. Chart 14-3 summarizes the conditions associated with DIC.

There is increasing evidence that the pathogenesis of DIC lies in the release of endotoxins that generate or release tissue factors from endothelial cells or directly activate

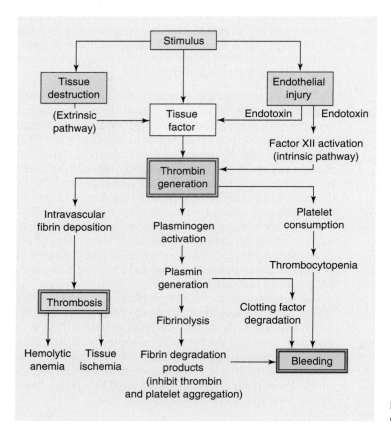

FIGURE 14-6 Pathophysiology of disseminated intravascular coagulation.

factor XII.[15] They may be the common mediating trigger in the events that cause DIC. There is also evidence that the fibrinolytic system is involved in the pathogenesis of DIC. It may be suppressed and thereby contribute to the formation of microthrombi, or it may be the source of fibrin degradation products that contribute to the bleeding that occurs. Finally, regardless of the inciting event, DIC may be a systemic inflammatory disorder with release of proinflammatory cytokines that mediate the derangement of coagulation and fibrin breakdown.[16]

Although coagulation and formation of microemboli initiate the events that characterize DIC, its acute manifestations usually are more directly related to the bleeding problems that occur. The bleeding may be present as petechiae, purpura, oozing from puncture sites, or severe hemorrhage. Cardiovascular shock is a common complication. Uncontrolled postpartum bleeding may indicate DIC. Microemboli may obstruct blood vessels and cause tissue hypoxia and necrotic damage to organ structures, such as the kidneys, heart, lungs, and brain. As a result, common clinical signs may be due to renal, circulatory, or respiratory failure or convulsions and coma. A form of hemolytic anemia may develop as red cells are damaged as they pass through vessels partially blocked by thrombus.

The treatment of DIC is directed toward managing the primary disease, replacing clotting components, and preventing further activation of clotting mechanisms. Transfusions of fresh-frozen plasma, platelets, or fibrinogen-containing cryoprecipitate may correct the clotting factor deficiency. Heparin may be given to decrease blood coagulation, thereby interrupting the clotting process. Heparin therapy is controversial, however, and the risk of hemorrhage may limit its use to severe cases. It typically is given as a continuous intravenous infusion that can be interrupted promptly if bleeding is accentuated. Tissue factor pathway inhibitors and protein C concentrates are being evaluated as potential future therapies.[16]

VASCULAR DISORDERS

Bleeding from small blood vessels may result from vascular disorders. These disorders may occur because of structurally weak vessel walls or because of damage to vessels by inflammation or immune responses. Among the vascular disorders that cause bleeding are hemorrhagic telangiectasia, an uncommon autosomal dominant disorder characterized by thin-walled, dilated capillaries and arterioles; vitamin C deficiency (*i.e.*, scurvy), resulting in poor collagen synthesis and failure of the endothelial cells to be cemented together properly, which causes a fragile wall; Cushing's disease, causing protein wasting and loss of vessel tissue support because of excess cortisol; and senile purpura (*i.e.*, bruising in elderly persons) caused by the aging process. Vascular defects also occur in the course of DIC as a result of the presence of microthrombi and corticosteroid therapy.

CHART 14-3

Conditions That Have Been Associated With DIC

Obstetric Conditions

Abruptio placentae
Dead fetus syndrome
Preeclampsia and eclampsia
Amniotic fluid embolism

Cancers

Metastatic cancer
Leukemia

Infections

Acute bacterial infections (*e.g.*, meningococcal meningitis)
Acute viral infections
Rickettsial infections (*e.g.*, Rocky Mountain spotted fever)
Parasitic infection (*e.g.*, malaria)

Shock

Septic shock
Severe hypovolemic shock

Trauma or Surgery

Burns
Massive trauma
Surgery involving extracorporeal circulation
Snake bite
Heatstroke

Hematologic Conditions

Blood transfusion reactions

Vascular disorders are characterized by easy bruising and the spontaneous appearance of petechiae and purpura of the skin and mucous membranes. In persons with bleeding disorders caused by vascular defects, the platelet count and results of other tests for coagulation factors are normal.

> In summary, bleeding disorders or impairment of blood coagulation can result from defects in any of the factors that contribute to hemostasis: platelets, coagulation factors, or vascular integrity. The number of circulating platelets can be decreased (*i.e.*, thrombocytopenia) or platelet function can be impaired (*i.e.*, thrombocytopathia). Impairment of blood coagulation can result from deficiencies of one or more of the known clotting factors. Deficiencies can arise because of defective synthesis (*i.e.*, liver disease or vitamin K deficiency), inherited diseases (*i.e.*, hemophilia A or von Willebrand disease), or increased consumption of the clotting factors (DIC). Bleeding may also occur from structurally weak vessels that result from impaired syn-

thesis of vessel wall components (*i.e.*, vitamin C deficiency, excessive cortisol levels as in Cushing's disease, or the aging process) or from damage by genetic mechanisms (*i.e.*, hemorrhagic telangiectasia) or the presence of microthrombi.

References

1. Kaushansky K. (1998). Thrombopoietin. *New England Journal of Medicine* 339, 746–754.
2. Kohler H.P., Grant P. J. (2000). Plasminogen-activator inhibitor type 1 and coronary artery disease. *New England Journal of Medicine* 342, 1792–1801.
3. Goldfien A. (1995). The gonadal hormones and inhibitors. In Katzung B.G. (Ed.), *Basic and clinical pharmacology* (6th ed., p. 623). Norwalk, CT: Appleton & Lange.
4. Alving B.M. (1993). The hypercoagulable states. *Hospital Practice* 28(2), 109–121.
5. Mitchell R.N., Cotran R.S. (1999). Hemodynamic disorders, thrombosis, and shock. In Cotran R.S., Kumar V., Collins T. (Eds.), *Robbins pathologic basis of disease* (6th ed., p. 125). Philadelphia: W.B. Saunders.
6. Harris E.N. (1994). Diagnosis and management of antiphospholipid syndrome. *Hospital Practice* 29(4), 65–76.
7. Warkentin T.E., Chong B.H., Greinacher A. (1998). Heparin-induced thrombocytopenia: Towards consensus. *Thrombosis and Haemostasis* 79, 1–7.
8. Andersen J. (1994). Response of resistant idiopathic thrombocytopenic purpura to pulsed high-dose dexamethasone therapy. *New England Journal of Medicine* 330, 1560–1564.
9. George J.N., Shattil S.J. (2000). Acquired disorders of platelet function. In Hoffman R., Benz E.J., Shattil S.J., Furie B., Cohen H.J., Silberstein L.E., McGlave P. (Eds.), *Hematology* (3rd ed., p. 2176). New York: Churchill Livingstone.
10. Steering Committee Physicians' Health Study Research Group. (1989). Final report on the aspirin component of the ongoing physicians' health study. *New England Journal of Medicine* 321, 129–135.
11. Cotran R.S. (1999). Red cells and bleeding disorders. In Cotran R.S., Kumar V., Collins T. (Eds.), *Robbins pathologic basis of disease* (6th ed., pp. 638, 639). Philadelphia: W.B. Saunders.
12. Soucie J.M., Richardson L.C., Evans B.L., Linden J.V., Ewenstein B.M., Stein S.F., et al. (2001). Risk factors for infection with HBV and HCV in a large cohort of hemophiliac males. *Transfusion* 41 (3), 338–343.
13. Feinstein D.I. (2000). Inhibitors in hemophilia. In Hoffman R., Benz E.J., Shattil S.J., Furie B., Cohen H.J., Silberstein L.E., McGlave P. (Eds.), *Hematology* (3rd ed., p. 1904). New York: Churchill Livingstone.
14. Mannucci P.M. (1997). Desmopressin (DDAVP) in the treatment of bleeding disorders: The first 20 years. *Blood* 90, 2515–2521.
15. Seligsohn U. (1995). Disseminated intravascular coagulation. In Buetler E., Lichtman M.A., Coller B. S., Kipps T.J. (Eds.), *Williams' hematology* (5th ed., p. 1497). New York: McGraw-Hill.
16. Levi M., ten Cate H. (1999). Disseminated intravascular coagulation. *New England Journal of Medicine* 341, 586–592.

Chapter 15

The Red Blood Cell and Alterations in Oxygen Transport

Kathryn J. Gaspard

Although the lungs provide the means for gas exchange between the external and internal environment, it is the hemoglobin in the red blood cells that transports oxygen to the tissues. The red blood cells also function as carriers of carbon dioxide and participate in acid-base balance. The function of the red blood cells, in terms of oxygen transport, is discussed in Chapter 27, and acid-base balance is covered in Chapter 32. This chapter focuses on the red blood cell, anemia, and polycythemia.

The Red Blood Cell

After you have completed this section of the chapter, you should be able to meet the following objectives:

✦ Trace the development of a red blood cell from erythroblast to erythrocyte
✦ Discuss the function of iron in the formation of hemoglobin
✦ Describe the formation, transport, and elimination of bilirubin
✦ Explain the function of the enzyme glucose-6-phosphate dehydrogenase in the red blood cell

✦ State the meaning of the red blood cell count, percentage of reticulocytes, hemoglobin, hematocrit, mean corpuscular volume, and mean corpuscular hemoglobin concentration as it relates to the diagnosis of anemia

The mature red blood cell, the erythrocyte, is a nonnucleated, biconcave disk (Fig. 15-1). This shape increases the surface area available for diffusion of oxygen and allows the cell to change in volume and shape without rupturing its membrane. A cytoskeleton of proteins attached to the lipid bilayer provides this unique shape and flexibility. The biconcave form presents the plasma with a surface 20 to 30 times greater than if the red blood cell were an absolute sphere. The erythrocytes, 500 to 1000 times more numerous than other blood cells, are the most common type of blood cell.

The function of the red blood cell, facilitated by the hemoglobin molecule, is to transport oxygen to the tissues. Hemoglobin also binds some carbon dioxide and carries it from the tissues to the lungs. The hemoglobin molecule is composed of two pairs of structurally different polypeptide chains determined by genes (Fig. 15-2). Alterations in these genes can result in abnormal hemoglobins. Each of the four polypeptide chains is attached to a heme unit, which

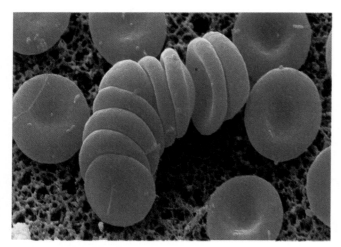

FIGURE 15-1 Scanning micrograph of normal red blood cells shows their normal concave appearance (× 3000). (© Andrew Syred, Science Photo Lab, Science Source/Photo Researchers)

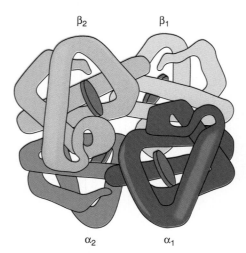

FIGURE 15-2 Structure of the hemoglobin molecule, showing the four subunits.

surrounds an atom of iron that binds oxygen. Four molecules of oxygen can be carried by one hemoglobin molecule.

The two major types of normal hemoglobin are adult hemoglobin (HbA) and fetal hemoglobin (HbF). HbA consists of a pair of α chains and a pair of β chains. HbF is the predominant hemoglobin in the fetus from the third through the ninth month of gestation. It has a pair of γ chains substituted for the β chains. Because of this chain substitution, HbF has a high affinity for oxygen. This facilitates the transfer of oxygen across the placenta. HbF is replaced within 6 months of birth with HbA.

The rate at which hemoglobin is synthesized depends on the availability of iron for heme synthesis. A lack of iron results in relatively small amounts of hemoglobin in the red blood cells. The amount of iron in the body is approximately 35 to 50 mg/kg of body weight for males and less for females. Body iron is found in several compartments. Most iron (80%) is complexed to heme in hemoglobin, with small amounts found in myoglobin and plasma. Approximately 20% is stored in the bone marrow, liver, spleen, and other organs. Iron in the hemoglobin compartment is recycled. When red blood cells age and are destroyed in the spleen, macrophages store the iron to be released and returned to the bone marrow for incorporation into new cells.

Dietary iron also helps to maintain body stores. Iron, principally derived from meat, is absorbed in the small intestine, especially the duodenum (Fig. 15-3). When body stores of iron are diminished or erythropoiesis is stimulated, absorption is increased. In iron overload, excretion of iron is accelerated. Normally, some iron is sequestered in the intestinal epithelial cells and is lost in the feces as these cells slough off. The iron that is absorbed enters the circulation, where it immediately combines with a β-globulin, apotransferrin, to form *transferrin*, which is then transported in the plasma. From the plasma, iron can be deposited in tissues such as liver, where it is stored as *ferritin*, a protein–iron complex, which can easily return to the circulation. Serum ferritin levels, which can be measured in the laboratory, provide an index of body iron stores. Clinically, decreased ferritin levels indicate the need for prescription of iron supplements. Transferrin can also deliver iron to the developing red cell in bone marrow by binding to membrane receptors. The iron is taken up by the developing red cell, where it is used in heme synthesis.

RED CELL PRODUCTION

Erythropoiesis is the production of red blood cells. After birth, red cells are produced in the red bone marrow. Until age 5 years, almost all bones produce red cells to meet growth needs. After this period, bone marrow activity gradually declines. After 20 years of age, red cell production takes place

 Red Blood Cells

➤ The function of red blood cells, facilitated by the iron-containing hemoglobin molecule, is to transport oxygen from the lungs to the tissues.

➤ The production of red blood cells, which is regulated by erythropoietin, occurs in the bone marrow and requires iron, vitamin B$_{12}$, and folate.

➤ The red blood cell, which has a life span of approximately 120 days, is broken down in the spleen; the degradation products such as iron and amino acids are recycled.

➤ The heme molecule, which is released from the red blood cell during the degradation process, is converted to bilirubin and transported to the liver, where it is removed and rendered water soluble for elimination in the bile.

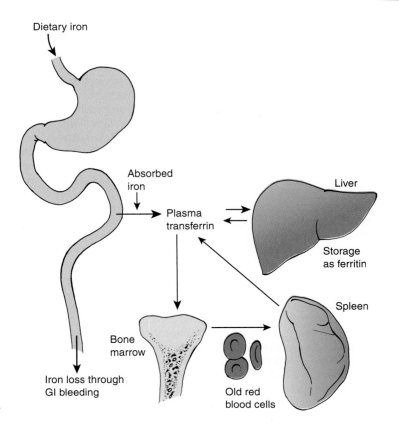

FIGURE 15-3 Iron cycle.

mainly in the membranous bones of the vertebrae, sternum, ribs, and pelvis. With this reduction in activity, the red bone marrow is replaced with fatty yellow bone marrow.

The red cells are derived from the erythroblasts, which are continuously being formed from the pluripotent stem cells in the bone marrow (Fig. 15-4). In developing into a mature red cell, the red cell precursors move through a series of divisions, each producing a smaller cell. Hemoglobin synthesis begins at the erythroblast stage and continues until the cell becomes an erythrocyte. During its transfor-

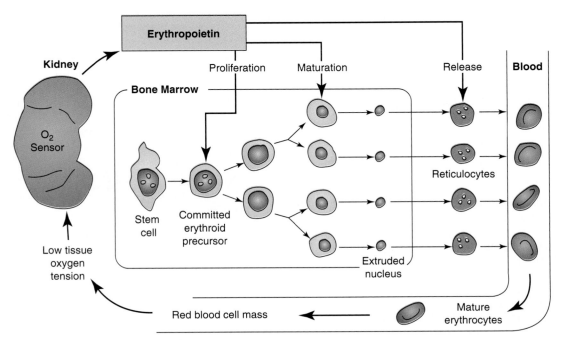

FIGURE 15-4 Red blood cell development.

mation from normoblast to reticulocyte, the red blood cell accumulates hemoglobin as the nucleus condenses and is finally lost. The period from stem cell to emergence of the reticulocyte in the circulation normally takes approximately 1 week. Maturation of reticulocyte to erythrocyte takes approximately 24 to 48 hours. During this process, the red cell loses its mitochondria and ribosomes, along with its ability to produce hemoglobin and engage in oxidative metabolism. Most maturing red cells enter the blood as reticulocytes. Approximately 1% of the body's total complement of red blood cells is generated from bone marrow each day, and the reticulocyte count therefore serves as an index of the erythropoietic activity of the bone marrow.

Erythropoiesis is governed for the most part by tissue oxygen needs. Any condition that causes a decrease in the amount of oxygen that is transported in the blood produces an increase in red cell production. The oxygen content of the blood does not act directly on the bone marrow to stimulate red blood cell production. Instead, the decreased oxygen content is sensed by the kidneys, which then produce a hormone called *erythropoietin*. Normally approximately 90% of erythropoietin is produced by the kidneys; the remaining 10% is released by the liver. In the absence of erythropoietin, as in kidney failure, hypoxia has little or no effect on red blood cell production. Erythropoietin takes several days to effect the release of red blood cells from the bone marrow, and only after 5 days or more does red blood cell production reach a maximum.

Erythropoietin acts in the bone marrow by binding to receptors on committed stem cells. It functions on many levels to promote hemoglobin synthesis, increase production of membrane proteins, and cause differentiation of erythroblasts. Human erythropoietin can be produced by recombinant deoxyribonucleic acid (DNA) technology. It is used for the management of anemia in cases of chronic renal failure, for anemias induced by chemotherapy for malignancies, and in the treatment of human immunodeficiency virus (HIV)–infected patients treated with zidovudine.

Because red blood cells are released into the blood as reticulocytes, the percentage of these cells is higher when there is a marked increase in red blood cell production. In some severe anemias, for example, the reticulocytes may account for as much as 30% of the total red cell count. In some situations, red cell production is so accelerated that numerous erythroblasts appear in the blood.

RED CELL DESTRUCTION

Mature red blood cells have a life span of approximately 4 months, or 120 days. As the red blood cell ages, a number of changes occur. Metabolic activity in the cell decreases, enzyme activity falls off, and adenosine triphosphate (ATP), potassium, and membrane lipids decrease. The rate of red cell destruction (1% per day) normally is equal to red cell production, but in conditions such as hemolytic anemia, the cell's life span may be shorter.

The destruction of red blood cells is accomplished by a group of large phagocytic cells found in the spleen, liver, bone marrow, and lymph nodes. These phagocytic cells recognize old and defective red cells and then ingest and destroy them in a series of enzymatic reactions. During these reactions, the amino acids from the globulin chains and iron from the heme units are salvaged and reused (Fig. 15-5). The bulk of the heme unit is converted to bilirubin, the pigment of bile, which is insoluble in plasma and attaches to the plasma proteins for transport. Bilirubin is removed from the blood by the liver and conjugated with glucuronide to render it water soluble so that it can be excreted in the bile. The plasma-insoluble form of bilirubin is referred to as *unconjugated bilirubin*; the water-soluble form is referred to as *conjugated bilirubin*. Serum levels of conjugated and unconjugated bilirubin can be measured in the laboratory and are reported as direct and indirect, respectively. If red cell destruction and consequent bilirubin production are excessive, unconjugated bilirubin accumulates in the blood. This results in a yellow discoloration of the skin, called *jaundice*.

When red blood cell destruction takes place in the circulation, as in hemolytic anemia, the hemoglobin remains in the plasma. The plasma contains a hemoglobin-binding protein called *haptoglobin*. Other plasma proteins, such as albumin, can also bind hemoglobin. With extensive intravascular destruction of red blood cells, hemoglobin levels may exceed the hemoglobin-binding capacity of haptoglobin. When this happens, free hemoglobin appears in the blood (*i.e.*, hemoglobinemia) and is excreted in the urine (*i.e.*, hemoglobinuria). Because excessive red blood cell

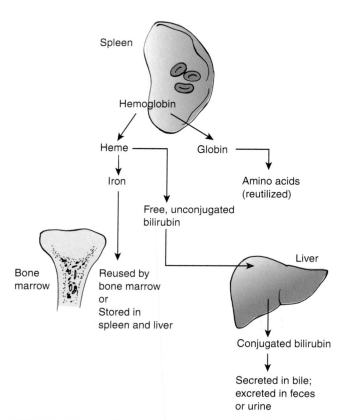

FIGURE 15-5 Destruction of red blood cells and fate of hemoglobin.

destruction can occur in hemolytic transfusion reactions, urine samples are tested for free hemoglobin after a transfusion reaction.

RED CELL METABOLISM AND HEMOGLOBIN OXIDATION

The red blood cell, which lacks mitochondria, relies on glucose and the glycolytic pathway for its metabolic needs. The enzyme-mediated anaerobic metabolism of glucose generates the ATP needed for normal membrane function and ion transport. The depletion of glucose or the functional deficiency of one of the glycolytic enzymes leads to the premature death of the red blood cell. An offshoot of the glycolytic pathway is the production of 2,3-diphosphoglycerate (2,3-DPG), which binds to the hemoglobin molecule and reduces the affinity of hemoglobin for oxygen. This facilitates the release of oxygen at the tissue level. An increase in the concentration of 2,3-DPG occurs in conditions of chronic hypoxia such as chronic lung disease, anemia, and high altitudes.

The oxidation of hemoglobin—the combining of hemoglobin with oxygen—can be interrupted by certain chemicals (*e.g.*, nitrates and sulfates) and drugs that oxidize hemoglobin to an inactive form. For example, the nitrite ion reacts with hemoglobin to produce *methemoglobin*, which has a low affinity for oxygen. Large doses of nitrites can result in high levels of methemoglobin, causing pseudocyanosis and tissue hypoxia. For example, sodium nitrate, which is used in curing meats, can produce methemoglobin when taken in large amounts. In nursing infants, the intestinal flora is capable of converting significant amounts of inorganic nitrate (*e.g.*, from well water) to nitrite. This inadvertent exposure to nitrates can cause serious toxic effects. A hereditary deficiency of glucose-6-phosphate dehydrogenase (G6PD; to be discussed) predisposes to oxidative denaturation of hemoglobin, with resultant red cell injury and lysis. Hemolysis occurs as the result of oxidative stress generated by either an infection or exposure to certain drugs.

LABORATORY TESTS

Red blood cells can be studied by means of a sample of blood (Table 15-1). In the laboratory, automated blood cell counters rapidly provide accurate measurements of red cell content and cell indices. The *red blood cell count* (RBC) measures the total number of red blood cells in 1 mm³ of blood. The *percentage of reticulocytes* (normally approximately 1%) provides an index of the rate of red cell production. The *hemoglobin* (grams per 100 mL of blood) measures the hemoglobin content of the blood. The major components of blood are the red cell mass and plasma volume. The *hematocrit* measures the volume of red cell mass in 100 mL of plasma volume. To determine the hematocrit, a sample of blood is placed in a glass tube, which is then centrifuged to separate the cells and the plasma. The hematocrit may be deceptive, because it varies with the quantity of extracellular fluid, rising with dehydration and falling with overexpansion of extracellular fluid volume.

Red cell indices are used to differentiate types of anemias by size or color of red cells. The *mean corpuscular volume* (MCV) reflects the volume or size of the red cells. The MCV falls in microcytic (small cell) anemia and rises in macrocytic (large cell) anemia. Some anemias are normocytic (*i.e.*, cells are of normal size or MCV). The *mean corpuscular hemoglobin concentration* (MCHC) is the concentration of hemoglobin in each cell. Hemoglobin accounts for the color of red blood cells. Anemias are described as *normochromic* (normal color or MCHC) or *hypochromic* (decreased color or MCHC). *Mean cell hemoglobin* (MCH) refers to the mass of the red cell and is less useful in classifying anemias.

A stained blood smear provides information about the size, color, and shape of red cells and the presence of immature or abnormal cells. If blood smear results are abnormal, examination of the bone marrow may be important.

TABLE 15-1 ✦ Standard Laboratory Values for Red Blood Cells

Test	Normal Values	Significance
Red blood cell count (RBC)		
Men	$4.2–5.4 \times 10^6/\mu L$	Number of red cells in the blood
Women	$3.6–5.0 \times 10^6/\mu L$	
Reticulocytes	1.0%–1.5% of total RBC	Rate of red cell production
Hemoglobin		
Men	14–16.5 g/dL	Hemoglobin content of the blood
Women	12–15 g/dL	
Hematocrit		
Men	40%–50%	Volume of cells in 100 mL of blood
Women	37%–47%	
Mean corpuscular volume	85–100 fL/red cell	Size of the red cell
Mean corpuscular hemoglobin concentration	31–35 g/dL	Concentration of hemoglobin in the red cell
Mean cell hemoglobin	27–34 pg/cell	Red cell mass

Marrow commonly is aspirated with a special needle from the posterior iliac crest or the sternum. The aspirate is stained and observed for number and maturity of cells and abnormal types.

In summary, the red blood cell provides the means for transporting oxygen from the lungs to the tissues. Red cells develop from stem cells in the bone marrow and are released as reticulocytes into the blood, where they become mature erythrocytes. Red blood cell production is regulated by the hormone erythropoietin, which is produced by the kidney in response to a decrease in oxygen levels. The life span of a red blood cell is approximately 120 days. Red cell destruction normally occurs in the spleen, liver, bone marrow, and lymph nodes. In the process of destruction, the heme portion of the hemoglobin molecule is converted to bilirubin. Bilirubin, which is insoluble in plasma, attaches to plasma proteins for transport in the blood. It is removed from the blood by the liver and conjugated to a water-soluble form so that it can be excreted in the bile.

The red blood cell, which lacks mitochondria, relies on glucose and the glycolytic pathway for its metabolic needs. The end product of the glycolytic pathway, 2,3-DPG, increases the release of oxygen to the tissues during conditions of hypoxia by reducing hemoglobin's affinity for oxygen.

In the laboratory, automated blood cell counters rapidly provide accurate measurements of red cell content and cell indices. A stained blood smear provides information about the size, color, and shape of red cells and the presence of immature or abnormal cells. If blood smear results are abnormal, examination of the bone marrow may be important.

resulting in diminished oxygen-carrying capacity. Anemia usually results from excessive loss (*i.e.*, bleeding) or destruction (*i.e.*, hemolysis) of red blood cells or from deficient red blood cell production because of a lack of nutritional elements or bone marrow failure.

MANIFESTATIONS

Anemia is not a disease, but an indication of some disease process or alteration in body function. The manifestations of anemia can be grouped into three categories: impaired oxygen transport, alterations in red cell structure, and signs and symptoms associated with the pathologic process that is causing the anemia. The manifestations of anemia also depend on its severity, the rapidity of its development, and the patient's age, health status, and compensatory mechanisms. With rapid blood loss, circulatory shock and circulatory collapse may occur. Because the body adapts to slowly developing anemia, the amount of red cell mass lost may reach 50% without the occurrence of signs and symptoms.[1]

In anemia, the oxygen-carrying capacity of hemoglobin is reduced, causing tissue hypoxia. Tissue hypoxia can give rise to angina, night cramps, fatigue, weakness, and dyspnea. Brain hypoxia results in headache, faintness, and dim vision. The redistribution of the blood from cutaneous tissues or a lack of hemoglobin causes pallor of the skin, mucous membranes, conjunctiva, and nail beds. Tachycardia and palpitations may occur as the body tries to compensate with an increase in cardiac output. A flow-type systolic murmur may result from changes in blood viscosity. Ventricular hypertrophy and high-output heart failure may develop in persons with severe anemia, particularly those with preexisting heart disease. Erythropoiesis is ac-

Anemia

After you have completed this section of the chapter, you should be able to meet the following objectives:

- ✦ Describe the manifestations of anemia and their mechanisms
- ✦ Explain the difference between intravascular and extravascular hemolysis
- ✦ Compare the hemoglobinopathies associated with sickle cell anemia and thalassemia
- ✦ Explain the cause of sickling in sickle cell anemia
- ✦ Cite common causes of iron-deficiency anemia in infancy, adolescence, and adulthood
- ✦ Describe the relation between vitamin B_{12} deficiency and megaloblastic anemia
- ✦ List three causes of aplastic anemia
- ✦ Compare characteristics of the red blood cells in acute blood loss, hereditary spherocytosis, sickle cell anemia, iron-deficiency anemia, and aplastic anemia

Anemia is defined as an abnormally low number of circulating red blood cells or hemoglobin level, or both,

Anemia

➤ Anemia, which is a deficiency of red cells or hemoglobin, results from excessive loss (blood loss anemia), increased destruction (hemolytic anemia), or impaired production of red blood cells (iron-deficiency, megaloblastic, and aplastic anemias).

➤ Blood loss anemia is characterized by loss of iron-containing red blood cells from the body; hemolytic anemia involves destruction of red blood cells in the body with iron being retained in the body.

➤ Manifestations of anemia are caused by the decreased presence of hemoglobin in the blood (pallor), tissue hypoxia due to deficient oxygen transport (weakness and fatigue), and recruitment of compensatory mechanisms (tachycardia and palpitations) designed to increase oxygen delivery to the tissues.

celerated and may be recognized by diffuse bone pain and sternal tenderness. The production of 2,3-DPG is a compensatory mechanism that reduces the hemoglobin affinity for oxygen, as evidenced by a shift to the right in the oxygen–hemoglobin saturation curve; this causes more oxygen to be released to the tissues rather than remaining bound to hemoglobin. In addition to the common anemic manifestations, hemolytic anemias are accompanied by jaundice caused by increased blood levels of bilirubin. In aplastic anemia, petechiae and purpura (*i.e.*, red spots caused by small-vessel bleeding) are the result of reduced platelet function.

BLOOD LOSS ANEMIA

With anemia caused by bleeding, iron and other components of the erythrocyte are lost from the body. Blood loss may be acute or chronic. Acute blood loss carries a risk of hypovolemia and shock (see Chapter 26). The red cells are normal in size and color. A fall in the red blood cell count, hematocrit, and hemoglobin results from hemodilution caused by movement of fluid into the vascular compartment. The hypoxia that results from blood loss stimulates red cell production by the bone marrow. If the bleeding is controlled and sufficient iron stores are available, the red cell concentration returns to normal within 3 to 4 weeks. Chronic blood loss does not affect blood volume but instead leads to iron-deficiency anemia when iron stores are depleted. Because of compensatory mechanisms, patients are commonly asymptomatic until the hemoglobin level is less than 8 g/dL. The red cells that are produced have too little hemoglobin, giving rise to microcytic hypochromic anemia.

HEMOLYTIC ANEMIAS

Hemolytic anemia is characterized by the premature destruction of red cells, with retention in the body of iron and the other products of red cell destruction. Almost all types of hemolytic anemia are distinguished by normocytic and normochromic red cells. Because of the red blood cell's shortened life span, the bone marrow usually is hyperactive, resulting in an increase in the number of reticulocytes in the circulating blood. As with other types of anemias, the person experiences easy fatigability, dyspnea, and other signs and symptoms of impaired oxygen transport. The person may have mild jaundice. In hemolytic anemia, red cell breakdown can occur in the vascular compartment, or it can result from phagocytosis by the reticuloendothelial system. Intravascular hemolysis occurs as a result of complement fixation in transfusion reactions, mechanical injury, or toxic factors. It is characterized by hemoglobinemia and hemoglobinuria. Extravascular hemolysis occurs when abnormal red cells are phagocytized in the spleen. A common example is sickle cell anemia.

The cause of hemolytic anemia can be intrinsic or extrinsic to the red blood cell. Intrinsic causes include defects of the red cell membrane, the various hemoglobinopathies, and inherited enzyme defects. Acquired forms of hemolytic anemia are caused by agents extrinsic to the red blood cell, such as drugs, bacterial and other toxins, antibodies, and physical trauma. Although all these factors can cause premature and accelerated destruction of red cells, they cannot all be treated in the same way. Some respond to splenectomy, others respond to treatment with corticosteroid hormones, and still others do not resolve until the primary disorder is corrected.

Inherited Disorders of the Red Cell Membrane

Hereditary spherocytosis, transmitted as an autosomal dominant trait, is the most common inherited disorder of the red cell membrane. The disorder is a deficiency of membrane proteins (*i.e.*, spectrin and ankyrin) that leads to gradual loss of the membrane surface during the life span of the red blood cell, resulting in a tight sphere instead of a concave disk. Although the spherical cell retains its ability to transport oxygen, it is poorly deformable and susceptible to destruction as it passes through the venous sinuses of the splenic circulation. Clinical signs are variable but typically include mild anemia, jaundice, splenomegaly, and bilirubin gallstones. A life-threatening aplastic crisis may occur when a sudden disruption of red cell production (in most cases from a viral infection) causes a rapid drop in hematocrit and the hemoglobin level. The disorder usually is treated with splenectomy to reduce red cell destruction.

Hemoglobinopathies

Abnormalities in hemoglobin structure can lead to accelerated red cell destruction. Two main types of hemoglobinopathies can cause red cell hemolysis: the abnormal substitution of an amino acid in the hemoglobin molecule, as in sickle cell anemia, and the defective synthesis of one of the polypeptide chains that form the globin portion of hemoglobin, as in the thalassemias.

Sickle Cell Anemia. Sickle cell disease affects approximately 50,000 (0.1% to 0.2%) black Americans. Approximately 8% of black Americans carry the trait.[2] Sickle cell anemia results from a defect in the β chain of the hemoglobin molecule, with an abnormal substitution of a single amino acid, valine, for glutamic acid. Sickle hemoglobin (HbS) is transmitted by recessive inheritance and can manifest as sickle cell trait (*i.e.*, heterozygote) or sickle cell disease (*i.e.*, homozygote). In the heterozygote, only approximately 40% of the hemoglobin is HbS, but in the homozygote, almost all the hemoglobin is HbS. Variations in proportions exist, and the concentration of HbS correlates with the risk of sickling.

In the homozygote, the HbS becomes sickled when deoxygenated or at an oxygen tension of approximately 40 mm Hg.[3] The deoxygenated hemoglobin aggregates and polymerizes, creating a semisolid gel that changes the shape and deformability of the cell (Fig. 15-6). After repeated episodes of deoxygenation, the cells remain permanently sickled. These sickled red cells are abnormally adhesive, attach to the vessel wall, and cause accumulation of more cells that obstruct blood flow in the microcirculation, leading to tissue hypoxia.[4] Premature destruction of the cells causes hemolysis. The person with sickle cell trait who has less HbS has little tendency to sickle except during severe

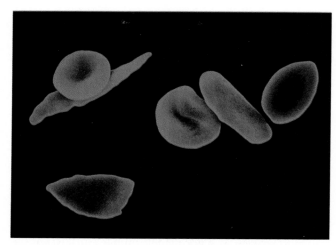

FIGURE 15-6 Photograph of a sickled cell and a normal red blood cell. (© Dr. Gopal Murti, Science Photo Library, Science Source/Photo Researchers)

hypoxia and is virtually asymptomatic. HbF does not interact with HbS or sickle; therefore, most children with sickle cell anemia do not begin to experience the effects of the sickling until sometime after 4 to 6 months of age, when the HbF has been replaced by HbS. The factors associated with sickling and consequent vaso-occlusive crisis include cold, stress, exertion; infection; illnesses that may cause hypoxia, acidosis, or dehydration; or even such trivial incidents as reduced oxygen tension induced by sleep.

Sickle cell anemia is a chronic disorder resulting in organ failure and premature death. Affected persons experience severe hemolytic anemia, chronic hyperbilirubinemia, and vaso-occlusive crises. Children may experience growth retardation and susceptibility to osteomyelitis. The hyperbilirubinemia that results from the breakdown products of hemoglobin often leads to jaundice and the production of pigment stones in the gallbladder.

An acute painful episode results from vessel occlusion and can occur suddenly in almost any part of the body. The frequency ranges from daily to yearly. Common sites obstructed by sickled cells include the abdomen, chest, bones, and joints. Infarctions caused by sluggish blood flow may cause chronic damage to the liver, spleen, heart, kidneys, retina, and other organs. Acute chest syndrome is an atypical pneumonia resulting from pulmonary infarction. It affects approximately 40% of persons with sickle cell disease and is characterized by fever, chest pain, and cough.[5] The syndrome can cause chronic respiratory insufficiency and is a leading cause of death in sickle cell disease. The most serious complication is stroke resulting from cerebral occlusion. Stroke associated with vessel occlusion occurs in children 1 to 15 years of age and may recur in two thirds of those afflicted.

The spleen is especially susceptible to damage by sickle cell hemoglobin. Because of the spleen's sluggish blood flow and low oxygen tension, hemoglobin is deoxygenated and causes ischemia. Splenic injury begins as early as 3 to 6 months of age with intense congestion and is usually asymptomatic.[6] The congestion causes functional asplenia and predisposes the person to life-threatening infections by encapsulated organisms such as *Streptococcus pneumoniae*, *Haemophilus influenzae* type b, and *Klebsiella* species. Neonates and small children have not had time to create antibodies to these organisms and rely on the spleen for their removal. In the absence of specific antibody to the polysaccharide capsular antigens of these organisms, splenic activity is essential for removing these organisms when they enter the blood. One study showed that 28% of children with sickle cell disease were functionally asplenic at 1 year, 58% at 2 years, and 94% at 5 years.[7]

Most children with sickle cell disease are at risk for fulminant septicemia and death during the first 3 years of life, when bacteremia from encapsulated organisms occurs commonly even in normal children. Neonatal screening and early diagnosis of sickle cell disease has facilitated prophylactic administration of penicillin. Prophylactic penicillin should be begun before 3 months of age and continued until at least 5 years of age. Routine immunizations, including *H. influenzae* vaccine and pneumococcal vaccine, should be administered at 2 and 5 years of age.[6] Parents and caregivers need to be educated regarding the manifestations of sickle cell complications and the importance of early medical evaluation of all febrile illnesses and other complications. There is no known cure for sickle cell anemia, so treatment to reduce symptoms includes pain control, hydration, and management of complications. The patient is advised to avoid situations that precipitate sickling episodes, such as infections, cold exposure, severe physical exertion, acidosis, and dehydration. Infections are aggressively treated, and blood transfusions may be warranted in a crisis or given chronically in severe disease.

Hydroxyurea is a promising new treatment for the prevention of complications. The drug allows synthesis of more HbF and less HbS, thereby decreasing sickling. Hydroxyurea administered to adults reduced painful crises, and initial studies in children show similar results.[8] Long-term effects on organ damage, growth and development, and risk of malignancies are unknown. Bone marrow and umbilical cord blood transplantation have been tried with good results but remain experimental and carry the risk of graft-versus-host disease. Drugs that inhibit sickle cell adherence or gene therapy to alter the HbS or activate the HbF genes may be future options.[4]

Neonatal diagnosis of sickle cell disease is made on the basis of clinical findings and hemoglobin solubility results, which are confirmed by hemoglobin electrophoresis. Prenatal diagnosis is done by the analysis of fetal DNA obtained by amniocentesis.[2]

In the United States, screening programs have been implemented to detect newborns with sickle cell disease and other hemoglobinopathies. Cord blood or heel stick samples are subjected to electrophoresis to separate the HbF from the small amount of HbA and HbS. Other hemoglobins may be detected and quantified by further laboratory evaluation. Many states mandate neonatal screening of all newborns, regardless of ethnic origin. Ideally, the effective screening program also includes expert genetic counseling and education about pregnancy options.

Thalassemias. In contrast to sickle cell anemia, the thalassemias result from absent or defective synthesis of the α or the β chains of hemoglobin. The β-thalassemias represent a defect in β-chain synthesis, and the α-thalassemias represent a defect in α-chain synthesis. The defect is inherited as a mendelian trait, and a person may be heterozygous for the trait and have a mild form of the disease or be homozygous and have the severe form of the disease. Like sickle cell anemia, the thalassemias occur with high degree of frequency in certain populations. The β-thalassemias, sometimes called *Cooley's anemia* or *Mediterranean anemia*, are most common in the Mediterranean populations of southern Italy and Greece, and the α-thalassemias are most common among Asians. Both α- and β-thalassemias are common in Africans and black Americans.

Two factors contribute to the anemia that occurs in thalassemia: reduced hemoglobin synthesis and an imbalance in globin chain production. In α- and β-thalassemia, defective globin chain production leads to deficient hemoglobin production and the development of a hypochromic microcytic anemia. The unaffected type of chain continues to be synthesized, accumulates in the red cell, interferes with normal maturation, and contributes to red cell destruction and anemia. In β-thalassemia, the excess α chains are denatured to form precipitates (*i.e.*, Heinz bodies) in the bone marrow red cell precursors. These Heinz bodies impair DNA synthesis and cause damage to the red cell membrane. Severely affected red cell precursors are destroyed in the bone marrow, and those that escape intramedullary death are at increased risk of destruction in the spleen.

The clinical manifestations of β-thalassemias are based on the severity of the anemia. The presence of one normal gene in heterozygous persons usually results in sufficient normal hemoglobin synthesis to prevent severe anemia. Persons who are homozygous for the trait have severe, transfusion-dependent anemia evident at 6 to 9 months of age. Severe growth retardation affects children with the disorder. Increased hematopoiesis in response to erythropoietin causes bone marrow expansion, impairs bone growth, and causes abnormalities. In addition, there is increased iron absorption, and splenomegaly and hepatomegaly result from increased red cell destruction. Bone marrow expansion leads to thinning of the cortical bone, with new bone formation evident on the maxilla and frontal bones of the face (*i.e.*, chipmunk facies). The long bones, ribs, and vertebrae may become vulnerable to fracture. Excess iron stores, which accumulate from increased dietary absorption and repeated transfusions, are deposited in the myocardium, liver, and pancreas and induce organ injury and congestive heart failure. Frequent transfusions prevent most of the complications, and iron chelation therapy can reduce the iron overload and extend life into the third decade.[9] Bone marrow transplantation is a potential cure for some patients. In the future, stem cell gene replacement may provide a cure for many with the disease.

Synthesis of the α-globin chains of hemoglobin is controlled by two pairs of genes; hence, α-thalassemia shows great variations in severity. Silent carriers who have deletion of a single α-globin gene and those with deletion of two genes are asymptomatic. The most severe form of α-thalassemia occurs in infants in whom all four α-globin genes are deleted. Such a defect results in a hemoglobin molecule (Hb Bart's) that is formed exclusively from the chains of HbF. Hb Bart's, which has an extremely high oxygen affinity, cannot release oxygen in the tissues. Affected infants suffer from severe hypoxia and are stillborn or die shortly after birth unless intrauterine transfusions are given. Deletion of three of the four α-chain genes leads to unstable aggregates of β chains called *hemoglobin H* (HbH). The β chains are more soluble than the α chains, and their accumulation is less toxic to the red cells, so that senescent, rather than precursor, red cells are affected. Most persons with HbH have only mild to moderate hemolytic anemia, and manifestations of ineffective erythropoiesis (*i.e.*, bone marrow expansion and iron overload) are absent.

Inherited Enzyme Defects

The most common inherited enzyme defect that results in hemolytic anemia is a deficiency of G6PD. The gene that determines this enzyme is located on the X chromosome, and the defect is expressed only in males and homozygous females. There are many genetic variants of this disorder. The African variant has been found in 10% of black Americans.[2] The disorder makes red cells more vulnerable to oxidants and causes direct oxidation of hemoglobin to methemoglobin and the denaturing of the hemoglobin molecule to form Heinz bodies, which are precipitated in the red blood cell. Hemolysis usually occurs as the damaged red blood cells move through the narrow vessels of the spleen, causing hemoglobinemia, hemoglobinuria, and jaundice. The hemolysis is short-lived, occurring 2 to 3 days after the trigger event. In blacks, the defect is mildly expressed and is not associated with chronic hemolytic anemia unless triggered by oxidant drugs, acidosis, or infection.

The antimalarial drug primaquine, the sulfonamides, nitrofurantoin, aspirin, phenacetin, some chemotherapeutics, and other drugs cause hemolysis. Free radicals generated by phagocytes during infections also are possible triggers. A more severe deficiency of G6PD is found in people of Mediterranean descent (*e.g.*, Sardinians, Sephardic Jews, Arabs). In some of these persons, chronic hemolysis occurs in the absence of exposure to oxidants. The disorder can be diagnosed through the use of a G6PD assay or screening test.

Acquired Hemolytic Anemias

Several acquired factors exogenous to the red blood cell produce hemolysis by direct membrane destruction or by antibody-mediated lysis. Various drugs, chemicals, toxins, venoms, and infections such as malaria destroy red cell membranes. Hemolysis can also be caused by mechanical factors such as prosthetic heart valves, vasculitis, and severe burns. Obstructions in the microcirculation, as in disseminated intravascular coagulation, thrombotic thrombocytopenic purpura, and renal disease, may traumatize the red cells by producing turbulence and changing pressure gradients.

Many hemolytic anemias are immune mediated, caused by antibodies that destroy the red cell. Autoantibodies may be produced by a person in response to drugs and disease.

Alloantibodies come from an exogenous source and are responsible for transfusion reactions and hemolytic disease of the newborn.

The autoantibodies that cause red cell destruction are of two types: warm-reacting antibodies of the immunoglobulin G (IgG) type, which are maximally active at 37°C, and cold-reacting antibodies of the immunoglobulin M (IgM) type, which are optimally active at or near 4°C. The warm-reacting antibodies cause no morphologic or metabolic alteration in the red cell. Instead, they react with antigens on the red cell membrane, causing destructive changes that lead to spherocytosis, with subsequent phagocytic destruction in the spleen or reticuloendothelial system. They lack specificity for the ABO antigens but may react with the Rh antigens. The hemolytic reactions associated with the warm-reacting antibodies occur with an incidence of approximately 10 per 1 million. The reactions have a rapid onset, and persons usually have mild jaundice and manifestations of anemia. There are varied causes; approximately 50% are idiopathic, and 50% are drug induced or are related to cancers of the lymphoproliferative system (*e.g.,* chronic lymphocytic leukemia, lymphoma) or collagen diseases (*e.g.,* systemic lupus erythematosus).[2] The antihypertensive drug α-methyldopa, penicillin, and the cephalosporins account for a small number of cases.[10]

The cold-reacting antibodies activate complement. Chronic hemolytic anemia caused by cold-reacting antibodies occurs with lymphoproliferative disorders and as an idiopathic disorder of unknown cause. The hemolytic process occurs in distal body parts, where the temperature may fall below 30°C. Vascular obstruction by red cells results in pallor, cyanosis of the body parts exposed to cold temperatures, and Raynaud's phenomenon (see Chapter 22). Hemolytic anemia caused by cold-reacting antibodies develops in only a few persons and is rarely severe.

Coombs' test, or the antiglobulin test, is used to diagnose immune hemolytic anemias. It detects the presence of antibody or complement on the surface of the red cell. The direct antiglobulin test (DAT) detects the antibody on red blood cells. In this test, red cells that have been washed free of serum are mixed with anti-human globulin reagent. The red cells agglutinate if the reagent binds to and bridges the antibody or complement on adjacent red cells. The DAT result is positive in cases of autoimmune hemolytic anemia, erythroblastosis fetalis (*i.e.,* Rh disease of the newborn), transfusion reactions, and drug-induced hemolysis. The indirect antiglobulin test detects antibody in the serum, and the result is positive for specific antibodies. It is used for antibody detection and crossmatching before transfusion.

ANEMIAS OF DEFICIENT RED CELL PRODUCTION

Anemia may result from the decreased production of erythrocytes by the bone marrow. A deficiency of nutrients for hemoglobin synthesis (iron) or DNA synthesis (cobalamin or folic acid) may reduce red cell production by the bone marrow. A deficiency of red cells also results when the marrow itself fails or is replaced by nonfunctional tissue.

Iron-Deficiency Anemia

Iron deficiency is a common worldwide cause of anemia affecting persons of all ages. The anemia results from dietary deficiency, loss of iron through bleeding, or increased demands. Because iron is a component of heme, a deficiency leads to decreased hemoglobin synthesis and consequent impairment of oxygen delivery.

Body iron is used repeatedly. When red cells become senescent and are broken down, their iron is released and reused in the production of new red cells. Despite this efficiency, small amounts of iron are lost in the feces and need to be replaced by dietary uptake. Iron balance is maintained by the absorption of 0.5 to 1.5 mg daily to replace the 1 mg lost in the feces. The average Western diet supplies this amount. The absorbed iron is more than sufficient to supply the needs of most individuals, but may be barely adequate in women and young children. Dietary deficiency of iron is not common in developed countries except in certain populations. Most iron is derived from meat, and when meat is not available, as for deprived populations, or is not a dietary constituent, as for vegetarians, iron deficiency may occur.

The usual reason for iron deficiency in adults is chronic blood loss because iron cannot be recycled to the pool. In men and postmenopausal women, blood loss may occur from gastrointestinal bleeding because of peptic ulcer, intestinal polyps, hemorrhoids, or cancer. Excessive aspirin intake may cause undetected gastrointestinal bleeding. In women, menstruation may account for an average of 1.5 mg of iron lost per day, causing a deficiency.[11] Although cessation of menstruation removes a major source of iron loss in the pregnant woman, iron requirements increase at this time, and deficiency is common. The expansion of the mother's blood volume requires approximately 500 mg of additional iron, and the growing fetus requires approximately 360 mg during pregnancy. In the postnatal period, lactation requires approximately 1.0 mg of iron daily.[11]

A child's growth places extra demands on the body. Blood volume increases, with a greater need for iron. Iron requirements are proportionally higher in infancy (3 to 24 months) than at any other age, although they are also increased in childhood and adolescence. In infancy, the two main causes of iron-deficiency anemia are low iron levels at birth because of maternal deficiency and a diet consisting mainly of cow's milk, which is low in absorbable iron. Adolescents are also susceptible to iron deficiency because of high requirements due to growth spurts, dietary deficiencies, and menstrual loss.[12]

Iron deficiency is characterized by a low hemoglobin and hematocrit, decreased iron stores, and low serum iron and ferritin. The red cells are decreased in number and are microcytic, hypochromic, and often malformed (*i.e.,* poikilocytosis). The laboratory values indicate reduced MCHC and MCV. Membrane changes may predispose to hemolysis, causing further loss of red cells.

The manifestations of iron-deficiency anemia are related to impaired oxygen transport and lack of hemoglobin. Depending on the severity of the anemia, fatigability, palpitations, dyspnea, angina, and tachycardia may occur. Epithelial atrophy is common and results in waxy pallor, brittle hair and nails, smooth tongue, sores in the corners of the mouth, and sometimes in dysphagia and decreased acid secretion. A poorly understood symptom that sometimes is seen is pica, the bizarre compulsive eating of ice, dirt, or other abnormal substances.

The treatment of iron-deficiency anemia is directed toward controlling chronic blood loss, increasing dietary intake of iron, and administering supplemental iron. Ferrous sulfate, which is the usual oral replacement therapy, replenishes iron stores in several months. Parenteral iron (iron dextran) therapy may be used when oral forms are not tolerated or are ineffective. Because of the possibility of severe hypersensitivity reactions, an initial test dose should be administered before administration of the first therapeutic dose of the drug. It is recommended that the test dose be administered in an environment equipped for treatment of severe allergic or anaphylactic reactions. Iron dextran can be given intravenously or injected deep intramuscularly using the "Z track" injection method in which the skin is pulled to one side before inserting the needle to prevent leakage into the tissues, with subsequent skin discoloration. In the future, gastric delivery systems may provide good therapy without side effects.

Megaloblastic Anemias

Megaloblastic anemias are caused by abnormal nucleic acid synthesis that results in enlarged red cells (MCV >100 fL) and deficient nuclear maturation. Cobalamin (vitamin B_{12}) and folic acid deficiencies are the most common megaloblastic anemias. Because megaloblastic anemias develop slowly, there are often few symptoms until the anemia is far advanced.

Cobalamin (Vitamin B_{12})-Deficiency Anemia.

Vitamin B_{12} serves as a cofactor for two important reactions in humans. It is essential for the synthesis of DNA. When it is deficient, nuclear maturation and cell division, especially of the rapidly proliferating red cells, fail to occur. It is also involved in a reaction that prevents abnormal fatty acids from being incorporated into neuronal lipids. This abnormality may predispose to myelin breakdown and produce some of the neurologic complications of vitamin B_{12} deficiency.

Vitamin B_{12} is found in all foods of animal origin. Dietary deficiency is rare and usually found only in strict vegetarians who avoid all dairy products as well as meat and fish. It is absorbed by a unique process. After release from the animal protein, vitamin B_{12} is bound to intrinsic factor, a protein secreted by the gastric parietal cells (Fig. 15-7). The vitamin B_{12}–intrinsic factor complex travels to the ileum, where membrane receptors allow the binding of the complex and transport of B_{12} across the membrane. From there it is bound to its carrier protein, transcobalamin II, which carries vitamin B_{12} in the circulation to its storage and tissue sites. Any defects in this pathway may cause a deficiency. An important cause of vitamin B_{12} deficiency is pernicious anemia, resulting from a hereditary atrophic gastritis. As discussed in Chapter 37, immune-mediated chronic atrophic gastritis is a disorder that destroys the gastric mucosa, with loss of parietal cells and production of antibodies that inter-

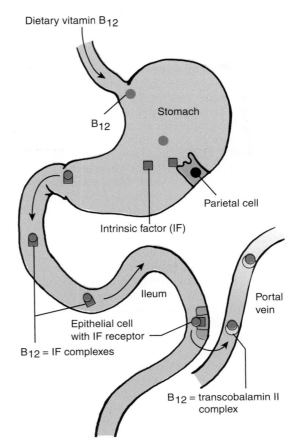

FIGURE 15-7 Absorption of vitamin B_{12}.

fere with the binding of intrinsic factor. This abnormality leads to pernicious anemia. Other causes of vitamin B_{12} deficiency anemia include gastrectomy, ileal resection, and malabsorption syndromes in which vitamin B_{12} and other vitamin B compounds are poorly absorbed.

The hallmark of vitamin B_{12} deficiency is megaloblastic anemia. When vitamin B_{12} is deficient, the red cells that are produced are abnormally large because of excess ribonucleic acid production of hemoglobin and structural protein. They have flimsy membranes and are oval rather than biconcave. These oddly shaped cells have a short life span that can be measured in weeks rather than months. The MCV is elevated, and the MCHC is normal.

Neurologic changes that accompany the disorder are caused by deranged methylation of myelin protein. Demyelination of the dorsal and lateral columns of the spinal cord causes symmetric paresthesias of the feet and fingers, loss of vibratory and position sense, and eventual spastic ataxia. In more advanced cases, cerebral function may be altered. In some cases, dementia and other neuropsychiatric changes may precede hematologic changes.

Diagnosis of vitamin B_{12} deficiency is made by finding an abnormally low vitamin B_{12} serum level. The Schilling test, which measures the 24-hour urinary excretion of radiolabeled vitamin B_{12} administered orally, is used to document decreased absorption of vitamin B_{12}. Lifelong treatment consisting of intramuscular injections of vitamin B_{12} reverses the anemia and improves the neurologic changes.

Folic Acid–Deficiency Anemia.   Folic acid is also required for DNA synthesis and red cell maturation, and its deficiency produces the same type of red cell changes that occur in vitamin B_{12} deficiency anemia (*i.e.,* increased MCV and normal MCHC). Symptoms are also similar, but the neurologic manifestations are not present.

Folic acid is readily absorbed from the intestine. It is found in vegetables (particularly the green leafy types), fruits, cereals, and meats. Much of the vitamin, however, is lost in cooking. The most common causes of folic acid deficiency are malnutrition or dietary lack, especially in the elderly or in association with alcoholism, and malabsorption syndromes such as sprue or other intestinal disorders. In neoplastic disease, tumor cells compete for folate, and deficiency is common. Some drugs used to treat seizure disorders (*e.g.,* primidone, phenytoin, phenobarbital) and triamterene, a diuretic, predispose to a deficiency by interfering with folic acid absorption. Methotrexate, a folic acid analog used in the treatment of cancer, impairs the action of folic acid by blocking its conversion to the active form.

Because pregnancy increases the need for folic acid 5- to 10-fold, a deficiency commonly occurs. Poor dietary habits, anorexia, and nausea are other reasons for folic acid deficiency during pregnancy. Studies also show an association between folate deficiency and neural tube defects, which suggests routine supplementation of approximately 1 mg folate daily to pregnant women and those of childbearing age and 4 mg to high-risk women. It is estimated that 75% of neural tube defects could thus be prevented.[13] To ensure adequate folate consumption, the U.S. Food and Drug Administration has issued a recommendation for the addition of folate to cereal grain products.[14]

Aplastic Anemia

Aplastic anemia (*i.e.,* bone marrow depression) describes a primary condition of bone marrow stem cells that results in a reduction of all three hematopoietic cell lines—red blood cells, white blood cells, and platelets—with fatty replacement of bone marrow. Pure red cell aplasia, in which only the red cells are affected, rarely occurs.

Anemia results from the failure of the marrow to replace senescent red cells that are destroyed and leave the circulation, although the cells that remain are of normal size and color. At the same time, because the leukocytes, particularly the neutrophils, and the thrombocytes have a short life span, a deficiency of these cells usually is apparent before the anemia becomes severe.

The onset of aplastic anemia may be insidious, or it may strike with suddenness and great severity. It can occur at any age. The initial presenting symptoms include weakness, fatigability, and pallor caused by anemia. Petechiae (*i.e.,* small, punctate skin hemorrhages) and ecchymoses (*i.e.,* bruises) often occur on the skin, and bleeding from the nose, gums, vagina, or gastrointestinal tract may occur because of decreased platelet levels. The decrease in the number of neutrophils increases susceptibility to infection.

Among the causes of aplastic anemia are exposure to high doses of radiation, chemicals, and toxins that suppress hematopoiesis directly, or through immune mechanisms. Chemotherapy and irradiation commonly result in bone marrow depression, which causes anemia, thrombocytopenia, and neutropenia. Identified toxic agents include benzene, the antibiotic chloramphenicol, and the alkylating agents and antimetabolites used in the treatment of cancer (see Chapter 8). Aplastic anemia caused by exposure to chemical agents may be an idiosyncratic reaction because it affects only certain susceptible persons. It typically occurs weeks after a drug is initiated. Such reactions often are severe and sometimes irreversible and fatal. Aplastic anemia can develop in the course of many infections and has been reported most often as a complication of viral hepatitis, mononucleosis, and other viral illnesses, including acquired immunodeficiency syndrome (AIDS). In two thirds of cases, the cause is unknown, and these are called *idiopathic aplastic anemia.*

Therapy for aplastic anemia in the young and severely affected includes stem cell replacement by bone marrow or peripheral blood transplantation. Histocompatible donors supply the stem cells to replace the patient's destroyed marrow cells. Graft-versus-host disease, rejection, and infections are major risks of the procedure, yet 70% or more survive.[15] For those who are not transplantation candidates, immunosuppressive therapy with lymphocyte immune globulin (*i.e.,* antithymocyte globulin) prevents suppression of proliferating stem cells, producing remission in up to 50% of patients.[15] Patients with aplastic anemia should avoid the offending agents and be treated with antibiotics for infection. Red cell transfusions to correct the anemia and platelets and corticosteroid therapy to minimize bleeding may also be required.

Chronic Disease Anemias

Anemia often occurs as a complication of chronic infections, inflammation, and cancer. Chronic diseases commonly associated with anemia include AIDS, osteomyelitis, rheumatoid arthritis, and Hodgkin's disease. It is theorized that the short life span, deficient red cell production, and low serum iron are caused by actions of macrophages and lymphocytes in response to cell injury. Macrophages sequester iron in the spleen and contribute to red cell destruction, and the lymphocytes release cytokines that suppress erythropoietin production and action.[16] The mild to moderate anemia is usually reversed when the underlying disease is treated.

Chronic renal failure almost always results in a normocytic, normochromic anemia, primarily because of a deficiency of erythropoietin. Uremic toxins also interfere with the actions of erythropoietin and red cell production. They also cause hemolysis and bleeding tendencies, which contribute to the anemia. Until recently, dialysis and red cell transfusions constituted the only therapy. Recombinant erythropoietin injected several times each week for 10 or more weeks dramatically elevates the hemoglobin level and hematocrit to a range of 32% to 38% and eliminates the need for transfusions.[17] Oral iron is usually required for a good response.

In summary, anemia is a condition of an abnormally low number of circulating red blood cells or hemoglobin level, or both. It is not a disease, but manifestation of a disease process or alteration in body function. Anemia can result from excessive blood loss, red cell destruction due to hemolysis, or deficient hemoglobin or red cell production. Blood loss anemia can be acute or chronic. With bleeding, iron and other components of the erythrocyte are lost from the body. Hemolytic anemia is characterized by the premature destruction of red cells, with retention in the body of iron and the other products of red cell destruction. Hemolytic anemia can be caused by defects in the red cell membrane, hemoglobinopathies (sickle cell anemia or thalassemia), or inherited enzyme defects (G6PD deficiency). Acquired forms of hemolytic anemia are caused by agents extrinsic to the red blood cell, such as drugs, bacterial and other toxins, antibodies, and physical trauma. Iron-deficiency anemia, which is characterized by decreased hemoglobin synthesis, can result from dietary deficiency, loss of iron through bleeding, or increased demands for red cell production. Vitamin B_{12} and folic acid deficiency impair red cell production by interfering with DNA synthesis. Aplastic anemia is caused by bone marrow suppression and usually results in a reduction of white blood cells and platelets, as well as red blood cells.

The manifestations of anemia are those associated with impaired oxygen transport; alterations in red blood cell number, hemoglobin content, and cell structure; and the signs and symptoms of the underlying process causing the anemia.

Transfusion Therapy

After you have completed this section of the chapter, you should be able to meet the following objectives:

✦ Differentiate red cell antigens from antibodies in persons with type A, B, AB, or O blood
✦ Explain the determination of the Rh factor
✦ List the signs and symptoms of a blood transfusion reaction

Anemias of various causes are treated with transfusions of whole blood or red blood cells only when oxygen delivery to the tissues is compromised, as evidenced by measures of oxygen transport and use, hemoglobin, and hematocrit. Current recommendations suggest transfusion for patients with hemoglobin levels of 8 to 10 g/dL, depending on risk factors and surgical procedures.[18] Acute massive blood loss usually is replaced with whole-blood transfusion. Most anemias, however, are treated with transfusions of red cell concentrates, which supply only the blood component that is deficient. Since the 1960s, devices that mechanically separate a unit of blood into its constituents provide red cell components, platelets, fresh-frozen plasma, cryoprecipitate, and clotting factor concentrates. In this way, a unit of blood can be used efficiently for several recipients to correct specific deficiencies.

Several red cell components that are used for transfusion are prepared and stored under specific conditions and have unique uses, as described in Table 15-2. These red cell components are derived principally from voluntary blood donors. In the future, red cell substitutes, such as hemoglobin solutions, may be used, particularly in the trauma setting.[19] The potential advantages are better storage, longer shelf life, and no risk of transfusion reaction.

The use of autologous donation and transfusion has been advocated since the early 1980s. Autologous transfusion refers to the procedure of receiving one's own blood—usually to replenish a surgical loss—thereby eliminating the risk of blood-borne disease or transfusion reaction. In 1992, a reported 8.5% of transfusions were autologous.[18] Autologous blood can be provided by several means: predeposit, hemodilution, and intraoperative salvage. A patient who is anticipating elective orthopedic, vascular, or open heart surgery may predeposit blood (*i.e.*, have the blood collected up to 6 weeks in advance and stored) for later transfusion during the surgery. Hemodilution involves phlebotomy before surgery with transfusion of the patient's blood at the completion of surgery. The procedure requires the use of fluid infusions to maintain blood volume and is commonly used in open heart surgery. Intraoperative blood salvage is the collection of blood shed from the operative site for reinfusion into the patient. Semiautomated devices are used to collect, anticoagulate, wash, and resuspend red cells for reinfusion during many procedures, including vascular, cardiac, and orthopedic surgery. Potential risks of autologous transfusion may include bacterial and other contamination, volume overload, and administrative errors.[19]

Before a red cell or whole-blood transfusion from a volunteer donor source can occur, a series of procedures are required to ensure a successful transfusion. Donor samples are first tested for blood-borne diseases, such as hepatitis B and hepatitis C, HIV types 1 and 2, human T-cell lymphocytic viruses (HTLV-I and -II), and syphilis. Donor and recipient samples are typed to determine ABO and Rh groups and screened for unexpected red cell antibodies. The crossmatch is performed by incubating the donor cells with the recipient's serum and observing for agglutination. If none appears, the donor and recipient blood types are compatible.

ABO BLOOD GROUPS

ABO compatibility is essential for effective transfusion therapy and requires knowledge of ABO antigens and antibodies. There are four major ABO blood groups as determined by the presence or absence of two red cell antigens (A and B). Persons who have neither A nor B antigens are classified as having type O blood; those with A antigens are classified as having type A blood; those with B antigens, as having type B blood; and those with A and B antigens, as having type AB blood (Table 15-3). The ABO blood groups are genetically determined. The type O gene

TABLE 15-2 ◆ Red Blood Cell Components Used in Transfusion Therapy

Component	Preparation	Use	Limitations
Whole blood	Drawn from donor Anticoagulant–preservative solutions added, usually citrate-phosphate-dextrose (CPDA-1) adenine; stored at 1°–6°C until expiration, up to 35 days	Replacement of blood volume and oxygen-carrying capacity lost in massive bleeding	Contains few viable platelets or granulocytes and is deficient in coagulation factors V and VIII; may cause hypervolemia, febrile and allergic reactions and infectious disease (*i.e.,* hepatitis and AIDS)
Red blood cells	Removal of two thirds of plasma by centrifugation; additive solution contains adenine and dextrose to extend shelf life up to 42 days and maintain ATP levels	Standard transfusion to increase oxygen-carrying capacity in chronic anemia and slow hemorrhage; reduce danger of hypervolemia	Contains no viable platelets or granulocytes; risk of reactions and infectious disease
Leukocyte-reduced red blood cells	Removal of 99% of leukocytes, platelets, and debris by centrifugation or filtration	Reduces risk of nonhemolytic febrile reactions in susceptible persons	Preparation may reduce red cell mass to 80%; 24-hr outdate and infectious disease risk
Washed red blood cells	Red cells are washed in normal saline solution and centrifuged several times to remove plasma and constituents.	Reduces risk of febrile and allergic reactions	Loss of red cell mass, 24-hr outdate, costly preparation, and infectious disease risk
Frozen red blood cells	Red cells are mixed with glycerol to prevent ice crystals from forming and rupturing the cell membrane; cells must be thawed, deglycerolized, and washed before transfusing.	Reduces risk of severe febrile reactions; preserves rare and autologous (self-donated) units for transfusion up to 10 yr	Costly and lengthy preparation; loss of red cell mass, 24-hr outdate, and infectious disease risk

ATP, adenosine triphosphate.
(Data from Vengelen-Tyler V. [Ed.] [1996]. *Technical manual.* [12th ed., pp. 135–142]. Bethesda, MD: American Association of Blood Banks)

is apparently functionless in production of a red cell antigen. Each of the other genes is expressed by the presence of a strong antigen on the surface of the red cell. Six genotypes, or gene combinations, result in four phenotypes, or blood type expressions. ABO antibodies predictably develop in the serum of persons whose red cells lack the corresponding antigen. Persons with type A antigens on their red cells develop type B antibodies; persons with type B antigens develop type A antibodies in their serum; persons with type O blood develop type A and type B antibodies; and persons with type AB blood develop neither A nor B antibodies. The ABO antibodies usually are not present at birth but begin to develop at 3 to 6 months of age and reach maximum levels between the ages of 5 and 10 years.[20]

Rh TYPES

The D antigen of the Rh system is also important in transfusion compatibility and is routinely tested. The Rh type is coded by three gene pairs: C, c; D, d; and E, e. Each allele, with the exception of d, codes for a specific antigen. The D antigen is the most immunogenic. Persons who express the D antigen are designated Rh positive, and those who do not express the D antigen are Rh negative. Unlike serum antibodies for the ABO blood types, which develop spontaneously after birth, Rh antibodies develop after exposure to one or more of the Rh antigens. More than 80% of Rh-negative persons develop the antibody to D antigen if they are exposed to Rh-positive blood.[10] Because it takes several weeks to produce antibodies, a reaction may be delayed and

TABLE 15-3 ◆ ABO System for Blood Typing

Genotype	Red Cell Antigens	Blood Type	Serum Antibodies
OO	None	O	AB
AO	A	A	B
AA	A	A	B
BO	B	B	A
BB	B	B	A
AB	AB	AB	None

usually is mild. If subsequent transfusions of Rh-positive blood are given to a person who has become sensitized, the person may have a severe, immediate reaction.

BLOOD TRANSFUSION REACTIONS

The seriousness of blood transfusion reactions prompts the need for extreme caution when blood is administered. Because most transfusion reactions result from administrative errors or misidentification, care should be taken to correctly identify the recipient and the transfusion source.[18] The recipient's vital signs should be monitored before and during the transfusion, and careful observation for signs of transfusion reaction is imperative. The most feared and lethal transfusion reaction is the destruction of donor red cells by reaction with antibody in the recipient's serum. This immediate hemolytic reaction usually is caused by ABO incompatibility. The signs and symptoms of such a reaction include sensation of heat along the vein where the blood is being infused, flushing of the face, urticaria, headache, pain in the lumbar area, chills, fever, constricting pain in the chest, cramping pain in the abdomen, nausea, vomiting, tachycardia, hypotension, and dyspnea. If any of these adverse effects occur, the transfusion should be stopped immediately. Access to a vein should be maintained because it may be necessary to infuse intravenous solutions to ensure diuresis, administer medications, and take blood samples. The blood must be saved for studies to determine the cause of the reaction.

Hemoglobin that is released from the hemolyzed donor cells is filtered in the glomeruli of the kidneys. Two possible complications of a blood transfusion reaction are oliguria and renal shutdown because of the adverse effects of the filtered hemoglobin on renal tubular flow. The urine should be examined for the presence of hemoglobin, urobilinogen, and red blood cells. Delayed hemolytic reactions may occur more than 10 days after transfusion and are caused by undetected antibodies in the recipient's serum. The reaction is accompanied by a fall in hematocrit and jaundice, but most recipients are asymptomatic.

A febrile reaction, the most common transfusion reaction, occurs in approximately 2% of transfusions. Recipient antibodies directed against the donor's white cells or platelets cause chills and fever. Antipyretics are used to treat this reaction. Future febrile reactions may be avoided by the use of leukocyte-reduced blood.

Allergic reactions are caused by patient antibodies against donor proteins, particularly immunoglobulin G. Urticaria and itching occur and can be relieved with antihistamines. Susceptible persons may be transfused with washed red cells to prevent reactions.

> In summary, transfusion therapy provides the means for replacement of red blood cells and other blood components. Red blood cells contain surface antigens, and reciprocal antibodies are found in the serum. Four major ABO blood types are determined by the presence or absence of two red cell antigens: A and B. The D antigen determines the Rh-positive type; absence of the D antigen determines the Rh-negative type. ABO and Rh types must be determined in recipient and donor blood before transfusion to ensure

Polycythemia

After you have completed this section of the chapter, you should be able to meet the following objectives:

✦ Define the term *polycythemia*
✦ Compare polycythemia vera and secondary polycythemia

Polycythemia is an abnormally high total red blood cell mass with a hematocrit greater than 55%. It is categorized as relative, primary, or secondary. In relative polycythemia, the hematocrit rises because of a loss of plasma volume without a corresponding decrease in red cells. This may occur with water deprivation, excess use of diuretics, or gastrointestinal losses. Relative polycythemia is corrected by increasing the vascular fluid volume.

Primary polycythemia, or polycythemia vera, is a proliferative disease of the pluripotent cells of the bone marrow characterized by an absolute increase in total red blood cell mass accompanied by elevated white cell and platelet counts. It most commonly is seen in men between the ages of 40 and 60 years. In polycythemia vera, the manifestations are related to an increase in the red cell count, hemoglobin level, and hematocrit with increased blood volume and viscosity. This gives rise to hypertension. There may be complaints of headache, inability to concentrate, and some difficulty with hearing and vision because of decreased cerebral blood flow. Venous stasis gives rise to a plethoric appearance or dusky redness—even cyanosis—particularly of the lips, fingernails, and mucous membranes. Because of the increased concentration of blood cells, the person may experience itching and pain in the fingers or toes, and the hypermetabolism may induce night sweats and weight loss. With the increased blood viscosity and stagnation of blood flow, thrombosis and hemorrhage are possible complications and are associated with manifestations of anginal pain, deep vein thrombosis, or cerebral insufficiency with transient ischemic attacks. The goal of treatment in primary polycythemia is to reduce blood viscosity. This can be done by withdrawing blood by means of periodic phlebotomy to reduce red cell volume. Control of platelet and white cell counts is accomplished by suppressing bone marrow function with chemotherapy or radiation therapy.

Secondary polycythemia results from a physiologic increase in the level of erythropoietin, commonly as a compensatory response to hypoxia. This elevation is related to living at high altitudes, chronic heart and lung disease, and smoking, all of which are causes of hypoxia. Treatment of secondary polycythemia focuses on relieving hypoxia. For example, continuous low-flow oxygen therapy can be used to correct the severe hypoxia that occurs in some persons with chronic obstructive lung disease. This form of treatment is thought to relieve the pulmonary hypertension and polycythemia and to delay the onset of cor pulmonale.

> In summary, polycythemia describes a condition in which the red blood cell mass is increased. It can present as a relative, primary, or secondary disorder. Relative polycythemia results from a loss of vascular fluid and is corrected by replacing the fluid. Primary polycythemia, or polycythemia vera, is a proliferative disease of the bone marrow with an absolute increase in total red blood cell mass accompanied by elevated white cell and platelet counts. Secondary polycythemia results from increased erythropoietin levels caused by hypoxic conditions such as chronic heart and lung disease. Many of the manifestations of polycythemia are related to increased blood volume and viscosity that lead to hypertension and stagnation of blood flow.

Age-Related Changes in Red Blood Cells

After you have completed this section of the chapter, you should be able to meet the following objectives:

- ✦ Cite the function of hemoglobin F in the neonate and describe the red blood cell changes that occur during the early neonatal period
- ✦ Cite the factors that predispose to hyperbilirubinemia in the infant
- ✦ Describe the pathogenesis of hemolytic disease of the newborn

- ✦ Compare conjugated and unconjugated bilirubin in terms of production of encephalopathy in the neonate
- ✦ Explain the action of phototherapy in the treatment of hyperbilirubinemia in the neonate
- ✦ State the changes in the red blood cells that occur with aging

RED CELL CHANGES IN THE NEONATE

At birth, changes in the red blood cell indices reflect the transition to extrauterine life and the need to transport oxygen from the lungs (Table 15-4). Hemoglobin concentrations at birth are high, reflecting the high synthetic activity in utero to provide adequate oxygen delivery.[21] Toward the end of the first postnatal week, hemoglobin concentration begins to decline, gradually falling to a minimum value at approximately age 2 months. The red cell count, hematocrit, and MCV likewise fall. The factors responsible for the decline include reduced red cell production and plasma dilution caused by increased blood volume with growth. Neonatal red cells also have a shorter life span of 50 to 70 days and are thought to be more fragile than those of older persons. During the early neonatal period, there is also a switch from HbF to HbA. The amount of HbF in term infants varies from 53% to 95% of the total hemoglobin and decreases by approximately 3% per week after birth.[22] At 6 months of age, HbF usually accounts for less than 2% of total hemoglobin. The switch to HbA provides greater unloading of oxygen to the tissues because HbA has a lower affinity for oxygen compared with HbF. Infants who are small for gestational age or born to diabetic or smoking mothers or who experienced hypoxia in utero have higher total hemoglobin levels, higher HbF levels, and a delayed switch to HbA.

TABLE 15-4 ✦ Red Cell Values for Term Infants				
Age	RBC × 10^6/μL Mean ± SD	Hb (g/dL) Mean ± SD	Hct (%) Mean ± SD	MCV (fL) Mean ± SD
Days				
1	5.14 ± 0.7	19.3 ± 2.2	61 ± 7.4	119 ± 9.4
4	5.00 ± 0.6	18.6 ± 2.1	57 ± 8.1	114 ± 7.5
7	4.86 ± 0.6	17.9 ± 2.5	56 ± 9.4	118 ± 11.2
Weeks				
1–2	4.80 ± 0.8	17.3 ± 2.3	54 ± 8.3	112 ± 19.0
3–4	4.00 ± 0.6	14.2 ± 2.1	43 ± 5.7	105 ± 7.5
8–9	3.40 ± 0.5	10.7 ± 0.9	31 ± 2.5	93 ± 12.0
11–12	3.70 ± 0.3	11.3 ± 0.9	33 ± 3.3	88 ± 7.9

Hb, hemoglobin; Hct, hematocrit; MCV, mean corpuscular volume.
(Adapted from Matoth Y., Zaizor R., Varsano I. [1971]. Postnatal changes in some red cell parameters. *Acta Paediatrica Scandinavica 60*, 317)

A physiologic anemia of the newborn develops at approximately 2 months of age. It seldom produces symptoms and cannot be altered by nutritional supplements. Anemia of prematurity, an exaggerated physiologic response in low–birth-weight infants, is thought to result from a poor erythropoietin response. The hemoglobin level rapidly declines after birth to a low of 7 to 10 g/dL at approximately 6 weeks of age. Signs and symptoms include apnea, poor weight gain, pallor, decreased activity, and tachycardia. In infants born before 33 weeks' gestation or those with hematocrits below 33%, the clinical features are more evident. One study suggests that the protein content of breast milk may not be sufficient for hematopoiesis in the premature infant. Protein supplementation significantly increases the hemoglobin concentrations between the ages of 4 and 10 weeks.[21]

Anemia at birth, characterized by pallor, congestive heart failure, or shock, usually is caused by hemolytic disease of the newborn. Bleeding from the umbilical cord, internal hemorrhage, congenital hemolytic disease, or frequent blood sampling are other possible causes of anemia. The severity of symptoms and presence of coexisting disease may warrant red cell transfusion.

Hyperbilirubinemia in the Neonate

Hyperbilirubinemia, an increased level of serum bilirubin, is a common cause of jaundice in the neonate. A benign, self-limited condition, it most often is related to the developmental state of the neonate. Rarely, cases of hyperbilirubinemia are pathologic and may lead to kernicterus and serious brain damage.

In the first week of life, approximately 60% of term and 80% of preterm neonates are jaundiced.[23] This physiologic jaundice appears in term infants on the second or third day of life, and bilirubin levels peak at less than 12 mg/dL. This complication probably is related to the increased red cell breakdown and the inability of the immature liver to conjugate bilirubin. Premature infants exhibit a similar rise in serum bilirubin level, perhaps because of poor hepatic uptake and reduced albumin binding of bilirubin. The rise is slower, appearing at day 3 or 4, and peak levels of bilirubin are higher (>15 mg/dL). Most neonatal jaundice resolves within 1 week and is untreated.

When jaundice appears at atypical times (*i.e.*, at birth or after 1 week), the cause is sought to prevent exaggerated hyperbilirubinemia and its toxic consequences. Many factors cause elevated bilirubin levels in the neonate: breast-feeding, hemolytic disease of the newborn, hypoxia, infections, acidosis, and albumin-binding drugs (*e.g.*, furosemide, hydrocortisone, gentamicin, digoxin).[24] Bowel or biliary obstruction and liver disease are less common causes. Associated risk factors include prematurity, Asian ancestry, and maternal diabetes. Breast milk jaundice occurs in approximately 1 in 200 breast-fed infants.[23] These neonates accumulate significant levels of unconjugated bilirubin 4 to 7 days after birth and reach maximum levels in the third week of life. It is thought that the breast milk contains fatty acids that inhibit bilirubin conjugation in the neonatal liver. A factor in breast milk is also thought to increase the absorption of bilirubin in the duodenum. This type of jaundice disappears if breast-feeding is discontinued. Nursing can be resumed in 3 to 4 days without any hyperbilirubinemia ensuing.

Hyperbilirubinemia places the neonate at risk for development of a neurologic syndrome called *kernicterus*. This condition is caused by the accumulation of unconjugated bilirubin in brain cells. Unconjugated bilirubin is lipid soluble, crosses the permeable blood–brain barrier of the neonate, and is deposited in cells of the basal ganglia, causing brain damage. Symptoms may appear 2 to 7 days after birth or later in the neonatal period. Lethargy, poor feeding, and short-term behavioral changes may be evident in mildly affected infants. Severe manifestations include rigidity, tremors, ataxia, and hearing loss. Extreme cases cause seizures and death. Most survivors are seriously damaged and by 3 years of age exhibit involuntary muscle spasm, seizures, mental retardation, and deafness. The potential for development of kernicterus is related to the level of unconjugated bilirubin in the serum, regardless of cause, and predisposing factors such as gestational age and weight. Signs and symptoms of kernicterus in term infants occur at indirect bilirubin levels of 25 to 30 mg/dL; less mature or ill infants are susceptible at lower levels.[25] Infants at risk for development of kernicterus are those with clinically apparent jaundice in the first 24 hours, an increase in total serum bilirubin of more than 5 mg/dL per day, a total bilirubin concentration higher than 12 mg/dL in term or 14 mg/dL in preterm infants, direct serum bilirubin levels higher than 1 mg/dL, and visible jaundice lasting for more than 1 week in term infants or 2 weeks in premature infants.[23]

Hyperbilirubinemia in the neonate is treated with phototherapy or exchange transfusion. Phototherapy is more commonly used to treat jaundiced infants and reduce the risk of kernicterus. Exposure to fluorescent light in the blue range of the visible spectrum (420- to 470-nm wavelength) reduces bilirubin levels. Bilirubin in the skin absorbs the light energy and is converted to a structural isomer that is more water soluble and can be excreted in the stool and urine. Effective treatment depends on the area of skin exposed and the infant's ability to metabolize and excrete bilirubin. Frequent monitoring of bilirubin levels, body temperature, and hydration is critical to the infant's care. Exchange transfusion is considered when signs of kernicterus are evident or hyperbilirubinemia is sustained or rising and unresponsive to phototherapy.

Hemolytic Disease of the Newborn

Erythroblastosis fetalis, or hemolytic disease of the newborn, occurs in Rh-positive infants of Rh-negative mothers who have been sensitized. The mother can produce anti-Rh antibodies from pregnancies in which the infants are Rh positive or by blood transfusions of Rh-positive blood. The Rh-negative mother usually becomes sensitized during the first few days after delivery, when fetal Rh-positive red cells from the placental site are released into the maternal circulation. Because the antibodies take several weeks to develop, the first Rh-positive infant of an Rh-negative mother usually is not affected. Infants with Rh-negative blood have no antigens on their red cells to react with the maternal antibodies and are not affected.

After an Rh-negative mother has been sensitized, the Rh antibodies from her blood are transferred to subsequent infants through the placental circulation. These antibodies react with the red cell antigens of the Rh-positive infant, causing agglutination and hemolysis. This leads to severe anemia with compensatory hyperplasia and enlargement of the blood-forming organs, including the spleen and liver, in the fetus. Liver function may be impaired, with decreased production of albumin causing massive edema, called *hydrops fetalis*. If blood levels of unconjugated bilirubin are abnormally high because of red cell hemolysis, there is danger of kernicterus developing in the infant, resulting in severe brain damage or death.

Several advances have served to significantly decrease the threat to infants born to Rh-negative mothers: prevention of sensitization, antenatal identification of the at-risk fetus, and intrauterine transfusion to the affected fetus. The injection of Rh immune globulin (*i.e.*, gamma-globulin–containing Rh antibody) prevents sensitization in Rh-negative mothers who have given birth to Rh-positive infants if administered at 28 weeks' gestation and within 72 hours of delivery, abortion, genetic amniocentesis, or fetal-maternal bleeding. After sensitization has developed, the immune globulin is of no value. Since 1968, the year Rh immune globulin was introduced, the incidence of sensitization of Rh-negative women has dropped dramatically. Early prenatal care and screening of maternal blood continue to be important in reducing immunization. Efforts to improve therapy are aimed at production of monoclonal anti-D, the Rh antibody.

In the past, approximately 20% of erythroblastotic fetuses died in utero. Fetal Rh phenotyping can now be performed to identify at-risk fetuses in the first trimester using fetal blood or amniotic cells.[26] Hemolysis in these fetuses can be treated by intrauterine transfusions of red cells through the umbilical cord. Exchange transfusions are administered after birth by removing and replacing the infant's blood volume with type O Rh-negative blood. The exchange transfusion removes most of the hemolyzed red cells and some of the total bilirubin, treating the anemia and hyperbilirubinemia.

RED CELL CHANGES WITH AGING

Aging is associated with red cell changes. Bone marrow cellularity declines with age, from approximately 50% cellularity at age 65 to approximately 30% at age 75 years. The decline may reflect osteoporosis rather than a decrease in hematopoietic cells.[27]

Hemoglobin levels decline after middle age. In studies of men older than 60 years of age, mean hemoglobin levels ranged from 15.3 to 12.4 g/dL, with the lowest levels found in the oldest persons. The decline is less in women, with mean levels ranging from 13.8 to 11.7 mg/dL.[27] In most asymptomatic elderly persons, lower hemoglobin levels result from iron deficiency and anemia of chronic disease. Orally administered iron is poorly used in older adults, despite normal iron absorption. Underlying neoplasms also may contribute to anemia in this population.

In summary, hemoglobin concentrations at birth are high, reflecting the in utero need for oxygen delivery; toward the end of the first postnatal week, these levels begin to decline, gradually falling to a minimum value at approximately 2 months of age. During the early neonatal period, there is a shift from fetal to adult hemoglobin. Many infants have physiologic jaundice because of hyperbilirubinemia during the first week of life, probably related to increased red cell breakdown and the inability of the infant's liver to conjugate bilirubin. The term *kernicterus* describes elevated levels of lipid-soluble, unconjugated bilirubin, which can be toxic to brain cells. Depending on severity, it is treated with phototherapy or exchange transfusions (or both). Hemolytic disease of the newborn occurs in Rh-positive infants of Rh-negative mothers who have been sensitized. It involves hemolysis of infant red cells in response to maternal Rh antibodies that have crossed the placenta. Administration of Rh immune globulin to the mother within 72 hours of delivery of an Rh-positive infant, abortion, or amniocentesis prevents sensitization. Aging is associated with red cell changes. Bone marrow cellularity decreases, and there is a decrease in hemoglobin.

Related Web Sites

Emory University Sickle Cell Information Center (source of up-to-date information on sickle cell anemia) www.emory.edu/PEDS/SICKLE/toc.htm#pharm
National Heart Lung and Blood Institute. (Rich source of information on sickle cell anemia and thalassemia) www.nhlbi.nih.gov/health/public/blood/sickle
Sickle Cell Anemia Organization www.4sicklecellanemia.org/Sickle
Sickle Cell Disease Association of America www.sicklecelldisease.org/

References

1. Beck W.S. (1991). Erythropoiesis and introduction to the anemias. In Beck W. S. (Ed.), *Hematology* (5th ed., pp. 27, 29). Cambridge, MA: MIT Press.
2. Cotran R.S., Kumar V., Collins T. (Eds.). (1999). *Robbins pathologic basis of disease* (6th ed., pp. 610, 611, 614). Philadelphia: W.B. Saunders.
3. Beutler E. (1995). The sickle cell diseases and related disorders. In Beutler E., Lichtman A., Coller B. S., Kipps T.J. (Eds.), *Williams' hematology* (5th ed., p. 616). New York: McGraw-Hill.
4. Hebbel R.P. (2000). Blockade of adhesion of sickle cells to endothelium by monoclonal antibodies. *New England Journal of Medicine* 342, 1910–1912.
5. Steinberg M.H. (1999). Management of sickle cell disease. *New England Journal of Medicine* 340, 1021–1030.
6. Lane P. (1996). Sickle cell disease. *Pediatric Clinics of North America* 43, 639–666.
7. Brown A.K., Sleeper L.A., Miller S.T., Pegelow C.H., Gill F.M., Waclawiw M.A. (1994). Reference values and hematologic changes from birth to 5 years in patients with sickle cell disease. *Archives of Pediatric and Adolescent Medicine* 148, 796–804.

8. Steinberg M.H. (1999). Management of sickle cell disease. *New England Journal of Medicine* 340, 1021–1030.

9. Olivieri N.F. (1999). The β-Thalassemias. *New England Journal of Medicine* 344, 99–109.

10. Vengelen-Tyler V. (Ed.). (1996). *Technical manual* (12th ed., pp. 135–142, 256). Bethesda, MD: American Association of Blood Banks.

11. Brittenham G.M. (2000). Disorders of iron metabolism: Iron deficiency and overload. In Hoffman R., Benz E.J., Shattil S. J., Furie B., Cohen H.J., Silberstein L.E., McGlave P. (Eds.), *Hematology: Basic principles and practice* (3rd ed., pp. 405, 413). New York: Churchill Livingstone.

12. Schwartz E. (1996). Anemia of inadequate production. In Behrman R.E., Kliegman R.M., Nelson W.E., Vaughan V.C. (Eds.), *Nelson textbook of pediatrics* (15th ed., pp. 1387–1389), Philadelphia: W.B. Saunders.

13. Hoffbrand A.V., Herbert V. (1999). Nutritional anemias. *Seminars in Hematology* 36 (Suppl. 7), 13–23.

14. Antony A.C. (2000). Megaloblastic anemias. In Hoffman R., Benz E.J., Shattil S.J., Furie B., Cohen H.J., Silberstein L.E., McGlave P. (Eds.), *Hematology: Basic principles and practice* (3rd ed., p. 476). New York: Churchill Livingstone.

15. Young N.S., Maciejewski J.P. (2000). Aplastic anemias. In Hoffman R., Benz E.J., Shattil S.J., Furie B., Cohen H.J., Silberstein L. E., McGlave P. (Eds.), *Hematology: Basic principles and practice* (3rd ed., pp. 316, 318). New York: Churchill Livingstone.

16. Means R.T. Jr. (1999). Advances in the anemia of chronic disease. *International Journal of Hematology* 70, 7–12.

17. Caro J., Erslev A.J. (1995). Anemia of chronic renal failure. In Beutler E., Lichtman A., Coller B.S., Kipps T.J. (Eds.), *Williams' hematology* (5th ed., p. 456). New York: McGraw-Hill.

18. Goodnough L.T., Brecher M.E., Kanter M.H., AuBuchon J.P. (1999). Blood transfusion. *New England Journal of Medicine* 340, 438–447.

19. Goodnough L.T., Brecher M.E., Kanter M.H., AuBuchon J.P. (1999). Blood conservation. *New England Journal of Medicine* 340, 525–533.

20. Pittiglio D.H. (Ed.). (1983). *Modern blood banking and transfusion practices* (pp. 91–92). Philadelphia: F.A. Davis.

21. Brown M.S. (1988). Physiologic anemia of infancy: Nutritional factors and abnormal states. In Stockman J.A., Pochedly C. (Eds.), *Developmental and neonatal hematology* (pp. 252, 274). New York: Raven Press.

22. Segel G.B. (1995). Hematology of the newborn. In Beutler E., Lichtman A., Coller B.S., Kipps T.J. (Eds.), *Williams' hematology* (5th ed., p. 59). New York: McGraw-Hill.

23. Kliegman R.M. (1996). The fetus and neonatal infant. In Behrman R.E., Kliegman R.M., Nelson W.E., Vaughan V.C. (Eds.), *Nelson textbook of pediatrics* (15th ed., pp. 493–499). Philadelphia: W.B. Saunders.

24. Hazinski M.F. (1992). *Nursing care of the critically ill child* (2nd ed., p. 739). St. Louis: Mosby–Year Book.

25. Cashore W.J. (1994). Neonatal hyperbilirubinemia. In Oski F.A., DeAngelis C.D., Feigin R.D., Warshaw J.B. (Eds.), *Principles and practice of pediatrics* (2nd ed., pp. 445–447). Philadelphia: J.B. Lippincott.

26. Kramer K., Cohen H.J. (2000). Antenatal diagnosis of hematologic disorders. In Hoffman R., Benz E.J., Shattil S.J., Furie B., Cohen H.J., Silberstein L.E., McGlave P. (Eds.), *Hematology: Basic principles and practice* (3rd ed., p. 2495). New York: Churchill Livingstone.

27. Williams W.J. (1995). Hematology in the aged. In Beutler E., Lichtman A., Coller B.S., Kipps T.J. (Eds.), *Williams' hematology* (5th ed., p. 73). New York: McGraw-Hill.

Chapter 16

Disorders of White Blood Cells and Lymphoid Tissues

Kathryn Ann Caudell

The white blood cells protect the body against invasion by foreign agents. They include phagocytic cells (*i.e.,* granulocytes and monocytes), which mediate innate immune responses, and the lymphocytes (*i.e.,* B cells and T cells), which are involved in acquired immunity. Disorders of white blood cells fall into two broad categories: deficiency disorders and proliferative disorders. This chapter focuses on disorders of white blood cell deficiency; infectious mononucleosis, a self-limiting benign lymphoproliferative disorder; the leukemias and myeloproliferative disorders; malignant lymphomas; and multiple myeloma. The origin and differentiation of the white blood cells are discussed in Chapter 13. The lymphoid system is presented in Chapter 18.

Hematopoietic and Lymphoid Tissues

After you have completed this section of the chapter, you should be able to meet the following objectives:

✦ List the cells and tissues of the hematopoietic system
✦ Trace the development of the different blood cells from their origin in the pluripotent bone marrow stem cell to their circulation in the bloodstream

The hematopoietic system encompasses all the blood cells, their precursors, and their derivatives: the red blood cells, the thrombocytes or platelets, and the white blood cells. It includes the myeloid or bone marrow tissue in which the white blood cells are formed, and the lymphoid tissues of the lymph nodes, thymus, and spleen, in which the white blood cells circulate and mature. The development of different cell lineages depends on cellular interactions and exposure to cytokines.

WHITE BLOOD CELLS

The white blood cells include the granulocytes (*i.e.,* neutrophils, eosinophils, and basophils), the monocyte and macrophage lineage, and the lymphocytes. Granulocytes and monocytes are derived from the myeloid stem cell in the bone marrow and circulate in the blood. T lymphocytes (T cells) and B lymphocytes (B cells) originate in the bone marrow and migrate between the blood and the lymph. T lymphocytes mature in the thymus, and B lymphocytes mature in the bone marrow, the mammalian equivalent of the avian bursa of Fabricius. Another population of lymphocytes includes the large granular lymphocytes, or *natural killer cells,* which do not share characteristics of the

T lymphocytes or the B lymphocytes, but have the ability to lyse target cells.[1]

BONE MARROW AND HEMATOPOIESIS

The entire hematopoietic system, in all its complexity, arises from a small number of stem cells that differentiate to form blood cells and replenish bone marrow by a process of self-renewal. All the hematopoietic precursors, including the erythroid (red blood cell), myelocyte (granulocyte and monocyte), lymphocyte (T cell and B cell), and megakaryocyte (platelet) series, are derived from a small population of cells called the *pluripotent stem cells.* These cells are capable of providing *progenitor cells (i.e.,* parent cells) for lymphopoiesis and myelopoiesis, processes by which lymphoid and myeloid blood cells are made, respectively. Several levels of differentiation lead to the development of committed *unipotent cells,* which are the progenitors for each of the blood cell types. The progenitor cells lose their capacity for self-renewal but retain the potential to differentiate into erythrocytes, monocytes, megakaryocytes, or lymphocytes. This regulation of blood cells is thought to be at least partially controlled by protein messenger molecules, called *cytokines,* that regulate the function of other cells, in this case the blood cell precursors.[1]

The different committed stem cells, when grown in culture, produce colonies of specific types of blood cells. A committed stem cell that forms a specific type of blood cell is called a *colony-forming unit.* The *hematopoietic growth factors* are a family of glycoproteins that support hematopoietic colony formation. These growth factors can be categorized into three functional groups: those that are involved in the development of a specific cell lineage, those that affect the early multipotential progenitor cells, and those that indirectly regulate hematopoiesis by inducing the expression of growth factor genes in other cells.[2]

There are several lineage-specific growth factors: erythropoietin, granulocyte macrophage-stimulating factor (GM-CSF), and monocyte-macrophage colony-stimulating factor (M-CSF). Although the hematopoietic growth factors act at different points in the proliferation and differentiation pathway, their functions overlap. Other cytokines, such as interleukin (IL)-1, IL-4, IL-6, and interferon, act synergistically to support the functions of the growth factors.[3]

Many of the hematopoietic growth factors have multiple functions and affect a variety of cells. For example, GM-CSF stimulates the erythropoietic burst-forming units, stimulates the growth and function of granulocyte, macrophage, and eosinophil progenitor cells, and induces IL-1 gene expression in neutrophils and peripheral mononuclear leukocytes. Other growth factors, such as IL-3, act on the most immature marrow progenitor cells, thereby promoting the development of cells that can differentiate into a number of cell types. Stem cell factor (also called *c-kit ligand*) mediates the activation of stem cells and stimulates their differentiation into various cell lineages.[2]

The identification and characterization of the various cytokines and growth factors have led to their use in treating a wide range of diseases, including bone marrow failure, hematopoietic neoplasms, infectious diseases, and congenital and myeloproliferative disorders. Many of these uses are investigational.

 Hematopoiesis

➤ White blood cells are formed partially in the bone marrow (granulocytes, monocytes, and some lymphocytes) and partially in the lymph system (lymphocytes and plasma cells).

➤ They are formed from hematopoietic stem cells that differentiate into committed progenitor cells that in turn develop into the myelocytic and lymphocytic lineages needed for the formation of the different types of white blood cell.

➤ The growth and reproduction of the different stem cells is controlled by multiple hematopoietic growth factors or inducers.

➤ The life span of white blood cells is relatively short so that constant renewal is necessary to maintain normal blood levels. Any conditions that decrease the availability of stem cells or hematopoietic growth factors produce a decrease in white blood cells.

LYMPHOID TISSUES

The body's lymphatic system, which consists of the lymphatic vessels, lymph nodes, spleen, and thymus, is made up of lymphoid tissue (see Chapter 18). Lymph is body fluid that originates as excess fluid from the capillaries. It is returned to the vascular compartment and the right side of the heart through lymphatic vessels.

The lymph nodes, which are situated along the lymphatic channels, filter the lymph before it is returned to the circulation (Fig. 16-1). Lymph enters a lymph node through afferent lymphatic channels, percolates through a labyrinthine system of minute channels lined with endothelial and phagocytic cells, and then emerges through efferent lymphatic vessels. A number of efferent vessels join to form collecting trunks. Each collecting trunk drains a definite area of the body. By filtering bacteria and other particulate matter, the lymph nodes serve as a secondary line of defense even when clinical disease is not present. In the event of malignant neoplasm development, cancer cells are filtered and retained by the lymph nodes for a period before being disseminated to other parts of the body. Because of their contribution to the development of the immune system, lymph nodes are relatively large at birth and progressively atrophy throughout life.

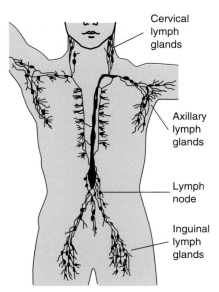

FIGURE 16-1 Location of a portion of the lymph nodes in the human body. (*What you need to know about Hodgkin's disease.* [1981]. Washington, DC: Department of Health and Human Services)

> In summary, the hematopoietic system consists of a number of cells derived from the pluripotent stem cells originating in the bone marrow. These cells differentiate into committed cell lines that mature into red blood cells, platelets, and a variety of white blood cells. The lymphoid system consists of a network of lymphatic vessels, nodes, and tissues whose function is to drain lymph fluid from specific areas of the body and to filter particular matter such as bacteria and cancer cells.

Disorders of White Blood Cell Deficiency

After you have completed this section of the chapter, you should be able to meet the following objectives:

✦ Define the terms *leukopenia, neutropenia, granulocytopenia,* and *aplastic anemia*
✦ Cite two general causes of neutropenia
✦ Describe the mechanism of symptom production in neutropenia

The number of leukocytes, or white blood cells, in the peripheral circulation normally ranges from 5000 to 10,000/μL of blood. Approximately 50% to 70% of the leukocytes are granulocytes (50% to 70% neutrophils, 1% to 4% eosinophils, and 0.4% basophils), 20% to 30% are lymphocytes, and 2% to 8% are monocytes. The term *leukopenia* describes an absolute decrease in white blood cell numbers. The disorder may affect any of the specific types of white blood cells, but most often it affects the neutrophils, which are the predominant type of granulocyte.

NEUTROPENIA

Neutropenia refers specifically to a decrease in neutrophils. It commonly is defined as a circulating neutrophil count of less than 1500 cells/μL. Agranulocytosis, which denotes a severe neutropenia, is characterized by a circulating neutrophil count of less than 200 cells/μL.[4]

Neutropenia can be acquired or congenital. It usually is the result of one or more of the following: a decrease in the production of neutrophils (*i.e.,* granulopoiesis) by the bone marrow, peripheral destruction, a shift from the circulatory system to the peripheral tissue, or a combination of these.[4] The causes of neutropenia are summarized in Table 16-1.

Acquired Neutropenia

Granulopoiesis may be impaired due to complications of certain procedures such as chemotherapy and irradiation or disease conditions such as aplastic anemia, systemic lupus erythematosus, rheumatoid arthritis, or infectious mononucleosis, which interfere with the formation of all blood cells. Infections by viruses or bacteria may drain neutrophils from the blood faster than they can be replaced, thereby depleting the neutrophil storage pool in the bone marrow.[4] Overgrowth of neoplastic cells in cases of non-myelocytic leukemia and lymphoma also may suppress the function of neutrophil precursors. Because of the neutrophil's short life span of approximately 1 day in the peripheral blood, neutropenia occurs rapidly when granulopoiesis is impaired. Under these conditions, neutropenia usually is accompanied by thrombocytopenia (*i.e.,* platelet deficiency).

In *aplastic anemia,* all of the myeloid stem cells are affected, resulting in anemia, thrombocytopenia, and agranulocytosis. Autoimmune disorders or idiosyncratic drug reactions may cause increased and premature destruction of neutrophils. In splenomegaly, neutrophils may be trapped in the spleen along with other blood cells. In Felty's syndrome, a variant of rheumatoid arthritis, there is increased destruction of neutrophils in the spleen. Most cases of neutropenia are drug related. Chemotherapeutic drugs used in the treatment of cancer (*e.g.,* alkylating agents, antimetabolites) cause predictable dose-dependent suppression of bone marrow function.

The term *idiosyncratic* is used to describe drug reactions that are different from the effects obtained in most persons and that cannot be explained in terms of allergy. A number of drugs, such as chloramphenicol (an antibiotic), phenothiazine tranquilizers, sulfonamides, propylthiouracil (used in the treatment of hyperthyroidism), and phenylbutazone (used in the treatment of arthritis), may cause idiosyncratic depression of bone marrow function. Some drugs, such as hydantoin derivatives and primidone (used in the treatment of seizure disorders), can cause intramedullary destruction of granulocytes and thereby impair production. Many idiosyncratic cases of drug-induced neutropenia are thought to be caused by immunologic mechanisms, with the drug or its metabolites acting as antigens (*i.e.,* haptens) to incite the production of antibodies reactive against the neutrophils. Neutrophils possess human leukocyte antigens (HLA) and other antigens specific to a given leukocyte line. Antibodies

TABLE 16-1 ✦ Causes of Neutropenia

Cause	Mechanism
Accelerated removal (*e.g.*, inflammation and infection)	Removal of neutrophils from the circulation exceeds production
Drug-induced granulocytopenia	
Defective production	
Cytotoxic drugs used in cancer therapy	Predictable damage to precursor cells, usually dose dependent
Phenothiazine, thiouracil, chloramphenicol, phenylbutazone, and others	Idiosyncratic depression of bone marrow function
Hydantoinates, primidone, and others	Intramedullary destruction of granulocytes
Immune destruction	Immunologic mechanisms with cytolysis or leukoagglutination
Aminopyrine and others	
Periodic or cyclic neutropenia (occurs during infancy and later)	Unknown
Neoplasms involving bone marrow (e.g., leukemias and lymphomas)	Overgrowth of neoplastic cells, which crowd out granulopoietic precursors
Idiopathic neutropenia that occurs in the absence of other disease or provoking influence	Autoimmune reaction
Felty's syndrome	Intrasplenic destruction of neutrophils

to these specific antigens have been identified in some cases of drug-induced neutropenia.[4]

Congenital Neutropenia

A decreased production of granulocytes is a feature of a number of hereditary disorders, including cyclic neutropenia and Kostmann's syndrome. *Periodic* or *cyclic neutropenia* is an autosomal dominant disorder with variable expression that begins in infancy and persists for decades. It is characterized by periodic neutropenia that develops every 21 to 30 days and lasts approximately 3 to 6 days. Although the cause is undetermined, it is thought to result from impaired feedback regulation of granulocyte production and release. *Kostmann's syndrome,* which occurs sporadically or as an autosomal recessive disorder, causes severe neutropenia while preserving the erythroid and megakaryocyte cell lineages. The total white blood cell count may be within normal limits, but the neutrophil count is less than 200/µL. Monocyte and eosinophil levels may be elevated.

A transient neutropenia may occur in neonates whose mothers have hypertension. It usually lasts from 1 to 60 hours but can persist for 3 to 30 days. This type of neutropenia, which is associated with increased risk of nosocomial infection, is thought to result from transiently reduced neutrophil production.[4]

Manifestations and Treatment

Because the neutrophil is essential to the cellular phase of inflammation, infections are common in persons with neutropenia, and extreme caution is needed to protect them from exposure to infectious organisms. Infections that may go unnoticed in a person with a normal neutrophil count could prove fatal in a person with neutropenia.

The clinical features of neutropenia usually depend on the severity of neutropenia and the cause. The primary problem is effectively managing infectious complications. These infections commonly are caused by organisms that colonize the skin and the gastrointestinal tract. However, the most common site of serious infection is the respiratory tract. Bacteria, fungi, and protozoa frequently colonize the upper and lower respiratory tracts.

The signs and symptoms initially include malaise, chills, and fever, followed by extreme weakness and fatigue. The white blood cell count often is reduced to 1000/µL and, in certain cases, may fall to 200 to 300/µL. Ulcerative necrotizing lesions of the mouth are common in neutropenia. Ulcerations of the skin, vagina, and gastrointestinal tract also may occur.[4]

Antibiotics are used to treat infections in those situations in which neutrophil destruction can be controlled or the neutropoietic function of the bone marrow can be recovered. Hematopoietic growth factors such as GM-CSF are being used more commonly to stimulate the maturation and differentiation of the polymorphonuclear cell lineage. Treatment with these biologic response modifiers has reduced the period of neutropenia and the risk for development of potentially fatal septicemia.[4]

In summary. neutropenia, a marked reduction in the number of circulating neutrophils, is one of the major disorders of the white blood cells. It can be acquired or congenital, and can result from a combination of mechanisms. Severe neutropenia can occur as a complication of lymphoproliferative diseases, in which neoplastic cells crowd out neutrophil precursor cells, or of radiation therapy or treatment with cytotoxic drugs, which destroy neutrophil precursor cells. Neutropenia also may be encountered as an idiosyncratic reaction to various drugs. Because the neutrophil is essential to the cellular stage of inflammation, severe and often life-threatening infections are common in persons with neutropenia.

Infectious Mononucleosis

After you have completed this section of the chapter, you should be able to meet the following objectives:

✦ Name the virus that causes infectious mononucleosis and describe how it is spread

✦ Describe the pathogenesis and manifestations of infectious mononucleosis

✦ List the signs and symptoms of infectious mononucleosis

Infectious mononucleosis is a self-limiting lympho-proliferative disorder caused by the Epstein-Barr virus (EBV). One of the herpesviruses, EBV is ubiquitous in all human populations. Infectious mononucleosis is most prevalent in adolescents and young adults in the upper socioeconomic classes in developed countries. This is probably because the disease, which is relatively asymptomatic when it occurs during childhood, confers complete immunity to the virus. In families from upper socioeconomic classes, exposure to the virus may be delayed until late adolescence or early adulthood. In such persons, the mode of infection, size of the viral pool, and physiologic and immunologic condition of the host may determine whether the infection occurs.

Evidence suggests that exposure to EBV-contaminated saliva is one of the main modes of transfer. In countries where family members practice the mastication of food for infants, most infants younger than 1 year of age are infected with EBV. By age 2 years, approximately 81% have had a primary EBV infection.[5]

The virus undergoes a replicative cycle in the oropharyngeal epithelium and then invades the blood by selectively infecting B cells, a cell population that has specific surface receptors for the virus. It is shed from the oropharynx for as long as 18 months after primary infection; thereafter, it may be spread intermittently by persons who are EBV seropositive despite the absence of clinical disease.[6] Immunosuppressed persons shed the virus more frequently. Asymptomatic shedding of EBV by healthy persons accounts for most of the spread of infectious mononucleosis, despite the fact that it is not a highly contagious disease.

PATHOGENESIS

Infectious mononucleosis is characterized by fever, generalized lymphadenopathy, and sore throat. The hallmark of infectious mononucleosis is the appearance in the blood of atypical lymphocytes that are primarily activated cytotoxic (CD8+) T cells and natural killer cells.[7] In the course of infection, EBV invades the B cells of oropharyngeal lymphoid tissues. Replication of the virus ensues, with the subsequent death of the B cells and release of the virus into the blood, causing the febrile reaction and specific immunologic responses. Concurrent with the febrile reaction, antiviral antibodies (*i.e.,* immunoglobulin M [IgM] and immunoglobulin G [IgG]) appear, and the virus disappears from the blood. Other virus-determined antibodies develop, including the well-known *heterophil* (*i.e.,* the Paul-Bunnel antibody) that is used in the diagnosis of infectious mononucleosis.[6]

Although infectious B cells and free virions disappear from the blood, some EBV-transformed B cells remain in the circulation with the genome of the virus integrated into their genetic structure. These B cells display virus-directed membrane antigens. These B-cell antigens stimulate production of cytotoxic (CD8+) and suppressor (CD4+) T cells. Together, the suppressor-cytotoxic T cells are the atypical lymphocytes seen in the blood of patients with infectious mononucleosis. The proliferation of atypical lymphocytes throughout the body is responsible for the lymphadenopathy and hepatosplenomegaly. The progressive increase in the number of EBV-specific antibodies and cytotoxic (CD8+) T cells eventually brings the disease under control and eliminates the latently infected B cells.[6]

MANIFESTATIONS

The onset of infectious mononucleosis usually is insidious. The incubation period lasts 4 to 8 weeks. A prodromal period, which lasts for several days, follows and is characterized by malaise, anorexia, and chills. The prodromal period precedes the onset of fever, pharyngitis, and lymphadenopathy. Occasionally, the disorder comes on abruptly with a high fever. Most persons seek medical attention for severe pharyngitis, which usually is most severe for 5 to 7 days and persists for 7 to 14 days. Severe toxic pharyngotonsillitis may cause airway obstruction.

Lymphadenopathy affects 90% of patients, who have symmetrically enlarged and often tender lymph nodes. Its duration is variable but seldom exceeds 3 weeks. Hepatitis and splenomegaly are common manifestations of infectious mononucleosis and are thought to be immune mediated. Hepatitis is characterized by hepatomegaly, nausea, anorexia, and jaundice. Although discomforting, it usually is a benign condition that resolves without causing permanent liver damage. The spleen may be enlarged two to three times its normal size, and rupture of the spleen is an infrequent complication. A rash that resembles rubella develops in 10% to 15% of cases.[6] Treatment with amoxicillin or ampicillin frequently produces skin eruptions.[7] The reason for this is unknown. In less than 1% of cases, mostly in the adult age group, complications of the central nervous system (CNS) develop. These complications include cranial nerve palsies, encephalitis, meningitis, transverse myelitis, and Guillain-Barré syndrome.

The peripheral blood usually shows an increase in the number of leukocytes, with a white blood cell count between 12,000 and 18,000/μL, 95% of which are lymphocytes. The rise in white blood cells begins during the first week, rises even higher during the second week of the infection, and then returns to normal around the fourth week. Although leukocytosis is common, leukopenia may be seen in some persons during the first 3 days of the illness. Atypical lymphocytes are common, constituting more than 20% of the total lymphocyte count. Heterophil antibodies usually appear during the second or third week and decline after the acute illness has subsided. They may, however, be detectable for up to 9 months after onset of the disease.

Most persons with infectious mononucleosis recover without incident. The acute phase of the illness usually lasts for 2 to 3 weeks, after which recovery occurs rapidly. Some degree of debility and lethargy may persist for 2 to 3 months.

DIAGNOSIS AND TREATMENT

Diagnosis is based on the clinical features of fever, pharyngitis, and lymphadenopathy, coupled with the presence of atypical lymphocytes and heterophil antibodies. EBV-specific antibody studies may facilitate diagnosis in heterophil-negative cases. Treatment is primarily symptomatic and supportive. It includes bed rest and analgesics such as aspirin to relieve the fever, headache, and sore throat. In severe pharyngotonsillitis, corticosteroids are given to reduce inflammation.[8]

A meta-analysis was performed on five randomized, controlled studies that evaluated the efficacy of acyclovir in reducing viral shedding and improving clinical outcomes. Although there was a trend toward clinical improvement, no statistically significant clinical results were achieved. A significant reduction in viral shedding was observed at the end of treatment, but there was no difference in shedding 3 weeks after discontinuation of therapy.[9]

In summary, infectious mononucleosis is a self-limited lymphoproliferative disorder caused by the B-lymphocytotropic EBV, a member of the herpesvirus family. The highest incidence of infectious mononucleosis is found in adolescents and young adults, and it is seen more frequently in the upper socioeconomic classes of developed countries. The disease is characterized by fever, generalized lymphadenopathy, sore throat, and the appearance in the blood of atypical lymphocytes and several antibodies, including the well-known heterophil antibodies that are used in the diagnosis of infectious mononucleosis. Treatment is largely symptomatic and supportive; however, corticosteroids are given to reduce inflammation in cases with severe pharyngotonsillitis.

unregulated, proliferating, immature neoplastic cells. In most cases, the leukemic cells spill out into the blood, where they are seen in large numbers. The term *leukemia* (i.e., "white blood") was first used by Virchow to describe a reversal of the usual ratio of red blood cells to white blood cells. Leukemia is thought to arise after the malignant transformation of a single hematopoietic cell line. The leukemic cells proliferate mainly in the bone marrow, circulate in the blood, and infiltrate the spleen, lymph nodes, and other tissues.

Leukemia strikes approximately 31,000 persons in the United States each year. In 2000, approximately 30,800 new cases were diagnosed, and approximately 21,700 persons died of this disease.[10] More children are stricken with leukemia than with any other form of cancer, and it is the leading cause of death in children between the ages of 3 and 14 years. Although leukemia commonly is thought of as a childhood disease, it strikes more adults than children.

Advances in molecular biology have contributed greatly to an understanding of leukemic cell types, including the early stages of cell differentiation and gene function. This information has greatly influenced the diagnosis, treatment, and prognosis of patients with leukemia.

CLASSIFICATION

The leukemias commonly are classified according to their predominant cell type (i.e., lymphocytic or myelocytic) and whether the condition is acute or chronic. A rudimentary classification system divides leukemia into four types: acute lymphocytic (lymphoblastic) leukemia (ALL), chronic lymphocytic leukemia (CLL), acute myelocytic (myeloblastic) leukemia (AML), and chronic myelocytic leukemia (CML). The *lymphocytic leukemias* involve immature lymphocytes

Neoplastic Disorders of Hematopoietic and Lymphoid Origin

After you have completed this section of the chapter, you should be able to meet the following objectives:

- ✦ Use the predominant white blood cell type and classification of acute or chronic to describe the four general types of leukemia
- ✦ State the warning signs of acute leukemia
- ✦ Explain the manifestations of leukemia in terms of altered cell differentiation
- ✦ Describe the following complications of acute leukemia and its treatment: leukostasis, tumor lysis syndrome, hyperuricemia, and blast crisis
- ✦ State the difference between syngeneic, allogeneic, and autologous bone marrow transplantation

The leukemias are malignant neoplasms of cells originally derived from the hematopoietic stem cell. They are characterized by diffuse replacement of bone marrow with

 Leukemias

- ➤ Leukemias are malignant neoplasms arising from the transformation of a single blood cell line derived from hematopoietic stem cells.

- ➤ The leukemias are classified as lymphocytic (lymphocytes) or myelocytic (granulocytes, monocytes) according to their cell lineage. Leukemic cells proliferate mainly in the bone marrow, circulate in the blood, and infiltrate the spleen, lymph nodes, and other tissues.

- ➤ Because leukemic cells are immature and poorly differentiated, they proliferate rapidly and have a long life span, they do not function normally, they interfere with the maturation of normal blood cells, and they circulate in the bloodstream, cross the blood-brain barrier, and infiltrate many body organs.

and their progenitors that originate in the bone marrow but infiltrate the spleen, lymph nodes, CNS, and other tissues. The *myelocytic leukemias,* which involve the pluripotent myeloid stem cells in bone marrow, interfere with the maturation of all blood cells, including the granulocytes, erythrocytes, and thrombocytes.

ALL is the most common leukemia in childhood, comprising 80% to 85% of leukemia cases.[11] The peak incidence occurs between 2 and 4 years of age. Approximately 2000 children are diagnosed with ALL in the United States yearly, whereas roughly 500 children are diagnosed with AML.[12] CLL affects older persons; fewer than 10% of those in whom the disease develops are younger than 50 years of age. AML is seen most often between the ages of 13 and 39 years, and CML between the ages of 30 and 50 years.

CAUSES

The causes of leukemia are unknown. The incidence of leukemia among persons who have been exposed to high levels of radiation is unusually high. The number of cases of leukemia reported in the most heavily exposed survivors of the atomic blasts at Hiroshima and Nagasaki during the 20-year period from 1950 to 1970 was nearly 30 times the expected rate.[13] An increased incidence of leukemia also is associated with exposure to benzene and the use of antitumor drugs (*i.e.,* mechlorethamine, procarbazine, cyclophosphamide, chloramphenicol, and the epipodophyllotoxins).[14] Leukemia may occur as a second cancer after aggressive chemotherapy for other cancers, such as Hodgkin's disease,[15] gastrointestinal cancers,[16] ovarian cancer,[17] and ALL.[18,19] AML is the most common type of secondary cancer.

A significant number of cases of leukemia have been reported in identical twins. An identical twin of a person with acute leukemia has a 25% chance for development of the disease, whereas a fraternal twin has little excess risk. Leukemia is relatively frequently associated with congenital chromosomal abnormalities such as Down syndrome, Klinefelter's syndrome, and Turner's syndrome.

Advances in cytogenetic studies have made it increasingly evident that many forms of leukemia are associated with nonrandom chromosomal changes (usually translocations). For example, the Philadelphia chromosome (*i.e.,* translocation from chromosome 22 to chromosome 9) is present in approximately 90% of persons with CML.[20] In many cases, these chromosomal aberrations, which are present at diagnosis, disappear with treatment and remission and then reappear with relapse. The underlying cause of these chromosomal changes is unknown. It is possible, however, to try to correlate the chromosomes that are affected with the genes involved. This may lead to increased understanding of the pathogenesis of leukemia and to the discovery of new methods of diagnosis and treatment.

CLINICAL MANIFESTATIONS

A leukemic cell is an immature type of white blood cell. As explained in Chapter 8, differentiation of a cell line deter-mines its structure, function, and life span. Because leukemic cells are immature and poorly differentiated, they are capable of an increased rate of proliferation and have a prolonged life span. They cannot perform the functions of mature leukocytes and therefore are ineffective as phagocytes. Because they proliferate rapidly, leukemic cells interfere with the maturation of normal bone marrow cells, including the erythroblasts (red blood cells) and the megakaryoblasts (platelets). The mobile cells can travel throughout the circulatory system, cross the blood-brain barrier, and infiltrate many body organs.[20]

ACUTE LEUKEMIAS

Acute leukemia is a cancer of the hematopoietic stem cells. It usually has a sudden and stormy onset with signs and symptoms related to depressed bone marrow function (Table 16-2). Most patients present for medical evaluation within 3 months of the onset of symptoms. The patients may complain of malaise, lethargy, weight loss, fever, night sweats, bone or joint pain, dyspnea, bruising, and genitourinary manifestations such as cystitis. They may have mild pancytopenia (*i.e.,* anemia, thrombocytopenia, and neutropenia), a normal leukocyte count and absence of blast cells, or leukocytosis and circulating blast cells. Generalized lymphadenopathy, splenomegaly, and hepatomegaly caused by infiltration of leukemic cells occur in all acute leukemias but are more common in ALL. Patients may exhibit hematuria, renal failure, hyperuricemia, uric acid nephropathy, and testicular involvement.[17,21]

The warning signs and symptoms of acute leukemia are fatigue, pallor, weight loss, repeated infections, easy bruising, and nosebleeds and other types of hemorrhage.[22] These features may appear suddenly in children. Both ALL and AML are characterized by fatigue resulting from anemia; bleeding because of a decreased platelet count; and bone marrow involvement, including subperiosteal infiltration, marrow expansion, and bone resorption, which causes bone tenderness and pain. Infection results from neutropenia, with the risk of infection becoming high as the neutrophil count falls below 500/µL.

A definitive diagnosis of acute leukemia is based on blood and bone marrow studies; it requires the demonstration of leukemic cells in the peripheral blood, bone marrow, or extramedullary tissue. Laboratory findings reveal the presence of immature white blood cells (blasts) in the circulation and bone marrow, where they may constitute 60% to 100% of the cells.[14] As these cells proliferate and begin to crowd the bone marrow, the development of other cell lineages in the marrow is suppressed. Consequently, there is a loss of mature myeloid cells, such as erythrocytes, granulocytes, and platelets. Anemia almost always is present, and the platelet count is decreased.

Signs and symptoms of CNS involvement occur in ALL and AML and include headache, nausea, vomiting, cranial nerve palsies, papilledema, and occasionally seizures and coma. The latter two are more common in children than in adults and in ALL than in AML. Leukostasis, a condition in which the circulating blast count is markedly elevated (usu-

TABLE 16-2 ✦ Clinical Manifestations of Leukemia and Their Pathologic Basis*	
Clinical Manifestations	**Pathologic Basis**
Bone marrow depression	
Malaise, easy fatigability	Anemia
Fever	Infection or increased metabolism by neoplastic cells
Bleeding	Decreased thrombocytes
Petechiae	
Ecchymosis	
Gingival bleeding	
Epistaxis	
Bone pain and tenderness upon palpation	Subperiosteal bone infiltration, bone marrow expansion, and bone resorption
Headache, nausea, vomiting, papilledema, cranial nerve palsies, seizures, coma	Leukemic infiltration of central nervous system
Abdominal discomfort	Generalized lymphadenopathy, hepatomegaly, splenomegaly due to leukemic cell infiltration
Increased vulnerability to infections	Immaturity of the white cells and ineffective immune function
Hematologic abnormalities	Physical and metabolic encroachment of leukemia cells on red blood cell and thrombocyte precursors
Anemia	
Thrombocytopenia	
Hyperuricemia and other metabolic disorders	Abnormal proliferation and metabolism of leukemic cells

*Manifestations vary with the type of leukemia.

ally >100,000/μL), leading to impaired circulation, presents as headache, confusion, and dyspnea. Once identified, this condition requires immediate and effective treatment, including leukapheresis (*i.e.,* removal of white blood cells) and chemotherapy.

Hyperuricemia occurs as the result of increased proliferation or increased purine breakdown secondary to leukemic cell death that results from chemotherapy. It may increase before and during treatment. Prophylactic therapy with allopurinol is routinely administered to prevent renal complications secondary to uric acid crystallization in the urine. Chemotherapy and selective irradiation (*e.g.,* CNS irradiation) are used in the treatment of acute leukemia. Chemotherapy includes induction therapy designed to elicit a remission, intensification therapy after a remission is achieved to reduce further the leukemic cell population, and maintenance therapy to maintain remission. Remission is defined as eradication of leukemic cells as detectable by conventional technology. Massive necrosis of malignant cells can occur during the initial phase of treatment. This phenomenon, known as *tumor lysis syndrome,* can lead to life-threatening metabolic disorders, including hyperkalemia, hyperphosphatemia, hyperuricemia, hypomagnesemia, hypocalcemia, and acidosis, with the potential for causing acute renal failure. Aggressive prophylactic hydration with alkaline solutions and administration of allopurinol to reduce uric acid levels are undertaken to counteract these effects.[14]

Bone marrow transplantation (BMT) from an identical twin (*i.e.,* syngeneic transplantation) or an HLA-matched sibling or unrelated donor (*i.e.,* allogeneic transplantation) has proved effective in treating ALL and AML. BMT usually is considered after the patient has achieved remission with the induction therapy. The BMT procedure involves first treating the recipient of the transplant with lethally high doses of chemotherapy alone or with irradiation (the conditioning regimen) to eliminate all the leukemic cells, followed by infusion of the bone marrow from the donor. Potential complications that can result from the conditioning regimen include gastrointestinal side effects such as nausea, vomiting, diarrhea, mucositis, and anorexia; hemorrhagic cystitis from high-dose cyclophosphamide, syndrome of inappropriate antidiuretic hormone from cyclophosphamide, tumor lysis syndrome, veno-occlusive disease, diffuse lung damage, and irreversible cardiac damage.[22]

A complication unique to allogeneic transplantation is graft-versus-host disease (see Chapter 19), in which the donor's immune system engrafts in the recipient and proceeds to recognize the recipient's tissues as foreign, subsequently mounting an immune response. Autologous (self) transplantation also has been used in the treatment of acute leukemia. In this approach, the leukemic patient's own bone marrow is collected during remission, cryopreserved, and then reinfused after treatment has destroyed all the leukemic cells. One of the problems with autologous BMT is the probable contamination of the bone marrow with leukemic cells. Various chemotherapeutic and immunologic agents have been used to eradicate residual tumor cells. One method under investigation involves purging the marrow with monoclonal antibodies that specifically bind to and destroy the leukemic cells.

Acute Lymphocytic Leukemia

Acute lymphocytic leukemia primarily strikes children and young adults, accounting for 80% of childhood acute leukemias. The peak incidence occurs at approximately 4 years of age. The French-American-British (FAB) group has developed a classification system for acute leukemias based on morphology and cytochemistry. Three types of acute lymphoid leukemias have been identified, L1, L2, and L3. L1, characterized by a small cell size, minimal cytoplasm with no granules, and rare nucleoli is the most common subtype in children. L2 is the most common subtype in adults (*i.e.*, 65% of adult ALL) and is characterized by larger cells, moderate amounts of cytoplasm, and prominent nucleoli. L3 is the Burkitt's or B-cell leukemia subtype and is associated with a poor prognosis when treated with standard ALL treatment protocols.[14]

Treatment of ALL usually consists of four phases, induction therapy; consolidation therapy; maintenance therapy, in which combination chemotherapy is administered; and CNS prophylaxis. Induction therapy usually consists of regimens of myeloid-sparing chemotherapeutic agents. Consolidation therapy consists of high doses of chemotherapy given to patients who have achieved remission with their induction therapy. Maintenance therapy usually is lower doses of chemotherapy given over a longer time (*e.g.*, 2 years) to patients after consolidation therapy. Because systemic chemotherapeutic agents cannot cross the blood-brain barrier and eradicate leukemic cells that have entered the CNS, CNS prophylaxis is administered concurrent with systemic chemotherapy.[14] The long-term effects of treatment on childhood cancer survivors are discussed in Chapter 8. Although CNS involvement is a major problem in children, the incidence in adults at the time of diagnosis is less than 10%.

ALL is one of the outstanding examples of a once-fatal disease that is now treatable and potentially curable with combination chemotherapy. Current chemotherapy regimens produce long-term survival in approximately 70% of children with ALL. Most recurrences are due to marrow relapse. Usually, a second complete response can be achieved in 70% to 90% of children with ALL of the B-lineage subtype and in 60% with the T-lineage subtype.[23] The prognosis for adults is more variable.

Acute Myelocytic Leukemia

Acute myelocytic leukemia, also called *acute nonlymphocytic leukemia,* is chiefly an adult disease, with more than 50% of cases occurring in patients older than 60 years of age. However, it also is seen in children and young adults. Complete remission rates for younger patients are higher than 70%, with 30% experiencing a prolonged disease-free survival. However, survival rates for the elderly seldom exceed 30% to 50%.[14]

Of all the leukemias, AML is most strongly linked with toxins and underlying congenital and hematologic disorders. It is the type of leukemia associated with Down syndrome and is the most frequent second cancer seen in persons who have been treated for other types of cancer.[24]

The AMLs are an extremely heterogeneous group of disorders. Some arise from the pluripotent stem cells in which myeloblasts predominate, and others arise from the monocyte-granulocyte precursor, which is the cell of origin for myelomonocytic leukemia. Based on the line of differentiation and the maturity of the cells, AMLs have been divided into seven subtypes in the widely used FAB classification system (Table 16-3). In addition to the common manifestations of acute leukemia (*e.g.*, fatigue, weight loss, fever, easy bruising), certain presentations are distinctive for the subtypes. Infiltration of malignant cells in the skin, gums, and other soft tissue is particularly common in the monocytic form (M5) of leukemia, whereas disseminated intravascular coagulation is a serious complication of promyelocytic leukemia (M3).

AML is treated with intensive chemotherapy to effect aplasia of the bone marrow. Treatment usually consists of induction therapy followed by intensive consolidations. During this period, supportive transfusion and antibiotic therapy often are needed. If remission is achieved, some type of continuing chemotherapy is used. In some cases, BMT may be performed. Chemotherapy induces complete remission in 70% of persons with AML, approximately one fourth of whom achieve long-term, disease-free survival or cure. In contrast to the treatment for ALL, several randomized trials have shown that prolonged maintenance therapy for AML is inferior to more intensive consolidation therapy.[14]

CHRONIC LEUKEMIAS

Chronic leukemias have a more insidious onset than acute leukemias and may be discovered during a routine medical examination by a blood count. CLL is a disorder of older adults. CML is predominantly a disorder of adults, but it can affect children as well.

Chronic Lymphocytic Leukemia

Mainly a disease of older persons, CLL typically follows a slow, chronic course. For these persons, reassurance that they can live a normal life for many years is important. Complications such as autoimmune thrombocytopenia and hemolytic anemia may be managed with corticosteroid treatment, or a splenectomy may be necessary. CLL is a disorder characterized by the proliferation and accumulation of relatively mature lymphocytes that are immunologically incompetent. The malignant cell lineage is predominantly the B lymphocyte in the United States and the T lymphocyte

TABLE 16-3 ✦ FAB Classification of Acute Myelogenous Leukemias

Class	Type of Leukemia	Percentage of AML
M0	Minimally differentiated AML	2–3
M1	AML without differentiation	20
M2	AML with maturation	30–40
M3	Acute promyelocytic leukemia	5–10
M4	Acute myelomonocytic leukemia	15–20
M5	Acute monocytic leukemia	10
M6	Acute erythroleukemia	5
M7	Acute megakaryoblastic leukemia	1

FAB, French-American-British; AML, acute myelocytic leukemia.
(Developed from information in Cotran R.S., Kumar V., Collins T. [1999] *Robbins pathologic basis of disease* [6th ed., p. 676]. Philadelphia: W.B. Saunders)

in Asia. Affected individuals initially experience fatigue and reduced exercise tolerance, enlargement of superficial lymph nodes, or splenomegaly. The onset of CLL is insidious, with approximately 25% of the cases diagnosed on a routine examination when enlarged lymph nodes are discovered. As the disease progresses, lymph nodes gradually increase in size and new nodes are involved, sometimes in unusual areas such as the scalp, orbit, pharynx, pleura, gastrointestinal tract, liver, prostate, and gonads. Severe fatigue, recurrent or persistent infections, pallor, edema, thrombophlebitis, and pain also are experienced. As the malignant cell population increases, the proportion of normal marrow precursors is reduced until only lymphocytes remain in the marrow.[21] The treatment of CLL is variable. Most early cases require no specific treatment. Indications for chemotherapy include progressive fatigue, troublesome lymphadenopathy, anemia, and thrombocytopenia.

Hairy cell leukemia (HCL), a rare leukemia of B-lymphocyte origin, is characterized by the presence of leukemic cells that have fine, hairlike cytoplasmic projections. It occurs mainly in older men. The most common physical finding is splenomegaly, which commonly is massive and may be the only presenting sign. Pancytopenia occurs from failure of the bone marrow, and splenic sequestration of cells is seen in more than 50% of cases. The course of the disease is chronic, and the median survival has been approximately 6 years. In the past, the treatment of choice was splenectomy, which has produced beneficial results in approximately two thirds of patients. This procedure raises the blood count and relieves symptoms in many persons. Interferon-α (IFN-α) produces responses in 67% to 90% of cases and has led to the disappearance of the disease for some time. Several new treatments demonstrate efficacy in the treatment of HCL. Pentostatin, a purine antimetabolite, produces complete responses in 60% to 90% of patients.[25] Cladribine, a purine analog, demonstrates efficacy in both HCL and an HCL variant.[26]

Chronic Myelocytic Leukemia

A myeloproliferative disorder, CML involves expansion of all bone marrow elements and accounts for 15% of all leukemias. The bone marrow cells from which CML is derived express the Philadelphia chromosome formed by the translocation between chromosomes 9 and 22. This translocation produces the BCR/ABL fusion gene from which a protein is made that has deregulated protein tyrosine kinase activity.[27,28] The deregulated tyrosine kinase activity is essential for malignant transformation. CML is divided into three stages: chronic or stable, accelerated, and acute or blast crisis. Early in the course, the clinical features are mild and nonspecific. CML usually progresses to a more aggressive phase within 30 to 40 months, at which time patients experience leukocytosis, weakness, splenomegaly, and weight loss.

The finding of abnormal blood counts on routine testing frequently leads to the diagnosis of CML. The most characteristic laboratory finding at presentation is leukocytosis with immature cell types in the peripheral blood. Anemia and, eventually, thrombocytopenia develop. Anemia causes weakness, easy fatigability, and exertional dys-

pnea. Splenomegaly is present in 50% of cases at the time of diagnosis; hepatomegaly is less common, and lymphadenopathy is relatively uncommon. Splenomegaly often causes a feeling of abdominal fullness and discomfort. Bleeding and easy bruising may arise from dysfunctional platelets.

Within an average of 3 to 4 years, most cases undergo transformation to the blast phase, which is heralded by the accelerated phase. During the accelerated phase, constitutional symptoms such as low-grade fever, night sweats, and weight loss develop because of rapid proliferation and hypermetabolism of the leukemic cells. Erratic fluctuations in white blood cell and platelet counts may accompany the accelerated phase. The blast crisis represents evolution to acute leukemia and is characterized by an increasing number of myeloid precursors, especially blast cells. Constitutional symptoms become more pronounced during this period, and splenomegaly may increase significantly. Isolated infiltrates of leukemic cells can involve the skin, lymph nodes, bones, and CNS. With very high blast counts (100,000/μL), symptoms of leukostasis may occur. The prognosis for patients who are in the blast crisis phase is poor, with survival averaging 2 to 4 months.

The treatment of chronic leukemia varies with the type of leukemic cell, the stage of the disease, other health problems, and the person's age. Often, the treatment is palliative. The median survival is 3 to 4 years, with fewer than 30% of persons living 5 years after diagnosis. Standard treatment for CML in the chronic phase has consisted of single-agent chemotherapy, producing remissions in 70% to 80% of patients. However, more than 90% of these patients continue to express Philadelphia chromosome–positive cells. During the blast crisis phase, combination therapy frequently used to treat AML is administered, although response rates are low (20% to 30%) and remissions vary from 2 to 12 months. Allogeneic BMT provides the only cure for CML, yielding a 5-year survival for 50% to 60% of patients. IFN-α has been evaluated in the treatment of the chronic phase of CML and has been found to produce complete responses in 50% to 75% of patients, with 20% to 40% exhibiting eradication of the Philadelphia chromosome.[29] However, treatment with IFN-α is limited because of side effects with resulting poor patient compliance. A novel therapy, STI571, has demonstrated significant activity in inhibiting BCR/ABL, thereby inhibiting the myeloid expansion that occurs with deregulation.[28]

In summary, leukemias are malignant neoplasms of the hematopoietic stem cells with diffuse replacement of bone marrow. Leukemias are classified according to cell type (*i.e.,* lymphocytic or myelocytic) and whether the disease is acute or chronic. The lymphocytic leukemias, most common in children, involve the lymphoid precursors that originate in bone marrow but infiltrate the spleen, lymph nodes, CNS, and other tissues. The myelocytic leukemias, which are seen more often in adults, involve the pluripotent myeloid stem cells in the bone marrow and interfere with the maturation of all blood cells, including granulocytes, erythrocytes, and thrombocytes. The warning signs and symptoms of acute leukemia are fatigue, paleness, weight loss, repeated infections, easy bruising, and nosebleeds and other hemorrhages. In children, these symptoms may appear suddenly.

Malignant Lymphomas

After you have completed this section of the chapter, you should be able to meet the following objectives:

✦ Compare the lymphoproliferative disorders associated with Hodgkin's disease and non-Hodgkin's lymphoma

✦ Contrast and compare the signs and symptoms of Hodgkin's disease and non-Hodgkin's lymphoma

The lymphomas, Hodgkin's disease and non-Hodgkin's lymphoma, represent malignant neoplasms of cells derived from lymphoid tissue (i.e., lymphocytes and histiocytes) and their precursors or derivatives.[7] The seventh most common cancer in the United States, the lymphomas are among the most studied human tumors and among the most curable.

HODGKIN'S DISEASE

Hodgkin's disease is a malignant neoplasm of the lymphatic structures. An English physician, Thomas Hodgkin, first described the disease in 1832. It was estimated that approximately 7400 new cases of Hodgkin's disease would be diagnosed in 2000, with 1400 deaths.[10] Distribution of the disease is bimodal; the incidence rises sharply after 10 years of age, peaks in the early 20s, and then declines until 50 years of age. After 50 years of age, the incidence again increases steadily with age. The younger adult group consists equally of men and women, but after age 50 years, the incidence is higher among men.[30] In 60% to 90% of persons with localized Hodgkin's disease, the possibility exists of a definitive cure, defined as normal life expectancy for the patient's age for 10 or more years after treatment.

The cause of Hodgkin's disease is unknown. There is a long-standing suspicion that the disease may begin as an inflammatory reaction to an infectious agent, possibly a virus. This belief is supported by epidemiologic data that include the clustering of the disease among family members and among students who have attended the same school. A suspected etiologic agent is EBV because a significant percentage of biopsy specimens have exhibited EBV DNA. In a number of studies that assessed the relationship between Hodgkin's disease and an infectious etiology, a threefold increased incidence of Hodgkin's disease was found in patients with a previous history of mononucleosis. Findings contradictory to the proposed viral hypothesis include an absence of occurrence in marital partners. There also seems to be an association between the presence of the disease and a deficient immune state. As with other forms of cancer, it is likely that no single agent is responsible for the development of Hodgkin's disease.

Manifestations

Hodgkin's disease is characterized by painless and progressive enlargement of a single node or group of nodes. It is believed to originate in one area of the lymphatic system, and if unchecked, it spreads throughout the lymphatic network. The initial lymph node involvement typically is above the level of the diaphragm, and the cervical chain or supraclavicular nodes most commonly are affected. An exception is in elderly persons, in whom the subdiaphragmatic lymph nodes may be the first to be involved. Involvement of the retroperitoneal lymph nodes, liver, spleen, and bone marrow occurs after the disease becomes generalized.

A distinctive tumor cell, called the *Reed-Sternberg cell,* is considered to be the true neoplastic element in Hodgkin's disease. The malignant proliferating cells may invade almost any area of the body and may produce a wide variety of signs and symptoms. The spleen is involved in one third of the cases at the time of diagnosis. A common symptom is the development of a progressive, painless, rubbery, lymph node enlargement that is predominantly found in the neck area in 60% to 80% of patients. Persons with Hodgkin's disease are commonly designated as stage A if they lack constitutional symptoms and stage B if significant weight loss, fever, or night sweats are present. Approximately 40% of persons with Hodgkin's disease exhibit the "B" symptoms.[30] Other symptoms such as fatigue, pruritus, and anemia are indicative of disease spread. In the advanced stages of Hodgkin's disease, liver, lungs, digestive tract, and, occasionally, the CNS may be involved. As the disease progresses, the rapid proliferation of abnormal lymphocytes leads to an immunologic defect, particularly in cell-mediated responses, rendering the person more susceptible to bacterial, viral, fungal, and protozoal infections. Neutrophilic leukocytosis and mild normocytic normochromic anemia are common. Eosinophilia also may occur. Leukopenia usually is a late manifestation. Hypergammaglobulinemia is common during the early stages of the disease, and hypogammaglobulinemia may develop in advanced disease.

Diagnosis and Treatment

A definitive diagnosis of Hodgkin's disease requires that the Reed-Sternberg cell be present in a biopsy specimen of lymph node tissue. The classic Reed-Sternberg cell is a binucleated cell with mirror-image nuclei that contain clear chromatin and a large eosinophilic nucleolus in each lobe (Fig. 16-2). Although the question of neoplastic lineage remains unclear, evidence suggests that the Reed-Sternberg cell is derived from the macrophage-monocyte line. This cell also may be found in other disorders, such as infectious mononucleosis.

Computed tomographic scans of the abdomen commonly are used in screening for involvement of abdominal and pelvic lymph nodes. Radiologic visualization of the abdominal and pelvic lymph structures can be achieved through the use of bipedal lymphangiography. In this diagnostic test, radiopaque dye is injected into the lymphatic channels of the lower leg, enabling visualization of the iliac and para-aortic nodes. Nuclear studies, such as a gallium scan in which the tumor takes up the radionuclide, or a stag-

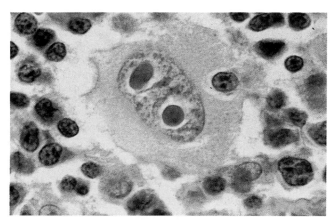

FIGURE 16-2 Classic Reed-Sternberg cell. Mirror-image nuclei contain large eosinophilic nucleoli. (Rubin E., Farber J.L. [1999]. *Pathology* [3rd ed., p. 1144]. Philadelphia: Lippincott Williams & Wilkins)

ing laparotomy to detect abdominal nodes and inspect the liver may be done.

The staging of Hodgkin's disease is of great clinical importance because the choice of treatment and the prognosis ultimately are related to the distribution of the disease. Staging is determined by the number of lymph nodes that are involved, whether the lymph nodes are on one or both sides of the diaphragm, and whether there is disseminated disease involving the bone marrow and liver. The Cotswold Classification, a modification of the frequently used Ann Arbor Classification of Hodgkin's Disease, includes extent of disease, location, bulk, and number of anatomic locations of involvement. Patients are designated stage A if they lack constitutional symptoms and stage B if they experience significant weight loss, fever, and night sweats.[30]

Irradiation and chemotherapy are used in treating the disease. Most patients with localized disease are treated with radiation therapy. As the accuracy of staging techniques, delivery of radiation, and curative efficacy of combination chemotherapy regimens have improved, the survival of patients with Hodgkin's disease also has improved. Nonetheless, long-term survivors of Hodgkin's disease are at increased risk of dying from cardiac disease caused primarily by mediastinal radiation, infections resulting from immunosuppressive chemotherapy and intensive irradiation, and secondary malignancies caused by the use of alkylating chemotherapy agents used in the chemotherapy protocols. These risks have prompted the development of clinical trials to evaluate the reduction of aggressive therapy with the intent of decreasing the risk of long-term complications.[30]

NON-HODGKIN'S LYMPHOMAS

The non-Hodgkin's lymphomas are a heterogeneous group of neoplastic disorders of the lymphoid tissue, usually the lymph nodes. Unlike Hodgkin's disease, which initially is localized to a single group of lymph nodes, the non-Hodgkin's lymphomas typically are multicentric in origin and spread early to various tissues throughout the body, especially the liver, spleen, and bone marrow. Non-Hodgkin's lymphomas occur three times more frequently than Hodgkin's disease. In 2000, approximately 54,900 new cases were diagnosed in the United States, and approximately 26,100 deaths resulted from these disorders.[10] Non-Hodgkin's lymphoma is the fifth most common malignancy, and its incidence and mortality rates have increased considerably during the last several decades.[31]

A viral cause is suspected in at least some of the lymphomas. Cell cultures and immunologic studies of one type of lymphoma, Burkitt's lymphoma, which is found in some parts of Africa, have implicated EBV without proving a causal association. Serologic studies also have demonstrated an association between the human T-lymphotropic retrovirus types I and II and T-cell leukemia or lymphoma. Non-Hodgkin's lymphomas also are seen with increased frequency in persons with acquired immunodeficiency syndrome, in those who have received chronic immunosuppressive therapy after kidney or liver transplantation, and in individuals with acquired or congenital immunodeficiencies. An association between hepatitis C virus and the incidence of non-Hodgkin's lymphoma is inconclusive.[31]

As tumors of the immune system, non-Hodgkin's lymphomas may originate from B cells (70% to 80%), T cells, or histiocytes (*i.e.,* macrophage-monocytes). Histiocytic forms of lymphoma are rare, accounting for less than 1% of cases. Non-Hodgkin's lymphomas commonly are divided into three groups, depending on the grade of the tumor: low-grade lymphomas, which are predominantly B-cell tumors; intermediate-grade lymphomas, which include B-cell and some T-cell lymphomas; and high-grade lymphomas, which are largely immunoblastic (B-cell), lymphoblastic (T-cell), Burkitt's, and non-Burkitt's lymphomas.

Manifestations

The signs and symptoms of non-Hodgkin's lymphomas are similar to those of Hodgkin's disease. The most frequently occurring clinical manifestations in Hodgkin's and non-Hodgkin's lymphoma are painless, superficial lymphadenopathy. Differences between the two conditions include the noncontiguous nodal spread of the disease, more common extranodal disease, more frequent involvement of the gastrointestinal tract, liver, testes, and bone marrow, and less frequent involvement of the mediastinum in non-Hodgkin's lymphoma as compared to Hodgkin's disease. The "B" symptoms are less common in non-Hodgkin's lymphoma.

The most frequently occurring clinical manifestation in persons with low-grade non-Hodgkin's lymphoma is a painless, superficial lymphadenopathy that may be isolated or widespread. Involved lymph nodes may be present in the retroperitoneum, mesentery, and pelvis. The low-grade lymphomas are often disseminated at the time of diagnosis and involvement of the bone marrow is frequent. Persons with intermediate or high-grade lymphomas may present with rapidly enlarging lymph node masses or with constitutional symptoms such as fever, drenching night sweats, or weight loss. Extranodal involvement is common and can include the gastrointestinal tract, skin, bone marrow, and central nervous system. Lymph node masses may cause lymphedema, ureteral obstruction, or vascular obstructions. Persons with Burkitt's lymphoma frequently present with abdominal pain or abdominal fullness because of the predilection of the disease for the abdomen.

Leukemic transformation with high peripheral lymphocytic counts occurs in approximately 13% of persons with non-Hodgkin's lymphoma. Patients have increased susceptibility to bacterial, viral, and fungal infections associated with hypogammaglobulinemia and a poor humoral antibody response, rather than the impaired cellular immunity seen with Hodgkin's disease.

Diagnosis and Treatment

As with Hodgkin's disease, a lymph node biopsy is used to confirm the diagnosis. Bone marrow biopsy, blood studies, abdominal computed tomographic scans, and nuclear medicine studies often are used to determine the stage of the disease.

For early-stage disease, radiation therapy is used as a single treatment. However, because most persons present with late-stage disease, combination chemotherapy, combined adjuvant radiation therapy, or both are recommended. Combination regimens frequently include aggressive multiple chemotherapy agents that result in a variety of distressing symptoms such as nausea, vomiting, infection, and alopecia. For rapidly progressive intermediate- or high-grade lymphoma, CNS prophylaxis is achieved with high doses of chemotherapeutic agents that can cross the blood-brain barrier such as methotrexate, intrathecal chemotherapy (administered by spinal tap), or cranial irradiation. The standard treatment for non-Hodgkin's lymphoma continues to be a combination of cyclophosphamide, doxorubicin, vincristine, and prednisone (CHOP). The anti-CD20 antibody, rituximab, is undergoing evaluation as an added therapeutic benefit to the standard CHOP therapy for its ability to convert the bcl2D2/Ig translocation from positive to negative.[32]

A radioimmunotherapy using iodine-131 tositumomab, which targets CD20, also has demonstrated early efficacy in producing frequent and durable responses in patients with B-cell non-Hodgkin's lymphoma.[33]

Bone marrow and peripheral stem cell transplantation are being investigated as potentially curative treatment modalities in patients with highly resistant disease. These treatments have been found to produce increases in disease-free survival rates, with complete remission rates of 60%.[34,35]

In summary, the lymphomas, Hodgkin's disease and non-Hodgkin's lymphoma, represent malignant neoplasms of cells native to lymphoid tissue (*i.e.,* lymphocytes and histiocytes) and their precursors or derivatives. They are among the best studied human tumors and among the most curable. Hodgkin's disease is characterized by painless and progressive enlargement of a single node or group of nodes. It is believed to originate in one area of the lymphatic system and, if unchecked, spreads throughout the lymphatic network. Non-Hodgkin's lymphomas are a group of neoplastic disorders of the lymphoid tissue, usually the lymph nodes. Unlike Hodgkin's disease, which initially is localized to a single group of lymph nodes, most non-Hodgkin's lymphomas are multicentric in origin and spread early to various tissues throughout the body, especially the liver, spleen, and bone marrow.

Multiple Myeloma

After you have completed this section of the chapter, you should be able to meet the following objectives:

✦ Describe the lymphoproliferative disorder that occurs with multiple myeloma
✦ Explain the origin of the Bence Jones protein that appears in the urine of a patient with multiple myeloma

Multiple myeloma is a plasma cell cancer of the osseous tissue and accounts for 10% to 15% of all hematologic malignancies. In the course of its dissemination, it also may involve nonosseous sites. It is characterized by the uncontrolled proliferation of an abnormal clone of plasma cells, which secrete primarily IgG or IgA. In 2000, approximately 13,600 new cases were diagnosed and more than 11,200 deaths resulted from this disease in the United States.[10] Fewer than 3% of cases occur before the age of 40 years, with the median age of patients with multiple myeloma being 65 years. The cause of multiple myeloma is unknown, but several risk factors have been associated with the disease. Occupational exposure to iron compounds, metal, aluminum, petroleum, welding fumes; exposure to high- and low-dose ionizing radiation; recurrent infections; and drug allergies have all been associated with its pathogenesis.[36]

In multiple myeloma, there is an atypical proliferation of one of the immunoglobulins, called the *M protein*, a monoclonal antibody. Although there is an abundance of immunoglobulin, it is not effective in maintaining humoral immunity. Myeloma cells secrete osteoclast-activating factors that stimulate the proliferation and activation of osteoclasts and lead to bone destruction and resorption (Fig. 16-3). This increased bone resorption predisposes the individual to pathologic fractures and hypercalcemia. Paraproteins secreted by the plasma cells may cause a hyperviscosity of body fluids and may break down into amyloid, a proteinaceous substance deposited between cells, causing heart failure and neuropathy. In some forms of multiple myeloma, the plasma cells produce only Bence Jones proteins, abnormal proteins that consist of the light chains of the immunoglobulin molecule. Because of their low molecular weight, Bence Jones proteins are partially excreted in the urine. Many of these abnormal proteins are directly toxic to renal tubular structures, which may lead to tubular destruction and, eventually, to renal failure. The malignant plasma cells also can form tumors (*i.e.,* plasmacytomas) that have a tendency to cause spinal cord compression.

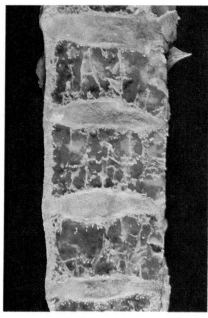

FIGURE 16-3 Multiple myeloma. Multiple lytic lesions of the vertebrae are present. (Rubin E., Farber J.L. [1999]. *Pathology* [3rd ed., p. 1148]. Philadelphia: Lippincott Williams & Wilkins)

Dysregulation of several oncogenes and tumor suppressor genes contributes to the pathogenesis of multiple myeloma. The retinoblastoma (RB) gene, p53 tumor suppressor gene, P21/Ras, bcl-2 proto-oncogene, and C-myc mutations are associated with disturbances in cellular proliferation, growth arrest, and apoptosis (see Chapter 8).[36]

Bone pain is one of the first symptoms to occur and one of the most common, occurring in approximately 80% of all individuals diagnosed with multiple myeloma. Bone destruction also impairs the production of erythrocytes and leukocytes and predisposes the patient to anemia and recurrent infections. Many patients experience weight loss and weakness. Renal insufficiency occurs in 50% of patients. Neurologic manifestations caused by neuropathy or spinal cord compression also may be present.

Although numerous treatments for multiple myeloma have been attempted since the early 1970s, the results have been disappointing. With standard chemotherapy, the median survival may reach 2 to 3 years. Multiple myeloma is a radiosensitive disease, but most radiation therapy is used primarily for palliation, specifically to treat lytic bone lesions and compression fractures and to decrease pain. IFN-α has produced response rates of 15% when used alone and 68% when used with chemotherapy. Some investigators discourage the use of IFN-α because it has been found in vitro to stimulate myeloma cells by inducing the autocrine production of IL-6. Syngeneic, allogeneic, or autologous BMT has produced complete remission rates of 50% to 60%, but 5-year survival rates are predicted to be approximately 40% to 50%. Melphalan-based conditioning regimens followed by peripheral stem cell transplantation have shown efficacy in producing 5-year complete response rates up to 52%.[37] Donor lymphocyte infusions administered to patients after

allogeneic peripheral stem cell transplantation is another novel treatment approach that produces a T-cell and natural killer cell alloimmune reaction leading to a graft-versus-myeloma response.[38]

In summary, multiple myeloma results in the uncontrolled proliferation of immunoglobulin-secreting plasma cells, usually a single clone of IgG- or IgA-producing cells, that results in increased bone resorption, leading to pathologic bone lesions.

Related Web Sites

American Bone Marrow Registry   www.abmdr.org
National Cancer Institute   www.nci.nih.gov
American Cancer Society   www.cancer.org
American Society of Hematology   www.hematology.org
National Marrow Donor Program   www.marrow.org

References

1. Delves P.J., Roitt I.M. (2000). The immune system. *Advances in Immunology* 343, 37–49.
2. Bagby G.C., Jr., Heinrich M.C. (1999). Cytokines, growth factors and hematopoiesis. In Wingard J.R., Demetri G.D. (Eds.), *Clinical applications of cytokines and growth factors* (pp. 2–55). Norwell, MA: Kluwer Academic Publishers.
3. Abbas A.K., Lichtman A.H., Pober J.S. (Eds.). (1994). Cytokines. In *Cellular and molecular immunology* (2nd ed., pp. 240–260). Philadelphia: W.B. Saunders.
4. Curnutte J.T., Coates T.D. (2000). Disorders of phagocyte function and number. In Hoffman R., Benz E.K., Shattil S.J., Furie B., Cohen H.J., Silberstein L.E., McGlave P. (Eds.), *Hematology: Basic principles and practice* (3rd ed., pp. 720–762). New York: Churchill Livingstone.
5. Sullivan J.L. (2000). Infectious mononucleosis and other Epstein-Barr virus-associated diseases. In Hoffman R., Benz E.K., Shattil S.J., Furie B., Cohen H.J., Silberstein L.E., McGlave P. (Eds.), *Hematology: Basic principles and practice* (3rd ed., pp. 812–821). New York: Churchill Livingstone.
6. Schooley R.T. (1994). Epstein-Barr virus infections, including infectious mononucleosis. In Isselbacher K.J., Braunwald E., Wilson J.D., Martin J.B., Fauci A.S., Kasper D.L. (Eds.), *Harrison's principles of internal medicine* (2nd ed., pp. 790–793). New York: McGraw-Hill.
7. Cotran R.S., Kumar V., Robbins S.L. (Eds.). (1994). Diseases of white cells, lymph nodes, and spleen. In *Pathologic basis of disease* (5th ed., pp. 629–672). Philadelphia: W.B. Saunders.
8. Godshall S.E., Krichner J.T. (2000). Infectious mononucleosis: Complexities of a common syndrome. *Postgraduate Medicine* 107, 175–186.
9. Torre D., Tambini R. (1999). Acyclovir for treatment of infectious mononucleosis: A meta-analysis. *Scandinavian Journal of Infectious Diseases* 31, 543–547.
10. Greenlee R.T., Murray T., Bolden S., Wingo P.A. (2000). Cancer statistics, 2000. *CA: A Cancer Journal for Clinicians, 50,* 7–33.
11. Khouri I., Sanchez F.G., Deisseroth A. (1997). Leukemias. In DeVita V.T., Hellman S., Rosenberg S.A. (Eds.), *Cancer: Principles and practice of oncology* (5th ed., pp. 2285–2293). Philadelphia: Lippincott-Raven.
12. Pui C.H. (1995). Childhood leukemias. *New England Journal of Medicine* 332, 1618–1630.

13. Jablon S., Kato H. (1972). Studies of the mortality of A-bomb survivors. *Radiation Research* 50, 649–698.

14. Scheinberg D.A., Maslak P., Weiss M. (1997). Acute leukemias. In DeVita V.T., Hellman S., Rosenberg S.A. (Eds.), *Cancer: Principles and practice of oncology* (5th ed., pp. 2293–2321). Philadelphia: Lippincott-Raven.

15. Kaldor J.M., Day N.E., Clarke E.A., Pettersson F., Clarke E.A., Pederson D., Mehnert W., et al. (1990). Leukemia following Hodgkin's disease. *New England Journal of Medicine* 322, 1–6.

16. Boise J.D., Greene M.H., Killen I.Y., Ellenberg S.S., Keehn R.J., McFadden E., et al. (1983). Leukemia and preleukemia after adjuvant treatment of gastrointestinal cancer with semustine. *New England Journal of Medicine* 309, 1079–1084.

17. Collman C.A., Dahlberg S. (1990). Treatment-related leukemia. *New England Journal of Medicine* 322, 52–53.

18. Pui C., Behm F.G., Raimondi S. (1989). Secondary acute myeloid leukemia in children treated for acute lymphoid leukemia. *New England Journal of Medicine* 321, 136–142.

19. Negalia J.P., Meadows A.T., Robison L.L. (1991). Secondary neoplasms after acute lymphoblastic leukemia in children. *New England Journal of Medicine* 325, 1330–1336.

20. Thijsen S.F.T., Schuurhuis G.J., van Oostveen J.W., Ossenkippele G.J. (1999). Chronic myeloid leukemia from basics to bedside. *Leukemia* 13, 1646–1674.

21. Callaghan M.E. (1996). Leukemia. In McCorkle R., Grant M., Frank-Stromborg M., Baird S. B. (Eds.), *Cancer nursing: A comprehensive textbook* (2nd ed., pp. 752–771). Philadelphia: W.B. Saunders.

22. Horowitz M.M., Howe C.W.S. (2000). Bone marrow transplantation using unrelated donors. In Armitage J.O., Antman K.H. (Eds.), *High-dose cancer therapy: Pharmacology, hematopoietins, stem cells* (3rd ed., pp. 221–242). Philadelphia: Lippincott Williams & Wilkins.

23. Silverman L.B., Billett A.L. (2000). High-dose therapy in acute lymphoblastic leukemia. In Armitage J.O., Antman K.H. (Eds.), *High-dose cancer therapy: Pharmacology, hematopoietins, stem cells.* (3rd ed., pp. 691–703). Philadelphia: Lippincott Williams & Wilkins.

24. Mitus A.J., Rosenthal D.S. (1991). Adult leukemias. In Hollieb A.L., Fink D.J., Murphy G. (Eds.), *American Cancer Society textbook of clinical oncology* (pp. 410–432). Atlanta: American Cancer Society.

25. Kraut E.H. (2000). Phase II trials of pentostatin (Nipent) in hairy cell leukemia. *Seminars in Oncology* 27 (Suppl. 5), 27–31.

26. Tetreault S.A., Robbins B.A., Saven A. (1999). Treatment of hairy cell leukemia-variant with cladribine. *Leukemia and Lymphoma* 35, 347–354.

27. Weisberg E., Griffin J.D. (2000). Mechanism of resistance to the ABL tyrosine kinase inhibitor STI571 in BCR/ABL-transformed hematopoietic cell lines. *Blood* 95, 3498–3505.

28. Marley S.B., Deininger M.W.N., Davidson R.J., Goldman J.M., Gordon M.Y. (2000). The tyrosine kinase inhibitor STI571, like interferon-α, preferentially reduces the capacity for amplification of granulocyte-macrophage progenitors from patients with chronic myeloid leukemia. *Experimental Hematology* 28, 551–557.

29. Carson C. (1996). Hodgkin's disease and non-Hodgkin's lymphomas. In McCorkle R., Grant M., Frank-Stromborg M., Baird S.B. (Eds.), *Cancer nursing: A comprehensive textbook* (2nd ed., pp. 729–751). Philadelphia: W.B. Saunders.

30. DeVita V.T., Mauch P.M., Harris N.L. (1997). Hodgkin's disease. In DeVita V.T., Hellman S., Rosenberg S.A. (Eds.), *Cancer: Principles and practice of oncology* (5th ed., pp. 2242–2283). Philadelphia: Lippincott-Raven.

31. Groves F.D., Linet M.S., Travis L.B., Devesa S.S. (2000). Cancer surveillance series: Non-Hodgkin's lymphoma incidence by histologic subtype in the United States from 1978 through 1995. *Journal of the National Cancer Institute* 92, 1240–1251.

32. Vose J.M., Link B.K., Grossbard M.L., Czuczman M., Grillo-Lopez A., Gilman P., Lowe A., Kunkel L.A., Fisher R.I. (2000). Phase II study of rituximab in combination with CHOP chemotherapy in patients with previously untreated, aggressive non-Hodgkin's lymphoma. *Journal of Clinical Oncology* 19, 389–397.

33. Kaminski M.S., Estes J., Zasadny K.R., Francis I.R., Ross C.W., Tuck M., Regan D., Fisher S., Gutierrez J., Kroll S., Stagg R., Tidmarsh G., Wahl R.L. (2000). Radio-immunotherapy with iodine 131 tositumomab for relapse or refractory B-cell non-Hodgkin lymphoma: Updated results and long-term follow-up of the University of Michigan experience. *Blood* 96, 1259–1266.

34. Keating A. (2000). Autologous bone marrow transplantation. In Armitage J.O., Antman K.H. (Eds.), *High-dose cancer therapy: Pharmacology, hematopoietins, stem cells* (3rd ed., pp. 243–272), Philadelphia: Lippincott Williams & Wilkins.

35. Chakraverty R.K., Goldstone A.H., McMillan A.K., Chopra R. (2000). High-dose therapy for the treatment of non-Hodgkin's lymphoma. In Armitage J.O., Antman K.H. (Eds.), *High-dose cancer therapy: Pharmacology, hematopoietins, stem cells* (3rd ed., pp. 779–795), Philadelphia: Lippincott Williams & Wilkins.

36. Triko G. (2000). Multiple myeloma and other plasma cell disorders. In Hoffman R., Benz E.K., Shattil S.J., Furie B., Cohen H.J., Silberstein L.E., McGlave P. (Eds.), *Hematology: Basic principles and practice* (3rd ed., pp. 1398–1416). New York: Churchill Livingstone.

37. Deskian R., Barlogie B., Sawyer J., Ayers D., Triscot G., Badros A., et al. (2000). Results of high-dose therapy for 1000 patients with multiple myeloma: Durable complete remissions and superior survival in the absence of chromosome 13 abnormalities. *Blood* 95, 4008–4010.

38. Lokhorst H.M., Schattenberg A., Cornelissen J.J., Van Oers M.H., Fibbe W., Russell I., et al. (2000). Donor lymphocyte infusions for relapsed multiple myeloma after allogeneic stem-cell transplantation: Predictive factors for response and long-term outcome. *Journal of Clinical Oncology* 18, 3031–3037.

Infection, Immunity, and Inflammation

The quest to understand the mechanism of disease and ways to prevent it permeates humankind's history. Many civilizations contributed to the storehouse of knowledge. Among the early accomplishments of the Chinese are a number of practices they developed to prevent disease, one of which took the form of inoculation.

The deadly smallpox had been one of the world's most dreaded diseases. During the Middle Ages, epidemics were frequent; they swept across Asia and other parts of the world, leaving widespread death in their wake. In the 1400s, the Chinese created a technique to protect themselves during an epidemic. They collected the crusts of smallpox sores and allowed them to dry. The dried material was ground into powder and inhaled. The procedure was found to be hazardous, but it remains one of the first attempts at vaccination.

Chapter 17

Mechanisms of Infectious Disease

W. Michael Dunne, Jr.

All living creatures share two basic objectives in life—survival and reproduction. This tenet applies equally to humans and to members of the microbial world, including bacteria, viruses, fungi, and protozoa. To satisfy these goals, organisms must extract from the environment nutrients essential for growth and proliferation; for countless microscopic organisms, that environment is the human body. Normally, the contact between humans and microorganisms is incidental and, in certain situations, may actually benefit both organisms. Under extraordinary circumstances, however, the invasion of the human body by microorganisms can produce harmful and potentially lethal consequences. The consequences of these invasions are collectively called *infectious diseases*.

Infectious Disease

After you have completed this section of the chapter, you should be able to meet the following objectives:

✦ Define the terms *host, infectious disease, colonization, microflora, virulence, pathogen,* and *saprophyte*
✦ Describe the concept of host–microorganism interaction using the concepts of commensalism, mutualism, and parasitic relationships

✦ Describe the structural characteristics and mechanisms of reproduction for prions, viruses, bacteria, rickettsiae, chlamydiae, fungi, and parasites

TERMINOLOGY

All scientific disciplines evolve with a distinct vocabulary, and the study of infectious diseases is no exception. The most appropriate way to approach this subject is with a brief discussion of the terminology used to characterize interactions between humans and microbes.

Any organism capable of supporting the nutritional and physical growth requirements of another is called a *host*. Throughout this chapter, the term *host* most often refers to humans supporting the growth of microorganisms. The term *infection* describes the presence and multiplication of a living organism on or in the host. Occasionally, the terms *infection* and *colonization* are used interchangeably.

One common misconception should be dispelled: not all interactions between microorganisms and humans are detrimental. The internal and external exposed surfaces of the human body are normally and harmlessly inhabited by a multitude of bacteria, collectively referred to as the *normal microflora* (Table 17-1). Although the colonizing bacteria acquire nutrition and shelter, the host is not adversely affected by the relationship. An interaction such as this is

TABLE 17-1 ◆ Location and Variety of Nonpathogenic Normal Human Microflora

Area	Sites	Bacteria	
		Gram-positive	Gram-negative
Upper respiratory tract	Mouth, nose	+++	+++
	Nasopharynx	(Aerobes and anaerobes)	Aerobes and anaerobes)
	Throat		
Lower respiratory tract	Larynx	0	0
	Trachea	0	0
	Lungs	0	0
External surfaces	Skin	++++	+
	Outer ear	(Aerobes and anaerobes)	(Transient)
	Eyes		0
Upper gastrointestinal tract	Stomach	+	+
	Duodenum	(Transient)	(Transient)
	Esophagus	0	0
	Jejunum	0	0
Lower gastrointestinal tract	Ileum	+++	++++
	Colon	(Predominantly anaerobes)	(Predominantly anaerobes)
External genitourinary tract	Vagina	++	++
	Anterior urethra	0	0
Internal genitourinary tract	Cervix, ovaries	0	0
	Fallopian tubes	0	0
	Uterus, prostate	0	0
	Bladder, kidney	0	0
	Testes, epididymis	0	0
Body fluids	Blood, urine	0	0
	Spinal fluid	0	0
	Synovial fluid	0	0
	Peritoneal fluid	0	0

Key: 0, none; +, rare; ++, few; +++, moderate; ++++, many.

called *commensalism* and the colonizing microorganisms are sometimes referred to as *commensal flora*. The term *mutualism* is applied to an infection in which the microorganism and the host derive benefits from the interaction. For example, certain inhabitants of the human intestinal tract extract nutrients from the host and secrete essential vitamin by products of metabolism (*e.g.*, vitamin K), which are absorbed and used by the host. A parasitic relationship is one in which only the infecting organism benefits from the relationship. If the host sustains injury or pathologic damage in response to a parasitic infection, the process is called an *infectious disease*.

The severity of an infectious disease can range from mild to life threatening, depending on many variables, including the health of the host at the time of infection and the *virulence* (disease-producing potential) of the microorganism. A select group of microorganisms called *pathogens* are so virulent that they rarely are found in the absence of disease. Fortunately, there are few human pathogens in the microbial world. Most microorganisms are harmless *saprophytes*, which are free-living organisms that grow on dead or decaying organic material in the environment. All microorganisms, even saprophytes and members of the normal flora, can be *opportunistic pathogens*, capable of producing an infectious disease when the health and immunity of the host have been severely weakened by illness, famine, or medical therapy.

AGENTS OF INFECTIOUS DISEASE

The agents of infectious disease include prions, viruses, bacteria, rickettsiae, chlamydiae, fungi, and parasites.

Prions

Can a protein alone cause a transmissable infectious disease? Until recently, microbiologists have always assumed that all infectious agents must possess a genetic master plan (a genome of either RNA or DNA) to code for production of the essential proteins and enzymes that are necessary for survival and reproduction. Prions, protein particles that lack any kind of demonstrable genome, appear to be an exception to this rule because they are infectious and capable of duplication. A number of prion-associated diseases have been identified, the most famous of which include Creutzfeld-Jakob disease and kuru in humans and scrapie and bovine spongiform encephalopathy, or mad cow disease, in animals.

Mycobacteria	Parasites	Mycoplasmas	Fungi	Chlamydia/Rickettsia	Spirochetes
+	+	+	+	0	+
0	(Protozoans)	0	(Yeast)	0	0
0	0	0	0	0	0
0	0	0	0	0	0
0	0	0	0	0	0
+	0	0	+	0	0
0	0	0	(Yeast)	0	0
0	0	0	0	0	0
+	0	0	0	0	0
(Transient)					
0	0	0	0	0	0
0					
+	+	0	+	0	+
0	(Protozoans)	0	(Yeast)	0	0
0	0	+	+	0	0
0	0	0	(Yeast)	0	0
0	0	0	0	0	0
0	0	0	0	0	0
0	0	0	0	0	0
0	0	0	0	0	0
0	0	0	0	0	0
0	0	0	0	0	0
0	0	0	0	0	0
0	0	0	0	0	0

The various prion-associated diseases produce very similar symptoms and pathologies in the host and are collectively called *transmissable neurodegenerative diseases*. All are characterized by a slowly progressive, neuronal, non-inflammatory degeneration leading to loss of coordination (ataxia), dementia, and death over a period ranging from months to years. In fact, recent studies indicate that *prion proteins* (called *PrP*SC) actually are altered or mutated forms of a normal host protein called *PrP*C. The mutated protein accumulates to a high concentration in neurons, leading to a toxic condition and cell death.

Studies of the transmission of prion disease in animals clearly demonstrate that prions replicate, leading researchers to question how proteins can reproduce in the absence of genetic material. One theory proposes that the interaction between a normal PrPC and an abnormal PrPSC leads to a structural change in the normal protein, resulting in two PrPSC molecules. PrPSC then accumulates and spreads in the axons of the nerve cells, causing progressively greater damage to host neurons and the eventual incapacitation of the host. Because prions lack reproductive and metabolic functions, current antibacterial and antiviral agents are useless against them.

Viruses

Viruses are the smallest obligate intracellular pathogens. They are incapable of replication outside of a living cell. They have no organized cellular structures, but instead consist of a protein coat, or capsid, surrounding a nucleic acid core, or genome, of RNA or DNA—never both (Fig. 17-1). Some viruses are enclosed in a lipoprotein envelope derived from the cytoplasmic membrane of the parasitized host cell. Certain viruses are continuously shed from the infected cell surface enveloped in buds pinched from the cytoplasmic membrane. Enveloped viruses include members of the herpesvirus group and paramyxoviruses, such as influenza virus.

Viruses must penetrate a susceptible living cell and use the biosynthetic machinery of the cell to produce viral progeny. The process of viral replication is shown in Figure 17-2. Not all viral agents cause lysis and death of the host cell during the course of replication. Some viruses enter the host cell and insert their genome into the host cell chromosome, where the genome remains in a latent, nonreplicating state for long periods without causing disease. Under the appropriate stimulation, the virus undergoes active replication and produces symptoms of disease months to years later.

Agents of Infectious Disease

➤ The agents of infectious disease represent a diversity of microorganisms that are not visible to the human eye.

➤ Microorganisms can be separated into eukaryotes (fungi) organisms containing a membrane-bound nucleus, and prokaryotes (bacteria), organisms in which the nucleus is not separated.

➤ Eukaryotes and prokaryotes are organisms because they contain all the enzymes required for their replication and possess all the biologic equipment necessary for exploiting metabolic energy.

➤ Viruses, which are the smallest pathogens, have no organized cellular structure, but consist of protein coat surrounding a nucleic acid core of DNA or RNA. Unlike eukaryotes and prokaryotes, viruses are incapable of replication outside of a living cell.

➤ Parasites (protozoa, helminths, and arthropods) are members of the animal kingdom that infect and cause disease in other animals, which then transmit them to humans.

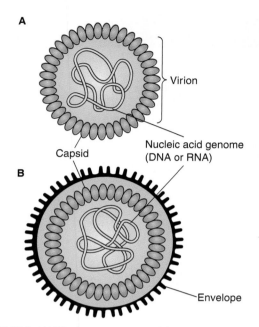

FIGURE 17-1 (**A**) The basic structure of a virus includes a protein coat surrounding an inner core of nucleic acid (DNA or RNA). (**B**) Some viruses may also be enclosed in a lipoprotein outer envelope.

Members of the herpesvirus group and adenovirus are the best examples of latent viruses. Herpesviruses include the viral agents of chickenpox and herpes zoster (shingles), genital herpes, cytomegalovirus infections, infectious mononucleosis, fever blisters, and possibly Kaposi's sarcoma. In each of these, the resumption of the latent viral replication may produce symptoms of primary disease (*e.g.*, genital herpes) or cause an entirely different symptomatology (*e.g.*, shingles instead of chickenpox).

Since the early 1980s, members of the retrovirus group have received considerable attention after identification of the human immunodeficiency virus (HIV) as the causative agent of acquired immunodeficiency syndrome (AIDS). The retroviruses have a unique mechanism of replication. After entry into the host cell, the viral RNA genome is first translated into DNA by a viral enzyme called *reverse transcriptase*. The viral DNA copy is integrated into the host chromosome and exists in a latent state, similar to the herpesviruses. Reactivation and replication require a reversal of the entire process. Some retroviruses lyse the host cell during the process of replication. In the case of HIV, the infected cells regulate the immunologic defense system of the host and

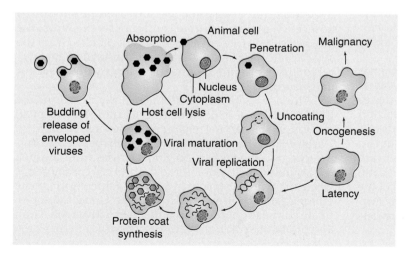

FIGURE 17-2 Schematic representation of the many possible consequences of viral infection of host cells, including cell lysis (poliovirus), continuous release of budding viral particles, or latency (herpesviruses) and oncogenesis (papovaviruses).

their lysis leads to a permanent suppression of the immune response.

In addition to causing infectious diseases, certain viruses also have the ability to transform normal host cells into malignant cells during the replication cycle. This group of viruses is referred to as *oncogenic* and includes certain retroviruses and DNA viruses, such as the herpesviruses, adenoviruses, and papovaviruses.

The viruses of humans and animals have been categorized somewhat arbitrarily according to various characteristics, including the type of viral genome (single-stranded or double-stranded DNA or RNA), the mechanism of replication (*e.g.*, retroviruses), the mode of transmission (*e.g.*, arthropod-borne viruses, enteroviruses), and the type of disease produced (*e.g.*, hepatitis A, B, C, D, and E viruses), to name just a few.

Bacteria

Bacteria are autonomously replicating unicellular organisms known as *prokaryotes* because they lack an organized nucleus. Compared with nucleated eukaryotic cells (see Chapter 4), the bacterial cell is small and its structure relatively primitive (Fig. 17-3). Bacteria approximate the size of the eukaryotic mitochondria (approximately 1 μm in diameter) and may be the evolutionary ancestors of mitochondria.

Bacteria usually have no organized intracellular organelles, and the genome consists of only a single chromosome of DNA. Many bacteria transiently harbor smaller extrachromosomal pieces of circular DNA called *plasmids*. Occasionally, plasmids contain genetic information that increases the virulence of the organism. Similar to eukaryotic cells, but unlike viruses, bacteria contain DNA and RNA.

The prokaryotic cell is organized into an internal compartment called the *cytoplasm*, which contains the reproductive and metabolic machinery of the cell (Fig. 17-4). The cytoplasm is surrounded by a flexible lipid membrane, called the *cytoplasmic membrane*, which is enclosed in a rigid cell wall. The structure and synthesis of the cell wall determine whether the microscopic shape of the bacterium is spherical (cocci), helical (spirilla), or elongate (bacilli). Most bacteria produce a cell wall composed of a distinctive polymer known as *peptidoglycan*. This polymer is produced only by prokaryotes and is therefore an ideal target for antibacterial therapy. Several bacteria synthesize an extracellular capsule composed of protein or carbohydrate. The capsule protects the organism from environmental hazards such as the immunologic defenses of the host.

Certain bacteria are motile as the result of external whip-like appendages called *flagella*. The rotary action of the flagella transports the organism through a liquid environment

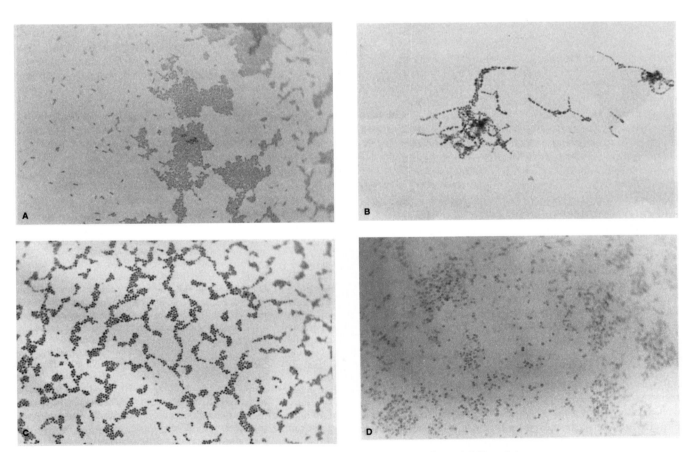

FIGURE 17-3 A sampling of the microscopic morphology of bacteria demonstrating the variability of size and shape including bacilli (**A**), streptococci (**B**), staphylococci (**C**), and diplococci (**D**).

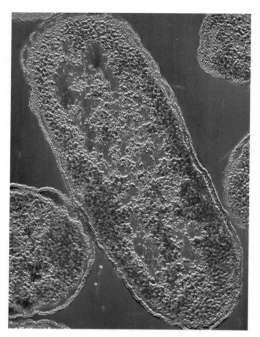

FIGURE 17-4 False-color transmission electron micrograph of the rod-shaped, gram-negative bacterium *Escherichia coli*, showing the simple procaryotic cell structure including the cytoplasm, the cytoplasmic membrane, and the rigid cell wall. (© Science Source/Photo Researchers)

like a propeller. Bacteria also can produce hairlike structures projecting from the cell surface called *pili* or *fimbriae*, which enable the organism to adhere to surfaces such as mucous membranes or other bacteria.

Most prokaryotes reproduce asexually by simple cellular division. The number of planes in which an organism divides can influence the microscopic morphology. For instance, when the cocci divide in chains, they are called *streptococci*; in pairs, *diplococci*; and in clusters, *staphylococci*. The growth rate of bacteria varies significantly among different species and depends greatly on physical growth conditions and the availability of nutrients. In the laboratory, a single bacterium placed in a suitable growth environment, such as an agar plate, reproduces to the extent that it forms a visible colony composed of millions of bacteria within a few hours. The physical appearance of the colony can be distinctive for each type of bacteria.

Some bacteria produce highly resistant spores when faced with an unfavorable environment. The spores exist in a quiescent state almost indefinitely until suitable growth conditions are encountered. The spores germinate, and the organism resumes normal metabolism and replication.

Bacteria are extremely adaptable life forms. They inhabit almost every environmental niche on earth, including humans. However, each individual bacterial species has a well-defined set of growth parameters, including nutrition, temperature, light, humidity, and atmosphere. Bacteria with extremely strict growth requirements are called *fastidious*. For example, *Neisseria gonorrhoeae*, the bacterium that causes gonorrhea, cannot live for extended periods outside the

human body. Some bacteria require oxygen for growth and metabolism and are called *aerobes*; others cannot survive in an oxygen-containing environment and are called *anaerobes*. An organism capable of adapting its metabolism to aerobic or anaerobic conditions is called *facultatively anaerobic*.

In the laboratory, bacteria usually are classified according to the microscopic appearance and staining properties of the cell. Gram's stain, originally developed in 1884 by the Danish bacteriologist Christian Gram, is still the most widely used staining procedure. Bacteria are designated as *gram-positive* organisms if they are stained purple by a primary basic dye (usually crystal violet); those that are not stained by the crystal violet but are counterstained a red color by a second dye (safranin) are called *gram-negative* organisms. Staining characteristics and microscopic morphology are used in combination to describe bacteria. For example, *Streptococcus pyogenes*, the agent of scarlet fever and rheumatic fever, is a gram-positive streptococcal organism that is spherical, grows in chains, and stains purple by Gram's stain. *Legionella pneumophila*, the bacterium responsible for Legionnaire's disease, is a gram-negative rod.

Another means of classifying bacteria according to microscopic staining properties is the acid-fast stain. Because of their unique cell membrane fatty acid content and composition, certain bacteria are resistant to the decolorization of a primary stain (either carbol fuchsin or a combination of auramine and rhodamine) when treated with a solution of acid alcohol. These organisms are termed *acid-fast* and include a number of significant human pathogens, most notably *Mycobacterium tuberculosis* (the cause of tuberculosis) and other mycobacteria and a variety of filamentous bacteria, including several species of *Nocardia* (*N. asteroides* complex and *N. braziliensis*).

For purposes of taxonomy, identification, and classification, each member of the bacterial kingdom is categorized into a small group of biochemically and genetically related organisms called the *genus* and further subdivided into distinct individuals within the genus called *species*. The genus and species assignment of the organism is reflected in its name (*e.g.*, *Staphylococcus* [genus] *aureus* [species]).

Spirochetes. The spirochetes are an eccentric category of bacteria that are mentioned separately because of their unusual cellular morphology and distinctive mechanism of motility. Technically, the spirochetes are gram-negative rods, but they are unique in that the cell's shape is helical and the length of the organism is many times its width. A series of filaments are wound about the cell wall and extend the entire length of the cell. These filaments propel the organism through an aqueous environment in a corkscrew motion.

Spirochetes are anaerobic or facultatively anaerobic organisms and comprise three genera: *Leptospira*, *Borrelia*, and *Treponema*. Each genus has saprophytic and pathogenic strains. The pathogenic leptospires infect a wide variety of wild and domestic animals. Infected animals shed the organisms into the environment through the urinary tract. Transmission to humans occurs by contact with infected animals or urine-contaminated surroundings. Leptospires gain access to the host directly through mucous membranes or breaks in the skin and can produce a severe and potentially fatal illness called *Weil's disease*. In contrast, the borreliae are transmitted from infected animals to humans through the bite of an arthropod vector such as lice or ticks. Included among the genus *Borrelia* are the agents of relapsing fever (*B. recurrentis*) and Lyme disease (*B. burgdorferi*). Pathogenic *Treponema* species require no intermediates and are spread from person to person by direct contact. The most important member of the genus is *Treponema pallidum*, the cause of syphilis.

Mycoplasmas. The mycoplasmas are unicellular prokaryotes capable of independent replication. These organisms are less than one-third the size of bacteria and contain a small DNA genome approximately one-half the size of the bacterial chromosome. The cell is composed of cytoplasm surrounded by a membrane, but, unlike bacteria, the mycoplasmas do not produce a rigid peptidoglycan cell wall. As a consequence, the microscopic appearance of the cell is highly variable, ranging from coccoid forms to filaments, and the mycoplasmas are resistant to cell wall–inhibiting antibiotics such as penicillins and cephalosporins.

The mycoplasmas of humans are divided into three genera: *Mycoplasma*, *Ureaplasma*, and *Acholeplasma*. The first two of these require cholesterol from the environment to produce the cell membrane; the *Acholeplasma* do not. In the human host, mycoplasmas are commensals. However, a number of species are capable of producing serious diseases, including pneumonia (*Mycoplasma pneumoniae*), genital infections (*Mycoplasma hominis* and *Ureaplasma urealyticum*), and maternally transmitted respiratory infections to low–birth-weight infants (*U. urealyticum*).

Rickettsiae, Chlamydiae, Ehrlichieae, and *Coxiella*

This interesting group of organisms combines the characteristics of viral and bacterial agents to produce disease in humans. All are obligate intracellular pathogens like the viruses, but they produce a rigid peptidoglycan cell wall, reproduce asexually by cellular division, and contain RNA and DNA, similar to the bacteria.

The rickettsiae depend on the host cell for essential vitamins and nutrients, but the chlamydiae appear to scavenge intermediates of energy metabolism such as adenosine triphosphate (ATP). The rickettsiae infect but do not produce disease in the cells of certain arthropods such as fleas, ticks, and lice. The organisms are accidentally transmitted to humans through the bite of the arthropod, or vector, and produce a number of potentially lethal diseases, including Rocky Mountain spotted fever and epidemic typhus.

The chlamydiae are slightly smaller than the rickettsiae but are structurally similar. Unlike the rickettsiae, chlamydiae are transmitted directly between susceptible vertebrates without an intermediate arthropod host. Transmission and replication of chlamydiae occur through a defined life cycle. The infectious form, called an *elementary body*, attaches to and enters the host cell, where it transforms into a *larger reticulate body*. The latter undergoes active replication into multiple elementary bodies, which then are shed into the extracellular environment to initiate another infectious cycle. Chlamydial diseases of humans include sexually transmitted genital infections (see Chapter 46); ocular infections and pneumonia of newborns (*Chlamydia trachomatis*); upper and lower respiratory tract infections in children, adolescents, and young adults (*Chlamydia pneumoniae*); and respiratory disease acquired from infected birds (*Chlamydia psittaci*).

The ehrlichieae also are obligate intracellular organisms that resemble the rickettsiae in structure and produce a variety of veterinary and human diseases, some of which have a tick vector. These organisms target host mononuclear and polymorphonuclear white blood cells for infection and, similar to the chlamydiae, multiply inside the cytoplasm of infected leukocytes in vacuoles called *morulae*. Unlike the chlamydiae, however, the ehrlichieae do not have a defined life cycle and are independent of the host cell for energy production. In eastern Asia, *Ehrlichia sennetsu* produces a disease in humans called *sennetsu fever* that resembles infectious mononucleosis. In the United States, the most frequent manifestation of *Ehrlichia* infection is human monocytotropic ehrlichiosis—a disease caused by *Ehrlichia chaffeensis* that is easily confused with Rocky Mountain spotted fever.

The genus *Coxiella* contains only one species, *C. burnetii*. Like its rickettsial counterparts, it is a gram-negative intracellular organism that infects a variety of animals, including cattle, sheep, and goats. In humans, *Coxiella* infection produces a disease called *Q fever*, characterized by a nonspecific febrile illness often accompanied by headache, chills, arthralgias, and mild pneumonia. The organism produces a highly resistant spore stage that is transmitted to humans when animal tissue is aerosolized, such as during meat processing, or by ingestion of contaminated milk.

Fungi

The fungi are free-living, eukaryotic saprophytes found in every habitat on earth. Some are members of the normal human microflora. Fortunately, few fungi are capable of causing diseases in humans, and most of these are incidental, self-limited infections of skin and subcutaneous tissue. Serious fungal infections are rare and usually initiated through puncture wounds or inhalation. Despite their normally harmless nature, fungi can cause serious life-threatening opportunistic diseases when host defense capabilities have been disabled.

The fungi can be separated into two groups, yeasts and molds, based on rudimentary differences in their morphology (Fig. 17-5). The yeasts are single-celled organisms, approximately the size of a red blood cell, that reproduce by a budding process. The buds separate from the parent cell and mature into identical daughter cells. Molds produce long, hollow, branching filaments called *hyphae*. Some molds produce cross walls, which segregate the hyphae into compartments, and others do not. A limited number of fungi are capable of growing as yeasts at one temperature and as molds at another. These organisms are called *dimorphic fungi* and include a number of human pathogens such as the agents of blastomycosis, histoplasmosis, and coccidioidomycosis (San Joaquin fever).

The appearance of a fungal colony tends to reflect its cellular composition. Colonies of yeast usually are smooth with a waxy or creamy texture. Molds tend to produce cottony or powdery colonies composed of mats of hyphae

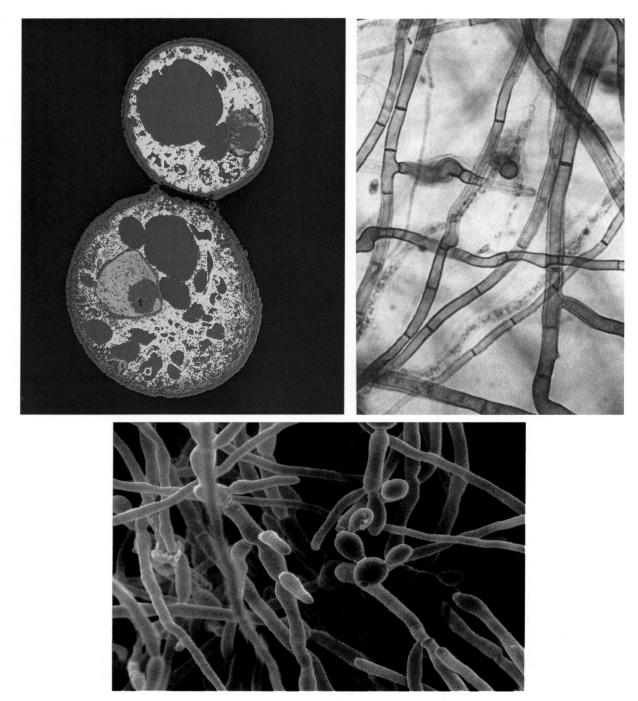

FIGURE 17-5 The microscopic morphology of fungal pathogens in humans. The yeasts are single-celled organisms that reproduce by the budding process (**upper left**). The molds (**right**) produce long branched or unbranched filaments called hyphae. *Candida albicans* (**lower left**) is a budding yeast that produces pseudohyphae both in culture and in tissues and exudates. (Upper left and lower left © Science Source/Photo Researchers)

collectively called a *mycelium*. The mycelium can penetrate the growth surface or project above the colony like the roots and branches of a tree. Yeasts and molds produce a rigid cell wall layer that is chemically unrelated to the peptidoglycan of bacteria and therefore is not susceptible to the effects of penicillin-like antibiotics.

Most fungi are capable of sexual or asexual reproduction. The former process involves the fusion of zygotes with the production of a recombinant zygospore. Asexual reproduction involves the formation of highly resistant spores called *conidia* or *sporangiospores*, which are borne by specialized structures that arise from the hyphae. Molds are identified in the laboratory by the characteristic microscopic appearance of the asexual fruiting structures and spores.

Just like the bacterial pathogens of humans, fungi can produce disease in the human host only if they can grow at the temperature of the infected body site. For example, a number of fungal pathogens called the *dermatophytes* are incapable of growing at core body temperature (37°C), and the infection is limited to the cooler cutaneous surfaces. Diseases caused by these organisms, including ringworm, athlete's foot, and jock itch, are collectively called *superficial mycoses*. Systemic mycoses are serious fungal infections of deep tissues and, by definition, are caused by organisms capable of growth at 37°C. Yeasts such as *Candida albicans* are commensal flora of the skin, mucous membranes, and gastrointestinal tract and are capable of growth at a wider range of temperatures. Intact immune mechanisms and competition for nutrients provided by the bacterial flora normally keep colonizing fungi in check. Alterations in either of these components by disease states or antibiotic therapy can upset the balance, permitting fungal overgrowth and setting the stage for opportunistic infections.

Parasites

In a strict sense, any organism that derives benefits from its biologic relationship with another organism is a parasite. In the field of clinical microbiology, however, the term *parasite* has evolved to designate members of the animal kingdom that infect and cause disease in other animals; these include protozoa, helminths, and arthropods.

The protozoa are unicellular animals with a complete complement of eukaryotic cellular machinery, including a well-defined nucleus and organelles. Reproduction may be sexual or asexual, and life cycles may be simple or complicated with several maturation stages requiring more than one host for completion. Most are saprophytes, but a few have adapted to the accommodations of the human environment and produce a variety of diseases, including malaria, amebic dysentery, and giardiasis. Protozoan infections can be passed directly from host to host, such as through sexual contact, indirectly through contaminated water or food, or by way of an arthropod vector. Direct or indirect transmission results from the ingestion of highly resistant cysts or spores that are shed in the feces of an infected host. When the cysts reach the intestine, they mature into vegetative forms called *trophozoites*, which are capable of asexual reproduction or cyst formation. Most trophozoites are motile by means of flagella, cilia, or ameboid motion.

The helminths are a group of wormlike parasites that include the roundworms (*i.e.*, nematodes), tapeworms (cestodes), and flukes (trematodes). The helminths reproduce sexually in the definitive host, and some require an intermediate host for the development and maturation of offspring. Humans can serve as the definitive or intermediate host and, in certain diseases such as trichinosis, as both. Transmission of helminth diseases occurs primarily through the ingestion of fertilized eggs (ova) or the penetration of infectious larval stages through the skin—directly or with the aid of an arthropod vector. Helminth infections can involve many organ systems and sites, including the liver and lung, urinary and intestinal tracts, circulatory and central nervous systems, and muscle. Although most helminth diseases have been eradicated from the United States, they are still a major health concern of developing nations.

The parasitic arthropods of humans and animals include the vectors of infectious diseases (*e.g.*, ticks, mosquitoes, biting flies) and the ectoparasites. The ectoparasites infest external body surfaces and cause localized tissue damage or inflammation secondary to the bite or burrowing action of the arthropod. The most prominent human ectoparasites are mites (scabies), chiggers, lice (head, body, and pubic), and fleas. Transmission of ectoparasites occurs directly by contact with immature or mature forms of the arthropod or its eggs found on the infested host or the host's clothing, bedding, or grooming articles (combs, brushes). Many of the ectoparasites are vectors of other infectious diseases, including endemic typhus and bubonic plague (fleas) and epidemic typhus (lice). A summary of the salient characteristics of human microbial pathogens is presented in Table 17-2.

TABLE 17-2 ✦ Comparison of Characteristics of Human Microbial Pathogens

Organism	Defined Nucleus	Genomic Material	Size*	Intracellular or Extracellular	Motility
Viruses	No	DNA or RNA	0.02–0.3	I	–
Bacteria	No	DNA	0.5–15	I/E	±
Mycoplasmas	No	DNA	0.2–0.3	E	–
Spirochetes	No	DNA	6–15	E	+
Rickettsiae	No	DNA	0.2–2	I	–
Chlamydiae	No	DNA	0.3–1	I	–
Yeasts	Yes	DNA	2–60	I/E	–
Molds	Yes	DNA	2–15 (hyphal width)	E	–
Protozoans	Yes	DNA	1–60	I/E	+
Helminths	Yes	DNA	2 mm–> 1 m	E	+

*Micrometers unless indicated.

In summary, throughout life, humans are continuously and harmlessly exposed to and colonized by a multitude of microscopic organisms. This relationship is kept in check by the intact defense mechanisms of the host (*e.g.*, mucosal and cutaneous barriers, normal immune function) and the innocuous nature of most environmental microorganisms. Those factors that weaken the resistance of the host or increase the virulence of colonizing microorganisms can disturb the equilibrium of the relationship and cause disease. The degree to which the balance is shifted in favor of the microorganism determines the severity of illness.

There is an extreme diversity of eukaryotic and protokaryotic microorganisms capable of causing infectious disease in humans. Eukaryotes and prokaryotes contain all of the enzymes required for their replication and possess the biologic equipment necessary for the production of metabolic energy. Thus, eukaryotes and prokaryotes differ from viruses, which depend on host cells for these necessary functions. Prions are protein particles that are infectious and capable of causing diseases such Creutzfeld-Jakob disease in humans and mad cow disease in animals. With the advent of immunosuppressive medical therapy and immunosuppressive diseases such as AIDS, the number and type of potential microbic pathogens, the so-called opportunistic pathogens, have increased dramatically. However, most infectious illnesses in humans continue to be caused by only a small fraction of the organisms that comprise the microscopic world.

Mechanisms of Infection

After you have completed this section of the chapter, you should be able to meet the following objectives:

✦ Differentiate between incidence and prevalence and among endemic, epidemic, and panepidemic

✦ Use the concepts of incidence, portal of entry, source of infection, symptomatology, disease course, site of infection, agent, and host characteristics to explain the mechanisms of infectious diseases

✦ Describe the stages of an infectious disease after the potential pathogen enters the body

✦ List the systemic manifestations of infectious disease

EPIDEMIOLOGY OF INFECTIOUS DISEASES

Epidemiology, in the context of this chapter, is the study of factors, events, and circumstances that influence the transmission of infectious diseases among humans. The ultimate goal of the epidemiologist is to devise strategies that interrupt or eliminate the spread of an infectious agent. To accomplish this, infectious diseases must be classified according to incidence, portal of entry, source, symptoms, disease course, site of infection, and virulence factors so that potential outbreaks may be predicted and averted or appropriately treated. Each of these categories is discussed in

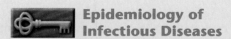

Epidemiology of Infectious Diseases

➤ Epidemiology is the study of factors, events, and circumstances that influence the transmission of infectious diseases in human populations.

➤ Epidemiology focuses on the incidence (number of new cases) and prevalence (number of active cases at any given time) of an infectious disease; the source of infection, its portal of entry, site of infection, and virulence factors of the infecting organism; and the signs and symptoms of the infection and its course.

➤ The ultimate goals of epidemiologic studies are the interruption of the spread of infectious diseases and their eradication.

detail, with the exception of agents and host, which already have been reviewed.

Epidemiology is a science of rates. The expected frequency of any infectious disease must be calculated so that gradual or abrupt changes in frequency can be observed. The term *incidence* is used to describe the number of new cases of an infectious disease that occur in a defined population (*e.g.*, per 100,000 persons) over an established period (*e.g.*, monthly, quarterly, yearly). Disease *prevalence* indicates the number of active cases at any given time. A disease is considered *endemic* in a particular geographic region if the incidence and prevalence are expected and relatively stable. An *epidemic* describes an abrupt and unexpected increase in the incidence of disease over endemic rates. A *pandemic* refers to the spread of disease beyond continental boundaries. The advent of rapid worldwide travel increased the likelihood of pandemic transmission of pathogenic microorganisms.

As an illustration of these principles, an outbreak of a suspected arboviral (virus transmitted by an insect) encephalitis (inflammation of the brain) was recognized in the New York City metropolitan area in the fall of 1999. Beginning in August, local health officials noted an increased incidence of encephalitis; by the end of September, 17 confirmed and 20 probable cases with 4 deaths were reported in the area. Studies of antibodies produced by the infected individuals suggested that the illnesses were caused by St. Louis encephalitis virus, which is classified as a flavivirus, is endemic in the United States, and is transmitted from infected birds and rodents to humans by mosquitoes. During the same period, public health workers also noted increased deaths among several New York City bird populations, particularly crows. The birds also had meningoencephalitis and myocarditis (inflammation of the heart). Tissue samples from the birds were sent to the National Veterinary Services Laboratory in Ames, Iowa, and to the Centers for Disease Control and Prevention in Atlanta. Much to the researchers' surprise, the virus isolated from the patients and birds in

New York City appeared to be West Nile virus (WNV), a virus endemic to Europe, Africa, and the Middle East that had never been isolated in the United States before. Therefore, the outbreak of WNV encephalitis was not only an epidemic but a pandemic because the disease crossed continental borders for the first time.

PORTAL OF ENTRY

The portal of entry refers to the process by which a pathogen enters the body, gains access to susceptible tissues, and causes disease. Among the potential modes of transmission are penetration, direct contact, ingestion, and inhalation.

Penetration

Any disruption in the integrity of the body's surface barrier, such as skin or mucous membranes, is a potential site for invasion of microorganisms. The break may be the result of an accidental injury resulting in abrasions, burns, or penetrating wounds; medical procedures such as surgery or catheterization; a primary infectious process that produces surface lesions such as chickenpox or impetigo; or direct inoculation from intravenous drug use or from animal or arthropod bites. The latter mode of transmission can be extremely dangerous because large numbers of organisms can gain direct access to vital sites, thus bypassing the host's primary immune defense systems.

Direct Contact

Some pathogens are transmitted directly from infected tissue or secretions to exposed, intact mucous membranes without a prerequisite for damaged mucosal barriers. This is especially true of certain sexually transmitted diseases (STDs) such as gonorrhea, syphilis, chlamydia, and herpes, for which exposure of uninfected membranes to pathogens occurs during intimate contact.

The transmission of STDs is not limited to sexual contact. Vertical transmission of these agents, from mother to child, can occur across the placenta or during birth when the mucous membranes of the child come in contact with infected vaginal secretions of the mother. When an infectious disease is transmitted from mother to child during gestation or birth, it is classified as a *congenital infection*. The most frequently observed congenital infections include the parasite *Toxoplasma gondii*, other infectious diseases, rubella, cytomegalovirus, and herpes simplex viruses (the so-called *TORCH* infections); as well as varicella-zoster (chickenpox), parvovirus B19, group B streptococci (*Streptococcus agalactiae*), and HIV. Of these, cytomegalovirus is by far the most common cause of congenital infection in the United States, affecting nearly 1% of all newborns. However, more than 6000 HIV-infected women give birth each year in the United States, and the numbers are likely to be far greater in developing nations. With a 13% to 30% chance of vertical transmission, HIV is rapidly gaining in stature as a congenitally transmitted infection.

The severity of congenital defects associated with these infections depends greatly on the gestational age of the fetus when transmission occurs, but most of these agents can cause profound mental retardation and neurosensory deficits, including blindness and hearing loss. HIV rarely produces overt signs and symptoms in the infected newborn, and it sometimes takes years for the effects of the illness to manifest.

Ingestion

The entry of pathogenic microorganisms or their toxic products through the oral cavity and gastrointestinal tract represents one of the more efficient means of disease transmission in humans. Many bacterial, viral, and parasitic infections, including cholera, typhoid fever, dysentery (amebic and bacillary), food poisoning, traveler's diarrhea, cryptosporidiosis, and hepatitis A, are initiated through the ingestion of contaminated food and water. This mechanism of transmission necessitates that an infectious agent survive the low pH and enzyme activity of gastric secretions and the peristaltic action of the intestines in numbers sufficient to establish infection (infectious dose). Ingested pathogens also must compete successfully with the normal bacterial flora of the bowel for nutritional needs. Persons with reduced gastric acidity (called *achlorhydria*) due to disease or medication are more susceptible to infection by this route because the number of ingested microorganisms surviving the gastric environment is greater. Ingestion also has been postulated as a means of transmission of HIV infection from mother to child through breast-feeding.

Inhalation

The respiratory tract of healthy persons is equipped with a multitiered defense system to prevent potential pathogens from entering the lungs. The surface of the respiratory tree is lined with a layer of mucus that is continuously swept up and away from the lungs and toward the mouth by the beating motion of ciliated epithelial cells. Humidification of inspired air increases the size of aerosolized particles, which are effectively filtered by the mucous membranes of the upper respiratory tract. Coughing also aids in the removal of particulate matter from the lower respiratory tract. Respiratory secretions contain antibodies and enzymes capable of inactivating infectious agents. Particulate matter and microorganisms that ultimately reach the lung are cleared by phagocytic cells.

Despite this impressive array of protective mechanisms, a number of pathogens can invade the human body through the respiratory tract, including agents of bacterial pneumonia (*Streptococcus pneumoniae, L. pneumophila*), meningitis and sepsis (*Neisseria meningitidis* and *Haemophilus influenzae*), and tuberculosis, and the viruses responsible for measles, mumps, chickenpox, influenza, and the common cold. Defective pulmonary function or mucociliary clearance caused by noninfectious processes such as cystic fibrosis, emphysema, or smoking can increase the risk of inhalation-acquired diseases.

The portal of entry does not dictate the site of infection. Ingested pathogens may penetrate the intestinal mucosa, disseminate through the circulatory system, and cause diseases in other organs such as the lung or liver. Whatever the mechanisms of entry, the transmission of infectious agents is directly related to the number of infectious agents absorbed by the host.

SOURCE

The source of an infectious disease refers to the location, host, object, or substance from which the infectious agent was acquired: essentially the who, what, where, and when of disease transmission. The source may be endogenous (acquired from the host's own microbial flora, as would be the case in an opportunistic infection) or exogenous (acquired from sources in the external environment such as water, food, soil, or air). The infectious agent can originate from another human being, as from mother to child during gestation (congenital infections) or birth (perinatal infections). Zoonoses are a category of infectious diseases passed from other animal species to humans. Examples of zoonoses include cat-scratch disease, rabies, and visceral or cutaneous larval migrans. The spread of infectious diseases, including Lyme disease, malaria, trypanosomiasis, and arboviral encephalitis (West Nile and St. Louis encephalitis viruses), through biting arthropod vectors already has been mentioned.

Source can denote a place. For instance, infections that develop in patients while they are hospitalized are called *nosocomial*, and those that are acquired outside of health care facilities are called *community acquired*. The source also may pertain to the body substance that is the most likely vehicle for transmission, such as feces, blood, body fluids, respiratory secretions, and urine. Infections can be transmitted from person to person through shared inanimate objects (fomites) contaminated with infected body fluids. An example of this mechanism of transmission would include the spread of HIV and the hepatitis B virus through the use of shared syringes by intravenous drug users. Infection also can be spread through a complex combination of source, portal of entry, and vector. The well-publicized 1993 outbreak of hantavirus pulmonary syndrome in the southwestern United States is a prime example. This viral illness was transmitted to humans by inhalation of dust contaminated with saliva, feces, and urine of infected rodents.

SYMPTOMATOLOGY

The term *symptomatology* refers to the collection of signs and symptoms expressed by the host during the disease course. This also is known as the *clinical picture* or *disease presentation* and can be characteristic of any given infectious agent. In terms of pathophysiology, symptoms are the outward expression of the struggle between invading organisms and the retaliatory inflammatory and immune responses of the host (see Chapter 18). The symptoms of an infectious disease may be specific and reflect the site of infection (*e.g.*, diarrhea, rash, convulsions, hemorrhage, pneumonia). Conversely, symptoms such as fever, myalgia, headache, and lethargy are relatively nonspecific and can be shared by a number of diverse infectious diseases. The symptoms of a diseased host can be obvious, as in the cases of chickenpox or measles. Other, covert symptoms, such as hepatitis or an increased white blood cell count, may require laboratory testing to detect. Accurate recognition and documentation of symptomatology can aid in the diagnosis of an infectious disease.

DISEASE COURSE

The course of any infectious disease can be divided into several distinguishable stages after the potential pathogen has entered the host. These stages are the incubation period, the prodromal stage, the acute stage, the convalescent stage, and the resolution stage (Fig. 17-6). The stages are based on the progression and intensity of the host's symptoms over time. The duration of each phase and the pattern of the overall illness can be specific for different pathogens, thereby aiding in the diagnosis of an infectious disease.

The *incubation period* is the phase during which the pathogen begins active replication without producing recognizable symptoms in the host. The incubation period may be short, as in the case of salmonellosis (6 to 24 hours), or prolonged, such as that of hepatitis B (50 to 180 days) or HIV (months to years). The duration of the incubation period can be influenced by additional factors, including the general health of the host, the portal of entry, and the infectious dose of the pathogen.

The hallmark of the *prodromal stage* is the initial appearance of symptoms in the host, although the clinical presentation during this time may be only a vague sense of malaise. The host may experience mild fever, myalgia, headache, and fatigue. These are constitutional changes shared by a great number of disease processes. The duration of the prodromal stage can vary considerably from host to host.

The *acute stage* is the period during which the host experiences the maximum impact of the infectious process, corresponding to rapid proliferation and dissemination of the pathogen. During this phase, toxic byproducts of microbial metabolism, cell lysis, and the immune response mounted by the host combine to produce tissue damage and inflammation. The host's symptoms are pronounced and

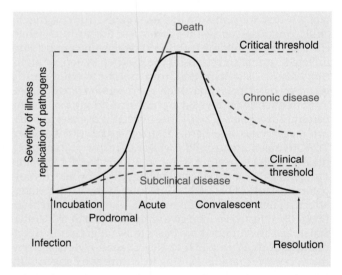

FIGURE 17-6 The stages of a primary infectious disease as they appear in relation to the severity of symptoms and the numbers of infectious agents. The clinical threshold corresponds with the initial expression of recognizable symptoms whereas the critical threshold represents the peak of disease intensity.

more specific than in the prodromal stage, usually typifying the pathogen and sites of involvement.

The *convalescent period* is characterized by the containment of infection, progressive elimination of the pathogen, repair of damaged tissue, and resolution of associated symptoms. Similar to the incubation period, the time required for complete convalescence may be days, weeks, or months, depending on the type of pathogen and the voracity of the host's immune response. The *resolution* is the total elimination of a pathogen from the body without residual signs or symptoms of disease.

Several notable exceptions to the classic presentations of an infectious process have been recognized. Chronic infectious diseases have a markedly protracted and sometimes irregular course. The host may experience symptoms of the infectious process continuously or sporadically for months or years without a convalescent phase. In contrast, *subclinical* or *subacute illness* progresses from infection to resolution without clinically apparent symptoms. A disease is called *insidious* if the prodromal phase is protracted; a *fulminant illness* is characterized by abrupt onset of symptoms with little or no prodrome. Fatal infections are variants of the typical disease course.

SITE OF INFECTION

Inflammation of an anatomic location usually is designated by adding the suffix *-itis* to the name of the involved tissue (*e.g.*, bronchitis, infection of the bronchi and bronchioles; encephalitis, brain infection; carditis, infection of the heart). These are general terms, however, and they apply equally to inflammation from infectious and noninfectious causes. The suffix *-emia* is used to designate the presence of a substance in the blood; the terms *bacteremia*, *viremia*, and *fungemia* describe the presence of these infectious agents in the bloodstream. The term *sepsis*, or *septicemia*, refers to the presence of microbial toxins in the blood.

The site of an infectious disease is determined ultimately by the type of pathogen, the portal of entry, and competence of the host's immunologic defense system. Many pathogenic microorganisms are restricted in their capacity to invade the human body. *M. pneumoniae*, influenza viruses, and *L. pneumophila* rarely cause disease outside the respiratory tract; infections caused by *N. gonorrhoeae* usually are confined to the genitourinary tract; and shigellosis and giardiasis seldom extend beyond the gastrointestinal tract. These are considered localized infectious diseases. The bacterium *Helicobacter pylori* is an extreme example of a site-specific pathogen. *H. pylori* is a significant cause of gastric ulcers and has not been implicated in disease processes elsewhere in the human body. Bacteria such as *N. meningitidis*, a prominent pathogen of children and young adults, *Salmonella typhi*, the cause of typhoid fever, and *B. burgdorferi*, the agent of Lyme disease, tend to disseminate from the primary site of infection to involve other locations and organ systems. These are examples of systemic pathogens. Most systemic infections disseminate throughout the body by way of the circulatory system.

An *abscess* is a localized pocket of infection composed of devitalized tissue, microorganisms, and the host's phagocytic white blood cells—in essence, a stalemate in the infectious process. The spread of the pathogen has been contained by the host, but white cell function in the toxic environment of the abscess is hampered, and the elimination of microorganisms is retarded. Abscesses usually must be surgically drained to effect a complete cure. Similarly, infections of biomedical implants such as catheters, artificial heart valves, and prosthetic bone implants seldom are cured by the host's immune response and antimicrobial therapy. The infecting organism colonizes the surface of the implant, producing a dense matrix of cells, host proteins, and capsular material called a *biofilm*, necessitating the removal of the device.

VIRULENCE FACTORS

Virulence factors are substances or products generated by infectious agents that enhance their ability to cause disease. Although there are many different types of microbial products that fit this description, they can be grouped into four general categories: toxins, adhesion factors, evasive factors, and invasive factors (Table 17-3).

TABLE 17-3 ◆ Examples of Virulence Factors Produced by Pathogenic Microorganisms

Factor	Category	Organism	Effect on Host
Cholera toxin	Exotoxin	*Vibrio-cholerae* (bacterium)	Secretory diarrhea
Diphtheria toxin	Exotoxin	*Corynebacterium diphtheriae* (bacterium)	Inhibits protein synthesis
Lipopolysaccharide	Endotoxin	Many gram-negative bacteria	Fever, hypotension, shock
Toxic shock toxin	Enterotoxin	*Staphylococcus aureus* (bacterium)	Rash, diarrhea, vomiting, hepatitis
Hemagglutinin	Adherence	Influenza virus	Establishment of infection
Pili	Adherence	*Neisseria gonorrhoeae* (bacterium)	Establishment of infection
Leukocidin	Evasive	*S. aureus*	Kills phagocytes
IgA protease	Evasive	*Haemophilus influenzae* (bacterium)	Inactivates antibody
Capsule	Evasive	*Cryptococcus neoformans* (yeast)	Prevents phagocytosis
Collagenase	Invasive	*Pseudomonas aeruginosa* (bacterium)	Penetration of tissue
Protease	Invasive	*Aspergillus* (mold)	Penetration of tissue
Phospholipase	Invasive	*Clostridium perfringens* (bacterium)	Penetration of tissue

Toxins

Toxins are substances that alter or destroy the normal function of the host or host's cells. Toxin production is a trait chiefly monopolized by bacterial pathogens, although certain fungal and protozoan pathogens also elaborate substances toxic to humans. Bacterial toxins have a diverse spectrum of activity and exert their effects on a wide variety of host target cells. For classification purposes, however, the bacterial toxins can be divided into two main types: *exotoxins* and *endotoxins*.

Exotoxins are proteins released from the bacterial cell during growth. Bacterial exotoxins enzymatically inactivate or modify key cellular constituents, leading to cell death or dysfunction. Diphtheria toxin, for example, inhibits cellular protein synthesis; botulism toxin decreases the release of neurotransmitter from cholinergic neurons, causing flaccid paralysis; tetanus toxin decreases the release of neurotransmitter from inhibitory neurons, producing spastic paralysis; and cholera toxin induces fluid secretion into the lumen of the intestine, causing diarrhea. Other examples of exotoxin-induced diseases include pertussis (whooping cough), anthrax, traveler's diarrhea, toxic shock syndrome, and a host of foodborne illnesses (*i.e.*, food poisoning).

Bacterial exotoxins that produce vomiting and diarrhea are sometimes referred to as *enterotoxins*. There has been a resurgent interest in streptococcal pyrogenic exotoxin A, an exotoxin produced by certain strains of group A, beta-hemolytic streptococci (*S. pyogenes*) that causes a life-threatening toxic shock–like syndrome similar to the disease associated with tampon use produced by *S. aureus*. The streptococcal form of intoxication is sometimes called *Henson's disease* because it was this infection that caused the death of the famous puppeteer Jim Henson. Other exotoxins that have gained notoriety include the Shiga toxins produced by *Escherichia coli* O157:H7 and other select strains. The ingestion of undercooked hamburger meat or unpasteurized fruit juices contaminated with this organism produces hemorrhagic colitis and a sometimes fatal illness called *hemolytic-uremic syndrome* (HUS), characterized by vascular endothelial damage, acute renal failure, and thrombocytopenia. HUS occurs primarily in infants and young children who have not developed antibodies to the Shiga toxins.

Endotoxins do not contain protein, are not actively released from the bacterium during growth, and have no enzymatic activity. Rather, endotoxins are complex molecules composed of lipid and polysaccharides found in the cell wall of gram-negative bacteria. Studies of different endotoxins have indicated that the lipid portion of the endotoxin confers the toxic properties to the molecule. Endotoxins are potent activators of a number of regulatory systems in humans. A small amount of endotoxin in the circulatory system (*i.e.*, endotoxemia) can induce clotting, bleeding, inflammation, hypotension, and fever. The sum of the physiologic reactions to endotoxins is sometimes called *endotoxic shock*.

Adhesion Factors

No interaction between microorganisms and humans can progress to infection or disease if the pathogen is unable to attach to and colonize the host. The process of microbial attachment may be site specific (*e.g.*, mucous membranes, skin surfaces), cell specific (*e.g.*, T lymphocytes, respiratory epithelium), or nonspecific (*e.g.*, moist areas, charged surfaces). In any of these cases, adhesion requires a positive interaction between the surfaces of host cells and the infectious agent.

The site to which microorganisms adhere is called a *receptor*, and the reciprocal molecule or substance that binds to the receptor is called a *ligand* or *adhesin*. Receptors may be proteins, carbohydrates, lipids, or complex molecules composed of all three. Similarly, ligands may be simple or complex molecules and, in some cases, highly specific structures. Ligands that bind to specific carbohydrates are called *lectins*. Certain bacteria produce hairlike structures protruding from the cell surface called *pili* or *fimbriae*, which anchor the organism to receptors on host cell membranes to establish an infection. Many viral agents, including influenza, mumps, measles, and adenovirus, produce filamentous appendages or spikes called *hemagglutinins*, which recognize carbohydrate receptors on the surfaces of specific cells in the upper respiratory tract of the host.

After initial attachment, a number of bacterial agents become embedded in a gelatinous matrix of polysaccharides called a *slime* or *mucous layer*. The slime layer serves two purposes: it anchors the agent firmly to host tissue surfaces and it protects the agent from the immunologic defenses of the host.

Evasive Factors

A number of factors produced by microorganisms enhance virulence by evading various components of the host's immune system. Extracellular polysaccharides, including capsules, slime, and mucous layers, discourage engulfment and killing of pathogens by the phagocytic white blood cells (*i.e.*, neutrophils and macrophages) of the host. Encapsulated organisms such as *S. agalactiae*, *S. pneumoniae*, *N. meningitidis*, and (before the vaccine) *H. influenzae* type b are a cause of significant morbidity and mortality in neonates and children who lack protective anticapsular antibodies. Certain bacterial, fungal, and parasitic pathogens avoid phagocytosis by excreting leukocidins—toxins that deplete the host of neutrophils and macrophages by causing specific and lethal damage to the cytoplasmic membrane of white blood cells. Other pathogens, such as the bacterial agents of listeriosis and Legionnaire's disease, are adapted to survive and reproduce within phagocytic white blood cells after ingestion, avoiding or neutralizing the usually lethal products contained in the lysosomes of the cell.

Other unique strategies used by pathogenic microbes to evade immunologic surveillance have evolved solely to avoid recognition by host antibodies. Strains of *S. aureus* produce a surface protein (protein A) that immobilizes immunoglobulin G (IgM), holding the antigen-binding region harmlessly away from the organisms. This pathogen also secretes a unique enzyme called *coagulase*. Coagulase converts soluble human coagulation factors into a solid clot, which envelops and protects the organism from phagocytic host cells and antibodies. *H. influenzae* and *N. gonorrhoeae* secrete enzymes that cleave and inactivate secretory IgA, neutralizing the primary defense of the respiratory and genital tracts at the site of infection. *H. pylori*, the infectious cause of gastritis and gastric ulcers, produces a urease enzyme on its outer cell wall. The urease converts gastric urea into ammonia, thus neutralizing the acidic environment of the stomach and allowing the organism to survive in this hostile environment.

Borrelia species, including the agents of Lyme disease and relapsing fever, alter surface antigens during the disease course to avoid immunologic detection. It appears that the capacity to devise strategic defense systems and stealth technologies is not limited to humans. Viruses such as HIV impair the function of immunoregulatory cells. Although this property increases the virulence of these agents, it is not considered a virulence factor in the true sense of the definition.

Invasive Factors

Invasive factors are products produced by infectious agents that facilitate the penetration of anatomic barriers and host tissue. Most invasive factors are enzymes capable of destroying cellular membranes (*e.g.*, phospholipases), connective tissue (*e.g.*, elastases, collagenases), intercellular matrices (*e.g.*, hyaluronidase), and structural protein complexes (*e.g.*, proteases). It is the combined effects of invasive factors, toxins, and antimicrobial and inflammatory substances released by host cells to counter infection that mediate the tissue damage and pathophysiology of infectious diseases.

Epidemiology is the study of factors, events, and circumstances that influence the transmission of disease. *Incidence* refers to the number of new cases of an infectious disease that occur in a defined population and *prevalence* to the number of active cases that are present at any given time. Infectious diseases are considered endemic in a geographic area if the incidence and prevalence are expected and relatively stable. An epidemic refers to an abrupt and unexpected increase in the incidence of a disease over endemic rates, and a pandemic to the spread of disease beyond continental boundaries.

The ultimate goal of epidemiology and epidemiologic studies is to devise strategies to interrupt or eliminate the spread of infectious disease. To accomplish this, infectious diseases are classified according to incidence, portal of entry, source, symptoms, disease course, site of infection, and virulence factors.

Diagnosis and Treatment of Infectious Diseases

After you have completed this section of the chapter, you should be able to meet the following objectives:

✦ State the two criteria used in the diagnosis of an infectious disease

✦ Explain the differences in culture, serology, and antigen, metabolite, or molecular detection methods for diagnosis of infectious disease

✦ Cite three general intervention methods that can be used in treatment of infectious illnesses

✦ State four basic mechanisms by which antibiotics exert their action

✦ Differentiate bactericidal from bacteriostatic

✦ Describe mechanisms and significance of antimicrobial and antiviral drug resistance

✦ Explain the actions of intravenous immunoglobulin and cytokines in treatment of infectious illnesses

DIAGNOSIS

The diagnosis of an infectious disease requires two criteria: the recovery of a probable pathogen or evidence of its presence from the infected sites of a diseased host, and accurate documentation of clinical signs and symptoms (symptomatology) compatible with an infectious process. In the laboratory, the diagnosis of an infectious agent is accomplished using three basic techniques: culture; serology, or the detection of characteristic antigens; and genomic sequences, or metabolites produced by the pathogen.

Culture refers to the propagation of a microorganism outside of the body, usually on or in artificial growth media such as agar plates or broth (Fig. 17-7). The specimen from the diseased host is inoculated into broth or placed on the surface of an agar plate, and the culture is placed in a controlled environment such as an incubator until the growth of microorganisms becomes detectable. In the case of a bacterial pathogen, identification is based on microscopic appearance and Gram's stain reaction, shape, texture, and color (*i.e.*, morphology) of the colonies, and by a panel of reactions that "fingerprint" salient biochemical characteristics of the organism. Certain bacteria such as *Mycobacterium leprae*, the agent of leprosy, and *T. pallidum*, the syphilis spirochete, do not grow on artificial media and require additional methods of identification. Fungi and mycoplasmas

 Diagnosis and Treatment of Infectious Diseases

➤ The definitive diagnosis of an infectious disease requires recovery and identification of the infecting organism by microscopic identification of the agent in stains of specimens or sections of tissue, culture isolation and identification of the agents, demonstration of antibody- or cell-mediated immune responses to an infectious agent, or DNA or RNA identification of infectious agents.

➤ Treatment of infectious disease is aimed at eliminating the infectious organism and promoting recovery of the infected person. Treatment is provided through the use of antimicrobial agents, immunotherapy, and, when necessary, surgical interventions.

➤ Prevention of infectious disease is accomplished through the use of immunization methods.

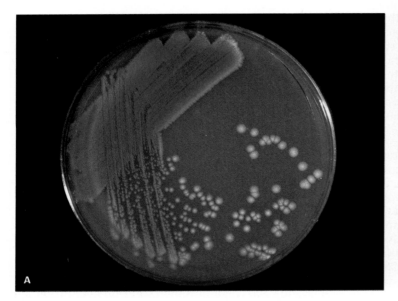

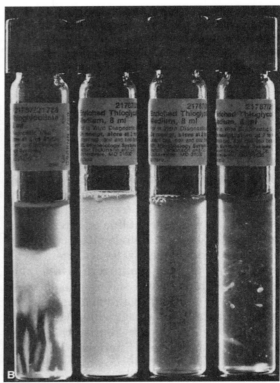

FIGURE 17-7 Variability of the macroscopic appearance of bacteria cultured on solid, agar-containing medium (**A**) and liquid broth medium (**B**). On solid surfaces, bacteria form distinct colonies as demonstrated by the β-hemolytic streptococcus (*Streptococcus pyogenes*) on sheep blood agar (**A**). Bacteria cultured in broth form a variety of growth patterns, ranging from particulate to homogenous, turbid suspensions. Anaerobic bacteria cultured in liquid medium tend to grow best at the bottom of the tube, where the concentration of molecular oxygen is lowest. (**A** © Science Source/Photo Researchers)

are cultured in much the same way as bacteria but with more reliance on microscopic and colonial morphology for identification.

Chlamydiae, rickettsiae, and all human viruses are obligate intracellular pathogens. As a result, the propagation of these agents in the laboratory requires the inoculation of eukaryotic cells grown in culture (cell cultures). A cell culture consists of a flask containing a single layer, or monolayer, of eukaryotic cells covering the bottom and overlaid with broth containing essential nutrients and growth factors. When a virus infects and replicates in cultured eukaryotic cells, it produces pathologic changes in the appearance of the cell called the *cytopathic effect* (Fig. 17-8). The cytopathic effect can be detected microscopically, and the pattern and extent of cellular destruction often are characteristic of a particular virus.

Although culture media have been developed for the growth of certain human protozoa and helminths in the laboratory, the diagnosis of parasitic infectious diseases traditionally has relied on microscopic, or in the case of worms, visible identification of organisms, cysts, or ova directly from infected patient specimens.

Serology, the study of serum, is an indirect means of identifying infectious agents by measuring serum antibodies in the diseased host. A tentative diagnosis can be made if the antibody level, also called *antibody titer*, against a specific pathogen rises during the acute phase of the disease and falls during convalescence. Serologic identification of an infectious agent is not as accurate as culture, but it may be a useful adjunct, especially for the diagnosis of diseases caused by pathogens that cannot be cultured, such as the hepatitis B virus. The measurement of antibody titers has another advantage in that specific antibody types such as IgM and IgG are produced by the host during different phases of an infectious process; IgM-specific antibodies usually rise and fall during the acute phase, whereas the synthesis of the IgG class of antibodies increases during the acute phase and remains elevated until or beyond resolution. Measurements of class-specific antibodies also are useful in the diagnosis of congenital infections. IgM antibodies do not cross the placenta, but certain IgG antibodies are transferred passively from mother to child during the final trimester of gestation. Consequently, an elevation of pathogen-specific IgM antibodies found in the serum of a neonate must have originated from the child and therefore indicates congenital infection. A similarly increased IgG titer in the neonate does not differentiate congenital from maternal infection.

The technology of *direct antigen detection* has evolved rapidly since the early 1990s and in the process has revolutionized the diagnosis of certain infectious diseases. Antigen

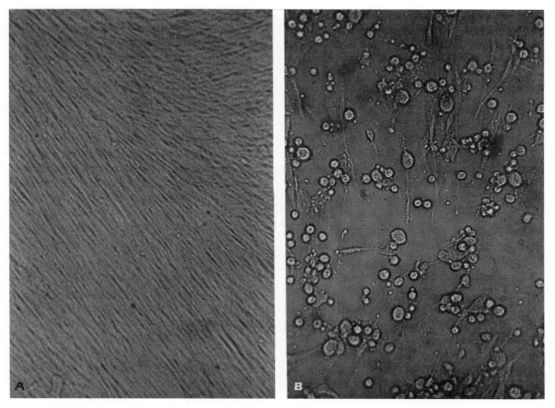

FIGURE 17-8 The microscopic appearance of a monolayer of uninfected human fibroblasts grown in cell culture (**A**) and the same cells after infection with herpes simplex virus (**B**), demonstrating the cytopathic effect caused by viral replication and concomitant cell lysis.

detection incorporates features of culture and serology but greatly reduces the time required for diagnosis. In principle, this method relies on purified antibodies to detect antigens of infectious agents in specimens obtained from the diseased host. The source of antibodies used for antigen detection can be animals immunized against a particular pathogen or *hybridomas*. Hybridomas are created by fusing normal antibody-producing spleen cells from an immunized animal with malignant myeloma cells, which synthesize large quantities of antibody. The result is a cell that produces an antibody called a *monoclonal antibody*, which is highly specific for a single antigen and a single pathogen. Regardless of the source, the antibodies are labeled with a substance that allows microscopic or overt detection when bound to the pathogen or its products. The three types of labels usually used for this purpose are fluorescent dyes, enzymes, and particles such as latex beads. Fluorescent antibodies allow visualization of an infectious agent with the aid of a fluorescence microscope. Depending on the type of fluorescent dye used, the organism may appear bright green or orange against a black background, making detection extremely easy. Enzyme-labeled antibodies function in a similar manner. The enzyme is capable of converting a colorless compound into a colored substance, thereby permitting detection of antibody bound to an infectious agent without the use of a fluorescence microscope. Particles coated with

antibodies clump together, or agglutinate, when the appropriate antigen is present in a specimen. Particle agglutination is especially useful when examining infected body fluids such as urine, serum, or spinal fluid.

The identification of infectious agents through the detection of sequences of DNA or RNA unique to a single agent has undergone rapid development and use during recent years. Several techniques have been devised to accomplish this goal, each having different degrees of sensitivity regarding the number of organisms that need to be present in a specimen for detection. The first of these methods is called *DNA probe hybridization*. Small fragments of DNA are cut from the genome of a specific pathogen and labeled with compounds (photoemitting chemicals or antigens) that allow detection. The labeled DNA "probes" are added to specimens from an infected host. If the pathogen is present, the probe attaches to the complementary strand of DNA on the genome of the infectious agent, permitting rapid diagnosis. The use of labeled probes has allowed visualization of particular agents in and around individual cells in histologic sections of tissue.

A second and more sensitive method of DNA detection is the *polymerase chain reaction* (PCR) (Fig. 17-9). This method incorporates two unique reagents: a specific pair of oligonucleotides (usually more than 25 nucleotides long) called *primers* and a heat-stable DNA polymerase. To perform the

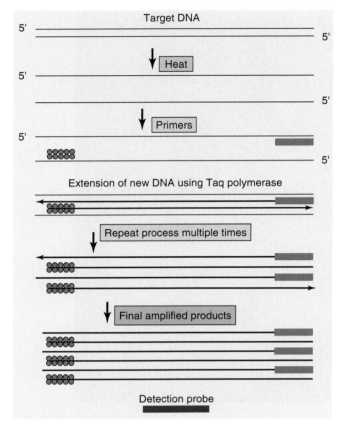

Target DNA

FIGURE 17-9 The polymerase chain reaction is depicted. The target DNA is first melted using heat (generally around 94°C) to separate the strands of DNA. Primers that recognize specific sequences within the target DNA are allowed to bind as the reaction cools. Using a unique, thermostable DNA polymerase called Taq and an abundance of deoxynucleoside triphosphates, new DNA strands are amplified from the point of the primer attachment. The process is repeated many times (called cycles) until millions of copies of DNA are produced, all of which have the same length defined by the distance (in base pairs) between the primer binding sites. These copies are then detected by electrophoresis and staining or through the use of labeled DNA probes that, similar to the primers, recognize a specific sequence located within the amplified section of DNA.

assay, the primers are added to the specimen containing the suspect pathogen, and the sample is heated to melt all the DNA in the specimen and then allowed to cool. The primers locate and bind only to the complementary target DNA of the pathogen in question. The heat-stable polymerase begins to replicate the DNA from the point at which the primers attached, similar to two trains approaching one another on separate but converging tracks. After the initial cycle, DNA polymerization ceases at the point where the primers were located, producing a strand of DNA with a distinct size, depending on the distance separating the two primers. The specimen is heated again, and the process starts anew. After many cycles of heating, cooling, and polymerization, a large number of uniformly sized DNA fragments are produced only if the specific pathogen (or its DNA) is

present in the specimen. The polymerized DNA fragments are separated by electrophoresis and visualized with a dye or identified by hybridization by a specific probe.

PCR is an extremely useful and powerful tool. In some circumstances, this method can detect as little as one virus or bacterium in a single specimen. This method also allows laboratorians to diagnose infections caused by microorganisms that are impossible or difficult to grow in culture.

Several variations of molecular gene detection techniques in addition to PCR have been developed and incorporated into diagnostic kits for use in the clinical laboratory, including ligase chain reaction, transcription-mediated amplification, strand displacement amplification, branched-chain DNA signal amplification, and Hybrid Capture assays. Many of the newer gene detection technologies have been adapted for quantitation of the target DNA or RNA in patient specimens, such as HIV and hepatitis C virus in serum or plasma of the infected patient. If the therapy is effective, viral replication is suppressed and the viral load (level of viral genome) in the peripheral blood is low. Conversely, if mutations in the viral genome lead to resistant strains or if the antiviral therapy is ineffective, viral replication and the patient's viral load rises, indicating a need to change the therapeutic approach.

TREATMENT

The goal of treatment for an infectious disease is complete removal of the pathogen from the host and restoration of normal physiologic function to damaged tissues. Most infectious diseases of humans are self-limiting (*i.e.*, they require little or no medical therapy for a complete cure). When an infectious process gains the upper hand and therapeutic intervention is essential, the choice of treatment may be medicinal, through the use of antimicrobial agents; immunologic with antibody preparations, vaccines, or substances that stimulate and improve the host's immune function; or surgical by removal of infected tissues. The decision of which therapeutic modality or combination of therapies to use is based on the extent, urgency, and location of the disease process, the pathogen, and the availability of effective antimicrobial agents.

Antimicrobial Agents

The use of chemicals, potions, and elixirs in the treatment of infectious diseases dates back to the earliest records of human medicine. More than 2000 years ago, Greek and Chinese physicians recognized that certain substances were useful for preventing or curing wound infections. Although the biologic activity of these compounds was not understood, some may have inadvertently contained byproducts of molds that resemble modern antibiotics. From that time until the late 1800s, when the relation between infection and microorganisms was finally accepted, the evolution of anti-infective therapy was less than explosive. It was not until the advent of World War II, after the introduction of sulfonamides and penicillin, that the development of antimicrobial compounds matured into a science of great consequence. Today, the comprehensive list of effective anti-infective agents is burgeoning. Most antimicrobial compounds can be categorized roughly according to mechanism of anti-infective activity, chemical structure, and target pathogen (*e.g.*, antibacterial, antiviral, antifungal, or antiparasitic agents).

Antibacterial Agents. Antibacterial agents are referred to as *antibiotics* or *antimicrobial drugs*. However, the formal definition of these terms is not identical. Antibiotics are compounds that are produced by other microorganisms—primarily bacteria and fungi—as byproducts of metabolism and usually are effective only against other prokaryotic organisms. Under this definition, only those agents that actually are produced by microorganisms could be called *antibiotics,* and drugs such as the sulfonamides, which are produced in the laboratory, would not be considered antibiotics. In contrast, *antimicrobial drugs* are defined as any agent, natural or synthetic, that has the ability to kill or suppress microorganisms. An antimicrobial drug is considered *bactericidal* if it causes irreversible and lethal damage to the bacterial pathogen and *bacteriostatic* if its inhibitory effects on bacterial growth are reversed when the agent is eliminated. Antimicrobial drugs can be classified into families of compounds with related chemical structure and activity (Table 17-4).

Not all antibiotics are effective against all pathogenic bacteria. Some agents are effective only against gram-negative bacteria, and others are specific for gram-positive organisms. The so-called broad-spectrum antibiotics, such as the newest class of cephalosporins, are active against a wide variety of gram-positive and gram-negative bacteria.

Members of the *Mycobacterium* genus, including *M. tuberculosis*, are extremely resistant to the effects of the major classes of antibiotics and require an entirely different spectrum of agents for therapy. The four basic mechanisms of the antibiotics are disruption of the bacterial cell wall through inhibition of peptidoglycan synthesis (*e.g.*, penicillins, cephalosporins, glycopeptides, monobactams, carbapenems); inhibition of bacterial protein synthesis (*e.g.*, aminoglycosides, macrolides, tetracyclines, chloramphenicol, oxyzolidinones, streptogramins, and rifampin); interruption of nucleic acid synthesis (*e.g.*, fluoroquinolones, nalidixic acid); and interference with normal metabolism (*e.g.*, sulfonamides, trimethoprim).

Despite lack of antibiotic activity against eukaryotic cells, many agents cause unwanted or toxic side effects in humans, including allergic responses (*e.g.*, penicillins, cephalosporins, sulfonamides, glycopeptides), hearing and kidney impairment (*e.g.*, aminoglycosides), and liver or bone marrow toxicity (chloramphenicol, fluoroquinolones). Of greater concern is the increasing prevalence of bacteria resistant to the effects of antibiotics. The ways in which bacteria acquire resistance to antibiotics are becoming as numerous as the number of antibiotics. Bacterial resistance mechanisms include the production of enzymes that inactivate antibiotics such as β-lactamases, genetic mutations that alter antibiotic binding sites, alternative metabolic pathways that bypass antibiotic activity, and changes in the filtration qualities of the bacterial cell wall that prevent access of antibiotics to the target site in the organism. It is the continuous search for a "better mousetrap" that makes anti-infective therapy such a fascinating aspect of the study of infectious diseases.

TABLE 17-4 ✦ Classification and Activity of Antibacterial Agents (Antibiotics)

Family	Example	Target Site	Side Effects
Penicillins	Ampicillin	Cell wall	Allergic reactions
Cephalosporins	Cephalexin	Cell wall	Allergic reactions
Monobactams	Aztreonam	Cell wall	Rash
Aminoglycosides	Tobramycin	Ribosomes (protein synthesis)	Hearing loss Nephrotoxicity
Tetracyclines	Doxycycline	Ribosomes (protein synthesis)	Gastrointestinal irritation Allergic reactions Teeth and bone dysplasia
Macrolides	Clindamycin	Ribosomes (protein synthesis)	Colitis Allergic reactions
Sulfonamides	Sulfadiazine	Folic acid synthesis	Allergic reactions Anemia Gastrointestinal irritation
Glycopeptides	Vancomycin	Ribosomes (protein synthesis)	Allergic reactions Hearing loss Nephrotoxicity
Quinolones	Ciprofloxacin	DNA synthesis	Gastrointestinal irritation
Miscellaneous	Chloramphenicol	Ribosomes (protein synthesis)	Anemia Hepatotoxicity
	Rifampin	Ribosomes (protein synthesis)	Allergic reactions
	Trimethoprim	Folic acid synthesis	Same as sulfonamides

Antiviral Agents.   Until relatively recently, few effective antiviral agents were available for treating human infections. The reason for this is host toxicity; viral replication requires the use of eukaryotic host cell enzymes, and the drugs that effectively interrupt viral replication are likely to interfere with host cell reproduction as well. However, in response to the AIDS epidemic, there has been massive, albeit delayed, development of antiretroviral agents. Almost all antiviral compounds are synthetic, and with few exceptions, the primary target of antiviral compounds is viral RNA or DNA synthesis. Agents such as acyclovir, ganciclovir, vidarabine, and ribavirin mimic the nucleoside building blocks of RNA and DNA. During active viral replication, the nucleoside analogs inhibit the viral DNA polymerase, preventing duplication of the viral genome and spread of infectious viral progeny to other susceptible host cells. Similar to the specificity of antibiotics, antiviral agents may be active against RNA viruses only, DNA viruses only, or occasionally both. The *nucleoside reverse transcriptase inhibitors* such as zidovudine, lamivudine, didanosine, stavudine, and zalcitabine and the *non-nucleoside inhibitors,* including nevirapine, efavirenz, and delavirdine, were developed specifically for the treatment of HIV/AIDS by targeting the HIV-specific enzyme, reverse transcriptase. This key enzyme is essential for viral replication and has no counterpart in the infected eukaryotic host cells.

Another class of antiviral agents developed solely for the treatment of HIV infections is the *protease inhibitors,* which include indinavir, ritonavir, and saquinavir. These drugs inhibit an HIV-specific enzyme that is necessary for late maturation events in the viral life cycle.

Experimental approaches to antiviral therapy include compounds that inhibit viral attachment to susceptible host cells, drugs that prevent uncoating of the viral genome once inside the host cell, and agents, such as foscarnet, that directly inhibit viral DNA polymerase. More recently, a new class of antiviral agent has been developed and released that specifically inhibits influenza virus neuraminidase, an essential enzyme for viral replication. Two agents in this class, zanamivir and oseltamivir, have been approved for treatment of both influenza A and B. Although the treatment of viral infections with antimicrobial agents is a relatively recent endeavor, reports of viral mutations resulting in resistant strains have become increasingly common. This is especially troubling in the case of HIV, in which resistance to relatively new antiviral agents, including nucleoside analogs and protease inhibitors, has already been described, prompting the need for combination or alternating therapy with multiple antiretroviral agents.

Antifungal Agents.   The target site of the two most important families of antifungal agents is the cytoplasmic membranes of yeasts or molds. Fungal membranes differ from human cell membranes in that they contain the sterol ergosterol instead of cholesterol. The polyene family of antifungal compounds (*e.g.,* amphotericin B, nystatin) preferentially binds to ergosterol and forms holes in the cytoplasmic membrane, causing leakage of the fungal cell contents and, eventually, lysis of the cell. The imidazole class of drugs (*e.g.,* fluconazole, itraconazole, ketoconazole) inhibit the synthesis of ergosterol, thereby damaging the integrity of the fungal cytoplasmic membrane. Both types of drugs bind to a certain extent to the cholesterol component of host cell membranes and elicit a variety of toxic side effects in treated patients. The nucleoside analog 5-fluorocytosine (5-FC) disrupts fungal RNA and DNA synthesis but without the toxicity associated with the polyene and imidazole drugs. Unfortunately, 5-FC demonstrates little or no antifungal activity against molds or dimorphic fungi and is primarily reserved for infections caused by yeasts.

A novel class of antifungal compounds called *pneumocandins* has received considerable attention because they inhibit the synthesis of β-1,3-glucan, a major cell wall polysaccharide that is found in fungi, including *C. albicans, Aspergillus,* and *Pneumocystis carinii.*

Antiparasitic Agents.   Because of the extreme diversity of human parasites and their growth cycles, a review of antiparasitic therapies and agents would be highly impractical and lengthy. Similar to other infectious disease caused by eukaryotic microorganisms, treatment of parasitic illnesses is based on exploiting essential components of the parasite's metabolism or cellular anatomy that are not shared by the host. Any relatedness between the target site of the parasite and the cells of the host increases the likelihood of toxic reactions in the host.

Continued development of improved antiparasitic agents suffers greatly from economic considerations. Parasitic diseases of humans are primarily the scourge of poor, developing nations of the world. As a result, financial incentives to produce more effective therapies are nonexistent. Resistance among human parasites to standard, effective therapy also is a major concern. In Africa, Asia, and South America, the incidence of chloroquine-resistant malaria (*Plasmodium falciparum*) is on the rise. Resistant strains require more complicated, expensive, and potentially toxic therapy with a combination of agents.

Immunotherapy

An exciting approach to the treatment of infectious diseases is immunotherapy. This strategy involves supplementing or stimulating the host's immune response so that the spread of a pathogen is limited or reversed. Several products are available for this purpose, including intravenous immunoglobulin (IVIG) and cytokines. IVIG is a pooled preparation of antibodies obtained from normal, healthy immune human donors that is infused as an intravenous solution. In theory, pathogen-specific antibodies present in the infusion facilitate neutralization, phagocytosis, and clearance of infectious agents above and beyond the capabilities of the diseased host. Hyperimmune immunoglobulin preparations, which also are commercially available, contain high titers of antibodies against specific pathogens, including hepatitis B virus, cytomegalovirus, rabies virus, and varicella-zoster virus.

Cytokines are substances produced by human white blood cells that, in small quantities, stimulate white cell replication, phagocytosis, antibody production, and the induction of fever, inflammation, and tissue repair—all of which counteract infectious agents and hasten recovery.

With the advent of genetic engineering and cloning, many cytokines, including interferons and interleukins, have been produced in the laboratory and are being evaluated experimentally as anti-infective agents. As we learn more about the action of cytokines, we are beginning to appreciate that some of the adverse reactions associated with infectious processes result from our own inflammatory response. Interventional therapies designed to inactivate certain cytokines (*e.g.*, tumor necrosis factor) have proven to be helpful in animal models of infection. It is not unlikely that therapies based on the regulation of the inflammatory response will become widely used in human medicine over the next few years.

One of the most efficient but often overlooked means of preventing infectious diseases is immunization. Proper and timely adherence to recommended vaccination schedules in children and boosters in adults effectively reduces the senseless spread of vaccine-preventable illnesses such as measles, mumps, pertussis, and rubella, which still occur in the United States with alarming frequency. New strategies for the development of vaccines carried by harmless viral vectors are being developed that, someday, might lead to inexpensive and effective oral immunization against HIV, hepatitis C, and other potentially lethal infectious diseases.

Surgical Intervention

Before the discovery of antimicrobial agents, surgical removal of infected tissues, organs, or limbs was occasionally the only option available to prevent the death of the infected host. Today, medicinal therapy with antibiotics and other anti-infective agents is an effective solution for most infectious diseases. However, surgical intervention is still an important option for cases in which the pathogen is resistant to available treatments; containment of a rapidly progressing infectious process is the only means of saving the patient (*e.g.*, gas gangrene); or access to an infected site by antimicrobial agents is limited and surgical drainage (*e.g.*, abscesses), cleaning of the site (debridement), or removal of organs or necrotic tissue (*e.g.*, appendectomy) can hasten the recovery process. In certain situations, surgery may be the only means of effecting a complete cure, as in the case of endocarditis (*i.e.*, infected heart valves), in which the diseased valve must be replaced with a mechanical or biologic valve to restore normal function.

In summary, the ultimate outcome of any interaction between microorganisms and the human host is decided by a complex and ever-changing set of variables that take into account the overall health and physiologic function of the host and the virulence and infectious dose of the microbe. In many instances, disease is an inevitable consequence, but with continued advancement of science and technology, the vast number of cases can be eliminated or rapidly cured with appropriate therapy. It is the intent of those who study infectious diseases to thoroughly understand the pathogen, the disease course, the mechanisms of transmission, and the host response to infection. This knowledge will lead to development of improved diagnostic techniques, revolutionary approaches to anti-infective therapy, and eradication or control of microscopic agents that cause frightening devastation and loss of life throughout the world.

Bibliography

Bush K., Jacoby G.A., Medeiros A.A. (1995). A functional classification scheme for β-lactamases and its correlation with molecular structure. *Antimicrobial Agents and Chemotherapy* 39, 1211–1233.

Butler J.C., Peters C.J. (1994). Hantaviruses and hantavirus pulmonary syndrome. *Clinical Infectious Diseases* 19, 387–395.

Carpenter C.C.J., Fischl M.A., Hammer S.M., Hirsch M.S., Jacobsen D.M., Katzenstein D.A., et al. (1996). Antiviral therapy for HIV infection in 1996. *Journal of the American Medical Association* 276, 146–154.

Centers for Disease Control and Prevention. (1999). Outbreak of West Nile-like viral encephalitis. *Morbidity and Mortality Weekly Report* 48, 845–849.

Dumler J.S., Bakken J.S. (1995). Ehrlichial diseases in humans: Emerging tick-borne infections. *Clinical Infectious Diseases* 20, 1102–1110.

Gold H.S., Moellering R.C., Jr. (1996). Drug resistance: Antimicrobial-drug resistance. *New England Journal of Medicine* 335, 1445–1453.

Jacobsen H., Hanggi M., Ott M., Duncan I.B., Owen S., Andreoni M., et al. (1996). In vivo resistance to a human immunodeficiency virus type 1 proteinase inhibitor: Mutations, kinetics, and frequencies. *Journal of Infectious Diseases* 173, 1379–1387.

Krogfelt K.A. (1991). Bacterial adhesion: Genetics, biogenetics, and role in pathogenesis of fimbrial adhesions of *Escherichia coli*. *Review of Infectious Disease* 13, 721–735.

Livermore D.M. (1995). β-Lactamases in laboratory and clinical resistance. *Clinical Microbiology Review* 8, 557–584.

Moore S.S. (1996). Pattern and predictability of emerging infections. *Hospital Practice* 31, 85–108.

Rosenthal N. (1994). Tools of the trade—recombinant DNA. *New England Journal of Medicine* 331, 315–317.

Tang Y.-W., Persing D.H. (1999). Molecular detection and identification of microorganisms. In Murray P.R., Baron E.J., Pfaller M.A., Tenover F.C., Yolken R.H. (Eds.), *Manual of Clinical Microbiology* (7th ed., pp. 215–244). Washington, DC: American Society for Microbiology.

Tyler K.L. (2000). Prions and prion diseases of the central nervous system (neurodegenerative diseases). In Mandell G.L., Bennett J.E., Dolin R. (Eds.), *Mandell, Douglas, and Bennett's principles and practice of infectious diseases* (5th ed., pp. 1971–1985). Philadelphia: Churchill Livingstone.

White N.J. (1996). Current concepts: The treatment of malaria. *New England Journal of Medicine* 335, 800–806.

Immunity and Inflammation

Cynthia Sommer

The human body constantly defends itself against bacteria, viruses, and other foreign substances it encounters. It also must detect and respond to abnormal cells and molecules that periodically develop in the body so that diseases such as cancers do not occur. These external and internal threats are efficiently handled by two cooperative defense systems. One system is our *nonspecific* or *innate defenses,* which can protect us from most pathogens and does not distinguish one type of pathogen from another (Table 18-1). These general defenses produce the same level of response on each encounter with the pathogen. The second defense system, the *specific* or *acquired immune system,* responds specifically to each type of foreign invader or molecule and develops during an individual's lifetime. Acquired immunity has the ability to produce an enhanced response on re-exposure to a pathogen because of memory cells. White cells called *lymphocytes* are key players in this response.

Nonspecific or innate resistance results from two lines of general defenses. Microorganisms encounter the first line of resistance on exposure to the epithelial layers that line our skin and mucous membranes. The second line of non-specific defenses involves chemical signals, antimicrobial substances, phagocytic cells, and fever associated with the inflammatory response. These two lines of nonspecific de-

fense mechanisms are important for excluding pathogens from our body and removing them if they enter. They also aid in proper signaling of the second defense system—specific immunity.

The major focus of this chapter is to present an overview of the immune cells, molecules, and tissues and to describe the normal mechanisms used to protect the body against foreign invaders.

Immune System

After you have completed this section of the chapter, you should be able to meet the following objectives:

✦ State the properties associated with specific or acquired immunity
✦ Define and describe the characteristics of an antigen or immunogen
✦ Characterize the significance and function of major histocompatibility complex molecules
✦ Describe the functions of the macrophage
✦ Contrast and compare the development and function of the T and B lymphocytes from stem cells to regulator or effector immune cells

TABLE 18-1 ✦ Immune Defenses

First Line of Defense	Second Line of Defense	Third Line of Defense
Intact skin Mucous membranes and their secretions	Phagocytic white blood cells Inflammation and fever Antimicrobial substances Natural killer cells	Specialized lymphocytes Antibodies

✦ Describe the function and characteristics of natural killer cells
✦ State the function of the five classes of immunoglobulins
✦ Differentiate between the central and peripheral lymphoid structures
✦ Describe the properties of cytokines and how they influence an immune response
✦ Compare passive and active immunity
✦ Characterize the role of the complement system in the immune response

The immune system consists of the immune cells and the central and peripheral lymphoid tissues. A variety of white blood cells and molecules is produced that can recognize and remove the myriad of intruders we encounter. These components interact to form a dynamic network that protects the body from harmful foreign invaders.

Fundamental to the appropriate functioning of the specific defense system is the ability to regulate the recognition, amplification, and response of the immune cells to the microbe. The immune system must recognize and differentiate one foreign pathogen from another, while simultaneously distinguishing these foreign molecules from normal cells and proteins in the body. This phenomenal ability to differentiate nonself or dangerous agents from self or nonharmful agents is unique to this system. An evolutionary adaptation that is unique to the immune system is a memory response—the ability to recall and quickly produce a heightened immune response on subsequent exposure to the same foreign agents. For example, after a person has had the mumps, the immune system "remembers" the experience and protects the person against having the disease again. Although the immune response normally is protective, it also can produce undesirable effects such as when the response is excessive, as in allergies, or when it recognizes self-tissue as foreign, as in autoimmune disease. Regulation of the immune response is important because of the tremendous energy requirements needed to produce new cells and molecules and because inappropriate or excessive responses can lead to permanent tissue damage.

ANTIGENS

Before discussing the cells and responses inherent to immunity, it is important to understand the substances that elicit a response from the host. *Antigens* or *immunogens* are substances foreign to the host that can stimulate an immune response. These foreign molecules are recognized by receptors on immune cells and by proteins, called *antibodies* or *immunoglobulins*, that are generated in response to the antigen. Antigens include bacteria, fungi, viruses, protozoans, and parasitic worms. Antigens also can include substances such as pollen, poison ivy plant resin, insect venom, and transplanted organs. Most antigens are macromolecules such as proteins and polysaccharides, although lipids and nucleic acids occasionally can serve as antigens. Chemically complex molecules tend to be good stimulators of immunity.

Antigens, which in general are large and complex, are biologically degraded into smaller chemical units or peptides.

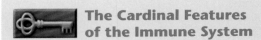

The Cardinal Features of the Immune System

➤ The immune system is a dynamic network of immune organs and immune cells that recognizes self from nonself and protects against foreign agents such as microorganisms and abnormal cells that arise within the body.

➤ The immune system responds in distinct and different ways to different foreign agents. The protection conferred by the immune system can be innate or nonspecific in that it does not differentiate among agents, or acquired and specific in that it differentiates among agents.

➤ The immune response consists of an interaction between an antigen or agent that is recognized as foreign and an antibody or immune cell.

➤ The memory capacity of the immune system enables it to "remember" previous exposures to a foreign agent so that it can rapidly and effectively respond on subsequent exposures.

➤ Communication between immune cells and recognition of antigen depend on an elaborate system of membrane molecules, such as the major histocompatibility complex, which distinguishes self from nonself, and the cytokines, which form a communication link between immune cells and other tissues and organs of the body.

These discrete, immunologically active sites on antigens are called *antigenic determinants* or *epitopes* (Fig. 18-1). It is the unique molecular shape of an epitope that is recognized by a specific receptor found on the surface of the lymphocyte or by the antigen-binding site of an antibody. A single antigen may contain several antigenic determinants; each can stimulate a distinct clone of lymphocytes to respond. For example, different proteins that comprise a virus may function as unique antigens, each of which contains several antigenic determinants. Hundreds of antigenic determinants are found on complex structures such as the bacterial cell wall.

Smaller substances (molecular masses <10,000 daltons) usually are unable to stimulate an adequate immune response by themselves. When these low–molecular-weight compounds, known as *haptens,* combine with larger protein molecules, they function as antigens. The proteins act as carrier molecules for the haptens to form antigenic hapten-carrier complexes. An allergic response to the antibiotic penicillin is an example of a hapten-carrier complex that has medical importance. Penicillin (molecular mass of approximately 350 daltons) is incapable of causing an immune response by itself. However, penicillin can chemically combine with body proteins to form larger complexes that can then generate in some individuals an immune response to the penicillin epitope.

IMMUNE CELLS

The primary cells of the specific immune system are white blood cells, called *lymphocytes* (Fig. 18-2). Other accessory cells, such as macrophages and dendritic cells, aid in the processing of antigen and activation of lymphocytes. Functionally, there are two types of immune cells: regulatory cells and effector cells. The *regulatory cells* assist in orchestrating and controlling the immune response. For example, helper

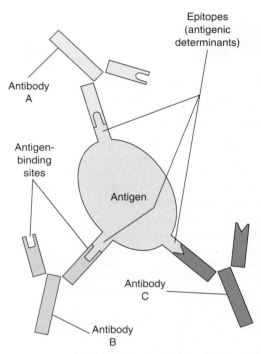

FIGURE 18-1 Multiple epitopes on a complex antigen being recognized by their respective (A, B, C) antibodies.

T lymphocytes activate other lymphocytes and phagocytes. The final stages of the immune response are aided by *effector cells* such as cytotoxic T lymphocytes, which efficiently kill virus-infected cells. Various types of effector cells help in causing destruction and removal of the antigen.

Lymphocytes represent 25% to 35% of blood leukocytes, and 99% of the cells reside in the lymph. Like other

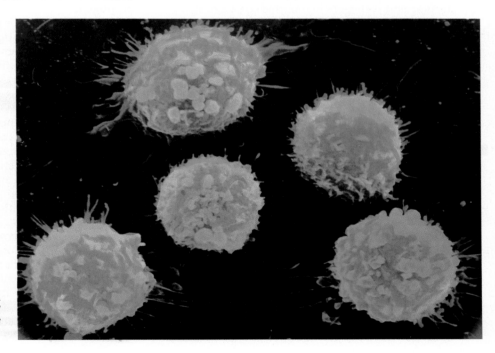

FIGURE 18-2 A scanning electron micrograph of lymphocytes. (© CNRI/ Science Photo Library, Science Source/ Photo Researchers)

Immune Cells

➤ Functionally, there are two types of immune cells: the regulatory cells that orchestrate and control the immune response, and the effector cells that destroy the offending agent.

➤ The cells of the immune system consist of the lymphocytes, which are the primary cells of the immune system, and the accessory cells such as the macrophages, which aid in processing of antigen and activation.

➤ There are two types of lymphocytes: the T lymphocytes, which provide cellular immunity and protect against intracellular pathogens such as viruses, and the B lymphocytes, which produce antibodies that travel in the blood and interact with circulating and cell surface antigens.

➤ The immune cells express membrane proteins called *clusters of differentiation* (CD) that serve as phenotypic markers for different types and generations of T and B lymphocytes.

➤ There are two main types of T lymphocytes: the CD4+ or helper T cells serve as the master switch for the immune system, and the CD8+ cytotoxic T cells selectively identify and destroy abnormal or virus-infected cells.

➤ The B lymphocytes differentiate into plasma cells that secrete five classes of immunoglobulins: IgM and IgG, which circulate in the blood to protect against bacteria, toxins, and viruses; IgA, which is a secretory immunoglobulin that protects against pathogens in bronchial, gastrointestinal, and other secretions; IgD, which serves as the antigen receptor for initiating differentiation of B cells; and IgE, which is implicated in hypersensitivity and allergic reactions.

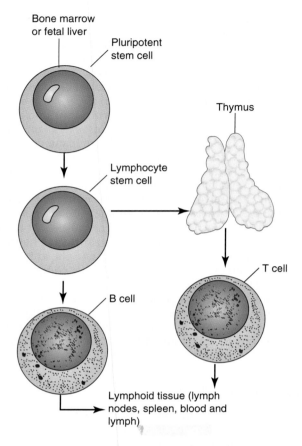

FIGURE 18-3 Pathway for T- and B-cell differentiation.

blood cells, lymphocytes are generated from stem cells in the bone marrow (Fig. 18-3). These undifferentiated cells congregate in the central lymphoid tissues, where they mature into distinct types of lymphocytes. One class of lymphocyte, the *B lymphocytes* (B cells), matures in the bone marrow and is essential for humoral or antibody-mediated immunity. The other class of lymphocyte, the *T lymphocytes* (T cells), completes its maturation in the thymus and functions in the peripheral tissues to produce cell-mediated immunity, as well as aiding with antibody production. Approximately 60% to 70% of blood lymphocytes are T cells, and 10% to 20% are B cells. The various types of lymphocytes are distinguished by their function and response to antigen, their cell membrane molecules and receptors, their types of secreted proteins, and their tissue location. High concentra-

tions of mature T and B lymphocytes are found in the lymph nodes, spleen, and mucosal tissues, where they can respond to antigen.

The key trigger for activation of B and T cells is the recognition of the antigen by unique surface receptors. The B-cell antigen receptor consists of membrane-bound immunoglobulin proteins that can bind a specific antigen. The T-cell receptor recognizes the antigen peptide in association with a self-recognition protein, called a *major histocompatibility complex* (MHC) molecule. The appropriate recognition of MHC and self-peptides or MHC associated with foreign peptides is essential for lymphocytes to differentiate "self" from "foreign."

The immune system enlists specialized *antigen-presenting cells* (APCs), such as macrophage and dendritic cells, to ensure the appropriate processing and presentation of antigen. On recognition of antigen and after additional stimulation by various secreted signaling molecules called *cytokines*, the B and T lymphocytes divide several times to form populations or clones of cells that continue to differentiate into effector cells and memory cells. Several types of effector cells and molecules defend the body in an immune response (Fig. 18-4). In humoral or antibody-mediated immunity, activated B cells produce effector cells called *plasma cells*, which secrete protein molecules called *antibodies* or *immunoglobulins*. Antibodies bind and aggregate foreign cells

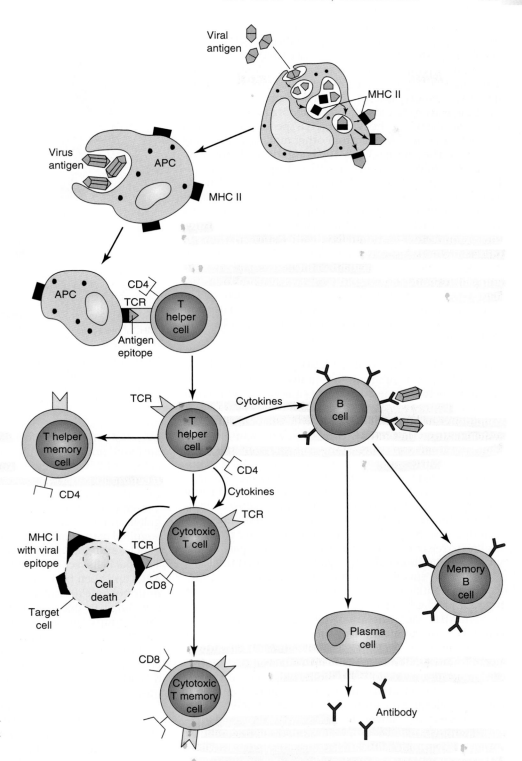

FIGURE 18-4 Pathway for immune cell participation in an immune response.

and molecules to ensure their removal. Phagocytic cells can more efficiently bind, engulf, and digest antigen–antibody aggregates or immune complexes than they can antigen alone.

Mature T and B cells display surface recognition molecules called *clusters of differentiation* (CD). These molecules serve to define functionally distinct T-cell subsets such as

CD4+ T helper cells and CD8+ T cytotoxic cells. The many cell surface CD molecules detected on immune cells have allowed scientists to identify cells and learn the normal and abnormal processes displayed by these cells. In cell-mediated immunity, regulatory CD4+ helper T cells enhance the response of other T and B cells, and effector cytotoxic T cells (CD8+) kill tumor cells and virus-infected cells (see

Fig. 18-4). The human immunodeficiency virus (HIV) that causes acquired immunodeficiency syndrome (AIDS) infects and destroys the CD4+ helper T cell (see Chapter 20).

T and B lymphocytes possess all of the key properties associated with the specific immune response—specificity, diversity, memory, and self–nonself recognition. These cells can exactly recognize a particular microorganism or foreign molecule. Each lymphocyte targets a specific antigen and differentiates that invader from other molecules that may be similar. The approximately 10^{12} lymphocytes in the body have tremendous diversity. They can respond to the millions of different kinds of antigens encountered daily. This diversity occurs because an enormous variety of lymphocyte populations have been programmed during development, each to respond to a particular antigen. After the lymphocytes are stimulated by their antigen, they acquire a memory response. The memory T and B lymphocytes that are generated remain in the body for a long time and can respond more rapidly on repeat exposure than naive cells (see Fig. 18-4). Because of this heightened state of immune reactivity, the immune system usually can respond to commonly encountered microorganisms so efficiently that we are unaware of the response.

Major Histocompatibility Complex Molecules

An essential feature of specific immunity is the ability to discriminate between the body's own molecules and foreign antigens. Failure to distinguish self from nonself can lead to conditions such as autoimmune disease where the immune system destroys the body's own cells. Key recognition molecules essential for distinguishing self from nonself are the cell surface MHC antigens. These molecules, which in humans are coded by closely linked genes on chromosome 6, were first identified because of their role in organ and tissue transplantation. When cells are transplanted between individuals who are not identical for their MHC molecules, the immune system produces a vigorous immune response leading to rejection of the transferred cells or organs. MHC molecules did not evolve to reject transplanted tissues, a situation not encountered in nature. Rather, these molecules are essential for correct cell-to-cell interactions among immune and body cells.

The MHC molecules involved in self-recognition and cell-to-cell communication fall into two classes, class I and class II (Fig. 18-5). *Class I MHC* molecules are cell surface glycoproteins that interact with antigen receptors and the CD8 molecule on T cytotoxic lymphocytes. They are found on nearly all nucleated cells in the body and thereby are capable of alerting the immune system of any cell changes due to viruses and cancer. The class I MHC molecule contains a groove that accommodates a peptide fragment of antigen. T cytotoxic cells can become activated only when they are presented with the foreign antigen peptide associated with the class I MHC molecule. Antigen peptides associate with class I molecules in cells that are infected by intracellular pathogens such as a virus. As the virus multiplies, small peptides from degraded virus proteins complex with class I MHC molecules and are then transported to the infected cell membrane. This complex communicates to the T cytotoxic cell that the cell must be destroyed for the

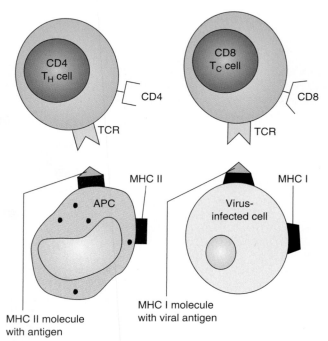

FIGURE 18-5 Interaction of a T-cell receptor (TCR) on a CD4 helper T (T_H) cell with class II MHC molecule on an antigen-presenting (APC) cell and CD8 cytotoxic (T_C) T cell with class I MHC molecule on a virus-infected cell.

overall survival of the host. *Class II MHC* molecules, which are found primarily on APCs such as macrophages, dendritic cells, and B lymphocytes, communicate with an antigen receptor and a CD4 molecule on T helper lymphocytes. Class II MHC molecules also have a groove or cleft that binds a fragment of antigen from pathogens that have been engulfed and digested during the process of phagocytosis. The engulfed pathogen is degraded into peptide in cytoplasmic vesicles and then complexed with class II MHC molecules. T helper cells recognize these complexes on the surface of APCs and then become activated. These triggered T cells multiply quickly and direct the need for a response to the invading pathogen through the secretion of cytokines. A third group of genes located on the same chromosome as the class I and II MHC genes encode other proteins involved in the immune response. Complement and cytokines important for signaling an immune response are examples of this third type of MHC molecule. These are structurally and functionally unrelated to the class I and II MHC molecules.

Each individual has a unique collection of several MHC proteins, and a variety of MHC molecules can exist in a population. Thus, MHC molecules are both polygenic and polymorphic. The MHC genes are the most polymorphic genes known. Because of the number of MHC genes and the possibility of several alleles for each gene, it is almost impossible for any two individuals to be identical, except if they are identical twins. The uniqueness of these genes is essential for the immune system to distinguish self from nonself. In contrast to the receptors on T and B lymphocytes that bind a unique antigen molecule, each MHC protein can bind a broad spectrum of antigen peptides. The bound antigen

TABLE 18-2 ✦ Properties of MHC Class I and MHC Class II Molecules

Properties	MHC Class I	MHC Class II
HLA antigens	HLA-A, HLA-B, HLA-C	HLA-DR, HLA-DP, HLA-DQ
Distribution	Virtually all nucleated cells	Restricted to immune cells, antigen-presenting cells, B cells, and macrophages
Functions	Present processed antigen to cytotoxic CD8+ T cells; restrict cytolysis to virus-infected cells, tumor cells, transplanted cells	Present processed antigenic fragments to CD4+ T cells; necessary for effective interaction among immune cells

HLA, human leukocyte antigen; MHC, major histocompatibility complex.

fragments then allow for proper recognition of self/nonself by immune cells and an appropriate immune response.

Human MHC proteins are called *human leukocyte antigens* (HLA) because they were first detected on white blood cells. Because these molecules play a role in transplant rejection and are detected by immunologic tests, they are commonly called *antigens*. More recently, analysis of the genes for the HLA molecules has ensured a more complete identification of the potential antigens present in an individual. The human class I MHC molecules are divided into types called HLA-A, HLA-B, and HLA-C, and the class II MHC molecules are identified as HLA-DR, HLA-DP, and HLA-DQ (Table 18-2). Additional, less well-defined class I and II MHC genes also have been described. Each of the gene loci that describe an HLA molecule can be occupied by multiple alleles or alternate genes. For example, there are more than 120 possible genes for the A locus and 250 genes for the B locus. Each of the gene products or antigens is designated by a number, such as HLA-B27.

Because the class I and II MHC genes are closely linked on one chromosome, the combination of HLA genes usually is inherited as a unit, called a *haplotype*. Each person inherits a chromosome from each parent and therefore has two HLA haplotypes. The identification or typing of HLA molecules is important in tissue or organ transplantation, forensics, and paternity evaluations. In organ or tissue transplantation, the closer the matching of HLA types, the greater is the probability of identical antigens and the lower the chance of rejection.

Monocytes, Macrophages, and Dendritic Cells

Monocytes and tissue macrophages are a part of the mononuclear phagocyte system, which in turn is part of the reticuloendothelial system. All of the cells of the mononuclear phagocytic system arise from common precursors in the bone marrow that produce the blood monocytes. The monocytes migrate to various tissues where they mature into macrophages. Macrophages are characterized as large cells with extensive cytoplasm and numerous vacuoles. As the general scavenger cells of the body, the macrophage can be fixed in a tissue or can be free to migrate from an organ to lymphoid tissues. The tissue macrophages are scattered in connective tissue or clustered in organs such as the lung (*i.e.,* alveolar macrophages), liver (*i.e.,* Kupffer's cells), spleen, lymph nodes, peritoneum, central nervous system (*i.e.,* microglial cells), and other areas.

Macrophages serve several important functions in an immune response. Macrophages are activated by the presence of antigen to engulf and digest foreign particles (Fig. 18-6). The ingestion process can be aided by the presence of antibody. The phagocytic destruction of microorganisms helps to contain infectious agents until specific immunity can be marshaled. Early in the host response, the macrophage functions as an accessory cell to ensure amplification of the inflammatory response and initiation of specific immunity. Macrophages also secrete cytokines (*e.g.,* tumor necrosis factor [TNF], interleukin-1 [IL-1]) that produce fever and prime T and B lymphocytes that have recognized

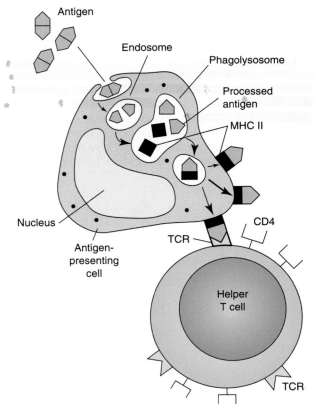

FIGURE 18-6 Presentation of antigen to helper T cell by an antigen-presenting cell (APC).

antigen. Activated macrophages act as APCs that break down complex antigens into peptide fragments that can associate with class II MHC molecules. Macrophages can then present these complexes to the helper T cell so that nonself–self-recognition and activation of the immune response can occur. The macrophages also can serve as phagocytic effector cells in humoral and cell-mediated immune responses. They can remove antigen–antibody aggregates or, under the influence of T-cell cytokines, they can destroy virus-infected cells or tumor cells.

Dendritic cells share with the macrophage the important task of presenting antigen to T lymphocytes. These distinctive, star-shaped cells with long extensions of their cytoplasmic membrane provide an extensive surface rich in class II MHC molecules, which is essential for initiation of an acquired immune response. Dendritic cells are found in lymphoid tissues and other body areas where antigen enters the body. In these different environments, dendritic cells can acquire specialized functions and appearances, as do macrophages. Langerhans' cells are specialized dendritic cells in the skin, whereas follicular dendritic cells are found in the lymph nodes. Langerhans' cells are constantly surveying the skin for antigen and can transport foreign material to a nearby lymph node. Skin dendritic cells and macrophages also are involved in cell-mediated immune reactions of the skin such as delayed allergic contact hypersensitivity.

B Lymphocytes

The B lymphocytes are responsible for humoral immunity. Humoral immunity provides for elimination of bacterial invaders, neutralization of bacterial toxins, prevention of viral infection, and immediate allergic responses (see Chapter 19).

B lymphocytes can be identified by the presence of surface immunoglobulin that functions as the antigen receptor, class II MHC proteins, complement receptors, and specific CD molecules. During the maturation of B cells, which occurs in the bone marrow, stem cells change into immature precursor (pre-B) cells. A rearrangement of immunoglobulin genes produces a unique receptor and type of effector antibody (*e.g.,* immunoglobulin M [IgM] or IgD). This stage of maturation is programmed into the B cells and does not require antigen; it is an antigen-independent process. The various stages of maturation can be defined by the presence of a partial (heavy chain only) or complete immunoglobulin receptor. CD molecules also change as the B cell matures. The CD surface markers are useful for defining B-cell malignancies. The mature B cell leaves the bone marrow, enters the circulation, and migrates to the various peripheral lymphoid tissues, where it is stimulated to respond to a specific antigen.

The commitment of a B-cell line to a specific antigen is evident by the expression of the surface immunoglobulin antigen receptor molecule. B cells that encounter antigen complementary to their surface immunoglobulin receptor and receive T-cell help undergo a series of changes that transform the B cells into antibody-secreting plasma cells or into memory B cells (Fig. 18-7). B lymphocytes also can function as APCs by ingesting the surface immunoglobulin–antigen complex, processing it into small peptides, and recycling the peptide, now complexed to the class II MHC molecules, to its surface. The antigen peptide–class II MHC complex is recognized by helper T cells, which then are stimulated to secrete various cytokines. These cytokines trigger the multiplication and maturation of antigen-activated B and T cells. The activated B cell divides and undergoes terminal maturation into a plasma cell, which can produce thousands of antibody molecules per second. The antibodies are released into the blood and lymph, where they bind and remove their unique antigen with the help of other immune cells and molecules. Longer-lived memory B cells are generated and distributed into the peripheral tissues in preparation for subsequent antigen exposure.

Immunoglobulins

Antibodies comprise a class of proteins called *immunoglobulins*. The immunoglobulins have been divided into five classes: IgG, IgA, IgM, IgD, and IgE (Table 18-3), each with a different role in the immune defense strategy. Immunoglobulins have a characteristic four-polypeptide structure consisting of at least two identical antigen-binding sites (Fig. 18-8). Each immunoglobulin is composed of two identical light (L) chains and two identical heavy (H) chains

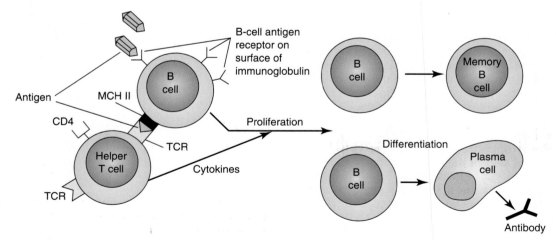

FIGURE 18-7 Pathway for B-cell differentiation.

TABLE 18-3 ✦ Classes and Characteristics of Immunoglobulins

Figure	Class	Percentage of Total	Characteristics
	IgG	75.0	Displays antiviral, antitoxin, and antibacterial properties; only Ig that crosses the placenta; responsible for protection of newborn; activates complement and binds to macrophages
	IgA	15.0	Predominant Ig in body secretions, such as saliva, nasal and respiratory secretions, and breast milk; protects mucous membranes
	IgM	10.0	Forms the natural antibodies such as those for ABO blood antigens; prominent in early immune responses; activates complement
	IgD	0.2	Found on B lymphocytes; needed for maturation of B cells
	IgE	0.004	Binds to mast cells and basophils; involved in parasitic infections, allergic and hypersensitivity reactions

to form a Y-shaped molecule. The two forked ends of the immunoglobulin molecule bind antigen and are called *Fab* (*i.e.,* antigen-binding) fragments, and the tail of the molecule, which is called the *Fc* fragment, determines the biologic properties that are characteristic of a particular class of immunoglobulins. The amino acid sequence of the heavy and light chains shows constant (C) regions and variable (V) regions. The *constant regions* have sequences of amino acids that vary little among the antibodies of a particular class of immunoglobulin. The constant regions allow separation of immunoglobulins into classes (*e.g.,* IgM, IgG) and allows each class of antibody to interact with certain effectors cells and molecules. For example, IgG can tag an antigen for recognition and destruction by phagocytes. The *variable regions* contain the antigen-binding sites of the molecule. The wide variation in the amino acid sequence of the variable regions

seen from antibody to antibody allows this region to serve as the antigen-binding site. A unique amino acid sequence in this region determines a distinctive three-dimensional pocket that is complementary to the antigen, allowing recognition and binding of the antigen. Each B-cell clone produces antibody with one specific antigen-binding variable region or domain. During the course of the immune response, class switching (*e.g.,* from IgM to IgG) can occur, causing the B-cell clone to produce any of the following antibody types.

IgG (gamma globulin) is the most abundant of the circulating immunoglobulins. It is present in body fluids and readily enters the tissues. IgG is the only immunoglobulin that crosses the placenta and can transfer immunity from the mother to the fetus. This class of immunoglobulin protects against bacteria, toxins, and viruses in body fluids and

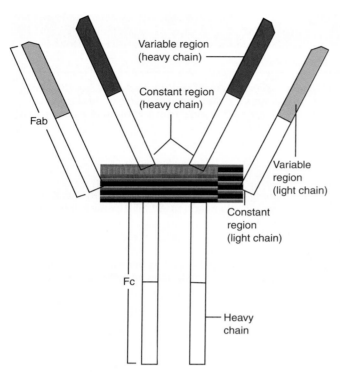

FIGURE 18-8 Schematic model of an IgG molecule showing the constant and variable regions of the light and dark chains.

activates the complement system. There are four subsets of IgG (*i.e.,* IgG1, IgG2, IgG3, and IgG4) that have some restrictions in their response to certain types of antigens. For example, IgG2 appears to be responsive to bacteria that are encapsulated with a polysaccharide covering, such as *Streptococcus pneumoniae, Haemophilus influenzae,* and *Neisseria meningitidis.*

IgA, a secretory immunoglobulin, is found in saliva, tears, colostrum (*i.e.,* first milk of a nursing mother), and in bronchial, gastrointestinal, prostatic, and vaginal secretions. This dimeric secretory immunoglobulin is considered a primary defense against local infections in mucosal tissues. IgA prevents the attachment of viruses and bacteria to epithelial cells.

IgM is a macromolecule that forms a polymer of five basic immunoglobulin units. It cannot cross the placenta and does not transfer maternal immunity. It is the first circulating immunoglobulin to appear in response to an antigen and is the first antibody type made by a newborn. This is diagnostically useful because the presence of IgM suggests a current infection by a specific pathogen. The identification of newborn IgM rather than maternally transferred IgG to a specific pathogen is indicative of an in utero or newborn infection.

IgD is found primarily on the cell membranes of B lymphocytes. It serves as an antigen receptor for initiating the differentiation of B cells.

IgE is involved in inflammation, allergic responses, and combating parasitic infections. It binds to mast cells and basophils. The binding of antigen to mast cell- or basophil-bound IgE triggers these cells to release histamine and other mediators important in inflammation and allergies.

T Lymphocytes

T lymphocytes function in the activation of other T cells and B cells, in the control of viral infections, in the rejection of foreign tissue grafts, and in delayed hypersensitivity reactions (see Chapter 19). Collectively, these immune responses are called *cell-mediated* or *cellular immunity.* Besides the ability to respond to cell-associated antigens, the T cell is integral to immunity because it regulates self-recognition and amplifies the response of B and T lymphocytes.

T lymphocytes arise from bone marrow stem cells, but unlike B cells, pre-T cells migrate to the thymus for their maturation. There, the immature T lymphocytes undergo rearrangement of the genes needed for expression of a unique T-cell antigen receptor similar to but distinct from the B-cell receptor. The T-cell receptor (TCR) is composed of two polypeptides that fold to form a groove that recognizes processed antigen peptide–MHC complexes. The TCR is associated with other surface molecules known as the *CD3 complex* that aid cell signaling. Maturation of subpopulations of T cells (*i.e.,* CD4+ and CD8+) also occurs in the thymus. Mature T cells migrate to the peripheral lymphoid tissues and, on encountering antigen, multiply and differentiate into memory T cells and various effector T cells.

Helper T Cells. The CD4+ helper T cell (T_H) serves as a master switch for the immune system. Activation of helper T cells depends on the recognition of antigen in association with class II MHC molecules. Activated helper T cells secrete cytokines that influence the function of nearly all other cells of the immune system. These cytokines activate and regulate B cells, cytotoxic T cells, natural killer (NK) cells, macrophages, and other immune cells. Distinct subpopulations of helper T cells (*i.e.,* T_H1 and T_H2) have been identified and shown to secrete different patterns of cytokines. The pattern of cytokine production determines whether an antibody- or cell-mediated immune response develops. This differential expression of cytokines can influence expressions of some diseases (*i.e.,* lepromatous and tuberculoid leprosy).

T Cytotoxic Cells. Activated CD8+ T cytotoxic cells become cytotoxic T cells after recognition of class I MHC–antigen complexes on target cell surfaces such as body cells infected by viruses or transformed by cancer (Fig. 18-9). The recognition of class I MHC–antigen complexes on infected target cells ensures that neighboring uninfected host cells, which express class I MHC molecules alone or with self-peptide, are not indiscriminately destroyed. The CD8+ T cells destroy target cells by releasing cytolytic enzymes, toxic cytokines, and pore-forming molecules (*i.e.,* perforins) or by triggering programmed cell death (apoptosis) in the target cell. The perforin proteins produce pores in the target cell membrane, allowing entry of toxic molecules and loss of cell constituents. The CD8+ T cells are especially important in controlling replicating viruses and intracellular bacteria because antibody cannot penetrate living cells.

Cell-mediated immunity involves CD4+ and CD8+ T lymphocytes. Activated CD4+ helper T cells release vari-

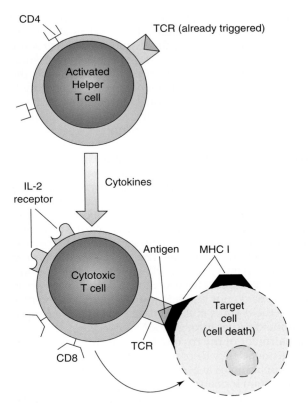

FIGURE 18-9 Destruction of target cell by cytotoxic T cell. Cytokines released from the activated helper T cell enhance final destruction of the target cell by the cytotoxic T cell.

ous cytokines that recruit and activate other lymphocytes, macrophages, and inflammatory cells. Cytokines can induce positive migration or chemotaxis of several types of inflammatory cells, including macrophages, granulocytes, and basophils. Activation of macrophages enhances their phagocytic, metabolic, and enzymatic potential, resulting in more efficient destruction of infected cells. This type of defense is important against intracellular pathogens such as *Mycobacterium* species and *Listeria monocytogenes*.

A similar sequence of T-cell and macrophage activation, but with sometimes excessive inflammation, can be elicited in delayed hypersensitivity reactions. Contact dermatitis due to a poison ivy reaction or dye sensitivity are examples of delayed hypersensitivity caused by hapten–carrier complexes.

Natural Killer Cells

Natural killer cells are lymphocytes that are functionally, genotypically, and phenotypically distinct from T cells, B cells, and monocyte-macrophages. The NK cell is a nonspecific effector cell that can kill tumor cells and virus-infected cells. They are called *natural killer cells* because, unlike T cytotoxic cells, they do not need to recognize a specific antigen before being activated. Both NK cells and T cytotoxic cells kill after contact with a target cell. The NK cell is programmed automatically to kill foreign cells, in contrast to the CD8+ T cells, which need to be activated

to become cytotoxic. However, programmed killing is inhibited if the NK cell membrane molecules contact MHC self-molecules on normal host cells.

NK cells appear as large, granular lymphocytes with an indented nucleus and abundant, pale cytoplasm containing red granules. These cells characteristically express CD16 and CD56 cell surface molecules but lack the typical T-cell markers (*i.e.*, TCR, CD4). The mechanism of NK cytotoxicity is similar to T-cell cytotoxicity in that it depends on production of pore-forming proteins (*i.e.*, NK perforins), enzymes, and toxic cytokines. NK cell activity can be enhanced in vitro on exposure to interleukin-2 (IL-2), a phenomenon called *lymphokine-activated killer* activity. NK cells also participate in *antibody-dependent cellular cytotoxicity*, a mechanism by which a cytotoxic effector cell can kill an antibody-coated target cell. The role of NK cells probably is one of immune surveillance for cancerous or virally infected cells.

LYMPHOID ORGANS

The cells of the immune system are present in large numbers in the central and peripheral lymphoid organs. These organs and tissues are widely distributed in the body and provide different, but often overlapping, functions (Fig. 18-10). The

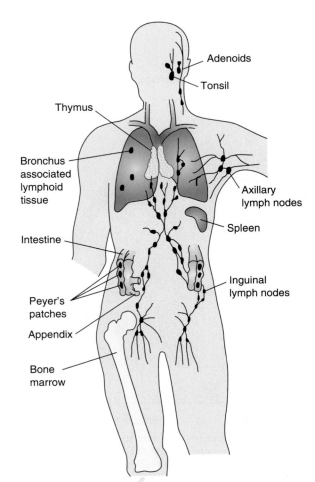

FIGURE 18-10 Central and peripheral lymphoid organs and tissues.

central lymphoid organs, the bone marrow and the thymus, provide the environment for immune cell production and maturation. The peripheral lymphoid organs function to trap and process antigen and promote its interaction with mature immune cells. Lymph nodes, spleen, tonsils, appendix, Peyer's patches in the intestine, and mucosa-associated lymphoid tissues in the respiratory, gastrointestinal, and reproductive systems comprise the peripheral lymphoid organs. The lymphoid organs are connected by networks of lymph channels, blood vessels, and capillaries. The immune cells continuously circulate through the various tissues and organs to seek out and destroy foreign material.

Thymus

The thymus is an elongated, bilobed structure that is located in the neck region above the heart. Each lobe is surrounded by a connective tissue capsule layer and is divided into lobules. Each lobule is composed of two compartments: an outer area or cortex, which is densely packed with thymocytes or immature T lymphocytes, and an inner, less dense area or medulla that contains few lymphocytes but more dendritic cells, macrophages, and the distinctive morphologic structure of the thymus, Hassall's corpuscles (Fig. 18-11).

The function of the thymus is central to the development of the immune system because it generates mature immunocompetent T lymphocytes. The thymus is a fully developed organ at birth, weighing approximately 15 to 20 g. At puberty, when the immune cells are well established in peripheral lymphoid tissues, the thymus begins regressing and is replaced by adipose tissue. Nevertheless, some thymus tissue persists into old age. Precursor T (pre-T) cells enter the thymus as functionally and phenotypically immature T cells. They progressively differentiate into mature T cells as they transverse the organ from the cortical to medullary areas. Rapid cell multiplication and maturation occur in the cortex under the influence of the microenvironment, thymic hormones, and cytokines. Cortical thymocytes undergo TCR gene rearrangement and TCR and CD4+/CD8+ surface expression. More than 95% of the thymocytes die in the cortex and never leave the thymus because in the random rearrangement of genes, cells are produced with inappropriate receptors. Only those T cells able to recognize foreign antigen and not react to self (*i.e.,* MHC or self-antigens) are allowed to mature. This process is called *thymic selection.* The thymus must be extremely thorough in eliminating self-reactive cells to ensure that autoimmune reactivity and disease do not result. Mature immunocompetent T cells leave the thymus in 2 to 3 days and enter the peripheral lymphoid tissues through the bloodstream.

Impairment of the thymic function can occur in immunologic deficiency disorders. If the thymus is removed from certain animals at birth or is congenitally absent, as is seen in certain human conditions, the result is a decrease in the number of lymphocytes in the blood and a marked depletion or absence of T lymphocytes in the circulation and peripheral lymphoid tissues.

Lymph Nodes

Lymph nodes are small aggregates of lymphoid tissue located along lymphatic vessels throughout the body. Each lymph node processes lymph from a discrete, adjacent anatomic site. Many lymph nodes are in the axillae, groin, and along the great vessels of the neck, thorax, and abdomen. These tissues are located along the lymph ducts, which lead from the tissues to the thoracic duct. Lymph nodes have two functions: removal of foreign material from lymph before it enters the bloodstream and serving as centers for proliferation of immune cells.

A lymph node is a bean-shaped tissue surrounded by a connective tissue capsule. Lymph enters the node through afferent channels that penetrate the capsule, and the lymph leaves through the efferent lymph vessels located in the deep indentation of the hilus. Lymphocytes and macrophages flow slowly through the node, which allows trapping and interaction of antigen and immune cells. The reticular meshwork serves as a surface on which macrophages can more easily phagocytose antigens. Dendritic cells, which also permeate the lymph node, aid antigen presentation.

A lymph node is divided into several specialized areas, an outer cortex, a paracortex, and inner medulla (Fig. 18-12). The T lymphocytes are more abundant in the paracortex of the node, and the B lymphocytes are more abundant in the follicles and germinal centers located in the outer cortex. The T lymphocytes proliferate on antigenic stimulation and migrate to the follicles, where they interact with B lymphocytes. These activated follicles become germinal centers,

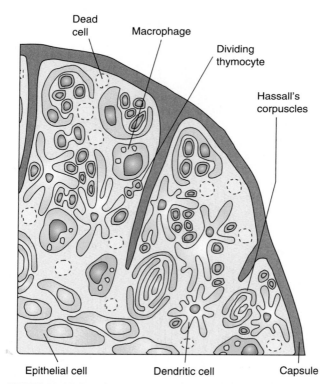

FIGURE 18-11 Structural features of the thymus gland. The thymus gland is divided into lobules containing an outer cortex densely packed with dividing thymocytes or premature T cells and an inner medulla that contains macrophages, dendritic cells, and Hassall's corpuscles.

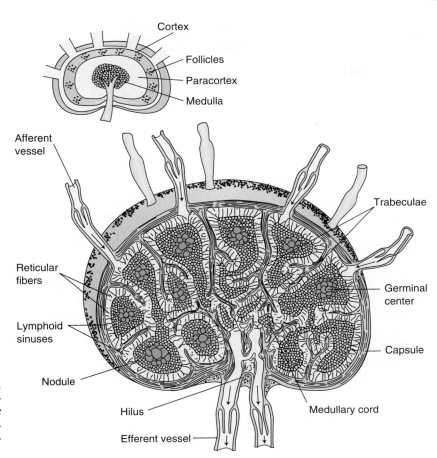

FIGURE 18-12 Structural features of a lymph node. Bacteria that gain entry to the body are filtered out of the lymph as it flows through the node. (From Chaffee E.E., Lytle I.M. [1980]. *Basic physiology and anatomy* [4th ed., p. 356]. Philadelphia: J. B. Lippincott)

containing macrophages, follicular dendritic cells, and maturing T and B cells. Activated B cells then migrate to the medullary area, where they complete their maturation into plasma cells. These cells stay localized in the lymph node but release large quantities of antibodies into the circulation.

Spleen
The spleen is a large, ovoid organ located high in the left abdominal cavity. The spleen filters antigens from the blood and is important in response to systemic infections. The spleen is composed of red and white pulp. The red pulp is well supplied with arteries and is the area where senescent and injured red blood cells are destroyed. The white pulp contains concentrated areas of B and T lymphocytes permeated by macrophages and dendritic cells. The lymphocytes (primarily T cells) that surround the central arterioles form the area called the *periarterial lymphoid sheath.* The diffuse marginal zone contains follicles and germinal centers rich in B cells and separates the white pulp from the red pulp. A sequence of activation events similar to that seen in the lymph nodes occurs in the spleen.

Other Secondary Lymphoid Tissues
Other secondary lymphoid tissues include the *mucosa-associated lymphoid tissues.* These nonencapsulated clusters of lymphoid tissues are located around membranes lining the respiratory, digestive, and urogenital tract. These gateways into the body must contain the immune cells needed to respond to a large and diverse population of microorganisms. In some tissues, the lymphocytes are organized in loose clusters, but in other tissues such as the tonsils, Peyer's patches in the intestine, and the appendix, organized structures are evident. These tissues contain all the necessary cell components (*i.e.,* T cells, B cells, macrophages, and dendritic cells) for an immune response. Because of the continuous stimulation of the lymphocytes in these tissues by microorganisms constantly entering the body, large numbers of plasma cells are evident. Immunity at the mucosal layers helps to protect the vulnerable internal organs.

CYTOKINES AND THE IMMUNE RESPONSE

Cytokines are low–molecular-weight regulatory proteins that are produced during all phases of an immune response. Cytokines are made primarily by and act predominantly on immune cells. These intercellular signal molecules are very potent, act at very low concentrations, and usually regulate neighboring cells. Cytokines modulate reactions of the host to foreign antigens or injurious agents by regulating the movement, proliferation, and differentiation of leukocytes and other cells (Table 18-4). Cytokines are synthesized by many cell types but are made primarily by activated T_H lymphocytes and macrophages.

TABLE 18-4 ✦ Characteristic Biologic Properties of Human Cytokines

Cytokine	Biologic Activity
Interleukin-1 (alpha and beta)	Activates resting T cells; is cofactor for hematopoietic growth factor; induces fever, sleep, adrenocorticotropic hormone release, neutropenia, and other systemic acute-phase responses; stimulates synthesis of cytokines, collagen, and collegenases; activates endothelial and macrophagic cells; mediates inflammation, catabolic processes, and nonspecific resistance to infection
Interleukin-2	Growth factor for activated T cells; induces synthesis of other cytokines, activates cytotoxic lymphocytes
Interleukin-3	Support growth of pluripotent (multilineage) bone marrow stem cells; is growth factor for mast cells
Interleukin-4	Growth factor for activated B cells, resting T cells, and mast cells; induces MHC class I antigen expression on B cells; enhances cytotoxic T cells; activates macrophages
Interleukin-5	B-cell differentiating and growth factor; promotes differentiation of eosinophils; promotes antibody production (IgA)
Interleukin-6	Acts as cofactor for immunoglobulin production by B cells; stimulates hepatocytes to produce acute-phase proteins
Interleukin-7	Stimulates pre-B cells and thymocytes; stimulates myeloid precursors and megakaryocytes
Interleukin-8	Chemoattracts neutrophils and T lymphocytes; regulates lymphocyte homing and neutrophil infiltration
Interleukin-10	Suppresses cytokine production by T helper cells; inhibits antigen presentation
Interleukin-12	Enhances activation of cytotoxic T, NK, and macrophages; acts opposite to IL-10
Interferon-gamma (γ)	Induces MHC class I, class II, and other surface antigens on a variety of cells; activates macrophages and endothelial cells; augments or inhibits other cytokine activities; augments NK cell activity; exerts antiviral activity
Interferon (alpha and beta) (α and β)	Exerts antiviral activity; induces class I antigen expression; augments NK cell activity; has fever-inducing and antiproliferative properties
Tumor necrosis factor (alpha) (α)	Direct cytotoxin for some tumor cells; induces fever, sleep, and other acute-phase responses; stimulates the synthesis of other cytokines, collagen and collagenases; activates endothelial and macrophagic cells; mediates inflammation, catabolic processes, and septic shock.
Colony-stimulating factor (CSF) Granulocyte–macrophage CSF	Promotes neutrophilic, eosinophilic, and macrophagic bone marrow colonies; activates mature granulocytes
Granulocyte CSF	Promotes neutrophilic colonies
Macrophage CSF	Promotes macrophagic colonies

MHC, major histocompatibility complex; NK, natural killer.

These regulator molecules can be named for the general cell type that produces them (*e.g.,* lymphokines, monokines). More specifically, they are named by an international nomenclature (*i.e.,* interleukins 1 through 18) or for the biologic property that was first ascribed to them. For example, *interferons* (IFNs) were named because they interfered with virus multiplication. Cytokines commonly affect more than one cell type and have more than one biologic effect. For example, IFN-γ inhibits virus replication and is a potent activator of macrophages and NK cells. Specific cytokines can have biologic activities that overlap. Maximization of the immune response and protection against detrimental mutations in a single cytokine are possible benefits of redundancy.

The production of cytokines often occurs in a cascade in which one cytokine affects the production of subsequent cytokines or cytokine receptors. Some cytokines function as antagonists to inhibit the biologic effects of earlier cytokines. This pattern of expression and feedback ensures appropriate control of cytokine synthesis and subsequently of the immune response. Excessive cytokine production can have serious adverse effects, including those associated with septic shock, food poisoning, and types of cancer.

Cytokines generate their responses by binding to specific receptors on their target cells. Many cytokine receptors share a common structural shape and a cytoplasmic tail that interacts with a family of cytoplasmic signaling proteins (JAKs) responsible for the induction of the genes for cell responses. The biologic responses associated with cytokines are partially regulated by the time of expression of the cell receptor. Most cytokines are released at cell-to-cell interfaces, where they bind to receptors on nearby cells. The short half-life of cytokines ensures that excessive immune responses and systemic activation do not occur.

The biologic properties of cytokines fall into several major groups. One group of cytokines (*e.g.,* IL-1, IL-6, TNF) mediates inflammation by producing fever and the acute-phase response and by attracting and activating phagocytes (*e.g.,* IL-8, IFN-γ). Other cytokines are maturation factors for the hematopoiesis of white or red blood cells (*e.g.,* IL-3, granulocyte–macrophage colony-stimulating factor [GM-CSF]). Recombinant CSF molecules are being used to increase the success rates of bone marrow transplantations. Most of the interleukin cytokines function as cell communication molecules among T cells, B cells, macrophages, and other immune cells. The availability of recombinant cytokines offers the possibility of several clinical therapies where stimulation or inhibition of the immune response is desirable. IL-2 therapy for several malignancies has led to some clinical success.

Interleukin-1

The major function of IL-1 is as a mediator of the inflammatory response. In concert with IL-6 and TNF-α, IL-1 can stimulate the production of an acute-phase response, mobilize neutrophils, produce a fever, and activate the vascular epithelium. IL-1 also can serve as a priming signal in the activation of CD4+ T cells and the growth and differentiation of B cells. The major source of IL-1 is the macrophage, although it also is produced by keratinocytes, Langerhans' cells, normal B cells, cultured T cells, fibroblasts, neutrophils, and smooth muscle cells.

Interleukin-2

The presence of IL-2, formerly known as *T-cell growth factor,* is necessary for the proliferation and function of helper T, cytotoxic T, B, and NK cells. IL-2 interacts with T lymphocytes by binding to specific membrane receptors that are present on activated T cells but not on resting T cells. The expression of high-affinity IL-2 receptors can be triggered by specific antigen and other stimulatory signals. Sustained T-cell proliferation relies on the presence of IL-2 and IL-2 receptors; if either is missing, cell proliferation ceases, and the cell dies. This cytokine ensures maximum amplification of immune responses if antigen is present. Severe combined immunodeficiency diseases have been associated with mutations in IL-2 and the IL-2 receptor, thereby documenting the importance of these molecules. Cyclosporine and tacrolimus, drugs used to prevent rejection of heart, kidney, and liver transplants, function primarily by inhibiting the synthesis of IL-2.

Interferons

The IFNs are a family of cytokines that protect neighboring cells from invasion by intracellular parasites, including viruses, rickettsiae, malarial parasites, and other organisms. Bacterial toxins, complex polysaccharides, and several other chemical substances can induce IFN production. Not all the substances that induce IFN are antigenic.

There are three types of IFN: IFN-α, produced by leukocytes; IFN-β, produced by fibroblasts; and IFN-γ, produced by T and NK cells. IFN-α and IFN-β are grouped as type I IFNs to distinguish them from IFN-γ (type II). Type I secreted IFNs interact with receptors on neighboring cells to stimulate the translation of an antiviral protein that affects viral synthesis and its spread to uninfected cells. The actions of IFNs are not pathogen specific; they are effective against different types of viruses and intracellular parasites. They are, however, species specific. Animal IFNs do not provide protection in humans. The IFN produced during immune reactions is primarily IFN-γ. IFN-γ functions to activate macrophages, generate cytotoxic lymphocytes, and enhance NK cell activity.

Tumor Necrosis Factor

Like IL-1, TNF-α is a cytokine with multiple immunologic and inflammatory effects. It was first described as an activity in serum that induced hemorrhagic necrosis in certain tumors, and can function as a circulating mediator of wasting disease. TNF is produced by activated macrophages and other activated cells, such as T cells. Besides functioning as a major chemical mediator in the inflammatory response and indirectly affecting the fever response, TNF may function as a costimulator of T cells. This cytokine is an especially potent stimulator of IL-1, IL-6, and IL-8. In bacterial sepsis, high serum levels of TNF may mediate endotoxic shock. TNF is primarily responsible for the tissue wasting seen in cases of chronic inflammation. New inhibitors of TNF or its receptors have been used to control the chronic inflammation associated with rheumatoid arthritis.

Hematopoietic Colony-Stimulating Factors

Colony-stimulating factors are cytokines that stimulate bone marrow pluripotent stem and progenitor or precursor cells to produce large numbers of platelets, erythrocytes, neutrophils, monocytes, eosinophils, and basophils. The CSFs were named according to the type of target cell on which they act (see Table 18-4). GM-CSF acts on the granulocyte–monocyte progenitor cells to produce monocytes, neutrophils and dendritic cells; G-CSF more specifically induces neutrophil proliferation; and M-CSF specifically directs the mononuclear phagocyte progenitor. Other cytokines, including IL-1, IL-2, IL-3, IL-4, IL-5, IL-6, IL-7, and IL-11, also may influence hematopoiesis.

IMMUNITY AND THE IMMUNE RESPONSE

Immunity is a normal adaptive response designed to protect the body against potentially harmful foreign substances, infections, and other sources of nonself-antigens. Immunity can be innate or acquired. *Innate* or *nonspecific immunity* is the natural resistance with which a person is born. General factors such as heredity, age, health, species, race, and sex can influence innate immunity. For example, humans get mumps but dogs do not because their cells lack virus-specific binding sites needed for infection. Natural or innate resistance also depends on internal and external surface barriers, chemicals, and cell responses that are grouped as anatomic, physiologic, phagocytic, and inflammatory. Innate immunity serves to contain an infection while the specific or acquired immune responses are being produced.

Acquired or *specific immunity* is the protection that a person gains through exposure to antigens or through transfer of protective antibodies against an antigen. The process of acquiring the ability to respond to an antigen after administration by vaccines is known as *immunization*. An acquired immune response can improve on repeated exposures to an injected antigen or a natural infection. The immune response describes the interaction between an antigen (*i.e.,* immunogen) and an antibody (*i.e.,* immunoglobulin) or reactive T lymphocyte.

Active immunity is acquired through immunization or actually having a disease. It is called *active immunity* because it depends on a response by the person's immune system. Active immunity, although long lasting once established, does require a few days to weeks after a first exposure before the immune response is sufficiently developed to contribute to the destruction of the pathogen. However, the immune system usually is able to react within hours to subsequent exposure to the same agent because of the presence of memory B and T lymphocytes.

Passive immunity is immunity transferred from another source. An infant receives passive immunity naturally from the transfer of antibodies from its mother in utero and through a mother's breast milk. Maternal IgG crosses the placenta and protects the newborn during the first few months of life. Normally, an infant has few infectious diseases during the first 3 to 6 months owing to the protection provided by the mother's antibodies. Passive immunity also can be artificially provided by the transfer of antibodies produced by other people or animals. Some protection against infectious disease can be provided by the injection of hyperimmune serum, which contains high concentrations of antibodies for a specific disease, or immune serum or gamma- globulin, which contains a pool of antibodies for many infectious agents. Passive immunity produces only short-term protection that lasts weeks to months.

Humoral Immunity

Humoral immunity depends on maturation of B lymphocytes into plasma cells, which produce and secrete antibodies. The combination of antigen with antibody can result in several effector responses, such as precipitation of antigen–antibody complexes, agglutination or clumping of cells, neutralization of bacterial toxins and viruses, lysis and destruction of pathogens or cells, adherence of antigen to immune cells, facilitation of phagocytosis, and complement activation. For example, antibodies can neutralize a virus by blocking the sites on the virus that it uses to bind to the host cell, thereby negating its ability to infect the cell.

Two types of responses occur in the development of humoral immunity: a primary and a secondary response (Fig. 18-13). A *primary immune response* occurs when the antigen is first introduced into the body. During this primary response, there is a latent period or lag before the antibody can be detected in the serum. This latent period involves the processing of antigen by the APCs and recognition by helper T cells. The antigen receptors on helper T cells recognize the antigenic peptide–class II MHC complex, become activated, and produce cytokines to further stimulate and direct the immune system. In humoral immunity, activated helper T cells trigger B cells to proliferate and differentiate into a clone of plasma cells that produce antibody. This activation process takes 1 to 2 weeks, but once generated, detectable

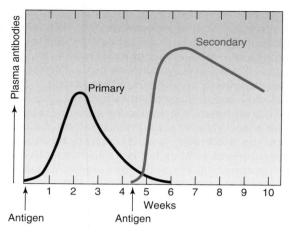

FIGURE 18-13 Primary and secondary phases of the humoral immune response to the same antigen.

antibody continues to rise for a few weeks. Recovery from many infectious diseases occurs at the time during the primary response when the antibody concentration is reaching its peak. The *secondary* or *memory response* occurs on second or subsequent exposures to the antigen. During the secondary response, the rise in antibody occurs sooner and reaches a higher level because of the available memory cells.

During the primary response, B cells are activated to proliferate and differentiate into antibody-secreting plasma cells. A fraction of activated B cells does not differentiate into plasma cells but forms a pool of memory B cells. During the secondary response, the memory cells recognize the antigen and respond more efficiently to produce the specific antibody. The booster immunization given for some diseases, such as tetanus, makes use of the secondary or memory response. For a person who has been previously immunized, administration of a booster shot causes an almost immediate rise in antibody to a level sufficient to prevent development of the disease.

Cell-Mediated Immunity

Cell-mediated immunity provides protection against viruses, intracellular bacteria, and cancer cells. In cell-mediated immunity, the actions of T lymphocytes and macrophages predominate. The most aggressive phagocyte, the macrophage, becomes activated after exposure to T-cell cytokines, especially IFN-γ. As in humoral immunity, the initial stages of cell-mediated immunity are directed by an APC displaying the antigen peptide–class II MHC complex to the helper T cell. Helper T cells become activated after recognition by the TCR of the antigen–MHC complex and by priming with IL-1. The activated helper T cell then synthesizes IL-2 and the IL-2 receptor. These molecules drive the multiplication of clones of helper T cells, which amplify the response. Further differentiation of the helper T cells leads to production of additional cytokines (*e.g.,* IFN-γ, TNF, IL-12), which enhance the activity of cytotoxic T cells and effector macrophages. A cell-mediated immune response usually occurs through the cytotoxic activity of cytotoxic T cells and the enhanced engulfment and killing by macrophages.

Complement System

The complement system is a primary mediator of the humoral immune response that enables the body to produce an inflammatory response, lyse foreign cells, and increase phagocytosis. The complement system, like the blood coagulation system, consists of a group of proteins that normally are present in the circulation as functionally inactive precursors (Fig. 18-14). These proteins make up 10% to 15% of the plasma protein fraction. For a complement reaction to occur, the complement components must be activated in the proper sequence. Uncontrolled activation of the complement system is prevented by inhibitor proteins and the instability of the activated complement proteins at each step of the process. There are three parallel but independent mechanisms for recognizing microorganisms that result in the activation of the complement system: the classic, the alternate, and the lectin-mediated pathways. All three pathways of activation generate a series of enzymatic reactions that proteolytically cleave successive complement proteins in the pathway. The consequence is the deposition of some complement protein fragments on the pathogen sur-face, thereby producing tags for better recognition by the phagocytic cells. Other complement fragments are released into the tissue fluids to stimulate further the inflammatory response.

The classic pathway of complement activation is initiated by antibody bound to antigens on the surface of microbes or through soluble immune complexes (Fig. 18-15). The alternate and the lectin pathways do not use antibodies and are part of the innate immune defenses. The alternate pathway of complement activation is initiated by the interaction with certain polysaccharide molecules characteristic of bacterial surfaces. The lectin-mediated pathway is initiated following the binding of a mannose-binding protein to mannose-containing molecules commonly present on the surface of bacteria and yeast.

The activation of the three pathways produces similar effects on C3 and subsequent complement proteins. The classic pathway of complement activation was the first discovered and is the best studied. The major proteins of the classic system are designated by a numbering system from C1 to C9. The classic pathway is triggered when

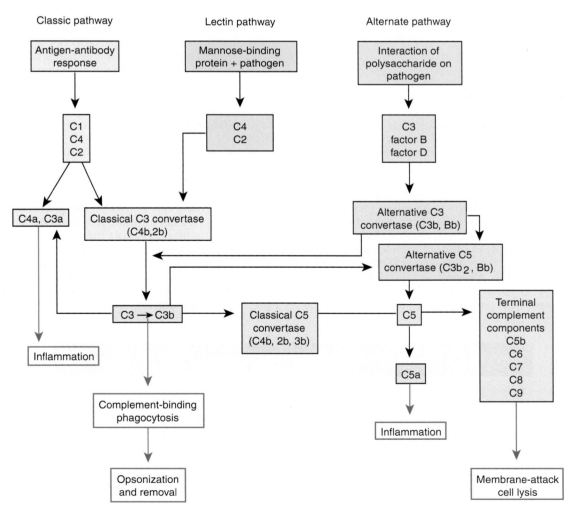

FIGURE 18-14 Classic, lectin, and alternative complement pathways.

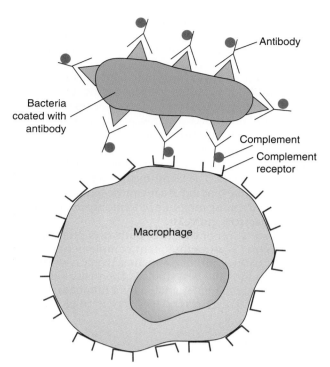

FIGURE 18-15 Complement-mediated interaction between macrophage and bacterium.

complement-fixing antibodies, such as IgG or IgM, bind to antigens. The immune complexes trigger a series of enzyme reactions that act in a cascade fashion. Modified or split complement proteins (*e.g.,* C3b, C3a, C5a) released during activation function in the next step of the pathway or are released into the tissue fluid to produce biologic effects important in inflammation. C3 has a central role in the complement pathway because it is integral to all three pathways. The triggering of C3 initiates several mechanisms for microbial destruction. One result of activation of C3 is the formation of the membrane attack complex formed by C5 to C9. Several structurally modulated complement proteins bind to form pores in the membrane of foreign cells that lead to eventual cell lysis. The alternate and lectin pathways are activated by microbial surface molecules and substitute other molecules for the proteins in the first two steps of the

classic complement pathway. The alternate pathway uses proteins B, D, and P for activation, whereas the lectin pathway uses mannose-binding protein and accessory proteins. Both pathways require the presence of C3b and subsequent complement proteins to generate biologic effects similar to those of the classic complement pathway. Whatever the mechanism of activation of the complement system, effects produced range from lysis of a variety of different cells to direct mediation of the inflammatory process. Table 18-5 lists immune responses that occur as the result of complement fixation or activation. First, complement has been shown to mediate the lytic destruction of many kinds of cells, including red blood cells, platelets, bacteria, and lymphocytes. All complement pathways may induce cytolysis. Second, a major biologic function of complement activation is opsonization—the coating of antigen–antibody complexes such that antigens are engulfed and cleared more efficiently by macrophages. Third, chemotactic complement products (C3a and C5a) can trigger an influx of leukocytes. These white blood cells remain fixed in the area of complement activation through attachment to specific sites on C3b and C4b molecules. Fourth, production of anaphylatoxin (C3a and C5a) can lead to contraction of smooth muscle, increased vascular permeability, and edema.

Regulation of the Immune Response

Self-regulation is an essential property of the immune system. An inadequate immune response may lead to immunodeficiency, but an inappropriate or excessive response may lead to conditions varying from allergic reactions to autoimmune diseases. This regulation is not well understood and involves all aspects of the immune response—antigen, antibody, cytokines, regulatory T cells, and the neuroendocrine system.

With each exposure to antigen, the immune system must determine the branch of the immune system to be activated and the extent and duration of the immune response. After exposure to an antigen, the immune response to that antigen develops after a brief lag, reaches a peak, and then recedes. Normal immune responses are self-limited because the response eliminates the antigen, and the products of the response, such as cytokines and antibodies, have a short or limited life span and are secreted only for brief periods after antigen recognition. Evidence suggests that cytokine feedback from the helper T cell controls several aspects of the immune response.

TABLE 18-5 ✦ **Complement-Mediated Immune Responses**	
Response	**Effects**
Cytolysis	Lysis and destruction of cell membranes of body cells or pathogens
Opsonization	Targeting of the antigen so it can be easily engulfed and digested by the macrophages and other phagocytic cells
Chemotaxis	Chemical attraction of neutrophils and phagocytic cells to the antigen
Anaphylaxis	Activation of mast cells and basophils with release of inflammatory mediators that produce smooth muscle contraction and increased vascular permeability

Another facet of immune self-regulation is inhibition of immune responses by tolerance. The term *tolerance* is used to define the ability of the immune system to be nonreactive to self-antigens while producing immunity to foreign agents. Tolerance to self-antigens protects an individual from harmful autoimmune reactions. Exposure of an individual to foreign antigens may lead to tolerance and the inability to respond to potential pathogens that cause infection. Tolerance exists not only to self-tissues, but to maternal-fetal tissues. Special regulation of the immune system also is evident in defined privileged sites such as the brain, testes, ovaries, and eyes. Immune damage in these areas could result in serious consequences to the individual and the species.

> In summary, immunity is the resistance to a disease that is provided by the immune system. It can be acquired actively through immunization or having a disease, or passively by receiving antibodies or immune cells from another source. Antigens have antigenic determinant sites or epitopes, which the immune system recognizes with specific receptors that distinguish the antigens as nonself and as unique foreign molecules. Immune mechanisms can be classified into two types: specific or acquired and nonspecific or innate immunity. Specific or acquired immunity involves humoral and cellular mechanisms whereby the immune cells differentiate self from nonself and recognize and respond to a unique antigen. The humoral immune response involves antibodies produced by activated B lymphocytes. Cell-mediated immunity depends on T-cell responses to cellular antigens. Nonspecific immune mechanisms can distinguish between self and nonself but cannot differentiate among antigens. They include the complement system, cytokines, and the phagocytic activities of neutrophils and macrophages. The cytokines, produced largely by T cells, function as intercellular signals that regulate immune and inflammatory responses.

Developmental Aspects of the Immune System

After you have completed this section of the chapter, you should be able to meet the following objectives:

✦ Explain the transfer of passive immunity from mother to fetus and from mother to infant during breast-feeding
✦ Characterize the development of active immunity in the infant and small child
✦ Describe changes in the immune response that occur with aging

Embryologically, the immune system develops in several stages, beginning at 5 to 6 weeks as the fetal liver becomes active in hematopoiesis. Development of the primary lymphoid organs (*i.e.*, thymus and bone marrow) begins during the middle of the first trimester and proceeds rapidly. Secondary lymphoid organs (*i.e.*, spleen, lymph nodes, and tonsils) develop soon after. These secondary lymphoid organs are rather small but well developed at birth and mature rapidly during the postnatal period. The thymus at birth is the largest lymphoid tissue relative to body size and normally is approximately two thirds its mature weight, which it achieves during the first year of life.

TRANSFER OF IMMUNITY FROM MOTHER TO INFANT

Protection of a newborn against antigens occurs through transfer of maternal antibodies. Maternal IgG antibodies cross the placenta during fetal development and remain functional in the newborn for the first months of life (Fig. 18-16). IgG is the only class of immunoglobulins to cross the placenta. Levels of maternal IgG decrease significantly during the first 3 to 6 months of life while infant synthesis of immunoglobulins increases. Maternally transmitted IgG is effective against most microorganisms and viruses. The largest amount of IgG crosses the placenta during the last weeks of pregnancy and is stored in fetal tissues, and infants born prematurely may be deficient. Because of transfer of IgG antibodies to the fetus, an infant born to a mother infected with HIV has a positive HIV antibody test result, although he or she may not be infected with the virus.

Cord blood does not normally contain IgM or IgA. If present, these antibodies are of fetal origin and represent exposure to intrauterine infection. The infant begins producing IgM antibodies within a few months after birth, in response to the immense antigenic stimulation of his or her new environment. Premature infants appear to be able to produce IgM as well as term infants. At approximately 6 days of age the IgM rises sharply, and this rise continues until approximately 1 year of age, when the adult level is achieved.

Serum IgA normally is first detected at approximately 13 days after birth. The level increases during early childhood until adult levels are reached between the sixth and

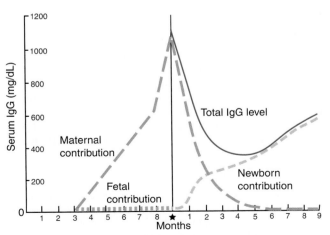

FIGURE 18-16 Maternal/neonatal serum immunoglobulin levels. (From Allansmith M., McClellan B.H., Butterworth M., Maloney, J.R. [1968]. *Journal of Pediatrics 72*, 289)

seventh year. Maternal IgA also is transferred to the infant in colostrum or milk by breast-feeding. These antibodies provide local immunity for the intestinal system and have been shown to decrease diarrheal infections in underdeveloped countries. These evolutionary adaptations of the immune system have increased the survival of our species and optimized the development of other important organs in the early months of life.

IMMUNE RESPONSE IN THE ELDERLY

Aging is characterized by a declining ability to adapt to environmental stresses. One of the factors thought to contribute to this problem is a decline in immune responsiveness. This includes changes in cell-mediated and antibody-mediated immune responses. Elderly persons tend to be more susceptible to infections, have more evidence of autoimmune and immune complex disorders than younger persons, and have a higher incidence of cancer. Experimental evidence suggests that vaccination is less successful in inducing immunization in older persons than younger adults. However, the effect of altered immune function on the health of elderly persons is clouded by the fact that age-related changes or disease may affect the immune response.

The alterations in immune function that occur with advanced age are not fully understood. There is a decrease in the size of the thymus gland, which is thought to affect T-cell function. The size of the gland begins to decline shortly after sexual maturity, and by 50 years of age, it usually has diminished to 15% or less of its maximum size. There are conflicting reports regarding age-related changes in the peripheral lymphocytes. Some researchers have reported a decrease in the absolute number of lymphocytes, and others have found little if any change. The most common finding is a slight decrease in the proportion of T cells to other lymphocytes and a decrease in CD4+ and CD8+ cells.

More evident are altered responses of the immune cells to antigen stimulation; increasing proportions of lymphocytes become unresponsive, while the remainder continue to function relatively normally. T and B cells show deficiencies in activation. In the T-cell types, the CD4+ subset is most severely affected. Evidence indicates that aged T cells have a decreased rate of synthesis of the cytokines that drive the proliferation of lymphocytes and a diminished expression of the receptors that interact with those cytokines. For example, it has been shown that IL-2 synthesis decreases markedly with aging. Although B-cell function is compromised with age, the range of antigens that can be recognized is not diminished. If anything, the repertoire is increased to the extent that B cells begin to recognize some self-antigens as foreign antigens. This may be the basis for the increased incidence of autoimmune disease in the elderly.

> In summary, a newborn is protected against antigens in early life by passive transfer of maternal antibodies through the placenta (IgG) and in colostrum (IgA) through breast-feeding. Some changes are seen with aging, including an increase in autoimmune diseases. The impact of alterations in immune function that occur with aging is not fully understood.

The Inflammatory Response

After you have completed this section of the chapter, you should be able to meet the following objectives:

- ◆ State the purpose of inflammation
- ◆ State the five cardinal signs of acute inflammation and describe the physiologic mechanisms involved in production of these signs
- ◆ Compare the hemodynamic and cellular phases of the inflammatory response
- ◆ Contrast acute and chronic inflammation
- ◆ List four types of inflammatory mediators and state their function
- ◆ Name and describe the five types of inflammatory exudates
- ◆ Define the characteristics of an acute-phase response

Inflammation is the reaction of vascularized tissue to local injury. Although the effects of inflammation often are viewed as undesirable because they are unpleasant and cause discomfort, the process is essentially a beneficial one that allows a person to live with the effects of everyday stress. Without the inflammatory response, wounds would not heal and minor infections would become overwhelming. However, inflammation also produces undesirable effects. The crippling effects of rheumatoid arthritis, for example, result from inflammation.

The causes of inflammation are many and varied. Inflammation commonly results because of an immune response to infectious microorganisms. Other causes of inflammation are trauma, surgery, caustic chemicals, extremes of heat and cold, and ischemic damage to body tissues.

Although the inflammatory response can be initiated by a variety of injurious agents and the extent can vary, the sequence of events that follows is remarkably similar. The body, however, uses only those responses that are needed to minimize tissue damage. A small area of local swelling and redness may be sufficient to prevent injury from a mosquito bite, whereas more serious conditions, such as appendicitis, may incite fever, leukocytosis, and body fluid and protein influx.

Inflammatory conditions are named by adding the suffix *-itis* to the affected organ or system. For example, *appendicitis* refers to inflammation of the appendix, *pericarditis* to inflammation of the pericardium, and *neuritis* to inflammation of a nerve. More descriptive expressions of the inflammatory process might indicate whether the process was acute or chronic and what type of exudate was formed (*e.g.,* acute fibrinous pericarditis).

ACUTE INFLAMMATION

The classic description of acute inflammation has been handed down through the ages. In the first century AD, the Roman physician Celsus described the local reaction of injury in terms known as the cardinal signs of inflammation. These signs are *rubor* (redness), *tumor* (swelling), *calor* (heat), and *dolor* (pain). In the second century AD, the Greek physician Galen added a fifth cardinal sign, *functio laesa,* or loss of function. An acute inflammatory response is characterized by a rapid onset and the resolution of the tissue changes

The Inflammatory Response

➤ Inflammation represents the response of body tissue to immune reactions, injury, or ischemic damage.

➤ The classic response to inflammation includes redness, swelling, heat, pain or discomfort, and loss of function.

➤ The inflammatory response can be acute and self-limited or chronic and self-perpetuating.

➤ The manifestations of an acute inflammatory response can be attributed to the immediate vascular changes that occur (vasodilation and increased capillary permeability), the influx of inflammatory cells such as neutrophils, and, in some cases, the widespread effects of inflammatory mediators, which produce fever and other systemic signs and symptoms.

➤ The manifestations of chronic inflammation are due to infiltration with macrophages, lymphocytes, and fibroblasts, leading to persistent inflammation, fibroblast proliferation, and scar formation.

and damage in a short period. Changes occur locally at the site of injury as well as systemically. A general alarm and recruitment system sent throughout the body is known as the *acute-phase response*. A rapid increase and decrease in several plasma proteins is characteristic of the acute-phase component of inflammation. C-reactive protein and mannose-binding protein are two types of acute-phase proteins that function to increase inflammation through activation of complement.

The manifestation of acute inflammation can be divided into two categories: vascular and cellular blood responses. At the biochemical level, many of the responses that occur during acute inflammation are associated with the release of chemical mediators. The hemodynamic and white blood cell responses contribute to the inflammatory exudates, the extravascular influx of fluid containing high concentrations of proteins, salts, cells, and cellular debris.

Vascular Response

The vascular, or hemodynamic, changes that occur with inflammation begin almost immediately after injury and are initiated by a momentary constriction of small vessels in the area. This vasoconstriction is followed immediately by vasodilation of the arterioles and venules that supply the area. As a result, the area become congested, causing the redness (erythema) and warmth associated with acute inflammation. Accompanying this hyperemic response is an increase in capillary permeability, which allows fluid to escape into the tissue and cause swelling (*i.e.,* edema). Pain and impaired function follow as a result of tissue swelling and release of chemical mediators.

These responses benefit the host by controlling the effects of the injurious agent. The movement of the fluid out of the capillaries and into the tissue spaces dilutes the toxic and irritating agent. As fluid moves out of the capillaries, stagnation of flow and clotting of blood in the small capillaries occurs at the site of injury. This aids in localizing the spread of infectious microorganisms.

Depending on the severity of injury, the hemodynamic changes that occur with inflammation follow one of three patterns of responses. The first is an immediate transient response, which occurs with minor injury. The second is an immediate sustained response, which occurs with more serious injury and continues for several days and damages the vessels in the area. The third type of response is a delayed hemodynamic response; the increase in capillary permeability occurs 4 to 24 hours after injury. A delayed response often accompanies radiation types of injuries, such as sunburn.

Cellular Responses

The cellular stage of acute inflammation is marked by movement of white blood cells (leukocytes) into the area of injury. The phagocytic cells that respond early are primarily neutrophils and possibly other granulocytes. As the process continues, monocytes exit the blood and mature into macrophages in the tissue environment. These longer-lived phagocytes help to destroy the causative agent, aid in the signaling processes of specific immunity, and serve to resolve the inflammatory process. The cellular response of the phagocytes includes the margination or pavementing of white blood cells to capillary walls due to increased expression of adhesion molecules, emigration of the white blood cells, chemotaxis or positive migration of the cells to the site of injury, and phagocytosis.

Granulocytes. Granulocytes are identifiable because of their characteristic cytoplasmic granules. These white blood cells have distinctive multilobed nuclei. The granulocytes are divided into three types (*i.e.,* neutrophils, eosinophils, and basophils) according to the staining properties of the granules (see Chapter 13).

The *neutrophil* is the primary phagocyte that arrives early at the site of inflammation, usually within 90 minutes of injury. Their cytoplasmic granules contain enzymes and other antibacterial substances that are used in destroying and degrading the engulfed particles. They also have oxygen-dependent metabolic pathways that generate toxic oxygen (*e.g.,* hydrogen peroxide) and nitrogen (*e.g.,* nitric oxide) products. Because these white blood cells have nuclei that are divided into three to five lobes, they often are called *polymorphonuclear neutrophils* or *segmented neutrophils*. The neutrophil count in the blood often increases greatly during the inflammatory process, especially with bacterial infections. After being released from the bone marrow, circulating neutrophils have a life span of only approximately 10 hours and therefore must be constantly replaced if their numbers are to remain adequate. This requires an increase in circulating white blood cells, a condition called *leukocytosis*. With excessive demand for phagocytes, immature forms of neutrophils are released from the bone marrow. These immature cells often are called *bands* because of the horseshoe shape of their nuclei. The phrase *a shift to the left* in a white blood cell differential count refers to the increase in immature neutrophils seen in severe infections.

The characteristic reddish-staining cytoplasmic granules of the *eosinophils* identifies these granulocytes. These leukocytes increase in the blood during allergic reactions and parasitic infections. For large parasitic worms that cannot be phagocytized, eosinophils are activated to release their granule armament. They also regulate inflammation and allergic reactions by controlling the release of specific chemical mediators during these processes. The dark purple–staining granules of the *basophils* contain histamine and other bioactive mediators of inflammation. The basophils are involved in producing the symptoms associated with inflammation and allergic reactions. They also may play a role in parasitic infections. The mast cell, which is found in the tissues, is very similar in many of its properties to the basophil.

Mononuclear Phagocytes.

The monocytes are the largest of the white blood cells and constitute 3% to 8% of the total blood leukocytes. The circulating life span of the monocyte is three to four times longer than that of the granulocytes, and these cells survive for a longer time in the tissues. The monocytes, which migrate in increased numbers into the tissues in response to inflammatory stimuli, mature into macrophages. Within 5 hours, mononuclear cells arrive at the inflammatory site, and by 48 hours, monocytes and macrophages are the predominant cell types. The macrophages engulf larger and greater quantities of foreign material than the neutrophils. They also migrate to the local lymph nodes to prime specific immunity. These leukocytes play an important role in chronic inflammation, where they can surround and wall off foreign material that cannot be digested.

Margination and Emigration of Leukocytes.

During the early stages of the inflammatory response, fluid leaves the capillaries, causing blood viscosity to increase. The release of chemical mediators (*i.e.,* histamine, leukotrienes, and kinins) and cytokines affects the endothelial cells of the capillaries and causes the leukocytes to increase their expression of adhesion molecules. The cells slow their migration and then pause owing to the increased stickiness of the capillary endothelial cells. The leukocytes begin to marginate, or move to and along the periphery of the blood vessels. The cobblestone appearance of the vessel lining due to margination of leukocytes has led to the term *pavementing.* After adherence of the phagocyte to the endothelial cells, emigration occurs.

Emigration is a mechanism by which the leukocytes extend pseudopodia, pass through the capillary walls by ameboid movement, and migrate into the tissue spaces (Fig. 18-17). The movement of white blood cells through the capillary walls occurs by a process called *diapedesis.* The emigration of leukocytes may be accompanied by an escape of red blood cells.

Chemotaxis.

The leukocytes wander through the tissue guided by secreted cytokines (chemokines; IL-8), bacterial

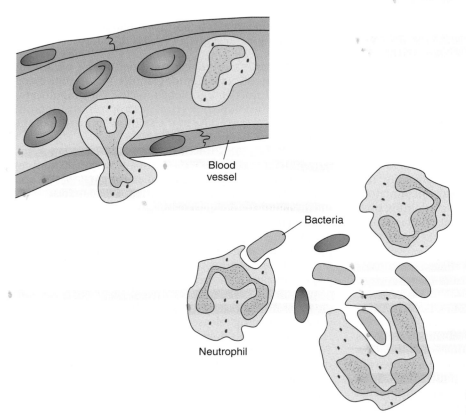

Blood vessel

Bacteria

Neutrophil

FIGURE 18-17 Neutrophil emigration and phagocytosis.

and cellular debris, and complement fragments (C3a, C5a). This process by which leukocytes migrate in response to a chemical signal is called *chemotaxis*. The positive movement up the concentration gradient of chemical mediators to the site of injury increases the probability of a sufficiently localized cellular response.

Phagocytosis.   In the next stage of the cellular response, the neutrophils and macrophages engulf and degrade the bacteria and cellular debris in a process called *phagocytosis* (see Fig. 18-17). Phagocytosis involves four distinct steps: chemotaxis, adherence plus opsonization, engulfment, and intracellular killing. Neutrophil and macrophage chemotaxis can be stimulated by many factors, including complement, chemotactic factors produced by leukocytes, and even bacteria. Contact of the bacteria or antigen with the phagocyte cell membrane is essential for trapping the agent and triggering the final steps of phagocytosis. If the antigen is coated with antibody or complement, its adherence is increased because of binding to Fc or complement receptors. These receptors recognize the constant part (Fc fragment) of the antibody molecule or the products of processed complement (C3b molecule). This process of enhanced binding of an antigen due to antibody or complement is called *opsonization*. Engulfment follows the recognition of the agent as foreign. Cytoplasmic extensions (pseudopods) surround and enclose the particle in a membrane-bounded phagocytic vesicle or phagosome. In the cell cytoplasm, the phagosome merges with a lysosome containing antibacterial molecules and enzymes that can digest the microbe.

Intracellular killing of pathogens is accomplished through several mechanisms, including enzymes, defensins, and toxic oxygen and nitrogen products produced by oxygen-dependent metabolic pathways. The metabolic burst pathways that generate toxic oxygen and nitrogen products (*i.e.*, nitric oxide, peroxyonitrites, hydrogen peroxide, and hypochlorous acid) require oxygen and metabolic enzymes such as myeloperoxidase, NADPH oxidase, and nitric oxide synthetase. Individuals born with genetic defects in some of these enzymes have immunodeficiency conditions that make them susceptible to repeated bacterial infection.

Acute-Phase Response

Along with the cellular responses, a constellation of systemic effects called the *acute-phase response* occurs. The acute-phase response, which usually begins within hours or days of the onset of inflammation or infection, includes changes in the concentrations of plasma proteins, increased erythrocyte sedimentation rate (ESR), fever, increased numbers of leukocytes, skeletal muscle catabolism, and negative nitrogen balance. These responses are generated after the release of the cytokines, IL-1, TNF-α, and IL-6. These cytokines affect the thermoregulatory center in the hypothalamus to produce fever, the most obvious sign of the acute-phase response. IL-1 and other cytokines induce an increase in the number and immaturity of circulating neutrophils by stimulating their production in the bone marrow. Lethargy, a common feature of the acute-phase response, results from the effects of IL-1 and TNF-α on the central nervous system.

During the acute-phase response, the liver dramatically increases the synthesis of acute-phase proteins such as fibrinogen and C-reactive protein that serve several different nonspecific host defense functions. The change in the types of plasma proteins contributes to the increased ESR (see Chapter 13). The metabolic changes, including skeletal muscle catabolism, provide amino acids that can be used in the immune response and for tissue repair. The total systemic process coordinates various activities in the body to enable an optimum host response.

Inflammatory Mediators

Although inflammation is precipitated by injury, its signs and symptoms are produced by chemical mediators. Mediators can be classified by function: those with vasoactive and smooth muscle–constricting properties such as histamine, prostaglandins, leukotrienes, and platelet-activating factor (PAF); chemotactic factors such as complement fragments (C5a) and cytokines (IL-8); plasma proteases that can activate complement and components of the clotting system; and reactive molecules and cytokines liberated from leukocytes, which when released into the extracellular environment can damage the surrounding tissue. Table 18-6

TABLE 18-6 ✦ Signs of Inflammation and Corresponding Chemical Mediator

Inflammatory Response	Chemical Mediator
Swelling, redness, and tissue warmth (vasodilation and increased capillary permeability)	Histamine, prostaglandins, leukotrienes, bradykinin, platelet-activating factor
Tissue damage	Lysosomal enzymes and products released from neutrophils, macrophages, and other inflammatory cells
Chemotaxis	Complement fragments
Pain	Prostaglandins Bradykinin
Fever	Interleukin-1 and interleukin-6
Leukocytosis	Tumor necrosis factor and interleukin-8

describes some chemical mediators and their major impact on inflammation.

Histamine. Histamine is widely distributed throughout the body. It is found in high concentration in platelets, basophils, and mast cells. Histamine causes dilation and increased permeability of capillaries. It is one of the first mediators of an inflammatory response. Antihistamine drugs inhibit this immediate, transient response.

Plasma Proteases. The plasma proteases consist of the kinins, activated complement proteins, and clotting factors. One kinin, bradykinin, causes increased capillary permeability and pain. The clotting system (see Chapter 14) contributes to the vascular phase of inflammation, mainly through fibrinopeptides that are formed during the final steps of the clotting process.

Prostaglandins. The prostaglandins are ubiquitous, lipid-soluble molecules derived from arachidonic acid, a fatty acid liberated from cell membrane phospholipids. Several prostaglandins are synthesized from arachidonic acid through the cyclooxygenase metabolic pathway. Prostaglandins contribute to vasodilation, capillary permeability, and the pain and fever that accompany inflammation. The stable prostaglandins (PGE_1 and PGE_2) induce inflammation and potentiate the effects of histamine and other inflammatory mediators. The prostaglandin thromboxane A_2 promotes platelet aggregation and vasoconstriction. Aspirin reduces inflammation by inactivating the first enzyme in the cyclooxygenase pathway for prostaglandin synthesis. The glucocorticoid hormones or drugs curtail the availability of arachidonic acid needed for prostaglandin synthesis.

Leukotrienes. The leukotrienes are chemical mediators first discovered in leukocytes and chemically have a triene structure. Like the prostaglandins, the leukotrienes are formed from arachidonic acid, but through the lipoxygenase pathway. Histamine and leukotrienes are complementary in action in that they have similar functions. Histamine is produced rapidly and transiently while the more potent leukotrienes are being synthesized. One leukotriene causes slow and sustained constriction of the bronchioles and is an important inflammatory mediator in bronchial asthma and immediate hypersensitivity reactions (see Chapters 19 and 29). The leukotrienes also have been reported to affect the permeability of the postcapillary venules, the adhesion properties of endothelial cells, and the chemotaxis and extravascularization of neutrophils, eosinophils, and monocytes.

Platelet-Activating Factor. Generated from a complex lipid stored in cell membranes, PAF affects a variety of cell types and induces platelet aggregation. It activates neutrophils and is a potent eosinophil chemoattractant. When injected into the skin, PAF causes a wheal-and-flare reaction and the leukocyte infiltrate characteristic of immediate hypersensitivity reactions. When inhaled, PAF causes bronchospasm, eosinophil infiltration, and nonspecific bronchial hyperreactivity.

Inflammatory Exudates

Characteristically, the acute inflammatory response involves production of exudates. These exudates can vary in terms of fluid, plasma protein, and cell content. Acute inflammation can produce serous, fibrinous, membranous, purulent, and hemorrhagic exudates. Inflammatory exudates often are composed of a combination of these types. *Serous exudates* are watery exudates low in protein content that result from plasma entering the inflammatory site. *Fibrinous exudates* contain large amounts of fibrinogen and form a thick and sticky meshwork, much like the fibers of a blood clot. *Membranous* or *pseudomembranous exudates* develop on mucous membrane surfaces and are composed of necrotic cells enmeshed in a fibrinopurulent exudate. A *purulent* or *suppurative exudate* contains pus, which is composed of degraded white blood cells, proteins, and tissue debris. An abscess and cellulitis are examples of purulent exudates. *Hemorrhagic exudates* occur where severe tissue injury causes damage to blood vessels or when there is significant leakage of red cells from the capillaries.

CHRONIC INFLAMMATION

Acute infections usually are self-limiting and rapidly controlled by the host defenses. In contrast, chronic inflammation is self-perpetuating and may last for weeks, months, or even years. It may develop during a recurrent or progressive acute inflammatory process or from low-grade, smoldering responses that fail to evoke an acute response. Characteristic of chronic inflammation is an infiltration by mononuclear cells (macrophages and lymphocytes) instead of the influx of neutrophils commonly seen in acute inflammation. Chronic inflammation also involves the proliferation of fibroblasts instead of exudates. As a result, the risk of scarring and deformity usually is considered greater than in acute inflammation. Agents that evoke chronic inflammation typically are low-grade, persistent irritants that are unable to penetrate deeply or spread rapidly. Among the causes of chronic inflammation are foreign bodies such as talc, silica, asbestos, and surgical suture materials. Many viruses provoke chronic inflammatory responses, as do certain bacteria, fungi, and larger parasites of moderate to low virulence. Examples are the tubercle bacillus, the treponema of syphilis, and the actinomyces. The presence of injured tissue such as that surrounding a healing fracture also may incite chronic inflammation. Immunologic mechanisms are thought to play an important role in chronic inflammation. The two patterns of chronic inflammation are a nonspecific chronic inflammation and granulomatous inflammation.

Nonspecific chronic inflammation involves a diffuse accumulation of macrophages and lymphocytes at the site of injury. Ongoing chemotaxis causes macrophages to infiltrate the inflamed site, where they accumulate owing to prolonged survival and immobilization. These mechanisms lead to fibroblast proliferation, with subsequent scar formation that in many cases replaces the normal connective tissue or the functional parenchymal tissues of the involved structures. For example, scar tissue resulting from chronic inflammation of the bowel causes narrowing of the bowel lumen.

A granulomatous lesion results from chronic inflammation. A *granuloma* typically is a small, 1- to 2-mm lesion in which there is a massing of macrophages surrounded by lymphocytes. These modified macrophages resemble epithelial cells and sometimes are called *epithelioid cells*. Like other macrophages, these epithelioid cells are derived originally from blood monocytes. Granulomatous inflammation is associated with foreign bodies such as splinters, sutures, silica, and asbestos and with microorganisms that cause tuberculosis, syphilis, sarcoidosis, deep fungal infections, and brucellosis. These types of agents have one thing in common: they are poorly digested and usually are not easily controlled by other inflammatory mechanisms. The epithelioid cells in granulomatous inflammation may clump in a mass (granuloma) or coalesce, forming a large, multinucleated giant cell that attempts to surround the foreign agent. A dense membrane of connective tissue eventually encapsulates the lesion and isolates it.

A *tubercle* is a granulomatous inflammatory response to *Mycobacterium tuberculosis* infection. Peculiar to the tuberculosis granuloma is the presence of a caseous (cheesy) necrotic center.

In summary, inflammation describes a local response to tissue injury and can present as an acute or chronic condition. Acute inflammation is the local response of tissue to a nonspecific form of injury. The classic signs of inflammation are redness, swelling, local heat, pain, and loss of function. The inflammatory response is orchestrated by chemical mediators such as histamine, prostaglandins, PAF, complement fragments, and reactive molecules that are liberated by leukocytes. Acute inflammation involves a hemodynamic phase during which blood flow and capillary permeability are increased, and a cellular phase during which phagocytic white blood cells move into the area to engulf and degrade the inciting agent. Cytokines also influence the cellular responses. Acute inflammation involves the production of exudates containing serous fluid (serous exudate), red blood cells (hemorrhagic exudate), fibrinogen (fibrinous exudate), mucous membrane and fibrinogen breakdown products (membranous exudate), and tissue debris and white blood cell breakdown products (purulent exudate).

In contrast to acute inflammation, which is self-limiting, chronic inflammation is prolonged and usually is caused by persistent irritants, most of which are insoluble and resistant to phagocytosis and other inflammatory mechanisms. Chronic inflammation involves the presence of mononuclear cells (lymphocytes and macrophages) rather than granulocytes. Instead of the exudates formed in acute inflammation, the proliferation of fibroblasts in chronic inflammation can cause scarring and deformity.

Related Web Site

AEGIS web site with extensive information and links on HIV/AIDS   http://www.aegis.com/
Biology Project web site with information on Immunology, antibodies and HIV   http://www.biology.arizona.edu/immunology/immunology.html
Cells Alive! web site with animations on various concepts of the immune system   http://www.cellsalive.com/
Immunization Gateway—multiple resources on vaccines and immunization recommendations   http://www.immunofacts.com/
National Institutes of Health Web site on the immune system   http://rex.nci.nih.gov/PATIENTS/INFO_TEACHER/bookshelf/NIH_immune/index.html
R&D Systems site contains many mini-reviews on cytokines and their receptors   http://www.rndsystems.com/
Kimball's biology pages: A description of T and B cells with some illustrations   http://www.ultranet.com/~jkimball/BiologyPages/B/B_and_Tcells.html

Bibliography

Abbas A.K., Litchman A.H., Pober J.H., Abbas A.K. (2000). *Cellular and molecular immunology* (4th ed.). Philadelphia: W.B. Saunders.

Ahmed R., Gray D. (1996). Immunological memory and protective immunity: Understanding their relation. *Science* 272, 54–60.

Baumann H., Gauldie J. (1994). The acute phase response. *Immunology Today* 15, 74–80.

Benjamini E., Sunshine G., Leskowitz S. (2000). *Immunology: A short course* (4th ed.). New York: John Wiley & Sons.

Cotran R.S., Kumar V., Robbins S.L. (1994). *Pathologic basis of disease* (5th ed., pp. 51–92, 171–178). Philadelphia: W.B. Saunders.

Delves P.J., Roitt I.M. (2000). The immune system: Parts I and II. *New England Journal of Medicine* 343, 37–49, 108–117.

Fearon D., Locksley R.M. (1996). The instructive role of innate immunity in the acquired immune response. *Science* 272, 50–54.

Galli S.J. (1993). New concepts about the mast cells. *New England Journal of Medicine* 328, 257–265.

Gallin J.I., Goldstein I.M., Snyderman R. (Eds.). (1992). *Inflammation: Basic principles and clinical correlates* (2nd ed.). New York: Raven Press.

Janeway C.A., Jr., Travers P. (1999). *Immunobiology: The immune system in health and disease* (4th ed.). New York: Garland Publishing.

Goldsby R.A., Kindt T.J., Osborne B.A. (2000). *Kuby immunology* (4th ed.). San Francisco: W.H. Freeman.

Miller R. A. (1996). The aging immune system: Primer and prospectus. *Science* 273, 70–73.

Moretta L. (1996). Receptors for HLA class-I molecules in human natural killer cells. *Annual Review of Immunology* 14, 619–648.

Parham P. (2000). *The immune system.* New York: Garland Publishing.

Roitt I., Brostoff J., Male D. (1998). *Immunology* (5th ed.). St. Louis: Mosby.

Sell S., Berkower I., Max E. (1996). *Immunology, immunopathology and immunity* (5th ed.). East Norwalk, CT: Appleton & Lange.

Stites D., Terr A., Parslow T.G. (Eds.). (1997). *Medical immunology* (9th ed.). East Norwalk, CT: Appleton & Lange.

Alterations in the Immune Response

The human immune network is a multifaceted defense system that has evolved to protect against invading microorganisms, prevent the proliferation of cancer cells, and mediate the healing of damaged tissue. Under normal conditions, the immune response deters or prevents disease. Occasionally, however, the inadequate, inappropriate, or misdirected activation of the immune system can lead to debilitating or life-threatening illnesses, typified by immunodeficiency states, allergic or hypersensitivity reactions, transplantation pathophysiology, and autoimmune disorders. The various immunologic disorders that directly or indirectly lead to pathologic conditions in humans are discussed in this chapter.

Immunodeficiency Disease

After you have completed this section of the chapter, you should be able to meet the following objectives:

♦ List the most important categories of immunodeficiency disease

♦ State the difference between primary and secondary immunodeficiency states

♦ Compare and contrast immunodeficiency disorders caused by B-cell and T-cell disorders

♦ State the function of the complement system and relate to the manifestations of hereditary angioneurotic edema

♦ State the proposed mechanisms of dysfunction and manifestations in primary disorders of phagocytosis

Immunodeficiency can be defined as an abnormality in one or more branches of the immune system that renders a person susceptible to diseases normally prevented by an intact immune system. Four major categories of immune mechanisms defend the body against infectious or neoplastic disease: humoral or antibody-mediated immunity (*i.e.,* B lymphocytes), cell-mediated immunity (*i.e.,* T lymphocytes and lymphokines), the complement system, and phagocytosis (*i.e.,* neutrophils and macrophages). Although not usually included in a discussion of the immune system, disorders that breach the integrity of natural barriers such as skin, mucous membranes, and secretory antimicrobial enzymes (*e.g.,* lysozyme in tears, the hydrolytic enzymes in saliva) also can produce a state of immunodeficiency.

Abnormalities of the immune system can be classified as primary (*i.e.,* congenital or inherited) or secondary if the immunodeficiency is acquired later in life. Secondary immunodeficiency can be the result of infection (*e.g.,* acquired immunodeficiency syndrome [AIDS]), neoplastic disease (*e.g.,* lymphoma), or immunosuppressive therapy (*e.g.,* corticosteroids or transplant rejection medications). Regardless of the cause, primary and secondary deficiencies can produce the same spectrum of disease. The severity and symptomatology of the various immunodeficiencies depend on the disorder and extent of immune system involvement. The various categories of immunodeficiency are summarized in Chart 19-1. AIDS is discussed in Chapter 20.

Until recently, little was known about the causes of primary immunodeficiency diseases. As a result of recent advances in mapping the human genome, the genetic origin of many of the defects has been identified.[1,2] Also, previous classifications of the disorders were based on specific clinical manifestations and alterations in immune function. Advances in molecular genetics now allow many of these disorders to be grouped according to types of genetically altered molecules that are involved. Although genes essential to immune function are located throughout the genome, a large number are located on the X chromosome. Thus, there is a clear dominance of X-linked immunodeficiencies in males due to hemizygosity.[2] Also, spontaneous mutations in these X-linked genes are relatively common.

HUMORAL (B-CELL) IMMUNODEFICIENCIES

Humoral immunodeficiency can range from a transient decrease in immunoglobulin levels during early infancy to inherited disorders that interrupt the production of one or all of the immunoglobulins. During the first few months of life, infants are protected from infection by immunoglobulin G (IgG) class antibodies that have been transferred from the maternal circulation during fetal life. IgA, IgM, IgD, and IgE do not normally cross the placenta. The presence of elevated levels of IgA or IgM in the infant cord blood suggests premature antibody production in response to an intrauterine infection. An infant's level of maternal IgG gradually declines over a period of approximately 6 months (see Fig. 18-16, Chapter 18). Concomitant with the loss of maternal antibody, the infant's immature humoral immune system begins to function, and between the ages of 1 and 2 years, the child's antibody production reaches adult levels.

Antibody production depends on the differentiation of B-lymphocyte stem cells in the bone marrow to mature, immunoglobulin-producing plasma cells. This maturation cycle initially involves the production of surface IgM, migration from the marrow to the peripheral lymphoid tissue, and switching to the specialized production of IgG, IgA, IgD, IgE, or IgM antibodies after antigenic stimulation (Fig. 19-1).

CHART 19-1

Immunodeficiency States

Humoral (B-Cell) Immunodeficiency

Primary
  Transient hypogammaglobulinemia of infancy
  X-linked hypogammaglobulinemia
  Common variable immunodeficiency
  Selective deficiency of IgG, IgA, IgM
Secondary
  Increased loss of immunoglobulins (nephrotic syndrome)*

Cellular (T-Cell) Immunodeficiency

Primary
  Congenital thymic aplasia (DiGeorge syndrome)
  Abnormal T-cell production (Nezelof syndrome)
Secondary
  Malignant disease (Hodgkin's disease and others)
  Transient suppression of T-cell production and function due to an acute viral infection such as measles
  AIDS
  Purine nucleoside phosphorylase or adenosine deaminase deficiency

Combined B-Cell and T-Cell Immunodeficiency

Primary
  Severe combined immunodeficiency (autosomal or sex-linked recessive)
  Wiskott-Aldrich syndrome (immunodeficiency, thrombocytopenia, and eczema)
  Ataxia-telangiectasia
Secondary
  Irradiation
  Immune suppressant and cytotoxic drugs
  Aging

Complement Disorders

Primary
  Angioneurotic edema (complement 1 inactivator deficiency)
  Selective deficiency in a complement component
Secondary
  Acquired disorders that involve complement utilization

Phagocytic Dysfunction

Primary
  Chronic granulomatous disease
  Glucose-6-phosphate dehydrogenase deficiency
  Job syndrome
  Chédiak-Higashi syndrome
  CD11/CD18 deficiency
Secondary
  Drug induced (corticosteroid and immunosuppressive therapy)
  Diabetes mellitus

*Examples are not inclusive.

Primary Immunodeficiency Disorders

➤ Primary immunodeficiency disorders are congenital or inherited abnormalities of immune function that render a person susceptible to diseases normally prevented by an intact immune system.

➤ Disorders of B-cell function impair the ability to produce antibodies and defend against microorganisms and toxins that circulate in body fluids (IgM and IgG) or enter the body through the mucosal surface of the respiratory or gastrointestinal tract (IgA). Persons with primary B-cell immunodeficiency are particularly prone to infections due to encapsulated organisms.

➤ Disorders of T-cell function impair the ability to orchestrate the immune response (CD4+ helper T cells) and to protect against fungal, protozoan, viral, and intracellular bacterial infections (CD8+ cytotoxic T cells).

➤ Combined T-cell and B-cell immunodeficiency states affect all aspects of immune function. Severe combined immunodeficiency represents a life-threatening absence of immune function that requires bone marrow transplantation for survival.

Defects in B-cell function increase the risk of recurrent pyogenic infections, including those caused by *Streptococcus pneumoniae, Haemophilus influenzae,* and *Staphylococcus aureus,* and by gram-negative organisms such as *Pseudomonas* species. Humoral immunity usually is not as important in defending against intracellular bacteria (mycobacteria), fungi, and protozoa. Viruses usually are handled normally, except for the enteroviruses that cause gastrointestinal infections.

Transient Hypogammaglobulinemia of Infancy

Any abnormality that blocks or prevents the maturation of B-lymphocyte stem cells can produce a state of immunodeficiency. For example, certain infants may experience a delay in the maturation process of B cells that leads to a prolonged deficiency in IgG levels (IgM and IgA levels are normal) beyond 6 months of age. The total number and antigenic response of circulating B cells is normal, but the chemical communication between B and T cells that leads to clonal proliferation of antibody-producing plasma cells seems to be reduced.[3] This condition is referred to as *transient hypogammaglobulinemia of infancy.* The result of this condition usually is limited to repeated bouts of upper respiratory and middle ear infections. This condition usually resolves by the time the child is 2 to 4 years of age.

Primary B-Cell Immunodeficiencies

Primary B-cell immunodeficiencies are genetic disorders of the B lymphocytes. They account for 70% of primary immunodeficiencies and are manifested by decreased IgG production.[4]

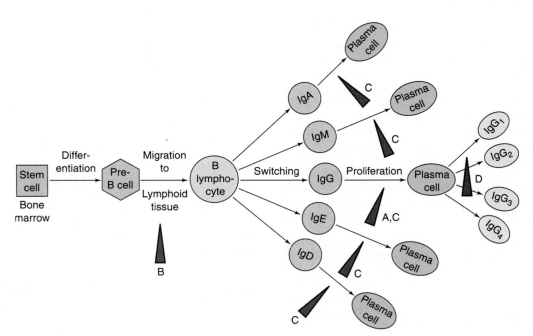

FIGURE 19-1 Stem cells to mature immunoglobulin-secreting plasma cells. *Arrows* indicate the stage of the maturation process that is interrupted in (**A**) transient hypoglobulinemia, (**B**) X-linked hypogammaglobulinemia, (**C**) common variable immunodeficiency, and (**D**) IgG subclass deficiency.

X-linked Agammaglobulinemia. X-linked or Bruton's agammaglobulinemia is a recessive trait that affects only males.[2–6] As the name implies, persons with this disorder have essentially undetectable levels of all serum immunoglobulins. Therefore, they are susceptible to meningitis and recurrent otitis media and to sinus and pulmonary infections with encapsulated organisms such as *S. pneumoniae, H. influenzae* type b, *S. aureus,* and *Neisseria meningitidis.*[2] Many boys with this disorder have severe tooth decay.

The central defect in this syndrome is a genetic mutation that blocks the differentiation of pre-B cells, creating an absence of mature circulating B cells and plasma cells. T lymphocytes, however, are normal in number and function. Symptoms of the disorder usually coincide with the loss of maternal antibodies. A clue to the presence of the disorder is failure of an infection to respond completely and promptly to antibiotic therapy. Diagnosis is based on demonstration of low or absent serum immunoglobulins. Therapy consists of prophylaxis with intravenous immunoglobulin and prompt antimicrobial therapy for suspected infections. The prognosis of this condition depends on the prompt recognition and treatment of infections. Chronic pulmonary disease is an ever-present danger.

Common Variable Immunodeficiency. Another disorder of B-cell maturation, which is similar to X-linked agammaglobulinemia, is a condition called *common variable immunodeficiency.* In this syndrome, the terminal differentiation of mature B cells to plasma cells is blocked. The result is markedly reduced serum immunoglobulin levels, normal numbers of circulating B lymphocytes, and a complete absence of germinal centers and plasma cells in lymph nodes and the spleen.

The symptomatology of common variable immunodeficiency is similar to that of X-linked agammaglobulinemia (*i.e.,* recurrent otitis media and sinus and pulmonary infections with encapsulated organisms), but the onset of symptoms occurs much later, usually between the ages of 15 and 35 years, and distribution of disease between the sexes is equal. Persons with late-onset hypogammaglobulinemia also have an increased tendency toward development of chronic lung disease, autoimmune disorders, hepatitis, gastric carcinoma, and chronic diarrhea with associated intestinal malabsorption. Approximately one half of persons with the disorder have evidence of abnormal T-cell immunity, suggesting that this syndrome is a complex immunodeficiency. Treatment methods for late-onset hypogammaglobulinemia are similar to those used for X-linked hypogammaglobulinemia.

Selective Immunoglobulin A Deficiency. Selective IgA deficiency is the most common type of immunoglobulin deficiency, affecting 1 in 400 to 1 in 1000 persons.[2] The syndrome is characterized by moderate to marked reduction in levels of serum and secretory IgA. It is likely that the cause of this deficiency is a block in the pathway that promotes terminal differentiation of mature B cells to IgA-secreting plasma cells.

Approximately two thirds of persons with selective IgA deficiency have no overt symptoms, presumably because IgG and IgM levels are normal and compensate for the defect. At least 50% of affected children overcome the deficiency by the age of 14 years. Persons with markedly reduced levels of IgA often experience repeated upper respiratory and gastrointestinal infections and have increased incidence of allergies such as asthma and autoimmune disorders. It has been estimated that as many as 50% of persons with selective IgA deficiency have some form of allergy.[6] It has been suggested that the lack of IgA allows inhaled and ingested antigens to cross the mucosal epithelium and elicit antibody responses in the gastrointestinal and bronchial lymphoid tissues. Persons with IgA deficiency also can develop antibodies against IgA, which can lead to an anaphylactic response when blood components containing IgA are given.[5]

There is no treatment available for selective IgA deficiency unless there is a concomitant reduction in IgG levels. Administration of IgA is of little benefit because it has a short half-life and is not secreted across the mucosa. There also is the risk associated with IgA antibodies.

Immunoglobulin G Subclass Deficiency. An IgG subclass deficiency can affect one or more of IgG subtypes, despite normal levels or elevated serum concentrations of IgG. As discussed in Chapter 18, IgG immunoglobulins can be divided into four subclasses (IgG1 through IgG4) based on structure and function. Most circulating IgG belongs to the IgG1 (70%) and IgG2 (20%) subclasses. In general, antibodies directed against protein antigens belong to the IgG1 and IgG3 subclasses, and antibodies directed against carbohydrate and polysaccharide antigens are primarily IgG2 subclass. As a result, persons who are deficient in IgG2 subclass antibodies can be at greater risk for development of sinusitis, otitis media, and pneumonia caused by polysaccharide-encapsulated microorganisms such as *S. pneumoniae, H. influenzae* type b, and *N. meningitidis.* Children with mild forms of the deficiency can be treated with prophylactic antibiotics to prevent repeated infections. Intravenous immune globulin can be given to children with severe manifestations of this deficiency. The use of polysaccharide vaccines conjugated to protein carriers can provide protection against some of these infections because protein conjugated to protein carriers stimulates an IgG1 response.

Secondary B-Cell Immunodeficiencies

Secondary deficiencies in humoral immunity can develop as a consequence of selective loss of immunoglobulins through the gastrointestinal or genitourinary tracts. Such is the case in persons with nephrotic syndrome who, because of abnormal glomerular filtration, lose serum IgA and IgG in their urine. Because of its larger molecular size, IgM is not filtered into the urine, and serum levels remain normal.

CELLULAR (T-CELL) IMMUNODEFICIENCIES

Unlike the B-cell lineage, in which a well-defined series of differentiation steps ultimately leads to the production of immunoglobulins, mature T lymphocytes are composed of distinct subpopulations whose immunologic assignments are diverse. T cells can be functionally divided into helper and cytotoxic subtypes and a population of T cells that promote delayed hypersensitivity reactions. Collectively, T lymphocytes protect against fungal, protozoan, viral, and intracellular bacterial infections; control malignant cell proliferation; and are responsible for coordinating the overall immune response.

Primary T-Cell Immunodeficiencies

There are few primary forms of T-cell immunodeficiency, probably because persons with defects in this branch of the immune response rarely survive beyond infancy or childhood. However, exceptions are being recognized as newer T-cell defects, such as the X-linked hyper-IgM syndrome, are identified. Other primary T-cell immunodeficiency disorders result from defective expression of the T-cell receptor (TCR) complex, defective cytokine production, and defects in T-cell activation.

DiGeorge Syndrome. DiGeorge syndrome stems from an embryonic developmental defect. The defect is thought to occur before the 12th week of gestation, when the thymus gland, parathyroid gland, and parts of the head, neck, and heart are developing. The disorder affects both sexes. Because familial occurrence is rare, it is not likely that the disorder is inherited. Formerly thought to be caused by a variety of factors, including extrinsic teratogens, this defect has been traced to a gene on chromosome 22 (22q11).[1,4,6,7]

Infants born with this defect have partial or complete failure of development of the thymus and parathyroid glands and have congenital defects of the head, neck, and heart. The extent of immune and parathyroid abnormalities is highly variable, as are the other defects. Occasionally, a child has no heart defect. In some children, the thymus is not absent but is in an abnormal location and is extremely small. These infants can have partial DiGeorge syndrome, in which hypertrophy of the thymus occurs with development of normal immune function. The facial disorders can include hypertelorism (*i.e.,* increased distance between the eyes); mi-

crognathia (*i.e.,* fish mouth); low-set, posteriorly angulated ears; split uvula; and high-arched palate (Fig. 19-2). Urinary tract abnormalities also are common. The most frequent presenting sign is hypocalcemia and tetany that develops in the first 24 hours of life. It is caused by the absence of the parathyroid gland and is resistant to standard therapy.

Children who survive the immediate neonatal period may have recurrent or chronic infections because of impaired T-cell immunity. Children also may have an absence of immunoglobulin production, caused by a lack of helper T-cell function. For children who do require treatment, thymus transplantation can be performed to reconstitute T-cell immunity. Bone marrow transplantation also has been successfully used to restore normal T-cell populations. If blood transfusions are needed, as during corrective heart surgery, special processing is required to prevent graft-versus-host disease.

X-Linked Immunodeficiency With Hyper-IgM. The X-linked immunodeficiency of hyper-IgM, also known as the *hyper-IgM syndrome,* is characterized by low IgG and IgA levels with normal or, more frequently, high IgM concentrations. Being X-linked, the disorder is confined to males. Formerly classified as a B-cell defect, it now has been traced to a T-cell defect. The disorder results from the inability of T cells to signal B cells to undergo isotype switching to IgG and IgA; thus, they produce only IgM.[5]

Like boys with X-linked agammaglobulinemia, affected boys become symptomatic during the first and second years of life. They have recurrent pyogenic infections, including otitis media, sinusitis, tonsillitis, and pneumonia. They are also more susceptible to *Pneumocystis carinii* infection. Thymic-dependent lymphoid tissues and T-cell function usually are normal, as are B-cell counts. Hemolytic anemia and thrombocytopenia may occur, and transient, persistent, or cyclic neutropenia is a common feature.[5] The frequency of autoimmune disorders is higher than with other immunoglobulin deficiency disorders.[5]

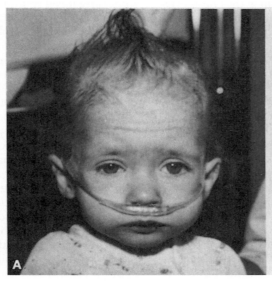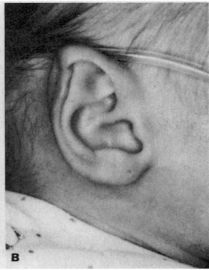

FIGURE 19-2 (A) Facial abnormalities in a child with DiGeorge syndrome, as illustrated by hypertelorism, defective low-set ears, hypoplastic mandible, and bowing upward of the upper lip and (**B**) by a closeup of the ears showing a notched pinna and deficient helix formation. (From Oski F.A. [Ed.]. [1990]. *Principles and practice of pediatrics.* Philadelphia: J.B. Lippincott)

Secondary T-Cell Immunodeficiencies

Secondary deficiencies of T-cell function are more common than primary deficiencies and have been described in conjunction with acute viral infections (*e.g.,* measles virus, cytomegalovirus) and with certain malignancies such as Hodgkin's disease and other lymphomas. In the case of viruses, direct infection of specific T-lymphocyte subpopulations (*e.g.,* helper cells) by lymphotropic viruses such as the human immunodeficiency virus (HIV) and human herpesvirus type 6 can lead to loss of cellular function and selective subtype depletion with a concomitant loss of immunologic function associated with that subtype. Persons with neoplastic disorders can have impaired T-cell function based on unregulated multiplication or dysfunction of one particular subclone of T cells. The outward expression of this may be an increased susceptibility to infections caused by normally harmless pathogens (*i.e.,* opportunistic infections) or failure to generate delayed-type hypersensitivity reactions (*i.e.,* anergy). Persons with anergy have a diminished or absent reaction to a battery of skin test antigens, including *Candida* and the tuberculin test, even when infected with *Mycobacterium tuberculosis.* In persons with anergy, a negative skin test result for tuberculosis can mean a true lack of exposure to tuberculosis or indicate the person's inability to mount an appropriate T-cell response (see Chapter 28).

COMBINED T-CELL AND B-CELL IMMUNODEFICIENCIES

Disorders of the immune response that have elements of B-cell and T-cell dysfunction fall under the broad classification of combined immunodeficiency syndrome (CIDS) and include a spectrum of inherited (autosomal recessive and X-linked) conditions. A single mutation in any one of the many genes that influence lymphocyte development or response, including lymphocyte receptors, cytokines, or major histocompatibility antigens, could lead to combined immunodeficiency. Regardless of the affected gene, the net result is a disruption in the normal communication system of B and T lymphocytes and deregulation of the immune response. The spectrum of disease resulting from CIDS ranges from mild to severe to ultimately fatal forms.

Severe Combined Immunodeficiency

The most severe form of T- and B-cell deficiency often is referred to as *severe combined immunodeficiency syndrome* (SCIDS). SCIDS is caused by diverse genetic mutations that lead to absence of all immune function.[5,6] A family history of similarly affected relatives occurs in approximately 50% of cases.[6] Both autosomal recessive and X-linked inheritance are involved. Infants with SCIDS have a disease course that resembles AIDS, with failure to thrive, chronic diarrhea, and opportunistic infections that usually lead to death by the age of 2 years. If recognized at birth or within the first 3 months of life, 95% of infants can be successfully treated with human leukocyte antigen (HLA)-identical or T-cell–depleted bone marrow stem cell transplantation.[5]

Approximately 50% of persons with the autosomal recessive form of SCIDS have an associated deficiency in the enzyme adenosine deaminase (ADA).[3] Absence of this enzyme leads to accumulation of toxic metabolites that kill dividing and resting T cells. Bone marrow and stem cell transplantation has been successful in treating children with ADA-negative SCIDS.[1,5,6,8] Gene therapy has been used to insert the missing gene into stem cells from cord blood of neonates who were diagnosed prenatally with the disease.[8,9] The gene-treated stem cells, which are then infused into the infant, home to the bone marrow, where they begin producing ADA-containing T cells. Only a limited number of children have been treated with gene therapy, and those results have been somewhat disappointing.[8] Repeated transfusions of gene-treated cells are needed, and only a small percentage of normal ADA activity is achieved. Enzyme replacement therapy also may be used in the management of persons with this form of SCIDS.[8]

Ataxia-Telangiectasia

Ataxia-telangiectasia is a complex syndrome of neurologic, immunologic, endocrinologic, hepatic, and cutaneous abnormalities. It is an autosomal recessive disorder that is thought to result from the mutation of a single gene located on the long arm of chromosome 11 (11q22-23).[5] As the name implies, this syndrome is heralded by worsening cerebellar ataxia (*i.e.,* poor muscle coordination) and the appearance of telangiectases (*i.e.,* lesions consisting of dilated capillaries and arterioles) on skin and conjunctival surfaces (Fig. 19-3). The ataxia usually goes unnoticed until the toddler begins to walk; the telangiectases develop thereafter, especially on skin surfaces exposed to the sun. The ataxia progresses slowly and relentlessly to severe disability. Intellectual development is normal at first but seems to stop at the 10-year level in many of these children. Children with this syndrome have associated deficiencies in cellular and humoral components of the immune response, including reduced levels of IgA, IgE, and IgG2, absolute lymphopenia, and a decrease in the ratio of CD4+ helper T cells to CD8+ suppressor T cells. Approximately 70% have an IgA deficiency, and approximately half also have an IgG subclass deficiency. There is increased susceptibility to recurrent upper and lower respiratory tract infections (particularly those caused by encapsulated bacteria) and an increased risk for the development of malignancies. Death from malignant lymphoma is common.

Wiskott-Aldrich Syndrome

The Wiskott-Aldrich syndrome is an X-linked recessive disorder that becomes symptomatic during the first year of life.[5] Infants with this syndrome are plagued by eczema, recurrent infections, and low platelet counts. Bleeding episodes or symptoms due to infection usually begin within the first 6 months of life. Abnormalities of humoral immunity include decreased serum levels of IgM and markedly elevated serum IgA and IgE concentrations. T-cell dysfunction initially is mild but progressively deteriorates, and patients become increasingly susceptible to development of malignancies of the mononuclear phagocytic system, including Hodgkin's lymphoma and leukemia. Children with Wiskott-Aldrich syndrome typically are unable to produce antibody to polysaccharide antigens and therefore are susceptible to

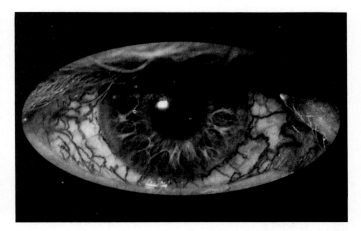

FIGURE 19-3 Striking telangiectasis on the bulbar conjunctiva of a 22-year-old patient with ataxia-telangiectasia. These dilated vessels typically appear between the ages of 2 and 5. (From Oski F.A. [Ed.]. [1990]. *Principles and practice of pediatrics*. Philadelphia: J.B. Lippincott)

infections caused by encapsulated microorganisms. They also are prone to septicemia and meningitis with these organisms. Varicella infection can be lethal to children with this condition. Bone marrow transplantation has been successful in children with Wiskott-Aldrich syndrome. Splenectomy may be used to control the thrombocytopenia in situations in which bone marrow transplantation cannot be done.

DISORDERS OF THE COMPLEMENT SYSTEM

The complement system is an integral part of the normal immune response (see Chapter 18). The activation of the complement network through the classic, lectin-mediated, or alternative pathways promotes chemotaxis, opsonization, and phagocytosis of invasive pathogens, bacteriolysis, and anaphylactic reactions. Thus, alterations in normal levels of complement or the absence of a particular complement component can lead to enhanced susceptibility to infectious diseases and immune-mediated disorders such as hemolytic anemia and collagen vascular disorders. As with B- and T-cell deficiencies, complement disorders can be classified as primary if the deficiency is inherited or secondary if the condition develops because of another disease process.

Primary Disorders of the Complement System

Most primary disorders of the complement system are transmitted as autosomal recessive traits and can involve one or more complement components (the complement components are designated by "C" and enzyme subcomponents by "q," "r," and "s"). Deficiencies of C1r, C1rs, C4, C2, C3, C5, C6, C7, C8, and C9 are transmitted as autosomal codominant traits, in which each parent transmits a gene that codes for half the serum level of the component.[10,11] Because 50% activity is sufficient to prevent disease, persons who are heterozygous and have one normally functioning gene seldom have problems.

In general, persons with deficiencies in factors C1 (C1q, r, and s) and C4 are not necessarily at increased risk for recurrent infections because the lectin-mediated and alternative pathways can be activated normally through C3.

However, many of them acquire autoimmune diseases, particularly lupus-like syndromes. Most persons with primary deficiency of C1q have had systemic lupus erythematosus (SLE), an SLE-like syndrome without typical SLE serology, a chronic rash with underlying vasculitis on biopsy, or membranoproliferative glomerulonephritis.[10,11] Like persons with C1q deficiency, persons with C1r, C1r/C1s, C4, C2, and C3 deficiencies have a high incidence of vasculitis syndromes, especially SLE or SLE-like syndrome. A C2 deficiency causes a susceptibility to multiple and potentially life-threatening infections caused by encapsulated bacteria, especially *S. pneumoniae*. Similarly, persons with C3 deficiency are predisposed to infections that trigger the lectin-mediated or alternate pathway (*e.g.*, those caused by encapsulated bacteria and *S. aureus*) because of their inability to opsonize and lyse bacteria. Although persons with deficiencies in the terminal components of complement (C5 through C9) are susceptible to repeated episodes of meningitis and sepsis caused by *N. meningitidis* or systemic gonococcal disease, they are less likely to have autoimmune disorders than persons with other complement deficiencies.[10]

Only supportive measures are available for treatment of primary disorders of the complement system. Measures to prevent bacterial infections are important. The affected person and close contacts should be immunized with vaccines for *S. pneumoniae*, *H. influenzae*, and *N. meningitidis*.

Hereditary Angioneurotic Edema. Hereditary angioneurotic edema is a particularly interesting form of complement deficiency.[12,13] Persons with this disorder do not produce a functional C1 inhibitor. Activation of the classic complement pathway is uncontrolled, leading to increased breakdown of C4 and C2 with concomitant release of C-kinin, a vasodilator. This causes episodic attacks of localized edema involving the face, neck, joints, abdomen, and sites of trauma. Swelling of the subcutaneous tissues, especially of the face, can be disfiguring, and swelling of the gastric mucosa causes nausea, vomiting, and diarrhea. If the trachea or larynx is involved, the episode can prove fatal. The attacks associated with this inherited disease usually begin before the age of 2 years and become progressively worse with age. Symptoms can last from 1 to 4 days, and most persons with the disorder have more than one attack a month. Adults with hereditary angioneurotic edema can be treated with danazol, a synthetic androgen with weak virilizing and mild anabolic potential. The drug, given orally, increases C1 inhibitor levels and prevents attacks.[10] A vapor-heated C1 inhibitor concentrate has been developed. This concentrate can be used to prevent and treat an acute attack of hereditary angioneurotic edema.[13,14]

Secondary Disorders of the Complement System

Secondary complement deficiencies also can occur in persons with functionally normal complement systems because of rapid activation and turnover of complement components (as is seen in immune complex disease) or reduced synthesis of components, as would be the case in chronic cirrhosis of the liver or malnutrition.

DISORDERS OF PHAGOCYTOSIS

The phagocytic system is composed primarily of polymorphonuclear leukocytes (*i.e.*, neutrophils and eosinophils) and mononuclear phagocytes (*i.e.*, circulating monocytes and tissue and fixed [spleen] macrophages). The primary purpose of phagocytic cells is to migrate to the site of infection (*i.e.*, chemotaxis), aggregate around the affected tissue (*i.e.*, adherence), envelope invading microorganisms or foreign substances (*i.e.*, phagocytosis), and generate microbicidal substances (*e.g.*, enzymes or byproducts of metabolism) to kill the ingested pathogens. A defect in any of these functions or a reduction in the absolute number of available cells can disrupt the phagocytic system. Patients with phagocytic disorders are particularly prone to infections by bacteria and often by *Candida* species and filamentous fungi, although the types of pathogens vary with different disorders.[15] As with other alterations in immune function, defects in phagocytosis can be primary or secondary disorders.

Primary Disorders of Phagocytosis

The best-known disorders of phagocytosis are the *chronic granulomatous diseases* (CGD). The CGD are a group of inherited disorders (X-linked or autosomal recessive) that greatly reduce or inactivate the ability of phagocytic cells to produce the so-called *respiratory burst* that results in the generation of toxic derivatives of oxygen (superoxide anion and hydrogen peroxide).[15–17] These oxygen species participate in creating an intracellular environment that kills ingested microorganisms. Recurrent infections, along with granulomatous lesions, in persons with CGD are thought to be due to persistence of viable microorganisms in impaired phagocytic cells. Other aspects of phagocyte function, such as engulfment of microorganisms, are normal.

Children with CGD are subject to chronic and acute infections of the skin, liver, lung, and other soft tissues despite aggressive antibiotic therapy. Severe facial acne and painful inflammation of the nares is common. Organisms responsible for the infections include *S. aureus, Serratia marcescens, Pseudomonas cepacia, Escherichia coli, Candida albicans,* and *Aspergillus* species.[16,17] These infections usually begin during the first 2 years of life. The disorder is diagnosed by examining the ability of a person's phagocytes to reduce a yellow dye (*i.e.*, nitroblue tetrazolium) to a blue compound during active respiration. Treatment of the disorder usually is limited to the use of prophylactic antibiotics or white blood cell infusions. Other disorders of phagocyte metabolism include myeloperoxidase deficiency, glucose-6-phosphate dehydrogenase deficiency, and glutathione peroxidase deficiency. Each of these metabolic disorders promotes an increased rate of infection in affected persons, but usually not with the frequency or severity seen in CGD.

Job Syndrome. Job syndrome is a multisystem disorder that is inherited as an autosomal dominant trait. It is characterized by unregulated IgE synthesis, delayed or diminished polymorphonuclear neutrophil chemotaxis, recurrent infections of the skin and respiratory tract, and chronic eczema. The manifestations of the disorder become apparent early in infancy with the development of chronic mucocutaneous candidiasis and "cold" cutaneous abscesses (*i.e.*, without the usual symptoms of warmth, redness, and pain). Similar to CGD, the most common pathogen is *S. aureus,* but children with the disorder also are susceptible to a multitude of bacterial and fungal infections. In addition to elevated IgE levels and poor chemotactic response, children with Job syndrome frequently have coarse facial features, red hair, retarded growth, a broad nasal bridge, eosinophilia, and osteoporosis

Chédiak-Higashi Syndrome. Chédiak-Higashi syndrome is an autosomal recessive disorder in which the central defect in phagocytic function is thought to be caused by abnormal cell membrane fluidity, poor cytoskeletal coordination, and poor fusion of neutrophilic granules with phagocytosed microorganisms. The end result is poor mobility of the phagocytes and delayed killing of ingested bacteria. As with other disorders of phagocytosis, children with Chédiak-Higashi syndrome are subject to repeated cutaneous and respiratory tract infections, usually caused by beta-hemolytic streptococci (*e.g., S. pyogenes*) and *S. aureus.* Other characteristics of the syndrome include partial albinism and bleeding disorders. Giant granules in the cytoplasm of neutrophils are pathognomonic of the condition.

Secondary Disorders of Phagocytosis

Secondary deficiencies of the phagocytic system can be caused by a number of circumstances, such as deficiencies of opsonins, which are factors such as antibody and complement that coat the surface of a foreign substance and enhance phagocytosis, and deficiencies of chemotactic factors, such as antibody and complement that coat the surface of microorganisms and promote increased migration of phagocytes to the site of infection and stimulate phagocytosis. Deficiencies of either of these factors reduce the overall effectiveness of phagocytes. Drugs that impair or prevent inflammation and T-cell function such as corticosteroids or cyclosporine also alter phagocytic response through modulation of cytokines.

Persons with diabetes mellitus also demonstrate poor phagocytic function, primarily because of altered chemotaxis. The reason for this dysfunction is not understood, but it is unrelated to the person's age or the severity of the metabolic disorder. Apparently, this is a separate genetic disorder that is coinherited at a higher frequency among persons with diabetes and among family members.

HIV infection and AIDS represent another form of acquired or secondary deficiency of phagocytic function. However, in this case, the deficiency is due to direct infection and destruction of helper T cells and monocytes–macrophages by the virus (see Chapter 20).

STEM CELL TRANSPLANTATION

Many of the primary immunodeficiency disorders in which the defect has been traced to the stem cell can be cured with allogeneic stem cell transplantation from an unaffected donor.[18] These include disorders such as SCID, Wiskott-Aldrich syndrome, chronic granulomatous disease, and Chédiak-Higashi syndrome.

It has been shown that stem cells can repopulate the bone marrow and reestablish hematopoiesis. For the procedure to be effective, the bone marrow cells of the host are destroyed by myeloablative doses of chemotherapy. The exception is children with SCID. Because of the profound cellular immune defect that is present in children with SCID, pretransplantation myeloablation may not be necessary.[18] After transplantation, a lineage-specific chimeric state usually develops in these children, in which the T-cell component is of donor origin and the B-cell component, although variable, remains largely of host origin.[18] Chronic immunoglobulin therapy may be necessary for transplant recipients who primarily retain B cells of host origin.

Stem cells can be collected from the bone marrow or peripheral blood. Donors with identical HLA types (*i.e.,* matched for at least three of the six HLA loci) are associated with the least risk of graft-versus-host disease or graft rejection. HLA-matched siblings usually produce the best results. Stem cell aspiration from the bone marrow is the most common form of allograft collection. Only a few (<1 in 100,000) nucleated bone marrow cells are true hematopoietic stem cells. These stem cells are separated from other bone marrow cells before transplantation. Peripheral blood offers a less invasive method for obtaining stem cells. Hematopoietic growth factors, such as granulocyte colony-stimulating factor, often are used to induce stem cells to move out of the bone marrow into the blood. Many of these stem cells can be collected from the blood using leukapheresis, a process that separates the stem cells from other blood cells. A third potential source of stem cells is umbilical cord blood. Umbilical cord blood is a rich source of primitive hematopoietic blood. Up to 250 mL of umbilical cord blood can be collected at the time of delivery without producing detrimental effects to the mother and newborn. Although reliable engraftment of bone marrow can be achieved in children, it is uncertain whether cord blood contains enough stem cells to engraft adult recipients.[18]

> In summary, an immunodeficiency is defined as an absolute or partial loss of the normal immune response, which places a person in a state of compromise and increases the risk for development of infections or malignant complications. Immunodeficiency states can affect one or more of the four main components of the immune response: antibody or humoral (B-cell) immunity, cellular or T-cell immunity, the complement system, and the phagocytic system. The variety of defects known to involve the immune response can be classified as primary (*i.e.,* endogenous or inherited) or secondary (*i.e.,* caused by exogenous factors such as drugs or infection). The extent to which any or all of these components are compromised dictates the severity of the immunodeficiency.

Allergic and Hypersensitivity Disorders

After you have completed this section of the chapter, you should be able to meet the following objectives:

- Compare the causes of immediate and delayed-type immune responses
- Describe the immune mechanisms involved in a type I, type II, type III, and type IV hypersensitivity reaction
- State the difference between an atopic and nonatopic hypersensitivity response
- Describe the pathogenesis of allergic rhinitis, food allergy, serum sickness, Arthus reaction, contact dermatitis, and hypersensitivity pneumonitis
- Characterize the differences in latex allergy caused by a type I, IgE-mediated hypersensitivity response and that caused by a type IV, cell-mediated response

Allergic or hypersensitivity disorders are caused by immune responses to environmental antigens that produce inflammation and cause tissue injury. In the context of an allergic response, these antigens usually are referred to as *allergens.* Allergens are any foreign substances capable of inducing an immune response. Many different chemicals of natural and synthetic origin are known allergens. Complex natural organic chemicals, especially proteins, are more likely to cause an immediate hypersensitivity response, whereas simple organic compounds, inorganic chemicals, and metals more commonly cause delayed hypersensitivity reactions. Exposure to the allergen can be through inhalation, ingestion, injection, or skin contact. Sensitization of a specific individual to a specific allergen is the result of a particular interplay between the chemical or physical properties of the allergen, the mode and quantity of exposure, and the unique genetic makeup of the person.

The manifestations of allergic responses reflect the effect of an immunologically induced inflammatory response in the organ or tissue involved. These manifestations usually are independent of the agent involved. For example, the symptoms of hay fever are the same whether the allergy is caused by ragweed pollen or mold spores. The diversity of allergic responses derives from the different immunologic effector pathways that are involved (*e.g.,* hay fever vs. allergic dermatitis).

Historically, allergic disorders have been categorized as two basic types: immediate and delayed-type hypersensitivity. The criteria for this classification involve the time

TABLE 19-1 ✦ Classification of Hypersensitivity Responses

Type	Mechanism	Examples
I—Anaphylactic (immediate) hypersensitivity	IgE-mediated—mast cell degranulation	Hay fever, asthma, anaphylaxis
II—Cytotoxic	Formation of antibodies (IgG, IgM) against cell surface antigens. Complement usually is involved.	Autoimmune hemolytic anemia, hemolytic disease of the newborn, Goodpasture's disease
III—Immune complex disease	Formation of antibodies (IgG, IgM, IgA) that interact with exogenous or endogenous antigens to form antigen-antibody complexes.	Arthus reaction, autoimmune diseases (systemic lupus erythematosus, rheumatoid arthritis), certain forms of acute glomerulosclerosis
IV— Cell-mediated (delayed-type) hypersensitivity	Sensitized T lymphocytes release cytokines and produce T-cell–mediated cytotoxicity.	Tuberculosis, contact dermatitis, transplant rejection

between exposure to the inducing antigen or allergen and the appearance of symptoms. The term *immediate hypersensitivity* is used to describe antibody-mediated allergy, and the term *delayed-type hypersensitivity* is used to describe T-lymphocyte–mediated responses.[19,20]

Allergic reactions can be divided into four categories: type I, IgE-mediated disorders; type II, antibody-mediated (cytotoxic) disorders; type III, complement-mediated immune disorders; and type IV, T-cell–mediated hypersensitivity reactions (Table 19-1).

Allergic and Hypersensitivity Disorders

➤ Allergic and hypersensitivity disorders result from immune responses to exogenous and endogenous antigens that produce inflammation and cause tissue damage.

➤ Type I hypersensitivity is an IgE-mediated immune response that leads to the release of inflammatory mediators for sensitized mast cells.

➤ Type II disorders involve humoral antibodies that participate directly in injuring cells by predisposing them to phagocytosis or lysis.

➤ Type III disorders result in generation of immune complexes in which humoral antibodies bind antigen and activate complement. The fractions of complement attract inflammatory cells that release tissue-damaging products.

➤ Type IV disorders involve tissue damage in which cell-mediated immune responses with sensitized T lymphocytes cause cell and tissue injury.

TYPE I, IGE-MEDIATED DISORDERS

Type I reactions are immediate-type hypersensitivity reactions that are triggered by binding of an allergen to a specific IgE that is found on the surface of a mast cell or basophil. In addition to its role in allergic responses, IgE is involved in acquired immunity to parasitic infections. Serum IgE levels may be elevated in response to the presence of either a parasitic infection or an allergy.

The mast cells, which are tissue cells, and basophils, which are blood cells, are derived from hematopoietic (blood) precursor cells. Mast cells normally are distributed throughout connective tissue, especially in areas beneath the skin and mucous membranes of the respiratory, gastrointestinal, and genitourinary tracts, and adjacent to blood and lymph vessels.[21] This location places mast cells near surfaces that are exposed to environmental antigens and parasites. Mast cells in different parts of the body and even in a single site can have significant differences in mediator content and sensitivity to agents that produce mast cell degranulation. For example, skin mast cells differ from lung mast cells in being more sensitive to morphine, substance P, and other neuropeptides and in the ideal temperature at which degranulation occurs (30°C in skin vs. 37°C in the lungs).[19]

Mast cells and basophils have granules that contain potent mediators of allergic reactions. These mediators are preformed in the cell or activated through enzymatic processing. During the sensitization or priming stage, the allergen-specific IgE antibodies attach to receptors on the surface of these mast cells and basophils. With subsequent exposure, the sensitizing allergen binds to the cell-associated IgE and triggers a series of events that ultimately leads to degranulation of the sensitized mast cells or basophils, causing release of their allergy-producing mediators (Fig. 19-4).

The most notable mediators of allergic reactions include histamine, acetylcholine, adenosine, chemotactic mediators, enzymes such as chymase and trypsin that lead to generation of kinins and complement, the leukotrienes, platelet-activating factor, and cytokines involved in the in-

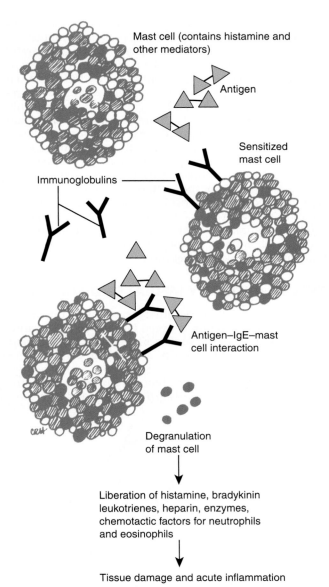

Mast cell (contains histamine and other mediators)

Antigen

Sensitized mast cell

Immunoglobulins

Antigen–IgE–mast cell interaction

Degranulation of mast cell

Liberation of histamine, bradykinin leukotrienes, heparin, enzymes, chemotactic factors for neutrophils and eosinophils

Tissue damage and acute inflammation

FIGURE 19-4 Type I, IgE-mediated hypersensitivity reaction. Exposure to the antigen causes sensitization of the mast cell; subsequent binding of the antigen to the sensitized degranulation of mast cell with release of potent inflammatory mediators, such as histamine, that are responsible for the hypersensitivity reactions.

flammatory response (see Chapter 18). Histamine is a potent vasodilator that increases the permeability of capillaries and venules and causes smooth muscle contraction and bronchial constriction. Complement, when activated, leads to further release of histamine, stimulates the inflammatory response, and promotes leukocyte chemotaxis with secondary release of cytokines. Acetylcholine produces bronchial smooth muscle contraction and dilation of small blood vessels. The leukotrienes and prostaglandins produce responses similar to histamine and acetylcholine, although their effects are delayed and prolonged by comparison. The kinins, which are a group of potent inflammatory peptides, require acti-

vation through enzymatic modification. Once activated, these peptide mediators produce vasodilatation, smooth muscle contraction, leukocyte chemotaxis, and increased vascular permeability. Eosinophil chemotactic factor prompts influx of eosinophils and leukocytes to the site of allergen contact, contributing to the inflammatory response.

There are two types of IgE-mediated allergic reactions—atopic and nonatopic disorders. The immunologic pathogenesis of the two disorders is the same, but predisposing factors and manifestations are different. The atopic diseases are characterized by a hereditary predisposition and production of a local reaction to IgE antibodies produced in response to common environmental agents. The nonatopic disorders lack the genetic component and organ specificity of the atopic disorders.

Atopic Disorders

The term *atopic* refers to a genetically determined hypersensitivity to common environmental allergens mediated by an IgE–mast cell reaction. Persons with atopic disorders commonly are allergic to more than one, and often many, environmental allergens. The disorder tends to run in families and affects approximately 1 in 10 persons in the United States. The most common atopic disorders are allergic rhinitis and allergic asthma. Atopic dermatitis is less common, and food allergy even less common. The discussion in this section focuses on allergic rhinitis and food allergy. Allergic asthma is discussed in Chapter 29 and atopic dermatitis in Chapter 61. Latex allergy is a newly emerging disorder that can result from an IgE-mediated or T-cell–mediated hypersensitivity response. It is discussed separately at the end of this section.

The cause of atopic disorders is complex and involves a genetic component and environmental allergen exposure. Persons with atopic allergic conditions tend to have high serum levels of IgE and increased numbers of basophils and mast cells. Although the IgE-triggered response is likely a key factor in the pathophysiology of atopic allergic disorders, it is not the only factor and may not be responsible for conditions such as atopic dermatitis and certain forms of asthma. Many stimuli can induce conditions that are indistinguishable from atopic disorders yet bypass the immune response. It is possible that persons with atopic disorders are exquisitely responsive to the chemical mediators of allergic reactions rather than having hyperactive IgE immunity.

Allergic Rhinitis. Allergic rhinitis (*i.e.*, allergic rhinoconjunctivitis) is characterized by symptoms of sneezing, itching, and watery discharge from the eyes and nose. Allergic rhinitis not only produces nasal symptoms but frequently is associated with other chronic airway disorders, such as sinusitis and bronchial asthma.[22] Severe attacks may be accompanied by systemic malaise, fatigue, and muscle soreness from sneezing. Fever is absent. Sinus obstruction may cause headache. Typical allergens include pollens from ragweed, grasses, trees, and weeds; fungal spores; house dust mites; animal dander; and feathers. Allergic rhinitis can be divided into perennial and seasonal allergic rhinitis depending on the chronology of symptoms. Persons with the perennial type of allergic rhinitis experience symptoms throughout the year, but those with seasonal allergic rhinitis (*i.e.*, hay fever) are plagued with intense symptoms in conjunction with periods of high allergen (*e.g.*, pollens, fungal spores) exposure. Symptoms that become worse at night suggest a household allergen, and symptoms that disappear on weekends suggest occupational exposure.

Diagnosis depends on a careful history and physical examination, microscopic identification of nasal eosinophilia, and skin testing to identify the offending allergens.

Treatment is symptomatic in most cases and includes the use of oral antihistamines and decongestants.[23] Intranasal corticosteroids often are effective when used appropriately. Intranasal cromolyn, a drug that stabilizes mast cells and prevents their degranulation, may be useful, especially when administered before expected contact with an offending allergen. The anticholinergic agent ipratropium, which is available as a nasal spray, also may be used. When possible, avoidance of the offending allergen is recommended. A program of desensitization may be used when symptoms are particularly bothersome. Desensitization involves frequent (usually weekly) injections of the offending antigens. The antigens, which are given in increasing doses, stimulate production of high levels of IgG, which acts as a blocking antibody by combining with the antigen before it can combine with the cell-bound IgE antibodies. Recent studies suggest a possible role of sublingual-swallow immunotherapy or local specific nasal immunotherapy.[23]

Food Allergies. Virtually any food can produce atopic or nonatopic allergies. The primary target of food allergy may be the skin, the gastrointestinal tract, and the respiratory system. The foods most commonly causing these reactions in children are milk, eggs, peanuts, soy, tree nuts, fish, and shellfish foods (*i.e.*, crustaceans and mollusks).[24] In adults, they are peanuts, shellfish, and fish.[24] The allergenicity of a food may be changed by heating or cooking. A person may be allergic to drinking milk but may not have symptoms when milk is included in cooked foods. Both acute reactions (hives and anaphylaxis) and chronic reactions (asthma, atopic dermatitis, and gastrointestinal disorders) can occur. Anaphylaxis occurs as a multiorgan response associated with IgE-mediated hypersensitivity. The foods most responsible for anaphylaxis are peanuts, tree nuts (*e.g.*, walnuts, almonds, pecans, cashews, hazelnuts), and shellfish. One form of food-associated anaphylaxis occurs with exercise.[24,25] Food-associated, exercise-induced anaphylaxis may occur when exercise follows ingestion of a particular food to which IgE sensitivity has been demonstrated, or it may occur after ingestion of any food. Exercise without ingestion of the incriminated food does not produce symptoms.

Food allergies can occur at any age but, similar to atopic dermatitis and rhinitis, they tend to manifest during childhood. The allergic response is thought to occur after contact between specific food allergens and sensitizing IgE found in the intestinal mucosa causes local and systemic release of histamine and other mediators of the allergic response. In this disorder, allergens usually are food proteins and partially digested food products. Carbohydrates, lipids, or food additives, such as preservatives, colorings, or flavorings, also are potential allergens. Closely related food groups can contain common cross-reacting allergens. For example, some persons are allergic to all legumes (*i.e.*, beans, peas, and peanuts).

Diagnosis of food allergies usually is based on careful food history and provocative diet testing. Provocative testing involves careful elimination of a suspected allergen from the diet for a time to see if the symptoms disappear and reintroducing the food to see the symptoms reappear. Only one food should be tested at a time. Treatment focuses on avoidance of the food or foods responsible for the allergy. However, avoidance may be difficult for persons who are exquisitely sensitive to a particular food protein because foods may be contaminated with the protein during processing or handling of the food. For example, contamination may occur when chocolate candies without peanuts are processed with the same equipment used for making candies with peanuts. Even using the same spatula to serve cookies with and without peanuts can cause enough contamination to produce a reaction.

TYPE II, ANTIBODY-MEDIATED DISORDERS

Type II (cytotoxic) hypersensitivity reactions are the end result of direct interaction between IgG and IgM class antibodies and tissue or cell surface antigens, with subsequent activation of complement- or antibody-dependent cell-mediated cytotoxicity (Fig. 19-5). Examples of type II reactions include mismatched blood transfusion reactions, hemolytic disease of the newborn due to ABO or Rh incom-

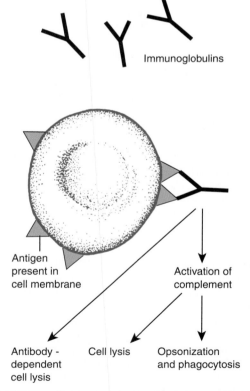

FIGURE 19-5 Type II, cytotoxic hypersensitivity reactions involve formation of immunoglobins (IgG and IgM) against cell surface antigens. The antigen-antibody response leads to (1) complement-mediated mechanisms of cell injury or to (2) antibody cytotoxicity that does not require the complement system.

patibility, and certain drug reactions. In the latter, the binding of certain drugs to the surface of red or white blood cells elicits an antibody and complement response that lyses the drug-coated cell. Lytic drug reactions can produce transient anemia, leukopenia, or thrombocytopenia, which are corrected by the removal of the offending drug.

TYPE III, IMMUNE COMPLEX ALLERGIC DISORDERS

Immune complex allergic disorders are mediated by the formation of insoluble antigen-antibody complexes that activate complement (Fig. 19-6). Activation of complement by the immune complex generates chemotactic and vasoactive mediators that cause tissue damage by a variety of mechanisms, including alterations in blood flow, increased vascular permeability, and the destructive action of inflammatory cells. Immune complexes formed in the circulation produce damage when they come in contact with the ves-

sel lining or are deposited in tissues, including the renal glomerulus, skin venules, the lung, and joint synovium. Once deposited, the immune complexes elicit an inflammatory response by activating complement, thereby leading to chemotactic recruitment of neutrophils and other inflammatory cells. Type III reactions are responsible for the vasculitis seen in certain autoimmune diseases such as SLE or the kidney damage seen with acute glomerulonephritis. Unlike type II reactions, in which the damage is caused by direct and specific binding of antibody to tissue, the harmful effects of type III reactions are indirect (*i.e.,* secondary to the inflammatory response induced by activated complement). Immune complex disorders can present with local manifestations, as in the Arthus reaction, or serum sickness, which is a systemic disorder.

Arthus Reaction

The *Arthus reaction* is a term used by pathologists and immunologists to describe localized tissue necrosis (usually in the skin) caused by immune complexes. In the laboratory, an Arthus reaction can be produced by injecting an antigen preparation into the skin of an immune animal with high levels of circulating antibody. Within 4 to 10 hours, a red, raised lesion appears on the skin at the site of the injection. An ulcer often forms in the center of the lesion. Unlike type I immune reactions, the Arthus reaction is not caused by IgE. It is thought that the injected antigen diffuses into local blood vessels, where it comes in contact with specific antibody (IgG) to incite a localized vasculitis (*i.e.,* inflammation of a blood vessel). Tissue sections of Arthus lesions show deposited immunoglobulin, complement, and fibrinolytic products in blood vessels. If the blood vessel bursts, hemorrhage into surrounding tissue occurs. If the blood vessel is occluded by fibrinolytic products, the oxygen supply to surrounding tissue is interrupted, causing cell death and tissue necrosis.

Serum Sickness

The term *serum sickness* was originally coined to describe a syndrome consisting of rash, lymphadenopathy, arthralgias, and occasionally neurologic disorders that appeared 7 or more days after injections of horse antisera (tetanus). Although this therapy is not used today, the name remains. The most common contemporary causes of this allergic disorder include antibiotics (especially penicillin), various foods, drugs, and insect venoms. Serum sickness is triggered by the deposition of insoluble antigen-antibody (IgM and IgG) complexes in blood vessels, joints, heart, and kidney tissue. The deposited complexes activate complement, increase vascular permeability, and recruit phagocytic cells, all of which can promote focal tissue damage and edema. The signs and symptoms include urticaria, patchy or generalized rash, extensive edema (usually of the face, neck, and joints), and fever. In most cases, the damage is temporary, and symptoms resolve within a few days. However, a prolonged and continuous exposure to the sensitizing antigen can lead to irreversible damage. In previously sensitized persons, severe and even fatal forms of serum sickness may occur immediately or within several days after the sensitizing drug or serum is administered.

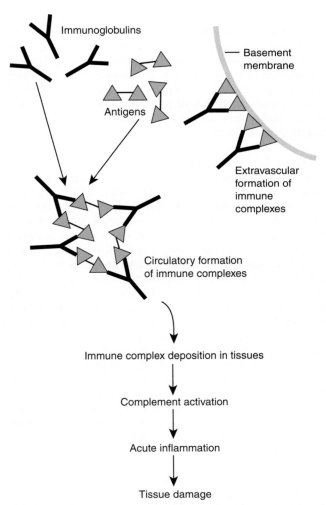

FIGURE 19-6 Type III, immune complex reactions involve complement-activating IgG and IgM immunoglobulins with formation of blood-borne immune complexes that are eventually deposited in tissues. Complement activation at the site of immune complex deposition leads to recruitment of leukocytes, which are eventually responsible for tissue injury.

Treatment of serum sickness usually is directed toward removal of the sensitizing antigen and providing symptom relief. This may include aspirin for joint pain and antihistamines for pruritus. Epinephrine or systemic corticosteroids may be used for severe reactions.

TYPE IV, CELL-MEDIATED HYPERSENSITIVITY DISORDERS

Unlike other hypersensitivity reactions, type IV, delayed hypersensitivity, is mediated by cells, not antibodies. Type IV hypersensitivity reactions usually occur 24 to 72 hours after exposure of a sensitized individual to the offending antigen. They are mediated by T lymphocytes that are directly cytotoxic (CD8+ T cells) or that secrete lymphokines (CD4+ T cells) that cause tissue changes (Fig. 19-7). The reaction is initiated by antigen-specific CD4+ helper T cells, which release numerous immunoregulatory and proinflammatory cytokines into the surrounding tissue. These substances attract antigen-specific and antigen-nonspecific T or B lymphocytes as well as monocytes, neutrophils, eosinophils, and basophils. Some of the cytokines promote differentiation and activation of macrophages that function as phagocytic and antigen-presenting cells (APCs). Activation of the coagulation cascade leads to formation and deposition of fibrin.

The best-known type of delayed hypersensitivity response is the reaction to the tuberculin test, in which inactivated tuberculin or purified protein derivative is injected under the skin. In a previously sensitized person, redness and induration of the area develop within 8 to 12 hours, reaching a peak in 24 to 72 hours. A positive tuberculin test indicates that a person has had sufficient exposure to the *M. tuberculosis* organism to incite a hypersensitivity reaction; it does not mean that the person has tuberculosis. Certain types of antigens induce cell-mediated immunity with an especially pronounced macrophage response. This type of delayed hypersensitivity commonly develops in response to particulate antigens that are large, insoluble, and difficult to eliminate. The accumulated macrophages are often transformed into so-called *epithelioid cells* because they resemble epithelium. A microscopic aggregation of epithelioid cells, which usually are surrounded by a layer of lymphocytes, is called a *granuloma*. Inflammation that is characterized by this type of type IV hypersensitivity is called *granulomatous inflammation* (see Chapter 18).

Direct T-cell–mediated cytotoxicity, which causes necrosis of antigen-bearing cells, is believed to be important in eradication of virus-infected cells, autoimmune diseases such as Hashimoto's thyroiditis, and host-versus-graft or graft-versus-host transplant rejection. Allergic contact dermatitis and hypersensitivity pneumonitis are presented as examples of cell-mediated hypersensitivity reactions.

Allergic Contact Dermatitis

Allergic contact dermatitis denotes an inflammatory response confined to the skin that is initiated by reexposure to an allergen to which a person had previously become sensitized (*e.g.*, cosmetics, hair dyes, metals, topical drugs). Contact dermatitis usually consists of erythematous macules, papules, and vesicles (*i.e.*, blisters). The affected area often becomes swollen and warm, with exudation, crusting, and development of a secondary infection. The location of the lesions often provides a clue about the nature of the antigen causing the disorder. The most common form of this condition is the dermatitis that follows an intimate encounter with poison ivy or poison oak antigens, although many other substances can trigger a reaction.

The mechanism of events leading to prior sensitization to an antigen is not completely understood. It is likely that sensitization follows transdermal transport of an antigen, with subsequent presentation to T lymphocytes. Subpopulations of sensitized lymphocytes are distributed throughout the body so that subsequent cutaneous exposure to the offending antigen promotes a localized reaction regardless of the initial site of contact. The severity of the reaction associated with contact dermatitis ranges from mild to intense, depending on the person and the allergen. Because this condition follows the mechanism of a delayed hypersensitivity response, the reaction does not become apparent for at least 12 hours and usually more than 24 hours after exposure. Depending on the antigen and the duration of exposure, the reaction may last from days to weeks and is typified by ery-

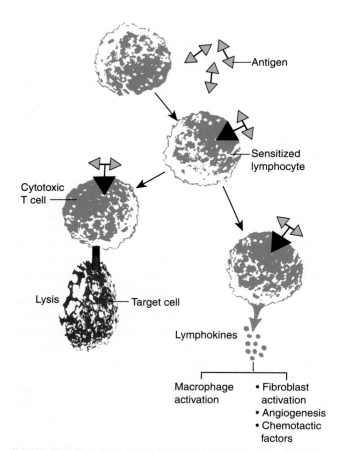

FIGURE 19-7 Type IV, cell-mediated or delayed-type hypersensitivity reactions involve sensitization of T lymphocytes with the subsequent formation of cytotoxic T cells that lyse target cells or T cells that release cell-damaging lymphokines.

thematous, vesicular, or papular lesions associated with intense pruritus and weeping.

Diagnosis of contact dermatitis is made by observing the distribution of lesions on the skin surface and associating a particular pattern with exposure to possible allergens. If a particular allergen is suspected, a patch test can be used to confirm the suspicion. For this, the suspected allergen is applied to a gauze or patch that is taped to a hair-free surface for 48 hours. The patch is removed, and the surface is inspected daily for a response. Treatment usually is limited to removal of the irritant and application of topical preparations (*e.g.*, ointments, corticosteroid creams) to relieve symptomatic skin lesions and prevent secondary bacterial infections. Severe reactions may require systemic corticosteroid therapy.

Hypersensitivity Pneumonitis

Hypersensitivity pneumonitis or allergic alveolitis is associated with exposure to inhaled organic dusts or related occupational antigens. The disorder is thought to involve a susceptible host and activation of pulmonary T cells, followed by the release of cytokine mediators of inflammation.[26] The inflammatory response that ensues (usually several hours after exposure) produces labored breathing, dry cough, chills and fever, headache, and malaise. The symptoms usually subside within hours after the sensitizing antigens are removed. A primary example of hypersensitivity pneumonitis is "farmer's lung," a condition resulting from exposure to moldy hay. Other sensitizing antigens include tree bark, sawdust, animal danders, and *Actinomycetes* bacteria that are occasionally found in humidifiers, hot tubs, and swimming pools. Exposure to small amounts of antigen for a long period may lead to chronic lung disease with minimal reversibility. This can happen to persons exposed to avian or animal antigens or a contaminated home air humidifier.[26]

The most important element in the diagnosis of hypersensitivity pneumonitis is to obtain a good history (occupational and otherwise) of exposure to possible antigens. Skin tests, when available, and serum tests for precipitating antibody can be done. Occasionally, direct observation of the person's work and other environments may help to establish a diagnosis. Treatment consists of identifying and avoiding the offending antigens. Severe forms of the disorder may be treated with systemic corticosteroid therapy.

LATEX ALLERGY

With the advent of HIV and other blood-borne diseases, the use of natural latex gloves has spiraled. Between 1988 and 1992, an estimated 11.8 billion examining gloves and 1.8 billion surgical gloves were used in the United States.[27] Along with the expanded use of latex gloves have come increased reports of latex allergy among health care workers. It has been estimated that 10% to 17% of health care workers have already been sensitized, and over 2% have occupational asthma as a result of exposure.[27] Other persons at high risk of sensitization are those with prolonged exposure to latex, including persons who have undergone repeated

surgeries. Exposure to latex may occur by cutaneous, mucous membrane, inhalation, internal tissue, or intravascular routes. Most severe reactions have resulted from latex proteins coming in contact with the mucous membranes of the mouth, vagina, urethra, or rectum. Children with meningomyelocele (spina bifida) who undergo frequent examinations and treatments involving the mucosal surface of the bladder or rectum are at particular risk for development of latex allergy.[27–30] A large number of latex products are used in dentistry, and oral mucosal contact is common during dental procedures. Anaphylactic reactions have been caused by exposure of the internal organs to the surgeon's gloves during surgery.

Natural rubber latex is derived from the milky sap of the *Heva brasiliensis* plant or rubber tree. Various accelerants, curing agents, antioxidants, and stabilizers are added to the liquid latex during the manufacturing process. Cornstarch powder is applied to the gloves during the manufacturing process to prevent stickiness and give the gloves a smooth feel. Allergic reactions to latex products can be triggered by the latex proteins or by the additives used in the manufacturing process. The cornstarch glove powder has an important role in the allergic response. Latex proteins are readily absorbed by glove powder and become airborne during removal of the gloves. High-exposure areas such as operating rooms where powdered gloves are used contain sufficiently high levels of aerosolized latex to produce symptoms in sensitized persons.

Latex allergy can involve a type I, IgE-mediated, hypersensitivity reaction or a type IV, T cell-mediated response.[29–31] The distinction between the type I and type IV reactions to latex products is not always clear. Affected individuals may experience both types of reactions. Persons with latex allergy commonly show cross-sensitivity to bananas, avocado, kiwi, tomatoes, and chestnuts, probably because latex proteins are similar to proteins in these products.[27,29] These foods have been responsible for anaphylactic reactions in latex-sensitive persons.

The most common type of allergic reaction to latex gloves is a contact dermatitis caused by a type IV, delayed hypersensitivity reaction to rubber additives. It usually develops 48 to 96 hours after direct contact with latex additives. It often affects the dorsum of the hands and is characterized by a vesicular rash. When latex contact is continued, the area becomes crusted and thickened. The type I, IgE-mediated hypersensitivity reactions that occur in response to the latex proteins are less common but far more serious. They may manifest as urticaria, rhinoconjunctivitis, asthma, or anaphylaxis.

Diagnosis of latex allergy often is based on careful history and evidence of skin reactions due to latex exposure. Symptoms after use of a rubber condom or diaphragm should raise suspicion of latex allergy. Because many of the reported reactions to latex gloves have been the result of a nonimmunologic dermatitis, it is important to differentiate between nonallergic and allergic types of dermatitis. Latex skin-prick testing can be done, but it should be done in an allergy center familiar with the test and with equipment available to treat possible anaphylactic reactions.

Serum tests for latex-specific IgE antibodies also can be done. However, these tests may give false-positive or false-negative results. Thus, at this time, diagnosis usually is based on latex-specific symptoms of IgE-mediated reactions to latex exposure.[28]

Treatment of latex allergy consists of avoiding latex exposure. Use of powder-free gloves can reduce the amount of airborne latex particles. Health care workers with severe and life-threatening allergy may be forced to change employment. Patients at high risk for latex allergy (*e.g.,* children with spina bifida, health care workers with atopy) should be offered clinical testing for latex allergy before undergoing procedures that expose them to natural rubber latex. All surgical or other procedures on persons with latex allergy should be done in a latex-free environment.

> In summary, hypersensitivity and allergic disorders are responses to environmental, food, or drug antigens that would not affect most of the population. There are four basic categories of hypersensitivity responses: type I responses, which are mediated by the IgE-class immunoglobulins and include anaphylactic shock, hay fever, angioedema, and bronchial asthma; type II cytotoxic reactions, which are characterized by hemolytic transfusion reactions and caused by immunoglobulin (IgG and IgM) activation of complement; type III reactions, which result from the formation of insoluble antigen-antibody complexes that become deposited in blood vessels or in the kidney and cause localized tissue injury; and type IV, cell-mediated responses in which sensitized T lymphocytes promote an inflammatory response when presented with the sensitizing antigen.

Transplantation Immunopathology

After you have completed this section of the chapter, you should be able to meet the following objectives:

✦ Discuss the rationale for matching of human leukocyte antigen and major histocompatibility complex types in organ transplantation

✦ Compare the immune mechanisms involved in host-versus-graft and graft-versus-host transplant rejection

Not long ago, transplantation of solid organs (*e.g.,* liver, kidney, heart) and bone marrow was considered experimental and reserved for persons for whom alternative methods of therapy were exhausted and survival was unlikely. However, with a greater understanding of humoral and cellular immune regulation, the development of immunosuppressive drugs such as cyclosporine, and an appreciation of the role of the major histocompatibility complex (MHC) antigens, transplantation has become nearly routine, and the subsequent success rate has been greatly enhanced.

Regardless of the type of transplant, the cell surface antigens that determine whether transplanted tissue is recognized as foreign or native are the MHC, also called *human leukocyte antigen* in humans (see Chapter 18). Transplanted

tissue can be categorized as *allogeneic* if the donor and recipient are related or unrelated but share similar HLA types, *syngeneic* if the donor and recipient are identical twins, and *autologous* if donor and recipient are the same person. Donors of solid organ transplants can be living or dead (cadaver) and related or nonrelated (heterologous). When cells bearing foreign MHC antigens are transplanted, the recipient's immune system attempts to eliminate the donor cells, a process referred to as *host-versus-graft disease* (HVGD). Conversely, the cellular immune system of the transplanted tissue can attack unrelated recipient tissue, causing a *graft-versus-host disease* (GVHD). The likelihood of rejection varies indirectly with the degree of HLA or MCH relatedness between donor and recipient. The 1-year graft survival rate for kidney transplants (1992 to 1994) was 94% for cadaver graft transplants and 97.3% for live donor graft transplants.[31]

HOST-VERSUS-GRAFT DISEASE

In HVGD, the immune cells of the transplant recipient attack the donor cells of the transplanted organ. HVGD usually is limited to allogeneic organ transplants, although even HLA-identical siblings may differ in some minor HLA loci, which can evoke slow rejection. Rejection due to HVGD is a complex process that involves cell-mediated and circulating antibodies. Although many cells may participate in the process of acute transplant rejection, only the T lymphocytes seem to be absolutely required.[32] The activation of CD8+ cytotoxic T cells and CD4+ helper T cells is triggered in response to the donor's HLA antigens. Activation of CD4+ helper cells leads to proliferation of B-cell–mediated antibody production and delayed-type hypersensitivity reaction. The initial target of the recipient antibodies is graft vasculature. The antibodies can produce injury to the transplanted organ by complement-mediated cytotoxicity, generation of antigen-antibody complexes, or through antibody-mediated cytolysis.[20]

There are three basic patterns of transplant rejection: hyperacute, acute, and chronic.[20] A hyperacute reaction occurs almost immediately after transplantation; in kidney transplants, it can often be seen at the time of surgery. As soon as blood flow from the recipient to the donor organ begins, it takes on a cyanotic, mottled appearance. Sometimes, the reaction takes hours to days to develop. The hyperacute response is produced by existing recipient antibodies to graft antigens that initiate an Arthus-type reaction in the blood vessels of the graft. These antibodies usually have developed in response to previous blood transfusions, pregnancies in which the mother makes antibodies to fetal antigens, or infections with bacteria or viruses possessing antigens that mimic MHC antigens.

Acute rejection usually occurs within the first few months after transplantation. It also may occur suddenly months or even years later, after immunosuppression has been used and terminated. In the patient with an organ transplant, acute rejection is evidenced by signs of organ failure. Acute rejection often involves humoral and cell-mediated immune responses. Histologically, humoral rejection is associated with vasculitis, whereas cellular rejection is marked by interstitial infiltration by mononuclear cells. Acute rejection vasculitis is mediated primarily by anti-donor antibodies and is characterized by lesions that lead to arterial narrowing or obliteration.

Chronic host-versus-graft rejection occurs over a prolonged period. It manifests with dense intimal fibrosis of blood vessels of the transplanted organ. In renal transplantation, it is characterized by a gradual rise in serum creatinine over a period of 4 to 6 months. The actual mechanism of this type of response is unclear but may include release of cytokines such as interleukin-1 and platelet-derived growth factor.

GRAFT-VERSUS-HOST DISEASE

Three basic requirements are necessary for GVHD to develop: the transplant must have a functional cellular immune component; the recipient tissue must bear antigens foreign to the donor tissue; and the recipient immunity must be compromised to the point that it cannot destroy the transplanted cells.[33] The primary agents of GVHD are T cells, and the antigens they recognize and attack are HLA. The greater the difference in tissue antigens between the donor and recipient, the greater is the likelihood of GVHD. If the recipient has a normally functioning immune system, it quickly eradicates HLA-mismatched transplants, making immunosuppression a necessity. Without appropriate therapy, most allogeneic (and even syngeneic or autologous) bone marrow transplant recipients acquire some form of GVHD.

If GVHD occurs, the primary targets of the acute illness are the skin, liver, intestine, and cells of the immune system. Acute GVHD is characterized by a pruritic, maculopapular rash, which begins on the palms and soles and frequently extends over the entire body, with subsequent desquamation. The epithelial layer is the primary site of injury. When the intestine is involved, symptoms include nausea, bloody diarrhea, and abdominal pain. GVHD of the liver can lead to bleeding disorders and coma. GVHD is considered chronic if symptoms persist or begin 100 days or more after transplantation. Chronic GVHD is characterized by abnormal humoral and cellular immunity, severe skin disorders, and liver disease.

The pathogenesis of acute GVHD is initiated in three stages: recognition and presentation by donor T cells of foreign recipient antigens, activation of T cells through cytokines, and multiplication of activated T cells. The actual tissue pathology observed with GVHD is produced directly by the action of cytotoxic T cells or indirectly through the release of inflammatory mediators such as tumor necrosis factor-α, interleukins, and complement. Conversely, chronic GVHD has all the markings of an autoimmune disorder in which activated T cells recognize minor MHC antigens common to all persons and that therefore are not foreign.

A third type of GVHD has been recognized that follows the transplantation of genetically identical tissue (*i.e.,* syngeneic or autologous). This variety of GVHD stems from the pretreatment conditioning regimen (*e.g.,* total-body irradiation) or treatment with cytotoxic drugs. The conditioning therapy disrupts the normal immune surveillance system and allows "rogue" autoreactive T cells to proliferate and attack native tissue. Syngeneic GVHD usually is self-limited and not severe.

GVHD can be prevented by blocking any of the three steps of pathogenesis. For example, donor T cells can be selectively removed from the transplanted tissue or destroyed using various treatments such as monoclonal antibodies with attached toxins, equivalent to heat-seeking missiles. Alternatively, immunosuppressive or anti-inflammatory drugs such as cyclosporine and tacrolimus or glucocorticoids can be used to block T-cell activation and the action of cytokines.

In summary, organ and bone marrow transplantation has been enhanced by a greater understanding of humoral and cellular immune regulation, the development of immunosuppressive drugs such as cyclosporine or tacrolimus, and an appreciation of the role of the MHC antigens. The likelihood of rejection varies with the degree of HLA (or MHC) relatedness between donor and recipient. A rejection can involve an attempt by the recipient's immune system to eliminate the donor cells, as in HVGD, or an attack by the cellular immunity of the transplanted tissue on the unrelated recipient tissue, as in GVHD.

Autoimmune Disease

After you have completed this section of the chapter, you should be able to meet the following objectives:

+ Relate the mechanisms of self-tolerance to the possible explanations for development of autoimmune disease
+ Name four or more diseases attributed to autoimmunity
+ Describe three or more postulated mechanisms underlying autoimmune disease
+ State the criteria for establishing an autoimmune basis for a disease

To function properly, the immune system must be able to differentiate foreign antigens from self-antigens. Normally, there is a high degree of immunologic tolerance to self-antigens, which prevents the immune system from destroying the host. Autoimmune disorders result from the breakdown in the integrity of immune tolerance such that a humoral or cellular immune response can be mounted against host tissue or antigens, leading to localized or systemic injury.

Autoimmune diseases can affect almost any cell or tissue in the body. There are known or suspected hematologic, rheumatologic, neurologic, and endocrine disorders associated with autoimmunity. Some autoimmune disorders, such as Hashimoto's thyroiditis, are tissue specific; others, such as SLE, affect multiple organs and systems. Chart 19-2 lists some of the probable autoimmune diseases. Many of these disorders are discussed elsewhere in this book.

IMMUNOLOGIC TOLERANCE

The ability of the immune system to differentiate self from nonself is called *self-tolerance.* It is the HLA antigens encoded by MHC genes that serve as recognition markers of

CHART 19-2

*Probable Autoimmune Disease**

Systemic
Mixed connective tissue disease
Polymyositis-dermatomyositis
Rheumatoid arthritis
Scleroderma
Sjögren's syndrome
Systemic lupus erythematosus

Blood
Autoimmune hemolytic anemia
Autoimmune neutropenia and lymphopenia
Idiopathic thrombocytopenic purpura

Other Organs
Acute idiopathic polyneuritis
Atrophic gastritis and pernicious anemia
Autoimmune adrenalitis
Goodpasture's syndrome
Hashimoto's thyroiditis
Insulin-dependent diabetes mellitus
Myasthenia gravis
Premature gonadal (ovarian) failure
Primary biliary cirrhosis
Sympathetic ophthalmia
Temporal arteritis
Thyrotoxicosis (Grave's disease)
Ulcerative colitis

*Examples are not inclusive.

 Immunologic Tolerance

➤ Immunologic tolerance is the ability of the immune system to differentiate self from nonself. It results from central and peripheral mechanisms that delete self-reactive immune cells that cause autoimmunity or render their response ineffective in destroying self-cells and self-tissue.

➤ Central tolerance involves the elimination of self-reactive T and B cells in the central lymphoid organs. Self-reactive T cells are deleted in the thymus and self-reactive B cells in the bone marrow.

➤ Peripheral tolerance derives from the deletion or inactivation of self-reactive T and B cells that escaped deletion in the central lymphoid organs. It involves mechanisms such as receptor editing, absence of necessary costimulatory signals, production of immunologic ignorance by separating self-reactive immune cells from target tissues, and the presence of suppressor immune cells.

self and nonself for the immune system (see Chapter 18). To elicit an immune response, an antigen must first be processed by an antigen-presenting cell (APC), such as a macrophage, which then presents the antigenic determinants along with an MHC II molecule to a CD4+ helper T cell for binding to its T-cell receptor (TCR). The dual recognition of the MHC–antigen complex by the TCR acts like a security check that affects all T cells, including CD4+ helper T cells that orchestrate T- and B-cell immune responses, and CD8+ cytotoxic T cells that act directly to destroy target cells. A number of chemical messengers (*e.g.,* interleukins) and costimulatory signals are essential to the activation of immune responses and the preservation of self-tolerance. These pathways are being rigorously studied in an effort to understand the mechanisms of autoimmunity.

Several mechanisms have been postulated to explain the tolerant state: central tolerance and peripheral tolerance.[20] Central tolerance refers to the elimination of self-reactive T cells and B cells in the central lymphoid organs (*i.e.,* the thymus for T cells and the bone marrow for B cells). Peripheral tolerance derives from the deletion or inactivation of autoreactive T cells or B cells that escaped elimination in the central lymphoid organs. *Clonal anergy* refers to a state of acquired immunologic tolerance to a specific allergen or autoantigen. Clonal anergy can affect both B-cell and T-cell tolerance.

B-Cell Tolerance

Loss of self-tolerance with development of autoantibodies is characteristic of a number of autoimmune disorders. For example, hyperthyroidism in Graves' disease is due to auto-antibodies to the thyroid-stimulating hormone receptor (see Chapter 40). Several mechanisms are available to filter autoreactive B cells out of the B-cell population: clonal deletion of immature B cells in the bone marrow, deletion of autoreactive B cells in the spleen or lymph nodes, functional inactivation or anergy, and receptor editing, a process that changes the specificity of a B-cell receptor when autoantigen is encountered.[34] There is increasing evidence that B-cell tolerance is predominantly due to help from T cells.[34]

Central T-Cell Tolerance

The central mechanisms of T-cell tolerance involve the deletion of self-reactive T cells in the thymus. T cells develop from bone marrow–derived progenitor cells that migrate to the thymus, where they encounter self-peptides bound to MHC molecules. T cells that display the host's MHC antigens and TCRs for a nonself-antigen are allowed to mature in the thymus (*i.e.,* positive selection) and those that have a high affinity for host cells are sorted out and destroyed (*i.e.,* negative selection).

Peripheral T-Cell Tolerance

The deletion of self-reactive T cells in the thymus requires the presence of autoantigens. Because many autoantigens are not present in the thymus, self-reactive T cells escape the thymus and are found in the peripheral circulation. Fortunately, a number of peripheral mechanisms control the responsiveness of the self-reactive T cells in the periphery.

Sometimes the host antigens are not available in the appropriate immunologic form or are separated from the T cells (*e.g.*, by the blood-brain barrier) so that corresponding T cells remain *immunologically ignorant* of their presence. In other cases, the T cell encounters its corresponding antigen in the absence of necessary costimulatory signals, resulting in anergy. For example, T cells that do not produce interleukin-2 on encountering their antigen cannot be completely activated and are anergic.[34] In other cases, the T-cell response may be suppressed or directed along a more harmless pathway, rather than leading to disease. Suppressor T cells with the ability to down-regulate the function of autoreactive T cells are thought to play an essential role in peripheral T-cell tolerance.[20] These cells are believed to be a distinct subset of CD8+ T cells. The mechanism by which these T cells exert their suppressor function is unclear. They may secrete cytokines that suppress the activity of self-reactive immune cells.

MECHANISMS OF AUTOIMMUNE DISEASE

There are multiple explanations for the formation of autoantibodies or failure to recognize host antigens as self. Among the possible mechanisms responsible for development of autoimmune disease are aberrations of MHC–antigen complex/receptor interactions, disorders of immune regulatory or surveillance function, cross-reactivity or molecular mimicry, and superantigens. Heredity and gender may play a role in the development of autoimmunity. Because of the complexity of the immune system, it seems unlikely that autoimmune disorders arise from a single defect.

Heredity and Gender

Genetic factors can increase the incidence and severity of autoimmune diseases,[35] as shown by the familial clustering of several autoimmune diseases and the observation that certain inherited HLA types occur more frequently in persons with a variety of immunologic and lymphoproliferative disorders. For example, 90% of persons with ankylosing spondylitis carry the HLA-B27 antigen, but only 7% of a control group without the disease have the antigen. Other HLA-associated diseases are Reiter's syndrome and HLA-B27, rheumatoid arthritis and HLA-DR4, and SLE and HLA-DR3. The molecular basis for these associations is unknown. In the case of SLE, as many as six potentially abnormal gene loci may be involved in providing a veritable matrix of disease patterns. Because autoimmunity does not develop in all persons with genetic predisposition, it appears that other factors such as a "trigger event" interact to precipitate the altered immune state. The event or events that trigger the development of an autoimmune response are unknown. It has been suggested that the "trigger" may be a virus or other microorganism, a chemical substance, or a self-antigen from a body tissue that has been hidden from the immune system during development.

A number of autoimmune disorders such as SLE occur more commonly in women than men, suggesting that estrogens may play a role in the development of autoimmune disease. Evidence suggests that estrogens stimulate and androgens suppress the immune response.[36]

Aberrations in MHC–Antigen Complex/Receptor Interactions

The immune system recognizes antigen in the context of MHC–antigen complex and TCR interactions. Aberrations in any of these three stages of the immune response—antigen structure, TCR function, or MHC antigen presentation—have the potential for initiating an autoimmune response. Because B-cell immunity requires support of CD4+ helper T cells, the development of autoantibodies also depends on these interactions. Cytokines that function as mediators in the immune response also may be involved. For example, estrogen stimulates a DNA sequence that promotes the production of interferon-γ, which is thought to assist in the induction of an autoimmune response.

Antigen Structure.   There are many ways in which chemical or microbial antigens can be modified to evoke an altered immune response, leading to an autoimmune disorder. Autoantigenic drugs and viruses can be complexed to a carrier that is recognized by nontolerant CD4+ helper T cells as foreign. Virus-encoded antigens expressed on the cell surface can serve as carriers for self-antigens. In this case, the self-antigen would appear as a hapten for which an immune response could be induced.

Partial degradation of self-antigens also may occur. For example, partially degraded collagen or enzymatically altered thyroglobulin or gamma globulin may be sufficiently foreign to promote an autoimmune response.

T-Cell Receptor and Major Histocompatibility Complex Interactions.   Activation of antigen-specific CD4+ T cells requires two signals: recognition of the antigen in association with class II MHC molecules on the surface of the APCs and a set of costimulatory signals provided by the APCs. One of the functions of the costimulatory signals provided by the APCs is to initiate clonal anergy to self-reactive T cells.[37] The costimulatory signal requires a special binding ligand that is present on the APC and the T cell. The possibility for development of autoimmune disorders arises when self-reactive antigens are presented to the TCRs by the MHC molecules of the APC. The costimulatory signal also may be defective, preventing the development of anergy in self-reactive T cells.

One of the more interesting aspects of the TCR and MHC interaction is research designed to develop mechanisms for interrupting the process as a means of treating autoimmune disease.[37] For example, monoclonal antibodies that would target the TCR are being investigated, as is the development of strategies to block the binding part of the responsible MHC molecule.

Failure of T-Cell–Mediated Suppression

Disorders of immune regulatory or surveillance function can result from failure to delete autoreactive immune cells or suppress the immune response.[20] Because T cells regulate the immune response, an increasing ratio of helper T to suppressor T cells may lead to the development of autoimmune disorders.

Molecular Mimicry

It is possible that certain autoimmune disorders are caused by molecular mimicry, in which a foreign antigen so closely resembles a self-antigen that antibodies produced against the former react with the latter.[37,38] A humoral or cellular response can be mounted against antigenically altered or injured tissue, creating an immune process. In rheumatic fever and acute glomerulonephritis, for example, a protein in the cell wall of group A β-hemolytic streptococci has considerable homology with antigens in heart and kidney tissue, respectively. After infection, antibodies directed against the microorganism cause a classic case of mistaken identity, which leads to inflammation of the heart or kidney. Certain drugs, when bound to host proteins or glycoproteins, form a complex to which a humoral response is directed with substantial cross-reactivity to the original self-protein. The antihypertensive agent methyldopa can bind to surface antigens on red cells to induce an antibody-mediated hemolytic anemia.

Not everyone exposed to group A β-hemolytic streptococci has an autoimmune reaction. The reason that only certain persons are targeted for autoimmune reactions to a particular self-mimicry molecule may be determined by differences in HLA types. The HLA type determines exactly which fragments of a pathogen are displayed on the cell surface for presentation to T cells. One individual's HLA may bind self-mimicry molecules for presentation to T cells, and another's HLA type may not. In the spondyloarthropathies, particularly Reiter's syndrome and reactive arthritis, there is a clear relationship between arthritis and an antecedent bacterial infection, combined with the inherited HLA-B27 antigens.[38]

Superantigens

Superantigens are a family of related substances, including staphylococcal and streptococcal exotoxins, that can short-circuit the normal sequence of events in an immune response, leading to inappropriate activation of CD4+ helper T cells. Superantigens do not require processing and presentation of antigen by APCs to induce a T-cell response.[39] Instead, they are able to interact with a TCR outside the normal antigen-binding site. Normally, only a small percentage of the T-cell population (0.01%) is stimulated by the presence of processed antigens on the surface of macrophages; superantigens, however, can interact with 5% to 30% of T cells.[39] Superantigens directly link the MHC II complex molecules of APCs such as macrophages to TCRs, causing a massive release of T-cell inflammatory cytokines, primarily interleukin-2 and tumor necrosis factor, and an uncontrolled proliferation of T cells. At least one disease in adults, toxic shock syndrome, is mediated by superantigens (see Chapter 26). Kawasaki's disease in children (see Chapter 24) probably has a similar cause. Superantigens also may participate in other autoimmune diseases such as rheumatoid arthritis.[39]

DIAGNOSIS AND TREATMENT OF AUTOIMMUNE DISEASE

Suggested criteria for determining that a disorder is an autoimmune disorder are evidence of an autoimmune reaction, determination that the immunologic findings are not secondary to another condition, and the lack of other identified causes for the disorder. Currently, the diagnosis of autoimmune disease is based primarily on clinical findings and serologic testing. In the future, it is likely that autoimmune disorders will be diagnosed by directly identifying the genes responsible for the condition.

The basis for most serologic assays is the demonstration of antibodies directed against tissue antigens or cellular components. For example, a child with chronic or acute history of fever, arthritis, and a macular rash along with high levels of antinuclear antibody has a probable diagnosis of SLE. The detection of autoantibodies in the laboratory usually is accomplished by one of three methods: indirect fluorescent antibody assays (IFA), enzyme-linked immunosorbent assay (ELISA), or particle agglutination of some kind. The rationale behind each of these methods is similar: the patient's serum is diluted and allowed to react with an antigen-coated surface (*i.e.,* whole, fixed cells for the detection of antinuclear antibodies). In the case of IFA and ELISA, a second "labeled" antibody is added, which binds to the patient's antibody and forms a visible reaction. Particle agglutination assays are much simpler. The binding of the patient's antibody to antigen-coated particles causes a visible agglutination reaction. For most serologic assays, the patient's serum is serially diluted until it no longer produces a visible reaction (*e.g.,* 1 : 100 dilution). This is called a *positive titer.* Healthy persons sometimes have low titers of antibody against cellular and tissue antigens, but the titers usually are far lower than in patients with autoimmune disease.

Treatment of autoimmune disease is based on the tissue or organ that is involved, the effector mechanism involved, and the magnitude and chronicity of the effector processes. Ideally, treatment should focus on the mechanism underlying the autoimmune disorder. Research into the development of vaccines to target critical pathways in the emergence of autoimmune responses is ongoing.

Intravenous IgG has been effectively used in treatment of some autoimmune disorders such as platelet depletion in immune thrombocytopenia. The mechanisms responsible for its effectiveness are not precisely known, but the effect is thought to occur because the exogenous antibodies bind to macrophages, which are prevented from attacking host cells coated with autoantibodies.[40]

In summary, autoimmune diseases represent a disruption in self-tolerance that results in damage to body tissues by the immune system. Autoimmune diseases can affect almost any cell or tissue of the body. The ability of the immune system to differentiate self from nonself is called *self-tolerance.* Normally, self-tolerance is maintained through central and peripheral mechanisms that delete autoreactive B or T cells or otherwise suppress or inactivate immune responses that would be destructive to host tissues. Defects in any of these mechanisms could impair self-tolerance and predispose to development of autoimmune disease.

The ability of the immune system to differentiate foreign from self-antigens is the responsibility of HLA encoded by MHC genes. Antigen is presented to receptors of T cells in combination with MHC molecules. Among the possible mechanisms responsible for development of autoimmune disease are aberrations in MHC–antigen–TCR interactions; failure of T-cell–mediated immune suppression; molecular mimicry; and superantigens.

Suggested criteria for determining that a disorder results from an autoimmune disorder are evidence of an autoimmune reaction, determination that the immunologic findings are not secondary to another condition, and the lack of other identified causes for the disorder.

Related Web Site

Primary Immunodeficiency: National Institute of Child Health and Human Development   www.nichd.nih.gov/publications/pubs/primaryimmunobooklet.htm.

References

1. Shyur S., Hill H.R. (1996). Recent advances in the genetics of primary immunodeficiency syndromes. *Journal of Pediatrics* 129, 8–24.
2. Buckley R.H. (2000). Primary immunodeficiency diseases due to defects in lymphocytes. *New England Journal of Medicine* 343, 1313–1324.
3. Sorensen R.U., Moore C. (2000). Antibody deficiency syndromes. *Pediatric Clinics of North America* 47, 1225–1252.
4. Ten R.M. (1998). Primary immunodeficiencies. *Mayo Clinic Proceedings* 73, 865–872.
5. Buckley R. (2000). T-, B-, and NK-cell systems. In Behrman R.E., Kliegman R.M., Jenson H.B. (Eds.), *Nelson textbook of pediatrics* (16th ed., pp. 590–606). Philadelphia: W.B. Saunders.
6. Johnson K.B., Oski F.A. (1997). *Oski's essential pediatrics.* (pp. 532–539). Philadelphia: Lippincott-Raven.
7. Elder M.E. (2000). T-cell immunodeficiencies. *Pediatric Clinics of North America* 47, 1253–1274.
8. Candotti F. (2000). The potential for therapy of immune disorders with gene therapy. *Pediatric Clinics of North America* 47, 1389–1405.
9. Blaese R.M. (1995). Steps toward gene therapy. *Hospital Practice* 30 (11), 33–40.
10. Johnston R.B. (2000). The complement system. In Behrman R.E., Kliegman R.M., Jensen H.B. (Eds.), *Nelson textbook of pediatrics* (16th ed., pp. 628–634). Philadelphia: W.B Saunders.
11. Frank M.M. (2000). Complement deficiencies. *Pediatric Clinics of North America* 47, 1339–1353.
12. Cotten H.R. (1987). Hereditary angioneurotic edema, 1887–1987. *New England Journal of Medicine* 317, 43–45.
13. Cicardi M., Agostoni A. (1996). Hereditary angioedema. *New England Journal of Medicine* 334, 1666–1667.
14. Waytes A.T., Rosen F.S., Frank M.M. (1996). Treatment of hereditary angioedema with a vapor-heated C1 inhibitor concentrate. *New England Journal of Medicine* 334, 1630–1634.
15. Segal B.H., Holland S.M. (2000). Primary phagocytic disorders of childhood. *Pediatric Clinics of North America* 47, 1311–1333.
16. Boxer L.A. (2000). Disorders of phagocyte function. In Behrman R.E., Kliegman R.M., Jensen H.B. (Eds.), *Nelson textbook of pediatrics* (16th ed., pp. 615–621). Philadelphia: W.B. Saunders.
17. Lekstrom-Himes J.A., Gallin J.I. (2000). Immunodeficiency diseases caused by defects in phagocytes. *New England Journal of Medicine* 343, 1703–1714.
18. Horwitz M.E. (2000). Stem-cell transplantation for inherited immunodeficiency disorders. *Pediatric Clinics of North America* 47, 1371–1384.
19. Johnson K.J., Chensue S.W., Ward P.A. (1999). In Rubin E., Farber J.L. (Eds.), *Pathology* (3rd ed., pp. 114–127). Philadelphia: Lippincott Williams & Wilkins.
20. Cotran R.S., Kumar V., Collins T. (1999). *Pathologic basis of disease* (6th ed., pp. 195–216). Philadelphia: W.B. Saunders.
21. Galli S.J. (1993). New concepts about the mast cell. *New England Journal of Medicine* 328, 257–265.
22. Jackler R.K., Kaplan M.J. (2001). Ear, nose, and throat. In Tierney L.M., McPhee S.J., Papadakis M.A. (Eds.), *Current medical diagnosis and treatment* (40th ed., pp. 236–238). New York: Lange Medical Books/McGraw-Hill.
23. Rachelefsky G.S. (1999). National guidelines need to manage rhinitis and prevent complications. *Annals of Allergy, Asthma, and Immunology* 82, 296–305.
24. Sicherer S.H. (1999). Manifestations of food allergy: Evaluation and management. *American Family Physician* 57, 93–102.
25. Sampson H.A. (1998). Fatal food-induced anaphylaxis. *Allergy* 53 (Suppl. 46), 125–130.
26. Salvaggio J.E. (1995). The identification of hypersensitivity pneumonitis. *Hospital Practice* 30 (5), 57–66.
27. Sussman G.L. (1995). Allergy to latex rubber. *Annals of Internal Medicine* 122, 43–46.
28. Reddy S. (1998). Latex allergy. *American Family Physician* 57, 93–102.
29. Poley G.E., Slater J.E. (2000). Latex allergy. *Journal of Allergy and Clinical Immunology* 105, 1054–1062.
30. Sussman G.L., Beezhold D.H. (1996). Safe use of natural rubber latex. *Allergy and Asthma Proceedings* 17, 101–102.
31. Lin H., Kauffman M., McBride M.A., Rosedale J.D., Smith C.M., Edwards E.B., Daily P., Kirklin J., Shield C.F., Hunsicker L.G. (1998). Center-specific graft and patient survival rate. *Journal of the American Medical Association* 280, 1153–1160.
32. Saveigh M.H., Turka L.A. (1998). The role of T-cell costimulatory activation pathways in transplant rejection. *New England Journal of Medicine* 338, 1813–1821.
33. Ferrara J.L.M., Deeg H.J. (1991). Graft-versus-host disease. *New England Journal of Medicine* 324, 667–674.
34. Kamradt T., Mitchison N.A. (2001). Advances in immunology: Tolerance and autoimmunity. *New England Journal of Medicine* 344, 655–664.
35. Theofilopoulos A.N. (1995). The basis of autoimmunity: Part II: Genetic predisposition. *Immunology Today* 16, 150–158.
36. Cutolo M., Sulli A., Seriolo S., Accardo S., Masi A.T. (1995). Estrogens, the immune response and autoimmunity. *Clinical and Experimental Rheumatology* 13, 217–226.
37. Rose N.R. (1997). Autoimmune disease: Tracing the shared threads. *Hospital Practice* 32(4), 147–154.
38. Albert L.J., Inman R.D. (1999). Molecular mimicry and autoimmunity. *New England Journal of Medicine* 341, 2068–2074.
39. Kotzin B.L. (1994). Superantigens and their role in disease. *Hospital Practice* 29 (11), 59–70.
40. Schenkein D.E. (1992). Intravenous IgG for treatment of autoimmune disease. *Hospital Practice* 27(10A), 29–51.

Chapter 20

Acquired Immunodeficiency Syndrome

Kathleen A. Sweeney and Cyril Llamoso

While we have come a long way in the struggle to overcome the personal, social, and economic impact of this epidemic, the battle is far from over. Last year (1999), 2.8 million deaths from HIV/AIDS were recorded—the highest global total since the epidemic began. In the United States alone, we have an unacceptably high number of new HIV infections every year. Every hour in our nation two new cases of HIV are reported in young people under the age of 25. Racial and ethnic minority communities, women, and youth are being particularly hard hit.

HIV has reached catastrophic proportions in some areas of the globe and is about to explode in others. AIDS threatens the economies of the poorest countries, the stability of friendly nations, and the future of fragile democracies. We do not live in isolation from our global neighbors, and it is imperative that the United States join together with all nations to mobilize a greatly expanded world response to stem the rising tide of this disease. We must also continue our efforts to make care and treatment, including drugs—which are increasing the life span and improving the quality of life of many infected with HIV— accessible to all who need them.

As we observe World AIDS Day 2000, our task must be to work in cooperation and solidarity here in the United States and with our neighbors around the world to stop the spread of this devastating disease. The future of the world's children depends on our ability to achieve this goal together.

—Bill Clinton,
Former President of the United States,
in his address to the Association of World Health,
December 1, 2000[1]

Human immunodeficiency virus, or HIV, is the virus that causes AIDS, or acquired immunodeficiency syndrome. HIV is a retrovirus that selectively attacks and destroys the immune system. At the end of 2000, nearly 36.1 million people worldwide were living with HIV/AIDS, 22 million had died of the infection, and 5.3 million people had become newly infected during the year[2] (Fig 20-1). In the United States, there had been over 750,000 cases of AIDS, and there had been over 430,000 deaths.[3] Most of the new infections are in people younger than 25 years of age who live in developing countries.[2] Sub-Saharan Africa has been hardest hit by HIV, with close to 70% of the world's infections, although it is home to only 10% of the world's population.[1] Because of the large number of infected people in Africa, the life expectancy is expected to drop from 59 years to 45 years by 2005.[2] In the United States, racial and ethnic minority populations are disproportionately affected by this epidemic. Although blacks and Hispanics represent a minority of the population in the United States, they account for 55% of HIV infections.[3]

The AIDS Epidemic and Transmission of HIV Infection

After you have completed this section of the chapter, you should be able to meet the following objectives:

✦ Briefly trace the history of the AIDS epidemic
✦ State the virus responsible for AIDS and explain how it differs from most other viruses

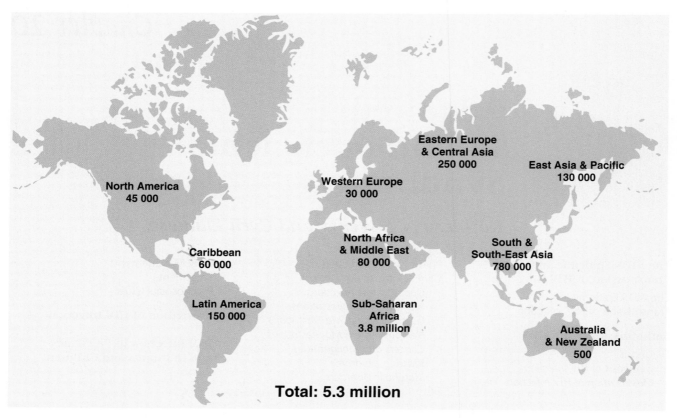

North America
45 000

Eastern Europe & Central Asia
250 000

East Asia & Pacific
130 000

Western Europe
30 000

Caribbean
60 000

North Africa & Middle East
80 000

South & South-East Asia
780 000

Latin America
150 000

Sub-Saharan Africa
3.8 million

Australia & New Zealand
500

Total: 5.3 million

FIGURE 20-1 Estimated number of adults and children newly infected with HIV during 2000. (Data from UNAIDS: Report on the global HIV/AIDS epidemic—December 2000. Available online at: www.unaids.org/epidemic_update/report_dec00/index_dec.html)

✦ Describe the mechanisms of HIV transmission and relate them to the need for public awareness and concern regarding the spread of AIDS

THE AIDS EPIDEMIC

In 1981, clinicians in New York, San Francisco, and Los Angeles recognized a new immunodeficiency syndrome in homosexual men. Initially, the syndrome was called GRIDS, for "gay-related immunodeficiency syndrome." By the end of 1981, there had been several hundred cases reported and the name was changed to acquired immunodeficiency syndrome, or AIDS.[2] It soon became apparent that this disease was not confined to one segment of the population, but was also occurring in intravenous drug users, hemophiliacs, blood transfusion recipients, infants born to infected mothers, and high-risk heterosexuals. Studies of these diverse groups led to the conclusion that AIDS is an infectious disease spread by blood, by sexual contact, and perinatally from mother to child.

An understanding of the virology of AIDS progressed with amazing efficiency; within 3 years of the first cases being recognized, the virus that caused AIDS was identified. The virus was initially known by various names, including human T-cell lymphotropic virus type 3 (HTLV-III), lymphadenopathy-associated virus (LAV), and AIDS-associated retrovirus (ARV).[4] In 1986, the name *human immunodeficiency virus* became internationally accepted.[5] HIV is a retrovirus that selectively attacks the CD4+ T lymphocytes, the immune cells responsible for orchestrating and coordinating the immune response to infection. As a consequence, persons with HIV infection have a deteriorating immune system, and thus are more susceptible to severe infections with ordinarily harmless organisms.

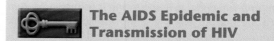

The AIDS Epidemic and Transmission of HIV

➤ HIV causes AIDS.

➤ AIDS occurs worldwide.

➤ There is no cure for AIDS.

➤ HIV is transmitted through blood, semen, vaginal fluids, and breast milk.

➤ HIV is not spread by casual contact or insects.

➤ HIV is infectious even if the person is asymptomatic.

Because HIV and AIDS occur throughout the world and affect an exceptionally high proportion of the population, it is often referred to as a *pandemic*. As of December 31, 2000, almost 60 million cases of HIV had been reported worldwide.[2] Because reporting of cases is not uniform throughout the world, many countries may not be accurately represented in this number.

The virus responsible for most HIV infection worldwide is called *HIV type 1* (HIV-1). A second type of human immunodeficiency virus, *HIV type 2* (HIV-2), is endemic in many countries in West Africa but in general is much rarer in other parts of the world.[6] HIV-2 appears to be transmitted in the same manner as HIV-1. HIV-2 also can cause immunodeficiency evidenced by a reduction in the number of CD4+ T cells and the development of AIDS. Although the spectrum of disease for HIV-2 is similar to that of HIV-1, it spreads more slowly and causes disease more slowly than HIV-1.[6] Long-term consequences of HIV-2 infection will depend on its spread in the population.

TRANSMISSION OF HIV INFECTION

Human immunodeficiency virus is transmitted from one person to another through sexual contact, blood, or perinatally. HIV is not transmitted through casual contact. Several studies involving more than 1000 uninfected, nonsexual household contacts with persons with HIV infection (including siblings, parents, and children) have shown no evidence of casual transmission.[7] HIV is not spread by mosquitoes or other insect vectors.[5] Transmission can occur when infected blood, semen, or vaginal secretions from one person are deposited onto a mucous membrane or into the bloodstream of another person.

Sexual contact is the most frequent way that HIV is transmitted. Worldwide, 75% to 85% of HIV infections are transmitted through unprotected sex.[8] HIV is present in semen and vaginal fluids. There is risk of transmitting HIV when these fluids come in contact with a part of the body that lets them enter the bloodstream. This can include the vaginal mucosa, anal mucosa, and wounds or a sore on the skin.[8] Contact with semen occurs during vaginal and anal sexual intercourse, oral sex (*i.e.,* fellatio), and donor insemination. Exposure to vaginal or cervical secretions occurs during vaginal intercourse and oral sex (*i.e.,* cunnilingus). Condoms are highly effective in preventing transmission of HIV. In most cities in the United States, sexual transmission of HIV is primarily related to vaginal or anal intercourse. In the United States, 47% of HIV infections are among men who have sex with men, and 10% are from heterosexual contact.[3] In the developing world, heterosexual transmission is the major route of HIV infection.[4]

Because HIV is found in blood, the use of needles, syringes, and other drug injection paraphernalia is a direct route for transmission. Of the reported cases of AIDS in the United States, 25% occurred among persons who injected drugs.[3] HIV-infected injecting drug users can pass the virus to their needle-sharing and sex partners and, in the case of pregnant women, to their offspring.[5] Although alcohol, cocaine, and other noninjected drugs do not directly transmit infection, their use alters perception of risk and reduces inhibitions about engaging in behaviors that pose a high risk of transmitting HIV infection.

Transfusions of whole blood, plasma, platelets, or blood cells before 1985 resulted in the transmission of HIV. Since 1985, all blood donations in the United States have been screened for HIV, so this is no longer a transmission risk. The clotting factor used by persons with hemophilia is derived from the pooled plasma of hundreds of donors. Before HIV testing of plasma donors was implemented in 1985, the virus was transmitted to persons with hemophilia through infusions of these clotting factors.[5] Seventy percent to 80% of hemophiliacs who were treated with factor before 1985 became infected. Other blood products, such as gamma globulin or hepatitis B immune globulin, have not been implicated in the transmission of HIV.[5]

HIV may be transmitted from infected women to their offspring in utero, during labor and delivery, or through breast-feeding.[9] Transmission from mother to infant is the most common way that children become infected with HIV. Ninety percent of infected children acquired the virus from their mother. The risk of transmission of HIV from mother to infant is approximately 25%, with estimates ranging from 15% to 45% depending on what country they live in.[10]

Occupational HIV infection among health care workers is uncommon. Through December 1996, the Centers for Disease Control and Prevention (CDC) had recorded only 52 documented occupational HIV infections.[11] Fewer than 20 additional cases of occupational infections have been reported from outside the U.S.[11] Universal Blood and Body Fluid Precautions should be used in encounters with all patients in the health care setting because HIV status is not always known. Occupational risk of infection for health care workers most often is associated with percutaneous inoculation (*i.e.,* needle stick) of blood from a patient with HIV. Transmission also is associated with the size of the needle, amount of blood present, depth of the injury, type of fluid contamination, stage of illness of the patient, and viral load of the patient.[11] The average risk for HIV infection from percutaneous exposure to HIV-infected blood is 0.3%.[12]

People with other sexually transmitted diseases (STDs) are at increased risk for HIV infection. The risk of HIV transmission is increased in the presence of genital ulcerative STDs (*i.e.,* syphilis, herpes simplex virus infection, and chancroid) and nonulcerative STDs (*i.e.,* gonorrhea, chlamydial infection, and trichomoniasis). HIV increases the duration and recurrence of STD lesions, treatment failures, and atypical presentation of genital ulcerative diseases due to the suppression of the immune system.

The HIV-infected person is infectious even when no symptoms are present. The point at which an infected person converts from being negative for the presence of HIV antibodies in the blood to being positive is called *seroconversion*. Seroconversion typically occurs within 1 to 3 months after exposure to HIV but can take up to 6 months.[13] An HIV-infected person can transmit the virus to others even before seroconversion. The time after infection and before seroconversion is known as the *window period*. During the window period, a person's HIV antibody test will be negative.

Rarely, infection can occur from transfused blood that was screened for HIV antibody and found negative because the donor was recently infected and still in the window period. Consequently, the U.S. Food and Drug Administration (FDA) requires blood collection centers to screen potential donors through interviews designed to identify behaviors known to present risk for HIV infection.

In summary, AIDS is an infectious disease of the immune system caused by the retrovirus HIV. First described in June 1981, the disease is prevalent worldwide and is one of the leading causes of death among young adults in the United States. The severity of the clinical disease and the absence of a cure or preventive vaccine have increased public awareness and concern. HIV is transmitted from one person to another through sexual contact, through blood exchange, or perinatally. Transmission occurs when the infected blood, semen, or vaginal secretions from one person are deposited onto a mucous membrane or into the bloodstream of another person. The primary routes of transmission are through sexual intercourse, intravenous drug use, and from mother to infant. Transmission used to occur with blood transfusions and other blood products. Occupational exposure in a health care setting accounts for only a tiny percentage of HIV transmission. HIV infection is not transmitted through casual contact or by insect vectors. There is growing evidence of an association between HIV infection and other STDs. Infected persons can transmit the virus to others before their own infections can be detected by antibody tests.

Pathophysiology of AIDS

After you have completed this section of the chapter, you should be able to meet the following objectives:

✦ Describe diagnosis of AIDS using the CDC AIDS case definition

✦ Describe the alterations in immune function that occur in persons with AIDS

✦ Relate the altered immune function in persons with HIV infection and AIDS to the development of opportunistic infections

✦ Explain the possible significance of a positive antibody test for HIV infection

✦ Differentiate between the enzyme immunoassay (enzyme-linked immunosorbent assay) and Western blot antibody detection tests for HIV infection

✦ List the three stages of HIV infection and describe the symptoms, psychosocial issues, and management concerns for each stage

Since the first description of AIDS, considerable strides have been made in understanding the pathophysiology of the disease. The virus and its mechanism of action, HIV antibody screening tests, and some treatment methods were discovered within a few years after the recognition of the

first cases. Further progress in understanding the pathophysiology of AIDS and the development of more powerful treatments continues to be made.

HIV belongs to a class of viruses called *retroviruses,* which carry their genetic information in ribonucleic acid (RNA) rather than deoxyribonucleic acid (DNA). HIV infects a limited number of cell types in the body, including a subset of lymphocytes called *CD4*[+] T lymphocytes (also known as *T helper cells, T4 lymphocytes,* or *CD4*[+] T cells)[5] and macrophages. The CD4[+] T cells are necessary for normal immune function (see Chapter 18). Among other functions, the CD4[+] T cell recognizes foreign antigens and infected cells and helps activate the antibody-producing B lymphocytes. The CD4[+] T cells also orchestrate cell-mediated immunity, in which cytotoxic CD8[+] T cells and natural killer cells directly destroy virus-infected cells and foreign antigens. Phagocytic monocytes and macrophages also are influenced to fight infection by CD4[+] T cells.

Replication of HIV occurs in eight steps (Fig. 20-2). Once HIV has entered the bloodstream, it attaches to the surface of a CD4[+] T cell by binding to the CD4 T-cell receptor and the chemokine coreceptor. This is known as *attachment.* HIV then unlocks these receptors, enters the cell, and injects its protein coat into the cell along with two single strands of viral RNA. This RNA carries the instructions to produce more HIV. This stage is called *uncoating.* For HIV to reproduce, it must change its RNA into DNA. It does this during reverse transcription, using an enzyme called *reverse transcriptase.* Reverse transcriptase makes a copy of the viral RNA, and then in reverse makes another copy, like a mirror image. The result is double-stranded DNA. During integration, the new DNA enters the nucleus of the CD4[+] T cell and, with the help of the enzyme *integrase,* combines with the cell's original DNA. Integrase inserts the HIV DNA into the cellular DNA. Next, in transcription, the viral DNA reprograms the CD4[+] T cell to produce viral RNA and viral messenger RNA (mRNA) that help form new viruses. During translation, ribosomal RNA (rRNA) uses the instructions in the mRNA to create a chain of proteins and enzymes called a *polyprotein.* These polyproteins are the components for the construction of new viruses in the next stages. During cleavage, *protease,* one of the enzymes in the polypeptide chain, cuts the chain into individual proteins, which will make up the new HIV vir-

 Pathophysiology of AIDS

➤ HIV destroys the body's immune system by taking over the CD4[+] T cells.

➤ HIV tests look for antibodies to the virus.

➤ The three phases of HIV are primary HIV, latency, and overt AIDS.

➤ As the CD4[+] T-cell count decreases, the body becomes susceptible to opportunistic infections.

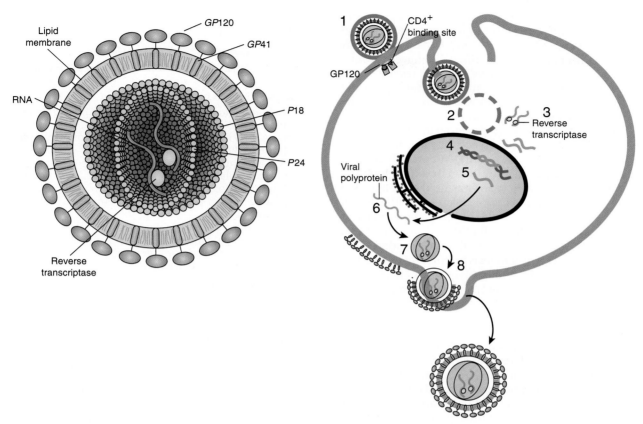

FIGURE 20-2 Life cycle of the HIV-1: (**1**) Attachment of the HIV virus to CD4+ receptor; (**2**) internalization and uncoating of the virus with viral RNA and reverse transcriptase; (**3**) reverse transcription, which produces a mirror image of the viral RNA and double-standard DNA molecule; (**4**) integration of viral DNA into host DNA using the integrase enzyme; (**5**) transcription of the inserted viral DNA to produce viral messenger RNA; (**6**) translation of viral messenger RNA to create viral polyprotein; (**7**) cleavage of viral polyprotein into individual viral proteins that make up the new virus; and (**8**) assembly and release of the new virus from the host cell.

uses. Finally, the proteins and the new RNA are assembled into new HIV viruses and released from the cell.

In some cells, the infection enters a latent phase that serves as a reservoir from which the virus can continue to be released for several years.[14] In other cells, the virus replicates, killing the cell and releasing copies of HIV into the bloodstream. These viral particles, or *virions*, invade other CD4+ T cells, allowing the infection to progress. Every day, millions of infected CD4+ T cells are destroyed, releasing billions of viral particles into the bloodstream, but each day nearly all the CD4+ T cells are replaced and nearly all the viral particles are destroyed. Over years, however, the CD4+ count gradually decreases through this process, and the number of viruses detected in the blood of persons infected with HIV increases.[14]

Until the CD4+ count falls to a very low level, infected persons can remain asymptomatic, although there is active viral replication[15] and serologic tests can identify antibodies to HIV. These antibodies, unfortunately, do not convey protection against the virus. Although symptoms are not evident, the infection proceeds on a microbiologic level, including the invasion and selective destruction of CD4+ T cells. The continual decline of CD4+ T cells, which are pivotal cells in the immune response, strips the person with AIDS of protection against common organisms and cancerous cells.[14]

DIAGNOSIS

The diagnostic methods used in HIV infection include laboratory methods to indicate infection and clinical methods to evaluate the progression of the disease.

Diagnosis of HIV Infection

The most accurate and inexpensive method for identifying HIV is the HIV antibody test. The first commercial assays for HIV were introduced in 1985 to screen donated blood. Since then, use of antibody detection tests has been expanded to include evaluating persons at increased risk for HIV infection. The HIV antibody test procedure consists of screening with an *enzyme immunoassay (EIA)*, also known as *enzyme-linked immunosorbent assay (ELISA)*, followed by a confirmatory test, the *Western blot* assay, which is performed if the EIA is positive.[16] EIA tests are used first because they are less expensive and are quicker to perform. In light of the psychosocial issues related to HIV and AIDS, sensitivity and confidentiality must be maintained whenever testing is implemented. Counseling before and after testing to allay fears, to provide accurate information, to ensure appropriate follow-up testing, and to provide referral to needed medical and psychosocial services is essential.

The EIA detects antibodies produced in response to HIV infection. In an EIA test, when blood is added, antibodies to HIV bind to HIV antigens. The antigen-antibody complex is then detected using an antihuman immunoglobulin G (IgG) antibody conjugated to an enzyme like alkaline phosphatase. A substrate is then added from which the enzyme produces a color reaction. Color development, indicating the amount of HIV antibodies found, is measured. The test is considered reactive, or positive, if color is produced, and negative, or nonreactive, if there is no color.[15] EIA tests have high false-positive and false-negative rates, so samples that are repeatedly reactive are tested by a confirmatory test such as the Western blot.[15]

The Western blot test is more specific than the EIA, and in the case of a false-positive EIA test result, the Western blot test can identify the person as uninfected. The Western blot is a more sensitive assay that looks for the presence of antibodies to specific viral antigens. For the test, HIV antigens are separated by electrophoresis based on their weight, and then transferred to nitrocellulose paper and arranged in strips, with larger proteins at the top and smaller proteins at the bottom. The serum sample is then added. If HIV antibodies are present, they bind with the specific viral antigen on the paper. An enzyme and substrate then are added to produce a color reaction as in the EIA test. If there are no colored bands present, the test is negative. A test is positive when certain combinations of bands are present. A test can be indeterminate if there are bands present but they do not meet the criteria for a positive test result. An indeterminate or false-positive test result can occur during the window period before seroconversion.[15] When a serum antibody test result is reactive or borderline by EIA and positive by Western blot, the person is considered to be infected with HIV, and when an EIA is reactive, and the Western blot is negative, the person in not infected with HIV. Both tests are important because, in some situations, misinformation can be generated by EIA testing alone because there are many situations that can produce a false-positive or a false-negative ELISA result (Chart 20-1). The Western blot test therefore is essential to determine which persons with positive EIA tests are truly infected.

Millions of HIV antibody tests are performed in the United States each year. New technology has led to new forms of testing, like the oral test and home kits. Oral fluids contain antibodies to HIV. In the late 1990s, the FDA approved the Orasure test. The Orasure uses a cotton swab, which is inserted into the mouth for 2 minutes, placed in a transport container with preservative, and then sent to a laboratory for EIA and Western blot testing.[15] Home HIV testing kits can be bought over the counter. The kits, approved by the FDA, allow persons to collect their own

---

CHART 20-1

Causes of False-Positive or False-Negative HIV ELISA Test Results

False-Positive Results
- Hematologic malignant disorders (*e.g.,* malignant melanoma)
- DNA viral infections (*e.g.,* infectious mononucleosis [Epstein-Barr virus])
- Autoimmune disorders
- Primary biliary cirrhosis
- Immunizations (influenza, hepatitis)
- Passive transfer of HIV antibodies (mother to infant)
- Antibodies to class II leukocytes
- Chronic renal failure/renal transplant
- Stevens-Johnson syndrome
- Positive rapid plasma reagin test

False-Negative Results
- "Window" period after infection
- Immunosuppression therapy
- Replacement transfusion
- B-cell dysfunction
- Bone marrow transplant
- Contamination of specimen with starch powder from gloves
- Use of kits that detect primary antibody to the p24 viral core protein

---

blood sample through a finger-stick process, mail the specimen to a laboratory for EIA and confirmatory tests, and receive results by telephone in 3 to 7 days.[15]

Polymerase chain reaction (PCR) is a technique for detecting HIV DNA (see Chapter 17). PCR detects the presence of the virus rather than the antibody to the virus, which the EIA and Western blot tests detect.[17] PCR is useful in diagnosing HIV infection in infants born to infected mothers because these infants have their mothers' HIV antibody regardless of whether the children are infected.[17] Because the amount of viral DNA in the HIV-infected cell is small compared with the amount of human DNA, direct detection of viral genetic material is difficult.[17] PCR is a method for amplifying the viral DNA up to 1 million times or more to increase the probability of detection.

Classification of HIV Infection

Effective January 1, 1993, the CDC implemented a new classification system for HIV infection and a new AIDS case definition for adolescents and adults that emphasizes the clinical importance of the CD4+ count in the categorization of HIV-related clinical conditions.[18] The new classification system defines three categories that correspond to CD4+ counts per microliter (μL) of blood:

- Category 1: >500 cells/μL
- Category 2: 200 to 499 cells/μL
- Category 3: <200 cells/μL

There also are three clinical categories. *Clinical category A* includes persons who are asymptomatic or have persistent generalized lymphadenopathy or symptoms of primary HIV infection (*i.e.,* acute seroconversion illness). *Clinical category B* includes persons with symptoms of immune deficiency not serious enough to be AIDS defining. *Clinical category C* includes AIDS-defining illnesses that are listed in the AIDS surveillance case definition shown in Chart 20-2.[18] Each HIV-infected person has a CD4+ T-cell category and a clinical category (Fig. 20-3). The combination of these two categorizations, CD4+ T-cell categories 1, 2, and 3 and clinical categories A, B, and C, can guide clinical and therapeutic actions in the management of HIV infection. According to the 1993 case definition, persons in category 3 or category C are considered to have AIDS (see Chart 20-2).

		Category 1 >500 cells u/L	Category 2 200–499 cells u/L	Category 3 <200 cells u/L
AIDS-defining clinical category	Category A No AIDS-defining symptoms			
	Category B Symptoms not severe enough to be AIDS defining			
	Category C AIDS-defining illnesses present			

CD4+ count category

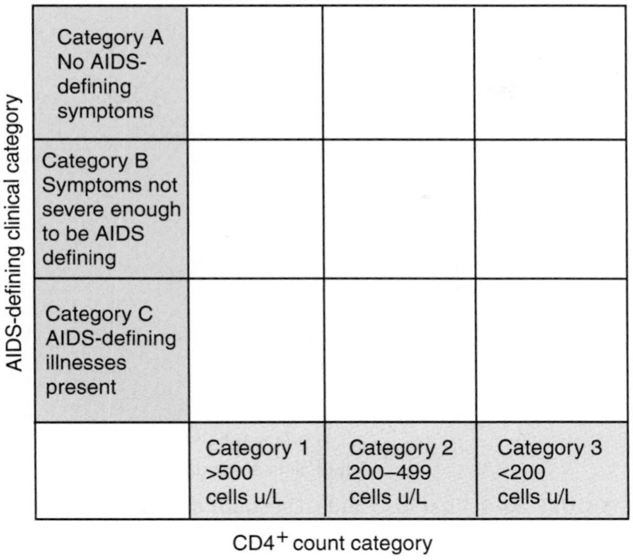

FIGURE 20-3 CD4 category and clinical category.

CHART 20-2

Conditions Included in the 1993 AIDS Surveillance Case Definition

Candidiasis of bronchi, trachea, or lungs
Candidiasis, esophageal
Cervical cancer, invasive*
Coccidioidomycosis, disseminated or extrapulmonary
Cryptococcosis, extrapulmonary
Cryptosporidiosis, chronic intestinal (>1 month's duration)
Cytomegalovirus disease (other than liver, spleen, or nodes)
Cytomegalovirus retinitis (with loss of vision)
Encephalopathy, HIV-related
Herpes simplex: chronic ulcer(s) (>1 month's duration) or bronchitis, pneumonitis, or esophagitis
Histoplasmosis, disseminated or extrapulmonary
Isosporiasis, chronic intestinal (>1 month's duration)
Kaposi's sarcoma
Lymphoma, Burkitt's (or equivalent term)
Lymphoma, immunoblastic (or equivalent term)
Lymphoma, primary, of brain
Mycobacterium avium-intracellulare complex or *M. kansasii,* disseminated or extrapulmonary
Mycobacterium tuberculosis, any site (pulmonary* or extrapulmonary)
Mycobacterium, other species or unidentified species, disseminated or extrapulmonary
Pneumocystis carinii pneumonia
Pneumonia, recurrent*
Progressive multifocal leukoencephalopathy
Salmonella septicemia, recurrent
Toxoplasmosis of brain
Wasting syndrome due to HIV

Added to the 1993 expansion of the AIDS surveillance case definition.
(Centers for Disease Control and Prevention. [1992]. 1993 Revised classification system for HIV infection and expanded surveillance case definition for AIDS among adolescents and adults. *Morbidity and Mortality Weekly Report* 41 [RR-17], 19)

PHASES OF HIV INFECTION

The typical course of HIV is defined by three phases, which usually occur over a period of 8 to 12 years. The three stages are primary infection, chronic asymptomatic phase or latency, and overt AIDS[19] (Fig. 20-4).

Many persons, when they are initially infected with HIV, have an acute mononucleosis-like syndrome known as primary infection. This acute phase may include fever, fatigue, myalgias, sore throat, night sweats, gastrointestinal problems, lymphadenopathy, maculopapular rash, and headache[19] (Chart 20-3). During this time, there is an increase in viral replication, which leads to very high viral loads, sometime greater than 1,000,000 copies/mL, and a decrease in the CD4+ count. The signs and symptoms of primary HIV infection usually appear 2 to 4 weeks after exposure to HIV, and last for a few days to 2 weeks.[19] After several weeks, the immune system acts to control viral replication and reduces it to a lower level, where it remains for several years.

The primary phase is followed by a latent period during which the person has no signs or symptoms of illness. The median time of the latent period is 10 years. During this time, the CD4+ count falls gradually from the normal range (800 to 1000 cells/μL) to 200 cells/μL or lower.[19] Lymphadenopathy develops in some persons with HIV infection during this phase. Persistent generalized lymphadenopathy usually is defined as lymph nodes that are chronically swollen for more than 3 months in at least two locations, not including the groin. The lymph nodes may be sore or visible externally.[20]

The third phase, overt AIDS, occurs when a person has a CD4+ count of less than 200 cells/μL or an AIDS-defining illness (see Fig. 20-4). Without antiretroviral therapy, this phase leads to death within 2 to 3 years. The risk of death

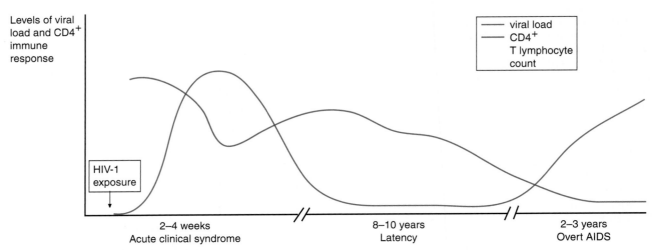

FIGURE 20-4 Viral load and CD4 count during the phases of HIV.

and opportunistic infection increases significantly when the CD4+ count reaches this level.[19]

CLINICAL COURSE

The clinical course of HIV varies from person to person. Most—60% to 70%—of those infected with HIV acquire AIDS 10 to 11 years after infection. These people are the *typical progressors*.[19] Another 10% to 20% of those infected progress rapidly. They acquire AIDS in less than 5 years and are called *rapid progressors*.[19] The final 5% to 15% are *slow progressors*, who do not progress to AIDS for more than 15 years. There is a subset of slow progressors, called *long-term nonprogressors*, who account for 1% of all HIV infections. These people have been infected for at least 8 years, are antiretroviral naive, have high CD4+ counts, and usually have very low viral loads[19] (Fig. 20-5). The opportunistic infections and manifestations of HIV include opportunistic diseases of the respiratory, gastrointestinal, and nervous systems; wasting syndrome; and metabolic disorders.

Opportunistic Infections

When the immune system becomes severely compromised, an opportunistic infection or malignancy may occur. The number of CD4+ T cells directly correlates with the risk of developing opportunistic infections. Once the CD4+ count drops below 200 cells/μL, the risk for developing an opportunistic infection is 33% after 1 year and 58% after 2 years.[21] Opportunistic infections involve common organisms that normally do not produce infection unless there is impaired immune function. Although a person with AIDS may live for many years after the first serious illness, as the immune system fails, these opportunistic illnesses become progressively more severe and difficult to treat.

In the United States, the most common opportunistic infections are *Pneumocystis carinii* pneumonia (PCP), oropharyngeal or esophageal candidiasis (thrush), cytomegalovirus (CMV), and infections caused by *Mycobacterium aviumintracellulare* complex (MAC).[21]

Respiratory Manifestations

The most common causes of respiratory disease in persons with HIV infection are PCP and pulmonary tuberculosis (TB). Other organisms that cause opportunistic pulmonary infections in persons with AIDS include CMV, MAC, *Toxoplasma gondii*, and *Cryptococcus neoformans*. Pneumonia also may occur because of more common pulmonary pathogens, including *Streptococcus pneumoniae*, *Haemophilus influenzae*, and *Legionella pneumophila*. Some persons may be infected with multiple organisms. Kaposi's sarcoma (KS) also can occur in the lungs.[22]

CHART 20-3

Signs and Symptoms of Acute HIV Infection

- Fever
- Fatigue
- Rash
- Headache
- Lymphadenopathy
- Pharyngitis
- Arthralgia
- Myalgia
- Night sweats
- Gastrointestinal problems
- Aseptic meningitis
- Oral or genital ulcers

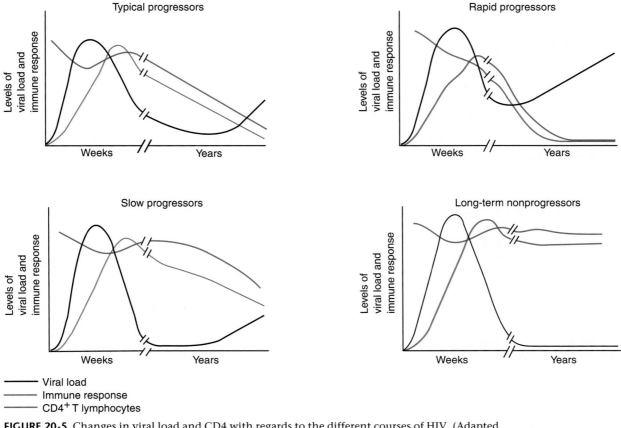

FIGURE 20-5 Changes in viral load and CD4 with regards to the different courses of HIV. (Adapted from Rizzardi G.P., Pantaleo G. [1999]. *The immunopathogenesis of HIV-1 infection.* In Armstrong D., Cohen J. [Eds.], *Infectious diseases.* London: Harcourt Publishers Ltd.)

P. carinii *Pneumonia.* *P. carinii* pneumonia was the most common presenting manifestation of AIDS during the first decade of the epidemic. Since highly active antiretroviral therapy (HAART) and prophylaxis for PCP were instituted, the incidence has decreased.[23] PCP still is common in people who do not know their HIV status, those who choose not to treat their HIV, and in those with poor access to health care.[23] The best predictor of PCP is a CD4+ T-cell count below 200 cell/µL,[24] and it is at this point that prophylaxis with trimethoprim-sulfamethoxazole (*e.g.,* Bactrim, Septra, generic) is started.[23] PCP is caused by *P. carinii,* an organism that is common in soil, houses, and many other places in the environment (see Chapter 28). In persons with healthy immune systems, *P. carinii* does not cause infection or disease. In persons with AIDS, *P. carinii* can multiply quickly in the lungs and cause pneumonia. The symptoms of PCP may be acute or gradually progressive. Patients may present with complaints of a mild cough, fever, shortness of breath, and weight loss. Physical examination may demonstrate only fever and tachypnea, and breath sounds may be normal. The chest x-ray film may show interstitial infiltrates, but in 5% of cases, the x-ray may be negative.[24] Diagnosis of PCP is made on recognition of the organism in pulmonary secretions. This can be done through examination of in-duced sputum, bronchoalveolar lavage, occasionally bronchoscopy, and, rarely, lung biopsy.[23]

Mycobacterium tuberculosis. Tuberculosis is the leading cause of death for people with HIV worldwide. There are over 80,000 people coinfected with HIV and TB in North America, and another 5 million in the rest of the world.[25] TB cases in the United States decreased from the 1950s until 1985; then, in 1986, the number of TB cases began to increase (see Chapter 28). A number of factors contributed to this increase, including changes in immigration patterns and increased numbers of people living in group settings like prisons, shelters, and nursing homes, but the most profound is HIV infection.[25] TB often is the first manifestation of HIV infection.

The lungs are the most common site of *M. tuberculosis* infection, but extrapulmonary infection of the kidney, bone marrow and other organs also occurs in people with HIV. Whether a person has pulmonary or extrapulmonary TB, most patients present with fever, night sweats, cough, and weight loss.[25] Persons infected with *M. tuberculosis* (*i.e.,* those with positive tuberculin skin tests) are more likely to develop reactivated TB if they become infected with HIV; if they are coinfected, they are more likely to have a rapidly progressive form of TB.[25] Equally important, HIV-infected persons with

TB coinfection usually have an increase in viral load, which decreases the success of TB therapy. They also have an increased number of other opportunistic infections and an increased mortality rate.[25]

Since the late 1960s, most persons with TB have responded well to therapy. However, in 1991, there were outbreaks of multidrug-resistant (MDR) TB. Many cases of drug-resistant TB occur in HIV-infected persons. A recent survey of MDR TB in eight metropolitan areas in the U.S. found that 38% of HIV-infected people with TB in New York had MDR TB, as compared with 18% of HIV-uninfected individuals with TB. Originally, mortality rates from MDR TB among HIV-infected persons were high and the survival time was only approximately 2 months. Now, because of earlier recognition and therapy, the survival time is approximately 7 months.[25]

Gastrointestinal Manifestations

Diseases of the gastrointestinal tract are some of the most frequent complications of HIV and AIDS. Esophageal candidiasis (thrush), CMV infection, and herpes simplex virus infection are common opportunistic infections that cause esophagitis in people with HIV. Persons experiencing these infections usually complain of painful swallowing or retrosternal pain. The clinical presentation can range from asymptomatic to a complete inability to swallow and dehydration. Endoscopy or barium esophagography is required for definitive diagnosis.[26]

Diarrhea or gastroenteritis is a common complaint in persons with HIV. The most common protozoal infection that causes diarrhea is that with *Cryptosporidium parvum*. The clinical features of cryptosporidiosis can range from mild diarrhea to severe, watery diarrhea with a loss of up to several liters of water per day. The most severe form usually occurs in persons with a CD4+ count of less than 50 cells/μL, and also can include malabsorption, electrolyte disturbances, dehydration, and weight loss.[19] Other organisms that cause gastroenteritis and diarrhea are *Salmonella*, CMV, *Clostridium difficile*, *Escherichia coli*, *Shigella*, *Giardia*, and microsporida. These organisms are identified by examination of stool cultures or endoscopy.[26]

Nervous System Manifestations

Human immunodeficiency virus infection, particularly in its late stages of severe immunocompromise, leaves the nervous system vulnerable to an array of neurologic disorders, including AIDS dementia complex (ADC), toxoplasmosis, and progressive multifocal leukoencephalopathy (PML). These disorders can affect the peripheral or central nervous system (CNS) and contribute to the morbidity and mortality of persons with HIV.

AIDS Dementia Complex. AIDS dementia complex is a syndrome of cognitive and motor dysfunction. ADC is caused by HIV itself, rather than an opportunistic infection, and usually is a late complication of HIV. The clinical features of ADC are impairment of attention and concentration, slowing of mental speed and agility, slowing of motor speed, and apathetic behavior. The diagnosis of ADC can be based on these clinical findings. Treatment of ADC con-

sists of HAART therapy to decrease symptoms, but this is not a cure.[27]

Toxoplasmosis. Toxoplasmosis is a common opportunistic infection in persons with AIDS. The organism responsible, *T. gondii*, is a parasite that most often affects the CNS. Toxoplasmosis usually is a reactivation of a latent *T. gondii* infection that has been dormant in the CNS.[28] The typical presentation includes fever, headaches, and neurologic dysfunction, including confusion and lethargy, visual disturbances, and seizures. Computed tomography scans or magnetic resonance imaging should be performed immediately to detect the presence of neurologic lesions. Prophylactic treatment with trimethoprim-sulfamethoxazole is effective against *T. gondii* when the CD4+ T-cell count falls below 200 cells/μL.[28] Since the use of trimethoprim-sulfamethoxazole and HAART was put into practice, the incidence of toxoplasmosis has decreased.[27]

Progressive Multifocal Leukoencephalopathy. Progressive multifocal leukoencephalopathy is a demyelinating disease of the white matter of the brain caused by the JC virus, a DNA papovavirus that attacks the oligodendrocytes. PML advance slowly, and it can be weeks to months before the patient seeks medical care.[27] It is characterized by progressive limb weakness, sensory loss, difficulty controlling the digits, visual disturbances, subtle alterations in mental status,[29] hemiparesis, ataxia, diplopia, and seizures.[30] The mortality rate is high, and the average survival time is 2 to 4 months.[30] Diagnosis is based on clinical findings and an MRI, and confirmed by the presence of the JC virus.[29] There is no proven cure for PML, but improvement can occur after starting HAART.[30]

Cancers and Malignancies

Persons with AIDS have a high incidence of certain malignancies, especially KS, non-Hodgkin's lymphoma, and non-invasive cervical carcinoma. It has been reported that KS or lymphoma is likely to develop in as many as 30% to 40% of people with HIV.[31] The increased incidence of malignancies probably is a function of impaired cell-mediated immunity.

Kaposi's Sarcoma. Kaposi's sarcoma is a malignancy of endothelial cells that line small blood vessels. An opportunistic cancer, KS occurs in immunosuppressed persons (*e.g.*, transplant recipients or persons with AIDS). KS was one of the first opportunistic cancers associated with AIDS, and still is the most frequent malignancy related to HIV.[32] It is 2000 times more common in people infected with HIV than in the rest of the population.[31] Before 1981, most cases of KS were found in North America among elderly men of Mediterranean or Eastern European Jewish descent and in Africa among young black adults and children.[33]

There is evidence linking KS to a herpesvirus (herpesvirus 8, also called KS-associated herpesvirus [KSHV]).[33] Over 95% of KS lesions, regardless of the source or clinical subtype, have reportedly been found to be infected with KSHV.[33] The virus is readily transmitted through homosexual and heterosexual activities. Maternal–infant transmission also occurs. The virus has been detected in saliva from infected persons, and other modes of transmission are suspected.

Kaposi's sarcoma can be found on the skin and in the oral cavity, gastrointestinal tract, and the lungs. More than 50% of people with skin lesions also have gastrointestinal lesions. The disease usually begins as one or more macules, papules, or violet skin lesions that enlarge and become darker. They may enlarge to form raised plaques or tumors. These irregularly shaped tumors can be from one eighth of an inch to silver dollar size. Tumor nodules frequently are located on the trunk, neck, and head, especially the tip of the nose. They usually are painless in the early stages, but discomfort may develop as the tumor ages. Invasion of internal organs, including the lungs, gastrointestinal tract, and lymphatic system, commonly occurs. Gastrointestinal tract KS often is asymptomatic, but can cause pain, bleeding, or obstruction.[31] Pulmonary KS usually is a late development of the disease. Pulmonary KS causes dyspnea, cough, and hemoptysis.[32] The tumors may obstruct organ function or rupture and cause internal bleeding. The progression of KS may be slow or rapid.

A presumptive diagnosis of KS usually is made based on visual identification of red or violet skin or oral lesions. Biopsy of at least one lesion must be done to establish the diagnosis and to distinguish the KS from other skin lesions that may resemble it. Diagnosis of gastrointestinal or pulmonary KS is more difficult because endoscopy and bronchoscopy are needed for diagnosis.[31] Effective HAART, local therapy with liquid nitrogen or vinblastine, chemotherapy, radiation, and interferon injections are the most common therapies. These therapies only are palliative and are not a cure.[32] However, with evidence that links KS to a herpesvirus, there is hope that effective therapies will be developed for preventing KS in persons at risk.[33]

Non-Hodgkin's Lymphoma.   Non-Hodgkin's lymphoma develops in 3% to 4% of people with HIV infection. The clinical features are fever, night sweats, and weight loss. Because the manifestations of non-Hodgkin's lymphoma are similar to those of other opportunistic infections, diagnosis often is difficult. Diagnosis can be made by biopsy of the affected tissue. Treatment includes aggressive combination chemotherapy that includes intrathecal chemotherapy. The prognosis for those with non-Hodgkin's lymphoma is poor, with survival ranging from 4 to 20 months.[31]

Noninvasive Cervical Carcinoma.   Women with HIV infection experience a higher incidence of cervical dysplasia than non–HIV-infected women.[34] These lesions, usually a slowly developing precursor to cervical carcinoma, progress rapidly in women with HIV infection.[34] Cervical carcinoma results from infection with human papillomavirus.[35] In addition to the rapid progression from mild dysplasia to carcinoma in situ, women with HIV infection may be less responsive to standard treatments and have a poorer prognosis than uninfected women.[34] Occurrence of cervical dysplasia is detected by Papanicolaou smear and cervical colposcopy.

Wasting Syndrome

In 1997, wasting became an AIDS-defining illness. The syndrome is common in persons with HIV infection or AIDS. Wasting is characterized by involuntary weight loss of at least 10% of baseline body weight in the presence of diarrhea, more than two stools per day, or chronic weakness and a fever. This diagnosis is made when no other opportunistic infections or neoplasms can be identified as causing these symptoms. Factors that contribute to wasting are anorexia, metabolic abnormalities, endocrine dysfunction, malabsorption, and cytokine dysregulation. Treatment for wasting includes nutritional interventions like oral supplements, or enteral or parenteral nutrition. There also are numerous pharmacologic agents used to treat wasting, including appetite stimulants, cannabinoids, and megestrol acetate.[36]

Metabolic Disorders

A wide range of metabolic disorders is associated with HIV infection, including lipodystrophy and mitochondrial disorders.

Lipodystrophy.   A metabolic disorder called *lipodystrophy* is one of the newest group of problems for those infected with HIV. Lipodystrophy related to HIV includes symptoms that fall into two categories: changes in body appearance and metabolic changes. The alterations in body appearance are an increase in abdominal girth, buffalo humps (abnormal distribution of fat in the supraclavicular area), wasting of fat from the face and extremities, and breast enlargement in men and women. The metabolic changes include elevated serum cholesterol and triglyceride levels and insulin resistance. Originally attributed to the use of protease inhibitors, the pathogenesis of lipodystrophy still is not understood. It may be due to protease inhibitor therapy or nucleoside reverse transcriptase inhibitor therapy, or may arise simply because people are living longer with HIV.

Diagnosis of lipodystrophy is based on patient complaints, clinical monitoring of triglycerides and cholesterol, and body shape.[37] Physical alterations can be assessed through changes in hip and waist circumference and, for women, bra size.[38] Management of lipodystrophy is controversial because the etiology is unknown. Some authorities recommend switching to a non–protease inhibitor-based HAART regimen. The problem with this is that although triglycerides and cholesterol decrease,[37] and there is some resolution to the fat redistribution, viral load often increases and becomes detectable.[38] Liposuction has been used with some success for patients with breast enlargement.[37] Currently, there are no guidelines for intervention in HIV-infected individuals who develop hyperlipidemia, but many clinicians initiate lipid-lowering therapy.[39] The long-term consequences of these metabolic changes need to be carefully evaluated and management guidelines need to be made.

Mitochondrial Disorders.   The mitochondria control many of the oxidative chemical reactions that release energy from glucose and other organic molecules. The mitochondria transform this newly released energy into adenosine triphosphate, which cells use as an energy source. In the absence of normal mitochondrial function, cells revert to anaerobic metabolism with generation of lactic acid. Mitochondrial disorders are metabolic disorders due to antiretroviral therapy, in particular, nucleoside reverse transcriptase inhibitors.[37] Patients often present with non-specific gastrointestinal symptoms, including nausea, vomiting, and abdominal pain. On examination, they can have hepatomegaly with normal liver function test results. The only laboratory abnormality may be lactic acidosis.[37] Mitochondrial dysfunction is the most feared complication of antiretroviral therapy. This fear is due to the condition's unpredictability, its fatality in half the presenting patients, the nonspecific presenting symptoms, and the prevalence of elevated lactate levels in 8% to 22% of patients who are asymptomatic.[40]

EARLY MANAGEMENT

The management of HIV infection has changed dramatically since the mid-1990s. This change is due to better understanding of the pathogenesis of HIV, the emergence of viral load testing, and the increased number of medications available to fight the virus. After HIV infection is confirmed, a baseline evaluation should be done. This evaluation should include a complete history and physical examination and baseline laboratory tests. Routine follow-up care of a stable, asymptomatic HIV-infected patient should include a history and physical examination along with CD4+ count and viral load testing every 3 to 4 months. Symptomatic patients and those with an AIDS diagnosis should be seen once a month.[41]

Therapeutic interventions are determined by the level of disease activity based on the viral load, the degree of immunodeficiency based on the CD4+ count, and the appearance of specific opportunistic infections. As HIV progresses, prophylaxis and treatment of opportunistic infections become very important.[41] Prophylaxis is different for every opportunistic infection and depends on the person's CD4+ T-cell level. Early recognition of HIV is becoming more common, and medical intervention in the early stages may delay life-threatening symptoms and slow the spread of disease.

Because of frequent advances in the management of HIV infection, primary care providers must be prepared to update their knowledge of diagnosis, testing, evaluation, and medical intervention. The CDC, the Department of Health and Human Services, and the United States Public Health Service regularly issue guidelines to assist clinicians in caring for persons with HIV disease.

TREATMENT

There is no cure for AIDS. Although many companies are working on a vaccine to prevent HIV infection, none has been approved. The first drug that was approved by the FDA for the treatment of HIV was zidovudine, which came out in 1987. Since then, an increasing number of therapeutics have been approved by the FDA for treatment of HIV infection.[42] Many other drugs aimed at stopping the replication of HIV in cells are under investigation. Actions of these drugs vary from interfering with HIV attachment to the host

cell to the phase when new virions are released. There currently are three different types of HIV antiretroviral medications: nucleoside reverse transcriptase inhibitors, non-nucleoside reverse transcriptase inhibitors, and protease inhibitors (Table 20-1). Each type of agent attempts to interrupt viral replication at a different point.

Reverse transcriptase inhibitors inhibit HIV replication by acting on the enzyme reverse transcriptase. There are two types of HIV medications that work on this enzyme, nucleoside reverse transcriptase inhibitors and non-nucleoside reverse transcriptase inhibitors. *Nucleoside reverse transcriptase inhibitors* act by blocking the elongation of the DNA chain by stopping more nucleosides from being added. *Nonnucleoside reverse transcriptase* inhibitors work by binding to the reverse transcriptase enzyme so it cannot copy the virus's RNA into DNA[43] (see Fig. 20-2).

Protease inhibitors bind to the protease enzyme and inhibit its action. This inhibition prevents the cleavage of the polyprotein chain into individual proteins, which would be used to construct the new virus. Because the information inside the nucleus is not put together properly, the new viruses that are released into the body are immature and noninfectious[43] (see Fig. 20-2).

The treatment of HIV is one of the most rapidly evolving fields in medicine. Optimal treatment of HIV includes a combination of drugs because different drugs act on different stages of the replication cycle.[42] The goal of HAART is a sustained suppression of HIV replication, resulting in an undetectable viral load and an increasing CD4+ count.[42] In general, antiviral therapies are prescribed to improve the overall survival time of persons with HIV infection and to slow the progression to AIDS.

Opportunistic infections occur as a consequence of immunodeficiency, which is caused by the progressive loss of CD4+ T cells. Drugs and vaccines commonly are used for the prevention and treatment of opportunistic infections and conditions, including PCP, toxoplasmosis, MAC,[44] candidiasis, CMV infection, influenza, hepatitis B, and *S. pneumoniae* infections.[45,46] Prophylactic medications are used once an individual's CD4+ count has dropped below a certain level that indicates his or her immune system is no longer able to fight off the opportunistic infections.

Persons with HIV should be advised to avoid infections as much as possible and seek evaluation promptly when they occur. Immunization is important because persons infected with HIV are at risk for contracting many infectious diseases. Some of these diseases can be avoided by vaccination while the immune system's responsiveness is relatively intact. Persons with asymptomatic HIV infection should be vaccinated against measles, mumps, and rubella. Pneumococcal vaccine should be given once, as soon as possible after HIV infection is diagnosed, and influenza vaccine should be given yearly.[47] Live-virus vaccines should not be given to persons with HIV infection or AIDS.

PSYCHOSOCIAL ISSUES

The psychological effects of HIV infection or AIDS may be just as significant as the physical effects. The dramatic impact of this catastrophic illness is compounded by complex reactions on the part of the person with HIV or AIDS;

TABLE 20-1 ✦ Antiviral Medications Used in Treatment of HIV Infections

Medication (Generic Name)	Medication (Trade Name)	Frequency of Dosage (in hr)
Nucleoside Reverse Transcriptase Inhibitors (NRTI)		
Zidovudine (AZT)	Retrovir	12
Didanosine (ddl)	Videx	12
Lamivudine (3TC)	Epivir	12
Stavudine (d4T)	Zerit	12
Abacavir	Ziagen	12
Zalcitabine (ddC)	Hivid	8
Non-nucleoside Reverse Transcriptase Inhibitors (NNRTI)		
Nevirapine (NVP)	Viramune	24 × 2 wk, then 12
Efavirenz (EFV)	Sustiva	24
Delavirdine (DLV)	Rescriptor	8
Protease Inhibitors		
Saquinavir (SAQ)	Invirase	8
	Fortovase	8
Ritonavir (RTV)	Norvir	12
Indinavir (IDV)	Crixivan	8
Nelfinavir (NLF)	Viracept	8 or 12
Combination Drugs		
Retrovir and lamivudine	Combivir	12
Retrovir, lamivudine, abacavir	Trizivir	12
Lopinavir, ritonavir	Kaletra	12

his or her partner, friends, and family; members of the health care team; and the community. These reactions may be influenced by inadequate information, fear of contagion, shame, prejudices, and condemnation of risk behaviors.[48] In addition to the fear and grief associated with death, the person with HIV or AIDS also may experience guilt, anger, and uncertainty.[48] Questioning and self-examination are common as the person attempts to cope with the disease.[48] Pre-existing mental health conditions may include alcohol and drug abuse. Appropriate treatment should be made available when alcohol or other drug dependence is evident.

The person with HIV infection or AIDS may feel helpless, hopeless, stigmatized, and out of control.[49] HIV and AIDS affect all spheres of life. Isolated from peers and with a threatened sense of identity, the person may be anxious, depressed, and miserable.[49] Acknowledging a diagnosis of AIDS may be the first indication to family and colleagues of an otherwise hidden lifestyle (*i.e.,* homosexuality or drug use). This increases the strain on relationships with important support persons.

Diagnosis and treatment of cognitive and affective disorders are essential parts of ongoing care for the HIV-infected person.[49] The emotional stress, feelings of isolation, and sadness experienced by the person with HIV or AIDS can be overwhelming. Most persons, however, manage to learn to cope and live with their HIV infection. Persons with the disease must have as much information and control over activities as possible. They should be encouraged to direct their energies in a positive manner and continue with their social and group activities as long as such activities are helpful. Appropriate social support systems (*e.g.,* AIDS service organizations, community groups, religious organizations) should be called on to assist whenever possible. When they learn they can live with HIV infection, often for several years, many persons acquire a positive outlook based on living their lives to the fullest.

To deal with these complex issues, the health care team must recognize and accept their own fears, prejudices, and emotions concerning those with HIV or AIDS. Personal feelings must not prevent caregivers from acknowledging the intrinsic human worth of all persons and their right to be treated with dignity and respect. Members of the health care team should have adequate support for their own emotional needs generated from working with persons with AIDS. Grief, anxiety, and concern over stigmatization are normal feelings and should be acknowledged and dealt with through peer support or professional counseling to reduce burnout and emotional strain of members of the health care provider team.

In summary, HIV is a retrovirus that infects the body's CD4+ T cells and macrophages. HIV genetic material becomes integrated into the host cell DNA, so new HIV can be made. Manifestations of infection, such as acute mononucleosis-like symptoms, may occur shortly after infection, and this is followed by a latent phase that may last for many years. The end of the latent period is marked by the onset of opportunistic infections and cancers as the person moves toward an AIDS diagnosis. The complications of these infections, manifested throughout the respiratory, gastrointestinal, and nervous systems, include pneumonia, esophagitis, diarrhea, gastroenteritis, tumors, wasting syndrome, altered mental status, seizures, motor deficits, and metabolic disorders. HIV is diagnosed using the EIA together with the Western blot assay antibody detection tests. The emotional stress, feelings of isolation, and sadness experienced by the person with HIV or AIDS can be overwhelming, but most persons adjust to living with HIV infection. Diagnosis and treatment of cognitive and affective disorders are an essential part of ongoing care for the HIV-infected person. Appropriate treatment should be made available when alcohol or other drug dependence is noted.

Prevention of HIV Infection

After you have completed this section of the chapter, you should be able to meet the following objectives:

✦ Discuss the transmission of HIV
✦ Describe preventive strategies to decrease the transmission of HIV

Because there is no cure for HIV or AIDS, adopting risk-free or low-risk behavior is the best protection against the disease. Abstinence or long-term, mutually monogamous sexual relationships between two uninfected partners are the best ways to avoid HIV infection and other STDs. Correct and consistent use of latex condoms can provide protection from the disease by not allowing contact with semen or vaginal secretions during intercourse.[8] Natural or lambskin condoms do not provide the same protection from HIV as latex because of the larger pores in the material. Only water-based lubricants should be used with condoms; petroleum (oil-based) products weaken the structure of the latex.

Injection of drugs provides another opportunity for HIV transmission. Avoiding recreational drug use and particularly avoiding the practice of using syringes that may have been used by another person are important to AIDS prevention. Medical and public health authorities recommend that persons who inject drugs use a new sterile syringe for each injection, or if this is not possible, clean their syringes thoroughly with full-strength household bleach.

Substances that alter inhibitions can lead to risky sexual behavior. For example, smoking cocaine (*i.e.*, "crack") heightens the perception of sexual arousal, and this can influence the user to practice unsafe sexual behavior.[50] The addictive nature of many recreational drugs can lead to an increase in the frequency of unsafe sexual behavior and the number of partners as the user engages in sex exchanged for money or drugs.[50] Persons concerned about their risk should be encouraged to get information and counseling about their infection status.

Public health programs in the United States have been profoundly affected by the HIV epidemic. Although standard methods for disease intervention and statistical analysis are applied to HIV, public health programs have become more responsive to community concerns, confidentiality, and long-term follow-up of clients as a direct result of the HIV epidemic. Testing for HIV antibodies and counseling have become widely available in the United States. Whenever HIV testing is performed, counseling should be offered. HIV prevention counseling should be culturally competent, sensitive to issues of sexual identity, developmentally appropriate, and linguistically relevant.[10]

The essential elements of any HIV prevention/ counseling interaction include a personalized risk assessment and prevention plan.[51] Education and behavioral intervention continue to be the mainstays of HIV prevention programs. Individual risk assessment and education regarding HIV transmission and possible prevention techniques or skills are delivered to persons in clinical settings and to those at high risk of infection in community settings. Community-wide education is provided in schools, in the workplace, and in the media. Training for professionals can have an impact on HIV spread and is an important element of prevention. The constant addition of new information on HIV makes prevention an ever-changing and challenging endeavor.

> In summary, risk-free or low-risk behavior is the best protection against HIV infection, because there is no cure for AIDS. Abstinence or long-term, mutually monogamous sexual relationships between two uninfected partners, use of condoms, avoiding drug use, and the use of sterile syringes are essential to stopping the spread of HIV.

HIV Infection in Pregnancy and in Infants and Children

After you have completed this section of the chapter, you should be able to meet the following objectives:

✦ Discuss the vertical transmission of HIV from mother to child and recommended prevention measures
✦ Cite problems with diagnosis of HIV infection in the infant
✦ Compare the progress of HIV infection in infants and children with HIV infection in adults

Early in the epidemic, children who contracted HIV could have become infected through blood products or perinatally. Now, almost all of the children who become infected with HIV at a young age in the United States get HIV perinatally. Infected women may transmit the virus to their offspring in utero, during labor and delivery, or through breast milk.[12] The risk of transmission is increased if the mother has advanced HIV disease as evidenced by low CD4+ counts, high levels of HIV in the blood (high viral load), prolonged time from rupture of membranes to delivery, if the mother breast-feeds the child,[10] or if there is increased exposure of the fetus to maternal blood.[52]

Diagnosis of HIV infection in children born to HIV-infected mothers is complicated by the presence of maternal HIV IgG antibody, which crosses the placenta to the fetus.

HIV Infection in Pregnancy and in Infants and Children

➤ HIV can be passed from mother to infant during labor and delivery or through breast-feeding.

➤ The course of HIV infection is different for children than adults.

In summary, infected women may transmit the virus to their offspring in utero, during labor and delivery, or through breast milk. Diagnosis of HIV infection in children born to HIV-infected mothers is complicated by the presence of maternal HIV antibody, which crosses the placenta to the fetus. This antibody usually disappears within 18 months in uninfected children. Administration of zidovudine to the mother during pregnancy and labor and delivery and to the infant when it is born can decrease perinatal transmission.

Consequently, infants born to HIV-infected women can be HIV antibody positive by ELISA for up to 18 months of age even though they are not HIV infected.[10] PCR testing for HIV DNA is used most often to diagnose HIV in infants younger than 18 months of age. Two positive PCR tests for HIV DNA are needed to diagnose a child with HIV. Children born to mothers with HIV infection are considered uninfected if they become HIV antibody negative after 6 months of age, have no other laboratory evidence of HIV infection, and have not met the surveillance case definition criteria for AIDS in children.[10]

Perinatal transmission can be lowered by two thirds, from 26% to 8%, by administering zidovudine to the mother during pregnancy and labor and delivery and to the infant when it is born.[9] The U.S. Public Health Service therefore recommends that HIV counseling and testing should be offered to all pregnant women and women of childbearing age in the United States.[12] The recommendations also stress that women who test positive for HIV antibodies should be informed of the perinatal prevention benefits of zidovudine therapy and offered treatment that includes zidovudine alone, or HAART therapy.[53] Benefits of voluntary testing for mothers and newborns include reduced morbidity because of intensive treatment and supportive health care, the opportunity for early antiviral therapy for mother and child, and information regarding the risk of transmission from breast milk.[12]

Because pregnant women in less developed countries do not always have access to zidovudine, studies are being conducted in Africa to determine if any other simple and less expensive antiretroviral regimen can be used to decrease transmission from mother to infant. One such study, HIVNET 012, looked at single-dose nevirapine compared with zidovudine. It found that nevirapine lowered the risk of HIV transmission by almost 50%.[54]

Children have a very different pattern of HIV infection than adults. Failure to thrive, CNS abnormalities, and developmental delays are the most prominent primary manifestations of HIV infection in children.[10] Children born infected with HIV usually weigh less and are shorter than noninfected infants.[10] A major cause of early mortality for HIV-infected children is PCP. As opposed to adults, in whom PCP occurs in the late stages, PCP occurs early in children, with the peak age of onset at 3 to 6 months. For this reason, prophylaxis with trimethoprim-sulfamethoxazole is started by 4 to 6 weeks for all infants born to HIV-infected mothers, regardless of their CD4+ count or infection status.[10]

Related Web Sites

AIDS Clinical Trial Information Service—includes drug information search www.actis.org
AIDS.ORG www.immunet.org
AIDS Treatment News www.aidsnews.org
Centers for Disease Control and Prevention, Divisions of HIV/AIDS Prevention—basic statistics www.cdc.gov/hiv/stats.htm
Centers for Disease Control and Prevention, Divisions of HIV/AIDS Prevention—brochures www.cdc.gov/hiv/pubs/brochure.htm
HIV/AIDS Treatment Information Service—DHHS Treatment Guidelines www.hivatis.org
HIV InSite hivinsite.ucsf.edu
Infectious Diseases Society of America www.idsociety.org
International Association of Physicians in AIDS Care www.iapac.org
Johns Hopkins AIDS Service www.hopkins-aids.edu
Kaiser Daily HIV/AIDS Report report.kff.org/aidshiv
Medscape—HIV/AIDS hiv.medscape.com
National Center for Infectious Diseases www.cdc.gov/ncidod
National Institute of Allergy and Infectious Diseases www.niaid.nih.gov
National Minority AIDS Council www.nmac.org
Project Inform www.projectinform.org

References

1. American Association for World Health. (2000). *AIDS: All men make a difference.* Washington, DC: Author.
2. Quinn T.C. (2001). The global HIV pandemic: Lessons from the past and glimpses into the future. *The Hopkins HIV Report* 13 (1), 4–5, 16.
3. Wisconsin Department of Health and Family Services. (2000). *Wisconsin AIDS/HIV update.* Madison, WI: Author.
4. Montagnier L., Alizon M. (1986). The human immune deficiency virus (HIV): An update. In Gluckman J.C., Vilmer E. (Eds.), *Proceedings of the Second International Conference on AIDS* (p. 13). Paris: Elsevier.
5. Friedland G.H., Klein R.S. (1987). Transmission of the human immunodeficiency virus. *New England Journal of Medicine* 317, 1125–1135.
6. O'Brien T.R., George J.R., Holmberg S.D. (1992). Human immunodeficiency virus type-2 infection in the United States: Epidemiology, diagnosis, and public health implications. *Journal of the American Medical Association* 267, 2775–2779.
7. Gershon R.R.M., Vlahov D., Nelson K.E. (1990). The risk of transmission of HIV-1 through non-percutaneous, non-sexual modes: A review. *AIDS* 4, 645–650.

8. Colpin H. (1999). Prevention of HIV transmission through behavioral changes and sexual means. In Armstrong D., Cohen J. (Eds.), *Infectious diseases* (Section 5, Chapter 2, pp. 1–4). London: Harcourt.

9. Connor E.M., Sperling R.S., Gelber R., Kiselev P., Scott G., O'Sullivan M., VanDyke R., Bey M., Sheaere W., Jacobson R., Jimenez E., O'Neil E., Bazin B., Delfraissey J., Culane M., Coombs R., Elkins M., Moye J., Stratton P., Balsey J. (1994). Reduction of maternal-infant transmission of human immunodeficiency virus type 1 with zidovudine treatment. *New England Journal of Medicine* 331, 1173–1180.

10. Havens P.L. (1999). Pediatric AIDS. In Armstrong D., Cohen J. (Eds.), *Infectious diseases* (Section 5, Chapter 20). London: Harcourt.

11. Henderson D.K. (1999). Preventing occupational infections with HIV in health care settings. In Armstrong D., Cohen J. (Eds.), *Infectious diseases* (Section 5, Chapter 3, pp. 1–10). London: Harcourt.

12. U.S. Public Health Service. (2000). *Revised public health service recommendations for human immunodeficiency virus screening of pregnant women.* Washington, DC: Author.

13. Hirschel B. (1999). Primary HIV infection. In Armstrong D., Cohen J. (Eds.), *Infectious diseases* (Section 5, Chapter 8, pp. 1–4). London: Harcourt.

14. Fauci A.S. (1988). The human immunodeficiency virus: Infectivity and mechanisms of pathogenesis. *Science* 239, 617–622.

15. Holodniy M. (1999). Establishing the diagnosis of HIV infection. In Dolin R., Masur H., Saag M.S. (Eds.), *AIDS therapy* (pp. 3–14). Philadelphia: Churchill Livingstone.

16. Brun-Vezinet F., Simon F. (1999). Diagnostic tests for HIV infection. In Armstrong D., Cohen J. (Eds.), *Infectious diseases* (Section 5, Chapter 23, pp. 1–10). London: Harcourt.

17. Rogers M.F., Ou C.Y., Kilbourne B., Schochetman G. (1991). Advances and problems in the diagnosis of human immunodeficiency virus infection in infants. *Pediatric Infectious Disease Journal* 10, 523–531.

18. Centers for Disease Control and Prevention. (1992). 1993 Revised classification system for HIV infection and expanded surveillance case definition for AIDS among adolescents and adults. *Morbidity and Mortality Weekly Report* 41 (RR-17), 1–23.

19. Rizzardi G.P., Pantaleo G. (1999). The immunopathogenesis of HIV-1 infection. In Armstrong D., Cohen J. (Eds.), *Infectious diseases* (Section 5, Chapter 6, pp. 1–12). London: Harcourt.

20. Pantaleo G., Graziosi C., Fauci A.S. (1993). The immunopathogenesis of human immunodeficiency virus infection. *New England Journal of Medicine* 328, 327–335.

21. Clumeck N., Dewit S. (1999). Prevention of opportunistic infections in the presence of HIV infection. In Armstrong D., Cohen J. (Eds.), *Infectious diseases* (Section 5, Chapter 9). London: Harcourt.

22. Dolin R., Masur H., Saag M.S. (Eds.). (1999). *AIDS therapy.* Philadelphia: Churchill Livingstone.

23. Masur H. (1999). *Pneumocystis.* In Dolin R., Masur H., Saag M.S. (Eds.), *AIDS therapy* (pp. 291–306). Philadelphia: Churchill Livingstone.

24. Girard P.M. (1999). *Pneumocystis carinii* pneumonia. In Armstrong D., Cohen J. (Eds.), *Infectious diseases* (Section 5, Chapter 10, pp. 1–4). London: Harcourt.

25. Gordin F. (1999). *Mycobacterium tuberculosis.* In Dolin R., Masur H., Saag M.S. (Eds.), *AIDS therapy* (pp. 359–374). Philadelphia: Churchill Livingstone.

26. Wilcox C.M., Monkemuller K.E. (1999). Gastrointestinal disease. In Dolin R., Masur H., Saag M.S. (Eds.), *AIDS therapy* (pp. 752–765). Philadelphia: Churchill Livingstone.

27. Price, R.W. (1999). Neurologic disease. In Dolin R., Masur H., Saag M.S. (Eds.), *AIDS therapy* (pp. 620–638). Philadelphia: Churchill Livingstone.

28. Katlama C. (1999). Parasitic infections. In Armstrong D., Cohen J. (Eds.), *Infectious diseases* (Section 5, Chapter 13, pp. 1–4). London: Harcourt.

29. Hall C.D. (1999). JC virus neurologic infection. In Dolin R., Masur H., Saag M.S. (Eds.), *AIDS therapy* (pp. 565–572). Philadelphia: Churchill Livingstone.

30. Murphy M.E., Polisky B. (1999). Viral infection. In Armstrong D., Cohen J. (Eds.), *Infectious diseases* (Section 5, Chapter 11). London: Harcourt.

31. Tirelli U., Vaccher E. (1999). Neoplastic disease. In Armstrong D., Cohen J. (Eds.), *Infectious diseases* (Section 5, Chapter 15, pp. 1–4). London: Harcourt.

32. Krown S.E. (1999). Kaposi sarcoma. In Dolin R., Masur H., Saag M.S. (Eds.), *AIDS therapy* (pp. 580–591). Philadelphia: Churchill Livingstone.

33. Anteman K., Chang Y. (2000). Kaposi's sarcoma. *New England Journal of Medicine* 342, 1027–1038.

34. Centers for Disease Control. (1990). Risk of cervical disease in HIV infected women. *Morbidity and Mortality Weekly Report* 39, 846–849.

35. Bonnez W. (1999). Sexually transmitted human papillomavirus infection. In Dolin R., Masur H., Saag M.S. (Eds.), *AIDS therapy* (pp. 530–564). Philadelphia: Churchill Livingstone.

36. Von Ruenn J.H., Mulligan K. (1999). Wasting syndrome. In Dolin R., Masur H., Saag M.S. (Eds.), *AIDS therapy* (pp. 607–619). Philadelphia: Churchill Livingstone.

37. Chaisson R.E., Triesman G.J. (2000). *Antiretroviral therapy in perspective: Managing drug side effects to improve patient outcomes* (Vol. I). Connecticut: Scientific Exchange.

38. Lyon D., Truban E. (2000). HIV-related lipodystrophy: A clinical syndrome with implications for nursing practice. *Journal of the Association of Nurses in AIDS Care* 11 (2), 36–42.

39. Lo J.C., Schambelan M. (1999). Endocrine disease. In Dolin R., Masur H., Saag M.S. (Eds.), *AIDS therapy* (pp. 740–751). Philadelphia: Churchill Livingstone.

40. Lucas, G.M. (2000). Report from the 38th IDSA: Preserving the immune response to HIV, HAART, and long-term toxicities. *The Hopkins HIV Report* 12 (5), 1, 6, 12.

41. Montaner J.S.G., Montesorri V. (1999). Principles of management. In Armstrong D., Cohen J. (Eds.), *Infectious diseases* (Section 5, Chapter 25, pp. 1–2). London: Harcourt.

42. Vella S., Floridia M. (1999). Antiretroviral therapy. In Armstrong D., Cohen J. (Eds.), *Infectious diseases* (Section 5, Chapter 26, pp. 1–10). London: Harcourt.

43. Merck & Co., Inc. (1999). *The HIV life cycle* (brochure). West Point, PA: Author.

44. Powderly W.G. (1999). Opportunistic infection prophylaxis in the era of highly active antiretroviral therapy. In Armstrong D., Cohen J. (Eds.), *Infectious diseases* (Section 5, Chapter 19, pp. 1–2). London: Harcourt.

45. Sande M.A., Gilbert D.N., Moellering, R.C. (Eds.). (2000). *The Sanford guide to HIV/AIDS therapy* (9th ed.). Hyde Park, VT: Antiretroviral Therapy.

46. Bartlett J.G., Gallant J.E. (2000). *2000–2001 Medical management of HIV infection.* Baltimore, MD: Johns Hopkins University Press.

47. Maenza J.R., Chaisson R.E. (1999). Bacterial infections in HIV disease. In Armstrong D., Cohen J. (Eds.), *Infectious diseases* (Section 5, Chapter 14, pp. 1–6). London: Harcourt.

48. Lippman S.W., James W.A., Frierson R.L. (1993). AIDS and the family: Implications for counselling. *AIDS Care* 5, 71–78.

49. O'Brien A.M., Oerlemans-Bunn M., Blachfield J.C. (1987). Nursing the AIDS patient at home. *AIDS Patient Care* 1, 21.

50. Edlin B.R., Irwin K.L., Faruque S., McCoy C.B., Word C., Serrano Y., et al., and the Multicenter Crack Cocaine and HIV Infection Study Team. (1994). Intersecting epidemics: Crack cocaine use and HIV infection among inner-city young adults. *New England Journal of Medicine* 331, 1422–1427.

51. Centers for Disease Control and Prevention. (1998). Public health service task force recommendations for the use of antiretroviral drugs in pregnant women infected with HIV-1 for maternal health and for reducing perinatal HIV-1 transmission in the United States. *Morbidity and Mortality Weekly Report* 47 (RR-2), 1–30.

52. Boyer P., Dillon M., Navaie M., Deveikis A., Keller M., O'Rourke S., Bryson Y. (1994). Factors predictive of maternal-fetal transmission of HIV-1. *Journal of the American Medical Association* 271, 1925–1930.

53. Centers for Disease Control and Prevention. (1998). Public health service guidelines for the management of health care worker exposures to HIV and recommendations for post exposure prophylaxis. *Morbidity and Mortality Weekly Report* 47 (RR-7), 1–33.

54. Guay L., Muskoe P., Fleming T., Bagenda D., Allen M., Nakabiito C., et. al. (1999). Intrapartum and neonatal single-dose nevirapine compared with zidovudine for prevention of mother-to-child transmission of HIV-1 in Kampala, Uganda: HIVNET 012 randomised trial. *Lancet* 354, 795–802.

Cardiovascular Function

Of all body systems, the heart and circulation presented the most difficult puzzle to solve. From the fifth century BC, theories about blood and its movement were linked to the concept of the four elements (fire, earth, air, and water) and the *pneuma*, or life force. According to the Greek physician Galen (AD 130–200), the starting point of the circulatory system was the gut, where food was made into "chyle" and then carried to the liver where it was converted into blood. From the liver, which was believed to be the center of the circulation, a small amount of blood was sent to the heart and lungs where heat from the heart and pneuma from the air were added, producing an ultimate concoction of "vital spirits" that was carried in the arteries to all parts of the body.

It was not until the work of the English physician William Harvey (1578–1657) that answers to the mysteries of the circulation began to emerge. It was he who first proposed that blood traveled in a circuitous route through the body, being pumped by the active phase of the heart's contraction, not relaxation as had previously been believed. In his studies, Harvey showed that a cut artery in an animal spurts during the heart's contraction. He also demonstrated that the atria of the heart had the same relationship to the ventricles as the ventricles do to the arteries and that blood from the heart was circulated through the lungs, where it was oxygenated. As strange as it may seem today, these concepts were so revolutionary to Harvey's contemporaries that the world's basic understanding of how the body functions was thrown into turmoil.

Control of the Circulation

The main function of the *circulatory system*, which consists of the heart and blood vessels, is transport. The circulatory system delivers oxygen and nutrients needed for metabolic processes to the tissues, carries waste products from cellular metabolism to the kidneys and other excretory organs for elimination, and circulates electrolytes and hormones needed to regulate body function. This process of nutrient delivery is carried out with exquisite precision so that the blood flow to each tissue of the body is exactly matched to tissue need. The circulatory system also plays an important role in body temperature regulation, which relies on the circulatory system for transport of core heat to the periphery, where it can be dissipated into the external environment. Transport of various immune substances that contribute to the body's defense mechanisms is also an important circu-latory function. The purpose of this chapter is to discuss the organization of the circulatory system, the function of the heart as a pump, the anatomy and circulatory function of the blood vessels, neural control of circulatory function, and the microcirculation and lymphatic system.

Organization of the Circulatory System

After you have completed this section of the chapter, you should be able to meet the following objectives:

✦ Compare the functions and distribution of blood flow and blood pressure in the systemic and pulmonary circulations

✦ State the relation between blood volume and blood pressure in the circulatory system

PULMONARY AND SYSTEMIC CIRCULATIONS

The circulatory system can be divided into two parts: the *pulmonary circulation*, which moves blood through the lungs and creates a link with the gas exchange function of the respiratory system, and the *systemic circulation*, which supplies all the other tissues of the body (Fig. 21-1). The blood that is in the heart and pulmonary circulation is sometimes referred to as the *central circulation*, and that outside the central circulation as the *peripheral circulation*.

Both the pulmonary and systemic circulations have a pump, an arterial system, capillaries, and a venous system. Arteries and arterioles function as a distribution system to move blood to the tissues. Capillaries serve as an exchange system where transfer of gases, nutrients, and wastes takes place. Venules and veins serve as collection and storage vessels that return blood to the heart. The pulmonary circulation consists of the right heart, the pulmonary artery, the pulmonary capillaries, and the pulmonary veins. The large pulmonary vessels are unique in that the pulmonary artery is the only artery that carries venous blood and the pulmonary veins, the only veins that carry arterial blood. The systemic circulation consists of the left heart, the aorta and its branches, the capillaries that supply the brain and peripheral tissues, and the systemic venous system and

the vena cava. The veins from the lower portion of the body converge into the inferior vena cava and those from the head and upper extremities converge into the superior vena cava. The inferior vena cava and superior vena cava empty into the right heart.

Although the pulmonary and systemic systems function similarly, they have some important differences. The pulmonary circulation is the smaller of the two and functions with a much lower pressure. Because the pulmonary circulation is located in the chest near to the heart, it functions as a low-pressure system with a mean arterial pressure of approximately 12 mm Hg. The low pressure of the pulmonary circulation allows blood to move through the lungs more slowly, which is important for gas exchange. Because the systemic circulation must transport blood to distant parts of the body, often against the effects of gravity, it functions as a high-pressure system, with a mean arterial pressure of 90 to 100 mm Hg.

The circulatory system is a closed system in which the heart consists of two pumps in series: one to propel blood through the lungs (*i.e.*, pulmonary circulation) and the other to propel blood to all other tissues of the body (*i.e.*, systemic circulation). Unidirectional flow through the heart is ensured by the heart valves. Both sides of the heart are further divided into two chambers, an *atrium* and a *ventricle*. The atria function as collection chambers for blood returning to the heart and as auxiliary pumps that assist in filling the ventricles. The ventricles are the main pumping chambers of the heart. The right ventricle pumps blood through the pulmonary artery to the lungs and the left ventricle pumps blood through the aorta into the systemic circulation. The ventricular chambers of the right and left heart have inlet and outlet valves that act reciprocally (*i.e.*, one set of valves is open while the other is closed) to control the direction of blood flow through the cardiac chambers.

The effective function of the circulatory system requires that the outputs of both sides of the heart pump the same amount of blood over time. If the output of the left heart were to fall below that of the right heart, blood would accumulate in the pulmonary circulation. Likewise, if the right heart were to pump less effectively than the left heart, blood would accumulate in the systemic circulation. However, the left and right heart seldom eject exactly the same amount of blood with each beat. This is because blood return to the heart is affected by activities of daily living such as taking a deep breath or moving from the seated to standing position. These beat-by-beat variations in cardiac output are accommodated by the storage capabilities of the venous system that allow for temporary changes in volume. Fluid accumulation occurs only when the storage capacity of the venous system has been exceeded.

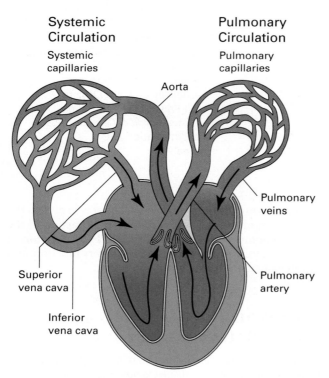

Systemic Circulation
Systemic capillaries

Pulmonary Circulation
Pulmonary capillaries

Aorta

Pulmonary veins

Pulmonary artery

Superior vena cava

Inferior vena cava

FIGURE 21-1 Systemic and pulmonary circulations. The right side of the heart pumps blood to the lungs, and the left side of the heart pumps blood to the systemic circulation.

VOLUME AND PRESSURE DISTRIBUTION

Blood flow in the circulatory system depends on a blood volume that is sufficient to fill the blood vessels and a pressure difference across the system that provides the force to move blood forward. The total blood volume is a function of age and body weight, ranging from 85 to 90 mL/kg in the neonate and from 70 to 75 mL/kg in the adult. As shown in Figure 21-2, approximately 4% of the blood at any given time is in the left heart, 16% is in the arteries and arterioles, 4% is in the capillaries, 64% is in the venules and veins, and 4% is in the right heart. The arteries and arterioles, which have thick, elastic walls and function as a distribution system, have the highest pressure. The capillaries are small, thin-walled vessels that link the arterial and venous sides of the circulation. Because of their small size and large surface area, the capillaries contain the smallest amount of blood. The venules and veins, which contain the largest amount of blood, are thin-walled, distensible vessels that function as a reservoir to collect blood from the capillaries and return it to the right heart.

Blood moves from the arterial to the venous side of the circulation along a pressure difference, moving from an area of higher pressure to one of lower pressure. The pressure distribution in the different parts of the circulation is almost an inverse of the volume distribution (see Fig. 21-2). The pressure in the arterial side of the circulation, which contains only approximately one sixth of the blood volume, is much greater than the pressure on the venous side of the circulation, which contains approximately two thirds of the blood. This pressure and volume distribution is due in large part to the structure and relative elasticity of the arteries and veins. It is the pressure difference between the arterial and venous sides of the circulation (approximately 84 mm Hg) that provides the driving force for flow of blood in the systemic circulation. The pulmonary circulation has a similar arterial-venous pressure difference, albeit of a lesser magnitude, that facilitates blood flow.

Because the pulmonary and systemic circulations are connected and function as a closed system, blood can be shifted from one circulation to the other. In the pulmonary circulation, the blood volume (approximately 450 mL in the adult) can vary from as low as 50% of normal to as high as 200% of normal. An increase in intrathoracic pressure, which impedes venous return to the right heart, can produce a transient shift from the central to the systemic circulation of as much as 250 mL of blood. Body position also affects the distribution of blood volume. In the recumbent position, approximately 25% to 30% of the total blood volume is in the central circulation. On standing, this blood is rapidly displaced to the lower part of the body because of the forces of gravity. Because the volume of the systemic circulation is approximately seven times that of the pulmonary circulation, a shift of blood from one system to the other has a much greater effect in the pulmonary than in the systemic circulation.

In summary, the circulatory system functions as a transport system that circulates nutrients and other materials to the tissues and removes waste products. The circulatory system can be divided into two parts: the systemic and the pulmonary circulation. The heart pumps blood throughout the system, and the blood vessels serve as tubes through which blood flows. The arterial system carries fluids from the heart to the tissues, and the veins carry them back to the heart. The cardiovascular system is a closed system with a right and left heart connected in series. The systemic circulation, which is served by the left heart, supplies all the tissues except the lungs, which are served by the right heart and the pulmonary circulation. Blood moves throughout the circulation along a pressure gradient, moving from the high-pressure arterial system to the low-pressure venous system. In the circulatory system, pressure is inversely related to volume. The pressure on the arterial side of the circulation, which contains only approximately one sixth of the blood volume, is much greater than the pressure on the venous side of the circulation, which contains approximately two thirds of the blood.

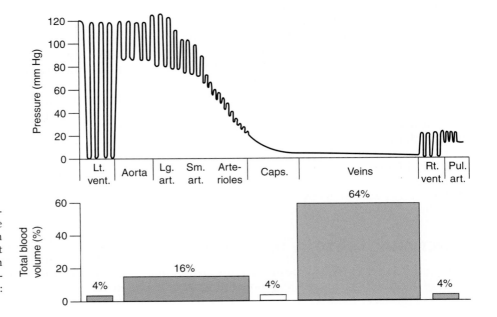

FIGURE 21-2 Pressure and volume distribution in the systemic circulation. The graphs show the inverse relation between internal pressure and volume in different portions of the circulatory system. (Smith J.J., Kampine J.P. [1990]. *Circulatory physiology: The essentials* [3rd ed.]. Baltimore: Williams & Wilkins)

Functional Organization of the Circulatory System

➤ The circulatory system consists of the heart, which pumps blood; the arterial system, which distributes oxygenated blood to the tissues; the venous system, which collects deoxygenated blood from the tissues and returns it to the heart; and the capillaries, where exchange of gases, nutrients, and wastes takes place.

➤ The circulatory system is divided into two parts: the low-pressure pulmonary circulation, linking circulation and gas exchange in the lungs, and the high-pressure systemic circulation, providing oxygen and nutrients to the tissues.

➤ Blood flows down a pressure gradient from the high-pressure arterial circulation to the low-pressure venous circulation.

➤ The circulation is a closed system, so the output of the right and left heart must be equal over time for effective functioning of the circulation.

The Heart as a Pump

After you have completed this section of the chapter, you should be able to meet the following objectives:

✦ Describe the structural components and function of the pericardium, myocardium, endocardium, and the heart valves and fibrous skeleton

✦ Draw a figure of the cardiac cycle, incorporating volume, pressure, phonocardiographic, and electrocardiographic changes that occur during atrial and ventricular systole and diastole

✦ Define the terms *preload* and *afterload*

✦ State the formula for calculating the cardiac output and explain the effects that venous return, cardiac contractility, and heart rate have on cardiac output

✦ Describe the cardiac reserve and relate it to the Frank-Starling mechanism

The heart is a four-chambered muscular pump approximately the size of a man's fist that beats an average of 70 times each minute, 24 hours each day, 365 days each year for a lifetime. In 1 day, this pump moves more than 1800 gallons of blood throughout the body, and the work performed by the heart over a lifetime would lift 30 tons to a height of 30,000 ft.

FUNCTIONAL ANATOMY OF THE HEART

The heart is located between the lungs in the mediastinal space of the intrathoracic cavity in a loose-fitting sac called the *pericardium*. It is suspended by the great vessels, with its broader side (*i.e.,* base) facing upward and its tip (*i.e.,* apex) pointing downward, forward, and to the left. The heart is positioned obliquely, so that the right side of the heart is almost fully in front of the left side of the heart, with only a small portion of the lateral left ventricle on the frontal plane of the heart (Fig. 21-3). When the hand is placed on the thorax, the main impact of the heart's contraction is felt against the chest wall at a point between the fifth and sixth ribs, a little below the nipple and approximately 3 inches to the left of the midline. This is called the *point of maximum impulse.*

The wall of the heart is composed of an outer epicardium, which lines the pericardial cavity; the myocardium or muscle layer; and the smooth endocardium, which lines the chambers of the heart. A fibrous skeleton supports the valvular structures of the heart. The interatrial and interventricular septa divide the heart into a right and a left pump, each composed of two muscular chambers: a thin-walled atrium, which serves as a reservoir for blood coming into the heart, and a thick-walled ventricle, which pumps blood out of the heart. The increased thickness of the left ventricular wall results from the additional work this ventricle is required to perform.

Pericardium

The pericardium forms a fibrous covering around the heart, holding it in a fixed position in the thorax and providing physical protection and a barrier to infection. The pericardium consists of a tough outer fibrous layer and a thin inner serous layer. The outer fibrous layer is attached to the great vessels that enter and leave the heart, the sternum, and the diaphragm. The fibrous pericardium is highly resistant to distention; it prevents acute dilatation of the heart chambers and exerts a restraining effect on the left ventricle. The inner serous layer consists of a visceral layer and a parietal layer. The visceral layer, also known as the *epicardium*, covers the entire heart and great vessels and then folds over to form the parietal layer that lines the fibrous pericardium (Fig. 21-4). Between the visceral and parietal layers is the *pericardial cavity*, a potential space that contains 30 to 50 mL of serous fluid. This fluid acts as a lubricant to minimize friction as the heart contracts and relaxes.

Myocardium

The myocardium, or muscular portion of the heart, forms the wall of the atria and ventricles. Cardiac muscle cells, like skeletal muscle, are striated and composed of *sarcomeres* that contain actin and myosin filaments (see Fig. 4-25). They are smaller and more compact than skeletal muscle cells and contain many large mitochondria, reflecting their continuous energy needs. The extracellular matrix of cardiac muscle is filled with a loose connective tissue, called the *endomysium*, containing numerous capillaries that support the function of the contracting muscle cells.

Cardiac muscle contracts much like skeletal muscle, except the contractions are involuntary and the duration of contraction is much longer (see Chapter 4). Unlike the

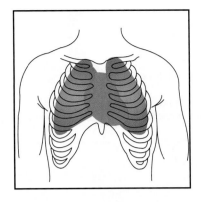

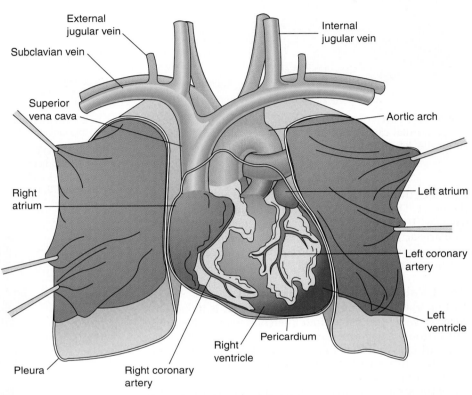

FIGURE 21-3 Anterior view of the heart and great vessels and their relationship to lungs and skeletal structures of the chest cage (*upper left box*).

orderly longitudinal arrangement of skeletal muscle fibers, cardiac muscle cells are arranged as an interconnecting latticework, with their fibers dividing, recombining, then dividing again (Fig. 21-5). The fibers are separated from neighboring cardiac muscle cells by dense structures called *intercalated disks*. The intercalated disks, which are unique to cardiac muscle, contain gap junctions consisting of intramembrane proteins surrounding a core channel that serves as a low-resistance pathway for the passage of ions and electrical impulses from one cardiac cell to another (Fig. 21-6). The myocardium therefore behaves as a single unit, or *syncytium*, rather than as a group of isolated units, as does skeletal muscle. When one myocardial cell becomes excited, the impulse travels rapidly so the heart can beat as a unit.

As in skeletal muscle, cardiac muscle contraction involves actin and myosin filaments, which interact and slide along one another during muscle contraction. However, compared with skeletal muscle cells, cardiac muscle cells have less well-defined sarcoplasmic reticulum for storing calcium, and the distance from the cell membrane to the myofibrils is shorter. Because less calcium can be stored in the muscle cells, cardiac muscle relies more heavily than skeletal muscle on an influx of extracellular calcium ions for contraction. Extracellular calcium, which enters through channels in the cell membrane and T tubules of the muscle cell, triggers the release of intracellular calcium from the sarcoplasmic reticulum, and it participates in muscle contraction. Muscle relaxation results from cessation of calcium release, its removal from the actin-myosin sites, and its energy-dependent reuptake from the cytoplasm into the sarcoplasmic reticulum and other storage sites.

Endocardium

The endocardium is a thin, three-layered membrane that lines the heart. The innermost layer consists of smooth endothelial cells supported by a thin layer of connective tissue. The endothelial lining of the endocardium is contin-

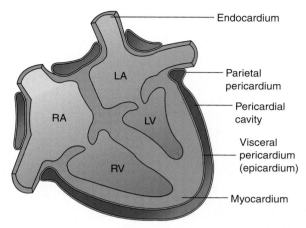

FIGURE 21-4 Layers of the heart, showing the visceral pericardium, the pericardial cavity, and the parietal pericardium. RA, right atrium; LA, left atrium; RV, right ventricle; LV, left ventricle.

uous with the lining of the blood vessels that enter and leave the heart. The middle layer consists of dense connective tissue with elastic fibers. The outer layer, composed of irregularly arranged connective tissue cells, contains blood vessels and branches of the conduction system and is continuous with the myocardium.

Heart Valves and Fibrous Skeleton

An important structural feature of the heart is its fibrous skeleton, which consists of four interconnecting valve rings and surrounding connective tissue. It separates the atria and ventricles and forms a rigid support for attachment of the valves and insertion of the cardiac muscle (Fig. 21-7). The tops of the valve rings are attached to the muscle tissue of the atria, pulmonary trunks, aorta, and valve rings. The bottoms are attached to the ventricular walls. For the heart to function effectively, blood must move through its chambers in an *orthograde* (forward) direction. This unidirectional flow is provided by the heart's two atrioventricular (*i.e.*, tricuspid and mitral) valves and two semilunar (*i.e.*, pulmonic and aortic) valves (Fig. 21-8).

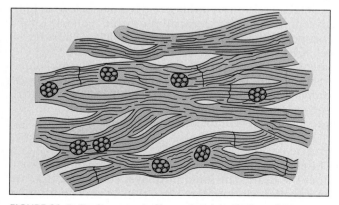

FIGURE 21-5 Cardiac muscle fibers, showing the branching structure and intercalated disks.

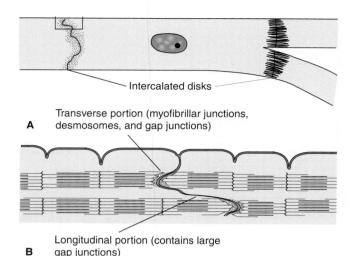

A Transverse portion (myofibrillar junctions, desmosomes, and gap junctions)

B Longitudinal portion (contains large gap junctions)

FIGURE 21-6 (**A**) Cardiac muscle with an intercalated disk at each end. (**B**) Area indicated in **A**, showing where cell junctions lie in the intercalated disks. (Cormack D.H. [1987]. *Ham's histology* [9th ed.]. Philadelphia: J.B. Lippincott)

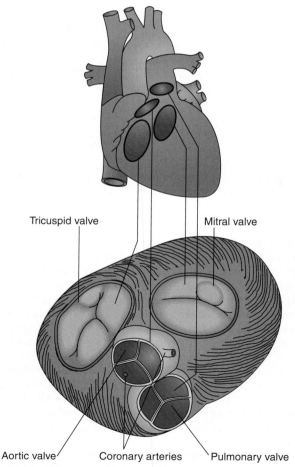

Tricuspid valve   Mitral valve

Aortic valve   Coronary arteries   Pulmonary valve

FIGURE 21-7 Fibrous skeleton of the heart, which forms the four interconnecting valve rings and support for attachment of the valves and insertion of cardiac muscle. (Chaffee E.E., Lytle I.M. [1980]. *Basic physiology and anatomy* [4th ed.]. Philadelphia: J.B. Lippincott)

The atrioventricular (AV) valves control the flow of blood between the atria and the ventricles. The thin edges of the AV valves form cusps, two on the left side of the heart (*i.e., bicuspid valve*) and three on the right side (*i.e., tricuspid valve*). The bicuspid valve is also known as the *mitral* valve. The AV valves are supported by the papillary muscles, which project from the wall of the ventricles, and the chordae tendineae, which attach to the valve. Contraction of the papillary muscles at the onset of systole ensures closure by producing tension on the leaflets of the AV valves before the full force of ventricular contraction pushes against them. The chordae tendineae are cordlike structures that support the AV valves and prevent them from everting into the atria during systole.

The *semilunar* valves control the movement of blood out of the ventricles. The *aortic* valve controls the flow of blood into the aorta; the *pulmonic* valve, also known as the pulmonary valve, controls blood flow into the pulmonary artery. The aortic and pulmonic valves often are referred to as the semilunar valves because their flaps are shaped like half-moons. The pulmonic and the aortic valve have three small, teacup-shaped leaflets. These cuplike structures collect the *retrograde*, or backward, flow of blood that occurs toward the end of systole, enhancing closure. For the development of a perfect seal along the free edges of the semilunar valves, each valve cusp must have a triangular shape, which is facilitated by a nodular thickening at the apex of each leaflet (Fig. 21-9). The openings for the coronary arteries are located in the aorta just above the aortic valve.

There are no valves at the atrial sites (*i.e.*, venae cavae and pulmonary veins) where blood enters the heart. This means that excess blood is pushed back into the veins when the atria become distended. For example, the jugular veins typically become prominent in severe right-sided heart failure when they normally should be flat or collapsed. Likewise, the pulmonary venous system becomes congested when outflow from the left atrium is impeded.

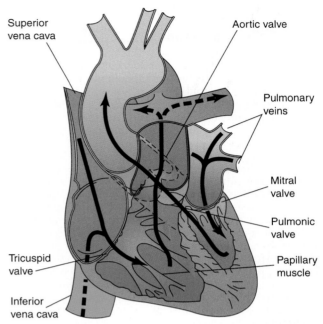

FIGURE 21-8 Valvular structures of the heart. The atrioventricular valves are in an open position, and the semilunar valves are closed. There are no valves to control the flow of blood at the inflow channels (*i.e.*, vena cava and pulmonary veins) to the heart.

CARDIAC CYCLE

The term *cardiac cycle* is used to describe the rhythmic pumping action of the heart. The cardiac cycle is divided into two parts: *systole*, the period during which the ventricles are contracting, and *diastole*, the period during which the ventricles are relaxed and filling with blood. Simultaneous changes occur in left atrial pressure, left ventricular pressure, aortic pressure, ventricular volume, the electro-

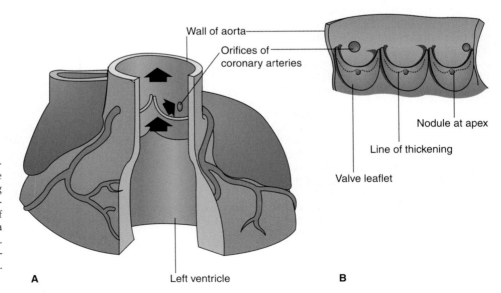

FIGURE 21-9 Diagram of the aortic valve. (**A**) The position of the aorta at the base of the ascending aorta is indicated. (**B**) The appearance of the three leaflets of the aortic valve when the aorta is cut open and spread out, flat. (Cormack D.H. [1987]. *Ham's histology* [9th ed.]. Philadelphia: J.B. Lippincott)

Heart Sounds

Closure of the heart valves produces vibrations of the surrounding heart tissues and blood that can be detected as the audible "lub-dup" sounds heard with a stethoscope during cardiac auscultation. There are four heart sounds (see Fig. 21-10). The first and second sounds are heard in all healthy individuals. The third and fourth heart sounds usually are not heard and may or may not indicate pathology.

The first and second heart sounds represent closure of the atrioventricular and semilunar valves, respectively. The first heart sound ("lub"), which has a lower pitch and lasts longer (approximately 0.14 second) than the second sound, marks the onset of systole and the closure of the atrioventricular valves. The second heart sound ("dup") occurs with the closure of the semilunar valves; it is shorter (0.10 second) and has a higher pitch than the first heart sound. The second heart sound is a composite sound resulting from the closure of both the aortic and the pulmonic valves. The aortic valve normally closes slightly before the pulmonic valve, causing a separation of the two components of the second heart sound. During expiration, aortic valve closure precedes pulmonic valve closure by 0.02 to 0.04 second. During inspiration, this difference is increased to 0.04 to 0.06 second because there is an increase in venous return to the right heart, and it takes longer for the right ventricle to empty and the pulmonic valve to close. At the same time, less blood is returning to the left ventricle, causing the aortic valve to close slightly earlier. An audible widening of the second heart sound that occurs with inspiration is a normal finding. It often is referred to as a *physiologic splitting* and can be heard only in the left second intercostal space.

The third heart sound is low pitched and occurs during rapid filling of the ventricles early in diastole, approximately 0.12 second after the second heart sound. It usually is heard only in young persons or in patients with heart failure. The fourth heart sound is produced by atrial contraction during the last third of diastole; it is audible only in conditions in which resistance to ventricular filling occurs during late diastole. The heart sounds and their relation to the cardiac cycle are shown in Figure 21-10.

Heart murmurs are caused by abnormal vibrations produced by turbulent blood flow. In the heart, turbulence occurs when the velocity of blood flow is increased, the valve diameter is decreased, or the viscosity of the blood is decreased. For example, very high velocities of flow may be reached when blood is ejected through a narrowed, or stenotic, heart valve. Severe anemia may reduce blood viscosity to the point at which turbulence occurs. Auscultation to detect murmurs or abnormalities of the heart sounds is a valuable diagnostic procedure. Although auscultation of the heart does not involve the use of expensive equipment, it does require a trained ear and a thorough understanding of the physiologic events associated with valvular function and the cardiac cycle.

cardiogram (ECG), and heart sounds during the cardiac cycle (Fig. 21-10).

The electrical activity, recorded on the ECG, precedes the mechanical events of the cardiac cycle. The small, rounded P wave of the ECG represents depolarization of the sinoatrial node (*i.e.*, pacemaker of the heart), the atrial conduction tissue, and the atrial muscle mass. The QRS complex registers the depolarization of the ventricular conduction system and the ventricular muscle mass. The T wave on the ECG occurs during the last half of systole and represents repolarization of the ventricles. The cardiac conduction system and the ECG are discussed in detail in Chapter 25.

Ventricular Systole and Diastole

Ventricular systole is divided into two periods: the isovolumetric contraction period and the ejection period. The *isovolumetric contraction period*, which begins with the closure of the AV valves and occurrence of the first heart sound, heralds the onset of systole. Immediately after closure of the AV valves, there is an additional 0.02 to 0.03 second during which the semilunar outlet (pulmonic and aortic) valves remain closed. During this period, the

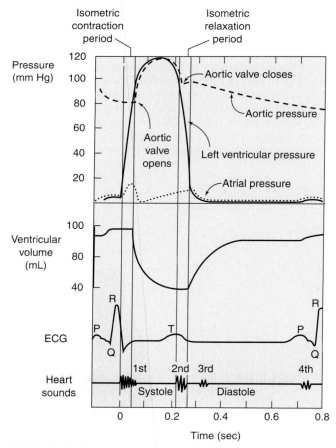

FIGURE 21-10 Events in the cardiac cycle, showing changes in aortic pressure, left ventricular pressure, atrial pressure, left ventricular volume, the electrocardiogram (ECG), and heart sounds.

volume remains the same but the ventricles are contracting. The ventricular pressures rise abruptly during this time because no blood is leaving the heart; the ventricles continue to contract until left ventricular pressure is slightly higher than aortic pressure, and right ventricular pressure is higher than pulmonary artery pressure. At this point, the semilunar valves open, signaling the onset of the *ejection period*. Approximately 60% of the stroke volume is ejected during the first quarter of systole, and the remaining 40% is ejected during the next two quarters of systole. Little blood is ejected from the heart during the last quarter of systole, although the ventricle remains contracted. At the end of systole, the ventricles relax, causing a precipitous fall in intraventricular pressures. As this occurs, blood from the large arteries flows back toward the ventricles, causing the aortic and pulmonic valves to snap shut—an event that is marked by the second heart sound.

The aortic pressure reflects changes in the ejection of blood from the left ventricle. There is a rise in pressure and stretching of the elastic fibers in the aorta as blood is ejected into the aorta at the onset of the ejection period. The aortic pressure continues to rise and then begins to fall during the last quarter of systole as blood flows out of the aorta into the peripheral vessels.

Diastole represents the period of ventricular relaxation. At the end of systole, the left ventricle begins to relax and its pressure falls below that in the aorta, at which point the aortic valve closes, giving rise to the second heart sound. The *incisura*, or notch, in the aortic pressure tracing represents closure of the aortic valve. The aorta is highly elastic and as such stretches during systole to accommodate the blood that is being ejected from the left heart during systole. During diastole, recoil of the elastic fibers in the aorta serves to maintain the arterial pressure.

Ventricular diastole is marked by ventricular filling. After closure of the semilunar valves, the ventricles continue to relax for another 0.03 to 0.06 second (the *isovolumetric relaxation period*). During this time, ventricular volume remains the same but ventricular pressure drops until it becomes less than atrial pressure. As this happens, the AV valves open, and the blood that has been accumulating in the atria during systole flows into the ventricles. Most of ventricular filling occurs during the first third of diastole, which is called the *rapid filling period*. During the middle third of diastole, inflow into the ventricles is almost at a standstill. The last third of diastole is marked by atrial contraction, which gives an additional thrust to ventricular filling. When audible, the third heart sound is heard during the rapid filling period of diastole as blood flows into a distended or noncompliant ventricle. A fourth heart sound can occur during the last third of diastole as the atria contract.

During diastole, the ventricles increase their volume to approximately 120 mL (*i.e.*, the *end-diastolic volume*), and at the end of systole, approximately 50 mL of blood (*i.e.*, the *end-systolic volume*) remains in the ventricles (Fig. 21-11). The difference between the end-diastolic and end-systolic volumes (approximately 70 mL) is called the *stroke volume*. The *ejection fraction*, which is the stroke volume divided by

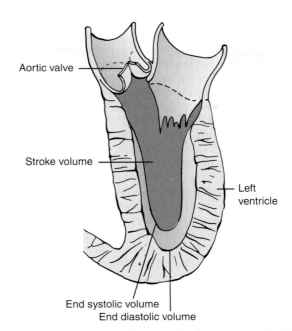

FIGURE 21-11 The ejection fraction, which represents the difference between the end-diastolic and end-systolic volumes.

the end-diastolic volume, represents the fraction or percentage of the diastolic volume that is ejected from the heart during systole.

Atrial Filling and Contraction

Atrial contraction occurs during the last third of diastole. There are three main atrial pressure waves that occur during the cardiac cycle. The *a* wave is caused by atrial contraction. The *c* wave occurs as the ventricles begin to contract, and their increased pressure causes the AV valves to bulge into the atria. The *v* wave results from a slow buildup of blood in the atria toward the end of systole when the AV valves are still closed. The right atrial pressure waves are transmitted to the internal jugular veins as pulsations. These pulsations can be observed visually and may be used to assess cardiac function. For example, exaggerated *a* waves occur when the volume of the right atrium is increased because of impaired emptying into the right ventricle.

Because there are no valves between the junctions of the central veins (*i.e.*, venae cavae and pulmonary veins) and the atria, atrial filling occurs during both systole and diastole. During normal quiet breathing, right atrial pressure usually varies between −2 and +2 mm Hg. It is this low atrial pressure that maintains the movement of blood from the systemic circulation into the right atrium and from the pulmonary veins into the left atrium. Right atrial pressure is regulated by a balance between the ability of the heart to move blood out of the right heart and through the left heart into the systemic circulation and the tendency of blood to flow from the peripheral circulation into the right atrium.

When the heart pumps strongly, right atrial pressure is decreased and atrial filling is enhanced. Right atrial pressure is also affected by changes in intrathoracic pressure. It is decreased during inspiration when intrathoracic pressure becomes more negative, and it is increased during coughing or forced expiration when intrathoracic pressure becomes more positive. Venous return is a reflection of the amount of blood in the systemic circulation that is available for return to the right heart and the force that moves blood back to the right side of the heart. Venous return is increased when the blood volume is expanded or when right atrial pressure falls and is decreased in hypovolemic shock or when right atrial pressure rises.

Although the main function of the atria is to store blood as it enters the heart, these chambers also act as pumps that aid in ventricular filling. This function becomes more important during periods of increased activity when the diastolic filling time is decreased because of an increase in heart rate or when heart disease impairs ventricular filling. In these two situations, the cardiac output would fall drastically were it not for the action of the atria. It has been estimated that atrial contraction can contribute as much as 30% to cardiac reserve during periods of increased need, while having little or no effect on cardiac output during rest.

REGULATION OF CARDIAC PERFORMANCE

The efficiency of the heart as a pump often is measured in terms of *cardiac output* or the amount of blood the heart pumps each minute. The cardiac output (CO) is the product of the *stroke volume* (SV) and the *heart rate* (HR) and can be expressed by the equation: $CO = SV \times HR$. The cardiac output varies with body size and the metabolic needs of the tissues. It increases with physical activity and decreases during rest and sleep. The average cardiac output in normal adults ranges from 3.5 to 8.0 L/minute. In the highly trained athlete, this value can increase to levels as high as 32 L/minute during maximum exercise.

The *cardiac reserve* refers to the maximum percentage of increase in cardiac output that can be achieved above the normal resting level. The normal young adult has a cardiac reserve of approximately 300% to 400%. The heart's ability to increase its output according to body needs mainly depends on four factors: the *preload*, or ventricular filling; the *afterload*, or resistance to ejection of blood from the heart; *cardiac contractility*; and the *heart rate*. Cardiac performance is influenced by the work demands of the heart and the ability of the coronary circulation to meet its metabolic needs (see Chapter 24).

Preload

The preload represents the volume work of the heart. It is called the *preload* because it is the work imposed on the heart before the contraction begins. Preload represents the amount of blood that the heart must pump with each beat and is largely determined by the venous return to the heart and the accompanying stretch of the muscle fibers.

The anatomic arrangement of the actin and myosin filaments in the myocardial muscle fibers is such that the tension or force of contraction is greatest when the muscle fibers are stretched just before the heart begins to contract. The maximum force of contraction and cardiac output is achieved when venous return produces an increase in left ventricular end-diastolic filling (*i.e.*, preload) such that the muscle fibers are stretched approximately two and one-half times their normal resting length (Fig. 21-12, *curve B*). When the muscle fibers are stretched to this degree, there is optimal overlap of the actin and myosin filaments and number of *crossbridge attachments* needed for maximal contraction.

The increased force of contraction that accompanies an increase in ventricular end-diastolic volume is referred to as the *Frank-Starling mechanism* or Starling's law of the heart. The Frank-Starling mechanism allows the heart to adjust its pumping ability to accommodate various levels of venous return. Cardiac output is less when decreased filling causes excessive overlap of the actin and myosin filaments or when the filaments are pulled too far apart because of excessive filling.

Afterload

The afterload is the pressure or tension work of the heart. It is the pressure that the heart must generate to move blood

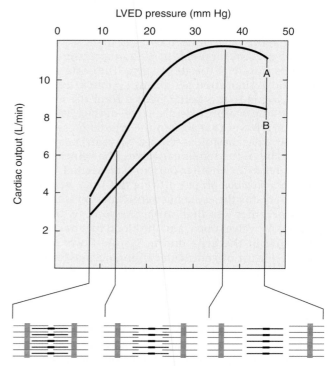

FIGURE 21-12 (Top) Starling ventricular function curve. An increase in left ventricular end-diastolic (LVED) pressure produces an increase in cardiac output (*curve B*) by means of the Frank-Starling mechanism. The maximum force of contraction and increased stroke volume are achieved when diastolic filling causes the muscle fibers to be stretched about two and one half times their resting length. In *curve A*, an increase in cardiac contractility produces an increase in cardiac output without a change in LVED volume and pressure. **(Bottom)** Stretching of the actin and myosin filaments at the different LVED filling pressures.

The Heart

➤ The heart is a four-chambered pump consisting of two atria (the right atrium, which receives blood returning to the heart from the systemic circulation, and the left atrium, which receives oxygenated blood from the lungs) and two ventricles (a right ventricle, which pumps blood to the lungs, and a left ventricle, which pumps blood into the systemic circulation).

➤ Heart valves control the direction of blood flow from the atria to the ventricles (the atrioventricular valves), from the right side of the heart to the lungs (pulmonic valve), and from the left side of the heart to the systemic circulation (aortic valve).

➤ The myocardium, or muscle layer of the atria and ventricles, produces the pumping action of the heart. Intercalated disks between cardiac muscle cells contain gap junctions that allow for immediate communication of electrical signals from one cell to another so the cardiac muscle acts as a single unit, or syncytium.

➤ The cardiac cycle is divided into two major periods: systole, when the ventricles are contracting, and diastole, when the ventricles are relaxed and filling.

➤ The cardiac output or amount of blood that the heart pumps each minute is determined by the amount of blood pumped with each beat (stroke volume) and the number of times the heart beats each minute (heart rate). Cardiac reserve refers to the maximum percentage of increase in cardiac output that can be achieved above the normal resting level.

➤ The work of the heart is determined by the volume of blood it pumps out (preload) and the pressure that it must generate to pump the blood out of the heart (afterload).

into the aorta. It is called the *afterload* because it is the work presented to the heart after the contraction has commenced. The systemic arterial blood pressure is the main source of afterload work on the left heart and the pulmonary arterial pressure is the main source of afterload work for the right heart. The afterload work of the left ventricle is increased with narrowing (*i.e.*, stenosis) of the aortic valve. For example, in the late stages of aortic stenosis, the left ventricle may need to generate systolic pressures up to 300 mm Hg to move blood through the diseased valve.

Cardiac Contractility

Cardiac contractility refers to the ability of the heart to change its force of contraction without changing its resting

(*i.e.*, diastolic) length. The contractile state of the myocardial muscle is determined by biochemical and biophysical properties that govern the actin and myosin interactions in the myocardial cells. It is strongly influenced by the number of calcium ions that are available to participate in the contractile process.

An *inotropic* influence is one that modifies the contractile state of the myocardium independent of the Frank-Starling mechanism (see Fig. 21-12, *curve A*). For instance, sympathetic stimulation produces a positive inotropic effect by increasing the calcium that is available for interaction between the actin and myosin filaments. Hypoxia exerts a negative inotropic effect by interfering with the generation of adenosine triphosphate (ATP), which is needed for muscle contraction.

Heart Rate

The heart rate determines the frequency with which blood is ejected from the heart. Therefore, as heart rate increases, cardiac output tends to increase. As the heart rate increases, the time spent in diastole is reduced, and there is less time for the filling of the ventricles before the onset of systole. At a heart rate of 75 beats per minute, one cardiac cycle lasts 0.8 second, of which approximately 0.3 second is spent in systole and approximately 0.5 second in diastole. As the heart rate increases, the time spent in systole remains approximately the same, whereas that spent in diastole decreases. This leads to a decrease in stroke volume; at high heart rates, it may cause a decrease in cardiac output. One of the dangers of ventricular tachycardia is a reduction in cardiac output because the heart does not have time to fill adequately.

In summary, the heart is a four-chambered muscular pump that lies in the pericardial sac within the mediastinal space of the intrathoracic cavity. The wall of the heart is composed of an outer epicardium, which lines the pericardial cavity; a fibrous skeleton; the myocardium, or muscle layer; and the smooth endocardium, which lines the chambers of the heart. The four heart valves control the direction of blood flow.

The cardiac cycle describes the pumping action of the heart. It is divided into two parts: systole, during which the ventricles contract and blood is ejected from the heart, and diastole, during which the ventricles are relaxed and blood is filling the heart. The stroke volume (approximately 70 mL) represents the difference between the end-diastolic volume (approximately 120 mL) and the end-systolic volume (approximately 50 mL). The electrical activity of the heart, as represented on the ECG, precedes the mechanical events of the cardiac cycle. The heart sounds signal the closing of the heart valves during the cardiac cycle. Atrial contraction occurs during the last third of diastole. Although the main function of the atria is to store blood as it enters the heart, atrial contraction acts to increase cardiac output during periods of increased activity when the filling time is reduced or in disease conditions in which ventricular filling is impaired.

The heart's ability to increase its output according to body needs depends on the preload, or filling of the ventricles (*i.e.*, end-diastolic volume); the afterload, or resistance to ejection of blood from the heart; cardiac contractility, which is determined by the interaction of the actin and myosin filaments of cardiac muscle fibers; and the heart rate, which determines the frequency with which blood is ejected from the heart. The maximum force of cardiac contraction occurs when an increase in preload stretches muscle fibers of the heart to approximately two and one-half times their resting length (*i.e.*, Frank-Starling mechanism).

Blood Vessels and the Systemic Circulation

After you have completed this section of the chapter, you should be able to meet the following objectives:

+ Compare the structure and function of arteries, arterioles, veins, and capillaries
+ Describe the structure and function of vascular smooth muscle
+ Use the term *compliance* to describe the characteristics of arterial and venous blood vessels
+ Define the term *hemodynamics* and describe the effects of blood pressure; vessel radius, length, and cross-sectional area; and blood viscosity on the characteristics of blood flow
+ Use Laplace's law to explain the effect of radius size on the pressure and wall tension in a vessel
+ Use the equation blood pressure = cardiac output × peripheral vascular resistance to explain the regulation of arterial blood pressure
+ Describe mechanisms involved in short-term and long-term regulation of blood pressure
+ Define autoregulation and characterize mechanisms responsible for short-term and long-term regulation of blood flow

The vascular system functions in the delivery of oxygen and nutrients and removal of wastes from the tissues. It consists of arteries and arterioles, the capillaries, and the venules and veins. Although blood vessels are often compared with a system of plumbing pipes, this analogy serves only as a starting point. Blood vessels are dynamic structures that constrict and relax to adjust blood pressure and flow to meet the varying needs of the many different tissue types and organ systems. Structures such as the heart, brain, liver, and kidneys require a large and continuous flow to carry out their vital functions. In other tissues such as the skin and skeletal muscle, the need for blood flow varies with the level of function. For example, there is a need for increased blood flow to the skin during fever and for increased skeletal muscle blood flow during exercise.

BLOOD VESSELS

All blood vessels, except the capillaries, have walls composed of three layers, or coats, called *tunicae* (Fig. 21-13). The *tunica externa*, or *tunica adventitia*, is the outermost covering of the vessel. This layer is composed of fibrous and connective tissues that support the vessel. The *tunica media*, or middle layer, is largely a smooth muscle layer that constricts to regulate and control the diameter of the vessel. The *tunica intima*, or inner layer, has an elastic layer that joins the media and a thin layer of endothelial cells that lie adjacent to the blood. The endothelial layer provides a smooth and slippery inner surface for the vessel. This smooth inner lining, as long as it remains intact, prevents platelet adherence and blood clotting. The layers of the different types of blood vessels vary with vessel function. The walls of the arterioles, which control blood pressure, have large amounts of smooth muscle. Veins are thin-walled, distensible, and collapsible vessels. Capillaries are single-cell–thick vessels designed for the exchange of gases, nutrients, and waste materials.

Arteries and Arterioles

The arterial system consists of the large and medium-sized arteries and the arterioles. Arteries are thick-walled vessels with large amounts of elastic fibers. The elasticity of these vessels allows them to stretch during cardiac systole, when the heart contracts and blood enters the circulation, and to recoil during diastole, when the heart relaxes. The arterioles, which are predominantly smooth muscle, serve as resistance vessels for the circulatory system. They act as control valves through which blood is released as it moves into the capillaries. Changes in the activity of sympathetic fibers

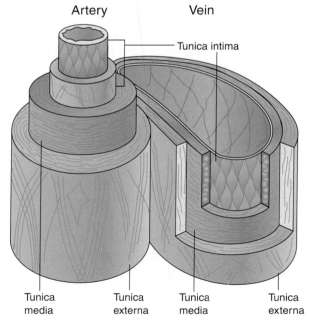

FIGURE 21-13 Medium-sized artery and vein, showing the relative thickness of the three layers. (Chaffee E.E., Lytle I.M. [1980]. *Basic physiology and anatomy* [4th ed.]. Philadelphia: J.B. Lippincott)

Capillaries

Capillaries are microscopic, single-cell–thick vessels that connect the arterial and venous segments of the circulation. In each person, there are approximately 10 billion capillaries, with a total surface area of 500 to 700 m². The capillary wall is composed of a single layer of endothelial cells surrounded by a basement membrane (Fig. 21-14).

Intracellular junctions join the capillary endothelial cells; these are called the *capillary pores*. Lipid-soluble materials diffuse directly through the capillary cell membrane. Water and water-soluble materials leave and enter the capillary through the capillary pores. The size of the capillary pores varies with capillary function. In the brain, the endothelial cells are joined by tight junctions that form the blood-brain barrier. This prevents substances that would alter neural excitability from leaving the capillary. In organs that process blood contents, such as the liver, capillaries have large pores so that substances can pass easily through the capillary wall. In the kidneys, the glomerular capillaries have small openings called *fenestrations* that pass directly through the middle of the endothelial cells. Fenestrated capillary walls are consistent with the filtration function of the glomerulus.

Veins and Venules

The veins and venules are thin-walled, distensible, and collapsible vessels. The venules collect blood from the capillaries, and the veins transport blood back to the heart. The veins are capable of enlarging and storing large quantities of blood, which can be made available to the circulation as needed. Even though the veins are thin walled, they are muscular. This allows them to contract or expand to accommodate varying amounts of blood. Veins are innervated by the sympathetic nervous system. When blood is lost from the circulation, the veins constrict as a means of maintaining intravascular volume.

The venous system is a low-pressure system, and when a person is in the upright position, blood flow in the venous

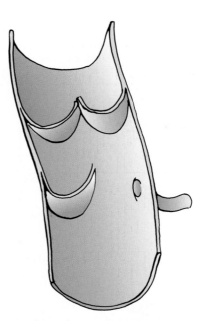

FIGURE 21-15 Portion of a femoral vein opened, to show the valves. The direction of flow is upward.

system must oppose the effects of gravity. Valves in the veins of extremities prevent retrograde flow (Fig. 21-15), and with the help of skeletal muscles that surround and intermittently compress the veins in a milking manner, blood is moved forward to the heart. Their pressure ranges from approximately 10 mm Hg at the end of the venules to approximately 0 mm Hg at the entrance of the vena cava into the heart. There are no valves in the abdominal or thoracic veins, and blood flow in these veins is heavily influenced by the pressure in the abdominal and thoracic cavities, respectively.

Vascular Smooth Muscle

Smooth muscle contracts slowly and generates high forces for long periods with low energy requirements; it uses only 1/10 to 1/300 the energy of skeletal muscle. These characteristics are important in structures, such as blood vessels, that must maintain their tone day in and day out.

Although vascular smooth muscle contains actin and myosin filaments, these contractile filaments are not arranged in striations as they are in skeletal and cardiac muscle. The smooth muscle fibers are instead linked together in a strong, cable-like system that generates a circular pull as it contracts. Smooth muscle also lacks the regulatory protein, troponin, which initiates crossbridge formation in skeletal and cardiac muscle (see Chapter 4). Instead, smooth muscle has a regulatory protein called *calmodulin* that binds calcium. The calcium-calmodulin complex activates myosin kinase, a phosphorylating enzyme that initiates crossbridge formation (Fig. 21-16).

Compared with skeletal and cardiac muscle, smooth muscle has less well-developed sarcoplasmic reticulum for storing intracellular calcium, and it has very few fast sodium channels. Depolarization of smooth muscle instead relies

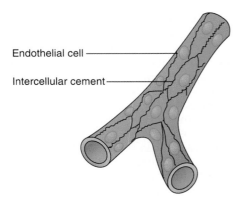

FIGURE 21-14 Endothelial cells and intercellular cement in a section of capillary.

Endothelial cell

Intercellular cement

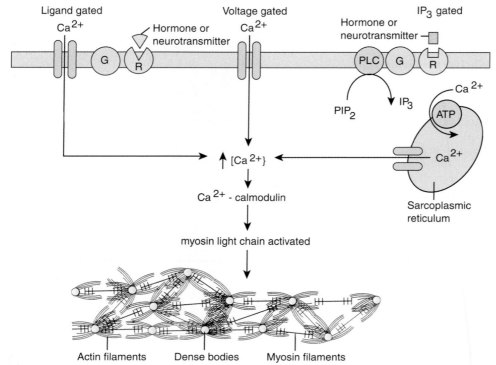

FIGURE 21-16 Mechanism of vascular smooth muscle contraction. Calmodulin binds calcium that enters through calcium channels in the cell membrane or is released from the sarcoplasmic reticulum. The calcium-calmodulin complex, in turn, activates myosin kinase, a phosphorylating enzyme, which initiates cross-bridge formation. Smooth muscle, which lacks the striations of cardiac and skeletal muscle, relies on the dense bodies to form a cable-like structure that produces a circular pull as the muscle contracts.

largely on extracellular calcium, which enters through calcium channels in the muscle membrane.

Smooth muscle has voltage-gated calcium channels that respond to changes in membrane potential and receptor-activated calcium channels. Receptor-activated channels respond to chemical messengers such as norepinephrine that can act in an excitatory manner that causes the channels to remain closed. Sympathetic nervous system control of vascular smooth muscle tone occurs by way of receptor-activated channels. In general, α-adrenergic receptors are excitatory and produce vasoconstriction, and β-adrenergic receptors are inhibitory and produce vasodilation. Calcium channel blocking drugs cause vasodilation by blocking calcium entry through the calcium channels.

Smooth muscle contraction and relaxation also occur in response to local tissue factors such as lack of oxygen, increased hydrogen ion concentrations, and excess carbon dioxide. Nitric oxide, formerly known as the *endothelial relaxing factor*, acts locally to produce smooth muscle relaxation and regulate blood flow. These factors are discussed more fully in the section on Local Control of Blood Flow.

PRINCIPLES OF BLOOD FLOW

The term *hemodynamics* (*hemo* means "blood," and *dynamic* refers to the relation between motion and forces) describes the physical principles governing pressure, flow, and resistance as they relate to the cardiovascular system. The hemodynamics of the circulatory system are complex. The heart is an intermittent pump, and as a result, blood flow in the arterial circulation is pulsatile. The blood vessels are branched, distensible tubes of various dimensions. The blood is a suspension of blood cells, platelets, lipid globules, and plasma proteins. Despite this complexity, the function of the circulatory system can be explained by the principles of basic fluid mechanics that apply to nonbiologic systems, such as household plumbing systems.

Pressure, Flow, and Resistance

The most important factors governing the function of the circulatory system are *volume*, *pressure*, *resistance*, and *flow*. Optimal function requires a volume that is sufficient to fill the vascular compartment and a pressure that is sufficient to ensure blood flow to all body tissues.

Blood flow is determined by two factors: a pressure difference between the two ends of a vessel or group of vessels and the resistance that blood must overcome as it moves through the vessel or vessels (Fig. 21-17). The relation between pressure, resistance, and flow is expressed by the equation $F = P/R$, in which F is the blood flow, P is the difference in pressure between the two ends of the system, and R is the resistance to flow through the system.

The total resistance that the blood encounters as it flows through the systemic circulation is referred to as the *sys-*

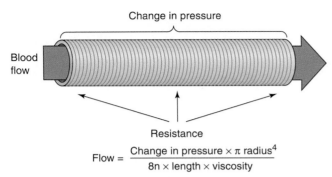

$$\text{Flow} = \frac{\text{Change in pressure} \times \pi \text{ radius}^4}{8n \times \text{length} \times \text{viscosity}}$$

FIGURE 21-17 Factors that affect blood flow (Poiseuille's law). Increasing the pressure difference between the two ends of the vessel increases flow. Flow diminishes as resistance increases. Resistance is directly proportional to blood viscosity and the length of the vessel and inversely proportional to the fourth power of the radius.

temic vascular resistance (SVR). In the systemic circulation, blood flow is represented by the cardiac output (CO) and SVR. The SVR cannot be measured directly. Instead, it is estimated by rearranging the variables in the previous equation ($SVR = P/CO$), in which P represents the pressure difference between the aortic or mean arterial pressure (approximately 100 mm Hg) and right atrial pressure (approximately 0 mm Hg). The flow (F) or cardiac output is approximately 100 mL/second at rest. The SVR is therefore 100/100 or 1 peripheral resistance unit (PRU). The total resistance in the pulmonary circulation is only approximately 0.12 PRU. In this case, the blood flow is the same as in the systemic circulation, but the pressure difference between the pulmonary artery and left atrium (16 − 4 mm Hg) is much less.

A helpful equation for understanding factors that affect blood flow ($F = \Delta P \times \pi \times r^4/8n \times L \times \text{viscosity}$) was derived by the French physician Poiseuille more than a century ago (see Fig. 21-17). According to this equation, the two most important determinants of flow in the circulatory system are a difference in pressure (ΔP) and the vessel radius to the fourth power (r^4). The length (L) of vessels does not usually change and 8n is a constant that does not change. Because flow is directly related to the fourth power of the radius, small changes in vessel radius can produce large changes in flow to an organ or tissue. For example, if the pressure difference remains constant, the rate of flow is 16 times greater in a vessel with a radius of 2 mm than in a vessel with a radius of 1 mm. The reader is asked to consider the consequences of a 25%, 50%, and 75% narrowing of a coronary artery in terms of blood flow to the myocardium.

According to Poiseuille's equation, blood flow is also affected by the viscosity of blood. Viscosity is the resistance to flow caused by the friction of molecules in a fluid. The viscosity of a fluid is largely related to its thickness. The more particles that are present in a solution, the greater the frictional forces that develop between the molecules. Unlike water that flows through plumbing pipes, blood is a nonhomogeneous liquid. It contains blood cells, platelets, fat globules, and plasma proteins that increase its viscosity. The red blood cells, which constitute 40% to 45% of the formed elements of the blood, largely determine the viscos-

ity of the blood. When measured in relation to water, the relative viscosity of plasma is 1.5, and at a normal hematocrit of 42% to 45%, that of whole blood is 3.0. Under special conditions, temperature may affect viscosity. There is a 2% rise in viscosity for each 1°C decrease in body temperature, a fact that helps explain the sluggish blood flow seen in persons with hypothermia.

Cross-sectional Area and Velocity of Flow

Velocity is a distance measurement; it refers to the speed or linear movement with time (centimeters per second) with which blood flows through a vessel. *Flow* is a volume measurement (milliliters per second); it is determined by the cross-sectional area of a vessel and the velocity of flow (Fig. 21-18). When the flow through a given segment of the circulatory system is constant—as it must be for continuous flow—the velocity is inversely proportional to the cross-sectional area of the vessel (*i.e.*, the smaller the cross-sectional area, the greater the velocity of flow). This phenomenon can be compared with cars moving from a two-lane to a single-lane section of a highway. To keep traffic moving at its original pace, cars would have to double their speed in the single-lane section of the highway. So it is with flow in the circulatory system.

The linear velocity of blood flow in the circulatory system varies widely from 30 to 35 cm/second in the aorta to 0.2 to 0.3 mm/second in the capillaries. This is because even though each individual capillary is very small, the total cross-sectional area of all the systemic capillaries greatly exceeds the cross-sectional area of other parts of the circulation. As a result of this large surface area, the slower movement of blood allows ample time for exchange of nutrients, gases, and metabolites between the tissues and the blood.

Laminar and Turbulent Flow

Blood flow normally is *laminar*, with the blood components arranged in layers so that the plasma is adjacent to the smooth, slippery endothelial surface of the blood vessel and the blood cells, including the platelets, are in the center or *axis* of the bloodstream (Fig. 21-19). This arrangement reduces friction by allowing the blood layers to slide smoothly over one another, with the axial layer having the most rapid rate of flow.

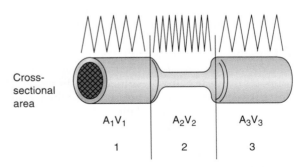

FIGURE 21-18 Effect of cross-sectional area (A) on velocity (V) of flow. In section 1, velocity is low because of an increase in cross-sectional area. In section 2, velocity is increased because of a decrease in cross-sectional area. In section 3, velocity is again reduced because of an increase in cross-sectional area. Flow is assumed to be constant.

Vessel A

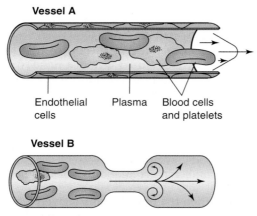

Endothelial   Plasma   Blood cells
cells   and platelets

Vessel B

FIGURE 21-19 Laminar and turbulent flow in blood vessels. Vessel A shows streamlined or laminar flow in which the plasma layer is adjacent to the vessel endothelial layer and blood cells are in the center of the bloodstream. Vessel B shows turbulent flow in which the axial location of the platelets and other blood cells is disturbed.

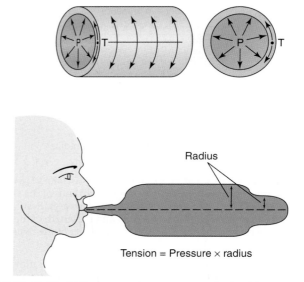

Radius

Tension = Pressure × radius

FIGURE 21-20 (**A**) Pressure and tension in a cylindric blood vessel. The tension (T) tends to open an imaginary slit along the length of the blood vessel. Laplace's law relates pressure, radius, and tension as described in the text. (**B**) Effect of the radius of a cylinder on tension. In a balloon, the tension in the wall is proportional to the radius because the pressure is the same everywhere inside the balloon. The tension is lower in the portion of the balloon with the smaller radius. (Rhoades R.A., Tanner G.A. [1996]. *Medical physiology* [p. 627]. Boston: Little, Brown)

Under certain conditions, blood flow switches from laminar to turbulent flow (see Fig. 21-19). *Turbulent* flow is flow in which blood moves crosswise and lengthwise along a vessel in a manner similar to the eddy currents seen in a rapidly flowing river at a point of obstruction. Turbulent flow is influenced by a number of conditions, including high velocity of flow, change in vessel diameter, and low blood viscosity. The tendency for turbulence to occur increases in direct proportion to the velocity of flow. Imagine the chaos as cars from a two- or three-lane highway converge on a single-lane section of the highway. The same type of thing happens in blood vessels that have been narrowed by disease processes, such as atherosclerosis. Low blood viscosity allows the blood to move faster and accounts for the transient occurrence of heart murmurs in some persons who are severely anemic. Turbulent flow predisposes to clot formation as platelets and other coagulation factors come in contact with the endothelial lining of the vessel. Turbulent flow often can be heard through a stethoscope. An audible murmur in a blood vessel experiencing turbulent flow is referred to as a *bruit*.

Wall Tension, Radius, and Pressure

In a blood vessel, *wall tension* is the force in the vessel wall that opposes the distending pressure inside the vessel. The relation between wall tension, pressure, and the radius of a vessel or sphere was described more than 200 years ago by the French astronomer and mathematician Pierre de Laplace. This relation, which has come to be known as *Laplace's law*, can be expressed by the equation, $P = T/r$, in which T is wall tension, P is the intraluminal pressure, and r is vessel radius. Using Laplace's law, wall tension can also be expressed as the product of vessel pressure times its radius (Fig. 21-20). In this case, the internal pressure expands the vessel until it is exactly balanced by wall tension. The larger the radius, the greater is the tension needed to balance

a particular pressure. This correlation can be compared with a partially inflated long balloon, in which the tension in the more inflated part of the balloon with the larger radius is greater than in the less inflated section with the smaller radius, because the pressure is the same throughout the balloon. These same principles apply to the increased radius of an arterial aneurysm, which is characterized by an outpouching of a segment of the arterial wall. Because of the increased wall tension, an aneurysm tends to progress and may eventually rupture (see Chapter 22).

Laplace's law was later expanded to include wall thickness ($T = P \times r/wall\ thickness$). Wall tension is inversely related to wall thickness, such that the thicker the vessel wall, the lower the tension, and vice versa. In hypertension, arterial vessel walls hypertrophy and become thicker, thereby minimizing wall stress. Laplace's law ($P = T/r$) can also be applied to the pressure required to maintain the patency of small blood vessels. Providing that the thickness of a vessel wall and its tension remain constant, it takes more pressure to overcome wall tension and keep a vessel open as its radius decreases in size. The critical closing pressure refers to the point at which vessels collapse so that blood can no longer flow through them. In circulatory shock, for example, there is a decrease in blood volume and vessel radii, along with a drop in blood pressure. As a result, many of the small vessels collapse as blood pressure drops to the point where it can no longer overcome the wall tension. The collapse of peripheral veins often makes it difficult to insert venous lines that are needed for fluid and blood replacement.

Distention and Compliance

Compliance refers to the total quantity of blood that can be stored in a given portion of the circulation for each millimeter rise in pressure. Compliance (C) is defined by the equation, $C = V/P$, in which V is the change in volume and P is the change in distending pressure. The distending pressure is the difference between the pressure inside the vessel minus the pressure outside the vessel. This is called the *transmural pressure*. As compliance increases, there is less change in transmural pressure with any given change in volume.

Compliance reflects the *distensibility* of the blood vessel (*i.e.*, increase in volume/increase in pressure × original volume). The distensibility of the arteries allows them to accommodate the pulsatile output of the heart. The most distensible of all vessels are the veins, which can increase their volume with only slight changes in pressure, allowing them to function as a reservoir for storing large quantities of blood that can be returned to the circulation when it is needed. The compliance of a vein is approximately 24 times that of its corresponding artery, because it is eight times as distensible and has a volume three times as great.

ARTERIAL BLOOD PRESSURE

Arterial Pulse Pressure

The arterial blood pressure, often referred to simply as the *blood pressure*, results from the intermittent ejection of blood from the left ventricle into the aorta at the onset of systole. It rises during systole as the left ventricle contracts and falls as the heart relaxes during diastole. This creates an *impulse* or *pressure wave* that is transmitted from molecule to molecule along the length of the vessel (Fig. 21-21). In the aorta, this pressure wave is transmitted at a velocity of 4 to

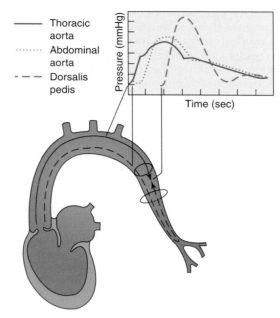

FIGURE 21-21 Amplification of the arterial pressure wave as it moves forward in the peripheral arteries. This amplification occurs as a forward-moving pressure wave merges with a backward-moving reflected pressure wave. (**Inset**) The amplitude of the pressure pulse increases in the thoracic aorta, abdominal aorta, and dorsalis pedis.

6 m/second, which is approximately 20 times faster than the flow of blood. These pressure waves are similar to those created by splashing water in a basin or tub. When taking a pulse, it is the pressure pulses that are felt, and it is the pressure pulses that produce the Korotkoff sounds heard during blood pressure measurement. The tip or maximum deflection of the pressure pulse coincides with the systolic blood pressure, and the minimum point of deflection coincides with the diastolic pressure.

As the pressure wave moves out through the aorta into the arteries, it changes as it collides with reflected waves from the periphery. Just as the waves created by splashing water in a tub increase in amplitude as they hit the edge of the tub and reverse their direction of movement, the pressure pulse increases as it moves to the peripheral arteries. This is why the systolic pressure is higher in the medium-sized arteries than in the aorta even though the diastolic pressure is lower. With peripheral arterial disease, resistance to transmission of the pressure wave increases and a delay occurs in the transmission of the reflected wave, so that the pulse decreases rather than increases in amplitude.

After its initial amplification, the pressure pulse becomes smaller and smaller as it moves through the smaller arteries and arterioles, until it disappears almost entirely in the capillaries. This damping of the pressure pulse is caused by the resistance and distensibility characteristics of these vessels. The increased resistance of these small vessels impedes the transmission of the pressure waves. The distensibility of these vessels is great enough, however, that any small change in flow does not cause a pressure change.

Hemodynamics

➤ Blood flow is directly related to the difference in pressure between the inlet and outlet of a vessel and is inversely related to the resistance to flow through that vessel. Resistance to flow through a vessel is inversely related to the fourth power of the vessel radius (r^4). Small decreases in vessel diameter cause large increases in resistance to flow.

➤ At any given intraluminal pressure, the tension in a vessel wall (the force that opposes the intraluminal pressure) is greater in the vessel with the greater radius.

➤ Compliance (C) is defined by the equation $C = V/P$. A given change in volume (V) causes less of an increase in transmural pressure (P) in a more compliant vessel. A vein is 24 times more compliant than its corresponding artery.

Although the pressure pulses usually are not transmitted to the capillaries, there are situations in which this does occur. For example, injury to a finger or other area of the body often results in a throbbing sensation. In this case, extreme dilatation of the small vessels in the injured area produces a reduction in the dampening of the pressure pulse. Capillary pulsations also occur in conditions that cause exaggeration of aortic pressure pulses, such as aortic regurgitation or patent ductus arteriosus (see Chapter 24).

Two major factors affect the pressure pulse in the arterial system and thereby affect the arterial blood pressure. These two factors are the cardiac output and the resistance that the blood encounters as it moves through the peripheral circulation. The cardiac output is determined by the stroke volume and heart rate (*i.e.*, stroke volume × heart rate). The peripheral vascular resistance reflects the resistance of the arterial vessels, mainly the arterioles. Blood pressure (BP) can be viewed as the product of the cardiac output (CO) and the total peripheral resistance (TPR) or SVR and can be represented by the equation, $BP = CO \times TPR$.

In healthy adults, the pressure at the height of the pressure pulse, called the *systolic pressure*, normally is approximately 120 mm Hg, and the lowest pressure, called the *diastolic pressure*, is approximately 80 mm Hg. The difference between the systolic and diastolic pressure (approximately 40 mm Hg) is called the *pulse pressure*. It reflects the magnitude or height of the pressure pulse. The mean arterial pressure (approximately 90 to 100 mm Hg) represents the average pressure in the arterial system during ventricular contraction and relaxation.

Regulation of Arterial Blood Pressure

Under ordinary conditions, there are moment-by-moment variations in blood pressure related to activities of daily living such as moving from the lying to standing position, exercise, and emotional stress. Normally, blood pressure is regulated at levels sufficient to ensure adequate tissue perfusion. Blood pressure regulation requires the use of short-term and long-term mechanisms.

Short-Term Regulation. Neural and hormonal mechanisms function in the short-term regulation of blood pressure. The short-term adjustments occurring over seconds, minutes, or hours are intended to correct temporary imbalances that occur during the performance of everyday activities such as physical exercise and changes in body position. These mechanisms also are responsible for maintenance of blood pressure at survival levels during life-threatening situations.

Neural Mechanisms. The neural control of blood pressure is mediated by the autonomic nervous system (ANS) through control mechanisms that include intrinsic circulatory reflexes, extrinsic reflexes, and higher neural control centers. The *intrinsic reflexes*, including the *baroreflex* and *chemoreceptor-mediated reflex*, are located in the circulatory system and are essential for rapid and short-term regulation of blood pressure (discussed under Neural Control of Circulatory Function). The *extrinsic reflexes* are found outside the circulation. They include blood pressure responses associated with factors such as pain, cold, and isometric handgrip exercise. The neural pathways for these reactions are largely unknown, and their responses are less consistent than those of the intrinsic reflexes. Among higher-center responses are the central nervous system (CNS) ischemic response and those caused by changes in mood and emotion.

Humoral Mechanisms. A number of hormones and humoral mechanisms contribute to blood pressure regulation, including the *renin-angiotensin-aldosterone* mechanism and *vasopressin*. The renin-angiotensin-aldosterone system plays a central role in blood pressure regulation. Renin is an enzyme that is synthesized, stored, and released from the juxtaglomerular cells of the kidneys in response to a decrease in blood pressure, sympathetic stimulation, or decreased extracellular sodium concentration. Most of the renin that is released leaves the kidney and enters the bloodstream, where it acts enzymatically to convert an inactive circulating plasma protein called *angiotensinogen* to angiotensin I (Fig. 21-22). Angiotensin I travels to the small blood vessels of the lung, where it is converted to angiotensin II by the angiotensin-converting enzyme that is present in the endothelium of the lung vessels. Although angiotensin II has a half-life of several minutes, renin persists in the circulation for 30 minutes to 1 hour and continues to cause production of angiotensin II during this time.

Angiotensin II functions in short-term and long-term regulation of blood pressure. It is a strong vasoconstrictor, particularly of arterioles and to a lesser extent of veins. The vasoconstrictor effect raises peripheral vascular resistance (and blood pressure) and functions in the short-term regulation of blood pressure. For example, the renin-angiotensin system, which is activated during blood loss, produces an increase in TPR even before the blood pressure starts to fall. A second major function of angiotensin II, stimulation of secretion of aldosterone from the adrenal gland, contributes to the long-term regulation of blood pressure by increasing salt and water retention by the kidney. It also acts directly on the kidney to decrease the elimination of salt and water. Angiotensin II plays a significant role in maintaining blood volume in persons on a low-sodium diet.

Vasopressin, or antidiuretic hormone, is released from the posterior pituitary gland in response to decreases in blood volume and blood pressure, an increase in the osmolality of body fluids, and other stimuli. The antidiuretic actions of vasopressin are discussed in Chapter 31. Vasopressin has a direct vasoconstrictor effect on blood vessels, particularly those of the splanchnic circulation. However, long-term increases in vasopressin cannot maintain volume expansion or hypertension, and it does not enhance hypertension produced by sodium-retaining hormones or other vasoconstricting substances. It has been suggested that vasopressin plays a permissive role in hypertension through its fluid-retaining properties or as a neurotransmitter that serves to modify ANS function.

Long-Term Regulation. Neural and hormonal regulation of blood pressure are short-term mechanisms that act rapidly to restore blood pressure. They are, however, ineffective in the long-term regulation of blood pressure. Instead, responsibility for the long-term regulation of blood

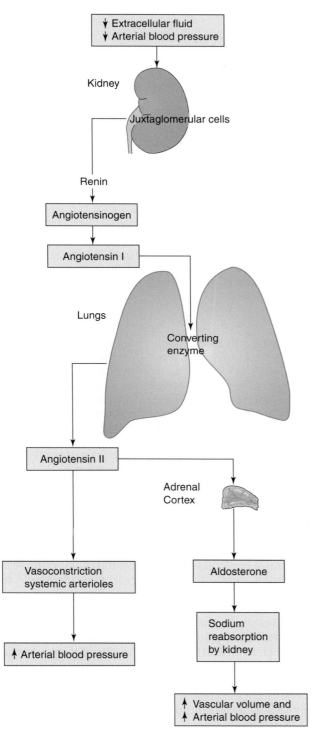

FIGURE 21-22 Control of blood pressure by the renin-angiotensin-aldosterone system. Renin enzymatically converts the plasma protein angiotensinogen to angiotensin I; angiotensin-converting enzyme in the lung converts angiotensin I to angiotensin II; and angiotensin II produces vasoconstriction and increases salt and water retention through direct action on the kidney and through increased aldosterone secretion by the adrenal cortex.

pressure appears to be vested in the kidneys' regulation of the extracellular fluid volume.

Renal–Body Fluid System. According to Arthur Guyton, a noted physiologist, the long-term regulation of blood pressure is vested in the renal–body fluid system that regulates extracellular fluid volume. Accordingly, when the body contains too much extracellular fluid, the arterial pressure increases; when too little fluid is present, blood pressure decreases. For example, an increase in arterial pressure greatly increases the rate at which water (*i.e., pressure diuresis*) and sodium (*i.e., pressure natriuresis*) are excreted by the kidney.

Figure 21-23 illustrates the control of blood pressure by the renal–body fluid system. This graph consists of two intersecting curves: the renal output curve and the straight line that represents the net salt and water intake or level at which the blood pressure is regulated. The only point on the graph at which the intake and output are balanced is at the equilibrium point, which in this case is 100 mm Hg.

As an example of how the renal–body fluid mechanism works, first assume that the blood pressure rises to 150 mm Hg; when this happens, the renal output of water and salt increases and blood pressure returns to the equilibrium point. However, if the blood pressure were to decrease to 70 mm Hg, the kidneys would decrease their output of water

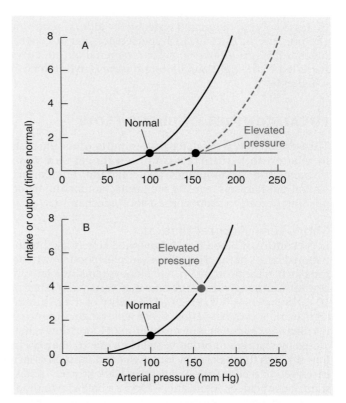

FIGURE 21-23 Two ways in which the arterial pressure can be increased: (**A**) by shifting the renal output curve in the right-hand direction toward a higher pressure level and (**B**) by increasing the intake level of salt and water. (Guyton A.C., Hall J.E. [1996]. *Textbook of medical physiology* [9th ed., p. 223]. Philadelphia: W.B. Saunders)

and salt, causing the blood pressure to rise. The kidneys continue to increase or decrease their elimination of water and salt until the blood pressure has returned to the equilibrium point.

The only way to change the long-term regulation of blood pressure using the concept of the renal–body fluid control system is to change the level of the water and salt line or the pressure range of the renal output curve. For example, a defect in pressure diuresis or natriuresis can shift the curve to the right so that blood pressure is maintained at a higher level. Likewise, a shift in the water and salt intake line raises the equilibrium point to a higher level of pressure.

Increased Fluid Volume. Increased extracellular volume elevates blood pressure through an increase in cardiac output. There are two different ways in which cardiac output increases blood pressure: one is through a direct effect on blood pressure, and the second is an indirect effect resulting from local autoregulation of blood flow. When blood flows through a tissue in excess of its metabolic needs, local blood vessels constrict and return the flow to normal. When cardiac output is increased, all of the tissues of the body are exposed to increased blood flow and autoregulation constricts blood vessels throughout the body; this increases the TPR, producing an increase in blood pressure (see discussion later). Normally, an increase in blood pressure should produce pressure diuresis and natriuresis with an increased output of salt and water by the kidney, returning the pressure to normal. In hypertension, renal control mechanisms are altered such that the renal output curve is shifted to the right and blood pressure is maintained at a higher level.

LOCAL CONTROL OF BLOOD FLOW

Tissue blood flow is regulated on a minute-to-minute basis in relation to tissue needs and on a longer-term basis through the development of collateral circulation. Neural mechanisms regulate the cardiac output and blood pressure needed to support these local mechanisms.

Short-Term Autoregulation

Local control of blood flow is governed largely by the nutritional needs of the tissue. For example, blood flow to organs such as the heart, brain, and kidneys remains relatively constant, although blood pressure may vary over a range of 60 to 180 mm Hg (Fig. 21-24). The ability of the tissues to regulate their own blood flow over a wide range of pressures is called *autoregulation*. Autoregulation of blood flow is mediated by changes in blood vessel tone due to changes in flow through the vessel or by local tissue factors, such as lack of oxygen or accumulation of tissue metabolites (*i.e.*, potassium, lactic acid, or adenosine, which is a breakdown product of ATP). Local control is particularly important in tissues such as skeletal muscle, which has blood flow requirements that vary according to the level of activity.

An increase in local blood flow is called *hyperemia*. The ability of tissues to increase blood flow in situations of increased activity, such as exercise, is called *functional hyper-*

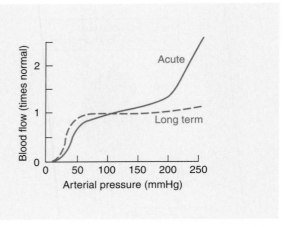

FIGURE 21-24 Effect of increasing arterial pressure on blood flow through a muscle. The *solid curve* shows the effect if pressure is raised over a few minutes. The *dashed curve* shows the effect if the arterial pressure is raised slowly over many weeks. (Guyton A.C., Hall J.E. [1996]. *Textbook of medical physiology* [9th ed., p. 203]. Philadelphia: W.B. Saunders)

emia. When the blood supply to an area has been occluded and then restored, local blood flow through the tissues increases within seconds to restore the metabolic equilibrium of the tissues. This increased flow is called *reactive hyperemia.* The transient redness seen on an arm after leaning on a hard surface is an example of reactive hyperemia. Local control mechanisms rely on a continuous flow from the main arteries; therefore, hyperemia cannot occur when the arteries that supply the capillary beds are narrowed. For example, if a major coronary artery becomes occluded, the opening of channels supplied by that vessel cannot restore blood flow.

Tissue Factors Contributing to Local Control of Blood Flow. Vasodilator substances, formed in tissues in response to a need for increased blood flow, also aid in the local control of blood flow. The most important of these are histamine, serotonin (*i.e.*, 5-hydroxytryptamine), the kinins, and the prostaglandins.

Histamine increases blood flow. Most blood vessels contain histamine in mast cells and nonmast cell stores; when these tissues are injured, histamine is released. In certain tissues, such as skeletal muscle, the activity of the mast cells is mediated by the sympathetic nervous system; when sympathetic control is withdrawn, the mast cells release histamine. Vasodilation then results from increased histamine and the withdrawal of vasoconstrictor activity.

Serotonin is liberated from aggregating platelets during the clotting process; it causes vasoconstriction and plays a major role in control of bleeding. Serotonin is found in brain and lung tissues, and there is some speculation that it may be involved in the vascular spasm associated with some allergic pulmonary reactions and migraine headaches.

The kinins (*i.e.*, kallidins and bradykinin) are liberated from the globulin kininogen, which is present in body fluids. The kinins cause relaxation of arteriolar smooth muscle, increase capillary permeability, and constrict the venules. In exocrine glands, the formation of kinins contributes to the vasodilation needed for glandular secretion.

Prostaglandins are synthesized from constituents of the cell membrane (*i.e.*, the long-chain fatty acid *arachidonic acid*). Tissue injury incites the release of arachidonic acid from the cell membrane, which initiates prostaglandin synthesis. There are several prostaglandins (*e.g.*, E_2, F_2, D_2), which are subgrouped according to their solubility; some produce vasoconstriction and some produce vasodilation. As a rule of thumb, those in the E group are vasodilators, and those in the F group are vasoconstrictors. The adrenal glucocorticoid hormones produce an anti-inflammatory response by blocking the release of arachidonic acid, preventing prostaglandin synthesis.

Endothelial Control of Vasodilation and Vasoconstriction. The *endothelium*, which lies between the blood and the vascular smooth muscle, serves as a physical barrier for vasoactive substances that circulate in the blood. Once thought to be nothing more than a single layer of cells that line blood vessels, it is now known that the endothelium plays an active role in controlling vascular function. In capillaries, which are composed of a single layer of endothelial cells, the endothelium is active in transporting cell nutrients and wastes. In addition to its function in capillary transport, the endothelium removes vasoactive agents such as norepinephrine from the blood, and it produces enzymes that convert precursor molecules to active products (*e.g.*, angiotensin I to angiotensin II in lung vessels).

One of the important functions of the normal endothelium is to synthesize and release factors that control vessel dilation. Of particular importance was the discovery, first reported in the early 1980s, that the intact endothelium was able to produce a factor that caused relaxation of vascular smooth muscle. This factor was originally named *endothelium-derived relaxing factor* and is now known to be *nitric oxide*. Many other cell types produce nitric oxide. In these tissues, nitric oxide has other functions, including modulation of nerve activity in the nervous system.

The normal endothelium maintains a continuous release of nitric oxide, which is formed from L-arginine through the action of an enzyme called *nitric oxide synthase* (Fig. 21-25). The production of nitric oxide can be stimulated by a variety of endothelial *agonists*, including acetylcholine, bradykinin, histamine, and thrombin. *Shear stress* on the endothelium resulting from an increase in blood flow or blood pressure also stimulates nitric oxide production and vessel relaxation. Nitric oxide also inhibits platelet aggregation and secretion of platelet contents, many of which cause vasoconstriction. The fact that nitric oxide is released into the vessel lumen (to inactivate platelets) and away from the lumen (to relax smooth muscle) suggests that it protects against both thrombosis and vasoconstriction. It has been suggested that the tendency toward vasoconstriction that characterizes atherosclerotic vessels may be related to impaired vasodilator function due to disruption of the vessel endothelial layer.

In addition to nitric oxide, the endothelium also produces other vasodilating substances such as the prosta-

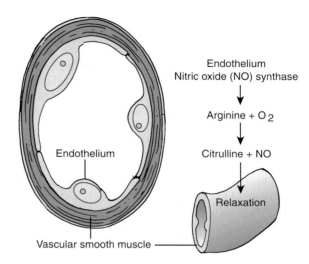

FIGURE 21-25 Function of nitric oxide in smooth muscle relaxation.

glandin, *prostacyclin*, which produces vasodilation and inhibits platelet aggregation. Endothelium-derived vessel relaxation may also be due to a number of other factors that have not been completely characterized and have been collectively called *endothelial-derived hyperpolarizing factor* (EDHF). The hyperpolarization is due to increased potassium efflux.

The endothelium also produces a number of vasoconstrictor substances, including *angiotensin II*, vasoconstrictor prostaglandins, and a family of peptides called *endothelins*. There are at least three endothelins. Endothelin-1, made by human endothelial cells, is the most potent endogenous vasoconstrictor known. Receptors for endothelins also have been identified.

Long-Term Regulation

Collateral circulation is a mechanism for the long-term regulation of local blood flow. In the heart and other vital structures, anastomotic channels exist between some of the smaller arteries. These channels permit perfusion of an area by more than one artery. When one artery becomes occluded, these anastomotic channels increase in size, allowing blood from a patent artery to perfuse the area supplied by the occluded vessel. For example, persons with extensive obstruction of a coronary blood vessel may rely on collateral circulation to meet the oxygen needs of the myocardial tissue normally supplied by that vessel. As with other long-term compensatory mechanisms, the recruitment of collateral circulation is most efficient when obstruction to flow is gradual rather than sudden.

In summary, the walls of all blood vessels, except the capillaries, are composed of three layers: the tunica externa, tunica media, and tunica intima. The layers of the vessel vary with its function. Arteries are thick-walled vessels with large amounts of elastic fibers. The walls of the arterioles, which control blood pressure, have large amounts of smooth muscle. Veins are thin-walled, distensible, and collapsible vessels. Venous flow is designed to return blood to the heart. It is a low-pressure system and relies on venous valves and the action of muscle pumps to offset the effects of gravity. Capillaries are single-cell–thick vessels designed for the exchange of gases, nutrients, and waste materials.

Blood flow is controlled by many of the same mechanisms that control fluid flow in nonbiologic systems. It is influenced by vessel length, pressure differences, vessel radius, blood viscosity, cross-sectional area, and wall tension. The rate of flow is directly related to the pressure difference between the two ends of the vessel and the vessel radius and inversely related to vessel length and blood viscosity. The cross-sectional area of a vessel influences the velocity of flow; as the cross-sectional area decreases, the velocity is increased, and vice versa. Laminar blood flow is flow in which there is layering of blood components in the center of the bloodstream. This reduces frictional forces and prevents clotting factors from coming in contact with the vessel wall. In contrast to laminar flow, turbulent flow is disordered flow, in which the blood moves crosswise and lengthwise in blood vessels. The relation between wall tension, transmural pressure, and radius is described by Laplace's law, which states that wall tension becomes greater as the radius increases. Wall tension is also affected by wall thickness; it increases as the wall becomes thinner and decreases as the wall becomes thicker.

Blood pressure is determined by the cardiac output and peripheral vascular resistance. Normally, blood pressure is regulated at levels sufficient to ensure adequate tissue perfusion. Blood pressure regulation requires the use of short-term and long-term mechanisms. Short-term regulation of blood pressure involves neural and hormonal mechanisms; it occurs over minutes and hours and is intended to correct temporary imbalances in blood pressure, such as those caused by postural changes, exercise, or hemorrhage. Long-term mechanisms control the daily, weekly, and monthly regulation of blood pressure and involve a change in the excretion of salt and water by the kidneys (*i.e.*, the renal–body fluid pressure control system).

The mechanisms that control blood flow are designed to ensure adequate delivery of blood to the capillaries in the microcirculation, where the exchange of cellular nutrients and wastes occurs. Local control is governed largely by the needs of the tissues and is regulated by local tissue factors such as lack of oxygen and the accumulation of metabolites. Hyperemia is a local increase in blood flow that occurs after a temporary occlusion of blood flow. It is a compensatory mechanism that decreases the oxygen debt of the deprived tissues. Collateral circulation is a mechanism for long-term regulation of local blood flow that involves the development of collateral vessels.

Neural Control of Circulatory Function

After you have completed this section of the chapter, you should be able to meet the following objectives:

◆ Describe the distribution of sympathetic and parasympathetic nervous system in innervation of the circulatory system and their effects on heart rate and cardiac contractility

◆ List the types of sympathetic and parasympathetic receptors and characterize their neurotransmitters in terms of circulatory function

◆ Describe the role of the CNS in terms of regulating circulatory function

◆ Explain the role of the ANS in the circulatory response to postural stress, increased intrathoracic pressure, and face immersion

The neural control of the circulatory system occurs primarily through the *sympathetic* and *parasympathetic* divisions of the ANS. The ANS contributes to the control of cardiovascular function through modulation of cardiac (*i.e.*, heart rate and cardiac contractility) and vascular (*i.e.*, peripheral vascular resistance) function.

The neural control centers for the integration and modulation of cardiac function and blood pressure are located bilaterally in the medulla oblongata. The medullary cardiovascular neurons are grouped into three distinct pools that lead to sympathetic innervation of the heart and blood vessels and parasympathetic innervation of the heart. The first two, which control sympathetic-mediated acceleration of heart rate and blood vessel tone, are called the *vasomotor center*. The third, which controls parasympathetic-mediated slowing of heart rate, is called the *cardioinhibitory center*. These brain stem centers receive information from many areas of the nervous system, including the hypothalamus. The arterial baroreceptors and chemoreceptors provide the medullary cardiovascular center with continuous information regarding the function of the circulatory system.

BARORECEPTORS

Baroreceptors are pressure-sensitive receptors located in the walls of blood vessels and the heart. The carotid and aortic baroreceptors are located in strategic positions between the heart and the brain (Fig. 21-26). The baroreceptors respond to a change in the stretch of the vessel wall by sending impulses to cardiovascular centers in the brain stem to effect appropriate changes in heart rate and vascular smooth muscle tone. For example, the fall in blood pressure that occurs on moving from the lying to the standing position produces a decrease in the stretch of the aortic and carotid baroreceptors with a resultant increase in heart rate and sympathetically induced vasoconstriction that causes an increase in peripheral vascular resistance. The rapidity with which the baroreflex response occurs is such that an increase

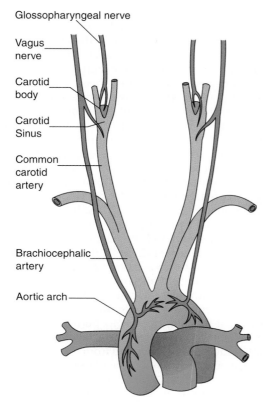

Glossopharyngeal nerve

Vagus nerve

Carotid body

Carotid Sinus

Common carotid artery

Brachiocephalic artery

Aortic arch

FIGURE 21-26 Location and innervation of the aortic arch and carotid sinus baroreceptors and the carotid body chemoreceptors. (Chaffee E.E., Lytle I.M. [1980]. *Basic physiology and anatomy* [4th ed.]. Philadelphia: J.B. Lippincott)

function of the chemoreceptors is to regulate ventilation, they also communicate with the vasomotor center and can induce widespread vasoconstriction. Whenever the arterial pressure drops below a critical level, the chemoreceptors are stimulated because of diminished oxygen supply and a buildup of carbon dioxide and hydrogen ions. In persons with chronic lung disease, systemic and pulmonary hypertension may develop because of hypoxemia (see Chapter 29).

AUTONOMIC REGULATION OF CARDIAC FUNCTION

The heart is innervated by the parasympathetic and sympathetic nervous systems. Parasympathetic innervation of the heart is achieved by means of the *vagus nerve.* The parasympathetic outflow to the heart originates from the vagal nucleus in the medulla. The axons of these neurons pass to the heart in the cardiac branches of the vagus nerve. The effect of vagal stimulation on heart function is largely limited to heart rate, with increased vagal activity producing a slowing of the pulse. Sympathetic outflow to the heart and blood vessels arises from neurons located in the reticular formation of the brain stem. The axons of these neurons descend in the intermediolateral columns of the spinal cord; they exit from the upper thoracic segments of the spinal cord and synapse in the paravertebral ganglia with the postganglionic neurons that innervate the heart. Cardiac sympathetic fibers are widely distributed to the sinoatrial and AV nodes and the myocardium. Increased sympathetic activity produces an increase in the heart rate and the velocity and force of cardiac contraction.

in heart rate usually can be observed within several heartbeats, and the adjustment of blood pressure is usually complete within 1 to 2 minutes. This rapid response is needed to prevent orthostatic hypotension that can result in dizziness and even fainting (see Chapter 23).

The carotid and aortic baroreceptors are often referred to as the *high-pressure baroreceptors* because they are located in the high-pressure arterial side of the circulation. There are also *low-pressure baroreceptors,* which are located in the right atria and pulmonary artery (*i.e.,* the low-pressure side of the circulation). As with other neural receptors, the baroreceptors adapt to prolonged changes in blood pressure and are probably of limited importance in the long-term regulation of blood pressure.

CHEMORECEPTORS

The chemoreceptors are sensitive to changes in the oxygen, carbon dioxide, and hydrogen ion content of the blood. The arterial chemoreceptors are located in the carotid bodies, which lie in the bifurcation of the two common carotids, and in the aortic bodies of the aorta (see Fig. 21-26). Because of their location, these chemoreceptors are always in close contact with the arterial blood. Although the main

AUTONOMIC REGULATION OF VASCULAR FUNCTION

The sympathetic nervous system serves as the final common pathway for controlling the smooth muscle tone of the blood vessels. Most of the sympathetic preganglionic fibers that control vessel function originate in the vasomotor center of the brain stem and travel in the intermediolateral column of the spinal cord and exit with the ventral nerves. They then synapse with postganglionic fibers in the paravertebral ganglia. The sympathetic neurons that supply the blood vessels maintain them in a state of tonic activity, so that even under resting conditions, the blood vessels are partially constricted. Vessel constriction and relaxation are accomplished by altering this basal input. Increasing sympathetic activity causes constriction of some vessels, such as those of the skin, the gastrointestinal tract, and the kidneys. Some blood vessels are supplied by vasoconstrictor and vasodilator fibers. Both types of fibers innervate vessels of skeletal muscle; activation of sympathetic vasodilator fibers provides the muscles with increased blood flow during exercise. Although the parasympathetic nervous system contributes to the regulation of heart function, it has little or no control over blood vessels.

AUTONOMIC NEUROTRANSMITTERS

The actions of the ANS are mediated by chemical neurotransmitters. *Acetylcholine* is the postganglionic neurotransmitter for parasympathetic neurons and *norepinephrine* is the main neurotransmitter for postganglionic sympathetic neurons. Sympathetic neurons also respond to epinephrine, which is released into the bloodstream by the adrenal medulla. The neurotransmitter *dopamine* can also act as a neuromediator for some sympathetic neurons. The sympathetic neurotransmitters are called *catecholamines*.

The catecholamines are synthesized in the axoplasm of sympathetic nerve terminal endings from the amino acid tyrosine (Fig. 21-27). In the process of catecholamine synthesis, tyrosine is hydroxylated (*i.e.*, has a hydroxyl group added) to form DOPA. DOPA is decarboxylated (*i.e.*, has a carboxyl group removed) to form dopamine, and dopamine is hydroxylated to form norepinephrine. In the adrenal

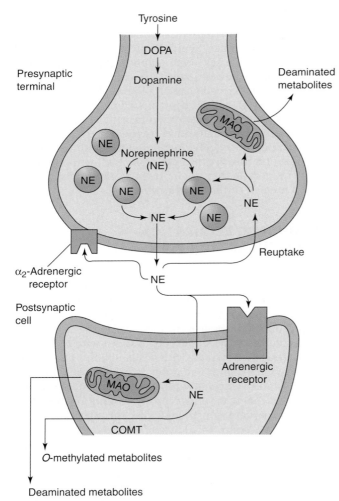

FIGURE 21-27 Mechanisms of norepinephrine synthesis, release, metabolism, and reuptake. Presynaptic α₂-adrenergic receptors act in the feedback regulation of norepinephrine synthesis and release. Norepinephrine is both removed from the synapse by the uptake process and degraded by monoamine oxidase (MAO) and catechol-*O*-methyltransferase (COMT).

gland, an additional step occurs during which norepinephrine is methylated (*i.e.*, a methyl group is added) to form epinephrine. Epinephrine is also called *adrenaline*, and sympathetic neurons are also called *adrenergic* neurons.

Each of the steps in neurotransmitter synthesis requires a different enzyme, and the type of neurotransmitter that is produced depends on the type of enzymes that are available in a nerve terminal. For example, the postganglionic sympathetic neurons that supply blood vessels synthesize norepinephrine, whereas postganglionic neurons in the adrenal medulla produce epinephrine or norepinephrine. Epinephrine accounts for approximately 80% of the catecholamines released from the adrenal gland. The synthesis of epinephrine by the adrenal medulla is influenced by glucocorticoid secretion from the adrenal cortex. These hormones are transported by way of an intra-adrenal vascular network from the adrenal cortex to the adrenal medulla, where they cause the sympathetic neurons to increase their production of epinephrine by way of increased enzyme activity. Thus, any stress situation sufficient to evoke increased levels of glucocorticoids also increases epinephrine levels.

As the catecholamines are synthesized, they are stored in vesicles. The final step of norepinephrine synthesis occurs in these vesicles. During an action potential, the neurotransmitter molecules are released from the storage vesicles. The storage vesicles not only provide a means for concentrated storage of the catecholamines, but they protect them from the cytoplasmic enzymes that are capable of degrading the neurotransmitter. In addition to neuronal synthesis, there is a second major mechanism for replenishment of norepinephrine in sympathetic nerve terminals. This mechanism consists of the active recapture or reuptake of the released neurotransmitter into the nerve terminal. From 50% to 80% of the norepinephrine that is released during an action potential is removed from the synaptic area by an active reuptake process. This process terminates the action of the neurotransmitter and allows it to be reused by the neuron. The remainder of the released catecholamines diffuses into the surrounding tissue fluids or is degraded by two special enzymes: catechol-*O*-methyltransferase (COMT), which is diffusely present in all tissues, and monoamine oxidase (MAO), which is found in the nerve endings themselves.

Autonomic Receptors

The neuromediators exert their effect through membrane proteins called *receptors*. The neuromediators and receptors interact in a lock-and-key fashion, which ensures specificity of action. Receptors that interact with acetylcholine are called *cholinergic receptors*, and those that interact with the sympathetic neuromediators are called *adrenergic receptors*. There are two types of adrenergic receptors: *alpha* (α) and *beta* (β) receptors. In vascular smooth muscle, stimulation of α receptors produces vasoconstriction; stimulation of β receptors causes vasodilatation. The α receptors have been further subdivided into α₁ and α₂ receptors. The *α₁ receptors* are found primarily at postsynaptic effector sites such as vascular smooth muscle. The *α₂ receptors* are abundant in the CNS and act at presynaptic sites to produce feedback inhibition of sympathetic outflow. The β₁ receptors are found primarily in the heart, and β_2 receptors are found in the bronchioles and in other sites that have β-mediated functions. In many tissues, the response that occurs is determined by the presence of a particular receptor type, which can vary from tissue to tissue. For example, in vascular smooth muscle that has α_1 receptors, sympathetic stimulation produces vasoconstriction; similar stimulation produces vasodilatation in other vessels that have β_2 receptors.

The role of the ANS in control of blood pressure is only beginning to be understood. For example, central α_2-adrenergic receptors are known to inhibit sympathetic outflow from the brain. Several antihypertensive medications exert their effect at this level. The α- and β-adrenergic receptors respond to endogenous catecholamines or exogenous pharmacologic agents (*e.g.*, drugs). Drugs that can selectively activate or block specific types of adrenergic receptors have been developed to treat high blood pressure.

Central Nervous System Responses

It is not surprising that the CNS, which plays an essential role in regulating vasomotor tone and blood pressure, would have a mechanism for controlling the blood flow to the cardiovascular centers that control circulatory function. When the blood flow to the brain has been sufficiently interrupted to cause ischemia of the vasomotor center, these vasomotor neurons become strongly excited, causing mas-

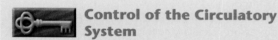

Control of the Circulatory System

➤ Arterial blood pressure equals the product of cardiac output and total peripheral resistance.

➤ Arterial blood pressure is regulated in the short term by neural (autonomic nervous) and hormonal (renin-angiotensin-aldosterone-vasopressin) systems and in the long term by the ability of the kidney to regulate extracellular water and sodium balance.

➤ Local control of blood flow is regulated by local mechanisms that match blood flow to the metabolic needs of the tissue. Over the short term, the tissues autoregulate flow through the synthesis of vasodilators and vasoconstrictors derived from the tissue, smooth muscle, or endothelial cells, and over the long term by creation of a collateral circulation.

➤ Neural control of blood flow and cardiac function and, therefore, blood pressure occurs through the sympathetic and parasympathetic divisions of the autonomic nervous system. Sympathetic stimulation increases heart rate, cardiac contractility, and vessel tone (vascular resistance), whereas parasympathetic stimulation decreases heart rate.

sive vasoconstriction as a means of raising the blood pressure to levels as high as the heart can pump against. This response is called the *CNS ischemic response*, and it can raise the blood pressure to levels as high as 270 mm Hg for as long as 10 minutes. The CNS ischemic response is a last-ditch stand to preserve the blood flow to vital brain centers; it does not become activated until blood pressure has fallen to at least 60 mm Hg, and it is most effective in the range of 15 to 20 mm Hg. If the cerebral circulation is not reestablished within 3 to 10 minutes, the neurons of the vasomotor center cease to function, so that the tonic impulses to the blood vessels stop and the blood pressure falls precipitously.

The *Cushing reflex* is a special type of CNS reflex resulting from an increase in intracranial pressure. When the intracranial pressure rises to levels that equal intra-arterial pressure, blood vessels to the vasomotor center become compressed, initiating the CNS ischemic response. The purpose of this reflex is to produce a rise in arterial pressure to levels above intracranial pressure so that the blood flow to the vasomotor center can be reestablished. Should the intracranial pressure rise to the point that the blood supply to the vasomotor center becomes inadequate, vasoconstrictor tone is lost, and the blood pressure begins to fall. The elevation in blood pressure associated with the Cushing reflex is usually of short duration and should be considered a protective homeostatic mechanism. The brain and other cerebral structures are located within the rigid confines of the skull, with no room for expansion, and any increase in intracranial pressure tends to compress the blood vessels that supply the brain.

AUTONOMIC RESPONSE TO CIRCULATORY STRESSES

The response of the cardiovascular system to the stresses of everyday living is mediated largely through the ANS. These stresses include postural stress, Valsalva's maneuver, and face immersion.

Postural Stress

During movement from the supine to the standing position, approximately 20% of the blood in the heart and lungs is displaced into the legs. The venous return to the heart is decreased, the stroke volume falls, and blood pressure decreases. As the blood pressure drops, the baroreceptors are stimulated and produce a reflex-mediated increase in heart rate and peripheral vascular resistance. These responses prevent the blood pressure from falling excessively when the standing position is assumed. With prolonged standing, an increase in plasma volume and the action of the skeletal muscle pumps aid in the return of blood to the heart. Decreased tolerance of the upright position causes *orthostatic hypotension*, which is discussed in Chapter 23.

Valsalva's Maneuver

Valsalva's maneuver, which involves forced expiration against a closed glottis, incites a sequence of rapid changes in preload and afterload stresses along with autonomically mediated changes in the heart rate and peripheral vascular resistance. Valsalva's maneuver is a normal accompaniment of many everyday activities. It is used in coughing, lifting, pushing, vomiting, and straining at stool. The pushing that occurs during the final stages of childbirth makes extensive use of the maneuver.

The rise in intrathoracic pressure (often to levels of ≥40 mm Hg) during the strain of Valsalva's maneuver causes a decrease in venous return to the heart, with a resultant decrease in cardiac output, a decrease in systolic and pulse pressures, and a baroreflex-mediated increase in the heart rate and peripheral vascular resistance. After the release of the strain, venous return is suddenly reestablished; stroke volume and arterial blood pressure undergo marked but transient elevations. The sudden rise in arterial pressure that occurs at a time when reflex vasoconstriction is still present causes a vagal slowing of the heart rate that normally lasts for several beats. Valsalva's maneuver may be used as a method of testing circulatory reflexes, because the increase in heart rate and total peripheral resistance that occur during Valsalva's strain and the bradycardia that follows its release are mediated through the baroreceptors and the ANS.

Face Immersion

The *diving reflex* (*i.e.*, face immersion) is a potent protective mechanism against asphyxia in birds and submerged vertebrates; it allows for gross redistribution of the circulation to ensure the oxygenation of the brain and heart. The diving response has three main features: apnea, an intense vagal slowing of heart rate, and a powerful peripheral vasoconstriction. Except for the coronary and cerebral blood vessels, there is massive vasoconstriction to the extent that the circulation becomes in effect a heart-brain circuit. Because of the severe vasoconstriction, arterial pressure remains relatively unchanged.

In humans, application of cold water to the face produces a similar reduction in the heart rate and in the skin and muscle blood flow. The slowing of the heart rate is greater with ice water than with cool water and greater with cool water than with cool air. Immersion of the face in ice water may be used clinically to terminate supraventricular paroxysmal tachycardia. Because the reflex is potent in the neonate, it may protect against asphyxia during the birth process. It has also been credited with increasing the chance of survival of children who have accidentally fallen into cold water and remained submerged for longer periods than are normally associated with survival.

In summary, the neural control centers for the regulation of cardiac function and blood pressure are located in the reticular formation of the lower pons and medulla of the brain stem, where the integration and modulation of ANS responses occur. These brain stem centers receive information from many areas of the nervous system, including the hypothalamus. Both the parasympathetic and sympathetic nervous systems innervate the heart. The parasympathetic nervous system functions in regulating heart rate through the vagus nerve, with increased vagal activity producing a

slowing of heart rate. The sympathetic nervous system has an excitatory influence on heart rate and contractility, and it serves as the final common pathway for controlling the smooth muscle tone of the blood vessels.

Autonomic control of the circulatory system occurs through neurotransmitters that exert their effect through membrane receptors. There are two types of adrenergic receptors: α and β receptors. In vascular smooth muscle, stimulation of α receptors produces vasoconstriction; stimulation of β receptors causes vasodilatation. Alpha receptors have been further subdivided into α_1 and α_2 receptors. The α_1 receptors are found primarily at postsynaptic effector sites such as vascular smooth muscle.

The response of the cardiovascular system to the stresses of everyday living such as postural stress, Valsalva's maneuver, and face immersion is mediated largely through the ANS. Many of these stresses can be used to evaluate the function of the ANS.

The Microcirculation and Lymphatic System

After you have completed this section of the chapter, you should be able to meet the following objectives:

+ Describe the structure and function of the microcirculation
+ Relate the effects of the capillary pressure, interstitial fluid pressure, capillary colloidal osmotic pressure, and interstitial colloidal osmotic pressure to the exchange of fluids at the capillary level
+ Describe the structures of the lymphatic system and relate them to the role of the lymphatics in controlling interstitial fluid volume
+ Define the term *edema*

The capillaries, venules, and arterioles of the circulatory system are collectively referred to as the *microcirculation*. It is here that exchange of gases, nutrients, and metabolites takes place between the tissues and the circulating blood.

THE MICROCIRCULATION

Blood enters the microcirculation through an arteriole, passes through the capillaries, and leaves by way of a small venule. The metarterioles serve as thoroughfare channels that link arterioles and capillaries (Fig. 21-28). Small cuffs of smooth muscle, the precapillary sphincters, are positioned at the arterial end of the capillary. The smooth muscle tone of the arterioles, venules, and precapillary sphincters serves to control blood flow through the capillary bed. Depending on venous pressure, blood flows through the capillary channels when the precapillary sphincters are open.

Blood flow through capillary channels, designed for exchange of nutrients and metabolites, is called *nutrient flow*.

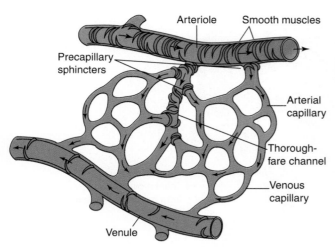

FIGURE 21-28 Capillary bed. Precapillary sphincters control the flow of blood through the capillary network. Thoroughfare channels (*i.e.*, arteriovenous shunts) allow blood to move directly from the arteriole into the venule without moving through nutrient channels of the capillary. (Chaffee E.E., Lytle I.M. [1980]. *Basic physiology and anatomy* [4th ed.]. Philadelphia: J.B. Lippincott)

In some parts of the microcirculation, blood flow bypasses the capillary bed, moving through a connection called an *arteriovenous shunt*, which directly connects an arteriole and a venule. This type of blood flow is called *nonnutrient flow* because it does not allow for nutrient exchange. Nonnutrient channels are common in the skin and are important in terms of heat exchange and temperature regulation.

The lymphatic system represents an accessory system that removes excess fluid, including osmotically active proteins, and large particles from the interstitial spaces and returns them to the circulation. Because of their size, these proteins and large particles cannot be reabsorbed into the venous capillaries. The removal of proteins from the interstitial spaces is an essential function, without which death would occur in approximately 24 hours.

CAPILLARY–INTERSTITIAL FLUID EXCHANGE

Approximately one sixth of the body consists of spaces between body cells called the *interstitium*. The interstitium is supported by *collagen* and *elastin* fibers and filled with *proteoglycan* (sugar-protein) molecules that combine with water to form a tissue gel. The tissue gel acts like a sponge to entrap the interstitial fluid and provide for even distribution of the fluid to all the cells, even those that are most distant from the capillary. Although most of the fluid is entrapped in the tissue gel, small "trickles" of free fluid develop between the proteoglycan molecules. Normally, only a small amount of free fluid is present. In a condition called *edema* in which excess fluid is present in the interstitial spaces, the amount of free fluid can expand tremendously.

Four forces determine the movement of fluid between capillaries and the interstitial spaces: (1) the *intracapillary fluid pressure*, (2) the *interstitial fluid pressure*, (3) the *plasma colloidal osmotic pressure*, and (4) the *interstitial colloidal osmotic pressure*. Water moves between the capillary and the tissue by the processes of filtration and osmosis. *Filtration* is the movement of water across the capillary wall due to differences in fluid pressures between the capillary and the tissue. *Osmosis* is the movement of water across the capillary wall due to differences in osmotic pressure between the capillary and the tissue.

The intracapillary and tissue pressures can be viewed as pushing pressures that force fluid out of the capillary or interstitial space and the osmotic pressures as pulling pressures that draw fluid into the capillary or interstitium. The intracapillary pressure causes fluids to move through the capillary pores into the interstitial spaces and the capillary colloidal osmotic pressure pulls the fluids back into the capillary. Also important to this exchange mechanism is the lymphatic system, which returns osmotically active proteins and excess interstitial fluids to the circulatory system.

Normally, the movement of fluid between the capillary bed and the interstitial spaces is continuous. A state of equilibrium exists as long as equal amounts of fluid enter and leave the interstitial spaces (Fig. 21-29). The approximate average forces at the arterial and venous ends of a capillary in the systemic circulation that cause fluid movement across the capillary membrane are shown in Figure 21-30. In the diagram, the capillary fluid pressure is 28 mm Hg. The capillary pressure, along with a negative interstitial pressure (3 mm Hg) and an interstitial colloidal osmotic pressure (8 mm Hg), contributes to the outward movement of fluid. Plasma proteins and other nondiffusible particles that remain in the capillary exert an osmotic pressure (28 mm Hg) that pulls fluids back into the venous end of the capillary. This yields a total outward pushing pressure of approximately 39 mm Hg and an inward pulling pressure of 28 mm Hg at the arterial end of the capillary. On the venous end, the outward pushing pressures drop to 21 mm Hg, and the inward pulling forces remain at 28 mm Hg. A slight imbalance in forces (*i.e.*, 11 mm Hg outward forces and 7 mm Hg inward forces) causes slightly more filtration of fluid into interstitial spaces than is pulled back into the capillary; it is this fluid that is returned to the circulation by the lymphatic system.

Capillary Filtration Pressure

The intracapillary fluid pressure, also called the *capillary filtration pressure*, is the force that pushes water through the capillary pores into the interstitial spaces. Capillary filtration pressure reflects the arterial pressure, the venous pressure, and the hydrostatic effects of gravity. The pressure at the arterial end of the capillary is normally higher than the pressure at its venous end, because arterial pressure decreases as blood moves away from the heart. If arterial pressure changes, capillary pressure changes, which in turn affects the movement of water across the membrane. For example, if arterial pressure falls owing to hemorrhage, the movement of water out of the capillaries into the tissues decreases, helping to maintain vascular volume. Capillary pressure also reflects changes in capillary volume. For example, intracapillary fluid pressure can be expected to increase when the tone of the precapillary sphincters and the

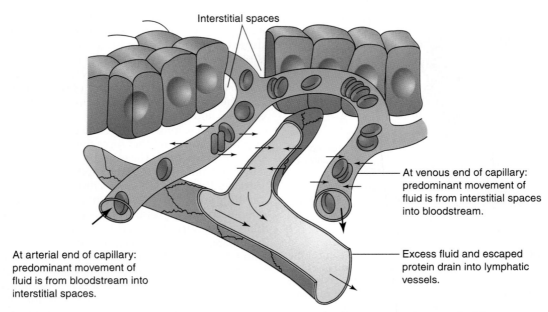

Interstitial spaces

At venous end of capillary: predominant movement of fluid is from interstitial spaces into bloodstream.

At arterial end of capillary: predominant movement of fluid is from bloodstream into interstitial spaces.

Excess fluid and escaped protein drain into lymphatic vessels.

FIGURE 21-29 Exchanges through capillary membranes in the formation and removal of interstitial fluid. (Chaffee E.E., Lytle I.M. [1980]. *Basic physiology and anatomy* [4th ed.]. Philadelphia: J.B. Lippincott)

arterioles that supply the capillary bed is decreased. The swelling that occurs with inflammation develops because of a histamine-induced dilatation of the precapillary sphincters and arterioles that supply the affected area. Venous pressure can be transmitted back to the capillary, thereby increasing intracapillary fluid pressure and the outward movement of fluid. For example, venous thrombosis can obstruct venous flow, producing an increase in venous and capillary pressures.

The pressure due to gravity is called the *hydrostatic pressure*. In a person in the standing position, the weight of the blood in the vascular column causes an increase of 1 mm Hg in pressure for every 13.6 mm of distance below the level of the heart. The hydrostatic pressure in the veins of an adult man can reach a level of 90 mm Hg. This pressure is then transmitted to the capillary bed. Gravity has no effect on blood pressure in a person in the recumbent position because the blood vessels are then at the level of the heart.

Outward Forces

Capillary pressure	28 mm Hg
Negative interstitial pressure	3 mm Hg
Interstitial colloidal osmotic pressure	8 mm Hg
Total forces	39 mm Hg

Inward Forces

| Plasma colloidal osmotic pressure | 28 mm Hg |
| Total forces | 28 mm Hg |

Summation of Forces

Outward	39 mm Hg
Inward	28 mm Hg
Net outward force	11 mm Hg

Inward Forces

| Plasma colloidal osmotic pressure | 28 mm Hg |
| Total forces | 28 mm Hg |

Outward Forces

Capillary pressure	10 mm Hg
Negative interstitial pressure	3 mm Hg
Interstitial colloidal osmotic pressure	8 mm Hg
Total forces	21 mm Hg

Summation of Forces

Inward	28 mm Hg
Outward	21 mm Hg
Net inward force	7 mm Hg

FIGURE 21-30 Inward and outward forces in the capillary.

Because of the passive nature of pressure in the capillary bed, the terms *capillary fluid pressure* and *hydrostatic pressure* are often used interchangeably.

Interstitial Fluid Pressure

The interstitial fluid pressure reflects the pressure exerted on the interstitial fluids. It can be positive or negative. In some organs, such as the kidneys, which are encased in a tough fibrous capsule, the interstitial fluid pressure is positive, thereby opposing filtration of fluid out of the capillaries. Atmospheric pressure is usually negative in relation to capillary pressure. In the skin exposed to atmospheric pressure, the interstitial pressure is usually several millimeters of mercury less than capillary pressures. A negative interstitial fluid pressure increases the outward forces that influence the movement of fluid out of the capillary into the interstitium.

Capillary Colloidal Osmotic Pressure

The capillary colloidal osmotic pressure reflects the osmotic effect of the plasma proteins in drawing fluid into the capillary. Osmosis is the movement of water across a semipermeable membrane along its concentration gradient, moving from the side of the membrane that has the greatest number of particles to the one that has the least number. A colloid solution is one in which there are evenly dispersed particles, much as cream particles become dispersed when milk is homogenized. The term *colloidal osmotic pressure* is used to differentiate the osmotic effects of the particles in a colloidal solution from those of the dissolved crystalloids such as sodium. The pressure units (millimeters of mercury) used for measuring osmotic pressure represent the mechanical pressure or force that would be needed to oppose the osmotic movement of water.

The plasma proteins are large molecules that disperse in the blood and occasionally escape into the tissue spaces. Because the capillary membrane is almost impermeable to the plasma proteins, these particles exert a force that draws fluid into the capillary and offsets the pushing force of the capillary filtration pressure. The plasma contains a mixture of plasma proteins, including albumin, the globulins, and fibrinogen. Albumin, which is the smallest and most abundant of the plasma proteins, accounts for approximately 70% of the total osmotic pressure. It is the number, not the size, of the particles in solution that controls the osmotic pressure. One gram of albumin (molecular weight of 69,000) contains almost six times as many molecules as 1 g of fibrinogen (molecular weight of 400,000). (Normal values for the plasma proteins are albumin, 4.5 g/dL; globulins, 2.5 g/dL; and fibrinogen, 0.3 g/dL.)

Tissue Colloidal Osmotic Pressure

Although the size of the capillary pores prevents most plasma proteins from leaving the capillary, small amounts do leak into the interstitial spaces to exert an osmotic force that favors movement of capillary fluid into the interstitium. This amount is often increased in conditions such as inflammation that increase capillary permeability. The lymphatic system is responsible for removing proteins from the interstitium. In the absence of a functioning lymphatic system, tissue colloidal osmotic pressure increases, causing fluid to accumulate. Normally, a few white blood cells, plasma proteins, and other large molecules enter the interstitial spaces; these cells and molecules, which are too large to reenter the capillary, rely on the loosely structured wall of the lymphatic vessels for return to the vascular compartment.

THE LYMPHATIC SYSTEM

The lymphatic system, commonly called the *lymphatics*, serves almost all body tissues, except cartilage, bone, epithelial tissue, and tissues of the CNS. Most of these tissues, however, have prelymphatic channels that eventually flow into areas supplied by the lymphatics. Lymph is derived from interstitial fluids that flow through the lymph channels. It contains plasma proteins and other osmotically active particles that rely on the lymphatics for movement back into the circulatory system. When lymph flow is obstructed, a condition called *lymphedema* occurs. Involvement of lymph structures by malignant tumors and removal of lymph nodes at the time of cancer surgery are common causes of lymphedema. The lymphatic system is also the main route for absorption of nutrients, particularly fats, from the gastrointestinal tract. The lymph system also filters the fluid at the lymph nodes and removes foreign particles such as bacteria.

The lymphatic system is made up of vessels similar to those of the circulatory system. These vessels commonly travel along with an arteriole or venule or with its companion artery and vein. The terminal lymphatic vessels are made up of a single layer of connective tissue with an endothelial lining and resemble blood capillaries. The lymphatic vessels lack tight junctions and are loosely anchored to the surrounding tissues by fine filaments (Fig. 21-31). The loose junctions permit the entry of large particles, and the filaments hold the vessels open under conditions of edema,

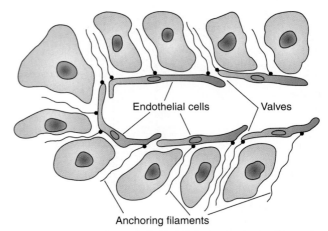

FIGURE 21-31 Special structure of the lymphatic capillaries that permits passage of substances of high molecular weight back into the lymph. (Guyton A.C., Hall J.E. [1996]. *Textbook of medical physiology* [9th ed., p. 194]. Philadelphia: W.B. Saunders)

when the pressure of the surrounding tissues would otherwise cause them to collapse. The lymph capillaries drain into larger lymph vessels that ultimately empty into the right and left thoracic ducts (Fig. 21-32). The thoracic ducts empty into the circulation at the junctions of the subclavian and internal jugular veins.

Although the divisions are not as distinct as in the circulatory system, the larger lymph vessels show evidence of having intimal, medial, and adventitial layers similar to blood vessels. The intima of these channels contain elastic tissue and an endothelial layer, and the larger collecting lymph channels contain smooth muscle in their medial layer. Contraction of this smooth muscle assists in propelling lymph fluid toward the thorax. External compression of the lymph channels by pulsating blood vessels in the vicinity and active and passive movements of body parts also aid in forward propulsion of lymph fluid. The rate of flow through the lymphatic system by way of all of the various lymph channels, approximately 120 mL per hour, is determined by the interstitial fluid pressure and the activity of lymph pumps.

EDEMA

Edema refers to excess interstitial fluid in the tissues (see Chapter 31). Edema can result from an imbalance of any of the factors that control movement of water between the vascular compartment and the tissue spaces. It can occur because of a disproportionate increase in capillary fluid pressure or permeability, decreased capillary colloidal osmotic pressure, or impaired lymph flow. Edema is not a disease but rather the manifestation of altered physiologic function, and can occur in healthy and sick individuals. In hot weather, the superficial blood vessels dilate, and sodium and water retention increase, which causes swelling of the hands and feet. Edema of the ankles and feet becomes more pronounced during prolonged periods of standing, when the forces of gravity are superimposed on the heat-induced vasodilatation and increased extracellular fluid volume.

> In summary, exchange of fluids between the vascular compartment and the interstitial spaces occurs at the capillary level. The capillary filtration pressure pushes fluids out of the capillaries, and the colloidal osmotic pressure exerted by the plasma proteins pulls fluids back into the capillaries. Albumin, which is the smallest and most abundant of the plasma proteins, provides the major osmotic force for return of fluid to the vascular compartment. Normally, slightly more fluid leaves the capillary bed than can be reabsorbed. This excess fluid is returned to the circulation by way of the lymphatic channels.

Related Web Sites

Anatomy of the Human Circulatory System   www.ultranet.com/~jkimball/BiologyPages/C/Circulation.html
Circulatory Dynamics in the Human   www.columbia.edu/~kj3/menu.html
Human Physiologic Systems   http//bio.rpi.edu/Parsons/HPS/Syllabus/syllabus.html
Human Physiology Illustration Resource   www1.oup.co.uk/best.textbooks/medicine/humanphys/illustrations/

Bibliography

Berne R.M., Levy M.N. (2000). *Principles of physiology* (3rd ed., pp. 201–275). St. Louis: C.V. Mosby.
Feletou M., Vanhoutte P.M. (1999). The alternative: EDHF. *Journal of Molecular and Cellular Cardiology* 31, 15–22.
Guyton A.C., Hall J.E. (2000). *Medical physiology* (10th ed., pp. 144–222). Philadelphia: W.B. Saunders.
Johansen K. (1982). Aneurysms. *Scientific American* 247 (1), 110–118.
Katz A.M. (1992). *Physiology of the heart*. New York: Raven Press.
McCormack D.H. (1987). *Ham's histology* (9th ed., p. 448). Philadelphia: J.B. Lippincott.
Porth C.J.M., Bamrah V.S., Tristani F.E., Smith J.J. (1984). The Valsalva: Mechanisms and clinical implications. *Heart and Lung* 13, 507.
Rhoades R.S., Tanner G.A. (1996). *Medical physiology* (pp. 207–301). Boston: Little, Brown.
Shepard J.T., Vanhoutte P.M. (1979). *The human cardiovascular system*. New York: Raven Press.
Smith J.J., Kampine J.P. (1989). *Circulatory physiology* (3rd ed.). Baltimore: Williams & Wilkins.
Vanhoutte P.M. (1999). How to assess endothelial function in human blood vessels. *Journal of Hypertension* 17, 1047–1058.

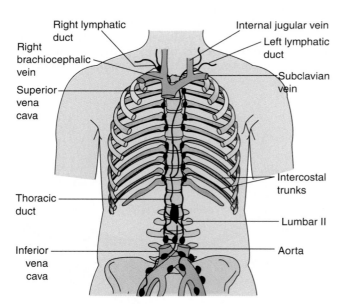

FIGURE 21-32 This diagram shows the course of the thoracic duct and right lymphatic duct. Deep lymphatic vessels and nodes are also shown. (Chaffee E.E., Lytle I.M. [1980]. *Basic physiology and anatomy* [4th ed.]. Philadelphia: J.B. Lippincott)

Chapter 22

Alterations in Blood Flow in the Systemic Circulation

Blood flow in the arterial and venous systems depends on a system of patent blood vessels and adequate perfusion pressure. A disturbance in blood flow in the arterial or venous system disrupts the delivery of oxygen and nutrients, removal of waste products, and the return of blood to the heart. Unlike disorders of the respiratory system or central circulation that cause hypoxia and impair oxygenation of tissues throughout the body, the effects of blood vessel disease usually are limited to local tissues supplied by a particular vessel or group of vessels. With arterial disorders, there is decreased blood flow to the tissues along with impaired delivery of oxygen and nutrients. Venous disorders interfere with the outflow of blood from the capillaries, removal of tissue wastes, and return of blood to the heart. Arterial and venous disorders can lead to tissue injury and death.

Disturbances in blood flow can result from pathologic changes in the vessel wall (*i.e.*, atherosclerosis and vasculitis), acute vessel obstruction due to thrombus or embolus, vasospasm (*i.e.*, Raynaud's phenomenon), abnormal vessel dilation (*i.e.*, arterial aneurysms or varicose veins), or compression of blood vessels by extravascular forces (*i.e.*, tumors, edema, or firm surfaces such as those associated with pressure ulcers).

This chapter is organized into three sections: disorders of the arterial circulation, disorders of the venous circulation, and disorders of blood vessel compression.

Disorders of the Arterial Circulation

After you have completed this section of the chapter, you should be able to meet the following objectives:

✦ List the five types of lipoproteins and state their function in terms of lipid transport and development of atherosclerosis

✦ Describe the role of low-density lipoprotein receptors in removal of cholesterol from the blood

✦ Cite the criteria for diagnosis of hypercholesterolemia

✦ List the vessels most commonly affected by atherosclerosis and describe the vessel changes that occur

✦ Describe possible mechanisms involved in the development of atherosclerosis

✦ List risk factors in atherosclerosis

✦ State the signs and symptoms of acute arterial occlusion

- ✦ Describe the pathology associated with the vasculitides and relate it to four disease conditions associated with vasculitis
- ✦ Compare the mechanisms and manifestations of ischemia associated with atherosclerotic peripheral vascular disease, Raynaud's phenomenon, and thromboangiitis obliterans (*i.e.*, Buerger's disease)
- ✦ Distinguish among berry aneurysms, aortic aneurysms, and dissecting aneurysms
- ✦ Compare the pathology and manifestations of thoracic or abdominal and dissecting aneurysms

The arterial system distributes blood to all the tissues in the body. There are three types of arteries: large elastic arteries, including the aorta and its distal branches; medium-sized arteries, such as the coronary and renal arteries; and small arteries and arterioles that pass through the tissues. The large arteries function mainly in transport of blood. The medium-sized arteries are composed predominantly of circular and spirally arranged smooth muscle cells. Distribution of blood flow to the various organs and tissues of the body is controlled by contraction and relaxation of the smooth muscle of these vessels. The small arteries and arterioles regulate capillary blood flow. Each of these different types of arteries tends to be affected by different disease processes.

Pathology of the arterial system affects body function by impairing blood flow. The effect of impaired blood flow on the body depends on the structures involved and the extent of altered flow. The term *ischemia* (*i.e.*, holding back of blood) denotes a reduction in arterial flow to a level that is insufficient to meet the oxygen demands of the tissues. *Infarction* refers to an area of ischemic necrosis in an organ produced by occlusion of its arterial blood supply or its venous drainage. The discussion in this section focuses on hypercholesterolemia, hyperlipidemia, atherosclerosis, vasculitis, arterial disease of the extremities, and arterial aneurysms.

HYPERLIPIDEMIA

Triglycerides, phospholipids, and cholesterol, which are classified as lipids, are chemical substances composed of long-chain hydrocarbon fatty acids. Triglycerides, which are used in energy metabolism, are combinations of three fatty acids condensed with a single glycerol molecule. Phospholipids, which contain a phosphate group, are important structural constituents of lipoproteins, blood clotting components, the myelin sheath, and cell membranes. Although cholesterol is not composed of fatty acids, its steroid nucleus is synthesized from fatty acids and thus its chemical activity is similar to that of other lipid substances.[1]

Elevated levels of blood cholesterol (*hypercholesterolemia*) are implicated in the development of atherosclerosis. This is a major public health issue that is underscored by striking statistics released by the American Heart Association. An estimated 39.9 million Americans have high cholesterol levels that could contribute to a heart attack, stroke, or other cardiovascular event associated with atherosclerosis,[2] and 99.5 million Americans have cholesterol levels that are considered borderline high.

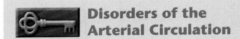

Disorders of the Arterial Circulation

- ➤ The arterial system delivers oxygen and nutrients to the tissues.

- ➤ Disorders of the arterial circulation produce ischemia owing to narrowing of blood vessels, thrombus formation associated with platelet adhesion, and weakening of the vessel wall.

- ➤ Atherosclerosis is a progressive disease characterized by the formation of fibrofatty plaques in the intima of large and medium-sized vessels, including the aorta, coronary arteries, and cerebral vessels. A major risk factor for atherosclerosis is hypercholesterolemia.

- ➤ Vasculitis is an inflammation of the blood vessel wall resulting in vascular tissue injury and necrosis. Arteries, capillaries, and veins may be affected. The inflammatory process may be initiated by direct injury, infectious agents, or immune processes.

- ➤ Aneurysms represent an abnormal localized dilatation of an artery due to a weakness in the vessel wall. As the aneurysm increases in size, the tension in the wall of the vessel increases and it may rupture. The increased size of the vessel also may exert pressure on adjacent structures.

Lipoproteins

Because cholesterol and triglyceride are insoluble in plasma, they are encapsulated by special fat-carrying proteins called *lipoproteins* for transport in the blood. There are five types of lipoproteins, classified by their densities as measured by ultracentrifugation: chylomicrons, very–low-density lipoprotein (VLDL), intermediate-density lipoprotein (IDL), low-density lipoprotein (LDL), and high-density lipoprotein (HDL). VLDL carries large amounts of triglycerides that have a lower density than cholesterol. LDL is the main carrier of cholesterol, whereas HDL actually is 50% protein.

Each type of lipoprotein consists of a large molecular complex of lipids combined with proteins called *apoproteins*.[3-5] The major lipid constituents are cholesterol esters, triglycerides, nonesterified cholesterol, and phospholipids. The insoluble cholesterol esters and triglycerides are located in the hydrophobic core of the lipoprotein macromolecule, surrounded by the soluble phospholipids, nonesterified cholesterol, and apoproteins (Fig. 22-1). Nonesterified cholesterol and phospholipids provide a negative charge that allows the lipoprotein to be soluble in plasma.

There are four major classes of apoproteins: A (*i.e.*, A-I, A-II, and A-IV), B (*e.g.*, B-48, B-100), C (*i.e.*, C-I, C-II, and C-III), and E.[3,4] The apoproteins control the interactions and ultimate metabolic fate of the lipoproteins. Some of the

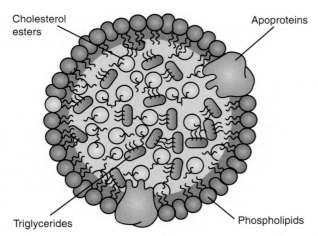

FIGURE 22-1 General structure of a lipoprotein. The cholesterol esters and triglycerides are located in the hydrophobic core of the macromolecule, surrounded by phospholipids and apoproteins.

apoproteins activate the lipolytic enzymes that facilitate the removal of lipids from the lipoproteins; others serve as a reactive site that cellular receptors can recognize and use in the endocytosis and metabolism of the lipoproteins. The major apoprotein in LDL is B-100. HDL is associated with A-I and A-II. Research findings suggest that genetic defects in apoproteins may be involved in hyperlipidemia and accelerated atherosclerosis.[3,4,6]

There are two sites of lipoprotein synthesis: the small intestine and the liver. The chylomicrons, which are the largest of the lipoprotein molecules, are synthesized in the wall of the small intestine. They are involved in the transport of dietary (exogenous pathway) triglycerides and cholesterol that have been absorbed from the gastrointestinal tract. Chylomicrons transfer their triglycerides to the cells of adipose and skeletal muscle tissue. The remnant chylomicron particles, which contain cholesterol, are then taken up by the liver and the cholesterol used in the synthesis of VLDL or excreted in the bile.

The liver synthesizes and releases VLDL and HDL. The VLDLs contain large amounts of triglycerides and lesser amounts of cholesterol esters.[7] They provide the primary pathway for transport of the endogenous triglycerides produced in the liver, as opposed to those obtained from the diet. Like chylomicrons, VLDLs carry their triglycerides to fat and muscle cells, where the triglycerides are removed. The resulting IDL fragments are reduced in triglyceride content and enriched in cholesterol. They are taken to the liver and recycled to form VLDL, or converted to LDL in the vascular compartment. IDLs are the main source of LDL. The exogenous and endogenous pathways for triglyceride and cholesterol transport are shown in Figure 22-2.

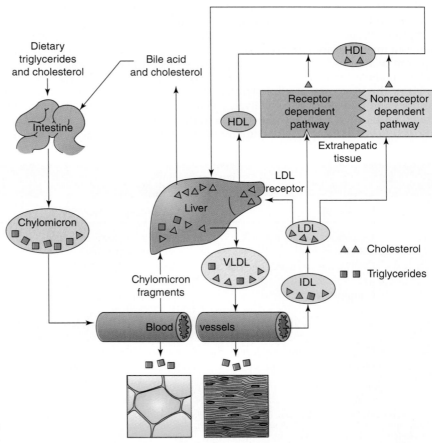

FIGURE 22-2 Schematic representation of the exogenous and endogenous pathways for triglyceride and cholesterol transport.

LDL, sometimes called the *bad cholesterol*, is the main carrier of cholesterol. LDL is removed from the circulation by receptor-dependent and non–receptor-dependent mechanisms. Receptor-mediated removal involves binding of LDL to cell surface receptors, followed by *endocytosis*, a phagocytic process in which LDL is engulfed and moved into the cell in the form of a membrane-covered endocytic vesicle. Within the cell, the endocytic vesicles fuse with lysosomes, and the LDL molecule is enzymatically degraded, causing free cholesterol to be released into the cytoplasm.

Approximately 70% of LDL is removed by way of the receptor-dependent pathway in the liver. Other, nonhepatic tissues (*i.e.*, adrenal glands, smooth muscle cells, endothelial cells, and lymphoid cells) also use the receptor-dependent pathway to obtain cholesterol needed for membrane and hormone synthesis. These tissues can control their cholesterol intake by adding or removing LDL receptors. The remaining LDL is removed by non–receptor-dependent mechanisms, including ingestion by phagocytic monocytes. Macrophage uptake of LDL in the arterial wall can result in the accumulation of insoluble cholesterol ester, the formation of foam cells, and the development of atherosclerosis. When there is a decrease in LDL receptors or when LDL levels exceed receptor availability, the amount of LDL that must be removed by the non–receptor-dependent mechanisms is increased.

HDL is synthesized in the liver and often is referred to as the *good cholesterol*. HDL participates in the reverse transport of cholesterol, that is, carrying cholesterol from the peripheral tissues back to the liver. Epidemiologic studies show an inverse relation between HDL levels and the development of atherosclerosis.[8,9] It is thought that HDL, which is low in cholesterol and rich in surface phospholipids, facilitates the clearance of cholesterol from atheromatous plaques and transports it to the liver, where it may be excreted rather than reused in the formation of VLDL. HDL also is believed to inhibit cellular uptake of LDL. It has been

observed that regular exercise and moderate alcohol consumption increase HDL levels. Smoking and diabetes, which are in themselves risk factors for atherosclerosis, are associated with decreased levels of HDL.[7]

Hypercholesterolemia

According to the guidelines published in the *Third Report of the National Cholesterol Education Program (NCEP) Expert Panel on Detection, Evaluation, and Treatment of High Blood Cholesterol in Adults*, a total serum cholesterol level <200 mg/dL is considered desirable; levels of 200–239 mg/dL are borderline high; and ≥240 mg/dL are high. LDL cholesterol levels <100 mg/dL are considered optimal; 100–129 mg/dL are near or above optimal; 130–159 mg/dL are borderline high; 160–189 mg/dL are high; and ≥190 mg/dL is very high.[10] HDL mg/dL cholesterol levels <40 mg/dL are considered low and levels ≥60 mg/dL are high.[10]

Serum cholesterol levels may be elevated as a result of an increase in any of the lipoproteins—the chylomicrons, VLDL, IDL, LDL, or HDL. The commonly used classification system for hyperlipidemia is based on the type of lipoprotein involved (Table 22-1). Three factors—nutrition, genetics, and metabolic diseases—can raise blood lipid levels. Most cases of elevated levels of cholesterol are probably multifactorial. Some persons may have increased sensitivity to dietary cholesterol, others have a lack of LDL receptors, and still others have an altered synthesis of the apoproteins, including oversynthesis of apoprotein B-100, the major apoprotein in LDL.

Hypercholesterolemia can be classified as primary or secondary hypercholesterolemia. *Primary hypercholesterolemia* describes elevated cholesterol levels that develop independent of other health problems or lifestyle behaviors. *Secondary hypercholesterolemia* is associated with other health problems and behaviors.

Many types of primary hypercholesterolemia have a genetic basis. There may be a defective synthesis of the apo-

---

TABLE 22-1 ✦ Classification of Hyperlipoproteinemias and Their Genetic Basis

Type	Familiar Name	Lipoprotein Abnormality	Known Underlying Genetic Defects
1	Exogenous dietary hyper-triglyceridemia	Elevated chylomicrons and triglycerides	Mutation in lipoprotein lipase gene
2a	Familial hypercholesterolemia	Elevated LDL cholesterol	Mutation in LDL receptor gene or in apoprotein B gene
2b	Combined hyperlipidemia	Elevated LDL, VLDL, and triglycerides	Mutation in LDL receptor gene or apoprotein B gene
3	Remnant hyperlipidemia	Increased remnants (chylomicrons), IDL triglycerides, and cholesterol	Mutation in apolipoprotein E gene
4	Endogenous hypertriglyceridemia	Elevated VLDL and triglycerides	Unknown
5	Mixed hypertriglyceridemia	Elevated VLDL, chylomicrons, and cholesterol; triglycerides greatly elevated	Mutation in apolipoprotein C-II gene

IDL, intermediate-density lipoprotein; LDL, low-density lipoprotein; VLDL, very–low-density lipoprotein.
(Data developed from Cotran R.S., Kumar V., Robbins S.L. [1994]. *Robbins pathologic basis of disease* [5th ed., pp. 481–482]. Philadelphia: W.B. Saunders; and Gotto A.M. [1988]. Lipoprotein metabolism and etiology of hyperlipidemia. *Hospital Practice*, 23[Suppl. 1], 4)

proteins, a lack of receptors, defective receptors, or defects in the handling of cholesterol in the cell that are genetically determined.[3,6] For example, the LDL receptor is deficient or defective in the genetic disorder known as *familial hyper-cholesterolemia (type IIA)*. This autosomal dominant type of hyperlipoproteinemia results from a mutation in the gene specifying the receptor for LDL. Because most of the circulating cholesterol is removed by receptor-dependent mechanisms, blood cholesterol levels are markedly elevated in persons with this disorder. The disorder is probably one of the most common of all mendelian disorders; the frequency of heterozygotes is 1 in 500 persons in the general population.[3] Plasma LDL levels in heterozygotes range between 250 and 500 mg/dL, whereas in homozygotes LDL cholesterol levels may rise to 1000 mg/dL. Although heterozygotes commonly have an elevated cholesterol level from birth, they do not develop symptoms until adult life, when they develop *xanthomas* (*i.e.*, cholesterol deposits) along the tendons and atherosclerosis appears (Fig. 22-3). Myocardial infarction before 40 years of age is common. Homozygotes are much more severely affected; they have cutaneous xanthomas in childhood and may experience myocardial infarction by 20 years of age.[3]

Causes of secondary hyperlipoproteinemia include obesity with high-calorie intake and diabetes mellitus. High-calorie diets increase the production of VLDL, with triglyceride elevation and high conversion of VLDL to LDL. Excess ingestion of cholesterol may reduce the formation of LDL receptors and thereby decrease LDL removal. Diets that are high in triglycerides and saturated fats increase cholesterol synthesis and suppress LDL receptor activity. In diabetes mellitus, metabolic derangements cause an elevation of lipoproteins.[11,12]

Measures to Control Blood Cholesterol Levels. The *Third Report of the NCEP Expert Panel on Detection, Evaluation, and Treatment of High Blood Cholesterol in Adults* recommends that all adults 20 years of age and older have a fasting lipoprotein profile (total cholesterol, LDL cholesterol, HDL cholesterol, and triglycerides) obtained once every 5 years. If testing is done in the nonfasting state, only the total cholesterol and HDL cholesterol are considered usable. Follow-up lipoprotein profiles should be done on persons with nonfasting total cholesterol levels ≥200 mg/dL or HDL levels >40 mg/dL.[10] Lipoprotein measurements are particularly important in persons at high risk for coronary heart disease (CHD).

Management of Hyperlipidemia. The NCEP continues to identify reduction in LDL cholesterol as the primary target for cholesterol-lowering therapy, particularly in people at risk for CHD. The major risk factors for CHD, exclusive of LDL cholesterol levels, that modify LDL cholesterol goals include cigarette smoking, hypertension, family history of premature CHD in a first-degree relative, age (men ≥45 years; women ≥55 years), and HDL cholesterol <40 mg/dL (see Chart 22-1). Accordingly, the NCEP recommends that persons with CHD or CHD equivalents (other forms of atherosclerotic disease or diabetes) should have a LDL cholesterol goal of <100 mg/dL; those with two or more of the major risk factors should have a LDL cholesterol goal of 130 mg/dL; and those with zero or no risk major factors should have a LDL cholesterol goal of ≤160 mg/dL.[10] The management of hypercholesteremia focuses on dietary and lifestyle modification, and when these are unsuccessful, pharmacologic treatment may be necessary. Lifestyle modification includes an increased emphasis on physical activity, dietary measures to reduce LDL cholesterol levels, and weight reduction for people who are overweight.

Three elements affect dietary cholesterol and its lipoprotein fractions: excess calorie intake, saturated fats, and cholesterol. Excess calories consistently lower HDL and less consistently elevate LDL. Saturated fats in the diet can strongly influence cholesterol levels. Each 1% of saturated fat relative to caloric intake increases the cholesterol level an average of 2.8 mg/dL.[13] Depending on individual differences, it raises the VLDL and the LDL. Dietary cholesterol

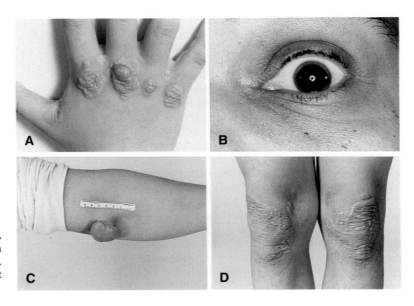

FIGURE 22-3 Xanthomas in the skin and tendons (**A, C, D**). Arcus lipoides represents the deposition of lipids in the peripheral cornea (**B**). (Rubin E., Farber J.L. [1999]. *Pathology* [3rd ed., p. 506]. Philadelphia: Lippincott Williams & Wilkins)

tends to increase LDL cholesterol. On average, each 100 mg/dL of ingested cholesterol raises the serum cholesterol 8 to 10 mg/dL.[13]

The aim of dietary therapy is to reduce total and LDL cholesterol levels and increase HDL cholesterol by reduction in total calories, and to reduce the percentage of total calories from saturated fat and cholesterol. The American Heart Association (AHA) has issued new dietary guidelines that focus on an overall plan of healthy food choices and increased physical activity to decrease the risk for development of cardiovascular disease.[14] The specific guidelines are intended to assist the general public in the maintenance of a body mass index lower than 25 (weight in kilograms divided by body surface area in square meters), to achieve and maintain a low total cholesterol and LDL and a high HDL, and to maintain a blood pressure within normal limits. In general, the dietary guidelines emphasize an increased intake of fruits, vegetables, and fish, and decreased intake of fat, cholesterol and salt. For persons who already have an elevated LDL, the AHA recommends that the upper limit of saturated fat intake be less than 7% of the total daily intake. However, even with strict adherence to the diet, drug therapy may be necessary. Clinical data suggest that drug therapy may be efficacious even for those with mild to moderate LDL cholesterol.[15]

Lipid-lowering drugs ultimately work by affecting cholesterol production, increasing intravascular breakdown, or removing cholesterol from the bloodstream. Drugs that act directly to decrease cholesterol levels also have the beneficial effect of further lowering cholesterol levels by stimulating the production of additional LDL receptors. Unless lipid levels are severely elevated, it is recommended that a minimum of 6 months of intensive diet therapy be undertaken before drug therapy is considered.[12]

Four types of medications are available for treating hypercholesterolemia: bile acid–binding resins, niacin and its congeners, HMG-CoA reductase inhibitors (statins), and fibric acid agents. Estrogen replacement therapy may be used as a possible alternative or adjunct to drug therapy in postmenopausal women. The bile acid–binding resins, cholestyramine and colestipol, bind and sequester cholesterol-containing bile acids in the intestine and prevent the reabsorption of cholesterol by way of the chylomicrons. When bile acid–binding resins are used in combination with statin therapy, serum HDL levels rise 0.5 mg/dL. Nicotinic acid, a niacin congener, blocks the synthesis and release of VLDL by the liver, thereby lowering not only VLDL levels but IDL and LDL levels. Nicotinic acid also increases HDL concentrations up to 30%. Inhibitors of HMG-CoA reductase (*e.g.*, atorvastatin, cerivastatin, fluvastatin, lovastatin, provastatin, simvastatin), a key enzyme in the cholesterol biosynthetic pathway, can reduce or block the hepatic synthesis of cholesterol. Statins also reduce triglyceride levels. The fibric acid derivatives, clofibrate and gemfibrozil, decrease the synthesis of VLDL from chylomicron fragments and enhance the intravascular lipolysis of VLDL and IDL. Because many of these drugs have significant adverse effects, they usually are used only in persons with significant hyperlipidemia that cannot be controlled by other means, such as diet.[16,17]

ATHEROSCLEROSIS

Atherosclerosis is a type of arteriosclerosis or hardening of the arteries. The term *atherosclerosis*, which comes from the Greek words *atheros* (meaning "gruel" or "paste") and *sclerosis* (meaning "hardness"), denotes the formation of fibrofatty lesions in the intimal lining of the large and medium-sized arteries such as the aorta and its branches, the coronary arteries, and the large vessels that supply the brain. Of these, the coronaries are the most commonly affected arteries (Fig. 22-4).

Although there has been a gradual decline in deaths from atherosclerosis over the past several decades, coronary heart disease remains the leading cause of death among men

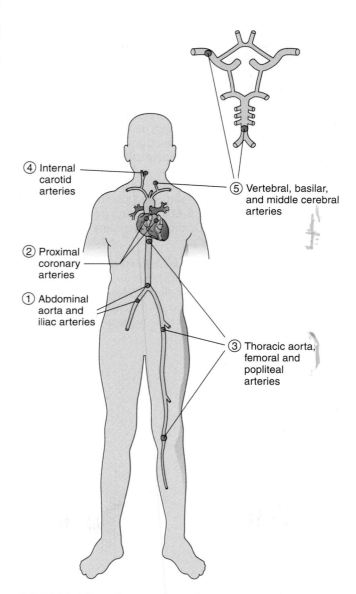

FIGURE 22-4 Sites of severe atherosclerosis in order of frequency. (Rubin E., Farber J.L. [1999]. *Pathology* [3rd ed., p. 508]. Philadelphia: Lippincott Williams & Wilkins)

and women in the United States.[2] The reported decline in death rate probably reflects new and improved methods of medical treatment and improved health care practices resulting from an increased public awareness of the factors that predispose to the development of this disorder.

Atherosclerosis begins as an insidious process, and clinical manifestations of the disease typically do not become evident for 20 to 40 years or longer. Fibrous plaques commonly begin to appear in the arteries of Americans in their twenties. Necropsy findings from 300 American soldiers (average age of 22 years) killed during the Korean War indicated that 77% had gross evidence of atherosclerosis.[18]

Risk Factors

The cause or causes of atherosclerosis have not been determined with certainty. Epidemiologic studies have, however, identified predisposing risk factors, which are listed in Chart 22-1.[3,19,20] In terms of health care behaviors, some of these risk factors can be affected by a change in behavior, and others cannot.

The major risk factor for atherosclerosis is hypercholesterolemia. Nonlipid risk factors such as increasing age, family history of premature coronary heart disease, and male sex cannot be changed. The tendency to development of atherosclerosis appears to run in families. Persons who come from families with a strong history of heart disease or stroke due to atherosclerosis are at greater risk for developing atherosclerosis than those with a negative family history. Several genetically determined alterations in lipoprotein and cholesterol metabolism have been identified, and it seems likely that others will be identified in the future. The incidence of atherosclerosis increases with age. Men (after 45 years of age) are at greater risk for developing coronary heart disease than are women; even though the death rate of women increases after menopause (after age 55 years without estrogen replacement therapy), it never reaches that of men.

The major risk factors that can be affected by a change in health care behaviors include cigarette smoking, hypertension, high blood cholesterol levels, and diabetes mellitus. Cigarette smoking is closely linked with coronary heart disease and sudden death. One hypothesis is that components of cigarette smoke may be toxic, causing oxidative insult and damage to the endothelial lining of blood vessels.[21] Endothelial dysfunction may be worsened by cigarette smoke, which is why cessation of smoking by high-risk individuals often is followed within a few years by reduced risk of ischemic heart disease.

High blood pressure and high blood cholesterol levels often can be controlled with a change in health care behaviors and medications. There is evidence that elevated serum cholesterol not only contributes to development of atherosclerotic lesions that block arteries, but interferes with vessel relaxation.[21,22] Observational research indicates that a linear relation exists between serum cholesterol levels and coronary heart disease; a 10% decrease in serum cholesterol is associated with a 20% decrease in coronary heart disease.[23] The association between coronary heart disease and contributing or "soft" factors is not as convincing as for the established risk factors. These soft risk factors commonly are linked with the established and other contributing risk factors. For example, obesity and physical inactivity often are observed in the same person. Both conditions are reported to bring about elevations in blood lipid levels. Likewise, major risk factors such as cigarette smoking are closely associated with stress and personality patterns. Diabetes mellitus (type 2) typically develops in middle-aged persons and those who are overweight. Diabetes elevates blood lipid levels and otherwise increases the risk of atherosclerosis (see Chapter 41). Controlling other risk factors is particularly important in those with diabetes.

Not all atherothrombotic vascular disease can be explained by the established genetic and environmental risk factors. Other factors that may be associated with an increased risk for developing atherosclerosis include serum homocysteine, serum lipoprotein (a), C-reactive protein (CRP), and infectious agents.[3,19,20]

Homocysteine is derived from the metabolism of dietary methionine, an amino acid that is abundant in animal protein. The normal metabolism of homocysteine requires adequate levels of folate, vitamin B_6, vitamin B_{12}, and riboflavin. Evidence is growing that an increased plasma level of homocysteine (>15 μmol/L) is an independent and dose-related risk factor for development of atherosclerosis. Homocysteine inhibits elements of the anticoagulant cascade and is associated with endothelial damage, which is thought to be an important first step in the development of atherosclerosis.[3,20,24] Factors tending to increase plasma levels of

---

CHART 22-1

Risk Factors in Coronary Heart Disease Other Than Low-Density Lipoproteins

Positive Risk Factors

Age
  Men: ≥45 years
  Women: ≥55 years or premature menopause without estrogen replacement therapy
Family history of premature coronary heart disease (definite myocardial infarction or sudden death before 55 years of age in father or other male first-degree relative, or before 65 years of age in mother or other female first-degree relative)
Current cigarette smoking
Hypertension (≥140/90 mm Hg* or on antihypertensive medication)
Low HDL cholesterol (<40 mg/dL*)
Diabetes mellitus

Negative Risk Factor

High HDL cholesterol (≥60 mg/dL)

HDL, high-density lipoprotein.
*Confirmed by measurements on several occasions.
(Modified from National Institute of Health Expert Panel [2001]. *Third Report of the National Cholesterol Program [NCEP] Expert Panel on Detection, Evaluation, and Treatment of High Blood Cholesterol in Adults* [Adult Treatment Panel III]. [NIH Publication No. 01-3670]. Bethesda, MD: National Institutes of Health.)

homocysteine include lower serum levels of folate and vitamins B_6 and B_{12}, genetic defects in homocysteine metabolism, renal impairment, malignancies, increasing age, male sex, and menopause.[14,24] There are several clinical studies in progress to determine the efficacy of vitamin supplementation (with folic acid, vitamin B_6, and vitamin B_{12}) as a means of lowering plasma homocysteine levels.[24]

Lipoprotein (a) is similar to LDL in composition and is an independent risk factor for the development of premature coronary heart disease in men. The mechanism by which lipoprotein (a) increases atherogenesis is unclear but may be similar to that of LDL. Lipoprotein (a) levels should be determined in persons who have premature coronary artery disease or a positive family history.[20] CRP is a serum marker for systemic inflammation. Several prospective studies have indicated that elevated CRP levels are associated with vascular disease. The pathophysiologic role of CRP in atherosclerosis has not been defined, but it may increase the likelihood of thrombus formation.[20] There also has been increased interest in the possible connection between infectious agents (*Chlamydia pneumoniae*, herpesvirus hominis, cytomegalovirus) and the development of vascular disease. The presence of these organisms in atheromatous lesions has been demonstrated by immunocytochemistry, but no cause-and-effect relationship has been established. The organisms may play a role in atherosclerotic development by initiating and enhancing the inflammatory response.[25]

Mechanisms of Development

Fatty streaks are thin, flat, yellow streaks in the intima. They consist of macrophages and smooth muscle cells that have become distended with lipid to form foam cells. Fatty streaks often are found in children at autopsy in the thoracic aorta as well as other parts of the arterial tree.[3] This occurs regardless of geographic setting, sex, or race. Fatty streaks in the coronary arteries begin to appear in adolescence. There is controversy about whether fatty streaks are precursors of atherosclerotic lesions.

Atherosclerotic lesions are characterized by the accumulation of intracellular and extracellular lipids, proliferation of vascular smooth muscle cells, and formation of scar tissue and connective tissue proteins. The lesions begin as a gray to pearly white, elevated thickening of the vessel intima with a core of extracellular lipid (mainly cholesterol, which usually is complexed to proteins) covered by a fibrous cap of connective tissue and smooth muscle (Fig. 22-5). More advanced lesions are characterized by hemorrhage, ulceration, and scar tissue deposits. As the lesions increase in size, they encroach on the lumen of the artery and eventually may occlude the vessel or predispose to thrombus formation, causing a reduction of blood flow. Because blood flow is related to the fourth power of the radius, reduction in blood flow becomes more severe as the disease progresses.

Although the risk factors associated with atherosclerosis have been identified through epidemiologic studies, many unanswered questions remain regarding the mechanisms by which these risk factors contribute to the development of atherosclerosis. There is increasing evidence suggesting that atherosclerosis is at least partially the result of endothelial injury, lipid (*i.e.*, LDL and cholesterol) infiltration, recruitment of inflammatory cells (*i.e.*, predominantly monocytes and T lymphocytes), and smooth muscle proliferation. The vascular endothelial layer, which consists of a single layer of cells with cell-to-cell attachments, normally serves as a selective barrier that protects the subendothelial layers by interacting with blood cells and other blood components.

One hypothesis of plaque formation is that injury to the endothelial vessel layer is the initiating factor in the development of atherosclerosis. Endothelial injury allows monocytes, platelets, cholesterol, and other blood components to come in contact with and stimulate abnormal proliferation of smooth muscle cells and connective tissue within the vessel wall. A number of factors are regarded as possible injurious agents, including products associated with smoking, immune mechanisms, and mechanical stress such as that associated with hypertension. If the injury is a single event, the damage usually is reversible. However, if the factors that led to vessel damage persist, there is less time for healing to occur, and the lesion may become chronic.

Evidence also suggests that LDLs that become trapped in the arterial wall are locally modified and may act as cofactors necessary for growth and proliferation of vascular smooth muscle cells.[6,19,26] Interactions between the endothelial layer of the vessel wall and white blood cells, particularly the monocytes (blood macrophages), normally occur throughout life; these interactions increase when blood cholesterol levels are elevated. One of the earliest responses to elevated cholesterol levels is the attachment of monocytes to the endothelium.[6] The monocytes have been observed to move through the cell-to-cell attachments of the endothelial layer into the subendothelial spaces, where they ingest lipid and in the process become foam cells (Fig. 22-6). Foam cells, which are present in all stages of atherosclerotic plaque formation, are thought to promote growth factors that modulate the proliferation of smooth muscle cells and deposition of extracellular matrix in the lesions.[6,19,26]

Clinical Manifestations

The clinical manifestations of atherosclerosis depend on the vessels involved and the extent of vessel obstruction. Atherosclerotic lesions produce their effects through narrowing of the vessel and production of ischemia; sudden vessel obstruction due to plaque hemorrhage or rupture; thrombosis and formation of emboli resulting from damage to the vessel endothelium; and aneurysm formation due to weakening of the vessel wall.[7] In larger vessels such as the aorta, the important complications are those of thrombus formation and weakening of the vessel wall. In medium-sized arteries such as the coronary and cerebral arteries, ischemia and infarction due to vessel occlusion are more common. Although atherosclerosis can affect any organ or tissue, the arteries supplying the heart, brain, kidneys, lower extremities, and small intestine are most frequently involved.

VASCULITIS

The vasculitides are a group of vascular disorders that cause inflammatory injury and necrosis of the blood vessel wall (*i.e.*, vasculitis). The vasculitides, which are a common pathway for tissue and organ involvement in many different dis-

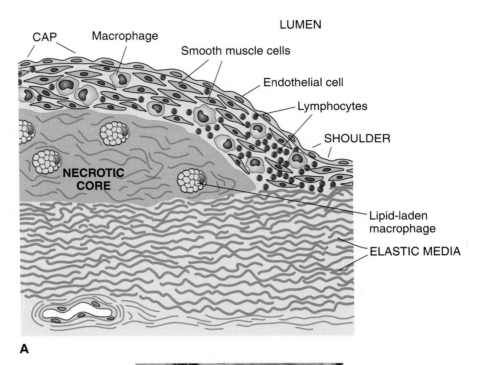

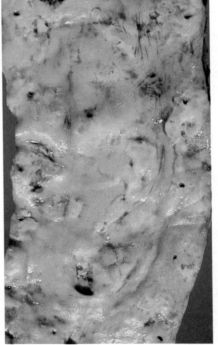

FIGURE 22-5 Fibrofatty plaque of atherosclerosis. (**A**) In this fully developed fibrous plaque, the core contains lipid-filled macrophages and necrotic smooth muscle cell debris. The "fibrous" cap is composed largely of smooth muscle cells, which produce collagen, small amounts of elastin, and glycosaminoglycans. Also shown are infiltrating macrophages and lymphocytes. Note that the endothelium over the surface of the fibrous cap frequently appear intact. (**B**) The aorta shows discrete raised, tan plaques. Focal plaque ulcerations are also evident. (Rubin E., Farber J.L. [1999]. *Pathology* [3rd ed., p. 497]. Philadelphia: Lippincott Williams & Wilkins)

ease conditions, involve the endothelial cells and smooth muscle cells of the arterial wall.[27,28] Because they also may affect veins and capillaries, the terms *vasculitis*, *angiitis*, and *arteritis* often are used interchangeably. Vasculitis may result from direct injury to the vessel, infectious agents, or immune processes, or may be secondary to other disease states such as systemic lupus erythematosus. Physical agents such as cold (*i.e.*, frostbite), irradiation (*i.e.*, sunburn), me-

chanical injury, and toxins may secondarily cause vessel damage, often leading to necrosis of the vessels. Small vessel vasculitides are sometimes associated with anti-neutrophil cytoplasmic antibodies. These autoantibodies may cause endothelial damage.[3]

The vasculitides are commonly classified based on clinical findings, pathologic findings, and prognosis. One classification system divides the conditions into four groups[3,27,28]

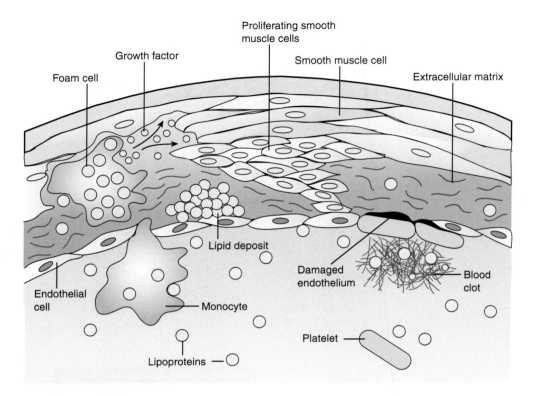

FIGURE 22-6 Role of excess lipoprotein and monocyte in the pathogenesis of atherosclerosis. Elevated levels of cholesterol-carrying lipoproteins cause monocytes to attach to and move through cell-to-cell attachments in the endothelium. Monocytes that consume excess lipoproteins become foam cells, which release growth factors that encourage proliferation of smooth muscle cells and extracellular matrix, leading to atherosclerotic plaque formation, endothelial injury, and blood clot formation.

(Table 22-2). Group I vasculitides produce necrotizing damage to small and medium-sized muscular arteries of major organ systems. Group II vasculitides involve hypersensitivity reactions that produce a venulitis. They commonly involve the skin and are often a complication of an underlying disease (*i.e.,* vasculitis associated with neoplasms or connective tissue disease) and exposure to environmental agents (*i.e.,* serum sickness and urticarial vasculitis; see Chapter 19). Group III vasculitides involve large elastic arteries; they are called *giant cell arterides* because they involve infiltration of the vessel wall with giant cells and mononuclear cells. Group IV consists of miscellaneous vasculitides; it includes conditions such as Kawasaki syndrome (see Chapter 24) and thromboangiitis obliterans (discussed in the section on arterial diseases of the extremities). Two examples of vasculitides are included in this section: polyarteritis nodosa and giant cell temporal arteritis.

Polyarteritis Nodosa

Polyarteritis nodosa, so named because of the numerous nodules found along the course of muscular arteries, is a primary multisystem inflammatory disease of small and medium-sized blood vessels, especially those of the kidney, liver, in-testine, peripheral nerve, skin, and muscle. The disease is seen more commonly in men than women.

The cause of polyarteritis nodosa remains unknown. It can occur in drug abusers and may be associated with use of certain drugs such as allopurinol and the sulfonamides. There is an association between polyarteritis nodosa and hepatitis B infection, with 10% to 40% of persons with the disease having antibodies to hepatitis in their serum. Other associations include serous otitis media, hairy cell leukemia, and hyposensitization therapy for allergies. Persons with connective tissue diseases such as systemic lupus erythematosus, rheumatoid arthritis, and primary Sjögren's syndrome may have manifestations similar to those of primary polyarteritis nodosa.

Manifestations. The onset of polyarteritis nodosa usually is abrupt, with complaints of anorexia, weight loss, fever, and fatigue often accompanied by signs of organ involvement. The kidney is the most frequently affected organ, and hypertension is a common manifestation of the disorder. Gastrointestinal involvement may manifest as abdominal pain, nausea, vomiting, or diarrhea. Myalgia, arthralgia, and arthritis are common, as are peripheral neuropathies such

TABLE 22-2 ◆ Examples of Vasculitides Classified by Group and Characteristics

Group	Examples	Characteristics
Group I—systemic necrotizing vasculitides	Polyarteritis nodosa Rheumatoid vasculitis Allergic angiitis and granulomatosis (Churg-Strauss syndrome)	Affects medium-sized vessels of major organ systems; usually associated with an underlying disease or environmental agent Churg-Strauss syndrome involves eosinophil-rich and granulomatous inflammation that affects the respiratory tract and is associated with asthma and allergic rhinitis.
Group II—hypersensitivity vasculitides	Serum sickness Vasculitis associated with infectious diseases (*e.g.*, bacterial endocarditis) Hepatitis B Vasculitis associated with neoplasms Vasculitis associated with connective tissue disease Urticarial vasculitis	Produces a venulitis with endothelial swelling, red blood cell extravasation, and fibrinoid necrosis Predominance of skin involvement with sporadic damage to major organ systems Thought to be mediated by immunologic mechanisms
Group III—giant cell arteritis	Temporal arteritis Takayasu's arteritis	Affects large elastic arteries; infiltration of vessel wall with giant cells and mononuclear cells, producing periarteritis with dramatic ischemic consequences Temporal arteritis affects extracranial branches of the carotid artery and often affects the temporal artery. Takayasu's arteritis affects the aorta and its branches.
Group IV—miscellaneous	Thromboangiitis obliterans Kawasaki syndrome	Kawasaki syndrome is an arteritis involving large, medium-sized, and small arteries (frequently the coronaries) and is associated with mucocutaneous lymph node syndrome, usually in young children.

(Developed from Pariser K.M., Wolff S.M. [1992]. The clinical spectrum of vasculitis. In Loscalzo J., Creager M.A., Dzau V.J. [Eds.], *Vascular medicine: A textbook of vascular biology and disease* [pp. 1012–1013]. Boston: Little, Brown; and Cotran R.S., Kumar V., Robbins S.L. [1994]. *Pathologic basis of disease* [4th ed., pp. 489–499]. Philadelphia: W.B. Saunders.)

as paresthesias, pain, and weakness. Central nervous system complications include thrombotic and hemorrhagic stroke. Cardiac manifestations result from involvement of the coronary arteries. Skin lesions also may occur and are highly variable. They include reddish blue, mottled areas of discoloration of the skin of the extremities called *livedo reticularis*, purpura (*i.e.*, black and blue discoloration from bleeding into the skin), urticaria (*i.e.*, hives), and ulcers.

Diagnosis and Treatment. Laboratory findings, although variable, include an elevated erythrocyte sedimentation rate, leukocytosis, anemia, and signs of organ involvement such as hematuria and abnormal liver function tests. The diagnosis is confirmed through biopsy specimens demonstrating necrotizing vasculitis of the small and large arteries. Treatment involves use of high-dose corticosteroid therapy and often cytotoxic immunosuppressant agents (*e.g.*, azathioprine, cyclophosphamide). Before the availability of corticosteroids and immunosuppressive agents, the disease commonly was fatal. With the use of these agents, the 5-year survival rate is greater than 50%.[29] After the disease is under control, treatment usually is continued for 18 to 24 months and then gradually tapered.[27] Intravenous immunoglobulin is being used with increasing frequency and very promising results.

Giant Cell Temporal Arteritis

Temporal arteritis (*i.e.*, giant cell arteritis) is a focal inflammatory condition of medium-sized and large arteries. It predominantly affects branches of arteries originating from the aortic arch, including the superficial temporal, vertebral, ophthalmic, and posterior ciliary arteries. The disorder progresses to involve the entire artery wall with focal necrosis and granulomatous inflammation involving multinucleated giant cells. It is more common in elderly persons, with a 2:1 female-to-male ratio. The cause is unknown, although an autoimmune origin has been suggested.

Manifestations. The disorder often is insidious in onset and may be heralded by the sudden onset of headache, tenderness over the artery, swelling and redness of the overlying skin, blurred vision or diplopia, and facial pain. Almost one half of affected persons have systemic involvement in the form of polymyalgia rheumatica.

Diagnosis and Treatment. Diagnosis is based on the clinical manifestations, a characteristically elevated erythrocyte sedimentation rate, and temporal artery biopsy. Treatment includes use of high-dose corticosteroids. Before persons with the disorder were treated with corticosteroids, blindness developed in almost 80% of cases.

ARTERIAL DISEASE OF THE EXTREMITIES

Disorders of the circulation in the extremities often are referred to as *peripheral vascular disorders*. In many respects, the disorders that affect arteries in the extremities are the same as those affecting the coronary and cerebral arteries in that they produce ischemia, pain, impaired function, and in some cases infarction and tissue necrosis. Not only are the effects similar, but the pathologic conditions that impair circulation in the extremities are identical. This section focuses on acute arterial occlusion of the extremities, atherosclerotic occlusive disease, thromboangiitis obliterans, and Raynaud's disease and phenomenon.

Acute Arterial Occlusion

Acute arterial occlusion is a sudden event that interrupts arterial flow to the affected tissues or organ. Most acute arterial occlusions are the result of an embolus or a thrombus. Rarely, the tips of catheters that have been inserted into a vessel can break off and become emboli. Although much less common than emboli and thrombus, trauma or arterial spasm caused by arterial cannulation can be another cause of acute arterial occlusion.

An embolus is a freely moving particle such as a blood clot that breaks loose and travels in the larger vessels of the circulation until lodging in a smaller vessel and occluding blood flow. Most emboli arise in the heart and are caused by conditions that cause blood clots to develop on the wall of a heart chamber or valve surface. Emboli usually are a complication of heart disease: ischemic heart disease with or without infarction, atrial fibrillation, or rheumatic heart disease. Prosthetic heart valves can be another source of emboli. Other types of emboli are fat emboli that originate from bone marrow of fractured bones, air emboli from the lung, and amniotic fluid emboli that develop during childbirth.

A thrombus is a blood clot that forms on the wall of a vessel and continues to grow until reaching a size that obstructs blood flow. These thrombi often arise as the result of rupture of the fibrous cap of an arteriosclerotic plaque.

Manifestations. The signs and symptoms of acute arterial occlusion depend on the artery involved and the adequacy of the collateral circulation. Emboli tend to lodge in bifurcations of the major arteries, including the aorta and iliac, femoral, and popliteal arteries. Occlusion in an extremity causes sudden onset of acute pain with numbness, tingling, weakness, pallor, and coldness. There often is a sharp line of demarcation between the oxygenated tissue above the line of obstruction and that below the line of obstruction. Pulses are absent below the level of the occlusion. These changes are followed rapidly by cyanosis, mottling, and loss of sensory, reflex, and motor function. Tissue dies unless blood flow is restored.

Diagnosis and Treatment. Diagnosis of acute arterial occlusion is based on signs of impaired blood flow. It uses visual assessment, palpation of pulses, and methods to assess blood flow. Treatment of acute arterial occlusion is aimed at restoring blood flow. Thrombolytic therapy (*i.e.,* streptokinase or tissue plasminogen activator) may be used in an attempt to dissolve the clot. Anticoagulant therapy (*i.e.,* heparin) usually is given to prevent extension of the embolus. Application of heat and cold should be avoided, and the extremity should be protected from injury resulting from hard surfaces and overlying bedclothes. An embolectomy—surgical removal of the embolus—may be indicated.

Atherosclerotic Occlusive Disease

Atherosclerosis is an important cause of peripheral vascular disease and is seen most commonly in the vessels of the lower extremities. The condition is sometimes referred to as *arteriosclerosis obliterans*. The superficial femoral and popliteal arteries are the most commonly affected vessels. When lesions develop in the lower leg and foot, the tibial, common peroneal, or pedal vessels are the arteries most commonly affected. The disease is seen most commonly in men in their sixties and seventies.[30–32] The risk factors for this disorder are similar to those for atherosclerosis. Cigarette smoking contributes to the progress of the atherosclerosis of the lower extremities and to the development of symptoms of ischemia. Persons with diabetes mellitus develop more extensive and rapidly progressive vascular disease than do nondiabetic individuals.

Manifestations. As with atherosclerosis in other locations, the signs and symptoms of vessel occlusion are gradual. Usually, there is at least a 50% narrowing of the vessel before symptoms of ischemia arise. The primary symptom of chronic obstructive arterial disease is *intermittent claudication* or pain with walking.[30,32] Typically, persons with the disorder complain of calf pain because the gastrocnemius muscle has the highest oxygen consumption of any muscle group in the leg during walking. Some persons may complain of a vague aching feeling or numbness, rather than pain. Other activities such as swimming, bicycling, and climbing stairs use other muscle groups and may not incite the same degree of discomfort as walking. Other signs of ischemia include atrophic changes and thinning of the skin and subcutaneous tissues of the lower leg and diminution in the size of the leg muscles. The foot often is cool, and the popliteal and pedal pulses are weak or absent. Limb color blanches with elevation of the leg because of the effects of gravity on perfusion pressure and becomes deep red when the leg is in the dependent position because of an autoregulatory increase in blood flow and a gravitational increase in perfusion pressure.

When blood flow is reduced to the extent that it no longer meets the minimal needs of resting muscle and nerves, ischemic pain at rest, ulceration, and gangrene develop. As tissue necrosis develops there typically is severe pain in the region of skin breakdown, which is worse at night with limb elevation and is improved with standing.[30]

Diagnosis and Treatment. Diagnostic methods include inspection of the limbs for signs of chronic low-grade ischemia such as subcutaneous atrophy, brittle toenails, hair loss, pallor, coolness, or dependent rubor. Palpation of the femoral, popliteal, posterior tibial, and dorsalis pedis pulses allows for an estimation of the level and degree of obstruction. The ratio of ankle to arm (*i.e.*, tibial and brachial arteries) systolic blood pressure is used to detect significant obstruction, with a ratio of less than 0.9 indicating occlusion. Normally, systolic pressure in the ankle exceeds that in the brachial artery because systolic pressure and pulse pressure tend to increase as the pressure wave moves away from the heart (see Chapter 21). Blood pressures may be taken at various levels on the leg to determine the level of obstruction. A Doppler ultrasound stethoscope may be used for detecting pulses and measuring blood pressure. Ultrasound imaging, radionuclide imaging, and contrast angiography also may be used as diagnostic methods.[30–32]

The tissues of extremities affected by atherosclerosis are easily injured and slow to heal. Treatment includes measures directed at protection of the affected tissues and preservation of functional capacity. Walking (slowly) to the point of claudication usually is encouraged because it increases collateral circulation.

Surgery (*i.e.*, femoropopliteal bypass grafting using a section of saphenous vein) may be indicated in severe cases. In persons with diabetes, the peroneal arteries between the knees and ankles commonly are involved, making revascularization difficult. Thromboendarterectomy with removal of the occluding core of atherosclerotic tissue may be done if the section of diseased vessel is short. Percutaneous transluminal angioplasty, in which a balloon catheter is inserted into the area of stenosis and the balloon inflated to increase vessel diameter, is another form of treatment.[30–32]

Thromboangiitis Obliterans

Thromboangiitis obliterans (*e.g.*, Buerger's disease) is an inflammatory (*i.e.*, vasculitis) arterial disorder that causes thrombus formation. The disorder affects the medium-sized arteries, usually the plantar and digital vessels in the foot and lower leg. Arteries in the arm and hand also may be affected. Although primarily an arterial disorder, the inflammatory process often extends to involve adjacent veins and nerves. It usually is a disease of men between the ages of 25 and 40 years who are heavy cigarette smokers, but it can occur in women. The pathogenesis of Buerger's disease remains speculative, although cigarette smoking and in some instances tobacco chewing seem to be involved. It has been suggested that the tobacco may trigger an immune response in susceptible persons or it may unmask a clotting defect, either of which could incite an inflammatory reaction of the vessel wall.[33]

Manifestations. Pain is the predominant symptom of the disorder. It usually is related to distal arterial ischemia. During the early stages of the disease, there is intermittent claudication in the arch of the foot and the digits. In severe cases, pain is present even when the person is at rest. The impaired circulation increases sensitivity to cold. The peripheral pulses are diminished or absent, and there are changes in the color of the extremity. In moderately advanced cases,

---

Assessment of Arterial Flow in the Extremities

The methods for assessing arterial blood flow and detecting arterial disease include monitoring of capillary refill time and peripheral pulses. Angiography, Doppler ultrasound flow studies, and magnetic resonance imaging (MRI) may be used for a more definitive diagnosis.

Capillary refill time is an indicator of the efficiency of the microcirculation. It is measured by depressing the nail bed of a finger or toe until the underlying skin blanches. The refill time is normal if the capillary vessels refill within 3 seconds after pressure is released. The volume of the peripheral pulses and capillary refill time are useful indirect methods for assessing peripheral perfusion. Peripheral pulses can be palpated over vessels in the head, neck (*i.e.*, carotid), and extremities. In situations associated with potential vessel spasm or thrombosis, it may be necessary to check only for the presence of pulses. In many situations, however, the pulse volume (weak and thready to strong and bounding) provides useful information about vascular volume and the condition of the arterial circulation. Arterial auscultation is used to listen to the flow of blood with a stethoscope. The term *bruit* is used to describe an audible murmur heard over a peripheral artery. It is caused by turbulent blood flow and is suggestive of obstructive arterial disease.

Doppler ultrasound flow studies use reflected ultrasound waves, which are transmitted back to the skin surface from a blood vessel, to determine the direction and velocity of blood flow. Doppler studies can be used to assess the patency of a given blood vessel. They are useful in studying blood flow in the carotid arteries, abdominal vessels, fetal blood vessels, and peripheral blood vessels.

MRI is a noninvasive technique that can be used to study blood flow. The method uses a magnetic field to align the charges on blood components as they move through blood vessels. The aligned charges emit measurable radiofrequency signals, which can be detected electronically and recorded.

---

the extremity becomes cyanotic when the person assumes a dependent position, and the digits may turn reddish blue even when in a nondependent position. With lack of blood flow, the skin assumes a thin, shiny look and hair growth and skin nutrition suffer. Chronic ischemia causes thick, malformed nails. If the disease continues to progress, tissues eventually ulcerate and gangrenous changes arise that may necessitate amputation.

Diagnosis and Treatment. Diagnostic methods are similar to those for atherosclerotic disease of the lower extremities. As part of the treatment program for thromboangiitis obliterans, it is mandatory that the person stop smoking cigarettes or using tobacco. Other treatment measures are of secondary importance and focus on methods for producing vasodilation and preventing tissue injury. Sympathectomy may be done to alleviate the vasospastic manifestations of the disease.

Raynaud's Disease and Phenomenon

Raynaud's disease or phenomenon is a functional disorder caused by intense vasospasm of the arteries and arterioles in the fingers and, less often, the toes. The disorder is divided into two types: the primary type, called *Raynaud's disease*, occurs without demonstrable cause, and the secondary type, called *Raynaud's phenomenon*, is associated with other disease states or known causes of vasospasm.[34–36]

Vasospasm implies an excessive vasoconstrictor response to stimuli that normally produce only moderate vasoconstriction. In contrast to other regional circulations that are supplied by vasodilator and vasoconstrictor fibers, the cutaneous vessels of the fingers and toes are innervated only by sympathetic vasoconstrictor fibers. In these vessels, vasodilation occurs by withdrawal of sympathetic stimulation. Cooling of specific body parts such as the head, neck, and trunk produces a sympathetic-mediated reduction in digital blood flow, as does emotional stress.

Raynaud's disease is seen in otherwise healthy young women, and it often is precipitated by exposure to cold or by strong emotions and usually is limited to the fingers. It also follows a more benign course than Raynaud's phenomenon, seldom causing tissue necrosis. The cause of vasospasm in primary Raynaud's disease is unknown. Hyperreactivity of the sympathetic nervous system has been suggested as a contributing cause.[34] Raynaud's phenomenon is associated with previous vessel injury, such as frostbite, occupational trauma associated with the use of heavy vibrating tools, collagen diseases, neurologic disorders, and chronic arterial occlusive disorders. Another occupation-related cause is the exposure to alternating hot and cold temperatures such as that experienced by butchers and food preparers.[34] Raynaud's phenomenon often is the first symptom of collagen diseases. It occurs in persons with scleroderma with systemic lupus erythematosus.[36]

Manifestations.   In Raynaud's disease and Raynaud's phenomenon, ischemia due to vasospasm causes changes in skin color that progress from pallor to cyanosis, a sensation of cold, and changes in sensory perception, such as numbness and tingling. The color changes usually are first noticed in the tips of the fingers, later moving into one or more of the distal phalanges (Fig. 22-7). After the ischemic episode, there is a period of hyperemia with intense redness, throbbing, and paresthesias. The period of hyperemia is followed by a return to normal color. Although all of the fingers usually are affected symmetrically, the involvement may affect only one or two digits. In some cases, only a portion of the digit is affected.

In severe, progressive cases usually associated with Raynaud's phenomenon, trophic changes may develop. The nails may become brittle, and the skin over the tips of the affected fingers may thicken. Nutritional impairment of these structures may give rise to arthritis. Ulceration and superficial gangrene of the fingers, although infrequent, may occur.

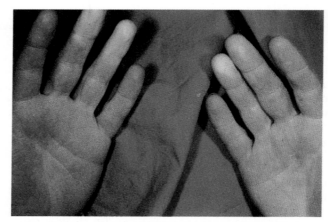

FIGURE 22-7 Raynaud's phenomenon. The tips of the fingers show marked pallor. (Rubin E., Farber J.L. [1999]. *Pathology* [3rd ed., p. 514]. Philadelphia: Lippincott Williams & Wilkins)

Diagnosis and Treatment.   The initial diagnosis is based on history of vasospastic attacks supported by other evidence of the disorder. Immersion of the hand in cold water may be used to initiate an attack as an aid to diagnosis. Laser Doppler flow velocimetry may be used to quantify digital blood flow during changes in temperature. Serial computed thermography (finger skin temperature) also may be a useful tool in diagnosing the extent of disease. Raynaud's disease is differentiated from Raynaud's phenomenon by excluding secondary disorders known to cause vasospasm.[36]

Treatment measures are directed toward eliminating factors that cause vasospasm and protecting the digits from trauma during an ischemic episode. Abstinence from smoking and protection from cold are priorities. The entire body must be protected from cold, not just the extremities. Avoidance of emotional stress is another important factor in controlling the disorder because anxiety and stress may precipitate a vascular spasm in predisposed persons. Biofeedback training may be helpful in persons with Raynaud's disease but does not seem to be as effective for those with Raynaud's phenomenon. Vasoconstrictor medications, such as the decongestants contained in allergy and cold preparations, should be avoided. Treatment with vasodilator drugs may be indicated, particularly if episodes are frequent, because frequency encourages the potential for development of thrombosis and gangrene. The calcium channel blocking drugs (*e.g.*, diltiazem, nifedipine, and nicardipine) decrease the severity and frequency of attacks. Prazosin, an α-adrenergic receptor blocking drug, also may be used. Analogues of prostacyclin (prostaglandin vasodilator) are being investigated as well. Surgical interruption of sympathetic nerve pathways (sympathectomy) may be used for persons with severe symptoms.[36]

ANEURYSMS

An *aneurysm* is an abnormal localized dilatation of a blood vessel. Aneurysms can occur in arteries and veins, but they are most common in the aorta. There are two types of aneurysms: *true aneurysms* and *false aneurysms*. A true aneurysm is one in which the aneurysm is bounded by a complete vessel wall and an increase in diameter of 50%.[37] The blood in a true aneurysm remains within the vascular compartment. A false aneurysm or pseudoaneurysm represents a localized rupture or tear in the inner wall of the artery with formation of an extravascular hematoma that causes vessel enlargement. Unlike true aneurysms, false aneurysms are bounded only by the outer layers of the vessel wall or supporting tissues.

Aneurysms can assume several forms and may be classified according to their cause, location, and anatomic features (Fig. 22-8). A *berry aneurysm* consists of a small, spherical dilatation of the vessel at a bifurcation.[3] This type of aneurysm usually is found in the circle of Willis in the cerebral circulation. A *fusiform aneurysm* involves the entire circumference of the vessel and is characterized by a gradual and progressive dilatation of the vessel. These aneurysms, which vary in diameter (up to 20 cm) and length, may involve the entire ascending and transverse portions of the thoracic aorta or may extend over large segments of the abdominal aorta. A *saccular aneurysm* extends over part of the circumference of the vessel and appears saclike. A *dissecting aneurysm* is a false aneurysm resulting from a tear in the intimal layer of the vessel that allows blood to enter the vessel wall, dissecting its layers to create a blood-filled cavity.

The weakness that leads to aneurysm formation may be caused by several factors, including congenital defects, trauma, infections, and atherosclerosis. Once initiated, the aneurysm grows larger as the tension in the vessel increases. This is because the tension in the wall of a vessel is equal to the pressure multiplied by the radius (*i.e.,* tension = pressure × radius; see Chapter 21). In this case, the pressure in the segment of the vessel affected by the aneurysm does not change but remains the same as that of adjacent portions of the vessel. As an aneurysm increases in diameter, the tension in the wall of the vessel increases in direct proportion to its increased size. If untreated, the aneurysm may rupture because of the increased tension. Even an unruptured aneurysm can cause damage by exerting pressure on adjacent structures and interrupting blood flow.

Aortic Aneurysms

Aortic aneurysms may involve any part of the aorta: the ascending aorta, aortic arch, descending aorta, thoracoabdominal aorta, or abdominal aorta. Multiple aneurysms may be present. The two most common causes of aortic aneurysms are atherosclerosis and degeneration of the vessel media. Aortic aneurysms are more common after 50 years of age and affect men more often than women.

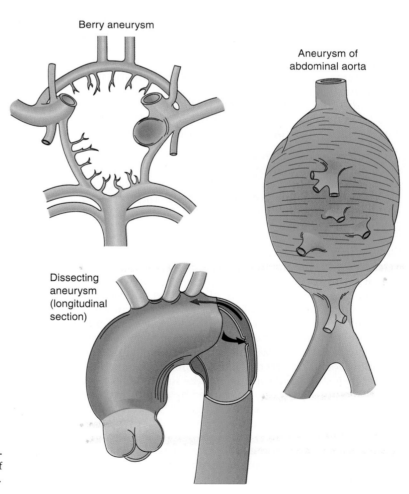

FIGURE 22-8 Three forms of aneurysms—berry aneurysm in the circle of Willis, fusiform-type aneurysm of the abdominal aorta, and a dissecting aortic aneurysm.

Manifestations. The signs and symptoms of aortic aneurysms depend on the size and location. An aneurysm also may be asymptomatic, with the first evidence of its presence being associated with vessel rupture. With aneurysms of the thoracic aorta, substernal, back, and neck pain may occur. There also may be dyspnea, stridor, or a brassy cough caused by pressure on the trachea. Hoarseness may result from pressure on the recurrent laryngeal nerve, and there may be difficulty swallowing because of pressure on the esophagus.[38] The aneurysm also may compress the superior vena cava, causing distention of neck veins and edema of the face and neck.

Abdominal aortic aneurysms are located most commonly below the level of the renal artery and involve the bifurcation of the aorta and proximal end of the common iliac arteries. Most abdominal aneurysms are asymptomatic. Because an aneurysm is of arterial origin, a pulsating mass may provide the first evidence of the disorder. Typically, aneurysms larger than 4 cm are palpable. The mass may be discovered during a routine physical examination or the affected person may complain of its presence. Calcification, which frequently exists on the wall of the aneurysm, may be detected during abdominal radiologic examination. Pain may be present and varies from mild mid-abdominal or lumbar discomfort to severe abdominal and back pain. As the aneurysm expands, it may compress the lumbar nerve roots, causing lower back pain that radiates to the posterior aspects of the legs. The aneurysm may extend to and impinge on the renal, iliac, mesenteric arteries, or vertebral arteries that supply the spinal cord. An abdominal aneurysm also may cause erosion of vertebrae. Stasis of blood favors thrombus formation along the wall of the vessel, and peripheral emboli may develop, causing symptomatic arterial insufficiency.

With thoracic and abdominal aneurysms, the most dreaded complication is rupture. The likelihood of rupture correlates with increasing aneurysm size.

Diagnosis and Treatment. Diagnostic methods include use of ultrasound imaging, computed tomographic (CT) scans, and magnetic resonance imaging (MRI). Surgical repair, in which the involved section of the aorta is replaced with a synthetic graft of woven Dacron, frequently is the treatment of choice.[37,39]

Dissecting Aneurysms

A dissecting aneurysm is an acute, life-threatening condition. It involves hemorrhage into the vessel wall with longitudinal tearing (*i.e.*, dissection) of the vessel wall to form a blood-filled channel. Unlike atherosclerotic aneurysms, dissecting aneurysms often occur without evidence of previous vessel dilatation. They can originate anywhere along the length of the aorta. Two thirds of dissections involve the ascending aorta.[39] The second most common site is the thoracic aorta just distal to the origin of the subclavian artery.

Dissecting aneurysms are caused by conditions that weaken or cause degenerative changes in the elastic and smooth muscle of the layers of the aorta. They are most common in the 40- to 60-year-old age group and more prevalent in men than in women.[7] There are two risk factors that predispose to a dissecting aneurysm: hypertension and degeneration of the medial layer of the vessel wall. There is

a history of hypertension in most cases.[7] Dissecting aneurysms also are associated with connective tissue diseases, such as Marfan's syndrome. Aortic dissection also may occur during pregnancy because of histochemical changes in the aorta that occur during this time. Other factors that predispose to aortic dissection are congenital defects of the aortic valve (*i.e.*, bicuspid or unicuspid valve structures) and aortic coarctation. Aortic dissection is a potential complication of cardiac surgery or catheterization. Surgically related dissection may occur at the points where the aorta has been incised or cross-clamped; it also has been reported at the site where the saphenous vein was sutured to the aorta during coronary artery bypass surgery.

There are several systems for classifying dissecting aortic aneurysms. The DeBakey system uses two classifications, type A and type B.[7] Those in the ascending aorta, regardless of the site of the primary tear, are designated type A (IA and IIA), and those not involving the ascending aorta are designated type B (Fig. 22-9). Dissections usually extend distally from the intimal tear. When the ascending aorta is involved, expansion of the wall of the aorta may impair closure of the aortic valve. There also is risk of aortic rupture with blood moving into the pericardium and compressing the heart. Although the length of dissection varies, it is possible for the abdominal aorta to be involved with progression into the renal, iliac, or femoral arteries. Partial or complete occlusion of the arteries that arise from the aortic arch or the intercostal or lumbar arteries may lead to stroke, ischemic peripheral neuropathy, or impaired blood flow to the spinal cord.

Manifestations. A major symptom of a dissecting aneurysm is the abrupt presence of excruciating pain, described

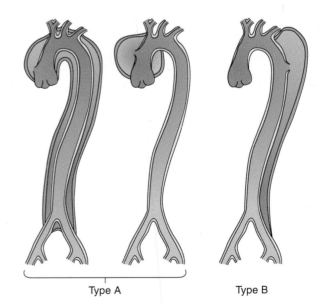

FIGURE 22-9 Classification of dissecting aneurysms into type A (proximal), affecting the ascending aorta, and type B (distal), which does not involve the ascending aorta. (Cotran R.S., Kumar V., Collins T. [1999]. *Robbins pathologic basis of disease* [6th ed., p. 529]. Philadelphia: WB Saunders)

Type A   Type B

as tearing or ripping. The location of the pain may point to the site of dissection.[7] Pain associated with dissection of the ascending aorta frequently is located in the anterior chest, and pain associated with dissection of the descending aorta often is located in the back. In the early stages, blood pressure typically is moderately or markedly elevated. Later, the blood pressure and the pulse rate become unobtainable in one or both arms as the dissection disrupts arterial flow to the arms. Syncope, hemiplegia, or paralysis of the lower extremities may occur because of occlusion of blood vessels that supply the brain or spinal cord. Heart failure may develop when the aortic valve is involved.

Diagnosis and Treatment.   Diagnosis of aortic dissection is based on history and physical examination. Aortic angiography, transesophageal echocardiography, CT scans, and MRI studies aid in the diagnosis.

The treatment of dissecting aortic aneurysm may be medical or surgical. Aortic dissection is a life-threatening emergency situation; persons with a probable diagnosis are stabilized medically even before the diagnosis is confirmed. Two important factors that participate in propagating the dissection are high blood pressure and the steepness of the pulse wave. Without intervention, these forces continue to cause extension of the dissection. Medical treatment therefore focuses on control of hypertension and the use of drugs that lessen the force of systolic blood ejection from the heart. Two commonly used drugs are intravenous sodium nitroprusside and a β-adrenergic blocking drug, given in combination. Surgical treatment consists of resection of the involved segment of the aorta and replacement with a prosthetic graft. The mortality rate due to untreated dissecting aneurysm is high, exceeding 50% within the first 48 hours, and 80% within 6 weeks.[40]

In summary, the arterial system distributes blood to all the tissues of the body, and lesions of the arterial system exert their effects through ischemia or impaired blood flow. There are two types of arterial disorders: diseases such as atherosclerosis, vasculitis, and peripheral arterial diseases that obstruct blood flow, and disorders such as aneurysms that weaken the vessel wall.

Atherosclerosis, a leading cause of death in the United States, affects large and medium-sized arteries, such as the coronary and cerebral arteries. It has an insidious onset, and its lesions usually are far advanced before symptoms appear. Although the mechanisms of atherosclerosis are uncertain, risk factors associated with its development have been identified. These include factors such as heredity, sex, and age, which cannot be controlled; factors such as smoking, high blood pressure, high serum cholesterol levels, and diabetes, which can be controlled; and other contributing factors such as obesity, lack of exercise, and stress. Cholesterol relies on lipoproteins (LDLs and HDLs) for transport in the blood. The LDLs, which are atherogenic, carry cholesterol to the peripheral tissues. The HDLs, which are protective, remove cholesterol from the tissues and carry it back to the liver for disposal. LDL receptors play a major role in removing cholesterol from the blood; persons with reduced numbers of receptors are at particularly high risk for development of atherosclerosis. The vasculitides are a group of vascular disorders characterized by vasculitis or inflammation and necrosis of the blood vessels in various tissues and organs of the body. They can be caused by injury to the vessel, infectious agents, or immune processes, or can occur secondary to other disease states such as systemic lupus erythematosus.

Occlusive disorders interrupt arterial flow of blood and interfere with the delivery of oxygen and nutrients to the tissues. Occlusion of flow can result from a thrombus, emboli, vessel compression, vasospasm, or structural changes in the vessel. Peripheral arterial diseases affect blood vessels outside the heart and thorax. They include Raynaud's disease or phenomenon, caused by vessel spasm, and thromboangiitis obliterans (Buerger's disease), characterized by an inflammatory process that involves medium-sized arteries. Aneurysms are localized areas of vessel dilation caused by weakness of the arterial wall. A berry aneurysm, most often found in the circle of Willis in the brain circulation, consists of a small, spherical vessel dilation. Fusiform and saccular aneurysms, most often found in the thoracic and abdominal aorta, are characterized by gradual and progressive enlargement of the aorta. They can involve part of the vessel circumference (saccular) or extend to involve the entire circumference of the vessel (fusiform). A dissecting aneurysm is an acute, life-threatening condition. It involves hemorrhage into the vessel wall with longitudinal tearing (dissection) of the vessel wall to form a blood-filled channel. The most serious consequence of aneurysms is rupture.

Disorders of the Venous Circulation

After you have completed this section of the chapter, you should be able to meet the following objectives:

✦ Describe venous return of blood from the lower extremities, including the function of the muscle pumps and the effects of gravity, and relate to the development of varicose veins
✦ Differentiate primary from secondary varicose veins
✦ Characterize the pathology of venous insufficiency and relate to the development of stasis dermatitis and venous ulcers
✦ Cite risk factors associated with venous thrombosis and describe the manifestation of the disorder and its treatment

Veins are low-pressure, thin-walled vessels that rely on the ancillary action of skeletal muscle pumps and changes in abdominal and intrathoracic pressure to return blood to the heart. Unlike the arterial system, the venous system is equipped with valves that prevent retrograde flow of blood. Although its structure enables the venous system to serve as a storage area for blood, it also renders the system susceptible to problems related to stasis and venous insufficiency. This section focuses on three common problems of the venous system: varicose veins, venous insufficiency, and venous thrombosis.

VENOUS CIRCULATION OF THE LOWER EXTREMITIES

The venous system in the legs consists of two components: the superficial veins (*i.e.*, saphenous vein and its tributaries) and the deep venous channels (Fig. 22-10). Perforating or communicating veins connect these two systems. Blood from the skin and subcutaneous tissues in the leg collects in the superficial veins and is then transported across the communicating veins into the deeper venous channels for return to the heart. Venous valves prevent the retrograde flow of blood and play an important role in the function of the venous system. Although these valves are irregularly located along the length of the veins, they almost always are found at junctions where the communicating veins merge with the larger deep veins and where two veins meet. The number of venous valves differs somewhat from one person to another, as does the structural competence, factors that may help to explain the familial predisposition to development of varicose veins.

The action of the leg muscles assists in moving venous blood from the lower extremities back to the heart. When

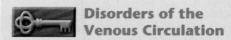

Disorders of the Venous Circulation

➤ Veins are thin-walled, distensible vessels that collect blood from the tissues and return it to the heart. The venous system is a low-pressure system that relies on the pumping action of the skeletal muscles to move blood forward and the presence of venous valves to prevent retrograde flow.

➤ Disorders of the venous system produce congestion of the affected tissues and predispose to clot formation because of stagnation of flow and activation of the clotting system.

➤ Varicose veins are dilated and tortuous veins that result from a sustained increase in pressure that causes the venous valves to become incompetent, allowing for reflux of blood and vein engorgement.

➤ Thrombophlebitis refers to thrombus formation in a vein and the accompanying inflammatory response in the vessel wall as a result of conditions that obstruct or slow blood flow, increase the activity of the coagulation system, or cause vessel injury. Deep vein thrombosis may be a precursor to pulmonary embolism.

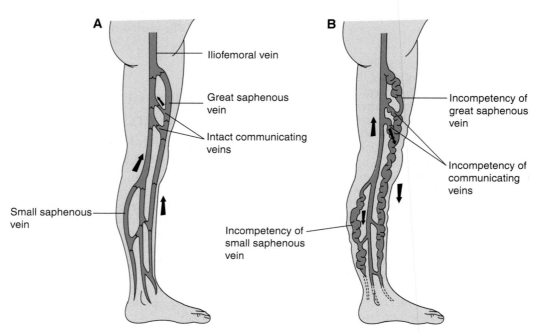

FIGURE 22-10 Superficial and deep venous channels of the leg. (**A**) Normal venous structures and flow patterns. (**B**) Varicosities in the superficial venous system are the result of incompetent valves in the communicating veins. The arrows in both views indicate the direction of blood flow. (Modified from Abramson D.I. [1974]. *Vascular disorders of the extremities* [2nd ed.]. New York: Harper & Row)

a person walks, the action of the leg muscles serves to increase flow in the deep venous channels and return venous blood to the heart (Fig. 22-11). The function of the so-called *muscle pump*, located in the gastrocnemius and soleus muscles of the lower extremities, can be compared with pumping action of the heart.[41] During muscle contraction, which is similar to systole, valves in the communicating channels close to prevent backward flow of blood into the superficial system, as blood in the deep veins is moved forward by the action of the contracting muscles. During relaxation, which is similar to diastole, the communicating valves open, allowing blood from the superficial veins to move into the deep veins.

VARICOSE VEINS

Varicose, or dilated, tortuous veins of the lower extremities are common and often lead to secondary problems of venous insufficiency. Varicose veins are described as being primary or secondary. Primary varicose veins originate in the superficial saphenous veins, and secondary varicose veins result from impaired flow in the deep venous channels. Approximately 80% to 90% of venous blood from the lower extremities is transported through the deep channels. The development of secondary varicose veins becomes inevitable when flow in these deep channels is impaired or blocked. The most common cause of secondary varicose veins is deep vein thrombosis (DVT). Other causes include congenital or acquired arteriovenous fistulas, congenital venous malformations, and pressure on the abdominal veins caused by pregnancy or a tumor.

It has been estimated that 10% to 20% of persons develop primary varicose veins in the lower extremities. The condition is more common after 50 years of age and in obese persons, and it occurs more often in women than men, probably because of venous stasis caused by pregnancy.[3] More than 50% of persons with primary varicose veins have a family history of the disorder, suggesting that heredity may play a role.

Mechanisms of Development

Prolonged standing and increased intra-abdominal pressure are important contributing factors in the development of primary varicose veins. Prolonged standing increases venous pressure and causes dilatation and stretching of the vessel wall. One of the most important factors in the elevation of venous pressure is the hydrostatic effect associated with the standing position. When a person is in the erect position, the full weight of the venous columns of blood is transmitted to the leg veins. The effects of gravity are compounded in persons who stand for long periods without using their leg muscles to assist in pumping blood back to the heart.

Because there are no valves in the inferior vena cava or common iliac veins, blood in the abdominal veins must be supported by the valves located in the external iliac or femoral veins. When intra-abdominal pressure increases, as it does during pregnancy, or when the valves in these two veins are absent or defective, the stress on the saphenofemoral junction is increased. The high incidence of varicose veins in women who have been pregnant also suggests a hormonal effect on venous smooth muscle contributing to venous dilatation and valvular incompetence. Lifting also increases intra-abdominal pressure and decreases flow of blood through the abdominal veins. Occupations that require repeated heavy lifting also predispose to development of varicose veins.

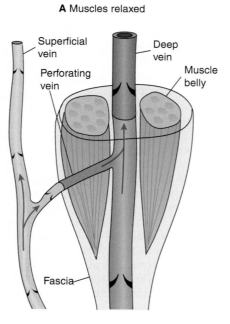
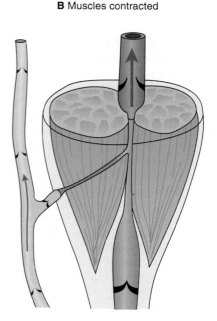

A Muscles relaxed

Superficial vein
Perforating vein
Deep vein
Muscle belly
Fascia

B Muscles contracted

FIGURE 22-11 The skeletal muscle pumps and their function in promoting blood flow in the deep and superficial calf vessels of the leg. The majority of perforating veins lie below the knee. When the calf muscle is relaxed (**A**), blood moves from the superficial to the deep veins. Muscle contraction (**B**) propels blood in the deep veins toward the heart, and closure of the venous valves prevents backflow. (Margolis D.J. [1992]. Management of venous ulcerations. *Hospital Practice* 27 [5], 37. © 1992, The McGraw-Hill Companies).

Prolonged exposure to increased pressure causes the venous valves to become incompetent so they no longer close properly. When this happens, the reflux of blood causes further venous enlargement, pulling the valve leaflet apart and causing more valvular incompetence in sections of adjacent distal veins. Another consideration in the development of varicose veins is the fact that the superficial veins have only subcutaneous fat and superficial fascia for support, but the deep venous channels are supported by muscle, bone, and connective tissue. Obesity reduces the support provided by the superficial fascia and tissues, increasing the risk for development of varicose veins.

Manifestations

The signs and symptoms associated with primary varicose veins vary. Most women with superficial varicose veins complain of their unsightly appearance. In many cases, aching in the lower extremities and edema, especially after long periods of standing, may occur. The edema usually subsides at night when the legs are elevated. When the communicating veins are incompetent, symptoms are more common.

Diagnosis and Treatment

The diagnosis of varicose veins often can be made after physical inspection. Several procedures are used to assess the extent of venous involvement associated with varicose veins. In one of these, Trendelenburg's test, a tourniquet is applied to the affected leg while it is elevated and the veins are empty. The person then assumes the standing position, and the tourniquet is removed. If the superficial veins are involved, the veins distend quickly. To assess the deep channels, the tourniquet is applied while the person is standing and the veins are filled. The person then lies down and the affected leg is elevated. Emptying of the superficial veins indicates that the deep channels are patent. The Doppler ultrasonic flow probe also may be used to assess the flow in the large vessels. Angiographic studies using a radiopaque contrast medium also are used to assess venous function.

After the venous channels have been repeatedly stretched and the valves rendered incompetent, little can be done to restore normal venous tone and function. Ideally, measures should be taken to prevent the development and progression of varicose veins. These measures center on avoiding activities such as continued standing that produce prolonged elevation of venous pressure. Treatment measures for varicose veins focus on improving venous flow and preventing tissue injury. When correctly fitted, elastic support stockings or leggings compress the superficial veins and prevent distention. The most precise control is afforded by prescription stockings, measured to fit properly. These stocking should be applied before the standing position is assumed, when the leg veins are empty.

Sclerotherapy, which often is used in treatment of small residual varicosities, involves the injection of a sclerosing agent into the collapsed superficial veins to produce fibrosis of the vessel lumen. Surgical treatment consists of removing the varicosities and the incompetent perforating veins, but it is limited to persons with patent deep venous channels.

CHRONIC VENOUS INSUFFICIENCY

The term *venous insufficiency* refers to the physiologic consequences of DVT, valvular incompetence, or a combination of both conditions. The most common cause is DVT, which causes deformity of the valve leaflets, rendering them incapable of closure. In the presence of valvular incompetence, effective unidirectional flow of blood and emptying of the deep veins cannot occur. The muscle pumps also are ineffective, often driving blood in retrograde directions. Secondary failure of the communicating and superficial veins subjects the subcutaneous tissues to high pressures.

With venous insufficiency, there are signs and symptoms associated with impaired blood flow. In contrast to the ischemia caused by arterial insufficiency, venous insufficiency leads to tissue congestion, edema, and eventual impairment of tissue nutrition. The edema is exacerbated by long periods of standing. Necrosis of subcutaneous fat deposits occurs, followed by skin atrophy. Brown pigmentation of the skin caused by hemosiderin deposits resulting from the breakdown of red blood cells is common. Secondary lymphatic insufficiency occurs, with progressive sclerosis of the lymph channels in the face of increased demand for clearance of interstitial fluid.

In advanced venous insufficiency, impaired tissue nutrition causes stasis dermatitis and the development of stasis or venous ulcers. Stasis dermatitis is characterized by the presence of thin, shiny, bluish brown, irregularly pigmented desquamative skin that lacks the support of the underlying subcutaneous tissues. Minor injury leads to relatively painless ulcerations that are difficult to heal. The lower part of the leg is particularly prone to development of stasis dermatitis and venous ulcers. Most lesions are located medially over the ankle and lower leg, with the highest frequency just above the medial malleolus. Persons with long-standing venous insufficiency may experience stiffening of the ankle joint and loss of muscle mass and strength.

VENOUS THROMBOSIS

The term *venous thrombosis*, or *thrombophlebitis*, describes the presence of thrombus in a vein and the accompanying inflammatory response in the vessel wall. Thrombi can develop in the superficial or the deep veins. DVT most commonly occurs in the lower extremities. DVT of the lower extremity is a serious disorder, complicated by pulmonary embolism (see Chapter 29), recurrent episodes of DVT, and development of chronic venous insufficiency. Most postoperative thrombi arise in the soleal sinuses or the large veins draining the gastrocnemius muscles.[42] Isolated calf thrombi often are asymptomatic. If left untreated, they may extend to the larger, more proximal veins, with an increased risk of pulmonary emboli.

In 1846, Virchow described the triad that has come to be associated with venous thrombosis: stasis of blood, increased blood coagulability, and vessel wall injury.[43] Risk factors for venous thrombosis are summarized in Chart 22-2. Stasis of blood occurs with immobility of an extremity or the entire body. Bed rest and immobilization are associated with decreased blood flow, venous pooling in the lower

CHART 22-2

*Risk Factors Associated With Venous Thrombosis**

Venous Stasis

Bed rest
Immobility
Spinal cord injury
Acute myocardial infarction
Congestive heart failure
Shock
Venous obstruction

Hyperreactivity of Blood Coagulation

Stress and trauma
Pregnancy
Childbirth
Oral contraceptive use
Dehydration
Cancer

Vascular Trauma

Indwelling venous catheters
Surgery
Massive trauma or infection
Fractured hip
Orthopedic surgery

*Many of these disorders involve more than one mechanism.

extremities, and increased risk of DVT. Persons who are immobilized by a hip fracture, joint replacement, or spinal cord injury are particularly vulnerable to DVT. The risk of DVT is increased in situations of impaired cardiac function. This may account for the relatively high incidence in persons with acute myocardial infarction and congestive heart failure. Elderly persons are more susceptible than younger persons, probably because disorders that produce venous stasis occur more frequently in older persons. Long airplane travel poses a particular threat in persons predisposed to DVT because of prolonged sitting and increased blood viscosity due to dehydration.[44]

Hypercoagulability is a homeostatic mechanism designed to increase clot formation, and conditions that increase the concentration or activation of clotting factors predispose to DVT. Thrombosis also can be caused by deficiencies in certain plasma proteins that normally inhibit thrombus formation, such as antithrombin III, protein C, and protein S.[45] The postpartum state is associated with increased levels of fibrinogen, prothrombin, and other coagulation factors. The use of oral contraceptives appears to increase coagulability and predispose to venous thrombosis, a risk that is further increased in women who smoke. Certain cancers are associated with increased clotting tendencies, and although the reason for this is largely unknown, substances that promote blood coagulation may be released from the tissues because of the cancerous growth. When body fluid is lost because of injury or disease, the resulting hemoconcentration causes clotting factors to become more concentrated.

Vessel injury can result from a trauma situation or from surgical intervention. It also may occur secondary to infection or inflammation of the vessel wall. Persons undergoing hip surgery and total hip replacement are at particular risk because of trauma to the femoral and iliac veins, and in the case of hip replacement, thermal damage from heat generated by the polymerization of the acrylic cement that is used in the procedure.[42] Venous catheters are another source of vascular injury.

Manifestations

Many persons with venous thrombosis are asymptomatic, probably because the vein is not totally occluded or because of collateral circulation.[46] When present, the most common signs and symptoms of venous thrombosis are those related to the inflammatory process: pain, swelling, and deep muscle tenderness. Fever, general malaise, and an elevated white blood cell count and sedimentation rate are accompanying indications of inflammation. There may be tenderness and pain along the vein. Swelling may vary from minimal to maximal. As much as 50% of persons with DVT are asymptomatic.

The site of thrombus formation determines the location of the physical findings. The most common site is in the venous sinuses in the soleus muscle and posterior tibial and peroneal veins (Fig. 22-12). Swelling in these cases involves the foot and ankle, although it may be slight or absent. Calf pain and tenderness are common. Femoral vein thrombosis with calf thrombosis produces pain and tenderness in the distal thigh and popliteal area. Thrombi in ileofemoral veins produce the most profound manifestations, with swelling, pain, and tenderness of the entire extremity. With DVT in the calf veins, active dorsiflexion produces calf pain (Homans' sign). Another assessment measure, Bancroft's sign, involves compression of the anterior calf muscles against the interosseous membrane. When tenderness is reported, the test result is positive.

Diagnosis and Treatment

The risk of pulmonary embolism emphasizes the need for early detection and treatment of DVT. Several tests are useful for this purpose: ascending venography, impedance plethysmography, and ultrasonography (*e.g.*, real-time, B-mode, duplex).

Whenever possible, venous thrombosis should be prevented in preference to being treated. Early ambulation after childbirth and surgery is one measure that decreases the risk of thrombus formation. Exercising the legs and wearing support stockings improve venous flow. A further precautionary measure is to avoid assuming body positions that favor venous pooling. Antiembolism stockings of the proper fit and length should be used routinely in persons at risk for DVT. Another strategy used for immobile persons at risk for developing DVT is a sequential pneumatic compression device. This consists of a plastic sleeve that encircles the legs and provides alternating periods of compression on the lower extremity. When properly used, these devices enhance venous emptying to augment flow and

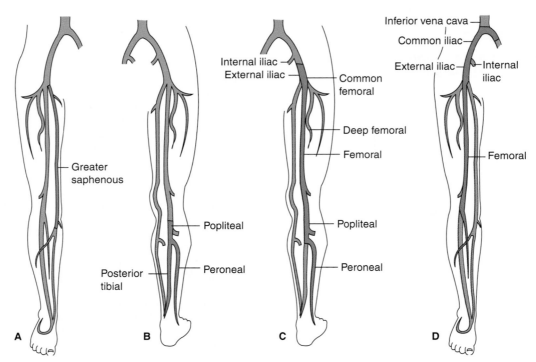

FIGURE 22-12 Common sites of venous thrombosis. (**A**) Superficial thrombophlebitis. (**B**) Most common form of deep thrombophlebitis. (**C** and **D**) Deep thrombophlebitis from the calf to iliac veins. (Haller J.A. Jr. [1967]. *Deep thrombophlebitis: Pathophysiology and treatment.* Philadelphia: W.B. Saunders)

reduce stasis. Prophylactic anticoagulation often is used in persons who are at high risk for development of venous thrombi.

The objectives of treatment of venous thrombosis are to prevent formation of additional thrombi, prevent extension and embolization of existing thrombi, and minimize venous valve damage. A 15- to 20-degree elevation of the legs prevents stasis. It is important that the entire lower extremity or extremities be carefully extended to avoid acute flexion of the knee or hip. Heat often is applied to the leg to relieve venospasm and to aid in the resolution of the inflammatory process. Bed rest usually is maintained until local tenderness and swelling have subsided. Gradual ambulation with elastic support is then permitted. Standing and sitting increase venous pressure and are to be avoided. Elastic support is needed for 3 to 6 months to permit recanalization and collateralization and to prevent venous insufficiency.

Anticoagulation therapy (*i.e.*, heparin and warfarin) is used to treat and prevent venous thrombosis. Treatment typically is initiated with continuous infusion or subcutaneous injections of heparin. Subcutaneous injections of low–molecular-weight heparin may be given on an outpatient basis. This usually is followed by prophylactic therapy with oral anticoagulants to prevent further thrombus formation. The mechanisms of action of the anticoagulant drugs are discussed in Chapter 14. Thrombolytic therapy (*i.e.*, streptokinase, urokinase, or tissue plasminogen activator) may be used in an attempt to dissolve the clot.

Surgical removal of the thrombus may be undertaken in selected cases. Surgical interruption of the vena cava may be done in persons at high risk of developing pulmonary emboli. This procedure involves ligating the vena cava with a suture or clamp or in creating a filter-like insertion to prevent large clots from moving through the vessel. Percutaneous (through the skin) insertion of intracaval devices has largely replaced direct surgical procedures.

In summary, the storage function of the venous system renders it susceptible to venous insufficiency, stasis, and thrombus formation. Varicose veins occur with prolonged distention and stretching of the superficial veins owing to venous insufficiency. Varicosities can arise because of defects in the superficial veins (*i.e.*, primary varicose veins) or because of impaired blood flow in the deep venous channels (*i.e.*, secondary varicose veins). Venous insufficiency reflects chronic venous stasis resulting from valvular incompetence. It is associated with stasis dermatitis and stasis or venous ulcers. Venous thrombosis describes the presence of thrombus in a vein and the accompanying inflammatory response in the vessel wall. It is associated with vessel injury, stasis of venous flow, and hypercoagulability states. Thrombi can develop in the superficial or the deep veins (*i.e.*, DVT). Thrombus formation in deep veins is a precursor to venous insufficiency and embolus formation.

Disorders of Blood Flow Due to Extravascular Forces

After you have completed this section of the chapter, you should be able to meet the following objectives:

✦ State five possible causes of compartment syndrome
✦ Explain why pulses and capillary refill time are not good assessment measures for compartment syndrome
✦ Cite two causes of pressure ulcers
✦ Explain how shearing forces contribute to ischemic skin damage
✦ List four measures that contribute to the prevention of pressure ulcers

Blood flow occurs along a pressure gradient, moving from the arterial to the venous side of the circulation. For blood to move through the vessels of the systemic circulation, arterial pressure must be greater than venous pressure, and the arterial and venous pressures must be greater than the external pressure of the surrounding tissues. Injury or infections that cause tissue swelling can compromise blood flow, particularly in parts of the body where the skin or other supporting tissues cannot expand to accommodate the increased volume. In other situations, external pressure may compress the tissues and the blood vessels. Two conditions that compromise blood flow because of increased external pressure are compartment syndrome and pressure ulcers.

Disorders of Blood Flow Due to Extravascular Forces

➤ Blood flow requires that arterial pressure is greater than venous pressure, and that arterial, venous, and capillary pressures are greater than the pressure surrounding the vessels.

➤ Compartment syndrome describes a condition of increased pressure in an anatomic space that cannot expand. The increased pressure may compromise blood flow to the tissue, resulting in ischemic damage. Causes include decreases in compartment size (*i.e.*, cast) or increases in compartment volume (*i.e.*, internal bleeding or edema).

➤ Pressure ulcers are ischemic lesions of the skin and underlying tissues caused by compression of blood vessels due to external pressure, such as that exerted by the weight of the body on the bed or chair surface. Prevention of pressure ulcers is preferable to treatment. Frequent position changes and meticulous skin care are essential components of prevention.

COMPARTMENT SYNDROME

The muscles and nerves of an extremity are enclosed in a tough, inelastic fascial envelope called a *muscle compartment* (Fig. 22-13). *Compartment syndrome* describes a condition of increased pressure in a limited anatomic space, usually a muscle compartment, that impairs circulation and produces ischemic tissue injury.[47] If the pressure in the compartment is sufficiently high, tissue circulation is compromised, causing death of nerve and muscle cells. Permanent loss of function and limb contracture may occur. The amount of pressure required to produce a compartment syndrome depends on many factors, including the duration of the pressure elevation, the metabolic rate of the tissues, vascular tone, and local blood pressure. Less tissue pressure is required to stop circulation when hypotension or vasoconstriction is present.

Intracompartmental pressures of 30 to 40 mm Hg (normal is approximately 6 mm Hg) are considered sufficient to impair capillary blood flow.[48] Nerve dysfunction (*i.e.*, paresthesia and hypoesthesia) develops within 30 minutes of ischemia, and muscle dysfunction within 2 to 4 hours; irreversible loss of function (*e.g.*, contractures, sensory aberrations, muscle weakness) begins after 12 to 24 hours of total ischemia.[49] Prompt diagnosis and decompression are essential to reinstate capillary pressure and prevent permanent disability.

Causes

Compartment syndrome can result from a decrease in compartment size or an increase in the volume of its contents (Chart 22-3). The most common causes are crushing injuries, fractures, contusions, snake bites, postischemic swelling after arterial injury or thrombosis, severe exercise, limb compression due to drug or alcohol overdose, and venous occlusion.

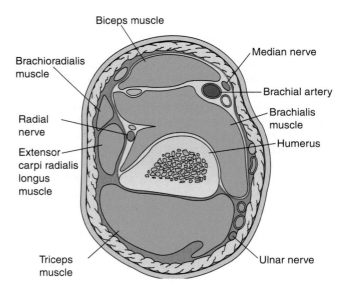

FIGURE 22-13 Distal anterior arm muscle compartment, showing the location of fascia, muscles, nerves, and blood vessels.

> ### CHART 22-3
>
> ### *Causes of Compartment Syndrome*
>
> ***Decreased Compartment Size***
> Constrictive dressings and casts
> Infiltration of intravenous fluids
> Thermal injury and frostbite
> Surgical closure of fascial defects
>
> ***Increased Compartment Volume***
> Fractures and orthopedic surgery
> Trauma and bleeding
> Postischemic injury
> Severe exercise
> Prolonged immobilization with limb compression
>   (*e.g.,* drug overdose)
> Thermal injury and frostbite
> Intravenous infiltration

Decreased Compartment Size.   Among the causes of decreased compartment size are constrictive dressings and casts, closure of fascial defects, and thermal injuries or frostbite. Splitting a cast or releasing the dressing usually is sufficient to relieve most of the pressure. The appearance of a muscle hernia or fascial defect may be the result of increased compartmental pressure. This commonly is seen in persons with chronic exercise-related compartment syndrome. Surgical closure of the hernia decreases compartmental size and may result in an acute compartment syndrome. In persons with circumferential third-degree burns, the inelastic and constricting eschar decreases the size of the underlying compartments. Burns also are associated with the formation of massive edema and an increase in compartment volume. The combination of the two problems may lead to necrosis of the underlying neuromuscular tissues. Frostbite produces neuromuscular injury for similar reasons.

Increased Compartment Volume.   Increased compartment volume can be caused by postischemic swelling, trauma, vascular injury and bleeding, infiltration of intravenous infusions, and venous obstruction. One of the most important causes of compartment syndrome is bleeding and edema caused by fractures and osteotomies (see Chapter 57). Contusions and soft tissue injury also are common causes of compartment syndrome. Bleeding can occur as a complication of arterial punctures, particularly in persons with bleeding disorders or those who are receiving anticoagulant drugs. Infiltration of intravenous fluids also can restrict compartment size and cause compartment ischemia and postischemic swelling. Increased compartment volume may follow ischemic events, such as arterial occlusion, that are of sufficient duration to produce capillary damage, causing increased capillary permeability and edema. During unattended coma caused by drug overdose or carbon monoxide poisoning, high compartment pressures are produced when an extremity is compressed by the weight of the overlying head or torso. Exercise may produce acute or chronic elevations in compartment pressure.

Diagnosis and Treatment

It is important that a person at risk for development of compartment syndrome be identified and that proper assessment methods be instituted. Assessment should include pain assessment, examination of sensory (*i.e.,* light touch and two-point discrimination) and motor function (*i.e.,* movement and muscle strength), test of passive stretch, and palpation of the muscle compartments.

The most important symptom of compartment syndrome is unrelenting pain, usually described as a deep, throbbing sensation, that is greater than that expected for the primary problem, such as fracture or contusion. Pain with passive stretch is a common finding. Tenseness and tenderness of the involved compartment are specific symptoms of compartment syndrome. The skin over the compartment may become taut, shiny, warm, and red. Paresthesias progressing to anesthesia occur secondary to nerve involvement. Muscle weakness results from muscle ischemia. Although peripheral pulses and capillary refill time are parts of a complete assessment, they frequently are normal in the presence of compartment syndrome because the major arteries are located outside the muscle compartments. Although edema may make it difficult to palpate the pulse, the increased compartment pressure seldom is sufficient to occlude flow in a major artery. Doppler methods usually confirm the existence of a pulse. Direct measurements of tissue pressure can be obtained using a needle or wick catheter inserted into the muscle compartment. This method is particularly useful in persons who are unresponsive and in those with nerve deficits. Compartment decompression is recommended when pressures rise to 30 mm Hg.

Treatment consists of reducing compartmental pressures. This entails cast splitting or removal of restrictive dressings. These procedures often are sufficient to relieve most of the underlying pressure and symptoms. Limb elevation is not recommended when compartment syndrome is suspected. Although elevation is widely used to promote venous drainage of an injured extremity, it may be detrimental in compartment syndrome. Because venous pressure must exceed tissue pressure, elevation of an extremity cannot augment venous drainage after intracompartmental pressures are elevated. When an extremity is elevated, its arterial pressure falls because of the effects of gravity. Blood flow to an extremity can be arrested because of diminution of arterial pressure in the elevated extremity.

When compartment syndrome cannot be relieved by the measures described, a fasciotomy may become necessary. During this procedure, the fascia is incised longitudinally and separated so that the compartment volume can expand and blood flow can be reestablished. Because of potential problems with wound infection and closure, this procedure is performed as a last resort.

PRESSURE ULCERS

Pressure ulcers are ischemic lesions of the skin and underlying structures caused by external pressure that impairs the flow of blood and lymph. Pressure ulcers often are referred to as *decubitus ulcers* or *bedsores*. The word *decubitus* comes from the Latin term meaning "lying down." A pressure ulcer, however, may result from pressure exerted in the seated or the lying position. Pressure ulcers are most likely to develop over a bony prominence, but they may occur on any part of the body that is subjected to external pressure, friction, or shearing forces.

The reported incidence and prevalence of pressure ulcers in hospital settings has ranged from 2.7% to 29.5%,[50–52] and in skilled care and nursing home settings, from 2.4% to 23%.[52,53] Several subpopulations are at particular risk, including persons with quadriplegia, elderly persons with restricted activity and hip fractures, and persons in the critical care setting. The prevention and treatment of pressure ulcers is a public health issue and is addressed in *Healthy People 2010*, a national public health policy statement, which has set a target of a 50% decrease in prevalence of pressure ulcers in nursing home residents.[54]

Mechanisms of Development

Two factors contribute to the development of pressure ulcers—external pressure that compresses blood vessels and friction and shearing forces that tear and injure blood vessels.

External pressure that exceeds capillary pressure interrupts blood flow in the capillary beds. When the pressure between a bony prominence and a support surface exceeds the normal capillary filling pressure of approximately 32 mm Hg, capillary flow essentially is obstructed.[55] If this pressure is applied constantly for 2 hours, oxygen deprivation coupled with an accumulation of metabolic end products leads to irreversible tissue damage. The same amount of pressure causes more damage when it is distributed over a small area than when it is distributed over a larger area. Approximately 7 lb of pressure per square inch of tissue surface is sufficient to obstruct blood flow. If a person weighing 70 kg with a total surface area of 1.8 m² were in the supine position, with pressure evenly distributed, the pressure at any given point would be 5.7 mm Hg.[56]

Whether a person is sitting or lying down, the weight of the body is borne by tissues covering the bony prominences. Ninety-six percent of pressure ulcers are located on the lower part of the body, most often over the sacrum, the coccygeal areas, the ischial tuberosities, and the greater trochanter.[57] Pressure over a bony area is transmitted from the surface to the underlying dense bone, compressing all of the intervening tissue. As a result, the greatest pressure occurs at the surface of the bone and dissipates outward in a conelike manner toward the surface of the skin (Fig. 22-14). Thus, extensive underlying tissue damage can be present when a small superficial skin lesion is first noticed.

Altering the distribution of pressure from one skin area to another prevents tissue injury. Pressure ulcers most commonly occur in persons with conditions in which normal sensation and movement to effect redistribution of body weight are impaired, such as spinal cord injury. Normally, persons unconsciously shift their weight to redistribute pressure on the skin and underlying tissues. During the night, for example, they turn in their sleep, preventing ischemic injury of tissues that overlie the bony prominences that support the weight of the body; the same is true for sitting for any length of time. The movements needed to shift the body weight are made unconsciously, and only when movement is restricted do they become aware of discomfort.

Shearing forces are caused by the sliding of one tissue layer over another with stretching and angulation of blood vessels, causing injury and thrombosis. Injury caused by shearing forces commonly occurs when the head of the bed is elevated, causing the torso to slide down toward the foot of the bed. When this happens, friction and perspiration cause the skin and superficial fascia to remain fixed against the bed linens while the deep fascia and skeleton slide downward. The same thing can happen when a person sitting up in a chair slides downward. Another source of shearing forces is pulling rather than lifting a person up in bed. In this case, the skin remains fixed to the sheet while the fascia and muscles are pulled upward.

Prevention

The prevention of pressure ulcers is preferable to treatment. In 1992, a special panel of the Agency for Health Care Policy and Research (AHCPR; now the Agency for Healthcare Research and Quality), the Panel for the Prediction and Prevention of Pressure Ulcers in Adults, released the *Clinical Practice Guidelines for Pressure Ulcers in Adults*.[58] The recommendations developed by the panel target four overall goals: identifying at-risk persons who need prevention and the specific factors placing them at risk; maintaining and improving tissue tolerance to pressure to prevent injury;

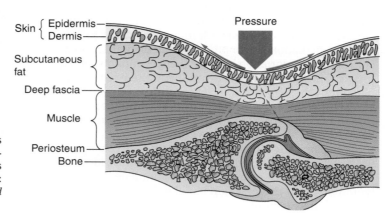

FIGURE 22-14 Pressure over a bony prominence compresses all intervening soft tissue, with a resulting wide, three-dimensional pressure gradient that causes various degrees of ischemia and damage. (Shea J.D. [1975]. Pressure sores: Classification and management. *Clinical Orthopaedics and Related Research* 112, 90)

protecting against the adverse effects of external mechanical forces (*i.e.*, pressure, friction, and shear); and reducing the incidence of pressure ulcers through educational programs.[58]

In 1994, a panel of the AHCPR released another document concerning the treatment of pressure ulcers.[59] The guidelines include specific recommendations for assessment of the patient and pressure ulcer, management of tissue load, ulcer care, managing bacterial colonization and infection, operative repair, and education and quality control.

Risk Factor Assessment.
Risk factors identified as contributing to the development of pressure ulcers were those related to sensory perception (*i.e.*, ability to respond meaningfully to pressure-related discomfort), level of skin moisture, urine and fecal continence, nutrition and hydration status, mobility, circulatory status, and presence of shear and friction forces.

Numerous risk assessment tools exist; however, only the Braden Scale and the Norton Scale have been extensively tested. The Norton Scale ranks risk according to physical condition, mental condition, activity, mobility, and incontinence,[60] and the Braden Scale ranks sensory perception, moisture, activity, nutrition, and friction and shear.[61] Identifying persons who are at risk for development of pressure ulcers allows health care facilities to focus prevention measures on this group to reduce the incidence of pressure ulcers.

Skin Care and Early Treatment.
Methods for preventing pressure ulcers include frequent position change, meticulous skin care, and frequent and careful observation to detect early signs of skin breakdown. All persons at risk for pressure ulcers should have systematic skin inspection done at least once each day, with particular attention to bony prominences.[58] The bed linens should be kept clean, dry, and wrinkle free. The skin should be cleaned at the time of urine and fecal soiling with a mild cleaning agent that minimizes irritation and skin dryness. When soiling of the skin cannot be controlled, it is recommended that absorbent underpads or briefs be used to present a quick-drying surface for the skin. Topical agents that act as moisture barriers also can be used.

Adequate hydration of the stratum corneum appears to protect the skin against mechanical insult.[58] The skin should be kept clean and protected from environmental factors that cause drying. The level of skin hydration decreases with decreasing ambient air temperature, particularly when the relative humidity of the ambient air is low.[58] Dry skin should be treated with moisturizers. The prevention of dehydration also improves the circulation. It also decreases the concentration of urine, thereby minimizing skin irritation in persons who are incontinent, and it reduces urinary problems that contribute to incontinence.

Maintenance of adequate nutrition is important. Anemia and malnutrition contribute to tissue breakdown and delay healing after tissue injury has occurred.

The panel also recommended that the age-old practice of massaging over the bony prominences be avoided. Research suggests that using massage to stimulate blood and lymph flow may decrease skin blood flow and increase the risk of deep tissue injury.

Protection Against Mechanical Forces.
Frequent change of position prevents tissue injury due to pressure. Persons who are in bed and at risk for development of pressure ulcers should be repositioned at least every 2 hours if this is consistent with the overall treatment goals. It is recommended that persons who are in a chair or wheelchair be repositioned every hour or put back to bed. Persons who are able to shift their weight should be advised to do so every 15 minutes.

Special pads and mattresses that distribute weight more evenly may be used. Silicone-filled pads, egg-crate cushions, turning frames, flotation pads, and other devices minimize contact pressure. Adequate exposure of the skin to air is necessary to avoid the buildup of heat and perspiration. Care should be taken to maintain the person at a position of 30 to 40 degrees to minimize slipping and shearing forces from sliding against the sheets. It also is important that the person be lifted and not dragged across the sheet. A lifting sheet works well for this purpose. Elevation of the ankles and heels off the sheets with foam pads can reduce skin breakdown in these areas of the body. The use of air cushions (*i.e.*, donuts) is not recommended. Casts, braces, and splints can exert extreme pressure on underlying tissues, and persons with these devices require special attention to avoid skin breakdown.

Staging and Treatment

Pressure ulcers can be staged according to the following four categories recommended by the Panel for Prediction and Prevention of Pressure Sores in Adults[58] and the National Pressure Ulcer Advisory Panel[62]:

- *Stage I*: observable pressure-related alteration of intact skin whose indicators as compared to the adjacent or opposite area on the body may include changes in one or more of the following: skin temperature, tissue consistency, and/or sensation. The ulcer appears as a defined area of persistent redness in lightly pigmented skin, whereas in darker skin tones, the ulcer may appear with persistent red, blue, or purple hues.[63]
- *Stage II*: partial-thickness skin loss involving epidermis or dermis, or both. The ulcer is superficial and presents clinically as an abrasion, a blister, or a shallow crater.
- *Stage III*: full-thickness skin loss involving damage and necrosis of subcutaneous tissue that may extend down to but not through underlying fascia. The ulcer manifests as a deep crater with or without undermining of adjacent tissue.
- *Stage IV*: full-thickness skin loss with extensive destruction, skin necrosis, or damage to muscle, bone, or supporting structures (*e.g.*, tendon or joint capsule). Undermining and sinus tracts may also be associated with stage IV pressure ulcers.

These staging criteria have limitations. Identification of stage I pressure ulcers may be difficult in persons with darkly pigmented skin, and when eschar is present. Accurate staging of the pressure ulcer may be difficult until the eschar has sloughed or the wound has been debrided.

After skin breakdown has occurred, special treatment measures are needed to prevent further ischemic damage, reduce bacterial contamination and infection, and promote healing. A major advance in the treatment of pressure ulcers has occurred in the area of wound dressings that offer moist wound healing. Dry dressings favor the formation of a dry crust over the wound, through which granulation tissue and advancing epithelium must burrow as it heals the area. Moist dressings, on the other hand, encourages formation of granulation and epithelialization.[64]

Treatment methods are selected based on the stage of the ulcer.[55,59] Stage I ulcers usually are treated with frequent turning and measures to remove pressure. Stage II or III ulcers with little exudate are treated with petroleum gauze, semipermeable, or occlusive dressings to maintain a moist healing environment. Transparent semipermeable dressings (*e.g.*, Op-Cit, Tegaderm) allow wound visibility and seal in the body's own defenses against invasion—leukocytes, plasma, fibrin, and growth factors. Stage III ulcers usually require debridement (*i.e.*, removal of necrotic tissue and eschar). This can be done surgically, with wet-to-dry dressings, through the use of proteolytic enzymes (*e.g.*, fibrinolysin-desoxyribonuclease [Elase], streptokinase-streptodornase [Varidase]), or autolytic debridement, which involves the use of synthetic dressings to cover the wound and allow devitalized tissues to self-digest from enzymes normally present in wound fluids.[55] Stage IV wounds often require packing to obliterate dead space and are covered with nonadherent dressings. Care is taken to avoid over-packing the wound because it may produce pressure and cause additional tissue damage. Dressings usually are changed every 8 to 12 hours, depending on severity, degree of infection, and amount of exudate. Stage IV ulcers may require surgical interventions, such as skin grafts or myo-cutaneous flaps.

There has been recent interest in the use of growth factors in healing of pressure ulcers.[65,66] Growth factors provide a means by which cells communicate with each other and can have profound effects on cell proliferation, migration, and extracellular matrix synthesis.[65] Becaplermin, a topical preparation of recombinant human platelet-derived growth factor, was approved by the U.S. Food and Drug Administration in 1997 for use in treatment of neuropathic lower extremity ulcers. There is hope that growth factors may prove beneficial in treatment of pressure ulcers.

In summary, blood flow in the circulatory system is brought about by pressure differences between the arterial and venous systems and a transmural pressure (*i.e.*, internal minus external) that holds the vessel open. Under certain conditions, such as compartment syndrome and pressure ulcers, increases in external pressures can exceed intravascular pressure and interrupt blood flow. Compartment syndrome is a condition of increased pressure in a muscle compartment that compromises blood flow and potentially leads to death of nerve and muscle tissue. It can result from a decrease in compartment size (*e.g.*, constrictive dressings, closure of fascial defects, thermal injury, frostbite) or an increase in compartment volume (*e.g.*, postischemic swelling, fractures, contusion and soft tissue trauma, bleeding caused by vascular injury, venous congestion).

Pressure ulcers are caused by ischemia of the skin and underlying tissues. They result from external pressure, which disrupts blood flow, or shearing forces, which cause stretching and injury to blood vessels. Pressure ulcers are divided into four stages, according to the depth of tissue involvement. The prevention of pressure ulcers is preferable to treatment. The goals of prevention should include identifying at-risk persons who need prevention and the specific factors placing them at risk; maintaining and improving tissue tolerance to pressure to prevent injury; protecting against the adverse effects of external mechanical forces (*i.e.*, pressure, friction, and shear), and reducing the incidence of pressure ulcers through educational programs.

Related Web Sites

HealthlinkUSA—health-related search site
   www.healthlinkusa.com
How You Can Lower Your Cholesterol Levels
   www.nhlbisupport.com/chd1/how.htm
National Cholesterol Education Program   www.nhlbi.nih.gov/about/ncep
National Pressure Ulcer Association   www.npuap.org
Skin and Wound Care—full-text journal articles
   www.woundcarenet.com

References

1. Guyton A., Hall J.E. (2000). *Textbook of medical physiology* (10th ed., pp. 781–790). Philadelphia: W.B. Saunders.
2. American Heart Association. (2000). Cholesterol statistics for professionals. [On-line]. Available: www.americanheart.org/cholesterol.
3. Rubin E., Farber J.L. (Eds.) (1999). *Pathology* (3rd ed., pp. 491–509, 520–522). Philadelphia: Lippincott Williams & Wilkins.
4. Beisiegel U. (1998). Lipoprotein metabolism. *European Heart Journal* 19 (Suppl. A), A20–A23.
5. Gwynne J.T. (1988). Lipoprotein structure and metabolism. *Consultant* 28 (6), 6–10.
6. Lusis A.J. (2000). Atherosclerosis. *Nature* 407, 233–241.
7. Schoen F.J., Cotran R.S. (1999). Blood vessels. In Cotran R.S., Kumar V., Collins T. (Eds.), *Pathologic basis of disease* (6th ed., pp. 498–514). Philadelphia: W.B. Saunders.
8. Harper C.R., Jacobson T.A. (1999). New perspectives on the management of low levels of high-density lipoprotein cholesterol. *Archives of Internal Medicine* 159, 1049–1057.
9. Steinberg D., Gotto A.M. (1999). Preventing coronary artery disease by lowering cholesterol levels. *JAMA* 282, 2043–2050.
10. National Institute of Health Expert Panel (2001). *Third Report of the National Cholesterol Education Program (NCEP) Expert Panel on Detection, Evaluation, and Treatment of High Blood Cholesterol in Adults (Adult Treatment Panel III)*. (NIH Publication No. 01–3670). Bethesda, MD: National Institutes of Health.
11. Verges B.L. (1999). Dyslipidemia in diabetes mellitus: Review of the main lipoprotein abnormalities and their consequences on the development of atherogenesis. *Diabetes and Metabolism* 25 (Suppl. 3), 32–40.

12. Lamarche B. (1998). Abdominal obesity and its metabolic complications: Implications for the risk of ischaemic heart disease. *Coronary Artery Disease* 9, 473–481.

13. Goldberg R.B. (1988). Dietary modification of cholesterol levels. *Consultant* 28 (Suppl. 6), 35–41.

14. AHA Dietary Guidelines. (2000). Revision 2000: A statement for healthcare professionals from the Nutrition Committee of the American Heart Association. *Circulation* 102, 2284–2299.

15. Ballantyne C.M., Grundy S.M., Oberman A., Kreisberg R.A., Havel R.J., Frost P.H., Haffner S.M. (2000). Hyperlipidemia: Diagnostic and therapeutic perspectives. *Journal of Clinical Endocrinology and Metabolism* 85, 2089–2092.

16. Knopp R. (1999). Drug therapy: Drug treatment of lipid disorders. *New England Journal of Medicine* 341, 498–511.

17. Ahmed S.M., Clasen M.E., Donnelly J.F. (1998). Management of dyslipidemia in adults. *American Family Physician* 57 (9), 2192–2208.

18. Enos W.F., Beyer J.C., Holmes R.F. (1955). Pathogenesis of coronary artery disease in American soldiers killed in Korea. *JAMA* 158, 912.

19. Ross R. (1999). Mechanisms of disease: Atherosclerosis—an inflammatory disease. *New England Journal of Medicine* 340, 115–126.

20. Kullo I.J., Gau G.T., Tajik A.J. (2000). Novel risk factors for atherosclerosis. *Mayo Clinic Proceedings* 75, 369–380.

21. Glasser S.P., Selwyn A.P., Ganz P. (1996). Atherosclerosis: Risk factors and the vascular endothelium. *American Heart Journal* 31, 379–384.

22. Levine G.N., Keaney J.F., Vita J.A. (1995). Cholesterol reduction in cardiovascular disease. *New England Journal of Medicine* 332, 512–521.

23. Gaziano J.M., Hebert P.R., Hennekens C.H. (1996). Cholesterol reduction: Weighing the benefits and risks. *Annals of Internal Medicine* 124, 914–918.

24. Hankey G.J., Eikelboom J.W. (1999). Homocysteine and vascular disease. *Lancet* 354, 407–413.

25. Fong I.W. (2000). Emerging relations between infectious diseases and coronary artery disease and atherosclerosis. *Canadian Medical Association Journal* 163, 49–56.

26. Libby P. (2000). Changing concepts of atherogenesis. *Journal of Internal Medicine* 247, 349–358.

27. Savage C.O.S., Harper L., Cockwell P., Adu D., Howie A.J. (2000). Vasculitis. Clinical review: ABC of arterial and vascular disease. *British Medical Journal* 320, 1325–1328.

28. Gross W.L., Trabandt A., Reinhold-Keller E. (2000). Diagnosis and evaluation of vasculitis. *Rheumatology* 39, 245–252.

29. Jayne D. (2000). Evidence-based treatment of systemic vasculitis. *Rheumatology* 39, 585–595.

30. Bartholomew J.R., Gray B.H. (1999). Large artery occlusive disease. *Rheumatic Disease Clinics of North America* 25, 669–686.

31. Carter S.A. (1999). Peripheral arterial disease. *Canadian Journal of Cardiology* 15 (Suppl. G), 106G–109G.

32. Hilleman D.E. (1998). Management of peripheral arterial disease. *American Journal of Health-System Pharmacy* 55 (Suppl. 1), S21–S27.

33. Tanaka K. (1998). Pathology and pathogenesis of Buerger's disease. *International Journal of Cardiology* 66 (Suppl. 1), S237–S242.

34. Belch, J. (1997). Raynaud's phenomenon. *Cardiovascular Research* 33, 25–30.

35. Cerinic M.M., Generini S., Pignone A. (1997). New approaches to the treatment of Raynaud's phenomenon. *Current Opinion in Rheumatology* 9, 544–556.

36. Ho M., Belch J. (1998). Raynaud's phenomenon: State of the art. *Scandinavian Journal of Rheumatology* 27, 319–322.

37. Thompson M.M., Bell P.R.F. (2000). Arterial aneurysms. Clinical review: ABC of arterial and venous disease. *British Medical Journal* 320, 1193–1196.

38. Creager M.A., Halperin J.L., Whittemore A.D. (1992). Aneurysm disease of the aorta and its branches. In Loscalzo J., Creager M.A., Dzau V.J. (Eds.), *Vascular medicine: A textbook of vascular biology and diseases* (pp. 903–923). Boston: Little, Brown.

39. Coady M.A., Rizzo J.A., Goldstein L.J., Elefteriades J.A. (1999). Natural history, pathogenesis, and etiology of thoracic aortic aneurysms and dissections. *Cardiology Clinics of North America* 17, 615–635.

40. House-Fancher M.A. (1996). Aortic dissection. Pathophysiology, diagnosis, and acute care management. *AACN Clinical Issues* 6 (3), 602–614.

41. Alguire P.C., Mathes B.M. (1997). Chronic venous insufficiency and venous ulceration. *Journal of General Internal Medicine* 12, 374–383.

42. Weinmann E.E., Salzman E.W. (1994). Deep-vein thrombosis. *New England Journal of Medicine* 331, 1630–1641.

43. Virchow R. (1846). Weinere untersuchungen uber die verstropfung der lungenrarterie und ihre folgen. *Beitrage zur Experimentelle Pathologie und Physiologie* 2, 21.

44. Hirsch J., Williams W.J. (1995). Deep vein thrombosis. Recovery or recurrence? *Hospital Practice* 30 (3), 71–79.

45. Sheppard D.R. (2000). Activated protein C resistance: The most common risk factor for venous thromboembolism. *Journal of the American Board of Family Practice* 13, 111–115.

46. Gorman W.P., Davis K.R., Donnelly R. (2000). Swollen lower limb—1: General assessment and deep vein thrombosis: Clinical review: ABC of arterial and venous disease. *British Medical Journal* 320, 1453–1456.

47. Kalb R.L. (1999). Preventing the sequelae of compartment syndrome. *Hospital Practice* 34 (1), 105–107.

48. Matsen F. (1975). Compartment syndrome: A unified concept. *Clinical Orthopaedics and Related Research* 113, 8–13.

49. Ashton H. (1962). Critical closing pressure in human peripheral vascular beds. *Clinical Science* 22, 79.

50. Clark M., Kadhom H.M. (1988). The nursing prevention of pressure sores in hospital and community patients. *Journal of Advanced Nursing* 13, 365–373.

51. Meehan M. (1990). Multisite pressure sore prevalence survey. *Decubitus* 3 (4), 14–17.

52. Langema D.K., Olson B., Hunter S., Burd C., Hansen D., Cathcart-Silberg T. (1989). Incidence and prediction of pressure ulcers in five patient care settings, extended care, home health, and hospice in one locale. *Decubitus* 2 (2), 42.

53. Young L. (1989). Pressure ulcer prevalence and associated patient characteristics in one long-term facility. *Decubitus* 2 (2), 52.

54. National Institutes of Health. *Healthy people 2010*. [On-line]. Available: www.health.gov/healthypeople.

55. Patterson J.A., Bennett R.G. (1995). Prevention and treatment of pressure sores. *Journal of the American Geriatric Society* 43, 919–927.

56. Beland I., Passos J.Y. (1981). *Clinical nursing* (4th ed., p. 1112). New York: Macmillan.

57. Reuler J.B., Cooney T.G. (1981). The pressure sore: Pathophysiology and principles of management. *Annals of Internal Medicine* 94, 661–666.

58. Panel for the Prediction and Prevention of Pressure Ulcers in Adults. (1992). *Pressure ulcers in adults: Prediction and prevention.* Clinical practice guideline. no. 3. AHCPR publication no. 92-0047. Rockville, MD: Agency for Health Care Policy and Research, Public Health Service, U.S. Department of Health and Human Services.
59. Bergstrom N., Bennett M.A., Carlson C.E., et al. (1994). *Treatment of pressure ulcers.* Clinical practice guideline. no. 15. AHCPR Publication No. 95-0652. Rockville, MD: U.S. Department of Health and Human Services. Public Health Service, Agency for Health Care Policy and Research.
60. Norton D. (1989). Calculating the risk: Reflections on the Norton Scale. *Decubitus* 2 (3), 24–31.
61. Braden B.J. (1989). Clinical utility of the Braden scale for predicting pressure ulcer risk. *Decubitus* 2 (3), 44–46, 50–51.
62. National Pressure Ulcer Advisory Panel. (1989). Pressure ulcers, incidence, economics, and risk assessment: Consensus Development Conference Statement. *Decubitus* 2 (2), 24–28.
63. National Pressure Ulcer Advisory Panel. (1998, February). *Task Force on Darkly Pigmented Skin and Stage I Pressure Ulcers: Stage I assessment in darkly pigmented skin.*
64. Findlay D. (1996). Practical management of pressure ulcers. *American Family Physician* 54, 1519–1528.
65. Bernabei R., Landi F., Bonini S., Onder G., Lambiase A., Pola R., Aloe L. (1999). Effect of topical application of nerve-growth factor on pressure ulcers. *Lancet* 354, 307.
66. National Pressure Ulcer Advisory Panel. (1998). *Task Force on Darkly Pigmented Skin and Stage I Pressure Ulcers: State I Assessment in Darkly Pigmented Skin.* Reston, VA. [On-line]. Available: www.npuap.org.

Chapter 23

Alterations in Blood Pressure: Hypertension and Orthostatic Hypotension

Clarence E. Grim and Carlene M. Grim

Blood pressure is one of the most variable but best regulated of all physiologic parameters. The "purpose" of the control of blood pressure is to keep blood flow constant to the heart, brain, and kidneys—for without constant flow to these organs, death ensues in seconds, minutes, or days. Because of the critical importance of keeping blood flow constant to each of these critical tissues, a number of backup systems have evolved so that if one fails, another may take over to protect the organism. Thus, the key to understanding the disorders of blood pressure regulation (hypertension and hypotension) is to understand the mechanisms by which the body regulates blood pressure from microsecond to microsecond, second to second, minute to minute, and day to day. Each limb of the blood pressure control system must have sensors that monitor the arterial pressure as well as effector mechanisms that increase and decrease the blood pressure. Thus, a thorough knowledge of the mechanisms of blood pressure control is needed to understand the person who presents with blood pressure–related illness. Furthermore, because high blood pressure is the most common contributor to premature disability and death, there also is a need for methods to detect and treat high blood pressure in a reliable and effective manner. Fortunately, the diagnosis and treatment of high blood pressure is, for the most part, relatively simple and inexpensive.

The discussion in this chapter focuses on determinants of blood pressure and conditions of altered arterial pressure—hypertension and orthostatic hypotension.

Arterial Blood Pressure

After you have completed this section of the chapter, you should be able to meet the following objectives:

✦ Define the terms *arterial blood pressure, systolic blood pressure, diastolic blood pressure, pulse pressure,* and *mean arterial blood pressure*
✦ Explain how cardiac output and peripheral vascular resistance interact in determining systolic and diastolic blood pressure
✦ Describe the requirements for accurate and reliable blood pressure measurement in terms of cuff size, method for determining cuff inflation pressure, deflation rate, and need for observer preparation in measurement methods
✦ State the rationale for use of self-measurement and ambulatory measurement of blood pressure

Blood flow in the circulatory system depends on a series of patent vessels and the continuous pumping of blood into the arterial vascular system. It is the rise in blood pressure that occurs with each heart beat and ejection of blood into the arterial system that drives the flow of blood to all of the tissues of the body.

DETERMINANTS OF BLOOD PRESSURE

The arterial blood pressure reflects the rhythmic ejection of blood from the left ventricle into the aorta. It rises during systole as the left ventricle contracts, and falls as the heart relaxes during diastole, giving rise to a pressure pulse (see Chapter 21). The contour of the arterial pressure tracing shown in Figure 23-1 is typical of the pressure changes that occur in the large arteries of the systemic circulation. There is a rapid rise in the pulse contour during left ventricular contraction, followed by a slower rise to peak pressure. Approximately 70% of the blood that leaves the left ventricle is ejected during the first one third of systole; this accounts for the rapid rise in the pressure contour. The end of systole is marked by a brief downward deflection and formation of the dicrotic notch, which occurs when ventricular pressure falls below that in the aorta. The sudden closure of the aortic valve is associated with a small rise in pressure caused by continued contraction of the aorta and other large vessels against the closed valve. As the ventricles relax and blood flows into the peripheral vessels during diastole, the arterial pressure falls rapidly at first and then declines slowly as the driving force decreases.

In healthy adults, the pressure at the height of the pressure pulse, called the *systolic pressure,* ideally is less than

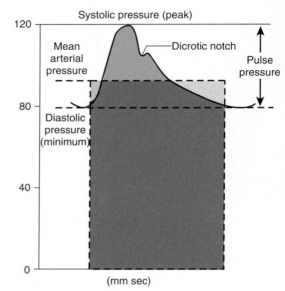

FIGURE 23-1 Intra-arterial pressure tracing made from the brachial artery. Pulse pressure is the difference between systolic and diastolic pressures. The darker area represents the mean arterial pressure, which can be calculated by using the formula of mean arterial pressure = diastolic pressure + pulse pressure/3.

120 mm Hg, and the lowest pressure, called the *diastolic pressure,* is less than 80 mm Hg. The difference between the systolic and diastolic pressure (approximately 40 mm Hg) is called the *pulse pressure.* It reflects the magnitude or height of the pressure pulse. The *mean arterial pressure* represents the average pressure in the arterial system during ventricular contraction and relaxation (approximately 90 to 100 mm Hg) and is depicted by the darker area under the pressure tracing in Figure 23-1.

In hypertension and disease conditions that affect blood pressure, changes in blood pressure usually are described in terms of systolic, diastolic, and pulse pressure and mean arterial pressure. Each of these pressures contributes individually and collectively to blood flow in the various tissue beds of the body. The levels to which these pressures rise and fall is influenced by the stroke volume, the rapidity with which blood is ejected from the heart, the elastic properties of the aorta and large arteries and their ability to accept various amounts of blood as it is ejected from the heart, and the properties of the resistance blood vessels that control the runoff of blood into the smaller vessels and capillaries that connect the arterial and venous circulations.

Systolic Blood Pressure

The systolic blood pressure reflects the rhythmic ejection of blood into the aorta (Fig. 23-2). As blood is ejected into the aorta, it stretches the vessel wall and produces a rise in aortic pressure. The extent to which the systolic pressure rises or falls with each cardiac cycle is determined by the amount of blood ejected into the aorta with each heart beat (*i.e.,* stroke volume), the velocity of ejection, and the elastic properties of the aorta. Systolic pressure increases when there is a rapid ejection of a large stroke volume or

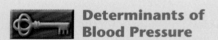

Determinants of Blood Pressure

➤ The arterial blood pressure represents the pressure of the blood as it moves through the arterial system. It reaches its peak (systolic pressure) as blood is ejected from the heart during systole and its lowest level (diastolic pressure) as the heart relaxes during diastole.

➤ Blood pressure is determined by the cardiac output (stroke volume × heart rate) and the resistance that the blood encounters as it moves through the peripheral vessels (peripheral vascular resistance).

➤ The systolic blood pressure is largely determined by the characteristics of the stroke volume being ejected from the heart and the ability of the aorta to stretch and accommodate the stroke volume.

➤ The diastolic pressure is largely determined by the energy that is stored in the aorta as its elastic fibers are stretched during systole and by the resistance to the runoff of blood from the peripheral blood vessels.

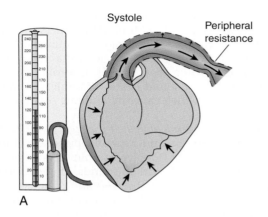

Systole

Peripheral resistance

A

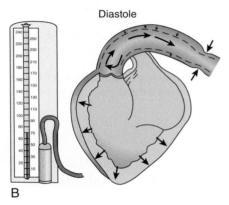

Diastole

B

FIGURE 23-2 Diagram of the left side of the heart. (**A**) Systolic blood pressure represents the ejection of blood into the aorta during ventricular systole; it reflects the stroke volume, the distensibility of the aorta, and the velocity with which blood is ejected from the heart. (**B**) Diastolic blood pressure represents the pressure in the arterial system during diastole; it is largely determined by the peripheral vascular resistance.

when the stroke volume is ejected into a rigid aorta. Only approximately one third of the ejected blood leaves the aorta during ventricular systole. The elastic walls of the aorta normally stretch to accommodate the varying amounts of blood that are ejected into the aorta; this prevents the pressure from rising excessively during systole and maintains pressure during diastole. In some elderly persons, the elastic fibers of the aorta lose some of their resiliency, and the aorta becomes more rigid. When this occurs, the aorta is less able to stretch and buffer the pressure that is generated as blood is ejected into the aorta, resulting in an elevated systolic pressure.

Diastolic Blood Pressure

The diastolic blood pressure is maintained by the energy that has been stored in the elastic walls of the aorta during systole (see Fig. 23-2). The level at which the diastolic pressure is maintained depends on the condition of the aorta and large arteries and their ability to stretch and store energy, the competency of the aortic valve, and the resistance of the arterioles that control the outflow of blood into the microcirculation. The larger arteries are located between

the outlet of the aorta and the arterioles, which control the runoff of blood from the arterial circulation. The arterioles often are referred to as the *resistance vessels* because they can selectively constrict or relax to control the resistance to outflow of blood into the capillaries. When there is an increase in peripheral vascular resistance, as with sympathetic stimulation, diastolic blood pressure rises. With arteriosclerosis, the smaller arteries may become rigid and unable to accept the runoff of blood from the aorta without producing an increase in diastolic pressure. Closure of the aortic valve at the onset of diastole is essential to the maintenance of the diastolic pressure. When there is incomplete closure of the aortic valve, as in aortic regurgitation (see Chapter 24), the diastolic pressure drops as blood flows backward into the left ventricle rather than moving forward into the arterial system.

Pulse Pressure

The pulse pressure is the difference between the systolic and diastolic pressures. It reflects the pulsatile nature of arterial blood flow and is an important component of blood pressure. During the rapid ejection period of ventricular systole, the volume of blood that is ejected into the aorta exceeds the amount that exits the arterial system. The pulse pressure reflects this difference. The pulse pressure rises when additional amounts of blood are ejected into the arterial circulation, and it falls when the resistance to outflow is decreased. In hypovolemic shock, the pulse pressure declines because of a decrease in stroke volume and systolic pressure. This occurs despite an increase in peripheral vascular resistance, which maintains the diastolic pressure. There is increasing evidence that elevations in pulse pressure play an important role in the morbidity and mortality associated with hypertension (to be discussed).

Mean Arterial Pressure

The mean arterial blood pressure represents the average blood pressure in the systemic circulation. The mean arterial pressure (MABP) is determined by the cardiac output (CO) or amount of blood that the heart pumps each minute (*i.e.,* stroke volume × heart rate), and the peripheral vascular resistance (PVR) or the resistance that the blood encounters as it is being pumped through the peripheral circulation: MABP = CO/PVR.

Mean arterial pressure can be estimated by adding one third of the pulse pressure to the diastolic pressure (*i.e.,* diastolic blood pressure + pulse pressure/3). Hemodynamic monitoring equipment in intensive and coronary care units measures or computes mean arterial pressure automatically. Because it is a good indicator of tissue perfusion, the mean arterial pressure often is monitored, along with systolic and diastolic blood pressures, in critically ill patients.

BLOOD PRESSURE MEASUREMENT

Arterial blood pressure measurements usually are obtained by the *indirect auscultatory method,* which uses a sphygmomanometer and a stethoscope. In the measurement of blood pressure, a cuff that contains an inflatable rubber bladder is placed around the upper arm. It is important that the bladder of the cuff be appropriate for the arm size. The width of the bladder should be at least 40% of arm circumference and the length at least 80% of arm circumference.[1-3] Undercuffing (using a cuff with a bladder that is small) can cause an overestimation of blood pressure.[4] This is because a cuff that is too small results in an uneven distribution of pressure across the arm, such that a greater cuff pressure is needed to occlude blood flow. Likewise, overcuffing (using a cuff with a bladder that is too large) can cause an underestimation of blood pressure.

The bladder of the cuff is inflated to a point at which its pressure exceeds that of the artery, occluding the blood flow. This should be done by palpation before the actual pressure is measured to get the palpated systolic pressure. By inflating the pressure in the cuff to a level of 30 mm Hg above the palpated pressure, the observer can be certain that the cuff pressure is high enough to avoid missing the auscultatory gap. This pressure (palpated pressure + 30 mm Hg) is called the *maximum inflation level*.[1] The cuff is then slowly deflated at 2 mm/second. The accuracy of the reading can be no greater than the rate of deflation. At the point where the pressure in the vessel again exceeds the pressure in the cuff, a small amount of blood squirts through the partially obstructed artery. The sounds generated by the turbulent flow are called the *Korotkoff (K) sounds* (Chart 23-1). These low-pitched sounds are best heard with the bell of the stethoscope.

Accurate and reliable blood pressure measurements are essential to the diagnosis and treatment of hypertension as well as other disease conditions.[1-3] This requires that the blood equipment be properly maintained and calibrated and that the persons taking the blood pressures are adequately prepared in blood pressure measurement. Research has shown that many health professionals who measure blood pressure were not taught or do not practice the proper skills and techniques needed to obtain accurate and reliable blood pressure measurements. This serious deficit in preventive health care practices may well be traced to the initial training and mastery of this basic skill. Fortunately, detailed curriculums that teach and document mastery of the key knowledge, skills, and behaviors needed for accurate and reliable blood pressure are available.[2]

Blood pressure is recorded in terms of systolic and diastolic pressures (*e.g.,* 120/70 mm Hg) unless sounds are heard to zero when three readings are required (122/64/0 or K1/K4/K5). Systolic pressure is defined as the first of at least two regular Korotkoff sounds. Diastolic pressure is recorded as the last sound heard (K5) unless sounds are heard to zero; in which case, the muffling sound of K4 is used.

Automated or *semiautomated methods* of blood pressure measurement use a microphone, pulse sensor (oscillometric method), or Doppler equipment for detecting the equivalent of the Korotkoff sounds. These devices are less accurate than trained observers and their use should be limited to situations in which frequent and less accurate blood pressure trends are important, not for diagnosis and monitoring hypertension. It is important that automated devices have been certified as accurate and reliable because not all devices on the market are considered acceptable.[5,6] Ambulatory monitoring, using automated systems, provide a means for assessing blood pressure over a 24-hour period.

Intra-arterial methods provide for direct measurement of blood pressure. Intra-arterial measurement requires the

Ambulatory and Home Blood Pressure Monitoring

The use of ambulatory and home (self) blood pressure monitoring equipment has grown dramatically. Ambulatory and self blood pressure monitoring equipment should meet the testing standards of the Association for Advancement of Medical Instrumentation or the British Hypertension Society.[6] Ambulatory blood pressure units are fully automatic, small, and easy to use. Typically, they take a blood pressure reading every 15 to 30 minutes throughout the day and night while the person goes about her or his normal activities. The readings are stored and then downloaded into a personal computer for analysis. Many of the ambulatory blood pressure measuring devices are equipped with "event buttons" that allow persons to obtain a blood pressure reading when they feel dizzy or have other symptoms associated with blood pressure changes. Home monitoring equipment is sold in pharmacies and medical supply stores throughout the country and is available in many styles and prices. The equipment should be a validated electronic device or an anaeroid monitor, should use an appropriate-sized inflatable cuff, and should be checked once each year for accuracy. The ambulatory and home blood pressure monitoring devices provide a means for measuring blood pressure at different times throughout the day and away from the clinical setting. This is important because some patients experience elevated pressures when having their blood pressure measured in a clinic or physician's office, a phenomenon called *white coat hypertension*.

CHART 23-1

Korotkoff Sounds

Phase I	Period marked by the first tapping sounds, which gradually increase in intensity
Phase II	Period during which a murmur or swishing sound is heard
Phase III	Period during which sounds are crisper and greater in intensity
Phase IV	Period marked by distinct, abrupt muffling or by a soft blowing sound
Phase V	Point at which sounds disappear

insertion of a catheter into a peripheral artery, or may be obtained at the time of cardiac catheterization in the aortic root. The arterial catheter is connected to a pressure transducer, which converts pressure into a digital signal that can be measured, displayed, and recorded. This type of blood pressure monitoring usually is restricted to intensive care units.

Self-measurement of blood pressure may provide valuable information outside the clinician's office regarding a person's blood pressure and response to treatment. Self-measurement has four general advantages: (1) it can help distinguish "white coat hypertension," a condition in which the blood pressure is consistently elevated in the health care provider's office but normal at other times; (2) it can be used to assess the response to treatment methods for hypertension; (3) it can motivate adherence to treatment regimens; and (4) it can potentially reduce health care costs.[7]

> In summary, the alternating contraction and relaxation of the heart produce a pressure pulse that moves the blood through the circulatory system. The elastic walls of the aorta stretch during systole and relax during diastole to maintain the diastolic pressure. The pressure pulse is responsible for the Korotkoff sounds heard when blood pressure is measured using a blood pressure cuff, and it is this impulse that is felt when the pulse is taken. Systolic pressure denotes the highest point of the pulse pressure, and diastolic denotes the lowest point. The pulse pressure is the difference between these two pressures. The mean arterial pressure reflects the average pressure throughout the cardiac cycle. It can be estimated by adding one third of the pulse pressure to the diastolic pressure.
>
> Physical (*i.e.,* blood volume and the elastic properties of the blood vessels) and physiologic factors (*i.e.,* cardiac output and peripheral vascular resistance) influence mean arterial blood pressure. Systolic pressure is determined primarily by the characteristics of the stroke volume, whereas diastolic pressure is determined largely by the conditions of the arteries and arterioles and their abilities to accept the runoff of blood from the aorta. The pulse pressure reflects the pulsatile nature of the arterial blood flow and is an important component of blood pressure. The mean arterial blood pressure represents the average blood pressure in the systemic circulation. It can be estimated by adding one third the pulse pressure to the diastolic blood pressure.
>
> The diagnosis and treatment of hypertension requires accurate and reliable measurement of blood pressure. It requires that persons taking the pressure be properly trained in blood pressure measurement; use accurately calibrated equipment and a properly fitted cuff; inflate the cuff to 30 mm Hg above the palpated pressure and deflate the cuff at a rate of 2 mm Hg/second; and accurately identify and record the Korotkoff sounds representative of the systolic and diastolic pressures.

Hypertension

After you have completed this section of the chapter, you should be able to meet the following objectives:

+ Describe the effect of small increases in blood pressure on the causes of premature disability and death based on the experience of the life insurance industry
+ Cite the definition of hypertension put forth by the sixth report of the Joint National Committee on Detection, Evaluation, and Treatment of Hypertension
+ Differentiate essential, systolic, secondary, and malignant forms of hypertension
+ Describe the possible influence of genetics, age, race, obesity, sodium and other cation (*i.e.,* potassium, calcium, and magnesium) intake, alcohol consumption, and stress on development of essential hypertension
+ Cite the risks of hypertension in terms of target organ damage
+ Define systolic hypertension and characterize the effect of increased systolic and pulse pressure on the production of target-organ damage
+ Describe behavior modification strategies used in prevention and treatment of hypertension
+ List the different categories of drugs used to treat hypertension and state their mechanisms of action in treatment of high blood pressure
+ Explain the changes in blood pressure that accompany normal pregnancy and describe the four types of hypertension that can occur during pregnancy
+ Cite the criteria for the diagnosis of high blood pressure in children
+ Define systolic hypertension and relate the circulatory changes that occur with aging that predispose to the development of systolic hypertension

Hypertension, or high blood pressure, is probably the most common of all health problems in adults and is the leading risk factor for cardiovascular disorders. In the United States, approximately 25% of all adults older than 18 years of age have high blood pressure.[7] It has been estimated that as many as 60 million adults have cardiovascular disease. In 50 million of these people (83%), the cause of cardiovascular disease is high blood pressure.

Hypertension is more common in younger men compared with younger women, in blacks compared with whites, in persons from lower socioeconomic groups, and in older persons. Men have higher blood pressures than women up until the time of menopause, at which point women quickly lose their protection. Although hypertension occurs in all geographic areas of the country, the Southeast clearly has a greater frequency of hypertension and its major consequences, stroke and renal failure. The prevalence of hypertension increases with age. With the aging "baby boomer" population, the problem of hypertension will become much more common.

The importance of high blood pressure levels with regard to health has been known since the early 1900s. The first strong evidence came from Janeway, who reported on the markedly shortened lives of patients who present with symptomatic hypertension (headaches, shortness of breath, congestive heart failure, edema, or uremia).[8] The life insurance industry quickly learned that the measurement of blood pressure was the single most important predictor of premature disability and death and early death in men, and by 1913 a person could not purchase life insurance if his or her blood pressure was greater than 150/100 mm Hg.[9]

In 1972, the National Institutes of Health founded the National High Blood Pressure Education Program. The purpose of the program was to increase awareness among health professionals and the public about the importance of detecting and treating hypertension. This program was followed by the formation of a multidisciplinary committee called the *Joint National Committee on Detection, Evaluation, and Treatment of High Blood Pressure,* which has met every 4 years, beginning in 1977, to update and refine the criteria for diagnosis and treatment of hypertension in persons 18 years of age and older. From the 1976 to 1980 National Health and Nutrition Examination Survey (NHANES II) to the 1988 to 1991 survey (NHANES III), the percentage of Americans who were aware that they had high blood pressure increased from 51% to 73%.[7] During the same period, treatment of persons with hypertension increased from 31% to 55%, the age-adjusted mortality rate from coronary heart disease decreased approximately 53%, and that from stroke fell by nearly 60% (Fig. 23-3). Despite these trends, hypertension remains one of the most frequently encountered chronic health problems and continues as one of the most significant risk factors for morbidity and mortality from coronary heart disease, congestive heart failure, chronic renal failure, and stroke.

Hypertension commonly is divided into the categories of primary and secondary hypertension. In primary hypertension, often called *essential hypertension,* the chronic elevation in blood pressure occurs without evidence of other disease. In secondary hypertension, the elevation of blood pressure results from some other disorder, such as kidney disease. Malignant hypertension, as the name implies, is an accelerated form of hypertension.

ESSENTIAL HYPERTENSION

The sixth report of the Joint National Committee on Detection, Evaluation, and Treatment of High Blood Pressure (JNC-VI) of the National Institutes of Health was published in 1997.[7] According to the JNC-VI recommendations, a systolic pressure of less than 120 mm Hg and diastolic pressure less than 80 mm Hg is optimal; systolic pressure less than 130 mm Hg systolic and diastolic pressure less than 80 mm Hg is normal; and systolic pressure of 130 to 139 mm Hg and diastolic pressure of 85 to 89 mm Hg is high-normal (Table 23-1). For adults with diabetes mellitus, the blood pressure goal has been lowered to less than 130/80 mm Hg.[10] A diagnosis of hypertension is made if the systolic blood pressure is 140 mm Hg or higher and diastolic blood pressure is 90 mm Hg or higher. Hypertension is further di-

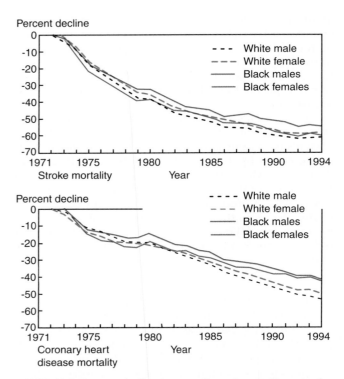

FIGURE 23-3 Percent decline in age adjusted mortality rates for stroke (**top**) and coronary heart disease (**bottom**) by sex and race: United States, 1972–94. (From the National Heart, Lung, and Blood Institute using data from *Vital Statistics of the United States,* National Center for Health Statistics.)

vided into stages 1, 2, and 3 based on systolic and diastolic blood pressure measurements (see Table 23-1).

The JNC-VI report emphasizes that obtaining one elevated blood pressure reading should not constitute the diagnosis of hypertension. The diagnosis of hypertension in a person who is not taking antihypertensive medications should be based on the average of at least two or more blood pressure readings taken at each of two or more visits after an initial screening visit.[7] Blood pressure measurements should be taken when the person is relaxed and has rested for at least 5 minutes and has not smoked or ingested caffeine within 30 minutes. At least two measurements should be made at each visit in the same arm while the person is seated. If the first two readings differ by more than 5 mm Hg, additional readings should be taken. Both the systolic and diastolic pressures should be recorded. The appearance of the first K sound (phase 1) is used to define systolic pressure, and the disappearance of the K sounds (phase V) is used to define the diastolic pressure.[2] Because blood pressure in many individuals is highly variable, blood pressure should be measured on different occasions over a period of several months before a diagnosis of hypertension is made unless the pressure is extremely elevated or associated with symptoms (see Table 23-1).

Hypertension

➤ Hypertension represents an elevation in systolic and/or diastolic blood pressure.

➤ Essential hypertension is characterized by a chronic elevation in blood pressure that occurs without evidence of other disease, and secondary hypertension by an elevation of blood pressure that results from some other disorder, such as kidney disease.

➤ The pathogenesis of essential hypertension is thought to reside with the kidney and its role regulating vascular volume through salt and water elimination; the renin-angiotensin-aldosterone system through its effects on blood vessel tone, regulation of renal blood flow, and salt metabolism; and the sympathetic nervous system, which regulates the tone of the resistance vessels. The medications that are used in the treatment of hypertension exert their effects through one or more of these regulatory mechanisms.

➤ Uncontrolled hypertension produces increased demands on the heart, resulting in left ventricular hypertrophy and heart failure, and on the vessels of the arterial system, leading to atherosclerosis, kidney disease, and stroke.

Aside from an elevation in blood pressure, essential hypertension is typically an asymptomatic disorder and the condition often is detected during screening procedures or when a person seeks medical care for other purposes. Although headache often is considered to be an early symptom of hypertension, it affects only a small number of hypertensive people at the time of diagnosis. When present, the headache associated with hypertension is believed to result from intense vasodilatation. It occurs most frequently on awakening and is usually felt in the back of the head or neck. A common early symptom of target-organ damage in long-term hypertension is nocturia, which indicates that the kidneys are losing their ability to concentrate urine. Other signs and symptoms commonly attributed to hypertension are probably related to the long-term effects of blood pressure elevation on other organ systems in the body, such as the eyes, heart, and blood vessels.

Mechanisms of Blood Pressure Elevation

Several factors, including hemodynamic, neural, humoral, and renal mechanisms, are thought to interact in producing long-term elevations in blood pressure. As with other disease conditions, it is improbable that there is a single cause responsible for the development of essential hypertension or that the condition is a single disease. Because arterial blood pressure is the product of cardiac output and peripheral vascular resistance, all forms of hypertension involve hemodynamic mechanisms—an increase in cardiac output or peripheral vascular resistance, or a combination of the two. Other factors, such as sympathetic nervous system activity, kidney function in terms of salt

TABLE 23-1 ✦ Classification and Follow-up of Blood Pressure Measurements for Adults 18 Years of Age and Older*

Category*	Systolic Blood Pressure (mm Hg)		Diastolic Blood Pressure (mm Hg)	Follow-up Recommended
Optimal†	<120	*and*	<80	Recheck in 2 years
Normal	<130	*and*	<85	Recheck in 2 years
High-Normal	130–139	*or*	85–89	Recheck in 1 year
Hypertension‡				
Stage 1	140–159	*or*	90–99	Confirm within 2 months
Stage 2	160–179	*or*	100–109	Evaluate or refer to source of care within 1 month
Stage 3	≥180	*or*	≥110	Evaluate or refer to source of care immediately or within 1 week, depending on clinical situation

*Not taking antihypertensive drugs and not acutely ill. When systolic and diastolic pressures fall into different categories, the higher category should be selected to classify the individual's blood pressure status. For instance, 160/92 should be classified as stage 2 and 174/120 should be classified as stage 3. Isolated systolic hypertension (ISH) is defined as systolic blood pressure ≥140 mm Hg and diastolic blood pressure <90 mm Hg and staged appropriately (*e.g.,* 170/82 mm Hg is defined as stage 2 ISH). In addition to classifying stages of hypertension on the basis of average blood pressure levels, clinicians should specify presence or absence of target-organ disease and additional risk factors. This specificity is important for risk classification and treatment.
†Optimal blood pressure with respect to cardiovascular risk is below 120/80 mm Hg. However, unusually low readings should be evaluated for clinical significance.
‡Based on the average of two or more readings taken at each of two or more visits after an initial screening.
(Adapted from the National Heart, Lung, and Blood Institute. [1997]. *The sixth report of the National Committee on Detection, Evaluation, and Treatment of High Blood Pressure* [pp. 11, 13]. NIH publication no. 98-4080. Bethesda, MD: National Institutes of Health. Available: http://www.nhlbi.nih.gov/guidelines/hypertension/jncintro.htm)

and water retention, the electrolyte composition of the intracellular and extracellular fluids, cell membrane transport mechanisms, and humoral influences such as the renin-angiotensin-aldosterone mechanism, play an active or permissive role in regulating the hemodynamic mechanisms that control blood pressure. Blood pressure regulation is discussed in Chapter 21.

Considerable evidence suggests that the kidney is directly or indirectly involved in most and perhaps all forms of hypertension.[11,12] Normally, the kidney maintains blood pressure within a very narrow range by regulating blood volume through the conservation or elimination of sodium and water. The relation between arterial pressure and the elimination of sodium and water has been called *pressure natriuresis* (see Chapter 21, Fig. 21-23). When blood pressure rises, the kidney normally responds by increasing its excretion of salt and water. Evidence suggests that persons in whom hypertension develops require a higher arterial pressure to regulate the elimination of salt and water by the kidney.[11] This does not mean that the abnormality leading to hypertension is internal to the kidney. For example, excess sympathetic nerve activity or the release of vasoconstrictor substances that alter the transmission of pressure to the kidney could initiate hypertension. Similarly, changes in neural and humoral control of kidney function can shift the pressure natriuresis relation to higher pressures and initiate hypertension. The renin-angiotensin-aldosterone system plays an essential role in regulating blood volume and blood pressure by means of salt and water retention by the kidney (Fig. 23-4). The role of the kidney in the development of essential hypertension is supported further by the fact that many hypertension medications produce their blood pressure–lowering effects by increasing salt and water excretion.

Contributing Factors

Although the cause or causes of essential hypertension are largely unknown, several factors have been implicated as contributing to its development. These risk factors include family history of hypertension, race, and age-related increases in blood pressure. Lifestyle factors can contribute to the development of hypertension by interacting with the risk factors. These lifestyle factors include high sodium intake, excessive calorie intake and obesity, physical inactivity, excessive alcohol consumption, and low intake of potassium. Oral contraceptive drugs also may increase blood pressure in predisposed women. Although stress can raise blood pressure acutely, there is less evidence linking it to chronic elevations in blood pressure. It also has been suggested that a diet that is low in calcium and magnesium may contribute to long-term elevations in blood pressure; however, there is no convincing evidence to justify increased intake of either of these minerals for the purpose of preventing or treating hypertension. Although dietary fats and cholesterol are independent risk factors for coronary heart disease, there is no evidence that they raise blood pressure. Although not identified as a primary risk factor in hypertension, smoking is an independent risk factor in coronary heart disease and should be avoided.

Family History. The inclusion of heredity as a contributing factor in the development of hypertension is supported by the fact that hypertension is seen most frequently among persons with a family history of hypertension. Persons with two or more first-degree relatives with hypertension before age 55 years have a 3.8 times greater risk for development of hypertension before age 50 years than persons without a family history.[13] The inherited predisposition does not seem to rely on other risk factors, but when they are present, the risk apparently is additive. The pattern of heredity is unclear; it is unknown whether a single gene or multiple genes are involved. Whatever the explanation, the high incidence of hypertension among close family members seems significant enough to be presented as a case for recommending that persons from these high-risk families be encouraged to participate in hypertensive screening programs on a regular basis.

Age-Related Changes in Blood Pressure. Maturation and growth are known to cause predictable increases in blood pressure. For example, in the newborn, arterial blood pressure normally is only approximately 50 mm Hg systolic and 40 mm Hg diastolic. Sequentially, blood pressure increases with physical growth from a value of 78 mm Hg systolic at 10 days of age to 120 mm Hg at the end of adolescence. Systolic blood pressure continues to undergo a slow rate of increase throughout adult life, whereas diastolic pressure increases until 50 years of age and then declines from the sixth decade onward.[14,15]

Race. Hypertension not only is more prevalent in African Americans than whites, it is more severe. The NHANES II (1988 to 1991) reported that diastolic blood pressures were significantly greater for African Americans than for white men and women 35 years of age and older, and that systolic pressures of African-American women at every age were greater than those of white women.[15,16] Hypertension tends to occur earlier in African Americans than in whites, and it often is not treated early enough or aggressively enough. Blacks also tend to experience greater cardiovascular and renal damage at any level of pressure.[17]

The reasons for the increased incidence of hypertension among African Americans are unknown. Studies have shown that many African-American persons with hypertension have lower renin levels than white persons with hypertension.[18] They also do not respond to increased salt intake by increasing their renal excretion of sodium at normal levels of arterial blood pressure. Instead, sodium elimination requires a higher level of blood pressure. These changes in sodium excretion have been linked to what has been called a *salt-thrifty gene*. It has been suggested that the genetic trait may have developed as an evolutionary adaptation to the severe demands for sodium conservation in the western African environment and the slavery environment of the Western Hemisphere. In both environments, survival under conditions of heavy exertion in a warm climate along with salt and water deprivation depended on the body's ability to conserve sodium.[19]

Evidence suggests that blacks, when provided equal access to diagnosis and treatment, can achieve overall

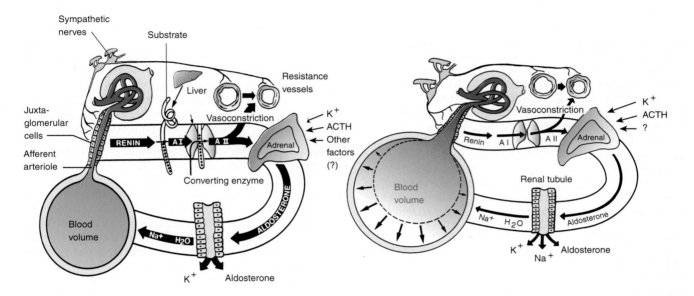

A   Normal sodium intake

B   Saline infusion

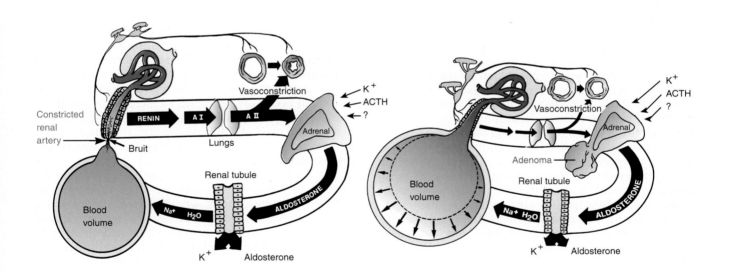

C   Secondary hyperaldosteronism
    renovascular hypertension

D   Primary hyperaldosteronism

FIGURE 23-4 Role of the renin-angiotensin-aldosterone system in regulation of blood pressure and pathogenesis of hypertension. (**A**) Function of the renin-angiotensin system with normal sodium intake. The release of renin by juxtaglomerular cells acts to convert angiotensinogen (substrate) to angiotensin I (AI), which is converted to angiotensin II (AII) in the lungs by angiotensin-converting enzyme. AII functions both as vasoconstrictor and as a mediator for the release of aldosterone by the adrenal gland. Aldosterone, in turn, regulates blood volume by increasing renal tubular reabsorption of sodium and water. (**B**) The effect of a rapid increase in sodium (saline infusion) on renin-angiotensin-aldosterone–mediated changes in blood volume. (**C**) The role of the secondary hyperaldosteronism in the pathogenesis of renovascular hypertension. (**D**) The role of primary aldosteronism in the pathogenesis of secondary hypertension. (Permission courtesy of Dr. Clarence E. Grim)

reductions in blood pressure and experience fewer cardio-vascular complications similar to whites.[7] Barriers that limit access to the health care system include inadequate financial support, inconveniently located health care fa-cilities, long waiting times, and inaccessibility to culturally relevant health education about hypertension. With the high prevalence of salt sensitivity, obesity, and smoking among blacks, health education and lifestyle modifica-tions are particularly important. Because of their increased salt sensitivity and low-renin profile, African Americans are reported to respond better to drugs, such as diuretics and calcium channel–blocking drugs, that do not exert their primary actions through renin mechanisms.[7]

Unfortunately, there is less information regarding hypertension in other racial groups, including Native Americans, Asians and Pacific Islanders, and Hispanics.

High Salt Intake. Increased salt intake has long been suspected as an etiologic factor in the development of hypertension. The relation between body levels of sodium and hypertension is based, at least partially, on the find-ing of a decreased incidence of hypertension among prim-itive, unacculturated people from widely different parts of the world.[20,21] For example, among the Yanomamo Indi-ans of northern Brazil, who excrete only approximately 1 mEq of sodium per day, the average blood pressure in men 40 to 49 years of age was 107/67 mm Hg, and 98/62 mm Hg in women of the same age.[20]

At present, salt intake among adults in the United States and United Kingdom averages at least 9 g/day, with large numbers of people consuming 12 g/day or more.[22] The American Heart Association recommends the daily salt in-take for adults in the general population should not exceed 6 g/day.[23] Approximately 75% of salt intake comes from salt added in processing and manufacturing of food; 15% from the discretionary addition in cooking and at the table; and 10% from the natural sodium content of food.[22,24,25]

Just how increased salt intake contributes to the devel-opment of hypertension is still unclear. It may be that salt causes an elevation in blood volume, increases the sensi-tivity of cardiovascular or renal mechanisms to adrenergic influences, or exerts its effects through some other mech-anism such as the renin-angiotensin-aldosterone mecha-nism. Regardless of the mechanism, numerous studies have shown that a reduction in salt intake can lower blood pres-sure.[24] The strongest data come from the INTERSALT study, which measured 24-hour urine sodium excretion (an indi-rect measure of salt intake) in 10,079 men and women 20 to 59 years of age in 52 places around the world. In all 52 sites, there was a positive correlation between sodium excretion and both systolic and diastolic blood pressure. Furthermore, the association of sodium and blood pres-sure was greatest for older (40 to 59 years) compared with younger (20 to 39 years) subjects in the study.[22] The DASH (Dietary Approaches to Stop Hypertension) diet is a nutri-tional plan that emphasizes fruits, vegetables, low-fat dairy products, whole grains, poultry, fish, and nuts, and is re-duced in fat, red meat, sweets, and sugar-containing bever-ages. Results from studies using the low-sodium DASH diet

have shown significant reductions in systolic and diastolic blood pressures.[26,27]

Despite the results of research relating salt and hyper-tension, the impact of a long-term restriction of sodium consumption in the normotensive population is unknown. It could, for example, create problems in persons who re-spond poorly to volume-depleting stresses in the absence of readily available sodium in their diet. Nevertheless, for people with hypertension, it seems that lowering salt intake along with other healthy lifestyle changes can be beneficial.

Obesity. Excessive weight commonly is associated with hypertension. Weight reduction of as little as 4.5 kg (10 lb) can produce a decrease in blood pressure in a large pro-portion of overweight people with hypertension.[7] It has been suggested that fat distribution might be a more criti-cal indicator of hypertension risk than actual overweight. The waist-to-hip ratio commonly is used to differentiate central or upper body obesity (*i.e.,* fat cell deposits in the abdomen) from peripheral or lower body obesity with fat cell deposits in the buttocks and legs (see Chapter 11). Studies have found an association between hypertension and increased waist-to-hip ratio (*i.e.,* central obesity) even when body mass index and skinfold thickness are taken into account.[7,28,29] Abdominal or visceral fat seems to be more insulin resistant than fat deposited over the buttocks and legs.

Hyperinsulinemia. Insulin resistance and an accompa-nying compensatory hyperinsulinemia have been sug-gested as possible etiologic links to the development of hypertension and associated metabolic disturbances such as hyperlipidemia and obesity.[30] Although insulin resis-tance is common in obesity and type 2 diabetes mellitus, it also has been observed in nonobese persons and those without type 2 diabetes. In persons with obesity and type 2 diabetes and in those with hypertension, the defect appears to be in the ability of insulin to stimulate the uptake and disposal of glucose by skeletal muscle.[31]

At least four mechanisms have been proposed for the effects of hyperinsulinemia on blood pressure: acti-vation of the sympathetic nervous system and its effects on cardiac output, peripheral vascular resistance, and renal sodium retention; insulin-stimulated changes in growth of vascular smooth muscle that result in an in-crease in peripheral vascular resistance; the effect of in-sulin on salt and water retention by the kidney; and changes in sodium and calcium transport across the cell membrane of vascular smooth muscle, thereby sensitiz-ing blood vessels to vasopressor stimuli.[32]

It has been suggested that the insulin-mediated in-crease in sympathetic activity is directed at increasing the metabolic rate as a means of burning the calories that can-not be stored because of insulin resistance. Unfortunately, the increase in sympathetic activity also contributes to the development of hypertension by stimulating the heart, the blood vessels, and the kidney. Hyperinsulinemia also is associated with high plasma triglyceride levels and low concentrations of high-density lipoproteins.

Insulin resistance may be a genetic or acquired trait. For example, it has been shown that insulin-mediated glucose disposal declines by 30% to 40% in persons who are 40% over ideal weight. Nonpharmacologic interventions, such as caloric restriction, weight loss, and exercise, tend to decrease insulin resistance, sympathetic nervous system activity, and blood pressure.[31]

Excess Alcohol Consumption. Regular alcohol drinking plays a role in the development of hypertension. The effect is seen with different types of alcoholic drinks, in men and women, and in a variety of ethnic groups.[33,34] One of the first reports of a link between alcohol consumption and hypertension came from the Oakland–San Francisco Kaiser Permanente Medical Care Program study of 84,000 persons that correlated known drinking patterns and blood pressure levels.[35] This study revealed that the regular consumption of three or more drinks per day increased the risk of hypertension. Systolic pressures were more markedly affected than diastolic pressures. Blood pressure may improve or return to normal when alcohol consumption is decreased or eliminated. The mechanism whereby alcohol exerts its effect on blood pressure is unclear. It has been suggested that lifestyle factors such as obesity and lack of exercise may be accompanying factors.

Intake of Potassium, Calcium, and Magnesium. Low levels of dietary potassium have been linked to increased blood pressure.[36–38] The strongest evidence comes from the previously described INTERSALT study. In this study, a 60 mmol/day higher urinary potassium excretion was associated with a decrease in systolic pressure of 3.4 mm Hg lower and a decrease in diastolic pressure of 1.9 mm Hg.[38] Various mechanisms have been proposed to explain the influence of potassium on blood pressure. These include a purported change in the ratio of sodium to potassium in the diet, a direct natriuretic effect, and suppression of the renin-angiotensin system. In terms of food intake, a diet high in potassium usually is low in sodium. One of the major benefits of increased potassium intake is increased elimination of sodium (natriuretic effect) through the renin-angiotensin-aldosterone mechanism. Other effects include a dampening of vasoconstrictor responses that are induced by norepinephrine and other vasoactive agents. A high-potassium diet does not appear to alter blood pressure in normotensive persons, nor is there evidence to suggest a significant effect from use of potassium supplements in hypertensive persons with normal potassium levels. The use of potassium supplements is expensive and possibly hazardous for some persons. Instead, it is recommended that high-potassium, low-sodium foods be substituted for high-sodium, low-potassium foods in the diet.

The associations between high blood pressure and calcium and magnesium levels have been investigated. Although there have been reports of high blood pressure in persons with low calcium intake or lowering of blood pressure with increased calcium intake, the link between low calcium and magnesium intake and hypertension is inconclusive.[39]

Stress. Physical and emotional stress undoubtedly contributes to transient alterations in blood pressure. Studies in which arterial blood pressure was continually monitored on a 24-hour basis as persons performed their normal activities showed marked fluctuations in pressure associated with normal life stresses—increasing during periods of physical discomfort and family crisis and declining during rest and sleep.[40,41] As with other risk factors, the role of stress-related episodes of transient hypertension in producing the chronically elevated pressures seen in essential hypertension is speculative. It may be that vascular smooth muscle hypertrophies with increased activity in a manner similar to that of skeletal muscle, or that the central integrative pathways in the brain become adapted to the frequent stress-related input.

Psychological techniques involving biofeedback, relaxation, and transcendental meditation have emerged as possible methods for controlling blood pressure. It still is too early to tell whether these techniques offer information about the role of stress in the production of hypertension or will prove useful in its treatment.[7]

Circadian Variations (Dippers vs. Nondippers). Normal changes in blood pressure follow a characteristic pattern. Blood pressure tends to highest in the early morning, shortly after arising from sleep, then decreases gradually throughout the day, reaching its lowest point at approximately 2 to 5 AM. In healthy normotensive people, mean intra-arterial pressure falls by approximately 20% from waking to sleeping hours.[42] The term *dippers* is used to refer to persons with a normal circadian blood pressure profile in which blood pressure falls during the night, and *nondippers* for persons whose 24-hour blood pressure profile is flattened. Ambulatory blood pressure monitoring can be used to determine alterations in a person's circadian blood pressure profile. Changes in the normal circadian blood pressure profile may occur in a number of conditions, including malignant hypertension, Cushing's syndrome, preeclampsia, orthostatic hypotension, congestive heart failure, and sleep apnea.[42] There is increasing evidence that alterations in the normal nocturnal decline in blood pressure may contribute to the development of target-organ disease in persons with hypertension.

Oral Contraceptive Drugs. Oral contraceptives cause a mild increase in blood pressure in many women and overt hypertension in approximately 5%.[43] Why this occurs is largely unknown, although it has been suggested that estrogen and progesterone are responsible for the effect. Various contraceptive drugs contain different amounts and combinations of estrogen and progestational agents, and these differences may contribute to the occurrence of hypertension in some women but not others. Fortunately, the hypertension associated with oral contraceptives usually disappears after the drug has been discontinued, although it may take as long as 6 months for this to happen. However, in some women the blood pressure may not return to normal; they may be at risk for developing hypertension.

The risk of hypertension-associated cardiovascular complications is found primarily in women older than 35 years of age and in those who smoke.[7]

Systolic Hypertension

Essential hypertension may be classified as systolic/diastolic hypertension in which both the systolic and diastolic pressures are elevated; as diastolic hypertension in which the diastolic pressure is selectively elevated; or as systolic hypertension in which the systolic pressure is selectively elevated. The JNC-VI report defined systolic hypertension as a systolic pressure of 140 mm Hg or greater and a diastolic pressure less than 90 mm Hg, indicating a need for increased recognition and control of isolated systolic hypertension.[7] Historically, diastolic hypertension was thought to confer a greater risk for cardiovascular events than systolic hypertension.[7] However, there is mounting evidence that elevated systolic blood pressure is at least as important, if not more so, than diastolic hypertension.[44-46] In a recent study that used data from the Framingham Offspring cohort to arrive at a hypertension classification based on the JNC-VI stages, it was found that systolic pressure alone correctly classified 95% of persons 60 years of age or younger and 99% of those older than 60 years of age.[47] Thought to be equally important as systolic pressure is the pulse pressure, which "hammers away" at the vessel wall.[46,48,49]

Systolic blood pressure rises almost linearly between 30 and 84 years of age, whereas diastolic pressure rises until 50 years of age and then levels off or decreases[15] (Fig. 23-5). This rise in systolic pressure is thought to be related to increased stiffness of the large arteries. With aging, the elastin fibers in the walls of the arteries are gradually replaced by collagen fibers that render the vessels stiffer and less compliant. Differences in the central and peripheral arteries relate to the fact that the larger vessels contain more elastin, whereas the peripheral resistance vessels have more smooth muscle and less elastin. Because of increased wall stiffness, the aorta and large arteries are less able to buffer the rise in systolic pressure that occurs as blood is ejected from the left heart and they are less able to store the energy needed to maintain the diastolic pressure. As a result, the systolic pressure rises, the diastolic pressure remains unchanged or actually decreases, and the pulse pressure or difference between the systolic pressure and diastolic pressure widens.

There are two aspects of systolic hypertension that confer increased risk of cardiovascular events—one is the actual elevation in systolic pressure and the other is the disproportionate rise in pulse pressure. Elevated pressures during systole favor the development of left ventricular hypertrophy, increased myocardial oxygen demands, and eventual left heart failure. At the same time, the absolute or relative lowering of diastolic pressure is a limiting factor in coronary perfusion because coronary perfusion is greatest during diastole. Elevated levels of pulse pressure produce greater stretch of arteries, causing damage to the elastic elements of the vessel and thus predisposing to

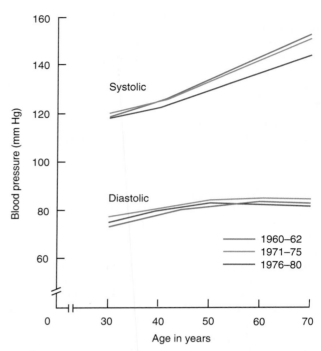

FIGURE 23-5 Mean systolic and diastolic blood pressures in adults ages 25–74 years in the United States (From Rowland M., Roberts J. [1982]. Blood pressure levels and hypertension in persons ages 6–74 years: United States, 1976–80. *NCHS Advancedata*, 84, 3)

aneurysms and development of the intimal damage that leads to atherosclerosis and thrombosis.

Target-Organ Damage

The 1997 JNC-VI report uses the term *target-organ disease* to describe the cardiac, cerebrovascular, peripheral vascular, renal, and retinal complications associated with hypertension.[7] The excess morbidity and mortality related to hypertension is progressive over the whole range of systolic and diastolic pressures. Target-organ damage varies markedly among persons with similar levels of hypertension.

Hypertension is a major risk factor for atherosclerosis; it predisposes to all major atherosclerotic cardiovascular disorders, including heart failure, stroke, coronary artery disease, and peripheral artery disease. The risk of coronary artery disease and stroke depends to a great extent on other risk factors such as obesity, smoking, and elevated cholesterol levels. If all else is favorable, the risk of a coronary event in persons with mild hypertension is no greater than in the average population of the same age. However, if a cluster of risk factors exists, the risk is greatly increased.[50] The same is true for stroke. The risk of stroke occurring in persons with hypertension occurs over an eightfold range, depending on the number of associated risk factors. Cerebrovascular complications are more closely related to systolic than diastolic hypertension. The incidence of these complications is greatly reduced by antihypertensive therapy.

Hypertension increases the workload of the left ventricle by increasing the pressure against which the heart must pump as it ejects blood into the systemic circulation. As the workload of the heart increases, the left ventricular wall hypertrophies to compensate for the increased pressure work. The prevalence of left ventricular hypertrophy increases with age and is highest in persons with blood pressures over 160/95 mm Hg. It was observed in 12% to 20% of persons with mild hypertension and in 50% of asymptomatic persons with mild to moderate hypertension.[51] Despite its adaptive advantage, left ventricular hypertrophy is a major risk factor for ischemic heart disease, cardiac dysrhythmias, sudden death, and congestive heart failure. Hypertensive left ventricular hypertrophy regresses with therapy. Regression is most closely related to systolic pressure reduction and does not appear to reflect the particular type of medication used.

Hypertension also can lead to nephrosclerosis, a common cause of renal insufficiency (see Chapter 33). Hypertensive kidney disease is more common in blacks than whites. Hypertension also plays an important role in accelerating the course of other types of kidney disease, particularly diabetic nephropathy. Because of the risk of diabetic nephropathy, the American Diabetes Association recommends that persons with diabetes maintain their blood pressure at levels less than 130/80 mm Hg (see Chapter 41).

Diagnosis and Treatment

Aside from measurements of elevated blood pressure, few diagnostic tests are useful in detecting and diagnosing essential hypertension. The increased availability of hypertensive screening clinics provides one of the best means for early detection. Laboratory tests, x-ray films, and other diagnostic tests usually are done to exclude secondary hypertension and determine the presence or extent of target-organ disease.

The main objective for treatment of essential hypertension is to achieve and maintain arterial blood pressure below 140/90 mm Hg, with the goal of preventing morbidity and mortality. For persons with secondary hypertension, efforts are made to correct or control the disease condition causing the hypertension. Antihypertensive medications and other measures supplement the treatment for the underlying disease. The JNC-VI report contains a treatment algorithm for hypertension that includes lifestyle modification and, when necessary, guidelines for the use of pharmacologic agents to achieve and maintain systolic pressure below 140 mm Hg and diastolic pressure below 90 mm Hg[7] (Fig. 23-6).

Lifestyle Modification. Lifestyle modification, previously referred to as *nonpharmacologic therapy*, includes weight reduction, reduction of sodium intake, regular physical activity, modification of alcohol intake, and smoking cessation. The DASH study showed that a combination diet rich in fruits and vegetables and in which saturated fat was replaced with low-fat dairy products produced a greater reduction of blood pressure than did most other dietary interventions.[26,27] Other lifestyle modification strategies, such as increased intake of potassium, calcium, and magnesium or the use of relaxation and biofeedback, were not included in the JNC-VI report because of a lack of convincing data to justify recommendation.[7] For persons with stage 1 hypertension, an attempt to control blood pressure with weight loss and other lifestyle modifications should be tried for at least 3 to 6 months before initiating pharmacologic treatment.

Recognizing obesity as a major risk factor in essential hypertension, the committee recommended that all obese hypertensive adults be encouraged to participate in weight reduction programs with the goal of achieving a body weight within 15% of their desirable weight.

A high-salt diet may play a critical role in maintaining blood pressure elevation, and it may limit the effectiveness of some antihypertensive drugs. The JNC-VI report recommends that persons with hypertension limit their salt

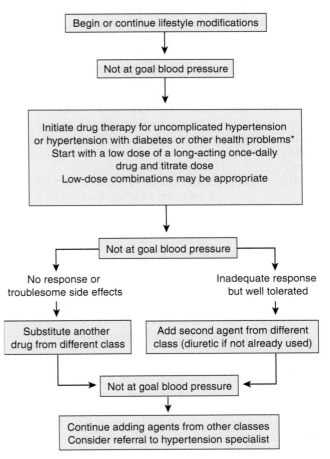

FIGURE 23-6 Algorithm for treatment of hypertension. *Drug choices should be based on randomized controlled trials or specific indications cited in JNC guidelines. A diuretic or a β-blocker is usually used as initial therapy for uncomplicated hypertension unless there is compelling or specific indications for another drug. (Modified from National Heart, Lung, and Blood Institute. [1997]. *The sixth report of the National Committee on Detection, Evaluation, and Treatment of High Blood Pressure.* Publication No. 98–4080. Bethesda, MD: NIH)

intake to 6 g/day.[7] Because many prepared foods are high in sodium, merely refraining from use of the salt shaker usually is not sufficient. Instead, it was recommended that persons consult package labels for the sodium content of canned foods, frozen foods, soft drinks, and other foods and beverages to reduce sodium intake adequately.

A sedentary lifestyle has been cited as a risk factor in cardiovascular disease. A regular program of physical exercise (*e.g.*, walking, biking, swimming) is protective, especially for those at increased risk for cardiovascular disease because of hypertension. Exercise may have further indirect benefits, such as weight loss or motivation for changing other risk factors. Persons with hypertension should be evaluated before beginning an exercise program of appropriate types of exercise. Weight lifting and other forms of isometric exercise can raise blood pressure acutely and should be done with caution.

Because of alcohol's association with high blood pressure, the JNC-VI report recommended restriction of alcohol consumption to no more than 1 oz (30 mL) ethanol per day (equal to 2 oz of 100-proof whiskey, approximately 10 oz of wine, or 24 oz of beer).[7] Significant hypertension may develop during withdrawal from heavy alcohol consumption, but the pressor effects of alcohol withdrawal usually subside within a few days after alcohol consumption is reduced.

Although nicotine has not been associated with long-term elevations in blood pressure as in essential hypertension, it has been shown to increase the risk of heart disease. The fact that smoking and hypertension are major cardiovascular risk factors should be reason enough to encourage the hypertensive smoker to quit.

There is conflicting evidence about the direct effects of dietary fats on blood pressure. As with smoking, however, the interactive effects of saturated fats and high blood pressure as cardiovascular risk factors would seem to warrant dietary modification to reduce the intake of foods high in cholesterol and saturated fats.

Pharmacologic Treatment. The decision to initiate pharmacologic treatment is based on the severity of the hypertension, the presence of target-organ disease, and the existence of other conditions and risk factors. Drug selection is based on the stage of hypertension. Among the drugs used in the treatment of hypertension are diuretics, β-adrenergic–blocking drugs, angiotensin-converting enzyme (ACE) inhibitors or angiotensin II receptor blockers, the calcium channel–blocking drugs, central α_2-adrenergic agonists, α_1-adrenergic receptor blockers, and vasodilators. Only diuretics and β-adrenergic–blocking drugs have been shown to reduce mortality and morbidity rates related to coronary heart disease in major clinical trials. However, such clinical trials require considerable time to complete, and these are two of the older drugs used in hypertension treatment. A brief discussion of the physiologic action of the commonly used antihypertensive drugs is provided.

Diuretics, such as the thiazides, loop diuretics, and the aldosterone antagonist (potassium-sparing) diuretics, lower blood pressure initially by decreasing vascular volume (by suppressing renal reabsorption of sodium and increasing salt and water excretion) and cardiac output (see Chapter 30). With continued therapy, a reduction in peripheral resistance becomes a major mechanism of blood pressure reduction.

β-Adrenergic–blocking drugs are effective in hypertension because they decrease heart rate and cardiac output. The β blockers also decrease renin release. There are two types of β-adrenergic receptors: β_1 and β_2. The β_1-blocking drugs are cardioselective, exerting their effects on the heart, whereas the β_2-adrenergic receptor–blocking drugs affect bronchodilation, relaxation of skeletal blood vessels, and other β-mediated functions. Both cardioselective (β_1) and nonselective (β_1 and β_2) β-adrenergic–blocking drugs are used in the treatment of hypertension.

The ACE inhibitors act by inhibiting the conversion of angiotensin I to angiotensin II, thus decreasing angiotensin II levels and reducing its effect on vasoconstriction, aldosterone levels, intrarenal blood flow, and the glomerular filtration rate. They also inhibit bradykinin degradation and stimulate prostaglandin synthesis, and sometimes reduce sympathetic nervous system activity. The latter effects may explain why they work in some persons with low-renin hypertension. The ACE inhibitors are increasingly used as the initial medication in mild to moderate hypertension. Because of their effect on the renin-angiotensin system, these drugs are contraindicated in persons with renal artery stenosis, in which the renin-angiotensin mechanism functions as a compensatory mechanism to maintain adequate renal perfusion. Because they inhibit aldosterone secretion, these agents also can increase serum potassium levels and cause hyperkalemia. A relative newcomer to the field of antihypertensive medications is the angiotensin II receptor–blocking drug class. These drugs have no effect on bradykinin levels and therefore are more selective blockers of angiotensin II than the ACE inhibitors. Because they do not affect bradykinin levels, they are less likely to produce a cough, which is a frequent side effect of ACE inhibitors.

The calcium channel receptor–blocking drugs inhibit the movement of calcium into cardiac and vascular smooth muscle. Each of the different agents in this group acts in a slightly different way. They probably reduce blood pressure by several mechanisms, including a reduction of smooth muscle tone in the venous and arterial systems. Some calcium blockers have a direct myocardial effect that reduces the cardiac output through a decrease in cardiac contractility and heart rate. Other calcium channel–blocking drugs influence venous tone and reduce the cardiac output through a decrease in venous return. Still others influence arterial vascular smooth muscle by inhibiting calcium transport across the cell membrane channels or inhibiting the vascular response to norepinephrine or angiotensin.

The centrally acting α-adrenergic inhibitors block sympathetic outflow from the central nervous system. These agents are α_2-adrenergic agonists that act in negative-feedback manner to decrease sympathetic outflow from presynaptic sympathetic neurons in the central nervous system. The α_2-adrenergic agonists are effective as single therapy for some persons, but they often are used as second- or third-line agents because of the high incidence of side effects. One of the agents, clonidine, is available as a transdermal patch that is replaced weekly.

The α_1-adrenergic receptor antagonists block postsynaptic α_1 receptors and reduce the effect of the sympathetic nervous system on the vascular smooth muscle tone of the blood vessels that regulate the peripheral vascular resistance. These drugs produce a pronounced decrease in blood pressure after the first dose; therefore, treatment is initiated with a smaller dose given at bedtime. Postdosing palpitations, headache, and nervousness may continue with chronic treatment. These agents usually are more effective when used in combination with other agents.

The direct-acting smooth muscle vasodilators promote a decrease in peripheral vascular resistance by producing relaxation of vascular smooth muscle, particularly of the arterioles. These drugs often produce initial stimulation of the sympathetic nervous system and tachycardia and salt and water retention as a result of the decreased filling of the vascular compartment. Vasodilators work best in combination with other antihypertensive drugs that oppose the compensatory cardiovascular responses.

Treatment Strategies. The pharmacologic treatment of stage 1 and 2 hypertension usually is initiated when blood pressure remains elevated after 3 to 6 months of vigorous encouragement of lifestyle modification (see Fig. 23-6). Drug therapy usually is initiated with a single drug, usually a diuretic or a β blocker. The alternative drugs—calcium antagonists, ACE inhibitors, angiotensin II receptor blockers and α or α-β blockers—may be used in selected cases. Some drugs, such as the central α_2-adrenergic agonists, α_1-adrenergic receptor blockers, and vasodilators, are not well suited to initial monotherapy because of their potential side effects.

Hypertension treatment usually is initiated with a low-dose therapy, slowly titrating upward at a schedule dependent on the person's age, needs, and desired response.[7] The optimal formulation should provide 24-hour drug action with once-daily dosing. Long-acting formulations usually are preferred because they enhance compliance; the control of hypertension is more consistent than intermittent; and protection is provided against risk for sudden death, heart attack, and stroke due to abrupt increases in blood pressure that occur after arising from overnight sleep.[7] For some agents, once-daily dosing requires fewer tablets and may be less costly than more frequent dosing.

If the response to the initial drug is not adequate after 1 to 3 months, one of three approaches is used: the dose can be increased if the initial dose was below the maximum recommended; an agent from another class can be added; or the initial drug can be discontinued and another drug substituted. Combining antihypertensive drugs with different modes of action often allows smaller doses of drugs to be used to achieve blood pressure control, minimizing the possibility of dose-dependent side effects from any one drug. In treating stage 3 or 4 hypertension, it often is necessary to add a second or third drug after a short interval if the treatment goal is not achieved.

Factors considered when hypertensive drugs are prescribed are the person's lifestyle (*i.e.,* someone with a busy schedule may have problems with medications that must be taken three times each day); demographics (*e.g.,* some drugs are more effective in elderly or African-American persons); motivation for adhering to the drug regimen (*e.g.,* some drugs can produce undesirable and even life-threatening consequences if discontinued abruptly); other disease conditions and therapies; and potential for side effects (*e.g.,* some drugs may impair sexual functioning or mental acuity; others have not been proved safe for women of childbearing age). Another factor to be considered is the cost of the drug in relation to financial resources. There is a wide variation in the prices of antihypertensive medications that should be considered when medications are prescribed. This is particularly important for low-income persons with moderate to severe hypertension, because keeping costs at an affordable level may be the key to compliance.

For persons with mild hypertension who have satisfactorily controlled their blood pressure through treatment for at least 1 year, reduction of medication using a reverse stepwise approach may be used, particularly if there has been successful adherence to nonpharmacologic methods of treatment.

SECONDARY HYPERTENSION

Only 5% to 10% of hypertensive cases are classified as secondary hypertension (*i.e.,* hypertension due to another disease condition). Unlike essential hypertension, many of the conditions causing secondary hypertension can be corrected or cured by surgery or specific medical treatment. Secondary hypertension tends to be seen in persons younger than 30 and older than 50 years of age.[52] Renal artery stenosis and coarctation of the aorta are more common in younger persons. Cocaine and cocaine-like substances can cause significant hypertension. In older persons, the sudden onset of secondary hypertension often is associated with atherosclerotic disease of the renal blood vessels.

Among the most common causes of secondary hypertension are kidney disease (*i.e.,* renovascular hypertension), adrenal cortical disorders, pheochromocytoma, and coarctation of the aorta. To avoid duplication in descriptions, the mechanisms associated with elevations of blood pressure in these disorders are discussed briefly, and a more detailed discussion of specific disease disorders is reserved for other sections of this book.

Renal Hypertension

With the dominant role that the kidney assumes in blood pressure regulation, it is not surprising that the largest single cause of secondary hypertension is renal disease. Most acute kidney disorders result in decreased urine formation, retention of salt and water, and hypertension. This includes acute glomerulonephritis, acute renal failure, and acute urinary tract obstruction. Hypertension also is common among persons with chronic pyelonephritis, polycystic kidney disease, diabetic nephropathy, and end-stage renal disease, regardless of cause.

Renovascular hypertension refers to hypertension caused by reduced renal blood flow and activation of the renin-angiotensin-aldosterone mechanism (see Fig. 23-4). It is the most common cause of secondary hypertension, accounting for 1% to 2% of all cases of hypertension. The reduced renal blood flow that occurs with renovascular disease causes the affected kidneys to release excessive amounts of renin, increasing circulating levels of angiotensin II. Angiotensin II, in turn, acts as a vasoconstrictor to increase peripheral vascular resistance and as a stimulus for increasing aldosterone levels and sodium retention by the kidney. One or both of the kidneys may be affected. When the renal artery of only one kidney is involved, the unaffected kidney is subjected to the detrimental effects of the elevated blood pressure so that the affected kidney can maintain its function.

There are two major types of renovascular disease: atherosclerotic artery stenosis and fibromuscular dysplasia.[53,54] Atherosclerotic artery stenosis accounts for 70% to 90% of cases and is seen most often in older persons, particularly those with diabetes, aortoiliac occlusive disease, coronary artery, or hypertension. Fibromuscular dysplasia is more common in women and tends to occur in younger age groups, often persons in their third decade. Genetic factors may be involved, and the incidence tends to increase with risk factors such as smoking and hyperlipidemia.

Renal artery stenosis should be suspected when hypertension develops in a previously normotensive person older than 50 (*i.e.*, atherosclerotic form) or younger than 30 (*i.e.*, fibromuscular hyperplasia) years of age, or when accelerated hypertension occurs in a person with previously controlled hypertension. Hypokalemia (due to increased aldosterone levels), the presence of an abdominal bruit, the absence of a family history of hypertension, and a duration of hypertension of less than 1 year help to distinguish renovascular hypertension from essential hypertension. Because renal blood flow depends on the increased blood pressure generated by the renin-angiotensin system, administration of ACE inhibitors can cause a rapid decline in renal function.

Diagnostic tests may include studies to assess overall renal function, physiologic studies to assess the renin-angiotensin system, perfusion studies to assess renal blood flow, and imaging studies to identify renal artery stenosis.[53] Methods to assess the renin-angiotensin response include the measurement of renin and sodium levels before and after oral administration of captopril, an ACE inhibitor. The captopril renal scintigram (scan) also can be used to assess renal blood flow. This test is based on the assumption that captopril can decrease renal blood flow, thereby decreasing the uptake of the radionuclide by the affected kidney. Renal arteriography remains the definitive test for identifying renal artery disease. Renal artery duplex ultrasonography or contrast-enhanced magnetic resonance imaging (MRI) also may be used.

The goal of treatment is to control the blood pressure and stabilize renal function. Angioplasty or revascularization has been shown to be an effective long-term treatment for the disorder. ACE inhibitors may be used in medical management of renal stenosis. However, these agents must be used with caution because of their ability to produce marked hypotension and renal dysfunction.

Disorders of Adrenocorticosteroid Hormones

Increased levels of adrenocorticosteroid hormones also can give rise to hypertension. Primary hyperaldosteronism (excess production of aldosterone due to adrenocortical hyperplasia or adenoma [see Fig. 23-4]) and excess levels of glucocorticoid (Cushing's disease or syndrome) tend to raise the blood pressure (see Chapter 40). These hormones facilitate salt and water retention by the kidney; the hypertension that accompanies excessive levels of either hormone probably is related to this factor. For patients with primary hyperaldosteronism, a salt-restricted diet often produces a reduction in blood pressure. Because aldosterone acts on the distal renal tubule to increase sodium absorption in exchange for potassium elimination in the urine, persons with hyperaldosteronism usually have decreased potassium levels. Potassium-sparing diuretics, such as spironolactone, which is an aldosterone antagonist, often are used in the medical management of persons with the disorder.

Licorice is an extract from the roots of the *Glycyrrhiza glabra* plant that has been used in medicine since ancient times. European licorice (not licorice flavoring) is associated with sodium retention, edema, hypertension, and hypokalemia. Licorice is an effective analog of the steroid 11β-dehydrogenase enzyme that modulates access to the aldosterone receptor in the kidney.[55] It produces a syndrome similar to primary hyperaldosteronism.

Pheochromocytoma

A pheochromocytoma is a tumor of chromaffin tissue, which contains sympathetic nerve cells that stain with chromium salts. The tumor is most commonly located in the adrenal medulla but can arise in other sites, such as sympathetic ganglia, where there is chromaffin tissue.[56] Although only 0.1% to 0.5% of persons with hypertension have an underlying pheochromocytoma, the disorder can cause serious hypertensive crises. Eight percent to 10% of the tumors are malignant.

Like adrenal medullary cells, the tumor cells of a pheochromocytoma produce and secrete the catecholamines epinephrine and norepinephrine. The hypertension that develops results from the massive release of these catecholamines. Their release may be paroxysmal rather than continuous, causing periodic episodes of headache, excessive sweating, and palpitations. Headache is the most common symptom and can be quite severe. Nervousness, tremor, facial pallor, weakness, fatigue, and weight loss occur less frequently. Marked variability in blood pressure between episodes is typical. Approximately 50% of persons with pheochromocytoma have paroxysmal episodes of hypertension, sometimes to dangerously high levels. The other 50% have sustained hypertension, and some even may be normotensive.[56]

Several tests are available to differentiate hypertension due to pheochromocytoma from other forms of hypertension. The most commonly used diagnostic measure is the determination of urinary catecholamines and their metabolites, including vanillylmandelic acid. Although measurement of plasma catecholamines also may be used, other conditions can cause catecholamines to be elevated. After the presence of a pheochromocytoma has been established, the tumor needs to be located. Computed tomographic scans or MRI may be used for this purpose. Surgical removal of operable tumors is curative.[56]

Coarctation of the Aorta

Coarctation represents a narrowing of the aorta. In the adult form of coarctation, the narrowing most commonly occurs just distal to the origin of the subclavian arteries[57] (see Chapter 24). Because of the narrowing, blood flow to the lower parts of the body and kidneys is reduced. In the infantile form of coarctation, the narrowing occurs proximal to the ductus arteriosus, in which case heart failure and other problems may occur. Many affected children die within their first year of life.

In the adult form of coarctation, an increase in cardiac output may result from renal compensatory mechanisms. The ejection of a large stroke volume into a narrowed aorta with limited ability to accept the runoff results in an increase in systolic blood pressure and blood flow to the upper part of the body. Blood pressure in the lower extremities may be normal, although it frequently is low. It has been suggested that the increase in cardiac output and maintenance of the pressure to the lower part of the body is achieved through the renin-angiotensin-aldosterone mechanism in response to a decrease in renal blood flow. Pulse pressure in the legs almost always is narrowed, and the femoral pulses are weak. Because the aortic capacity is diminished, there usually is a marked increase in pressure (measured in the arms) during exercise, when the stroke volume and heart rate are exaggerated. For this reason, blood pressures in both arms and one leg should be determined; a 20 mm Hg or more higher pressure in the arms than in the legs suggests coarctation of the aorta. Involvement of the left subclavian artery or an anomalous origin of the right subclavian may produce decreased or absent left or right brachial pulses, respectively. Palpation of both brachial pulses and measurement of blood pressure in both arms are important.

Treatment consists of surgical repair or balloon angioplasty. Although balloon angioplasty is a relatively recent form of treatment, it has been used in children and adults with good results. However, there are few data on long-term follow-up.

MALIGNANT HYPERTENSION

A small number of persons with secondary hypertension develop an accelerated and potentially fatal form of the disease—malignant hypertension. This usually is a disease of younger persons, particularly young African-American men, women with toxemia of pregnancy, and persons with renal and collagen diseases.

Malignant hypertension is characterized by sudden marked elevations in blood pressure, with diastolic values above 120 mm Hg, renal disorders, vascular changes, and retinopathy. There may be intense arterial spasm of the cerebral arteries with hypertensive encephalopathy. Cerebral vasoconstriction probably is an exaggerated homeostatic response designed to protect the brain from excesses of blood pressure and flow. The regulatory mechanisms often are insufficient to protect the capillaries, and cerebral edema frequently develops. As it advances, papilledema (*i.e.*, swelling of the optic nerve at its point of entrance into the eye) ensues, giving evidence of the effects of pressure on the optic nerve and retinal vessels. The patient may have headache, restlessness, confusion, stupor, motor and sensory deficits, and visual disturbances. In severe cases, convulsions and coma follow.

Prolonged and severe exposure to exaggerated levels of blood pressure in malignant hypertension injures the walls of the arterioles, and intravascular coagulation and fragmentation of red blood cells may occur. The renal blood vessels are particularly vulnerable to hypertensive damage. Renal damage due to vascular changes probably is the most important prognostic determinant in malignant hypertension. Elevated levels of blood urea nitrogen and serum creatinine, metabolic acidosis, hypocalcemia, and proteinuria provide evidence of renal impairment.

The complications associated with a hypertensive crisis demand immediate and rigorous medical treatment in an intensive care unit with continuous monitoring of arterial blood pressure. With proper therapy, the death rate from this cause can be markedly reduced, as can additional episodes. Two drugs, diazoxide and sodium nitroprusside, often are used to treat hypertensive emergencies, although others also may be required to bring the blood pressure down to a safe level. Diazoxide, which causes arteriolar dilatation, and sodium nitroprusside, a vasodilator that also affects the venous system, are administered intravenously. Because chronic hypertension is associated with autoregulatory changes in cerebral blood flow, care is taken to avoid excessively rapid decreases in blood pressure, which can lead to cerebral hypoperfusion and brain injury.

HIGH BLOOD PRESSURE IN PREGNANCY

Hypertensive disorders complicate 6% to 8% of pregnancies. They are the second leading cause, after embolism, of maternal mortality in the United States, accounting for almost 15% of such deaths.[37] Hypertensive disorders also contribute to stillbirths and neonatal morbidity and mortality. Premature separation of the placenta (abruptio placentae) is reported to complicate up to 10% of hypertensive pregnancies.[58] The incidence of hypertensive disorders of pregnancy increases with maternal age and is more common in African-American women.[58]

Classification

The National Institutes of Health Working Group Report on High Blood Pressure in Pregnancy published a revised classification system for high blood pressure in pregnancy that included chronic hypertension, preeclampsia-eclampsia, preeclampsia superimposed on chronic hypertension, and gestational hypertension[59] (Table 23-2).

TABLE 23-2 ◆ Classification of High Blood Pressure in Pregnancy	
Classification	**Description**
Gestational hypertension	Blood pressure elevation, without proteinuria, that is detected for the first time during midpregnancy and returns to normal by 12 weeks postpartum.
Chronic hypertension	Blood pressure ≥140 mm Hg systolic or ≥90 mm Hg diastolic that is present and observable before the 20th week of pregnancy. Hypertension that is diagnosed for the first time during pregnancy and does not resolve after pregnancy also is classified as chronic hypertension.
Preeclampsia-eclampsia	Pregnancy-specific syndrome of blood pressure elevation (blood pressure ≥140 mm Hg systolic or ≥90 mm Hg diastolic) that occurs after the first 20 weeks of pregnancy and is accompanied by proteinuria (urinary excretion of 0.3 g protein in a 24-hour specimen).
Preeclampsia superimposed on chronic hypertension	Chronic hypertension (blood pressure ≥140 mm Hg systolic or ≥90 mm Hg diastolic prior to 20th week of pregnancy) with superimposed proteinuria and with or without signs of the preeclampsia syndrome

(Developed using information from National Institutes of Health. [2000]. *Working group report on high blood pressure in pregnancy*. NIH publication no. 00-3029. Bethesda, MD: Author. Available: http://www.nhlbi.gov/health/prof/heart/hbp/hbp_preg.htm)

Gestational Hypertension. Gestational hypertension represents a blood pressure elevation without proteinuria that is detected for the first time after midpregnancy. It includes women with preeclampsia syndrome who have not yet manifested proteinuria, as well as women who do not have the syndrome. The hypertension may be accompanied by other signs of the syndrome. The final determination that a woman does not have the preeclampsia syndrome is made only postpartum. If preeclampsia has not developed and blood pressure has returned to normal by 12 weeks postpartum, the condition is considered to be gestational hypertension. If blood pressure elevation persists, a diagnosis of chronic hypertension is made.

Chronic Hypertension. Chronic hypertension is considered as hypertension that is unrelated to the pregnancy. It is defined as a history of high blood pressure before pregnancy, identification of hypertension before 20 weeks of pregnancy, and hypertension that persists after pregnancy. Hypertension is defined as blood pressure of at least 140 mm Hg systolic or 90 mm Hg diastolic. Hypertension that is diagnosed for the first time during pregnancy and does not resolve after pregnancy also is classified as chronic hypertension.

In women with chronic hypertension, blood pressure often decreases in early pregnancy and increases during the last trimester (3 months) of pregnancy, resembling preeclampsia. Consequently, women with undiagnosed chronic hypertension who do not present for medical care until the later months of pregnancy may be incorrectly diagnosed as having preeclampsia. Women with chronic hypertension are at increased risk for development of preeclampsia.

Preeclampsia-Eclampsia. Preeclampsia-eclampsia is a pregnancy-specific syndrome that usually occurs after 20 weeks of gestation. It is defined as an elevation in blood pressure (systolic blood pressure ≥140 mm Hg or diastolic pressure ≥90 mm Hg) and proteinuria (≥300 g in 24 hours) developing after the 20th week of gestation. The Working Group recommends that K5 be used for determining diastolic pressure. Edema, which previously was included in definitions of preeclampsia, was excluded from this most recent definition. The presence of blood pressure greater than 160 mm Hg systolic or 110 mm Hg or more diastolic; hyperproteinuria greater than 2 g in 24 hours; increased serum creatinine (>1.2 mg/dL); platelet counts less than 100,000 cells/mm³; elevated liver enzymes (alanine aminotransferase [ALT] or aspartate aminotransferase [AST]); persistent headache or cerebral or visual disturbances; and persistent epigastric pain serve to reinforce the diagnosis.[59] Eclampsia is the occurrence, in a woman with preeclampsia, of seizures that cannot be attributed to other causes.[59]

Preeclampsia occurs primarily during first pregnancies and during subsequent pregnancies in women with multiple fetuses, diabetes mellitus, or coexisting renal disease. It is associated with a condition called a *hydatidiform mole* (*i.e.,* abnormal pregnancy caused by a pathologic ovum, resulting in a mass of cysts). Women with chronic hypertension who become pregnant have an increased risk of preeclampsia and adverse neonatal outcomes, particularly when associated with proteinuria early in pregnancy.[60] Of interest is the reversal of the diurnal pattern of blood pressure in preeclamptic hypertension; it often is highest during the night.[61]

Pregnancy-induced hypertension is thought to involve a decrease in placental blood flow leading to the release of toxic mediators that alter the function of endothelial cells in blood vessels throughout the body, including those of the kidney, brain, liver, and heart.[60,62,63] The endothelial changes result in signs and symptoms of preeclampsia and, in more severe cases, of intravascular clotting and hypoperfusion of vital organs. There is risk for development of disseminated intravascular coagulation, cerebral hemorrhage, hepatic failure, and acute renal failure. Thrombocytopenia is the most common hematologic complication of preeclampsia. Platelet counts below 100,000/mm³ signal serious disease. The cause of thrombocytopenia has been ascribed to platelet deposition at the site of endothelial injury. The renal changes that occur with preeclampsia include a decrease in glomerular filtration rate and renal blood flow. Sodium excretion may be impaired, although this is variable. Edema may or may not be present. Some of the severest forms of preeclampsia occur in the absence of edema. Even when there is extensive edema, the plasma volume usually is lower than that of normal pregnancy. Liver damage, when it occurs, may range from mild hepatocellular necrosis with elevation of liver enzymes to the more ominous hemolysis, elevated liver function tests, and low platelet count (HELLP) syndrome that is associated with significant maternal mortality. Eclampsia, the convulsive stage of preeclampsia, is a significant cause of maternal mortality. The pathogenesis of eclampsia remains unclear, and has been attributed to both increased coagulability and fibrin deposition in the cerebral vessels.

Defining the causes of pregnancy-induced hypertension is difficult because of the normal circulatory changes that occur during pregnancy. Blood pressure normally decreases during the first trimester, reaches its lowest point during the second trimester, and gradually rises during the third trimester. The fact that there is a 40% to 60% increase in cardiac output during early pregnancy suggests the decrease in blood pressure that occurs during the first part of pregnancy results from a decrease in peripheral vascular resistance. Because the cardiac output remains high throughout pregnancy, the gradual rise in blood pressure that begins during the second trimester probably represents a return of the peripheral vascular resistance to normal. Pregnancy normally is accompanied by increased levels of renin, angiotensin I and II, estrogen, progesterone, prolactin, and aldosterone, all of which may alter vascular reactivity. Women who develop preeclampsia are thought to be particularly sensitive to the vasoconstrictor responses of the renin-angiotensin-aldosterone system. They also are particularly responsive to other vasoconstrictors, including the catecholamines and vasopressin. It has been proposed that some of the sensitivity may be caused by a prostacyclin-thromboxane imbalance. Thromboxane is a prostaglandin with vasoconstrictor properties, and prostacyclin is a prostaglandin with vasodilator properties. Emerging evidence suggests that insulin resistance, including gestational diabetes, polycystic kidney ovary syndrome, and obesity, may predispose to hypertensive disorders in pregnancy.[64]

Preeclampsia Superimposed on Chronic Hypertension. Preeclampsia may occur in women who already are hypertensive, in which case the prognosis for the mother and fetus tends to be worse than for either condition alone.[48] Superimposed preeclampsia should be considered in women with hypertension before 20 weeks' gestation who develop new-onset proteinuria; women with hypertension and proteinuria before 20 weeks' gestation; women with previously well-controlled hypertension who develop a sudden increase in blood pressure; and

women with chronic hypertension who develop thrombocytopenia or an increase in serum ALT or AST to abnormal levels.

Diagnosis and Treatment

Early prenatal care is important in the detection of high blood pressure during pregnancy. It is recommended that all pregnant women, including those with hypertension, refrain from alcohol and tobacco use. Salt restriction usually is not recommended during pregnancy because pregnant women with hypertension tend to have lower plasma volumes than normotensive pregnant women and because the severity of hypertension may reflect the degree of volume contraction. The exception is women with pre-existing hypertension who have been following a salt-restricted diet.

In women with preeclampsia, delivery of the fetus is curative. The timing of delivery becomes a difficult decision in preterm pregnancies because the welfare of both the mother and the infant must be taken into account. Bed rest is a traditional therapy. Antihypertensive medications, when required, must be carefully chosen because of their potential effects on uteroplacental blood flow and on the fetus. For example, the ACE inhibitors can cause injury and even death of the fetus when given during the second and third trimesters of pregnancy.

HIGH BLOOD PRESSURE IN CHILDREN

Blood pressure is known to rise from infancy to late adolescence. The average systolic blood pressure at 1 day of age is approximately 70 mm Hg and increases to approximately 85 mm Hg at 1 month of age.[65,66] In premature infants, during the first 3 to 6 hours of life, the limits of systolic and diastolic blood pressure are shown to be independent of birth weight and gestational age, but tend to correlate with low Apgar scores and maternal hypertension.[65,66] During the preschool years, blood pressure begins to follow a pattern that tends to be maintained as the children grow older. This pattern continues into adolescence and adulthood, suggesting the roots of essential hypertension are established early in life. A familial influence on blood pressure often can be identified early in life. Children of parents with high blood pressure tend to have higher blood pressures than children with normotensive parents.

In 1977, the Task Force on Hypertension in Children published its first recommendations on blood pressure measurement and control in children. This report was updated in 1987 and again in 1996. In its update of the 1987 Task Force Report on High Blood Pressure in Children and Adolescents, the 1996 Task Force included height as a variable in determination of blood pressure.[67] They recommended continued classification of blood pressure into three ranges: normal (*i.e.*, systolic and diastolic pressures below the 90th percentile for age, height, and sex); high normal (*i.e.*, systolic or diastolic blood pressures between the 90th and 95th percentile for age, height, and sex); and high blood pressures or hypertension (*i.e.*, average systolic and diastolic blood pressures equal to or greater than the 95th percentile for age, height, and sex on at least three occasions).

High blood pressure in children has been further defined as significant hypertension (*i.e.*, blood pressure between the 95th and 99th percentile for age and sex) and severe hypertension (*i.e.*, blood pressure above the 99th percentile for age and sex). Table 23-3 presents percentiles of blood pressure for boys and girls 3 to 16 years of age according to height. The Task Force recommended that children 3 years of age through adolescence should have their blood pressure taken once each year. They recommended that phase V Korotkoff sounds be used for determining diastolic pressure for children of all ages. Systolic pressure is determined by the onset of the "tapping" Korotkoff sounds.[66] As with adults, blood pressure should be obtained using the proper-sized cuff and a well-functioning manometer. Repeated measurements over time, rather than a single, isolated determination, are required to establish consistent and significant observations. Accurate blood pressure measurements often are difficult to obtain in infants and children who are restless; errors are easily generated in Korotkoff sounds if heavy pressure is exerted on the stethoscope. The Task Force recommended the use of auscultatory methods of blood pressure measurement in children, rather than automated methods. Automated methods are acceptable in infants, in the intensive care unit, and in children in whom auscultation is difficult. Ambulatory blood pressure monitoring may be indicated in some children, particularly those suspected of having abnormalities in the circadian blood pressure pattern.[68]

Secondary hypertension is most the most common form of high blood pressure in infants and children. In later childhood and adolescence, essential hypertension is more common. Approximately 75% to 80% of secondary hypertension in children is caused by kidney abnormalities.[67] Coarctation of the aorta is another cause of hypertension in children and adolescents. Endocrine causes of hypertension such as pheochromocytoma and adrenal cortical disorders are rare. Hypertension in infants is associated most commonly with high umbilical catheterization and renal artery obstruction due to thrombosis.[69] Most cases of essential hypertension are associated with obesity or a family history of hypertension.

A number of drugs of abuse, therapeutic agents, and toxins also may increase blood pressure. Alcohol should be considered as a risk factor in adolescents. Oral contraceptives may be a cause of hypertension in adolescent females. The nephrotoxicity of the drug cyclosporine, an immunosuppressant used in transplant therapy, may cause hypertension in children after bone marrow, heart, kidney, or liver transplantation. The coadministration of glucocorticosteroid drugs appears to increase the incidence of hypertension.

Children with high blood pressure, significant high blood pressure, or severe high blood pressure should be referred for medical evaluation and treatment as indicated. Treatment includes nonpharmacologic methods and, if necessary, pharmacologic therapy. The Task Force suggested use of the stepped-care approach for drug treatment of children who require antihypertensive medications.[67]

HIGH BLOOD PRESSURE IN THE ELDERLY

The prevalence of hypertension in the elderly population (65 to 74 years of age) of the United States ranges from

TABLE 23-3 ♦ 95th Percentile Blood Pressure in Boys and Girls 1 to 16 Years of Age, According to Height*

Blood Pressure	Age (yr)	Height Percentile for Boys				Height Percentile for Girls			
		5th	25th	75th	95th	5th	25th	75th	95th
Systolic									
	1	98	101	104	106	101	103	105	107
	3	104	107	111	113	104	105	108	110
	6	109	112	115	117	108	110	112	114
	10	114	117	121	123	116	117	120	122
	13	121	124	128	130	121	123	126	128
	16	129	132	136	138	125	127	130	132
Diastolic									
	1	55	56	58	59	57	57	59	60
	3	63	64	66	67	65	65	67	68
	6	72	73	75	76	71	72	73	75
	10	77	79	80	82	77	77	79	80
	13	79	81	83	84	80	81	82	84
	16	83	84	86	87	83	83	85	86

*The height percentiles were determined with standard growth curves.
(Data adapted from National Heart, Lung, and Blood Institute. [1996]. Update of the 1987 Task Force Report of the Second Task Force on High Blood Pressure in Children and Adolescents: A working group report from the National High Blood Pressure Education Program. *Pediatrics* 98, 653–654. Available: http://www.nhlbi.nih.gov/health/prof/heart/hbp/hbp_ped.htm)

60% for whites to 71% for African Americans.[70] The most common type of hypertension in the elderly is isolated systolic hypertension, in which systolic pressure is elevated while diastolic pressure remains within normal range. The JNC-VI definition of isolated systolic hypertension (systolic pressure ≥140 mm Hg and diastolic pressure <90 mm Hg) has not been universally accepted, and the former definition, a systolic pressure of at least 160 mm Hg and a diastolic pressure of less than 90 mm Hg, continues to be used in some settings. A Clinical Advisory Statement intended to advance and clarify the JNC-VI guidelines on the importance of systolic pressure in older Americans, issued by the Coordinating Committee of the National High Blood Pressure Education Program in 2000, reaffirmed the importance of lifelong maintenance of a blood pressure of 140/90 mm Hg or less.[71] The Committee further emphasized that the use of age-adjusted blood pressure targets are inappropriate, including the unsubstantiated but persistent clinical folklore that it is acceptable for the systolic blood pressure to be 100 plus the person's age.

Among the aging processes that contribute to an increase in blood pressure are a stiffening of the large arteries, particularly the aorta; decreased baroreceptor sensitivity; increased peripheral vascular resistance; and decreased renal blood flow. The disproportionate rise in systolic pressure observed in some elderly persons is explained in terms of the increased rigidity of the aorta and peripheral arteries that accompanies the aging process. These changes largely are caused by a loss of elastin fibers in the wall of the aorta and larger blood vessels. Normally, the elastic properties of the aorta allow it to stretch during systole as a means of buffering the rise in pressure that occurs as blood is ejected from the heart. During diastole, the recoil of the elastin fibers transmits the stored pressure to the peripheral arterioles as a means of maintaining the diastolic blood pressure. As the aorta loses its elasticity and becomes more rigid as a result of the aging process, the pressure generated during ventricular systole is transmitted to the peripheral arteries practically unchanged, causing a rise in systolic pressure. At the same time, the rigid vessels are less able to store the energy needed to maintain the diastolic pressure. Thus, diastolic pressure does not change or undergoes a gradual decline (see Fig. 23-5).

Isolated systolic hypertension is recognized as an important risk factor for cardiovascular morbidity and mortality in older persons.[72,73] Stroke is two to three times more common in elderly hypertensive people than in age-matched normotensive subjects. Treatment of hypertension in the elderly has beneficial effects in terms of reducing the incidence of cardiovascular events such as stroke. The Systolic Hypertension in the Elderly Program (SHEP) showed a reduction of 36% in stroke and a 27% reduction in myocardial infarction in persons who were treated for hypertension compared with those who were not.[74]

The recommendations for measurement of blood pressure in the elderly are similar to those for the rest of the population. Blood pressure variability is particularly preva-lent among older persons, and it therefore is especially important to obtain six to nine measurements (*i.e.,* two or three readings on two or three occasions) to establish a diagnosis of hypertension. The effects of food, position, and other environmental factors also are exaggerated in older persons. Special care also is warranted when the blood pressure is being taken because blood pressure measurement methods can produce pressures that are too low (*i.e.,* auscultatory gap) or falsely elevated (*i.e.,* pseudohypertension). In some elderly persons with hypertension, a silent interval, called the *auscultatory gap,* may occur between the end of the first and beginning of the third phases of the Korotkoff sounds, providing the potential for underestimating the systolic pressure, sometimes by as high as 50 mm Hg. Because the gap occurs only with auscultation, it is recommended that a preliminary determination of systolic blood pressure be made by palpation and the cuff be inflated 30 mm Hg above this value for auscultatory measurement of blood pressure. It also is recommended that the cuff be deflated slowly to avoid missing the first Korotkoff sounds. In some older persons, the indirect measurement using a blood pressure cuff and the Korotkoff sounds has been shown to give falsely elevated reading compared with the direct intra-arterial method. This is because excessive cuff pressure is needed to compress the rigid vessels of older persons. Pseudohypertension should be suspected in older persons with hypertension in whom the radial or brachial artery remains palpable but pulseless at higher cuff pressures.

Although sitting has been the standard position for blood pressure measurement, it is recommended that blood pressure also be taken in the supine and standing positions in the elderly. There often is a transient decrease in blood pressure on standing, after which baroreflex-mediated increases in heart rate and peripheral vascular resistance (*i.e.,* vascular constriction) usually return blood pressure to normal values. Because these reflexes often are less responsive in the elderly and may be impaired by hypertensive medications, it has been recommended that blood pressure be measured in the supine position and at 2 to 5 minutes after assumption of the standing position. This should be done during pretreatment examinations and during follow-up examinations after treatment has been instituted. This approach can detect the complication of postural hypotension, which can occur with some medications.

Despite the proven benefits of reducing elevated systolic blood pressure levels, many older persons remain untreated or are inadequately treated. The treatment of hypertension in the elderly is similar to that for younger age groups. However, blood pressure should be reduced slowly and cautiously. When possible, appropriate lifestyle modification measures should be tried first. Antihypertensive medications should be prescribed carefully because the older person may have impaired baroreflex sensitivity and renal function. Usually, medications are initiated at smaller doses, and doses are increased more gradually. Health care providers must be alert to the hazards of adverse drug interactions in older persons, who may be on multiple medications, including over-the-counter drugs.

In summary, hypertension probably is one of the most common cardiovascular disorders. It may occur as a primary disorder (*i.e.*, essential hypertension) or as a symptom of some other disease (*i.e.*, secondary hypertension). Causes of secondary hypertension include renal disorders and adrenal cortical disorders such as hyperaldosteronism and Cushing's disease, which increase salt and water retention; pheochromocytomas, which increase catecholamine levels; and coarctation of the aorta, which produces a compensatory increase in blood pressure.

The incidence of essential hypertension increases with age, the condition is seen more frequently among African Americans, and it is linked to a family history of high blood pressure, obesity, and increased salt intake. Uncontrolled hypertension increases the risk of heart disease, renal complications, retinopathy, and stroke. Because hypertension occurs as a silent disorder, screening programs provide an effective means of early detection. The importance of screening lies in the fact that hypertension usually can be controlled and its complications can be prevented or minimized with appropriate treatment measures. Treatment of essential hypertension focuses on nonpharmacologic methods such as weight reduction, reduction of sodium intake, regular physical activity, modification of alcohol intake, and smoking cessation. The decision to initiate pharmacologic treatment is based on the severity of the hypertension, the presence of target-organ disease, and the existence of other conditions and risk factors. Among the drugs used in the treatment of hypertension are diuretics, adrenergic inhibitors, vasodilators, ACE inhibitors, and calcium channel–blocking drugs.

Hypertension that occurs during pregnancy can be divided into four categories: chronic hypertension, preeclampsia-eclampsia, chronic hypertension with superimposed preeclampsia-eclampsia, and gestational hypertension. Preeclampsia-eclampsia is hypertension that develops after 20 weeks' gestation and is accompanied by proteinuria. This form of hypertension, which is thought to result from impaired placental perfusion along with the release of toxic vasoactive substances that alter blood vessel tone and blood clotting mechanisms, poses a particular threat to the mother and the fetus.

Blood pressure is known to rise from infancy to late adolescence. During childhood, blood pressure is influenced by growth and maturation; therefore, blood pressure norms have been established using percentiles specific to age and height, race, and sex to identify children for further follow-up and treatment. Although hypertension occurs infrequently in children, it is recommended that children 3 years of age through adolescence should have their blood pressure taken once each year.

The most common type of hypertension in the elderly is isolated systolic hypertension (systolic pressure ≥140 mm Hg and diastolic pressure <90 mm Hg).

Its pathogenesis is related to the loss of elastin fibers in the aorta and the inability of the aorta to stretch during systole. Untreated systolic hypertension is recognized as an important risk factor for stroke and other cardiovascular morbidity and mortality in older persons. Indirect blood pressure measurements can be falsely elevated because of sclerotic blood vessels that require excessive cuff pressures, or blood pressure may be underestimated because of an auscultatory gap.

Orthostatic Hypotension

After you have completed this section of the chapter, you should be able to meet the following objectives:

✦ Define the term *orthostatic hypotension*
✦ Explain how fluid deficit, medications, aging, disorders of the autonomic nervous system, and bed rest contribute to the development of orthostatic hypotension

Orthostatic or postural hypotension is an abnormal drop in blood pressure on assumption of the standing position. In the absence of normal circulatory reflexes or blood volume, blood pools in the lower part of the body when the standing position is assumed, cardiac output falls, and blood flow to the brain is inadequate. Dizziness, syncope (*i.e.*, fainting), or both may occur.

After the assumption of the upright posture from the supine position, approximately 500 to 700 mL of blood is momentarily shifted to the lower part of the body, with an accompanying decrease in central blood volume and arterial pressure.[75] Normally, this decrease in blood pressure is transient, lasting through several cardiac cycles, because the baroreceptors located in the thorax and carotid sinus area sense the decreased pressure and initiate reflex constriction of the veins and arterioles and an increase in heart rate, which brings blood pressure back to normal. Within a few minutes of standing, blood levels of antidiuretic hormone and sympathetic neuromediators increase as a secondary means of ensuring maintenance of normal blood pressure in the standing position. Muscle movement in the lower extremities also aids venous return to the heart by pumping blood out of the legs.

In persons with healthy blood vessels and normal autonomic nervous system function, cerebral blood flow usually is not reduced on assumption of the upright position unless arterial pressure falls below 70 mm Hg. The strategic location of the arterial baroreceptors between the heart and brain is designed to ensure that the arterial pressure is maintained within a range sufficient to prevent a reduction in cerebral blood flow.

CLASSIFICATION

Although there is no firm agreement on the definition of orthostatic hypotension, many authorities consider a drop in systolic of 20 mm Hg or more or a drop in diastolic blood pressure of 10 mm Hg or more as diagnostic of the condition.[76] Some authorities regard the presence of orthostatic

Orthostatic Hypotension

➤ Orthostatic hypotension represents an abnormal decrease in blood pressure on assumption of the upright position that results from a decrease in venous return to the heart due to pooling of blood in the lower part of the body or from an inadequate circulatory response to decreased cardiac output and a decrease in blood pressure.

➤ Orthostatic hypotension is accompanied by a decrease in cerebral perfusion that causes a feeling of light-headedness, dizziness, and, in some cases, fainting. It poses a particular threat for falls in the elderly.

➤ It can be caused by conditions that decrease vascular volume (dehydration), impair muscle pump function (bed rest and spinal cord injury), or interfere with the cardiovascular reflexes (medications that decrease heart rate or cause vasodilation, disorders of the autonomic nervous system, effects of aging on baroreflex function).

symptoms (*e.g.*, dizziness, syncope) as being more relevant than the numeric decrease in blood pressure. Kochar developed a functional classification of orthostatic hypotension that uses the drop in blood pressure and orthostatic symptoms[77] (Chart 23-2).

CAUSES

A wide variety of conditions, acute and chronic, are associated with orthostatic hypotension. These include reduced

---

CHART 23-2

Functional Classification of Orthostatic Hypotension

Class 1	Asymptomatic postural hypotension (decrease in either systolic or diastolic blood pressure ≥20 mm Hg)
Class 2	Lightheadedness (dizziness, giddiness) associated with postural hypotension but no history of syncope
Class 3	History of syncope (fainting) accompanied with postural hypotension
Class 4	Incapacitated because of severe dizziness or frequent syncope due to documented postural hypotension

(Kochar M.S. [1990]. Orthostatic hypotension. In Smith J.J. [Ed.], *Circulatory response to the upright posture* [p. 171]. Boca Raton, FL: CRC Press)

---

blood volume, drug-induced hypotension, altered vascular responses associated with aging, bed rest, and autonomic nervous system dysfunction.

Reduced Blood Volume

Orthostatic hypotension often is an early sign of reduced blood volume or fluid deficit. When blood volume is decreased, the vascular compartment is only partially filled; although cardiac output may be adequate when a person is in the recumbent position, it often decreases to the point of causing weakness and fainting when the person assumes the standing position. Common causes of orthostatic hypotension related to hypovolemia are excessive use of diuretics, excessive diaphoresis, loss of gastrointestinal fluids through vomiting and diarrhea, and loss of fluid volume associated with prolonged bed rest.

Drug-Induced Hypotension

Antihypertensive drugs and psychotropic drugs are the most common cause of chronic orthostatic hypotension. In most cases, the orthostatic hypotension is well tolerated. If postural hypotension is of class 2 or more, it is recommended that the dosage of the drug be reduced or a different drug be used.[77] Table 23-4 lists some drugs that have the potential for causing orthostatic hypotension.

Aging

Weakness and dizziness on standing are common complaints of elderly persons. The Cardiovascular Health Study reports a 16.2% prevalence of asymptomatic orthostatic hypotension among persons 65 years of age and older.[78] Orthostatic hypotension was associated with systolic hypertension, major electrocardiographic abnormalities, and carotid artery stenosis.[78] Because cerebral blood flow primarily depends on systolic pressure, patients with impaired cerebral circulation may experience symptoms of weakness, ataxia, dizziness, and syncope when their arterial pressure falls even slightly. This may happen in older persons who are immobilized for brief periods or whose blood volume is decreased owing to inadequate fluid intake or overzealous use of diuretics.

Postprandial blood pressure often decreases in elderly persons.[79,80] The greatest postprandial changes occur after a high-carbohydrate meal.[81] Although the mechanism responsible for these changes is not fully understood, it is thought to result from glucose-mediated impairment of baroreflex sensitivity and increased splanchnic blood flow mediated by insulin and vasoactive gastrointestinal hormones.

Bed Rest

Prolonged bed rest promotes a reduction in plasma volume, a decrease in venous tone, failure of peripheral vasoconstriction, and weakness of the skeletal muscles that support the veins and assist in returning blood to the heart (see Chapter 12). Physical deconditioning follows even short periods of bed rest. After 3 to 4 days, the blood volume is decreased. Loss of vascular and skeletal muscle tone is less predictable but probably becomes maximal after ap-

TABLE 23-4 ✦ Drugs Known to Cause Orthostatic Hypotension

Drug Groups*	Specific Drugs	Mechanism of Action
Antihypertensive drugs	Pentolinium (Ansolysen) Trimetaphan (Arfonad) Guanethidine (Ismelin) Methyldopa (Aldomet) Clonidine (Catapres) Hydralazine (Apresoline) Prazosin (Minipres) Minoxidil (Loniten)	Blocks transmission of sympathetic impulses at the autonomic ganglia Blocks sympathetic impulses at the post-ganglionic sites Decreases sympathetic outflow from the central nervous system Direct vasodilator action
Antiparkinsonian drugs	Levodopa preparation Amantadine (Symmetrel)	Vasodilation due to β-adrenergic stimulation or α blockade of the peripheral vascular system
Antipsychotic drugs	Chlorpromazine (Thorazine) Thiethylperazine (Torecan) Thioridazine (Mellaril)	Loss of reflex vasoconstriction due to blocking of α receptors; these drugs also impair sympathetic outflow from the brain
Calcium channel blockers	Diltiazem (Cardizem) Nifedipine (Procardia) Verapamil (Calan, Isoptin)	Direct vasodilator action
Tricyclic and related antidepressant drugs	Amitriptyline (Elavil, Endep, Amitid, Amtril, others) Amoxapine (Asendin) Desipramine (Norepramine, Pertofrane) Doxepin (Adapin, Sinequan) Imipramine (Tofranil, Imavate, others) Nortriptyline (Aventyl, Pamelor) Maprotiline (Ludiomil) Traxodone (Desyrel)	Blocks norepinephrine uptake in central adrenergic neurons, with a resultant increase in stimulation of central α-adrenergic receptors, causing a decrease in peripheral sympathetic nervous system activity
Vasodilator drugs	Nitrates (nitroglycerin and long-acting nitrates)	Direct vasodilator action

*This list is not intended to be inclusive; it encompasses some of the widely prescribed drugs.

proximately 2 weeks of bed rest. Orthostatic intolerance is a recognized problem of space flight—a potential risk after reentry into the earth's gravitational field.

Disorders of Autonomic Nervous System Function

The sympathetic nervous system plays an essential role in adjustment to the upright position. Sympathetic stimulation increases heart rate and cardiac contractility and causes constriction of peripheral veins and arterioles. Orthostatic hypotension caused by altered autonomic function is common in peripheral neuropathies associated with diabetes mellitus, after injury or disease of the spinal cord, or as the result of a cerebral vascular accident in which sympathetic outflow from the brain stem is disrupted. The American Autonomic Society and the American Academy of Neurology have distinguished three forms of primary autonomic nervous system dysfunction: pure autonomic failure, defined as a sporadic, idiopathic cause of persistent orthostatic hypotension and other manifestations of autonomic failure such as urinary retention, impotence, or decreased sweating; Parkinson's disease with autonomic failure; and multiple-system atrophy (Shy-Drager syndrome).[82,83] The Shy-Drager syndrome usually develops in

middle to late life as orthostatic hypotension associated with uncoordinated movements, urinary incontinence, constipation, and other signs of neurologic deficits referable to the corticospinal, extrapyramidal, corticobulbar, and cerebellar systems.

DIAGNOSIS AND TREATMENT

Orthostatic hypotension can be assessed with the blood pressure cuff. A reading should be made when the patient is supine, immediately after assumption of the seated or upright position, and at 2- to 3-minute intervals for 5 minutes. Because it takes approximately 5 to 10 minutes for the blood pressure to stabilize after lying down, it is recommended that the patient be supine for this period before standing. It is strongly recommended that a second person be available when blood pressure is measured in the standing position to prevent injury should the patient become faint. A tilt table also can be used for this purpose. With a tilt table, the recumbent patient can be moved to a head-up position without voluntary movement when the table is tilted. The tilt table also has the advantage of rapidly and safely returning persons with a profound postural drop in blood pressure to the horizontal position.

Persons with a drop in blood pressure to orthostatic levels should be evaluated to determine the cause and seriousness of the condition. A history should be done to elicit information about symptoms, particularly dizziness and history of syncope and falls; medical conditions, particularly those such as diabetes mellitus that predispose to orthostatic hypotension; use of prescription and over-the-counter drugs; and symptoms of autonomic nervous system dysfunction, such as impotence or bladder dysfunction. A physical examination should document blood pressure in both arms and the heart rate while in the supine, sitting, and standing positions and should note the occurrence of symptoms. Noninvasive, 24-hour ambulatory blood pressure monitoring may be used to determine blood pressure responses to other stimuli of daily life, such as food ingestion and exertion.[76]

Treatment of orthostatic hypotension usually is directed toward alleviating the cause or, if this is not possible, toward helping people learn ways to cope with the disorder and prevent falls and injuries. Medications that predispose to postural hypotension should be avoided. Correcting the fluid deficit and trying a different antihypertensive medication are examples of measures designed to correct the cause. Measures designed to help persons prevent symptomatic orthostatic drops in blood pressure include gradual ambulation (*i.e.,* sitting on the edge of the bed for several minutes and moving the legs to initiate skeletal muscle pump function before standing) to allow the circulatory system to adjust; avoidance of situations that encourage excessive vasodilatation (*e.g.,* drinking alcohol, exercising vigorously in a warm environment); and avoidance of excess diuresis (*e.g.,* use of diuretics), diaphoresis, or loss of body fluids. Tight-fitting elastic support hose or an abdominal support garment may help prevent pooling of blood in the lower extremities and abdomen.

Pharmacologic treatment may be used when nonpharmacologic methods are unsuccessful. A number of types of drugs can be used for this purpose.[76] Mineralocorticoids (*e.g.,* fludrocortisone) can be used to reduce salt and water loss and probably increase α-adrenergic sensitivity. Vasopressin-2 receptor agonists (desmopressin as a nasal spray) may be used to reduce nocturnal polyuria. Sympathomimetic drugs that act directly on the resistance vessels (phenylephrine, noradrenaline, clonidine) or on the capacitance vessels (*e.g.,* dihydroergotamine) may be used. Many of these agents have undesirable side effects. Octreotide, a somatostatin analog that inhibits the release of vasodilatory gastrointestinal peptides, may prove useful in persons with postprandial hypotension.

In summary, orthostatic hypotension refers to an abnormal decrease in systolic and diastolic blood pressures that occurs on assumption of the upright position. An important consideration in orthostatic hypotension is the occurrence of dizziness and syncope. Among the factors that contribute to its occurrence are decreased fluid volume, medications, aging, defective function of the autonomic nervous system, and the effects of immobility. Diagnosis of orthostatic hypotension includes blood pressure measurement in the supine and upright positions, a history of symptomatology, medication use, and disease conditions that contribute to a postural drop in blood pressure. Treatment includes correcting the reversible causes and assisting the person to compensate for the disorder and prevent falls and injuries.

References

1. Grim C.E., Grim C.M. (2001). Accurate and reliable blood pressure measurement in the clinic and home: The key to hypertension control. In Hollenberg N. (Ed.), *Hypertension: Mechanisms and management* (3rd ed., pp. 315–324). Philadelphia: Current Medicine.
2. Grim C.M., Grim C.E. (1995). A curriculum for the training and certification of blood pressure measurement for health care providers. *Canadian Journal of Cardiology* 11 (Suppl. H), 38H–42H.
3. Grim C.M., Grim C.E. (2000). Manual blood pressure measurement: Still the gold standard. In Weber M.A. (Ed.), *Hypertension medicine* (pp. 131–145). Totowa, NJ: Humana Press.
4. O'Brien E. (1996). Review: A century of confusion; which bladder for accurate blood pressure measurement? *Journal of Human Hypertension* 10, 565–572.
5. American Society of Hypertension. (1992). Recommendations for routine blood pressure measurement by indirect cuff sphygmomanometry. *American Journal of Hypertension* 5, 207–209.
6. Pickering T. (1995). American Society for Blood Pressure Ad Hoc Panel: Recommendations for use of home (self) and ambulatory blood pressure monitoring. *Journal of Hypertension* 9, 1–11.
7. National Heart, Lung, and Blood Institute. (1997). The sixth report of the Joint National Committee on Detection, Evaluation, and Treatment of High Blood Pressure. *Archives of Internal Medicine* 157, 2413–2443.
8. Janeway T.C. (1913). A clinical study of hypertensive cardiovascular disease. *Archives of Internal Medicine* 12, 755–760.
9. Society of Actuaries. (1925). *Blood pressure: report of the Joint Committee on Mortality of the Association of Life Insurance Medical Directors and the Actuarial Society of America.* New York: Author.
10. American Diabetes Association. (2001). Summary of revisions for the 2001 clinical practice recommendations. *Diabetes Care* 24 (Suppl. 1), 1.
11. Guyton A.C., Hall J.E. (2000). *Textbook of medical physiology* (10th ed., pp. 195–209). Philadelphia: W.B. Saunders.
12. Cowley A.W., Roman R.J. (1996). The role of the kidney in hypertension. *Journal of the American Medical Association* 275, 1581–1589.
13. Williams R.R., Hunt S.C., Hasstedt S.J., Hopkins P.N., Wu L.L., Berry T.D. (1991). Are there interactions and relations between genetic and environmental factors predisposing to high blood pressure? *Hypertension* 18 (Suppl. I), S29–S37.
14. Franklin S.S., Milagros J.J., Wong N.D., L'Italien G.J., Lapuerta P. (2001). Predominance of isolated systolic hypertension among middle-aged and elderly US hypertensives. *Hypertension* 37, 869–874.
15. Burt V.L., Whelton P., Rocella E.J., Brown C., Cutler J.A., Higgins M., et al. (1995). Prevalence of hypertension in the US population: Results from the Third National Health and

Nutrition Examination Survey, 1988–91. *Hypertension* 25, 305–313.

16. Gillum R.F. (1996). Epidemiology of hypertension in African American women. *American Heart Journal* 131, 385–395.

17. Grim C.E., Henry J.P., Myers H. (1995). High blood pressure in blacks: Salt, slavery, survival, stress, and racism. In Laragh J.H., Brenner B.M. (Eds.), *Hypertension: Pathophysiology, diagnosis, and management* (pp. 171–207). New York: Raven Press.

18. Blaustein M.P., Grim C.E. (1991). The pathogenesis of hypertension: Black-white differences. *Cardiovascular Clinics* 21 (3), 97–114.

19. Wilson T.W., Grim C.E. (1991). Biohistory of slavery and blood pressure differences in blacks today: A hypothesis. *Hypertension* 17 (Suppl. I), I122–I128.

20. Oliver W.J., Cohen E.L., Neel J.V. (1975). Blood pressure, sodium intake, and sodium related hormones in the Yanomamo Indians, a "no-salt" culture. *Circulation* 52, 146.

21. Denton D. (1997). Can hypertension be prevented? *Journal of Human Hypertension* 11, 97–104.

22. Elliott P., Stamler S., Nichols R., Dyer A.R., Stamler R., Kestefoot H., Marmot M. (1996). Intersalt revisited: Further analyses of 24 hour sodium excretion and blood pressure within and across populations. *British Medical Journal* 312, 1249–1253.

23. Kotchen T.A., McCarron D.A. (1998). Dietary electrolytes and blood pressure: A statement for healthcare professionals from the American Heart Association Nutrition Committee. *Circulation* 98, 613–617.

24. Kaplan N.M. (2000). Evidence in favor of moderate dietary sodium reduction. *American Journal of Hypertension* 13 (9), 8–13.

25. Wilson T.W., Grim C.E. (2000). Sodium and hypertension. In Kiple K (Ed.), *The Cambridge world history of food and nutrition* (pp. 848–856). Cambridge: Cambridge University Press.

26. Conlin P.R., Chow D., Miller E.R. III, Svetky L.P., Pao-Hwa L., Harsha D.W., Moore T.H., Sachs F.M., Appel L.J. (2000). The effect of dietary pattern on blood pressure control in hypertensive patients: Results from the Dietary Approaches to Stop Hypertension (DASH) trial. *Journal of Hypertension* 13, 949–953.

27. Sacks F.M., Svetkey L.P., Vollmer W.M., Appel L.J., Bray G.A., Harsha D., Obarzanek E., Conlin P., Miller E.R., Simons-Morton D.G., Karanja N., Pao-Hwa L. (2001). Effects on blood pressure of reduced sodium and the Dietary Approaches to Stop Hypertension (DASH) diet. *New England Journal of Medicine* 344, 3–10.

28. Cassano P.A., Segal M.R., Vokonas P.S., Weiss S.T. (1990). Body fat distribution, blood pressure, and hypertension: A prospective study of men in the normative aging study. *Annals of Epidemiology* 1, 33–48.

29. Peiris A.N., Sothmann M.S., Hoffmann R.G., Hennes M.I., Wilson M.I., Wilson C.R., et al. (1989). Obesity, fat distribution, and cardiovascular risk. *Annals of Internal Medicine* 110, 867–872.

30. Ward K.D., Sparrow D., Landsberg L. (1996). Influence of insulin, sympathetic nervous system activity, and obesity on blood pressure: The Normative Aging Study. *Journal of Hypertension* 14, 301–306.

31. Reaven G.M., Lithell H., Landsberg L. (1996). Hypertension and associated metabolic abnormalities: The role of insulin resistance and the sympathoadrenal system. *New England Journal of Medicine* 334, 374–381.

32. Williams B. (1994). Insulin resistance: The shape of things to come. *Lancet* 344, 521–524.

33. Fuchs F.D., Chambless L.E., Whelton P.K., Nieto F.J., Heiss G. (2001). Alcohol consumption and the incidence of hypertension. *Hypertension* 37, 1242–1250.

34. Marmot M.G., Elliott P., Shipley M.J., Dyer A.R., Ueshima U., Beevers D.G., et. al. (1994). Alcohol and blood pressure: The INTERSALT study. *British Medical Journal* 308, 1263–1267.

35. Klatsky A.L., Freidman G.D., Siegelaub A.B. (1977). Alcohol consumption and blood pressure. *New England Journal of Medicine* 296, 1194–1200.

36. Langford H.G. (1983). Dietary potassium and hypertension: Epidemiologic data. *Annals of Internal Medicine* 98, 770–772.

37. Whelton P.K. (1999). Potassium and blood pressure. In Izzo J.L., Black H.R. (Eds.), *Hypertension primer* (2nd ed., pp. 250–252). Dallas, TX: American Heart Association.

38. Intersalt Cooperative Research Group. (1988). Intersalt: An international study of electrolyte excretion and blood pressure: Results of 24 hour urinary sodium and potassium excretion. *British Medical Journal* 297, 319–328.

39. Sacks F.M., Willett W.C., Smith A., Brown L.E., Rosner B., Moore T.J. (1998). Effect on blood pressure of potassium, calcium, and magnesium in women with low habitual intake. *Hypertension* 31, 131–138.

40. Bevan A.T., Hanour A.J., Stott F.H. (1969). Direct arterial pressure recording in unrestricted man. *Clinical Science and Molecular Medicine* 36, 329–334.

41. Pickering T., Harshfield G.A., Kleinert H.D., Blank J., Laragh J.H. (1982). Blood pressure during normal daily activities, sleep, and exercise. *Journal of the American Medical Association* 247, 992–996.

42. Verdecchia P., Schillaci G., Porcella C. (1991). Dippers versus non-dippers. *Hypertension* 9 (Suppl. 8), S42–S44.

43. Kaplan N.M. (1995). The treatment of hypertension in women. *Archives of Internal Medicine* 155, 563–567.

44. Black H.R., Kuller L.H., O'Rourke M.F., Weber M.A., Alderman M.H., Benetos A., et al. (1999). The first report of the Systolic and Pulse Pressure (SYPP) working group. *Journal of Hypertension* 17 (Suppl. 5), S3–S14.

45. Black H.R. (1999). The paradigm has shifted, to systolic pressure. *Hypertension* 34, 386–387.

46. Alderman M.H. (1999). A new model of risk implications of increasing pulse pressure and systolic blood pressure in cardiovascular disease. *Journal of Hypertension* 17 (Suppl. 5), S23–S28.

47. Lloyd-Jones D.M., Evans J.C., Larson M.G., O'Donnell C.J., Levy D. (1999). Differential impact of systolic and diastolic blood pressure level on JNC-VI staging. *Hypertension* 34, 381–385.

48. O'Rourke M., Frohlich E.D. (1999). Pulse pressure: Is this a clinically useful risk factor? *Hypertension* 34, 372–374.

49. Benetos A. (1999). Pulse pressure and cardiovascular risk. *Journal of Hypertension* 17 (Suppl. 5), S21–S24.

50. Kannel W.B. (1996). Blood pressure as a cardiovascular risk factor. *Journal of the American Medical Association* 275, 1571–1576.

51. Frohlich E.D., Chobanian A.B., Devereux R.G., Dustin H.P., Dzau V., Fauad-Taruzi F. (1992). The heart in hypertension. *New England Journal of Medicine* 327, 998–1008.

52. Ram C.V. (1994). Secondary hypertension: Workup and correction. *Hospital Practice* 4, 137–155.

53. Safian R.D., Textor S.C. (2001). Renal-artery stenosis. *New England Journal of Medicine* 344, 431–442.

54. Kaplan N.N. (1997). Systemic hypertension: Mechanisms and diagnosis. In Braunwald E. (Ed.), *Heart disease* (5th ed., pp. 824–834). Philadelphia: W.B. Saunders.

55. Gomez-Sanchez C.E., Gomez-Sanchez E.P., Yamakita N. (1995). Endocrine causes of hypertension. *Seminars in Nephrology* 15, 106–115.

56. Venkata C., Ram S., Fierro-Carrion G.A. (1995). Pheochromocytoma. *Seminars in Nephrology* 15, 126–137.

57. Roa P.S. (1995). Coarctation of the aorta. *Seminars in Nephrology* 15, 87–105.

58. Chames M.C., Sibal B.M. (2001). When chronic hypertension complicates pregnancy. *Contemporary OB/GYN Archive* April 2 [On-line.] Available: http://ahgyn.pdf.net/public.htm. Accessed 5/14/01/.

59. Gifford R.W. Jr. (Chair) (2000). *National High Blood Pressure Working Group report on high blood pressure in pregnancy.* NIH publication no. 00-3029. Bethesda, MD: National Institutes of Health.

60. Sibai B.M., Lindheimer M., Hauth J., Cartis S., VanDorsten P., Klebanoff M., MacPherson C., Landon M., Midovnik M., Paul R., Meis P., Dombrowski M. (1998). Risk factors for preeclampsia, abruptio placentae, and adverse neonatal outcomes among women with chronic hypertension. *New England Journal of Medicine* 339, 667–671.

61. Olofsson P. (1995). Characteristics of a reversed circadian blood pressure rhythm in pregnant women with hypertension. *Journal of Human Hypertension* 9, 565–570.

62. Duda J. (1996). Preeclampsia. *Western Journal of Medicine* 164, 315–320.

63. Lindheimer M.D., Katz A.I. (1985). Hypertension in pregnancy. *New England Journal of Medicine* 313, 675–680.

64. Solomon C.G. (2001). Hypertension in pregnancy: A manifestation of insulin resistance syndrome. *Hypertension* 37, 232–239.

65. Sinaiko A.R. (1996). Hypertension in children (Review). *New England Journal of Medicine* 335, 1968–1973.

66. Bartosh S.M., Aronson A.J. (1999). Childhood hypertension. *Pediatric Clinics of North America* 46, 235–251.

67. National Heart, Lung and Blood Institute. (1996). Update of the 1987 Task Force Report of the Second Task Force on High Blood Pressure in Children and Adolescents: A working group report from the National High Blood Pressure Education Program. *Pediatrics* 88, 649–658.

68. Sorof J.M., Portman R.J. (2000). Ambulatory blood pressure monitoring in the pediatric patient. *Journal of Pediatrics* 136, 578–586.

69. Behrman R.E., Kliegman R.M., Arvin A.M. (2000). Systemic hypertension. In Behrman R.E., Kliegman R.M., Jenson H.B. (Eds.), *Nelson textbook of pediatrics* (16th ed., pp. 1450–1455). Philadelphia: W.B. Saunders.

70. National High Blood Pressure Education Program Working Group. (1994). National High Blood Pressure Education Working Group report on hypertension in the elderly. *Hypertension* 23, 275–285.

71. Izzo J.L., Levy D., Black H.R. (2000). Clinical advisory statement: Importance of systolic blood pressure in older Americans. *Hypertension* 35, 1021–1024.

72. Black H.R. (1999). Isolated hypertension in the elderly: Lessons from clinical trials and future directions. *Journal of Hypertension* 17 (Suppl. 5), S49–S54.

73. Franklin S.S. (1999). Aging and hypertension: The assessment of blood pressure indices in predicting coronary heart disease. *Journal of Hypertension* 17 (Suppl. 5), S29–S36.

74. SHEP Cooperative Research Group. (1991). Prevention of stroke by antihypertensive drug treatment in older persons with isolated systolic hypertension. *Journal of the American Medical Association* 265, 3255–3264.

75. Smith J.J., Porth C.J.M. (1990). Age and the response to orthostatic stress. In Smith J.J. (Ed.), *Circulatory response to the upright posture* (pp. 121–138). Boca Raton, FL: CRC Press.

76. Mathias C.J., Kimber J.R. (1999). Postural hypotension: Causes, clinical features, investigation, and management. *Annual Review of Medicine* 50, 317–336.

77. Kochar M.S. (1990). Orthostatic hypotension. In Smith J.J. (Ed.), *Circulatory response to the upright posture* (pp. 170–179). Boca Raton, FL: CRC Press.

78. Rutan G.H., Hermanson B., Bild D.E., Kittner S.J., LaBaw F., Tell G.S. (1992). Orthostatic hypotension in older adults: The Cardiovascular Study. *Hypertension* 19, 508–519.

79. Jansen R.W.M.M., Lipsitz L.A. (1995). Postprandial hypotension: Epidemiology, pathophysiology, and clinical management. *Annals of Internal Medicine* 122, 286–295.

80. Lipsitz L.A., Lyquist R.P., Wei J.Y., Rowe J.W. (1983). Postprandial reduction in blood pressure in the elderly. *New England Journal of Medicine* 309, 81–86.

81. Potter J.F., Heseltine D., Matthews J., et al. (1989). Effects of meal composition on the postprandial blood pressure, catecholamine and insulin changes in elderly subjects. *Clinical Science* 77, 265–272.

82. American Autonomic Society and American Academy of Neurologists. (1996). Consensus statement of the definition of orthostatic hypotension, pure autonomic failure, and multiple system atrophy. *Neurology* 46, 1470.

83. Goldstein D.S., Holmes C., Cannon R.O. III, Eisenhofer G., Kopin I.J. (1997). Sympathetic cardioneuropathy in dysautonomias. *New England Journal of Medicine* 336, 696–702.

84. Porth C.J.M. (1996). Unpublished data from Orthostatic Hypotension in the Elderly.

Chapter 24

Alterations in Cardiac Function

Carol M. Porth and Candace L. Hennessy

Heart disease is the number one cause of death in the United States. One in five Americans has heart disease, stroke, or another form of cardiovascular disease. The American Heart Association (AHA) has stated that if cardiovascular disease were eliminated, life expectancy would increase by almost 7 years. Heart disease is also the leading cause of permanent disability in the U.S. labor force and accounts for 19% of Social Security disability payments.[1] Heart disease accounts for 43% of all deaths in women in the United States and is the leading killer of women in most developing countries. It is projected that by 2020, cardiovascular disease will, for the first time in human history, be the most common cause of death worldwide.[2]

In an attempt to focus on common heart problems that affect persons in all age groups, this chapter is organized into six sections: disorders of the pericardium, coronary heart disease, disorders of the myocardium, infectious and immunologic disorders, valvular heart disease, and heart disease in infants and children.

Disorders of the Pericardium

After you have completed this section of the chapter, you should be able to meet the following objectives:

- ✦ Describe the function of the pericardium
- ✦ Describe the physiology of pericardial effusion
- ✦ Compare the manifestations of acute pericarditis with those of chronic pericarditis with effusion and constrictive pericarditis
- ✦ Relate the cardiac compression that occurs with cardiac tamponade to the clinical manifestations of the disorder, including pulsus paradoxus

The pericardium is a double-layered serous membrane that isolates the heart from other thoracic structures, maintains its position in the thorax, and prevents it from overfilling. The pericardium also contributes to coupling the distensibility between the two ventricles during diastole so that they both fill equally.[3] The two layers of the pericardium are separated by a thin layer of serous fluid, which prevents frictional forces from developing as the inner visceral layer, or epicardium, comes in contact with the outer parietal layer of the fibrous pericardium. The mechanisms that control the movement of fluid between the capillaries and the pericardial space are the same as those that control fluid movement between the capillaries and the interstitial spaces of other body tissues (see Chapter 21).

TYPES OF PERICARDIAL DISORDERS

The pericardium is subject to many of the same pathologic processes (*e.g.*, congenital disorders, infections, trauma,

Disorders of the Pericardium

- ➤ The pericardium isolates the heart from other thoracic structures, maintains its position in the thorax, and prevents it from overfilling.

- ➤ The two layers of the pericardium are separated by a thin layer of serous fluid, which prevents frictional forces from developing between the visceral and parietal layers of the pericardium.

- ➤ Disorders that produce inflammation of the pericardium interfere with the friction-reducing properties of the pericardial fluid and produce pain.

- ➤ Disorders that increase the fluid volume of the pericardial sac interfere with cardiac filling and produce a subsequent reduction in cardiac output.

immune mechanisms, and neoplastic disease) that affect other structures of the body. Pericardial disorders frequently are associated with or result from another disease in the heart or the surrounding structures (Chart 24-1). The discussion in this section focuses on the pathologic processes associated with acute inflammation of the pericardium (*i.e.*, pericarditis), pericardial effusion, and constrictive pericarditis.

Acute Pericarditis

Acute pericarditis represents an acute inflammatory process of the pericardium.[3,4] It can result from a number of diverse causes. In many cases, the condition is self-limited, resolving in 2 to 6 weeks, but in other cases, pericarditis from the same cause may persist and produce recurrent subacute or chronic disease.

Acute pericarditis can be classified according to cause (*e.g.*, infections, trauma, rheumatic fever) or the nature of the exudate (*e.g.*, serous, fibrinous, purulent, hemorrhagic). Like other inflammatory conditions, acute pericarditis often is associated with increased capillary permeability. The cap-

---

CHART 24-1

Classification of Disorders of the Pericardium

Inflammation
Acute inflammatory pericarditis
1. Infectious
   Viral (echovirus, coxsackievirus, and others)
   Bacterial (*e.g.*, tuberculosis, *Staphylococcus*, *Streptococcus*)
   Fungal
2. Immune and collagen disorders
   Rheumatic fever
   Rheumatoid arthritis
   Systemic lupus erythematosus
3. Metabolic disorders
   Uremia and dialysis
   Myxedema
4. Ischemia and tissue injury
   Myocardial infarction
   Cardiac surgery
   Chest trauma
5. Physical and chemical agents
   Radiation therapy
   Untoward reactions to drugs, such as hydralazine, procainamide, and anticoagulants
Chronic inflammatory pericarditis
   Can be associated with most of the agents causing an acute inflammatory response

Neoplastic Disease
1. Primary
2. Secondary (*e.g.*, carcinoma of the lung or breast, lymphoma)

Congenital Disorders
1. Complete or partial absence of the pericardium
2. Congenital pericardial cysts

illaries that supply the serous pericardium become permeable, allowing plasma proteins, including fibrinogen, to leave the capillaries and enter the pericardial space. This results in an exudate that varies in type and amount according to the causative agent. Acute pericarditis frequently is associated with a fibrinous (fibrin-containing) exudate, which heals by resolution or progresses to deposition of scar tissue and formation of adhesions between the layers of the serous pericardium. Inflammation also may involve the superficial myocardium and the adjacent pleura.

Viral infections (especially infections with the coxsackieviruses and echoviruses, but also influenza, Epstein-Barr, varicella, hepatitis, mumps, and human immunodeficiency viruses) are the most common cause of acute pericarditis. Acute viral pericarditis is seen more frequently in men than in women and often is preceded by a prodromal phase during which fever, malaise, and other flu-like symptoms are present. In some cases, a well-defined infection elsewhere in the body, such as an upper respiratory tract infection, precedes the onset of pericarditis and is the primary site of infection. Although the acute symptoms usually subside in several weeks, easy fatigability often continues for several months.

Other causes of acute pericarditis are rheumatic fever, the postpericardiotomy syndrome, post-traumatic pericarditis, metabolic disorders (*e.g.*, uremia, myxedema), and pericarditis associated with connective tissue diseases (*e.g.*, systemic lupus erythematosus, rheumatoid arthritis). With the increased use of open heart surgery in the treatment of various heart disorders, the postpericardiotomy syndrome has become a commonly recognized form of pericarditis. Pericarditis with effusion is a common complication in persons with renal failure, in those with untreated uremia, and in those being treated with hemodialysis. Irradiation may initiate a subacute pericarditis, with an onset usually within the first year of therapy. It is most commonly associated with high doses of radiation delivered to areas near the heart.

The manifestations of acute pericarditis include a triad of chest pain, pericardial friction rub, and serial electrocardiographic (ECG) changes. The clinical findings and other manifestations may vary according to the causative agent.

Nearly all persons with acute pericarditis have chest pain. The pain usually is abrupt in onset, occurs in the precordial area, and is described as sharp. It may radiate to the neck, back, abdomen, or side. It typically is worse with deep breathing, coughing, swallowing, and positional changes because of changes in venous return and cardiac filling. Many persons seek relief by sitting up and leaning forward. Only a small portion of the pericardium, the outer layer of the lower parietal pericardium below the fifth and sixth intercostal spaces, is sensitive to pain. This means that pericardial pain probably results from inflammation of the surrounding structures, particularly the pleura. Pain is more common when a considerable amount of fluid is in the pericardial sac, probably because of the increased stretching of the lower parietal pericardium.

A pericardial friction rub, which is heard when a stethoscope is placed on the chest, results from the rubbing and friction between the inflamed pericardial surfaces. The sound associated with a friction rub has been described as leathery or close to the ear. It is heard best when the patient is leaning forward in the seated position and the diaphragm of the stethoscope is placed firmly along the left sternal border over the xiphoid process or near the lower border of the sternum.

Four stages of ECG changes occur during acute pericarditis.[3,4] Serial ECGs are useful in differentiating acute pericarditis from myocardial infarction. In stage I, there is an acute ST-segment elevation with an upward concavity that differentiates it from the ST-segment elevations seen in ischemic heart disease. These ECG changes accompany the onset of chest pain and are virtually diagnostic of acute pericarditis. Stage II changes occur several days later and represent return of the ST-segment to baseline accompanied by flattening of the T wave. Stage III is characterized by T-wave inversion. Stage IV represents the return of T-wave changes to normal, which may take up to weeks or months. However, only approximately half of persons with acute pericarditis display all four ECG changes, and variations are common.

Pericardial Effusion

Pericardial effusion refers to the accumulation of fluid in the pericardial cavity. It may develop as the result of injury, inflammation, or altered capillary filtration pressures. Its major threat is compression of the heart chambers. The amount of fluid, the rapidity with which it accumulates, and the elasticity of the pericardium determines the effect the effusion has on cardiac function. Small pericardial effusions may produce no symptoms or abnormal clinical findings. Even a large effusion that develops slowly may cause few or no symptoms, provided the pericardium is able to stretch and avoid compressing the heart. However, a sudden accumulation of even 200 mL may raise intracardiac pressure to levels that seriously limit the venous return to the heart. Symptoms of cardiac compression also may occur with relatively small accumulations of fluid when the pericardium has become thickened by scar tissue or neoplastic infiltrations.

Cardiac Tamponade. Cardiac tamponade represents an increase in intrapericardial pressure caused by an accumulation of fluid or blood in the pericardial sac. It can occur as the result of conditions such as trauma, cardiac surgery, cancer, uremia, or cardiac rupture due to myocardial infarction. The seriousness of cardiac tamponade results from increased intracardiac pressure, progressive limitation of ventricular diastolic filling, and reduction in stroke volume and cardiac output. The severity of the condition depends on the amount of fluid that is present and the rate at which it accumulated. A rapid accumulation of fluid results in an elevation of central venous pressure, jugular venous distention, a decline in venous return to the heart, a decrease in cardiac output despite an increase in heart rate, a fall in systolic blood pressure, and signs of circulatory shock. Persons in whom cardiac tamponade develops slowly usually appear acutely ill, but not to the extreme seen in those with rapidly developing tamponade, and the major complaint usually is dyspnea.

Pulsus paradoxus, which refers to an exaggeration of the normal 2- to 4-mm Hg decrease in systolic blood pressure that occurs during inspiration, is a clinical indicator of cardiac tamponade. The decreased intrathoracic pressure that occurs during inspiration normally accelerates venous flow, increasing right atrial and right ventricular filling. This causes the interventricular septum to bulge to the left, producing a decrease in left ventricular filling, stroke volume output, and systole blood pressure. In cardiac tamponade, the left ventricle is compressed from within by movement of the interventricular septum and from without by fluid in the pericardium (Fig. 24-1). This produces a marked decrease in left ventricular filling and left ventricular stroke volume output, often within a beat of the beginning of inspiration.

Pulsus paradoxus can be determined by palpation or cuff sphygmomanometry. In this condition, the arterial pulse, as palpated at the carotid or femoral artery, is reduced or absent during inspiration. Palpation provides only a gross estimate of the degree of pulsus paradoxus. It is more sensitively estimated when the blood pressure cuff is inflated to a value above the systolic pressure and then deflated slowly at a rate of 2 mm Hg per second until the first Korotkoff

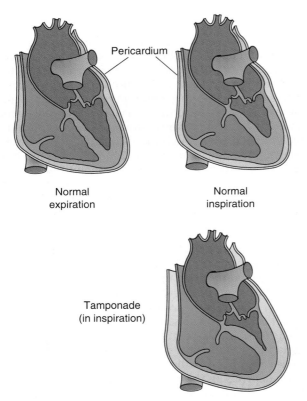

FIGURE 24-1 Effects of respiration and cardiac tamponade on ventricular filling and cardiac output. During inspiration venous flow into the right heart increases, causing the interventricular septum to bulge into the left ventricle. This produces a decrease in left ventricular volume, with a subsequent decrease in stroke volume output. In cardiac tamponade, the fluid in the pericardial sac produces further compression of the left ventricle, causing an exaggeration of the normal inspiratory decrease in stroke volume and systolic blood pressure.

sound is detected with expiration. After notation of this pressure, the cuff is deflated until the Korotkoff sounds can be heard throughout the respiratory cycle. A difference greater than 10 mm Hg between inspiration and expiration is indicative of pulsus paradoxus.[3,4] In cardiac tamponade, this implies a large reduction in diastolic volume and stroke volume output.

Chronic Pericarditis with Effusion.   Chronic pericarditis with effusion is characterized by an increase in inflammatory exudate that continues beyond the acute period. In some cases, the exudate persists for several years. In most cases of chronic pericarditis, no specific pathogen can be identified. The process commonly is associated with other forms of heart disease, such as rheumatic fever, congenital heart lesions, or hypertensive heart disease. Systemic diseases, such as lupus erythematosus, rheumatoid arthritis, scleroderma, and myxedema, also are causes of chronic pericarditis, as are metabolic disturbances associated with acute and chronic renal failure. Unlike with acute pericarditis, the signs and symptoms of chronic pericarditis often are minimal; often the disease is detected for the first time on routine chest x-ray films. As the condition progresses, the fluid may accumulate and compress the adjacent cardiac structures and impair cardiac filling.

Constrictive Pericarditis

In constrictive pericarditis, fibrous scar tissue develops between the visceral and parietal layers of the serous pericardium. In time, the scar tissue contracts and interferes with diastolic filling of the heart, at which point cardiac output and cardiac reserve become fixed. Ascites is a prominent early finding and may be accompanied by pedal edema, dyspnea on exertion, and fatigue. The jugular veins also are distended. Kussmaul's sign is an inspiratory distention of the jugular veins caused by the inability of the right atrium, encased in its rigid pericardium, to accommodate the increase in venous return that occurs with inspiration.

Diagnosis and Treatment

Various diagnostic tests are used to confirm the presence of pericardial disease. These measures include auscultation, chest radiology, ECG, echocardiography, radiation scanning procedures, computed tomography (CT), and magnetic resonance imaging (MRI). The echocardiogram is a rapid, accurate, and widely used method for evaluating pericardial effusion. Aspiration and laboratory analysis of the pericardial fluid may be used to identify the causative agent. Cardiac catheterization may used to determine the hemodynamic effects of pericardial effusion and cardiac tamponade.

Treatment depends on the cause. When infection is present, antibiotics specific for the causative agent usually are prescribed. Anti-inflammatory drugs such as aspirin and nonsteroidal anti-inflammatory agents may be given to minimize the inflammatory response and the accompanying undesirable effects. Pericardiocentesis, the removal of fluid from the pericardial sac, may be a lifesaving measure in severe cardiac tamponade. Surgical treatment may be required for traumatic lesions of the heart or for constrictive pericarditis in which cardiac filling is severely impaired.

> In summary, the pericardium is a two-layered membranous sac that isolates the heart from other thoracic structures, maintains its position in the thorax, and prevents it from overfilling. The mechanisms that control the movement of fluid between the capillaries and the space that separates the two layers of the pericardium are the same as those that control fluid movement between the capillaries and the interstitial spaces of other body tissues.
>
> Disorders of the pericardium include acute pericarditis, pericardial effusion, cardiac tamponade, and constrictive pericarditis. The major threat of pericardial disease is compression of the heart chambers. Acute pericarditis is characterized by chest pain, ECG changes, and a friction rub. Among its causes are infections, uremia, rheumatic fever, connective tissue diseases, and myocardial infarction. Pericardial effusion refers to the presence of an exudate in the pericardial cavity, and the condition can be acute or chronic. It can increase intracardiac pressure, compress the heart, and interfere with venous return to the heart. The amount of exudate, the rapidity with which it accumulates, and the elasticity of the pericardium determine the effect the effusion has on cardiac function. Cardiac tamponade is a life-threatening cardiac compression resulting from excess fluid in the pericardial sac. In constrictive pericarditis, scar tissue develops between the visceral and parietal layers of the serous pericardium. In time, the scar tissue contracts and interferes with cardiac filling.

Coronary Heart Disease

After you have completed this section of the chapter, you should be able to meet the following objectives:

+ Describe blood flow in the coronary circulation and relate it to the metabolic needs of the heart
+ Characterize the pathogenesis of atherosclerosis in terms of fixed atherosclerotic lesions, unstable plaque, and thrombosis with obstruction
+ Describe the use of the ECG, stress testing, nuclear imaging, and cardiac catheterization in assessment of the coronary circulation
+ Define the term *acute coronary syndromes* and distinguish among chronic stable angina, unstable angina, non–ST-segment elevation myocardial infarction, and ST-segment elevation myocardial infarction in terms of pathology, symptomatology, ECG changes, and serum cardiac markers
+ Compare the treatment goals for stable angina and the acute coronary syndromes
+ Explain the mechanisms, criteria for use, and benefits of thrombolytic therapy in patients with myocardial infarction
+ Compare the procedures used in percutaneous transluminal coronary angioplasty and coronary bypass surgery

The term *coronary heart disease* (CHD) describes heart disease caused by impaired coronary blood flow. In most cases, CHD is caused by atherosclerosis. Diseases of the coronary arteries can cause angina, myocardial infarction or heart attack, cardiac dysrhythmias, conduction defects, heart failure, and sudden death. In 1998, CHD caused approximately 459,800 deaths in the United States—1 of every 5 deaths.[1] Men are affected more often than women. Approximately 80% of persons who die of CHD are 65 years of age or older.

Over the past 50 years, there have been phenomenal advances in understanding the pathogenesis of CHD and in the development of diagnostic techniques and treatment methods for disease. However, declines in morbidity and mortality have failed to keep pace with these scientific advances, probably because many of the outcomes are more dependent on lifestyle factors and age than on scientific advances.

CORONARY CIRCULATION AND PATHOGENESIS OF CORONARY HEART DISEASE

Coronary Arteries and Control of Coronary Blood Flow

There are two main coronary arteries, the left and the right, which arise from the coronary sinus just above the aortic valve (Fig. 24-2). The left coronary artery extends for approximately 3.5 cm as the *left main coronary artery* and then divides into the *anterior descending* and *circumflex branches*. The left anterior descending artery passes down through the groove between the two ventricles, giving off diagonal branches, which supply the left ventricle, and perforating branches, which supply the anterior portion of the interventricular septum and the anterior papillary muscle of the left ventricle. The circumflex branch of the left coronary artery passes to the left and moves posteriorly in the groove that separates the left atrium and ventricle, giving off branches that supply the left lateral wall of the left ventricle. The *right coronary artery* lies in the right atrioventricular (AV) groove, and its branches supply the right ventricle. The right coronary artery usually moves to the back of the heart, where it forms the *posterior descending artery*, which supplies the posterior portion of the heart (the interventricular septum, AV node, and posterior papillary muscle). The sinoatrial node usually is supplied by the right coronary artery. In 10% to 20% of persons, the left circumflex rather than the right coronary artery moves posteriorly to form the posterior descending artery.

Because the openings for the coronary arteries originate in the root of the aorta just outside the aortic valve, the primary factor responsible for perfusion of the coronary arteries is the aortic blood pressure. Changes in aortic pressure produce parallel changes in coronary blood flow.

In addition to generating the aortic pressure that moves blood through the coronary vessels, the contracting heart muscle influences its own blood supply by compressing the intramyocardial and subendocardial blood vessels.[5] The large epicardial coronary arteries lie on the surface of the

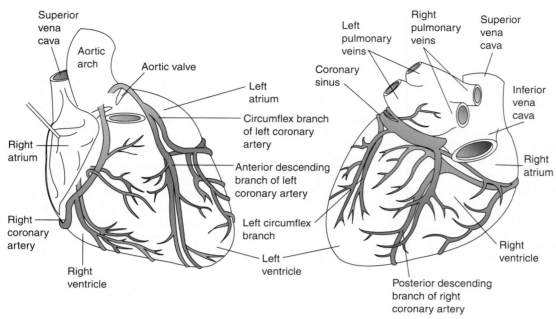

FIGURE 24-2 Coronary arteries and some of the coronary sinus veins.

heart, with the smaller intramyocardial coronary arteries branching off and penetrating the myocardium before merging with a network or plexus of subendocardial vessels. During systole, contraction of the cardiac muscle compresses the intramyocardial vessels that feed the subendocardial plexus and the increased pressure in the ventricle causes further compression of these vessels (Fig. 24-3). As a result, blood flow through the subendocardial vessels is less during systole than in the outer coronary vessels. To compensate, the subendocardial vessels are far more extensive than the outermost arteries, allowing a disproportionate increase in subendocardial flow during diastole. Because blood flow mainly occurs during diastole, there is a risk of subendocardial ischemia and infarction when diastolic pressure is low and when there is an elevation in diastolic intraventricular pressure sufficient to compress the vessels

in the subendocardial plexus.[5,6] Intramyocardial blood flow also is affected by heart rate because at rapid heart rates, the time spent in diastole is greatly reduced.

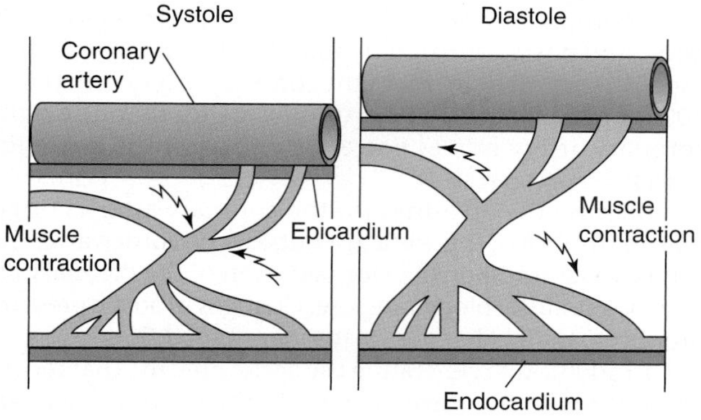

Metabolic Control of Coronary Blood Flow. Heart muscle relies primarily on fatty acids and aerobic metabolism to meet its energy needs. Although the heart can engage in anaerobic metabolism, this process relies on the continuous delivery of glucose and results in the formation of large amounts of lactic acid. Blood flow usually is regulated by the need of the cardiac muscle for oxygen. Even under normal resting conditions, the heart extracts and uses 60% to 80% of oxygen in blood flowing through the coronary arteries, compared with the 25% to 30% extracted by skeletal muscle. Because there is little oxygen reserve in the blood, the coronary arteries must increase their flow to meet the metabolic needs of the myocardium during periods of increased activity. The normal resting blood flow through the coronary arteries averages approximately 225 mL/minute.[5] During strenuous exercise, coronary flow may increase fourfold to fivefold to meet the energy requirements of the heart.

One of the major determinants of coronary blood flow is the metabolic activity of the heart. Although the link between cardiac metabolic rate and coronary blood flow remains unsettled, it appears to result from the release of metabolic mediators that are generated as a result of a decrease in the ratio of oxygen supply to oxygen demand. Numerous agents, referred to as *metabolites*, are thought to act as mediators for the vasodilation that accompanies increased cardiac work. These substances, which include potassium ions, lactic acid, carbon dioxide, and adenosine, are released from working myocardial cells. Of these substances, adenosine has the greatest vasodilator action.[5]

Endothelial Control of Coronary Vascular Tone. The endothelial cells that line blood vessels, including the

FIGURE 24-3 The compressing effect of the contracting myocardium on intramyocardial blood vessels and subendocardial blood flow during systole and diastole.

coronaries, normally present a barrier between the blood and the arterial wall, and they have antithrombogenic properties that inhibit platelet aggregation and clot formation. The endothelial cells also produce vasodilating and vasoconstricting factors that function in the control of blood flow.

Endothelial cells synthesize several substances that, when released, can affect the degree of relaxation or constriction of the smooth muscle in the vessel wall. The most important of these is the vasodilator substance called the *endothelium-derived relaxing factor* (EDRF), which is composed principally, if not entirely, of *nitric oxide* (see Chapter 21). Most vasodilators and vasodilating stimuli exert their effects through nitric oxide. The synthesis and release of nitric oxide is stimulated by products from aggregating platelets, thrombin, the products of mast cells, and increased shear force, which is responsible for the so-called flow-mediated vasodilation.[6] Only a few vasodilators act independently of the endothelium to produce vasodilation. These include the nitrate vasodilator drugs (*e.g.*, nitroglycerin and nitroprusside). Atherosclerotic lesions tend to disrupt the endothelial lining of blood vessels. It has been suggested that the tendency for vasospasm that occurs in atherosclerotic vessels may be related to impaired function of the endothelium in terms of EDRF synthesis.

The endothelium also is the source of vasoconstricting factors, the best known of which are the endothelins. Although there are several endothelins, endothelin-1 (ET-1) seems to be important in producing vasoconstriction. The formation of ET-1 is stimulated by thrombin, epinephrine, and vasopressin. Plasma levels of ET-1 are reportedly elevated in atherosclerosis, acute myocardial infarction, congestive heart failure, and hypertension. ET-1 also is reportedly produced by activated macrophages in atherosclerotic lesions of persons with acute ischemic coronary disease and plaque rupture.[6]

Collateral Circulation. Although there are no connections between the large coronary arteries, there are anastomotic channels that join the small arteries (Fig. 24-4). With gradual occlusion of the larger vessels, the smaller collateral vessels increase in size and provide alternative channels for blood flow.[7] One of the reasons CHD does not produce symptoms until it is far advanced is that the collateral channels develop at the same time the atherosclerotic changes are occurring.

Assessment of Coronary Blood Flow

Among the methods used in evaluation of coronary blood flow and myocardial perfusion are ECG, exercise and pharmacologic stress tests, and cardiac catheterization.

Electrocardiography. Electrocardiography is the most frequently used method for detecting myocardial ischemia, injury, or infarction due to CHD (see Chapter 25). During the period of impaired blood flow, injured and ischemic cells revert to anaerobic metabolism, with a resultant increase in lactic acid production, much of which is released into the local extracellular fluid. With myocardial infarc-

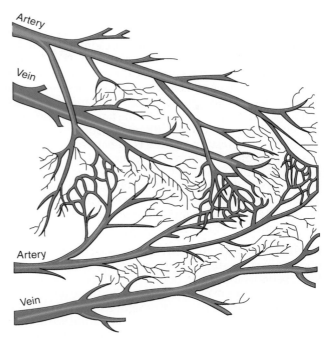

FIGURE 24-4 Anastomoses of the smaller coronary arterial vessels. (Guyton A.C., Hall J.E. [1996]. *Textbook of medical physiology* [9th ed., p. 260]. Philadelphia: W.B. Saunders)

tion, the necrotic cells become electrically inactive, and their membranes become disrupted, such that their intracellular contents, including potassium, are released into the surrounding extracellular fluid. This causes local areas of hyperkalemia, which can affect the resting membrane potentials of functioning myocardial cells. As a result of membrane injury and local changes in extracellular potassium and pH levels, some parts of the infarcted myocardium are unable to conduct or generate impulses, other areas are more difficult to excite, and still others are overly excitable. These different levels of membrane excitability in the necrotic, injured, and ischemic zones of the infarcted area set the stage for development of dysrhythmias and conduction defects after myocardial infarction. Each of these zones in the infarcted area conducts impulses differently. These changes in impulse conduction can be detected on the ECG and are the basis for determining whether an infarct has occurred and the area of the heart in which it is located.

The ECG pattern also is used to detect dysrhythmias that manifest as a result of myocardial ischemia due to CHD, and it can provide evidence of old myocardial infarction.

Continuous ambulatory ECG monitoring can be done using a Holter monitor. Ambulatory ECG monitoring often is done to detect transient ST-segment and T-wave changes that occur and are not accompanied by symptoms (*i.e.*, silent ischemia).

Another method, called *signal-averaged* or *high-resolution ECG*, accentuates the QRS complex so that low-amplitude afterpotentials that correlate with high risk of ventricular dysrhythmias and sudden death can be detected.

Exercise Stress Testing.   Stress testing is a means of observing cardiac function under stress. Three types of tests commonly are used: the motorized treadmill, the bicycle ergometer, and pharmacologic stress testing. The treadmill test requires higher levels of myocardial performance than other forms of exercise. Bicycle exercise does not require as high a level of myocardial oxygen demand as treadmill walking, and the person can become fatigued before myocardial ischemia is reached. Blood pressure is monitored during exercise testing and the ECG pattern recorded for the purpose of determining heart rate and detecting myocardial ischemic changes. Chest pain, severe shortness of breath, dysrhythmias, ST-segment changes on the ECG, or a decrease in blood pressure suggests CHD, and if one or more of these signs or symptoms is present, the test usually is terminated.

Pharmacologic Stress Tests.   Some persons are unable to undergo exercise stress testing owing to orthopedic, neurologic, peripheral vascular, or other conditions that preclude use of the treadmill or exercise bicycle. These persons can be evaluated for the presence of significant CHD by use of pharmacologic vasodilation in combination with radionuclide myocardial imaging. The intravenous injection of either dipyridamole or adenosine can be used. The intravenous infusion of dipyridamole blocks the cellular reabsorption of adenosine, an endogenous vasodilator, and increases coronary blood flow three to five times above baseline levels. In persons with significant CHD, the resistance vessels distal to the stenosis already are maximally dilated to maintain normal resting flow. In these persons, further vasodilation does not produce an increase in blood flow. Intravenous injection of adenosine has comparable effects.

Dobutamine infusion can be used as an alternative agent in persons who have contraindications to dipyridamole or adenosine infusion (*e.g.*, those with bronchospastic pulmonary disease). Dobutamine increases myocardial oxygen demand by increasing cardiac contractility, heart rate, and blood pressure.

Nuclear Imaging.   Nuclear cardiology techniques involve the use of radionuclides (*i.e.*, radioactive substances) and essentially are noninvasive. Three types of nuclear cardiology tests commonly are used: myocardial perfusion imaging, infarct imaging, and radionuclide angiocardiography. With all three types of tests, a scintillation (gamma) camera is used to record the radiation emitted from the radionuclide. A computer processing system, which is linked to the scintillation camera, is an essential part of all nuclear imaging systems.

Myocardial perfusion imaging is used to visualize the regional distribution of blood flow. *Myocardial perfusion scintigraphy* uses thallim-201 or one of the newer technetium-based agents that are extracted from the blood and taken up by functioning myocardial cells. Thallium-201, an analog of potassium, is distributed to the myocardium in proportion to the magnitude of blood flow. After injection, an external detection device describes the distribution of the radioactive material. An ischemic area appears as a "cold spot" that lacks radioactive uptake. The most important application of this technique has been its use during stress testing for evaluation of ischemic heart disease.

Radionuclide angiocardiography provides actual visualization of the ventricular structures during systole and diastole and provides a means for evaluating ventricular function during rest and exercise stress testing. A radioisotope such as technetium-labeled albumin, which does not leave the capillaries but remains in the blood and is not bound to the myocardium, is used for this type of imaging. This type of nuclear imaging can be used to determine right and left ventricular volumes, ejection fractions, regional wall motion, and cardiac contractility. This method also is useful in the diagnosis of intracardiac shunts.

Acute infarct imaging uses a radionuclide such as technetium pyrophosphate that is taken up by the cells in the infarcted zone. With this method, the radionuclide becomes concentrated in the damaged myocardium, allowing its visualization as a "hot spot," or positive area, of increased uptake of the radionuclide. Its usefulness is limited by an 18- to 24-hour lag after acute infarction before the test becomes positive, and it has limited sensitivity for small, non-transmural infarcts.

Cardiac Catheterization.   Cardiac catheterization involves the passage of flexible catheters into the great vessels and chambers of the heart. In right heart catheterization, the catheters are inserted into a peripheral vein (usually the basilic or femoral) and then advanced into the right heart. The left heart catheter is inserted retrograde through a peripheral artery (usually the brachial or femoral) into the aorta and left heart. The cardiac catheterization laboratory, where the procedure is done, is equipped for viewing and recording fluoroscopic images of the heart and vessels in the chest and for measuring pressures in the heart and great vessels. It also has equipment for cardiac output studies and for obtaining samples of blood for blood gas analysis. Angiographic studies are made by injecting a radiographic contrast medium into the heart so that an outline of the moving structures can be visualized and filmed. Coronary arteriography involves the injection of a radiographic contrast medium into the coronary arteries; this permits visualization of lesions in these vessels.

Coronary Atherosclerosis and the Pathogenesis of Coronary Artery Disease

Atherosclerosis (discussed in Chapter 22) is by far the most common cause of CHD, and atherosclerotic plaque disruption the most frequent cause of myocardial infarction and sudden death. More than 90% of persons with CHD have coronary atherosclerosis.[8] Most, if not all, have one or more lesions causing at least 75% reduction in cross-sectional area, the point at which augmented blood flow provided by compensatory vasodilation no longer is able to keep pace with even moderate increases in metabolic demand.[8]

Atherosclerosis can affect one or all three of the major epicardial coronary arteries and their branches (*i.e.*, one-, two-, or three-vessel disease). Clinically significant lesions may be located anywhere in these vessels, but tend to predominate in the first several centimeters of the left anterior descending and left circumflex or the entire length of the right coronary artery.[8] Sometimes the major secondary branches also are involved.

Stable Versus Nonstable Plaque.   There are two types of atherosclerotic lesions: the fixed or stable plaque, which obstructs blood flow, and the unstable or vulnerable plaque, which can rupture and cause platelet adhesion and thrombus formation. The fixed or stable plaque is commonly implicated in stable angina and the unstable plaque in unstable angina and myocardial infarction. There are three major determinants of plaque vulnerability to rupture: (1) the size of the lipid-rich core and the stability and thickness of its fibrous cap, (2) the presence of inflammation with plaque degradation, (3) and the lack of smooth muscle cells with impaired healing and plaque stabilization[9–11] (Fig. 24-5). Plaques with a thin fibrous cap overlaying a large lipid core are at high risk for rupture. Inflammation and immune responses are thought to play an important role in plaque instability. The influx of activated macrophages and T lymphocytes, with the subsequent elaboration of cytokines and matrix-degrading proteins, leads to weakening of the connective tissue matrix of the plaque wall and fibrous cap. The antigens that elicit these responses are not yet known and both autoantigens (*e.g.*, against oxidized low-density lipoproteins [LDL]) and microorganisms (*e.g.*, *Chlamydia pneumoniae*) have been proposed to play a role.[10]

Although plaque rupture may occur spontaneously, it also may be triggered by hemodynamic factors such as blood flow characteristics and vessel tension. For example, a sudden surge of sympathetic activity with an increase in blood pressure, heart rate, force of cardiac contraction, and coronary blood flow is thought to increase the risk of plaque disruption.[9] Indeed, many people with myocardial infarction report a trigger event, most often emotional stress or physical activity.[9,11] Plaque rupture also has a diurnal variation, occurring most frequently during the first hour of arising, suggesting that physiologic factors such as surges in coronary artery tone and blood pressure may promote atherosclerotic plaque disruption and subsequent platelet deposition.[11] It has been suggested that the sympathetic nervous system is activated on arising, resulting in changes in platelet aggregation and fibrinolytic activity that tend to favor thrombosis. The diurnal variation in plaque rupture is minimized by β-adrenergic blockers and aspirin.[11] Vasoconstricting factors (*i.e.*, thromboxane, serotonin, and platelet-derived growth factor) are released from platelets that aggregate at the site of injury. These platelet factors contribute, even at rest, to episodes of reduced coronary blood flow and silent or symptomatic myocardial ischemia.

Thrombosis and Vessel Occlusion.   Plaque disruption may occur with or without thrombosis. When the plaque injury is mild, intermittent thrombotic occlusions may occur and cause episodes of anginal pain at rest. More extensive thrombus formation can progress until the coronary artery becomes occluded, leading to myocardial infarction.

Local thrombosis occurring after plaque disruption results from complex interactions among the lipid core, smooth muscle cells, macrophages, and collagen. The lipid core provides a stimulus for platelet aggregation and thrombus formation.[12] Both smooth muscle and foam cells in the

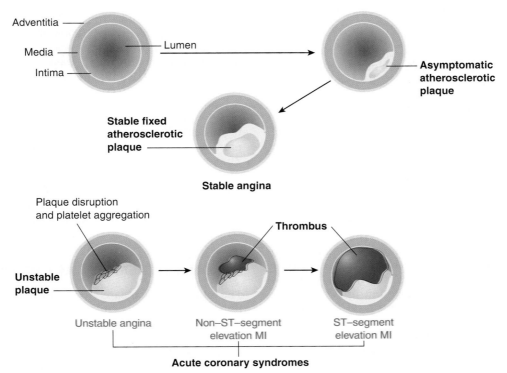

FIGURE 24-5 Atherosclerotic plaque. Stable fixed atherosclerotic plaque in stable angina and the unstable plaque with plaque disruption and platelet aggregation in the acute coronary syndromes.

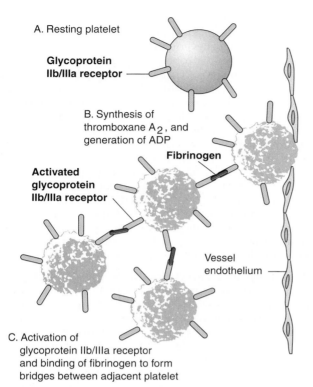

A. Resting platelet

Glycoprotein IIb/IIIa receptor

B. Synthesis of thromboxane A$_2$, and generation of ADP

Fibrinogen

Activated glycoprotein IIb/IIIa receptor

Vessel endothelium

C. Activation of glycoprotein IIb/IIIa receptor and binding of fibrinogen to form bridges between adjacent platelet

FIGURE 24-6 Steps in development of the platelet clot: (**A**) Resting platelet; (**B**) synthesis of thromboxane A$_2$ (inhibited by aspirin) and generation of adenosine diphosphate (ADP) (inhibited by ticlopidine and clopidogrel) that leads to platelet adhesion and aggregation; and (**C**) activation of glycoprotein IIb/IIIa receptors, which bind fibrinogen, form bridges between adjacent platelet (blocked by glycoprotein receptor IIa/IIIb antagonists).

lipid core contribute to the expression of tissue factor in unstable plaques. Once exposed to blood, tissue factor initiates the extrinsic coagulation pathway, resulting in the local generation of thrombin and deposition of fibrin (see Chapter 14).

Platelets play an important role in linking plaque disruption to acute CHD. As a part of the response to plaque disruption, platelets adhere to the endothelium and release substances that promote further aggregation of platelets and thrombus formation. Platelets have enzyme systems capable of forming adenosine diphosphate (ADP) and the prostaglandin, thromboxane A$_2$, which play an essential role in platelet aggregation. The cell membrane of platelets contains glycoprotein receptors that bind fibrinogen and link platelets together. Platelet adhesion and aggregation occurs in several steps. First, release of ADP, thromboxane A$_2$, and thrombin initiates the aggregation process. Second, glycoprotein IIb/IIIa receptors on the platelet surface are activated. Third, fibrinogen binds to the activated glycoprotein receptors, forming bridges between adjacent platelets. Each of these steps is amenable to pharmacologic inhibition.

There are two types of thrombi formed as a result of plaque disruption—white platelet-containing thrombi and red fibrin-containing thrombi. The thrombi in unstable angina have been characterized as grayish-white and presumably platelet rich.[13] Red thrombi, which develop with vessel occlusion in myocardial infarction, are rich in fibrin and red blood cells superimposed on the platelet component and extended by the stasis of blood flow.

Antiplatelet and Anticoagulant Therapy. Studies relating plaque disruption, platelet aggregation, and thrombus formation to CHD have led to the use of antiplatelet drugs for preventing platelet aggregation at the site of plaque disruption. The actions of antiplatelet drugs are illustrated in Figure 24-6. Anticoagulation therapy, which targets the coagulation pathway and formation of the fibrin clot, involves the use of unfractionated and low–molecular-weight heparin (see Chapter 14).

Aspirin is the preferred antiplatelet agent for preventing platelet aggregation in persons with CHD. Aspirin acts by inhibiting synthesis of the prostaglandin, thromboxane A$_2$. The actions of aspirin (*i.e.,* acetylsalicylic acid) are related to the presence of the acetyl group, which irreversibly acetylates the critical platelet enzyme, cyclooxygenase, that is required for thromboxane A$_2$ synthesis. Because the action is irreversible, the effect of aspirin on platelet function lasts for the lifetime of the platelet—approximately 8 to 10 days. The recommended doses of aspirin range from 80 to 325 mg / day.[12] Higher doses of aspirin do not increase its efficacy but do increase gastric irritation. Aspirin also has anti-inflammatory actions, which may prove beneficial.

Ticlopidine and *clopidogrel* are other antiplatelet agents that may be used when aspirin is contraindicated.[14] Ticlopidine and clopidogrel achieve their antiplatelet effects by irreversibly inhibiting the binding of ADP to its receptor on the platelets. Unlike aspirin, these drugs have no effect on prostaglandin synthesis. Ticlopidine can cause rash and diarrhea. Although rare, it can cause severe neutropenia; frequent blood counts may be needed.

Another class of antiplatelet agents are the platelet receptor antagonists. In contrast to aspirin and ticlopidine or clopidogrel, which target a single step in the aggregation process, the platelet glycoprotein IIb/IIIa receptor antagonists block the receptor involved in the final common pathway for platelet adhesion, activation, and aggregation. Three classes of glycoprotein IIb/IIIa antagonists have been developed: murine–human monoclonal antibodies (abciximab), synthetic forms (eptifibatide), and synthetic nonpeptide forms (tirofiban and lamifiban). The agents are used most commonly in treatment of the acute coronary syndromes.

CHRONIC ISCHEMIC HEART DISEASE

The term *ischemia* means "to suppress or withhold blood flow." Myocardial ischemia occurs when the ability of the coronary arteries to supply blood is inadequate to meet the metabolic demands of the heart. Limitations in coronary blood flow most commonly are the result of atherosclerosis, with vasospasm and thrombosis as contributing factors. The metabolic demands of the heart are increased with everyday activities such as mental stress, exercise, and exposure to cold. In certain disease states such as thyrotoxicosis, the metabolic demands may be so excessive that the blood flow may be inadequate despite normal coronary arteries. In other situations, such as aortic stenosis, the coronary arteries may not be diseased, but the perfusion pressure may be insufficient to provide adequate blood flow.

Coronary heart disease is commonly divided into two types of disorders: chronic ischemic heart disease and the acute coronary syndromes (Fig. 24-7). There are three types of chronic ischemic heart disease: chronic stable angina, variant or vasospastic angina, and silent myocardial ischemia. The acute coronary syndromes represent the spectrum of ischemic coronary disease ranging from unstable angina through myocardial infarction.

Stable Angina

The term *angina* is derived from a Latin word meaning "to choke." Angina pectoris is a symptomatic paroxysmal chest pain or pressure sensation associated with transient myocardial ischemia. Chronic stable angina is associated with a fixed coronary obstruction that produces a disparity between coronary blood flow and metabolic demands of the myocardium. Stable angina is the initial manifestation of ischemic heart disease in approximately half of persons with CHD.[14] Although most persons with stable angina have atherosclerotic heart disease, angina does not develop in a considerable number of persons with advanced coronary atherosclerosis. This probably is because of their sedentary lifestyle, the development of adequate collateral circulation, or the inability of these persons to perceive pain. In many instances, myocardial infarction occurs without a history of angina.

Angina pectoris usually is precipitated by situations that increase the work demands of the heart, such as physical exertion, exposure to cold, and emotional stress. The pain typically is described as a constricting, squeezing, or suffocating sensation. It usually is steady, increasing in intensity only at the onset and end of the attack. The pain of angina commonly is located in the precordial or substernal area of the chest; it is similar to myocardial infarction in that it may radiate to the left shoulder, jaw, arm, or other areas of the chest (Fig. 24-8). In some persons, the arm or shoulder pain may be confused with arthritis; in others, epigastric pain is confused with indigestion. Angina commonly

Ischemic Heart Disease

➤ The term *ischemic heart disease* refers to disorders due to stable or unstable coronary atherosclerotic plaques.

➤ Stable atherosclerotic plaques produce fixed obstruction of coronary blood flow with myocardial ischemia occurring during periods of increased metabolic need, such as in stable angina.

➤ Unstable atherosclerotic plaques tend to fissure or rupture, causing platelet aggregation and potential for thrombus formation with production of a spectrum of acute coronary syndromes of increasing severity, ranging from unstable angina, to non–ST-segment elevation myocardial infarction, to ST-segment elevation myocardial infarction.

is categorized according to whether it occurs with exercise, during rest, is of new onset, or of increasing severity. The Canadian Cardiovascular Society Classification (CCSC) system can be used to grade the severity of anginal pain and discomfort[15] (Table 24-1).

Typically, chronic stable angina is provoked by exertion or emotional stress and relieved within minutes by rest or the use of nitroglycerin. A delay of more than 5 to 10 minutes before relief is obtained suggests that the symptoms are not due to ischemia or that they are due to severe ischemia.[16] Angina that occurs at rest, is of new onset, or is increasing in intensity or duration denotes an increased risk for myocardial infarction and should be evaluated using the criteria for acute coronary syndromes (discussed later).

Diagnosis and Treatment. The diagnosis of stable angina is based on a detailed pain history and the presence of risk factors. Noncoronary causes of chest pain, such as that due to esophageal or musculoskeletal disorders, are ruled out. ECG, echocardiography, exercise stress testing or pharma-

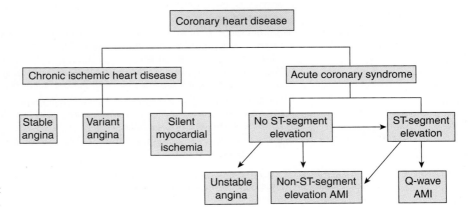

FIGURE 24-7 Types of coronary heart disease. AMI, acute myocardial infarction.

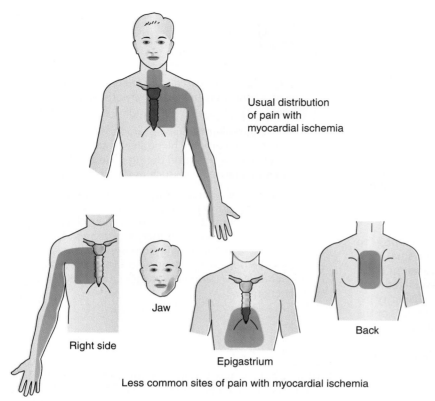

Usual distribution
of pain with
myocardial ischemia

Jaw

Right side

Epigastrium

Back

Less common sites of pain with myocardial ischemia

FIGURE 24-8 Pain patterns with myocardial ischemia. The usual distribution is referral to all or part of the sternal region, the left side of the chest, the neck, and down the ulnar side of the left forearm and hand. With severe ischemic pain, the right chest and right arm are often involved as well, although isolated involvement of these areas is rare. Other sites sometimes involved, either alone or together with pain in other sites, are the jaw, epigastrium, and back. (Horowitz L.D., Groves B.M. [1985]. *Signs and symptoms in cardiology*. Philadelphia: J.B. Lippincott)

cologic imaging studies, and coronary angiography may be used to confirm the diagnosis and describe the type of angina (exercise vs. vasospastic).

The treatment goals for stable angina are directed toward prevention of myocardial infarction and symptom reduction.[14] Both nonpharmacologic and pharmacologic treatment methods are used. Coronary artery bypass surgery or percutaneous transluminal coronary angioplasty (PTCA) may be indicated in persons with significant coronary artery occlusion.

Nonpharmacologic Treatment Methods. Nonpharmacologic methods are aimed at symptom control and lifestyle modifications to lower risk factors for coronary disease.

TABLE 24-1 ✦ Canadian Cardiovascular Society Classification for Angina	
Class	**Description of Stage**
Class I	Ordinary physical activity, such as walking or climbing stairs, does not cause angina. Angina occurs with strenuous, rapid, or prolonged exertion at work or recreation.
Class II	Slight limitation of ordinary activity. Angina occurs on walking or climbing stairs rapidly, walking uphill, walking or stair climbing after meals, or in cold, in wind, under emotional stress, or only during the few hours after awakening. Walking more than two blocks on the level and climbing more than one flight of ordinary stairs at a normal pace and in normal conditions can elicit angina.
Class III	Marked limitations of ordinary physical activity. Angina occurs on walking one to two blocks on the level and climbing one flight of stairs in normal conditions and at a normal pace.
Class IV	Inability to carry on any physical activity without discomfort—anginal symptoms may be present at rest.

(From Campeau L. [1976]. Grading of angina pectoris [letter]. *Circulation* 54, 522–523. Copyright 1976, American Heart Association, Inc. Used with permission.)

They include smoking cessation in persons who smoke, stress reduction, a regular exercise program, limiting dietary intake of cholesterol and saturated fats, weight reduction if obesity is present, and avoidance of cold or other stresses that produce vasoconstriction. Immediate cessation of activity often is sufficient to abort an anginal attack. Sitting down or standing quietly may be preferable to lying down because these positions decrease preload by producing pooling of blood in the lower extremities.

Pharmacologic Treatment Methods. Pharmacologic methods include the use antiplatelet drugs, β-adrenergic–blocking drugs in the absence of contraindications, calcium antagonists or long-acting nitrates when β-adrenergic blockers are contraindicated, sublingual nitroglycerin or nitroglycerin spray for immediate relief of anginal pain, and lipid-lowering therapy in persons with elevated LDL cholesterol levels.[14]

The β-*adrenergic–blocking drugs* act as antagonists that block β-receptor–mediated functions of the sympathetic nervous system. There are two types of β receptors, β_1 and β_2. The β_1 receptors are found primarily in the heart, and β_2 receptors are found in smooth muscle in other parts of the body (*e.g.*, bronchial smooth muscle and skeletal muscle blood vessels). In angina, the primary benefits of β-adrenergic–blocking drugs are derived from their effects on β_1 receptors in the heart that decrease cardiac work and myocardial oxygen consumption.

The *calcium channel–blocking drugs* sometimes are called *calcium antagonists*. Free intracellular calcium serves to link many membrane-initiated events with cellular responses, such as action potential generation and muscle contraction. Vascular smooth muscle lacks the sarcoplasmic reticulum and other structures necessary for adequate intracellular storage of calcium; instead, it relies on the influx of calcium from the extracellular fluid into the cell to initiate and sustain contraction. In cardiac muscle, the slow inward calcium current contributes to the plateau of the action potential and to cardiac contractility. The slow calcium current is particularly important in the pacemaker activity of the sinoatrial node and the conduction properties of the AV node. The therapeutic effect of the calcium antagonists results from coronary and peripheral artery dilatation and decreased myocardial metabolism associated with the decrease in myocardial contractility.

Nitroglycerin (glycerol trinitrate) and *long-acting nitrates* (*e.g.*, isosorbide dinitrate and isosorbide mononitrate) are used to relieve anginal pain and silent myocardial ischemia. They are vasodilating drugs that relax venous and arterial vessels. Venous dilation decreases venous return to the heart (*i.e.*, preload), thereby reducing ventricular volume and compression of the subendocardial vessels. These drugs also decrease the tension in the wall of the left ventricle so that less pressure is needed to pump blood. Relaxation of the arteries reduces the pressure against which the heart must pump (*i.e.*, afterload). In addition to their vasodilator effects, the nitrates are thought to have an inhibitory effect on platelet activation and aggregation that may contribute to their beneficial effects in persons with CHD.

Nitroglycerin is absorbed into the portal circulation and destroyed by the liver when it is taken orally; therefore, it is administered by methods such as sublingual pills or sprays or with topical ointments or patches that bypass the portal circulation. Sublingual absorption is rapid, and pain relief usually begins in 30 seconds. Topical ointments have a duration of action of 4 to 6 hours. The adhesive patches have a longer duration of action (24 hours). Two long-acting oral nitrate preparations are available: isosorbide dinitrate and isosorbide mononitrate. These medications are given two to three times each day. Administration of any of the nitrates leads to drug tolerance, a condition in which larger doses of the drug are needed or the drug no longer is effective in relieving angina. The only effective method for preventing the development of tolerance is to use an intermittent dosing that provides for an 8- to 10-hour drug-free period. This can be accomplished by measures such as removing nitroglycerin patches at night or using an asymmetric dosing regimen (*e.g.*, 8 AM and 3 PM) for administration of the long-acting nitrates.

Lipid-lowering agents or statins, such as simvastatin and pravastatin, may be used to reduce LDL cholesterol (see Chapter 22). Use of these agents is reported to decrease CHD by 24% to 31% in patients with prevalent CHD.[17]

Variant or Vasospastic Angina

The syndrome of variant angina or *Prinzmetal's angina* was first described by Prinzmetal and associates in 1959.[18] Subsequent evidence indicated variant angina is caused by spasms of the coronary arteries; hence, the condition is referred to a *vasospastic angina*.[19] In most instances, the spasms occur in the presence of coronary artery stenosis; however, variant angina has occurred in the absence of visible disease. Unlike stable angina that occurs with exertion or stress, variant angina usually occurs during rest or with minimal exercise and frequently occurs nocturnally. It may be associated with the rapid eye movement stage of sleep. It commonly follows a cyclic or regular pattern of occurrence (*e.g.*, it happens at the same time each day). The mechanism of coronary vasospasm is uncertain. It has been suggested that it may result from hyperactive sympathetic nervous system responses, from a defect in the handling of calcium in vascular smooth muscle, or from a reduced production of prostaglandin I_2 (prostacyclin), which promotes vasodilation.

Dysrhythmias often occur when the pain is severe, and most persons are aware of their presence during an attack. ECG changes are significant if recorded during an attack. These abnormalities include ST-segment elevation or depression, T-wave peaking, inversion of U waves, and rhythm disturbances. Persons with variant angina who have serious dysrhythmias during spontaneous episodes of pain are at a higher risk of sudden death. The ECG abnormalities may be recorded by continuous ECG monitoring or ambulatory Holter monitoring and are reversed by nitroglycerin. Ergonovine, a nonspecific vasoconstrictor, may be administered during cardiac catheterization to evoke an anginal attack and demonstrate the presence and location of coronary vasospasm.

Persons with variant angina usually respond to treatment with calcium antagonists. These agents, along with short- and long-term nitrates, are the mainstay of treatment of variant angina. Because the two drugs act through different mechanisms, their beneficial effects may be additive.

Silent Myocardial Ischemia

Silent myocardial ischemia occurs in the absence of anginal pain. The factors that cause silent myocardial ischemia appear to be the same as those responsible for angina: impaired blood flow from the effects of coronary atherosclerosis or vasospasm. Silent myocardial ischemia affects three populations—persons who are asymptomatic without other evidence of CHD, persons who have had a myocardial infarct and continue to have episodes of silent ischemia, and persons with angina who also have episodes of silent ischemia.[20] The reason for the painless episodes of ischemia is unclear. The episodes may be shorter and involve less myocardial tissue than those producing pain. Another explanation is that persons with silent angina have defects in pain threshold or pain transmission, or autonomic neuropathy with sensory denervation. There is evidence of an increased incidence of silent myocardial ischemia in persons with diabetes mellitus, probably the result of autonomic neuropathy, which is a common complication of diabetes.[21]

ACUTE CORONARY SYNDROMES

The term *acute coronary syndromes* (ACS) has recently been accepted to describe the spectrum of acute ischemic heart diseases that include unstable angina, non–ST-segment elevation (non–Q-wave) myocardial infarction, and ST-segment elevation (Q-wave) myocardial infarction[22–24] (Fig. 24-9). Elevation of the ST segment usually indicates acute myocardial injury. The diagnosis of myocardial infarction usually is made by the presence of significant Q waves. When the ST segment is elevated without associated Q waves, it called a *non–Q-wave infarction*. A non–Q-wave infarction is a small infarct that may herald an impending larger infarct.

Persons with an ACS are routinely classified as low risk or high risk based on presenting characteristics, ECG variables, serum cardiac markers, and the timing of presentation. Persons with ST-segment elevation on ECG are usually found to have complete coronary occlusion on angiography, and many ultimately have Q-wave myocardial infarction. This type of ACS has been labeled reperfusion-eligible acute myocardial infarction (AMI). Persons without ST-segment elevation usually represent a group in whom thrombotic coronary occlusion is subtotal or intermittent, and most experience unstable angina or are found on the basis of elevated cardiac markers to have non–ST-segment elevation AMI. In this type of ACS, thrombolytic therapy is reportedly of little clinical benefit,[13] probably because the intracoronary thrombus is composed largely of platelets rather than the fibrin-rich occlusive thrombin associated with Q-wave myocardial infarction.[25]

Unstable Angina/Non–ST-Segment Elevation Myocardial Infarction

Guidelines developed by the American College of Cardiology and AHA (ACC/AHA) Task Force on Practice Guidelines for Management of Patients with Unstable Angina and Non–ST-Segment Elevation Myocardial Infarction indicate that the two conditions are similar but of different severity. They differ primarily in whether the ischemia is severe enough to cause sufficient myocardial damage to release detectable quantities of serum cardiac markers (discussed later). Persons who have no evidence of serum markers for myocardial damage are considered to have unstable angina, whereas a diagnosis of non–ST-segment elevation myocardial infarction is indicated if a serum marker of myocardial injury is present.

Unstable angina is considered to be a clinical syndrome of myocardial ischemia ranging between stable angina and myocardial infarction. Unlike chronic stable angina, which is caused by a fixed obstruction, unstable angina most frequently results from atherosclerotic plaque disruption and repair. Abnormal constriction of the coronary arteries also may play a role.

The Agency for Healthcare Research and Quality Clinical Practice Guideline defines unstable angina as having three presentations: symptoms at rest (usually prolonged, *i.e.*, >20 minutes); new-onset (<2 months) exertional angina as evidenced by an increase in severity of at least one CCSC class to at least CCSC class III; or recent (<2 months) acceleration of angina to at least CCSC class III.[26] Most cases of unstable angina are caused by significant CHD. Classic angina and variant angina may progress to unstable angina. Cocaine has been implicated as a risk factor for unstable angina. Cocaine is thought to induce myocardial ischemia through increased myocardial oxygen demand, decreased oxygen supply from coronary artery spasm or thrombosis, or direct myocardial toxicity.[26]

The diagnosis of unstable angina/non–ST-segment elevation myocardial infarction is based on pain severity

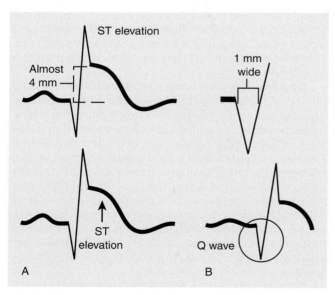

FIGURE 24-9 Illustration of an ECG tracing showing ST-segment elevation (**A**) and Q wave in acute coronary syndromes (**B**).

and presenting symptoms, hemodynamic stability, ECG findings, and serum cardiac markers. When chest pain has been unremitting for longer than 20 minutes, the possibility of ST-segment elevation myocardial infarction usually is considered.[22]

ST-Segment Elevation Myocardial Infarction

Acute myocardial infarction or ST-segment elevation myocardial infarction, also known as a *heart attack*, is characterized by the ischemic death of myocardial tissue associated with atherosclerotic disease of the coronary arteries. Heart attack is the largest killer of American men and women, claiming more than 218,000 lives annually.[1] Each year, 1.5 million Americans have new or recurrent heart attacks, and one third of those die within the first hour, usually as the result of cardiac arrest resulting from ventricular fibrillation.

The area of infarction is determined by the coronary artery that is affected and by its distribution of blood flow. Approximately 30% to 40% of infarcts affect the right coronary artery, 40% to 50% affect the left anterior descending artery, and the remaining 15% to 20% affect the left circumflex artery.[8]

Diagnosis of AMI is based on presenting signs and symptoms, ECG, and serum cardiac markers. ECG changes may not be present immediately after the onset of symptoms, except as dysrhythmias. Premature ventricular contractions are common dysrhythmias after myocardial infarction. The occurrence of other dysrhythmias and conduction defects depends on the areas of the heart and conduction pathways that are included in the infarct. Typical ECG changes include ST-segment elevation, prolongation of the Q wave, and inversion of the T wave.

Manifestations. ST-segment elevation myocardial infarction may occur as an abrupt-onset event or as progression from unstable angina/non–ST-segment myocardial infarction of the ACS. The onset of myocardial infarction usually is abrupt, with pain as the significant symptom. The pain typically is severe and crushing, often described as being constricting, suffocating, or like "someone sitting on my chest." The pain usually is substernal, radiating to the left arm, neck, or jaw, although it may be experienced in other areas of the chest. Unlike that of angina, the pain associated with myocardial infarction is more prolonged and not relieved by rest or nitroglycerin, and narcotics frequently are required. Women often experience atypical ischemic-type chest discomfort, whereas the elderly may complain of shortness of breath more frequently than chest pain.[27]

Serum Cardiac Markers

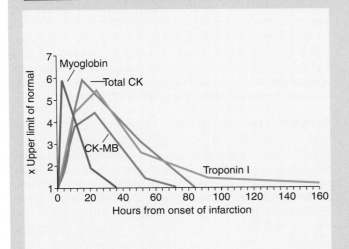

The relative timing, rate of rise, peak values, and duration of cardiac marker elevation above the upper limit of normal for multiple serum markers following AMI. (Modified from Antman E.M. [1994]. General hospital management. In Julian D.G. & Braunwald E. [Eds.], *Management of acute myocardial infarction* [p. 63]. London: W.B. Saunders Ltd.).

- *Myoglobin* is an oxygen-carrying protein, similar to hemoglobin, that is normally present in cardiac and skeletal muscle. It is a small molecule that is released quickly from infarcted myocardial tissue and becomes elevated within 1 hour after myocardial cell death, with peak levels reached within 4 to 8 hours. Because myoglobin is present in both cardiac and skeletal muscle, it is not cardiac specific.

- *Creatine kinase* (CK), formerly called *creatinine phosphokinase,* is an intracellular enzyme found in muscle cells. Muscles, including cardiac muscle, use adenosine triphosphate (ATP) as their energy source. Creatine, which serves as a storage form of energy in muscle, uses CK to convert ADP to ATP. CK exceeds normal range within 4 to 8 hours of myocardial injury and declines to normal within 2 to 3 days. There are three isoenzymes of CK, with the MB isoenzyme (CK-MB) being highly specific for injury to myocardial tissue.

- *The troponin complex* consists of three subunits (*i.e.,* troponin C, troponin I, and troponin T) that regulate calcium-mediated contractile process in striated muscle. These subunits are released during myocardial infarction. Cardiac muscle forms of both troponin T and troponin I are used in diagnosis of myocardial infarction. Troponin I (and troponin T; not shown) rises more slowly than myoglobin and may be useful for diagnosis of infarction, even up to 3 to 4 days after the event. It is thought that cardiac troponin assays are more capable of detecting episodes of myocardial infarction in which cell damage is below that detected by CK-MB level.

Gastrointestinal complaints are common. There may be a sensation of epigastric distress; nausea and vomiting may occur. These symptoms are thought to be related to the severity of the pain and vagal stimulation. The epigastric distress may be mistaken for indigestion, and the patient may seek relief with antacids or other home remedies, which only delays getting medical attention. Complaints of fatigue and weakness, especially of the arms and legs, are common. Pain and sympathetic stimulation combine to give rise to tachycardia, anxiety, restlessness, and feelings of impending doom. The skin often is pale, cool, and moist. The impaired myocardial function may lead to hypotension and shock.

Sudden death from AMI is death that occurs within 1 hour of symptom onset. It usually is attributed to fatal dysrhythmias, which may occur without evidence of infarction. Approximately 30% to 50% of persons with AMI die of ventricular fibrillation within the first few hours after symptoms begin. Early hospitalization after onset of symptoms greatly improves chances of averting sudden death because appropriate resuscitation facilities are immediately available when the ventricular dysrhythmia occurs.

Pathologic Changes. The extent of the infarct depends on the location and extent of occlusion, amount of heart tissue supplied by the vessel, duration of the occlusion, metabolic needs of the affected tissue, extent of collateral circulation, and other factors such as heart rate, blood pressure, and cardiac rhythm. A myocardial infarct may involve the endocardium, myocardium, epicardium, or a combination of these. *Transmural infarcts* involve the full thickness of the ventricular wall and most commonly occur when there is obstruction of a single artery. *Subendocardial infarcts* involve the inner one third to one half of the ventricular wall and occur more frequently in the presence of severely narrowed but still patent arteries. Most infarcts are transmural, involving the free wall of the left ventricle and the interventricular septum (Fig. 24-10).

The principal biochemical consequence of AMI is the conversion from aerobic to anaerobic metabolism with inadequate production of energy to sustain normal myocardial function. As a result, a striking loss of contractile function occurs within 60 seconds of AMI onset. Changes in cell structure (*i.e.*, glycogen depletion and mitochondrial swelling) develop within several minutes. These early changes are reversible if blood flow is restored.

Although gross tissue changes are not apparent for hours after onset of an AMI, the ischemic area ceases to function within a matter of minutes, and irreversible damage to cells occurs in approximately 40 minutes. Irreversible myocardial cell death (necrosis) occurs after 20 to 40 minutes of severe ischemia.[8] Microvascular injury occurs in approximately 1 hour and follows irreversible cell injury. The term *reperfusion* refers to reestablishment of blood flow through use of thrombolytic therapy. Early reperfusion (within 15 to 20 minutes) after onset of ischemia can prevent necrosis. Reperfusion after a longer interval can salvage some of the myocardial cells that would have died owing to longer periods of ischemia. It also may prevent microvas-

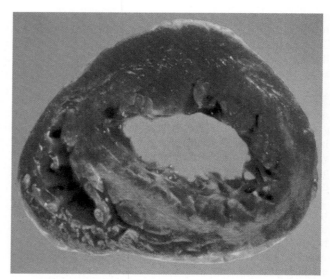

FIGURE 24-10 Acute myocardial infarct. A cross-section of the ventricles of a man who died a few days after the onset of severe chest pain shows a transmural infarct in the posterior and septal regions of the left ventricle. The necrotic myocardium is soft, yellowish, and sharply demarcated. (Rubin E., Farber J.L. [1999]. *Pathology* [3rd ed., p. 558]. Philadelphia: Lippincott Williams & Wilkins)

cular injury that occurs over a longer period. Even though much of the viable myocardium existing at the time of reflow ultimately recovers, critical abnormalities in biochemical function may persist, causing impaired ventricular function. The recovering area of the heart is often referred to as a *stunned myocardium*. Because myocardial function is lost before cell death occurs, a stunned myocardium may not be capable of sustaining life, and persons with large areas of dysfunctional myocardium may require life support until the stunned regions regain their function.[8]

Postinfarct Recovery Period. After a myocardial infarction, there usually are three zones of tissue damage: a zone of myocardial tissue that becomes necrotic because of an absolute lack of blood flow; a surrounding zone of injured cells, some of which will recover; and an outer zone in which cells are ischemic and can be salvaged if blood flow can be reestablished (Fig. 24-11). The boundaries of these zones may change with time after the infarction and with the success of treatment measures to reestablish blood flow. If blood flow can be restored within the 20- to 40-minute time frame, loss of cell viability does not occur or is minimal. The progression of ischemic necrosis usually begins in the subendocardial area of the heart and extends through the myocardium to involve progressively more of the transmural thickness of the ischemic zone.

Myocardial cells that undergo necrosis are gradually replaced with scar tissue (Table 24-2). An acute inflammatory response develops in the area of necrosis approximately 2 to 3 days after infarction. Thereafter, macrophages begin removing the necrotic tissue; the damaged area is gradually replaced with an ingrowth of highly vascularized granula-

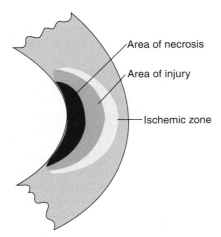

FIGURE 24-11 Areas of tissue damage after myocardial infarction.

Area of necrosis

Area of injury

Ischemic zone

tion tissue, which gradually becomes less vascular and more fibrous.[8] At approximately 4 to 7 days, the center of the infarcted area is soft and yellow; if rupture of the ventricle, interventricular septum, or valve structures occurs, it usually happens at this time. Replacement of the necrotic myocardial tissue usually is complete by the seventh week. Areas of the myocardium that have been replaced with scar tissue lack the ability to contract and initiate or conduct action potentials.

Complications.   The stages of recovery from AMI are closely related to the size of the infarct and the changes that have taken place in the infarcted area. Fibrous scar tissue lacks the contractile, elastic, and conductive properties of normal myocardial cells; the residual effects and the complications are determined essentially by the extent and location of the injury. Among the complications of AMI are sudden death, heart failure and cardiogenic shock, pericarditis and Dressler's syndrome, thromboemboli, rupture

of the heart, and ventricular aneurysms. Depending on its severity, myocardial infarction has the potential for compromising the pumping action of the heart. Heart failure and cardiogenic shock (see Chapter 26) are dreaded complications of AMI.

Pericarditis may complicate the course of AMI. It usually appears on the second or third day after infarction. The person experiences a new type of pain that is sharp and stabbing and is aggravated with deep inspiration and positional changes. A pericardial friction rub may or may not be heard in all persons who have postinfarction pericarditis, and it often is transitory, usually resolving uneventfully. Dressler's syndrome describes the signs and symptoms associated with pericarditis, pleurisy, and pneumonitis: fever, chest pain, dyspnea, and abnormal laboratory test results (*i.e.*, elevated white blood cell count and sedimentation rate) and ECG findings. The symptoms may arise between 1 day and several weeks after infarction and are thought to represent a hypersensitivity response to tissue necrosis. Anti-inflammatory agents or corticosteroid drugs may be used to reduce the inflammatory response.

Thromboemboli are a potential complication of AMI, arising as venous thrombi or occasionally as clots from the wall of the ventricle. Immobility and impaired cardiac function contribute to stasis of blood in the venous system. Elastic stockings, along with active and passive leg exercises, usually are included in the postinfarction treatment plan as a means of preventing thrombus formation. If a clot is detected on the wall of the ventricle (usually by echocardiography), treatment with anticoagulants is indicated.

Dreaded complications of AMI are rupture of the myocardium, the interventricular septum, or a papillary muscle. Myocardial rupture, occurring on the fourth to seventh day post-AMI when the injured ventricular tissue is soft and weak, often is fatal. Necrosis of the septal wall or papillary muscle may lead to the rupture of either of these structures,

TABLE 24-2 ✦ Tissues Changes After Myocardial Infarction	
Time After Onset	**Type of Injury and Gross Tissue Changes**
0–0.5 hours	Reversible injury
1–2 hours	Onset of irreversible injury
4–12 hours	Beginning of coagulation necrosis
18–24 hours	Continued coagulation necrosis; gross pallor of infarcted tissue
1–3 days	Total coagulation necrosis; continued gross pallor of infarcted area and sometimes hyperemia due to onset of acute inflammatory process
3–7 days	Infarcted area becomes soft with a yellow-brown center and hyperemic edges
7–10 days	Maximally soft and yellow with vascularized edges; fibroblastic activity at edges denotes beginning of scar tissue generation
8th week	Scar tissue replacement complete

(Developed from information in Cotran R.S., Kumar V., Collins T. [1999]. *Robbins pathologic basis of disease* [6th ed., pp. 555–560]. Philadelphia: W.B. Saunders.)

with worsening of ventricular performance. Surgical repair usually is indicated, but whenever possible, it is delayed until the heart has had time to recover from the initial infarction. Vasodilator therapy and the aortic balloon counterpulsation pump may provide supportive assistance during this period.

An aneurysm is an outpouching of the ventricular wall. Scar tissue does not have the characteristics of normal myocardial tissue; when a large section of ventricular muscle is replaced by scar tissue, an aneurysm may develop (Fig. 24-12). This section of the myocardium does not contract with the rest of the ventricle during systole. Instead, it diminishes the pumping efficiency of the heart and increases the work of the left ventricle, predisposing the patient to heart failure. Ischemia in the surrounding area predisposes the patient to development of dysrhythmias, and stasis of blood in the aneurysm can lead to thrombus formation. Surgical resection often is corrective.

Medical Management

The treatment of ACS depends on the extent of ischemia or infarction. Because the specific diagnosis of AMI often is difficult to make at the time of entry into the health care system, the immediate management of all ACSs in general is the same. Commonly indicated treatment regimens for all acute coronary ischemic syndromes include aspirin, β-adrenergic blockers, and nitrates. Persons with ECG evidence of infarction should receive immediate reperfusion therapy with thrombolytic agents or PTCA.[27]

The ACC/AHA Task Force Guidelines for Management of Acute Myocardial Infarction recommend that the initial emergency department management of myocardial infarction include administration of oxygen by nasal prongs; sublingual nitroglycerin (unless systolic blood pressure is <90 mm Hg or the heart rate is <50 or >100 beats/minute); adequate analgesia; and aspirin (160 to 325 mg).[27] ECG monitoring should be instituted, and a 12-lead ECG should be performed.

The administration of oxygen augments the oxygen content of inspired air and increases the oxygen saturation of hemoglobin. Arterial oxygen levels may fall precipitously after AMI, and oxygen administration helps to maintain the oxygen content of the blood perfusing the coronary circulation.

The severe pain of myocardial infarction gives rise to anxiety and recruitment of autonomic nervous system responses, both of which increase the work demands of the heart. Morphine often is given intravenously for pain relief because it has a rapid onset of action and the intravenous route does not elevate enzyme levels. The intravenous route also bypasses the variable rate of absorption of subcutaneous or intramuscular sites, which often are underperfused because of a decrease in cardiac output that occurs after infarction. Morphine has vasodilator properties and often is used as the narcotic of choice in treatment of AMI.[27] Vasodilating drugs decrease venous return (*i.e.*, reduce preload) and arterial blood pressure (*i.e.*, reduce afterload) and thereby reduce oxygen consumption. Sublingual nitroglycerin is given because of its vasodilating effect and ability to relieve coronary pain. Intravenous nitroglycerin may be given to limit infarction size and is most effective if given within 4 hours of symptom onset.

Because sympathetic nervous system activity increases the metabolic demands of the myocardium, β-adrenergic–blocking drugs may be used to reduce sympathetic stimulation of the heart after myocardial infarction. These drugs decrease myocardial contractility and cardiac workload, alter resting myocardial membrane potentials and decrease dysrhythmia frequency, and may aid in redistributing coronary artery blood flow and improving myocardial blood flow.

Aspirin inhibits platelet aggregation and is thought to promote reperfusion and reduce the likelihood of rethrombosis.[28] It has been suggested that because of its antiplatelet effects, aspirin also may help to stabilize arterial patency after thrombolytic therapy. The glycoprotein IIb/IIIa receptor inhibitors may be used in persons who have non–ST-segment elevation AMI provided they do not have a major contraindication due to bleeding risk. Low–molecular-weight heparin may be used to prevent thrombin generation.

Thrombolytic Therapy

Thrombolytic drugs dissolve blood and platelet clots and are used to reduce mortality and limit infarct size. The best results occur if treatment is initiated within 60 to 90 minutes of symptom onset.[29] The magnitude of benefit declines after this period, but it is possible that some benefit can be achieved for up to 12 hours after the onset of pain. The person must be a low-risk candidate for complications caused by bleeding.

The thrombolytic agents interact with plasminogen to generate plasmin, which lyses fibrin clots and digests clotting factors V and VIII, prothrombin, and fibrinogen (see Chapter 14). Several thrombolytic agents are ap-

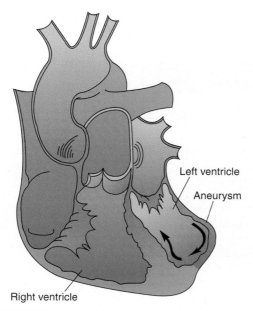

Left ventricle

Aneurysm

Right ventricle

FIGURE 24-12 Paradoxical movement of a ventricular aneurysm during systole.

proved by the U.S. Food and Drug Administration (FDA). Streptokinase and urokinase act indirectly via enzyme-catalyzed mechanisms to promote the conversion of plasminogen to plasmin. The tissue plasminogen activators (tPA) promote the selective activation of plasminogen that is bound to fibrin in thrombi. Anistrepase, an anisoylated derivative of the plasminogen-streptokinase activator complex (APSAC), is an inactive thrombolytic enzyme that is activated in the bloodstream or in the thrombus. The tPAs (alteplase, reteplase, and tenecteplase) are plasminogen activators that been developed using recombinant DNA technology. Studies that have compared the three types of thrombolytic agents (streptokinase, APSAC, and tPA) found no significant differences between them in relation to mortality, morbidity, and left ventricular function.[29]

Revascularization Interventions

Revascularization interventions, including PTCA, coronary stent implantation, and coronary artery bypass surgery, may be performed to relieve coronary artery obstruction caused by atherosclerotic lesions.

Percutaneous transluminal coronary angioplasty is used to reduce atherosclerotic plaque obstruction. Although angioplasty usually produces immediate relief of anginal symptoms, its use is associated with death or nonfatal myocardial infarction in approximately 5% of persons and with restenosis requiring repeated angioplasty or bypass surgery in approximately 30% of persons undergoing the procedure.[30] Implantation of coronary stents reduces the occurrence of restenosis. Measures to reduce thrombosis during angioplasty also decrease the risk of death and myocardial infarction.

PTCA involves balloon dilatation of a stenotic coronary vessel. The procedure is done under local anesthesia in the cardiac catheterization laboratory and is similar to cardiac catheterization for coronary angiography. With PTCA, a double-lumen balloon dilatation catheter is introduced percutaneously into the femoral or brachial artery and then advanced under fluoroscopic view to the coronary ostium. It is then directed into the affected coronary artery and advanced until the balloon segment is in the stenotic area of the vessel. When in place, the balloon is inflated for 15 seconds to 2 or 3 minutes using a pressure-controlled pump.[31] The mechanism of dilation is compression and rupture of the atherosclerotic plaque and stretching of the plaque-free vessel wall (Fig. 24-13). PTCA also can be used to dilate coronary artery bypass grafts. Acute complications of PTCA include thrombosis and vessel dissection; longer-term complications involve restenosis of the dilated vessel. Refinements in the balloon catheters have resulted in decreased risk of vessel perforation and ischemic complications.

Because of the risk of restenosis, a stent may be inserted into the dilated vessel at the time of PTCA. *Coronary stents* are fenestrated, stainless steel tubes that can be inserted into a coronary artery and then expanded to prevent vessel restenosis (Fig. 24-14). Stents also are used to prevent abrupt vessel closure caused by vessel dissection that occurs as a complication of PTCA. Stenting is used in high-risk situations that are not likely to be managed successfully

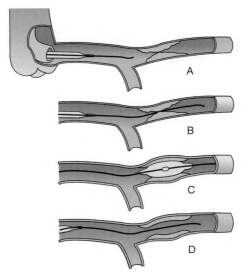

FIGURE 24-13 (**A**) PTCA dilation catheter and guidewire exiting the guiding catheter. (**B**) Guidewire advanced across the stenosis. (**C**) Dilation catheter advanced across the stenosis and inflated. (**D**) Dilation catheter pulled back to assess luminal diameter. (Reprinted with permission of Advanced Cardiovascular Systems [ACS], Inc., Santa Clara, CA)

by PTCA alone. Persons undergoing stent procedures are treated with antiplatelet and anticoagulant drugs to prevent thrombosis, which is a major risk after the procedure. Adjunctive blockade of the platelet glycoprotein IIb/IIIa receptor may be used to prevent thrombosis and complications associated with PTCA.

A new approach to the prevention of coronary restenosis after balloon angioplasty and stent placement is the use of localized intracoronary radiation. Two approaches to intracoronary radiation, endoluminal beta irradiation and localized intracoronary gamma radiation, were approved by the FDA in November 2000.[32,33] The procedure, also known as *brachytherapy*, is credited with inhibiting cell proliferation and vascular lesion formation and preventing constrictive arterial remodeling. The radiation source can be impregnated into stents, or the radiation can be delivered by a radiation catheter containing a sealed source of radiation (radioactive seeds, wire, or ribbon) that is inserted into the treatment site and then removed.[34]

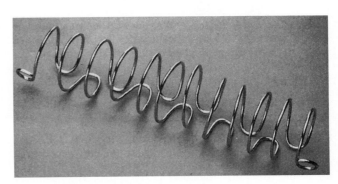

FIGURE 24-14 The Gianturco-Roubin Flex-Stent. (Courtesy of Cook, Inc., Bloomington, IN)

Atherectomy (*i.e.*, cutting of the atherosclerotic plaque with a high-speed circular blade from within the vessel) is being tested as a mechanical technique to remove atherosclerotic tissue during angioplasty. Laser angioplasty devices also are being tested.[30]

Coronary Artery Bypass Grafting. Coronary artery bypass grafting (CABG) may be the treatment of choice for people with significant CHD who do not respond to medical treatment and who are not suitable candidates for PTCA. It may also be indicated as a treatment for AMI, in which case the surgery should be done within 4 to 6 hours of symptom onset if possible.

Coronary artery bypass grafting involves revascularization of the affected myocardium by placing a saphenous vein graft between the aorta and the affected coronary artery distal to the site of occlusion, or by using the internal mammary artery as a means of revascularizing the left anterior descending artery or its branches. Figure 24-15 shows the placement of a saphenous vein graft and a mammary artery graft. One to five distal anastomoses commonly are done. Although it cannot be documented that this surgery significantly alters the progress of the disease, it does relieve pain, and patients may have more productive lives.[29]

Cardiac Rehabilitation Programs

Rehabilitation programs for persons with ACSs incorporate rest, exercise, and risk factor modification. Modifying the diet to include foods that are low in salt and cholesterol and easy to digest is another treatment measure used to decrease cardiac work. Stool softeners may be prescribed to prevent constipation and avoid straining with defecation.

An exercise program is an integral part of a cardiac rehabilitation program. It includes activities such as walking, swimming, and bicycling. These exercises involve changes in muscle length and rhythmic contractions of muscle groups. Most exercise programs are individually designed to meet each person's physical and psychological needs. The goal of the exercise program is to increase the maximal oxygen consumption by the muscle tissues, so that these persons are able to perform more work at a lower heart rate and blood pressure. In addition to exercise, cardiac risk factor modification incorporates strategies for smoking cessation, weight loss, stress reduction, and control of hypertension and diabetes.

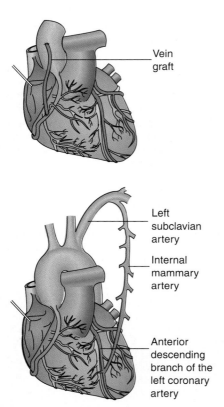

FIGURE 24-15 Coronary artery revascularization. (**Top**) Saphenous vein bypass graft. The vein segment is sutured to the ascending aorta and the right coronary artery at a point distal to the occluding lesion. (**Bottom**) Mammary artery bypass. The mammary artery is anastomosed to the anterior descending left coronary artery, bypassing the obstructing lesion.

Labels in figure: Vein graft; Left subclavian artery; Internal mammary artery; Anterior descending branch of the left coronary artery

> In summary, CHD is a disorder of impaired coronary blood flow, usually caused by atherosclerosis. Myocardial ischemia occurs when there is a disparity between coronary blood flow and the metabolic needs of the heart. Ischemia can be present as a chronic ischemic heart disease and as an ACS. Diagnostic methods for CHD include ECG methods, exercise testing, nuclear imaging studies, and angiographic studies in the cardiac catheterization laboratory.
>
> The chronic ischemic heart diseases include chronic stable angina, variant angina, and silent myocardial ischemia. Chronic stable angina is associated with a fixed atherosclerotic obstruction and pain that is precipitated by increased work demands on the heart and relieved by rest. Variant angina results from spasms of the coronary arteries. Silent myocardial ischemia occurs without symptoms. Treatment includes nonpharmacologic methods, such as pacing of activities and avoidance of activities that cause angina, and the use of pharmacologic agents, including aspirin, β-adrenergic blockers, calcium channel blockers, and nitrates. Revascularization procedures include PTCA along with the use of coronary artery stents and CABG.
>
> The ACSs result from unstable atherosclerotic plaques, platelet aggregation, and thrombus formation. They include unstable angina, non–ST-segment elevation AMI, and ST-segment elevation AMI. Unstable angina is an accelerated form of angina in which the pain occurs more frequently, is more severe, and lasts longer than chronic stable angina. AMI refers to the ischemic death of myocardial tissue associated with obstructed blood flow in the coronary arteries due to plaque disruption and occlusion of blood flow. Non–ST-segment and ST-segment elevation AMI differ in

terms of extent of myocardial damage. The complications of AMI include potentially fatal dysrhythmias, heart failure and cardiogenic shock, pericarditis, thromboemboli, rupture of cardiac structures, and ventricular aneurysms. Diagnostic methods include the use of ECG monitoring and serum cardiac markers. Treatment goals focus on reestablishment of myocardial blood flow through rapid recanalization of the occluded coronary artery, prevention of clot extension through use of aspirin and other antiplatelet and antithrombotic agents, alleviation of pain, measures such as administration of oxygen to increase the oxygen saturation of hemoglobin, and the use of vasodilators to reduce the work demands of the heart. Thrombolytic agents, PTCA, and CABG are measures used to recanalize or bypass the occluded artery.

Myocardial Disease

After you have completed this section of the chapter, you should be able to meet the following objectives:

✦ Define and cite selected causes of myocarditis
✦ Characterize the pathogenesis and possible outcomes of viral myocarditis
✦ Define the term *cardiomyopathy* and compare the heart changes that occur with dilated, hypertrophic, and constrictive cardiomyopathies, and arrhythmogenic right ventricular cardiomyopathy

Myocardial diseases, including myocarditis and the primary cardiomyopathies, are disorders originating in the myocardium, but not from cardiovascular disease. Both myocarditis and the cardiomyopathies are causes of sudden death and heart failure. Of the more than 3 million persons in the United States who have heart failure, approximately 25% of cases result from idiopathic dilated cardiomyopathy.[35]

MYOCARDITIS

The term *myocarditis* is used to describe an inflammation of the heart muscle and conduction system without evidence of myocardial infarction.[36,37] Viruses are the most important cause of myocarditis in North America and Europe.[37] *Coxsackieviruses A* and *B* and other enteroviruses probably account for most of the cases. Myocarditis is a frequent pathologic cardiac finding in persons with acquired immunodeficiency syndrome (AIDS), although it is unclear whether it is due to the human immunodeficiency virus itself or to a secondary infection. Other causes of myocarditis are radiation therapy, hypersensitivity reactions, or exposure to chemical or physical agents that induce acute myocardial necrosis and secondary inflammatory changes. A drug that is increasingly associated with myocarditis is cocaine, probably owing to its vasoconstrictor properties.[37]

Myocardial injury due to infectious agents is thought to result from necrosis caused by direct invasion of the offending organism, toxic effects of exogenous toxins or endotoxins produced by a systemic pathogen, or destruction of cardiac tissue by immunologic mechanisms initiated by the infectious agent. The immunologic response may be directed at foreign antigens of the infectious agent that share molecular characteristics with those of the host cardiac myocytes (*i.e.*, molecular mimicry; see Chapter 19), providing a continuous stimulus for the immune response even after the infectious agent has been cleared from the body.

The *manifestations of myocarditis* vary from an absence of symptoms to profound heart failure or sudden death. When viral myocarditis occurs in children or young adults, it often is asymptomatic. Acute symptomatic myocarditis typically manifests as a flulike syndrome with malaise, low-grade fever, and tachycardia that is more pronounced than would be expected for the level of fever present. There commonly is a history of an upper respiratory tract or gastrointestinal tract infection, followed by a latent period of several days. Cardiac auscultation may reveal an S_3 ventricular gallop rhythm and a transient pericardial or pleurocardial rub. In approximately one half of the cases, myocarditis is transient, and symptoms subside within 1 to 2 months. In other cases, fulminant heart failure and life-threatening dysrhythmias develop, causing sudden death. Still others progress to subacute and chronic disease.

The *diagnosis* of myocarditis can be suggested by clinical manifestations. The ECG changes of acute myocarditis include conduction disturbances such as ventricular dysrhythmias, AV junctional block, ST-segment elevation, T-wave inversion, and transient Q waves. Serum creatinine kinase often is elevated. Troponin T or troponin I, or both, may be elevated, providing evidence of myocardial cell damage.[37] Confirmation of active myocarditis requires endomyocardial biopsy.

Treatment measures focus on symptom management and prevention of myocardial damage. Bed rest is necessary, and activity restriction must be maintained until fever and cardiac symptoms subside to decrease the myocardial workload. Activity is gradually increased but kept at a sedentary level for 6 months to 1 year. The restriction includes the avoidance of swimming, jogging, weight lifting, and carrying heavy objects. The use of corticosteroids and immunosuppressant drugs such as azathioprine and cyclosporine remains controversial. There is some evidence that people with acute fulminant myocarditis may benefit from short-term circulatory support with left ventricular assist devices.[37] The use of the antiviral agent, interferon alfa, for treatment of enterovirus-positive forms of myocarditis is under study.[37] Although treatment of myocarditis is successful in many persons, some progress to congestive heart failure and can expect only a limited life span. For these persons, heart transplantation becomes an alternative.

CARDIOMYOPATHIES

The cardiomyopathies are a group of disorders that affect the heart muscle. They can develop as primary or secondary disorders. The primary cardiomyopathies, which are discussed in this chapter, are heart muscle diseases of unknown origin.

Secondary cardiomyopathies are conditions in which the cardiac abnormality results from another cardiovascular disease, such as myocardial infarction. The onset of the primary cardiomyopathies often is silent, and symptoms do not occur until the disease is well advanced. The diagnosis is suspected when a young, previously healthy, normotensive person experiences cardiomegaly and heart failure.

In 1989, the International Society and Federation of Cardiology and the World Health Organization categorized the primary cardiomyopathies into three groups: dilated, hypertrophic, and restrictive[38] (Fig. 24-16). This classification was enlarged in 1996 to include arrhythmogenic right ventricular cardiomyopathy.[39] Peripartum cardiomyopathy is a disorder of pregnancy.

Dilated Cardiomyopathies

Dilated cardiomyopathies are characterized by progressive cardiac hypertrophy and dilation and impaired pumping ability of one or both ventricles. Although all four chambers of the heart are affected, the ventricles are more dilated than the atria. Because of the wall thinning that accompanies dilation, the thickness of the ventricular wall often is less than would be expected for the amount of hypertrophy present.[40] Mural thrombi are common and may be a source of thromboemboli. The cardiac valves are intrinsically normal. Microscopically, there is evidence of scarring and atrophy of myocardial cells.

Dilated cardiomyopathy may result from a number of different myocardial insults, including infectious myocarditis, alcohol and other toxic agents, metabolic influences, neuromuscular diseases, and immunologic disorders. Genetic influences have been documented in some cases. One study found that 20% of affected persons have first-degree

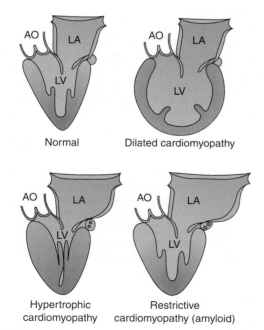

FIGURE 24-16 The various types of cardiomyopathies compared with the normal heart. (Roberts W.C., Ferrans V.J. [1975]. Pathologic anatomy of the cardiomyopathies. *Human Pathology* 6, 289)

relatives with myocardial dysfunction.[41] These disorders can be inherited in an autosomal dominant, autosomal recessive, or X-linked inheritance pattern. Often the cause is unknown; these cases are appropriately designated as *idiopathic dilated cardiomyopathy*.

The most common initial manifestations of dilated cardiomyopathy are those related to heart failure. There is a profound reduction in the left ventricular ejection fraction (*i.e.*, ratio of stroke volume to end-diastolic volume) to 40% or less, compared with a normal value of approximately 67%. After symptoms have developed, the course of the disorder is distinguished by worsening of heart failure, development of mural thrombi, and ventricular dysrhythmias. The most striking symptoms of dilated cardiomyopathy are dyspnea on exertion, paroxysmal nocturnal dyspnea, orthopnea, weakness, fatigue, ascites, and peripheral edema. On physical examination, an enlarged apical beat with the presence of a third and fourth heart sound and a murmur associated with regurgitation of one or both AV valves frequently are found. The systolic blood pressure is normal or low, and the peripheral pulses often are of low amplitude. Pulsus alternans, in which the pulse regularly alternates between weaker and stronger volume, may be present. Basilar rales frequently are detected. Sinus tachycardia, atrial fibrillation, and complex ventricular dysrhythmias leading to sudden cardiac death are common.

The treatment of dilated cardiomyopathy is directed toward relieving the symptoms of heart failure and reducing the workload of the heart (see Chapter 26). Digoxin, diuretics, and afterload-reducing drugs are used to improve myocardial contractility and decrease left ventricular filling pressures. Avoiding myocardial depressants, including alcohol, and pacing rest with asymptomatic levels of exercise or activity is imperative. Proper electrolyte balance and internal cardioverter-defibrillators are effective in controlling recurrent ventricular dysrhythmias associated with dilated cardiomyopathy. In persons with severe heart failure that is refractory to treatment, cardiac transplantation may be considered.

Hypertrophic Cardiomyopathies

Hypertrophic cardiomyopathy is characterized by left, right, or left and right ventricular hypertrophy and abnormal diastolic filling. Although the hypertrophy may be symmetric, the involvement of the ventricular septum often is disproportionate, producing intermittent left ventricular outflow obstruction.[42] Synonyms for this disorder include *idiopathic hypertrophic subaortic stenosis* and *asymmetric septal hypertrophy*.

Symptomatic hypertrophic cardiomyopathy commonly is a disease of young adulthood. The cause of the disorder is unknown, although it often is of familial origin, with the disorder being inherited as an autosomal dominant trait. Molecular studies of the genetic alterations responsible for hypertrophic cardiomyopathy suggest that the disease is caused by mutation in one of four genes encoding the proteins of the cardiac sarcomeres (*i.e.*, muscle fibers): the β-myosin heavy chain, cardiac troponin T, α-tropomyosin, and myosin-binding protein C.[42] More than 50 mutations in these proteins have been identified. The prognosis of persons with different myosin mutations varies greatly; some mutations are relatively benign, whereas others are associated with premature death.

A distinctive microscopic finding in hypertrophic cardiomyopathy is myofibril disarray. Instead of the normal parallel arrangement of myofibrils, the myofibrils branch off at random angles, sometimes at right angles to an adjacent fiber with which they connect. Small bundles of fibers may course haphazardly through normally arranged muscle fibers.[8] These disordered fibers may produce abnormal movements of the ventricles, with uncoordinated contraction and impaired relaxation. Arrhythmias and premature sudden death are common with this disorder. Study results have shown that 36% of young athletes who die suddenly have probable or definite hypertrophic cardiomyopathy.[1]

The manifestations of hypertrophic cardiomyopathy are variable; for reasons that are unclear, some persons with the disorder remain stable for many years and gradually acquire more symptoms as the disease progresses, but others experience sudden cardiac death as first evidence of the disease.[42] Atrial fibrillation is a common precursor to sudden death in those who die of dysrhythmias. Dyspnea is the most common symptom associated with a gradual elevation in left ventricular diastolic pressure resulting from impaired ventricular filling and increased wall stiffness due to ventricular hypertrophy. Because of the obstruction to outflow from the left ventricle, increasingly greater levels of ventricular pressure are needed to eject blood into the aorta, limiting cardiac output. Chest pain, fatigue, and syncope are common and worsen during exertion.

The treatment of hypertrophic cardiomyopathy includes medical and surgical management. The goal of medical management is to relieve the symptoms by lessening the pressure difference between the left ventricle and the aorta, thereby improving cardiac output. Drugs that block the β-adrenergic receptors may be used in persons with chest pain, dysrhythmias, or dyspnea.[40,42,43] These drugs reduce the heart rate and improve myocardial function by allowing more time for ventricular filling and reducing ventricular stiffness. The calcium channel–blocking drug verapamil may be used as an alternative to the β-adrenergic blockers. Increased calcium uptake and increased intracellular calcium content are associated with an increased contractile state, a characteristic finding in patients with hypertrophic cardiomyopathy.

Surgical treatment may be used if severe symptoms persist despite medical treatment. It involves incision of the septum (*i.e.*, myotomy) with or without the removal of part of the tissue (*i.e.*, myectomy). It is accompanied by all the risks of open heart surgery. Implantable cardioverter-defibrillators may be used to abort lethal arrhythmias.[43]

Restrictive Cardiomyopathies

Of the three categories of cardiomyopathies, the restrictive type is the least common in Western countries. With this form of cardiomyopathy, ventricular filling is restricted because of excessive rigidity of the ventricular walls, although the contractile properties of the heart remain relatively normal. The condition is endemic in parts of Africa, India, South and Central America, and Asia.[44] Outside the tropics, the most common causes of restrictive cardiomyopathy are endocardial infiltrations such as amyloidosis. Amyloid infiltrations of the heart are common in the elderly. The idiopathic form of the disorder may have a familial origin.

Symptoms of restrictive cardiomyopathy include dyspnea, paroxysmal nocturnal dyspnea, orthopnea, peripheral edema, ascites, fatigue, and weakness. The manifestations of restrictive cardiomyopathy resemble those of constrictive pericarditis. In the advanced form of the disease, all the signs of heart failure are present except cardiomegaly.

Arrhythmogenic Right Ventricular Cardiomyopathy

In arrhythmogenic right ventricular cardiomyopathy, right ventricular myocardium is replaced with a fibrofatty deposit. This condition frequently has a familial predisposition, with an autosomal dominant inheritance pattern. Sudden death due to arrhythmias is common, particularly in the young.[39]

Peripartum Cardiomyopathy

Peripartum cardiomyopathy refers to left ventricular dysfunction developing in the last month before delivery to 5 months postpartum. The condition is relatively rare, with an estimated incidence of 1 per 3000 to 4000 live births.[45] Risk factors for peripartum cardiomyopathy include advanced maternal age, African-American race, multifetal pregnancies, preeclampsia, and gestational hypertension.[45] The reported mortality rate ranges from 18% to 56%. Survivors may not recover completely and may require heart transplantation.

The cause of peripartum cardiomyopathy is uncertain. A number of causes have been proposed, including myocarditis, an abnormal immune response to pregnancy, maladaptive response to the hemodynamic stresses of pregnancy, or prolonged inhibition of contractions in premature labor. There is more evidence for myocarditis as a cause than for other purported etiologies.[46]

The signs and symptoms resemble those of dilated cardiomyopathy. Because many women experience dyspnea, fatigue, and pedal edema during the last month of normal pregnancy, the symptoms may be ignored and the diagnosis delayed. The diagnosis is based on echocardiography studies, ECG, and other tests of cardiac function. Treatment methods are similar to those used in dilated cardiomyopathy.

There are two possible outcomes of peripartum cardiomyopathy. In approximately one half of cases, the heart returns to normal within 6 months, and the chances for long-term survival are good. In these women, heart failure returns only during subsequent pregnancies. In the other one half of cases, cardiomegaly persists, and the prognosis is poor and death is probable if another pregnancy occurs. In women with cardiomyopathy from documented viral myocarditis, the likelihood of recurrence is low.

> In summary, myocardial disorders represent a diverse group of disorders of myocardial muscle cells, not related to coronary artery disease. Myocarditis is an acute inflammation of cardiac muscle cells, most often of viral

origin. Myocardial injury from myocarditis is thought to result from necrosis due to direct invasion of the offending organism, toxic effects of exogenous toxins or endotoxins produced by a systemic pathogen, and destruction of cardiac tissue by immunologic mechanisms initiated by the infectious agent. Although the disease usually is benign and self-limited, it can result in sudden death or chronic heart failure, for which heart transplantation may be considered.

The cardiomyopathies represent disorders of the heart muscle. Cardiomyopathies may manifest as primary or secondary disorders. There are four main types of primary cardiomyopathies: dilated cardiomyopathy, in which fibrosis and atrophy of myocardial cells produces progressive dilation and impaired pumping ability of the heart; hypertrophic cardiomyopathy, characterized by myocardial hypertrophy, abnormal diastolic filling, and in many cases intermittent left ventricular outflow obstruction; restrictive cardiomyopathy, in which there is excessive rigidity of the ventricular wall; and arrhythmogenic right ventricular cardiomyopathy. Peripartum cardiomyopathy occurs during pregnancy. The cause of many of the primary cardiomyopathies is unknown. The disease is suspected when cardiomegaly and heart failure develop in a young, previously healthy person.

Infectious and Immunologic Disorders

After you have completed this section of the chapter, you should be able to meet the following objectives:

✦ Distinguish between the role of infectious organisms and the immune system in rheumatic fever, infective endocarditis, and Kawasaki's disease

✦ Compare the effects of rheumatic fever, bacterial endocarditis, and Kawasaki's disease on cardiac structures and their function

✦ Describe the relation between the infective vegetations associated with infective endocarditis and the extracardiac manifestations of the disease

✦ Explain measures that can be used to prevent infective endocarditis

INFECTIVE ENDOCARDITIS

Infective endocarditis is a relatively uncommon, life-threatening infection of the endocardial surface of the heart, including the heart valves. It is characterized by colonization or invasion of the heart valves and the mural endocardium by a microbial agent, leading to the formation of bulky, friable vegetations and destruction of underlying cardiac tissues.[8] Because bacteria are the most frequent infecting organisms, the condition may be referred to as *bacterial endocarditis.* Despite important advances in antimicrobial therapy and improved ability to diagnose and treat complications, infective endocarditis continues to produce substantial morbidity and mortality.

Although anyone can contract infective endocarditis, the infection usually develops in people with preexisting heart defects. Heart valves are involved most commonly, but the lesions may affect a septal defect or the endocardial surface of the heart wall. Factors that determine the clinical presentation and outcome of infective endocarditis are the nature of the infecting organism and the presence of preexisting heart defects. Because endocarditis in intravenous drug users and infections acquired during heart surgery have special features, the source of the infection also is important.

Predisposing Factors

For infective endocarditis to develop, two independent factors normally are required: a damaged endocardial surface and a portal of entry by which the organism gains access to the circulatory system. The presence of valvular disease, prosthetic heart valves, or congenital heart defects provides an environment conducive to bacterial growth.[8,47,48] In persons with preexisting valvular or endocardial defects, simple gum massage or an innocuous oral lesion may afford the pathogenic bacteria access to the bloodstream. Transient bacteremia may emerge in the course of seemingly minor health problems, such as an upper respiratory tract infection, a skin lesion, or a dental procedure.

Although infective endocarditis usually occurs in persons with preexisting heart lesions, it also can develop in normal hearts of intravenous drug abusers. The risk of infective endocarditis is increased among intravenous drug users to an incidence of 2% to 5% per patient year, which is severalfold greater than that for persons with rheumatic heart disease and prosthetic heart valves.[47] The mode of infection is a contaminated drug solution or a needle contaminated with skin flora. Intravenous drug abuse is the most common source of right-sided (tricuspid) lesions. Although staphylococcal infections are common, intravenous drug users may be infected with unusual organisms, such as gram-negative bacilli, yeasts, and fungi.

In hospitalized patients, infective endocarditis may arise as a complication of infected intravascular or urinary tract catheters. Infective endocarditis also may complicate prosthetic heart valve replacement. It can develop as an early infection that follows surgery or as a later infection that results from the long-term presence of the prosthesis. Infections of prosthetic valves account for 10% to 20% of cases of infectious endocarditis.[47]

Depending on the duration of the disease, presenting manifestations, and complications, cases of infective endocarditis can be classified as acute, subacute, or chronic.[49] Acute infective endocarditis is thought primarily to affect persons with normal hearts and usually is caused by *Staphylococcus aureus, Streptococcus pneumoniae, Streptococcus pyogenes,* and *Neisseria* species. *S. aureus* in particular produces a rapidly progressive and destructive form of the disease. Subacute endocarditis is seen most frequently in patients with damaged hearts and usually is caused by less virulent organisms such as *Streptococcus viridans,* enterococci, and varieties of other gram-negative and gram-positive bacilli, yeasts, and fungi. Certain low-virulence organisms such as *Legionella* and *Brucella* may produce a chronic form of the disease.[49]

The pathophysiology of infective endocarditis involves the formation of intracardiac vegetative lesions that have local and distant systemic effects. The vegetative lesion that is characteristic of infective endocarditis consists of a collection of infectious organisms and cellular debris enmeshed in the fibrin strands of clotted blood. The infectious loci continuously release bacteria into the bloodstream and are a source of persistent bacteremia. These lesions may be singular or multiple, may grow to be as large as several centimeters, and usually are found loosely attached to the free edges of the valve surface (Fig. 24-17). As the lesions grow, they cause valve destruction, leading to valvular regurgitation, ring abscesses with heart block, and valve perforation. The loose organization of these lesions permits the organisms and fragments of the lesions to form emboli and travel in the bloodstream. The fragments may lodge in small blood vessels, causing small hemorrhages, abscesses, and infarction of tissue. The bacteremia also can initiate immune responses thought to be responsible for the skin manifestations, arthritis, glomerulonephritis, and other immune disorders associated with the condition.

Manifestations

The signs and symptoms of infective endocarditis include fever and signs of systemic infection, change in the character of an existing heart murmur, and evidence of embolic distribution of the vegetative lesions. In the acute form, the fever usually is spiking and accompanied by chills. In the subacute form, the fever usually is low grade, of gradual onset, and frequently accompanied by other systemic signs of inflammation, such as anorexia, malaise, and lethargy. Small petechial hemorrhages frequently result when emboli lodge in the small vessels of the skin, nail beds, and mucous membranes. Splinter hemorrhages (*i.e.*, dark red lines) under the nails of the fingers and toes are common. Cough, dyspnea, arthralgia or arthritis, diarrhea, and abdominal or flank pain may occur as the result of systemic emboli.

The clinical course of infective endocarditis is determined by the extent of heart damage, the type of organism involved, site of infection (*i.e.*, right or left side of the heart),

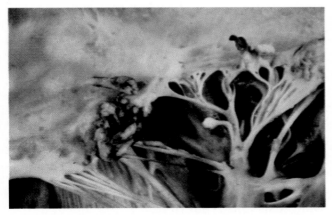

FIGURE 24-17 Bacterial endocarditis. The mitral valve shows destructive vegetations, which have eroded through the free margin of the valve leaflet. (Rubin E., Farber J.L. [1999]. *Pathology* [3rd ed., p. 572]. Philadelphia: Lippincott Williams & Wilkins)

and whether embolization from the site of infection occurs. Destruction of infected heart valves is common with certain forms of organisms, such as *S. aureus*. Peripheral embolization can lead to metastatic infections and abscess formation; these are particularly serious when they affect organs such as the brain and kidneys. In right-sided endocarditis, which usually involves the tricuspid valve, septic emboli travel to the lung, causing infarction and lung abscesses.

Diagnosis and Treatment

The blood culture is the most definitive diagnostic procedure and is essential to guide treatment. At least six cultures should be obtained to increase the probability of obtaining a positive culture. The optimal time to obtain cultures is during a chill, just before a temperature rise. Positive cultures usually are obtainable for infections caused by gram-positive cocci, but cultures may fail to grow gram-negative organisms or fungi. The echocardiogram is useful in detecting underlying valvular disease. Transesophageal echocardiography is rapid and noninvasive, and has proved useful for detecting vegetations.

The Duke University criteria can be used in making a definitive diagnosis of infective endocarditis. A diagnosis of infective endocarditis using the Duke criteria requires the presence of two major criteria, one major and three minor criteria, or five minor criteria.[48,50] The two major criteria are persistently positive blood cultures (at least two positive cultures separated by 12 hours, or all of three or the majority of four or more separate cultures, with the first and last drawn at least 1 hour apart) and evidence of endocardial involvement as demonstrated by a positive echocardiogram or new valvular regurgitation. The six minor criteria are a predisposing heart condition; fever; vascular phenomena such as emboli, mycotic aneurysm, or intracranial hemorrhage; immunologic phenomena such as glomerulonephritis or rheumatoid factor; positive blood cultures not meeting the major criteria; and a positive echocardiogram not meeting the major criteria.

Treatment of infective endocarditis focuses on identifying and eliminating the causative microorganism, minimizing the residual cardiac effects, and treating the pathologic effects of the emboli. Antibiotic therapy is used to eradicate the pathogen. Blood cultures are used to identify the causative organism and determine the most appropriate antibiotic regimen. Surgery may be indicated for moderate to severe heart failure, progressive renal failure, significant emboli, dysrhythmias, or left-sided endocarditis. Infected prosthetic valves may need to be replaced.

Of great importance is the prevention of infective endocarditis in persons with prosthetic heart valves, previous bacterial endocarditis, certain congenital heart defects, and other known risk factors.[51] Prevention can be accomplished largely through prophylactic administration of an antibiotic before dental and other procedures that may cause bacteremia.[51]

RHEUMATIC HEART DISEASE

Rheumatic fever is an acute, immune-mediated, multisystem inflammatory disease that follows a group A (β-hemolytic) streptococcal (GAS) throat infection. The most serious aspect of rheumatic fever is the development of chronic valvular disorders that produce permanent cardiac dysfunction and sometimes cause fatal heart failure years later. In the United States and other industrialized countries, the incidence of rheumatic fever and prevalence of rheumatic heart disease has markedly declined in the past 40 to 50 years. This decline has been attributed to the introduction of antimicrobial agents for improved treatment of GAS pharyngitis, increased access to medical care, and improved economic standards, along with better and less crowded housing. Unfortunately, rheumatic fever and rheumatic heart disease continue to be major health problems in many underdeveloped countries, where inadequate health care, poor nutrition, and crowded living conditions still prevail.

Rheumatic fever is primarily a disease of school-aged children. The incidence of acute rheumatic fever peaks between 5 and 15 years of age.[8] The disease usually follows an inciting GAS throat infection by 1 to 4 weeks. Rheumatic fever and its cardiac complications can be prevented by antibiotic treatment of the initial GAS throat infection.

The pathogenesis of rheumatic fever is unclear, and why only a small percentage of persons with uncomplicated streptococcal infections contract rheumatic fever remains to be answered. The time frame for development of symptoms in relation to the sore throat and the presence of antibodies to the GAS organism strongly suggest an immunologic origin. Like other immunologic phenomena, rheumatic fever requires an initial sensitizing exposure to the offending streptococcal agent, and the risk of recurrence is high after each subsequent exposure.

Manifestations

Rheumatic fever can manifest as an acute, recurrent, or chronic disorder. The *acute stage* of rheumatic fever includes a history of an initiating streptococcal infection and subsequent involvement of the mesenchymal connective tissue of the heart, blood vessels, joints, and subcutaneous tissues. Common to all is a lesion called the *Aschoff body*,[8] which is a localized area of tissue necrosis surrounded by immune cells. The *recurrent phase* usually involves extension of the cardiac effects of the disease. The *chronic phase* of rheumatic fever is characterized by permanent deformity of the heart valves and is a common cause of mitral valve stenosis. Chronic rheumatic heart disease usually does not appear until at least 10 years after the initial attack, sometimes decades later.

Most children with rheumatic fever have a history of sore throat, headache, fever, abdominal pain, nausea, vomiting, swollen glands (usually at the angle of the jaw), and other signs and symptoms of streptococcal infection. Other clinical features associated with an acute episode of rheumatic fever are related to the acute inflammatory process and the structures involved in the disease process.

Rheumatic fever is characterized by a constellation of findings that includes carditis, migratory polyarthritis of the large joints, erythema marginatum, subcutaneous nodules, and Sydenham's chorea.

Carditis. Acute rheumatic carditis, which complicates the acute phase of rheumatic fever, may progress to chronic valvular disorders. The carditis can affect the pericardium, myocardium, or endocardium, and all of these layers of the heart usually are involved. Both the pericarditis and myocarditis usually are self-limited manifestations of the acute stage of rheumatic fever. The involvement of the endocardium and valvular structures produces the permanent and disabling effects of rheumatic fever. Although any of the four valves can be involved, the mitral and aortic valves are affected most often. During the acute inflammatory stage of the disease, the valvular structures become red and swollen; small vegetative lesions develop on the valve leaflets. The acute inflammatory changes gradually proceed to development of fibrous scar tissue, which tends to contract and cause deformity of the valve leaflets and shortening of the chordae tendineae. In some cases, the edges or commissures of the valve leaflets fuse together as healing occurs.

The manifestations of acute rheumatic carditis include a heart murmur in a child without a previous history of rheumatic fever, change in the character of a murmur in a person with a previous history of the disease, cardiomegaly or enlargement of the heart, friction rub or other signs of pericarditis, and congestive heart failure in a child without discernible cause.

Arthritis, Erythema Marginatum, Subacute Nodes, and Chorea. Although not a cause of permanent disability, polyarthritis is the most common finding in rheumatic fever. The arthritis involves the larger joints, particularly the knees, ankles, elbows, and wrists, and almost always is migratory, affecting one joint and then moving to another. In untreated cases, the arthritis lasts approximately 4 weeks. A striking feature of rheumatic arthritis is the dramatic response (usually within 48 hours) to salicylates.

Erythema marginatum lesions are maplike, macular areas most commonly seen on the trunk or inner aspects of the upper arm and thigh. Skin lesions are present only in approximately 10% of patients who have rheumatic fever; they are transitory and disappear during the course of the disease.

The subcutaneous nodules are 1 to 4 cm in diameter. They are hard, painless, and freely movable and usually overlie the extensor muscles of the wrist, elbow, ankle, and knee joints. Subcutaneous nodules are rare, but when present, they occur most often in persons with carditis.

Chorea (i.e., Sydenham's chorea), sometimes called *St. Vitus' dance*, is the major central nervous system manifestation. It is seen most frequently in girls. There typically is an insidious onset of irritability and other behavior problems. The child often is fidgety, cries easily, begins to walk clumsily, and drops things. The choreic movements are spontaneous, rapid, purposeless, jerking movements that interfere with voluntary activities. Facial grimaces are common, and even speech may be affected. The chorea is self-limited, usually running its course within a matter of weeks or months.

Diagnosis and Treatment

Diagnosis. The diagnosis of rheumatic fever is based on the Jones criteria, which were initially proposed in 1955 and revised in 1984 and 1992 by a committee of the AHA.[52,53]

The criteria were developed because no single laboratory test, sign, or symptom is pathognomonic of the disease, although several combinations of them are diagnostic. The signs and symptoms of rheumatic fever are grouped into major and minor categories. The presence of two major signs (*i.e.*, carditis, polyarthritis, chorea, erythema marginatum, and subcutaneous nodules) or one major and two minor signs (*i.e.*, arthralgia, fever, elevated levels of acute-phase reactants, and prolonged PR interval) accompanied by evidence of a preceding GAS infection indicates a high probability of rheumatic fever.

Elevated levels of acute-phase reactants are not specific for rheumatic fever but provide evidence of an acute inflammatory response. The erythrocyte sedimentation rate, C-reactive protein, and white blood cell count commonly are used; unless corticosteroids or salicylates have been used, the results of these tests almost always are elevated in persons who present with polyarthritis, carditis, or chorea. These tests also are used to determine when the acute phase of the illness has subsided. A prolonged PR interval on the ECG is a nonspecific finding. It does not correlate with the ultimate development of chronic rheumatic heart disease. Echocardiography/Doppler ultrasound (echo-Doppler) may be used to identify cardiac lesions in persons who do not show typical signs of cardiac involvement during an attack of rheumatic fever.[54]

Prevention. Prevention of initial episodes of acute rheumatic fever requires accurate recognition and proper antibiotic treatment of GAS pharyngitis. Evidence of a streptococcal infection is established through the use of throat cultures, antigen tests, and antibodies to products liberated by the streptococci. Throat cultures taken at the time of the acute infection usually are positive for GAS infection. It takes several days to obtain the results of a throat culture. The development of rapid tests for direct detection of GAS antigens has provided at least a partial solution for this problem. These tests use latex agglutination or an enzyme immunoassay and can be completed in a few minutes. Both types of tests are highly specific for GAS infection but are limited in terms of their sensitivity (*e.g.*, the person may have a negative test result but have a streptococcal infection), and a negative antigen test result should be confirmed with a throat culture when a streptococcal infection is suspected.[55] GAS elaborate a large number of extracellular products, including streptolysin O and deoxyribonuclease B. The antibodies to these products are measured for retrospective confirmation of recent streptococcal infections in persons thought to have acute rheumatic fever.[53] Penicillin (or another antibiotic in penicillin-sensitive patients) is the treatment of choice for GAS infection.[55]

Treatment. Treatment of acute rheumatic fever is designed to control the acute inflammatory process and prevent cardiac complications and recurrence of the disease. During the acute phase, prevention of residual cardiac effects is of primary concern; antibiotics, anti-inflammatory drugs, and selective restriction of physical activities are prescribed. Penicillin also is the antibiotic of choice for treating the acute illness. Salicylates and corticosteroids also are widely used.

The person who has had an attack of rheumatic fever is at high risk for recurrence after subsequent GAS throat infections. Penicillin is the treatment of choice for secondary prophylaxis, but sulfadiazine or erythromycin may be used in penicillin-allergic individuals.[55] The duration of prophylaxis depends on whether residual valvular disease is present or absent. It is recommended that persons with persistent valvular disease receive prophylaxis for at least 10 years after the last episode of acute rheumatic fever.[55]

Secondary prevention and compliance with a plan for prophylactic administration of penicillin require that the patient and family understand the rationale for such measures and the measures themselves. Patients also need to be instructed to report possible streptococcal infections to their physicians. They should be instructed to inform their dentists about the disease so that they can be adequately protected during dental procedures that may traumatize the oral mucosa.

KAWASAKI'S DISEASE

Kawasaki's disease, also known as *mucocutaneous lymph node syndrome*, is an acute febrile disease of young children. First described in Japan in 1967 by Dr. Tomisaku Kawasaki, the disease affects the skin, brain, eyes, joints, liver, lymph nodes, and heart.[56–58] The disease can produce aneurysmal disease of the coronary arteries and is the most common cause of acquired heart disease in young children. More than 3500 children with Kawasaki's disease are hospitalized annually in the United States.[57] Although first reported in Japanese children, the disease affects children of many races, occurs worldwide, and is increasing in frequency.

The disease is characterized by a vasculitis (*i.e.*, inflammation of the blood vessels) that begins in the small vessels (*i.e.*, arterioles, venules, and capillaries) and progresses to involve some of the larger arteries, such as the coronaries. The cause of Kawasaki's disease is unknown, but it is thought to be of immunologic origin. Immunologic abnormalities that include increased activation of helper T cells and increased levels of immune mediators and antibodies that destroy endothelial cells have been detected during the acute phase of the disease. It has been hypothesized that some unknown antigen, possibly a common infectious agent, triggers the immune response in a genetically predisposed child.

Manifestations

The course of the disease is triphasic and includes an acute febrile phase that lasts approximately 7 to 14 days; a subacute phase that follows the acute phase and lasts from days 10 through 24; and a convalescent phase that follows the subacute stage and continues until the signs of the acute-phase inflammatory response have subsided and the signs of the illness have disappeared.

The *acute phase* begins with an abrupt onset of fever, followed by conjunctivitis, rash, involvement of the oral mucosa, redness and swelling of the hands and feet, and enlarged cervical lymph nodes. The fever typically is high, reaching 40°C (104°F) or more, has an erratic spiking pattern, is unresponsive to antibiotics, and persists for 5 or more days. The conjunctivitis, which is bilateral, begins shortly after the onset of fever, persists throughout the febrile course of the disease, and may last as long as 3 to 5 weeks. There is no exudate, discharge, or conjunctival ulceration, differentiating it from many other types of conjunctivitis. The rash usually is deeply erythematous and may take several forms, the most common of which is a nonpruritic urticarial rash with large erythematous plaques, or a measles-type rash. Although the rash usually is generalized, it may be accentuated centrally or peripherally. Some children have a perianal rash with a diaper-like distribution. Oropharyngeal manifestations include fissuring of the lips, diffuse erythema of the oropharynx, and hypertrophic papillae of the tongue, creating a "strawberry" appearance. The hands and feet become swollen and painful, and have reddened palms and soles. The rash, oropharyngeal manifestations, and changes in hands and feet appear within 1 to 3 days of fever onset and usually disappear as the fever subsides. Lymph node involvement is the least constant feature of the disease. It is cervical and unilateral, with a single, firm, enlarged lymph node mass that usually is larger than 1.5 cm in diameter.

The *subacute phase* begins with defervescence and lasts until all signs of the disease have disappeared. During the subacute phase, desquamation (*i.e.*, peeling) of the skin of the fingers and toe tips begins and progresses to involve the entire surface of the palms and soles. Patchy peeling of skin areas other than the hands and feet may occur in some children. The *convalescent stage* persists from the complete resolution of symptoms until all signs of inflammation have disappeared. This usually takes approximately 8 weeks.

In addition to the major manifestations that occur during the acute stage of the illness, there are several associated, less specific characteristics of the disease, including arthritis, urethritis and pyuria, gastrointestinal manifestations (*e.g.*, diarrhea, abdominal pain), hepatitis, and hydrops of the gallbladder. Arthritis or arthralgia occurs in approximately 30% of children with the disease, characterized by symmetric joint swelling that involves large and small joints. Central nervous system involvement occurs in almost all children and is characterized by pronounced irritability and lability of mood.

Cardiac involvement is the most important manifestation of Kawasaki's disease. Coronary vasculitis develops in between 10% and 40% of children within the first 2 weeks of the illness, manifested by dilatation and aneurysm formation in the coronary arteries, as seen on two-dimensional echocardiography. The manifestations of coronary artery involvement include signs and symptoms of myocardial ischemia or, rarely, overt myocardial infarction or rupture of the aneurysm. Pericarditis, myocarditis, endocarditis, heart failure, and dysrhythmias also may develop.

Diagnosis and Treatment

As with rheumatic fever, the diagnosis of Kawasaki's disease is based on clinical findings because no specific laboratory test for the disease exists. Clinical criteria developed by the Japan Kawasaki Disease Research Committee and subsequently by the AHA are used in establishing a diagnosis of Kawasaki's disease.[59] The diagnosis is confirmed by the presence of a fever that lasts 5 or more days without another more reasonable explanation and by at least four of the following five acute-stage manifestations of the disease: changes in the extremities (an acute erythema and edema of the hands, followed by membranous desquamation of fingertips during the convalescent period); polymorphous exanthem (skin eruption involving the trunk and extremities); bilateral painless bulbar conjunctival injection without exudate; oropharyngeal manifestations (*e.g.*, injected or fissured lips, injected pharynx, strawberry tongue); and cervical lymphadenopathy (≥1.5 cm in diameter). Chest radiographs, ECG tests, and two-dimensional echocardiography are used to detect coronary artery involvement and follow its progress. Coronary angiography may be used to determine the extent of coronary artery involvement.

Intravenous gamma globulin and aspirin are considered the best therapy for prevention of coronary artery abnormalities in children with Kawasaki's disease.[57,58] During the acute phase of the illness, aspirin usually is given in larger doses and for its anti-inflammatory and antipyretic effects.[57,58] After the fever is controlled, the aspirin dose is lowered, and the drug is given for its anti–platelet-aggregating effects.

Recommendations for cardiac follow-up evaluation (*i.e.*, stress testing and sometimes coronary angiography) are based on the level of coronary artery changes. Anticoagulant therapy may be recommended for children with multiple or large coronary aneurysms. Some restrictions in activities such as competitive sports may be advised for children with significant coronary artery abnormalities.

In summary, infective endocarditis involves the invasion of the endocardium by pathogens that produce vegetative lesions on the endocardial surface. The loose organization of these lesions permits the organisms and fragments of the lesions to be disseminated throughout the systemic circulation. The condition can be caused by several organisms. Two predisposing factors contribute to the development of infective endocarditis: a damaged endocardium and a portal of entry through which the organisms gain access to the bloodstream.

Rheumatic fever, which is associated with an antecedent GAS throat infection, is an important cause of heart disease. Its most serious and disabling effects result from involvement of the heart valves. Because there is no single laboratory test, sign, or symptom that is pathognomonic of acute rheumatic fever, the Jones criteria are used to establish the diagnosis during the acute stage of the disease.

Kawasaki's disease is an acute febrile disease of young children that affects the skin, brain, eyes, joints, liver, lymph nodes, and heart. The disease can produce aneurysmal disease of the coronary arteries and is the most common cause of acquired heart disease in young children.

Valvular Heart Disease

After you have completed this section of the chapter, you should be able to meet the following objectives:

✦ State the function of the heart valves and relate alterations in hemodynamic function of the heart that occur with valvular disease

✦ Compare the effects of stenotic and regurgitant mitral and aortic valvular heart disease on cardiovascular function

✦ Compare the methods of and diagnostic information obtained from cardiac auscultation, phonocardiography, and echocardiography as they relate to valvular heart disease

The function of the heart valves is to promote directional flow of blood through the chambers of the heart. Dysfunction of the heart valves can result from a number of disorders, including congenital defects, trauma, ischemic damage, degenerative changes, and inflammation. Although any of the four heart valves can become diseased, the most commonly affected are the mitral and aortic valves. Disorders of the pulmonary and tricuspid valves are uncommon, probably because of the low pressure in the right side of the heart.

HEMODYNAMIC DERANGEMENTS

The heart valves consist of thin leaflets of tough, flexible, endothelium-covered fibrous tissue firmly attached at the base to the fibrous valve rings (see Chapter 21). Capillaries and smooth muscle are present at the base of the leaflet but do not extend up into the valve. The leaflets of the heart valves may be injured or become the site of an inflammatory process that can deform their line of closure. Healing of the valve leaflets often is associated with increased collagen content and scarring, causing the leaflets to shorten and become stiffer. The edges of the valve leaflets can heal together so that the valve does not open or close properly.

Two types of mechanical disruptions occur with valvular heart disease: narrowing of the valve opening so it does not open properly and distortion of the valve so it does not close properly (Fig. 24-18). *Stenosis* refers to a narrowing of the valve orifice and failure of the valve leaflets to open

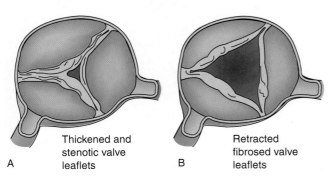

FIGURE 24-18 Disease of the aortic valve as viewed from the aorta. (**A**) Stenosis of the valve opening. (**B**) An incompetent or regurgitant valve that is unable to close completely.

A — Thickened and stenotic valve leaflets

B — Retracted fibrosed valve leaflets

normally. Blood flow through a normal valve can increase by five to seven times the resting volume; consequently, valvular stenosis must be severe before it causes problems. Significant narrowing of the valve orifice increases the resistance to blood flow through the valve, converting the normally smooth laminar flow to a less efficient turbulent flow. This increases the volume and work of the chamber emptying through the narrowed valve—the left atrium in the case of mitral stenosis and the left ventricle in aortic stenosis. Symptoms usually are noticed first during situations of increased flow, such as exercise. An *incompetent* or *regurgitant valve* permits backward flow to occur when the valve should be closed—flowing back into the left ventricle during diastole when the aortic valve is affected and back into the left atrium during systole when the mitral valve is diseased.

The effect that valvular heart disease has on cardiac function is related to alterations in blood flow across the valve and to the resultant increase in work demands on the heart that the disorder generates. Many valvular heart defects are characterized by heart murmurs resulting from turbulent blood flow through a diseased valve. Disorders in valve flow and heart chamber size for mitral and aortic valve disorders are illustrated in Figure 24-19.

MITRAL VALVE DISORDERS

The mitral valve controls the directional flow of blood between the left atrium and the left ventricle. The edges or cusps of the AV valves are thinner than those of the semilunar valves; they are anchored to the papillary muscles by the chordae tendineae. During much of systole, the mitral valve is subjected to the high pressure generated by the left ventricle as it pumps blood into the systemic circulation. During this period of increased pressure, the chordae

 Valvular Heart Disease

➤ The heart valves determine the direction of blood flow through the heart chambers.

➤ Valvular heart defects exert their effects by obstructing flow of blood (stenotic valve disorder) or allowing backward flow of blood (regurgitant valve disorders).

➤ Stenotic valvular defects produce distention of the heart chamber that empties blood through the diseased valve and impaired filling of the chamber that receives blood that moves through the valve.

➤ Regurgitant valves allow blood to move back through the valve when it should be closed. This produces distention and places increased work demands on the chamber ejecting blood through the diseased valve.

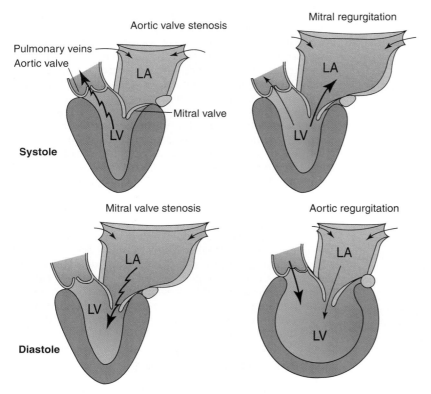

FIGURE 24-19 Alterations in hemodynamic function that accompany aortic valve stenosis, mitral valve regurgitation, mitral valve stenosis, and aortic valve regurgitation. *Thin arrows* indicate direction of normal flow, and *thick arrows* the direction of abnormal flow.

tendineae prevent the eversion of the valve leaflets into the left atrium.

Mitral Valve Stenosis

Mitral valve stenosis represents the incomplete opening of the mitral valve during diastole with left atrial distention and impaired filling of the left ventricle. Mitral valve stenosis most commonly is the result of rheumatic fever. Less frequently, the defect is congenital and manifests during infancy or early childhood.[60] Mitral valve stenosis is a continuous, progressive, lifelong disorder, consisting of a slow, stable course in the early years and progressive acceleration in later years. The 10-year survival rate for persons with untreated mitral stenosis is 50% to 60%, depending on symptoms at time of presentation.[60,61]

Mitral valve stenosis is characterized by fibrous replacement of valvular tissue, along with stiffness and fusion of the valve apparatus (Fig. 24-20). Typically, the mitral cusps fuse at the edges and involvement of the chordae tendineae causes shortening, which pulls the valvular structures more deeply into the ventricles. As the resistance to flow through the valve increases, the left atrium becomes dilated and left atrial pressure rises (see Fig. 24-19). The increased left atrial pressure eventually is transmitted to the pulmonary venous system, causing pulmonary congestion.

The rate of flow across the valve depends on the size of the valve orifice, the driving pressure (*i.e.*, atrial minus ventricular pressure), and the time available for flow during diastole. The normal mitral valve area is 4 to 5 cm². Narrowing of the valve area to less than 2.5 cm² must occur before symptoms begin to develop.[61] As the condition progresses, symptoms of decreased cardiac output occur during extreme

exertion or other situations that cause tachycardia and thereby reduce diastolic filling time. In the late stages of the disease, pulmonary vascular resistance increases with the development of pulmonary hypertension; this increases the pressure against which the right heart must pump and eventually leads to right-sided heart failure.

The signs and symptoms of mitral valve stenosis depend on the severity of the obstruction and are related to the elevation in left atrial pressure and pulmonary conges-

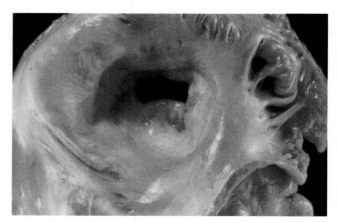

FIGURE 24-20 Chronic rheumatic valvulitis. A view of the mitral valve from the left atrium shows rigid, thickened, and fused leaflets with a narrow orifice, creating the characteristic "fish mouth" appearance of the rheumatic mitral stenosis. (Rubin E., Farber J.L. [1999]. *Pathology* [3rd ed., p. 570]. Philadelphia: Lippincott Williams & Wilkins)

tion, decreased cardiac output owing to impaired left ventricular filling, and left atrial enlargement with development of atrial arrhythmias and mural thrombi. The symptoms are those of pulmonary congestion, including nocturnal paroxysmal dyspnea and orthopnea. Palpitations, chest pain, weakness, and fatigue are common complaints. Premature atrial beats, paroxysmal atrial tachycardia, and atrial fibrillation may occur as a result of distention of the left atrium. Atrial fibrillation develops in 30% to 40% of persons with symptomatic mitral stenosis.[61] Together, the fibrillation and distention predispose to mural thrombus formation. The risk of arterial embolization, particularly stroke, is significantly increased in persons with atrial fibrillation.

The murmur of mitral valve stenosis is heard during diastole when blood is flowing through the constricted valve orifice; it is characteristically a low-pitched, rumbling murmur, best heard at the apex of the heart. The first heart sound often is accentuated and somewhat delayed because of the increased left atrial pressure; an opening snap may precede the diastolic murmur as a result of the elevation in left atrial pressure.

Medical treatment of mitral valve stenosis is aimed at relieving signs of decreased cardiac output and pulmonary congestion. Anticoagulation therapy is used to prevent systemic embolization in persons with atrial fibrillation. Three different procedures can be used to correct valve function: percutaneous mitral balloon valvuloplasty, mitral valve repair, and mitral valve replacement. Percutaneous balloon valvuloplasty, which emerged in the 1980s, has become an accepted alternative to surgical treatments in selected people.

Mitral Valve Regurgitation

Mitral valve regurgitation is characterized by incomplete closure of the mitral valve, with the left ventricular stroke volume being divided between the forward stroke volume that moves into the aorta and the regurgitant stroke volume that moves back into the left atrium during systole (see Fig. 24-19). Mitral valve regurgitation can result from many processes. Rheumatic heart disease is associated with a rigid and thickened valve that does not open or close completely. In addition to rheumatic disease, mitral regurgitation can result from rupture of the chordae tendineae or papillary muscles, papillary muscle dysfunction, or stretching of the valve structures due to dilatation of the left ventricle or valve orifice. Mitral valve prolapse is a common cause of mitral valve regurgitation.

Acute mitral valve regurgitation may occur abruptly, such as with papillary muscle dysfunction after myocardial infarction, valve perforation in infective endocarditis, or ruptured chordae tendineae in mitral valve prolapse. In acute severe mitral regurgitation, acute volume overload increases left ventricular preload, allowing a modest increase in left ventricular stroke volume. However, the forward stroke volume (that moving through the aorta into the systemic circulation) is reduced and the regurgitant stroke volume leads to a rapid rise in left atrial pressure and pulmonary edema. Acute mitral valve prolapse almost always is symptomatic; if severe, mitral valve replacement often is indicated.

The hemodynamic changes that occur with chronic mitral valve regurgitation occur more slowly, allowing for recruitment of compensatory mechanisms. An increase in left ventricular end-diastolic volume permits an increase in total stroke volume, with restoration of forward flow into the aorta. Augmented preload and reduced or normal afterload (provided by unloading the left ventricle into the left atrium) facilitates left ventricular ejection. At the same time, a gradual increase in left atrial size allows for accommodation of the regurgitant volume at a lower filling pressure.

The increased volume work associated with mitral regurgitation is relatively well tolerated, and many persons with the disorder remain asymptomatic for 10 to 20 years despite severe regurgitation.[60] The degree of left ventricular enlargement reflects the severity of regurgitation. As the disorder progresses, left ventricular function becomes impaired, the forward (aortic) stroke volume decreases, and the left atrial pressure increases, with the subsequent development of pulmonary congestion. Mitral regurgitation, like mitral stenosis, predisposes to atrial fibrillation.

A characteristic feature of mitral valve regurgitation is an enlarged left ventricle, a hyperdynamic left ventricular impulse, and a pansystolic (throughout systole) murmur. Valvular surgery may be indicated for persons with severe regurgitant disease.

Mitral Valve Prolapse

Sometimes referred to as the *floppy mitral valve syndrome,* mitral valve prolapse occurs in 2% to 6% of the population.[61] The disorder is seen more frequently in women than in men and may have a familial basis. Although the cause of the disorder usually is unknown, it has been associated with Marfan's syndrome, osteogenesis imperfecta, and other connective tissue disorders and with cardiac, hematologic, neuroendocrine, metabolic, and psychological disorders.

Pathologic findings in persons with mitral valve prolapse include a myxedematous (mucinous) degeneration of mitral valve leaflets that causes them to become enlarged and floppy so that they prolapse or balloon back into the left atrium during systole. Secondary fibrotic changes reflect the stresses and injury that the ballooning movements impose on the valve. Certain forms of mitral valve prolapse may arise from disorders of the myocardium that result in abnormal movement of the ventricular wall or papillary muscle; this places undue stress on the mitral valve.

Most persons with mitral valve prolapse are asymptomatic and the disorder is discovered during a routine physical examination. A minority of persons have chest pain mimicking angina, dyspnea, fatigue, anxiety, palpitations, and light-headedness. Unlike angina, the chest pain often is prolonged, ill defined, and not associated with exercise or exertion. The pain has been attributed to ischemia resulting from traction of the prolapsing valve leaflets. The anxiety, palpitations, and dysrhythmias may result from abnormal autonomic nervous system function that commonly accompanies the disorder. Rare cases of sudden death have been reported for persons with mitral valve prolapse, mainly those with a family history of similar occurrences. The disorder is characterized by a spectrum of auscultatory findings, ranging from a silent form to one or more mid-systolic clicks followed by a late systolic murmur. Various abnormal ECG changes can occur. Dysrhythmias may be brought out by exercise stress testing or detected on 24-hour ECG monitoring. Echocardiographic studies have become a method for the diagnosis of mitral valve prolapse, and the availability of this technique undoubtedly has contributed to increased recognition of the problem, particularly in its asymptomatic form.

The treatment of mitral valve prolapse focuses on the relief of symptoms and the prevention of complications.[61] Persons with palpitations and mild tachyarrhythmias or increased adrenergic symptoms and those with chest discomfort, anxiety, and fatigue often respond to therapy with the β-adrenergic–blocking drugs. In many cases, the cessation of stimulants such as caffeine, alcohol, and cigarettes may be sufficient to control symptoms. Infective endocarditis is an uncommon complication in persons with a murmur; antibiotic prophylaxis usually is recommended before dental or surgical procedures associated with bacteremia. Persons with severe valve dysfunction may require valve surgery.

AORTIC VALVE DISORDERS

The aortic valve is located between the aorta and left ventricle. The aortic valve has three cusps and sometimes is referred to as the *aortic semilunar valve* because its leaflets are crescent or moon shaped (see Chapter 21, Fig. 21-9). The aortic valve has no chordae tendineae. Although their structures are similar, the cusps of the aortic valve are thicker than those of the mitral valve. The middle layer of the aortic valve is thickened near the middle, where the three leaflets meet, ensuring a tight seal. Between the thickened tissue and their free margins, the leaflets are more thin and flimsy.

An important aspect of the aortic valve is the location of the orifices for the two main coronary arteries, which are located behind the valve and at right angles to the direction of blood flow. It is the lateral pressure in the aorta that propels blood into the coronary arteries (Fig. 24-21). During the ejection phase of the cardiac cycle, the lateral pressure is diminished by conversion of potential energy to kinetic energy as blood moves forward into the aorta. This process is grossly exaggerated in aortic stenosis because of the high flow velocities.

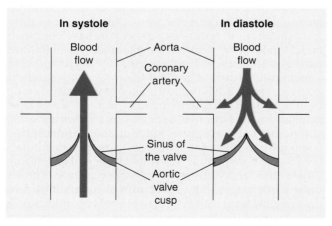

FIGURE 24-21 Location of the orifices for the coronary arteries and the direction of blood flow during systole and diastole.

Aortic Valve Stenosis

Aortic stenosis is characterized by increased resistance to ejection of blood from the left ventricle into the aorta (see Fig. 24-19). Because of the increased resistance, the work demands on the left ventricle are increased, and the volume of blood ejected into the systemic circulation is decreased. The most common causes of aortic stenosis are rheumatic fever and congenital valve malformations. Congenital malformations may result in unicuspid, bicuspid, or misshaped valve leaflets. In elderly persons, stenosis may be related to degenerative atherosclerotic changes of the valve leaflets. Approximately 25% of persons older than 65 and 35% of those older than 70 years of age have echocardiographic evidence of sclerosis, with 2% to 3% having evidence of aortic stenosis.[62]

The progression of aortic stenosis varies widely among individuals. The progression may be more rapid in persons with degenerative calcific disease than in those with congenital or rheumatic disease.[61] The aortic valve must be reduced to approximately one fourth its normal size before critical changes in cardiac function occur.[60] Significant obstruction to aortic outflow causes a decrease in stroke volume, along with a reduction in systolic blood pressure and pulse pressure. Because of the narrowed valve opening, it takes longer for the heart to eject blood; the heart rate often is slow, and the pulse is of low amplitude. There is a soft, absent, or paradoxically split S_2 sound and a harsh systolic ejection murmur that is heard best along the left sternal border.

Persons with aortic stenosis tend to be asymptomatic for many years despite severe obstruction. Eventually, symptoms of angina, syncope, and heart failure develop. Angina occurs in approximately two thirds of persons with advanced aortic stenosis and is similar to that observed in CHD. Syncope (fainting) is most commonly due to the reduced cerebral circulation that occurs during exertion when the arterial pressure declines consequent to vasodilation in the presence of a fixed cardiac output. Exertional hypotension may cause "graying out" spells or dizziness on exercise.[60] Dyspnea, marked fatigability, peripheral cyanosis, and other signs of low-output heart failure usually are not prominent until late in the course of the disease.

Both percutaneous balloon valvuloplasty and aortic valve replacement are used in the treatment of aortic stenosis. Percutaneous balloon valvuloplasty may be used to treat aortic stenosis in adolescents and young adults. In most adults with aortic valve stenosis, aortic valve replacement is the most effective treatment.

Aortic Valve Regurgitation

Aortic regurgitation is the result of an incompetent aortic valve that allows blood to flow back to the left ventricle during diastole (see Fig. 24-19). As a result, the left ventricle must increase its stroke volume to include blood entering from the lungs as well as that leaking back through the regurgitant valve. This defect may result from conditions that cause scarring of the valve leaflets or from enlargement of the valve orifice to the extent that the valve leaflets no longer meet. Rheumatic fever ranks first on the list of causes of aortic regurgitation; failure of a prosthetic valve is another cause.

Acute aortic regurgitation is characterized by the presentation of a sudden, large regurgitant volume to a left ventricle of normal size that has not had time to adapt to the volume overload. It is caused most commonly by disorders such as infective endocarditis, trauma, or aortic dissection. Although the heart responds with use of the Frank-Starling mechanisms and an increase in heart rate, these compensatory mechanisms fail to maintain the cardiac output. As a result, there is severe elevation in left ventricular end-diastolic pressure, which is transmitted to the left atrium and pulmonary veins, culminating in pulmonary edema. A decrease in cardiac output leads to sympathetic stimulation and a resultant increase in heart rate and peripheral vascular resistance that cause the regurgitation to worsen. Death from pulmonary edema, ventricular arrhythmias, or circulatory collapse are common in severe acute aortic regurgitation.[61]

Chronic aortic regurgitation, which usually has a gradual onset, represents a condition of combined left ventricular volume and pressure overload. As the valve deformity increases, regurgitant flow into the left ventricle increases, diastolic blood pressure falls, and the left ventricle progressively enlarges. Hemodynamically, the increase in left ventricular volume results in the ejection of a large stroke volume that usually is adequate to maintain the forward cardiac output until late in the course of the disease. Most persons remain asymptomatic during this compensated phase, which may last decades. The only sign for many years may be soft systolic aortic murmur.

As the disease progresses, signs and symptoms of left ventricular failure begin to appear. These include exertional dyspnea, orthopnea, and paroxysmal nocturnal dyspnea. In aortic regurgitation, failure of aortic valve closure during diastole causes an abnormal drop in diastolic pressure. Because coronary blood flow is greatest during diastole, the drop in diastolic pressure produces a decrease in coronary perfusion. Although angina is rare, it may occur when the heart rate and diastolic pressure fall to low levels. Persons with severe aortic regurgitation often complain of an uncomfortable awareness of heartbeat, particularly when lying down, and chest discomfort due to pounding of the heart against the chest wall. Tachycardia, occurring with emotional stress or exertion, may produce palpitations, head pounding, and premature ventricular contractions.

The major physical findings relate to the widening of the arterial pulse pressure. The pulse has a rapid rise and fall (Corrigan's pulse), with an elevated systolic pressure and low diastolic pressure owing to the large stroke volume and rapid diastolic runoff of blood back into the left ventricle. Korotkoff sounds may persist to zero, even though intra-arterial pressure rarely falls below 30 mm Hg.[60] The large stroke volume and wide pulse pressure may result in prominent carotid pulsations in the neck, throbbing peripheral pulses, and a left ventricular impulse that causes the chest to move with each beat. The hyperkinetic pulse of more severe aortic regurgitation, called a *water-hammer pulse*, is characterized by distention and quick collapse of the artery. In persons with severe aortic stenosis, the head may bob with each heartbeat (*i.e.*, de Musset's sign). The turbulence of flow across the aortic valve during diastole produces a high-pitched or blowing sound.

Treatment includes medical management of heart failure and associated problems. Surgery (valve replacement or repair) usually is indicated once aortic regurgitation causes symptoms.

DIAGNOSIS AND TREATMENT

Valvular defects usually are detected through cardiac auscultation (*i.e.*, heart sounds). Diagnosis is aided by phonocardiography, echocardiography, and cardiac catheterization. A phonocardiogram, a permanent recording of the heart sounds, is obtained by placing a high-fidelity microphone on the chest wall over the heart while a recording is made. An ECG tracing usually is made simultaneously for timing purposes.

The term *echocardiography* refers to a group of tests that use ultrasound to examine the heart and record information in the form of echoes. An ultrasound signal has a frequency greater than 20,000 Hz (cycles per second) and is inaudible to the human ear. Echocardiography uses ultrasound signals in the range of 2 million to 5 million Hz. The ultrasound signal is reflected (*i.e.*, echoes) whenever tissue resistance to the transmission of the sound beam changes. It is possible to create an image of the internal structures of the heart because the chest wall, blood, and different heart structures all reflect ultrasound differently. The echocardiogram is useful for determining ventricular dimensions and valve movements, obtaining data on the movement of the left ventricular wall and septum, estimating diastolic and systolic volumes, and viewing the motion of individual segments of the left ventricular wall during systole and diastole. It also can be used for studying valvular disease and detecting pericardial effusion.

There are several types of echocardiography tests: *M-mode*, two-dimensional, Doppler, and esophageal. The M-mode uses a stationary ultrasonic beam to produce a one-dimensional or "ice-pick" view of the heart. *Two-dimensional echocardiography* uses a moving ultrasonic beam to produce an integrated view of the heart comprising multiple pie-shaped images. *Doppler echocardiography* uses ultrasound to record blood flow within the heart. *Transesophageal echocardiography* uses a two-dimensional echocardiography transducer placed at the end of a flexible endoscope to obtain echocardiographic images from the esophagus. Placement of the transducer into the esophagus allows echocardiographic images of cardiac structures to be obtained from different viewpoints, rather than only from the surface of the chest. Transesophageal echocardiography is particularly useful in assessing valve function.

The treatment of valvular defects consists of medical management of heart failure and associated problems and surgical intervention to repair or replace the defective valve. Surgical valve repair or replacement depends on the valve that is involved and the extent of deformity. Valvular replacement with a prosthetic device or a homograft usually is reserved for severe disease because the ideal substitute valve has not yet been invented. Percutaneous balloon valvuloplasty involves the opening of a stenotic valve by guiding an inflated balloon through the valve orifice. The procedure is done in the cardiac catheterization laboratory and involves the insertion of a balloon catheter into the heart by way of a peripheral blood vessel.

> In summary, dysfunction of the heart valves can result from a number of disorders, including congenital defects, trauma, ischemic heart disease, degenerative changes, and inflammation. Rheumatic endocarditis is a common cause. Valvular heart disease produces its effects through disturbances of blood flow. A stenotic valvular defect is one that causes a decrease in blood flow through a valve, resulting in impaired emptying and increased work demands on the heart chamber that empties blood across the diseased valve. A regurgitant valvular defect permits the blood flow to continue when the valve is closed. Valvular heart disorders produce blood flow turbulence and often are detected through cardiac auscultation.

Heart Disease in Infants and Children

After you have completed this section of the chapter, you should be able to meet the following objectives:

✦ Trace the flow of blood in the fetal circulation, and state the function of the foramen ovale and ductus arteriosus

✦ State the changes in circulatory function that occur at birth

✦ Compare the effects of left-to-right and right-to-left shunts on the pulmonary circulation and production of cyanosis

✦ Describe the anatomic defects and altered patterns of blood flow in children with atrial septal defects, ventricular septal defects, endocardial cushion defects, pulmonary stenosis, tetralogy of Fallot, patent ductus arteriosus, transposition of the great vessels, and coarctation of the aorta

This section of the chapter provides an overview of congenital heart defects and includes the embryonic development of the heart, fetal and postnatal circulation, hemodynamic manifestations of congenital heart defects, and a description of the more common defects.

Approximately 40,000 infants are born each year with a congenital heart defect.[1] Approximately 25% of these have a severe defect that would cause death within the first year if not corrected. Premature infants have a higher incidence of congenital heart defects, most commonly patent ductus arteriosus and atrial septal defects. Depending on the type of defect, children with congenital heart disease experience various signs and symptoms associated with altered heart action, heart failure, pulmonary vascular disorders, and difficulty in supplying the peripheral tissues with oxygen and other nutrients. Advances in diagnostic methods and surgical treatment have greatly increased the long-term survival and outcomes for children born with congenital heart defects. From 1988 to 1998, death rates for congenital heart defects declined 26.1%.[1]

EMBRYONIC DEVELOPMENT OF THE HEART

The heart is the first functioning organ in the embryo; its first pulsatile movements begin during the third week after conception. This early development of the heart is essential to the rapidly growing embryo as a means of circulating nutrients and removing waste products. Most of the development of the heart and blood vessels occurs between the third and eighth weeks of embryonic life.

The developing heart begins as two endothelial tubes that fuse into a single tubular structure.[63,64] The early heart structures develop as the tubular heart elongates and forms alternate dilations and constrictions. A single atrium and ventricle along with the bulbus cordis develop first. This is followed by formation of the truncus arteriosus and the sinus venosus, a large venous sinus that receives blood from the embryo and developing placenta (Fig. 24-22). The early pulsatile movements of the heart begin in the sinus venosus and move blood out of the heart by way of the bulbus cordis, truncus arteriosus, and aortic arches.

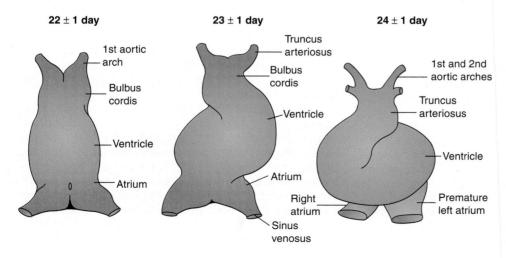

22 ± 1 day

- 1st aortic arch
- Bulbus cordis
- Ventricle
- Atrium

23 ± 1 day

- Truncus arteriosus
- Bulbus cordis
- Ventricle
- Atrium
- Right atrium
- Sinus venosus

24 ± 1 day

- 1st and 2nd aortic arches
- Truncus arteriosus
- Ventricle
- Premature left atrium

FIGURE 24-22 Ventral view of the developing heart (20–25 days). (Adapted from Moore K.L. [1977]. *The developing human* [2nd ed.]. Philadelphia: W.B. Saunders)

A differential growth rate in the early cardiac structures, along with fixation of the heart at the venous and arterial ends, causes the tubular heart to bend over on itself. As the heart bends, the atrium and the sinus venosus come to lie behind the bulbus cordis, truncus arteriosus, and ventricle. This looping of the primitive heart results in the heart's alignment in the left side of the chest with the atrium located behind the ventricle. Malrotation during formation of the ventricular loop can cause various malpositions, such as dextroposition of the heart.

The embryonic heart undergoes further development as partitioning of the chambers occurs. Partitioning of the AV canal, atrium, and ventricle begins in the fourth week and essentially is complete by the fifth week. The separation of the heart begins as tissue bundles, called the *endocardial cushions*, form in the midportion of the dorsal and ventral walls of the heart in the region of the AV canal and begin to grow inward. Until the separation begins, a single AV canal exists between the atria and the ventricles. As the endocardial cushions enlarge, they meet and fuse to form separate right and left AV canals (Fig. 24-23). The mitral and tricuspid valves develop in these canals. The endocardial cushions also contribute to formation of parts of the atrial and ventricular septum. Defects in endocardial cushion formation can result in atrial and ventricular septal defects, complete AV canal defects, and anomalies of the mitral and tricuspid valves.

Compartmentalization of the ventricles begins with the growth of the intraventricular septum from the floor of the ventricle moving upward toward the endocardial cushions. Fusion of the endocardial cushions with the intraventricular septum usually is completed by the end of the seventh week.

Partitioning of the atrial septum is more complex and occurs in two stages, beginning with the formation of a thin, crescent-shaped membrane called the *septum primum* that emerges from the anterosuperior portion of the heart and grows toward the endocardial cushions, leaving an opening called the *foramen primum* between its lower edge and the endocardial cushions. A second membrane, called *septum secundum*, also begins to grow from the upper wall of the atrium on the right side of the septum primum. As this membrane grows toward the endocardial cushions, it gradually overlaps an opening in the upper part of the septum primum, forming an oval opening with a flap-type valve called the *foramen ovale* (see Fig. 24-23). The upper part of the septum primum gradually disappears; the remaining part becomes the valve of the foramen ovale. The foramen ovale forms a communicating channel between the two upper chambers of the heart. This opening, which closes shortly after birth, allows blood from the umbilical vein to pass directly into the left heart, bypassing the lungs. An *ostium secundum defect*, which is one type of atrial septal defect, is thought to result from excessive absorption of the septum primum.

To complete the transformation into a four-chambered heart, provision must be made for separating the blood pumped from the right side of the heart, which is to be diverted into the pulmonary circulation, from the blood pumped from the left side of the heart, which is to be pumped to the systemic circulation. This separation of blood flow is accomplished by developmental changes in the outlet channels of the tubular heart, the *bulbus cordis* and the *truncus arteriosus*, which undergo spiral twisting and vertical partitioning (Fig. 24-24). As these vessels spiral and divide, the location of the aorta becomes posterior and to the right of the pulmonary artery. Impaired spiraling during this stage of development can lead to defects such as *transposition of the great vessels*.

In the process of forming a separate pulmonary trunk and aorta, a vessel called the *ductus arteriosus* develops. This vessel, which connects the pulmonary artery and the aorta, allows blood entering the pulmonary trunk to be shunted into the aorta as a means of bypassing the lungs. Like the foramen ovale, the ductus arteriosus usually closes shortly after birth.

FETAL AND PERINATAL CIRCULATION

The fetal circulation is different anatomically and physiologically from the postnatal circulation. Before birth, oxygenation of blood occurs by way of the placenta, and after birth, it occurs by way of the lungs. The fetus is maintained in a low-oxygen state (PO_2 to 30 to 35 mm Hg and 60% to 70% saturation).[63–65] To compensate, fetal cardiac output is higher than at any other time (400 to 500 mL/kg/minute).

In the fetus, blood enters the circulation through the umbilical vein and returns to the placenta by way of the two umbilical arteries (Fig. 24-25). A vessel called the *ductus venosum* allows blood from the umbilical vein to bypass the hepatic circulation and pass directly into the inferior vena cava. From the inferior vena cava, blood flows into the right atrium and then is directed through the foramen ovale into the left atrium. Blood then passes into the left ventricle and is ejected into the ascending aorta to perfuse the head and upper extremities. In this way, the best-oxygenated

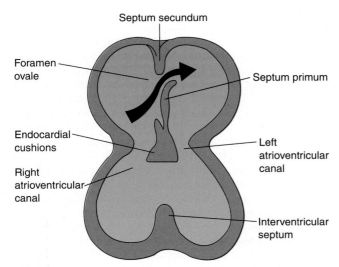

FIGURE 24-23 Development of the endocardial cushions, right and left atrioventricular canals, interventricular septum, and septum primum and septum secundum of the foramen ovale. Note that blood from the right atrium flows through the foramen ovale to the left atrium.

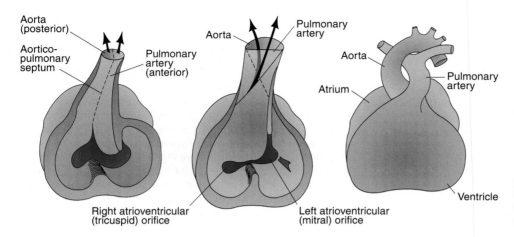

FIGURE 24-24 Separation and twisting of the truncus arteriosus to form the pulmonary artery and aorta.

blood from the placenta is used to perfuse the brain. At the same time, venous blood from the head and upper extremities returns to the right side of the heart by way of the superior vena cava, moves into the right ventricle, and is ejected into the pulmonary artery. The pulmonary vascular resistance is very high because the lungs are fluid filled and the resultant alveolar hypoxia contributes to intense vasoconstriction. Because of the high pulmonary vascular resistance, the blood that is ejected into the pulmonary artery is diverted through the ductus arteriosus into the descending aorta. This blood perfuses the lower extremities and is returned to the placenta by way of the umbilical arteries.

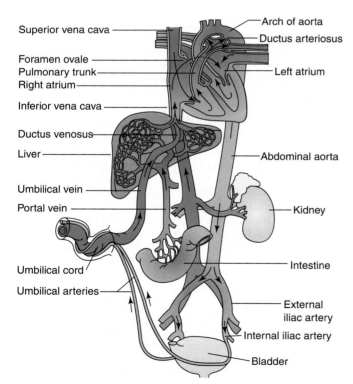

FIGURE 24-25 Fetal circulation. (Modified from Chaffee E.E., Lytle I.M. [1980]. *Basic physiology and anatomy* [4th ed.]. Philadelphia: J.B. Lippincott)

At birth, the infant takes its first breath and switches from placental to pulmonary oxygenation of the blood. The most dramatic alterations in the circulation after birth are the elimination of the low-resistance placental vascular bed and the marked pulmonary vasodilation that is produced by initiation of ventilation. The pressure in the pulmonary circulation and the right side of the heart fall as fetal lung fluid is replaced by air and as lung expansion decreases the pressure transmitted to the pulmonary blood vessels. With lung inflation, the alveolar oxygen tension increases, causing reversal of the hypoxemia-induced pulmonary vasoconstriction of the fetal circulation. Cord clamping and removal of the low-resistance placental circulation produce an increase in systemic vascular resistance and a resultant increase in left ventricular pressure. The resultant decrease in right atrial pressure and increase in left atrial pressure produce closure of the foramen ovale. Reversal of the fetal hypoxemic state also produces constriction of ductal smooth muscle, contributing to closure of the ductus arteriosus. The foramen ovale and the ductus arteriosus normally close within the first day of life, effectively separating the pulmonary and systemic circulations.

After the initial precipitous fall in pulmonary vascular resistance, a more gradual decrease in pulmonary vascular resistance is related to regression of the medial smooth muscle layer in the pulmonary arteries. During the first 2 to 9 weeks of life, gradual thinning of the medial smooth muscle layer of pulmonary arteries results in further decreases in pulmonary vascular resistance.[65] By the time a healthy, term infant is several weeks old, the pulmonary vascular resistance has fallen to adult levels.

Several factors, including prematurity, alveolar hypoxia, lung disease, and congenital heart defects, may affect postnatal pulmonary vascular development.[65] If an infant is born prematurely, the smooth muscle layers of the pulmonary vasculature may develop incompletely or regress in a shorter period. Much of the development of the smooth muscle layer in the pulmonary arterioles occurs during the latter part of gestation; as a result, infants who are born prematurely have less medial smooth muscle. These infants follow the same pattern of smooth muscle regression, but because less muscle exists, the muscle layer may regress in a shorter period. The pulmonary vascular smooth muscle in premature infants also may be less responsive to hypoxia. For these reasons, a premature infant may demonstrate a larger decrease in pulmonary vascular resistance and a resultant shunting of blood from the aorta through the ductus arteriosus to the pulmonary artery within hours of birth.

Hypoxia during the first days of life may delay or prevent the normal decrease in pulmonary vascular resistance. During this period, the pulmonary arteries remain reactive and can constrict in response to hypoxia, acidosis, hyperinflation of the alveoli, and hypothermia. Alveolar hypoxia is one of the most potent stimuli of pulmonary vasoconstriction and pulmonary hypertension in the neonate.

CONGENITAL HEART DEFECTS

The major development of the fetal heart occurs between the fourth and seventh weeks of gestation, and most congenital heart defects arise during this time. The development of the heart may be altered by environmental, genetic, and chromosomal influences.

Most congenital heart defects are thought to be multifactorial in origin, resulting from an interaction between a genetic predisposition toward development of a heart defect and environmental influences. Infants born to parents with congenital heart defects or with siblings who have congenital heart defects are at higher risk. Some heart defects, such as coarctation of the aorta, atrial septal defect of the secundum type, pulmonary valve stenosis, and certain ventricular septal defects, have a stronger familial predisposition than others.

Approximately 13% of children with congenital heart disease have an associated chromosomal abnormality. Heart disease is found in 90% of children with trisomy 18, 50% of those with trisomy 21, and 40% of those with Turner's syndrome.[64] Another 2% to 4% of cases result from adverse maternal conditions and teratogenic influences, including maternal diabetes, congenital rubella, maternal alcohol ingestion, and treatment with anticonvulsant drugs.[64]

Ultrasound technology now allows examination of fetal development and function in utero.[64,66] Diagnostic images of the fetal heart can be obtained as early as 16 weeks of gestation. Echocardiography of the fetus allows for differentiation among heart defects in the fetus. Among the disorders that can be diagnosed with certainty by fetal echocardiography are hypoplastic left heart syndrome, aortic valve stenosis, hypertrophic cardiomyopathy, pulmonic valve stenosis, AV septal defect, transposition of the great arteries, and patent ductus arteriosus.[66]

Acyanotic and Cyanotic Disorders

Congenital heart defects produce their effects through abnormal shunting of blood and alterations in pulmonary blood flow. They commonly are classified as congenital heart disease with cyanosis or congenital heart disease with little or no cyanosis.[65,67] Left-to-right shunts commonly are categorized as acyanotic disorders and right-to-left shunts with obstruction as cyanotic disorders. Of the congenital defects discussed in this chapter, patent ductus arteriosus, atrial and ventricular septal defects, endocardial cushion de-

fects, pulmonary valve stenosis, and coarctation of the aorta are considered defects with little or no cyanosis; tetralogy of Fallot and transposition of the great vessels are considered defects with cyanosis.

Shunting of blood refers to the diverting of blood flow from one system to the other—from the arterial to the venous system (*i.e.*, left-to-right shunt) or from the venous to the arterial system (*i.e.*, right-to-left shunt). The shunting of blood in congenital heart defects is determined by the presence of an abnormal opening between the right and left circulations and the degree of resistance to flow through the opening.

A right-to-left shunt results in unoxygenated blood moving from the right side of the heart into the left side of the heart and then being ejected into the systemic circulation. Cyanosis develops when sufficient unoxygenated blood mixes with oxygenated blood in the left side of the heart. In left-to-right shunt, blood intended for ejection into the systemic circulation is recirculated through the right side of the heart and back through the lungs; this increased volume distends the right side of the heart and pulmonary circulation and increases the workload placed on the right ventricle. A child with a septal defect that causes left-to-right shunting usually has an enlarged right side of the heart and pulmonary blood vessels.

The vascular resistance of the systemic and pulmonary circulations may influence the direction of shunting. Because of the high pulmonary vascular resistance in the neonate, atrial and septal defects usually do not produce significant shunt or symptoms during the first weeks of life. As the pulmonary vascular smooth muscle regresses in the neonate, the resistance in the pulmonary circulation normally falls below that of the systemic circulation; in uncomplicated atrial or ventricular septal defects, blood shunts from the left side of the heart to the right. In more complicated ventricular septal defects, increased resistance to outflow may affect the pattern of shunting. For example, defects that increase resistance to aortic outflow (*e.g.*, aortic valve stenosis, coarctation of the aorta) increase left-to-right shunting, and defects that obstruct pulmonary outflow (*e.g.*, pulmonary valve stenosis, increased pulmonary vascular resistance) increase right-to-left shunting. Crying may increase right-to-left shunting in infants with septal defects by increasing pulmonary vascular resistance. This may be one of the reasons some infants with congenital heart defects become cyanotic during crying.

Changes in Pulmonary Vascular Resistance and Blood Flow

In contrast to the arterioles in the systemic circulation, the mature pulmonary arterioles are thin-walled vessels, and they can accommodate various levels of stroke volume from the right heart. Many of the complications of congenital heart disorders result from their effect on the pulmonary circulation, which may be exposed to an increase or a decrease in blood flow.

In a term infant who has a congenital heart defect that produces markedly increased pulmonary blood flow (*e.g.*, ventricular septal defect), the increased flow stimulates pulmonary vasoconstriction and prevents normal thinning of pulmonary vascular smooth muscle. These conditions delay or reduce the normal decrease in pulmonary vascular resistance. As a result, symptoms related to increased pulmonary blood flow often are not apparent until the infant is 4 to 12 weeks of age.

Congenital heart defects that persistently increase pulmonary blood flow or pulmonary vascular resistance have the potential of causing pulmonary hypertension and producing pathologic changes in the pulmonary vasculature. When shunting of systemic blood flow into the pulmonary circulation threatens permanent injury to the pulmonary vessels, a surgical procedure may be done in an attempt to reduce the flow by increasing resistance to outflow from the right ventricle. This procedure, called *pulmonary banding*, consists of placing a constrictive band around the main pulmonary artery. The banding technique is used as a temporary measure to alleviate the symptoms and protect the pulmonary vessels in anticipation of later surgical repair of the defect. This procedure requires thoracotomy (*i.e.*, opening the chest cavity) but does not necessitate cardiopulmonary bypass (*i.e.*, use of the heart–lung machine).

Some congenital heart defects, such as pulmonary valve stenosis, decrease pulmonary blood flow, producing inadequate oxygenation of blood. The affected child may experience fatigue, exertional dyspnea, impaired growth, and even syncope.

Manifestations and Treatment

Congenital heart defects manifest with numerous signs and symptoms. Some defects, such as patent ductus arteriosus and small ventricular septal defects, close spontaneously, and in other, less severe defects, there are no signs and symptoms. The disorder typically is discovered during a routine health examination. Pulmonary congestion, cardiac failure, and decreased peripheral perfusion are the chief concerns in children with more severe defects. Such defects often cause problems shortly after birth or early in infancy. The child may exhibit cyanosis, respiratory difficulty, and fatigability and is likely to have difficulty with feeding and failure to thrive. A generalized cyanosis that persists longer than 3 hours after birth suggests congenital heart disease.

One technique for evaluating the infant consists of administering 100% oxygen for 10 minutes. If the infant "pinks up," the cyanosis probably was caused by respiratory problems. Because infant cyanosis may appear as a duskiness, it is important to assess the color of the mucous membranes, fingernails, toenails, tongue, and lips. Pulmonary congestion in the infant causes an increase in respiratory rate, orthopnea, grunting, wheezing, coughing, and rales. The infant whose peripheral perfusion is markedly decreased may appear to be in a shocklike state.

The manifestations and treatment of heart failure in the infant and young child are similar to those in the adult, but the infant's small size and limited physical reserve make the manifestations more serious and treatment more difficult. The treatment plan usually includes supportive therapy designed to help the infant compensate for the limitations in cardiac reserve and to prevent complications. Surgical intervention often is required for severe defects; it may be done in the early weeks of life or, conditions permitting,

delayed until the child is older. A discussion of congestive heart failure in children is presented in Chapter 26.

Most children with structural congenital heart disease and those who have had corrective surgery are at risk for development of infectious endocarditis. These children should receive prophylactic antibiotic therapy during periods of increased risk of bacteremia.

Types of Defects

Congenital heart defects can affect almost any of the cardiac structures or central blood vessels. Defects include communication between heart chambers, interrupted development of the heart chambers or valve structures, malposition of heart chambers and great vessels, and altered closure of fetal communication channels. The particular defect reflects the embryo's stage of development at the time it occurred. Some congenital heart disorders, such as tetralogy of Fallot, involve several defects. The development of the heart is simultaneous and sequential; a heart defect may reflect the multiple developmental events that were occurring simultaneously or sequentially. At least 35 types of defects have been identified, the most common being patent ductus arteriosus (6% to 11%), atrial septal defects (8% to 13%), and ventricular septal defects (20% to 25%).[1]

Patent Ductus Arteriosus. Patent ductus arteriosus results from persistence of the fetal ductus beyond the prenatal period. In fetal life, the ductus arteriosus is the vital link by which blood from the right side of the heart bypasses the lungs and enters the systemic circulation (Fig. 24-26G). After birth, this passage no longer is needed, and it usually closes during the first 24 to 72 hours. The physiologic stimulus and mechanisms associated with permanent closure of the ductus are not entirely known, but the fact that infant hypoxia predisposes to a delayed closure suggests that the increase in arterial oxygen levels that occurs immediately after birth plays a role. Additional factors that contribute to closure are a fall in endogenous levels of prostaglandins and adenosine and the release of vasoactive substances. After constriction, the lumen of the ductus becomes permanently sealed with fibrous tissue within 2 to 3 weeks. Ductal closure may be delayed or prevented in very premature infants, probably as a result of a combination of factors, including decreased medial muscle in the ductus wall, decreased constrictive response to oxygen, and increased circulating levels of vasodilating prostaglandins. Hemodynamically significant patent ductus arteriosus is observed in approximately one half of infants with birth weights less than 1000 g.[64] Ductal closure also may be delayed in infants with congenital heart defects that produce a decrease in oxygen tension.

As is true of other heart and circulatory defects, patency of the ductus arteriosus may vary; the size of the opening may be small, medium, or large. After the infant's pulmonary vascular resistance falls, the patent ductus arteriosus provides for a continuous runoff of aortic blood into the pulmonary artery, causing a decrease in aortic diastolic and mean arterial pressure and a widening of the pulse pressure. With a large patent ductus, the runoff is continuous, resulting in increased pulmonary blood flow, pulmonary congestion, and increased resistance against which the right

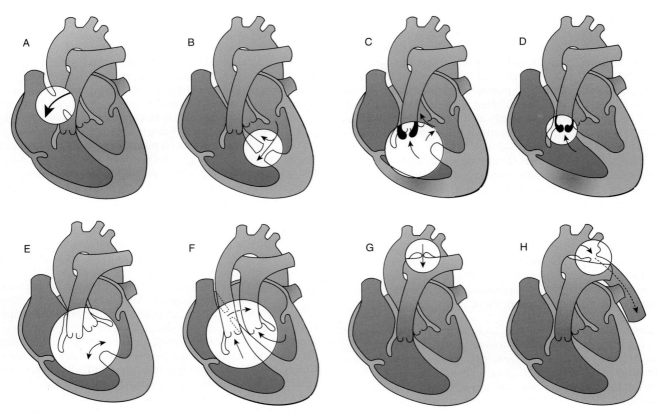

FIGURE 24-26 Congenital heart defects. (**A**) Atrial septal defect. Blood is shunted from left to right. (**B**) Ventricular septal defect. Blood is usually shunted from left to right. (**C**) Tetralogy of Fallot. This involves a ventricular septal defect, dextroposition of the aorta, right ventricular outflow obstruction, and right ventricular hypertrophy. Blood is shunted from right to left. (**D**) Pulmonary stenosis, with decreased pulmonary blood flow and right ventricular hypertrophy. (**E**) Endocardial cushion defects. Blood flows between the chambers of the heart. (**F**) Transposition of the great vessels. The pulmonary artery is attached to the left side of the heart and the aorta to the right side. (**G**) Patent ductus arteriosus. The high-pressure blood of the aorta is shunted back to the pulmonary artery. (**H**) Postductal coarctation of the aorta.

side of the heart must pump. Increased pulmonary venous return and increased work demands may lead to left ventricular failure.

Patent ductus arteriosus can be treated either pharmacologically or surgically. Indomethacin, an inhibitor of prostaglandin synthesis, is used to induce closure of a patent ductus arteriosus. Indomethacin has been associated with several adverse effects in newborns, including alterations in renal function and gastrointestinal complications. Recent studies suggest that ibuprofen, another prostaglandin inhibitor, may be equally effective in promoting closure and may produce fewer side effects.[68] Surgical closure can be accomplished using a transcatheter or a thoracoscopic approach. Transcatheter closure, using a Teflon plug, occlusive umbrella, or intravascular coil, is done in the cardiac catheterization laboratory.[64,66] The thoracoscopic surgical technique, which is used to ligate the ductus, allows closure to be accomplished without thoracotomy.

The function of the ductus arteriosus in providing a right-to-left shunt in prenatal life has prompted the surgical creation of an aortic-pulmonary shunt as a means of improving pulmonary blood flow in children with severe pulmonary outflow disorders. Research has focused on the role of type E prostaglandins in maintaining the patency of the ductus. By injecting prostaglandin E into the umbilical vein of infants who require a ductal shunt, closure has been delayed or prevented.

Atrial Septal Defects. In atrial septal defects, a hole in the atrial septum persists as a result of improper septal formation (see Fig. 24-26A). Two common types of atrial septal defects are those that involve the ostium secundum (most common) and the ostium primum (with endocardial cushion defects). The defect occurs more frequently in females than males. It may be single or multiple and varies from a small, asymptomatic opening to a large, symptomatic opening.

Most atrial septal defects are small and discovered inadvertently during a routine physical examination.[69] In the case of an isolated septal defect that is large enough to allow shunting, the flow of blood usually is from the left side to the right side of the heart because of the more compliant right ventricle and because the pulmonary vascular resistance is lower than the systemic vascular resistance. This produces right ventricular volume overload and increased pulmonary blood flow. The increased volume of blood that must be ejected from the right heart also prolongs closure of the pulmonary valve and produces a separation (*i.e.,* fixed splitting) of the aortic and pulmonary components of the second heart sound. Most children with atrial septal defects are asymptomatic. Adolescents and young adults may experience atrial fibrillation or atrial flutter and palpations because of atrial dilation.

Because spontaneous closure occurs in some children, surgical treatment usually is delayed until the child is of school age. Transcatheter closure in the cardiac catheterization laboratory has proved effective. This procedure uses a double-umbrella catheter, with an umbrella placed on each side of the defect.[65] It often is used in children who have complex congenital heart defects that require multistage surgical procedures. This approach can eliminate one surgical procedure. Surgical closure may be necessary when the defect does not close spontaneously or transcatheter closure is not deemed appropriate.

Ventricular Septal Defects. A ventricular septal defect is an opening in the ventricular septum that results from an imperfect separation of the ventricles during early fetal development (see Fig. 24-26B). Ventricular septal defects are the most common form of congenital heart defect, accounting for 20% to 25% of congenital heart disorders.[64,69] Ventricular septal defects may be the only cardiac defect, or they may be one of multiple cardiac anomalies.

The ventricular septum originates from two sources: the interventricular groove of the folded tubular heart that gives rise to the muscular part of the septum, and the endocardial cushions that extend to form the membranous portion of the septum. The upper membranous portion of the septum is the last area to close, and it is here that most defects occur.

Depending on the size of the opening, the signs and symptoms of a ventricular septal defect may range from an asymptomatic murmur to congestive heart failure. If the defect is small, it allows a small shunt and small increases in pulmonary blood flow. These defects produce few symptoms, and approximately one third close spontaneously.[65] With medium-sized defects, a larger shunt occurs, producing a larger increase in pulmonary blood flow (*i.e.,* twice as much blood may pass through the pulmonary circulation as through the systemic circulation). The increased pulmonary flow most often occurs under relatively low pressure. Most of the children with such defects are asymptomatic and have a low risk for development of pulmonary vascular disease.

Children with large defects have a large amount of pulmonary blood flow. Because the defect is nonrestrictive, the pressure in the left and right sides of the heart is equalized, and blood is shunted from the left side of the heart into the pulmonary artery under high pressures that are sufficient to produce pulmonary hypertension. In these children, left-to-right shunting through the ventricular defect is lessened when pulmonary and systemic circulations offer equal resistance to flow. The child's symptoms improve during this time.[65] As the child's pulmonary vascular resistance in-

creases further, a right-to-left shunt develops, and the child demonstrates cyanosis. This reversal of the direction of shunt flow is called *Eisenmenger's syndrome.*

Most infants with a ventricular septal defect are asymptomatic during early infancy because the higher pulmonary vascular resistance prevents shunting from occurring. After an infant's pulmonary vascular resistance falls and a shunt develops, a characteristic systolic murmur develops. The infant with a large, uncomplicated ventricular septal defect usually is asymptomatic until pulmonary vascular resistance begins to fall at approximately 4 to 25 weeks of age. After a large shunt develops, the mother reports that the infant breathes rapidly, feeds poorly, and is diaphoretic (*i.e.,* signs of congestive heart failure). Right-to-left shunting produces cyanosis.

The treatment of a ventricular septal defect depends on the size of the defect and accompanying hemodynamic derangements. Children with small or medium-sized defects are followed closely in the hope that the defect will close spontaneously. Prophylactic antibiotic therapy is given during periods of increased risk for bacteremia. Cardiac catheterization may be performed in children with medium-sized or large defects who become symptomatic to document the location of the lesion, identify any associated heart defects, and determine the pulmonary vascular resistance. Congestive heart failure is treated medically. Surgical intervention is required for infants who do not respond to medical management. When possible, surgical closure of the defect is performed. Pulmonary artery banding may be done in cases of complex congenital defects with the risk of pulmonary vascular involvement, in children with defects that are not amenable to medical or surgical treatment, or when the ventricular defect is only one of several defects present. The pulmonary band is removed when the ventricular defect is closed during open heart surgery at a later time.

Endocardial Cushion Defects. The endocardial cushions form the AV canals, the upper part of the ventricular septum, and the lower part of the atrial septum. Endocardial cushion defects are responsible for approximately 5% of all congenital heart defects. As many as 50% of children with Down syndrome have endocardial cushion defects.[65]

Because endocardial cushions contribute to multiple aspects of heart development, several variations with this type of defect are possible. The terms most commonly used to categorize endocardial cushion defects are *partial* and *complete AV canal defects.*[65] In partial AV canal defects, the two AV valve rings are complete and separate. The most common type of partial AV canal defect is an ostium primum defect, with a cleft in the mitral valve. In complete canal defect, there is a common AV valve orifice along with defects in both the atrial and ventricular septal tissue. Many variations of these two forms of endocardial cushion defect are possible (see Fig. 24-26E). Ebstein's anomaly is a defect in endocardial cushion development characterized by displacement of tricuspid valvular tissue into the ventricle. The displaced tricuspid leaflets are attached directly to the right ventricular endocardial surface or to shortened or malformed chordae tendineae.

The direction and magnitude of a shunt in a child with endocardial cushion defects are determined by the combination of defects and the child's pulmonary and systemic vascular resistance. The hemodynamic effects of an isolated ostium primum defect are those of the previously described atrial septal defect. These children are largely asymptomatic during childhood. If a ventricular septal defect is present, pulmonary blood flow is increased after pulmonary vascular resistance falls. Many children with ventricular septal defects have effort intolerance, easy fatigability, and recurrent infections, particularly when the shunt is large. The larger the defect, the greater is the shunt and the higher is the pressure in the pulmonary vascular system.

With complete AV canal defects, congestive heart failure and intercurrent pulmonary infections appear early in infancy. There is left-to-right shunting and transatrial and transventricular mixing of blood. Pulmonary hypertension and increased pulmonary vascular resistance are common. Cyanosis develops with progressive shunting.

The treatment for endocardial cushion defects is determined by the severity of the defect. With an ostium primum defect, surgical repair usually is planned on an elective basis before the child enters school. Palliative or corrective surgery is required in infants with complete AV canal defects who have congestive heart failure and do not respond to medical treatment. Total surgical repair of complete AV canal defects can be accomplished with low operative risk.

Pulmonary Stenosis. Pulmonary stenosis may occur as an isolated valvular lesion or in conjunction with more complex defects, such as tetralogy of Fallot. In isolated valvular defects, the pulmonary cusps may be absent or malformed, or they may remain fused at their commissural edges; all three abnormalities often coexist.

Pulmonary valvular defects usually cause some impairment of pulmonary blood flow and increase the workload imposed on the right side of the heart (see Fig. 24-26D). Most children with pulmonic valve stenosis have mild to moderate stenosis that does not increase in severity. These children are largely asymptomatic. Severe defects are manifested by marked impairment of pulmonary blood flow that begins during infancy and is likely to become more severe as the child grows. Cyanosis develops in approximately one third of children younger than 2 years of age.[65] The ductus arteriosus may provide the vital accessory route for perfusing the lungs in infants with severe stenosis. When pulmonary stenosis is extreme, increased pressures in the right side of the heart may delay closure of the foramen ovale.

Treatment measures designed to maintain the patency of the ductus arteriosus may be used as a palliative measure to maintain or increase pulmonary blood flow in infants with severe pulmonary stenosis. Pulmonary valvotomy often is the treatment of choice. Transcatheter balloon valvuloplasty may be used in some infants with moderate degrees of obstruction. Introduction of an expandable intravascular stent may be used to prevent restenosis.[64]

Tetralogy of Fallot. As the name implies, tetralogy of Fallot consists of four associated congenital heart defects: (1) a ventricular septal defect involving the membranous septum and the anterior portion of the muscular septum; (2) dextroposition or shifting to the right of the aorta, so that it overrides the right ventricle and is in communication with the septal defect; (3) obstruction or narrowing of the pulmonary outflow channel, including pulmonic valve stenosis, a decrease in the size of the pulmonary trunk, or both; and (4) hypertrophy of the right ventricle because of the increased work required to pump blood through the obstructed pulmonary channels[64,68,70] (see Fig. 24-26C).

Most children with tetralogy of Fallot display some degree of cyanosis—hence the term *blue babies*. The cyanosis develops as the result of decreased pulmonary blood flow and because the right-to-left shunt causes mixing of unoxygenated blood with the oxygenated blood, which is ejected into the peripheral circulation. Hypercyanotic attacks ("tet spells") may occur during the first months of life. These spells typically occur in the morning during crying, feeding, or defecating. These activities increase the infant's oxygen requirements. Crying and defecating may further increase pulmonary vascular resistance, thereby increasing right-to-left shunting and decreasing pulmonary blood flow. With the hypercyanotic spell, the infant becomes acutely cyanotic, hyperpneic, irritable, and diaphoretic. Later in the spell, the infant becomes limp and may lose consciousness. Placing the infant in the knee-chest position increases systemic vascular resistance, which increases pulmonary blood flow and decreases right-to-left shunting. During a hypercyanotic spell, toddlers and older children may spontaneously assume the squatting position, which functions like the knee-chest position to relieve the spell.[65]

Because of the hypoxemia that occurs in these children, palliative surgery designed to increase pulmonary blood flow often is needed during early infancy, with corrective surgery carried out at a later age. Palliative surgery involves the creation of a surgical shunt to increase pulmonary blood flow. The most popular procedures use the subclavian artery or prosthetic material to create a shunt between the aorta and pulmonary artery.

Transposition of the Great Vessels. In complete transposition of the great vessels, the aorta originates in the right ventricle, and the pulmonary artery originates in the left ventricle (see Fig. 24-26F). The defect is more common in infants whose mothers have diabetes and in boys. In infants born with this defect, survival depends on communication between the right and left sides of the heart in the form of a patent ductus arteriosus or septal defect. Prostaglandin E_1 may be administered in an effort to maintain the patency of the ductus arteriosus. Balloon atrial septostomy may be done to increase the blood flow between the two sides of the heart. In this procedure, a balloon-tipped catheter is inserted into the heart through the vena cava and then passed through the foramen ovale into the left atrium. The balloon is then inflated and brought back through the foramen ovale, enlarging the opening as it goes.

Corrective surgery is essential for long-term survival.[64] An arterial switch procedure (*i.e.*, Jatene operation) may be done. This procedure, which corrects the relation of the systemic and pulmonary blood flows, is preferably performed in the first 2 to 3 weeks of life, before postnatal reduction in pulmonary vascular resistance. An atrial switch procedure (*i.e.*, Mustard or Senning operation) is performed on older children. Both of these procedures reverse the blood flow at the atrial level by the surgical formation of intra-atrial baffles. The atrial switch procedures have a much higher long-term morbidity and are done when conditions prevent performance of the arterial switch procedure.

Coarctation of the Aorta.   Coarctation of the aorta is a localized narrowing of the aorta, proximal (preductal or coarctation of infancy) or distal (postductal) to the ductus (see Fig. 24-26H). Approximately 98% of coarctations are postductal. The anomaly occurs twice as often in males as in females. Coarctation of the aorta may be a feature of Turner's syndrome (see Chapter 7).

The classic sign of coarctation of the aorta is a disparity in pulsations and blood pressures in the arms and legs. The femoral, popliteal, and dorsalis pedis pulsations are weak or delayed compared with the bounding pulses of the arms and carotid vessels. The systolic blood pressure in the legs obtained by the cuff method normally is 10 to 20 mm Hg higher than in the arms.[64] In coarctation, the pressure is lower and may be difficult to obtain. The differential in blood pressure is common in children older than 1 year of age, approximately 90% of whom have hypertension in the upper extremities greater than the 95th percentile for age (see Chapter 23).

Children with significant coarctation should be treated surgically; the optimal age for surgery is 2 to 4 years. If untreated, most persons with coarctation of the aorta die between 20 and 40 years of age. The common serious complications are related to the hypertensive state. In some centers, balloon valvoplasty has been used for treatment of unoperated coarctation. This method is still being developed and ongoing clinical trials are needed to determine its long-term effectiveness and possible complications.[64]

In preductal or infantile coarctation, the ductus remains open and shunts blood from the pulmonary artery through the ductus arteriosus into the aorta. It frequently is seen with other cardiac anomalies and carries a high mortality rate. Because of the position of the defect, blood flow throughout the systemic circulation is reduced, and heart failure develops in the affected infant at an early age because of the increased workload imposed on the left ventricle. Medical and surgical methods are used to treat these infants.

In summary, the embryonic development of the heart occurs during weeks 3 through 8 after conception. During this time, development of the atrial and ventricular septa divides the embryonic tubular heart into a right and a left side. The endocardial cushions develop to form separate right and left AV canals, and the separation and spiraling of the bulbus cordis and truncus arteriosus separate the blood flow for the pulmonary and systemic circulations. At birth, the fetus takes its first breath and switches from placental to pulmonary oxygenation of blood. The foramen ovale and ductus arteriosus close, separating the pulmonary and systemic circulations. There is an almost immediate increase in systemic vascular resistance and left heart pressures and a decrease in pulmonary vascular resistance and right heart pressures. The smooth muscle layer in the pulmonary blood vessels undergoes grad-

ual thinning during the first weeks of life, producing a further decrease in pulmonary vascular resistance.

Congenital heart defects arise during fetal heart development and reflect the stage of development at the time the causative event occurred. Several factors contribute to the development of congenital heart defects, including genetic and chromosomal influences, viruses, and environmental agents such as drugs and radiation. The cause of the defect often is unknown. The defect may produce no effects, or it may markedly affect cardiac function. Congenital heart defects commonly produce shunting of blood from the right to the left side of the heart or from the left to the right side of the heart. Left-to-right shunts typically increase the volume of the right side of the heart and pulmonary circulation, and right-to-left shunts transfer unoxygenated blood from the right side of the heart to the left side, diluting the oxygen content of blood that is being ejected into the systemic circulation and causing cyanosis. The direction and degree of shunt depend on the size of the defect that connects the two sides of the heart and the difference in resistance between the two sides of the circulation. Congenital heart defects often are classified as defects that produce cyanosis and those that produce little or no cyanosis. Depending on the severity of the defect, congenital heart defects may be treated medically or surgically. Medical and surgical treatment often is indicated in children with severe defects.

Related Web Sites

American College of Cardiology—source of guidelines
    www.acc.org/clinical/statements.htm
American Heart Association—source of patient and professional
    education   www.americanheart.org

References

1. American Heart Association. (2000). *1999 Heart and stroke facts.* Dallas, TX: Author.
2. Hoyert D.L., Kochanek K.D., Murphy S.L. (1999). Deaths: Final data for 1997. *National Vital Statistics Report* 47 (19), 1–104.
3. Lorell B.H. (1997). Pericardial diseases. In Braunwald E. (Ed.), *Heart disease: A textbook of cardiovascular medicine* (5th ed., Vol. 2, pp. 1478–1505). Philadelphia: W.B. Saunders.
4. Hoit B.D. (1997). Pericardial heart disease. *Current Problems in Cardiology* 22, 359–397.
5. Guyton A., Hall J.E. (2000). *Textbook of medical physiology* (10th ed., pp. 226–229). Philadelphia: W.B. Saunders.
6. Ganz P., Braunwald E. (1997). Coronary blood flow and myocardial ischemia. In Braunwald E. (Ed.), *Heart disease: A textbook of cardiovascular medicine* (5th ed., Vol. 2, pp. 1164–1168). Philadelphia: W.B. Saunders.
7. Gregg D.E., Patterson R.E. (1980). Functional importance of coronary collaterals. *New England Journal of Medicine* 303, 1404–1406.
8. Cotran R.S., Kumar V., Collins T. (1999). *Robbins pathologic basis of disease* (6th ed., pp. 528, 566–656, 570–576). Philadelphia: W.B. Saunders.

9. Kullo I.J., Edwards W.D., Schwartz R.S. (1998). Vulnerable plaque: Pathophysiology and clinical implications. *Annals of Internal Medicine* 129, 1050–1060.

10. Falk E. (1999). Stable vs unstable atherosclerosis: Clinical aspects. *American Heart Journal* 138, S421–S425.

11. Forrester J.S. (2000). Role of plaque rupture in acute coronary syndromes. *American Journal of Cardiology* 86 (Suppl.) 15J–23J.

12. Yeghiazarians Y., Braunstein J.B., Askari A., Stone P.H. (2000). Unstable angina pectoris. *New England Journal of Medicine* 342, 101–114.

13. Ambrose J.A., Dangas G. (2000). Unstable angina: Current concepts of pathogenesis and treatment. *Archives of Internal Medicine* 160, 25–35.

14. Gibbons R.J., Chatterjee K., Daley J., Douglas J.S., Fihn D., Gardin J.M., et al., Committee Members. (1999). ACC/ACP-ASIM guidelines for the management of patients with chronic stable angina: Executive summary and recommendations. *Circulation* 99, 2829–2848.

15. Champeau L. (1976). Grading of angina pectoris [Letter]. *Circulation* 54, 522–523.

16. Gersh B.J., Braunwald E., Rutherford J.D. (1997). Chronic coronary artery disease. In Braunwald E. (Ed.), *Heart disease: A textbook of cardiovascular medicine* (5th ed., Vol. 2, pp. 1289–1316). Philadelphia: W.B. Saunders.

17. Sachs F.M., Pfeffer M.A., Moye L.A., et al. (1994). Scandinavian Simvastatin Survival Study Group. Randomized trial of cholesterol lowering in 4444 patients with coronary heart disease: The Scandinavian Simvastatin Survival Study. *Lancet* 334, 1383–1389.

18. Prinzmetal M., Kennamer, R., Merliss R., et al. (1959). A variant form of angina pectoris. *American Journal of Medicine* 27, 375–388.

19. Pepine C.J., El-Tamimi H., Lambert C.R. (1992). Prinzmetal's angina (variant angina). *Heart Disease and Stroke* 1, 281–286.

20. Cohn P.F. (1994). Silent myocardial ischemia: To treat or not to treat. *Hospital Practice* 29 (6), 107–116.

21. Chiariello M., Indolfi C. (1996). Silent myocardial ischemia in patients with diabetes mellitus. *Circulation* 93, 2089–2091.

22. Braunwald E., Antman E.M., Beasley J.W., Califf R.M., Cheitlin M.D., Hochman J.S., et al., Committee Members. (2000). ACC/AHA guidelines for the management of patients with unstable angina and non-ST-segment elevation myocardial infarction: Executive summary and recommendations. *Circulation* 102, 1193–1209.

23. Fullwood J., Butler G., Smith T., Cox M., Bride W., Mostaghimia Z., Cook P.S., Granger B.G. (2000). New strategies in management of acute coronary syndromes. *Nursing Clinics of North America* 35, 877–896.

24. Kong D.F., Blazing M.A., O'Connor C.M. (2000). Advances in the approach to acute coronary syndromes. *Hospital Practice* 35 (4), 61–82.

25. Lincoff A.M. (2000). Gusto IV: Expanding therapeutic options in acute coronary syndromes. *American Heart Journal* 140, S104–S114.

26. Unstable Angina Guideline Panel. (1994). *Unstable angina: Diagnosis and management.* AHCPR publication no. 94B0602. Rockville, MD: U.S. Department of Health and Social Services.

27. Ryan T.J., Antman E.M., Brooks N.H., Califf R.M., Hillis L.D., Hiratzka L.F., et al., Committee Members. (1999). 1999 update: ACC/AHA guidelines for the management of acute myocardial infarction: Executive summary and recommendation. A report of the American College of Cardiology/American Heart Association Task Force on Practice Guidelines (Committee on Management of Acute Myocardial Infarction). *Journal of the American College of Cardiology* 28, 1328–1428.

28. Eisenberg M.J., Topol E.J. (1996). Prehospital administration of aspirin in patients with unstable angina and acute myocardial infarction. *Archives of Internal Medicine* 156, 1506–1510.

29. Antman E.M., Braunwald E. (1997). Acute myocardial infarction. In Braunwald E. (Ed.), *Heart disease: A textbook of cardiovascular medicine* (5th ed., Vol. 2, pp. 1184–1288). Philadelphia: W.B. Saunders.

30. Bittl J.A. (1997). Advances in coronary angioplasty. *New England Journal of Medicine* 337, 1290–1302.

31. Lincoff A.M., Topol E.J. (1997). Interventional catheterization techniques. In Braunwald E. (Ed.), *Heart disease: A textbook of cardiovascular medicine* (5th ed., Vol. 2, pp. 1366–1383). Philadelphia: W.B. Saunders.

32. Shepard R., Eisenberg M.J. (2001). Intracoronary radiotherapy for restenosis. *New England Journal of Medicine* 344, 295–296.

33. Sapirstein W., Zuckerman B., Dillard J. (2001). FDA approval of coronary-artery brachytherapy. *New England Journal of Medicine* 344, 297–298.

34. Morris N.B. (1999). Brachytherapy. *Critical Care Clinics of North America* 11, 333–343.

35. Brown C.A., O'Connell J.B. (1995). Myocarditis and idiopathic dilated cardiomyopathy. *American Journal of Medicine* 99, 309–314.

36. Olinde K.D., O'Connell J.B. (1994). Inflammatory heart disease: Pathogenesis, clinical manifestations, and treatment of myocarditis. *Annual Review of Medicine* 45, 481–490.

37. Feldman A.M., McNamara D. (2000). Myocarditis. *New England Journal of Medicine* 343, 1388–1398.

38. Bradenburg R.O., Chazo J.E., Cherian G., Falase A.O., Grogogreat Y., Kawai C., et al. Committee Members. (1982). Report of WHO/ISF Task Force on the Definition and Classification of Cardiomyopathies. *British Heart Journal* 44, 672–673.

39. Richardson P., Rapporteur W., McKenna W., et al. (1996). Report of the 1995 World Health Organization/International Society and Federation of Cardiology Task Force on Definition and Classification of Cardiomyopathies. *Circulation* 93, 841–842.

40. Wyne J., Braunwald E. (1997). The cardiomyopathies and myocarditides. In Braunwald E. (Ed.), *Heart disease: A textbook of cardiovascular medicine* (5th ed., Vol. 2, pp. 1404–1451). Philadelphia: W.B. Saunders.

41. Dec G.W., Fuster V. (1994). Idiopathic dilated cardiomyopathy. *New England Journal of Medicine* 331, 1564–1575.

42. Spirito P., Seidman C.E., McKenna W.J., Maron B.J. (1997). The management of hypertrophic cardiomyopathy. *New England Journal of Medicine* 336, 775–783.

43. Golledge P., Knight C.J. (2001). Current management of hypertrophic cardiomyopathy. *Hospital Medicine* 62(2), 79–82.

44. Kushwaha S.S., Fallon J.T., Fuster V. (1997). Restrictive cardiomyopathy. *New England Journal of Medicine* 336, 267–274.

45. Pearson G.D., Veille J., Rahimtoola S., Hsia J., Oakley C.M., Hosenpud J.D., Ansari A., Baughman K.L. (2000). Peripartum cardiomyopathy: National Heart, Lung, and Blood Institute and Office of Rare Diseases (National Institutes of Health) Workshop Recommendations and Review. *Journal of the American Medical Association* 283, 83–88.

46. Felker G.M., Jaeger C.J., Kodas E., Thiemann D.R., Hare J.M., Hruban R.H., Kasper E.K., Baughman K.L. (2000). Myocarditis and long-term survival in peripartum cardiomyopathy. *American Heart Journal* 140, 785–791.

47. Karchmer A.W. (1997). Infective endocarditis. In Braunwald E. (Ed.), *Heart disease: A textbook of cardiovascular medicine* (5th ed., Vol. 2, pp. 1077–1099). Philadelphia: W.B. Saunders.

48. American Heart Association Advisory and Coordinating Committee. (1998). Diagnosis and management of infective endocarditis and its complications. *Circulation 98*, 2936–2948.

49. Bansal R.C. (1995). Infective endocarditis. *Medical Clinics of North America 79*, 1205–1239.

50. Durek D.T., Lukas A.S., Bright D.R. (1994). New criteria for diagnosis of infective endocarditis. *American Journal of Medicine 96*, 200.

51. Dajani A.S., Taubert K.A., Wilson W., et al. (1997). Prevention of bacterial endocarditis: Recommendations of the American Heart Association. *Journal of the American Medical Association 277*, 1794–1780.

52. Ad Hoc Committee to Revise Jones Criteria (Modified) of the Council on Rheumatic Fever and Congenital Heart Disease of the American Heart Association. (1984). Jones criteria (revised) for guidance in the diagnosis of rheumatic fever. *Circulation 69*, 203A–208A.

53. Committee on Rheumatic Fever, Endocarditis, and Kawasaki Disease of the Council on Cardiovascular Disease in the Young of the American Heart Association. (1993). Guidelines for the diagnosis of rheumatic fever. *Journal of the American Medical Association 268*, 2069–2073.

54. Narula J., Chandrasekhar Y., Rahimtoola S. (1999). Diagnosis of active rheumatic carditis. *Circulation 100*, 1576–1581.

55. Committee on Rheumatic Fever, Endocarditis, and Kawasaki Disease of the Council on Cardiovascular Disease in the Young of the American Heart Association. (1995). *Treatment of acute streptococcal pharyngitis and prevention of rheumatic fever.* Dallas, TX: American Heart Association.

56. Shulman S.T., DeInocencio J., Hirsch R. (1995). Kawasaki disease. *Pediatric Clinics of North America 42*, 1205–1222.

57. Taubert K.A., Stanford S.T. (1999). Kawasaki disease. *American Family Physician 59*, 3093–3108.

58. Lueng D.Y.M., Meissner H.C. (2001). The many faces of Kawasaki syndrome. *Hospital Practice 35* (1), 77–94.

59. American Heart Association. (1999). *Diagnostic guidelines for Kawasaki disease.* [On-line]. Available: http:/www.american heart.org/catalog/Kawasaki.html.

60. Braunwald E. (1997). Valvular heart disease. In Braunwald E. (Ed.), *Heart disease: A textbook of cardiovascular medicine* (5th ed., Vol. 2, pp. 1007–1076). Philadelphia: W.B. Saunders.

61. Bonow R.O., Carabello B., deLeon A.D. Jr., et. al., Committee on Management of Patients with Valvular Heart Disease. (1998). Guideline for the management of patients with valvular heart disease: Executive summary. A report of the American College of Cardiology/American Heart Association Task Force on Guidelines. *Circulation 98*, 1949–1984.

62. Massie B.M., Amidon T.M. (2001). Heart. In Tierney L.M., McPhee S.J., Papadakis M.A. (Eds.), *Current medical diagnosis and treatment* (40th ed., pp. 361–369). New York: Lange Medical Books/McGraw-Hill.

63. Moore K.L. (1998). *The developing human* (6th ed., pp. 350–371). Philadelphia: W.B. Saunders.

64. Bernstein D. (2000). The cardiovascular system. In Behrman R.E., Kliegman R.M., Jenson H.B. (Eds.), *Nelson textbook of pediatrics* (16th ed., pp. 1337–1413). Philadelphia: W.B. Saunders.

65. Hazinski M.F. (1992). *Nursing care of the critically ill child* (2nd ed., pp. 112–131, 271–361). St. Louis: Mosby-Year Book.

66. Friedman W.F. (1997). Congenital heart disease in infancy and childhood. In Braunwald E. (Ed.), *Heart disease: A textbook of cardiovascular medicine* (5th ed., Vol. 2, pp. 877–962). Philadelphia: W.B Saunders.

67. Nouri S. (1997). Congenital heart defects: Cyanotic and acyanotic. *Pediatric Annals 26*, 92–98.

68. Van Overmeire B., Smets K., Lecoutere D., Van De Broek H., Weyler J., DeGroot K., Langhendreis J. (2000). A comparison of ibuprofen and indomethacin for closure of patent ductus arteriosus. *New England Journal of Medicine 343*, 674–681.

69. Driscoll D.J. (1999). Left-to-right shunt lesions. *Pediatric Clinics of North America 46*, 355–368.

70. Waldman J.D., Wernly J.A. (1999). Cyanotic congenital heart disease with decreased pulmonary blood flow in children. *Pediatric Clinics of North America 46*, 385–404.

Chapter 25

Disorders of Cardiac Conduction and Rhythm

Jill M. White Winters

Heart muscle is unique among other muscles in that it is capable of generating and rapidly conducting its own action potentials (*i.e.,* electrical impulses). These action potentials result in excitation of muscle fibers throughout the myocardium. Impulse formation and conduction result in weak electrical currents that spread through the entire body. When electrodes are applied to various positions on the body and connected to an electrocardiographic machine, an electrocardiogram (ECG) can be recorded.

Cardiac Conduction System

After you have completed this section of the chapter, you should be able to meet the following objectives:

✦ Describe the cardiac conduction system and relate it to the mechanical functioning of the heart
✦ Characterize the four phases of a cardiac action potential and differentiate between the fast and slow responses
✦ Draw an ECG tracing and state the origin of the component parts of the tracing

In certain areas of the heart, the myocardial cells have been modified to form the specialized cells of the conduction system. Although most myocardial cells are capable of

initiating and conducting impulses, it is this specialized conduction system that maintains the pumping efficiency of the heart. Specialized pacemaker cells generate impulses at a faster rate than other types of heart tissue, and the conduction tissue transmits impulses at a faster rate than other types of heart tissue. Because of these properties, the conduction system usually controls the rhythm of the heart.

The sinoatrial (SA) node has the fastest intrinsic rate of firing (60 to 100 beats per minute) and normally is the pacemaker of the heart. It is located in the posterior wall of the right atrium near the entrance of the superior vena cava. Impulses originating in the SA node travel through the atria to the atrioventricular (AV) node (Fig. 25-1). Because of the anatomic location of the SA node, the progression of atrial depolarization occurs in an inferior, leftward, and somewhat posterior direction, and the right atrium is depolarized slightly before the left atrium.[1] There are three internodal pathways between the SA node and the AV node, including the anterior (Bachmann-James'), middle (Wenckebach's), and posterior (Thorel's) internodal tracts. These three tracts anastomose with each other proximally to the AV node. Interatrial conduction appears to be accomplished through Bachmann's bundle. This large muscle bundle originates along the anterior border of the SA node and travels posteriorly around the aorta to the left atrium.[2]

Cardiac Conduction System

➤ The cardiac conduction system controls the rate and direction of electrical impulse conduction in the heart.

➤ Normally, impulses are generated in the SA node, which has the fastest rate of firing, and travel to the Purkinje system in the ventricles.

➤ Cardiac action potentials are divided into five phases: phase 0, or the rapid upstroke of the action potential; phase 1, or early repolarization; phase 2, or the plateau; phase 3, or final repolarization period; and phase 4, or diastolic repolarization period.

➤ Cardiac muscle has two types of ion channels that function in producing the voltage changes that occur during the depolarization phase of the action potential: the fast sodium channels and the slow calcium channels.

➤ There are two types of cardiac action potentials: the fast response, which occurs in atrial and ventricular muscle cells and the Purkinje conduction system and uses the fast sodium channels; and the slow response of the SA and AV nodes, which uses the slow calcium channels.

The heart essentially has two conduction systems: one that controls atrial activity and one that controls ventricular activity. A structure called the *AV node* connects the two conduction systems and provides one-way conduction between the atria and ventricles. The AV node is located slightly beneath the right atrial endocardium, an-

terior to the ostium of the coronary sinus, and immediately above the insertion of the septal leaflet of the tricuspid valve.[2,3] In the adult, the AV node is a compact ovoid structure measuring approximately $1 \times 3 \times 5$ mm.[2] Within the AV node, atrial fibers connect with very small junctional fibers of the node itself. The velocity of conduction through these fibers is very slow (approximately one half that of normal cardiac muscle), which greatly delays transmission of the impulse into the AV node.[4] A further delay occurs as the impulse travels through the AV node into the transitional fibers and into the *bundle of His,* also called the *AV bundle.* This delay provides a mechanical advantage whereby the atria complete their ejection of blood before ventricular contraction begins. Under normal circumstances, the AV node provides the only connection between the two conduction systems. The atria and ventricles would beat independently of each other if the transmission of impulses through the AV node were blocked.

The *Purkinje system,* which supplies the ventricles, has large fibers that allow for rapid conduction and almost simultaneous excitation of the entire right and left ventricles (0.06 second).[4] This rapid rate of conduction throughout the Purkinje system is necessary for the swift and efficient ejection of blood from the heart. The Purkinje fibers originate in the AV node and proceed to form the bundle of His, which extends through the fibrous tissue between the valves of the heart and into the ventricular system. Because of its proximity to the aortic valve and the mitral valve ring, the bundle of His is predisposed to inflammation and deposits of calcified debris that can interfere with impulse conduction.[4,5] The bundle of His penetrates into the ventricles and almost immediately divides into *right and left bundle branches* that straddle the interventricular septum. The bundle branches move through the subendocardial tissues toward the papillary muscles and then subdivide into the Purkinje fibers, which branch out and supply the outer walls of the ventricles. The main trunk of the left bundle branch extends for approximately 1 to 2 cm before fanning out as it enters the septal area and divides further into two

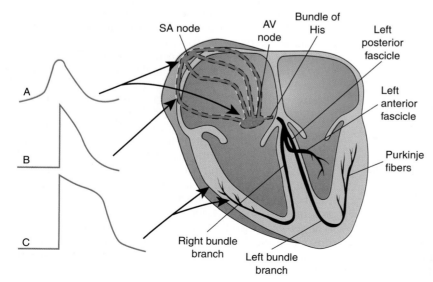

FIGURE 25-1 Conduction system of the heart and action potentials. (**A**) Action potential of sinoatrial (SA) and atrioventricular (AV) nodes; (**B**) atrial muscle action potential; (**C**) action potential of ventricular muscle and Purkinje fibers.

segments: the *left posterior* and *anterior fascicles*. The left bundle branch is supplied with blood from both the left anterior descending artery and the posterior descending right coronary arteries, whereas the right bundle branch receives its blood from both right and left anterior descending coronary arterial systems.[3]

ACTION POTENTIALS

A stimulus delivered to excitable tissues (*i.e.,* muscles, nerves) evokes an action potential that is characterized by a sudden change in voltage resulting from transient depolarization and subsequent repolarization. These action potentials are electrical currents involving the movement or flow of electrically charged ions at the level of the cell membrane (see Chapter 4). Action potentials are conducted throughout the heart and are responsible for initiating each cardiac contraction.

The inside of a cardiac cell, like all living cells, contains a negative electrical charge compared with the outside of the cell. During the resting state, the membrane is relatively permeable to potassium but much less so to sodium and calcium.[4] Charges of opposite polarity become aligned along the membrane (positive on the outside and negative on the inside; Fig. 25-2).

Depolarization occurs when the cell membrane suddenly becomes selectively permeable to current-carrying ions such as sodium. Sodium ions enter the cell and result in a sharp rise of the intracellular potential to positivity.

Repolarization is complex and poorly understood. It involves reestablishment of the resting potential. It is a somewhat slower process and involves the outward flow of electrical charges, and the membrane potential becomes reversed so that the inside becomes negative in relation to the outside.[6] The membrane conductance or permeability for potassium greatly increases, allowing the positively charged potassium ions to move outward across the membrane. This outward movement of potassium removes positive charges from inside the cell; thus, the membrane again becomes negative on the inside and positive on the outside. The sodium-potassium membrane pump also assists in repolarization by pumping positively charged

sodium ions out across the cell membrane. The sodium-potassium pump helps to preserve the intracellular negativity by moving three sodium ions out of the cell in exchange for two potassium ions.[7]

Action Potential Phases

The action potential of cardiac muscle is divided into five phases: *phase 0*—the upstroke or rapid depolarization, *phase 1*—early repolarization period, *phase 2*—plateau, *phase 3*—final rapid repolarization period, and *phase 4*—diastolic depolarization (Fig. 25-3). Cardiac muscle has three types of membrane ion channels that contribute to the voltage changes that occur during the phases of the cardiac action potential. They are the *fast sodium channels,* the *slow calcium channels,* and the *potassium channels.*

During *phase 0* in atrial and ventricular muscle and in the Purkinje system, the fast sodium channels in the cell membrane are stimulated to open, resulting in the rapid influx of sodium. The action potentials in the normal sinus and AV nodes have a much slower upstroke and are mediated predominantly by the slow calcium currents. The point at which the sodium gates open is called the *depolarization threshold*. When the cell has reached this threshold, a rapid influx of sodium occurs. The exterior of the cell now is negatively charged in relation to the highly positive interior of the cell. This rapid influx of

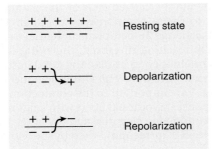

FIGURE 25-2 The flow of charge during impulse generation in excitable tissue. During the resting state, opposite charges are separated by the cell membrane. Depolarization represents the flow of charge across the membrane, and repolarization denotes the return of the membrane potential to its resting state.

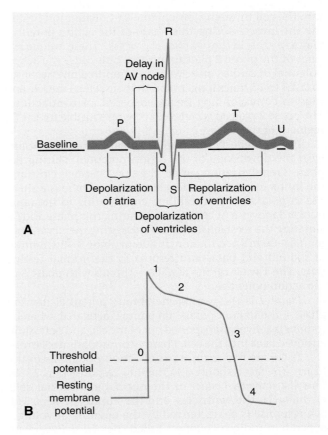

FIGURE 25-3 Relation between (**A**) the electrocardiogram and (**B**) ventricular action potential.

sodium produces a rapid, positively directed change in the transmembrane potential, resulting in the electrical spike and overshoot during phase 0 of the action potential.[6] The membrane potential shifts from a resting membrane potential of approximately –90 millivolts (mV) to +20 mV. The rapid depolarization that comprises phase 0 is responsible for the QRS complex on the ECG (see Fig. 25-3). Depolarization of a cardiac cell tends to cause adjacent cells to depolarize because the voltage spike of the cell's depolarization stimulates the sodium channels in nearby cells to open. Therefore, when a cardiac cell is stimulated to depolarize, a wave of depolarization is propagated across the heart, cell by cell.

Phase 1 occurs at the peak of the action potential and signifies inactivation of the fast sodium channels with an abrupt decrease in sodium permeability. The slight downward slope is thought to be caused by the influx of a small amount of negatively charged chloride ions and efflux of potassium.[3] The increase in intracellular negativity reduces the positive membrane voltage to a level near 0 mV, from which the plateau, or phase 2, arises.

Phase 2 represents the plateau of the action potential. If potassium permeability increased to its resting level at this time, as it does in nerve fibers or skeletal muscle, the cell would repolarize rapidly. Instead, potassium permeability is low, allowing the membrane to remain depolarized throughout the phase 2 plateau of the action potential. Contributing to the phase 2 plateau is an influx of calcium into the cell through slow channels.[6] Calcium ions entering the muscle during this phase of the action potential play a key role in the contractile process.[3] These unique features of the phase 2 plateau in these cells cause the action potential of cardiac muscle (several hundred milliseconds) to last 3 to 15 times longer than that of skeletal muscle and cause a corresponding increased period of contraction.[4] The phase 2 plateau is believed to be responsible for the ST segment of the ECG.

Phase 3 reflects final rapid repolarization and begins with the downslope of the action potential. During the phase 3 repolarization period, the slow channels close and the influx of calcium and sodium ceases. There is a sharp rise in potassium permeability, contributing to the rapid outward movement of potassium during this phase and facilitating the reestablishment of the resting membrane potential (–90 mV). At the conclusion of phase 3, distribution of sodium and potassium returns to the normal resting state. The T wave on the ECG corresponds with phase 3 of the action potential.

Phase 4 is the resting membrane potential. During phase 4, the sodium-potassium pump is activated, whereby sodium is actively transported out of the cell and potassium is moved back into the cell. Phase 4 corresponds to diastole.

There are two main types of action potentials in the heart—the fast response and the slow response (Fig. 25-4). The *fast response* occurs in the normal myocardial cells of the atria, the ventricles, and the Purkinje fibers. The fast response is characterized by the opening of voltage-dependent sodium channels called the *fast sodium channels*. The fast-response cardiac cells do not normally

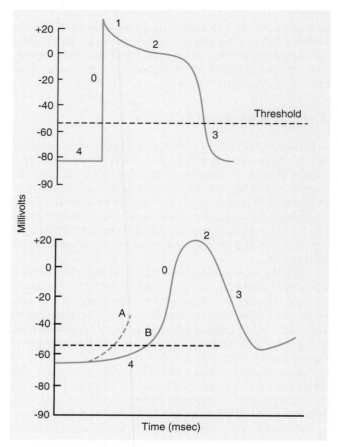

FIGURE 25-4 Changes in action potential recorded from a fast response in cardiac muscle cell (**top**) and from a slow response recorded in the sinoatrial and atrioventricular nodes (**bottom**). The phases of the action potential are identified by numbers: phase 4, resting membrane potential; phase 0, depolarization; phase 1, brief period of repolarization; phase 2, plateau; phase 3, repolarization. The slow response is characterized by a slow, spontaneous rise in the phase 4 membrane potential to threshold levels; it has a lesser amplitude and shorter duration than the fast response. Increased automaticity *(A)* occurs when the rate of phase 4 depolarization is increased.

initiate cardiac action potentials. Instead, these impulses originate in the specialized cells of the SA node and are conducted to the fast-response myocardial cells, where they effect a change in membrane potential to the threshold level. On reaching threshold, the voltage-dependent *sodium* channels open to initiate the rapid upstroke of the phase 1 action potential. The amplitude and the rate of rise of phase 1 are important to the conduction velocity of the fast response. Myocardial fibers with a fast response are capable of conducting electrical activity at relatively rapid rates (0.5 to 5.0 m/second), thereby providing a high safety factor for conduction.[8]

The *slow response* is found in the SA node, which is the natural pacemaker of the heart, and the conduction fibers of the AV node (see Fig. 25-4). The hallmark of these pacemaker cells is a spontaneous phase 4 depolarization. The membrane permeability of these cells allows a slow inward leak of current to occur through the slow channels during phase 4. This leak continues until the threshold for firing is reached, at which point the cell spontaneously depolarizes. Under normal conditions, the slow response, sometimes referred to as the *calcium current,* does not contribute significantly to depolarization. Its primary role in normal atrial and ventricular cells is to provide for the entrance of calcium during systole. The key role of calcium is in the excitation-contraction mechanism that couples the electrical activity with muscle contraction. The slow response may be the primary mode of depolarization in the presence of hyperkalemia.[9]

The rate of pacemaker cell discharge varies with the resting membrane potential and the slope of phase 4 depolarization (see Fig. 25-3). Catecholamines (*i.e.,* epinephrine and norepinephrine) increase the heart rate by increasing the slope or rate of phase 4 depolarization. Acetylcholine, which is released during vagal stimulation of the heart, slows the heart rate by decreasing the slope of phase 4.

The fast response of atrial and ventricular muscle can be converted to a slow pacemaker response under certain conditions. For example, such conversions may occur spontaneously in individuals with severe coronary artery disease, in areas of the heart where blood supply has been markedly compromised or curtailed. Impulses generated by these cells can lead to ectopic beats and serious dysrhythmias.

Absolute and Relative Refractory Periods

The pumping action of the heart requires alternating contraction and relaxation. There is a period in the action potential curve during which no stimuli can generate another action potential (Fig. 25-5). This period, which is known as the *absolute refractory period,* includes phases 0, 1, 2, and part of phase 3. During this time, the cell cannot depolarize again under any circumstances. When repolarization has returned the membrane potential to below threshold, although not yet at the resting membrane potential (–90 mV), the cell is capable of responding to a greater-than-normal stimulus. This condition is referred to as the *relative refractory period.* The relative refractory period begins when the transmembrane potential in phase 3 reaches the threshold potential level and ends just before the terminal portion of phase 3. After the relative refractory period is a short period, called the *supernormal excitatory period,* during which a weak stimulus can evoke a response. The supernormal excitatory period extends from the terminal portion of phase 3 until the beginning of phase 4. It is during this period that cardiac dysrhythmias develop.

In skeletal muscle, the refractory period is very short compared with the duration of contraction, such that a second contraction can be initiated before the first is over, resulting in a summated tetanized contraction. In cardiac muscle, the absolute refractory period is almost as long as the contraction, and a second contraction cannot be stimulated until the first is over. The longer length of the absolute refractory period of cardiac muscle is important in maintaining the alternating contraction and relaxation that is essential to the pumping action of the heart and for the prevention of fatal dysrhythmias.

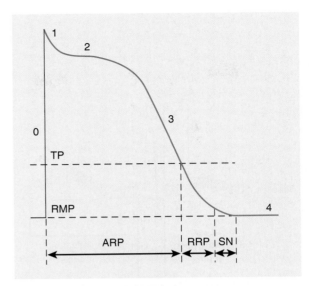

FIGURE 25-5 Diagram of an action potential of a ventricular muscle cell, showing the threshold potential (TP), resting membrane potential (RMP), absolute refractory period (ARP), relative refractory period (RRP), and supernormal (SN) period.

ELECTROCARDIOGRAPHY

The ECG is a recording of the electrical activity of the heart. The electrical currents generated by the heart spread through the body to the skin, where they can be sensed by appropriately placed electrodes, amplified, and viewed on an oscilloscope or chart recorder. The deflection points of an ECG are designated by the letters P, Q, R, S, and T. Figure 25-6 depicts the electrical activity of the conduction system on an ECG tracing. The P wave represents the SA node and atrial depolarization; the QRS complex (*i.e.,* beginning of the Q wave to the end of the S wave) depicts ventricular depolarization; and the T wave portrays ventricular repolarization. The isoelectric line between the P wave and the Q wave represents depolarization of the AV node, bundle branches, and Purkinje system (Fig. 25-7). Atrial repolarization occurs during ventricular depolarization and is hidden in the QRS complex.

The ECG records the potential difference in charge (in millivolts) between two electrodes as depolarization and repolarization waves move through the heart and are conducted to the skin surface. The shape of the recorder tracing is determined by the direction in which the impulse spreads through the heart muscle in relation to electrode placement. A depolarization wave that moves toward the recording electrode registers as a positive, or upward, deflection. Conversely, if the impulse moves away from the recording electrode, the deflection is downward, or negative. When there is no flow of charge between electrodes, the potential is zero, and a straight line is recorded at the baseline of the chart.

The ECG recorder is much like a camera in that it can record different views of the electrical activity of the heart, depending on where the recording electrode is placed. The

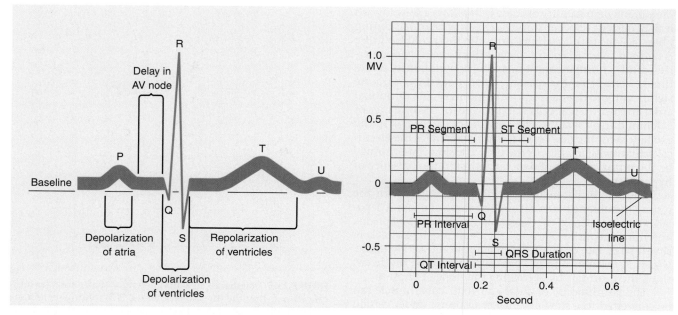

FIGURE 25-6 Diagram of the electrocardiogram (lead II) and representative depolarization and repolarization of the atria and ventricle. The P wave represents atrial depolarization, the QRS complex ventricular depolarization, and the T wave ventricular repolarization. Atrial repolarization occurs during ventricular depolarization and is hidden under the QRS complex.

horizontal axis of the ECG measures time (seconds), and the vertical axis measures the amplitude of the impulse (millivolts). Each heavy vertical line represents 0.2 second, and each thin line represents 0.04 second (see Fig. 25-6). The widths of ECG complexes are commonly referred to in terms of duration of time. On the vertical axis, each heavy horizontal line represents 0.5 mV. The connections of the ECG are arranged such that an upright deflection indicates

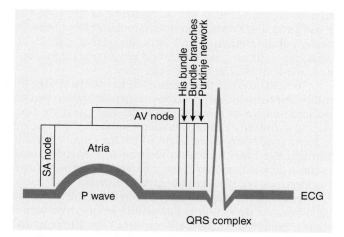

FIGURE 25-7 Tissues depolarized by a wave of activation commencing in the sinoatrial (SA) node are shown in a series of blocks superimposed on the deflections of the electrocardiogram (ECG). (Katz A.M. [1992]. *Physiology of the heart* [p. 483]. New York: Raven Press)

a positive potential and a downward deflection indicates a negative potential. Although the vertical axis determines amplitude in terms of voltage, these values frequently are communicated as millimeters of positive or negative deflection rather than in volts.

Conventionally, 12 leads are recorded for a diagnostic ECG, each providing a unique view of the electrical forces of the heart from a different position on the body's surface. Six limb leads view the electrical forces as they pass through the heart on the frontal or vertical plane. The electrodes are attached to the four extremities or representative areas on the body near the shoulders and lower chest or abdomen. The electrical potential recorded from any one extremity should be the same no matter where the electrode is placed on the extremity. Chest electrodes provide a view of the electrical forces as they pass through the heart on the horizontal plane. They are moved to different positions on the chest, including the right and left sternal borders and the left anterior surface. The right lower extremity lead is used as a ground electrode. When indicated, additional electrodes may be applied to other areas of the body, such as the back or right anterior chest.

The goals of continuous bedside cardiac monitoring have shifted from simple heart rate and dysrhythmia monitoring to identification of ST segment changes, advanced dysrhythmia identification, diagnosis, and treatment. Many diagnostic criteria are lead specific. The monitoring leads selected must maximize the potential for accurately identifying anticipated dysrhythmias and ischemic events on the basis of the patient's underlying clinical situation.

In summary, the rhythmic contraction and relaxation of the heart rely on the specialized cells of the heart's conduction system. Specialized cells in the SA node have the fastest inherent rate of impulse generation and act as the pacemaker of the heart. Impulses from the SA node travel through the atria to the AV node and then to the AV bundle and the ventricular Purkinje system. The AV node provides the only connection between the atrial and ventricular conduction systems. The atria and the ventricles function independently of each other when AV node conduction is blocked.

The action potential of cardiac muscle is divided into five phases: phase 0 represents depolarization and is characterized by the rapid upstroke of the action potential; phase 1 is characterized by a brief period of repolarization; phase 2 consists of a plateau, which prolongs the duration of the action potential; phase 3 represents repolarization; and phase 4 is the resting membrane potential. After an action potential, there is a refractory period during which the membrane is resistant to a second stimulus. During the absolute refractory period, the membrane is insensitive to stimulation. This period is followed by the relative refractory period, during which a more intense stimulus is needed to initiate an action potential. The relative refractory period is followed by a supernormal excitatory period, during which a weak stimulus can evoke a response.

Disorders of Cardiac Rhythm and Conduction

After you have completed this section of the chapter, you should be able to meet the following objectives:

✦ Describe the possible mechanisms for dysrhythmia generation
✦ Compare sinus dysrhythmias with atrial dysrhythmias
✦ Characterize the effects of atrial flutter and atrial fibrillation on heart rhythm
✦ Describe the characteristics of first-, second-, and third-degree heart block
✦ Compare the effects of premature ventricular contractions, ventricular tachycardia, and ventricular fibrillation on cardiac function
✦ Cite the types of cardiac conditions that can be diagnosed using the ECG
✦ Describe the methods used in diagnosis of cardiac dysrhythmias
✦ Explain the mechanisms, criteria for use, and benefits of antidysrhythmic drugs and internal cardioverter-defibrillator therapy in treatment of persons with recurrent, symptomatic dysrhythmias

The specialized cells in the conduction system manifest four inherent properties: automaticity, excitability, con-

ductivity, and refractoriness. Automaticity is the ability of certain cells of the conduction system to initiate repeated, spontaneous production of action potentials. Excitability refers to the ability of a cell to respond to external stimuli. These stimuli may be in the form of chemical, mechanical, or electrical input. All cardiac cells have the ability to conduct impulses. It is this ability that allows the heart to function in a synchronous fashion. Refractoriness is a protective mechanism that prevents the cells from responding to repeated, rapid external stimulation.

The term *dysrhythmia* refers to an alteration in cardiac rhythm. An alteration in any of the aforementioned four properties may produce dysrhythmias or conduction defects. There are many causes of altered cardiac rhythms, including congenital defects of the conduction system, degenerative changes, ischemia and myocardial infarction, fluid and electrolyte imbalances, and the effects of drug ingestion. Dysrhythmias are not necessarily pathologic; they can occur in both healthy and diseased hearts. Disturbances in cardiac rhythms exert their harmful effects by interfering with the heart's pumping ability. Rapid heart rates reduce the diastolic filling time, causing a subsequent decrease in the stroke volume output and in coronary perfusion while increasing the myocardial oxygen needs. Abnormally slow heart rates may impair the blood flow to vital organs such as the brain.

MECHANISMS OF DYSRHYTHMIAS AND CONDUCTION DISORDERS

The ability of certain cells of the conduction system spontaneously to initiate an impulse or action potential is

Physiologic Basis of Dysrhythmia Generation

➤ Cardiac dysrhythmias represent disorders of cardiac rhythm related to alterations in automaticity, excitability, conductivity, or refractoriness of specialized cells in the conduction system of the heart.

➤ Automaticity refers to the ability of pacemaker cells in the heart spontaneously to generate an action potential. Normally, the SA is the pacemaker of the heart because of its intrinsic automaticity.

➤ Excitability is the ability of cardiac tissue to respond to an impulse and generate an action potential.

➤ Conductivity and refractoriness represent the ability of cardiac tissue to conduct action potentials.

➤ Whereas conductivity relates to the ability of cardiac tissue to conduct impulses, refractoriness represents temporary interruptions in conductivity related to the repolarization phase of the action potential.

referred to as *automaticity*. The SA node has an inherent discharge rate of 60 to 100 times per minute. It normally acts as the pacemaker of the heart because it reaches the threshold for excitation before other parts of the conduction system have recovered sufficiently to be depolarized. If the SA node fires more slowly or SA node conduction is blocked, another site that is capable of automaticity takes over as pacemaker. Other regions that are capable of automaticity include the atrial fibers that have plateau-type action potentials, the AV node, the bundle of His, and the bundle branch Purkinje fibers. These pacemakers have a slower rate of discharge than the SA node. The AV node has an inherent firing rate of 40 to 60 times per minute, and the Purkinje system fires at a rate of 20 to 40 times per minute. The SA node may be functioning properly, but because of additional precipitating factors, other cardiac cells can assume accelerated properties of automaticity and begin to initiate impulses. These additional factors might include injury, hypoxia, electrolyte disturbances, enlargement or hypertrophy of the atria or ventricles, and exposure to certain chemicals or drugs.

An *ectopic pacemaker* is an excitable focus outside the normally functioning SA node. These pacemakers can reside in other parts of the conduction system or in muscle cells of the atria or ventricles. A premature contraction occurs when an ectopic pacemaker initiates a beat. Premature contractions do not follow the normal conduction pathways, they are not coupled with normal mechanical events, and they often render the heart refractory or incapable of responding to the next normal impulse arising in the SA node. They occur without incident in persons with healthy hearts in response to sympathetic nervous system stimulation or other stimulants such as caffeine. In the diseased heart, premature contractions may lead to more serious dysrhythmias.

Excitability describes the ability of a cell to respond to an impulse and generate an action potential. Myocardial cells that have been injured or replaced by scar tissue do not possess normal excitability. For example, during the acute phase of an ischemic event, involved cells become depolarized. These ischemic cells remain electrically coupled to the adjacent nonischemic area; current from the ischemic zone can induce reexcitation of cells in the nonischemic zone.

Conductivity is the ability to conduct impulses, and *refractoriness* refers to the extent to which the cell is able to respond to an incoming stimulus. The refractory period of cardiac muscle is the interval in the repolarization period during which an excitable cell has not recovered sufficiently to be reexcited. Disturbances in conductivity or refractoriness predispose to dysrhythmias.

Almost all tachydysrhythmias are the result of a phenomenon known as *reentry*.[6,10] Under normal conditions, an electrical impulse is conducted through the heart in an orderly, sequential manner. The electrical impulse then dies out and does not reenter adjacent tissue because that tissue has already been depolarized and is refractory to immediate stimulation. However, under certain abnormal conditions, an impulse can reenter an area of myocardium that was previously depolarized and depolarize it again.[10,11] This activity disrupts the normal conduction sequence. For reentry to occur, there must be areas of slow conduction and uni-

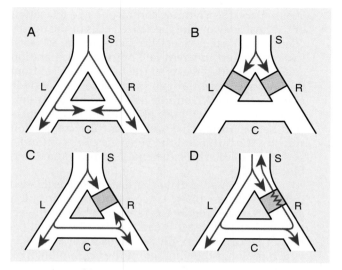

FIGURE 25-8 The role of unidirectional block in reentry. (**A**) An excitation wave traveling down a single bundle (S) of fibers continues down the left (L) and right (R) branches. The depolarization wave enters the connecting branch (C) from both ends and is extinguished at the zone of collision. (**B**) The wave is blocked in the L and R branches. (**C**) Bidirectional block exists in branch R. (**D**) The antegrade impulse is blocked, but the retrograde impulse is conducted through and reenters bundle S. (Berne R.M., Levy M.N. [1988]. *Physiology* [2nd ed., p. 417]. St. Louis: C.V. Mosby)

directional conduction block (Fig. 25-8). For previously depolarized areas to repolarize adequately to conduct an impulse again, slow conduction is necessary. Unidirectional block is necessary to provide a one-way route for the original impulse to reenter, thereby blocking other impulses entering from the opposite direction from extinguishing the reentrant circuit. Reentry requires a triggering stimulus such as an extrasystole. If sufficient time has elapsed for the refractory period in the reentered area to have ended, a self-perpetuating, circuitous movement can be initiated.

Reentry may occur anywhere in the conduction system. The functional components of a reentry circuit can be large and include an entire specialized conduction system, or the circuit can be microscopic. It can include myocardial tissue, AV nodal cells, or junctional tissue. Factors contributing to the development of a reentrant circuit include ischemia, infarct, and elevated serum potassium levels.[12] Scar tissue interrupts the normally low-resistance paths between viable myocardial cells, slowing conduction, promoting asynchronous myocardial activation, and predisposing to unidirectional conduction block. Specially filtered signal-averaged electrocardiography can be used to detect the resultant late potentials. Effects of drugs such as epinephrine can produce a shortened refractory period, thereby increasing the likelihood of reentrant dysrhythmias.

TYPES OF DYSRHYTHMIAS

Sinus Node Dysrhythmias

In a healthy heart driven by sinus node discharge, the rate ranges between 60 and 100 beats per minute. On the ECG, a P wave may be observed to precede every QRS complex.

Historically, normal sinus rhythm has been considered the "normal" rhythm of a healthy heart. In normal sinus rhythm, a P wave precedes each QRS complex and the RR intervals remain relatively constant over time (Fig. 25-9). Alterations in the function of the SA node lead to changes in rate or rhythm of the heartbeat.

Years ago, it was believed that sinus rhythm should be regular; that is, all RR intervals should be equal. Today, it is accepted that a more optimal rhythm is respiratory sinus dysrhythmia. Respiratory sinus dysrhythmia is a cardiac rhythm characterized by gradual lengthening and shortening of RR intervals (see Fig. 25-9). This variation in cardiac cycles is related to intrathoracic pressure changes that occur with respiration and resultant alterations in autonomic control of the SA node. Inspiration causes acceleration of the heart rate, and expiration causes slowing. Respiratory sinus dysrhythmia accounts for most heart rate variability in healthy individuals. Decreased heart rate variability has been associated with altered health states, including myocardial infarction, congestive heart failure, hypertension, diabetes mellitus, and prematurity in infants.

Sinus bradycardia describes a slow (<60 beats per minute) heart rate (see Fig. 25-9). In sinus bradycardia, a P wave precedes each QRS. A normal P wave and PR interval (0.12 to 0.20 second) indicates that the impulse originated in the SA node rather than in another area of the conduction system that has a slower inherent rate. Vagal stimulation decreases the firing rate of the SA node and conduction through the AV node to cause a decrease in heart rate. This rhythm may be normal in trained athletes, who maintain a large stroke volume, and during sleep. Sinus bradycardia may be an indicator of poor prognosis when it occurs in conjunction with acute myocardial infarction, particularly if associated with hypotension.

Sinus tachycardia refers to a rapid heart rate (>100 beats per minute) that has its origin in the SA node (see Fig. 25-9). A normal P wave and PR interval should precede each QRS complex. The mechanism of sinus tachycardia is enhanced automaticity related to sympathetic stimulation or withdrawal of vagal tone. Sinus tachycardia is a normal response during fever and exercise and in situations that incite sympathetic stimulation. It may be associated with congestive heart failure, myocardial infarction, and hyperthyroidism. Pharmacologic agents such as atropine, isoproterenol, epinephrine, and quinidine also can cause sinus tachycardia.

Sinus arrest refers to failure of the SA node to discharge and results in an irregular pulse. An escape rhythm develops as another pacemaker takes over. Sinus arrest may result in prolonged periods of asystole and often predisposes to other dysrhythmias. Causes of sinus arrest include disease of the SA node, digitalis toxicity, myocardial infarction, acute myocarditis, excessive vagal tone, quinidine, acetylcholine, and hyperkalemia or hypokalemia.[13]

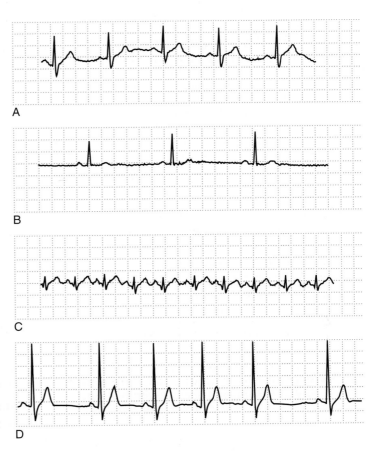

A

B

C

D

FIGURE 25-9 Electrocardiographic (ECG) tracings of rhythms originating in the sinus node. (**A**) Normal sinus rhythm (60 to 100 beats/minute). (**B**) Sinus bradycardia (<60 beats/minute). (**C**) Sinus tachycardia (>100 beats/minute). (**D**) Respiratory sinus dysrhythmia, characterized by gradually lengthening and shortening of RR intervals.

Sick sinus syndrome is a term that describes a number of forms of cardiac impulse formation and intra-atrial and AV conduction abnormalities.[14,15] Some of these types of dysfunction include spontaneous persistent sinus bradycardia that is not drug induced or appropriate for the physiologic circumstances, prolonged sinus pauses, combinations of SA and AV node conduction disturbances, or alternating paroxysms of rapid regular or irregular atrial tachydysrhythmias and periods of slow atrial and ventricular rates (bradycardia-tachycardia syndrome).[15] The most common use of the term is for bradycardia-tachycardia syndrome.[16] The bradycardia is caused by disease of the sinus node (or other intra-atrial conduction pathways), and the tachycardia is caused by paroxysmal atrial or junctional dysrhythmias. Individuals with this syndrome often are asymptomatic. Ironically, the development of atrial fibrillation may alleviate symptoms in persons who are symptomatic because heart rate can be controlled more consistently under these circumstances.[14] Sick sinus syndrome most frequently is the result of total or subtotal destruction of the SA node, areas of nodal-atrial discontinuity, inflammatory or degenerative changes of the nerves and ganglia surrounding the node, or pathologic changes in the atrial wall.[15] In addition, occlusion of the sinus node artery may be a significant contributing factor.[17]

Dysrhythmias That Originate in the Atria

Impulses from the SA node pass through the conductive pathways in the atria to the AV node. Dysrhythmias of atrial origin include premature atrial contractions, paroxysmal supraventricular tachycardia, atrial flutter, and atrial fibrillation (Fig. 25-10).

Premature Atrial Contractions. Premature atrial contractions can originate in the atrial conduction pathways or in atrial muscle cells, and they occur before the next expected sinus impulse. This impulse to contract usually is transmitted to the ventricle and back to the SA node. The location of the ectopic focus determines the configuration of the P wave. In general, the closer the ectopic focus is to the SA node, the more the ectopic complex resembles

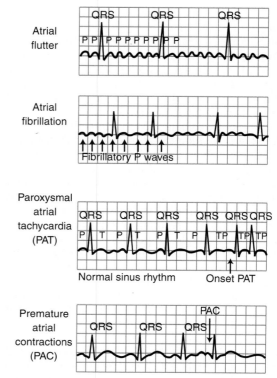

FIGURE 25-10 Electrocardiographic tracings of atrial dysrhythmias. Atrial flutter *(first tracing)* is characterized by the atrial flutter (P) waves occurring at a rate of 240 to 450 beats per minute. The ventricular rate remains regular because of the conduction of every sixth atrial contraction. Atrial fibrillation *(second tracing)* has grossly disorganized atrial electrical activity that is irregular with respect to rate and rhythm. The ventricular response is irregular, and no distinct P waves are visible. The *third tracing* illustrates paroxysmal atrial tachycardia (PAT), preceded by a normal sinus rhythm. The *fourth tracing* illustrates premature atrial complexes (PAC).

> ### 🔑 Supraventricular and Ventricular Dysrhythmias
>
> ➤ Supraventricular dysrhythmias represent disorders of atrial rhythm or conduction.
>
> ➤ Atrioventricular nodal and junctional dysrhythmias result from disruption in conduction of impulses from the atria to the ventricles.
>
> ➤ Ventricular dysrhythmias represent disorders of ventricular rhythm or conduction.
>
> ➤ Because the ventricles are pumping chambers of the heart, dysrhythmias that produce an abnormally slow (heart block) or rapid ventricular rate (*e.g.,* ventricular tachycardia or fibrillation) are potentially life threatening.

a normal sinus complex. The retrograde transmission to the SA node often interrupts the timing of the next sinus beat, such that a pause occurs between the two normally conducted beats. In healthy individuals, premature atrial contractions may be the result of stress, tobacco, or caffeine. They also have been associated with myocardial infarction, digitalis toxicity, low serum potassium or magnesium levels, and hypoxia.

Paroxysmal Supraventricular Tachycardia. Paroxysmal supraventricular tachycardia is sometimes referred to as *paroxysmal atrial tachycardia.* This term includes all tachycardias that originate above the bifurcation of the bundle of His and have a sudden onset and termination. They may be the result of AV nodal reentry, Wolff-Parkinson-White syndrome (caused by an accessory conduction pathway between the atria and ventricles), or intra-atrial or sinus node reentry. Paroxysmal supraventricular tachycardias tend to be recurrent and of short duration.

Atrial Flutter. Atrial flutter is a rapid atrial ectopic tachycardia, with a rate that ranges from 240 to 450 beats per minute. There are two types of atrial flutter.[14] Type I flutter (classic) is the result of a reentry mechanism in the right atrium and can be entrained and interrupted with atrial pacing techniques. The atrial rate in typical type I flutter usually is in the vicinity of 300 beats per minute, but it can range from 240 to 340 beats per minute. The mechanism of type II flutter is unknown. The atrial rate in type II flutter ranges between 350 and 450 beats per minute. On the ECG, atrial flutter generates a defined sawtooth pattern in leads II, III, aVF, and V_1.[18] The ventricular response rate and regularity are variable and depend on the AV conduction sequence. When regular, the ventricular response rate usually is a defined fraction of the atrial rate (*i.e.,* when conduction from the atria to the ventricles is 2:1, an atrial flutter rate of 300 would result in a ventricular response rate of 150 beats per minute). The QRS complex may be normal or abnormal, depending on the presence or absence of pre-existing intraventricular conduction defects or aberrant ventricular conduction.

Atrial flutter rarely is seen in normal, healthy individuals. It may be seen in persons of any age in the presence of underlying atrial abnormalities. Subgroups that are at particularly high risk for development of atrial flutter include children, adolescents, and young adults who have undergone corrective surgery for complex congenital heart diseases.[14]

Atrial Fibrillation. Atrial fibrillation is the result of chaotic current flow in the atria. When the atrial cells cannot repolarize in time for the next incoming stimulus, the ectopic current is rejected by the refractory cells and sent in another direction. These activities result in atrial fibrillation. It is characterized electrocardiographically by grossly disorganized atrial electrical activity that is irregular with respect to rate and rhythm. This conduction abnormality results in disorganized atrial depolarizations without effective atrial contraction. Conduction through the AV node occurs at random intervals, peripheral pulses are grossly irregular, and a pulse deficit can be observed. On ECG, there are no discernible P waves. Atrial activity is depicted by fibrillatory (f) waves of varying amplitude, duration, and morphology. These f waves appear as random oscillation of the baseline. Because of the random conduction through the AV node, QRS complexes appear in an irregular pattern. Atrial fibrillation may appear paroxysmally or be a chronic phenomenon.[18] Atrial fibrillation can be seen in persons without any apparent disease, or it may occur in individuals with coronary artery disease, mitral valve disease, ischemic heart disease, hypertension, myocardial infarction, pericarditis, congestive heart failure, digitalis toxicity, and hyperthyroidism. Atrial fibrillation is the most common atrial dysrhythmia in the elderly. It predisposes individuals to thrombus formation in the atria, with subsequent risk of formation of systemic emboli.

Junctional Dysrhythmias

The AV node can act as a pacemaker in the event the SA node fails to initiate an impulse. Junctional rhythms can be transient or permanent, and they usually have a rate of 40 to 60 beats per minute. Junctional fibers in the AV node or bundle of His also can serve as ectopic pacemakers, producing premature junctional complexes. Another rhythm originating in the junctional tissues is nonparoxysmal junctional tachycardia. This rhythm usually is of gradual onset and termination. However, it may occur abruptly if the dominant pacemaker slows sufficiently. The rate associated with junctional tachycardia ranges from 70 to 130 beats per minute, but it may be faster.[3] The P waves may precede, be buried in, or follow the QRS complexes, depending on the site of the originating impulses. The clinical significance of nonparoxysmal junctional tachycardia is the same as for atrial tachycardias. Catheter ablation therapy has been used successfully to treat some individuals with recurrent or intractable junctional tachycardia. Nonparoxysmal junctional tachycardia is observed most frequently in individuals with underlying heart disease, such as inferior wall myocardial infarction or myocarditis, or after open heart surgery. It also may be present in persons with digitalis toxicity.

Ventricular Conduction Defects

The junctional fibers in the AV node join with the bundle of His, which divides to form the right and left bundle branches. The bundle branches continue to divide and form the Purkinje fibers, which supply the walls of the ventricles (see Fig. 25-1). As the cardiac impulse leaves the junctional fibers, it travels through the AV bundle. Next, the impulse moves down the right and left bundle branches that lie beneath the endocardium on either side of the septum. It then spreads out through the walls of the ventricles. Interruption of impulse conduction through the bundle branches is called *bundle branch block*. These blocks usually do not cause alterations in the rhythm of the heartbeat. Instead, a bundle branch block interrupts the normal progression of depolarization, causing the ventricles to depolarize one after the other because the impulses must travel through muscle tissue rather than through the specialized conduction tissue.[19] This prolonged conduction causes the QRS complex to be wider than the normal 0.08 to 0.12 second. The left bundle branch bifurcates into the left anterior and posterior fascicles. An interruption of one of these fascicles is referred to as a *hemiblock*.

Ventricular Dysrhythmias

Dysrhythmias that arise in the ventricles commonly are considered more serious than those that arise in the atria because they afford the potential for interfering with the pumping action of the heart. A premature ventricular contraction (PVC) is caused by a ventricular ectopic pacemaker. After a PVC, the ventricle usually is unable to repolarize sufficiently to respond to the next impulse that arises in the SA node. This delay is commonly referred to as a *compensatory pause,* which occurs while the ventricle waits to reestablish its previous rhythm (Fig. 25-11). When a PVC occurs, the diastolic volume usually is insufficient for ejection of blood into the arterial system. As a result, PVCs usually do not produce a palpable pulse. In the absence of heart disease, PVCs typically are not clinically significant. The incidence of PVCs is greatest with ischemia, acute myocardial infarction, history of myocardial infarction, ventricular hypertrophy, infection, increased sympathetic nervous system activity, or increased heart rate.[20] PVCs also can be the result of electrolyte disturbances or medications.

A special pattern of PVC called *ventricular bigeminy* occurs in such a way that each normal beat is followed by or paired with a PVC. This pattern often is an indication of dig-

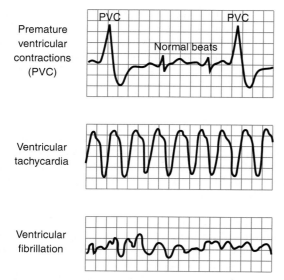

Premature ventricular contractions (PVC)

Ventricular tachycardia

Ventricular fibrillation

FIGURE 25-11 Electrocardiographic (ECG) tracings of ventricular dysrhythmias. Premature ventricular contractions (PVCs) *(top tracing)* originate from an ectopic focus in the ventricles, causing a distortion of the QRS complex. Because the ventricle usually cannot repolarize sufficiently to respond to the next impulse that arises in the sinoatrial node, a PVC frequently is followed by a compensatory pause. Ventricular tachycardia *(middle tracing)* is characterized by a rapid ventricular rate of 70 to 250 beats per minute and the absence of P waves. In ventricular fibrillation *(bottom tracing),* there are no regular or effective ventricular contractions, and the ECG tracing is totally disorganized.

italis toxicity or heart disease. The occurrence of frequent PVCs in the diseased heart predisposes one to the development of other, more serious dysrhythmias, including ventricular tachycardia and ventricular fibrillation.

Ventricular tachycardia describes a cardiac rhythm originating distal to the bifurcation of the bundle of His, in the specialized conduction system, in ventricular muscle, or both.[3] It is characterized by a ventricular rate of 70 to 250 beats per minute, and the onset can be sudden or insidious. Usually, ventricular tachycardia is exhibited electrocardiographically by wide, tall, bizarre-looking QRS complexes that persist longer than 0.12 second (see Fig. 25-11). QRS complexes can be uniform in appearance, or they can vary randomly, in a repetitive manner (*e.g.*, torsades de pointes), in an alternating pattern (*e.g.*, bidirectional), or in a stable but changing fashion. Ventricular tachycardia can be sustained, lasting more than 30 seconds and requiring intervention, or it can be nonsustained and stop spontaneously. This rhythm is dangerous because it eliminates atrial kick and can cause a reduction in diastolic filling time to the point at which cardiac output is severely diminished or nonexistent.

In ventricular fibrillation, the ventricle quivers but does not contract. When the ventricle does not contract, there is no cardiac output, and there are no palpable or audible pulses. The classic ECG pattern of ventricular fibrillation is that of gross disorganization without identifiable waveforms or intervals (see Fig. 25-11).

Disorders of Atrioventricular Conduction

Under normal conditions, the AV junction provides the only connection for transmission of impulses between the atrial and ventricular conduction systems. The AV junction comprises the atrial approaches to the AV node, the AV node, and the nonbranching portion of the common bundle of His. Junctional fibers in the AV node have high-resistance characteristics that cause a delay in the transmission of impulses from the atria to the ventricles. This delay provides optimal timing for atrial contribution to ventricular filling and protects the ventricles from abnormally rapid rates that arise in the atria. Conduction defects of the AV node are most commonly associated with fibrosis or scar tissue in fibers of the conduction system. Conduction defects also may result from medications, including digoxin, β-adrenergic blocking agents, calcium channel blocking agents, and class 1A antidysrhythmic agents.[21] Additional contributing factors include electrolyte imbalances, inflammatory disease, or cardiac surgery.

Heart Block.   Heart block refers to abnormalities of impulse conduction. It may be normal, physiologic (*e.g.*, vagal tone), or pathologic. It may occur in the AV nodal fibers or in the AV bundle (*i.e.*, bundle of His), which is continuous with the Purkinje conduction system that supplies the ventricles. The PR interval on the ECG corresponds with the time it takes for the cardiac impulse to travel from the SA node to the ventricular pathways. Normally, the PR interval ranges from 0.12 to 0.20 second.

First-degree AV block is characterized by a prolonged PR interval (exceeds 0.20 second) (Fig. 25-12). The prolonged PR interval indicates delayed AV conduction, but all atrial impulses are conducted to the ventricles. This condition usually produces a regular atrial and ventricular rhythm. Clinically significant PR interval prolongation can result from conduction delays in the AV node itself, the His-Purkinje system, or both.[3] When the QRS complex is normal in contour and duration, the AV delay almost always occurs in the AV node and rarely in the bundle of His. In contrast, when the QRS complex is prolonged, showing a bundle branch block pattern, conduction delays may be in the AV node or the His-Purkinje system. First-degree block may be the result of disease in the AV node such as ischemia or infarction, or of infections such as rheumatic fever or myocarditis.[22] Isolated first-degree heart block usually is not symptomatic, and temporary or permanent cardiac pacing is not indicated.

Second-degree AV block is characterized by intermittent failure of conduction of one or more impulses from the atria to the ventricles. The nonconducted P wave can appear intermittently or frequently. A distinguishing feature of second-degree AV block is that conducted P waves relate to QRS complexes with recurring PR intervals; that is, the association of P waves with QRS complexes is not random.[3] Second-degree AV block has been divided into two types: type I (*i.e.*, Mobitz type I or Wenckebach's phenomenon) and type II (*i.e.*, Mobitz type II). The Mobitz type I AV block is characterized by progressive lengthening of the PR interval until an impulse is blocked and the sequence begins again. It usually is associated with an adequate ventricular rate and rarely is symptomatic.[14] In Mobitz type II

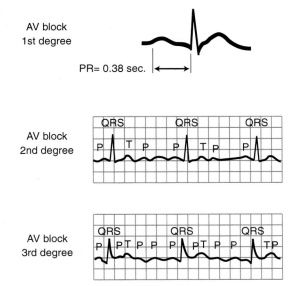

FIGURE 25-12 Electrocardiographic changes that occur with alterations in atrioventricular (AV) node conduction. The *top tracing* shows the prolongation of the PR interval, which is characteristic of first-degree AV block. The *middle tracing* illustrates Mobitz type II second-degree AV block, in which the conduction of one or more P waves is blocked. In third-degree AV block *(bottom tracing),* complete block in conduction of impulses through the AV node occurs, and the atria and ventricles develop their own rates of impulse generation.

AV block, an intermittent block of atrial impulses occurs, with a constant PR interval (see Fig. 25-12). The Mobitz type I block frequently occurs in persons with inferior wall myocardial infarction, particularly with concomitant right ventricular infarction.[3] This condition usually is transient and does not require temporary pacing. In contrast, Mobitz type II AV block frequently accompanies anterior wall myocardial infarction and can require temporary or permanent pacing. This condition is associated with a high mortality rate. In addition, Mobitz type II AV block is associated with other types of organic heart disease and often progresses to complete heart block.

Third-degree, or complete AV block, occurs when the conduction link between the atria and ventricles is lost and each is controlled by independent pacemakers (see Fig. 25-12). The atrial pacemaker can be sinus or ectopic in origin. The ventricular pacemaker usually is located just below the region of the block. The atria usually continue to beat at a normal rate and the ventricles develop their own rate, which normally is slow (30 to 40 beats per minute). The atrial and ventricular rates are regular but dissociated. Third-degree AV block can result from an interruption at the level of the AV node, in the bundle of His, or in the Purkinje system. Third-degree blocks at the level of the AV node usually are congenital, whereas blocks in the Purkinje system usually are acquired. Normal QRS complexes, with rates ranging from 40 to 60 complexes per minute, usually are displayed on the ECG when the block occurs proximal to the bundle of His. Complete heart block causes a decrease in cardiac output with possible periods of syncope, known as a *Stokes-Adams attack.*[3] Other symptoms include dizziness, fatigue, exercise intolerance, or episodes of acute heart failure. Most persons with complete heart block require a permanent cardiac pacemaker.

DIAGNOSTIC METHODS

The diagnosis of disorders of cardiac rhythm and conduction usually is made on the basis of the surface ECG. Further clarification of conduction defects and cardiac dysrhythmias can be obtained using electrophysiologic studies.

A resting surface ECG records the impulses originating in the heart as they are recorded at the body surface. These impulses are recorded for a limited time and during periods of inactivity. Although there are no complications related to the procedure, errors related to misdiagnosis may result in iatrogenic heart disease.[1] The resting ECG is the first approach to the clinical diagnosis of disorders of cardiac rhythm and conduction, but it is limited to events that occur during the period the ECG is being monitored.

Signal-Averaged Electrocardiogram

Signal-averaged ECG is a special type of ECG that is used to detect ventricular late action potentials that are thought to originate from slow-conducting areas of the myocardium. Ventricular late action potentials are low-amplitude, high-frequency waveforms in the terminal QRS complex, and they persist for tens of milliseconds into the ST segment.[23] These late potentials are detectable from leads of the surface ECG when signal averaging is performed. This technique averages together multiple samples of QRS waveforms and creates a tracing that is an average of all the repetitive signals. The presence of late potentials indicates high risk for development of ventricular tachycardia and sudden cardiac death.

Holter Monitoring

Holter monitoring is one form of long-term monitoring during which a person wears a device that digitally records two or three ECG leads for up to 48 hours. During this time, the person keeps a diary of his or her activities or symptoms, which later are correlated with the ECG recording. Most recording devices also have an event marker button that can be pressed when the individual experiences symptoms, which assists the technician or physician in correlating the diary, symptoms, and ECG changes during analysis. Holter monitoring is useful for documenting dysrhythmias, conduction abnormalities, and ST segment changes.

Intermittent ECG recorders also are used in the diagnosis of dysrhythmias and conduction defects. There are two basic types of recorders that perform this type of monitoring.[24] The first continuously monitors rhythm and is programmed to recognize abnormalities. In the second variety, the unit does not continuously monitor the ECG and therefore cannot automatically recognize abnormalities. This latter form relies on the person to activate the unit when he or she is symptomatic. The data are stored in memory or transmitted telephonically to an electrocardiographic receiver, where they are recorded. These types of ECG recordings are useful in persons who have transient symptoms.

Exercise Stress Testing

The exercise stress test elicits the body's response to measured increases in acute exercise (see Chapter 24).[22] This technique provides information about changes in heart rate, blood pressure, respiration, and perceived level of exercise. It is useful in determining exercise-induced alterations in hemodynamic response and ischemic-type ECG ST segment changes, and can detect and classify disturbances in cardiac rhythm and conduction associated with exercise. These changes are indicative of a poorer prognosis in persons with known coronary disease and recent myocardial infarction.

Electrophysiology Studies

An electrophysiologic study involves the passage of two or more electrode catheters into the right side of the heart. These catheters are inserted into the femoral, subclavian, internal jugular, or the antecubital veins and positioned with fluoroscopy into the high right atrium near the sinus node, the area of the His bundle, the coronary sinus that lies in the posterior AV groove, and into the right ventricle.[6] The electrode catheters are used to stimulate the heart and record intracardiac ECGs. During the study, overdrive pacing, cardioversion, or defibrillation may be necessary to terminate tachycardia induced during the stimulation procedures.

Electrophysiology studies are performed for diagnostic or therapeutic purposes. A diagnostic study is performed to determine a person's potential for dysrhythmia formation. Electrophysiologic testing also defines reproducible dysrhythmia induction characteristics and, as a result, can be used to evaluate the therapeutic efficacy of a particular treatment modality. Diagnostic studies can locate dysrhythmia foci for therapeutic intervention as well.

Therapeutic electrophysiology studies are used as interventions. These interventions may include pacing a person out of tachycardia or ablation therapy. Both types of electrophysiologic testing may be done repeatedly to test patient responses to drugs, devices such as implantable defibrillators, and surgical interventions used in the treatment of dysrhythmias.

TREATMENT

The treatment of cardiac rhythm or conduction disorders is directed toward controlling the dysrhythmia, correcting the cause, and preventing more serious or fatal dysrhythmias. Correction may involve simply adjusting an electrolyte disturbance or withholding a medication such as digitalis. Preventing more serious dysrhythmias often involves drug therapy, electrical stimulation, or surgical intervention.

Pharmacologic Treatment

Antidysrhythmic drugs act by modifying disordered formation and conduction of impulses that induce cardiac muscle contraction. These drugs are classified into four major groups according to the drug's effect on the action potential of the cardiac cells. Although drugs in one category have similar effects on conduction, they may vary significantly in their hemodynamic effects.

Class I drugs act by blocking the fast sodium channels. The drugs affect impulse conduction, excitability, and automaticity to various degrees and therefore have been divided further into three groups: IA, IB, and IC. Class IA drugs (*e.g.,* quinidine, procainamide, disopyramide, moricizine) decrease automaticity by depressing phase 4 of the action potential, decrease conductivity by moderately prolonging phase 0, and prolong repolarization by extending phase 3 of the action potential. Because these drugs are effective in suppressing ectopic foci and in treating reentrant dysrhythmias, they are used for supraventricular and ventricular dysrhythmias.[25] Class IB drugs (*e.g.,* lidocaine, phenytoin, tocainide, mexiletine, aprindine) decrease automaticity by depressing phase 4 of the action potential, have little effect on conductivity, decrease refractoriness by decreasing phase 2, and shorten repolarization by decreasing phase 3. Drugs in this group are used for treating ventricular dysrhythmias only and have little or no effect on myocardial contractility. Class IC drugs (*e.g.,* flecainide, encainide, propafenone, indecainide) decrease conductivity by markedly depressing phase 0 of the action potential but have little effect on refractoriness or repolarization. Drugs in this class are used for life-threatening ventricular dysrhythmias and supraventricular tachycardias.

Class II agents (*e.g.,* propranolol, nadolol, atenolol, timolol, acebutolol, metoprolol, pindolol, esmolol) are β-adrenergic blocking drugs that act by blunting the effect of sympathetic nervous system stimulation on the heart. These drugs decrease automaticity by depressing phase 4 of the action potential; they also decrease heart rate and cardiac contractility. These medications are effective for treatment of supraventricular dysrhythmias and tachydysrhythmias secondary to excessive sympathetic activity, but they are not very effective in treating severe dysrhythmias such as recurrent ventricular tachycardia.[26]

Class III drugs (*e.g.,* amiodarone, bretylium, sotalol, *N*-acetylprocainamide [NAPA]) act by extending the action potential and refractoriness. These agents are used in the treatment of serious ventricular dysrhythmias.[25]

Class IV drugs (*e.g.,* verapamil, diltiazem, nifedipine, bepridil, nitrendipine, felodipine, isradipine, nicardipine) act by blocking the slow calcium channels, thereby depressing phase 4 and lengthening phases 1 and 2. By blocking the release of intracellular calcium ions, these agents reduce the force of myocardial contractility, thereby decreasing myocardial oxygen demand. These drugs are used to slow the ventricular response in atrial tachycardias and to terminate reentrant paroxysmal supraventricular tachycardias when the AV node functions as a reentrant pathway.[25]

Two other types of antidysrhythmic drugs, the cardiac glycosides and adenosine, are not included in this classification schema. The cardiac glycosides (*i.e.,* digitalis drugs) slow the heart rate and are used in the management of dysrhythmias such as atrial tachycardia, atrial flutter, and atrial fibrillation. Adenosine, an endogenous nucleoside that is present in every cell, is used for emergency intravenous treatment of paroxysmal supraventricular tachycardia involving the AV node. It interrupts AV node conduction and slows SA node firing.

Electrical Interventions

The correction of conduction defects, bradycardias, and tachycardias can involve the use of an electronic pacemaker, cardioversion, or defibrillation. Electrical interventions can be used in emergency and elective situations.

Efforts directed at cardiac electrostimulation date back more than a century. During this time, tremendous strides have been made in the effectiveness of cardiac pacing. A cardiac pacemaker is an electronic device that delivers an electrical stimulus to the heart. It is used to initiate heartbeats in situations when the normal pacemaker of the heart is defective, with certain types of AV heart block, symptomatic bradycardia in which the rate of cardiac contraction and consequent cardiac output is inadequate to perfuse vital tissues, as well as other cardiac dysrhythmias. A pacemaker may be used as a temporary or a permanent measure. Pacemakers can pace the atria, the ventricles, or the atria and ventricles sequentially, or overdrive pacing can be used. Overdrive pacing is used to treat recurrent ventricular tachycardia and reentrant atrial or ventricular tachydysrhythmias, and to terminate atrial flutter.

Temporary pacemakers are useful for treatment of symptomatic bradycardias and to perform overdrive pacing. They can be placed transcutaneously, transvenously, or epicardially. External temporary pacing, also known as *transcutaneous pacing,* involves the placement of large patch electrodes on the anterior and posterior chest wall, which then are connected by a cable to an external pulse generator. Many defibrillators today have transcutaneous pacing capabilities, as well. Internal temporary pacing, also known as *transvenous pacing,* involves the passage of a venous catheter with electrodes on its tip into the right atrium or ventricle, where it is wedged against the endocardium. The electrode then is attached to an external pulse generator. This procedure is performed under fluoroscopic or electrocardiographic direction. During open thoracotomy procedures, epicardial pacing wires sometimes are placed. These wires are brought out directly through the chest wall and also can be attached to an external pulse generator, if necessary.

Permanent cardiac pacemakers may become necessary for a variety of reasons. Permanent pacemakers require implantation of pacing wires into the epicardium and a pulse generator. The pulse generator typically weighs approximately 25 to 40 g.[28] Ongoing evaluation of the pacemakers sensing and firing capabilities is necessary.

Defibrillation and synchronized cardioversion are two reliable methods for treating ventricular tachycardia, and defibrillation is the definitive treatment for atrial fibrillation. The discharge of electrical energy that is synchronized with the R wave of the ECG is referred to as *synchronized cardioversion,* and unsynchronized discharge is known as *defibrillation.* The goal of both of these techniques is to provide an electrical pulse to the heart in such a way as to depolarize the heart completely during passage of the current. This electrical current interrupts the disorganized impulses, allowing the SA node to regain control of the heart. Defibrillation and synchronized cardioversion can be delivered externally through large patch electrodes on the chest or internally through small paddle electrodes placed directly on the myocardium, patch electrodes sewn into the epicardium, or transvenous wires placed in the right ventricle. Electrical devices that combine antitachycardial pacing, cardioversion, defibrillation, and bradycardial pacing are under investigation.

Automatic implantable cardioverter-defibrillators (AICDs) are being used successfully to treat individuals with life-threatening ventricular tachydysrhythmias by the use of intrathoracic electrical countershock.[27] Reliable sensing and detection of ventricular tachydysrhythmias are essential for proper functioning of the AICD. Sensing and detection are accomplished by means of endocardial leads. The AICD responds to ventricular tachydysrhythmias by delivering an electrical shock between intrathoracic electrodes within 10 to 20 seconds of its onset. This time frame provides nearly a 100% likelihood of reversal of the dysrhythmia, supporting the utility of this device as a reliable and effective means of preventing sudden cardiac death in survivors of out-of-hospital cardiac arrest.

Ablation and Surgical Interventions

Ablation therapy is used for treating recurrent, life-threatening supraventricular and ventricular tachydysrhythmias. It involves localized destruction, isolation, or excision of cardiac tissue that is considered to be dysrhythmogenic.[6,25] Ablative therapy may be performed by catheter or surgical techniques. Radiofrequency ablation uses radiofrequency energy waves to destroy defective or aberrant electrical conduction pathways. Cryoablation is the direct application of an extremely cold probe to dysrhythmogenic cardiac tissue that causes freezing and necrosis of defective or aberrant electrical conduction pathways. The major complication with surgical ablation techniques is the perioperative mortality rate of 5% to 15%.[6] There also has been a high morbidity rate reported.

Additional surgical interventions such as coronary artery bypass surgery, ventriculotomy, and endocardial resection may be used to improve myocardial oxygenation, remove dysrhythmogenic foci, or alter electrical conduction pathways. Coronary artery bypass surgery improves myocardial oxygenation by increasing blood supply to the myocardium. Ventriculotomy involves the removal of aneurysm tissue and the resuturing of the myocardial walls to eliminate the paradoxical ventricular movement and the foci of dysrhythmias. In endocardial resection, endocardial tissue that has been identified as dysrhythmogenic through the use of electrophysiologic testing or intraoperative mapping is surgically removed. Ventriculotomy and endocardial resection have been performed with cryoablation or laser ablation as an adjunctive therapy.[25] Other surgical techniques, including transvenous electrocoagulation and laser ablation, are under investigation as potential treatment modalities for recurrent tachycardias.

In summary, disorders of cardiac rhythm arise as the result of disturbances in impulse generation or conduction in the heart. Normal sinus rhythm and respiratory sinus dysrhythmia (*i.e.,* heart rate speeds up and slows down in concert with respiratory cycle) are considered normal cardiac rhythms. Cardiac dysrhythmias are not necessarily pathologic; they occur in healthy and diseased hearts. Sinus dysrhythmias originate in the SA node. They include sinus bradycardia (heart rate <60 beats per minute); sinus tachycardia (heart rate >100 beats per minute); sinus arrest, in which there are prolonged periods of asystole; and sick sinus syndrome, a condition characterized by periods of bradycardia alternating with tachycardia.

Atrial dysrhythmias arise from alterations in impulse generation that occur in the conduction pathways or muscle of the atria. They include atrial premature contractions, atrial flutter (*i.e.,* atrial depolarization rate of 240 to 450 beats per minute), and atrial fibrillation (*i.e.,* grossly disorganized atrial depolarization that is irregular with regard to rate and rhythm). Atrial dysrhythmias often go unnoticed unless they are transmitted to the ventricles.

Alterations in the conduction of impulses through the AV node lead to disturbances in the transmission of impulses from the atria to the ventricles. There can be a delay in transmission (*i.e.,* first-degree heart block), failure to conduct one or more impulses (*i.e.,* second-degree heart block), or complete failure to conduct impulses between the atria and the ventricles (*i.e.,* third-degree heart block). Conduction disorders of the bundle of His and Purkinje system, called *bundle branch blocks,* cause a widening of and changes in the configuration of the QRS complex of the ECG. Because of their potential for interfering with the pumping action of the heart, dysrhythmias that arise in the ventricles usually are considered more serious than those that arise in the atria. A PVC is caused by a ventricular ectopic pacemaker. Ventricular tachycardia is characterized by a ventricular rate of 70 to 250 beats per minute. Ventricular fibrillation (*e.g.,* ventricular rate >350 beats per minute) is a fatal dysrhythmia unless it is successfully treated with defibrillation.

References

1. Castellanos A., Kessler K.M., Myerburg R.J. (1997). The resting electrocardiogram. In Alexander R.W., Schlant R.C., Ruster V., O'Rourke R.A., Roberts R., Sonnenblick E.H. (Eds.), *Hurst's The heart* (9th ed., pp. 351–385). New York: McGraw-Hill.
2. Waller B.F., Schlant R.C. (1997). Anatomy of the heart. In Alexander R.W., Schlant R.C., Ruster V., O'Rourke R.A., Roberts R., Sonnenblick E.H. (Eds.), *Hurst's The heart* (9th ed., pp. 19–79). New York: McGraw-Hill.
3. Zipes D.P. (1997). Genesis of cardiac arrhythmias: Electrophysiological considerations. In Braunwald E. (Ed.), *Heart disease: A textbook of cardiovascular medicine* (5th ed., pp. 548–592). Philadelphia: W.B. Saunders.
4. Guyton A.C. (2000). *Textbook of medical physiology* (10th ed., pp. 107–113). Philadelphia: W.B. Saunders.
5. Kernicki J.G., Weiler K.M. (1981). *Electrocardiography for nurses: Physiological correlates.* New York: John Wiley & Sons.
6. Fogoros R.N. (1999). *Electrophysiologic testing* (3rd ed.). Malden, MA: Blackwell Science.
7. Katz A.M. (1992). *Physiology of the heart* (2nd ed.). New York: Raven Press.
8. Wit A.L., Friedman P.L. (1975). Basis for ventricular arrhythmias accompanying myocardial infarction. *Archives of Internal Medicine* 135, 459–472.
9. Berne R.M., Levy M.N. (2001). *Cardiovascular physiology* (8th ed.). St. Louis: Mosby.
10. Waldo A.L., Wit A.L. (1997). Mechanisms of cardiac arrhythmias and conduction disturbances. In Alexander R.W.,

11. Moser D.K., Woo M.A. (1994). Recurrent ventricular tachycardia. *Critical Care Clinics of North America* 6, 15–26.
12. Kay G.N., Bubien R.S. (1992). *Clinical management of cardiac arrhythmias.* Gaithersburg, MD: Aspen.
13. Conover M. (1996). *Understanding electrocardiography* (7th ed.). St. Louis: Mosby-Year Book.
14. Myerburg R.J., Kessler K.M., Castellanos A. (1997). Recognition, clinical assessment, and management of arrhythmias and conduction disturbances. In Alexander R.W., Schlant R.C., Ruster V., O'Rourke R.A., Roberts R., Sonnenblick E.H. (Eds.), *Hurst's The heart* (9th ed., pp. 873–941). New York: McGraw-Hill.
15. Zipes D.P. (1997). Specific arrhythmias: Diagnosis and treatment. In Braunwald E. (Ed.), *Heart disease: A textbook of cardiovascular medicine* (5th ed., pp. 640–704). Philadelphia: W.B. Saunders.
16. Marriott H.J.L. (1988). *Practical electrocardiography* (8th ed.). Baltimore: Williams & Wilkins.
17. Alboni P., Baggioni G.F., Scarfo S., Cappata R., Percoco G.F., Paparella N., et al. (1991). Role of sinus node artery disease in sick sinus syndrome in inferior wall acute myocardial infarction. *American Heart Journal* 67, 1180–1184.
18. Chou T., Knilans T.K. (1996). *Electrocardiography in clinical practice* (4th ed.). Philadelphia: W.B. Saunders.
19. Menzel L.K., White J.M. (1996). Electrocardiogram interpretation. In Clochesy J.M., Breu C., Cardin S., Whittaker A.A., Rudy E.B. (Eds.), *Critical care nursing* (2nd ed., pp. 127–166). Philadelphia: W.B. Saunders.
20. Bigger Jr. J.T. (1994). Ventricular premature complexes. In Kastor J.A. (Ed.), *Arrhythmias* (pp. 310–325). Philadelphia: W.B. Saunders.
21. Moungey S.J. (1994). Patients with sinus node dysfunction or atrioventricular blocks. *Critical Care Nursing Clinics of North America* 6, 55–68.
22. Phillips R.E., Feeney M.A. (1990). *The cardiac rhythms: A systematic approach to interpretation* (3rd ed.). Philadelphia: W.B. Saunders.
23. Walter P.F. (1994). Technique of signal-averaged electrocardiography. In Schlant R.C., Alexander R.W., O'Rourke R.A., Roberts R., Sonnenblick E.H. (Eds.), *Hurst's The heart* (8th ed., pp. 893–904). New York: McGraw-Hill.
24. Noble R.J., Zipes D.P. (1997). Long-term continuous electrocardiographic recording. In Alexander R.W., Schlant R.C., Ruster V., O'Rourke R.A., Roberts R., Sonnenblick E.H. (Eds.), *Hurst's The heart* (9th ed., pp. 943–953). New York: McGraw-Hill.
25. Zipes D.P. (1997). Management of cardiac arrhythmias: Pharmacological, electrical, and surgical techniques. In Braunwald E. (Ed.), *Heart disease: A textbook of cardiovascular medicine* (5th ed., pp. 593–639). Philadelphia: W.B. Saunders.
26. Woosley R.L. (1997). Antiarrhythmic drugs. In Alexander R.W., Schlant R.C., Ruster V., O'Rourke R.A., Roberts R., Sonnenblick E.H. (Eds.), *Hurst's The heart* (9th ed., pp. 969–994). New York: McGraw-Hill.
27. O'Callaghan P.A., Ruskin J.N. (1997). The implantable cardioverter defibrillator. In Alexander R.W., Schlant R.C., Ruster V., O'Rourke R.A., Roberts R., Sonnenblick E.H. (Eds.), *Hurst's The heart* (9th ed., pp. 1007–1022). New York: McGraw-Hill.
28. Mitrani R.D., Myerburg R.J., Castellanos A. (1997). Cardiac pacemakers. In Alexander R.W., Schlant R.C., Ruster V., O'Rourke R.A., Roberts R., Sonnenblick E.H. (Eds.), *Hurst's The heart* (9th ed., pp. 1023–1055). New York: McGraw-Hill.

Chapter 26

Heart Failure and Circulatory Shock

Candace L. Hennessy and Carol M. Porth*

Adequate perfusion of body tissues depends on the pumping ability of the heart, a vascular system that transports blood to the cells and back to the heart, sufficient blood to fill the circulatory system, and tissues that are able to extract and use oxygen and nutrients from the blood. Impaired pumping ability of the heart and circulatory shock are separate conditions that reflect failure of the circulatory system. Both conditions exhibit common compensatory mechanisms even though they differ in terms of pathogenesis and causes.

Heart Failure

After you have completed this section of the chapter, you should be able to meet the following objectives:

 ✦ Explain the effect of the cardiac reserve on symptom development in heart failure

---

* In memory of Tim Hennessy.

 ✦ Define the terms *preload, afterload,* and *cardiac contractility*
 ✦ Explain how increased sympathetic activity, fluid retention, the Frank-Starling mechanism, and myocardial hypertrophy function as compensatory mechanisms in heart failure
 ✦ Differentiate high-output versus low-output heart failure, systolic versus diastolic heart failure, and right-sided versus left-sided heart failure
 ✦ Describe the physiologic mechanisms underlying the manifestations of congestive heart failure
 ✦ Describe the methods used in diagnosis and assessment of cardiac function in persons with heart failure
 ✦ Relate the actions of diuretics, digoxin, angiotensin-converting enzyme inhibitors, and β-adrenergic–blocking drugs to the treatment of heart failure
 ✦ Relate the effect of left ventricular failure to the development of and manifestations of pulmonary edema
 ✦ Describe the pathophysiology of cardiogenic shock
 ✦ Compare the indications for use of ventricular support devices, heart transplantation, and cardiomyoplasty in treatment of heart failure

The term *heart failure* denotes the failure of the heart as a pump. Although morbidity and mortality rates from other cardiovascular diseases have decreased over the past several decades, the incidence of heart failure is increasing at an alarming rate. This change undoubtedly reflects treatment improvements and survival from other forms of cardiac illness. It has been estimated that almost 5 million Americans have heart failure, with approximately 550,000 new cases diagnosed each year.[1] In a national survey, heart disease was the primary admitting diagnosis for 875,000 hospital admissions, accounting for 6.5 million hospital days at an estimated cost of $10 billion.[2] Despite advances in treatment, the 5-year survival rate for heart failure is only about 50%.[1] In its more advanced form, heart failure may progress to pulmonary edema and cardiogenic shock, which are immediately life-threatening forms of heart failure.

This section of the chapter is divided into four parts: physiology of heart failure, congestive heart failure, acute pulmonary edema, and cardiogenic shock.

PHYSIOLOGY OF HEART FAILURE

The heart has the amazing capacity to adjust its function to meet the varying needs of the body. During sleep, its output declines, and during exercise, it increases markedly. The ability to increase cardiac output during increased activity is called the *cardiac reserve*. For example, competitive swimmers and long-distance runners have large cardiac reserves. During exercise, the cardiac output of these athletes rapidly increases to as much as five to six times their resting level. In sharp contrast with healthy athletes, persons with heart failure often use their cardiac reserve at rest. For them, just climbing a flight of stairs may cause shortness of breath because they have exceeded their cardiac reserve.

The physiology of heart failure involves an interplay between two factors: the inability of the failing heart to maintain sufficient cardiac output to support body functions and the recruitment of compensatory mechanisms designed to maintain the cardiac reserve.

Cardiac Output

The cardiac output is the amount of blood that the heart pumps each minute. It reflects how often the heart beats each minute (heart rate) and how much blood the heart pumps with each beat (stroke volume) and can be expressed as the product of the heart rate and stroke volume: cardiac output = heart rate × stroke volume. Heart rate is regulated by balancing sympathetic, or adrenergic, activity, which accelerates heart rate, with parasympathetic, or vagal, activity, which slows it down. Stroke volume is a function of preload, afterload, and cardiac contractility.

Preload and Afterload. The work that the heart performs consists mainly of ejecting blood that has returned to the ventricles during diastole into the pulmonary or systemic circulations. As with skeletal muscle, the work of cardiac muscle is determined by what are called *loading conditions*—the stretch imposed by the load (*i.e.*, blood volume) and the force that the muscle must generate to move the load. The terms *preload* and *afterload* often are used to describe the workload of the heart.

Preload reflects the loading condition of the heart at the end of diastole just prior to the onset of systole. It is the volume of blood stretching the resting heart muscle and is determined mainly by the venous return to the heart. For any given cardiac cycle, the maximum volume of blood filling the ventricle is present at the end of diastole. Known as the *end-diastolic volume*, this volume causes the tension in the wall of the ventricles and the pressure in the ventricles to rise. End-diastolic pressure can be measured clinically, providing an estimate of preload status. Within limits, as end-diastolic volume or preload increases, the stroke volume increases in accord with the Frank-Starling mechanism (see Chapter 21, Fig. 21-12). In heart failure, the ventricles may become overstretched because of excessive filling. When this happens, intraventricular pressure rises, and stroke volume may decrease. Preload may be excessively elevated in conditions such as myocardial infarction, in which the ventricles become distended because of impaired pumping ability; in valvular heart disease, such as aortic regurgitation, in which a portion of the ejected systolic volume moves back into the ventricle and is added to the diastolic volume; and in renal failure, in which an increase in blood volume produces an increase in venous return.

Afterload represents the force that the contracting heart must generate to eject blood from the filled heart. The main components of afterload are ventricular wall tension and the systemic (peripheral) vascular resistance. The greater the systemic vascular resistance, the higher the wall tension and resulting intraventricular pressure that must be generated to open the semilunar (aortic and pulmonic) valves. As a result, excessive afterload may impair ventricular ejection if the ventricles cannot generate sufficient pressure. Both aortic stenosis and severe hypertension increase the afterload of the left ventricle by increasing the pressure needed to eject blood into the aorta.

Cardiac Contractility. Cardiac contractility refers to the mechanical performance of the heart—the ability of the contractile elements (actin and myosin filaments) of the heart muscle to interact and shorten against a load. The ejection of blood from the heart during systole depends on cardiac contractility. Contractility increases cardiac output independent of preload filling and muscle stretch.

An *inotropic influence* is one that increases cardiac contractility. Sympathetic stimulation increases the strength of cardiac contraction (*i.e.*, positive inotropic action), and hypoxia and ischemia decrease contractility (*i.e.*, negative inotropic effect). The drug digitalis, which is classified as an inotropic agent, increases cardiac contractility such that the heart is able to eject more blood at any level of preload filling. A decrease in cardiac contractility can result from loss of functional muscle tissue due to myocardial infarction or from conditions such as cardiomyopathy that diffusely affect the myocardium.

Compensatory Mechanisms

In heart failure, the cardiac reserve is largely maintained through compensatory mechanisms such as the Frank-

Starling mechanism, activation of neurohumoral mechanisms, and myocardial remodeling and hypertrophy.[3] The healthy and the failing heart may use the same compensatory mechanisms. In the failing heart, early decreases in cardiac function may go unnoticed because these compensatory mechanisms maintain the cardiac output (Fig. 26-1). This state is called *compensated heart failure.* Unfortunately, these mechanisms were not intended for long-term use. In severe and prolonged heart failure, the compensatory mechanisms are no longer effective and may themselves worsen the failure, causing *decompensated failure.*

Frank-Starling Mechanism. The Frank-Starling mechanism increases stroke volume by means of an increase in ventricular end-diastolic volume (Fig. 26-2). With increased diastolic filling, there is increased stretching of the myocardial fibers, more optimal approximation of the actin and myosin filaments, and a resultant increase in the force of the next contraction (see Chapter 21). In the normally functioning heart, the Frank-Starling mechanism serves to match the outputs of the two ventricles.

In heart failure, the Frank-Starling mechanism also helps to support the cardiac output. Cardiac output may be normal at rest in persons with heart failure because of increased ventricular end-diastolic volume and the Frank-Starling mechanism. However, this mechanism becomes ineffective when the heart becomes overfilled and the muscle fibers are overstretched. With deterioration of myocardial function, the ventricular function curve depicted in Figure 26-2 flattens, and when an increase in cardiac output is needed, as occurs with increased physical activity, there is a lesser increase in cardiac output at any given increase in left ventricular end-diastolic volume or pressure. The maximal increase in cardiac output that can be achieved may

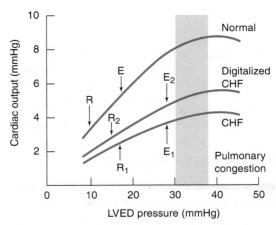

FIGURE 26-2 Frank-Starling curves. R, resting; E, exercise; LVED, left ventricular end-diastolic; CHF, congestive heart failure. (Iseri L.T., Benvenuti D.J. [1983]. Pathogenesis and management of congestive heart failure—revisited. *American Heart Journal* 105 [2], 346)

severely limit activity, while at the same time producing an elevation in left ventricular and pulmonary capillary pressure and development of dyspnea and pulmonary congestion. At the point where the heart becomes overfilled to the extent that actin and myosin filaments cannot produce an effective contraction, further increases in ventricular filling may produce a decrease in cardiac output.

An important determinant of myocardial energy consumption is ventricular wall tension. Overfilling of the ventricle produces a decrease in wall thickness and an increase in wall tension. Because increased wall tension increases myocardial oxygen requirements, it can produce ischemia and further impairment of cardiac function. The use of diuretics in persons with heart failure helps to reduce vascular volume and ventricular filling, thereby unloading the heart and reducing ventricular wall tension.

Increased Sympathetic Nervous System Activity. Stimulation of the sympathetic nervous system plays an important role in the compensatory response to decreased cardiac output and to the pathogenesis of heart failure.[3–6] The neurohormonal influence of heart failure leads to systemic vasoconstriction, which causes increased systemic vascular resistance and decreased blood flow to skeletal muscles.[4] Both cardiac sympathetic tone and catecholamine (epinephrine and norepinephrine) levels are elevated during the late stages of most forms of heart failure. By direct stimulation of heart rate and cardiac contractility and by regulation of vascular tone, the sympathetic nervous system helps to maintain perfusion of the various organs, particularly the heart and brain. In persons with more severe heart failure, blood is diverted to the more critical cerebral and coronary circulations.

The negative aspects of increased sympathetic activity include an increase in vascular resistance and the afterload against which the heart must pump. Excessive sympathetic stimulation also may result in decreased blood flow to skin, muscle, kidney, and abdominal organs. This not only decreases tissue perfusion, but contributes to an increase in

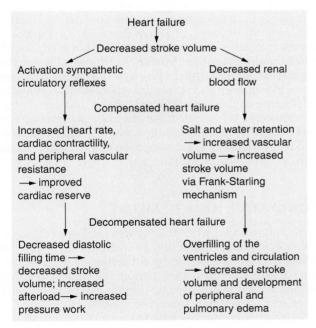

FIGURE 26-1 Sequence of events in compensated and decompensated heart failure.

systemic vascular resistance and afterload stress of the heart.

There also is evidence that prolonged sympathetic stimulation may exhaust myocardial stores of norepinephrine and may lead to down-regulation and a reduction in β-adrenergic receptors.[3] Moreover, these effects adversely affect the balance between oxygen supply and demand in persons in whom this ratio is precariously balanced. The catecholamines also may contribute to the high rate of sudden death by promoting dysrhythmias.[7]

Renin-Angiotensin Mechanism. One of the most important effects of a lowered cardiac output in heart failure is a reduction in renal blood flow and glomerular filtration rate, which leads to salt and water retention. Renal function can be used as an indicator of cardiovascular status in persons with heart failure. Normally, the kidneys receive approximately 25% of the cardiac output, but this may be decreased to as low as 8% to 10% in persons with heart failure. With decreased renal blood flow, there is a progressive increase in renin secretion by the kidneys along with parallel increases in circulating levels of angiotensin II. The increased concentration of angiotensin II contributes to a generalized and excessive vasoconstriction and provides a powerful stimulus for aldosterone production by the adrenal cortex (see Chapter 21). Aldosterone increases tubular reabsorption of sodium, with an accompanying increase in water retention. Because aldosterone is metabolized in the liver, its levels are further increased when heart failure causes liver congestion. Angiotensin II also increases the level of antidiuretic hormone (ADH), which serves as a vasoconstrictor and inhibitor of water excretion (see Chapter 31).

Angiotensin II is a growth factor for both cardiac muscle cells and fibroblasts and is thought to contribute to the myocardial hypertrophy that occurs in heart failure.[3,5,8] Angiotensin-converting enzyme (ACE) inhibitor drugs, which block the conversion of angiotensin I to angiotensin II, have become common therapy for heart failure.[3,5,7]

Atrial Natriuretic Peptide. Atrial natriuretic peptide (ANP), or atriopeptin, is a peptide hormone released from atrial cells in the heart in response to increased atrial stretch and pressure.[3,8] ANP produces rapid and transient natriuresis, diuresis, and moderate loss of potassium in the urine. It inhibits aldosterone and renin secretion and acts as an antagonist to angiotensin II. It also inhibits the release of norepinephrine from presynaptic nerve terminals. Increased ANP levels have been found in adults with CHF, but the role of ANP in compensating for alterations in cardiac function still is unclear. It has been suggested that ANP may act as a counter-regulatory hormone because of its diuretic, natriuretic, and vascular smooth muscle-relaxing properties.

Endothelin. Endothelin-1 (ET-1) is another peptide that is elevated in persons with heart failure.[3,8] ET-1 is released from arterial and venous endothelial cells and is a potent vasoconstrictor. Other actions of ET-1 include inducing vascular smooth muscle cell proliferation and myocyte hypertrophy. Plasma ET-1 levels correlate directly with pulmonary vascular resistance, and it is thought that the peptide may play a role in mediating pulmonary hypertension in persons with heart failure.[3]

Myocardial Hypertrophy. Myocardial hypertrophy is a long-term compensatory mechanism. Cardiac muscle, like skeletal muscle, responds to an increase in work demands by undergoing hypertrophy. Hypertrophy increases the number of contractile elements in myocardial cells as a means of increasing their contractile performance. There is increasing evidence that growth signals generated by the release of substances such as angiotensin II, ANP, and ET-1 may direct the development of ventricular hypertrophy in persons with heart failure.[9]

Myocardial hypertrophy occurs early in the course of heart failure, and is an important risk factor for subsequent morbidity and mortality. Although hypertrophy increases the systolic function of the heart, it also eventually can lead to diastolic dysfunction and myocardial ischemia. Some forms of hypertrophy may lead to abnormal remodeling of the ventricular wall with reduction in chamber size and reduced diastolic filling and increased wall tension. For example, untreated hypertension causes hypertrophy that may preserve systolic function for a time, but eventually the work performed by the ventricle exceeds the augmented muscle mass and the heart dilates.[3] The hypertrophied heart also has impaired coronary vascular reserve and susceptibility to ischemia. When the oxygen requirements of the increased muscle mass exceed the ability of the coronary vessels to bring blood to the area, myocardial hypertrophy is no longer beneficial and may result in ischemia with decreased contractility. Abnormal growth of nonmyocardial tissue (*e.g.*, fibrous tissue) may produce stiffness of the ventricle and further impair ventricular function

Recent interest has focused on the type of hypertrophy that develops in persons with heart failure. At the cellular level, cardiac muscle cells respond to stimuli from stress placed on the ventricular wall by pressure and volume overload by initiating several different processes that lead to hypertrophy. These include those that lead to a symmetric increase in muscle length and width, as occurs in athletes (*concentric hypertrophy*), and those that lead to a disproportionate increase in muscle length, as occurs in persons with dilated cardiomyopathies (*eccentric hypertrophy*).[9] When the primary stimulus to hypertrophy is *pressure overload*, the increase in wall stress leads to parallel replication of myofibrils, thickening of the individual myocytes, and concentric hypertrophy.[3] When the primary stimulus is *ventricular volume overload*, increased diastolic wall stress leads to replication of myofibrils in series, elongation of the cardiac muscle cells, and ventricular dilation.

CONGESTIVE HEART FAILURE

Heart failure occurs when the pumping ability of the heart becomes impaired. Congestive heart failure (CHF) is heart failure that is accompanied by congestion of body tissues. After an initial compensatory period, the clinical manifestations of heart failure become complicated by pulmonary congestion or systemic venous congestion.

Heart failure may be caused by a variety of conditions, including acute myocardial infarction, hypertension, or degenerative conditions of the heart muscle known collectively as *cardiomyopathies*. Heart failure also may occur because of excessive work demands, such as occurs with hypermetabolic states, or with volume overload, such as occurs with renal failure. Either of these states may exceed the work capacity of even a healthy heart. In persons with asymptomatic heart disease, heart failure may be precipitated by an unrelated illness or stress. Table 26-1 lists major causes of heart failure. Heart failure may be described as high-output or low-output failure, systolic or diastolic failure, and right-sided or left-sided failure.

High-Output Versus Low-Output Failure

High- and low-output failure are described in terms of cardiac output. *High-output failure* is an uncommon type of heart failure that is caused by an excessive need for cardiac output. With high-output failure, the function of the heart may be supranormal but inadequate owing to excessive metabolic needs. Causes of high-output failure include severe anemia, thyrotoxicosis, conditions that cause arteriovenous shunting, and Paget's disease. High-output failure tends to be specifically treatable.

Low-output failure is caused by disorders that impair the pumping ability of the heart, such as ischemic heart disease and cardiomyopathy. As a result, treatment options tend to be more limited and focus primarily on symptom management, with attempts to slow the natural progress of the etiologic disease state.

Systolic Versus Diastolic Failure

Until recently, CHF was viewed mainly in terms of backward and forward failure. *Backward failure* represented failure of one the ventricles to effectively empty the heart during diastole, such that blood backs up in the venous system, causing congestion. *Forward failure* was characterized by impaired forward movement of blood into the arterial system emerging from the heart.

A more recent classification separates the pathophysiology of congestive failure into two new categories—systolic

---

⚷ Heart Failure

> ► The function of the heart is to move deoxygenated blood from the venous system through the right heart into the pulmonary circulation, and to move the oxygenated blood from the pulmonary circulation through the left heart into the arterial system.

> ► To function effectively, the right and left hearts must maintain an equal output.

> ► Right heart failure represents failure of the right heart to pump blood forward into the pulmonary circulation; blood backs up in the systemic circulation, causing peripheral edema and congestion of the abdominal organs.

> ► Left heart failure represents failure of the left heart to move blood from the pulmonary circulation into the system circulation; blood backs up in the pulmonary circulation.

---

dysfunction and diastolic dysfunction. With systolic dysfunction, there is impaired ejection of blood from the heart during systole; with diastolic dysfunction, there is impaired filling of the ventricles during diastole (Fig. 26-3). Many persons with heart failure fall into an intermediate category, with combined elements of both systolic and diastolic failure. The most common form of heart failure, that caused by coronary atherosclerosis, is an example of combined systolic and diastolic failure.[10]

TABLE 26-1 ✦ Causes of Heart Failure

Impaired Cardiac Function	Excess Work Demands
Myocardial Disease	**Increased Pressure Work**
Cardiomyopathies	Systemic hypertension
Myocarditis	Pulmonary hypertension
Coronary insufficiency	Coarctation of the aorta
Myocardial infarction	
Valvular Heart Disease	**Increased Volume Work**
Stenotic valvular disease	Arteriovenous shunt
Regurgitant valvular disease	Excessive administration of intravenous fluids
Congenital Heart Defects	**Increased Perfusion Work**
	Thyrotoxicosis
	Anemia
Constrictive Pericarditis	

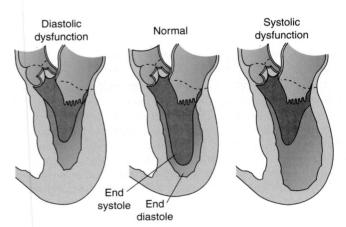

FIGURE 26-3 Congestive heart failure due to systolic and diastolic dysfunction. The ejection fraction represents the difference between the end-diastolic and end-systolic volumes. Normal systolic and diastolic function with normal ejection fraction (**middle**); diastolic dysfunction with decreased ejection fraction due to decreased diastolic filling (**left**); systolic dysfunction with decreased ejection fraction due to impaired systolic function (**right**).

Systolic Dysfunction. Systolic dysfunction involves a decrease in cardiac contractility and ejection fraction. It commonly results from conditions that impair the contractile performance of the heart (*e.g.,* ischemic heart disease and cardiomyopathy), produce a volume overload (*e.g.,* valvular insufficiency and anemia), or generate a pressure overload (*e.g.,* hypertension and valvular stenosis) on the heart.

A normal heart ejects approximately 65% of the blood that is present in the ventricle at the end of diastole when it contracts. This is called the *ejection fraction*. In systolic heart failure, the ejection fraction declines progressively with increasing degrees of myocardial dysfunction. In very severe forms of heart failure, the ejection fraction may drop to a single-digit percentage. With a decrease in ejection fraction, there is a resultant increase in diastolic volume, ventricular dilation, and ventricular wall tension and a rise in ventricular end-diastolic pressure. The symptoms of persons with systolic dysfunction result mainly from reductions in ejection fraction and cardiac output.

Diastolic Dysfunction. Diastolic dysfunction, which reportedly accounts for approximately 40% of all cases of CHF, is characterized by a smaller ventricular chamber size, ventricular hypertrophy, and poor ventricular compliance (*i.e.,* ability to stretch during filling).[11,12] Because of impaired filling, congestive symptoms tend to predominate in diastolic dysfunction. Among the conditions that cause diastolic dysfunction are those that restrict diastolic filling (*e.g.,* mitral stenosis), those that increase ventricular wall thickness and reduce chamber size (*e.g.,* myocardial hypertrophy due to lung disease and hypertrophic cardiomyopathy), and those that delay diastolic relaxation (*e.g.,* aging, ischemic heart disease). Aging often is accompanied by a delay in relaxation of the heart during diastole; diastolic filling begins while the ventricle is still stiff and resistant to stretching to accept an increase in volume.[13] A similar delay occurs with myocardial ischemia, resulting from a lack of energy to break the rigor bonds that form between the actin and myosin filaments of the contracting cardiac muscle.[14] Because tachycardia produces a decrease in diastolic filling time, persons with diastolic dysfunction often become symptomatic during activities and situations that increase heart rate.

Right-Sided Versus Left-Sided Heart Failure

Heart failure also can be classified according to the side of the heart (right or left) that is affected. An important feature of the circulatory system is that the right and left ventricles act as two pumps that are connected in series. To function effectively, the right and left ventricles must maintain an equal output. Although the initial event that leads to heart failure may be primarily right sided or left sided in origin, long-term heart failure usually involves both sides. To understand the physiologic mechanisms associated with heart failure, right- and left-sided failure are considered separately.

Right-Sided Heart Failure. The right heart pumps deoxygenated blood from the systemic circulation into the pulmonary circulation. Consequently, when the right heart fails, there is accumulation or damming back of blood in the systemic venous system. This causes an increase in right atrial, right ventricular end-diastolic, and systemic venous pressures.

A major effect of right-sided heart failure is the development of peripheral edema (Fig. 26-4). Because of the effects of gravity, the edema is most pronounced in the dependent parts of the body—in the lower extremities when the person is in the upright position and in the area over the sacrum when the person is supine. The accumulation of edema fluid is evidenced by a gain in weight (*i.e.,* 1 pint of accumulated fluid results in a 1-lb weight gain). Daily measurement of weight can be used as a means of assessing fluid accumulation in a patient with chronic CHF. As a rule, a weight gain of more than 2 lb in 24 hours or 5 lb in 1 week is considered a sign of worsening failure.

Right-sided heart failure also produces congestion of the viscera. As venous distention progresses, blood backs up in the hepatic veins that drain into the inferior vena cava, and the liver becomes engorged. This may cause hepatomegaly and right upper quadrant pain. In severe and prolonged right-sided failure, liver function is impaired and hepatic cells may die. Congestion of the portal circulation

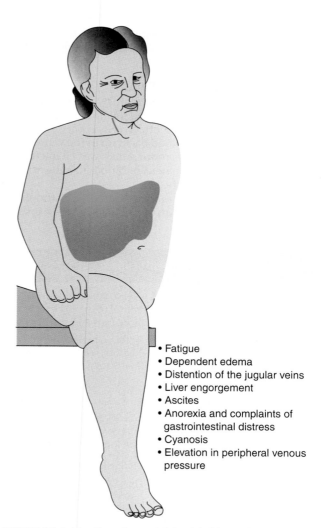

- Fatigue
- Dependent edema
- Distention of the jugular veins
- Liver engorgement
- Ascites
- Anorexia and complaints of gastrointestinal distress
- Cyanosis
- Elevation in peripheral venous pressure

FIGURE 26-4 Manifestations of right-sided heart failure.

also may lead to engorgement of the spleen and the development of ascites. Congestion of the gastrointestinal tract may interfere with digestion and absorption of nutrients, causing anorexia and abdominal discomfort. The jugular veins, which are above the level of the heart, are normally collapsed in the standing position or when sitting with the head at higher than a 30-degree angle. In severe right-sided failure, the external jugular veins become distended and can be visualized when the person is sitting up or standing.

The causes of right-sided heart failure include conditions that restrict blood flow into the lungs. Stenosis or regurgitation of the tricuspid or pulmonic valves, right ventricular infarction, cardiomyopathy, and persistent left-sided failure are common causes. Acute or chronic pulmonary disease, such as severe pneumonia, pulmonary embolus, or pulmonary hypertension, can cause right heart failure, referred to as *cor pulmonale*.

Left-Sided Heart Failure. The left side of the heart pumps blood from the low-pressure pulmonary circulation into the high-pressure arterial side of the systemic circulation.

With impairment of left heart function, there is a decrease in cardiac output; an increase in left atrial and left ventricular end-diastolic pressures; and congestion in the pulmonary circulation. When the pulmonary capillary filtration pressure (normally approximately 10 mm Hg) exceeds the capillary osmotic pressure (normally approximately 25 mm Hg), there is a shift of intravascular fluid into the interstitium of the lung and development of pulmonary edema (Fig. 26-5). An episode of pulmonary edema often occurs at night, after the person has been reclining for some time and the gravitational forces have been removed from the circulatory system. It is then that the edema fluid that had been sequestered in the lower extremities during the day is returned to the vascular compartment and redistributed to the pulmonary circulation. The manifestations of left-sided heart failure are illustrated in Figure 26-6.

The most common causes of left-sided heart failure are acute myocardial infarction and cardiomyopathy. Left-sided heart failure and pulmonary congestion can develop very rapidly in persons with acute myocardial infarction.

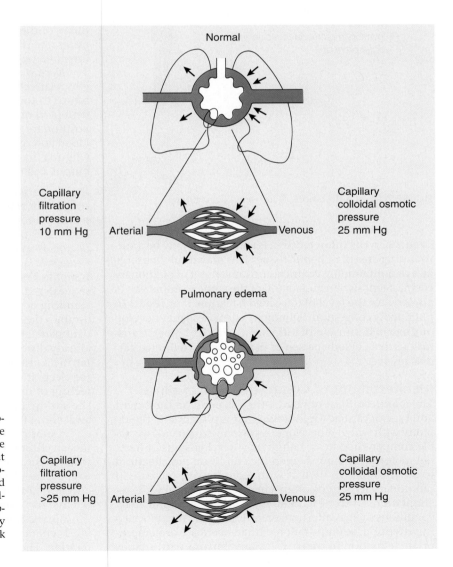

Normal

Capillary filtration pressure 10 mm Hg

Arterial   Venous

Capillary colloidal osmotic pressure 25 mm Hg

Pulmonary edema

Capillary filtration pressure >25 mm Hg

Arterial   Venous

Capillary colloidal osmotic pressure 25 mm Hg

FIGURE 26-5 Mechanism of respiratory symptoms in left-sided heart failure. Normal exchange of fluid in the pulmonary capillaries **(top)**. The capillary filtration pressure that moves fluid out of the capillary into the lung is less than the capillary colloidal osmotic pressure that pulls fluid back into the capillary. Development of pulmonary edema **(bottom)** occurs when the capillary filtration pressure exceeds the capillary colloidal osmotic pressure that pulls fluid back into the capillary.

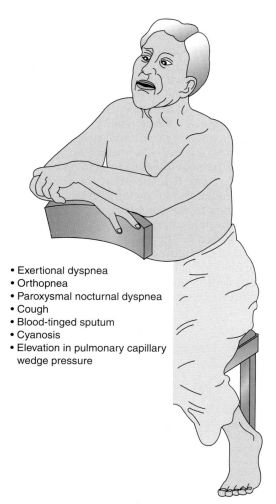

- Exertional dyspnea
- Orthopnea
- Paroxysmal nocturnal dyspnea
- Cough
- Blood-tinged sputum
- Cyanosis
- Elevation in pulmonary capillary wedge pressure

FIGURE 26-6 Manifestations of left-sided heart failure.

Even when the infarcted area is small, there may be a surrounding area of ischemic tissue. This may result in a large area of nonpumping ventricle and rapid onset of pulmonary edema. Stenosis or regurgitation of the aortic or mitral valves also creates the level of left-sided backflow that results in pulmonary congestion. Pulmonary edema also may develop during rapid infusion of intravenous fluids or blood transfusions in an elderly person or in a person with limited cardiac reserve.

Manifestations of Congestive Heart Failure

The manifestations of heart failure depend on the extent and type of cardiac dysfunction that is present and the rapidity with which it develops. A person with previously stable compensated heart failure may develop signs of heart failure for the first time when the condition has advanced to a critical point, such as with a progressive increase in pulmonary hypertension in a person with mitral valve regurgitation. Overt heart failure also may be precipitated by conditions such as infection, emotional stress, uncontrolled hypertension, administration of fluid overload, or inappropriate reduction in therapy.[10] Many persons with serious

underlying heart disease, regardless of whether they have previously experienced heart failure, may be relatively asymptomatic as long they carefully adhere to their treatment regimen. A dietary excess of sodium is a frequent cause of sudden cardiac decompensation.

The manifestations of heart failure reflect the physiologic effects of the impaired pumping ability of the heart, decreased renal blood flow, and activation of the sympathetic compensatory mechanisms. The severity and progression of symptoms depend on the extent and type of dysfunction that is present (systolic vs. diastolic failure). The signs and symptoms include fluid retention and edema, shortness of breath and other respiratory manifestations, fatigue and limited exercise tolerance, cyanosis, cachexia and malnutrition, and cyanosis. Distention of the jugular veins may be present in right-sided failure. Persons with severe heart failure may exhibit diaphoresis and tachycardia.

Fluid Retention and Edema.   Many of the manifestations of CHF result from the increased capillary pressures that develop in the peripheral circulation in right-sided heart failure and in the pulmonary circulation in left-sided heart failure. The increased capillary pressure reflects an overfilling of the vascular system because of increased salt and water retention and venous congestion resulting from the impaired pumping ability of the heart.[15]

Nocturia is a nightly increase in urine output that occurs relatively early in the course of CHF. It results from the return to the circulation of edema fluids from the dependent parts of the body when the person assumes the supine position for the night. As a result, the cardiac output, renal blood flow, glomerular filtration, and urine output increase. Oliguria is a late sign related to a severely reduced cardiac output and resultant renal failure.

Respiratory Manifestations.   Shortness of breath due to congestion of the pulmonary circulation is one of the major manifestations of left-sided heart failure. Perceived shortness of breath (*i.e.,* breathlessness) is called *dyspnea*. Dyspnea related to an increase in activity is called *exertional dyspnea*. *Orthopnea* is shortness of breath that occurs when a person is supine. The gravitational forces that cause fluid to become sequestered in the lower legs and feet when the person is standing or sitting are removed when a person with CHF assumes the supine position; fluid from the legs and dependent parts of the body is mobilized and redistributed to an already distended pulmonary circulation. *Paroxysmal nocturnal dyspnea* is a sudden attack of dyspnea that occurs during sleep. It disrupts sleep, and the person awakens with a feeling of extreme suffocation that resolves when he or she sits up. Initially, the experience may be interpreted as awakening from a bad dream.

A subtle and often overlooked symptom of heart failure is a chronic dry, nonproductive cough, which becomes worse when the person is lying down. Bronchospasm due to congestion of the bronchial mucosa may cause wheezing and difficulty in breathing. This condition is sometimes referred to as *cardiac asthma*.

Cheyne-Stokes respiration, also known as *periodic breathing,* is characterized by a slow waxing and waning of respiration. The person breathes deeply for a period when the arterial carbon dioxide pressure (PCO$_2$) is high and then slightly or not all when the PCO$_2$ falls. In persons with left-sided heart failure, the condition is thought to be caused by a prolongation of the heart-to-brain circulation, particularly in persons with hypertension and associated cerebral vascular disease. Cheyne-Stokes breathing may contribute to daytime sleepiness, and occasionally the person awakens at night with dyspnea precipitated by Cheyne-Stokes breathing.[10]

Fatigue and Limited Exercise Tolerance. Fatigue and limb weakness often accompany diminished output from the left ventricle. Cardiac fatigue is different from general fatigue in that it usually is not present in the morning but appears and progresses as activity increases during the day. In acute or severe left-sided failure, cardiac output may fall to levels that are insufficient for providing the brain with adequate oxygen, and there are indications of mental confusion and disturbed behavior. Confusion, impairment of memory, anxiety, restlessness, and insomnia are common in elderly persons with advanced heart failure, particularly in those with cerebral atherosclerosis. These very symptoms may confuse the diagnosis of heart failure in the elderly because of the myriad other causes associated with aging.

Cachexia and Malnutrition. Cardiac cachexia is a condition of malnutrition and tissue wasting that occurs in persons with end-stage heart failure. A number of factors probably contribute to its development, including the fatigue and depression that interfere with food intake, congestion of the liver and gastrointestinal structures that impairs digestion and absorption and produces feelings of fullness, and the circulating toxins and mediators released from poorly perfused tissues that impair appetite and contribute to tissue wasting.

Cyanosis. Cyanosis is the bluish discoloration of the skin and mucous membranes caused by excess desaturated hemoglobin in the blood; it often is a late sign of heart failure. Cyanosis may be central, caused by arterial desaturation resulting from impaired pulmonary gas exchange, or peripheral, caused by venous desaturation resulting from extensive extraction of oxygen at the capillary level. Central cyanosis is caused by conditions that impair oxygenation of the arterial blood, such as pulmonary edema, left heart failure, or right-to-left shunting. Peripheral cyanosis is caused by conditions such as low-output failure that cause delivery of poorly oxygenated blood to the peripheral tissues, or by conditions such as peripheral vasoconstriction that cause excessive removal of oxygen from the blood. Central cyanosis is best monitored in the lips and mucous membranes because these areas are not subject to conditions such as cold that cause peripheral cyanosis. Persons with right-sided or left-sided heart failure may develop cyanosis especially around the lips and in the peripheral parts of the extremities.

Diagnostic Methods

Diagnostic methods in heart failure are directed toward establishing the cause of the disorder and determining the extent of the dysfunction. Because heart failure represents the failure of the heart as a pump and can occur in the course of a number of heart diseases or other systemic disorders, the diagnosis of heart failure often is based on signs and symptoms related to the failing heart itself, such as shortness of breath and fatigue. The functional classification of the New York Heart Association is one guide to classifying the extent of dysfunction (Table 26-2).

The diagnostic methods include history and physical examination, laboratory studies, electrocardiography, chest radiography, and echocardiography.[16] The history should include information related to dyspnea, cough, nocturia, generalized fatigue, and other signs and symptoms of heart failure. A complete physical examination includes assessment of heart rate, heart sounds, blood pressure, jugular veins for venous congestion, lungs for signs of pulmonary congestion, and lower extremities for edema. Laboratory tests are used in the diagnosis of anemia and electrolyte imbalances, and to detect signs of chronic liver congestion.

Electrocardiographic findings may indicate atrial or ventricular hypertrophy, underlying disorders of cardiac rhythm, or conduction abnormalities such as right or left bundle branch block. Chest radiographs provide information about the size and shape of the heart and pulmonary vasculature. The cardiac silhouette can be used to detect cardiac hypertrophy and dilatation. X-ray films can indicate the relative severity of the failure by revealing if pulmonary edema is predominantly vascular, interstitial, or advanced to the alveolar and bronchial stages. Echocardiography plays

---

TABLE 26-2 ◆ New York Heart Association Functional Classification of Patients With Heart Disease

Classification	Characteristics
Class I	Patients with cardiac disease but without the resulting limitations in physical activity. Ordinary activity does not cause undue fatigue, palpitation, dyspnea, or anginal pain.
Class II	Patients with heart disease resulting in slight limitations of physical activity. They are comfortable at rest. Ordinary physical activity results in fatigue, palpitation, dyspnea, or anginal pain.
Class III	Patients with cardiac disease resulting in marked limitation of physical activity. They are comfortable at rest. Less than ordinary physical activity causes fatigue, palpitation, dyspnea, or anginal pain.
Class IV	Patients with cardiac disease resulting in inability to carry on any physical activity without discomfort. The symptoms of cardiac insufficiency or of the anginal syndrome may be present even at rest. If any physical activity is undertaken, discomfort increases.

(From Criteria Committee of the New York Heart Association. [1964]. *Diseases of the heart and blood vessels: Nomenclature and criteria for diagnosis* [6th ed., pp. 112–113]. Boston: Little, Brown)

a key role in assessing the anatomic and functional abnormalities in CHF, which include the size and function of cardiac valves, the motion of both ventricles, and the ventricular ejection fraction.[17] Radionuclide angiography and cardiac catheterization are other diagnostic tests used to detect the underlying causes of heart failure, such as heart defects and cardiomyopathy.

Invasive hemodynamic monitoring often is used in the management of acute, life-threatening episodes of heart failure. These monitoring methods include central venous pressure (CVP), pulmonary capillary wedge pressure (PCWP), thermodilution cardiac output measurements, and intraarterial measurements of blood pressure.

CVP reflects the amount of blood returning to the heart. Measurements of CVP are best obtained by means of a catheter inserted into the right atrium through a peripheral vein, or by means of the right atrial port (opening) in a pulmonary artery catheter. This pressure is decreased in hypovolemia and increased in right heart failure. The changes that occur in CVP over time usually are more significant than the absolute numeric values obtained during a single reading.

PCWP pressure is obtained by means of a flow-directed, balloon-tipped pulmonary artery (Swan-Ganz) catheter. This catheter is introduced through a peripheral or central vein and then advanced into the right atrium. The balloon is then inflated with air, enabling the catheter to float through the right ventricle into the pulmonary artery until it becomes wedged in a small pulmonary vessel (Fig. 26-7). After the catheter is in place, the balloon is inflated only when the PCWP is being measured. Continuous inflation of the balloon with its accompanying occlusion of a small pulmonary artery would cause necrosis of pulmonary tissue. With the balloon inflated, the catheter monitors pulmonary capillary pressures in direct communication with pressures from the left heart. The pulmonary capillary pressures provide a means of assessing the pumping ability of the left heart.

One type of pulmonary artery catheter is equipped with a thermistor probe to obtain *thermodilution measurements* of cardiac output. A known amount of solution of a known temperature (iced or room temperature) is injected into the right atrium through an opening in the catheter, and the temperature of the blood is measured downstream in the pulmonary artery by means of a thermistor probe located at the end of that catheter. A microcomputer calculates the cardiac output from the time-temperature curve resulting from the rate of change of the temperature of the blood that flows past the thermistor. Catheters with oximeters built into their tips that permit continuous monitoring of oxygen saturation (SvO_2) also are available, as are catheters that provide continuous output data.

Intra-arterial blood pressure monitoring provides a means for continuous monitoring of blood pressure. It is used in persons with acute heart failure when aggressive intravenous drug therapy or a mechanical assist device is required. Measurements are obtained through the use of a small catheter inserted into a peripheral artery, usually the radial artery. The catheter is connected to a pressure transducer, and beat-by-beat measurements of blood pressure are recorded. The monitoring system displays the contour of the pressure waveform and a digital reading of the systolic, diastolic, and mean arterial pressures along with heart rate and rhythm. Continuous digital display of respiratory rate and core temperature from the thermistor located at the end of the pulmonary artery catheter also may be warranted.

Treatment Methods

The goals of treatment for chronic heart failure are directed toward relieving the symptoms and improving the quality of life, with a long-term goal of slowing, halting, or reversing the cardiac dysfunction.[18,19] Treatment measures include correction of reversible causes such as anemia or thyrotoxicosis, surgical repair of a ventricular defect or an improperly functioning valve, pharmacologic and non-pharmacologic control of afterload stresses such as hypertension, modification of activities and lifestyle to a level consistent with the functional limitations of a reduced cardiac reserve, and the use of medications to improve cardiac function and limit excessive compensatory mechanisms. Restriction of salt intake and diuretic therapy facilitate the excretion of edema fluid. Counseling, health teaching, and ongoing evaluation programs help persons with heart failure to manage and cope with their treatment regimen.

In severe heart failure, restriction of activity, including bed rest if necessary, often facilitates temporary recompensation of cardiac function. However, there is no convincing evidence that continued bed rest is of benefit. Carefully designed and managed exercise programs for patients with CHF are well tolerated and beneficial to patients with stable New York Heart Association (NYHA) class I to III heart failure.[20]

Pharmacologic Treatment. Once heart failure is moderate to severe, polypharmacy becomes a management stan-

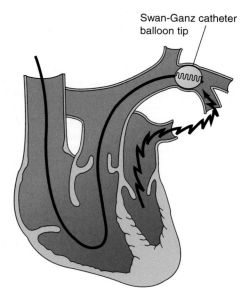

FIGURE 26-7 Swan-Ganz balloon-tipped catheter positioned in a pulmonary capillary. The pulmonary capillary wedge pressure, which reflects the left ventricular diastolic pressure, is measured with the balloon inflated.

Swan-Ganz catheter balloon tip

dard and often includes diuretics, digoxin, ACE inhibitors, and β-adrenergic–blocking agents.[21–23] The choice of pharmacologic agents is determined by problems caused by the disorder (*i.e.,* systolic or diastolic dysfunction) and those brought about by activation of compensatory mechanisms (*e.g.,* excess fluid retention, inappropriate activation of sympathetic mechanisms).

Diuretics are among the most frequently prescribed medications for heart failure. They promote the excretion of edema fluid and help to sustain cardiac output and tissue perfusion by reducing preload and allowing the heart to operate at a more optimal part of the Frank-Starling curve. Thiazide and loop diuretics are used. In emergencies, such as acute pulmonary edema, loop diuretics such as furosemide or bumetanide can be administered intravenously. When given intravenously, these drugs act quickly to reduce venous return through vasodilatation so that right ventricular output and pulmonary vascular pressures are decreased. This response to intravenous drug administration is extrarenal and precedes the onset of diuresis.

Digitalis has been a recognized treatment for CHF for over 200 years. The various forms of digitalis are called *cardiac glycosides.* They improve cardiac function by increasing the force and strength of ventricular contraction. By decreasing sinoatrial node activity and decreasing conduction through the atrioventricular node, they also slow the heart rate and increase diastolic filling time. Although not a diuretic, digitalis promotes urine output by improving cardiac output and renal blood flow. The digitalis drugs act by binding to sodium-potassium adenosine triphosphatase (ATPase) on the cell membrane and inhibiting the sodium-potassium pump. When intracellular sodium is increased because of inhibition of the sodium-potassium pump by digitalis, the exchange of intracellular calcium for extracellular sodium is inhibited; as a result, more calcium is available to activate the myocardial actin–myosin contractile apparatus. The role of digitalis in the treatment of heart failure is controversial and has been studied in clinical trials over the past several decades. Although the results of these studies remain controversial, there seems to be a growing consensus that although it does not necessarily reduce mortality rates, digitalis prevents clinical deterioration and hospitalization, and improves exercise tolerance.[24]

The *ACE inhibitors,* which prevent the conversion of angiotensin I to angiotensin II, have been effectively used in the treatment of heart failure. In heart failure, renin activity frequently is elevated because of decreased renal blood flow. The net result is an increase in angiotensin II, which causes vasoconstriction and increased aldosterone production with a subsequent increase in salt and water retention by the kidney. Both mechanisms increase the workload of the heart. Some studies have shown that the ACE inhibitors can relieve symptoms and increase survival in persons with symptomatic CHF.[25] The newer angiotensin II receptor blockers have the advantage of not causing a cough, which is a troublesome side effect of the ACE inhibitors for many persons.

Large clinical trials have shown that long-term therapy with β-adrenergic–blocking agents reduces morbidity and mortality in persons with chronic heart failure.[18,22,26]

Left ventricular dysfunction is associated with activation of the renin-angiotensin-aldosterone and sympathetic nervous systems. Chronic elevation of norepinephrine levels has been shown to cause cardiac muscle cell death and progressive left ventricular dysfunction, and is associated with poor prognosis in heart failure. Until recently, β blockers were thought to be contraindicated in left ventricular systolic dysfunction because of their negative inotropic effects. Large clinical trials involving more than 10,000 patients, most of whom had stable NYHA class II and III heart failure, have demonstrated significant reductions in the overall mortality rate with treatment with various β blockers. Several β blockers (*i.e.,* carvedilol, metoprolol, and bisoprolol) are used in the treatment of heart failure. The ongoing Carvedilol and Metoprolol European Trial (COMET) is designed to evaluate the relative benefits of these agents.[22]

ACUTE PULMONARY EDEMA

Acute pulmonary edema is the most dramatic symptom of left heart failure. It is a life-threatening condition in which capillary fluid moves into the alveoli. The accumulated fluid in the alveoli and respiratory airways causes lung stiffness, makes lung expansion more difficult, and impairs the gas exchange function of the lung. With the decreased ability of the lungs to oxygenate the blood, the hemoglobin leaves the pulmonary circulation without being fully oxygenated. Cyanosis and shortness of breath result.

Manifestations

Acute pulmonary edema usually is a terrifying experience. The person usually is seen sitting and gasping for air, in obvious apprehension. The pulse is rapid, the skin is moist and cool, and the lips and nail beds are cyanotic. As the lung edema worsens and oxygen supply to the brain drops, confusion and stupor appear. Dyspnea and air hunger are accompanied by a cough productive of frothy (resembling beaten egg whites) and often blood-tinged sputum—the effect of air mixing with serum albumin and red blood cells that have moved into the alveoli. The movement of air through the alveolar fluid produces fine crepitant sounds called *crackles,* which can be heard through a stethoscope placed on the chest. As fluid moves into the larger airways, the breathing becomes louder. The crackles heard earlier become louder and more coarse. In the terminal stage the breathing pattern is called the *death rattle.* Persons with severe pulmonary edema literally drown in their own secretions.

Treatment

Treatment of acute pulmonary edema is directed toward reducing the fluid volume in the pulmonary circulation. This can be accomplished by reducing the amount of blood that the right heart delivers to the lungs or by improving the work performance of the left heart. Several measures can decrease the blood volume in the pulmonary circulation; the seriousness of the pulmonary edema determines which are used. One of the simplest measures to relieve orthopnea is assumption of the seated position. For many persons, sitting up or standing is almost instinctive and may be sufficient to relieve the symptoms associated with mild accumulation of fluid.

Measures to improve left heart performance focus on decreasing the preload by reducing the filling pressure of the left ventricle and on reducing the afterload against which the left heart must pump. This can be accomplished through the use of diuretics, vasodilator drugs, treatment of arrhythmias that impair cardiac function, and improvement of the contractile properties of the left ventricle with digitalis. Rapid digitalization can be accomplished with intravenous administration of the drug.

Oxygen therapy increases the oxygen content of the blood and helps relieve anxiety. Positive-pressure breathing increases the intra-alveolar pressure, opposes the capillary filtration pressure in the pulmonary capillaries, and sometimes is used as a temporary measure to decrease the amount of fluid moving into the alveoli. Positive-pressure breathing can be administered through a specially designed, continuous positive airway pressure mask. In the most severe cases, however, endotracheal intubation and mechanical ventilation may be necessary. Although its mechanisms of action are unclear, morphine sulfate usually is the drug of choice in acute pulmonary edema. Morphine relieves anxiety and depresses the pulmonary reflexes that cause spasm of the pulmonary vessels. It also increases venous pooling by vasodilatation.

CARDIOGENIC SHOCK

Cardiogenic shock implies failure of the heart to pump blood adequately. Cardiogenic shock can occur relatively quickly because of the damage to the heart that occurs during myocardial infarction; ineffective pumping caused by cardiac dysrhythmias; mechanical defects that may occur as a complication of myocardial infarction, such as ventricular septal defect; ventricular aneurysm; acute disruption of valvular function; or problems associated with open heart surgery. Cardiogenic shock also may ensue as an end-stage condition of coronary artery disease or cardiomyopathy.

The most common cause of cardiogenic shock is myocardial infarction. Most patients who die of cardiogenic shock have lost at least 40% of the contracting muscle of the left ventricle because of a recent infarct or a combination of recent and old infarcts.[27] Cardiogenic shock can follow other types of shock associated with inadequate coronary blood flow, or it can develop because substances released from ischemic tissues impair cardiac function. One such substance, myocardial depressant factor, is thought to be released into the circulation during severe shock. Myocardial depressant factor produces reversible (although often severe) myocardial depression, ventricular dilation, and decreased left ventricular ejection fraction and diastolic pressure.[28]

In all cases of cardiogenic shock, there is failure to eject blood from the heart, hypotension, and inadequate cardiac output. Increased systemic vascular resistance often contributes to the deterioration of cardiac function by increasing afterload or the resistance to ventricular systole. The filling pressure, or preload of the heart, also is increased as blood returning to the heart is added to blood that previously was returned but not pumped forward, resulting in an increase in end-systolic ventricular volume. Increased resistance to ventricular systole (*i.e.,* afterload) combined with the decreased myocardial contractility causes the increased end-systolic ventricular volume and increased preload, which further complicate cardiac status.

Manifestations

The signs and symptoms of cardiogenic shock are consistent with those of extreme heart failure. The lips, nail beds, and skin are cyanotic because of stagnation of blood flow and increased extraction of oxygen from the hemoglobin as it passes through the capillary bed. The CVP and PCWP rise as a result of volume overload caused by the pumping failure of the heart.

Treatment

Treatment of cardiogenic shock requires a precarious balance between improving cardiac output, reducing the workload and oxygen needs of the myocardium, and preserving coronary perfusion. Fluid volume must be regulated within a level that maintains the filling pressure (*i.e.,* venous return) of the heart and maximum use of the Frank-Starling mechanism without causing pulmonary congestion.

Pharmacologic treatment includes the use of vasodilators such as nitroprusside and nitroglycerine. Nitroprusside causes arterial and venous dilatation, producing a decrease in venous return to the heart, with a reduction in arterial resistance against which the left heart must pump. Nitroglycerin focuses its effects on the venous vascular beds until, at high doses, it begins to dilate the arterial beds as well. The arterial pressure is maintained by an increased ventricular stroke volume ejected against a lowered systemic vascular resistance; this allows blood to be redistributed from the pulmonary vascular bed to the systemic circulation. Catecholamines increase cardiac contractility but must be used with caution because they also produce vasoconstriction and increase cardiac workload by increasing the afterload.

Treatment using hemofiltration or the intra-aortic balloon pump is an alternative for patients who do not respond to medical treatment. The use of extracorporeal membrane oxygenation, once considered effective only in infants and children, has been used with limited success in adults.[29]

Continuous hemofiltration is an external process for removing, filtering, and returning blood volume using a compact device and peripheral vascular access. When used early in the management of moderate to severe heart failure, hemofiltration can increase mean arterial pressure, reduce preload and afterload, reverse cardiac dysfunction, help restore renal function, and eliminate cardiopulmonary toxic metabolites from the plasma, all of which improve survival.[30]

The intra-aortic balloon pump provides a means of increasing aortic diastolic pressure and enhances coronary and peripheral blood flow without increasing systolic pressure and the afterload, against which the left ventricle must pump.[27] The device, which pumps in synchrony with the heart, consists of a 10-inch-long balloon that is inserted through a catheter into the descending aorta (Fig. 26-8). The balloon is positioned so that the distal tip lies approximately 1 inch from the aortic arch. The balloon is filled with helium and is timed to inflate during ventricular diastole and deflate just before ventricular systole. Diastolic inflation creates a pressure wave in the ascending aorta that increases coronary artery flow and a less intense wave in the lower aorta that enhances organ perfusion. The sudden balloon deflation at the onset of systole lowers the resistance to ejection of blood from the left ventricle, thereby increasing the heart's pumping efficiency and decreasing myocardial oxygen consumption.

When cardiogenic shock is caused by myocardial infarction, several aggressive interventions can be used successfully. The rapid and aggressive administration of a thrombolytic agent to dissolve intracoronary thrombi has been shown significantly to improve aortic pressure and survival.[31] Another alternative includes emergent direct percutaneous transluminal angioplasty (see Chapter 24).

MECHANICAL SUPPORT AND HEART TRANSPLANTATION

Refractory heart failure reflects deterioration in cardiac function that is unresponsive to medical or surgical interventions. With improved methods of treatment, more people are reaching a point where a cure is unachievable

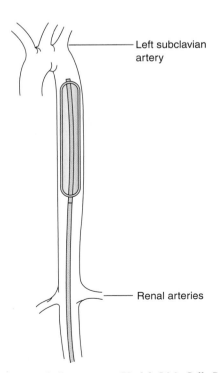

FIGURE 26-8 Aortic balloon pump. (Hudak C.M., Gallo B.M. [1994]. *Critical care nursing* [6th ed.]. Philadelphia: J.B. Lippincott)

Left subclavian artery

Renal arteries

and death is imminent without mechanical support or heart transplantation.

Since the early 1960s, significant progress has been made in improving the efficacy of *ventricular assist devices* (VADs), which are mechanical pumps used to support ventricular function. VADs are used to decrease the workload of the myocardium while maintaining cardiac output and systemic arterial pressure. This decreases the workload on the ventricle and allows it to rest and recover. Most VADs require an invasive open chest procedure for implantation. They may be used in patients who fail or have difficulty being weaned from cardiopulmonary bypass after cardiac surgery; those who develop cardiogenic shock after myocardial infarction; those with end-stage cardiomyopathy; and those who are awaiting cardiac transplantation. Earlier and more aggressive use of VADs as a bridge to transplantation has been shown to increase survival.[32] VADs that allow the patient to be mobile and managed at home are beginning to be considered as long-term or permanent support for treatment of end-stage heart failure, rather than simply as a bridge to transplantation.[32] VADs can be used to support the function of the left ventricle, right ventricle, or both.

Heart transplantation remains the treatment of choice for end-stage cardiac failure. The number of successful heart transplantations has been steadily climbing, with over 2800 procedures performed per year. Patients with heart transplants who are treated with triple-immunosuppressant therapy have a 5-year survival rate of 70% to 80%.[33] Despite the overall success of heart transplantation, donor availability and complications from infection, rejection, and immunosuppression drug therapy remain problems.

The current technique for orthotopic heart transplantation (the most common) was described in 1960 by Lower and Shumway.[34] The procedure is performed by placing the recipient on cardiopulmonary bypass and excising the diseased heart. The method involves retaining a large portion of the posterior wall of the right and left atrium in the recipient and attaching the donor heart with relatively long sutures (Fig. 26-9). Pacing wires are loosely attached to the right ventricle to assist with temporary pacing of the heartbeat in the event of bradycardia in the immediate postoperative phase.

An alternative to heart transplantation is a procedure called *cardiomyoplasty*.[35] This procedure involves fashioning one of the patient's latissimus dorsi back muscles into a wrap that embraces the heart. The muscle is native tissue; thus, rejection is not a problem. Because the proximal end of the muscle remains intact, perfusion is optimal with enhanced potential for healing and performance. A pacemaker, which is placed between the heart and the back muscle, stimulates the muscle to contract. After several weeks of rest and healing, the skeletal muscle is gradually stimulated by the pacemaker to condition it in a necessary transformation into a more fatigue-resistant type of muscle tissue. Although more work is needed to identify the optimal way to wrap the muscle and condition it for maximum ventricular assist, cardiomyoplasty provides an alternative to transplantation for some persons, particularly when a donor heart is not available.

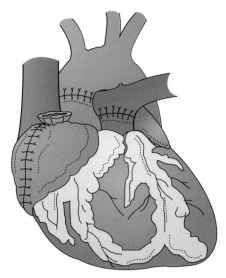

FIGURE 26-9 Orthotopic heart transplantation and sites of donor heart attachment.

In summary, heart failure occurs when the heart fails to pump sufficient blood to meet the metabolic needs of body tissues. The physiology of heart failure reflects an interplay between a decrease in cardiac output that accompanies impaired function of the failing heart and the compensatory mechanisms designed to preserve the cardiac reserve. Four compensatory mechanisms contribute to the cardiac reserve: increased activity of the sympathetic nervous system, salt and water retention, the Frank-Starling mechanism, and myocardial hypertrophy. In the failing heart, early decreases in cardiac function may go unnoticed because these compensatory mechanisms maintain the cardiac output. This is called *compensated heart failure.* Unfortunately, the mechanisms were not intended for long-term use, and in severe and prolonged decompensated heart failure, the compensatory mechanisms no longer are effective, and themselves further impair cardiac function. In CHF, there is a decrease in cardiac output along with fluid accumulation in body tissues.

Heart failure may be described as high-output or low-output failure, systolic or diastolic failure, and right-sided or left-sided failure. With high-output failure, the function of the heart may be supranormal but inadequate because of excessive metabolic needs, and low-output failure is caused by disorders that impair the pumping ability of the heart. With systolic dysfunction, there is impaired ejection of blood from the heart during systole; with diastolic dysfunction, there is impaired filling of the heart during diastole. Right-sided failure is characterized by congestion in the peripheral circulation, and left-sided failure by congestion in the pulmonary circulation.

The manifestations of heart failure include edema, nocturia, fatigue and impaired exercise tolerance, cyanosis, signs of increased sympathetic nervous sys-

tem activity, and impaired gastrointestinal function and malnutrition. In right-sided failure, there is dependent edema of the lower parts of the body, engorgement of the liver, and ascites. In left-sided failure, shortness of breath and chronic, nonproductive cough are common.

The diagnostic methods in heart failure are directed toward establishing the cause and extent of the disorder. Treatment is directed toward correcting the cause whenever possible, improving cardiac function, maintaining the fluid volume within a compensatory level, and developing an activity pattern consistent with individual limitations in cardiac reserve. Among the medications used in the treatment of heart failure are diuretics, digoxin, ACE inhibitors, and β blockers.

Acute pulmonary edema is a life-threatening condition in which the accumulation of fluid in the interstitium of the lung and alveoli interferes with lung expansion and gas exchange. It is characterized by extreme breathlessness, rales, frothy sputum, cyanosis, and signs of hypoxemia. In cardiogenic shock, there is failure to eject blood from the heart, hypotension, inadequate cardiac output, and impaired perfusion of peripheral tissues. Mechanical support devices, including the intra-aortic balloon pump (for acute failure) and the VAD, sustain life in persons with severe heart failure. Heart transplantation remains the treatment of choice for many persons with end-stage heart failure.

Circulatory Failure (Shock)

After you have completed this section of the chapter, you should be able to meet the following objectives:

✦ State a clinical definition of shock
✦ Describe the compensatory mechanisms that are activated in circulatory shock
✦ List the chief characteristics of hypovolemic shock, cardiogenic shock, obstructive shock, and distributive shock
✦ List and describe the four stages of hypovolemic shock
✦ Compare the pathophysiology of neurogenic shock, anaphylactic shock, and septic shock
✦ Characterize changes in thirst, skin blood flow, pulse rate, urine output, and sensorium that are indicative of shock
✦ Describe the complications of shock as they relate to the lung, kidney, gastrointestinal tract, and blood clotting
✦ State the rationale for treatment measures to correct and reverse shock
✦ Define multiple organ dysfunction syndrome and cite its significance in shock

The functions of the circulatory system are to perfuse body tissues and supply them with oxygen. *Circulatory shock* can be described as a failure of the vascular system to supply the peripheral tissues and organs of the body with an adequate blood supply. It is not a specific disease but can occur in the course of many life-threatening traumatic or disease states. Although circulatory shock produces hypotension, it should not be equated with a drop in blood pressure. Hypotension often is a late sign and indicates a failure of compensatory mechanisms.

PHYSIOLOGY OF SHOCK

Adequate perfusion of body tissues depends on the pumping ability of the heart, a vascular system that transports blood to the cells and back to the heart, sufficient blood to fill the vascular system, and tissues that are able to use and extract oxygen and nutrients from the blood. As with heart failure, circulatory shock produces compensatory physiologic responses that eventually decompensate into various shock states if the condition is not properly treated in a timely manner.

In severe and prolonged shock, the vascular system fails. When this occurs, there is relaxation of the arterioles and venules, a decrease in arterial pressure, and venous pooling of blood. At the capillary level, hypoxia and the products of cell damage cause increased capillary permeability, stagnation of blood flow, the formation of small blood clots, and shifting of intravascular volume into the interstitium, a condition called *third spacing*.

The delivery of oxygen and nutrients to cells and the removal of metabolic waste products depend on adequate blood flow throughout the capillaries of the microcirculation. There are two types of capillary flow: nutrient flow and non-nutrient flow. Nutrient flow describes flow in the true capillary pathways that supply cells with oxygen and nutrients. In non-nutrient flow, blood is shunted directly from the arterial to the venous side of the circulation without passing through the true capillary pathways. Non-nutrient flow provides warmth, but not oxygen and nutrients, to the tissues. In septic shock, non-nutrient flow often is increased, and the skin is warm and flushed. Both nutrient and non-nutrient flow are decreased in hypovolemic shock, and the skin is cool and clammy.

Compensatory Mechanisms

Without compensatory mechanisms to maintain cardiac output and blood pressure, the loss of vascular volume would result in a rapid progression from the initial to the progressive and irreversible stages of shock.

The most immediate of the compensatory mechanisms are the sympathetic-mediated responses designed to maintain cardiac output and blood pressure. Within seconds after the onset of hemorrhage or the loss of blood volume, tachycardia, increased cardiac contractility, vasoconstriction, and other signs of sympathetic and adrenal medullary activity appear (Fig. 26-10). The sympathetic vasoconstrictor response affects the arterioles and the veins. Arteriolar constriction helps to maintain blood pressure by increasing the systemic vascular resistance, and venous constriction mobilizes blood that has been stored in the capacitance side of the circulation as a means of increasing venous return to the heart. There is considerable capacity for blood storage in the large veins of the abdomen and liver. Approximately 350 mL of blood that can be mobilized in shock is stored in the liver. Sympathetic stimulation does not cause constriction of the cerebral and coronary vessels, and blood flow through the heart and brain is maintained at essentially normal levels as long as the mean arterial pressure remains above 70 mm Hg.[36]

During the early stages of hypovolemic shock, vasoconstriction causes a reduction in the size of the vascular compartment and an increase in systemic vascular resistance. This response usually is all that is needed when the injury is slight, and blood loss is arrested at this point. As hypovolemic shock progresses, there are further increases in heart rate and cardiac contractility, and vasoconstriction becomes more intense. There is vasoconstriction of the blood vessels that supply the skin, skeletal muscles, kidneys, and abdominal organs, with a resultant decrease in blood flow and conversion to anaerobic metabolism with lactic acid formation. When acidosis becomes evident, the arterial chemoreceptors are activated and contribute an additional vasoconstrictor effect.

Compensatory mechanisms designed to restore blood volume include absorption of fluid from the interstitial spaces, conservation of salt and water by the kidneys, and thirst. Extracellular fluid is distributed between the interstitial spaces and the vascular compartment. When there is a loss of vascular volume, capillary pressures decrease, and water is drawn into the vascular compartment from the interstitial spaces. The maintenance of vascular volume is further enhanced by renal mechanisms that conserve fluid. A decrease in renal blood flow, which results from sympathetic vasoconstriction, lowers the glomerular filtration rate and activates the renin-angiotensin mechanism, which increases the release of aldosterone by the adrenal cortex, producing a further increase in sodium reabsorption by the kidney tubules. The decrease in blood volume also stimulates centers in the hypothalamus that regulate ADH release and thirst. A decrease in blood volume by 10% is sufficient to stimulate ADH release and thirst.[37] ADH, also known as *vasopressin*, constricts the peripheral arteries and veins and greatly increases water retention by the kidneys.

The compensatory mechanisms that the body recruits in hypovolemic and other forms of circulatory shock were not intended for long-term use. When injury is severe or its effects prolonged, the compensatory mechanisms begin to exert their own detrimental effects. The intense vasoconstriction causes a decrease in tissue perfusion, impaired cellular metabolism, release of vasoactive inflammatory mediators such as histamine, liberation of lactic acid, and cell death. After circulatory function has been reestablished, whether the shock will be irreversible or the patient will survive is determined largely at the cellular level.

Cellular Changes

At the cellular level, oxygen and nutrients supply the energy needed to maintain cellular function. In the cell, oxygen and fuel substrates are converted to adenosine triphosphate (ATP), the cell's energy source. The cell uses ATP for a number of purposes, including operation of the sodium-potassium membrane pump that moves sodium out of the cell and potassium back into the cell.

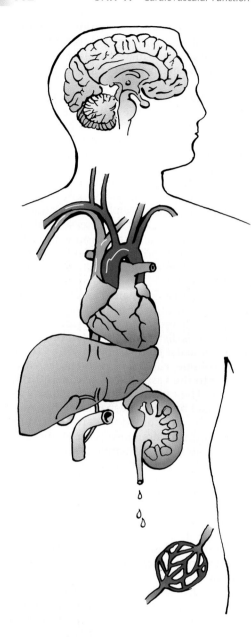

Brain
- Thirst
- Increased production and release ADH

Cardiovascular system
- Increased heart rate
- Increased force of cardiac contraction
- Increased systemic vascular resistance
- Decreased blood flow to the
  kidney
  gastrointestinal tract
  skin
  skeletal muscles
- Constriction of the veins

Adrenal gland
- Increased production and release of aldosterone by the adrenal cortex
- Increased production and release of the catecholamines (epinephrine and norepinephrine) by the adrenal medulla

Liver
- Constriction of veins and sinusoids with mobilization of blood stored in the liver

Kidney
- Increased retention of sodium and water
- Decreased urine output

Capillary bed
- Increased reabsorption of water into the capillary from the interstitial spaces due to constriction of the arterioles with a resultant decrease in capillary pressure

FIGURE 26-10 Compensatory mechanisms in hypovolemic shock.

The cell uses two pathways to convert nutrients to energy (see Chapter 4). The first is the anaerobic (nonoxygen) glycolytic pathway, which is located in the cytoplasm. Glycolysis converts glucose to ATP and pyruvate. The second pathway is the aerobic (oxygen-dependent) pathway, called the *citric acid cycle,* which is located in the mitochondria. When oxygen is available, pyruvate from the glycolytic pathway moves into the mitochondria and enters the citric acid cycle, where it is transformed into ATP and the metabolic byproducts carbon dioxide and water. Fatty acids and proteins also can be metabolized in the mitochondrial pathway. When oxygen is lacking, pyruvate does not enter the citric acid cycle; instead, it is converted to lactic acid. In severe shock, cellular metabolic processes are essen-

tially anaerobic, which means that excess amounts of lactic acid accumulate in the cellular and the extracellular compartment.

The anaerobic pathway, although allowing energy production to continue in the absence of oxygen, is relatively inefficient and produces significantly less ATP than does the aerobic pathway. Without sufficient energy production, normal cell function cannot be maintained, and the activity of the sodium-potassium membrane pump is impaired. As a result, sodium chloride accumulates in cells and potassium is lost from cells. The cells then swell, and their membranes become more permeable. Mitochondrial activity becomes severely depressed and lysosomal membranes rupture, resulting in the release of enzymes that cause further intracellular destruction. This is followed by cell death and the release of intracellular contents into the extracellular spaces. The resultant changes in the microcirculation reduce the chance of recovery.

CIRCULATORY SHOCK

Circulatory shock is used to describe a critical decrease in tissue perfusion due to a loss or redistribution of intravascular fluid. It can be classified as hypovolemic, obstructive, or distributive. These three main types of shock are summarized in Chart 26-1 and depicted in Figure 26-1. Cardiogenic shock, which results from failure of the heart as a pump, was discussed earlier in the chapter.

Hypovolemic Shock

Hypovolemic shock is characterized by diminished blood volume such that there is inadequate filling of the vascular compartment (see Fig. 26-10). It occurs when there is an acute loss of 15% to 20% of the circulating blood volume.

CHART 26-1

Classification of Circulatory Shock

Hypovolemic
Loss of whole blood
Loss of plasma
Loss of extracellular fluid

Obstructive
Inability of the heart to fill properly (cardiac tamponade)
Obstruction to outflow from the heart (pulmonary embolus, cardiac myxoma, pneumothorax, or dissecting aneurysm)

Distributive
Loss of sympathetic vasomotor tone
Presence of vasodilating substances in the blood (anaphylactic shock)
Presence of inflammatory mediators (septic shock)

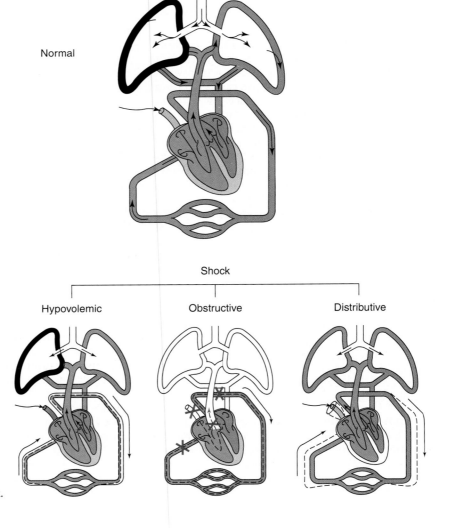

FIGURE 26-11 Types of shock.

Circulatory Shock

➤ Circulatory shock represents the inability of the circulation to adequately perfuse the tissues of the body.

➤ It can result from a loss of fluid from the vascular compartment, an increase in the size of the vascular compartment that interferes with the distribution of blood, or obstruction of flow through the vascular compartment.

➤ The manifestations of shock reflect both the impaired perfusion of body tissues and the body's attempt to maintain tissue perfusion through conservation of water by the kidney, translocation of fluid from extracellular to the intravascular compartment, and activation of sympathetic nervous systems mechanisms that increase heart rate and divert blood from less to more essential body tissues.

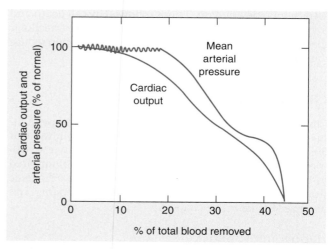

FIGURE 26-12 Effect of hemorrhage on cardiac output and arterial pressure. (Guyton A.C. [1986]. *Textbook of medical physiology* [7th ed.]. Philadelphia: W.B. Saunders)

The decrease may be caused by an external loss of whole blood (*e.g.*, hemorrhage), plasma (*e.g.*, severe burns), or extracellular fluid (*e.g.*, gastrointestinal fluids lost in vomiting or diarrhea). Hypovolemic shock also can result from an internal hemorrhage or from third-space losses, when extracellular fluid is shifted from the vascular compartment to the interstitial space or compartment.

Hypovolemic shock has been the most widely studied type of shock and usually serves as a prototype in discussions of the manifestations of shock. Figure 26-12 shows the effect of removing blood from the circulatory system during approximately 30 minutes.[36] Approximately 10% can be removed without changing the cardiac output or arterial pressure. The average blood donor loses a pint of blood without experiencing adverse effects. As increasing amounts of blood (10% to 25%) are removed, the cardiac output falls but the arterial pressure is maintained because of sympathetic-mediated increases in heart rate and vasoconstriction. Blood pressure is the product of cardiac output and systemic vascular resistance (BP = CO × SVR); an increase in systemic vascular resistance maintains blood pressure in the presence of decreased cardiac output for a short period. Cardiac output and tissue perfusion decrease before signs of hypotension occur. Cardiac output and arterial pressure fall to zero when approximately 35% to 45% of the total blood volume has been removed.[36]

Stages of Hypovolemic Shock.

The progression of hypovolemic shock can be divided into four stages. During the *initial stage,* the circulatory blood volume is decreased, but not enough to cause serious effects. The *second stage* is the compensatory stage; although the circulating blood volume is reduced, compensatory mechanisms are able to maintain blood pressure and tissue perfusion at a level sufficient

to prevent cell damage. The *third stage* is the progressive stage or stage of decompensated shock. At this point, unfavorable signs begin to appear: the blood pressure begins to fall, blood flow to the heart and brain is impaired, capillary permeability is increased, fluid begins to leave the capillaries, blood flow becomes sluggish, and the cells and their enzyme systems are damaged. The *fourth and final stage* is the irreversible stage. In irreversible shock, even though the blood volume may be restored and vital signs stabilized, death ensues eventually. Although the factors that determine recovery from severe shock have not been clearly identified, it appears that they are related to blood flow at the level of the microcirculation. The severity and clinical findings associated with hypovolemic shock are summarized in Table 26-3.

Manifestations.

The signs and symptoms of hypovolemic shock depend on shock stage and are closely related to low peripheral blood flow and excessive sympathetic stimulation. They include thirst, an increase in heart rate, cool and clammy skin, a decrease in arterial blood pressure, a decrease in urine output, and changes in mentation. Laboratory tests of hemoglobin and hematocrit provide information regarding the severity of blood loss or hemoconcentration due to dehydration. Serum lactate and arterial pH provide information about the severity of acidosis.

Thirst is an early symptom in hypovolemic shock. Although the underlying cause is not fully understood, it probably is related to decreased blood volume and increased serum osmolality (see Chapter 31). An increase in heart rate often is another early sign of shock. As shock progresses, the pulse becomes weak and thready, indicating vasoconstriction and a reduction in filling of the vascular compartment.

Arterial blood pressure is decreased in moderate to severe shock. However, controversy exists over the value of blood pressure measurements in the early diagnosis and management of shock. This is because compensatory mechanisms tend to preserve blood pressure until shock is rela-

TABLE 26-3 ✦ Correlation of Clinical Findings and the Magnitude of Volume Deficit in Hemorrhagic Shock

Severity of Shock	Clinical Findings	Percentage of Reduction in Blood Volume (mL)
None	None; normal blood donation	≤10 (500)*
Mild	Minimal tachycardia	15–25 (750–1250)
	Slight decrease in blood pressure	
	Mild evidence of peripheral vasoconstriction with cool hands and feet	
Moderate	Tachycardia, 100–120 beats per minute	25–35 (1250–1750)
	Decrease in pulse pressure	
	Systolic pressure, 90–100 mm Hg	
	Restlessness	
	Increased sweating	
	Pallor	
	Oliguria	
Severe	Tachycardia over 120 beats per minute	Up to 50 (2500)
	Blood pressure below 60 mm Hg systolic and frequently unobtainable by cuff	
	Mental stupor	
	Extreme pallor, cold extremities	
	Anuria	

*Based on blood volume of 7% in a 70-kg male of medium build.
(Adapted from Weil M., Shubin H. [1967]. *Diagnosis and treatment of shock* [p. 118]. Baltimore: Williams & Wilkins)

tively far advanced. Furthermore, an adequate arterial pressure does not ensure adequate perfusion and oxygenation of vital organs at the cellular level. This does not imply that blood pressure should not be closely monitored in patients at risk for development of shock, but it does indicate the need for other assessment measures by which shock may be detected at an earlier stage. Blood pressure often is measured intra-arterially in persons with severe shock because auscultatory (cuff and stethoscope) or oscillometric (automatic blood pressure machines) methods may not always provide an accurate measurement. The Doppler method, in which blood pressure is measured noninvasively by ultrasound, may provide a more accurate estimate of Korotkoff sounds when they are no longer audible through the stethoscope. In some instances, this method may be used as an alternative to continuous intra-arterial monitoring.

As shock progresses, the respirations become rapid and deep. Decreased intravascular volume results in decreased venous return to the heart and a decrease in CVP. When shock becomes severe, the peripheral veins collapse, making it difficult to insert peripheral venous lines. Sympathetic stimulation also leads to intense vasoconstriction of the skin vessels and activation of the sweat glands. As a result, the skin is cool and moist. When shock is caused by hemorrhage, the loss of red blood cells leaves the skin and mucous membranes looking pale.

Urine output decreases very quickly in hypovolemic and other forms of shock. Compensatory mechanisms decrease renal blood flow as a means of diverting blood flow to the heart and brain. Oliguria of 20 mL/hour or less indicates severe shock and inadequate renal perfusion. Continuous measurement of urine output is essential for assessing the circulatory status of the person in shock.

Restlessness and apprehension are common behaviors in early shock. As the shock progresses and blood flow to the brain decreases, restlessness is replaced by apathy and stupor. If shock is unchecked, the apathy progresses to coma. Coma caused by blood loss alone and not related to head injury or other factors is an unfavorable sign.

Treatment. The treatment of hypovolemic shock is directed toward correcting or controlling the underlying cause and improving tissue perfusion. Persons who have sustained blood loss are commonly placed in supine position with the legs elevated to maximize cerebral blood flow. Oxygen is administered to persons with signs of hypoxemia. Because subcutaneous administration is unpredictable, pain medications usually are administered intravenously. Frequent measurements of heart rate and cardiac rhythm, blood pressure, and urine flow are used to assess the severity of circulatory compromise and to monitor treatment.

In hypovolemic shock, the goal of treatment is to restore vascular volume. This can be accomplished through intravenous administration of fluids and blood. The crystalloids (*e.g.*, isotonic saline) are readily available for emergencies and mass casualties. They often are effective, at least temporarily, when given in adequate doses. Plasma expanders, including dextrans and colloidal albumin solutions, have a high molecular weight, do not necessitate blood typing, and remain in the circulation for longer periods than the crystalloids, such as glucose and saline. The dextrans must be used with caution because they may induce serious or fatal reactions, including anaphylaxis. Blood or blood products (packed or frozen red cells) are administered based on hematocrit and hemodynamic findings. Fluids and blood are best administered based on volume indicators such as CVP and PCWP. This is particularly important in pediatric patients, whose fluid balance allows less variation from normal before compromise to tissue perfusion results, and who may respond better to hypertonic saline than to other crystalloid or colloid solutions.[38]

Vasoactive drugs (*e.g.*, adrenergic agents) are agents capable of constricting or dilating blood vessels. Considerable controversy exists about the advantages or disadvantages related to the use of these drugs. There are two types of adrenergic receptors for the sympathetic nervous system: α and β. The β receptors are further subdivided into β_1 and β_2 receptors. In the cardiorespiratory system, stimulation of the α receptors causes vasoconstriction; stimulation of β_1 receptors causes an increase in heart rate and the force of myocardial contraction; and stimulation of β_2 receptors produces vasodilatation of the skeletal muscle beds and relaxation of the bronchioles.

As a general rule, the adrenergic drugs are not used as a primary form of therapy in shock. Simple blood pressure elevation produced by vasopressor drugs has little effect on the underlying cause of shock and in many cases may be detrimental. These agents are given only when hypotension persists after volume deficits have been corrected.

Dopamine, which induces a more favorable array of α- and β-receptor actions than many of the other adrenergic drugs, may be used in the treatment of severe and prolonged shock. Dopamine is thought to increase blood flow to the kidneys, liver, and other abdominal organs while maintaining vasoconstriction of less vital structures, such as the skin and skeletal muscles, when given in low doses. In severe shock, higher doses may be needed to maintain blood pressure. After dopamine administration exceeds this low-dose range, it has vasoconstrictive effects on blood flow to the kidneys and abdominal organs that are similar to those of epinephrine.

Obstructive Shock

The term *obstructive shock* is used to describe circulatory shock that results from mechanical obstruction of the flow of blood through the central circulation (great veins, heart, or lungs; see Fig. 26-11). Obstructive shock may be caused by a number of conditions, including dissecting aortic aneurysm, cardiac tamponade, pneumothorax, atrial myxoma, or evisceration of abdominal contents into the thoracic cavity because of a ruptured hemidiaphragm. The most frequent cause of obstructive shock is pulmonary embolism.

The primary physiologic results of obstructive shock are elevated right heart pressure and impaired venous return to the heart. The signs of right heart failure are seen, including elevation of CVP and jugular venous distention. Treatment modalities focus on correcting the cause of the disorder, frequently with surgical interventions such as pulmonary embolectomy, pericardiocentesis (*i.e.*, removal of fluid from the pericardial sac) for cardiac tamponade, or the insertion of a chest tube for correction of a tension pneumothorax or hemothorax. In select cases of pulmonary

embolus, thrombolytic drugs may be used to dissolve the clots causing the obstruction.

Distributive Shock

Distributive shock is characterized by loss of blood vessel tone, enlargement of the vascular compartment, and displacement of the vascular volume away from the heart and central circulation. With distributive shock, the capacity of the vascular compartment expands to the extent that a normal volume of blood does not fill the circulatory system (see Fig. 26-11). Loss of vessel tone has two main causes: a decrease in the sympathetic control of vasomotor tone and the presence of vasodilator substances in the blood. Venous return is decreased in distributive shock, which leads to a diminished cardiac output but not a decrease in total blood volume; this type of shock is also referred to as *normovolemic shock*. There are three shock states that share the basic circulatory pattern of distributive shock: neurogenic shock, anaphylactic shock, and septic shock.

Neurogenic Shock. Neurogenic shock describes shock caused by decreased sympathetic control of blood vessel tone due to a defect in the vasomotor center in the brain stem or the sympathetic outflow to the blood vessels. Output from the vasomotor center can be interrupted by brain injury, the depressant action of drugs, general anesthesia, hypoxia, or lack of glucose (*e.g.*, insulin reaction). Fainting due to emotional causes is a transient form of neurogenic shock. Spinal anesthesia or spinal cord injury above the midthoracic region can interrupt the transmission of outflow from the vasomotor center. The term *spinal shock* is used to describe the neurogenic shock that occurs in persons with spinal cord injury. Many general anesthetic agents can cause a neurogenic shock-like reaction, especially during induction, because of interference with sympathetic nervous system function. In contrast to hypovolemic shock, the heart rate in neurogenic shock often is slower than normal, and the skin is dry and warm. This type of distributive shock is rare and usually transitory.

Anaphylactic Shock. Anaphylactic shock is characterized by massive vasodilatation, pooling of blood in the peripheral blood vessels, and increased capillary permeability.[39] This type of shock, which is a manifestation of systemic anaphylaxis, is caused by an immunologically mediated reaction in which vasodilator substances such as histamine are released into the blood (see Chapter 19). These substances cause dilatation of arterioles and venules along with a marked increase in capillary permeability. The vascular response in anaphylactic shock is often accompanied by bronchospasm, contraction of gastrointestinal and uterine smooth muscle, and urticaria or angioedema.

Among the most frequent causes of anaphylactic shock are reactions to drugs, such as penicillin; foods, such as nuts and shellfish; and insect venoms. The most common cause is stings from insects of the order Hymenoptera (*i.e.*, bees, wasps, and fire ants). Latex allergy has caused life-threatening anaphylaxis in a growing segment of the population. Health care workers and others who are exposed to latex are developing latex sensitivities that range from mild urticaria, contact dermatitis, and mild respiratory distress to anaphylactic shock.[40] Children with spina bifida also are at extreme risk for this increasingly serious allergy (see Chapter 19).

The onset of anaphylaxis depends on the sensitivity of the person and the rate and quantity of antigen exposure. Anaphylactic shock often develops suddenly; death can occur within a matter of minutes unless appropriate medical intervention is promptly instituted. Signs and symptoms associated with impending anaphylactic shock include abdominal cramps, apprehension, burning and warm sensation of the skin, itching, urticaria (*i.e.*, hives), coughing, choking, wheezing, chest tightness, and difficulty in breathing. After blood begins to pool peripherally, there is a precipitous drop in blood pressure and the pulse becomes so weak that it is difficult to detect. Life-threatening airway obstruction may ensue as a result of laryngeal edema or bronchial spasm.

Treatment includes immediate discontinuance of the inciting agent or institution of measures to decrease its absorption (*e.g.*, application of ice); close monitoring of cardiovascular and respiratory function; and maintenance of adequate respiratory gas exchange, cardiac output, and tissue perfusion. Epinephrine constricts the blood vessels and relaxes the smooth muscle in the bronchioles; it usually is the first drug to be given to a patient believed to be experiencing an anaphylactic reaction. Other treatment measures include the administration of oxygen, antihistaminic drugs, and corticosteroids. Resuscitation measures may be required.

The prevention of anaphylactic shock is preferable to treatment. Once a person has been sensitized to an antigen, the risk of repeated anaphylactic reactions with subsequent exposure is high. All health care providers should question patients regarding previous drug reactions and inform patients as to the name of the medication they are to receive before it is administered or prescribed. Persons with known hypersensitivities should carry some form of medical identification to alert medical personnel if they become unconscious or unable to relate this information. Persons who are risk for anaphylaxis should be provided with emergency medications (*e.g.*, epinephrine autoinjector) and instructed in procedures to follow in case they are inadvertently exposed to the offending antigen. In some situations, it may be medically necessary to administer agents known to cause anaphylaxis. Protocols that have been developed to prevent or decrease the severity of the reaction involve pharmacologic pretreatment to block or blunt the reaction.

Sepsis and Septic Shock

Septic shock is associated with severe infection and the systemic response to infection. It is associated most frequently with gram-negative bacteremia, although it can be caused by gram-positive bacilli and other microorganisms such as fungi, which carry an even greater risk of mortality.[41] Unlike other types of shock, septic shock commonly is associated with pathologic complications, such as pulmonary insufficiency, disseminated intravascular coagulation, and multiple organ dysfunction syndrome.

Septic shock has become the most common type of distributive shock. There are approximately 400,000 to 500,000 septic episodes each year in the United States, which results in $5 to $10 billion in health care costs. The growing incidence has been attributed to an increased awareness of the diagnosis, increased numbers of immunocompromised patients, increased use of invasive procedures, increased number of resistant organisms, and an increased number of elderly patients.[42] Despite advances in treatment methods, the mortality rate is approximately 40%.[43]

Septic shock has been described in the context of the systemic inflammatory response. Although usually associated with infection, the systemic inflammatory response syndrome can be initiated by noninfectious disorders such as acute trauma and pancreatitis. To enable recognition, description, and classification of persons with sepsis, the American College of Chest Physicians and the Society of Critical Care Medicine published consensus terminology to describe and define the clinical manifestations and progression of sepsis[44] (Chart 26-2).

Mechanisms. The mechanisms of septic shock are thought to be related to mediators of the inflammatory response.[45,46] Although the immune system and the inflammatory response are designed to overcome infection and eliminate bacterial breakdown products, it has been proposed that the dysregulated release of cytokines or inflammatory mediators (see Chapter 18) may elicit toxic reactions, resulting in the potentially fatal sepsis syndrome. The most widely investigated cytokines are tumor necrosis factor (TNF), interleukin-1, and interleukin-8, which usually are proinflammatory, and interleukin-6 and interleukin-10, which tend to be anti-inflammatory. A trigger such as a microbial toxin stimulates the release of TNF and interleukin-1, which in turn promotes endothelial cell–leukocyte adhesion, release of cell-damaging proteases and prostaglandins, and activation of clotting. The prostaglandins, thromboxane A_2 (a vasoconstrictor), prostacyclin (a vasodilator), and prostaglandin E_2, participate in the generation of fever, tachycardia, ventilation-perfusion abnormalities, and lactic acidosis. Interleukin-8, a neutrophil chemotaxin, may have a particularly important role in perpetuating tissue inflammation. Interleukin-6 and interleukin-10, which have anti-inflammatory actions and perhaps are counter-regulatory, augment the acute-phase response and consequent generation of additional proinflammatory mediators.[47]

In addition to inducing the release of inflammatory mediators, endotoxins may themselves induce tissue damage by directly activating pathways such as the coagulation cascade, the complement cascade, vessel injury, or release of vasodilating prostaglandins.[46] Thus, the processes that result in the sepsis syndrome, with circulatory collapse, organ failure, and death, are complex consequences of microbial products that profoundly dysregulate inflammatory mediator release and regulation of several important pathways.

Manifestations. Septic shock typically manifests with fever, vasodilatation, and warm, flushed skin. Mild hyperventilation, respiratory alkalosis, and abrupt changes in personality and behavior due to reduction in cerebral blood flow may be the earliest signs and symptoms of septic shock. These manifestations, which are thought to be a primary response to the bacteremia, commonly precede the usual

CHART 26-2

Definitions of Sepsis and Septic Shock

Infection: Microbial phenomenon characterized by an inflammatory response to the presence of microorganisms and the invasion of normally sterile host tissue by these organisms.

Bacteremia: The presence of viable bacteria in the blood.

Systemic inflammatory response syndrome: The systemic inflammatory response to a variety of severe clinical insults. The response is manifested by two or more of the following conditions:
Temperature >38°C or <36°C
Heart rate >90 beats per minute
Respiratory rate >20 breaths per minute or $PaCO_2$ <32 mm Hg (pH <4.3)
WBC >12,000 cells/mm³, <4000 cells/mm³, or 10% immature (band) forms

Sepsis: The systemic response to infection. This systemic response is manifested by two or more of the above conditions (temperature, heart rate, respiratory rate, and WBC) as a result of infection.

Severe sepsis: Sepsis associated with organ dysfunction, hypoperfusion, or hypotension. Hypoperfusion and perfusion abnormalities may include, but are not limited to, lactic acidosis, oliguria, or an acute alteration in mental status.

Septic shock: Sepsis with hypotension, despite adequate fluid resuscitation, along with the presence of perfusion abnormalities that may include, but are not limited to, lactic acidosis, oliguria, or an acute alteration in mental status. Patients who are on inotropic or vasopressor agents may not be hypotensive at the time that perfusion abnormalities are measured.

Hypotension: A systolic blood pressure of <90 mm Hg or a reduction of >40 mm Hg from baseline in the absence of other causes of hypotension.

Multiple organ dysfunction syndrome: Presence of altered organ function in an acutely ill patient such that homeostasis cannot be maintained without intervention.

(From American College of Chest Physicians/Society of Critical Care Medicine Consensus Conference. [1992]. Definitions for sepsis and organ failure and guidelines for use of innovative therapies in sepsis. *Critical Care Medicine* 20 [6], 866)

signs and symptoms of sepsis by several hours or days. Unlike other forms of shock (*i.e.*, cardiogenic, hypovolemic, and obstructive) that are characterized by a compensatory increase in systemic vascular resistance, septic shock often presents with hypovolemia because of arterial and venous dilatation and leakage of plasma into the interstitial spaces.

Aggressive treatment of the hypovolemia in septic shock leads to a decrease in systemic vascular resistance and increased cardiac output and tachycardia. In the past, this hyperdynamic pattern of response was thought to be present early in shock and was called *warm shock*. A second pattern of *cold shock* accompanied by a low cardiac output

and cold extremities was thought to indicate the late stages of septic shock and a poor prognosis. With the development of refined resuscitation methods and better hemodynamic monitoring systems, approximately 90% of patients in septic shock demonstrate a hyperdynamic response with high cardiac output and low systemic vascular resistance.[46] Despite the fact that cardiac output is normal or increased, cardiac function is depressed, the heart becomes dilated, and the ejection fraction decreases.

Treatment. The treatment of septic shock focuses on the causative agent and support of the circulation. The administration of antibiotics specific to the infectious agent is essential. The cardiovascular status of the patient must be supported to maintain oxygen delivery to the cells. Swift and aggressive fluid administration is needed to compensate for third spacing, and equally aggressive use of vasopressors, such as epinephrine, norepinephrine bitartrate, and phenylephrine, is needed to counteract the vasodilation caused by endotoxins. Studies support the early and aggressive use of positive inotropic drugs, such as dobutamine, to increase cardiac contractility and maintain oxygen delivery.[48] Of particular interest has been the development of human monoclonal antibodies to the endotoxins produced by gram-negative sepsis. Supplemental immune globulins have been used to treat sepsis, but without great success unless used early or prophylactically in persons at risk for septic shock, such as high-risk cardiac surgery patients.[49]

COMPLICATIONS OF SHOCK

Wiggers, a noted circulatory physiologist, stated, "Shock not only stops the machine, but it wrecks the machinery."[50] Many body systems are wrecked by severe shock. Five major complications of severe shock are shock lung, acute renal failure, gastrointestinal ulceration, DIC, and MODS. The complications of shock are serious and often fatal.

Acute Respiratory Distress Syndrome

Acute respiratory distress syndrome (ARDS) is a potentially lethal form of respiratory failure that can follow severe shock (see Chapter 29). The mortality rate remains at greater than 50% despite advances in mechanical ventilation.[51]

The symptoms of ARDS usually do not develop until 24 to 48 hours after the initial trauma; in some instances, they occur later. The respiratory rate and effort of breathing increase. Arterial blood gas analysis establishes the presence of profound hypoxemia with hypercapnia, resulting from impaired matching of ventilation and perfusion and from the greatly reduced diffusion of blood gases across the thickened alveolar membranes.

The exact cause of ARDS is unknown. Neutrophils are thought to play a key role in the pathogenesis of ARDS. A cytokine-mediated activation and accumulation of neutrophils in the pulmonary vasculature and subsequent endothelial injury is thought to cause leaking of fluid and plasma proteins into the interstitium and alveolar spaces.[51,52] The fluid leakage impairs gas exchange and makes the lung stiffer and more difficult to inflate. Abnormalities in the production, composition, and function of surfactant may contribute to alveolar collapse and gas exchange abnormalities.[52]

Interventions for ARDS focus on increasing the oxygen concentration in the inspired air and supporting ventilation mechanically to optimize gas exchange while avoiding oxygen toxicity and preventing further lung injury.[51-53] Despite the delivery of high levels of oxygen using high-pressure mechanical ventilatory support and positive end-expiratory pressure, many persons with ARDS remain hypoxic, often with a fatal outcome.

Inhaled nitrous oxide is under investigation in the treatment of ARDS. Nitrous oxide appears to improve gas exchange but has not been demonstrated to significantly decrease mortality.[51,52] New interventions have focused on more aggressive treatment of the underlying cause, with the first line of treatment remaining supportive care.

Acute Renal Failure

The renal tubules are particularly vulnerable to ischemia, and acute renal failure is one important late cause of death in severe shock. Sepsis and trauma account for most cases of acute renal failure. The endotoxins implicated in septic shock are powerful vasoconstrictors that are capable of activating the sympathetic nervous system and causing intravascular clotting. They have been shown to trigger all the separate physiologic mechanisms that contribute to the onset of acute renal failure. The degree of renal damage is related to the severity and duration of shock. The normal kidney is able to tolerate severe ischemia for 15 to 20 minutes. The renal lesion most frequently seen after severe shock is acute tubular necrosis. Acute tubular necrosis usually is reversible, although return to normal renal function may require weeks or months (see Chapter 34). Continuous monitoring of urine output during shock provides a means of assessing renal blood flow. Frequent monitoring of serum creatinine and blood urea nitrogen levels also provides valuable information regarding renal status.

Gastrointestinal Complications

The gastrointestinal tract is particularly vulnerable to ischemia because of the changes in distribution of blood flow to its mucosal surface. In shock, there is widespread constriction of blood vessels that supply the gastrointestinal tract, causing a redistribution of blood flow that severely diminishes mucosal perfusion. Superficial mucosal lesions of the stomach and duodenum can develop within hours of severe trauma, sepsis, or burn.

Bleeding is a common symptom of gastrointestinal ulceration caused by shock. Hemorrhage has its onset usually within 2 to 10 days after the original insult and often begins without warning. Poor perfusion in the gastrointestinal tract has been credited with allowing intestinal bacteria to enter the bloodstream, thereby contributing to the development of sepsis and shock.[54]

Histamine type 2 receptor antagonists, proton pump inhibitors, or sucralfate may be given prophylactically to prevent gastrointestinal ulcerations caused by shock.[46] Nasogastric tubes, when attached to intermittent suction, also help to diminish the accumulation of hydrogen ions in the stomach.

Disseminated Intravascular Coagulation

Disseminated intravascular coagulation (DIC) is characterized by widespread activation of the coagulation system with resultant formation of fibrin clots and thrombotic occlusion of small and midsized vessels (see Chapter 14). The systemic formation of fibrin results from increased generation of thrombin, the simultaneous suppression of physiologic anticoagulation mechanisms, and the delayed removal of fibrin as a consequence of impaired fibrinolysis. Clinically overt DIC is reported to occur in as many as 30% to 50% of persons with sepsis and septic shock.[55] As with other systemic inflammatory responses, the derangement of coagulation and fibrinolysis is thought to be mediated by inflammatory mediators.

The contribution of DIC to morbidity and mortality in sepsis depends on the underlying clinical condition and the intensity of the coagulation disorder. Depletion of the platelets and coagulation factors increases the risk of bleeding. Deposition of fibrin in the vasculature of organs contributes to ischemic damage and organ failure. In a large number of clinical trials, the occurrence of DIC appeared to be associated with an unfavorable outcome and was an independent predictor of mortality.[55] However, it remains uncertain whether DIC was a predictor of unfavorable outcome, or merely a marker of the seriousness of the underlying condition causing the DIC.

The management of sepsis-induced DIC focuses on treatment of the underlying disorder and measures to interrupt the coagulation process. Anticoagulation therapy and administration of platelets and plasma may be used. The use of antithrombin III, a coagulation inhibitor, is under investigation. Clinical trails have shown modest to marked reductions in mortality based on the dose of antithrombin III that was used.[55] Other therapeutic options, aimed at interrupting the intrinsic coagulation pathway at the point where tissue factor complexes with factor VIIa, also are being investigated.[54]

Multiple Organ Dysfunction Syndrome

Multiple organ dysfunction syndrome (MODS) represents the presence of altered organ function in an acutely ill patient such that homeostasis cannot be maintained without intervention. As the name implies, MODS commonly affects multiple organ systems, including the kidneys, lungs, liver, brain, and heart. MODS is a particularly life-threatening complication of shock, especially septic shock. It has been reported as the most frequent cause of death in the noncoronary intensive care unit. Mortality rates vary from 30% to 100%, depending on the number of organs involved.[56] Mortality rates increase with an increased number of organs failing. A high mortality rate is associated with failure of the brain, liver, kidney, and lung. The pathogenesis of MODS is not clearly understood, and current management therefore is primarily supportive. Major risk factors for the development of MODS are sepsis, shock, prolonged periods of hypotension, hepatic dysfunction, trauma, infarcted bowel, advanced age, and alcohol abuse.[56] Interventions for multiple organ failure are focused on support of the affected organs.

In summary, circulatory shock is an acute emergency in which body tissues are deprived of oxygen and cellular nutrients or are unable to use these materials in their metabolic processes. Circulatory shock may develop because there is not enough blood in the circulatory system (*i.e.,* hypovolemic shock), blood flow or venous return is obstructed (*i.e.,* obstructive shock), or the tissues are unable to use oxygen and nutrients (*i.e.,* distributive shock). Three types of shock share the basic circulatory pattern of distributive shock: neurogenic shock, anaphylactic shock, and septic shock. Septic shock, which is the most common of these three types, is associated with a severe, overwhelming infection and has a mortality rate of approximately 40%.

The manifestations of circulatory shock are related to low peripheral blood flow and excessive sympathetic stimulation. The low peripheral blood flow produces thirst, changes in skin temperature, a decrease in blood pressure, an increase in heart rate, decreased venous pressure, decreased urine output, and changes in the sensorium. Signs and symptoms, such as changes in skin temperature (*i.e.,* increased in septic shock and decreased in hypovolemic and other forms of shock), may differ with the type of shock. The intense vasoconstriction that serves to maintain blood flow to the heart and brain causes a decrease in tissue perfusion, impaired cellular metabolism, liberation of lactic acid, and, eventually, cell death. Whether the shock will be irreversible or the patient will survive is determined largely by changes that occur at the cellular level.

The rapidity of support to regain perfusion and cellular oxygenation is critical to ensure cellular and patient survival. The treatment of shock is determined by the type of shock. It focuses on correcting or controlling the cause and improving tissue perfusion. In hypovolemic shock, the goal of treatment is to restore vascular volume. Vasoactive drugs capable of constricting or dilating blood vessels may be used.

The complications of shock result from the deprivation of blood flow to vital organs or systems, such as the lungs, kidneys, gastrointestinal tract, and blood coagulation system. ARDS produces lung changes that occur with shock. It is characterized by changes in the permeability of the alveolar-capillary membrane with the development of interstitial edema and severe hypoxia that does not respond to oxygen therapy. The renal tubules are particularly vulnerable to ischemia, and acute renal failure is an important complication of shock. Gastrointestinal ischemia may lead to gastrointestinal bleeding and increased permeability to the intestinal bacteria, which cause further sepsis and shock. DIC is characterized by formation of small clots in the circulation. It is thought to be caused by inappropriate activation of the coagulation cascade because of toxins or other products released as a result of the shock state. Multiple organ failure, perhaps the most ominous complication of shock, rapidly depletes the body's ability to compensate and recover from a shock state.

Circulatory Failure in Children and the Elderly

After you have completed this section of the chapter, you should be able to meet the following objectives:

✦ Describe the manifestations of heart failure in infants and children
✦ Cite how the aging process affects heart failure in the elderly
✦ State how the signs and symptoms of heart failure may differ between younger and older adults

HEART FAILURE IN INFANTS AND CHILDREN

As in adults, heart failure in infants and children results from the inability of the heart to maintain the cardiac output required to sustain metabolic demands.[57,58,59] Congenital heart defects are the most common cause of CHF during childhood. Surgical correction of congenital heart defects may cause CHF as a result of intraoperative manipulation of the heart and resection of heart tissue, with subsequent alterations in pressure, flow, and resistance relations.[57] Usually, the heart failure that results is acute and resolves after the effects of the surgical procedure have subsided. Chronic congestive failure occasionally is observed in children with severe chronic anemia, inflammatory heart disease, end-stage congenital heart disease, or cardiomyopathy. Chart 26-3 lists some of the more common causes of heart failure in children. Inflammatory heart disorders (*e.g.,* myocarditis, rheumatic fever, bacterial endocarditis, Kawasaki's disease), cardiomyopathy, and congenital heart disorders are discussed in Chapter 24.

Manifestations
Many of the signs and symptoms of heart failure in infants and children are similar to those in adults. They include fatigue, effort intolerance, cough, anorexia, and abdominal pain. A subtle sign of cardiorespiratory distress in infants and children is a change in disposition or responsiveness, including irritability or lethargy. Sympathetic stimulation produces peripheral vasoconstriction and diaphoresis. Decreased renal blood flow often results in a urine output of less than 0.5 to 1.0 mL/kg/hour, despite adequate fluid intake.[57] When right ventricular function is impaired, systemic venous congestion develops. Hepatomegaly due to liver congestion often is one of the first signs of systemic venous congestion in infants and children. However, dependent edema or ascites rarely is seen unless the CVP is extremely high. Because of their short, fat necks, jugular venous distention is difficult to detect in infants; it is not a reliable sign until the child is of school age or older.

A third heart sound, or gallop rhythm, is a common finding in infants and children with heart failure. It results from rapid filling of a noncompliant ventricle. However, it is difficult to distinguish at high heart rates.

Most commonly, children develop interstitial edema rather than alveolar pulmonary edema. This reduces lung compliance and increases the work of breathing, causing tachypnea and increased respiratory effort. Older children

CHART 26-3

Causes of Heart Failure in Children

Newborn Period

Congenital heart defects
    Severe left ventricular outflow disorders
        Hypoplastic left heart
        Critical aortic stenosis or coarctation of the aorta
    Large arteriovenous shunts
        Ventricular septal defects
        Patent ductus arteriosus
    Transposition of the great vessels
Heart muscle dysfunction (secondary)
    Asphyxia
    Sepsis
    Hypoglycemia
Hematologic disorders (*e.g.*, anemia)

Infants 1 to 6 Months

Congenital heart disease
    Large arteriovenous shunts (ventricular septal defect)
Heart muscle dysfunction
    Myocarditis
    Cardiomyopathy
Pulmonary abnormalities
    Bronchopulmonary dysplasia
    Persistent pulmonary hypertension

Toddlers, Children, and Adolescents

Acquired heart disease
    Cardiomyopathy
    Viral myocarditis
    Rheumatic fever
    Endocarditis
    Systemic disease
        Sepsis
        Kawasaki's disease
        Renal disease
        Sickle cell disease
Congenital heart defects
    Nonsurgically treated disorders
    Surgically treated disorders

display use of accessory muscles (*i.e.*, scapular and sternocleidomastoid). Head bobbing and nasal flaring may be observed in infants. Signs of respiratory distress often are the first and most noticeable indication of CHF in infants and young children. Pulmonary congestion may be mistaken for bronchiolitis or lower respiratory tract infection. The infant or young child with respiratory distress often grunts with expiration. This grunting effort (essentially, exhaling against a closed glottis) is an instinctive effort to increase end-expiratory pressures and prevent collapse of small airways and the development of atelectasis. Respiratory crackles (*i.e.*, rales) are uncommon in infants and usually suggest development of a respiratory tract infection. Wheezes may be heard, particularly if there is a large left-to-right shunt.

Infants with heart failure often have increased respiratory problems during feeding.[57,58] The history is one of prolonged feeding with excessive respiratory effort and fatigue.

Weight gain is slow owing to high energy requirements and low calorie intake. Other frequent manifestations of heart failure in infants are excessive sweating (due to increased sympathetic tone), particularly over the head and neck, and repeated lower respiratory tract infections. Peripheral perfusion usually is poor, with cool extremities; tachycardia is common (resting heart rate >150 beats per minute); and respiratory rate is increased (resting rate >50 breaths per minute).[57]

Diagnosis and Treatment

Diagnosis of congestive failure in infants and children is based on symptomatology, chest radiographic films, electrocardiographic findings, echocardiographic techniques to assess cardiac structures and ventricular function (*i.e.*, end-systolic and end-diastolic diameters), arterial blood gases to determine intracardiac shunting and ventilation-perfusion inequalities, and other laboratory studies to determine anemia and electrolyte imbalances.

Treatment of congestive failure in infants and children includes measures aimed at improving cardiac function and eliminating excess intravascular fluid. Oxygen delivery must be supported and oxygen demands controlled or minimized. Whenever possible, the cause of the disorder is corrected (*e.g.*, medical treatment of sepsis and anemia, surgical correction of congenital heart defects). With congenital anomalies that are amenable to surgery, medical treatment often is needed for a time before surgery and usually is continued in the immediate postoperative period. For many children, only medical management can be provided.

Medical management of heart failure in infants and children is similar to that in the adult, although it is tailored to the special developmental needs of the child. Inotropic agents such as digitalis often are used to increase cardiac contractility. Diuretics may be given to reduce preload and vasodilating drugs used to manipulate the afterload. Drug doses must be carefully tailored to control for the child's weight and conditions such as reduced renal function. Daily weighing and accurate measurement of intake and output are imperative during acute episodes of failure.

Most children feel better in the semiupright position. An infant seat is useful for infants with chronic CHF. Activity restrictions usually are designed to allow children to be as active as possible within the limitations of their heart disease. Infants with congestive failure often have problems feeding. Small, frequent feedings usually are more successful than larger, less frequent feedings. Severely ill infants may lack sufficient strength to suck and may need to be tube fed.

The treatment of heart failure in children should be designed to allow optimal physical and psychosocial development. It requires the full involvement of the parents, who often are the primary care providers; therefore, parent education and support is essential.

HEART FAILURE IN THE ELDERLY

Congestive heart failure is one of the most common causes of disability in the elderly and is the most frequent hospital discharge diagnosis for the elderly. More than 75% of patients with CHF are older than 65 years of age. It also is a major cause of chronic disability, and annual expenditures exceed $10 billion.[60] Among the factors that have contributed to the increased numbers of older people with CHF are the improved therapies for ischemic and hypertensive heart disease.[60] Thus, persons who would have died from acute myocardial disease 20 years ago are now surviving, but with residual left ventricular dysfunction. Similarly, improved blood pressure control has led to a 60% decline in stroke mortality rates, yet these same people remain at risk for CHF as a complication of hypertension. Also, advances in treatment of other diseases have contributed indirectly to the rising prevalence of CHF in the older population.

Coronary heart disease, hypertension, and valvular heart disease (particularly aortic stenosis and mitral regurgitation) are common causes of CHF in older adults.[60,61] Although the pathophysiology of CHF is similar in younger and older persons, elderly persons tend to develop cardiac failure when confronted with stresses that would not produce failure in younger persons. There are four principal changes associated with cardiovascular aging that impair the ability to respond to stress.[60] First, reduced responsiveness to β-adrenergic stimulation limits the heart's capacity maximally to increase heart rate and contractility. A second major effect of aging is increased vascular stiffness, which results in an increased resistance to left ventricular ejection (afterload) and contributes to the development of systolic hypertension in the elderly. Third, in addition to increased vascular stiffness, the heart itself becomes stiffer and less compliant with age. The changes in diastolic stiffness result in important alterations in diastolic filling and atrial function. A reduction in ventricular filling not only affects cardiac output, but produces an elevation in diastolic pressure that is transmitted back to the left atrium, where it stretches the muscle wall and predisposes to atrial ectopic beats and atrial fibrillation. The fourth major effect of cardiovascular aging is altered myocardial metabolism at the level of the mitochondria. Although older mitochondria may able to generate sufficient ATP to meet the normal energy needs of the heart, they may not be able to respond under stress.

Manifestations

The manifestations of CHF in the elderly often are masked by other disease conditions. Nocturia is an early symptom but may be caused by other conditions such as prostatic hypertrophy. Dyspnea on exertion may result from lung disease, lack of exercise, and deconditioning. Lower extremity edema commonly is caused by venous insufficiency.

Among the acute manifestations of CHF in the elderly are increasing lethargy and confusion, probably the result of impaired cerebral perfusion. Activity intolerance is common. Instead of dyspnea, the prominent sign may be restlessness. Impaired perfusion of the gastrointestinal tract is a common cause of anorexia and profound loss of lean body mass. Loss of lean body mass may be masked by edema.

The elderly also maintain a precarious balance between the managed symptom state and acute symptom exacerbation. During the managed symptom state, they are relatively symptom free while adhering to their treatment regimen. Acute symptom exacerbation, often requiring emergency medical treatment, can be precipitated by seemingly minor conditions such as poor compliance with sodium restriction, infection, or stress. Failure promptly to seek medical care is a common cause of progressive acceleration of symptoms.

Diagnosis and Treatment

The diagnosis of heart failure in the elderly is based on the history, physical examination, chest radiograph, and electrocardiographic findings. However, the presenting symptoms of CHF often are difficult to evaluate.

Treatment of CHF in the elderly involves many of the same methods as in younger persons. Activities are restricted to a level that is commensurate with the cardiac reserve. Seldom is bed rest recommended or advised. Bed rest causes rapid deconditioning of skeletal muscles and increases the risk of complications, such as orthostatic hypotension and thromboemboli. Instead, carefully prescribed exercise programs can help to maintain activity tolerance. Even walking around a room usually is preferable to continuous bed rest. Sodium restriction usually is indicated.

Age- and disease-related changes increase the likelihood of adverse drug reactions and drug interactions. Drug dosages and the number of drugs that are prescribed should be kept to a minimum. Compliance with drug regimens often is difficult; the simpler the regimen, the more likely it is that the older person will comply. In general, the treatment plan for elderly persons with CHF must be put in the context of the person's overall needs. An improvement in the quality of life may take precedence over increasing the length of survival.

In summary, the mechanisms of heart failure in children and the elderly are similar to those in adults. However, the causes and manifestations may differ because of age. In children, CHF is seen most commonly during infancy and immediately after heart surgery. It can be caused by congenital and acquired heart defects and is characterized by fatigue, effort intolerance, cough, anorexia, abdominal pain, and impaired growth. Treatment of CHF in children includes correction of the underlying cause whenever possible. For congenital anomalies that are amenable to surgery, medical treatment often is needed for a time before surgery and usually is continued in the immediate postoperative period. For many children, only medical management can be provided.

In the elderly, age-related changes in cardiovascular functioning contribute to CHF but are not in themselves sufficient to cause heart failure. The manifestations of congestive failure often are different and superimposed on other disease conditions; therefore, CHF often is more difficult to diagnose in the elderly than in younger persons. Because the elderly are more susceptible to adverse drug reactions and have more problems with compliance, the number of drugs that are prescribed is kept to a minimum, and the drug regimen is kept as simple as possible.

References

1. American Heart Association. (2001). American Heart Association 2000 Statistical Update. [On-line]. Available: http://www.americanheart.org/statistics/othercvd.html.
2. Graves E.J. (1995). *National hospital discharge survey: Annual summary, 1993*. Vital and Health Statistics, Series 13; Data from National Health Surveys (121) 1–63.
3. Colucci W.C., Braunwald E. (1997). Pathophysiology of heart failure. In Braunwald E. (Ed.), *Heart disease* (5th ed., pp. 394–420). Philadelphia: W.B. Saunders.
4. Mark A.L. (1995). Sympathetic dysregulation in heart failure: Mechanisms and therapy. *Clinical Cardiology* 18 (3 Suppl. I), I3–I8.
5. Braunwald E., Bristow M.R. (2000). Congestive heart failure: Fifty years of progress. *Circulation* 102, IV-14–V-23.
6. Schrier R.W., Abraham W.T. (1999). Hormones and hemodynamics in heart failure. *New England Journal of Medicine* 341, 577–584.
7. Schlant R.C., Sonnenblick E.H., Katz A.M. (1997). Physiology of heart failure. In Alexander R.W., Schlant R.C., Fuster V., O'Rourke R.A., Roberts R., Sonnenblick E.H. (Eds.), *Hurst's The heart* (9th ed., pp. 681–726). New York: McGraw-Hill.
8. Piano M.R., Bondmass M., Schwertz D.W. (1998). The molecular and cellular pathophysiology of heart failure. *Heart and Lung* 27, 3–19.
9. Hunter J.J., Chien K.R. (1999). Signaling pathways for cardiac hypertrophy and failure. *New England Journal of Medicine* 341, 1276–1284.
10. Braunwald E., Colucci W.S., Grossman W. (1997). Clinical aspects of high output heart failure: High output heart failure; pulmonary edema. In Braunwald E. (Ed.), *Heart disease* (5th ed., pp. 445–470). Philadelphia: W.B. Saunders.
11. Weinberger H.D. (1999). Diagnosis and treatment of diastolic heart failure. *Hospital Practice* 34 (3), 115–126.
12. Bonow R.O., Udelson J.E. (1992). Left ventricular diastolic dysfunction as a cause of congestive heart failure. *Annals of Internal Medicine* 117, 502–510.
13. Tresch D.D., McGough M.F. (1995). Heart failure with normal systolic function: A common disorder in older people. *Journal of the American Geriatric Society* 49(9), 1035–1042.
14. Katz A.M. (1991). Energetics and the failing heart. *Hospital Practice* 26 (8), 78–90.
15. Nava J.R., Martinez-Maldonado M. (1993). Pathophysiology of edema in congestive heart failure. *Heart Disease and Stroke* 2(4), 325–329.
16. Shamsham F., Mitchell J. (2000). Essentials of the diagnosis of heart failure. *American Family Physician* 61, 1319–1328.
17. Vitarelli A., Gheorghiade M. (2000). Transthoracic and transesophageal echocardiogram in the hemodynamic assessment of patients with CHF. *American Journal of Cardiology* 86, 366–406.
18. Parker W.R., Anderson A.S. (2001). Slowing the progression of CHF. *Postgraduate Medicine* 109 (3), 36–45.
19. Hoyt R.E., Bowling L.S. (2001). Reducing readmission for congestive heart failure. *American Family Physician* 63, 1593–1600.
20. Wielenga R.P., Huisveld A., Bol E., Dunselman R.H., Erdman P.A., Baselier M.R., et al. (1999). Safety and effects of physical training in chronic heart failure: Results of the chronic heart failure and graded exercise study. *European Heart Journal* 20(12), 872–879.
21. Stanek, B. (2000). Optimizing management of patients with advanced heart failure: The importance of preventing progression. *Drugs and Aging* 16, 87–106.
22. Fruedenberger R.S., Gottlieb S.S., Robinson S.W., Fisher M.L. (1999). A four-part regimen for clinical heart failure. *Hospital Practice* 34 (9), 51–64.
23. Katz A.M., Silverman D.I. (2000). Treatment of heart failure. *Hospital Practice* 35 (12B), 19–26.
24. Haji S.A., Movahed A. (2000). Update on digoxin therapy in congestive heart failure. *American Family Physician* 62, 409–416.
25. The SOLVD Investigators. (1991). Effect of enalapril on survival in patients with reduced left ventricular ejection fractions and congestive heart failure. *New England Journal of Medicine* 325, 293–302.
26. Ramahi T.M. (2000). Beta blocker therapy for chronic heart failure. *American Family Physician* 62, 2267–2274.
27. Califf R.M., Bengton J.R. (1994). Cardiogenic shock. *New England Journal of Medicine* 330, 1724–1730.
28. Bone R.C. (1991). The pathogenesis of sepsis. *Annals of Internal Medicine* 115, 457–469.
29. Muehrcke D.D., McCarthy P.M., Foster R.C., Ogella D.A., Borsch J.A., Cosgrove D.M. (1996). Extracorporeal membrane oxygenation post cardiotomy cardiogenic shock. *Annals of Thoracic Surgery* 61, 684–691.
30. Coraim F.E., Wolner E. (1995). Continuous hemofiltration for the failing heart. *New Horizons* 3, 725–731.
31. Garber P.J., Mathieson A.L., Ducas J., Patton J.N., Geddes J.S., Prewitt R.M. (1995). Thrombolytic therapy for cardiogenic shock: Effect of increased intrathoracic pressure and rapid tPA administration. *Canadian Journal of Cardiology* 11 (1), 30–36.
32. Mussivand T. (1999). Mechanical circulatory devices for the treatment of heart failure. *Journal of Cardiac Surgery* 14, 218–228.
33. The Registry of the International Society of Heart and Lung Transplant. (1992). Ninth official report. *Journal of Heart and Lung Transplantation* 11, 599–606.
34. Perlroth M.G., Reitz B.A. (1997). Heart and heart-lung transplantation. In Braunwald E. (Ed.), *Heart disease* (5th ed., pp. 515–520). Philadelphia: W.B. Saunders.
35. Futterman L.G., Lemberg L. (1996). Cardiomyoplasty: A potential alternative to cardiac transplantation. *American Journal of Critical Care* 5 (1), 80–86.
36. Guyton A.C., Hall J.E. (2000). *Textbook of medical physiology* (10th ed., pp. 253–262). Philadelphia: W.B. Saunders.
37. Whitman G. (1988). Tissue perfusion. In McKinney M., Packa D., Dunbar S. (Eds.), *ACCN clinical reference for critical-care nursing* (2nd ed., p. 119). New York: McGraw-Hill.
38. Taylor G., Myers S, Kurth C.D., Duhaime A.C., Yu H., McKernan M., et al. (1996). Hypertonic saline improves brain resuscitation in pediatric model of head injury and hemorrhagic shock. *Journal of Pediatric Surgery* 31(1), 65–70.
39. Bochner B.S., Lichtenstein L.M. (1991). Anaphylaxis. *New England Journal of Medicine* 324, 1785–1790.
40. Stankiewicz J., Ruta W., Gorski P. (1995). Latex allergy. *International Journal of Occupational Medicine and Environmental Health* 8, 139–148.
41. Leibovici L., Smara Z., Konigsberger H., Drucker M., Askenzi S., Pitlik S.D. (1995). Long-term survival following bacteremia or fungemia. *Journal of the American Medical Association* 274, 897–812.
42. Balk R.A. (2000). Severe sepsis and septic shock. *Critical Care Clinics* 16, 179–191.
43. Carcillo J.A., Cunnin R.E. (1997) Septic shock. *Critical Care Clinics* 13, 553–574.
44. Members of the American College of Chest Physicians/Society of Critical Care Medicine Consensus Conference Committee. (1992). American College of Chest Physicians/Society of Critical Care Medicine consensus conference: Definitions of sepsis and organ failure and guidelines for

the use of innovative therapies in sepsis. *Critical Care Medicine* 20, 864–874.

45. Glauser M.P. (2000). Pathologic basis of sepsis: Considerations for future strategies of intervention. *Critical Care Medicine* 28 (9 Suppl.), S4–S8.

46. Wheeler A.P., Bernard G.R. (1999). Treating patients with severe sepsis. *New England Journal of Medicine* 340, 207–214.

47. Parrillo J.E. (1995). Pathogenetic mechanisms of septic shock. *New England Journal of Medicine* 328, 1471–1477.

48. Wiessner W.H., Casey L.C., Zbilut J.P. (1995). Treatment of sepsis and septic shock: A review. *Heart and Lung* 24, 380–392.

49. Werdan K., Pilg G. (1996). Supplemental immune globulinsin sepsis: A critical appraisal. *Clinical and Experimental Immunology* 104 (Suppl. 1), 83–90.

50. Smith J.J., Kampine J.P. (1980). *Circulatory physiology* (p. 298). Baltimore: Williams & Wilkins.

51. Fein A.M., Calalang-Colucci M.G. (2000). Acute lung injury and acute respiratory distress syndrome in sepsis and septic shock. *Critical Care Clinics* 4, 289–317.

52. Ware L.B., Mattay M.A. (2000). The acute respiratory distress syndrome. *New England Journal of Medicine* 342, 1334–1349.

53. Sessler C.N. (1998). Mechanical ventilation of patients with acute lung injury. *Critical Care Clinics of North America* 14, 707–729.

54. Fink M. (1991). Gastrointestinal mucosal injury in experimental models of shock, trauma and sepsis. *Critical Care Medicine* 19, 627–641.

55. Levi M., Ten Cate H.T. (1999). Disseminated intravascular coagulation. *New England Journal of Medicine* 341, 586–592.

56. Balk R.A. (2000). Pathogenesis and management of multiple organ dysfunction or failure in severe sepsis and septic shock. *Critical Care Clinics* 16, 337–352.

57. Hazinski F.H. (1992). *Nursing care of the critically ill child* (2nd ed., pp. 156–170). St. Louis: C.V. Mosby.

58. Bernstein D. (2000). Heart failure. In Behrman R.E., Kliegman R.M., Nelson W., Jenson H.B. (Eds.). *Nelson textbook of pediatrics* (16th ed., pp. 1440–1444). Philadelphia: W.B. Saunders.

59. O'Laughlin M.P. (1999). Congestive heart failure in children. *Pediatric Clinics of North America* 46, 263–273.

60. Rich M.W. (1997). Epidemiology, pathophysiology, and etiology of congestive heart failure in older adults. *Journal of the American Geriatrics Society* 45, 968–974.

61. Duncan A.K., Vittone J., Fleming K.C., Smith H.C. (1996). Cardiovascular disease in elderly patients. *Mayo Clinic Proceedings* 71, 184–196.

Respiratory Function

In the early studies of the body, there is almost no mention of the lungs or respiratory passages. Although the pneuma, or "vital spirits," of the body were closely related to the air and vapors of the universe, the lungs and air passages were almost disregarded. It was not until the circulation of blood had been charted that real progress in understanding the respiratory system took place.

A major step in the understanding of respiration began with the work of Robert Boyle (1627–1691), an Irish scholar. Using an air pump, Boyle proved that a candle would not burn and a small bird or mouse could not live inside a jar from which the air had been removed. Scientists at this time believed that when something burned, air lost a mysterious substance called *phlogiston*. It was the British clergyman Joseph Priestley (1733–1804) who discovered that a gas made by heating oxide of mercury supported combustion. He called this gas, which later became known as oxygen, *dephlogisticated* air. Priestley showed that a mouse lived longer in a given volume of dephlogisticated air than it did in ordinary air. Antoine Lavoisier (1743–1794), a French chemist, confirmed that oxygen was present in inspired air and carbon dioxide in expired air and gave oxygen its name. In 1791, just 16 years after Priestley's discovery of oxygen, it was shown that blood contained both oxygen and carbon dioxide. From this point on, a detailed understanding of the respiratory system and its function proceeded rapidly.

Control of Respiratory Function

Respiration provides the body with a means of gas exchange. It is the process whereby oxygen from the air is transferred to the blood and carbon dioxide is eliminated from the body. Internal respiration provides for gas exchange at the cellular level.

Respiration can be divided into three parts: ventilation, or the movement of air between the atmosphere and the respiratory portion of the lungs; perfusion, or the flow of blood through the lungs; and diffusion, or the transfer of gases between the air-filled spaces in the lungs and the blood. The nervous system controls the movement of the respiratory muscles and adjusts the rate of breathing so that it matches the needs of the body during various levels of activity. The content in this chapter focuses on the structure and function of the respiratory system as it relates to these aspects of respiration. The function of the red blood cell in the transport of oxygen is discussed in Chapter 15.

Structural Organization of the Respiratory System

After you have completed this section of the chapter, you should be able to meet the following objectives:

✦ State the difference between the conducting and the respiratory airways
✦ Trace the movement of air through the airways, beginning in the nose and oropharynx and moving into the respiratory tissues of the lung
✦ Describe the function of the mucociliary blanket
✦ Define the term *water vapor pressure* and cite the source of water for humidification of air as it moves through the airways
✦ Compare the supporting structures of the large and small airways in terms of cartilaginous and smooth muscle support
✦ Differentiate the function of the bronchial and pulmonary circulations that supply the lungs
✦ State the function of the two types of alveolar cells

The respiratory system consists of the air passages and the lungs. Functionally, the respiratory system can be divided into two parts: the *conducting airways*, through which air moves as it passes between the atmosphere and the lungs, and the *respiratory tissues* of the lungs, where gas exchange takes place.

THE CONDUCTING AIRWAYS

The conducting airways consist of the nasal passages, mouth and pharynx, larynx, trachea, bronchi, and bronchioles (Fig. 27-1). The air we breathe is warmed, filtered, and moistened as it moves through these structures. Heat is transferred to the air from the blood flowing through the walls of the respiratory passages; the mucociliary blanket removes foreign materials; and water from the mucous membranes is used to moisten the air.

The conducting airways are lined with a pseudo-stratified columnar epithelium that contains a mosaic of mucus-secreting goblet cells and cells that contain hairlike projections called *cilia* (Fig. 27-2). The epithelial layer gradually becomes thinner as it moves from the pseudostratified epithelium of the bronchi to cuboidal epithelium of the bronchioles and then to squamous epithelium of the alveoli. The mucus produced by the goblet cells in the conducting airways forms a layer, called the *mucociliary blanket*, that protects the respiratory system by entrapping dust and other foreign particles that enter the airways. The cilia, which constantly are in motion, move the mucociliary blanket with its entrapped particles toward the oropharynx, from which it is expectorated or swallowed. The function of the mucociliary blanket in clearing the lower airways and alveoli is optimal at normal oxygen levels and is impaired in situations of low and high oxygen levels. Clearance is stimulated by coughing. It is impaired by drying, such as breathing heated but unhumidified indoor air during winter. Cigarette smoking slows down or paralyzes the motility of the cilia. This slowing allows the residue from tobacco smoke, dust, and other particles to accumulate in the lungs, decreasing the efficiency of this pulmonary defense system. There also is evidence that smoking causes hyperplasia of

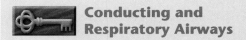

Conducting and Respiratory Airways

➤ Respiration requires ventilation, or movement of gases into and out of the lung; perfusion, or movement of blood through the lungs; and diffusion of gases between the lungs and the blood.

➤ Ventilation depends on conducting airways, including the nasopharynx and oropharynx, larynx, and tracheobronchial tree, which move air into and out of the lung but do not participate in gas exchange.

➤ Gas exchange takes place in the respiratory airways of the lung, where gases diffuse across the alveolar-capillary membrane as they are exchanged between lung and the blood that flows through the pulmonary capillaries.

the goblet cells, with a resultant increase in respiratory tract secretions and increased susceptibility to respiratory tract infections. As discussed in Chapter 29, these changes are thought to contribute to the development of chronic bronchitis and emphysema.

The airways are kept moist by water contained in the mucous layer. Moisture is added to the air as it moves through the conducting airways. The capacity of the air to contain moisture or water vapor without condensation increases as the temperature rises. Thus, the air in the alveoli, which is maintained at body temperature, usually contains considerably more water vapor than the atmospheric-temperature air that we breathe. The difference between the water vapor contained in the air we breathe and that found in the alveoli is drawn from the moist surface of the mucous membranes that line the conducting airways and is a source of insensible water loss (see Chapter 31). Under normal conditions, approximately 1 pint of water per day is lost in humidifying the air breathed. During fever, the water vapor in the lungs increases, causing more water to be lost from the respiratory mucosa. Also, fever usually is accompanied by an increase in respiratory rate so that more air passes through the airways, withdrawing moisture from its mucosal surface. As a result, respiratory secretions thicken, preventing free movement of the cilia and impairing the protective function of the mucociliary defense system. This is particularly true in persons whose water intake is inadequate.

Nasopharyngeal Airways

The nose is the preferred route for the entrance of air into the respiratory tract during normal breathing. As air passes through the nasal passages, it is filtered, warmed, and humidified. The outer nasal passages are lined with coarse hairs, which filter and trap dust and other large

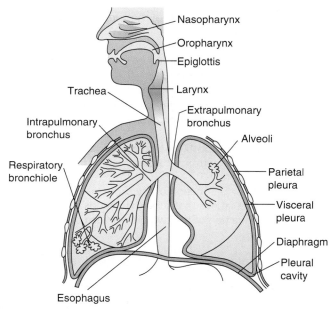

Nasopharynx
Oropharynx
Epiglottis
Trachea
Larynx
Extrapulmonary bronchus
Intrapulmonary bronchus
Alveoli
Respiratory bronchiole
Parietal pleura
Visceral pleura
Diaphragm
Pleural cavity
Esophagus

FIGURE 27-1 Structures of the respiratory system.

FIGURE 27-2 Airway wall structure: bronchus, bronchiole, and alveolus. The bronchial wall contains pseudostratified epithelium, smooth muscle cells, mucous glands, connective tissue, and cartilage. In smaller bronchioles, a simple epithelium is found, cartilage is absent, and the wall is thinner. The alveolar wall is designed for gas exchange, rather than structural support. (From Weibel E.R., Taylor R.C. [1988]. Design and structure of the human lung. In Fishman A.P. [ed.]. *Pulmonary diseases and disorders,* Vol. 1. [p. 14] New York: McGraw-Hill)

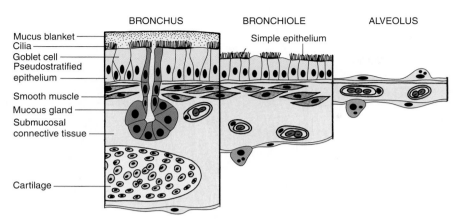

particles from the air. The upper portion of the nasal cavity is lined with mucous membrane that contains a rich network of small blood vessels; this portion of the nasal cavity supplies warmth and moisture to the air we breathe.

The mouth serves as an alternative airway when the nasal passages are plugged or when there is a need for the exchange of large amounts of air, as occurs during exercise. The oropharynx extends posteriorly from the soft palate to the epiglottis. The oropharynx is the only opening between the nose and mouth and the lungs. Both swallowed food on its way to the esophagus and air on its way to the larynx pass through it. Obstruction of the oropharynx leads to immediate cessation of ventilation. Neural control of the tongue and pharyngeal muscles may be impaired in coma and certain types of neurologic disease. In these conditions, the tongue falls back into the pharynx and obstructs the airway, particularly if the person is lying on his or her back. Swelling of the pharyngeal structures caused by injury, infection, or severe allergic reaction also predisposes a person to airway obstruction, as does the presence of a foreign body.

Laryngotracheal Airways

The larynx connects the oropharynx with the trachea. The walls of the larynx are supported by firm cartilaginous structures that prevent collapse during inspiration. The functions of the larynx can be divided into two categories: those associated with speech and those associated with protecting the lungs from substances other than air. The larynx is located in a strategic position between the upper airways and the lungs and sometimes is referred to as the "watchdog of the lungs."

The epiglottis, which is located above the vocal folds, is a large, leaf-shaped piece of cartilage that is covered with epithelium. The stemlike base of the epiglottis is attached to the anterior rim of the larynx, allowing the leaf-shaped portion to move up and down like a trapdoor. During swallowing, the free edges of the epiglottis move downward to cover the larynx, thus routing liquids and foods into the esophagus.

The cavity of the larynx is divided into two pairs of two-by-two folds of mucous membrane stretching from front to back with an opening in the midline (Fig. 27-3). The upper pair of folds, called the *vestibular folds*, has a protective function. The lower pair of folds has cordlike margins; they are termed the *vocal folds* because their vibrations are required for making vocal sounds. The vocal folds and the elongated opening between them are called the *glottis*. A complex set of muscles controls the opening and closing of the glottis. Speech involves the intermittent release of expired air and opening and closing of the glottis.

In addition to opening and closing the glottis for speech, the vocal folds of the larynx can perform a sphincter function in closing off the airways. When confronted with substances other than air, the laryngeal muscles contract and close off the airway. At the same time, the cough reflex is initiated as a means of removing a foreign substance from the airway. If the swallowing mechanism is partially or totally paralyzed, food and fluids can enter the airways instead of the esophagus when a person attempts to swallow. These substances are not easily removed; and when they are pulled into the lungs, they can cause a serious inflammatory condition called *aspiration pneumonia*.

During defecation and urination, inhaled air is temporarily held in the lungs by closing the glottis. The intra-abdominal muscles then contract, causing both intra-abdominal and intrathoracic pressures to rise. These collective actions are called *Valsalva's maneuver*. By producing an increase in intrathoracic pressure, Valsalva's maneuver decreases the return of blood to the heart, thereby inciting a series of circulatory reflexes. A tachycardia, or increase in heart rate, develops during the maneuver as the circulatory system compensates for the decrease in blood return to the heart. On termination of the maneuver, a short period of bradycardia, or decreased heart rate, occurs as blood that has been dammed back in the venous circulation returns to the heart.

The trachea, or windpipe, is a continuous tube that connects the larynx and the major bronchi of the lungs (Fig. 27-4). The walls of the trachea are supported by horse-

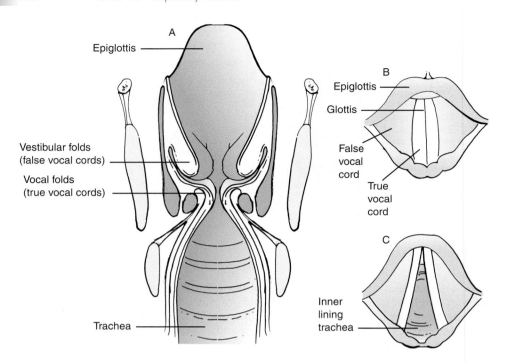

FIGURE 27-3 (**A**) Coronal section showing the position of the epiglottis, the vestibular folds (false vocal cords), the vocal folds (true vocal cords), and glottis. (**B**) Vocal cords viewed from above with the glottis closed and (**C**) with the glottis open.

shoe-shaped cartilages, which prevent it from collapsing when the pressure in the thorax becomes negative.

Tracheobronchial Tree

The tracheobronchial tree, which consists of the trachea, bronchi, and bronchioles, can be viewed as a system of branching tubes. It is similar to a tree whose branches become smaller and more numerous as they divide. There are approximately 23 levels of branching, beginning with the conducting airways and ending with the respiratory airways, where gas exchange takes place (Fig. 27-5).

The trachea divides to form the right and the left primary bronchi. Each bronchus enters the lung through a slit called the *hilus*. The point at which the trachea divides is called the *carina*. The carina is heavily innervated with sensory neurons, and coughing and bronchospasm result when this area is stimulated, as during tracheal suctioning. The right primary bronchus is shorter and wider and continues

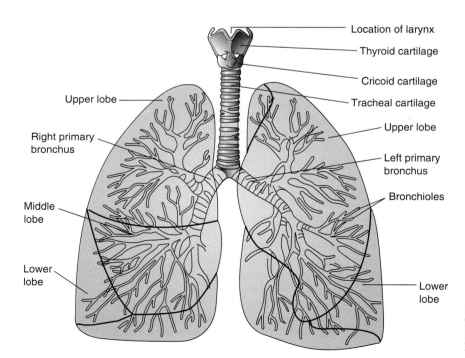

FIGURE 27-4 Larynx, trachea, and bronchial tree (anterior view). (Chaffee E.E., Lytle I.M. [1980]. *Basic physiology and anatomy* [4th ed.]. Philadelphia: J.B. Lippincott)

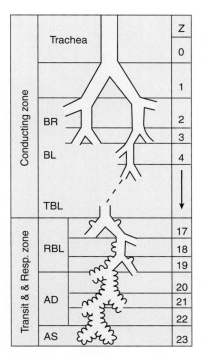

FIGURE 27-5 Idealization of the human airways. The first 16 generations of branching (Z) make up the conducting airways, and the last seven constitute the respiratory zone (or transitional and respiratory zone). BR, bronchus; BL, bronchiole; TBL, terminal bronchiole; RBL, respiratory bronchiole; AD, alveolar ducts; AS, alveolar sacs. (Weibel E.R. [1962]. *Morphometry of the human lung* [p. 111]. Berlin: Springer-Verlag)

at a more vertical angle with the trachea than the left primary bronchus, which is longer and narrower and forms a more acute angle with the trachea. The anatomic differences between the two bronchi also make it easier for foreign bodies to enter the right main bronchus than the left.

The right and left primary bronchi divide into secondary, or lobular, bronchi, which supply each of the lobes of the lungs. The bronchi continue to branch, forming smaller bronchi, until they become the terminal bronchioles, the smallest of the conducting airways.

The right middle lobe bronchus is of relatively small diameter and length and sometimes bends sharply near its bifurcation. It is surrounded by a collar of lymph nodes that drain the middle and the lower lobe and is particularly subject to obstruction. The secondary bronchi divide to form the segmental bronchi, which supply the bronchopulmonary segments of the lung. There are 10 segments in the right lung and 9 segments in the left lung (Fig. 27-6). These segments are identified according to their location in the lung (*e.g.*, the apical segment of the right upper lobe) and are the smallest named units in the lung. Lung lesions such as atelectasis and pneumonia often are localized to a particular bronchopulmonary segment.

The structure of the primary bronchi is similar to that of the trachea, in that these airways are supported by cartilaginous rings. As the bronchi move into the lungs, the horseshoe-shaped cartilage rings are replaced by irregular plates of cartilage. As these bronchi branch and become

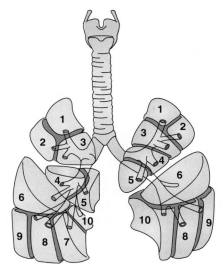

FIGURE 27-6 Bronchopulmonary segments of the human lung. Left and right upper lobes: (*1*) apical, (*2*) posterior, (*3*) anterior, (*4*) superior, lingular, and (*5*) inferior lingular segments. Right middle lobe: (*4*) lateral and (*5*) medial segments. Lower lobes: (*6*) superior (apical), (*7*) medial-basal, (*8*) anterior-basal, (*9*) lateral-basal, and (*10*) posterior-basal segments. The medial-basal segment (*7*) is absent in the left lung. (Fishman A.P. [1980]. *Assessment of pulmonary function* [p. 19]. New York: McGraw-Hill)

smaller, this cartilaginous support becomes thinner and then disappears at the level of the respiratory bronchioles. Between the cartilaginous support and the mucosal surface are two crisscrossing layers of smooth muscle that wind in opposite directions (Fig. 27-7). Bronchospasm, or contraction of these muscles, causes narrowing of the bronchioles

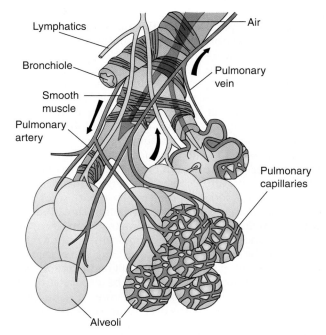

FIGURE 27-7 Lobule of the lung, showing the bronchial smooth muscle fibers, pulmonary blood vessels, and lymphatics.

and impairs air flow. The epithelial lining of conducting airways gradually becomes reduced from pseudostratified epithelium in the bronchi to a thin layer of tightly joined epithelial cells in the alveoli.

THE LUNGS AND RESPIRATORY AIRWAYS

The lungs are soft, spongy, cone-shaped organs located side by side in the chest cavity (see Fig. 27-1). They are separated from each other by the *mediastinum* (*i.e.*, the space between the lungs) and its contents—the heart, blood vessels, lymph nodes, nerve fibers, thymus gland, and esophagus. The upper part of the lung, which lies against the top of the thoracic cavity, is called the *apex*, and the lower part, which lies against the diaphragm, is called the *base*. The lungs are divided into lobes: three in the right lung and two in the left (see Fig. 27-4).

The lungs are the functional structures of the respiratory system. In addition to their gas exchange function, they inactivate vasoactive substances such as bradykinin; they convert angiotensin I to angiotensin II; and they serve as a reservoir for blood storage. Heparin-producing cells are particularly abundant in the capillaries of the lung, where small clots may be trapped.

Respiratory Lobules

The gas exchange function of the lung takes place in the lobules of the lungs. Each lobule, which is the smallest functional unit of the lung, is supplied by a branch of a terminal bronchiole, an arteriole, the pulmonary capillaries, and a venule (see Fig. 27-7). Gas exchange takes place in the terminal respiratory bronchioles and the alveolar ducts and sacs. Blood enters the lobules through a pulmonary artery and exits through a pulmonary vein. Lymphatic structures surround the lobule and aid in the removal of plasma proteins and other particles from the interstitial spaces.

Unlike larger bronchi, the respiratory bronchioles are lined with simple epithelium rather than ciliated pseudostratified epithelium. The respiratory bronchioles also lack the cartilaginous support of the larger airways. Instead, they are attached to the elastic spongework of tissue that contains the alveolar air spaces. When the air spaces become stretched during inspiration, the bronchioles are pulled open by expansion of the surrounding tissue.

The alveolar sacs are cup-shaped, thin-walled structures that are separated from each other by thin alveolar septa. Most of the septa are occupied by a single network of capillaries, so that blood is exposed to air on both sides. There are approximately 300 million alveoli in the adult lung, with a total surface area of approximately 50 to 100 m². Unlike the bronchioles, which are tubes with their own separate walls, the alveoli are interconnecting spaces that have no separate walls (Fig. 27-8). As a result of this arrangement, there is a continual mixing of air in the alveolar structures. Small holes in the alveolar walls, the pores of Kohn, probably contribute to the mixing of air under certain conditions.

The alveolar structures are composed of two types of cells: type I alveolar cells and type II alveolar cells (Fig. 27-9). The type I alveolar cells are flat squamous epithelial cells

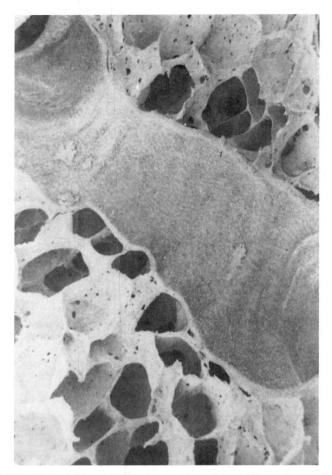

FIGURE 27-8 Close-up of a cross section of a small bronchus and surrounding alveoli. (Courtesy of Janice A. Nowell, University of California, Santa Cruz)

across which gas exchange takes place. The type II alveolar cells produce surfactant, a lipoprotein substance that decreases the surface tension in the alveoli. This action allows for greater ease of lung inflation and helps to prevent the collapse of smaller airways. The alveoli also contain alveolar macrophages, which are responsible for the removal of offending substances from the alveolar epithelium.

Lung Circulation

The lungs are provided with a dual blood supply, the pulmonary and bronchial circulations. The pulmonary circulation arises from the pulmonary artery and provides for the gas exchange function of the lungs. Deoxygenated blood leaves the right heart through the pulmonary artery, which divides into a left pulmonary artery that enters the left lung and a right pulmonary artery that enters the right lung. Return of oxygenated blood to the heart occurs by way of the pulmonary veins, which empty into the left atrium.

The bronchial circulation distributes blood to the conducting airways and supporting structures of the lung. The bronchial circulation has a secondary function of warming

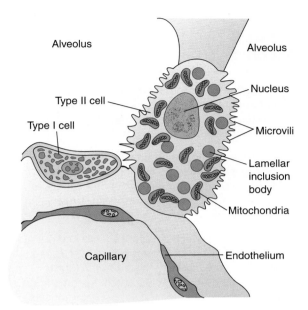

FIGURE 27-9 Schematic drawing of the two types of alveolar cells and their relation to alveoli and capillaries. Alveolar type I cells comprise most of the alveolar surface. Alveolar type II cells are located in the corner between two adjacent alveoli. Also shown are endothelial cells that line the pulmonary capillaries. (Rhoades R.A., Tanner G.A. [1996]. *Medical physiology* [p. 362]. Boston: Little, Brown)

and humidifying incoming air as it moves through the conducting airways. The bronchial arteries arise from the thoracic aorta and enter the lungs with the major bronchi, dividing and subdividing along with the bronchi as they move out into the lung, supplying them and other lung structures with oxygen. The capillaries of the bronchial circulation drain into the bronchial veins, the larger of which empties into the vena cava. The smaller of the bronchial veins empties into the pulmonary veins. This blood is unoxygenated because the bronchial circulation does not participate in gas exchange. As a result, this blood dilutes the oxygenated blood returning to the left side of the heart.

The bronchial blood vessels are the only ones that undergo angiogenesis (formation of new vessels) and develop collateral circulation when vessels in the pulmonary circulation are obstructed, as in pulmonary embolism. The development of new blood vessels helps to keep lung tissue alive until the pulmonary circulation can be restored.

PLEURA

A thin, transparent, double-layered serous membrane, called the *pleura*, lines the thoracic cavity and encases the lungs. The outer parietal layer lies adjacent to the chest wall, and the inner visceral layer adheres to the outer surface of the lung (see Fig. 27-1). The parietal pleura forms part of the mediastinum and lines the inner wall of the thoracic or chest cavity. A thin film of serous fluid separates the two pleural layers, and this allows the two layers to glide over each other and yet hold together, so there is no separation between the lungs and the chest wall. The pleural cavity is a potential space in which serous fluid or inflammatory exudate can accumulate. The term *pleural effusion* is used to describe an abnormal collection of fluid or exudate in the pleural cavity.

In summary, the respiratory system consists of the air passages and the lungs, where gas exchange takes place. Functionally, the air passages of the respiratory system can be structurally divided into two parts: the conducting airways, through which air moves as it passes into and out of the lungs, and the respiratory tissues, where gas exchange actually takes place. The conducting airways include the nasal passages, mouth and nasopharynx, larynx, and tracheobronchial tree. Air is warmed, filtered, and humidified as it passes through these structures.

The lungs are the functional structures of the respiratory system. In addition to their gas exchange function, they inactivate vasoactive substances such as bradykinin; they convert angiotensin I to angiotensin II; and they serve as a reservoir for blood. The lobules, which are the functional units of the lung, consist of the respiratory bronchioles, alveoli, and pulmonary capillaries. It is here that gas exchange takes place. Oxygen from the alveoli diffuses across the alveolar capillary membrane into the blood, and carbon dioxide from the blood diffuses into the alveoli.

The lungs are provided with a dual blood supply: the pulmonary circulation provides for the gas exchange function of the lungs and the bronchial circulation distributes blood to the conducting airways and supporting structures of the lung. The lungs are encased in a thin, transparent, double-layered serous membrane called the *pleura*. The pressure in the pleural space, which is negative in relation to alveolar pressure, prevents the lungs from collapsing.

Exchange of Gases Between the Atmosphere and the Lungs

After you have completed this section of the chapter, you should be able to meet the following objectives:

✦ Describe the basic properties of gases in relation to their partial pressures and their pressures in relation to volume and temperature

✦ State the definition of intrathoracic, intrapleural, and intra-alveolar pressures, and state how each of these pressures changes in relation to atmospheric pressure during inspiration and expiration

✦ State a definition of lung compliance

✦ Use Laplace's law to explain the need for surfactant in maintaining the inflation of small alveoli

✦ State the major determinant of airway resistance

✦ Explain why increasing lung volume (*e.g.*, taking deep breaths) reduces airway resistance

✦ Define inspiratory reserve, expiratory reserve, vital capacity, and residual volume

✦ Describe the method for measuring $FEV_{1.0}$

BASIC PROPERTIES OF GASES

The air we breathe is made up of a mixture of gases, mainly nitrogen and oxygen. These gases exert a combined pressure called the *atmospheric pressure*. The pressure at sea level is defined as 1 atmosphere, which is equal to 760 millimeters of mercury (mm Hg) or 14.7 pounds per square inch (PSI). When measuring respiratory pressures, atmospheric pressure is assigned a value of 0. A respiratory pressure of +15 mm Hg means that the pressure is 15 mm Hg above atmospheric pressure, and a respiratory pressure of −15 mm Hg is 15 mm Hg less than atmospheric pressure. Respiratory pressures often are expressed in centimeters of water (cm H_2O) because of the small pressures involved (1 mm Hg = 1.35 cm H_2O pressure).

The pressure exerted by a single gas in a mixture is called the *partial pressure*. The capital letter "P" followed by the chemical symbol of the gas (PO_2) is used to denote its partial pressure. The law of partial pressures states that the total pressure of a mixture of gases, as in the atmosphere, is equal to the sum of the partial pressures of the different gases in the mixture. If the concentration of oxygen at 760 mm Hg (1 atmosphere) is 20%, its partial pressure is 152 mm Hg (760×0.20).

Water vapor is different from other types of gases; its partial pressure is affected by temperature but not atmospheric pressure. The relative humidity refers to the percentage of moisture in the air compared with the amount that the air can hold without causing condensation (100% saturation). Warm air holds more moisture than cold air. This is the reason that precipitation in the form of rain or snow commonly occurs when the relative humidity is high and there is a sudden drop in atmospheric temperature. The air in the alveoli, which is 100% saturated at normal body temperature, has a water vapor pressure of 47 mm Hg. The water vapor pressure must be included in the sum of the total pressure of the gases in the alveoli (*i.e.*, the total pressure of the other gases in the alveoli is 760 − 47 = 713 mm Hg).

Air moves between the atmosphere and the lungs because of a pressure difference. According to the laws of physics, the pressure of a gas varies inversely with the volume of its container, provided the temperature remains constant. If equal amounts of a gas are placed in two different-sized containers, the pressure of the gas in the smaller container is greater than the pressure in the larger container. The movement of gases is always from the container with the greater pressure to the one with the lesser pressure. The chest cavity can be viewed as a volume container. During inspiration, the size of the chest cavity increases and air moves into the lungs; during expiration, air moves out as the size of the chest cavity decreases.

VENTILATION AND THE MECHANICS OF BREATHING

Ventilation is concerned with the movement of gases into and out of the lungs. There is nothing mystical about ventilation. It is purely a mechanical event that obeys the laws of physics as they relate to the behavior of gases. It relies on

Ventilation and Gas Exchange

➤ Ventilation refers to the movement of gases into and out of the lungs through a system of open airways and along a pressure gradient resulting from a change in chest volume.

➤ During inspiration, air is drawn into the lungs as the respiratory muscles expand the chest cavity; during expiration, air moves out of the lungs as the chest muscles recoil and the chest cavity becomes smaller.

➤ The ease with which air is moved into and out of the lung depends on the resistance of the airways, which is inversely related to the fourth power of the airway radius, and lung compliance, or the ease with which the lungs can be inflated.

➤ The minute volume, which is determined by the metabolic needs of the body, is the amount of air that is exchanged each minute. It is the product of the tidal volume or amount of air exchanged with each breath multiplied by the respiratory rate.

a system of open airways and the respiratory pressures created as the movements of the respiratory muscles change the size of the chest cage. The degree to which the lungs inflate and deflate depends on the respiratory pressures inflating the lung, compliance of the lungs, and airway resistance.

Respiratory Pressures

The pressure inside the airways and alveoli of the lungs is called the *intrapulmonary pressure* or *alveolar pressure*. The gases in this area of the lungs are in communication with atmospheric pressure (Fig. 27-10). When the glottis is open and air is not moving into or out of the lungs, as occurs just before inspiration or expiration, the intrapulmonary pressure is zero or equal to atmospheric pressure.

The pressure in the pleural cavity is called the *intrapleural pressure*. The intrapleural pressure is always negative in relation to alveolar pressure, approximately −4 mm Hg between breaths when the glottis is open and the alveolar spaces are open to the atmosphere. The lungs and the chest wall have elastic properties, each pulling in the opposite direction. If removed from the chest, the lungs would contract to a smaller size, and the chest wall, if freed from the lungs, would expand. The opposing forces of the chest wall and lungs create a pull against the visceral and parietal layers of the pleura, causing the pressure in the pleural cavity to become negative. During inspiration, the elastic recoil of the lungs increases, causing intrapleural pressure to become more negative than during expiration. Without the negative intrapleural pressure holding the lungs against the chest

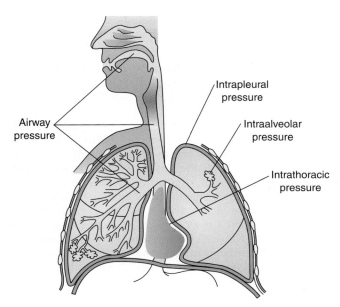

FIGURE 27-10 Partitioning of respiratory pressures.

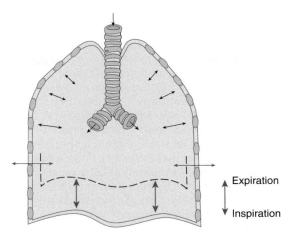

FIGURE 27-11 Frontal section of the chest showing the movement of the rib cage and diaphragm during inspiration and expiration.

wall, their elastic recoil properties would cause them to collapse. Although intrapleural pressure is negative in relation to alveolar pressure, it may become positive in relation to atmospheric pressure (*e.g.*, during forced expiration and coughing).

The *intrathoracic pressure* is the pressure in the thoracic cavity. It is essentially equal to intrapleural pressure and is the pressure to which the lungs, heart, and great vessels are exposed. Forced expiration against a closed glottis compresses the air in the thoracic cavity and produces marked increases in intrathoracic pressure and intrapleural pressure.

The Chest Cage and Respiratory Muscles

The lungs and major airways share the chest cavity with the heart, great vessels, and esophagus. The chest cavity is a closed compartment bounded on the top by the neck muscles and at the bottom by the diaphragm. The outer walls of the chest cavity are formed by 12 pairs of ribs, the sternum, the thoracic vertebrae, and the intercostal muscles that lie between the ribs. Mechanically, the act of breathing depends on the fact that the chest cavity is a closed compartment whose only opening to the exterior is the trachea.

Ventilation consists of inspiration and expiration. During *inspiration*, the size of the chest cavity increases, the intrathoracic pressure becomes more negative, and air is drawn into the lungs. *Expiration* occurs as the elastic components of the chest wall and lung structures that were stretched during inspiration recoil, causing the size of the chest cavity to decrease and the pressure in the chest cavity to increase. The diaphragm is the principal muscle of inspiration. When the diaphragm contracts, the abdominal contents are forced downward and the chest expands from top to bottom (Fig. 27-11). During normal levels of inspiration, the diaphragm moves approximately 1 cm, but this can be increased to 10 cm on forced inspiration. The diaphragm is

innervated by the phrenic nerve roots, which arise from the cervical level of the spinal cord, mainly from C4 but also from C3 and C5. Paralysis of one side of the diaphragm causes the chest to move up on that side rather than down during inspiration because of the negative pressure in the chest. This is called *paradoxical movement.*

The external intercostal muscles, which also aid in inspiration, connect to the adjacent ribs and slope downward and forward (Fig. 27-12). When they contract, they raise the ribs and rotate them slightly so that the sternum is pushed forward; this enlarges the chest from side to side and from front to back. The intercostal muscles receive their innervation from nerves that exit the central nervous system at the thoracic level of the spinal cord. Paralysis of these muscles usually does not have a serious effect on respiration because of the effectiveness of the diaphragm.

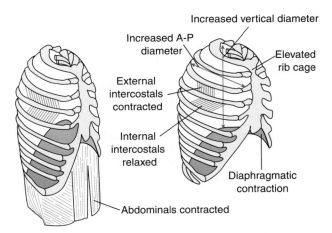

FIGURE 27-12 Expansion and contraction of the thoracic cage during expiration and inspiration, demonstrating especially diaphragmatic contraction, elevation of the rib cage, and function of the intercostals. (Guyton A.C., Hall J.E. [2000]. *Textbook of medical physiology* [10th ed., p. 433]. Philadelphia: W.B. Saunders)

The accessory muscles of inspiration include the scalene muscles and the sternocleidomastoid muscles. The scalene muscles elevate the first two ribs, and the sternocleidomastoid muscles raise the sternum to increase the size of the chest cavity. These muscles contribute little to quiet breathing but contract vigorously during exercise. For the accessory muscles to assist in ventilation, they must be stabilized in some way. For example, persons with bronchial asthma often brace their arms against a firm object during an attack as a means of stabilizing their shoulders so that the attached accessory muscles can exert their full effect on ventilation. The head commonly is bent backward so that the scalene and sternocleidomastoid muscles can elevate the ribs more effectively. Other muscles that play a minor role in inspiration are the alae nasi, which produce flaring of the nostrils during obstructed breathing.

Expiration is largely passive. It occurs as the elastic components of the chest wall and lung structures that were stretched during inspiration recoil, causing air to leave the lungs as the intrathoracic pressure increases. When needed, the abdominal and the internal intercostal muscles can be used to increase expiratory effort (see Fig. 27-12). The increase in intra-abdominal pressure that accompanies the forceful contraction of the abdominal muscles pushes the diaphragm upward and results in an increase in intrathoracic pressure. The internal intercostal muscles move inward, which pulls the chest downward, increasing expiratory effort.

Lung Compliance

Lung compliance refers to the ease with which the lungs can be inflated. It is determined by the elastin and collagen fibers of the lung, its water content, and surface tension. Compliance can be appreciated by comparing the ease of blowing up a new balloon that is stiff and resistant with one that has been previously blown up and stretched. Specifically, lung compliance (C) describes the change in lung volume (ΔV) that can be accomplished with a given change in respiratory pressure (ΔP).

$$C = \Delta V / \Delta P$$

The normal compliance of both lungs in the average adult is approximately 200 mL/cm H_2O. This means that every time the transpulmonary pressure increases by 1 cm/H_2O, the lung volume expands by 200 mL. It would take more pressure to move the same amount of air into a noncompliant lung.

Changes in Elastin/Collagen Composition of Lung Tissue. Lung tissue is made up of elastin and collagen fibers. The elastin fibers are easily stretched and increase the ease of lung inflation, whereas the collagen fibers resist stretching and make lung inflation more difficult. In lung diseases such as interstitial lung disease and pulmonary fibrosis, the lungs become stiff and noncompliant as the elastin fibers are replaced with scar tissue. Pulmonary congestion and edema produce a reversible decrease in pulmonary compliance.

Elastic recoil describes the ability of the elastic components of the lung to recoil to their original position after having been stretched. Overstretching the airways, as occurs with emphysema, causes the elastic components of the lung to lose their recoil, making the lung easier to inflate but more difficult to deflate because of its inability to recoil.

Surface Tension. An important factor in lung compliance is the *surface tension* in the alveoli. The alveoli are lined with a thin film of liquid, and it is at the interface between this liquid film and the alveolar air that surface tension develops. This is because the forces that hold the liquid film molecules together are stronger than those that hold the air molecules in the alveoli together. As an example, it is surface tension that holds the water molecules in a raindrop together. In the alveoli, excess surface tension causes the liquid film to contract, making lung inflation more difficult.

The pressure in the alveoli (which are modeled as spheres with open airways projecting from them) can be predicted using Laplace's law (pressure = 2 × surface tension/radius). If the surface tension were equal throughout the lungs, the alveoli with the smallest radii would have the greatest pressure, and this would cause them to empty into the larger alveoli (Fig. 27-13). The reason this does not occur is because of special surface tension–lowering molecules, called *surfactant*, that line the inner surface of the alveoli.

Surfactant is a complex mixture of lipoproteins (largely phospholipids) and small amounts of carbohydrates that is synthesized in the type II alveolar cells. The surfactant molecule has two ends: a hydrophobic (water-insoluble) tail and a hydrophilic (water-soluble) head (Fig. 27-14). The hydrophilic head of the surfactant molecule attaches to the liquid molecules and the hydrophobic tail to the gas molecules, interrupting the intermolecular forces that are responsible for creating the surface tension.

Surfactant exerts four important effects on lung inflation: it lowers the surface tension; it increases lung compliance and ease of inflation; it provides for stability and more even inflation of the alveoli; and it assists in preventing pulmonary edema by keeping the alveoli dry. Without surfactant, lung inflation would be extremely difficult, requiring intrapleural pressures of −20 to −30 mm Hg, compared with the pressures of −3 to −5 mm Hg that normally are needed. The surfactant molecules are more densely packed in the

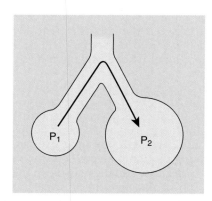

FIGURE 27-13 Law of Laplace (P = 2 T/r, P = pressure, T = tension, r = radius). The effect of the radius on the pressure and movement of gases in the alveolar structures is depicted. Air moves from P_1 with a small radius and higher pressure to P_2 with its larger radius and lower pressure.

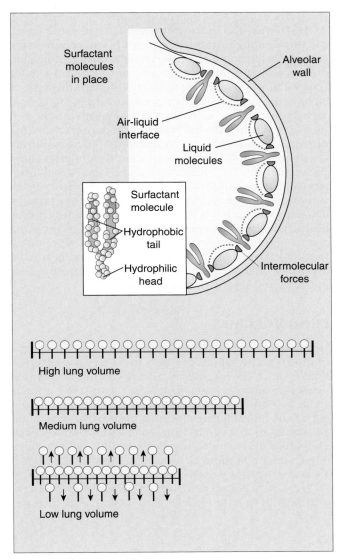

FIGURE 27-14 (**Top**) Alveolar wall depicting surface tension resulting from the intramolecular forces in the air–liquid film interface; the surfactant molecule with its hydrophobic tail and hydrophilic head; and its function in reducing surface tension by disrupting the intermolecular forces. (**Bottom**) The surface concentration of surfactant molecules at high, medium, and low lung volumes.

small alveoli than in larger alveoli, where the density of the molecules is less. Therefore, surfactant reduces the surface tension more effectively in the small alveoli, which have the greatest tendency to collapse, providing for stability and more even distribution of ventilation. Surfactant also helps to keep the alveoli dry and prevent pulmonary edema. This is because water is pulled out of the pulmonary capillaries into the alveoli when increased surface tension causes the alveoli to contract.

The type II alveolar cells that produce surfactant do not begin to mature until the 26th to 28th week of gestation; consequently, many premature infants have difficulty producing sufficient amounts of surfactant. This can

lead to alveolar collapse and severe respiratory distress. This condition, called *infant respiratory distress syndrome,* is the single most common cause of respiratory disease in premature infants. Surfactant dysfunction also is possible in the adult. This usually occurs as the result of severe injury or infection and can contribute to the development of a condition called *adult respiratory distress syndrome* (see Chapter 29).

Airway Resistance

The volume of air that moves into and out of the air exchange portion of the lungs is directly related to the pressure difference between the lungs and the atmosphere and inversely related to the resistance that the air encounters as it moves through the airways.

Airway resistance is the ratio of the pressure driving inspiration or expiration to airflow. The French physician Jean Léonard Marie Poiseuille first described the pressure-flow characteristics of laminar flow in a straight circular tube, a correlation that has become known as *Poiseuille's law.* According to Poiseuille's law, the resistance to flow is inversely related to the fourth power of the radius ($R = 1/r^4$). If the radius is reduced by one half, the resistance increases 16-fold ($2 \times 2 \times 2 \times 2 = 16$).

Airway resistance normally is so small that only small changes in pressure are needed to move large volumes of air into the lungs. For example, the average pressure change that is needed to move a normal breath of 500 mL of air into the lungs is approximately 1 to 2 cm H_2O. Because the resistance of the airways is inversely proportional to the fourth power of the radius, small changes in airway caliber, such as those caused by pulmonary secretions or bronchospasm, can produce a marked increase in airway resistance. For persons with these conditions to maintain the same rate of air flow as before the onset of increased airway resistance, an increase in driving pressure (*i.e.*, respiratory effort) is needed.

Airway resistance is greatly affected by lung volumes, being less during inspiration than during expiration. This is because elastic-type fibers connect the outside of the airways to the surrounding lung tissues. As a result, these airways are pulled open as the lungs expand during inspiration, and they become narrower as the lungs deflate during expiration (Fig. 27-15). This is one of the reasons why persons with conditions that increase airway resistance, such as bronchial asthma, usually have less difficulty during inspiration than during expiration.

Laminar Versus Turbulent Flow. Airflow can be laminar or turbulent, depending on the velocity and pattern of flow. Laminar, or streamlined, airflow occurs at low flow rates in which the airstream is parallel to the sides of the airway. With laminar flow, the air at the periphery must overcome the resistance to flow, and as a result, the air in the center of the airway moves faster. Turbulent flow is disorganized flow in which the molecules of the gas move laterally, collide with one another, and change their velocities. Whether turbulence develops depends on the radius of the airways, the interaction of the gas molecules, and the velocity of airflow. It is most likely to occur when the radius of the airways is large and the velocity of flow is high. Turbulent flow occurs regularly in the trachea. Turbulence of airflow ac-

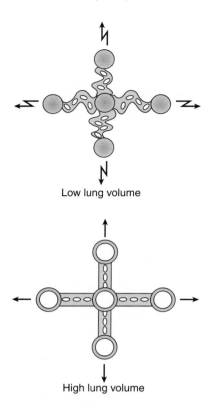

FIGURE 27-15 Interaction of tissue forces on airways during low and high lung volumes. At low lung volumes, the tissue forces tend to fold and place less tension on the airways and they become smaller; during high lung volumes, the tissue forces are stretched and pull the airways open.

counts for the respiratory sounds that are heard during chest auscultation (i.e., listening to chest sounds using a stethoscope).

In the bronchial tree with its many branches, laminar airflow probably occurs only in the very small airways, where the velocity of flow is low. Because the small airways contribute little resistance to airflow, they constitute a silent zone. In small airway disease (*e.g.,* chronic obstructive pulmonary disease), it is probable that considerable abnormalities are present before the usual measurements of airway resistance can detect them.

Airway Compression. Airflow through the collapsible airways in the lungs depends on the distending airway (intrapulmonary) pressures that hold the airways open and the external (intrapleural or intrathoracic) pressures that surround and compress the airways. The difference between these two pressures (intrathoracic pressure minus airway pressure) is called the *transpulmonary pressure*. For airflow to occur, the distending pressure inside the airways must be greater than the compressing pressure outside the airways.

During forced expiration, the transpulmonary pressure is decreased because of a disproportionate increase in the intrathoracic pressure compared with airway pressure. The resistance that air encounters as it moves out of

the lungs causes a further drop in airway pressure (Fig. 27-16). If this drop in airway pressure is sufficiently great, the surrounding intrathoracic pressure will compress the collapsible airways (*i.e.,* those that lack cartilaginous support), causing airflow to be interrupted and air to be trapped in the alveoli (Fig. 27-17). Although this type of airway compression usually is seen only during forced expiration in persons with normal respiratory function, it may occur during normal breathing in persons with lung diseases. For example, in conditions that increase airway resistance, such as emphysema, the pressure drop along the smaller airways is magnified, and an increase in intra-airway pressure is needed to maintain airway patency. Measures such as pursed-lip breathing increase airway pressure and improve expiratory flow rates in persons with chronic obstructive lung disease. This is also the basis for using positive end-expiratory pressure in persons who are on mechanical ventilators. Infants who are having trouble breathing often grunt to increase their expiratory airway pressures and keep their airways open.

LUNG VOLUMES

Lung volumes, or the amount of air exchanged during ventilation, can be subdivided into three components: the tidal volume, the inspiratory reserve volume, and the expiratory reserve volume. The *tidal volume* (TV), usually about 500 mL, is the amount of air that moves into and out of the lungs during a normal breath. The maximum amount of air that can be inspired in excess of the normal TV is called the *inspiratory reserve volume* (IRV), and the maximum amount that can be exhaled in excess of the normal TV is the *expiratory reserve volume* (ERV). Approximately 1200 mL of air always remains in the lungs after forced expiration; this air is the *residual volume* (RV). The RV increases

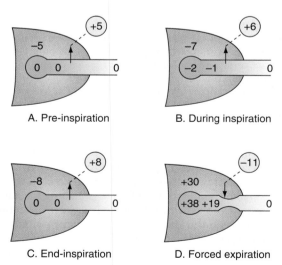

A. Pre-inspiration   B. During inspiration

C. End-inspiration   D. Forced expiration

FIGURE 27-16 Scheme showing why airways are compressed during forced expiration. The pressure difference across the airway is holding it open, except during a forced expiration. (West J.B. [2000]. *Respiratory physiology: The essentials* [p. 98]. Philadelphia: Lippincott Williams & Wilkins)

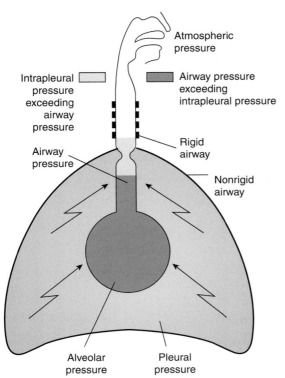

Intrapleural pressure exceeding airway pressure

Atmospheric pressure

Airway pressure exceeding intrapleural pressure

Airway pressure

Rigid airway

Nonrigid airway

Alveolar pressure

Pleural pressure

FIGURE 27-17 Mechanism that limits maximal expiratory flow rate. Forced expiration increases intrapleural pressure, causing airway compression of nonrigid airways where intrapleural pressure exceeds airway pressure.

with age because there is more trapping of air in the lungs at the end of expiration. These volumes can be measured using an instrument called a *spirometer*. With the type of spirometer shown in Figure 27-18, the bell, which is inverted over a water bath, moves down during inspiration and up during expiration, causing the pen to move up and down and mark the chart paper.

Lung capacities include two or more lung volumes. The *vital capacity* equals the IRV plus the TV plus the ERV and is the amount of air that can be exhaled from the point of maximal inspiration. The *inspiratory capacity* equals the TV plus the IRV. It is the amount of air a person can breathe in beginning at the normal expiratory level and distending the lungs to the maximal amount. The *functional residual capacity* is the sum of the RV and ERV; it is the volume of air that remains in the lungs at the end of normal expiration. The *total lung capacity* is the sum of all the volumes in the lungs. The RV cannot be measured with the spirometer because this air cannot be expressed from the lungs. It is measured by indirect methods, such as the helium dilution methods, the nitrogen washout methods, or body plethysmography. Lung volumes and capacities are summarized in Table 27-1.

Pulmonary Function Studies
The previously described lung volumes and capacities are anatomic or static measures, determined by lung volumes and measured without relation to time. The spirometer also is used to measure dynamic lung function (*i.e.*, ventilation with respect to time); these tests often are used in assessing pulmonary function. Pulmonary function measures include maximum voluntary ventilation, forced vital capacity, forced expiratory volumes and flow rates, and forced inspiratory flow rates (Table 27-2). Pulmonary function is measured for various clinical purposes, including diagnosis of respiratory disease, preoperative surgical and anesthetic risk evaluation, and symptom and disability evaluation for legal or insurance purposes. The tests also are used for evaluating dyspnea, cough, wheezing, and abnormal radiologic or laboratory findings.

The *maximum voluntary ventilation* measures the volume of air that a person can move into and out of the lungs during maximum effort lasting for 12 to 15 seconds. This measurement usually is converted to liters per minute. The *forced expiratory vital capacity* (FVC) involves full inspiration to total lung capacity followed by forceful maximal expiration. Obstruction of airways produces a FVC that is lower than that observed with more slowly performed vital capacity measurements. The *forced expiratory volume* (FEV) is the expiratory volume achieved in a given time period. The $FEV_{1.0}$ is the forced expiratory volume that can be exhaled in 1 second. The $FEV_{1.0}$ frequently is expressed as a percentage of the FVC. The $FEV_{1.0}$ and FVC are used in the diagnosis of obstructive lung disorders.

The *forced inspiratory vital flow* (FIF) measures the respiratory response during rapid maximal inspiration. Calculation of airflow during the middle half of inspiration ($FIF_{25\%-75\%}$) relative to the forced midexpiratory flow rate ($FEF_{25\%-75\%}$) is used as a measure of respiratory muscle dysfunction because inspiratory flow depends more on effort than does expiration.

EFFICIENCY AND THE WORK OF BREATHING

The *minute volume*, or total ventilation, is the amount of air that is exchanged in 1 minute. It is determined by the metabolic needs of the body. The minute volume is equal to the TV multiplied by the respiratory rate, which is normally about 6000 mL (500 mL TV × respiratory rate of 12 breaths per minute) during normal activity. The efficiency of breathing is determined by matching the TV and respiratory rate in a manner that provides an optimal minute volume while minimizing the work of breathing.

The work of breathing is determined by the amount of effort required to move air through the conducting airways and by the ease of lung expansion, or compliance. Expansion of the lungs is difficult for persons with stiff and noncompliant lungs; they usually find it easier to breathe if they keep their TV low and breathe at a more rapid rate (*e.g.*, 300 × 20 = 6000 mL) to achieve their minute volume and meet their oxygen needs. In contrast, persons with obstructive airway disease usually find it less difficult to inflate their lungs but expend more energy in moving air through the airways. As a result, these persons take deeper breaths and breathe at a slower rate (*e.g.*, 600 × 10 = 6000 mL) to achieve their oxygen needs.

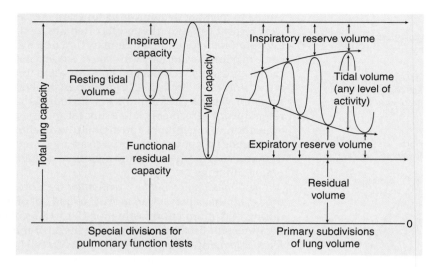

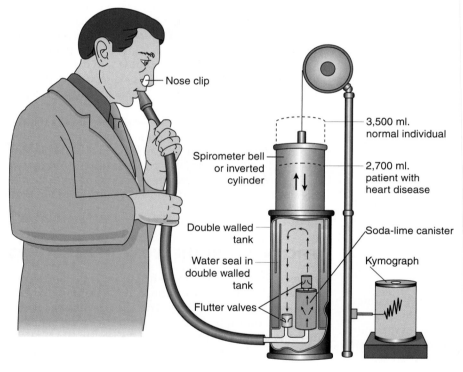

FIGURE 27-18 Measurement of vital capacity using a spirometer. (Chaffee E.E., Lytle I.M. [1980]. *Basic physiology and anatomy* [4th ed.]. Philadelphia: J.B. Lippincott)

In summary, the movement of air between the atmosphere and the lungs follows the laws of physics as they relate to gases. The air in the alveoli contains a mixture of gases, including nitrogen, oxygen, carbon dioxide, and water vapor. With the exception of water vapor, each gas exerts a pressure that is determined by the atmospheric pressure and the concentration of the gas in the mixture. Water vapor pressure is affected by temperature but not atmospheric pressure. Air moves into the lungs along a pressure gradient. The pressure inside the airways and alveoli of the lungs is called *intrapulmonary* (or *alveolar*) *pressure*; the pressure in the pleural cavity is called *pleural pressure*; and the pressure in the thoracic cavity is called *intrathoracic pressure*.

Breathing is the movement of gases between the atmosphere and the lungs. It requires a system of open airways and pressure changes resulting from the action of the respiratory muscles in changing the volume of the chest cage. The diaphragm is the principal muscle of inspiration, assisted by the external intercostal muscles. The scalene and sternocleidomastoid muscles elevate the ribs and act as accessory muscles for inspiration. Expiration is largely passive, aided by the elastic recoil of the respiratory muscles that were

TABLE 27-1 ✦ Lung Volumes and Capacities

Volume	Symbol	Measurement
Tidal volume (about 500 mL at rest)	TV	Amount of air that moves into and out of the lungs with each breath
Inspiratory reserve volume (about 3000 mL)	IRV	Maximum amount of air that can be inhaled from the point of maximal expiration
Expiratory reserve volume (about 1100 mL)	ERV	Maximum volume of air that can be exhaled from the resting end-expiratory level
Residual volume (about 1200 mL)	RV	Volume of air remaining in the lungs after maximal expiration. This volume cannot be measured with the spirometer; it is measured indirectly using methods such as the helium dilution method, the nitrogen washout technique, or body plethysmography.
Functional residual capacity (about 2300 mL)	FRC	Volume of air remaining in the lungs at end-expiration (sum of RV and ERV)
Inspiratory capacity (about 3500 mL)	IC	Sum of IRV and TV
Vital capacity (about 4600 mL)	VC	Maximal amount of air that can be exhaled from the point of maximal inspiration
Total lung capacity (about 5800 mL)	TLC	Total amount of air that the lungs can hold; it is the sum of all the volume components after maximal inspiration. This value is about 20% to 25% less in females than in males.

TABLE 27-2 ✦ Pulmonary Function Tests

Test	Symbol	Measurement*
Maximal voluntary ventilation	MVV	Maximum amount of air that can be breathed in a given time
Forced vital capacity	FVC	Maximum amount of air that can be rapidly and forcefully exhaled from the lungs after full inspiration. The expired volume is plotted against time.
Forced expiratory volume achieved in 1 second	$FEV_{1.0}$	Volume of air expired in the first second of FVC
Percentage of forced vital capacity	$FEV_{1.0}/FVC\%$	Volume of air expired in the first second, expressed as a percentage of FVC
Forced midexpiratory flow rate	$FEF_{25\%-75\%}$	The forced midexpiratory flow rate determined by locating the points on the volume-time curve recording obtained during FVC corresponding to 25% and 75% of FVC and drawing a straight line through these points. The slope of this line represents the average midexpiratory flow rate.
Forced inspiratory flow rate	$FIF_{25\%-75\%}$	FIF is the volume inspired from RV at the point of measurement. $FIF_{25\%-75\%}$ is the slope of a line between the points on the volume pressure tracing corresponding to 25% and 75% of the inspired volume.

*By convention, all the lung volumes and rates of flow are expressed in terms of body temperature and pressure and saturated with water vapor (BTPS), which allows for a comparison of the pulmonary function data from laboratories with different ambient temperatures and altitudes.

stretched during inspiration. When needed, the abdominal and internal intercostal muscles can be used to increase expiratory effort.

Lung compliance describes the ease with which the lungs can be inflated. It reflects the elasticity of the lung tissue and the surface tension in the alveoli. Surfactant molecules, produced by type II alveolar cells, reduce the surface tension in the lungs and thereby increase lung compliance. Airway resistance refers to the impediment to flow that the air encounters as it moves through the airways. The minute volume, which is determined by the metabolic needs of the body, is the amount of air that is exchanged in 1 minute (*i.e.*, respiratory rate and TV). The efficiency and work of breathing are determined by factors such as impaired lung compliance and airway diseases that increase the work involved in maintaining the minute volume. Lung volumes and lung capacities can be measured using a spirometer. Pulmonary function studies are used to assess ventilation with respect to time.

Exchange and Transport of Gases

After you have completed this section of the chapter, you should be able to meet the following objectives:

+ Trace the exchange of gases between the air in the alveoli and the blood in the pulmonary capillaries
+ Differentiate between pulmonary and alveolar ventilation
+ Explain why ventilation and perfusion must be matched
+ Cite the difference between dead air space and shunt
+ List four factors that affect the diffusion of gases in the alveoli
+ Explain the difference between PO_2 and hemoglobin-bound oxygen and O_2 saturation and content
+ Explain the significance of a shift to the right and a shift to the left in the oxygen-hemoglobin dissociation curve

The primary functions of the lungs are oxygenation of the blood and removal of carbon dioxide. Pulmonary gas exchange is conventionally divided into three processes: ventilation or the flow of gases into and out of the alveoli of the lungs, perfusion or flow of blood in the adjacent pulmonary capillaries, and diffusion or transfer of gases between the alveoli and the pulmonary capillaries. The efficiency of gas exchange requires that alveolar ventilation occur adjacent to perfused pulmonary capillaries.

VENTILATION

Ventilation refers to the exchange of gases in the respiratory system. There are two types of ventilation: pulmonary and alveolar. *Pulmonary ventilation* refers to the total exchange of gases between the atmosphere and the lungs. *Alveolar ventilation* is the exchange of gases within the gas exchange portion of the lungs. Ventilation requires a system of open airways and a pressure difference that moves air into and out of the lungs. It is affected by body position and lung vol-

ume as well as by disease conditions that affect the heart and respiratory system.

Distribution of Ventilation

The distribution of ventilation between the top (apex) and bottom (base) of the lung varies with body position and the weight of the lung and the effects of gravity on intrapleural pressure. Compliance reflects the change in volume that occurs with a change in pressure. It is less in fully expanded alveoli, which have difficulty accommodating more air, and greater in alveoli that are less inflated. In the seated or standing position, gravity exerts a downward pull on the lung, causing intrapleural pressure at the apex of the lung to become more negative than that at the base of the lung (Fig. 27-19). As a result, the alveoli at the apex of the lung are more fully expanded and less compliant than those at the base of the lung. The same holds true for lung compliance in the dependent portions of the lung in the supine or lateral position. In the supine position, ventilation in the lowermost (posterior) parts of the lung exceeds that in the uppermost (anterior) parts. In the lateral position (*i.e.*, lying on the side), the dependent lung is better ventilated.

The distribution of ventilation also is affected by lung volumes. During full inspiration in the seated or standing position, the airways are pulled open and air moves into the more compliant portions of the lower lung. At low lung volumes, the opposite occurs. At functional residual capacity, the pleural pressure at the base of the lung exceeds airway pressure compressing the airways so that ventilation is greatly reduced. In contrast, the airways in the apex of the lung remain open and this area of the lung is well ventilated.

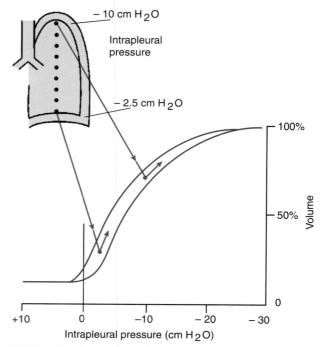

FIGURE 27-19 Explanation of the regional differences in ventilation down the lung; the intrapleural pressure is less negative at the base than at the apex. As a consequence, the basal lung is relatively compressed in its resting state but expands more on inspiration than the apex. (West J.B. [2001]. *Pulmonary physiology and pathophysiology* [p. 43]. Lippincott Williams & Wilkins)

Even at low lung volumes, some air remains in the alveoli of the lower portion of the lungs, preventing their collapse. According to Laplace's law (discussed previously), the pressure needed to overcome the tension in the wall of a sphere or an elastic tube is inversely related to its radius; therefore, the small airways close first, trapping some gas in the alveoli. There may be increased trapping of air in the alveoli of the lower part of the lungs in older persons and in those with lung disease (*e.g.*, emphysema). This condition is thought to result from a loss in the elastic recoil properties of the lungs, so that the intrapleural pressure, created by the elastic recoil of the lung and chest wall, becomes less negative. In these persons, airway closure occurs at the end of normal instead of low lung volumes, trapping larger amounts of air. The air trapping eventually causes an increase in the anteroposterior chest dimensions.

PERFUSION

The primary functions of the pulmonary circulation are to perfuse or provide blood flow to the gas exchange portion of the lung and to facilitate gas exchange. The pulmonary circulation serves several important functions in addition to gas exchange. It filters all the blood that moves from the right to the left side of the circulation; it removes most of the thromboemboli that might form; and it serves as a reservoir of blood for the left side of the heart.

The gas exchange function of the lungs requires a continuous flow of blood through the respiratory portion of the lungs. Deoxygenated blood enters the lung through the pulmonary artery, which has its origin in the right side of the heart and enters the lung at the hilus, along with the primary bronchus. The pulmonary arteries branch in a manner similar to that of the airways. The small pulmonary arteries accompany the bronchi as they move down the lobules and branch to supply the capillary network that surrounds the alveoli (see Fig. 27-7). The meshwork of capillaries in the respiratory portion of the lungs is so dense that the flow in these vessels often is described as being similar to a sheet of blood. The oxygenated capillary blood is collected in the small pulmonary veins of the lobules, and then it moves to the larger veins to be collected in the four large pulmonary veins that empty into the left atrium. The term *perfusion* is used to describe the flow of blood through the pulmonary capillary bed.

The pulmonary blood vessels are thinner, more compliant, and offer less resistance to flow than those in the systemic circulation, and the pressures in the pulmonary system are much lower (*e.g.*, 22/8 mm Hg versus 120/70 mm Hg). The low pressure and low resistance of the pulmonary circulation accommodate the delivery of varying amounts of blood from the systemic circulation without producing signs and symptoms of congestion. The volume in the pulmonary circulation is approximately 500 mL, with approximately 100 mL of this volume located in the pulmonary capillary bed. When the output of the right ventricle and input of the left ventricle are equal, pulmonary blood flow remains constant. Small differences between input and output can result in large changes in pulmonary volume if the differences continue for many heartbeats. The movement of blood through the pulmonary capillary bed requires that the mean pulmonary arterial pressure be greater than the mean pulmonary venous pressure. Pulmonary venous pressure increases in left-sided heart failure, allowing blood to accumulate in the pulmonary capillary bed and cause pulmonary edema. Acute pulmonary edema is discussed in Chapter 26.

Distribution of Blood Flow and Body Position

As with ventilation, the distribution of pulmonary blood flow is affected by body position and gravity. In the upright position, the distance of the upper apices of the lung above the level of the heart may exceed the perfusion capabilities of the mean pulmonary arterial pressure (approximately 12 mm Hg); therefore, blood flow in the upper part of the lungs is less than that in the base or bottom part of the lungs (Fig. 27-20). In the supine position, the lungs and the heart are at the same level, and blood flow to the apices and base of the lungs becomes more uniform. In this position, blood flow to the posterior or dependent portions (*e.g.*, bottom of the lung when lying on the side) exceeds flow in the anterior or nondependent portions of the lungs. In persons with left-sided heart failure, congestion develops in the dependent portions of the lungs exposed to increased blood flow.

Hypoxia

The blood vessels in the pulmonary circulation undergo marked vasoconstriction when they are exposed to hypoxia. The precise mechanism for this response is unclear. When alveolar oxygen levels drop below 60 mm Hg, marked vasoconstriction may occur, and at very low oxygen levels, the local flow may be almost abolished. In regional hypoxia, as occurs with atelectasis, vasoconstriction is localized to a specific region of the lung. Vasoconstriction has the effect of directing blood flow away from the hypoxic regions of the lungs. When alveolar hypoxia no longer exists, blood flow is restored.

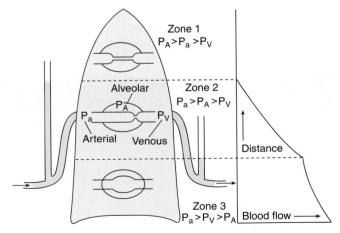

FIGURE 27-20 The uneven distribution of blood flow in the lung results from different pressures affecting the capillaries, which are affected by body position and gravity. (West J.B. [2000]. *Respiratory physiology: The essentials* [p. 29]. Philadelphia: Lippincott Williams & Wilkins)

Generalized hypoxia causes vasoconstriction throughout the lung. Generalized vasoconstriction occurs when the partial pressure of oxygen is decreased at high altitudes, or it can occur in persons with chronic hypoxia due to lung disease. Prolonged hypoxia can lead to pulmonary hypertension and increased workload on the right heart. A low blood pH also produces vasoconstriction, especially when alveolar hypoxia is present (*e.g.*, during circulatory shock).

DIFFUSION

There are two types of air movement in the lung: bulk flow and diffusion. Bulk flow occurs in the conducting airways and is controlled by pressure differences between the mouth and that of airways in the lung. Diffusion refers to the movement of gases in the alveoli and across the alveolar capillary membrane. Gas diffusion in the lung can be described by *Fick's law*. Fick's law states that the volume of a gas (Vgas) diffusing across the membrane per unit time is directly proportional to the partial pressure difference of the gas ($P_1 - P_2$), the surface area (SA) of the membrane, and the diffusion coefficient (D), and is inversely proportional to the thickness (T) of the membrane:

$$Vgas = \frac{(P_1 - P_2) \times SA \times D}{T}$$

Several factors influence diffusion of gases in the lung. The administration of high concentrations of oxygen increases the difference in partial pressure between the two sides of the membrane and increases the diffusion of the gas. Diseases that destroy lung tissue (*i.e.*, surface area for diffusion) or increase the thickness of the alveolar-capillary membrane adversely influence the diffusing capacity of the lungs. The removal of one lung, for example, reduces the diffusing capacity by one half. The thickness of the alveolar-capillary membrane and the distance for diffusion are increased in persons with pulmonary edema or pneumonia. The characteristics of the gas and its molecular weight and solubility constitute the diffusion coefficient and determine how rapidly the gas diffuses through the respiratory membranes. For example, carbon dioxide diffuses 20 times more rapidly than oxygen because of its greater solubility in the respiratory membranes. The factors that affect alveolar-capillary gas exchange are summarized in Table 27-3.

The diffusing capacity of the lung is a measure of the rate of transfer of gases through the alveolar-capillary membrane (measured in milliliters per minute). It is measured using a gas that readily diffuses across the membrane, is easily analyzed, and is affected by the same factors that influence oxygen diffusion. Carbon monoxide, which meets these criteria, commonly is used for this purpose. The test is done by having a person breathe a known concentration of carbon monoxide (usually for a 10-second breath hold). The volume of carbon monoxide that diffuses across the respiratory membranes is calculated from measurements of lung volume and changes in the carbon monoxide content of inspired and expired air. Because blood levels of carbon monoxide usually are zero, there is no "back diffusion" of the gas, and the difference between the inspired and the expired carbon monoxide reflects the diffusion of the gas. The diffusing capacity for oxygen can be calculated using the diffusing capacity of carbon monoxide and known information about the solubility of the two gases. Persons who smoke or are exposed to carbon monoxide may have appreciable amounts of the gas in their lungs, invalidating the test results. The diffusing capacity of the lung is affected by conditions that alter the permeability of the alveolar-capillary membrane and the ability of the red blood cells to bind and transport the gas.

MATCHING OF VENTILATION AND PERFUSION

The gas exchange properties of the lung depend on matching ventilation and perfusion, ensuring that equal amounts of air and blood are entering the respiratory portion of the lungs. Two factors may interfere with the matching of ventilation and perfusion: dead air space and shunt.

Dead Air Space

Not all inspired air reaches the alveoli. Dead space refers to the air that must be moved with each breath but does not participate in gas exchange. The movement of air through

---

TABLE 27-3 ◆ Factors Affecting Alveolar-Capillary Gas Exchange

Factors Affecting Gas Exchange	Examples
Surface area available for diffusion	Removal of a lung or diseases such as emphysema and chronic bronchitis, which destroy lung tissue or cause mismatching of ventilation and perfusion
Thickness of the alveolar-capillary membrane	Conditions such as pneumonia, interstitial lung disease, and pulmonary edema, which increase membrane thickness
Partial pressure of alveolar gases	Ascent to high altitudes where the partial pressure of oxygen is reduced. In the opposite direction, increasing the partial pressure of a gas in the inspired air (*e.g.*, oxygen therapy) increases the gradient for diffusion
Solubility and molecular weight of the gas	Carbon dioxide, which is more soluble in the cell membranes, diffuses across the alveolar-capillary membrane more rapidly than oxygen.

Matching of Ventilation and Perfusion

➤ Exchange of gases between the air in the alveoli and the blood in pulmonary capillaries requires a matching of ventilation and perfusion.

➤ Two factors interfere with matching of ventilation and perfusion: dead air space and shunt.

➤ Dead air space refers to air that is moved with each breath but is not ventilated. Anatomic dead space is that contained in the conducting airways that normally do not participate in gas exchange. Alveolar dead space results from alveoli that are ventilated but not perfused.

➤ Shunt refers to blood that moves from the right to the left side of the circulation without being oxygenated. With an anatomic shunt, blood moves from the venous to the arterial side of the circulation without going through the lungs. Physiologic shunting results from blood moving through unventilated parts of the lung.

➤ The blood oxygen level reflects the mixing of blood from alveolar dead space and physiologic shunting areas as it moves into the pulmonary veins.

logic shunt, there is mismatching of ventilation and perfusion, resulting in insufficient ventilation to provide the oxygen needed to oxygenate the blood flowing through the alveolar capillaries. In an *anatomic shunt*, blood moves from the venous to the arterial side of the circulation without moving through the lungs. Anatomic intracardiac shunting of blood due to congenital heart defects is discussed in Chapter 24. Physiologic shunting of blood usually results from destructive lung disease that impairs ventilation or from heart failure that interferes with movement of blood through sections of the lungs.

Mismatching of Ventilation and Perfusion

There are many causes of mismatched ventilation and perfusion, and the most obvious are shown in Figure 27-21. This figure depicts three groups of alveoli with low, normal, and high ventilation–perfusion ratios. The ventilation–perfusion ratio in the center alveoli is normal, resulting in normal gas exchange and oxygen concentrations. Perfusion without ventilation (left) results in a low ventilation–perfusion ratio. This is the type of situation that occurs in atelectasis (see Chapter 29). Ventilation without perfusion (right) results in a high ventilation–perfusion ratio. An example of this type of situation is pulmonary embolism, when a blood clot obstructs flow.

The arterial blood leaving the pulmonary circulation reflects mixing of the three alveolar-capillary units. Most of the situations in which ventilation and perfusion are mismatched are less obvious. In lung disease, for example, there may be altered ventilation in one area of the lung and altered perfusion in another area.

GAS TRANSPORT

The lungs enable inhaled air to come in contact with blood flowing through the pulmonary capillaries so that exchange of gases between the external environment and the internal environment of the body can take place. The lungs restore the oxygen content of the arterial blood and remove carbon dioxide from the venous blood.

The blood carries oxygen and carbon dioxide in the dissolved state and in combination with hemoglobin. Carbon dioxide also is converted to bicarbonate and transported in that form. The amount of a gas that can dissolve in plasma is determined by two factors: the solubility of the gas in the plasma and the partial pressure of the gas in the alveoli. Oxygen and carbon dioxide dissolve in plasma. The gases that are dissolved in plasma are similar to the carbon dioxide that is dissolved in a capped bottle of a carbonated drink. In the case of the carbonated drink, the gas is dissolved under increased pressure, which allows more gas to be dissolved. When the bottle cap is removed, the pressure is reduced, and less gas remains in the dissolved state. Tiny bubbles form as the gas moves from the dissolved to the gaseous state.

In the clinical setting, blood gas measurements are used to determine the level of the partial pressure of oxygen (PO_2) and carbon dioxide (PCO_2) in the blood. Arterial blood commonly is used for measuring blood gases. Venous blood is not used because venous levels of oxygen and carbon dioxide reflect the metabolic demands of the tissues rather than the gas exchange function of the lungs. The

dead space contributes to the work of breathing but not to gas exchange.

There are two types of dead space: that contained in the conducting airways, called the *anatomic dead space*, and that contained in the respiratory portion of the lung, called the *alveolar dead space*. The volume of anatomic airway dead space is fixed at approximately 150 to 200 mL, depending on body size. It constitutes air contained in the nose, pharynx, trachea, and bronchi. The creation of a tracheostomy decreases anatomic dead space ventilation because air does not have to move through the nasal and oral airways. Alveolar dead space, normally about 5 to 10 mL, constitutes alveolar air that does not participate in gas exchange. When alveoli are ventilated but deprived of blood flow, they do not contribute to gas exchange and thereby constitute alveolar dead space.

The *physiologic dead space* includes the anatomic dead space plus alveolar dead space. In persons with normal respiratory function, physiologic dead space is about the same as anatomic dead space. Only in lung disease does physiologic dead space increase. Alveolar ventilation is equal to the minute ventilation minus the physiologic dead space ventilation.

Shunt

Shunt refers to blood that moves from the right to the left side of the circulation without being oxygenated. There are two types of shunts: physiologic and anatomic. In a *physio-*

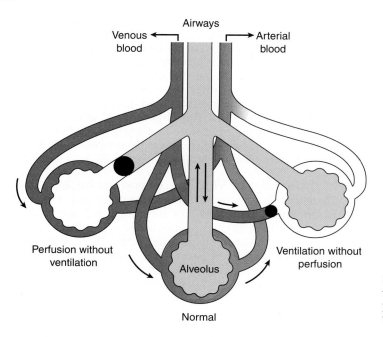

Airways

Venous blood

Arterial blood

Perfusion without ventilation

Ventilation without perfusion

Alveolus

Normal

FIGURE 27-21 Matching of ventilation and perfusion. (**Center**) Normal matching of ventilation and perfusion; (**left**) perfusion without ventilation (*i.e.,* shunt); (**right**) ventilation without perfusion (*i.e.,* dead air space).

PO$_2$ of arterial blood normally is above 80 mm Hg, and the PCO$_2$ is in the range of 35 to 45 mm Hg. Normally, the arterial blood gases are the same or nearly the same as the partial pressure of the gases in the alveoli. The arterial PO$_2$ often is written PaO$_2$, and the alveolar PO$_2$ as PAO$_2$, with the same types of designations being used for PCO$_2$. This text uses PO$_2$ and PCO$_2$ to designate both arterial and alveolar levels of the gases.

Oxygen Transport

Oxygen is transported in two forms: in chemical combination with hemoglobin and in the dissolved state. The hemoglobin in red blood cells serves as a transport vehicle for oxygen. It binds oxygen in the pulmonary capillaries and releases it in the tissue capillaries. As oxygen moves into or out of the red blood cells, it dissolves in the plasma. It is the dissolved form of oxygen that leaves the capillary, crosses cell membranes, and participates in cell metabolism. Only approximately 1% of the oxygen in the blood is carried in the dissolved state; the remainder is carried in combination with hemoglobin. The oxygen content of the blood (measured in milliliters per 100 milliliters of blood) includes the oxygen carried by hemoglobin and dissolved oxygen.

Dissolved Oxygen. The partial pressure of oxygen (PO$_2$) represents the level of dissolved oxygen in plasma. The amount of gas that can be dissolved in a liquid depends on the solubility of the gas and its pressure. The solubility of oxygen in plasma is fixed and very small. For every 1 mm Hg of PO$_2$ present in the alveoli, 0.003 mL of oxygen becomes dissolved in 100 mL of plasma. This means that at a normal alveolar PO$_2$ of 100 mm Hg, the blood carries only 0.3 mL of dissolved oxygen in each 100 mL of plasma. This amount is very small compared with the amount that can be carried in an equal amount of blood when oxygen is attached to hemoglobin.

Although the amount of oxygen carried in plasma under normal conditions is small, it can become a lifesaving mode of transport in carbon monoxide poisoning, when most of the hemoglobin sites are occupied by carbon monoxide and are unavailable for transport of oxygen. The use of a hyperbaric chamber, in which 100% oxygen can be administered at high atmospheric pressures, increases the amount of oxygen that can be carried in the dissolved state.

Hemoglobin Transport. Hemoglobin is a highly efficient carrier of oxygen, and approximately 98% to 99% of

 Oxygen Transport

➤ Oxygen is transported in chemical combination with hemoglobin and as a gas dissolved in the plasma.

➤ Hemoglobin, which is the main transporter for oxygen, binds oxygen as it passes through the lungs and releases it as it moves through the tissues.

➤ The amount of oxygen that is carried as a dissolved gas is determined by the partial pressure of the gas in the lungs.

➤ The oxygen content of the blood, or the amount of oxygen that is available to the tissues, represents the total amount of oxygen carried by the hemoglobin (hemoglobin concentration [g/dL] multiplied by its saturation) plus the amount of oxygen that is carried in the dissolved state.

the oxygen used by body tissues is carried in this manner. Hemoglobin with bound oxygen is called *oxyhemoglobin*, and when oxygen is removed, it is called *deoxygenated* or *reduced hemoglobin*. Each gram of hemoglobin carries approximately 1.34 mL of oxygen when it is fully saturated. This means that a person with a hemoglobin of 14 g/ 100 mL carries 18.8 mL of oxygen per 100 mL of blood. In the lungs, oxygen moves across the alveolar-capillary membrane, through the plasma, and into the red blood cell, where it forms a loose and reversible bond with the hemoglobin molecule. In normal lungs, this process is rapid, so that even with a fast heart rate, the hemoglobin is almost completely saturated with oxygen during the short time it spends in the pulmonary capillaries.

The oxygenated hemoglobin is transported in the arterial blood to the peripheral capillaries, where the oxygen is released and made available to the tissues for use in cell metabolism. As the oxygen moves out of the capillaries in response to the needs of the tissues, the hemoglobin saturation, which usually is approximately 95% to 97% as the blood leaves the left side of the heart, drops to approximately 75% as the mixed venous blood returns to the right side of the heart.

Oxygen-Hemoglobin Dissociation. Oxygen that remains bound to hemoglobin cannot participate in tissue metabolism. The efficiency of the oxygen dissociation transport system depends on the ability of the hemoglobin molecule to bind oxygen in the lungs and release it as it is needed in the tissues. The affinity of hemoglobin refers to its capacity to bind oxygen. Hemoglobin binds oxygen more readily when its affinity is increased and releases it more readily when its affinity is decreased. As described in Chapter 15, the hemoglobin molecule is composed of four polypeptide chains bound to an iron-containing heme group. Because oxygen binds to the iron atom, each hemoglobin molecule can bind four molecules of oxygen. Oxygen binds cooperatively with hemoglobin. After the first molecule of oxygen binds to hemoglobin, the molecule undergoes a change in shape. As a result, the second and third molecules bind more readily, and binding of the fourth molecule is even easier. When oxygen is bound to all four of the heme groups, the hemoglobin molecule is said to be fully *saturated*. Hemoglobin is partially saturated when it contains only one, two, or three molecules of oxygen. In a like manner, unloading of one oxygen molecule enhances the unloading of the next molecule, and so on. Thus, the affinity of hemoglobin for oxygen changes with oxygen saturation.

Hemoglobin's affinity for oxygen is influenced by pH, carbon dioxide concentration, and temperature. Hemoglobin binds oxygen more strongly under conditions of increased pH (alkalosis), decreased carbon dioxide concentration, and decreased body temperature, and releases it more readily under conditions of decreased pH (acidosis), increased carbon dioxide concentration, and fever. Conditions that decrease affinity and favor unloading of oxygen reflect the level of tissue metabolism and need for oxygen. For example, increased tissue metabolism generates carbon dioxide and metabolic acids and thereby decreases the affinity of hemoglobin for oxygen. Heat also is a byproduct of tissue metabolism, explaining the effect of fever on oxygen binding.

Red blood cells contain a metabolic intermediate called *2,3-diphosphoglycerate* (2,3-DPG) that also affects the affinity of hemoglobin for oxygen. An increase in 2,3-DPG enhances unloading of oxygen from hemoglobin at the tissue level. An increase in 2,3-DPG occurs with exercise and the hypoxia that occurs with high altitude and chronic lung disease.

The relation between the oxygen carried in combination with hemoglobin and the PO_2 of the blood is described by the *oxygen-hemoglobin dissociation curve*, which is shown in Figure 27-22. The x axis depicts the PO_2; the left y axis, hemoglobin saturation, and the right y axis, the oxygen content or total amount of oxygen in the blood, including the dissolved oxygen and that carried by the hemoglobin. There are three important things to observe about the relationships among PO_2, hemoglobin saturation, and oxygen content. First, PO_2 is the dissolved oxygen. It reflects the partial pressure of the gas in the lung (*i.e.*, the PO_2 is approximately 100 mm Hg when room air is being breathed, but can rise to 200 mm Hg or higher when oxygen-enriched air is breathed). Second, hemoglobin saturation reflects the amount of oxygen that is carried by the hemoglobin. Third, it is the oxygen content of the blood rather than the PO_2, or even hemoglobin saturation, that determines the amount of oxygen carried in the blood and delivered to the tissues. An anemic person may have a normal PO_2 and hemoglobin saturation level but decreased oxygen content because of the lower amount of hemoglobin for binding oxygen.

The "S"-shaped oxygen dissociation curve has a flat top portion representing binding of oxygen by the hemoglobin in the lungs and a steep portion representing its release into the tissue capillaries. The "S" shape of the curve reflects the effect that oxygen saturation has on the affinity of hemoglobin for oxygen. At approximately 100 mm Hg PO_2, a plateau occurs, at which point the hemoglobin is approximately 98% saturated. Increasing the alveolar PO_2 above this level does not increase the hemoglobin saturation. Even at high altitudes, when the partial pressure of oxygen is considerably decreased, the hemoglobin remains relatively well saturated. At 60 mm Hg PO_2, for example, the hemoglobin is still approximately 89% saturated.

The steep portion of the dissociation curve—between 60 and 40 mm Hg—represents the removal of oxygen from the hemoglobin as it moves through the tissue capillaries. This portion of the curve reflects the fact that there is considerable transfer of oxygen from hemoglobin to the tissues with only a small drop in PO_2, thereby ensuring a gradient for oxygen to move into body cells. The tissues normally remove approximately 5 mL of oxygen per 100 mL of blood, and the hemoglobin of mixed venous blood is approximately 75% saturated as it returns to the right side of the heart. In this portion of the dissociation curve (saturation <75%), the rate at which oxygen is released from hemoglobin is determined largely by tissue uptake. During strenuous exercise, for example, the muscle cells may remove as much as 15 mL of oxygen per 100 mL of blood from hemoglobin.

Hemoglobin can be regarded as an oxygen buffer system that regulates oxygen pressure in the tissues. Hemo-

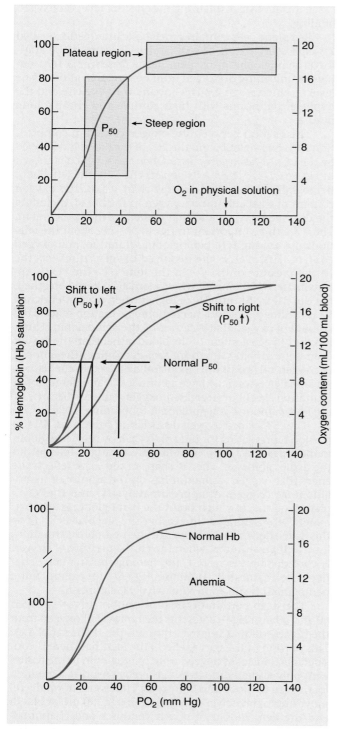

globin affinity for oxygen must change with the metabolic needs of the tissues. This change is represented by a shift to the right or left in the dissociation curve, as shown in Figure 27-22. A shift to the right indicates that the tissue PO_2 is greater for any given level of hemoglobin saturation and represents reduced affinity of the hemoglobin for oxygen at any given PO_2. It usually is caused by conditions such as fever or acidosis or by an increase in PCO_2, which reflects increased tissue metabolism. High altitude and conditions such as pulmonary insufficiency, heart failure, and severe anemia also cause the oxygen dissociation curve to shift to the right.

A shift to the left in the oxygen dissociation curve represents enhanced affinity of hemoglobin for oxygen and occurs in situations associated with a decrease in tissue metabolism, such as alkalosis, decreased body temperature, and decreased carbon dioxide levels. The degree of shift can be determined by the P_{50}, or the partial pressure of oxygen that is needed to achieve a 50% saturation of hemoglobin. Returning to Figure 27-22, the dissociation curve on the left has a P_{50} of approximately 20 mm Hg; the normal curve, a P_{50} of 26; and the curve on the right, a P_{50} of 39 mm Hg.

Carbon Dioxide Transport

Carbon dioxide is transported in the blood in three forms: as dissolved carbon dioxide (10%), attached to hemoglobin (30%), and as bicarbonate (60%). Acid-base balance is influenced by the amount of dissolved carbon dioxide and the bicarbonate level in the blood (see Chapter 32).

As carbon dioxide is formed during the metabolic process, it diffuses out of cells into the tissue spaces and then into the capillaries. The amount of dissolved carbon dioxide that can be carried in plasma is determined by the partial pressure of the gas and its solubility coefficient (0.03 mL/100 mL/1 mm Hg PCO_2). Carbon dioxide is 20 times more soluble in plasma than oxygen. Thus, the dissolved state plays a greater role in transport of carbon dioxide compared with oxygen.

Most of the carbon dioxide diffuses into the red blood cells, where it either forms carbonic acid or combines with hemoglobin. *Carbonic acid* (H_2CO_3) is formed when carbon dioxide combines with water ($CO_2 + H_2O = H^+ + HCO_3^-$). The process is expedited by an enzyme called *carbonic anhydrase*, which is present in large quantities in red blood cells. Carbonic anhydrase increases the rate of the reaction between carbon dioxide and water approximately 5000-fold. Carbonic acid readily ionizes to form a bicarbonate (HCO_3^-) and a hydrogen (H^+) ion. The hydrogen ion that is generated combines with the hemoglobin, which is a powerful acid-base buffer, and the bicarbonate ion diffuses into

FIGURE 27-22 Oxygen-hemoglobin dissociation curve. (**Top**) Left boxed area represents the steep portion of the curve where oxygen is released from hemoglobin (Hb) to the tissues, and the top boxed area the plateau of the curve where oxygen is loaded onto hemoglobin in the lung. P_{50} partial pressure of oxygen required to saturate 50% of hemoglobin with oxygen. (**Middle**) The effect of body temperature, arterial PCO_2, and pH on hemoglobin affinity for oxygen as indicated by a shift in the curve and position of the P_{50}. A shift of the curve to the right due to an increase in temperature, PCO_2, or decreased pH favors release of oxygen to the tissues. A decrease in temperature, PCO_2, or increase in pH shifts the curve to the left and has the opposite effect. (**Bottom**) Effect of anemia on the oxygen-carrying capacity of blood. The hemoglobin can be completely saturated, but the oxygen content of the blood is reduced. (**Top** and **bottom** adapted from Rhoades R.A., Tanner, G.A. [1996]. *Medical physiology*. Boston: Little, Brown)

plasma in exchange for a chloride ion. This exchange is made possible by a special bicarbonate-chloride carrier protein in the red blood cell membrane. As a result of the bicarbonate-chloride shift, the chloride and water content of the red blood cell is greater in venous blood than in arterial blood.

In addition to the carbonic anhydrase–mediated reaction with water, carbon dioxide reacts directly with hemoglobin to form *carbaminohemoglobin*. The combination of carbon dioxide with hemoglobin is a reversible reaction that involves a loose bond, which allows transport of carbon dioxide from tissues to the lungs, where it is released into the alveoli for exchange with the external environment. The release of oxygen from hemoglobin in the tissues enhances the binding of carbon dioxide to hemoglobin; in the lungs, the combining of oxygen with hemoglobin displaces carbon dioxide. The binding of carbon dioxide to hemoglobin is determined by the acidic nature of hemoglobin. Binding with carbon dioxide causes the hemoglobin to become a stronger acid. In the lungs, the highly acidic hemoglobin has a lesser tendency to form carbaminohemoglobin, and carbon dioxide is released from hemoglobin into the alveoli. In the tissues, the release of oxygen from hemoglobin causes hemoglobin to become less acid, thereby increasing its ability to combine with carbon dioxide and form carbaminohemoglobin.

In summary, the primary functions of the lungs are oxygenation of the blood and removal of carbon dioxide. Pulmonary gas exchange is conventionally divided into three processes: ventilation, or the flow of gases into the alveoli of the lungs; perfusion, or movement of blood through the adjacent pulmonary capillaries; and diffusion, or transfer of gases between the alveoli and the pulmonary capillaries.

Ventilation is the movement of air between the atmosphere and the lungs. Pulmonary ventilation refers to the total exchange of gases between the atmosphere and the lungs, and alveolar ventilation to ventilation in the gas exchange portion of the lungs. The distribution of alveolar ventilation and pulmonary capillary blood flow varies with lung volume and body position. In the upright position and at high lung volumes, ventilation is greatest in the lower parts of the lungs. The upright position also produces a decrease in blood flow to the upper parts of the lung, resulting from the distance above the level of the heart and the low mean arterial pressure in the pulmonary circulation.

The diffusion of gases in the lungs is influenced by four factors: the surface area available for diffusion; the thickness of the alveolar-capillary membrane, through which the gases diffuse; the differences in the partial pressure of the gas on either side of the membrane; and the characteristics of the gas. The efficiency of gas exchange requires matching of ventilation and perfusion, so that equal amounts of air and blood enter the respiratory portion of the lungs. Two factors—dead air space and shunt—interfere with matching of ventilation and perfusion and do not contribute to gas exchange. Dead air space occurs when areas of the lungs are ventilated but not perfused. Shunt is the condition under which areas of the lungs are perfused but not ventilated.

The blood transports oxygen to the cells and returns carbon dioxide to the lungs. Oxygen is transported in two forms: in chemical combination with hemoglobin and physically dissolved in plasma (PO_2). Hemoglobin is an efficient carrier of oxygen, and approximately 98% to 99% of oxygen is transported in this manner. Carbon dioxide is carried in three forms: carbaminohemoglobin (30%), dissolved carbon dioxide (10%), and bicarbonate (60%).

Control of Breathing

After you have completed this section of the chapter, you should be able to meet the following objectives:

- ✦ Compare the neural control of the respiratory muscles, which control breathing, with that of cardiac muscle, which controls the pumping action of the heart
- ✦ Describe the function of the chemoreceptors and lung receptors in the regulation of ventilation
- ✦ Trace the integration of the cough reflex from stimulus to explosive expulsion of air that constitutes the cough
- ✦ Describe the type of periodic breathing known as Cheyne-Stokes breathing
- ✦ Define dyspnea and list three types of conditions in which dyspnea occurs

Unlike the heart, which has inherent rhythmic properties and can beat independently of the nervous system, the muscles that control respiration require continuous input from the nervous system. Movement of the diaphragm, intercostal muscles, sternocleidomastoid, and other accessory muscles that control ventilation is integrated by neurons located in the pons and medulla. These neurons are collectively referred to as the *respiratory center* (Fig. 27-23).

RESPIRATORY CENTER

The respiratory center consists of two dense, bilateral aggregates of respiratory neurons involved in initiating inspiration and expiration and incorporating afferent impulses into motor responses of the respiratory muscles. The first, or dorsal, group of neurons in the respiratory center is concerned primarily with inspiration. These neurons control the activity of the phrenic nerves that innervate the diaphragm and drive the second, or ventral, group of respiratory neurons. They are thought to integrate sensory input from the lungs and airways into the ventilatory response. The second group of neurons, which contains inspiratory and expiratory neurons, controls the spinal motor neurons of the intercostal and abdominal muscles.

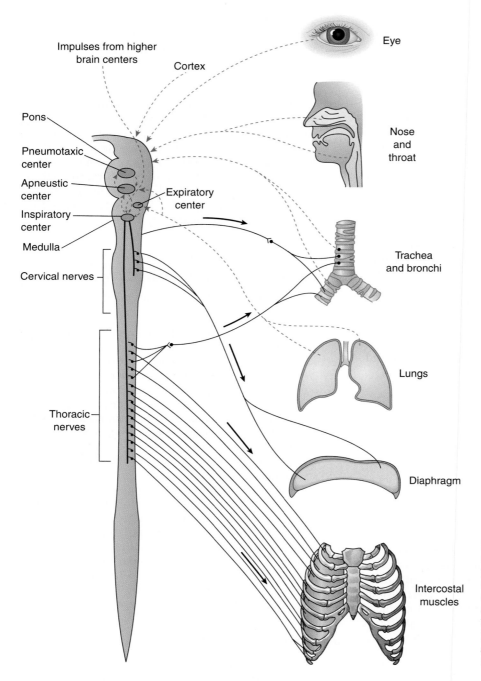

FIGURE 27-23 Schematic representation of activity in the respiratory center. Impulses traveling over afferent neurons activate central neurons, which activate efferent neurons that supply the muscles of respiration. Respiratory movements can be altered by a variety of stimuli. (Chaffee E.E., Lytle I.M. [1980]. *Basic physiology and anatomy* [4th ed.]. Philadelphia: J.B. Lippincott)

The pacemaker properties of the respiratory center result from the cycling of the two groups of respiratory neurons: the *pneumotaxic center* in the upper pons and the *apneustic center* in the lower pons. These two groups of neurons contribute to the function of the respiratory center in the medulla. The apneustic center has an excitatory effect on inspiration, tending to prolong inspiration. The pneumotaxic center switches inspiration off, assisting in the control of respiratory rate and inspiratory volume. Brain injury that damages the connection between the pneumotaxic and apneustic centers results in an irregular breathing pattern that

consists of prolonged inspiratory gasps interrupted by expiratory efforts.

Axons from the neurons in the respiratory center cross in the midline and descend in the ventrolateral columns of the spinal cord. The tracts that control expiration and inspiration are spatially separated in the cord, as are the tracts that transmit specialized reflexes (*i.e.,* coughing and hiccupping) and voluntary control of ventilation. Only at the level of the spinal cord are the respiratory impulses integrated to produce a reflex response. The neural control of ventilation is illustrated in Figure 27-23.

The control of breathing has automatic and voluntary components. The automatic regulation of ventilation is controlled by input from two types of sensors or receptors: chemoreceptors and lung receptors. Chemoreceptors monitor blood levels of oxygen, carbon dioxide, and pH and adjust ventilation to meet the changing metabolic needs of the body. Lung receptors monitor breathing patterns and lung function. Voluntary regulation of ventilation integrates breathing with voluntary acts such as speaking, blowing, and singing. These acts, initiated by the motor and premotor cortex, cause temporary suspension of automatic breathing. The automatic and voluntary components of respiration are regulated by afferent impulses that come to the respiratory center from a number of sources. Afferent input from higher brain centers is evidenced by the fact that a person can consciously alter the depth and rate of respiration. Fever, pain, and emotion exert their influence through lower brain centers. Vagal afferents from sensory receptors in the lungs and airways are integrated in the dorsal area of the respiratory center. It has been suggested that alterations in the control of automatic and voluntary regulation of breathing may contribute to various forms of sleep apnea (see Chapter 51).

CHEMORECEPTORS

Tissue needs for oxygen and the removal of carbon dioxide are regulated by chemoreceptors that monitor blood levels of these gases. Input from these sensors is transmitted to the respiratory center, and ventilation is adjusted to maintain the arterial blood gases within a normal range.

There are two types of chemoreceptors: central and peripheral. The most important chemoreceptors for sensing changes in blood carbon dioxide content are the *central chemoreceptors*. These receptors are located in chemosensitive regions near the respiratory center in the medulla and are bathed in cerebrospinal fluid. Although the central chemoreceptors monitor carbon dioxide levels, the actual stimulus for these receptors is provided by hydrogen ions in the cerebrospinal fluid. This fluid is separated from the blood by the blood-brain barrier, which permits free diffusion of carbon dioxide but not bicarbonate or hydrogen ions. The carbon dioxide combines rapidly with water to form carbonic acid, which dissociates into hydrogen and bicarbonate ions. The carbon dioxide content in the blood regulates ventilation through its effect on the pH of the extracellular fluid of the brain. The central chemoreceptors are extremely sensitive to short-term changes in carbon dioxide. The effect of an increase in plasma carbon dioxide levels on ventilation reaches its peak within a minute or so and then declines if the carbon dioxide level remains elevated. Long-term elevation of the carbon dioxide level prompts a compensatory increase in bicarbonate secretion into the cerebrospinal fluid, which acts as a buffer for the hydrogen ions. Thus, persons with chronically elevated levels of carbon dioxide no longer respond to this stimulus for increased ventilation but rely on the stimulus provided by a decrease in blood oxygen levels.

The *peripheral chemoreceptors* are located in the carotid and aortic bodies, which are found at the bifurcation of the common carotid arteries and in the arch of the aorta, respectively. These chemoreceptors monitor arterial blood oxygen levels. Although the peripheral chemoreceptors also monitor carbon dioxide, they play a much more important role in monitoring oxygen levels. These receptors exert little control over ventilation until the PO_2 has dropped below 60 mm Hg. Hypoxia is the main stimulus for ventilation in persons with chronic hypercapnia. If these patients are given oxygen therapy at a level sufficient to increase the PO_2 above that needed to stimulate the peripheral chemoreceptors, their ventilation may be seriously depressed.

LUNG RECEPTORS

Lung and chest wall receptors provide information on the status of breathing in terms of airway resistance and lung expansion. There are three types of lung receptors: stretch, irritant, and juxtacapillary receptors.

Stretch receptors are located in the smooth muscle layers of the conducting airways. They respond to changes in pressure in the walls of the airways. When the lungs are inflated, these receptors inhibit inspiration and promote expiration (*i.e., Hering-Breuer reflex*). They are important in establishing breathing patterns and minimizing the work of breathing by adjusting respiratory rate and TV to accommodate changes in lung compliance and airway resistance.

The *irritant receptors* are located between the airway epithelial cells. They are stimulated by noxious gases, cigarette smoke, inhaled dust, and cold air. Stimulation of the irritant receptors leads to airway constriction and a pattern of rapid, shallow breathing. This pattern of breathing probably protects respiratory tissues from the damaging effects of toxic inhalants. It also is thought that the mechanical stimulation of these receptors may ensure more uniform lung expansion by initiating periodic sighing and yawning. It is possible that these receptors are involved in the bronchoconstriction response that occurs in some persons with bronchial asthma.

The *juxtacapillary* or *J receptors* are located in the alveolar wall, close to the pulmonary capillaries. It is thought that these receptors sense lung congestion. These receptors may be responsible for the rapid, shallow breathing that occurs with pulmonary edema, pulmonary embolism, and pneumonia.

COUGH REFLEX

Coughing is a neurally mediated reflex that protects the lungs from accumulation of secretions and from entry of irritating and destructive substances. It is one of the primary defense mechanisms of the respiratory tract. The cough reflex is initiated by receptors located in the tracheobronchial wall; these receptors are extremely sensitive to irritating substances and to the presence of excess secretions. Afferent impulses from these receptors are transmitted through the vagus to the medullary center, which integrates the cough response.

Coughing itself requires the rapid inspiration of a large volume of air (usually about 2.5 L), followed by rapid closure of the glottis and forceful contraction of the abdominal and expiratory muscles. As these muscles contract, intrathoracic pressures are elevated to levels of 100 mm Hg or more. The rapid opening of the glottis at this point leads to an explosive expulsion of air.

Many conditions can interfere with the cough reflex and its protective function. The reflex is impaired in persons whose abdominal or respiratory muscles are weak. This problem can be caused by disease conditions that lead to muscle weakness or paralysis, by prolonged inactivity, or as an outcome of surgery involving these muscles. Bed rest interferes with expansion of the chest and limits the amount of air that can be taken into the lungs in preparation for coughing, making the cough weak and ineffective. Disease conditions that prevent effective closure of the glottis and laryngeal muscles interfere with production of the marked increase in intrathoracic pressure that is needed for effective coughing. The presence of a nasogastric tube, for example, may prevent closure of the upper airway structures and may fatigue the receptors for the cough reflex that are located in the area. The cough reflex also is impaired when there is depressed function of the medullary centers in the brain that integrate the cough reflex. Interruption of the central integration aspect of the cough reflex can arise as the result of disease of this part of the brain or the action of drugs that depress the cough center.

Although the cough reflex is a protective mechanism, frequent and prolonged coughing can be exhausting and painful and can exert undesirable effects on the cardiovascular and respiratory systems and on the elastic tissues of the lungs. This is particularly true in young children and elderly persons.

DYSPNEA

Dyspnea is a subjective sensation or a person's perception of difficulty in breathing that includes the perception of labored breathing and the reaction to that sensation. The terms *dyspnea*, *breathlessness*, and *shortness of breath* often are used interchangeably. Dyspnea is observed in at least three major cardiopulmonary disease states: primary lung diseases such as pneumonia, asthma, and emphysema; heart disease that is characterized by pulmonary congestion; and neuromuscular disorders such as myasthenia gravis and muscular dystrophy that affect the respiratory muscles. Although dyspnea commonly is associated with respiratory disease, it also occurs during exercise, particularly in untrained persons.

The cause of dyspnea is unknown. Four types of mechanisms have been proposed to explain the sensation: stimulation of lung receptors; increased sensitivity to changes in ventilation perceived through central nervous system mechanisms; reduced ventilatory capacity or breathing reserve; and stimulation of neural receptors in the muscle fibers of the intercostals and diaphragm and of receptors in the skeletal joints. The first of the suggested mechanisms is stimulation of lung receptors. These receptors are stimulated by the contraction of bronchial smooth muscle, the stretch of the bronchial wall, pulmonary congestion, and conditions that

decrease lung compliance. The second category of proposed mechanisms focuses on central nervous system mechanisms that transmit information to the cortex regarding respiratory muscle weakness or a discrepancy between the increased effort of breathing and inadequate respiratory muscle contraction. The third type of mechanism focuses on a reduction in ventilatory capacity or breathing reserve. A reduction in breathing reserve (*i.e.*, maximum voluntary ventilation not being used during a given activity) to less than 65% to 75% usually correlates well with dyspnea. The fourth possible mechanism is stimulation of muscle and joint receptors in the respiratory musculature because of a discrepancy in the tension generated by these muscles and the TV that results. These receptors, once stimulated, transmit signals that bring about an awareness of the breathing discrepancy. Like other subjective symptoms, such as fatigue and pain, dyspnea is difficult to quantify because it relies on a person's perception of the problem.

The most common method for measuring dyspnea is a retrospective determination of the level of daily activity at which a person experiences dyspnea. Several scales are available for this use. One of these uses four grades of dyspnea to evaluate disability. The visual analog scale may be used to assess breathing difficulty that occurs with a given activity, such as walking a certain distance. The visual analog scale consists of a line (often 10 cm in length) with descriptors such as "easy to breathe" on one end and "very difficult to breathe" on the other. The person being assessed selects a point on the scale that describes his or her perceived dyspnea. It also can be used to assess dyspnea over time.

The treatment of dyspnea depends on the cause. For example, persons with impaired respiratory function may require oxygen therapy, and those with pulmonary edema may require measures to improve heart function. Methods to decrease anxiety, breathing retraining, and energy conservation measures may be used to decrease the subjective sensation of dyspnea.

In summary, the respiratory system requires continuous input from the nervous system. Movement of the diaphragm, intercostal muscles, and other respiratory muscles is controlled by neurons of the respiratory center located in the pons and medulla. The control of breathing has automatic and voluntary components. The automatic regulation of ventilation is controlled by two types of receptors: lung receptors, which protect respiratory structures, and chemoreceptors, which monitor the gas exchange function of the lungs by sensing changes in blood levels of carbon dioxide, oxygen, and pH. There are three types of lung receptors: stretch receptors, which monitor lung inflation; irritant receptors, which protect against the damaging effects of toxic inhalants; and J receptors, which are thought to sense lung congestion. There are two groups of chemoreceptors: central and peripheral. The central chemoreceptors are the most important in sensing changes in carbon dioxide levels, and the peripheral chemoreceptors function in sensing arterial blood oxygen levels.

Breathing Patterns

The act of breathing normally is effortless and does not require conscious thought. In an adult, the normal rate of respiration is approximately 16 to 18 breaths per minute, with approximately 1 breath for every 4 heartbeats. The respiratory rate increases with exercise and other activities that raise the body's metabolism. In normal breathing, expiration is largely passive and accomplished within 4 to 6 seconds. Respiratory movements normally are smooth, with equal expansion of both sides of the chest. In men, respiratory movements are primarily diaphragmatic, but in women, there is greater movement of the intercostal muscles. When breathing becomes labored, the accessory muscles of the neck come into play, and the nostrils may flare.

The suffix *pnea* refers to breathing. *Tachypnea* is rapid breathing, and *hyperpnea* is an increase in the rate and the depth of respiration. Hyperpnea is normal during exercise. *Bradypnea* is an abnormally slow respiratory rate. *Hyperventilation* is ventilation in excess of that needed for normal elimination of carbon dioxide. It is associated with decreased partial pressure of carbon dioxide (PCO_2) in the arterial blood and respiratory alkalosis (see Chapter 32). *Hypoventilation* is ventilation that is inadequate for alveolar-capillary exchange of carbon dioxide and oxygen. Hypoventilation causes an increase in PCO_2 and respiratory acidosis and a decrease in the partial pressure of oxygen (PO_2) in the arterial blood.

Periodic breathing describes a pattern in which there are episodes of apnea, or absence of breathing. *Cheyne-Stokes breathing* is a type of periodic breathing characterized by periods of slowly waxing and waning respirations separated by a period of apnea that lasts as long as 30 seconds. Cheyne-Stokes breathing is thought to be caused by impaired function of the central feedback mechanisms that buffer the respiratory center's response to carbon dioxide. For Cheyne-Stokes respirations to occur, the hyperpneic and apneic phases of the breathing pattern must be long enough for sufficient changes in the carbon dioxide content of the blood to occur. During the hyperpneic phase of Cheyne-Stokes breathing, carbon dioxide levels falls, leading to a decreased stimulus for ventilation and, finally, to apnea. The period of apnea causes carbon dioxide to accumulate in the blood, and this leads to the hyperpneic phase of the respiratory pattern.

Two types of disease conditions predispose to Cheyne-Stokes breathing. One is congestive heart failure, in which there is a great delay in moving blood with its altered carbon dioxide content from the lungs to the chemoreceptors in the brain that control ventilation. The other is impaired function of the brain centers that regulate the feedback mechanisms that control respiration. An area of the brain stem controls the feedback gain of the respiratory center in response to changes in the carbon dioxide level. Cheyne-Stokes respirations may occur in patients who have brain lesions that affect this area. They also occur in healthy persons as an adaptive response to high altitudes, especially during sleep.

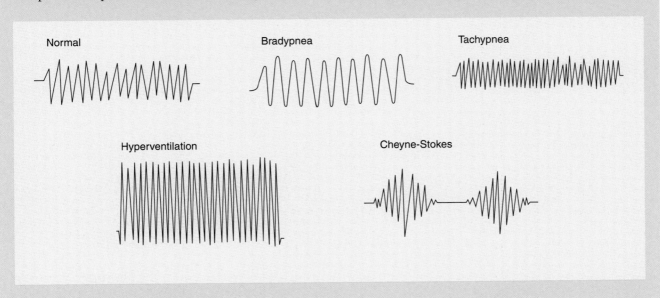

Voluntary respiratory control is needed for integrating breathing and actions such as speaking, blowing, and singing. These acts, which are initiated by the motor and premotor cortex, cause temporary suspension of automatic breathing. The cough reflex protects the lungs from the accumulation of secretions and from the entry of irritating and destructive substances; it is one of the primary defense mechanisms of the respiratory tract. Dyspnea is a subjective sensation of difficulty in breathing. Alterations in breathing patterns include tachypnea (rapid breathing), hyperpnea (increase in the rate and the depth of respiration), bradypnea (abnormally slow respiratory rate), hyperventilation (respiration in excess of that needed to maintain a normal level of PCO_2), and hypoventilation (inadequate ventilation).

Bibliography

Berne R.M., Levy M.N. (2000). *Principles of physiology* (3rd ed., pp. 302–352). St. Louis: C.V. Mosby.

Carrieri V.K., Jansen-Bjerklie S. (1984). The sensation of dyspnea: A critical review. *Heart and Lung* 13, 436–447.

Cormack D.H. (1987). *Ham's histology* (9th ed., pp. 541–563). Philadelphia: J.B. Lippincott.

Fishman A.P. (1980). *Assessment of pulmonary function*. New York: McGraw-Hill.

Guyton A., Hall J.E. (2000). *Textbook of medical physiology* (10th ed., pp. 432–482). Philadelphia: W.B. Saunders.

Reischman R.R. (1988). Review of ventilation and perfusion physiology. *Critical Care Nurse* 8 (7), 24–28.

Rhoades R.A., Tanner G.A. (1996). *Medical physiology* (pp. 341–414). Boston: Little, Brown.

West J.B. (2000). *Respiratory physiology: The essentials*. Philadelphia: Lippincott Williams & Wilkins.

Chapter 28

Alterations in Respiratory Function: Respiratory Tract Infections, Neoplasms, and Childhood Disorders

Respiratory illnesses represent one of the more common reasons for visits to the physician, admission to the hospital, and forced inactivity among all age groups. The common cold, although not usually serious, results in missed work and school days. Pneumonia is the sixth leading cause of death in the United States, particularly among the elderly and those with compromised immune function. Tuberculosis remains one of the deadliest diseases in the world. It has been estimated that between 19% and 43% of the world population is infected with tuberculosis. Although the rate of tuberculosis infection in the United States has declined slightly since its resurgence in the early 1990s, there remains a large number of people who are infected; without effective treatment for latent infection, new cases can be expected to emerge from within this group. Lung cancer remains the leading cause of cancer death in the United States.

Respiratory Tract Infections

After you have completed this section of the chapter, you should be able to meet the following objectives:

✦ Describe the transmission of the common cold from one person to another

✦ Explain why rest and drinking large amounts of liquids are helpful in treating influenza
✦ Describe the causes, manifestations, and treatment of acute and chronic sinusitis
✦ Differentiate among community-acquired pneumonia, hospital-acquired pneumonia, and pneumonia in immunocompromised persons in terms of pathogens, manifestations, and prognosis
✦ Differentiate between primary tuberculosis and reactivated tuberculosis on the basis of their pathophysiology
✦ State the mechanism for the transmission of fungal infections of the lung

Respiratory tract infections can involve the upper respiratory tract (*i.e.,* nose, oropharynx, and larynx), the lower respiratory tract (*i.e.,* lower airways and lungs), or the upper and lower airways. The discussion in this section of the chapter focuses on the common cold, influenza, pneumonia, tuberculosis, and fungal infections of the lung. Acute respiratory infections in children are discussed in the last section of the chapter.

The respiratory tract is susceptible to infectious processes caused by many different types of microorganisms.

For the most part, the signs and symptoms of respiratory tract infections depend on the function of the structure involved, the severity of the infectious process, and the person's age and general health status.

Viruses are the most frequent cause of respiratory tract infections. They can range from a self-limited cold to life-threatening pneumonia. Moreover, viral infections can damage bronchial epithelium, obstruct airways, and lead to secondary bacterial infections. Each viral species has its own pattern of respiratory tract involvement. The rhinoviruses grow best at 33°C to 35°C and remain strictly confined to the upper respiratory tract.[1] The influenza viruses can infect the upper and lower respiratory tracts. Measles and chickenpox viruses "pass through" the respiratory tract and do not cause respiratory symptoms until secondary viremic spread has occurred. Other microorganisms, such as bacteria (*e.g.,* pneumococci, staphylococci), mycobacteria (*e.g., Mycobacterium tuberculosis*), fungi (*e.g.,* histoplasmosis, coccidioidomycosis, blastomycosis), and opportunistic organisms (*e.g., Pneumocystis carinii*), also produce infections of the lung, many of which produce significant morbidity and mortality.

THE COMMON COLD

The common cold is a viral infection of the upper respiratory tract. It occurs more frequently than any other respiratory tract infection. Most adults have two to four colds per year; the average school child may have up to 10 per year.[2] The condition usually begins with a feeling of dryness and stuffiness affecting mainly the nasopharynx; it is accompanied by excessive production of nasal secretions and lacrimation, or tearing of the eyes. Usually, the secretions remain clear and watery. The mucous membranes of the upper respiratory tract become reddened, swollen, and bathed in secretions. Involvement of the pharynx and larynx causes sore throat and hoarseness. The affected person may experience headache and generalized malaise. In severe cases, there may be chills, fever, and exhaustion. The disease process is usually self-limited, lasting approximately 7 days.

Initially thought to be caused by either a single or group of "cold viruses," the common cold is now recognized to be associated with more than 200 viruses.[3,4] The most common of these are the rhinoviruses, parainfluenza viruses, respiratory syncytial virus, coronaviruses, and adenoviruses. The season of the year, age, and prior exposure are important factors in the type of virus causing the infection and the type of symptoms that occur. For example, outbreaks of colds due to rhinoviruses are most common in early fall and late spring; those due to respiratory syncytial virus peak in the winter and spring months; and infections due the adenoviruses and coronaviruses are more frequent during the winter and spring months. Infections resulting from respiratory syncytial virus and parainfluenza viruses are most common and severe in children younger than 3 years of age. Infections occur less frequently and with milder symptoms with increasing age. Parainfluenza viruses often produce lower respiratory symptoms with first infections, but less severe upper respiratory symptoms with reinfections. The rhinoviruses are the most common cause of colds in persons between 5 and 40 years of age. There are over 100 serotypes of rhinovirus. Although people acquire lifetime immunity to an individual serotype, it would take a long time to become immune to all serotypes.

The "cold viruses" are rapidly spread from person to person. Children are the major reservoir of cold viruses, often acquiring a new virus from another child in school or day care.[3] The first step in the spreading of the common cold is the shedding of viruses, the area of greatest potential being the nasal mucosa. The fingers are the greatest source of spread, and the nasal mucosa and conjunctival surface of the eyes are the most common portals of entry of the virus. The most highly contagious period is during the first 3 days after the onset of symptoms, and the incubation period is approximately 5 days. Cold viruses have been found to survive for more than 5 hours on the skin and hard surfaces, such as plastic countertops.[4,5] Aerosol spread of colds through coughing and sneezing is much less important than the spread by fingers picking up the virus from contaminated surfaces and carrying it to the nasal membranes and eyes.[4,5] This suggests that careful attention to hand washing is one of the most important preventive measures for avoiding the common cold. Host defenses also influence the development of the common cold. Psychological stress, which is thought to influence immune function, is reported to increase the risk for development of a cold.[6]

Many over-the-counter (OTC) remedies are available for treating the common cold. Because the common cold is an acute and self-limited illness in persons who are otherwise healthy, symptomatic treatment with rest and antipyretic drugs is usually all that is needed. Antibiotics are ineffective against viral infections and are not recommended. There is some controversy about the use of vitamin C to reduce the incidence and severity of colds and influenza. Some studies have found vitamin C intake to be beneficial and others have it to be of questionable value.[7] Zinc lozenges are also marketed as an OTC remedy for colds. As with vitamin C, some studies have shown the lozenges to be beneficial and others have not.[8, 9]

Antihistamines are popular OTC drugs because of their action in drying nasal secretions. However, they may dry up bronchial secretions and worsen the cough, and they may cause dizziness, drowsiness, and impaired judgment. As with vitamin C, there is no evidence that they shorten the duration of the cold. Decongestant drugs (*i.e.,* sympathomimetic agents) are available in OTC nasal sprays, drops, and oral cold medications. These drugs constrict the blood vessels in the swollen nasal mucosa and reduce nasal swelling. Rebound nasal swelling can occur with indiscriminate use of nasal drops and sprays. Oral preparations containing decongestants may cause systemic vasoconstriction and elevation of blood pressure when given in doses large enough to relieve nasal congestion, and they should be avoided by persons with hypertension, heart disease, hyperthyroidism, diabetes mellitus, or other health problems.

Efforts to develop vaccines against the cold viruses have been largely unsuccessful, mainly because of number of viruses involved and their large array of serotypes. Recently, investigators have isolated a receptor (intracellular adhesion molecule-1) on the respiratory epithelial cells that is the site of attachment for most of the rhinovirus serotypes. Identification of this receptor molecule provides a target for development of pharmacologic interventions. A recombinant, soluble form of a glycoprotein, known as *tremacamra*, has been developed to inhibit adhesion of the rhinovirus to the receptor and thus reduce the severity of infection in exposed persons.[10]

RHINITIS AND SINUSITIS

Rhinitis refers to inflammation of the nasal mucosa and sinusitis to inflammation of the paranasal sinuses. The paranasal sinuses are air cells that are connected by narrow openings or *ostia* with the superior, middle, and inferior nasal turbinates of the nasal cavity (Fig. 28-1). Each sinus is named for the bone in which it occurs—frontal, ethmoid, sphenoid, and maxillary. The *maxillary sinus* is inferior to the bony orbit and superior to the hard palate, and its opening is located superiorly and medially in the sinus, a location that impedes drainage. The *frontal sinuses* open into the middle meatus of the nasal cavity. The *sphenoid sinus* is just anterior to the pituitary fossa behind the posterior ethmoid sinuses, and its paired openings drain into the sphenoethmoidal recess at the top of the nasal cavity. The *ethmoid sinuses* comprise 3 to 15 air cells on each side, with each maintaining a separate path to the nasal chamber.

The sinus mucosa is similar to that of the respiratory tract and nasal passages. Ciliated mucous membranes help move fluid and microorganisms out of the sinuses and into the nasal cavity. Nasal swelling that obstructs the sinus openings and impairs mucociliary function is thought to be a major cause of sinus infections. The lower oxygen content in the sinuses facilitates the growth of organisms, impairs local defenses, and alters the function of immune cells.

The most common causes of sinusitis are conditions that obstruct the narrow ostia that drain the sinuses. Most commonly, sinusitis develops when upper respiratory tract infection or allergic rhinitis narrows the ostia and obstructs flow of mucus. Nasal polyps also can obstruct the sinus opening and facilitate sinus infection. Infections associated with nasal polyps can be self-perpetuating because constant irritation from infection can facilitate growth of the polyps. Barotrauma caused by changes in barometric pressure, as occurs in airline pilots and flight attendants, may lead to impaired sinus ventilation and clearance of secretions. Swimming, diving, and abuse of nasal decongestants are other causes of sinus irritation and impaired drainage. In approximately 10% of cases of maxillary sinusitis, the cause is a contiguous dental infection.

The paranasal sinuses normally are sterile. In adults, acute sinusitis most commonly results from infection with *Haemophilus influenza* or *Streptococcus pneumoniae*.[11,12] In chronic sinusitis, anaerobic organisms, including species of *Peptostreptococcus*, *Fusobacterium*, and *Prevotella*, tend to predominate, alone or in combination with aerobes such as the *Streptococcus* species or *Staphylococcus aureus*. In immunocompromised persons, such as those with human immunodeficiency virus (HIV) infection, the sinuses may become infected with gram-negative species and opportunistic fungi. In this group, particularly those with leukopenia, the disease may have a fulminant and even fatal course.

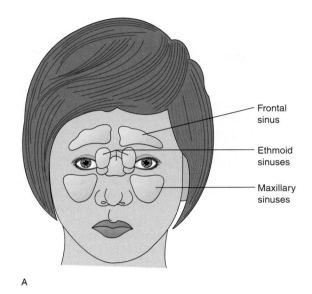

A

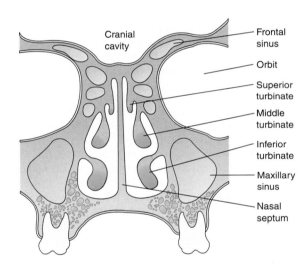

B

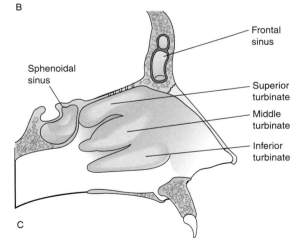

C

FIGURE 28-1 Paranasal sinuses. (**A**) Frontal view; (**B**) cross-section of nasal cavity, anterior view; (**C**) lateral wall, left nasal cavity. (Courtesy of Carole Russell Hilmer, C.M.I.)

Hospital-acquired sinusitis is more often caused by different microbial agents than community-acquired sinusitis. In the hospital, *S. aureus, Pseudomonas* species, *Klebsiella* species, and other gram-negative organisms predominate. Approximately 35% to 45% of hospital-acquired infections are polymicrobial.[12] Predisposing factors include irritation from endotracheal tubes, nasogastric tubes, and nasal packing, and the use of corticosteroids and other immunosuppressant drugs.

Acute and Chronic Sinusitis

Sinusitis can be classified as acute, subacute, or chronic. Acute suppurative sinusitis is any bacterial infection of the paranasal sinuses that lasts from 1 day to 3 weeks. Subacute sinusitis lasts from 3 weeks to 3 months. Chronic sinusitis lasts beyond 3 months.[12] Persons with chronic sinusitis may have superimposed bouts of acute sinusitis. The epithelial changes that occur during acute and subacute forms of sinusitis usually are reversible, but the mucosal changes that occur with chronic sinusitis often are irreversible.

The symptoms of acute sinusitis often are difficult to differentiate from those of the common cold and allergic rhinitis. They include facial pain, headache, purulent nasal discharge, decreased sense of smell, and fever. A history of a preceding common cold and the presence of purulent rhinitis, pain on bending, unilateral maxillary pain, and pain in the teeth are common findings in maxillary sinusitis.

In persons with chronic sinusitis, the only symptoms may be those such as nasal obstruction, a sense of fullness in the ears, postnasal drip, hoarseness, chronic cough, loss of taste and smell, or unpleasant breath.[13,14] Sinus pain often is absent; instead, the person may complain of a headache that is dull and constant. Persons who are immunocompromised, such as those with leukemia, aplastic anemia, a bone marrow transplant, primary immunodeficiency disease, or HIV infection, often present with fever of unknown origin, rhinorrhea, or facial edema. Often, other signs of inflammation such as purulent drainage are absent.

Diagnosis and Treatment. The diagnosis of sinusitis usually is based on symptom history and a physical examination that includes inspection of the nose and throat. Headache due to sinusitis needs to be differentiated from other types of headache. Sinusitis headache usually is exaggerated by bending forward, coughing, or sneezing. Transillumination may be used for detecting fluid in the maxillary or frontal sinus. It is done in a dark room and with a light source such as a light attached to an otoscope. Sinus radiographs and computed tomography (CT) scans may be used. CT scans usually are reserved for diagnosis of chronic sinusitis or to exclude complications. Diagnostic nasal endoscopy, which is done in the office of an otolaryngologist, provides a clear view of the anterior nasal cavity and sinus openings.[12] Magnetic resonance imagining (MRI) is expensive and reserved for cases of suspected neoplasms or intracranial lesions.[14]

Treatment of sinusitis includes appropriate antibiotic therapy, depending on whether the infection is community acquired or hospital acquired, or occurs in an immunocompromised person. The duration of antibiotic therapy is longer for chronic sinusitis than for acute sinusitis. In addition to antibiotic therapy, the treatment of acute sinusitis includes measures to promote adequate drainage by reducing nasal congestion. Oral and topical decongestants and antihistamines may be used for this purpose. Oral decongestants constrict nasal blood vessels, decrease tissue congestion, and facilitate drainage. The use of intranasal decongestants should be limited to 3 to 7 days to prevent rebound vasodilatation.[11] The use of antihistamines is controversial, particularly for acute sinusitis, because they can dry up secretions and thereby decrease drainage. Expectorants such as guaifenesin may be used to thin secretions. Topical corticosteroids may be used to decrease inflammation in persons with allergic rhinitis or sinusitis. Nonpharmacologic measures include saline nasal sprays and steam inhalations.

Surgical intervention directed at correcting obstruction of the ostiomeatal openings may be indicated in persons with chronic sinusitis that is resistant to other forms of therapy. Indications for surgical intervention include obstructive nasal polyps and obstructive nasal deformities.

Complications. Because of the sinuses' proximity to the brain and orbital wall, sinusitis can lead to intracranial and orbital wall complications. Intracranial complications are seen most commonly with infection of the frontal and ethmoid sinuses because of their proximity to the dura and drainage of the veins from the frontal sinus into the dural sinus. Sinusitis is the primary source of infection in as many as two thirds of intracranial abscesses and 5% of community-acquired cases of meningitis.[12] Orbital complications can range from edema of the eyelids to orbital cellulitis and subperiosteal abscess formation. Orbital involvement can result in exophthalmos, edema of the ocular conjunctiva, and visual impairment. Involvement of nerves supplying the extraocular muscles can lead to ophthalmoplegia. In persons with ethmoid sinusitis, infection can extend to the nasolacrimal gland, causing obstruction and tearing.

Allergic Rhinoconjunctivitis

Allergic sinusitis occurs in conjunction with allergic rhinitis. The mucosal changes are the same as those seen in allergic rhinitis. Symptoms usually consist of nasal stuffiness, itching and burning of the nose, frequent bouts of sneezing, recurrent frontal headache, and a watery nasal discharge. Headache located in the frontal area between the eyes is a common symptom. Allergic rhinitis can lead to nasal polyp formation, and similar polypoid lesions commonly are seen in persons with allergic sinusitis. Treatment include oral antihistamines, nasal decongestants, and intranasal cromolyn. Persistent symptoms may be treated with nasal corticosteroids and severe symptoms with oral corticosteroids.[15]

INFLUENZA

Influenza is a viral infection that can affect the upper and lower respiratory tracts. It usually occurs in epidemics or pandemics. Until the advent of acquired immunodeficiency syndrome (AIDS), it was the last uncontrolled pandemic killer of humans. More persons died in the 1918 and 1919 influenza pandemic than in World War I. In the United States, approximately 20,000 persons die each year of influenza-related illness during nonpandemic years.[16] Most deaths are caused by pneumonia or exacerbation of cardio-pulmonary or other conditions; 80% to 90% of those who die are 65 years of age or older.

There are two types of influenza viruses that cause epidemics in humans: types A and B. Infection with type A is most common and causes the most severe disease. Influenza A is further divided into subtypes based on two surface antigens: hemagglutinin (H) and neuraminidase (N). Influenza B has not been categorized into subtypes. Host antibodies to the surface antigens, which provide entrance in host cells, prevent future infection with influenza virus. New variants result from frequent mutations or antigenic shifts in the surface antigens.[16] Influenza B undergoes less frequent shifts than influenza A. The incubation period for influenza is 1 to 4 days with 2 days being the average. Persons become infectious starting 1 day before their symptoms begin and remain infectious through approximately 5 days after illness onset. Children can be infectious for a longer time.

The influenza viruses can cause three types of infections: an uncomplicated rhinotracheitis, a respiratory viral infection followed by a bacterial infection, and viral pneumonia. In the early stages, the symptoms of influenza often are indistinguishable from other viral infections. There is an abrupt onset of fever and chills, malaise, muscle aching, headache, profuse, watery nasal discharge, nonproductive cough, and sore throat. One distinguishing feature of an influenza viral infection is the rapid onset, sometimes in as little as 1 to 2 minutes, of profound malaise.[17] The infection causes necrosis and shedding of the serous and ciliated cells that line the respiratory tract, leaving gaping holes between the underlying basal cells and allowing extracellular fluid to escape. This is the reason for the "runny nose" that is characteristic of this phase of the infection. During recovery, the serous cells are replaced more rapidly than the ciliated cells. Mucus is produced, but the ciliated cells are unable to move it adequately; people recovering from influenza must continue to blow their nose to clear the sinuses and cough to clear the trachea.

The symptoms of uncomplicated rhinotracheitis usually peak by days 3 to 5 and disappear by days 7 to 10. Persons who have secondary complications usually report that they were beginning to feel better when they experienced a return of symptoms. Complications typically include sinusitis, otitis media, bronchitis, and bacterial pneumonia. The clinical course of influenza pneumonia progresses rapidly. It can cause hypoxemia and death within a few days of onset. The rapid onset is thought to be related to the mode of spread and the absence of an initial rhinotracheitis. If the virus is spread by fingers or large-droplet spray, as from sneezing or coughing, only the upper respiratory tract is involved. Infection of the upper respiratory tract is thought to give the immune system enough time to build the defenses needed to protect against viral pneumonia. When the virus is contained in small droplets, it can bypass the upper respiratory tract and travel directly into the lungs to establish infection.[17]

Diagnosis and Treatment

The goals of treatment for influenza are designed to limit the infection to the upper respiratory tract. The symptomatic approach, which uses rest, keeping warm, and drinking large amounts of liquids, helps to accomplish this. Rest decreases the oxygen requirements of the body and reduces the respiratory rate and the chance of spreading the virus from the upper to lower respiratory tract. Keeping warm helps maintain the respiratory epithelium at a core body temperature of 37°C (or higher if fever is present), thereby inhibiting viral replication, which is optimal at 35°C. Drinking large amounts of liquids ensures that the function of the epithelial lining of the respiratory tract is not further compromised by dehydration.

The appropriate pharmacologic treatment of people with influenza depends on accurate and timely diagnosis. The early diagnosis can reduce the inappropriate use of antibiotics and provide the opportunity for use of an antiviral drug. Rapid antigen detection tests are available to confirm a diagnosis of influenza A or B infection. These tests allow health care providers to monitor influenza type and its prevalence in their community, to diagnose influenza more accurately, and to consider treatment options more carefully.[18]

Antiviral Drugs. Four antiviral drugs are available for treatment of influenza: amantadine (Symmetrel), rimantadine (Flumadine), zanamivir (Relenza), and oseltamivir (Tamiflu).[18-20] The first-generation antiviral drugs amantadine and rimantadine are similarly effective against influenza A but not influenza B. These agents inhibit the uncoating of viral RNA in the host cells and prevent its replication. Both drugs are effective in prevention of influenza A in high-risk groups and in treatment of persons who acquire the disease. Unfortunately, resistance to the drugs develops rapidly and strains that are resistant to amantadine also are resistant to rimantadine. Amantadine stimulates release of catecholamines, which can produce central nervous system side effects such as anxiety, depression, and insomnia.

The second-generation antiviral drugs zanamivir and oseltamivir are inhibitors of neuraminidase, a viral glycoprotein that is necessary for viral replication and release. These drugs, which have been approved for treatment of acute uncomplicated influenza infection, are effective against both influenza A and B viruses. Zanamivir and oseltamivir result in less resistance than amantadine and rimantadine. Zanamivir is administered intranasally and oseltamivir is administered orally. Zanamivir can cause bronchospasm and is not recommended for persons with asthma or chronic obstructive lung disease. To be effective, the antiviral drugs should be initiated within 30 hours after onset of symptoms.

Influenza Immunization

Vaccines are available to protect against influenza infections. Immunization is recommended for high-risk groups who, because of their age or underlying health problems, are unable to cope well with the infection and often require medical attention, including hospitalization. The effectiveness of the influenza vaccine in preventing and lessening the effects of influenza infection depend primarily on the age and immunocompetence of the recipient and the match between the virus strains included in the vaccine and those that circulate during the influenza season.[17] When there is a good match, the vaccine is effective in preventing the illness in approximately 70% to 90% of healthy persons younger than 65 years of age.[17] Under similar circumstances, the vaccine is able to decrease the rate of hospitalization for pneumonia and influenza in elderly persons living in settings other than nursing homes by 30% to 70%.

Several strains of the influenza virus are responsible for epidemics of the disease. These strains undergo small changes over time that affect their antigenicity and the host protection afforded by previous immunization. Influenza's impact normally is greatest when new strains appear against which the population lacks immunity. The formulation of the influenza vaccine must be changed yearly in response to changes in the influenza virus. The Centers for Disease Control and Prevention (CDC) Advisory Committee on Immunization Practices (ACIP) annually updates its recommendations for the composition of the vaccine.

The ACIP recommends annual immunization using inactivated influenza vaccine to prevent or minimize the effect of influenza infections in any person 6 months of age or older who is at high risk for complications of influenza.[17] Groups at highest risk for complications include persons 50 years of age or older; residents of nursing homes or other chronic care facilities housing persons of any age with chronic medical conditions; adults or children with chronic disorders of the pulmonary or cardiovascular systems, including children with asthma; adults and children who have required regular medical follow-up or hospitalization during the preceding year because of chronic metabolic diseases (*e.g.,* diabetes mellitus), renal dysfunction, hemoglobinopathies (*e.g.,* sickle cell anemia), or immunosuppression (including immunosuppression caused by medications or by HIV infection); children or teenagers (6 months to 18 years) who are receiving long-term aspirin therapy (because of the risk of development of Reye's syndrome); and women who will be in the second or third trimester of pregnancy during the influenza season. Because the influenza vaccine is an inactivated vaccine, it is thought to be safe during pregnancy.[17] Immunization also is recommended for groups (*e.g.,* household members, health care workers) who live with or care for persons who are at high risk for development of influenza complications. It is believed that the protection of persons in the high-risk groups can be improved by reducing the chances of exposure to influenza from household contacts and health care providers. Vaccination is contraindicated for persons who have a history of anaphylactic hypersensitivity to egg or other components of the vaccine.

PNEUMONIAS

The term *pneumonia* describes inflammation of parenchymal structures of the lung, such as the alveoli and the bronchioles. An estimated 4 million cases occur annually in the United States, for a rate of 12 cases per 1000 persons per year.[21,22] Pneumonia is the sixth leading cause of death in the United States and the most common cause of death from infectious disease. Etiologic agents include infectious and noninfectious agents. Although much less common than infectious pneumonia, inhalation of irritating fumes or aspiration of gastric contents can result in severe pneumonia.

Although antibiotics have significantly reduced the mortality rate from pneumonias, these diseases remain an important immediate cause of death of the elderly and persons with debilitating diseases. There have been subtle changes in the spectrum of microorganisms that cause infectious pneumonias, including a decrease in pneumonias caused by *S. pneumoniae* and an increase in pneumonias caused by other microorganisms such as *Pseudomonas, Candida* and other fungi, and nonspecific viruses. Many of these pneumonias occur in persons with impaired immune defenses, including persons who are on immunosuppressant drugs to prevent rejection of a bone marrow or organ transplant. *P. carinii* pneumonia, a virulent type of infection, is associated with AIDS.

Pathogenesis

Bacteria commonly enter the lower airways but do not normally cause pneumonia because of extensive defense mechanisms. When pneumonia does occur, it usually is because of an exceedingly virulent organism, large inoculum, or impaired host defenses. In nonhospitalized persons, bacteria reach the lung by one of four routes: inhalation from the ambient air, aspiration from the previously colonized upper airway, direct spread from contiguous infected sites, or hematogenous spread. Critically ill patients may acquire organisms from colonized nasogastric tubes or from an endotracheal tube.

Pneumonias

➤ Pneumonias are respiratory disorders involving inflammation of the lung structures, such as the alveoli and bronchioles.

➤ Pneumonia can be caused by infectious agents such as bacteria and viruses and noninfectious agents such as gastric secretions that are aspirated into the lungs.

➤ The development of pneumonia is facilitated by an exceedingly virulent organism, large inoculum, and impaired host defenses.

➤ Pneumonias due to infectious agents commonly are classified according to the source of infection (community- vs. hospital-acquired) and according to the immune status of the host (pneumonia in the immunocompromised person).

Most of the agents that cause pneumonia and lower respiratory tract infections are aspirated from the tracheobronchial tree or inhaled into the lung along with the air breathed. Most persons unknowingly aspirate small amounts of organisms that have colonized their upper airways, particularly during sleep. Normally, these organisms do not cause infection because of the small numbers that are aspirated and because of the respiratory tract's defense mechanisms (Table 28-1). After bacteria reach the lower airways, they encounter a number of host defenses that prevent them from entering the lung and causing pneumonia. Loss of the cough reflex, damage to the ciliated endothelium that lines the respiratory tract, or impaired immune defenses predispose to colonization and infection of the lower respiratory system. Immune defenses include the bronchial-associated lymphoid tissue, phagocytic cells (*i.e.,* polymorphonuclear cells and macrophages), immunoglobulins (*i.e.,* IgA and IgG), and T-cell–mediated cellular immunity (see Chapter 18). Bacterial adherence also plays a role in colonization of the lower airways. The epithelial cells of critically and chronically ill persons are more receptive to binding microorganisms that cause pneumonia. Other clinical risk factors favoring colonization of the tracheobronchial tree include antibiotic therapy that alters the normal bacterial flora, diabetes, smoking, chronic bronchitis, and viral infection.

Until recently, pneumonias have been classified as typical (*i.e.,* bacterial) or atypical (*i.e.,* viral or mycoplasmal) pneumonias. Bacterial pneumonia results from infection by bacteria that multiply extracellularly in the alveoli and cause inflammation and exudation of fluid into the air-filled spaces of the alveoli (Fig. 28-2). They are characterized by chills and fever, severe malaise, purulent sputum, elevated white blood cell counts, and patchy or lobar infiltrates seen on the chest radiograph. Atypical pneumonias produce patchy inflammatory changes that are confined to the alveolar septum and the interstitium of the lung (see Fig. 28-2). They produce less striking symptoms and physical findings than bacterial pneumonia; there is a lack of alveolar infiltration and purulent sputum, leukocytosis, and lobar consolidation on the radiograph.

Because of the overlap in symptomatology and changing spectrum of infectious organisms involved, pneumonias are increasingly being classified as community-acquired and hospital-acquired pneumonias. Persons with compromised immune function constitute a special concern in both categories.

Community-Acquired Pneumonia

The term *community-acquired pneumonia* is used to describe infections from organisms found in the community rather than in the hospital or nursing home. It is defined as an infection that begins outside the hospital or is diagnosed within 48 hours after admission to the hospital in a person who has not resided in a long-term care facility for 14 days or more before admission.[21]

The most common cause of infection in all categories is *S. pneumoniae.*[21–23] Other common pathogens include *Haemophilus influenzae, S. aureus,* and gram-negative bacilli. Less common agents are *Moraxella catarrhalis, Klebsiella pneumoniae,* and *Neisseria meningitidis. Legionella* species, *Mycoplasma pneumoniae,* and *Chlamydia pneumoniae* (strain TWAR), sometimes called *atypical agents,* account for 10% to 20% of all cases of pneumonia. Common viral causes of community-acquired pneumonia include the influenza virus, respiratory syncytial virus, adenovirus, and parainfluenza virus.

There are several different systems for classifying community-acquired pneumonia based on factors such as age, preexisting health care status, and severity of illness. Guidelines developed by the American Thoracic Society divide persons with community-acquired pneumonia into four categories based on severity of illness, presence of coexisting disease and age, and need for hospitalization.[24] The categories are (1) persons younger than 60 years of age, who are without comorbidity and who can be treated on an outpatient basis; (2) persons with comorbidity who are 60 years of age and older and who can be treated on an outpatient

TABLE 28-1 ✦ Respiratory Defense Mechanisms and Conditions That Impair Their Effectiveness		
Defense Mechanism	**Function**	**Factors That Impair Effectiveness**
Nasopharyngeal defenses	Remove particles from the air; contact with surface lysosomes and immunoglobulins (IgA) protects against infection	IgA deficiency state, hay fever, common cold, trauma to the nose, others
Glottic and cough reflexes	Protect against aspiration into tracheobronchial tree	Loss of cough reflex due to stroke or neural lesion, neuromuscular disease, abdominal or chest surgery, depression of the cough reflex due to sedation or anesthesia, presence of a nasogastric tube (tends to cause adaptation of afferent receptors)
Mucociliary blanket	Removes secretions, microorganisms, and particles from the respiratory tract	Smoking, viral diseases, chilling, inhalation of irritating gases
Pulmonary macrophages	Remove microorganisms and foreign particles from the lung	Chilling, alcohol intoxication, smoking, anoxia

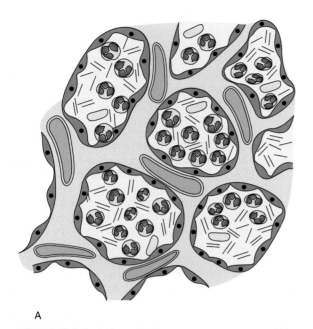

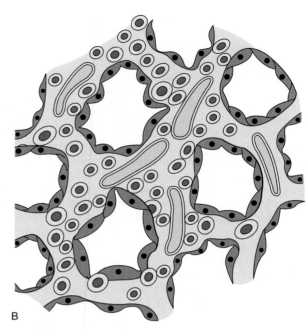

A B

FIGURE 28-2 Location of inflammatory processes in (**A**) typical and (**B**) atypical forms of pneumonia.

basis; (3) persons with community-acquired pneumonia who require hospitalization but not admission to the intensive care unit; and (4) persons with community-acquired pneumonia who require admission to the intensive care unit. The infecting organisms can remain confined to the lungs, as in persons in category 1, or they can cause bacteremia and sepsis. The mortality rate for persons in the first category is low (1% to 2%) compared with category 4, severe community-acquired pneumonia, which requires admission to the intensive care unit and for which the mortality rate can be as high as 50%.

The signs and symptoms of pneumonia vary from fever, general malaise, chest discomfort, and a cough to those of respiratory compromise with a respiratory rate above 30 breaths per minute, signs of hemoglobin desaturation and respiratory failure, and evidence of sepsis or shock (see Chapter 26).

The type and extent of tests used in diagnosis depend on the severity of illness. In persons younger than 65 years of age and without coexisting disease, the diagnosis usually is based on history and physical examination, chest radiographs, and knowledge of the microorganisms currently causing infections in the community. Sputum specimens may be obtained for staining procedures and culture. Blood cultures may be done for persons requiring hospitalization. Diagnostic measures may include procedures such as fiberoptic bronchoscopy, which is done to obtain samples of lower respiratory tract secretions for identifying the pathogen, particularly in severely ill persons and those who are unresponsive to antimicrobial therapy. Thoracentesis may be used to obtain specimens of pleural fluid when the infection extends into the pleural cavity.

Treatment involves the use of appropriate antibiotic therapy. Empiric therapy, based on knowledge regarding an antibiotic's spectrum of action and ability to penetrate bronchopulmonary secretions, often is used for persons with community-acquired pneumonia who do not require hospitalization. Hospitalization and more intensive care may be required depending on the person's age, preexisting health status, and severity of the infection.

Pneumococcal Pneumonia. *Streptococcus pneumoniae* (pneumococcus) remains the most common cause of bacterial pneumonia. *S. pneumoniae* colonizes the upper respiratory system and, in addition to pneumonia and lower respiratory tract infections, the organism is an important cause of upper respiratory infections, including sinusitis and otitis media, and of disseminated invasive infections such as bacteremia and meningitis.[25] It is among the leading causes of illness and death of young children, persons with other health problems, and the elderly worldwide.

S. pneumoniae are gram-positive diplococci, possessing a capsule of polysaccharide. There are 90 serologically distinct types of *S. pneumoniae* based on the antigenic properties of their capsular polysaccharides. The virulence of the pneumococcus is a function of its capsule, which prevents or delays digestion by phagocytes. The polysaccharide is an antigen that primarily elicits a B-cell response with antibody production. In the absence of antibody, clearance of the pneumococci from the body relies on the reticuloendothelial system, with the macrophages in the spleen playing a major role in elimination of the organism.[26] This, along with the spleen's role in antibody production, increases the risk of pneumococcal bacteremia in persons who are anatomically or functionally asplenic, such as children with sickle cell disease. The initial step in the pathogenesis of pneumococcal infection is the attachment and colonization of the organism to the mucus and cells of nasopharynx. Colonization does not equate with signs of infection. Perfectly healthy people can be colonized and carry the organism without evidence of infection. The spread of particular strains of pneumococci, particularly antibiotic-resistant strains, is largely by healthy colonized individuals. The factors that permit the pneumococci to spread beyond the nasopharynx vary depending on the virulence of organism, impaired host defense mechanisms, and the existence of preceding viral infection. Viral and other infections damage the surface cells or increase mucus production, which protect pneumococci from phagocytosis. In the alveoli, the pneumococci initially adhere to the alveolar wall, causing an outpouring of red cells and leukocytes, which results in consolidation of the lung. They reach the bloodstream through lymphatic drainage.

The signs and symptoms of pneumococcal pneumonia vary widely, depending on the age and health status of the infected person. In previously healthy persons, the onset usually is sudden and is characterized by malaise, a severe, shaking chill, and fever. The temperature may go as high as 106°F. During the initial or congestive stage, coughing brings up a watery sputum, and breath sounds are limited, with fine crackles. As the disease progresses, the character of the sputum changes; it may be blood tinged or rust colored to purulent. Pleuritic pain, a sharp pain that is more severe with respiratory movements, is common. With antibiotic therapy, fever usually subsides in approximately 48 to 72 hours, and recovery is uneventful. Elderly persons are less likely to experience marked elevations in temperature; in these persons, the only sign of pneumonia may be a loss of appetite and deterioration in mental status.

Treatment includes the use of antibiotics that are effective against *S. pneumoniae*. In the past, *S. pneumoniae* was uniformly susceptible to penicillin. However, penicillin-resistant and multidrug-resistant strains have been emerging in the United States and other countries.[27]

Pneumococcal pneumonia can be prevented through immunization. A 23-valent pneumococcal vaccine, composed of antigens from 23 types of *S. pneumoniae* capsular polysaccharides, is used. The capsular polysaccharides induce antibodies primarily by T-cell–independent mechanisms. Because their immune system is immature, the antibody response to most pneumococcal capsular polysaccharides usually is poor or inconsistent in children younger than 2 years of age.[25] The vaccine is recommended for persons 65 years of age or older and persons aged 2 to 65 years with chronic illnesses, particularly cardiovascular and pulmonary diseases, diabetes mellitus, and alcoholism, who sustain increased morbidity with respiratory infections. Immunization also is recommended for immunocompromised persons 2 years of age or older, including those with sickle cell disease, splenectomy, Hodgkin's disease, multiple myeloma, renal failure, nephrotic syndrome, organ transplantation, and HIV infection.[25] Immunization is recommended for residents in special environments or social settings in which the risk for invasive pneumococcal disease is increased (*e.g.,* Alaskan Natives, certain Native American populations) and for residents of nursing homes and long-term care facilities.

A single dose of pneumococcal vaccine usually confers some lifetime immunity. Serotype antibody levels decline after 5 to 10 years and decrease more rapidly in some groups than others.[25] Although not currently recommended for immunocompetent people who received the 23-valent vaccine, a second dose of vaccine is recommended for persons older than 65 years of age if 5 years or more have elapsed since the previous vaccine was given and if the person was younger than 65 years at the time of vaccination.[25] Revaccination also is recommended for immunocompromised persons 10 to 64 years of age and those with anatomic or functional asplenia (*i.e.,* splenectomy or sickle cell disease) if more than 5 years have elapsed since the previous dose and after 3 years if the person is younger than 10 years of age.[25]

In 2000, a 7-valent pneumococcal polysaccharide–protein conjugate vaccine (Prevnar) was licensed for use among infants and children.[28] Although the 23-valent vaccines are effective in older children, they do not prevent infection in children 2 years of age or younger, the age group with the highest rate of infection. With the success of *H. influenzae* type b vaccine, *S. pneumoniae* has become the leading cause of bacterial meningitis in the United States. *S. pneumoniae* also contributes substantially to noninvasive respiratory infections and is the most common cause of community-acquired pneumonia, acute otitis media, and sinusitis among young children. The ACIP recommends that vaccine be used for all children aged 2 to 23 months and for children aged 24 to 49 months who are at increased risk for pneumococcal disease (*e.g.,* children with sickle cell disease, HIV infection, and other immunocompromising or chronic medical conditions).[28]

Legionnaire's Disease. Legionnaire's disease is a form of bronchopneumonia caused by a gram-negative rod, *Legionella pneumophila*. It ranks among the three or four most common causes of community-acquired pneumonia.[21] Although more than 14 serotypes of *L. pneumophila* have been identified, serotype 1 accounts for more than 80% of reported cases of legionellosis.[29] The organism frequently is found in water, particularly in warm, standing water. The disease was first recognized and received its name after an epidemic of severe and, for some, fatal pneumonia that developed among delegates to the 1976 American Legion convention held in a Philadelphia hotel. The spread of infection was traced to a water-cooled air-conditioning system. Although healthy persons can contract the infection, the risk is greatest among smokers, persons with chronic diseases, and those with impaired cell-mediated immunity.[21,29,30]

Symptoms of the disease typically begin approximately 2 to 10 days after infection, with malaise, weakness, lethargy, fever, and dry cough. Other manifestations include disturbances of central nervous system function, gastrointestinal tract involvement, arthralgias, and elevation in body temperature, sometimes to more than 104°F. The presence of pneumonia along with diarrhea, hyponatremia, and confusion is characteristic of *Legionella* pneumonia. The disease causes consolidation of lung tissues and impairs gas exchange.

Diagnosis is based on clinical manifestations, radiologic studies, and specialized laboratory tests to detect the presence of the organism. Of these, the *Legionella* urinary antigen test is a relatively inexpensive, rapid test that detects antigens of *L. pneumophila* in the urine.[30] The urine test usually is easier to obtain because people with legionellosis often have a nonproductive cough and the results remain positive for weeks despite antibiotic therapy. The test is available as both a radioimmunoassay and an enzyme immunoassay and has sensitivity of 70% and a specificity approaching 100%.[29] The possible disadvantage of the test is that it detects only *L. pneumophila* serogroup 1. Culture methods permit identification of other serotypes.

Treatment consists of administration of antibiotics that are known to be effective against *L. pneumophila*. Delay in instituting antibiotic therapy significantly increases mortality rates; therefore, antibiotics known to be effective against *L. pneumophila* should be included in the treatment regimen for severe community-acquired pneumonia.[29]

Mycoplasma and Viral Pneumonias. Mycoplasmas and viruses tend to cause atypical or interstitial pneumonias.[1] The mycoplasmas are the smallest free-living agents of disease, having characteristics of viruses and bacteria. The influenza virus is the most common cause of viral pneumonia. Less common offenders are parainfluenza and respiratory syncytial viruses. Other viruses sometimes are implicated, including the measles and chickenpox viruses.

The clinical course among persons with mycoplasmal and viral pneumonias varies widely from a mild infection (*e.g.*, influenza types A and B, adenovirus) that masquerades as a chest cold to a more serious and even fatal outcome (*e.g.*, chickenpox pneumonia). The symptoms may remain confined to fever, headache, and muscle aches and pains. Cough, when present, is characteristically dry, hacking, and nonproductive. Viruses impair the respiratory tract defenses and predispose to secondary bacterial infections with the development of lobar or bronchopneumonia. Some viruses such as herpes simplex, varicella, and adenovirus may be associated with necrosis of the alveolar epithelium and acute inflammation.

Hospital-Acquired Pneumonia

Hospital-acquired, or nosocomial, pneumonia is defined as a lower respiratory tract infection that was not present or incubating on admission to the hospital. Usually, infections occurring 48 hours or more after admission are considered hospital acquired.[21,31] Hospital-acquired pneumonia is the second most common cause of hospital-acquired infection and has a mortality rate of 20% to 50%.[21] Persons requiring mechanical ventilation are particularly at risk, as are those with compromised immune function, chronic lung disease, and airway instrumentation, such as endotracheal intubation or tracheotomy.

Ninety percent of infections are bacterial. The organisms are those present in the hospital environment and include *Pseudomonas aeruginosa*, *S. aureus*, *Enterobacter* species, *Klebsiella* species, *Escherichia coli*, and *Serratia*. The organisms that are responsible for hospital-acquired pneumonias are different from those responsible for community-acquired pneumonia, and many of them have acquired antibiotic resistance and are more difficult to treat.

Pneumonia in Immunocompromised Persons

Pneumonia in immunocompromised persons remains a major source of morbidity and mortality. The term *immunocompromised host* usually is applied to persons with variety of underlying defects in host defenses. It includes persons with primary and acquired immunodeficiency states, those who have undergone bone marrow or organ transplantation, persons with solid organ or hematologic cancers, and those on corticosteroid and other immunosuppressant drugs.[32] Although almost all types of microorganisms can cause pulmonary infection in immunocompromised persons, certain types of immunologic defects tend to favor certain types of infections. Defects in humoral immunity predispose to bacterial infections against which antibodies play an important role; defects in cellular immunity predispose to infections with viruses, fungi, mycobacteria, and protozoa. Neutropenia and impaired granulocyte function, as occurs in persons with leukemia, chemotherapy, and bone marrow metaplasia, predispose to infections caused by *S. aureus*, *Aspergillus*, gram-negative bacilli, and *Candida*. The time course of infection often provides a hint to the type of agent involved. A fulminant pneumonia usually is caused by bacterial infection, but an insidious onset probably heralds viral, fungal, protozoal, or mycobacterial infection.

Pneumocystis carinii Pneumonia. *Pneumocystis carinii* pneumonia is an opportunistic, often fatal form of lung infection seen in debilitated persons and those with impaired immune function, particularly those with impaired cell-mediated immunity. *P. carinii* is a parasite of uncertain classification. Although the terminology applied to protozoa is used to describe the various stages of its life cycle, analysis suggests that it is a fungus.[33] The organism is widely distributed, but it does not produce disease in persons with a healthy immune system.

P. carinii pneumonia is seen in persons with severely impaired cell-mediated immunity due to AIDS or treatment with cytotoxic drugs or irradiation for management of organ transplantation or cancer. In the United States, *P. carinii* pneumonia develops in 60% to 80% of persons with AIDS during the course of their disease.[34] It is the most common opportunistic infection in children with AIDS. Because it occurs so regularly in persons with AIDS, it is used as a diagnostic criterion for the disease (see Chapter 20).

Although the source of infection is uncertain (*e.g.*, environment, animals, or infected humans), the organism is thought to be airborne and introduced into the lungs through inhalation. In persons with intact cell-mediated immunity, *P. carinii* infection is rapidly contained without producing symptoms.[33]

The onset of *P. carinii* pneumonia is abrupt, with high fever, tachypnea, shortness of breath, a mild, nonproductive cough, intercostal retractions, and cyanosis. In vulnerable hosts, the disease spreads rapidly throughout the lungs, producing involvement similar to that of acute respiratory distress syndrome (see Chapter 29). The infection produces an initial random and patchy involvement of the lungs. The *P. carinii* trophozoites attach and feed on alveolar epithelial cells but do not invade them.[33] As they divide, some form cup-shaped or boat-shaped cysts that can be detected microscopically. Microscopically, the walls of the involved alveoli become thickened and edematous, and the alveoli become filled with a foamy, protein-rich fluid. As the disease progresses, the gas exchange function of the lungs becomes severely impaired (Fig. 28-3).

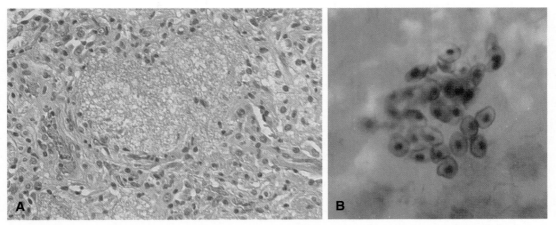

FIGURE 28-3 *Pneumocystis carinii* pneumonia. (**A**) The alveoli are filled with a foamy exudate, and the interstitium is thickened and contains a chronic inflammatory infiltrate. (**B**) A centrifuged broncho-alveolar lavage specimen impregnated with silver shows a cluster of *Pneumocystis carinii* cysts. (From Rubin E., Farber J.L. [1994]. *Pathology* [2nd ed.]. Philadelphia: J.B. Lippincott)

The diagnosis of the disease depends on microscopic methods that use specific stains to identify the organism.[33] Usually, sputum specimens obtained after inhalation of hypertonic saline produced by an ultrasonic nebulizer are required for this purpose. Other methods for obtaining specimens include bronchoalveolar lavage and transbronchial lung biopsy.

The mainstay of treatment for *P. carinii* pneumonia is trimethoprim-sulfamethoxazole (TMP-SMX) given intravenously or orally. Other drugs that may be used are pentamidine, trimethoprim and dapsone, clindamycin and primaquine, and atovaquone.[34] Because of the risk of *P. carinii* pneumonia, the CDC recommends that *P. carinii* prophylaxis (*i.e.,* TMP-SMX or, alternatively, dapsone, dapsone plus pyrimethamine plus leucovorin, aerosolized pentamidine, or atovaquone) be provided for all HIV-infected adults and adolescents (including pregnant women and those on highly active antiretroviral therapies [HAART]) who have a CD4+ T-cell count of less than 200/μL or a history of oral candidiasis.[35] Persons also should be considered for prophylaxis if they have a CD4+ T-cell percentage less than 14% of total lymphocytes or a history of AIDS-defining illness, but do not otherwise qualify for prophylactic treatment.[35] It is suggested that prophylaxis may be discontinued in persons who are on HAART with a sustained increase in the CD4+ T-cell count.[35] Patients who do not have HIV infection, but are at high risk for *P. carinii* pneumonia, including those receiving aggressive therapy for leukemia or lymphoma and transplant recipients, also should be considered for prophylaxis.[34]

Because most children with HIV infection contract *P. carinii* pneumonia before the age of 1 year, it is recommended that all infants born to HIV-infected mothers be started on a prophylaxis regimen at 4 to 6 weeks of age, regardless of their CD4+ T-cell count.[35] Infants who are identified as being exposed to HIV after 6 weeks of age should be started on prophylaxis at the time of identification. All HIV-infected infants whose infection status has not been determined should continue prophylaxis until 12 months of age. Treatment is discontinued for infants in whom the infection has been excluded. After 1 year of age, prophylaxis is determined by CD4+ T-cell count.

TUBERCULOSIS

Tuberculosis is the world's foremost cause of death from a single infectious agent, causing 25% of avoidable deaths in developing countries. In 1998, approximately 8 million cases and 2 million deaths were attributed to tuberculosis.[36] With the introduction of antibiotics in the 1950s, the United States and other Western countries enjoyed a long decline in the number of infections until the mid-1980s. Since that time, the rate of infection has increased, particularly among HIV-infected people. In the United States, the biggest increase in new cases was from 1985 to 1993, after which the rate of cases reported yearly has again declined. In part, this decline reflects the impact of resources to assist state and local control efforts, wider screening and prevention programs, and increased support for prevention programs among HIV-infected persons.[36] Tuberculosis is more common among foreign-born persons from countries with a high incidence of tuberculosis and among residents of high-risk congregate settings such as correctional facilities, drug treatment facilities, and homeless shelters. Outbreaks of a drug-resistant form of tuberculosis have occurred, complicating the selection of drugs and affecting the duration of treatment.

Tuberculosis is an infectious disease caused by the mycobacterium, *M. tuberculosis*. The mycobacteria are slender, rod-shaped, aerobic bacteria that do not form spores. They are similar to other bacterial organisms except for an outer waxy capsule that makes them more resistant to destruction; the organism can persist in old necrotic and calcified lesions and remain capable of reinitiating growth. The waxy coat also causes the organism to retain red dye when treated with acid in acid-fast staining.[1] Thus, the mycobacteria are often referred to as *acid-fast bacilli.* Although *M. tuberculosis* can infect practically any organ of the body, the lungs are most frequently involved. The tubercle bacilli are strict aerobes that thrive in an oxygen-rich environment. This explains their tendency to cause disease in the upper lobe or upper parts of the lower lobe of the lung, where ventilation is greatest.

Two forms of tuberculosis pose a particular threat to humans: *M. tuberculosis hominis* (human tuberculosis) and *M. tuberculosis bovis* (bovine tuberculosis). Human tuberculosis is an airborne infection spread by minute, invisible particles, called *droplet nuclei,* that are harbored in the respiratory secretions of persons with active tuberculosis.[37,38] Coughing, sneezing, and talking all create respiratory droplets; these droplets evaporate, leaving the organisms (droplet nuclei), which remain suspended in the air and are circulated by air currents. Living under crowded and confined conditions increases the risk for spread of the disease. Bovine tuberculosis is acquired by drinking milk from infected cows, and it initially affects the gastrointestinal tract. This form of tuberculosis has been virtually eradicated in North America and other developed countries as a result of rigorous controls on dairy herds and the pasteurization of milk.

There has been a recent increase in the United States of atypical mycobacterial infections, including that caused by *Mycobacterium avium-intracellulare* complex.[1] Opportunistic infection with *M. avium-intracellulare* complex occurs in severely immunosuppressed persons. The infection usually originates in the gastrointestinal tract but can begin in the lungs. It affects the reticuloendothelial system throughout the body, causing enlargement of the lymph nodes, spleen, and liver.

Primary Tuberculosis

The tubercle bacillus incites a distinctive chronic inflammatory response referred to as *granulomatous inflammation.* The destructiveness of the disease results from the hypersensitivity response that the bacillus evokes rather than its inherent destructive capabilities. Cell-mediated immunity and hypersensitivity reactions contribute to the evolution of the disease. Tuberculosis can manifest as a primary or reactivated infection.

Primary tuberculosis occurs in a person lacking previous contact with the tubercle bacillus. It typically is initiated as a result of inhaling droplet nuclei that contain the tubercle bacillus.[37,38] Inhaled droplet nuclei pass down the bronchial tree without settling on the epithelium and implant in a respiratory bronchiole or alveolus beyond the mucociliary system. Soon after entering the lung, the bacilli are surrounded and engulfed by macrophages. *M. tuberculosis* has no known endotoxins or exotoxins; therefore, there is no early immunoglobulin response to infection. The tubercle bacillus grows slowly, dividing every 25 to 32 hours in the macrophage.[38] As the bacilli multiply, the macrophages degrade some mycobacteria and present antigen to the T lymphocytes for development of a cell-mediated immune response. The organisms grow for 2 to 12 weeks until they reach sufficient numbers to elicit a cellular immune response. In persons with intact cell-mediated immunity, this

Tuberculosis

➤ Tuberculosis is an infectious disease caused by *Mycobacterium tuberculosis,* a rod-shaped, aerobic bacteria that is resistant to destruction and can persist in necrotic and calcified lesions for prolonged periods and remain capable of reinstating growth.

➤ The organism is spread by inhaling the mycobacterium-containing droplet nuclei that circulate in the air. Overcrowded living conditions increase the risk of tuberculosis spread.

➤ The tubercle bacillus has no known antigens to stimulate an early immunoglobulin response; instead, the host mounts a delayed-type cell-mediated immune response.

➤ The cell-mediated response plays a dominant role in walling off the tubercle bacilli and preventing the development of active tuberculosis. People with impaired cell-mediated immunity are more likely to develop active tuberculosis when infected.

➤ A positive tuberculin skin test results from a cell-mediated immune response and implies that a person has been infected with *M. tuberculosis* and has mounted a cell-mediated immune response. It does not mean that the person has active tuberculosis.

action is followed by the development of a single, gray-white, circumscribed granulomatous lesion, called a *Ghon's focus,* that contains the tubercle bacilli, modified macrophages, and other immune cells. Within 2 to 3 weeks, the central portion of the Ghon's focus undergoes soft, caseous (cheeselike) necrosis. This occurs at approximately the time that the tuberculin test result becomes positive, suggesting that the necrosis is caused by the cell-mediated hypersensitivity immune response (see Chapter 19). During this same period, tubercle bacilli, free or inside macrophages, drain along the lymph channels to the tracheobronchial lymph nodes of the affected lung and there evoke the formation of caseous granulomas. The combination of the primary lung lesion and lymph node granulomas is called *Ghon's complex* (Fig. 28-4).

The cell-mediated hypersensitivity response plays a dominant role in limiting further replication of the bacilli. The immune response also provides protection against additional tubercle bacilli that may be inhaled at a later time. People with HIV infection and others with disorders of cell-mediated immunity are more likely to acquire active tuberculosis if they become infected. Although people with HIV infection are more likely to contract the disease, they are no more likely to transmit *M. tuberculosis.*

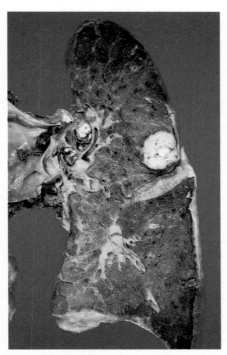

FIGURE 28-4 Primary tuberculosis. A healed Ghon's complex is represented by a subpleural nodule and involved hilar lymph nodes. (From Rubin E., Farber J.L. [1994]. *Pathology* [2nd ed.]. Philadelphia: J.B. Lippincott)

When the number of organisms inhaled is small and the body's resistance is adequate, scar tissue forms and encapsulates the primary lesion. In time, most of these lesions become calcified and are visible on a chest radiographs. Occasionally, primary tuberculosis may progress, causing more extensive destruction of lung tissue. Often, the granulomatous tissue erodes into a bronchus, and the necrotic inflammatory tissue is discharged into it. An air-filled cavity forms, permitting bronchogenic spread of the disease. Tubercle bacilli also enter the sputum, allowing the person to infect others. In rare instances, tuberculosis may erode into a blood vessel, giving rise to hematogenic dissemination. *Miliary tuberculosis* describes minute lesions, resembling millet seeds, resulting from this type of dissemination that can involve almost any organ, particularly the brain, meninges, liver, kidney, and bone marrow.

Reactivated Tuberculosis

Reactivated tuberculosis usually results from activation of a previously healed primary lesion. Less commonly, it develops because of reinfection. It often occurs in situations of impaired body defense mechanisms. The partial immunity that follows initial exposure affords protection against reinfection and to some extent aids in localizing the disease should reactivation occur. On the other hand, the hypersensitivity reaction is an aggravating factor in reactivation tuberculosis, as evidenced by the frequency of cavitation and bronchial dissemination. The cavities may coalesce to a size of up to 10 to 15 cm in diameter. Pleural effusion and tuberculous empyema are common as the disease progresses.

Manifestations

Primary tuberculosis usually is asymptomatic, with the only evidence of the disease being a positive tuberculin skin test result and calcified lesions seen on the chest radiograph. Uncommonly, the immune response is inadequate, and progressive primary tuberculosis develops. The person with progressive primary or reactivation tuberculosis presents with low-grade fevers, night sweats, easy fatigability, anorexia, and weight loss. A cough initially is dry but later becomes productive with purulent and sometimes blood-tinged sputum. Dyspnea and orthopnea develop as the disease advances.

Diagnosis

The most frequently used screening methods for pulmonary tuberculosis are the tuberculin skin tests and chest radiographic studies. The Mantoux test is the standard skin test for the diagnosis of tuberculosis. A second type of test, the multiple-puncture test, is available for population screening purposes. Because the quantity of tuberculin introduced under the skin using the multiple-puncture technique cannot be precisely controlled, this method of testing should not be used to screen high-risk populations.[38] The Mantoux test involves the intradermal injection of tuberculin (*i.e.*, purified protein derivative standard). The transverse width of induration at the test site is measured after 48 to 72 hours. A 5-mm or larger reaction is considered a positive test result for persons with or at high risk for HIV infection, close contacts of persons with tuberculosis, and persons with chest radiographic findings consistent with old, healed tuberculosis lesions.[38] In persons who are not immunosuppressed but belong to one of the high-risk groups, such as intravenous drug abusers, persons with other medical problems that increase the risk of moving from latent to active tuberculosis, residents of high-risk congregate settings, or foreign-born persons from countries with a high prevalence of tuberculosis, a positive reaction is evidenced by a skin elevation of 10 mm or more.[39] An induration of 15 mm is classified as positive in persons who do not belong to either of these groups.[38]

False-positive and false-negative reactions can occur. False-positive reactions often result from cross-reactions with nontuberculosis mycobacteria, such as *M. avium-intracellulare* complex. Because the hypersensitivity response to the tuberculin test depends on cell-mediated immunity, a false-negative test result can occur because of immunodeficiency states that result from HIV infection, immunosuppressive therapy, lymphoreticular malignancies, or aging. This is called *anergy*. In the immunocompromised person, a negative tuberculin test result can mean that the person has a true lack of exposure to tuberculosis or is unable to mount an immune response to the test. Because of the problem with anergy in persons with HIV infection and other immunocompromised states, the use of control tests is recommended. Three antigens that can be used for control testing are *Candida*, mumps virus, and tetanus toxoid. Most healthy persons in the population have been exposed to these antigens. The CDC recommends the use of control tests with two of these antigens when screening persons with HIV infection for tuberculosis. If a person reacts to at least one of the control antigens, a negative tuberculin test result usually means that the person is not infected with tuberculosis.

A two-step testing procedure, which uses a "boosting" phenomenon, may be used to increase the reaction to a subsequent tuberculin test in persons who have been infected with tuberculosis.[40] If the first test result of the two-step procedure is negative, a second test is administered 1 week later. If the second test result is negative, the person is considered to be uninfected or anergic. If the second test result is positive, it is assumed to have occurred because of a boosted response. The boosted effect can last for 1 year or longer. Use of the two-step test procedure for employee health or institutional screening can reduce the likelihood that a boosted response in a subsequent test will not be interpreted as a recent infection.

The tuberculin skin test was introduced by Robert Koch in the late 19th century. The test measures delayed hypersensitivity (*i.e.,* cell-mediated, type IV) that follows exposure to the tubercle bacillus. Persons who become tuberculin positive usually remain so for the remainder of their lives. A positive reaction to the skin test does not mean that a person has active tuberculosis, only that there has been exposure to the bacillus and that cell-mediated immunity to the organism has developed.

Diagnosis of active pulmonary tuberculosis requires identification of the organism in respiratory tract secretions. Bacteriologic studies (*i.e.,* acid-fast stain and cultures) of early-morning sputum specimens are used to determine the presence of the organism. Induced sputum collection methods (inhalation of an aerosol of sterile normal saline) may be used in persons who have difficulty producing sputum. Gastric aspirations may be necessary for persons, particularly children, who cannot produce sputum, even with aerosol inhalation. Multiple specimens often are necessary. Fiber-optic bronchoscopy may be used to obtain bronchial washings for bacteriologic studies. Cultures on solid media may take 6 to 8 weeks, delaying diagnosis. The polymerase chain reaction allows rapid detection of *M. tuberculosis* and differentiation from other mycobacteria (see Chapter 17). Automated radiometric culture systems such as the BACTEC 460 (Becton Dickinson Microbiology Systems, Sparks, MD) may allow for detection of *M. tuberculosis* in several days. Genotyping can be done to identify different strains of *M. tuberculosis*. It is useful in investigating outbreaks of tuberculosis, tracing the sources of infection, and determining whether new episodes of the disease are due to reinfection or reactivation. In addition, genotyping is useful in determining sites and patterns of *M. tuberculosis* transmission in communities.

Treatment

Two groups meet the criteria established for the use of antimycobacterial therapy for tuberculosis: persons with active tuberculosis and those who have had contact with cases of active tuberculosis and who are at risk for development of an active form of the disease.

The primary drugs used in the treatment of tuberculosis are isoniazid (INH), rifampin, pyrazinamide, ethambutol, and streptomycin.[39] INH is remarkably potent against the tubercle bacillus and probably is the most widely used drug for tuberculosis. Although its exact mechanism of action is unknown, it apparently combines with an enzyme that is needed by the INH-susceptible strains of the tubercle bacillus. Resistance to the drug develops rapidly, and combination with other effective drugs delays the development of resistance. Rifampin inhibits RNA synthesis in the bacillus. Although ethambutol and pyrazinamide are known to inhibit the growth of the tubercle bacillus, their mechanisms of action are largely unknown. Streptomycin, the first drug found to be effective against tuberculosis, must be given by injection, which limits its usefulness, particularly in long-term therapy. It remains an important drug in tuberculosis therapy and is used primarily in persons with severe, possibly life-threatening forms of tuberculosis.

Treatment of active tuberculosis requires the use of multiple drugs. Tuberculosis is an unusual disease in that chemotherapy is required for a relatively long period of time. The tubercle bacillus is an aerobic organism that multiplies slowly and remains relatively dormant in oxygen-poor caseous material. It undergoes a high rate of mutation and tends to acquire resistance to any one drug. For this reason, multidrug regimens are used for treating persons with active tuberculosis.

Based on the results of several trials, a marked change in chemotherapy for uncomplicated tuberculosis has developed. Short-course programs of therapy (usually for 6 to 12 months) have replaced the earlier 18- to 24-month multidrug regimens. Treatment may need to be prolonged in HIV-infected persons and in persons with drug-resistant strains of *M. tuberculosis*. Drug susceptibility tests are used to guide treatment in drug-resistant forms of the disease.

Prophylactic treatment is used for persons who are infected with *M. tuberculosis* but do not have active disease.[33,39] This group includes persons with a positive skin test who have had close contact with active cases of tuberculosis; have converted from a negative to positive skin test result within 2 years; have a history of untreated or inadequately treated tuberculosis; have chest radiographs with evidence of tuberculosis but no bacteriologic evidence of the active disease; have special risk factors such as silicosis, diabetes mellitus, prolonged corticosteroid therapy, immunosuppression therapy, end-stage renal disease, chronic malnutrition from any cause, or hematologic or reticuloendothelial cancers; have a positive HIV test result or have AIDS; or are 35 years of age or younger with a positive reaction of unknown duration. These persons harbor a small number of microorganisms and usually are treated with INH.

Outbreaks of multidrug-resistant tuberculosis have posed a problem for the prophylactic treatment of exposed persons, including health care workers.[40] Most exposed persons who have contracted active multidrug-resistant tuberculosis were infected with the HIV virus; the fatality rate among these persons is high, at 80%.[41] Various treatment protocols are recommended, depending on the type of resistant strain that is identified.

Success of chemotherapy for prophylaxis and treatment of tuberculosis depends on strict adherence to a lengthy drug regimen. This often is a problem, particularly for asymptomatic persons with tuberculosis infections and for poorly motivated groups such as intravenous drug abusers. Directly observed therapy, which requires that a health care worker observe while the person takes the antituberculosis drug, is recommended for some persons and for some types of treatment protocols.

First administered to humans in 1921, the bacillus Calmette-Guérin (BCG) vaccine is used to prevent the development of tuberculosis in persons who are at high risk for infection. BCG is an attenuated strain of *M. tuberculosis bovis*. The vaccine has been used worldwide to prevent tuberculosis.[42] It is administered only to persons who have a negative tuberculin skin test result. The vaccine, which is given intradermally, produces a local reaction that can last as long as 3 months and may result in scarring at the injection site. Persons who have been vaccinated with BCG usually have a positive tuberculin skin test result that wanes with time and is unlikely to persist beyond 10 years. The vaccine also has been used to increase the immune response in persons with some types of cancers. The CDC recommends that use of the BCG vaccine in the United States be reserved for high-risk groups such as infants and children who reside in settings in which the likelihood of *M. tuberculosis* transmission and infection is high and for health care workers where the risk of transmission of multidrug-resistant strains of the bacterium are high. The vaccine is not recommended for children and adults infected with HIV.[42]

FUNGAL INFECTIONS

Although the spores of fungi are constantly present in the air we breathe, only a few reach the lung and cause disease. The most common of these are histoplasmosis, coccidioidomycosis, and blastomycosis. These infections usually are mild and self-limited and seldom are noticed unless they produce local complications or progressive dissemination occurs. The signs and symptoms of these infections commonly resemble those of tuberculosis.

Histoplasmosis

Histoplasmosis is caused by the dimorphic fungus *Histoplasma capsulatum* and is the most common fungal infection in the United States. Skin testing surveys suggest that 18% to 20% of persons in the United States have been infected with the disease.[43] Most cases occur along the major river valleys of the Midwest—the Ohio, the Mississippi, and the Missouri. The organism grows in soil and other areas that have been enriched with bird excreta: old chicken houses, pigeon lofts, barns, and trees where birds roost. The infection is acquired by inhaling the fungal spores that are released when the dirt or dust from the infected areas is disturbed. The spores convert to the parasitic yeast phase when exposed to body temperature in the alveoli. The organisms are then carried to the regional lymphatics and from there are disseminated throughout the body in the bloodstream. They are removed from the circulation by fixed macrophages of the reticuloendothelial system. When delayed hypersensitivity develops (see Chapter 19), the macrophages usually are able to destroy the fungi.

The manifestations of histoplasmosis are strikingly similar to those of tuberculosis. Depending on the host's resistance and immunocompetence, the disease usually takes one of four forms: latent asymptomatic disease, self-limited primary disease, chronic pulmonary disease, or disseminated infection. The average incubation period for the infection is approximately 14 days. Only 40% of infected persons have symptoms, and only approximately 10% of these are ill enough to seek the care of a physician.[44]

Latent asymptomatic histoplasmosis is characterized by evidence of healed lesions in the lungs or hilar lymph nodes, accompanied by a positive histoplasmin skin test result (analogous to the tuberculin test). Primary pulmonary histoplasmosis occurs in otherwise healthy persons as a mild, self-limited, febrile respiratory infection. Its symptoms include muscle and joint pains and a nonproductive cough. Erythema nodosum (*i.e.*, subcutaneous nodules) or erythema multiforme (*i.e.*, hivelike lesions) sometimes appears. During this stage of the disease, chest radiographs usually show single or multiple infiltrates.

Chronic histoplasmosis resembles reactivation tuberculosis. Infiltration of the upper lobes of one or both lungs occurs with cavitation. This form of the disease is more common in middle-aged men who smoke and in persons with chronic lung disease. The most common manifestations are productive cough, fever, night sweats, and weight loss. In many persons, the disease is self-limited. In others, there is progressive destruction of lung tissue and dissemination of the disease.

Disseminated histoplasmosis can follow primary or chronic histoplasmosis but most often develops as an acute and fulminating infection in the very old or the very young or in persons with compromised immune function. Although the macrophages of the reticuloendothelial system can remove the fungi from the bloodstream, they are unable to destroy them. Characteristically, this form of the disease produces a high fever, generalized lymph node enlargement, hepatosplenomegaly, muscle wasting, anemia, leukopenia, and thrombocytopenia. There may be hoarseness, ulcerations of the mouth and tongue, nausea, vomiting, diarrhea, and abdominal pain. Often, meningitis becomes a dominant feature of the disease.

Absolute diagnosis of histoplasmosis requires identification of the organism on culture. The infection incites a delayed hypersensitivity immune response, and the histoplasmin skin test is used to test for exposure to the organism. This test result remains positive after the initial infection has occurred and does not indicate whether the disease is of recent or past origin. In addition to the delayed response, the humoral immune system responds to the acute infection by producing antibodies. Although these antibodies are not protective, they serve as markers of infection. These antibodies can be measured by means of the complement fixation test. An immunodiffusion test can also be used as a test for the antibodies. The complement fixation and immunodiffusion tests become positive 2 weeks after the onset of symptoms.

The antifungal drug, itraconazole, usually is the drug of choice for treatment of persons with disease severe enough to require treatment or those with compromised immune function who are at risk for development of disseminated disease.[45] Amphotericin B is given intravenously and usually is the drug of choice in severe disease.

Coccidioidomycosis

Coccidioidomycosis is a common fungal infection caused by inhaling the spores of *Coccidioides immitis*.[46,47] The disease resembles tuberculosis, and its mechanisms of infection are similar to those of histoplasmosis. It is most prevalent in the southwestern United States, principally in California, Arizona, and Texas. Because of its prevalence in the San Joaquin Valley, the disease is sometimes referred to as *San Joaquin fever* or *valley fever*. The *C. immitis* organism lives in soil and can establish new sites in the soil. Events such as dust storms and digging for construction have been associated with increased incidence of the disease.

The disease most commonly occurs as an acute, primary, self-limited pulmonary infection with or without systemic involvement, but in some cases, it progresses to a disseminated disease. Approximately 60% of exposed persons manifest only a positive skin test result (*i.e.,* coccidioidin skin test or spherulin skin test) and are unaware of the infection.[45] In the other 40%, the illness usually resembles influenza. There may be fever, cough, and pleuritic pain, accompanied by erythema multiforme or erythema nodosum. The skin lesions usually are accompanied by arthralgias or arthritis without effusion, particularly of the ankles and knees. The terms *desert bumps* and *desert arthritis* are used to describe these manifestations. The presence of skin and joint manifestations indicates strong host defenses because persons who have had such manifestations seldom acquire disseminated disease. Disseminated disease occurs in approximately 0.5% to 1% of infected persons. Commonly affected structures in disseminated disease are the lymph nodes, meninges, spleen, liver, kidney, skin, and adrenal glands. Meningitis is the most common cause of death. Persons with diabetes or compromised immune function, infants, and members of dark-skinned races tend to localize the disease poorly and are at higher risk for disseminated disease. In HIV-infected persons in endemic areas, coccidioidomycosis is now a common opportunistic infection.

Radiologic studies, including chest radiographic studies and bone scans, are useful in determining disease but cannot distinguish coccidioidomycosis from other pulmonary diseases. A definitive diagnosis requires microscopic or serologic evidence that *C. immitis* is present in body tissues or fluids. *C. immitis* spherules can be visualized in specially stained biopsy specimens. Serologic tests can be done for IgM and IgG antibody detection. Treatment depends on the severity of infection. Persons without associated risk factors such as HIV infection or without specific evidence of progressive disease usually can be managed without antifungal therapy. The oral antifungal drugs (ketoconazole, itraconazole, and fluconazole) or intravenous amphotericin B are used in the treatment of persons with progressive disease.

Blastomycosis

Blastomycosis is caused by the organism *Blastomyces dermatitidis*. It is characterized by local suppurative and granulomatous lesions of the lungs and skin. The disease is most commonly found in the southern and north central United States, especially in areas bordering the Mississippi and Ohio River basins, and the Great Lakes.[48] The symptoms of acute infection are similar to those of acute histoplasmosis, including fever, cough, aching joints and muscles, and, uncommonly, pleuritic pain. In contrast to histoplasmosis, the cough in blastomycosis often is productive, and the sputum is purulent. Acute pulmonary infections may be self-limited or progressive. In persons with overwhelming pulmonary disease, diffuse interalveolar infiltrates and evidence of acute respiratory distress syndrome may develop (see Chapter 29). Extrapulmonary spread most commonly involves the skin, bones, or the prostate. These lesions may provide the first evidence of the disease.

The diagnosis of blastomycosis is more difficult than that of histoplasmosis. Visualization of the yeast in the sputum after application of 10% potassium hydroxide provides a presumptive diagnosis. When this fails, cultural isolation of the fungus often is attempted. The blastomycin skin test lacked specificity and is no longer available.

Treatment of the progressive or disseminated form of the disease includes the use of amphotericin B, ketoconazole, or fluconazole. Most persons with blastomycosis are identified and treated before the development of overwhelming or fatal disease.[48]

In summary, respiratory infections are the most common cause of respiratory illness. They include the common cold, influenza, pneumonias, tuberculosis, and fungal infections. The common cold occurs more frequently than any other respiratory infection. The fingers are the usual source of transmission, and the most common portals of entry are the nasal mucosa and the conjunctiva of the eye. The influenza virus causes three syndromes: an uncomplicated rhinotracheitis, a respiratory viral infection followed by a bacterial infection, and viral pneumonia.

Pneumonia describes an infection of the parenchymal tissues of the lung. Loss of the cough reflex, damage to the ciliated endothelium that lines the respiratory tract, or impaired immune defenses predispose to pneumonia. Pneumonia is being increasingly classified as community acquired or hospital acquired. Persons with compromised immune function constitute a special concern in both categories. Community-acquired pneumonia involves infections from organisms that are present more often in the community than in the hospital or nursing home. The most common cause of community-acquired pneumonia is *S. pneumoniae*. Hospital-acquired (nosocomial) pneumonia is defined as a lower respiratory tract infection occurring 72 hours or more after admission. Hospital-acquired pneumonia is the second most common cause of hospital-acquired infection. Legionnaire's disease is a form of bronchopneumonia caused by the gram-negative bacillus *L. pneumophila.* Viral or atypical pneumonia can occur as a primary infection, such as that caused by influenza virus, or as a complication of other viral infections, such as measles or chickenpox. Viral and atypical pneumonias involve the interstitium of the lung and often masquerade as chest colds. *P. carinii* pneumonia is an opportunistic infection that occurs in debilitated persons with impaired immune function, including persons with HIV infection.

Tuberculosis is a chronic respiratory infection caused by *M. tuberculosis,* which is spread by minute, invisible particles called *droplet nuclei.* Tuberculosis is a particular threat among HIV-infected persons, foreign-born persons from countries with a high incidence of tuberculosis, and residents of high-risk congregate settings such as correctional facilities, drug treatment facilities, and homeless shelters. The tubercle bacillus incites a distinctive chronic inflammatory response referred to as *granulomatous inflammation.* The destructiveness of the disease results from the hypersensitivity response that the bacillus evokes rather than its inherent destructive capabilities. Cell-mediated immunity and hypersensitivity reactions contribute to the evolution of the disease. The treatment of tuberculosis has been complicated by outbreaks of drug-resistant forms of the disease.

Infections caused by the fungi *H. capsulatum* (histoplasmosis), *C. immitis* (coccidioidomycosis), and *B. dermatitidis* (blastomycosis) produce pulmonary manifestations that resemble tuberculosis. These infections are common but seldom serious unless they produce progressive destruction of lung tissue or the infection disseminates to organs and tissues outside the lungs.

Cancer of the Lung

After you have completed this section of the chapter, you should be able to meet the following objectives:

✦ Cite risk factors associated with lung cancer
✦ Describe the manifestations of lung cancer and list two symptoms of lung cancer that are related to the invasion of the mediastinum
✦ Define the term *paraneoplastic* and cite three paraneoplastic manifestations of lung cancer
✦ Characterize the 5-year survival rate for lung cancer

Lung cancer is the leading cause of cancer deaths among men and women in the United States, accounting for 25% of all cancer deaths. In 2000, it was responsible for the deaths of 89,300 men and 67,600 women.[49] The increases in lung cancer incidence and deaths over the past 50 years have coincided closely with the increase in cigarette smoking over the same period. It has been estimated that more than 80% of lung cancer cases are caused by cigarette smoking. Many studies have shown that the risk for development of lung cancer increases with the number of cigarettes smoked and that the average male smoker is 10 times more likely to have lung cancer than the nonsmoker.[1] Industrial hazards also contribute to the incidence of lung cancer. A commonly recognized hazard is exposure to asbestos, with the mean risk of lung cancer being significantly greater in asbestos workers than in the general population. Tobacco smoke contributes heavily to the development of lung cancer in persons exposed to asbestos; the risk in this population group is estimated to be 50 to 90 times greater than that for nonsmokers.[1]

Because cancer of the lung usually is far advanced before it is discovered, the prognosis in general is poor. The overall 5-year survival rate is 13% to 15%, a dismal statistic that has not changed since the late 1960s.[49]

BRONCHOGENIC CARCINOMA

Bronchogenic carcinoma, which has its origin in the bronchial or bronchiolar epithelium, constitutes 90% to 95% of all lung cancers. Bronchogenic carcinomas are aggressive, locally invasive, and widely metastatic tumors that arise from the epithelial lining of the major bronchi. These tumors begin as small mucosal lesions that may follow one of several patterns of growth. They may form intraluminal masses that invade the bronchial mucosa and infiltrate the peribronchial connective tissue, or they may form large, bulky masses that extend into the adjacent lung tissue. Some large tumors undergo central necrosis and acquire local areas of hemorrhage, and some invade the pleural cavity and chest wall and spread to adjacent intrathoracic structures.[1]

Bronchogenic carcinomas can be subdivided into four major categories: squamous cell lung carcinoma (25% to 40%), adenocarcinoma (20% to 40%), small cell carcinoma (20% to 25%), and large cell carcinoma (10% to 15%).[1] *Squamous cell carcinoma* is found most commonly in men and is closely correlated with a smoking history. Squamous cell carcinoma tends to originate in the central bronchi as an intraluminal growth and is thus more amenable to early detection through cytologic examination of the sputum than other forms of lung cancer. It tends to spread centrally into major bronchi and hilar lymph nodes and disseminates outside the thorax later than other types of bronchogenic cancers.

Adenocarcinoma is the most common type of lung cancer in women and nonsmokers. Its association with cigarette smoking is weaker than for squamous cell carcinoma. Adenocarcinomas can have their origin in either the bronchiolar or alveolar tissues of the lung. These tumors tend to be located more peripherally than squamous cell sarcomas and sometimes are associated with areas of scarring. The scars may be due to old infarcts, metallic foreign bodies, wounds, and granulomatous infections such as tuberculosis. In general, these tumors grow more slowly than squamous cell carcinomas.

The *small cell carcinomas* are characterized by a distinctive cell type—small round to oval cells that are approximately the size of a lymphocyte.[1] The cells grow in clusters that exhibit neither glandular nor squamous organization. Electron microscopic studies demonstrate the presence of neurosecretory granules in some of the tumor cells similar to those found in the bronchial epithelium of the fetus or neonate. The presence of these granules, the ability of some of these tumors to secrete polypeptide hormones, and presence of neuroendocrine markers such as neuron-specific enolase and parathormone-like and other hormonally active products suggest that these tumors may arise from the neuroendocrine cells of the bronchial epithelium. The small cell carcinomas are highly malignant, tend to infiltrate widely, disseminate early in their course, and rarely are resectable. These tumors are particularly sensitive to chemotherapy and irradiation, and newer protocols have improved the outlook somewhat. The small cell carcinomas have a strong relationship to smoking; only approximately 1% occur in nonsmokers. *Large cell carcinomas* have large polygonal cells. They constitute a group of neoplasms that are highly anaplastic and difficult to categorize as squamous or adenocarcinoma. They have a poor prognosis because of their tendency to spread to distant sites early in their course.

In general, adenocarcinoma and squamous cell carcinoma tend to remain localized longer and have a better prognosis than other, less differentiated cancers, which usually are far advanced at the time of diagnosis. All varieties of bronchogenic carcinomas, especially small cell lung carcinoma, have the capacity to synthesize bioactive products and produce paraneoplastic syndromes, including adrenocorticotropic hormone (ACTH), antidiuretic hormone (ADH), parathyroid-like hormone, gonadotropins, and gastrin-releasing peptide.

MANIFESTATIONS

Cancer of the lung develops insidiously, often giving little or no warning of its presence. Because its symptoms are similar to those associated with smoking and chronic bronchitis, they often are disregarded.

The manifestations of lung cancer can be divided into three categories: those due to involvement of the lung and adjacent structures, the effects of local spread and metastasis, and the nonmetastatic paraneoplastic manifestations involving endocrine, neurologic, and connective tissue function. As with other cancers, lung cancer also causes nonspecific symptoms such as anorexia and weight loss.

Many of the manifestations of lung cancers result from local irritation and obstruction of the airways and from invasion of the mediastinum and pleural space. The earliest symptoms usually are chronic cough, shortness of breath, and wheezing because of airway irritation and obstruction. Hemoptysis (*i.e.*, blood in the sputum) occurs when the lesion erodes blood vessels. Pain receptors in the chest are limited to the parietal pleura, mediastinum, larger blood vessels, and peribronchial afferent vagal fibers. Dull, intermittent, poorly localized retrosternal pain is common in tumors that involve the mediastinum. Pain becomes persistent, localized, and more severe when the disease invades the pleura.

Tumors that invade the mediastinum may cause hoarseness because of the involvement of the recurrent laryngeal nerve and cause difficulty in swallowing because of compression of the esophagus. An uncommon complication called the *superior vena cava syndrome* can occur in some persons with mediastinal involvement. Interruption of blood flow in this vessel usually results from compression by the tumor or involved lymph nodes. The disorder can interfere with venous drainage from the head, neck, and chest wall. The outcome is determined by the speed with which the disorder develops and the adequacy of the collateral circulation.

Tumors adjacent to the visceral pleura often insidiously produce pleural effusion. This effusion can compress the lung and cause atelectasis and dyspnea. It is less likely to cause fever, pleural friction rub, or pain than pleural effusion resulting from other causes.

Metastatic spread occurs by way of lymph channels and the vascular system. Metastases already exist in 50% of patients presenting with evidence of lung cancer and develop eventually in 90% of patients. The most common sites of these metastases are the brain, bone, and liver.

Paraneoplastic disorders are those that are unrelated to metastasis. These include hypercalcemia from secretion of parathyroid-like peptide, Cushing's syndrome from ACTH secretion, inappropriate secretion of ADH, neuromuscular syndromes (*e.g.*, myasthenic syndromes, peripheral neuropathy, polymyositis), and hematologic disorders (*e.g.*, migratory thrombophlebitis, nonbacterial endocarditis, disseminated intravascular coagulation). Neurologic or muscular symptoms can develop 6 months to 4 years before the lung tumor is detected. One of the more common of these problems is weakness and wasting of the proximal muscles of the pelvic and shoulder girdles, with decreased deep tendon reflexes but without sensory changes. Hypercalcemia is seen most often in persons with squamous cell carcinoma, hematologic syndromes in persons with adenocarcinomas, and the remaining syndromes in persons with small cell neoplasms.[1] Manifestations of the paraneoplastic syndrome may precede the onset of other signs of lung cancer and may lead to discovery of an occult tumor.

DIAGNOSIS AND TREATMENT

The diagnosis of lung cancer is based on a careful history and physical examination and other tests such as chest radiography, bronchoscopy, cytologic studies (Papanicolaou's test) of the sputum or bronchial washings, percutaneous needle biopsy of lung tissue, and scalene lymph node biopsy. CT scans, MRI studies, and ultrasonography are used to locate lesions and evaluate the extent of the disease. The carcinoembryonic antigen (CEA) is produced by undifferentiated lung tumor cells; high CEA titers usually correlate with extensive disease. This test often is used to follow the progress of the disease and its response to treatment.

Like other types of cancer, lung cancers are classified according to cell type (*i.e.*, squamous cell carcinoma, adenocarcinoma, and large cell carcinoma) and staged according to the TNM system, which was revised in 1996 (see Chapter 8). These classifications are used for treatment planning. Small cell carcinoma is not evaluated by the TNM system but staged as limited (confined to the one hemithorax and hilar, mediastinal, and supraclavicular nodes) and extensive (spread to more distant sites).[21,50]

Treatment methods for lung cancer include surgery, radiation therapy, and chemotherapy.[21] These treatments may be used singly or in combination. Surgery is used for the removal of small, localized tumors. It can involve a lobectomy, pneumonectomy, or segmental resection of the lung. Radiation therapy can be used as a definitive or main treatment modality, as part of a combined treatment plan, or for palliation of symptoms. Because of the frequency of metastases, chemotherapy often is used in treating lung cancer. Combination chemotherapy, which uses a regimen of several drugs, usually is used. Chemotherapy is the treatment of choice for small cell carcinoma. Advances in the use of combination chemotherapy have improved the outlook for persons with small cell carcinoma. National Cancer Institute studies report that 10% of persons with limited-stage disease and 5% of all persons with small cell carcinoma treated with combination chemotherapy have survived 10 years or longer.[51]

In summary, cancer of the lung is a leading cause of death among men and women between the ages of 50 and 75 years, and the death rate is increasing among women. In the United States, the increased death rate has coincided with an increase in cigarette smoking. Industrial hazards, such as exposure to asbestos, increase the risk for development of lung cancer. Of all forms of lung cancer, bronchogenic carcinoma is the most common, accounting for 90% to 95% of cases. Because lung cancer develops insidiously, it often is far advanced before it is diagnosed, a fact that is used to explain the poor 5-year survival rate.

The manifestations of lung cancer can be attributed to the involvement of the lung and adjacent structures, the effects of local spread and metastasis, and the nonmetastatic paraneoplastic manifestations involving endocrine, neurologic, and connective tissue function. As with other cancers, lung cancer causes nonspecific symptoms such as anorexia and weight loss. Treatment methods for lung cancer include surgery, irradiation, and chemotherapy.

Respiratory Disorders in Children

After you have completed this section of the chapter, you should be able to meet the following objectives:

♦ Trace the development of the respiratory tract through the five stages of embryonic and fetal development
♦ Cite the function of surfactant in lung function in the neonate
♦ Cite the possible cause and manifestations of bronchopulmonary dysplasia
♦ Describe the physiologic basis for sternal and chest wall retractions and grunting, stridor, and wheezing as signs of respiratory distress in infants and small children
♦ Compare croup, epiglottitis, and bronchiolitis in terms of incidence by age, site of infection, and signs and symptoms
♦ List the signs of impending respiratory failure in small children

Acute respiratory disease is the most common cause of illness in infancy and childhood, accounting for 50% of illness in children younger than 5 years of age and 30% of illness in children between 5 and 12 years of age.[52] This section focuses on (1) lung development, with an emphasis on the developmental basis for lung disorders in children; (2) respiratory disorders in the neonate; and (3) respiratory infections in children. A discussion of bronchial asthma in children and cystic fibrosis is included in Chapter 29.

LUNG DEVELOPMENT

Although other body systems are physiologically ready for extrauterine life as early as 25 weeks of gestation, the lungs require much longer. Immaturity of the respiratory system is a major cause of morbidity and mortality in infants born prematurely. Even at birth, the lungs are not fully mature, and additional growth and maturation continue well into childhood.

Lung development may be divided into five stages: embryonic period, pseudoglandular period, canicular period, saccular period, and alveolar period.[53,54] The development of the respiratory system begins with the embryonic period (weeks 4 to 6 of gestation), during which a rudimentary lung bud branches from the esophagus to begin formation of the airways and alveolar spaces (Fig. 28-5). The lung bud divides into two lung buds that grow laterally; the right bud gives rise to two secondary buds and the left bud to one secondary bud. Consequently, at maturity, there are three main (primary) bronchi and three lung lobes on the right and only two main bronchi and two lung lobes on the left. Each secondary lung bud subsequently undergoes continuous branching. The tertiary (segmental) bronchi (10 in the right lung and 8 or 9 in the left lung) begin to form during the seventh week.

During the glandular period (weeks 5 to 16), the lungs resemble a gland. During this period, the conducting airways are formed. At 17 weeks, all of the major elements of the lung have formed except the gas exchange structures. Respiration is not possible because the airways end in blind tubes.

The canicular period (weeks 17 to 27) marks the formation of the primitive alveoli. The lumina of the bronchi and bronchioles become much larger, and the lung tissue becomes more highly vascularized. By the 24th week, each bronchiole has given rise to two or more respiratory bronchioles. Respiration is possible at this time because some primitive alveoli have developed at the ends of the bronchioles.[53]

The saccular period (weeks 27 to 35) is devoted to the development of the terminal alveolar sacs, which facilitate gas exchange. During this period, the terminal sacs thin out, and capillaries begin to bulge into the terminal sacs. These thin cells are known as type I alveolar cells. By the 25th to 28th week, sufficient terminal sacs are present to permit survival. Before this time, the premature lungs are incapable of adequate gas exchange. It is not so much the presence of the thin alveolar epithelium as it is the adequate matching of pulmonary vasculature to it that is critical to survival.[53] Type II alveolar cells begin to develop at

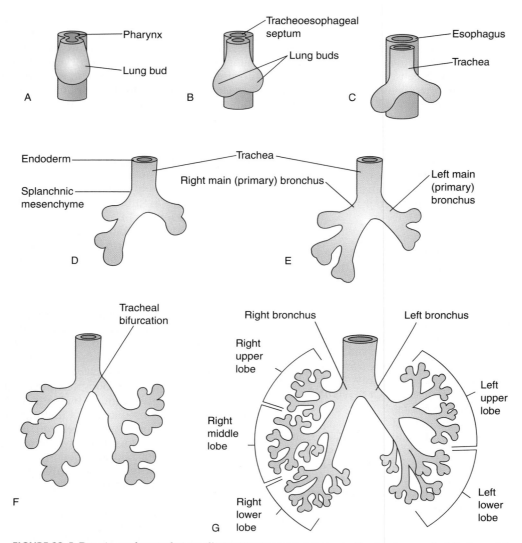

FIGURE 28-5 Drawings of ventral views illustrating successive stages in the development of the bronchi and lungs. (**A–C**) 4 weeks, (**D, E**) 5 weeks, (**F**) 6 weeks, (**G**) 8 weeks. (Moore K. [1993]. *The developing human* [5th ed.]. Philadelphia: W.B. Saunders)

approximately 24 weeks. These cells produce surfactant, a substance capable of lowering the surface tension of the air-alveoli interface (see Chapter 27). By the 28th to 30th week, sufficient amounts of surfactant are available to prevent alveolar collapse when breathing begins.

The alveolar period (late fetal to early childhood) marks the maturation and expansion of the alveoli. Starting as early as 30 weeks and usually by 36 weeks, the saccular structures become alveoli. Alveolar development is characterized by thinning of the pulmonary interstitium and the appearance of a single-capillary network, in which one capillary bulges into each terminal alveolar sac. By the late fetal period, the lungs are capable of respiration because the alveolar-capillary membrane is sufficiently thin to allow for gas exchange.

Although transformation of the lungs from glandlike structures to highly vascular, alveoli-like organs occurs dur-

ing the late fetal period, mature alveoli do not form for some time after birth. The growth of the lung during infancy and early childhood involves an increase in the number rather than the size of the alveoli. Only one eighth to one sixth of the adult number of alveoli are present at birth. There is a relative slowing of alveolar growth during the first 3 months after birth, and this is followed by a rapid increase in alveolar number during the rest of the first year of life, reaching approximately the adult number of 300 million alveoli by 8 years of age.[53]

Development of Breathing in the Fetus and Neonate

The fetal lung is a secretory organ, and fluids and electrolytes are secreted into the potential air spaces. This fluid appears to be important in stimulating alveolar development. For the fetus to complete the transition from intrauterine to extrauterine life, this fluid must be cleared from the lung soon after birth. Presumably with the onset of labor, the secretion of fluid ceases. During the birth process, pressure on the fetal thorax causes the fluid to be expelled from the mouth and nose. When the lungs expand after birth, the fluid moves into the tissues surrounding the alveoli and is then absorbed into the pulmonary capillaries or removed by the lymphatic system.

Fetal breathing movements occur in utero. These movements are irregular in rate and amplitude, ranging from 30 to 70 breaths per minute and become more rapid as gestation advances. Because they are rapid and shallow, these movements do not result in movement of fluid into or out of the fetal lung. Instead, they are thought to condition the respiratory muscles and stimulate lung development. The breathing movements in the fetus become more rapid in response to an increase in carbon dioxide levels and become slower in response to hypoxia.

The major difference between respiration in the fetus and the neonate is that there is complete separation between gas exchange and breathing movements in the fetus. The gas supply and exchange depend entirely on maternal mechanisms controlling placental circulation. At birth, dependence on the placental circulation is terminated, and the infant must integrate the two previously separate functions of gas exchange and respiratory movements. Within seconds of clamping the umbilical cord, the infant takes its first breath, and rhythmic breathing begins and persists for life.

Effective ventilation requires coordinated interaction between the muscles of the upper airways, including those of the pharynx and larynx, the diaphragm, and the intercostal muscles of the chest wall. In infants, a specific sequence of upper airway nerve and muscle activity occurs before and early in inspiration: the tongue moves forward to prevent airway obstruction and the vocal cord abducts, reducing laryngeal resistance. By moving downward, the action of the diaphragm increases chest volume in both the longitudinal and transverse direction. In the infant, the diaphragm inserts more horizontally than in the adult. As a result, contraction of the diaphragm tends to draw the lower ribs inward, especially if the infant is placed in the horizontal position. The function of the intercostal muscles is to lift the ribs during inspiration. In the infant, however, the intercostal muscles are not fully developed, so they function largely to stabilize the chest rather than lift the chest wall.

The chest wall of the neonate is highly compliant; although this is advantageous during the birth process in that it allows for marked distortion to occur without damaging chest structures, it has implications for ventilation during the postnatal period. A striking characteristic of neonatal breathing is the paradoxical inward movement of the upper chest during inspiration, especially during active sleep. This occurs because of decreased activity of the intercostal muscles during active sleep, which allows the contracting diaphragm to pull the highly compliant chest wall inward. Under circumstances such as crying, the intercostal muscles of the neonate function together with the diaphragm to splint the chest wall and prevent its collapse.

Normally, the infant's lungs also are compliant; this is advantageous to the infant with its compliant chest cage, because it takes only small changes in inspiratory pressure to inflate a compliant lung. When respiratory disease develops, lung compliance is reduced and it takes more effort to inflate the lungs. The diaphragm must generate more negative pressure; as a result, the compliant chest wall structures are sucked inward. *Retractions* are abnormal inward movements of the chest wall during inspiration; they may occur intercostally (between the ribs), in the substernal or epigastric area, and in the supraclavicular spaces. Because the chest wall of the infant is compliant, substernal retractions become more obvious with small changes in lung function. Retractions can indicate airway obstruction or atelectasis.

Also influencing the effectiveness of ventilation in the neonate are the intrinsic mechanical properties of the diaphragm. Although much uncertainty remains regarding the functioning of the respiratory muscles in the neonate, it seems that these muscles, particularly in the preterm infant, are undeveloped and poorly adapted for high workloads. The underdeveloped sarcoplasmic reticulum of the premature infant results in an increased contraction and relaxation time. This increased relaxation time may be an important factor in impeding blood flow and limiting oxidative metabolism during increased muscle function.[54]

Airway Resistance

Normal lung inflation requires uninterrupted movement of air through the extrathoracic airways (*i.e.,* nose, pharynx, larynx, and upper trachea) and intrathoracic airways (*i.e.,* bronchi and bronchioles). The neonate (0 to 4 weeks of age) breathes predominantly through the nose and does not adapt well to mouth breathing. Any obstruction of the nose or nasopharynx may increase upper airway resistance and increase the work of breathing.

The airways of the infant and small child are much smaller than those of the adult. Because the resistance to airflow is directly related to the fourth power of the radius (resistance = $1/r^4$), relatively small amounts of mucus secretion, edema, or airway constriction can produce marked changes in airway resistance and airflow (Fig. 28-6). Nasal flaring is a method that infants use to take in more air. This method of breathing increases the size of the nares and decreases the resistance of the small airways.

Normally, the extrathoracic airways in the infant narrow during inspiration and widen during expiration, and the intrathoracic airways widen during inspiration and narrow during expiration.[55] This occurs because the pressure inside the extrathoracic airways reflects the intrapleural pressures that are generated during breathing, whereas the pressure outside the airways is similar to atmospheric pressure. Thus, during inspiration, the pressure inside becomes more negative, causing the airways to narrow, and during expiration it becomes more positive, causing them to widen. In contrast to the extrathoracic airways, the pressure outside the intrathoracic airways is equal to the intrapleural pressure. These airways widen during inspiration as the surrounding intrapleural pressure becomes more negative and pulls them open, and they narrow during expiration as the surrounding pressure becomes more positive.

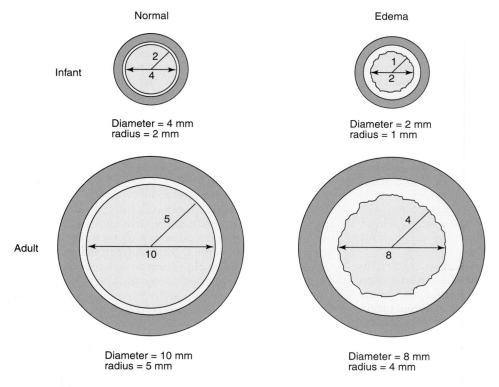

Normal   Edema

Infant

Diameter = 4 mm
radius = 2 mm

Diameter = 2 mm
radius = 1 mm

Adult

Diameter = 10 mm
radius = 5 mm

Diameter = 8 mm
radius = 4 mm

Resistance = 1/radius^4

FIGURE 28-6 Effect of airway swelling on airway radius in infant and adult.

Lung Volumes and Gas Exchange

The functional residual capacity, which is the air left in the lungs at the end of normal expiration, plays an important role in the gas exchange of the infant. In the infant, the functional residual capacity occurs at a higher lung volume than in the older child or adult.[56] This higher end-expiratory volume results from a more rapid respiratory rate, which leaves less time for expiration. However, the increased residual volume is important to the neonate because it holds the airways open throughout all phases of respiration; it favors the reabsorption of intrapulmonary fluids; and it maintains more uniform lung expansion and enhances gas exchange. During sleep, the tone of the upper airway muscles is reduced, so that the time spent in expiration is shorter and the intercostal activity that stabilizes the chest wall is less; this produces a lower end-expiratory volume and less optimal gas exchange during active sleep.[56]

Control of Ventilation

Fetal blood oxygen (PO$_2$) levels normally range from 25 to 30 mm Hg, and carbon dioxide (PCO$_2$) levels range from 45 to 50 mm Hg, independent of any respiratory movements. Any decrease in oxygen levels induces quiet sleep in the fetus with subsequent cessation of breathing movements, both of which lead to a decrease in oxygen consumption. Switching to oxygen derived from the aerated lung at birth causes an immediate increase in PO$_2$ to approximately 50 mm Hg; within a few hours, it increases to approximately 70 mm Hg.[55] These levels, which greatly exceed fetal levels, cause the chemoreceptors (see Chapter 27) to become silent

for several days. Although the infant's PO$_2$ may fluctuate during this critical time, the chemoreceptors do not respond appropriately. It is not until several days after birth that the chemoreceptors "reset" their PO$_2$ threshold; only then do they become the major controller of breathing. However, the response seems to be biphasic, with an initial hyperventilation followed by a decreased respiratory rate and even apnea. In normal neonates, particularly in preterm infants, breathing patterns and respiratory reflexes depend on the arousal state.[56] Periodic breathing and apnea are characteristic of premature infants and reflect patterns of fetal breathing. The fact that they occur with sleep and disappear during wakefulness underscores the importance of arousal.

ALTERATIONS IN BREATHING

Most lung diseases in children produce decreased lung compliance and manifestations of restrictive lung disease, or they increase airway resistance. Children with restrictive lung disease breathe at faster rates, and their respiratory excursions are shallow. Grunting is an audible noise emitted during expiration. An expiratory grunt is common as the child tries to raise the functional residual capacity by closing the glottis at the end of expiration. Grunting is a sign of labored breathing that usually is caused by decreased lung compliance or lung volume; it may serve as a compensatory mechanism for lung dysfunction by increasing lung volume and improving arterial oxygenation.

The pressure needed to overcome airway resistance depends on the rate of airflow as it moves into and out of the lungs; the need is greatest during periods of high flow. Because airway resistance increases the work of breathing, children with obstructive disease take slower, deeper breaths. When the obstruction is in the extrathoracic airways, inspiration is more prolonged than expiration, and an *inspiratory stridor* commonly is heard. When the obstruction is in the intrathoracic airways, expiration is prolonged, and the child makes use of the accessory expiratory muscles.

When obstruction of the extrathoracic airways occurs, as in croup, the pressures distal to the point of obstruction must become more negative to overcome the resistance; this causes collapse of the distal airways, and the increased turbulence of air moving through the obstructed airways produces an audible crowing sound called *stridor.* With intrathoracic airway obstruction as occurs with bronchiolitis and bronchial asthma, the intrapleural pressure becomes more positive during expiration because of air trapping; this causes collapse of intrathoracic airways and produces an audible wheezing or whistling sound during expiration.

RESPIRATORY DISORDERS IN THE NEONATE

The neonatal period is one of transition from placental dependency to air breathing. This transition requires functioning of the surfactant system, conditioning of the respiratory muscles, and establishment of parallel pulmonary and systemic circulations. Respiratory disorders develop in infants who are born prematurely or who have other problems that impair this transition. Among the respiratory disorders of the neonate are the respiratory distress syndrome (RDS), bronchopulmonary dysplasia (BPD), and persistent fetal circulation (*i.e.,* delayed closure of the ductus arteriosus and foramen ovale).

Respiratory Distress Syndrome

Respiratory distress syndrome, also known as *hyaline membrane disease,* is one of the most common causes of respiratory disease in premature infants. In these infants, pulmonary immaturity, together with surfactant deficiency, leads to alveolar collapse. The type II alveolar cells that produce surfactant do not begin to mature until approximately the 25th to 28th weeks of gestation, and consequently, many premature infants are born with poorly functioning type II alveolar cells and have difficulty producing sufficient amounts of surfactant. The incidence of RDS is higher among preterm male infants, white infants, infants of diabetic mothers, and those subjected to asphyxia, cold stress, precipitous deliveries, and delivery by cesarean section (when performed before the 38th week of gestation).

Surfactant synthesis is influenced by several hormones, including insulin and cortisol. Insulin tends to inhibit surfactant production; this explains why infants of insulin-dependent diabetic mothers are at increased risk for development of RDS. Cortisol can accelerate maturation of type II cells and formation of surfactant. The reason that premature infants born by cesarean section presumably are at greater risk for development of RDS is because they are not subjected to the stress of vaginal delivery, which is thought to increase the infants' cortisol levels. These observations have led to administration of corticosteroid drugs before delivery to mothers with infants at high risk for development of RDS.[57]

Surfactant reduces the surface tension in the alveoli, thereby equalizing the retractive forces in the large and small alveoli and reducing the amount of pressure needed to inflate and hold the alveoli open. Without surfactant, the large alveoli remain inflated while the small alveoli become difficult to inflate. At birth, the first breath requires high inspiratory pressures to expand the lungs. With normal levels of surfactant, the lungs retain up to 40% of the residual volume after the first breath, and subsequent breaths require far lower inspiratory pressures.[1] With a surfactant deficiency, the lungs collapse between breaths, making the infant work as hard with each successive breath as with the first breath. The airless portions of the lungs becomes stiff and noncompliant. A hyaline membrane forms inside the alveoli as protein- and fibrin-rich fluids are pulled into the alveolar spaces. The fibrin-hyaline membrane constitutes a barrier to gas exchange, leading to hypoxemia and carbon dioxide retention, a condition that further impairs surfactant production.

Infants with RDS present with multiple signs of respiratory distress, usually within the first 24 hours of birth. Central cyanosis is a prominent sign. Breathing becomes more difficult, and retractions occur as the infant's soft chest wall is pulled in as the diaphragm descends. Grunting sounds occur during expiration. As the tidal volume drops because of atelectasis, the respiration rate increases (usually to 60 to 120 breaths/minute) in an effort to maintain normal minute ventilation. Fatigue may develop rapidly because of the increased work of breathing. The stiff lung of infants with RDS also increases resistance to blood flow in the pulmonary circulation. As a result, a hemodynamically significant patent ductus arteriosus may develop in infants with RDS (see Chapter 24).

Infants with suspected RDS require continuous cardiorespiratory monitoring. Oxygen levels can be assessed through an arterial line (umbilical) or by an transcutaneous oxygen sensor. Treatment includes administration of supplemental oxygen, continuous positive airway pressure through nasal prongs, and often assisted mechanical ventilation. A neutral thermal environment and prevention of hypoglycemia are recommended.

Surfactant therapy is used to prevent and treat RDS. There are two types of surfactants available in the United States: surfactants prepared from animal sources and synthetic surfactants.[58] The surfactants are suspended in saline and administered into the airways, usually through an endotracheal tube. The treatment often is initiated soon after birth in infants who are at high risk for RDS.

Bronchopulmonary Dysplasia

Bronchopulmonary dysplasia is a chronic lung disease that develops in premature infants who were treated with mechanical ventilation, mainly for RDS. The condition is considered to be present if the neonate is oxygen dependent at 36 weeks after gestation. The disorder is thought to be a response of the premature lung to early injury. High inspired oxygen concentration and injury from positive-pressure ventilation (*i.e.,* barotrauma) have been implicated. Newer therapies such as administration of surfactants, high-frequency ventilation, and prenatal or postnatal administration of corticosteroids may have altered the severity of BPD, but the condition remains a major health problem.[59,60]

BPD is characterized by chronic respiratory distress, persistent hypoxemia when breathing room air, reduced lung compliance, increased airway resistance, and severe expiratory flow limitation. There is a mismatching of ventilation and perfusion with development of hypoxemia and hypercapnia. Pulmonary vascular resistance may be increased and pulmonary hypertension and cor pulmonale (*i.e.,* right heart failure associated with lung disease) may develop. The infant with BPD may have tachycardia, shallow breathing, chest retractions, cough, barrel chest, and poor weight gain. Clubbing of the fingers occurs in children with severe disease. In infants with right heart failure, tachycardia, tachypnea, hepatomegaly, and periorbital edema develop.

The treatment is mechanical ventilation and administration of adequate oxygenation. Weaning from ventilation is accomplished gradually, and some infants may require ventilation at home. Rapid lung growth occurs during the first year of life, and lung function usually improves. Adequate nutrition is essential for recovery of infants with BPD.

Most adolescents and young adults who had severe BPD during infancy have some degree of pulmonary dysfunction, consisting of airway obstruction, airway hyperreactivity, or hyperinflation.

RESPIRATORY INFECTIONS IN CHILDREN

In children, respiratory tract infections are common, and although they are troublesome, they usually are not serious. Frequent infections occur because the immune system of infants and small children has not been exposed to many common pathogens; consequently, they tend to contract infections with each new exposure. Although most such infections are not serious, the small size of an infant or child's airways tends to foster impaired airflow and obstruction. For example, an infection that causes only sore throat and hoarseness in an adult may result in serious airway obstruction in a small child.

Upper Airway Infections

Two serious upper respiratory tract infections are relatively common during early childhood—croup and epiglottitis. Croup is the more common one, and it usually is benign and self-limited. Epiglottitis is a rapidly progressive and life-threatening condition. The site of involvement is illustrated in Figure 28-7, and the characteristics of both infections are described in Table 28-2.

Obstruction of the upper airways because of infection tends to exert its greatest effect during the inspiratory phase of respiration. Movement of air through an obstructed upper airway, particularly the vocal cords in the larynx, causes stridor.[61] Impairment of the expiratory phase of respiration also can occur, causing wheezing. With mild to moderate obstruction, inspiratory stridor is more prominent than expiratory wheezing because the airways tend to dilate with expiration. When the swelling and obstruction become se-

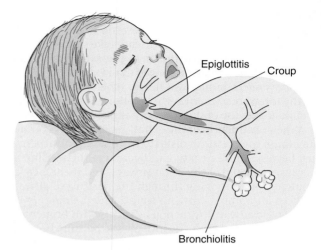

FIGURE 28-7 Location of airway obstruction in epiglottitis, acute laryngotracheobronchitis (croup), and bronchiolitis. (Courtesy of Carole Russell Hilmer, C.M.I.)

vere, the airways no longer can dilate during expiration, and both stridor and wheezing occur.

Cartilaginous support of the trachea and the larynx is poorly developed in infants and small children. These structures are soft and tend to collapse when the airway is obstructed and the child cries, causing the inspiratory pressures to become more negative. When this happens, the stridor and inspiratory effort are increased. The phenomenon of airway collapse in the small child is analogous to what happens when a thick beverage, such as a milkshake, is drunk through a soft paper straw. The straw collapses when the negative pressure produced by the sucking effort exceeds the flow of liquid through the straw.

Viral Croup. Croup is characterized by inspiratory stridor, hoarseness, and a barking cough. The British use the term *croup* to describe the cry of the crow or raven, and this is undoubtedly how the term originated.

Viral croup, more appropriately called *acute laryngotracheobronchitis,* is a viral infection that affects the larynx, trachea, and bronchi. The parainfluenza viruses account for approximately 75% all cases; the remaining 25% are caused by adenoviruses, respiratory syncytial virus, influenza A and B viruses, and measles virus.[61] Viral croup usually is seen in children 3 months to 5 years of age. The condition may affect the entire laryngotracheal tree, but because the subglottic area is the narrowest part of the respiratory tree in this age group, the obstruction usually is greatest in this area. For example, the subglottic airway in the 1- to 2-year-old child is approximately 6.5 mm in diameter, and 1 mm of edema can reduce the cross-sectional area by 50%.[52]

Although the respiratory manifestations of croup often appear suddenly, they usually are preceded by upper respiratory infections that cause rhinorrhea (*i.e.,* runny nose), coryza (*i.e.,* common cold), hoarseness, and a low-grade fever. In most children, the manifestation of croup advances only to stridor and slight dyspnea before they begin to recover. The symptoms usually subside when the child is

TABLE 28-2 ✦ Characteristics of Epiglottitis, Croup, and Bronchiolitis in Small Children			
Characteristics	**Epiglottitis**	**Croup**	**Bronchiolitis**
Common causative agent	*Haemophilus influenzae* type B bacterium	Mainly parainfluenza virus	Respiratory syncytial virus
Most commonly affected age group	2–7 years (peak 3–5 years)	3 months to 5 years	Less than 2 years (most severe in infants younger than 6 months)
Onset and preceding history	Sudden onset	Usually follows symptoms of a cold	Preceded by stuffy nose and other signs
Prominent features	Child appears very sick and toxic Sits with mouth open and chin thrust forward Low-pitched stridor, difficulty swallowing, fever, drooling, anxiety *Danger of airway obstruction and asphyxia*	Stridor and a wet, barking cough Usually occurs at night Relieved by exposure to cold or moist air	Breathlessness, rapid, shallow breathing, wheezing, cough, and retractions of lower ribs and sternum during inspiration
Usual treatment	Hospitalization Intubation or tracheotomy Treatment with appropriate antibiotic	Mist tent or vaporizer Administration of oxygen	Supportive treatment, administration of oxygen and hydration

exposed to moist air. For example, letting the bathroom shower run and then taking the child into the bathroom often brings prompt and dramatic relief of symptoms. Exposure to cold air also seems to relieve the airway spasm; often, the severe symptoms are relieved simply because the child is exposed to cold air on the way to the hospital emergency room. Viral croup does not respond to antibiotics; expectorants, bronchodilating agents, and antihistamines are not helpful. The child should be disturbed as little as possible and carefully monitored for signs of respiratory distress.

Airway obstruction may progress in some children. As obstruction increases, the stridor becomes continuous and is associated with nasal flaring with substernal and intercostal retractions. Agitation and crying aggravate the signs and symptoms, and the child prefers to sit up or be held upright. In the cyanotic, pale, or obstructed child, any manipulation of the pharynx, including use of a tongue depressor, can cause cardiorespiratory arrest and should be done only in a medical setting that has the facilities for emergency airway management. Other treatments may be required when a humidifier or mist tent is ineffective. One method is to administer a racemic mixture of epinephrine (L-epinephrine and D-epinephrine) by positive-pressure breathing through a face mask.[61] Establishment of an artificial airway may become necessary in severe airway obstruction.

Spasmodic Croup. Spasmodic croup manifests with symptoms similar to those of acute viral croup. Because the child is afebrile and lacks other manifestations of the viral prodrome, it is thought that it may have an allergic origin. Spasmodic croup characteristically occurs at night and tends to recur with respiratory tract infections. The episode usually lasts several hours and may recur several nights in a row.

Most children with spasmodic croup can be effectively managed at home. An environment of high humidification (*i.e.*, cold-water room humidifier or taking the child into a bathroom with a warm, running shower) lessens irritation and prevents drying of secretions.

Epiglottitis. Acute epiglottitis is a dramatic, potentially fatal condition most often caused by the *H. influenzae* type B bacterium. It is seen less commonly since the widespread use of immunization against *H. influenzae* type B. The condition usually occurs in children 2 to 7 years of age, with a peak incidence at approximately 3.5 years.[61] It is characterized by inflammatory edema of the supraglottic area, including the epiglottis and pharyngeal structures, that comes on suddenly, bringing danger of airway obstruction and asphyxia. Within a matter of hours, epiglottitis may progress to complete obstruction of the airway and death unless adequate treatment is instituted.

The child appears pale, toxic, and lethargic and assumes a distinctive position—sitting up with the mouth open and the chin thrust forward. The child has difficulty in swallowing, a muffled voice, drooling, fever, and extreme anxiety. Moderate to severe respiratory distress is evident. There is inspiratory and sometimes expiratory stridor, flaring of the nares, and inspiratory retractions of the suprasternal notch and supraclavicular and intercostal spaces. Usually, no other family members are ill with acute respiratory disease.

The child with epiglottitis requires immediate hospitalization. Immediate establishment of an airway by endotracheal tube or tracheotomy usually is needed. If epiglottitis is suspected, the child should never be forced to lie down because this causes the epiglottis to fall backward and may lead to complete airway obstruction. Examination of the throat with a tongue blade or other instrument may cause cardiopulmonary arrest and should be done only by medical personnel experienced in intubation of small children. It also is unwise to attempt any procedure, such as drawing blood, that would heighten the child's anxiety, because this also could precipitate airway spasm and cause death. Recovery from epiglottitis usually is rapid and uneventful after an adequate airway has been established and appropriate antibiotic therapy has been initiated.

Epiglottitis can occur in adults as well as children. The incidence is low (an estimated 9.7 cases per 1 million persons) but appears to be increasing. In adults, epiglottitis may present with acute respiratory compromise or as a milder form of disease. Although the causative agent or agents have not been identified, *H. influenzae* does not appear to be a primary causative agent in adults. Airway closure is less of a threat in adults; it does occur, however, and provision for emergency tracheotomy should be available.[62]

Lower Airway Infections

Lower airway infections produce air trapping with prolonged expiration. Wheezing results from bronchospasm, mucosal inflammation, and edema. The child presents with increased expiratory effort, increased respiratory rate, and wheezing. If the infection is severe, there also are marked intercostal retractions and signs of impending respiratory failure.

Acute bronchiolitis is a viral infection of the lower airways, most commonly caused by the respiratory syncytial virus.[63] Other viruses, such as parainfluenza 3 virus and some adenoviruses, as well as mycoplasma, also are causative. The infection produces inflammatory obstruction of the small airways and necrosis of the cells lining the lower airways. It occurs during the first 2 years of life, with a peak incidence between 3 to 6 months of age. The source of infection usually is a family member with a minor respiratory illness. Older children and adults tolerate bronchiolar edema much better than infants and do not manifest the clinical picture of bronchiolitis. Because the resistance to airflow in a tube is related to the fourth power of the radius, even minor swelling of bronchioles in an infant can produce profound changes in airflow.

Most affected infants in whom bronchiolitis develops have a history of a mild upper respiratory tract infection. These symptoms usually last several days and may be accompanied by fever and diminished appetite. There is then a gradual development of respiratory distress, characterized by a wheezy cough, dyspnea, and irritability. The infant usually is able to take in sufficient air but has trouble exhaling it. Air becomes trapped in the lung distal to the site of obstruction and interferes with gas exchange. Hypoxemia and, in severe cases, hypercapnia may develop. Airway obstruction may produce air trapping and hyperinflation of the lungs or collapse of the alveoli. Infants with acute bronchiolitis have a typical appearance, marked by breathlessness with rapid respirations, a distressing cough, and retractions of the lower ribs and sternum. Crying and feeding exaggerate these signs. Wheezing and rales may or may not be present, depending on the degree of airway obstruction. In infants with severe airway obstruction, wheezing decreases as the airflow diminishes. Usually, the most critical phase of the disease is the first 48 to 72 hours. Cyanosis, pallor, listlessness, and sudden diminution or absence of breath sounds indicate impending respiratory failure. The characteristics of bronchiolitis are described in Table 28-2.

Infants with respiratory distress usually are hospitalized. Treatment is supportive and includes administration of humidified oxygen to relieve hypoxia. Elevation of the head facilitates respiratory movements and avoids airway compression. Handling is kept at a minimum to avoid tiring. Because the infection is viral, antibiotics are not effective and are given only for a secondary bacterial infection. Dehydration may occur as the result of increased insensible water losses because of the rapid respiratory rate and feeding difficulties, and measures to ensure adequate hydration are needed. Recovery usually begins after the first 48 to 72 hours and usually is rapid and complete.

Signs of Impending Respiratory Failure

Respiratory problems of infants and small children often are of sudden origin, and recovery usually is rapid and complete. Children are at risk for the development of airway obstruction and respiratory failure resulting from obstructive disorders or lung infection. The child with epiglottitis is at risk for airway obstruction. The child with bronchiolitis is at risk for respiratory failure resulting from impaired gas exchange. Children with impending respiratory failure due to airway or lung disease have rapid breathing, exaggerated use of the accessory muscles, retractions, which are more pronounced in the child than in the adult because of more compliant chest, nasal flaring, and grunting during expiration.[64] The signs and symptoms of impending respiratory failure are listed in Chart 28-1.

Respiratory failure due to central nervous system conditions such as narcotic overdose or brain tumor usually cause a decreased ventilatory drive and hypoventilation.

In summary, acute respiratory disease is the most common cause of illness in infancy and childhood, accounting for 50% of illnesses in children younger than 5 years of age and 30% of illnesses in children between 5 and 12 years of age. Although other body systems are physiologically ready for extrauterine life as early as

---

CHART 28-1

Signs of Respiratory Distress and Impending Respiratory Failure in the Infant and Small Child

Severe increase in respiratory effort, including severe retractions or grunting, decreased chest movement
Cyanosis that is not relieved by administration of oxygen (40%)
Heart rate of 150 per minute or greater and increasing
Bradycardia
Very rapid breathing (rate 60 per minute in the newborn to 6 months or above 30 per minute in children 6 months to 2 years)
Very depressed breathing (rate 20 per minute or below)
Retractions of the supraclavicular area, sternum, epigastrium, and intercostal spaces
Extreme anxiety and agitation
Fatigue
Decreased level of consciousness

25 weeks of gestation, the lungs take longer. Immaturity of the respiratory system is a major cause of morbidity and mortality in premature infants.

Lung development may be divided into five stages: embryonic period, glandular period, canicular period, saccular period, and alveolar period. The first three phases are devoted to development of the conducting airways, and the last two phases are devoted to development of the gas exchange portion of the lung. By the 25th to 28th weeks of gestation, sufficient terminal air sacs are present to permit survival. It is also during this period that type II alveolar cells, which produce surfactant, begin to function. Lung development is incomplete at birth; an infant is born with only one eighth to one sixth the adult number of alveoli. Alveoli continue to be formed during early childhood, reaching the adult number of 300 million alveoli by 5 to 6 years of age.

Children with restrictive lung disease breathe at faster rates, and their respiratory excursions are shallow. An expiratory grunt is common as the child tries to raise the functional residual capacity by closing the glottis at the end of expiration. Obstruction of the extrathoracic airways often produces turbulence of airflow and an audible inspiratory crowing sound called *stridor*, and obstruction of the intrathoracic airways produces an audible expiratory wheezing or whistling sound. RDS is one of the most common causes of respiratory disease in premature infants. In these infants, pulmonary immaturity, together with surfactant deficiency, leads to alveolar collapse. BPD is a chronic pulmonary disease that develops in premature infants who were treated with mechanical ventilation.

Because of the smallness of the airway of infants and children, respiratory tract infections in these groups often are more serious. Infections that may cause only a sore throat and hoarseness in the adult may produce serious obstruction in the child. Among the respiratory tract infections that affect small children are croup, epiglottitis, and bronchiolitis. Epiglottitis is a life-threatening supraglottic infection that may cause airway obstruction and asphyxia.

References

1. Cotran R.S., Kumar V., Collins T. (Eds.). (1999). *Robbins' pathologic basis of disease* (6th ed., pp. 347–348, 471–473, 741–753). Philadelphia: W.B. Saunders.
2. Kirkpatrick G.L. (1996). The common cold. *Primary Care* 23, 657–673.
3. Herendeen N.E., Szilagy P.G. (2000). In Berhrman R.E., Kliegman R.M., Jenson H.B. (Eds.), *Nelson textbook of pediatrics* (16th ed., pp. 1261–1264). Philadelphia: W.B. Saunders.
4. Johnson K.B., Oski F.A. (Eds.). (1997). *Oski's essential pediatrics* (pp. 128–130). Philadelphia: Lippincott-Raven.
5. Goldman D.A. (2000). Transmission of viral respiratory tract infections in the home. *Pediatric Infectious Disease Journal* 19, S97–S107.
6. Cohen S., Tyrerell D.A.J., Smith A.P. (1991). Psychological stress and susceptibility to the common cold. *New England Journal of Medicine* 325, 606–612.
7. Mossad S.B. (1998). Treatment of the common cold. *British Medical Journal* 317, 33–36.
8. Potter Y.J., Hart L.L. (1993). Zinc lozenges for treatment of the common cold. *Annals of Pharmacotherapeutics* 27, 589–562.
9. Mossad S.B., Maknin M.L., Medendorp S.V., Mason P. (1996). Zinc gluconate lozenges for treating the common cold. *Annals of Internal Medicine* 125, 81–88.
10. Turner R.B., Wecker M.T., Pohl G., Witek T.J., McNally E., St George R., Winther B., Hayden F.G. (1999). Efficacy of tremacamra, a soluble intercellular adhesion molecule 1, for experimental rhinovirus infection. *Journal of the American Medical Association* 281, 1797–1804.
11. Fagnan L.J. (1998). Acute sinusitis: A cost-effective approach to diagnosis and treatment. *American Family Practitioner* 58(8), 1795–1806.
12. Reuler J.B., Lucas L.M., Kumar K.L. (1995). Sinusitis: A review for generalists. *Western Journal of Medicine* 163, 40–48.
13. Ferguson B.J. (1995). Acute and chronic sinusitis. *Postgraduate Medicine* 97 (5), 45–69.
14. Lockey R.F. (1996). Management of chronic sinusitis. *Hospital Practice* 31 (3), 141–151.
15. Hollingsworth H.M. (1996). Allergic rhinoconjunctivitis: Current therapy. *Hospital Practice* 31 (6), 61–73.
16. Advisory Committee on Immunization Practices. (2000). Prevention and control of influenza: Recommendations of the Advisory Committee on Immunization Practices (ACIP). *Morbidity and Mortality Weekly Report* 49 (RR-3), 1–38.
17. Small P.A. (1990). Influenza: Pathogenesis and host defenses. *Hospital Practice* 25 (11A), 51–62.
18. Montalto N.J., Gum K.D., Ashley J.V. (2000). Updated treatment for influenza A and B. *American Family Physician* 62, 2467–2476.
19. Wenzel R.P. (2000). Expanding the treatment options for influenza. *Journal of the American Medical Association* 283, 1057–1059.
20. Couch R.B. (2000). Drug therapy: Prevention and treatment of influenza. *New England Journal of Medicine* 343, 1778–1787.
21. Chestnutt M.S., Prendergast T.J. (2001). Lung. In Tierney L.M., McPhee S.J., Papadakis M.A. (Eds.), *Current medical diagnosis and treatment* (40th ed., pp. 291–313). New York: Lange Medical Books/McGraw-Hill.
22. Marrie T.J. (1998). Community-acquired pneumonia: Etiology, treatment. *Infectious Disease Clinics of North America* 12, 723–739.
23. Fine M.J., Chowdry T., Ketema A. (1998). Outpatient management of community-acquired pneumonia. *Hospital Practice* 33(6), 123–133.
24. American Thoracic Society. (1993). Guidelines for the initial management of adults with community-acquired pneumonia: Diagnosis, assessment of severity, and initial antimicrobial therapy. *American Review of Respiratory Disease* 148, 1418–1426.
25. Centers for Disease Control and Prevention. (1996). Prevention of pneumococcal disease: Recommendations of the Advisory Committee on Immunization Practices (ACIP). *Morbidity and Mortality Weekly Report* 46 (RR-8), 1–24.
26. Catterall J.R. (1999). *Streptococcus pneumoniae. Thorax* 54, 929–937.
27. Centers for Disease Control and Prevention. (1996). Defining the public health impact of drug-resistant *Streptococcus pneumoniae. Morbidity and Mortality Weekly Report* 45 (RR-1), 1–20.
28. Centers for Disease Control and Prevention. (2000). Preventing pneumococcal disease among infants and small

children: Recommendations of the Advisory Committee on Immunization Practices (ACIP). *Morbidity and Mortality Weekly Report* 46 (RR-9), 1–38.

29. Chambers H.F. (2001). Infectious diseases: Bacterial and chlamydial. In Tierney L.M., McPhee S.J., Papadakis M.A. (Eds.), *Current medical diagnosis and treatment* (40th ed., pp. 1368–1369). New York: Lange Medical Books/ McGraw-Hill.

30. Stout J.E., Yu V.C. (1997). Legionellosis. *New England Journal of Medicine* 337, 682–688.

31. McEachen R., Campbell G.D. (1998). Hospital-acquired pneumonia: Epidemiology, etiology, and treatment. *Infectious Disease Clinics of North America* 12 (3), 761–779.

32. Collin B.A., Ramphal R. (1998). Pneumonia in the compromised host including cancer patients and transplant patients. *Infectious Disease Clinics of North America* 12 (3), 781–801.

33. Genta R.M., Conner D.H. (1999). Infectious and parasitic diseases. In Rubin E., Farber J.L. (Eds.), *Pathology* (3rd ed., pp. 451–452). Philadelphia: Lippincott Williams & Wilkins.

34. Wilkin A., Feinberg J. (1999). *Pneumocystis carinii* pneumonia: A clinical review. *American Family Physician* 60 (16), 1699–1714.

35. U.S. Public Health Service (USPHS) and Infectious Diseases Society of America (IDSA). (1999). 1999 USPHS/IDSA guidelines for the prevention of opportunistic infections in persons infected with human immunodeficiency virus. *Morbidity and Mortality Weekly Report* 48 (RR-10), 1–59.

36. American Lung Association. (2000). Trends in tuberculosis morbidity and mortality. [On-line]. Available: http://www. lungusa.org.

37. Travis W.D., Farber J.L., Rubin E. (1999). The respiratory system. In Rubin E., Farber J.E. (Eds.), *Pathology* (3rd ed., pp. 606–608). Philadelphia: Lippincott Williams & Wilkins.

38. American Thoracic Society and Centers for Disease Control and Prevention. (2000). Diagnostic standards and classification of tuberculosis in adults and children. *American Review of Respiratory Disease* 161, 1376–1395.

39. American Thoracic Society and Centers for Disease Control and Prevention. (1994). Treatment of tuberculosis and tuberculosis infection in adults and children. *American Journal of Critical Care Medicine* 149, 1359–1374.

40. Spiegler P., Ilowitz J. (1999). Multiple-drug-resistant tuberculosis: Parts 1 and 2. *Emergency Medicine* 31 (6, 7), 10–23.

41. Havlir D.V., Barnes P.F. (1999). Tuberculosis in patients with human immunodeficiency virus infection. *New England Journal of Medicine* 380, 367–372.

42. Centers for Disease Control and Prevention. (1996). The role of BCG vaccine in the prevention and control of tuberculosis in the United States. *Morbidity and Mortality Weekly Report* 45 (RR-4), 1–19.

43. Dismukes W.E. (1996). Histoplasmosis. In Bennett J.C., Plum F. (Eds.), *Cecil textbook of medicine* (20th ed., pp. 1816–1820). Philadelphia: W.B. Saunders.

44. Hammarsten J.E., Hammarsten J.F. (1990). Histoplasmosis: Recognition and treatment. *Hospital Practice* 25 (6A), 95–126.

45. Hamill R.J. (2001). Infectious disease: Mycotic. In Tierney L.M., McPhee S.J., Papadakis M.A. (Eds.), *Current medical diagnosis and treatment* (40th ed., pp. 1482–1490). New York: Lange Medical Books/McGraw-Hill.

46. Galgiani J.N. (1999). Coccidioidomycosis: A regional disease of national importance. *Annals of Internal Medicine* 130, 293–300.

47. Vaz A., Pineda-Roman M., Thomas A.R., Carlson R.W. (1998). Coccidioidomycosis: An update. *Hospital Practice* 33 (9), 105–120.

48. Dismukes W.E. (1996). Blastomycosis. In Bennett J.C., Plum F. (Eds.), *Cecil textbook of medicine* (20th ed., pp. 1821–1822). Philadelphia: W.B. Saunders.

49. American Cancer Society. (2000). Lung cancer: Overview. [On-line]. Available: http://www3.cancer.org/cancerinfo/.

50. Petty T.L. (1997). Lung cancer. *Postgraduate Medicine* 101 (3), 121–122.

51. Matthay R.A., Carter D.C. (1995). Lung neoplasms. In George R.B., Light R.W., Matthay M.A., Matthay R.A. (Eds.), *Chest medicine* (3rd ed., pp. 393–422). Baltimore: Williams & Wilkins.

52. Zander J., Hazinski M.F. (1992). Pulmonary disorders. In Hazinski M.F. (Ed.), *Nursing care of the critically ill child* (2nd ed., pp. 395–407). Philadelphia: W.B. Saunders.

53. Moore K., Persaud T.V.N (1998). *The developing human* (6th ed., pp. 262–269). Philadelphia: W.B. Saunders.

54. Haddad G.G., Fontán J.J.P. (2000). Development of the respiratory system. In Behrman R.E., Kliegman R.M., Jensen H.L. (Eds.), *Nelson textbook of pediatrics* (16th ed., pp. 1235–1248). Philadelphia: W.B. Saunders.

55. Fontán J.J.P., Haddad G.G. (2000). Respiratory pathophysiology. In Behrman R.E., Kliegman R.M., Jensen H.L. (Eds.), *Nelson textbook of pediatrics* (16th ed., pp. 1237–1240). Philadelphia: W.B. Saunders.

56. Oski F.A. (Ed.). (1994). *Principles and practices of pediatrics* (2nd ed., pp. 336–339, 365–370). Philadelphia: J.B. Lippincott.

57. Stoll B.J., Kliegman R.M. (2000). The fetus and neonatal infant. In Behrman R.E., Kliegman R.M., Jensen H.L. (Eds.), *Nelson textbook of pediatrics* (16th ed., pp. 498–505). Philadelphia: W.B. Saunders.

58. *Drug Facts and Comparisons*. (2001). Lung surfactants (55th ed., pp. 704–710). St. Louis: Wolters Kluwer.

59. McColley S.A. (1998). Bronchopulmonary dysplasia. *Pediatric Clinics of North America* 45, 573–585.

60. Alexander K.C., Leung M.B.B.C., Cho H. (1999). Diagnosis of stridor in children. *American Family Physician* 60, 2289–2296.

61. Orenstein D.M. (2000). Acute inflammatory upper airway obstruction. In Behrman R.E., Kiegman R.M., Jensen H.L. (Eds.), *Nelson textbook of pediatrics* (16th ed., pp. 1274–1278). Philadelphia: W.B. Saunders.

62. Baker A.S., Eavey R.D. (1986). Adult supraglottitis (epiglottitis). *New England Journal of Medicine* 314, 1185–1186.

63. Orenstein D.M. (2000). Bronchitis. In Behrman R.E., Kliegman R.M., Jensen H.L. (Eds.), *Nelson textbook of pediatrics* (16th ed., pp. 1284–1287). Philadelphia: W.B. Saunders.

64. Derish M.T., Frankel L.R. (2000). Respiratory distress and failure. In Behrman R.E., Kliegman R.M., Jensen H.L. (Eds.), *Nelson textbook of pediatrics* (16th ed., pp. 266–268). Philadelphia: W.B. Saunders.

Chapter 29

Alterations in Respiration: Alterations in Ventilation and Gas Exchange

The major function of the lungs is to oxygenate and remove carbon dioxide from the blood as a means of supporting the metabolic functions of body cells. The gas exchange function of the lungs depends on a system of open airways, expansion of the lungs, an adequate area for gas diffusion, and blood flow that carries the gases to the rest of the body. This chapter focuses on diseases that disrupt ventilation and gas exchange and on respiratory failure and hyperventilation.

Disorders of Lung Inflation

After you have completed this section of the chapter, you should be able to meet the following objectives:

✦ State the characteristics of pleural pain and differentiate it from other types of chest pain

✦ Differentiate among the causes and manifestations of spontaneous pneumothorax, secondary pneumothorax, and tension pneumothorax

✦ Characterize the pathogenesis and manifestations of pleural effusion

✦ State the difference between a transudate and exudate as it relates to pleural effusion

✦ Describe the causes and manifestations of atelectasis

Air entering through the airways inflates the lung, and the negative pressure in the pleural cavity keeps the lung from collapsing. Disorders of lung inflation are caused by conditions that produce lung compression or lung collapse. There can be compression of the lung by an accumulation of fluid in the intrapleural space, complete collapse of an entire lung as in pneumothorax, or collapse of a segment of the lung as in atelectasis.

DISORDERS OF THE PLEURA

The pleura is a thin, double-layered membrane that encases the lungs. The inner visceral layer lies adjacent to the lung; the outer parietal layer lines the inner aspect of the chest wall, the superior aspect of the diaphragm, and the mediastinum. The visceral and parietal pleurae are separated by a thin layer of serous fluid, and the potential space between these two layers is called the *pleural* or *thoracic cavity* (Fig. 29-1). The right and left pleural cavities are separated by the mediastinum, which contains the heart and other thoracic structures.

Both the chest wall and the lungs have elastic properties. Because of these elastic properties, there is a tendency for the chest wall to expand and move outward and for the lungs to recoil or move inward and collapse (see Chapter 27). As a result of these two opposing forces, the pressure in the pleural cavity becomes negative in relation to alveolar pressure. It is the negative pressure in the pleural cavity that holds the lungs against the chest wall and keeps them from collapsing. Disorders of the pleura include pain, pleural effusion, and pneumothorax.

Pleural Pain

Pain is a frequent symptom of pleuritis, or inflammation of the pleura. Pleuritis is common in infectious processes such as viral respiratory infections or pneumonia that extend to involve the pleura. Most commonly the pain is abrupt in onset, such that the person experiencing it can cite almost to the minute when the pain started. It usually is unilateral and tends to be localized to the lower and lateral part of the chest. When the central part of the diaphragm is irritated, the pain may be referred to the shoulder. The pain is usually made worse by chest movements, such as deep breathing and coughing, that exaggerate pressure changes in the pleural cavity and increase movement of the inflamed or injured pleural surfaces. Because deep breathing is painful, tidal volumes usually are kept small, and breathing be-

Disorders of Pleura

➤ The pleura is a thin, double-layered membrane that encases the lungs.

➤ The two layers of the pleural membrane are separated by the pleural space, in which fluid can accumulate and interfere with lung function.

➤ The opposing forces of the chest wall and the lungs generate a negative pressure in the pleural space that separates the two membrane layers. The pressure in the pleural space, which is negative in relation to intra-alveolar pressure, holds the lungs against the chest wall and keeps them from collapsing. When air is allowed to enter the pleural space, the negative pressure holding the lung against the chest wall is lost and the lung collapses.

comes more rapid. Reflex splinting of the chest muscles may occur, causing a lesser respiratory excursion on the affected side.

It is important to differentiate pleural pain from pain produced by other conditions, such as musculoskeletal strain of chest muscles, bronchial irritation, and myocardial disease. Musculoskeletal pain may occur as the result of frequent, forceful coughing. This type of pain usually is bilateral and located in the inferior portions of the rib cage, where the abdominal muscles insert into the anterior rib cage. It is made worse by movements associated with contraction of the abdominal muscles. The pain associated with irritation of the bronchi usually is substernal and dull in character rather than sharp. It is made worse with coughing but is not affected by deep breathing. Myocardial pain, which is discussed in Chapter 24, usually is located in the substernal area and is not affected by respiratory movements.

Analgesics and nonsteroidal anti-inflammatory drugs (*e.g.*, indomethacin) may be used for pleural pain. Although these agents reduce awareness of pleural pain, they do not entirely relieve the discomfort associated with deep breathing and coughing.

Pleural Effusion

Pleural effusion refers to an abnormal collection of fluid in the pleural cavity (see Fig. 29-1). The fluid may be a transudate, exudate, purulent drainage (empyema), chyle, or blood. Normally, only a thin layer (<10 to 20 mL) of serous fluid separates the visceral and parietal layers of the pleural cavity. Like fluid developing in other transcellular spaces in the body, pleural effusion occurs when the rate of fluid formation exceeds the rate of its removal (see Chapter 31). Five mechanisms have been linked to the abnormal collection of fluid in the pleural cavity: (1) increased capillary

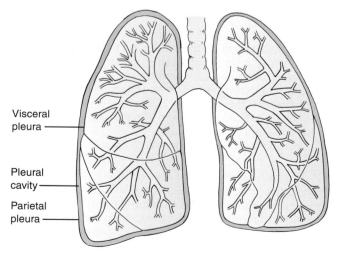

Visceral pleura —

Pleural cavity —

Parietal pleura —

FIGURE 29-1 The parietal and visceral pleura and site of fluid accumulation in pleural effusions.

pressure, as in congestive heart failure; (2) increased capillary permeability, which occurs with inflammatory conditions; (3) decreased colloidal osmotic pressure, such as the hypoalbuminemia occurring with liver disease and nephrosis; (4) increased negative intrapleural pressure, which develops with atelectasis; and (5) impaired lymphatic drainage of the pleural space, which results from obstructive processes such as mediastinal carcinoma.

A transudate consists of serous fluid. The accumulation of a serous transudate in the pleural cavity often is referred to as *hydrothorax*. The condition may be unilateral or bilateral. The most common cause of hydrothorax is congestive heart failure. Other causes are renal failure, nephrosis, liver failure, and malignancy.

An exudate is a pleural fluid having one or more of the following characteristics: a pleural fluid protein to serum protein ratio greater than 0.5; a pleural fluid lactate dehydrogenase (LDH) to serum LDH ratio greater than 0.6; and pleural fluid LDH greater than two thirds the upper limit of normal serum LDH.[1] LDH is an enzyme that is released from inflamed and injured pleural tissue. Because measurements of LDH are easily obtained from a sample of pleural fluid, it is a useful marker for diagnosis of exudative pleural disorders. Conditions that produce exudative pleural effusions are infections, pulmonary infarction, malignancies, rheumatoid arthritis, and lupus erythematosus.

Empyema refers to pus in the pleural cavity. It is caused by direct infection of the pleural space from an adjacent bacterial pneumonia, rupture of a lung abscess into the pleural space, invasion from a subdiaphragmatic infection, or infection associated with trauma.

Chylothorax is the effusion of lymph in the thoracic cavity.[2] Chyle, a milky fluid containing chylomicrons, is found in the lymph fluid originating in the gastrointestinal tract. The thoracic duct transports chyle to the central circulation. Chylothorax also results from trauma, inflammation, or malignant infiltration obstructing chyle transport from the thoracic duct into the central circulation. It is the most common cause of pleural effusion in the fetus and neonate, resulting from congenital malformation of the thoracic duct or lymph channels.[2] Chylothorax also can occur as a complication of intrathoracic surgical procedures and use of the great veins for total parenteral nutrition and hemodynamic monitoring.

Hemothorax is the presence of blood in the thoracic cavity. Bleeding may arise from chest injury, a complication of chest surgery, malignancies, or rupture of a great vessel such as an aortic aneurysm. Hemothorax may be classified as minimal, moderate, or large.[3] A minimal hemothorax involves the presence of 300 to 500 mL of blood in the pleural space. Small amounts of blood usually are absorbed from the pleural space, and a minimal hemothorax usually clears in 10 to 14 days without complication. A moderate hemothorax (500 to 1000 mL blood) fills approximately one third of the pleural space and may produce signs of lung compression and loss of intravascular volume. It requires immediate drainage and replacement of intravascular fluids. A large hemothorax fills one half or more of one side of the chest; it indicates the presence of 1000 mL or more of blood in the thorax and usually is caused by bleeding from a high-pressure vessel such as an intercostal or mammary artery. It requires immediate drainage and, if the bleeding continues, surgery to control the bleeding. One of the complications of untreated moderate or large hemothorax is fibrothorax—the fusion of the pleural surfaces by fibrin, hyalin, and connective tissue—and in some cases, calcification of the fibrous tissue, which restricts lung expansion.

Manifestations. The manifestations of pleural effusion vary with the cause. Hemothorax may be accompanied by signs of blood loss, and empyema by fever and other signs of inflammation. Fluid in the pleural cavity acts as a space-occupying mass; it causes a decrease in lung expansion on the affected side that is proportional to the amount of fluid collected. The effusion may cause a mediastinal shift toward the contralateral side of the chest with a decrease in lung volume on that side as well as the side with the pneumothorax. Characteristic signs of pleural effusion are dullness or flatness to percussion and diminished breath sounds. Dyspnea, the most common symptom, occurs when fluid compresses the lung, resulting in decreased ventilation. Pleuritic pain usually occurs only when inflammation is present, although constant discomfort may be felt with large effusions. Mild hypoxemia may occur and usually is corrected with supplemental oxygen.

Diagnosis and Treatment. Diagnosis of pleural effusion is based on chest radiographs, chest ultrasound, and computed tomography (CT). Thoracentesis is the aspiration of fluid from the pleural space. It can be used to obtain a sample of pleural fluid for diagnosis, or it can be used for therapeutic purposes. The treatment of pleural effusion is directed at the cause of the disorder. With large effusions, thoracentesis may be used to remove fluid from the intrapleural space and allow for reexpansion of the lung. A palliative method used for treatment of pleural effusions caused by a malignancy is the injection of a sclerosing agent into the pleural cavity. This method of treatment causes obliteration of the pleural space and prevents the reaccumulation of fluid. Open surgical drainage may be necessary in cases of continued effusion.

Pneumothorax

Normally, the pleural cavity is free of air and contains only a thin layer of fluid. When air enters the pleural cavity, it is called *pneumothorax*. Pneumothorax causes partial or complete collapse of the affected lung. Pneumothorax can occur without an obvious cause or injury (*i.e.*, spontaneous pneumothorax) or as a result of direct injury to the chest or major airways (*i.e.*, traumatic pneumothorax). Tension pneumothorax describes a life-threatening condition of excessive pressure in the pleural cavity.

Spontaneous Pneumothorax. Spontaneous pneumothorax occurs when an air-filled bleb, or blister, on the lung surface ruptures. Rupture of these blebs allows atmospheric air from the airways to enter the pleural cavity (Fig. 29-2). Because alveolar pressure normally is greater than pleural pressure, air flows from the alveoli into the pleural space, causing the involved portion of the lung to collapse as a result of its own recoil. Air continues to flow into the pleural

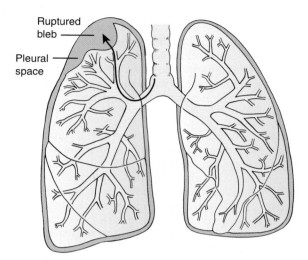

FIGURE 29-2 Mechanism for development of spontaneous pneumothorax.

space until a pressure gradient no longer exists or until the decline in lung size causes the leak to seal. Spontaneous pneumothoraces can be divided into primary and secondary pneumothoraces.[4] Primary spontaneous pneumothorax occurs in otherwise healthy persons. Secondary spontaneous pneumothorax occurs in persons with underlying lung disease.

What causes the air-filled blebs responsible for primary spontaneous pneumothorax and the reasons why they rupture are largely unknown. In primary spontaneous pneumothorax, these blebs usually are located at the top of the lungs. The condition is seen most often in tall boys and young men between 10 and 30 years of age.[4] It has been suggested that the difference in pleural pressure from the top to the bottom of the lung is greater in tall persons and that this difference in pressure may contribute to the development of blebs. Another factor that has been associated with primary spontaneous pneumothorax is smoking. Disease of the small airways related to smoking probably contributes to the condition.

Secondary spontaneous pneumothoraces usually are more serious because they occur in persons with lung disease. They are associated with many different types of lung conditions that cause trapping of gases and destruction of lung tissue, including asthma, tuberculosis, cystic fibrosis, sarcoidosis, bronchogenic carcinoma, and metastatic pleural diseases. The most common cause of secondary spontaneous pneumothorax is emphysema.

Catamenial pneumothorax occurs in relation to the menstrual cycle and usually is recurrent.[4] It typically occurs in women who are 30 to 40 years of age and have a history of endometriosis. It usually affects the right lung and develops within 72 hours of onset of menses. Although the cause of catamenial pneumothorax is unknown, it has been suggested that air may gain access to the peritoneal cavity during menstruation and then enter the pleural cavity through a diaphragmatic defect. Pleural and diaphragmatic endometriosis also have been implicated as causes of the condition.

Traumatic Pneumothorax.   Traumatic pneumothorax may be caused by penetrating or nonpenetrating injuries. Fractured or dislocated ribs that penetrate the pleura are the most common cause of pneumothorax from nonpenetrating chest injuries. Hemothorax often accompanies these injuries. Pneumothorax also may accompany fracture of the trachea or major bronchus or rupture of the esophagus. Persons with pneumothorax due to chest trauma frequently have other complications and may require chest surgery. Medical procedures such as transthoracic needle aspirations, intubation, and positive-pressure ventilation occasionally may cause pneumothorax. Traumatic pneumothorax also can occur as a complication of cardiopulmonary resuscitation.

Tension Pneumothorax.   Tension pneumothorax occurs when the intrapleural pressure exceeds atmospheric pressure. It is a life-threatening condition and occurs when injury to the chest or respiratory structures permits air to enter but not leave the pleural space (Fig. 29-3). This results in a rapid increase in pressure in the chest with compression atelectasis of the unaffected lung, a shift in the mediastinum to the opposite side of the chest, and compression of the vena cava with impairment of venous return to the heart.[5]

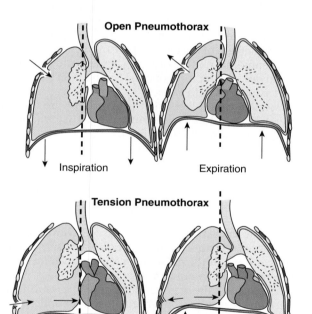

FIGURE 29-3 Open or communicating pneumothorax (**top**) and tension pneumothorax (**bottom**). In an open pneumothorax, air enters the chest during inspiration and exits during expiration. There may be slight inflation of the affected lung due to a decrease in pressure as air moves out of the chest. In tension pneumothorax, air can enter but not leave the chest. As the pressure in the chest increases, the heart and great vessels are compressed and the mediastinal structures are shifted toward the opposite side of the chest. The trachea is pushed from its normal midline position toward the opposite side of the chest, and the unaffected lung is compressed.

Although tension pneumothorax can develop in persons with spontaneous pneumothoraces, it is seen most often in persons with traumatic pneumothoraces. It also may result from mechanical ventilation.

Manifestations. The manifestations of pneumothorax depend on its size and the integrity of the underlying lung. In spontaneous pneumothorax, manifestations of the disorder include development of ipsilateral chest pain in an otherwise healthy person. There is an almost immediate increase in respiratory rate, often accompanied by dyspnea that occurs as a result of the activation of receptors that monitor lung volume. Heart rate is increased. Asymmetry of the chest may occur because of the air trapped in the pleural cavity on the affected side. This asymmetry may be evidenced during inspiration as a lag in the movement of the affected side, with inspiration being delayed until the unaffected lung reaches the same level of pressure as the lung with the air trapped in the pleural space. Percussion of the chest produces a more hyperresonant sound, and breath sounds are decreased or absent over the area of the pneumothorax. With tension pneumothorax, the structures in the mediastinal space shift toward the opposite side of the chest (see Fig. 29-3). When this occurs, the position of the trachea, normally located in the midline of the neck, deviates with the mediastinum. The position of the trachea can be used as a means of assessing for a mediastinal shift. There may be distention of the neck veins and subcutaneous emphysema (*i.e.*, air bubbles in the subcutaneous tissues of the chest and neck) and clinical signs of shock.

Hypoxemia usually develops immediately after a large pneumothorax, followed by vasoconstriction of the blood vessels in the affected lung, causing the blood flow to shift to the unaffected lung. In persons with primary spontaneous pneumothorax, this mechanism usually returns oxygen saturation to normal within 24 hours. Hypoxemia usually is more serious in persons with underlying lung disease in whom secondary spontaneous pneumothorax develops. In these persons, the hypoxemia caused by the partial or total loss of lung function can be life threatening.

Diagnosis and Treatment. Diagnosis of pneumothorax can be confirmed by chest radiograph or CT scan. Blood gas analysis may be done to determine the effect of the condition on blood oxygen levels.

Treatment of pneumothorax varies with the cause and extent of the disorder. Even without treatment, air in the pleural space usually reabsorbs after the pleural leak seals. In small spontaneous pneumothoraces, the air usually reabsorbs spontaneously, and only observation and follow-up chest radiographs are required. Supplemental oxygen may be used to increase the rate at which the air is reabsorbed. In larger pneumothoraces, the air is removed by needle aspiration or a closed drainage system used with or without an aspiration pump. This type of drainage system uses a one-way valve or a tube submerged in water to allow air to exit the pleural space and prevent it from reentering the chest. In secondary pneumothorax, surgical closure of the chest wall defect, ruptured airway, or perforated esophagus may be required.

Emergency treatment of tension pneumothorax involves the prompt insertion of a large-bore needle or chest tube into the affected side of the chest along with one-way valve drainage or continuous chest suction to aid in lung reexpansion. Sucking chest wounds, which allow air to pass in and out of the chest cavity, should be treated by promptly covering the area with an airtight covering (*e.g.*, Vaseline gauze, firm piece of plastic). Chest tubes are inserted as soon as possible.

Because of the risk of recurrence, persons with primary spontaneous pneumothorax should be advised against cigarette smoking, exposure to high altitudes, flying in nonpressurized aircraft, and scuba diving.

ATELECTASIS

Atelectasis means "imperfect expansion"; it refers to the incomplete expansion of a lung or portion of a lung. It can be caused by airway obstruction, lung compression such as occurs in pneumothorax or pleural effusion, or the increased recoil of the lung due to loss of pulmonary surfactant (see Chapter 27). The disorder may be present at birth (*i.e.*, primary atelectasis), or it may develop in the neonatal period or later in life (*i.e.*, acquired or secondary atelectasis).

Primary Atelectasis
Primary atelectasis of the newborn implies that the lung has never been inflated. It is seen most frequently in premature and high-risk infants (Fig. 29-4).

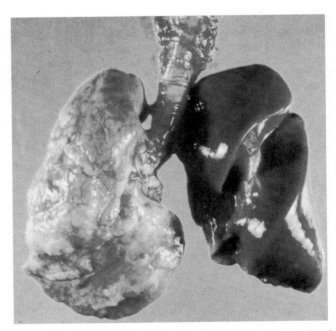

FIGURE 29-4 Atelectasis. The right lung of an infant (left side of photo) is pale and expanded by air, whereas the left lung is collapsed. (Rubin E., Farber J.L. [1994]. *Pathology* [2nd ed.]. Philadelphia: J.B. Lippincott)

Secondary Atelectasis

A secondary form of atelectasis can occur in infants who established respiration and subsequently experienced impairment of lung expansion. Among the causes of secondary atelectasis in the newborn are the respiratory distress syndrome associated with lack of surfactant and airway obstruction due to aspiration of amniotic fluid or blood.

Acquired atelectasis occurs mainly in adults. It is caused most commonly by airway obstruction and lung compression (Fig. 29-5). Obstruction can be caused by a mucus plug in the airway or by external compression by fluid, tumor mass, exudate, or other matter in the area surrounding the airway. A small segment of lung or an entire lung lobe may be involved in obstructive atelectasis. Complete obstruction of an airway is followed by the absorption of air from the dependent alveoli and collapse of that portion of the lung. Breathing high concentrations of oxygen, such as while on a ventilator, increases the rate at which gases are absorbed from the alveoli and predisposes to atelectasis.

The danger of obstructive atelectasis increases after surgery. Anesthesia, pain, administration of narcotics, and immobility tend to promote retention of viscid bronchial secretions and hence airway obstruction. Encouraging a patient to take deep breaths and cough, frequent changes of position, adequate hydration, and early ambulation decrease the likelihood of atelectasis developing.

Another cause of atelectasis is compression of lung tissue. It occurs when the pleural cavity is partially or completely filled with fluid, exudate, blood, a tumor mass, or air. It is observed most commonly in persons with pleural effusion from congestive heart failure or cancer. In compression atelectasis, the mediastinum shifts away from the affected lung.

Manifestations.   The clinical manifestations of atelectasis include tachypnea, tachycardia, dyspnea, cyanosis, signs of hypoxemia, diminished chest expansion, absence of breath sounds, and intercostal retractions. Fever and other signs of infection may develop. Both chest expansion and breath sounds are decreased on the affected side. There may be intercostal retraction (pulling in of the intercostal spaces) over the involved area during inspiration. If the collapsed area is large, the mediastinum and trachea shift to the affected side. Signs of respiratory distress are proportional to the extent of lung collapse.

Diagnosis and Treatment.   The diagnosis of atelectasis is based on signs and symptoms. Chest radiographs are used to confirm the diagnosis. CT scans may be used to show the exact location of the obstruction.

Treatment depends on the cause and extent of lung involvement. It is directed at reducing the airway obstruction or lung compression and at reinflating the collapsed area of the lung. Ambulation and body positions that favor increased lung expansion are used when appropriate. Administration of oxygen may be needed to treat the hypoxemia. Bronchoscopy may be used as a diagnostic and treatment method.

> In summary, disorders of the pleura include pleuritis and pain, pleural effusion, and pneumothorax. Pain is commonly associated with conditions that produce inflammation of the pleura. Characteristically, it is unilateral, abrupt in onset, and exaggerated by respiratory movements. Pleural effusion refers to the abnormal accumulation of fluid in the pleural cavity. The fluid may be a transudate (*i.e.*, hydrothorax), exudate (*i.e.*, empyema), blood (*i.e.*, hemothorax), or chyle (*i.e.*, chylothorax). Pneumothorax refers to an accumulation of air in the pleural cavity with the partial or complete collapse of the lung. It can result from rupture of an air-filled bleb on the lung surface or from penetrating or nonpenetrating injuries. A tension pneumothorax is a life-threatening event in which air progressively accumulates in the thorax, collapsing the lung on the injured side and progressively shifting the mediastinum to the opposite side of the thorax, producing severe cardiorespiratory impairment.
>
> Atelectasis refers to an incomplete expansion of the lung. The disorder may be present at birth (*i.e.*, primary atelectasis), or it may develop in the neonatal period or later in life (*i.e.*, acquired or secondary atelectasis). Primary atelectasis occurs most often in premature and high-risk infants. Acquired atelectasis occurs mainly in adults and is caused most commonly by a mucus plug in the airway or by external compression by fluid, tumor mass, exudate, or other matter in the area surrounding the airway.

▮ Obstructive Airway Disorders

After you have completed this section of the chapter, you should be able to meet the following objectives:

✦ Describe the physiology of bronchial smooth muscle as it relates to airway disease

✦ Explain the changes in pulmonary function studies that occur with airway disease

✦ Characterize the acute or early phase and late phase responses in the pathogenesis of bronchial asthma and

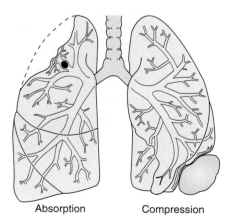

Absorption   Compression

FIGURE 29-5 Atelectasis caused by airway obstruction and absorption of air from the involved lung area on the *left* and by compression of lung tissue on the *right*.

relate them to current methods for treatment of the disorder

✦ Relate the pathologic changes that occur in bronchial asthma to the production of signs and symptoms

✦ Explain the distinction between chronic bronchitis and emphysema in terms of pathology and clinical manifestations

✦ State the chief manifestations of bronchiectasis

✦ Describe the genetic abnormality responsible for cystic fibrosis and state the disorder's effect on lung function

Obstructive airway disorders are caused by disorders that limit expiratory air flow. Bronchial asthma represents a reversible form of airway disease caused by narrowing of airways due to bronchospasm, inflammation, and increased airway secretions. Chronic obstructive airway disease can be caused by a variety of airway diseases, including chronic bronchitis, emphysema, bronchiectasis, and cystic fibrosis.

PHYSIOLOGY OF AIRWAY DISEASE

Air moves through the upper airways (*i.e.*, trachea and major bronchi) into the lower or pulmonary airways (*i.e.*, bronchi and alveoli), which are located in the lung. In the pulmonary airways, the cartilaginous layer that provides support for the trachea and major bronchi gradually disappears and is replaced with crisscrossing strips of smooth muscle (see Chapter 27). The contraction and relaxation of the smooth muscle layer, which is innervated by the autonomic nervous system, controls the diameter of the airways and consequent resistance to airflow. Parasympathetic stimulation, through the vagus nerve and cholinergic receptors, produces bronchial constriction, and sympathetic stimulation, through β_2-adrenergic receptors, increases bronchodilation. Normally, a slight vagally mediated bronchoconstrictor tone predominates. When there is need for increased airflow, as during exercise, the vagally mediated bronchoconstrictor tone is inhibited, and the bronchodilator effects of the sympathetic nervous system are stimulated.

Bronchial smooth muscle also responds to inflammatory mediators, such as histamine, that act directly on smooth muscle cells to produce bronchial constriction. During an antigen-antibody response, inflammatory mediators are released by a special type of cell, called the *mast cell*, which is present in the airways. The binding of immunoglobulin E (IgE) antibodies to specific receptors on mast cells prepares them for an allergic reaction when antigen appears (see Chapter 19).

BRONCHIAL ASTHMA

Bronchial asthma is a chronic inflammatory airway disease. According to 1998 data, an estimated 26 million Americans have been diagnosed with asthma, and 10.6 million have had an asthma episode in the past 12 months.[6] Of the 26 million Americans diagnosed with asthma, 8.6 million are younger than 18 years of age. In the general population, asthma prevalence rates have increased 102% between 1980

Airway Responsiveness

➤ Airway responsiveness refers to the reaction of the airways to various stimuli. Increased airway responsiveness leads to narrowing of the airways.

➤ Movement of gases through the respiratory airways depends on the pressure moving the gases and on the radius of the airways and their patency.

➤ The tone of the bronchial smooth muscles surrounding the airways determines airway radius, and the presence or absence of airway secretions influences airway patency.

➤ Bronchial smooth muscle is innervated by the autonomic nervous system—the parasympathetic nervous system through the vagus nerve produces bronchoconstriction and the sympathetic nervous system produces bronchodilation.

➤ Inflammatory mediators that are released in response to environmental irritants, immune responses, and infectious agents increase airway responsiveness by producing bronchospasm, increasing mucus secretion, and producing injury to the mucosal lining of the airways.

and 1994.[6] There also has been a reported increase in incidence and mortality from asthma over the past several decades. One suggested explanation for the growing morbidity and mortality is the increased exposure to indoor "aeroallergens" resulting from tighter houses with more carpets and soft furnishings, which retain dust mites, cockroach allergens, animal dander, and other allergens.[7] Also, people tend to spend more time indoors than they did in the past.

Pathophysiology

The National Heart, Lung, and Blood Institute's Second Expert Panel on the Management of Asthma defined bronchial asthma as "a chronic inflammatory disorder of the airways in which many cells and cellular elements play a role, in particular, mast cells, eosinophils, T lymphocytes, and epithelial cells."[8] This inflammatory process produces recurrent episodes of airway obstruction, characterized by wheezing, breathlessness, chest tightness, and a cough that often is worse at night and in the early morning. These episodes, which usually are reversible either spontaneously or with treatment, also cause an associated increase in bronchial hyperresponsiveness to a variety of stimuli.[8]

In susceptible persons, an asthma attack can be triggered by a variety of stimuli that do not normally cause symptoms. Based on their mechanism of response, these triggers can be divided into two categories—bronchospastic or inflammatory. Bronchospastic triggers depend on the existing level of airway responsiveness. They do not normally increase airway responsiveness but produce symptoms in persons who already are predisposed to bronchospasm. Bronchospastic triggers include cold air, exercise, emotional upset, and exposure to bronchial irritants such as cigarette smoke. Inflammatory triggers exert their effects through the inflammatory response. They cause inflammation and prime the sensitive airways so they are hyperresponsive to nonallergic stimuli. The mechanisms whereby these two types of triggers produce an asthmatic attack can be further described as the early or acute response versus the late phase response.[9]

The *acute* or *early response* results in immediate bronchoconstriction on exposure to an inhaled antigen or irritant. The symptoms of the acute response, which usually develop within 10 to 20 minutes, are caused by the release of chemical mediators from IgE-coated mast cells. In the case of airborne antigens, the reaction occurs when antigen binds to sensitized mast cells on the mucosal surface of the airways. Mediator release results in opening of the mucosal intercellular junctions and enhancement of antigen movement to the more prevalent submucosal mast cells (Fig. 29-6). In addition, there is bronchoconstriction due to direct stimulation of parasympathetic receptors, mucosal edema due to increased vascular permeability, and increased mucus secretions. The acute response usually can be inhibited or reversed by bronchodilators, such as β_2-adrenergic agonists, but not by the anti-inflammatory actions of the corticosteroids.

The *late phase response* develops 4 to 8 hours after exposure to an asthmatic trigger.[9] The late phase response involves inflammation and increased airway responsiveness that prolong the asthma attack and set into motion a vicious cycle of exacerbations. Typically, the response reaches a maximum within a few hours and may last for days or even weeks. An initial trigger in the late phase response causes the release of inflammatory mediators from mast cells, macrophages, and epithelial cells. These substances induce the migration and activation of other inflammatory cells (*e.g.*, basophils, eosinophils, neutrophils), which then produce epithelial injury and edema, changes in mucociliary function and reduced clearance of respiratory tract secretions, and increased airway responsiveness (see Fig. 29-6). Responsiveness to cholinergic mediators often is heightened, suggesting changes in parasympathetic control of airway function. Chronic inflammation can lead to airway remodeling, in which case airflow limitations may be only partially reversible.[8]

Causes of Asthma

A number of factors can contribute to an asthmatic attack, including allergens, respiratory tract infections, hyperventilation, cold air, exercise, drugs and chemicals, hormonal changes and emotional upsets, airborne pollutants, and gastroesophageal reflux.

Inhalation of allergens is a common cause of asthma. Usually, this type of asthma has its onset in childhood or

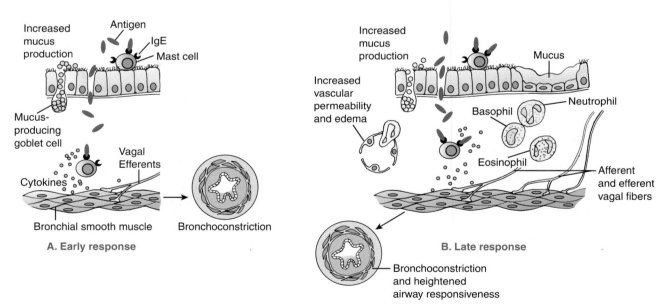

FIGURE 29-6 The pathogenesis of bronchial asthma. (**A**) The acute or early phase response. On exposure to an antigen, the immediate reaction is triggered by an IgE-mediated release of chemical mediators from sensitized mast cells. The release of chemical mediators results in increased mucus secretion, opening of mucosal intercellular junctions with increased antigen exposure of submucosal mast cells, and bronchoconstriction. Inhaled antigen produces release of chemical mediators from sensitized mast cells. (**B**) The late phase response involves release of inflammatory mediators from mast cells, macrophages, basophils, neutrophils, and eosinophils; epithelial cell injury and edema, decreased mucociliary function, and accumulation of mucus; and increased airway responsiveness.

adolescence and is seen in persons with a family history of atopic allergy. Persons with allergic asthma often have other allergic disorders, such as hay fever, hives, and eczema. Attacks are related to exposure to specific allergens. Among airborne allergens implicated in perennial (year-around) asthma are house dust mite allergens, cockroach allergens, animal danders, and the fungus *Alternaria*.

Respiratory tract infections, especially those caused by viruses, may produce their effects by causing epithelial damage and stimulating the production of IgE antibodies directed toward the viral antigens. In addition to precipitating an asthmatic attack, viral respiratory infections increase airway responsiveness to other asthma triggers that may persist for weeks beyond the original infection.

Exercise-induced asthma occurs in 40% to 90% of persons with bronchial asthma.[10] The cause of exercise-induced asthma is unclear. It has been suggested that during exercise, bronchospasm may be caused by the loss of heat and water from the tracheobronchial tree because of the need for conditioning (*i.e.*, warming and humidification) of large volumes of air.[11] The response is commonly exaggerated when the person exercises in a cold environment; wearing a mask over the nose and mouth often minimizes the attack or prevents it. A proper warm-up period also is important. An attack usually can be prevented by using an inhaled short-acting β_2-adrenergic agonist or anti-inflammatory agent (cromolyn, nedocromil) shortly before engaging in exercise.[8]

Inhaled irritants, such as tobacco smoke and strong odors, are thought to induce bronchospasm by way of irritant receptors and a vagal reflex. Exposure to parenteral smoking has been reported to increase asthma severity in children.[12] High doses of irritant gases such as sulfur dioxide, nitrogen dioxide, and ozone may induce inflammatory exacerbations of airway responsiveness (*e.g.*, smog-related asthma). Occupational asthma is stimulated by fumes and gases (*e.g.*, epoxy resins, plastics, toluene), organic and chemical dusts (*i.e.*, wood, cotton, platinum), and other chemicals (*e.g.*, formaldehyde) in the workplace.[13]

There is a small group of asthmatics in whom aspirin and nonsteroidal anti-inflammatory drugs are associated with asthmatic attacks, presence of nasal polyps, and recurrent episodes of rhinitis.[14,15] An addition to the list of chemicals that can provoke an asthmatic attack are the sulfites used in food processing and as a preservative added to beer, wine, and fresh vegetables. Nonselective β-blocking drugs (*e.g.*, propranolol), including those used in ophthalmic preparations (*e.g.* timolol, betaxolol), also can produce asthma symptoms by blocking the vasodilating effects of the sympathetic neurotransmitters.[8]

Both emotional factors and changes in hormone levels are thought to contribute to an increase in asthma symptoms. Emotional factors produce bronchospasm by way of vagal pathways. They can act as a bronchospastic trigger, or they can increase airway responsiveness to other triggers through noninflammatory mechanisms. The role of sex hormones in asthma is unclear, although there is much circumstantial evidence to suggest that they may be important. Up to 40% of women with asthma report a premenstrual increase in asthma symptoms.[16] Female sex hor-

mones have a regulatory role on β_2-adrenergic function, and it has been suggested that abnormal regulation may be a possible mechanism for premenstrual asthma.[16]

Symptoms of gastroesophageal reflux are common in both adults and children with asthma, suggesting that reflux of gastric secretions may act as a bronchospastic trigger. Reflux during sleep can contribute to nocturnal asthma.[8]

Manifestations

Persons with asthma exhibit a wide range of signs and symptoms, from episodic wheezing and feelings of chest tightness to an acute, immobilizing attack. The attacks differ from person to person, and between attacks, many persons are symptom free. Attacks may occur spontaneously or in response to various triggers, respiratory infections, emotional stress, or weather changes. Asthma is often worse at night. Nocturnal asthma attacks usually occur at approximately 4 AM because of the occurrence of the late response to allergens inhaled during the evening and because of circadian variations in bronchial reactivity.[17]

During an asthmatic attack, the airways narrow because of bronchospasm, edema of the bronchial mucosa, and mucus plugging. Expiration becomes prolonged because of progressive airway obstruction. The amount of air that can be forcibly expired in 1 second (forced expiratory volume [$FEV_{1.0}$]) and the peak expiratory flow rate (PEF), measured in liters per second, are decreased. A fall in the PEF to levels below 50% of the predicted value during an acute asthmatic attack indicates a severe exacerbation and the need for emergency room treatment.[8]

Air becomes trapped behind the occluded and narrowed airways during a prolonged attack, causing hyperinflation of the lungs. The residual volume is increased, and the inspiratory reserve capacity (tidal volume + inspiratory reserve volume) and forced vital capacity (FVC) are diminished so that the person breathes close to his or her functional residual capacity (residual volume + expiratory reserve volume) (Fig. 29-7). As a result, more energy is needed to overcome the tension already present in the lungs, and the accessory muscles (*i.e.*, sternocleidomastoid

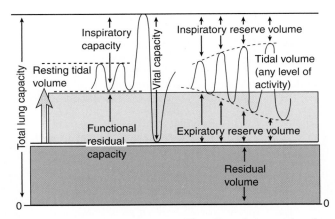

FIGURE 29-7 A spirometry tracing. The effect of air trapping during an asthmatic attack on lung volumes and inspiratory and expiratory reserve volumes.

muscles) are used to maintain ventilation and gas exchange. This causes dyspnea and fatigue. Because air is trapped in the alveoli and inspiration is occurring at higher residual lung volumes, the cough becomes less effective. As the condition progresses, the effectiveness of alveolar ventilation declines, and mismatching of ventilation and perfusion occurs, causing hypoxemia and hypercapnia. Pulmonary vascular resistance may increase as a result of the hypoxemia and hyperinflation, leading to a rise in pulmonary artery pressure and increased work demands on the right heart.

The physical signs of bronchial asthma vary with the severity of the attack. A mild attack may produce a feeling of chest tightness, a slight increase in respiratory rate with prolonged expiration, and mild wheezing. A cough may accompany the wheezing. More severe attacks are associated with use of the accessory muscles, distant breath sounds due to air trapping, and loud wheezing. As the condition progresses, fatigue develops, the skin becomes moist, and anxiety and apprehension are obvious. Dyspnea may be severe, and often the person is able to speak only one or two words before taking a breath. At the point where airflow is markedly decreased, breath sounds become inaudible with diminished wheezing and the cough becomes ineffective despite being repetitive and hacking. This point often marks the onset of respiratory failure.

With increased air trapping, a greater negative intrapleural pressure is needed to inflate the lungs. This negative pressure, which is transmitted to the heart and blood vessels, causes the systolic blood pressure to fall during inspiration, a condition called *pulsus paradoxus*. It can be detected by using a blood pressure cuff and a mercury manometer (see Chapter 24). Detection of pulsus paradoxus greater than 25 mm Hg suggests that the $FEV_{1.0}$ is reduced to less than 50% of the predicated value.[8]

Diagnosis

The diagnosis of asthma is based on a careful history and physical examination, laboratory findings, and pulmonary function studies. Spirometry provides a means for measuring FVC, $FEV_{1.0}$, PEF, tidal volume, expiratory reserve, and IRC. The level of airway responsiveness can be measured by inhalation challenge tests using methacholine (a cholinergic agonist), histamine, or exposure to a nonpharmacologic agent such as cold air. The Expert Panel of the National Education and Prevention Program of the National Heart, Lung, and Blood Institute has developed asthma classification systems intended for use in directing asthma treatment and identifying persons at high risk for development of life-threatening asthma attacks[8] (Table 29-1).

Small, inexpensive, portable meters that measure PEF are available. Although not intended for use in diagnosis of asthma, they can be used in clinics and physicians' offices and in the home to provide frequent measures of flow rates. Day–night (circadian) variations in asthma symptoms and PEF variability can be used to indicate the severity of bronchial hyperresponsiveness. The person's best performance is established from readings taken over several weeks. This often is referred to as the individual's *personal best* and is used as a reference to indicate changes in respiratory function.[8] The indicators for the functional levels have been adapted to resemble a traffic signal system to make the device easier to use. Green (80% to 100% of the personal best) signals an all clear and indicates that the

---

TABLE 29-1 ◆ Classification of Asthma Severity

	Symptoms	Nighttime Symptoms	Lung Function
Mild intermittent	Symptoms ≤2 times a week Asymptomatic and normal PEF between exacerbations Exacerbations brief (from a few hours to a few days); intensity may vary	≤2 times a month	$FEV_{1.0}$ or PEF ≥80% predicted PEF variability <20%
Mild persistent	Symptoms >2 times a week but <1 time a day Exacerbations may affect activity	>2 times a month	$FEV_{1.0}$ or PEF ≥80% predicted PEF variability 20%–30%
Moderate persistent	Daily symptoms Daily use of inhaled short-acting β₂-agonist Exacerbations affect activity Exacerbations ≥2 times a week; may last days	>1 time a week	$FEV_{1.0}$ or PEF >60%–<80% predicted PEF variability >30%
Severe persistent	Continual symptoms Limited physical activity Frequent exacerbations	Frequent	$FEV_{1.0}$ or PEF ≤60% predicted PEF variability >30%

$FEV_{1.0}$, forced expiratory volume in 1 second; PEF, peak expiratory flow rate.
(Adapted from National Education and Prevention Program. [1997]. *Expert Panel report 2: Guidelines for the diagnosis and management of asthma.* National Institutes of Health publication no. 97-4051. Bethesda, MD: National Institutes of Health.)

asthma is under control; yellow (50% to 80%) signals caution and indicates that the asthma is not under sufficient control and additional medication or treatment is needed; and red (50% or less) signals a medical alert and the immediate need for a bronchodilator, and the need to consult a health care provider if the person's PEF does not immediately return to the caution range.[8]

Treatment

The Expert Panel of the National Heart, Lung, and Blood Institute's National Asthma Education Program recommends two categories of treatment for management of asthma: control of factors contributing to asthma severity and pharmacologic treatment.[8]

Control of Factors Contributing to Asthma Severity.

Measures to control factors contributing to asthma severity are aimed at prevention of exposure to irritants and factors that increase asthma symptoms and precipitate asthma exacerbations. They include education of the patient and family regarding measures used in avoiding exposure to irritants and allergens that are known to induce or trigger an attack. A careful history often is needed to identify all the contributory factors. Factors such as nasal polyps, a history of aspirin sensitivity, and gastroesophageal reflux should be considered. Annual influenza vaccination is recommended for persons with persistent asthma.

Relaxation techniques and controlled breathing often help to allay the panic and anxiety that aggravate breathing difficulties. The hyperventilation that often accompanies anxiety and panic is known to act as an asthmatic trigger. In a child, measures to encourage independence as it relates to symptom control, along with those directed at helping to develop a positive self-concept, are essential.

A program of desensitization may be undertaken in persons with persistent asthma who react to allergens, such as house dust mites, that cannot be avoided. This involves the injection of selected antigens (based on skin tests) to stimulate the production of IgG antibodies that block the IgE response. A course of allergen immunotherapy is typically of 3 to 5 years' duration.[8]

Pharmacologic Treatment.

Pharmacologic treatment is used to prevent or treat reversible airway obstruction and airway hyperresponsiveness caused by the inflammatory process. The Expert Panel recommends a stepwise approach to pharmacologic therapy based on frequency and severity of disease symptoms.[8] The medications used in the treatment of asthma include those with bronchodilator and anti-inflammatory actions. They are categorized into two general categories: quick-relief medications and long-term–control medications.

The *quick-relief medications* include the short-acting β_2-adrenergic agonists, anticholinergic agents, and systemic corticosteroids. The short-acting β_2-adrenergic agonists (albuterol, bitolterol, pirbuterol, terbutaline) relax bronchial smooth muscle and provide prompt relief of symptoms, usually within 30 minutes. They are administered by inhalation (*i.e.*, metered-dose inhaler [MDI] or nebulizer). The short-acting β_2-agonists are used for treating acute attacks of asthma but are not recommended for daily use because of concern over safety.[8] The increasing use of short-acting β_2-agonists or use of more than one canister in a month indicates inadequate control of asthma. Ipratropium is an anticholinergic drug that blocks the postganglionic efferent vagal pathways that cause bronchoconstriction. The drug, which is administered by inhalation, produces bronchodilation by direct action on the large airways and does not change the composition or viscosity of the bronchial mucus. It is thought that ipratropium may provide some additive benefit for treatment of asthma exacerbations when administered with inhaled β_2-agonists.[8] A short course of systemic corticosteroids, administered orally or parenterally, may be used for treating the inflammatory reaction associated with the late phase response. Although their onset of action is slow (>4 hours), systemic corticosteroids often are used in the treatment of moderate to severe exacerbations because of their action in preventing the progression of the exacerbation, speeding recovery, and preventing early relapses.[8]

The *long-term medications* are taken on a daily basis to achieve and maintain control of persistent asthma symptoms. They include anti-inflammatory agents, long-acting bronchodilators, and leukotriene modifiers. The Expert Panel defines anti-inflammatory medications as "those that cause a reduction in markers of airway inflammation in airway tissues and airway secretions [*e.g.*, eosinophils, mast cells, activated lymphocytes, macrophages, cytokines or inflammatory mediators] and thus decrease the intensity of airway hyperresponsiveness."[8] The corticosteroids are considered the most effective anti-inflammatory agents for use in long-term treatment of asthma. Inhaled corticosteroids (*e.g.*, beclomethasone, triamcinolone, budesonide, flunisolide) that are administered by MDI usually are preferred because of minimal systemic absorption and degree of disruption in hypothalamic-pituitary-adrenal function. In severe cases, oral or parenterally administered corticosteroids may be necessary.

The anti-inflammatory agents sodium cromolyn and nedocromil are used to prevent an asthmatic attack. These agents act by stabilizing mast cells, thereby preventing release of the inflammatory mediators that cause an asthmatic attack. They are used prophylactically to prevent early and late responses. They are of no benefit when taken during an attack. Cromolyn is available as an MDI, a dry powder inhaler, or a solution for use with a nebulizer. Nedocromil is available as an MDI.

The long-acting β_2-agonists, which are available in inhalation (salmeterol) or oral (albuterol sustained release) forms, act by relaxing bronchial smooth muscle. They are used as an adjunct to anti-inflammatory medications for providing long-term control of symptoms, especially nocturnal symptoms, and to prevent exercise-induced bronchospasm. The long-acting β_2-agonists have a duration of action of at least 12 hours and should not be used to treat acute symptoms or exacerbations.[8]

Theophylline, a methylxanthine, is a bronchodilator that acts by relaxing bronchial smooth muscle. The sustained-release form of the drug is used as an adjuvant therapy and is particularly useful in relieving nighttime symptoms. It may be used as an alternative, but not pre-ferred, medication in long-term preventative therapy when there are issues concerning adherence with regimens using inhaled medications, or cost is a factor. Because elimination of the drug varies widely among persons, blood levels are required to ensure that the therapeutic, but not toxic dose, is achieved.[8]

A newer group of drugs called the *leukotriene modifiers* have become available for use in the treatment of asthma.[18] The leukotrienes are potent biochemical mediators released from mast cells that cause bronchoconstriction, increased mucus secretion, and attraction and activation of inflammatory cells in the airways of people with asthma. There are two types of leukotriene modifiers: (1) those that act by inhibiting 5-lipoxygenase (zileuton), an enzyme required for leukotriene synthesis; and (2) those that act as receptor antagonists (zafirlukast and montelukast) by inhibiting the binding of leukotrienes to their receptor in the target tissues. A particular advantage of the leukotriene modifiers is that they are taken orally. Montelukast has been approved for children as young as 6 years of age.

Administration of Aerosol Medications. A number of asthma medications are administered by inhalation using either the MDI or nebulizer. The MDI usually is the pre-ferred method for delivery of sympathomimetic, anti-cholinergic, and corticosteroid drugs. Various extension devices (*i.e.,* spacers) are available to facilitate use and enhance aerosol deposition in the lungs. This is difficult to achieve when the inhaler is held at the level of the mouth. In this position, large droplets tend to be delivered to the oropharynx and throat, rather than moving down into the small airways.

Nebulizers are specially constructed devices that use a high-pressure gas source to produce an aerosol drug mixture. They use a mouthpiece or mask for drug delivery and usually are powered by portable compressors or hospital gas supplies. Nebulizers also can be placed in mechanical ventilator circuits. Nebulizers often are the method of choice for administration of β_2-agonist drugs in the initial phase of acute asthma and are used to administer aerosol drugs to children and to persons who have difficulty using the MDI.

Status Asthmaticus and Fatal Asthma

Status asthmaticus is severe, prolonged asthma that is re-fractory to conventional methods of therapy. The death rate from asthma in the United States from 1980 through 1987 increased 31%, from 1.3 to 1.7 deaths per 100,000 per-sons.[19] African Americans have asthma-related mortality rates higher than those of whites, especially in young age groups.[19,20]

Most asthma deaths have occurred outside the hospital. Persons at highest risk are those with previous exacer-bations resulting in respiratory failure, respiratory acidosis, and the need for intubation. Risk factors for fatal asthma are described in Chart 29-1.[8] Although the cause of death during an acute asthmatic attack is largely unknown, both cardiac dysrhythmias and asphyxia due to severe airway obstruction have been implicated. It has been suggested that an underestimation of the severity of the attack may

---

> ## CHART 29-1
>
> ### *Risk Factors for Death From Asthma*
>
> - Past history of sudden severe exacerbations
> - Prior intubation for asthma
> - Two or more hospitalizations for asthma in the past year
> - Three or more emergency care visits for asthma in the past year
> - Hospitalization or an emergency care visit for asthma within the past month
> - Use of more than two canisters per month of inhaled short-acting β_2-agonist
> - Current use of systemic corticosteroids or recent withdrawal from systemic corticosteroids
> - Difficulty perceiving airflow obstruction or its severity
> - Comorbidity, as from cardiovascular diseases or chronic obstructive pulmonary disease
> - Serious psychiatric disease or psychosocial problems
> - Low socioeconomic status and urban residence
> - Illicit drug use
> - Sensitivity to *Alternaria*
>
> (From National Education and Prevention Program. [1997]. *Expert Panel report 2: Guidelines for the diagnosis and management of asthma.* National Institutes of Health publication no. 97-4051. Bethesda, MD: National Institutes of Health.)

---

be a contributing factor. Deterioration often occurs rapidly during an acute attack, and underestimation of its severity may lead to a life-threatening delay in seeking medical attention. Frequent and repetitive use of β_2-agonist inhalers (more than twice in a month) far in excess of the recommended doses may temporarily blunt symptoms and mask the severity of the condition. Lack of access to medical care is another risk factor associated with asthma-related death. Distance, as in rural areas, or lack of financial resources, as in the uninsured or underinsured, may limit access to emergency care.

Persons who have fatal or near-fatal asthmatic attacks may have impaired perception of dyspnea and its sever-ity.[21] It has been suggested that persons who have had a previous episode of sudden asphyxia be educated in the use of a peak flow meter as a means of determining the severity of their attack rather than relying on their per-ceptions of dyspnea.[21]

Bronchial Asthma in Children

Asthma is a leading cause of chronic illness in children and is responsible for a significant number of lost school days. It is the most frequent admitting diagnosis in children's hospitals. As many as 10% to 15% of boys and 7% to 10% of girls have asthma at some time during childhood.[22] Asthma may have its onset at any age; 30% of children are symptomatic by 1 year of age, and 80% to 90% are symptomatic by 4 to 5 years of age.[22] Data on inheritance of asthma are most consistent with polygenic or multifacto-rial determinants. A child with one affected parent has approximately a 25% risk of developing the disease, and this risk increases to 50% when both parents are affected.[22]

As with adults, asthma in children commonly is associated with an IgE-related reaction. It has been suggested that IgE directed against respiratory viruses in particular may be important in the pathogenesis of wheezing illnesses in infants (*i.e.*, bronchiolitis), which often precedes the onset of asthma. The respiratory syncytial virus and parainfluenza viruses are the most commonly involved.[22] Other contributing factors include exposure to environmental allergens such as pet danders, dust mite antigens, and cockroach allergens. Exposure to environmental tobacco smoke also may contribute to asthma in children. Of particular concern is the effect of in utero exposure to maternal smoking on lung function in infants and children.[23,24]

The signs and symptoms of asthma in infants and small children vary with the stage and severity of an attack. Because airway patency decreases at night, many children have acute signs of asthma at this time. Often, previously well infants and children develop what may seem to be a cold with rhinorrhea, rapidly followed by irritability, a tight and nonproductive cough, wheezing, tachypnea, dyspnea with prolonged expiration, and use of accessory muscles of respiration. Cyanosis, hyperinflation of the chest, and tachycardia indicate increasing severity of the attack. Wheezing may be absent in children with extreme respiratory distress. The symptoms may progress rapidly and require a trip to the emergency room or hospitalization.

The Expert Panel of the National Heart, Lung, and Blood Institute's National Asthma Education Program has developed guidelines for management of asthma in infants and children younger than 5 years of age and for adults and children older than 5 years of age.[8] As with adults and older children, the Expert Panel recommends a stepwise approach to diagnosing and managing asthma in infants and children younger than 5 years of age. The anti-inflammatory agents cromolyn and nedocromil are recommended as an initial therapy for mild to moderate persistent asthma in infants and children. More severe symptoms may require the use of inhaled corticosteroids. Inhaled short-acting β_2-agonists may be used for mild intermittent symptoms or exacerbations. Theophylline should be considered only if serum concentration levels can be carefully monitored. Sustained-release theophylline may have particularly adverse effects in infants who frequently have febrile illnesses that increase drug levels.[8] Systemic corticosteroids may be required during an episode of severe disease.

Special delivery systems for administration of inhalation medications are available for infants and small children, including nebulizers with face masks and spacers/holding chambers for use with an MDI. For children younger than 2 years of age, nebulizer therapy usually is preferred. Children between 3 and 5 years of age may begin using an MDI with a spacer/holding chamber. The child's caregiver should be carefully instructed in the appropriate use of these devices.

The Expert Panel recommends that adolescents (and younger children when appropriate) be directly involved in developing their asthma management plans. Active participation in physical activities, exercise, and sports should be encouraged. A written asthma management plan should be prepared for the student's school, including plans to ensure reliable, prompt access to medications.[8]

CHRONIC OBSTRUCTIVE PULMONARY DISEASE

Chronic obstructive pulmonary disease (COPD) denotes a group of respiratory disorders characterized by chronic and recurrent obstruction of air flow in the pulmonary airways. Airflow obstruction usually is progressive, may be accompanied by airway hyperreactivity, and may be partially reversible.[25] It has been estimated that approximately 14 million Americans have COPD. Grouped together, COPD and asthma now represent the fourth leading cause of death in the United States, with over 109,000 deaths reported in 1997.[26] The death rate from COPD is increasing, especially among older men.

The most common cause of COPD is smoking.[26,27] Thus, the disease is largely preventable. Unfortunately, clinical findings are almost always absent during the early stages of COPD, and by the time symptoms appear, the disease usually is far advanced. For smokers with early signs of airway disease, there is hope that early recognition, combined with appropriate treatment and smoking cessation, may prevent or delay the usually relentless progression of the disease.

The term *chronic obstructive pulmonary disease* encompasses two types of obstructive airway disease: *emphysema*, with enlargement of air spaces and destruction of lung tissue, and *chronic obstructive bronchitis*, with obstruction of small airways. The mechanisms involved in the pathogenesis of COPD usually are multiple and include inflammation and fibrosis of the bronchial wall, hypertrophy of the submucosal glands and hypersecretion of mucus, and loss of elastic lung fibers and alveolar tissue (Fig. 29-8).[27] Inflammation and fibrosis of the bronchial wall, along with excess mucus secretion, obstruct airflow and cause mismatching of ventilation and perfusion. Destruction of alve-

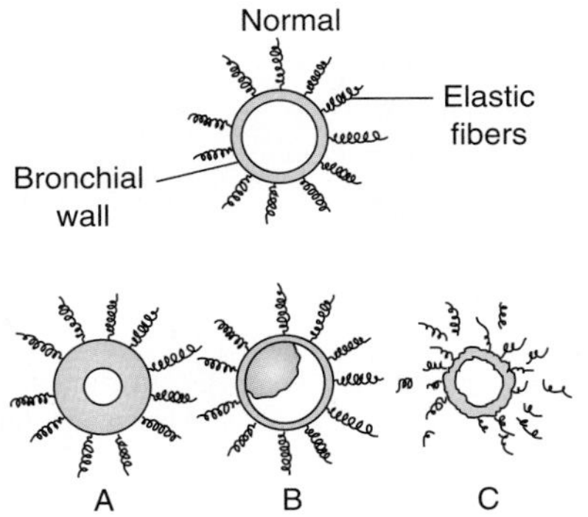

FIGURE 29-8 Mechanisms of airflow obstruction in chronic obstructive lung disease. (**Top**) The normal bronchial airway with elastic fibers that provide traction and hold the airway open. (**Bottom**) Obstruction of the airway caused by (**A**) hypertrophy of the bronchial wall, (**B**) inflammation and hypersecretion of mucus, and (**C**) loss of elastic fibers that hold the airway open.

olar tissue decreases the surface area for gas exchange, and loss of elastic fibers leads to airway collapse. Normally, recoil of the elastic fibers that were stretched during inspiration provides the force needed to move air out of the lung during expiration. Because the elastic fibers are attached to the airways, they also provide radial traction to hold the airways open during expiration. In persons with COPD, the loss of elastic fibers impairs the expiratory flow rate, increases air trapping, and predisposes to airway collapse.

Emphysema

Emphysema is characterized by a loss of lung elasticity and abnormal enlargement of the air spaces distal to the terminal bronchioles, with destruction of the alveolar walls and capillary beds (Fig. 29-9). Enlargement of the air spaces leads to hyperinflation of the lungs and produces an increase in TLC. Two of the recognized causes of emphysema are smoking, which incites lung injury, and an inherited deficiency of α_1-*antitrypsin*, an antiprotease enzyme that protects the lung from injury. Genetic factors, other than an inherited α_1-antitrypsin deficiency, also may play a role in smokers who develop COPD at an early age.[28]

Emphysema is thought to result from the breakdown of elastin and other alveolar wall components by enzymes, called *proteases*, that digest proteins. These proteases, particularly elastase, which is an enzyme that digests elastin, are released from polymorphonuclear leukocytes (*i.e.*, neutrophils), alveolar macrophages, and other inflammatory cells.[27] Normally, the lung is protected by antiprotease enzymes including α_1-antitrypsin. Cigarette smoke and other irritants stimulate the movement of inflammatory cells

into the lungs, resulting in increased release of elastase and other proteases. In smokers in whom COPD develops, antiprotease production and release may be inadequate to neutralize the excess protease production such that the process of elastic tissue destruction goes unchecked (Fig. 29-10).

A hereditary deficiency in α_1-antitrypsin accounts for approximately 1% of all cases of COPD and is more common in young persons with emphysema.[27] The type and amount of α_1-antitrypsin that a person has is determined by a pair of codominant genes referred to as PI (protein inhibitor) genes. An α_1-antitrypsin deficiency is inherited as an autosomal recessive disorder. There are more than 75 mutations of the gene. One of these, the PIZ variant, which occurs in 5% of the population, causes the most serious deficiency in α_1-antitrypsin. It is most common in persons of Scandinavian descent and is rare in Jews, blacks, and Japanese.[29] Homozygotes who carry two defective PIZ genes have only about 15% to 20% of the normal plasma concentration of α_1-antitrypsin. Almost all persons who have emphysema before the age of 40 years have an α_1-antitrypsin deficiency. Smoking and repeated respiratory tract infections, which also decrease α_1-antitrypsin levels, contribute to the risk of emphysema in persons with an α_1-antitrypsin deficiency. Laboratory methods are available for measuring α_1-antitrypsin levels. Human α_1-antitrypsin is available for replacement therapy in persons with a

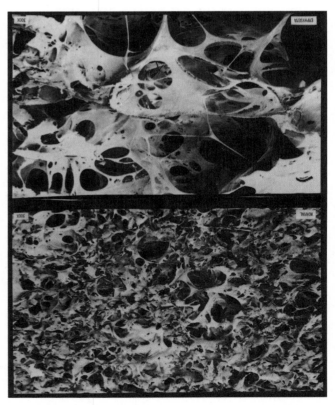

FIGURE 29-10 Scanning electron micrographs of lung tissue. (**Top**) Normal tissue; (**bottom**) emphysematous tissue (both at same magnification). Note the enlargement of air spaces in the emphysematous lung.

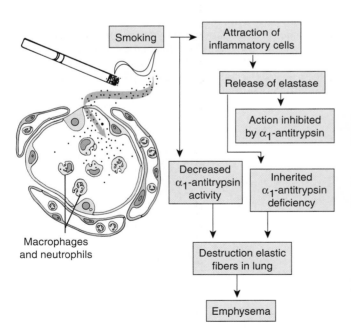

FIGURE 29-9 Smoking and protease–antiprotease mechanisms of emphysema. Smoking inhibits antielastase and favors the recruitment of leukocytes and release of elastase, with elastic tissue destruction in the lung and development of emphysema.

hereditary deficiency of the enzyme. The preparation is administered by intravenous infusion.

There are two commonly recognized types of emphysema: centriacinar and panacinar. The centriacinar type affects the bronchioles in the central part of the respiratory lobule, with initial preservation of the alveolar ducts and sacs[29] (Fig. 29-11). It is the most common type of emphysema and is seen predominantly in male smokers. The panacinar type produces initial involvement of the peripheral alveoli and later extends to involve the more central bronchioles. This type of emphysema is more common in persons with α_1-antitrypsin deficiency. It also is found in smokers in association with centrilobular emphysema. In such cases, panacinar changes are seen in the lower parts of the lung and the centriacinar changes in the upper parts of the lung.

Chronic Bronchitis

In chronic bronchitis, airway obstruction is caused by inflammation of the major and small airways. There is edema and hyperplasia of submucosal glands and excess mucus excretion into the bronchial tree.[29] A history of a chronic productive cough of more than 3 months' duration for more than 2 consecutive years is necessary for diagnosis of chronic bronchitis.[25,28] Typically, the cough has been present for many years, with a gradual increase in acute exacerbations that produce frankly purulent sputum. Chronic bronchitis without airflow obstruction often is referred to as *simple bronchitis* and chronic bronchitis with airflow obstruction as *chronic obstructive bronchitis*. The outlook for persons with simple bronchitis is good, compared with the premature morbidity and mortality associated with chronic obstructive bronchitis.

Chronic bronchitis is seen most commonly in middle-aged men and is associated with chronic irritation from smoking and recurrent infections. In the United States, smoking is the most important cause of chronic bronchitis. Viral and bacterial infections are common in persons with chronic bronchitis and are thought to be a result rather than a cause of the problem.

Manifestations

The mnemonics "pink puffer" and "blue bloater" have been used to differentiate the clinical manifestations of

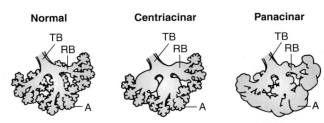

FIGURE 29-11 Centriacinar and panacinar emphysema. In centriacinar emphysema, the destruction is confined to the terminal (TB) and respiratory bronchioles (RB). In panacinar emphysema, the peripheral alveoli (A) are also involved. (West J.B. [1997]. *Pulmonary pathophysiology* [5th ed., p. 53]. Philadelphia: Lippincott-Raven)

emphysema and chronic obstructive bronchitis.[30] The important features of these two forms of COPD are described in Table 29-2. In practice, differentiation between the two types is not as vivid as presented here. This is because persons with COPD often have some degree of both emphysema and chronic bronchitis.

A major difference between the pink puffers and the blue bloaters is the respiratory responsiveness to the hypoxic stimuli. With pulmonary emphysema, there is a proportionate loss of ventilation and perfusion area in the lung. These persons are pink puffers, or fighters able to overventilate and thus maintain relatively normal blood gas levels until late in the disease. Chronic obstructive bronchitis is characterized by excessive bronchial secretions and airway obstruction that causes mismatching of ventilation and perfusion. Thus, persons with chronic bronchitis are unable to compensate by increasing their ventilation; instead, hypoxemia and cyanosis develop. These are the blue bloaters, or nonfighters.

Persons with emphysema have marked dyspnea and struggle to maintain normal blood gas levels with increased ventilatory effort, including prominent use of the accessory muscles. The seated position, which stabilizes chest structures and allows for maximum chest expansion and use of accessory muscles, is preferred. With loss of lung elasticity and hyperinflation of the lungs, the airways often collapse during expiration because pressure in surrounding lung tissues exceeds airway pressure. Air becomes trapped in lungs, producing an increase in the anteroposterior dimensions of the chest, the so-called *barrel chest* that is typical of persons with emphysema (Fig. 29-12). Expiration often is accomplished through pursed lips. Pursed-lip breathing, which increases the resistance to the outflow of air, helps to prevent airway collapse by increasing airway pressure. The work of breathing is greatly increased in persons with emphysema, and eating often is difficult. As a result, there often is considerable weight loss.

Chronic obstructive bronchitis is characterized by shortness of breath with a progressive decrease in exercise tolerance. As the disease progresses, breathing becomes increasingly more labored, even at rest. The expiratory phase of respiration is prolonged, and expiratory wheezes and crackles can be heard on auscultation. In contrast to persons with emphysema, those with chronic obstructive bronchitis are unable to maintain normal blood gases by increasing their breathing effort. Hypoxemia, hypercapnia, and cyanosis develop, reflecting an imbalance between ventilation and perfusion. Hypoxemia, in which arterial PO_2 levels fall below 55 mm Hg, causes reflex vasoconstriction of the pulmonary vessels and further impairment of gas exchange in the lung. Hypoxemia also stimulates red blood cell production, causing polycythemia. As a result, persons with chronic obstructive bronchitis develop pulmonary hypertension and, eventually, right-sided heart failure with peripheral edema (*i.e.*, cor pulmonale). A common finding in chronic obstructive bronchitis is clubbing of the fingers, a condition in which the tips of the fingers become bulbous, resembling drumsticks.

Persons with combined forms of COPD characteristically seek medical attention in the fifth or sixth decade of

TABLE 29-2 ✦ Characteristics of Chronic Bronchitis and Emphysematous Types of Chronic Obstructive Lung Disease

Characteristic	Type A Pulmonary Emphysema ("Pink Puffers")	Type B Chronic Bronchitis ("Blue Bloaters")
Smoking history	Usual	Usual
Age of onset	40 to 50 years of age	30 to 40 years of age; disability in middle age
Clinical features		
Barrel chest (hyperinflation of the lungs)	Often dramatic	May be present
Weight loss	May be severe in advanced disease	Infrequent
Shortness of breath	May be absent early in disease	Predominant early symptom, insidious in onset, exertional
Decreased breath sounds	Characteristic	Variable
Wheezing	Usually absent	Variable
Rhonchi	Usually absent or minimal	Often prominent
Sputum	May be absent or may develop late in the course	Frequent early manifestation, frequent infections, abundant purulent sputum
Cyanosis	Often absent, even late in the disease when there is low PO_2	Often dramatic
Blood gases	Relatively normal until late in the disease process	Hypercapnia may be present Hypoxemia may be present
Cor pulmonale	Only in advanced cases	Frequent Peripheral edema
Polycythemia	Only in advanced cases	Frequent
Prognosis	Slowly debilitating disease	Numerous life-threatening episodes due to acute exacerbations

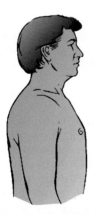
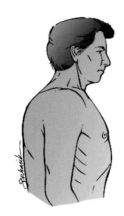

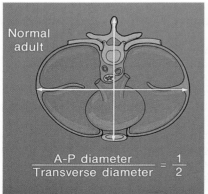
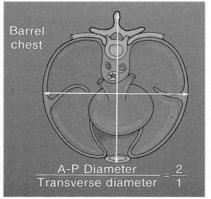

FIGURE 29-12 Characteristics of normal chest wall and chest wall in emphysema. The normal chest wall and its cross section are illustrated on the left (**A**). The barrel-shaped chest of emphysema and its cross section are illustrated on the right (**B**). (Smeltzer S.C., Bare B.G. [2000]. *Medical-surgical nursing*. [9th ed., p. 454]. Philadelphia: Lippincott Williams & Wilkins)

life, complaining of cough, sputum production, and shortness of breath. The symptoms typically have existed to some extent for 10 years or longer. The productive cough usually occurs in the morning. Dyspnea becomes more severe as the disease progresses. Frequent exacerbations of infection and respiratory insufficiency are common, causing absence from work and eventual disability. The late stages of COPD are characterized by pulmonary hypertension, cor pulmonale, recurrent respiratory infections, and chronic respiratory failure. Death usually occurs during an exacerbation of illness associated with infection and respiratory failure.

Diagnosis

The diagnosis of COPD is based on a careful history and physical examination, pulmonary function studies, chest radiographs, and laboratory tests. Airway obstruction prolongs the expiratory phase of respiration and affords the potential for impaired gas exchange because of mismatching of ventilation and perfusion. The FVC is the amount of air that can be forcibly exhaled after maximal inspiration (see Fig. 29-7). In an adult with normal respiratory function, this should be achieved in 4 to 6 seconds. In patients with chronic lung disease, the time required for FVC is increased, and the $FEV_{1.0}$ is decreased, and the ratio of $FEV_{1.0}$ to FVC is decreased. In severe disease, the FVC is markedly reduced. Lung volume measurements reveal a marked increase in residual volume (RV), an increase in TLC, and elevation of the RV to TLC ratio. These and other measurements of expiratory flow are determined by spirometry and are used in the diagnosis of COPD (see Chapter 27).

Treatment

The treatment of COPD depends on the stage of the disease and often requires an interdisciplinary approach. Smoking cessation is the only measure that slows the progression of the disease.[27] Nicotine replacement therapy (gum, transdermal patches, or inhaler) or the noradrenergic antidepressant drug bupropion may be used to reduce withdrawal symptoms. Persons in more advanced stages of the disease often require measures to maintain and improve physical and psychosocial functioning, pharmacologic interventions, and oxygen therapy. Lung volume reduction surgery may be used in some cases.

Avoidance of cigarette smoke and other environmental airway irritants is a must. Wearing a cold-weather mask often prevents dyspnea and bronchospasm due to cold air and wind exposure. Respiratory tract infections can prove life threatening to persons with severe COPD. A person with COPD should avoid exposure to others with known respiratory tract infections and should avoid attending large gatherings during periods of the year when influenza or respiratory tract infections are prevalent. Immunization for influenza and pneumococcal infections decreases the likelihood of their occurrence. Persons with COPD should be taught to monitor their sputum for signs of infection, so that treatment can be instituted at the earliest sign of infection. Although antibiotics are used to treat acute exacerbations of COPD due to bacterial infection, there is no evidence that the prophylactic use of antibiotics prevents acute exacerbations.[27]

Because persons with COPD expend so much effort on breathing, many find it difficult to chew their food and manage the effort of a large meal. This situation, combined with impaired diaphragm descent, air swallowing, and medications that cause anorexia and nausea, impairs nutrition and promotes weight loss. Undernutrition (body weight <90% of ideal weight) affects approximately 25% of persons with COPD.[30] It is associated with reduced respiratory muscle function and increased mortality rates. Small, frequent, nutritious, and easily swallowed feedings aid in maintaining good nutrition and preventing weight loss. Carbohydrates in the diet can increase carbon dioxide production and arterial carbon dioxide levels. However, it usually is not a problem unless a high-carbohydrate diet is followed.[31]

Measures to Improve Physical and Psychosocial Functioning. Maintaining and improving physical and psychosocial functioning is an important part of the treatment program for persons with COPD. A long-term pulmonary rehabilitation program can significantly reduce episodes of hospitalization and add measurably to a person's ability to manage and cope with his or her impairment in a positive way. Breathing exercises and retraining focus on restoring the function of the diaphragm, reducing the work of breathing, and improving gas exchange. Physical conditioning with appropriate exercise training increases maximal oxygen consumption and reduces ventilation and heart rate for a given workload. Work simplification and energy conservation strategies may be needed when impairment is severe.

Education of persons with COPD and their families is a key to successful management of the disease. Psychosocial rehabilitation must be individualized to meet the specific needs of persons with COPD and their families. These needs vary with age, occupation, financial resources, social and recreational interests, and interpersonal and family relationships.

Pharmacologic Treatment. Bronchodilators, including adrenergic drugs, the anticholinergic drug ipratropium, and theophylline preparations are probably the most widely prescribed medications for use in the treatment of COPD. Inhaled β_2-adrenergic agonists have been the mainstay of treatment for COPD for many years. It has been suggested that long-acting inhaled β_2-adrenergic agonists may be even more effective than the short-acting forms of the drug. In addition to their action as bronchodilators, the long-acting β_2-adrenergic agonists are thought to reduce the adherence of bacteria such as *Haemophilus influenzae* to airway epithelial cells, thereby reducing the risk of infective exacerbations.[27]

The anticholinergic drug ipratropium, which is administered by inhalation, produces bronchodilation by blocking parasympathetic cholinergic receptors that produce contraction of bronchial smooth muscle. Ipratropium also reduces the volume of sputum without altering its viscosity. Because the drug has a slower onset of action and longer duration of action, it usually is used on a regular basis rather than on an as-needed basis.

Oral theophylline may be used in treatment of persons who fail to respond to inhaled bronchodilators. The long-acting theophylline preparations may be used to reduce overnight declines in respiratory function. There also is evidence that theophylline may improve respiratory muscle function, increase mucociliary clearance, and improve central respiratory drive.[31] When theophylline is prescribed, blood levels are used as a guide in arriving at an effective dose schedule.

Although inhaled corticosteroids often are used in treatment of COPD, there is controversy regarding their usefulness. There is evidence that inflammation in COPD is not suppressed by inhaled or oral corticosteroids.[27] An explanation for this lack of effect may be related to the fact that corticosteroids prolong the action of neutrophils and hence do not suppress the neutrophilic inflammation seen in COPD. Because corticosteroids are useful in relieving asthma symptoms, they may benefit persons with asthma concomitant with COPD. Inhaled corticosteroids also may be beneficial in treating acute exacerbations of COPD, minimizing the undesirable effects that often accompany systemic use.

Although they are still in the developmental phases, interest has focused on inhibitors of enzymes that break down lung tissue. Several inhibitors of neutrophil elastase, one of the enzymes involved in the breakdown of lung tissue in persons with COPD, are now in clinical development. There also is interest in the development of new anti-inflammatory agents, particularly those capable of inhibiting neutrophilic inflammation.[27]

Oxygen Therapy. Oxygen therapy is prescribed for selected persons with significant hypoxemia (arterial PO_2 <55 mm Hg). Administration of continuous low-flow (1 to 2 L/minute) oxygen to maintain arterial PO_2 levels between 55 and 65 mm Hg decreases dyspnea and pulmonary hypertension and improves neuropsychological function and activity tolerance. The overall goal of oxygen therapy is to maintain a hemoglobin oxygen saturation above 90%.[32] Oxygen usually is administered using a nasal cannula. Portable oxygen administration units, which allow mobility and the performance of activities of daily living, usually are used. Transtracheal oxygen, delivered by a small-diameter percutaneous catheter placed in the trachea, can be used to increase oxygen delivery and ventilatory effort. It is particularly useful in persons with high oxygen requirements.[27,32] It also can be used to increase ambulation by eliminating the need to wear a nasal cannula. Oxygen administration in persons with severe COPD must be undertaken with a certain amount of caution. The flow rate (in liters per minute) usually is titrated to provide an arterial PO_2 of 55 to 65 mm Hg. Because the ventilatory drive associated with hypoxic stimulation of the peripheral chemoreceptors does not occur until the arterial PO_2 has been reduced to about 60 mm Hg or less, increasing the arterial PO_2 above 60 mm Hg tends to depress the hypoxic stimulus for ventilation and often leads to hypoventilation and carbon dioxide retention.

Surgical Treatment. Lung volume reduction surgery involves the resection of the most distended areas of the lung as a means of improving respiratory function. The procedure is designed to reduce the overall volume of the lung, reshape the configuration of the lung, and improve elastic recoil and its effects on the airways and the diaphragm.[33] Two surgical approaches are used: one in which the chest is opened through a median sternotomy, and the other through a thoracoscopic approach.[34] Although the procedure still is experimental, early results have demonstrated improvement in the 6-minute walk, dyspnea index, and quality-of-life assessment.[34] Bullectomy is a surgical procedure that involves the removal of large emphysematous bullae that compress adjacent lung tissue and cause dyspnea. The procedure can now be done thoracoscopically using a carbon dioxide laser.

Lung transplantation is becoming an alternative treatment for persons with severe lung disease, limited life expectancy without transplantation, adequate functioning of other organ systems, and a good social support system.

Bronchiectasis

Bronchiectasis is a chronic obstructive lung disease characterized by an abnormal dilatation of the large bronchi associated with infection and destruction of the bronchial walls (Fig. 29-13). To be diagnosed as bronchiectasis, the

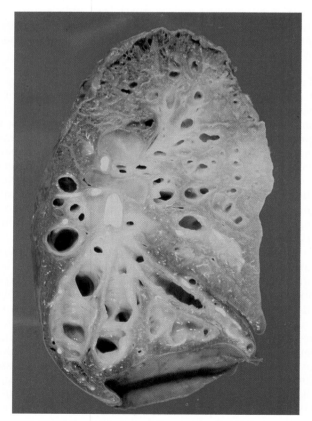

FIGURE 29-13 Bronchiectasis. The resected upper lobe shows widely dilated bronchi, with thickening of the bronchial walls and collapse and fibrosis of the pulmonary parenchyma. (Rubin E., Farber J.L. [1999]. *Pathology* [3rd ed., p. 601]. Philadelphia: Lippincott Williams & Wilkins)

dilatation must be permanent, as compared with the reversible bronchial dilatation that sometimes accompanies viral and bronchial pneumonias. With the advent of vaccinations to prevent respiratory infections and extended-spectrum antibiotics that more effectively treat respiratory infections, there has been a decrease in the prevalence of bronchiectasis.[35]

The pathogenesis of bronchiectasis can be either obstructive or nonobstructive.[29] Obstructive bronchiectasis is confined to a segment of the lung distal to a mechanical obstruction. It is caused by conditions such as tumors, foreign bodies, and mucus plugs in asthma. Nonobstructive bronchiectasis can be either localized or generalized. Use of immunizations and antibiotics has largely eliminated localized bronchiectasis due to childhood bronchopulmonary infections such as measles, pertussis, and other bacterial infections.

Generalized bronchiectasis is due largely to inherited impairments of host mechanisms or acquired disorders that permit introduction of infectious organisms into the airways. They include inherited conditions such as cystic fibrosis, in which airway obstruction is caused by impairment of normal mucociliary function; congenital and acquired immunodeficiency states, which predispose to respiratory tract infections; lung infection (*e.g.*, tuberculosis, fungal infections, lung abscess); and exposure to toxic gases that cause airway obstruction.

Generalized bronchiectasis usually is bilateral and most commonly affects the lower lobes. Localized bronchiectasis can affect any area of the lung, the area being determined by the site of obstruction or infection. As the disease progresses, airway obstruction leads to smooth muscle relaxation with dilatation and eventual destruction of the bronchial walls. Infection produces inflammation, impairs mucociliary function, and causes weakening and further dilatation of the walls of the bronchioles. Pooling of secretions produces a vicious cycle of chronic inflammation and development of new infections.

Bronchiectasis is associated with an assortment of abnormalities that profoundly affect respiratory function, including atelectasis, obstruction of the smaller airways, and diffuse bronchitis. Affected persons have fever, recurrent bronchopulmonary infection, coughing, production of copious amounts of foul-smelling, purulent sputum, and hemoptysis. Weight loss and anemia are common. The physiologic abnormalities that occur in bronchiectasis are similar to those seen in chronic bronchitis and emphysema. As in the latter two conditions, chronic bronchial obstruction leads to marked dyspnea and cyanosis. Clubbing of the fingers is common in moderate to advanced bronchiectasis and is not seen in other types of obstructive lung diseases.[35]

Diagnosis is based on history and imaging studies. The condition often is evident on chest radiographs. High-resolution CT scanning of the chest allows for definitive diagnosis. Treatment consists of early recognition and treatment of infection along with regular postural drainage and chest physical therapy. Persons with this disorder benefit from many of the rehabilitation and treatment measures used for chronic bronchitis and emphysema. Localized bronchiectasis may be treated surgically.

Cystic Fibrosis

Cystic fibrosis is an autosomal recessive disorder involving fluid secretion in the exocrine glands and epithelial lining of the respiratory, gastrointestinal, and reproductive tracts. Most of the clinical manifestations of the disease are related to abnormal secretions that result in obstruction of organ passages such as the respiratory airways and pancreatic ducts. The disease affects approximately 30,000 children and adults in the United States, and more than 10 million persons are asymptomatic carriers of the defective gene.[36] The gene is rare in African blacks and Asians. Homozygotes (*i.e.*, persons with two defective genes) have all or substantially all of the clinical symptoms of the disease, compared with heterozygotes, who are carriers of the disease but have no recognizable symptoms. The disease is the most common fatal hereditary disorder of whites in the United States and is the most common cause of chronic lung disease in children.

The cystic fibrosis gene was identified on the long arm of chromosome 7.[37–39] In most cases of cystic fibrosis, the mutation consists of the deletion of a single phenylalanine residue from the gene. The gene encodes the production of a single protein, the cystic fibrosis transmembrane conductance regulator (CFTR), which functions in chloride transport across membranes. In cystic fibrosis, chloride transport in airway epithelial cells is diminished. Because of the defective chloride transport, there is a threefold increase in sodium reabsorption. Water moves out of the extracellular fluid with the sodium, causing the exocrine secretions to become exceedingly viscid.

Clinically, cystic fibrosis is manifested by (1) chronic respiratory disease, (2) pancreatic exocrine deficiency, and (3) elevation of sodium chloride in the sweat. Nasal polyps, sinus infections, pancreatitis, and cholelithiasis also are common. Excessive loss of sodium in the sweat predisposes young children to salt depletion episodes. Most males with cystic fibrosis have congenital bilateral absence of the vas deferens with azoospermia.

Respiratory manifestations are caused by an accumulation of viscid mucus in the bronchi, impaired mucociliary clearance, and lung infections. Chronic bronchiolitis and bronchitis are the initial lung manifestations, but after months and years, structural changes in the bronchial wall lead to bronchiectasis. Widespread bronchiectasis is common by 10 years of age; large bronchiectic cysts and abscesses develop in later stages of the disease.[38] Infection and ensuing inflammation are causes of lung destruction in cystic fibrosis. *Staphylococcus aureus* and *Pseudomonas* infections occur. With advanced disease, 80% of persons harbor the *Pseudomonas* organism. New findings suggest that absence of CFTR predisposes to *Pseudomonas* infections, and once established, *Pseudomonas* is not easily cleared from the lungs, producing a cycle of chronic inflammation, tissue damage, and obstruction.

Pancreatic function is abnormal in approximately 80% to 90% of affected persons.[40] Steatorrhea, diarrhea, and abdominal pain and discomfort are common. In the newborn, meconium ileus may cause intestinal obstruction. The degree of pancreatic involvement is highly variable. In some children, the defect is relatively mild, and in others the involvement is severe and impairs intestinal absorption. In addition to exocrine pancreatic insufficiency, hyperglycemia may occur, especially after 10 years of age when approximately 8% of persons with cystic fibrosis develop diabetes mellitus.[41]

Early diagnosis and treatment are important in delaying the onset and severity of chronic illness. Diagnosis is based on the presence of respiratory and gastrointestinal manifestations typical of cystic fibrosis, a history of cystic fibrosis in a sibling, or a positive newborn screening test. Confirmatory laboratory tests include the sweat test, genetic tests for CFTR gene mutations, and measurement of nasal membrane potential differences.[41] *Newborn screening* consists of a test for determination of immunoreactive trypsinogen. The test can be done on blood spots collected for routine metabolic screening. Newborns with cystic fibrosis have elevated blood levels of immunoreactive trypsinogen, presumably because of secretory obstruction in the pancreas. This test has a sensitivity of approximately 95%. The *sweat test*, using pilocarpine iontophoresis to aid in the collection of a sweat sample, remains the standard approach to diagnosis. The test usually is done on sweat obtained from a child's forearm or from an infant's thigh. A small electric current is used to carry the drug pilocarpine, which increases sweat production, into the skin. Sweat is collected using an absorbent paper or gauze sponge and then analyzed in the laboratory. Two positive tests on two different days are required for accurate diagnosis. The test may be inaccurate in newborns because the quantity of sweat produced is insufficient for testing. The *nasal membrane potential difference* measures the electrical potential across the nasal epithelium. The loss of the potential difference with topical application of amiloride (a drug that inhibits active sodium transport) and the absence of a voltage response with application of a β-adrenergic agonist may be used to confirm a diagnosis of cystic fibrosis.[41]

Genetic tests can be used to detect mutations in the CFTR gene. At least 500 mutations of the CFTR gene have been identified; of these, only 70 have commercially available probes.[39] Although these 70 mutations account for 90% of all cases of cystic fibrosis, the probes cannot be used to exclude cystic fibrosis in persons without these mutant genes. Even if both genes are abnormal, it is possible for a neutralizing second gene to be present elsewhere. Thus, cystic fibrosis cannot be accurately diagnosed by genetic testing methods unless there are characteristic clinical manifestations or a family history of the disorder. Genetic tests also may be used to detect carriers of a mutant CFTR gene.

The treatment of cystic fibrosis usually consists of replacement of pancreatic enzymes, physical measures to improve the clearance of tracheobronchial secretions (*i.e.*, postural drainage and chest percussion), bronchodilator therapy, and prompt treatment of respiratory tract infections. The abnormal viscosity of airway secretions is attributed largely to the presence of polymorphonuclear white blood cells and their degradation products. A purified recombinant human deoxyribonuclease (rhDNase), an enzyme that breaks down these products, has been developed. Clinical trials have shown that the drug, which is adminis-

tered by inhalation, can improve pulmonary symptoms and reduce the frequency of respiratory exacerbations. Although many persons benefit from the therapy, the drug is costly, and recommendations for its use are evolving.

Treatment methods to manipulate the increased sodium reabsorption and decreased chloride secretion are being studied. Amiloride, a potassium-sparing diuretic that blocks sodium reabsorption, has been administered in aerosol form. In pilot studies that used the drug, there was a decrease in sputum viscosity and a slowing of the decline of pulmonary function. Agents such as adenosine triphosphate and uridine triphosphate that increase chloride secretion also are being studied.[39]

Progress of the disease is variable. Improved medical management has led to longer survival—approximately half of children live beyond 20 years, and approximately one third of the nearly 30,000 persons with cystic fibrosis are adults. Lung transplantation is being used as a treatment for persons with end-stage lung disease. Current hopes reside in the development of gene therapy. The complementary DNA for the CFTR gene has been successfully cloned and introduced into affected epithelial cells in the laboratory and in a limited number of persons with cystic fibrosis.[36] It is hoped that further research will make gene therapy a feasible alternative for persons with the disease.

In summary, obstructive ventilatory disorders are characterized by airway obstruction and limitation in expiratory airflow. Bronchial asthma is a chronic inflammatory disorder of the airways, characterized by airway hypersensitivity and episodic attacks of airway narrowing. An asthmatic attack can be triggered by a variety of stimuli. Based on their mechanism of response, these triggers can be divided into two types: bronchospastic and inflammatory. Bronchospastic triggers depend on the level of airway responsiveness. There are two types of responses in persons with asthma: the acute or early response and the late phase response. The acute response results in immediate bronchoconstriction on exposure to an inhaled antigen and usually subsides within 90 minutes. The late phase response usually develops 3 to 5 hours after exposure to an asthmatic trigger; it involves inflammation and increased airway responsiveness that prolong the attack and cause a vicious cycle of exacerbations.

COPD describes a group of conditions characterized by obstruction to airflow in the lungs. Among the conditions associated with COPD are emphysema, chronic bronchitis, and bronchiectasis. Emphysema is characterized by a loss of lung elasticity, abnormal, permanent enlargement of the air spaces distal to the terminal bronchioles, and hyperinflation of the lungs. Chronic bronchitis is caused by inflammation of major and small airways and is characterized by edema and hyperplasia of submucosal glands and excess mucus secretion into the bronchial tree. A history of a chronic productive cough that has persisted for at least 3 months and for at least 2 consecutive years in the absence of other disease is necessary for the diagnosis of chronic bronchitis. Emphysema and chronic bronchitis are manifested by eventual mismatching of ventilation and perfusion. As the condition advances, signs of respiratory distress and impaired gas exchange become evident, with development of hypercapnia and hypoxemia. Bronchiectasis is a form of COPD that is characterized by an abnormal dilatation of the large bronchi associated with infection and destruction of the bronchial walls.

Cystic fibrosis is an autosomal recessive genetic disorder manifested by chronic lung disease, pancreatic exocrine deficiency, and elevation of sodium chloride in the sweat. The disorder is caused by a mutation of the CFTR gene located on the long arm of chromosome 7. The gene functions in chloride transport across membranes; the defect increases sodium reabsorption, causing the exocrine secretions to become exceedingly viscid. Respiratory manifestations are caused by an accumulation of viscid mucus in the bronchi, impaired mucociliary clearance, lung infections, bronchiectasis, and dilatation. Mucus plugs can result in the total obstruction of an airway, causing atelectasis.

Interstitial Lung Diseases

After you have completed this section of the chapter, you should be able to meet the following objectives:

- ✦ State the difference between chronic obstructive pulmonary diseases and interstitial lung diseases
- ✦ Cite the characteristics of occupational dusts that determine their pathogenicity in terms of the production of pneumoconioses
- ✦ Characterize the organ involvement in sarcoidosis

The diffuse interstitial lung diseases are a diverse group of lung disorders that produce similar inflammatory and fibrotic changes in the interstitium or interalveolar septa of the lung. They include sarcoidosis, the occupational lung diseases, hypersensitivity pneumonitis, and lung diseases caused by exposure to toxic drugs (*e.g.*, amiodarone) and radiation. There is no universally accepted classification system for these disorders. In many cases, no specific cause can be found.[42,43]

The diffuse interstitial lung diseases produce various degrees of inflammation, fibrosis, and disability. The disorders may be acute or insidious in onset; they may be rapidly progressive, slowly progressive, or static in their course. Because they result in a stiff and noncompliant lung, they are commonly classified as fibrotic or restrictive lung disorders. The most common of the interstitial lung diseases are those caused by exposure to occupational and environmental inhalants, and sarcoidosis, the cause of which is unknown. Examples of interstitial lung diseases and their causes are listed in Table 29-3.

In contrast to the obstructive lung diseases, which primarily involve the airways of the lung, the interstitial lung disorders exert their effects on the collagen and elastic connective tissue found between the airways and the blood vessels of the lung. Many of these diseases also involve the airways, arteries, and veins. In general, these lung diseases share a pattern of lung dysfunction that includes diminished lung volumes, reduced diffusing capacity of the lung, and varying degrees of hypoxemia.

Current theory suggests that most interstitial lung diseases, regardless of the causes, have a common pathogenesis. It is thought that these disorders are initiated by some type of injury to the alveolar epithelium, followed by an inflammatory process that involves the alveoli and interstitium of the lung. An accumulation of inflammatory and immune cells causes continued damage of lung tissue and the replacement of normal, functioning lung tissue with fibrous scar tissue.

In general, the interstitial lung diseases are characterized by clinical changes consistent with restrictive rather than obstructive changes in the lung. Persons with interstitial lung diseases have dyspnea, tachypnea, and eventual cyanosis, without evidence of wheezing or signs of airway obstruction. Usually there is an insidious onset of breathlessness that initially occurs during exercise and may progress to the point that the person is totally incapacitated. Typically, a person with a restrictive lung disease breathes with a pattern of rapid, shallow respirations. This tachypneic pattern of breathing, in which the respiratory rate is increased and the tidal volume is decreased, reduces the work of breathing because it takes less work to move air through the airways at an increased rate than it does to stretch a stiff lung to accommodate a larger tidal volume. A nonproductive cough may develop, particularly with continued exposure to the inhaled irritant. Clubbing of the fingers and toes may develop.

Lung volumes, including vital capacity and TLC, are reduced in interstitial lung disease. In contrast to COPD, in which expiratory flow rates are reduced, the $FEV_{1.0}$ usually is preserved, even though the ratio between the $FEV_{1.0}$ and FVC may increase. Although resting arterial blood gases usually are normal early in the course of the disease, arterial oxygen levels may fall during exercise, and in cases of advanced disease, hypoxemia often is present, even at rest. In the late stages of the disease, hypercapnia and respiratory acidosis develop. The impaired diffusion of gases that occurs in persons with interstitial lung disease is thought to be caused by an increase in physiologic dead space resulting from unventilated regions of the lung.

The diagnosis of interstitial lung disease requires a careful personal and family history, with particular emphasis on exposure to environmental, occupational, and other injurious agents. Chest radiographs may be used as an initial diagnostic method, and serial chest films often are used to follow the progress of the disease. A biopsy specimen for histologic study and culture may be obtained by surgical incision or bronchoscopy using a fiberoptic bronchoscope. In bronchoalveolar lavage, fluid is instilled into the alveoli through a bronchoscope and then removed by suction to obtain inflammatory and immune cells for laboratory

TABLE 29-3 ✦ Causes and Examples of Interstitial Lung Diseases

Causes	Examples
Known	
Occupational and environmental inhalants	
Inorganic dusts	Silicosis
	Asbestosis
	Talcosis
	Coal miner's pneumoconiosis
	Berylliosis
Organic dusts	Farmer's lung (moldy hay)
	Pigeon breeder's lung (bird serum, excreta, and feathers)
	Air conditioner lung (bacteria found in humidifiers and air conditioners)
	Bagassosis (contaminated sugarcane)
Gases, fumes, aerosols	Silo filler's lung (nitrogen dioxide, chlorine, ammonia, phosgene, sulfur dioxide)
Drugs	Cancer therapeutic drugs (*e.g.*, bleomycin), nitrofurantoin, amiodarone
Radiation	External radiation, inhaled radioactive materials
Infections	Widespread tuberculosis
Poisons	Paraquat
Diseases of other organ systems	Chronic pulmonary edema
	Chronic uremia
Unknown	
	Sarcoidosis
	Idiopathic pulmonary fibrosis
	Connective tissue diseases, such as lupus erythematosus, scleroderma, and rheumatoid arthritis

study. Gallium lung scans often are used to detect and quantify the chronic alveolitis that occurs in interstitial lung disease. Gallium does not localize in normal lung tissue, but uptake of the radionuclide is increased in interstitial lung disease and other diffuse lung diseases.

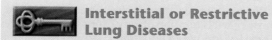

Interstitial or Restrictive Lung Diseases

➤ Expansion of the lung depends on the ability of lung tissues to stretch and accommodate an increase in lung volume.

➤ Interstitial lung diseases produce fibrosis of lung tissue, making the lung stiff and difficult to inflate.

➤ It takes more breathing work to inflate a stiff and noncompliant lung than it does one that is easy to inflate.

➤ Because of the increased effort needed to expand a lung that is stiff and difficult to inflate, persons with interstitial lung disease tend to take small but more frequent breaths.

The treatment goals for persons with interstitial lung disease focus on identifying and removing the injurious agent, suppressing the inflammatory response, preventing progression of the disease, and providing supportive therapy for persons with advanced disease. In general, the treatment measures vary with the type of lung disease. Corticosteroid drugs frequently are used to suppress the inflammatory response. Many of the supportive treatment measures used in the late stages of the disease, such as oxygen therapy and measures to prevent infection, are similar to those discussed for persons with COPD.

OCCUPATIONAL LUNG DISEASES

The occupational lung diseases can be divided into two major groups: the pneumoconioses and the hypersensitivity diseases. The *pneumoconioses* are caused by the inhalation of inorganic dusts and particulate matter. The *hypersensitivity diseases* result from the inhalation of organic dusts and related occupational antigens. A third type of occupational lung disease, byssinosis, a disease that affects cotton workers, has characteristics of the pneumoconioses and hypersensitivity lung disease.

Among the pneumoconioses are silicosis, found in hard-rock miners, foundry workers, sandblasters, pottery makers, and workers in the slate industry; coal miner's pneumoconiosis; asbestosis, found in asbestos miners, manufacturers of asbestos products, and installers and removers of asbestos insulation; talcosis, found in talc miners or millers and infants and small children who accidentally inhale powder containing talc; and berylliosis, found in ore extraction workers and alloy production workers. The danger of exposure to asbestos dust is not confined to the workplace. The dust pervades the general environment because it was used in the construction of buildings and in other applications before its health hazards were realized. It has been mixed into paints and plaster, wrapped around water and heating pipes, used to insulate hair dryers, and woven into theater curtains, hot pads, and ironing board covers.

Important etiologic determinants in the development of the pneumoconioses are the size of the dust particle, its chemical nature and ability to incite lung destruction, and the concentration of dust and the length of exposure to it. The most dangerous particles are those in the range of 1 to 5 μm.[43] These small particles are carried through the inspired air into the alveolar structures, whereas larger particles are trapped in the nose or mucous linings of the airways and removed by the mucociliary blanket. Exceptions are asbestos and talc particles, which range in size from 30 to 60 μm but find their way into the alveoli because of their density.

All particles in the alveoli must be cleared by the lung macrophages. Macrophages are thought to transport engulfed particles from the small bronchioles and the alveoli, which have neither cilia nor mucus-secreting cells, to the mucociliary escalator or to the lymphatic channels for removal from the lung. This clearing function is hampered when the function of the macrophage is impaired by factors such as cigarette smoking, consumption of alcohol, and hypersensitivity reactions. This helps to explain the increased incidence of lung disease among smokers exposed to asbestos. In silicosis, the ingestion of silica particles leads to the destruction of the lung macrophages and the release of substances that lead to inflammation and fibrosis.[43] Tuberculosis and other diseases caused by mycobacteria are common in persons with silicosis. Because the macrophages are responsible for protecting the lungs from tuberculosis, the destruction of macrophages accounts for the increased susceptibility of persons with silicosis to tuberculosis.

The concentration of some dusts in the environment strongly influences their effects on the lung. For example, acute silicosis is seen only in persons whose occupations entail intense exposure to silica dust over a short period. It is seen in sandblasters, who use a high-speed jet of sand to clean and polish bricks and the insides of corroded tanks, in tunnelers, and in rock drillers, particularly if they drill through sandstone. Acute silicosis is a rapidly progressive disease, usually leading to severe disability and death within 5 years of diagnosis. In contrast to acute silicosis, which is caused by exposure to extremely high concentrations of silica dust, the symptoms related to chronic, low-level exposure to silica dust often do not begin to develop until after many years of exposure, and then the symptoms often are insidious in onset and slow to progress.

The hypersensitivity occupational lung disorders (*e.g.,* hypersensitivity pneumonitis) are caused by intense and often prolonged exposure to inhaled organic dusts and related occupational antigens. Affected persons have a heightened sensitivity to the antigen. The most common forms of hypersensitivity pneumonitis are farmer's lung, which results from exposure to moldy hay; pigeon breeder's lung, provoked by exposure to the serum, excreta, or feathers of birds; bagassosis, from contaminated sugar cane; and humidifier or air conditioner lung, caused by mold in the water reservoirs of these appliances. Unlike bronchial asthma, this type of hypersensitivity reaction involves primarily the alveoli. These disorders cause progressive fibrotic lung disease, which can be prevented by the removal of the environmental agent.

SARCOIDOSIS

Sarcoidosis is a multisystem granulomatous disorder characterized by an exaggerated cellular immune response at the sites of involvement. The disease predominantly affects adults younger than 40 years of age, although it can occur in older persons.[44,45] The annual incidence of sarcoidosis in the United States is approximately 1 in 2500 to 1 in 10,000. It is more common among African Americans and whites living in the southeastern part of the country. The cause of sarcoidosis remains obscure. It is thought that the disorder may result from various antigens causing T-cell activation in genetically predisposed persons.[45]

Sarcoidosis has variable manifestations and an unpredictable course of progression in which any organ system can be affected. The three systems that most commonly manifest symptoms are the lungs, the skin, and the eyes. More than 40% of persons with sarcoidosis report nonspecific symptoms such as fever, sweating, anorexia, weight loss, fatigue, and myalgia. Although only approximately 60% of persons with sarcoidosis have respiratory symptoms, almost all have abnormalities on chest radiography. In approximately 25% of cases, the disease is detected first on a routine chest radiogram. Overall, approximately 50% have permanent pulmonary abnormalities, and 5% to 15% have progressive pulmonary fibrosis.[44] Pulmonary involvement in sarcoidosis is primarily an interstitial lung disease. Approximately one third to one half of persons with chronic sarcoidosis have skin lesions, most of which are granulomatous. Ocular disease, usually in the form of chorioretinitis, affects approximately 20% of persons with the disease. Hepatic involvement, due to the presence of granulomas, is present in approximately 20% of persons at some time during the course of the disease. Cardiac sarcoidosis occurs in approximately 3% to 5% of persons. It often manifests as bundle branch block, tachyarrhythmias, or bradyarrhythmias.[45] Bone sarcoidosis affects approximately 3% to 4% of persons and is associated with soft tissue swelling and joint stiffness and pain.[44] Kidney and liver involvement also are infrequent accompaniments of the disorder.

The diagnosis of sarcoidosis is based on history and physical examination, tests to exclude other diseases, chest radiography, and biopsy to obtain confirmation of noncaseating granuloma.[44] When treatment is indicated, corticosteroid drugs are used. These agents produce clearing of the lung, as seen on the chest radiograph, and improve pulmonary function, but it is not known whether they affect the long-term outcome of the disease.

> In summary, the interstitial lung diseases are characterized by fibrosis and decreased compliance of the lung. They include the occupational lung diseases, lung diseases caused by toxic drugs and radiation, and lung diseases of unknown origin, such as sarcoidosis. These disorders are thought to result from an inflammatory process that begins in the alveoli and extends to involve the interstitial tissues of the lung. Unlike COPD, which affects the airways, interstitial lung diseases affect the supporting collagen and elastic tissues that lie between the airways and blood vessels. These lung diseases decrease lung volumes, reduce the diffusing capacity of the lung, and cause various degrees of hypoxia. Because lung compliance is reduced, persons with this form of lung disease have a rapid, shallow breathing pattern.

Pulmonary Vascular Disorders

After you have completed this section of the chapter, you should be able to meet the following objectives:

- ✦ State the most common cause of pulmonary embolism and the clinical manifestations of the disorder
- ✦ Describe the physiology of pulmonary arterial hypertension and three causes of secondary pulmonary hypertension
- ✦ Describe the alterations in cardiovascular function that are characteristic of cor pulmonale
- ✦ Describe the pathologic lung changes that occur in acute respiratory distress syndrome and relate them to the clinical manifestations of the disorder

As blood moves through the lung, blood oxygen levels are raised, and carbon dioxide is removed. These processes depend on the matching of ventilation (*i.e.,* gas exchange) and perfusion (*i.e.,* blood flow). This section discusses three major problems of the pulmonary circulation: pulmonary embolism, pulmonary hypertension, and acute respiratory distress syndrome. Pulmonary edema, another major problem of the pulmonary circulation, is discussed in Chapter 26.

PULMONARY EMBOLISM

Pulmonary embolism develops when a blood-borne substance lodges in a branch of the pulmonary artery and obstructs the flow. The embolism may consist of a thrombus, air that has accidentally been injected during intravenous infusion, fat that has been mobilized from the bone marrow after a fracture or from a traumatized fat depot (see

Chapter 57), or amniotic fluid that has entered the maternal circulation after rupture of the membranes at the time of delivery. In the United States, as many as 250,000 hospitalizations and 50,000 deaths occur annually as the result of pulmonary emboli.[46,47] The overall mortality rate for pulmonary embolism continues to be high—15% to 17.5%.[46]

Almost all pulmonary emboli arise from deep vein thrombosis (DVT) in the lower extremities (see Chapter 22). The presence of thrombosis in the deep veins of the legs or pelvis often is unsuspected until embolism occurs. The effects of emboli on the pulmonary circulation are related to mechanical obstruction of the pulmonary circulation and neurohumoral reflexes causing vasoconstriction. Obstruction of pulmonary blood flow causes reflex bronchoconstriction in the affected area of the lung, wasted ventilation and impaired gas exchange, and loss of alveolar surfactant. Pulmonary hypertension and right heart failure may develop when there is massive vasoconstriction because of a large embolus. Although small areas of infarction may occur, frank pulmonary infarction is uncommon.

Persons at risk for developing DVT also are at risk for developing thromboemboli. Among the physiologic factors that contribute to venous thrombosis are venous stasis, venous endothelial injury, and hypercoagulability states.

Venous stasis and venous endothelial injury can result from prolonged bed rest, trauma, surgery, childbirth, fractures of the hip and femur, myocardial infarction and congestive heart failure, and spinal cord injury. Persons undergoing orthopedic surgery and gynecologic cancer surgery are at particular risk, as are bedridden patients in an intensive care unit. Cancer cells can produce thrombin and synthesize procoagulation factors, increasing the risk

Disorders of the Pulmonary Vascular System

➤ The pulmonary circulation, which links the peripheral venous system with the peripheral arterial system, functions as a conduit for gas exchange.

➤ Pulmonary emboli are blood clots that originate in the peripheral venous system and become lodged in the pulmonary vessels as they move through the lungs.

➤ The pulmonary circulation is a low-pressure system located between the right and left heart. The pulmonary arterial pressure is regulated by the pressure in the left heart, by vasoconstrictor reflexes that respond to stimuli such as hypoxia, and by vasoactive substances produced by the endothelial layer of the pulmonary vessels.

➤ Pulmonary hypertension can be caused by an elevation in left atrial pressure, increased pulmonary blood flow, or increased pulmonary vascular resistance resulting from stimuli such as hypoxia.

of thromboembolism. Use of oral contraceptive, pregnancy, and hormone replacement therapy are thought to increase the resistance to endogenous anticoagulants. The risk of pulmonary embolism among users of oral contraceptives is approximately three times the risk of nonusers.[46] Women who smoke are at particular risk. Hormone replacement therapy doubles the risk of venous thromboembolism.[46] The risk is higher at the start of therapy than after long-term use.

Manifestations

The manifestations of pulmonary embolism depend on the size and location of the obstruction. Chest pain, dyspnea, and increased respiratory rate are the most frequent signs and symptoms of pulmonary embolism. Pulmonary infarction often causes pleuritic pain that changes with respiration; it is more severe on inspiration and less severe on expiration. Moderate hypoxemia without carbon dioxide retention occurs as a result of impaired gas exchange. Small emboli that become lodged in the peripheral branches of the pulmonary artery may exert little effect and go unrecognized. However, repeated small emboli gradually reduce the size of the pulmonary capillary bed, resulting in pulmonary hypertension. Moderate-sized emboli often present with breathlessness accompanied by pleuritic pain, apprehension, slight fever, and cough productive of blood-streaked sputum. Tachycardia often is detected, and the breathing pattern is rapid and shallow. Patients with massive emboli usually present with sudden collapse, crushing substernal chest pain, shock, and sometimes loss of consciousness. The pulse is rapid and weak, the blood pressure is low, the neck veins are distended, and the skin is cyanotic and diaphoretic. Massive pulmonary emboli often are fatal.

Diagnosis

The diagnosis of pulmonary embolism is based on clinical signs and symptoms, blood gas determinations, venous thrombosis studies, D-dimer testing, lung scans, CT scans, and, in selected cases, pulmonary angiography. Laboratory studies and radiologic films are useful in ruling out other conditions that might give rise to similar symptoms. Because emboli can cause an increase in pulmonary vascular resistance, the electrocardiogram (ECG) may be used to detect signs of right heart strain. There has been recent interest in combining several noninvasive methods (lower limb compression ultrasonography, D-dimer measurements, and clinical assessment measures) as a means of establishing a diagnosis of pulmonary embolism.[47]

Because almost all pulmonary emboli originate from DVT, venous studies such as *lower limb compression ultrasonography, impedance plethysmography,* and *contrast venography* often are used as initial diagnostic procedures. Of these, lower limb compression ultrasonography has become an important noninvasive means for detecting DVT. The specificity of the test is as high as 97%.[47]

D-dimer testing involves the measurement of plasma D-dimer, a degradation product of coagulation factors that have been activated as the result of a thromboembolic event.[47] A normal test value indicates a high probability that the person does not have pulmonary embolism. Because a number of conditions such as inflammation, infection, necrosis, and cancer can elevate D-dimer levels, a positive test does not necessarily mean that pulmonary embolism is present.

The *ventilation-perfusion scan* uses radiolabeled albumin, which is injected intravenously, and a radiolabeled gas, which is inhaled. A scintillation (gamma) camera is used to scan the various lung segments for blood flow and distribution of the radiolabeled gas. Ventilation-perfusion scans are useful only when their results are either normal or indicate a high probability of pulmonary embolism. Because of difficulties in interpreting the results of a ventilation-perfusion scan, a definitive diagnosis of pulmonary embolism can be established on the basis of lung scan alone only in approximately 30% of cases.[47] *Helical (spiral) CT angiography* requires administration of an intravenous radio-contrast media. It is sensitive for the detection of emboli in the proximal pulmonary arteries and provides another method of diagnosis. To date, magnetic resonance imaging studies have found limited usefulness because of artifacts introduced by respiration and heart movement.

Pulmonary angiography involves the passage of a venous catheter through the right heart and into the pulmonary artery under fluoroscopy. Although it remains the most accurate method of diagnosis, it is an invasive procedure; therefore, its use is reserved for selected cases. An embolectomy sometimes is performed during this procedure.

Treatment

The treatment goals for pulmonary emboli focus on preventing DVT and the development of thromboemboli, protecting the lungs from exposure to thromboemboli when they occur, and in the case of large and life-threatening pulmonary emboli, sustaining life and restoring pulmonary blood flow. Prevention focuses on identification of persons at risk, avoidance of venous stasis and hypercoagulability states, and early detection of venous thrombosis.

For patients at risk, graded compression elastic stockings and intermittent pneumatic compression (IPC) boots can be used to prevent venous stasis. Both of these devices are safe and practical ways to prevent venous thrombosis. IPC boots provide intermittent inflation of air-filled sleeves that prevent venous stasis. Some devices produce sequential gradient compression that moves blood upward in the leg.

Pharmacologic prophylaxis involves the use of anticoagulant drugs. Anticoagulant therapy may be used to decrease the likelihood of deep vein thrombosis, thromboembolism, and fatal pulmonary embolism after major surgical procedures. Low–molecular-weight heparin, which can be administered subcutaneously on an outpatient basis, often is used. Warfarin, an oral anticoagulation drug, may be used for persons with long-term risk of developing thromboemboli.

Surgical interruption of the vena cava often is indicated when pulmonary embolism poses a life-threatening risk. There are two surgical procedures for protecting the lung from thromboemboli: venous ligation to prevent the embolus from traveling to the lung and vena caval plication. The plication, done with a suture or by insertion of a clip, filter, or sieve, permits blood to flow while trapping the embolus. Percutaneous transjugular placement of a filter has become the preferred mode of inferior vena caval interruption.

Thrombolytic therapy using streptokinase, urokinase, or recombinant tissue plasminogen activator may be indicated in persons with multiple or large emboli. Thrombolytic therapy is followed by administration of heparin and then warfarin. Restoration of blood flow in persons with life-threatening pulmonary emboli can be accomplished through the surgical removal of the embolus or emboli.

PULMONARY HYPERTENSION

The pulmonary circulation is a low-pressure system designed to accommodate varying amounts of blood delivered from the right heart and to facilitate gas exchange. The main pulmonary artery and major branches are relatively thin-walled, compliant vessels. The distal pulmonary arterioles also are thin walled and have the capacity to dilate, collapse, or constrict depending on the presence of vasoactive substances released from the endothelial cells of the vessel, neurohumoral influences, flow velocity, oxygen tension, and alveolar ventilation.

The term *pulmonary hypertension* describes the elevation of pressure in the pulmonary arterial system. The normal mean pulmonary artery pressure is approximately 15 mm Hg (*e.g.*, 28 systolic/8 diastolic). Pulmonary artery hypertension can be caused by an elevation in left atrial pressure, increased pulmonary blood flow, or increased pulmonary vascular resistance. Because of the increased pressure in the pulmonary circulation, pulmonary hypertension increases the workload of the right heart. Although pulmonary hypertension can develop as a primary disorder, most cases develop secondary to some other condition.

Secondary Pulmonary Hypertension

Secondary pulmonary hypertension refers to an increase in pulmonary pressures associated with other disease conditions, usually cardiac or pulmonary. Secondary causes, or mechanisms, of pulmonary hypertension can be divided into three major categories: pulmonary venous pressure elevation, increased pulmonary blood flow and pulmonary vascular obstruction, and hypoxemia.[48] Often more than one factor, such as COPD, heart failure, and sleep apnea, contributes to the elevation in pulmonary pressures.

Elevation of pulmonary venous pressure is common in conditions such as mitral valve stenosis and left ventricular heart failure, in which an elevated left atrial pressure is transmitted to the pulmonary circulation. Continued increases in left atrial pressure can lead to medial hypertrophy and intimal thickening of the small pulmonary arteries, causing sustained hypertension.

Increased pulmonary blood flow results from increased flow through left-to-right shunts in congenital heart diseases such as atrial or ventricular septal defects and patent ductus arteriosus. If the high-flow state is allowed to continue, morphologic changes occur in the pulmonary vessels, leading to sustained pulmonary hypertension. The pulmonary vascular changes that occur with congenital heart disorders are discussed in Chapter 24. Pulmonary emboli are common causes of obstructed flow in the pulmonary circulation. Once initiated, the pulmonary hypertension is self-perpetuating because of hypertrophy and proliferation of vascular smooth muscle.

Hypoxemia is a common cause of pulmonary hypertension. Unlike the vessels in the systemic circulation, most of which dilate in response to hypoxemia and hypercapnia, the pulmonary vessels constrict. The stimulus for constriction seems to originate in the air spaces near the smaller branches of the pulmonary arteries. In situations in which certain regions of the lung are hypoventilated, the response is adaptive in that it diverts blood flow away from the poorly ventilated areas to more adequately ventilated portions of the lung. This effect, however, becomes less beneficial as more and more areas of the lung become poorly ventilated. Pulmonary hypertension is a common problem in persons with advanced chronic bronchitis and emphysema. It also may develop at high altitudes in persons with normal lungs. Persons who experience marked hypoxemia during sleep (*i.e.*, those with sleep apnea) often experience marked elevations in pulmonary arterial pressure.

The signs and symptoms of secondary pulmonary hypertension reflect not only the underlying cause, but the effect that the elevated pressures have on right heart function and oxygen transport. Dyspnea and fatigue are common. Peripheral edema, ascites, and signs of right heart failure (cor pulmonale, to be discussed) develop as the condition progresses.

Diagnosis is based on radiographic findings, echocardiography, and Doppler ultrasonography. Precise measurement of pulmonary pressures can be obtained only through right heart cardiac catheterization. Treatment measures are directed toward the underlying disorder. Vasodilator therapy may be indicated for some persons.

Primary Pulmonary Hypertension

Primary pulmonary hypertension is a relatively rare and rapidly progressive form of pulmonary hypertension that leads to right ventricular failure and death within a few years. Estimates of incidence range from 1 to 2 cases per million people in the general population.[49] The disease can occur at any age, and familial occurrences have been reported. Persons with the disorder usually have a steadily progressive downhill course, with death occurring in 3 to 4 years. Overall, the 5-year survival rate of untreated primary pulmonary hypertension is approximately 20%.[50]

Primary pulmonary hypertension is thought to be associated with a number of factors, including an autosomal dominant genetic predisposition along with an exogenous trigger.[50] Triggers include low oxygen levels that occur at high altitudes, exposure to certain drugs, human immunodeficiency virus infection, and autoimmune disorders.

The disorder is characterized by endothelial damage, coagulation abnormalities, and marked intimal fibrosis leading to obliteration or obstruction of the pulmonary arteries and arterioles. Most of the manifestations of the disorder are attributable to increased work demands on the right heart and a decrease in cardiac output. Symptoms are the same as those for secondary hypertension. The most obvious are dyspnea and fatigue that is out of proportion to other signs of a person's well-being.

The diagnosis of primary pulmonary hypertension is based on an absence of disorders that cause secondary hypertension and mean pulmonary artery pressures greater than 25 mm Hg at rest or 30 mm Hg with exercise.

Treatment consists of measures to improve right heart function to reduce fatigue and peripheral edema. Supplemental oxygen may used to increase exercise tolerance. The most widely used drugs for long-term therapy are the calcium channel blockers (nifedipine and diltiazem). Anticoagulant (warfarin) therapy may be used to decrease the risk of thrombosis due to sluggish pulmonary blood flow. Epoprostenol, a short-acting (half-life, 3 to 5 minutes) analog of the naturally occurring vasodilator prostacyclin (prostaglandin I$_2$), is increasingly used in the long-term management of persons with the disorder. Because of its short half-life, the drug must be administered by continuous infusion, usually through an indwelling catcher (*e.g.*, subclavian Hickman) with an automatic ambulatory pump. Properties of the drug other than its vasodilating effects include inhibition of platelet aggregation and beneficial vascular remodeling effects. Epoprostenol therapy has markedly improved the quality of life for persons with primary pulmonary hypertension. It has been reported that several people have been receiving epoprostenol by continuous infusion for 10 years or more with sustained clinical and hemodynamic benefits.[49] Lung transplantation may be an alternative for persons who do not respond to other forms of treatment.

Cor Pulmonale

The term *cor pulmonale* refers to right heart failure resulting from primary lung disease and long-standing primary or secondary pulmonary hypertension. It involves hypertrophy and the eventual failure of the right ventricle. The manifestations of cor pulmonale include the signs and symptoms of the primary lung disease and the signs of right-sided heart failure (see Chapter 26). The patient has shortness of breath and a productive cough, which becomes worse during periods of heart failure. Failure of the right ventricle and elevation of intrathoracic pressure resulting from airway obstruction cause venous distention and peripheral edema. Plethora (*i.e.*, redness) and cyanosis and warm, moist skin may result from the compensatory polycythemia and desaturation of arterial blood that accompany chronic lung disease. Drowsiness and altered consciousness may occur as the result of carbon dioxide retention. Management of cor pulmonale focuses on the treatment of the lung disease and the heart failure. Low-flow oxygen therapy may be used to reduce the pulmonary hypertension and polycythemia associated with severe hypoxemia due to chronic lung disease.

ACUTE RESPIRATORY DISTRESS SYNDROME

Acute respiratory distress syndrome (ARDS), first described in 1967, is a devastating syndrome of acute lung injury. Initially called the *adult respiratory distress syndrome*, it is now called the *acute respiratory distress syndrome* because it also affects children. ARDS affects approximately 150,000 to 200,000 persons each year; at least 50% to 60% of these persons die, despite the most sophisticated intensive care.[51] The disorder is the final common pathway through which many serious localized and systemic disorders produce diffuse injury to the alveolar-capillary membrane.

ARDS may result from a number of conditions, including aspiration of gastric contents, major trauma (with or without fat emboli), sepsis secondary to pulmonary or nonpulmonary infections, acute pancreatitis, hematologic disorders, metabolic events, and reactions to drugs and toxins[51-53] (Chart 29-2). Although the pathogenesis of ARDS is unclear, it is hypothesized that neutrophils play a

---

CHART 29-2

*Conditions in Which Respiratory Distress Syndrome Can Develop**

Aspiration
Gastric acid
Near-drowning

Reaction to Drugs and Toxins
Chlordiazepoxide
Heroin
Methadone
Propoxyphene
Chloroform
Colchicine
Barbiturates
Inhaled gases
  Ammonia
  Phosgene
  Ozone
  Oxygen (high concentrations)
  Smoke

Hematologic Disorders
Multiple blood transfusions
Disseminated intravascular coagulation
Exposure to cardiopulmonary bypass

Infectious Causes
Bacterial pneumonia
Fungal and *Pneumocystis carinii* pneumonias
Gram-negative sepsis
Viral pneumonia

Immune Reactions
Anaphylactic shock
Allergic reactions to inhaled substances

Metabolic Disorders
Diabetic ketoacidosis
Uremia

Trauma
Burns
Fat embolus
Heat trauma
Chest trauma and lung injury
Shock

*This list is not intended to be inclusive.

central role. Neutrophils can synthesize and release products that are capable of tissue injury, including proteolytic enzymes, toxic oxygen species (free radicals; see Chapter 5), and phospholipid products.

Although a number of conditions may lead to ARDS, they all produce similar pathologic lung changes that include diffuse epithelial cell injury with increased permeability of the alveolar-capillary membrane. The increased permeability permits fluid, protein, and blood cells to move out of the vascular compartment into the interstitium and alveoli of the lung. The resultant pulmonary edema leads to intrapulmonary shunting of blood, impaired gas exchange, and profound hypoxia. Gas exchange is further compromised by alveolar collapse resulting from abnormalities in surfactant production. As the disease progresses, the work of breathing becomes greatly increased as the lung stiffens and becomes more difficult to inflate. When injury to the alveolar epithelium is severe, disorganized epithelial repair may lead to fibrosis.[52]

Clinically, the syndrome consists of progressive respiratory distress, an increase in respiratory rate, and signs of respiratory failure. Radiologic findings usually show extensive bilateral consolidation of the lung tissue. Severe hypoxia persists despite increased inspired oxygen levels.

The treatment goals in ARDS are to supply oxygen to vital organs and provide supportive care until the condition causing the pathologic process has been reversed and the lungs have had a chance to heal. Assisted ventilation using high concentrations of oxygen may be required to overcome the hypoxia. Positive end-expiratory pressure breathing, which increases the pressure in the airways during expiration, may be used to assist in reinflating the collapsed areas of the lung and to improve the matching of ventilation and perfusion.

An important advance aimed at understanding the pathogenesis and treatment of ARDS has been the establishment of the Acute Respiratory Distress Syndrome Network supported by the National Institutes of Health. The establishment of the network provides the infrastructure for well-designed, multicenter, randomized trials of existing and potential new therapies. Among the therapies that are being considered for investigation are ventilation methods, fluid and hemodynamic management, use of surfactant therapy, nitric oxide and other vasodilators, and the corticosteroids. Another area being explored is the use of growth factors to protect against lung injury and accelerate recovery from ARDS.

In summary, pulmonary vascular disorders include pulmonary embolism and pulmonary hypertension. Pulmonary embolism develops when a blood-borne substance lodges in a branch of the pulmonary artery and obstructs blood flow. The embolus can consist of a thrombus, air, fat, or amniotic fluid. The most common form is a thromboembolus arising from the deep venous channels of the lower extremities. Pulmonary hypertension is the elevation of pulmonary arterial pressure. It can be caused by an elevated left atrial pressure, increased pulmonary blood flow, or increased pulmonary vascular resistance secondary to lung disease. The term *cor pulmonale* describes right heart failure caused by primary pulmonary disease and longstanding pulmonary hypertension.

ARDS is a devastating syndrome of acute lung injury resulting from a number of serious localized and systemic disorders that damage the alveolar-capillary membrane of the lung. It results in interstitial edema of lung tissue, an increase in surface tension caused by inactivation of surfactant, collapse of the alveolar structures, a stiff and noncompliant lung that is difficult to inflate, and impaired diffusion of the respiratory gases with severe hypoxia that is resistant to oxygen therapy.

Respiratory Failure

After you have completed this section of the chapter, you should be able to meet the following objectives:

✦ Define the terms *hypoxia*, *hypoxemia*, and *hypercapnia*
✦ State a general definition for respiratory failure
✦ Characterize the mechanisms whereby respiratory disorders cause hypoxemia and hypercapnia
✦ Compare the manifestations of hypoxia and hypercapnia
✦ Describe the treatment of hypoxia and hypercapnia

The function of the respiratory system is to add oxygen to the blood and remove carbon dioxide. To accomplish this task, the respiratory system moves air into and out of the lung, provides for the transfer of the gases from the air to the blood, and moves blood through the lung so that gas exchange can take place. When respiratory function is impaired, the blood is not oxygenated and carbon dioxide is not removed.

The term *hypoxia* refers to a reduction in oxygen supply to the tissues; *hypoxemia*, to a low level of oxygen in the blood; and *hypercapnia* (sometimes referred to as *hypercarbia*), to excess carbon dioxide in the blood. The abbreviation PO_2 often is used to indicate the partial pressure of oxygen in arterial blood, and the abbreviation PCO_2, the partial pressure of carbon dioxide. Hypoxia and hypercapnia can manifest as acute and chronic conditions, and hypoxia may exist without hypercapnia, or the two conditions may coexist.

MECHANISMS

Respiratory failure is a condition in which the lungs fail to oxygenate the blood adequately and prevent carbon dioxide retention. It is not a specific disease, but the result of a number of conditions that impair ventilation, compromise the matching of ventilation and perfusion, or disrupt blood flow in the lung. These conditions include impaired ventilation caused by impaired function of the respiratory center, airway obstruction, weakness and paralysis of the respiratory muscles, chest wall deformities, and disease of the airways and lungs. It may occur in previously healthy persons as the result of acute disease or trauma involving the respiratory system, or it may develop in the course of a chronic neuromuscular or respiratory disease. The causes of respiratory failure are summarized in Table 29-4.

The common manifestations of respiratory failure are hypoxemia and hypercapnia. There is no absolute definition of the levels of PO_2 and PCO_2 that indicate respiratory failure. As a general rule, *respiratory failure* refers to a PO_2 level of 50 mm Hg or less and a PCO_2 level greater than 50 mm Hg (Table 29-5). These values are not reliable when dealing with persons who have chronic lung disease because many of these persons are alert and functioning with blood gas levels outside this range.

Various types of respiratory failure are associated with different degrees of hypoxemia or hypercapnia, as indicated in Figure 29-14. For example, pure hypoventilation, as occurs in conditions such as drug overdose, favors retention of CO_2 (line A, Fig. 29-14). Severe ventilation-perfusion mismatching with alveolar ventilation that is inadequate to maintain the PO_2 (line B) results in hypoxemia that is more severe in relation to hypercarbia than occurs with pure hypoventilation. This pattern of respiratory failure is seen most commonly in persons with advanced COPD. As noted by the broken lines in Figure 29-14, breathing high concentrations of oxygen increases both the PO_2 and the PCO_2. In interstitial lung disease (line C), there is severe hypox-

Disorders of Blood Gases in Respiratory Failure

➤ Respiratory failure represents failure of the lungs to adequately oxygenate the blood and prevent carbon dioxide retention.

➤ The carbon dioxide level in the arterial blood is proportional to carbon dioxide production and inversely related to alveolar ventilation. Carbon dioxide retention is characteristic of conditions such as depression of the respiratory center or musculoskeletal disorders that produce hypoventilation. Carbon dioxide diffuses more readily across the alveolar-capillary membrane than oxygen. Severe mismatching of ventilation and perfusion, such as that which occurs in conditions such as chronic obstructive pulmonary disease, produces a more profound effect on oxygenation of the blood than on carbon dioxide retention.

➤ Conditions such as acute respiratory distress syndrome that impede the diffusion of gases in the lung impair the oxygenation of blood but do not interfere with the elimination of carbon dioxide.

TABLE 29-4 ✦ Causes of Respiratory Failure

Category of Impairment	Examples
Impaired Ventilation	
Upper airway obstruction	Laryngospasm
	Foreign body aspiration
	Tumor of the upper airways
	Infection of the upper airways (*e.g.*, epiglottitis)
Weakness or paralysis of the respiratory muscles	Drug overdose
	Injury to the spinal cord
	Poliomyelitis
	Guillain-Barré syndrome
	Muscular dystrophy
	Disease of the brain stem
Chest wall injury	Rib fracture
	Burn eschar
Impaired Matching of Ventilation and Perfusion	
	Chronic obstructive lung disease
	Restrictive lung disease
	Severe pneumonia
	Atelectasis
Impaired Diffusion	
Pulmonary edema	Left heart failure
	Inhalation of toxic materials
Respiratory distress syndrome	Respiratory distress syndrome in the neonate
	Acute respiratory distress syndrome

Arterial Blood Gas Value	Normal Value	Respiratory Failure
PO_2	>80 mm Hg	≤50 mm Hg
PCO_2	35–45 mm Hg	≥50 mm Hg

TABLE 29-5 ✦ **Blood Gases in Respiratory Failure Compared With Normal Values**

emia but no hypercapnia because of increased ventilation. In ARDS (line D), the arterial PCO_2 is typically low, but hypoxemia is severe. In this case, administration of oxygen can produce an increase in PO_2 without producing an increase in PCO_2.

Hypoventilation

Hypoventilation occurs when the volume of "fresh" air moving into and out of the lung is significantly reduced. Hypoventilation is commonly caused by conditions outside the lung such as depression of the respiratory center (*e.g.*, drug overdose), diseases of the nerves supplying the respiratory muscles (*e.g.*, Guillain-Barré syndrome), disorders of the respiratory muscles (*e.g.*, muscular dystrophy), or thoracic cage disorders (*e.g.*, severe scoliosis or crushed chest).

Hypoventilation has two important effects on arterial blood gases. First, it always causes an increase in PCO_2. The rise in PCO_2 is directly related to the level of ventilation. If the alveolar ventilation is reduced by one half, the PCO_2 doubles. Thus, the PCO_2 level is a good diagnostic measure for hypoventilation. If the PCO_2 level is not elevated, a person is not hypoventilating.[54] Second, any hypoxemia caused by hypoventilation can be easily abolished by in-

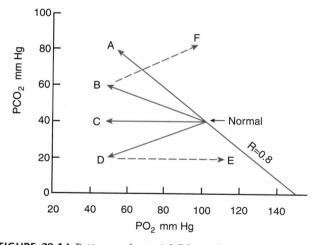

FIGURE 29-14 Patterns of arterial PO_2 and PCO_2 in different types of respiratory failure. Note that PCO_2 can be high, as in pure hypoventilation (A), or low, as in acute respiratory distress syndrome (D). The broken lines show the effects of oxygen breathing. (West J.B. [1997]. *Pulmonary pathophysiology* [5th ed., p. 132]. Philadelphia: Lippincott-Raven)

creasing the oxygen content of the inspired air.[54] In fact, pure hypoventilation does not cause large decreases in PO_2. The PO_2 falls by approximately 1 mm Hg for every 1 mm Hg rise in PCO_2. Hypoventilation sufficient to double the PCO_2 from 40 to 80 mm Hg decreases the PO_2 from 100 to 60 mm Hg.[54]

Ventilation-Perfusion Mismatching

The mismatching of ventilation and perfusion occurs when areas of the lung are ventilated but not perfused or when areas are perfused but not ventilated. Usually the hypoxemia seen in situations of ventilation-perfusion mismatching is more severe in relation to hypercapnia than that seen in hypoventilation. Severe mismatching of ventilation and perfusion often is seen in persons with advanced COPD. These disorders contribute to the retention of carbon dioxide by reducing the effective alveolar ventilation, even when total ventilation is maintained. This occurs because a region of the lung is not perfused and gas exchange cannot take place or because an area of the lung is not being ventilated. Maintaining a high ventilation rate effectively prevents hypercapnia but also increases the work of breathing.

The hypoxemia associated with ventilation-perfusion disorders often is exaggerated by conditions such as hypoventilation and decreased cardiac output. For example, sedation can cause hypoventilation in persons with severe COPD, resulting in further impairment of ventilation. Likewise, a decrease in cardiac output because of myocardial infarction can exaggerate the ventilation-perfusion impairment in a person with mild pulmonary edema.

The beneficial effects of oxygen administration on PO_2 levels in ventilation-perfusion disorders depends on the degree of mismatching that is present. Because oxygen administration increases the diffusion gradient in ventilated portions of the lung, it usually is effective in raising arterial PO_2 levels but may decrease the respiratory drive and produce an increase in PCO_2.

Impaired Diffusion

Diffusion impairment describes a condition in which gas exchange between the alveoli and the red blood cells is impeded because of an increase in the distance for diffusion or a decrease in the permeability of the alveolar capillary membrane to movement of gases.

Impaired diffusion is caused by conditions such as interstitial lung disease, ARDS, pulmonary edema, and pneumonia. These conditions alter the thickness or permeability of the alveolar capillary membrane, rather than the time that the blood spends in pulmonary capillaries. Movement of oxygen across the alveolar-capillary membrane normally is rapid, with equilibration occurring during the first third of the time that the blood spends in the pulmonary capillaries. Even under conditions of increased heart rate, as occurs during exercise, there usually is sufficient time for gas exchange to occur.

Hypoxemia resulting from impaired diffusion can be partially or completely corrected by the administration of 100% oxygen. This occurs because the increase in alveolar oxygen establishes a large alveolar-capillary diffusion gradient that overcomes the resistance to diffusion.

Shunt

Shunt occurs when blood reaches the arterial system without passing through the ventilated portion of the lung. Most shunts, such as those that occur with congenital heart disease, are extrapulmonary. However, a completely unventilated portion of the lung, as occurs with atelectasis, can result in the shunting of blood in the pulmonary circulation. Administration of oxygen usually increases arterial oxygen levels with intrapulmonary shunting, but not with extrapulmonary shunting, as occurs in children with intracardiac shunts. Because unoxygenated venous blood is being mixed with oxygenated blood in persons with intrapulmonary shunts, the rise in PO_2 levels depends on the degree of shunt.

CHART 29-3

Signs and Symptoms of Hypoxia

Arterial PO_2 <50 mm Hg	Loss of judgment
Tachycardia	Euphoria
Mild increase in blood pressure	Unruly or combative behavior
Cool and moist skin	Sensory impairment
Confusion	Mental fatigue
Delirium	Drowsiness
Difficulty in problem solving	Stupor and coma (late)
	Hypotension (late)
	Bradycardia (late)

HYPOXEMIA

Hypoxemia refers to a reduction in blood oxygen levels. Hypoxemia can result from an inadequate amount of oxygen in the air, disease of the respiratory system, or alterations in circulatory function. The mechanisms whereby respiratory disorders lead to a significant reduction in PO_2 are hypoventilation, impaired diffusion of gases, shunt, and mismatching of ventilation and perfusion.[54] Another cause of hypoxemia, reduction of the partial pressure of oxygen in the inspired air, occurs only under special circumstances, such as at high altitudes. Often more than one mechanism contributes to hypoxemia in a person with respiratory or cardiac disease.

Manifestations

Hypoxemia produces its effects through tissue hypoxia and the compensatory mechanisms that the body uses to adapt to the lowered oxygen level. Body tissues vary considerably in their vulnerability to hypoxia; those with the greatest need are the nervous system and heart. Cessation of blood flow to the cerebral cortex results in loss of consciousness within 10 to 20 seconds. If the PO_2 of the tissues falls below a critical level, aerobic metabolism ceases and anaerobic metabolism takes over, with formation and release of lactic acid.

The signs and symptoms of hypoxia, which are listed in Chart 29-3, can be grouped into two categories: those resulting from impaired function of vital centers and those resulting from activation of compensatory mechanisms. Mild hypoxemia produces few manifestations. There may be slight impairment of mental performance and visual acuity and sometimes hyperventilation. This is because hemoglobin saturation still is approximately 90% when the PO_2 is only 60 mm Hg (see Chapter 27, Fig. 27-22). More pronounced hypoxemia may produce personality changes, restlessness, agitated or combative behavior, muscle incoordination, euphoria, impaired judgment, delirium, and, eventually, stupor and coma. Tachycardia, cool skin (*i.e.*, peripheral vasoconstriction), diaphoresis, and a mild increase in blood pressure result from the recruitment of sympathetic nervous system compensatory mechanisms. Profound acute hypoxemia can cause convulsions, retinal hemorrhages, and permanent brain damage. Hypotension and bradycardia often are preterminal events in persons with hypoxemia, indicating the failure of compensatory mechanisms.

The body compensates for hypoxemia by increased ventilation, pulmonary vasoconstriction and increased production of red blood cells. Hyperventilation results from the hypoxic stimulation of the chemoreceptors. Increased production of red blood cells results from the release of erythropoietin from the kidneys in response to hypoxia (see Chapter 15). Polycythemia increases the red blood cell concentration and the oxygen-carrying capacity of the blood. Pulmonary vasoconstriction occurs as a local response to alveolar hypoxia; it increases pulmonary arterial pressure and improves the matching of ventilation and blood flow. Other adaptive mechanisms include a shift to the right in the oxygen dissociation curve as a means of increasing oxygen release to the tissues (see Chapter 27). Elevation of intracellular levels of oxidative enzymes increases the efficiency of oxygen use at the tissue level.

In conditions of chronic hypoxemia, the manifestations may be insidious in onset and attributed to other causes, particularly in chronic lung disease. Decreased sensory function, such as impaired vision or fewer complaints of pain, may be an early sign of worsening hypoxemia. This is probably because the involved sensory neurons have the same need for high levels of oxygen, as do other parts of the nervous system. Pulmonary hypertension is common because of associated alveolar hypoxia.

Cyanosis. Cyanosis refers to the bluish discoloration of the skin and mucous membranes that results from an excessive concentration of reduced or deoxygenated hemoglobin in the small blood vessels. It usually is most marked in the lips, nail beds, ears, and cheeks. The degree of cyanosis is modified by the amount of cutaneous pigment, skin thickness, and the state of the cutaneous capillaries. Cyanosis is more difficult to distinguish in persons with dark skin and in areas of the body with increased skin thickness.

Although cyanosis may be evident in persons with respiratory failure, it often is a late sign. A concentration of approximately 5 g/dL of deoxygenated hemoglobin is required in the circulating blood for cyanosis. The absolute quantity of reduced hemoglobin, rather than the relative quantity, is important in producing cyanosis. Persons with anemia and low hemoglobin levels are less likely to exhibit cyanosis (because they have less hemoglobin to deoxygenate), even though they may be relatively hypoxic because of their decreased ability to transport oxygen, than persons who have high hemoglobin concentrations. Someone with a high hemoglobin level because of polycythemia may be cyanotic without being hypoxic.

Cyanosis can be divided into two types: central or peripheral. *Central cyanosis* is evident in the tongue and lips. It is caused by an increased amount of deoxygenated hemoglobin or an abnormal hemoglobin derivative in the arterial blood. Abnormal hemoglobin derivatives include *methemoglobin*, in which the nitrite ion reacts with hemoglobin. Because methemoglobin has a low affinity for oxygen, large doses of nitrites can result in cyanosis and tissue hypoxia. Although nitrites are used in treating angina, the therapeutic dose is too small to cause cyanosis. Sodium nitrite is used as a curing agent for meat. In nursing infants, the intestinal flora is capable of converting significant amounts of inorganic nitrate (*e.g.*, from well water) into nitrite ion.[55]

Peripheral cyanosis occurs in the extremities and on the tip of the nose or ears. It is caused by slowing of blood flow to an area of the body, with increased extraction of oxygen from the blood. It results from vasoconstriction and diminished peripheral blood flow, as occurs with cold exposure, shock, congestive heart failure, and peripheral vascular disease. Acute arterial obstruction in an extremity, such as occurs with an embolus or arterial spasm (*i.e.*, Raynaud's phenomenon, discussed in Chapter 22), usually presents with pallor and coldness, although there may be cyanosis.

Diagnosis

Diagnosis of hypoxemia is based on clinical observation and diagnostic measures of oxygen levels. The analysis of arterial blood gases provides a direct measure of the oxygen content of the blood and is a good indicator of the lungs' ability to oxygenate the blood. Continuous mixed venous oxygen saturation ($S\bar{V}O_2$) can be monitored using a special type of pulmonary artery catheter.[56] This method, which measures the mixed venous blood that is being returned to the lungs, reflects the use of oxygen by the peripheral tissues. Arterial blood gases and $S\bar{V}O_2$ often are monitored in critically ill patients. Both measurements are invasive and require direct sampling of the patient's blood through a peripheral arterial catheter (for blood gases) or a pulmonary artery catheter (for $S\bar{V}O_2$).

There are two noninvasive methods for oxygen assessment: the transcutaneous sensor method and the pulse oximeter.[57] Transcutaneous oxygen monitoring uses an oxygen electrode. The electrode and covering membrane allow oxygen to diffuse through the skin and be measured. The pulse oximeter uses light-emitting diodes and combines plethysmography (*i.e.*, changes in light absorbance and vasodilatation) with spectrophotometry.[58] Spectrophotometry uses a red-wavelength light that passes through oxygenated hemoglobin and is absorbed by deoxygenated hemoglobin and an infrared-wavelength light that is absorbed by oxygenated hemoglobin and passes through deoxygenated hemoglobin. Sensors that can be placed on the ear, finger, toe, or forehead are available. These methods, although not as accurate as the invasive methods, provide a means for continuous monitoring of oxygen levels and are useful indicators of respiratory and circulatory status. The pulse oximeters cannot distinguish between oxygen-carrying hemoglobin and carbon monoxide–carrying hemoglobin. In addition, the pulse oximeter cannot detect elevated levels of methemoglobin.

HYPERCAPNIA

Hypercapnia refers to an increase in the carbon dioxide content of the blood. The diagnosis of hypercapnia is based on physiologic manifestations, arterial pH, and blood gas levels. The carbon dioxide level in the arterial blood, or PCO_2, is proportional to carbon dioxide production and inversely related to alveolar ventilation. The diffusing capacity of carbon dioxide is 20 times that of oxygen; therefore, hypercapnia is observed only in situations of hypoventilation sufficient to cause hypoxia.

Hypercapnia can occur in a number of disorders that cause hypoventilation or mismatching of ventilation and perfusion. Hypoventilation is a cause of hypercapnia in respiratory failure due to depression of the respiratory center in drug overdose, neuromuscular diseases such as Guillain-Barré syndrome, or chest wall deformities such as seen with severe scoliosis. Hypercapnia due to ventilation-perfusion inequalities is seen most commonly in persons with COPD. Conditions that increase carbon dioxide production, such as an increase in metabolic rate or a high-carbohydrate diet, can contribute to the degree of hypercapnia that occurs in persons with impaired respiratory function.

Mechanisms

Impaired Neural Control. The respiratory center, which controls the activity of the muscles of respiration, is a crucial determinant of ventilation and elimination of carbon dioxide. It is composed of widely dispersed groups of neurons located in the medulla oblongata and pons (see Chapter 27). The activity of the respiratory center is regulated by chemoreceptors that monitor changes in the chemical composition of the blood. The most important chemoreceptors in terms of the minute-by-minute control of ventilation are the central chemoreceptors that respond to changes in the hydrogen ion (H^+) concentration of the cerebrospinal fluid. Although the blood-brain barrier is impermeable to H^+ ions, CO_2 crosses it with ease. The CO_2, in turn, reacts with water to form carbonic acid, which dissociates to form H^+ and bicarbonate (HCO_3^-) ions. When the CO_2 content of the blood rises, CO_2 crosses the blood-brain barrier, liberating H^+ ions that stimulate the central chemoreceptors. The excitation of the respiratory center due to CO_2 is greatest during the first 1 to 2 days that blood levels are elevated, but it gradually declines over the next 1 to 2 days.[59] Part of this decline results from renal compensatory mechanisms that readjust the blood pH by increasing blood bicarbonate levels.

In persons with respiratory problems that cause chronic hypoxia and hypercapnia, the peripheral chemoreceptors become the driving force for ventilation. These chemoreceptors, which are located in the bifurcation of the common carotid arteries and in the aortic arch, respond to changes in PO_2. Administration of high-flow oxygen to these persons can abolish the input from these peripheral receptors, causing a decrease in alveolar ventilation and a further rise in PCO_2 levels.

Respiratory Muscle Fatigue. Respiratory muscle fatigue can contribute to carbon dioxide retention in persons with various primary respiratory diseases and in those with neuromuscular disorders. In these persons, respiratory muscle fatigue develops when energy requirements exceed the energy supply. A number of factors increase energy requirements or decrease the energy supply. The energy demands of the respiratory muscles are increased by high levels of ventilation or by factors that increase the work of breathing, such as high levels of airway resistance. The energy supply depends on blood flow and the oxygen content of the blood. Low cardiac output, anemia, and decreased oxygen saturation contribute to a decreased energy supply and increase the likelihood of respiratory muscle fatigue. With malnutrition, the energy stores of the muscles are diminished, and there may be structural changes in the muscle as well. Electrolyte imbalances, especially hypokalemia and hypophosphatemia, contribute to respiratory muscle weakness.[60]

Increased Carbon Dioxide Production. Disorders of carbon dioxide retention may be exaggerated by changes in metabolic rate or intake of carbon dioxide–generating foods. Changes in the metabolic rate resulting from an increase in activity level, fever, or disease can have profound effects on carbon dioxide production. Alveolar ventilation usually rises proportionally with these changes, and hypercapnia occurs only when this increase is inappropriate.

Interest has been focused on the effect of carbohydrate metabolism on carbon dioxide production. The respiratory quotient (RQ), which is the ratio of carbon dioxide production to oxygen consumption (RQ = CO_2 production/O_2 consumption), varies with the type of food metabolized. A characteristic of carbohydrate metabolism is an RQ of 1.0, with equal carbon dioxide being produced and oxygen being consumed. Because fats contain less oxygen than carbohydrates, their oxidation produces less carbon dioxide (RQ = 0.7). The metabolism of pure proteins (RQ = 0.81) results in the production of more carbon dioxide than the metabolism of fat but less than the metabolism of carbohydrates. The type of food that is eaten or the types of nutrients that are delivered through enteral feedings (*i.e.*, through a tube placed in the small intestine) or parenteral nutrition (*i.e.*, through a venous catheter placed in the central vena cava) may influence PCO_2 levels. Portable devices and metabolic carts that use indirect calorimetry to determine the RQ and energy requirements are available for use in the clinical setting.[61]

In persons who receive a high glucose load in association with total parenteral nutrition, the RQ can rise to a level of 1 or more.[59] Persons with adequate respiratory function can increase their alveolar ventilation proportional to the increased carbon dioxide production. Hypercapnic respiratory failure can occur in persons who cannot ade-

quately increase their ventilation. It has been suggested that such persons receive a larger proportion of nonprotein calories in the form of fat emulsions because these emulsions are associated with a lower rate of carbon dioxide production.[60]

Manifestations

Hypercapnia affects a number of body functions, including renal function, neural function, cardiovascular function, and acid-base balance. Elevated levels of PCO_2 produce a decrease in pH and respiratory acidosis (see Chapter 32). The body normally compensates for an increase in PCO_2 by increasing renal bicarbonate retention. As long as the pH is in an acceptable range, the main complications of hypercapnia are those resulting from the accompanying hypoxia. Because the body adapts to chronic increases in blood levels of carbon dioxide, persons with chronic hypercapnia may not have symptoms until the PCO_2 is markedly elevated.

Carbon dioxide has a direct vasodilatory effect on many blood vessels and a sedative effect on the nervous system. When the cerebral vessels are dilated, headache develops. The conjunctivae are hyperemic, and the skin flushed. Hypercapnia has nervous system effects similar to those of an anesthetic—hence the term *carbon dioxide narcosis*. There is progressive somnolence, disorientation, and, if the condition is untreated, coma. Mild to moderate increases in blood pressure are common. Air hunger and rapid breathing occur when alveolar PCO_2 levels rise to approximately 60 to 75 mm Hg; as PCO_2 levels reach 80 to 100 mm Hg, the person becomes lethargic and sometimes becomes semicomatose. Anesthesia and death can result when PCO_2 levels reach 100 to 150 mm Hg.[52] The signs and symptoms of hypercapnia are summarized in Chart 29-4.

Diagnosis of hypercapnia is based on blood gas measurements and end-tidal volume carbon dioxide tension (*i.e.*, capnometry).

TREATMENT

The treatment of respiratory failure focuses on correcting the problem causing impaired gas exchange when pos-

---

CHART 29-4

Signs and Symptoms of Hypercapnia

Increased PCO_2
Headache
Conjunctival hyperemia
Flushed skin
Increased sedation
  Drowsiness
  Disorientation
  Coma
Tachycardia
Diaphoresis
Mild to moderate increase in blood pressure

sible and on relieving the hypoxemia and hypercapnia. A number of treatment modalities are available, including the establishment of an airway, use of bronchodilating drugs, and antibiotics for respiratory infections. Controlled oxygen therapy and mechanical ventilation are used in treating blood gas abnormalities associated with respiratory failure.

Decreasing the Work of Breathing and Improving Respiratory Muscle Function

Therapy for hypercapnia is directed at decreasing the work of breathing and improving the ventilation-perfusion balance. Intermittent rest therapy, such as nocturnal negative-pressure ventilation, applied to hypercapnic patients with chronic obstructive disease or chest wall disease may be effective in increasing the strength and endurance of the respiratory muscle and improving the PCO_2. Respiratory muscle retraining aimed at improving the respiratory muscles, their endurance, or both has been used to improve exercise tolerance and diminish the likelihood of respiratory fatigue.

Oxygen Therapy

Oxygen may be delivered by nasal cannula or mask. It also may be administered directly into an endotracheal or tracheostomy tube in persons who are being ventilated. A high-flow administration system is one in which the flow rate and reserve capacity are sufficient to provide all the inspired air.[62] A low-flow oxygen system delivers less than the total inspired air.[62] The oxygen must be humidified as it is being administered. The concentration of oxygen that is being administered (usually determined by the flow rate) is based on the PO_2. The rate must be carefully monitored in persons with chronic lung disease because increases in PO_2 above 60 mm Hg are likely to depress the ventilatory drive. There also is the danger of oxygen toxicity with high concentrations of oxygen. Continuous breathing of oxygen at high concentrations can lead to diffuse parenchymal lung injury. Persons with healthy lungs begin to experience respiratory symptoms such as cough, sore throat, substernal distress, nasal congestion, and painful inspiration after breathing pure oxygen for 24 hours.[54]

Mechanical Ventilation

When alveolar ventilation is inadequate to maintain PO_2 or PCO_2 levels because of respiratory or neurologic failure, mechanical ventilation may be life saving. Usually a nasotracheal, orotracheal, or tracheotomy tube is inserted into the trachea to provide the patient with the airway needed for mechanical ventilation. There has been recent interest in noninvasive forms of mechanical ventilation that use a face mask to deliver positive-pressure ventilation.[63,64]

There are two basic types of positive-pressure mechanical ventilators: pressure-cycled units and volume-cycled units.[62] The pressure-cycled unit delivers a tidal volume determined by the airway pressure while the flow rate is being controlled. The volume-cycled ventilator delivers a preselected tidal volume while the pressure is monitored. The tidal volume and respiratory rate are adjusted to maintain ventilation at a given minute volume. Ventilators are capable of functioning in assist-control method, in which the ventilator delivers a breath triggered by the patient or independently if such an effort does not occur; an intermittent mandatory ventilation, in which the patient receives periodic positive-pressure ventilation from the ventilator at a preset volume and rate; and pressure-support ventilation, in which the ventilator delivers a set pressure rather than volume to augment each spontaneous respiratory effort.[54] Ventilators also can be programmed to supply positive end-expiratory pressure or continuous positive airway pressure in spontaneously breathing patients.

A third type of ventilator uses negative pressure to expand the chest. These ventilators do not require an artificial airway. The early negative-pressure ventilator, known as the *iron lung*, consisted of a large tank that enclosed all of the body except the head. They were used extensively to ventilate patients with bulbar poliomyelitis. A modification of the iron lung is the cuirass ventilator that fits over the thorax. Negative-pressure ventilators no longer are used in treatment of acute respiratory failure, but occasionally are used for persons with chronic neuromuscular disorders who need to be ventilated for months or years.

In summary, the lungs enable inhaled air to come in proximity to the blood flowing through the pulmonary capillaries, so that the exchange of gases between the internal environment of the body and the external environment can take place. Respiratory failure is a condition in which the lungs fail adequately to oxygenate the blood or prevent undue retention of carbon dioxide. The causes of respiratory failure are many. It may arise acutely in persons with previously healthy lungs, or it may be superimposed on chronic lung disease. Respiratory failure is defined as a PO_2 of 50 mm Hg or less and a PCO_2 of 50 mm Hg or more.

Hypoxia refers to an acute or chronic reduction in tissue oxygenation. It can occur as the result of hypoventilation, diffusion impairment, shunt, and ventilation-perfusion impairment. Acute hypoxia incites sympathetic nervous system responses such as tachycardia and produces symptoms that are similar to those of alcohol intoxication. In conditions of chronic hypoxia, the manifestations may be insidious in onset and attributed to other causes, particularly in chronic lung disease. The development of cyanosis requires a concentration of 5 g/dL of deoxygenated hemoglobin.

Hypercapnia refers to an increase in carbon dioxide levels. In the clinical setting, four factors contribute to hypercapnia: alterations in carbon dioxide production, disturbance in the gas exchange function of the lungs, abnormalities in respiratory function of the chest wall and respiratory muscles, and changes in neural control of respiration. The manifestations of hypercapnia consist of those associated with the vasodilation of blood vessels, including those in the brain, and depression of the central nervous system (*e.g.*, carbon dioxide narcosis).

Hyperventilation Syndrome

After you have completed this section of the chapter, you should be able to meet the following objectives:

✦ Cite four general causes of hyperventilation syndrome
✦ State the signs and symptoms of hyperventilation syndrome
✦ Describe the diagnostic and treatment methods used in sleep apnea and hyperventilation syndrome

Hyperventilation syndrome involves overbreathing, reduction in PCO_2, and respiratory alkalosis. In 1871, De Costa provided the first account of the syndrome in the medical literature when he reported on the cases of 300 Civil War soldiers affected with the disorder.[65,66] The disorder subsequently has been labeled *soldier's heart, irritable heart, De Costa's syndrome,* and *neurocirculatory asthenia.* Symptoms included palpitations, chest pain, shortness of breath, indigestion, headache, disturbed sleep, and dizziness.

The causes of hyperventilation syndrome have been categorized into four groups: organic, physiologic, emotional, and habitual (*i.e.,* faulty breathing habits). Organic causes include drug effects and central nervous system lesions, such as meningitis. Responses to high altitude, heat, and exercise constitute physiologic causes of hyperventilation. Emotional states that predispose to hyperventilation are hysteria, anxiety, depression, and anger. Faulty breathing habits such as rapid and shallow breathing often are linked to emotional states. Although stress may trigger the initial event, anxiety and fear over the symptoms may perpetuate the syndrome. Because the symptoms of hyperventilation syndrome commonly involve the heart and head, the person experiences intense anxiety, often accompanied by a fear of death or of losing control. The condition occurs in children and adults.

Hyperventilation syndrome commonly produces such symptoms as headache, dyspnea, numbness and tingling sensations, dizziness and light-headedness, chest pain, palpitations, and, sometimes, syncope. Many persons complain of dyspnea and of being unable to take a full, deep breath. Persons with the full constellation of the syndrome breathe with rapid, shallow breaths marked by irregularity in the depth and rate of respiration. Sighing is common. Those who hyperventilate are primarily thoracic rather than abdominal breathers. They tend to use their upper chest wall intercostal muscles to breathe, which may cause dull, aching soreness in the left precordial area, mimicking angina. It has been suggested that the alkalosis associated with hyperventilation syndrome can induce coronary artery spasm in persons with Prinzmetal's angina and in some persons with atherosclerotic coronary artery disease.[67] It also has been observed that ST-wave changes can occur with hyperventilation.

Many persons with hyperventilation syndrome do not have a continuously symptomatic state but rather recurrences of symptoms with or without recognizable provocative stresses. Others have a more chronic form of the disorder in which the respiratory center is reset to enable low levels of PCO_2 to persist despite a normal pH. This may explain the chronicity of the disorder and the ease with which symptoms associated with hyperventilation can be provoked in persons who are chronically hypocapnic. Sympathetic nervous system stimulation provokes a hyperventilatory response and may increase the occurrence of symptoms in persons with chronic hyperventilation problems.

Panic disorder and hyperventilation syndrome have similar manifestations. Hyperventilation has been demonstrated in persons with panic episodes, and panic is a frequent manifestation of hyperventilation. It has been suggested that some persons with either diagnosis have the same disorder and share a biologically and often genetically determined hypersensitivity of a central nervous system alarm system.[68]

A provocative test in which a person deliberately hyperventilates can be done to demonstrate occurrence of the symptoms. Arterial blood gases may be obtained to study the pH and carbon dioxide levels. ECG monitoring is done during the test on persons who have complained of chest pain, and caution should be used when performing the test on persons with known or suspected coronary artery disease.

Treatment focuses on educating the person and his or her family about the disorder, relaxation therapy, and training to overcome faulty breathing patterns. Rebreathing into a paper bag can be used to control the symptoms. For many persons, the realization that they can control their symptoms and nothing is seriously wrong reduces their anxiety and helps them to control the disorder. Adjunctive pharmacologic treatment may be useful in some cases. β-Adrenergic blocking agents lessen the peripheral symptoms of anxiety, such as palpitations and diaphoresis, and may lessen the respiratory stimulatory effect of the catecholamines released during periods of high anxiety.[68]

> Hyperventilation syndrome consists of overbreathing, reduction in PCO_2, and respiratory alkalosis. It can result from organic causes, such as drug effects and central nervous system lesions; physiologic changes caused by heat exposure and exercise; emotional states; or habit. It can cause headache, dizziness, dyspnea, numbness and tingling sensations, light-headedness, palpitations, and, sometimes, syncope.

Related Web Sites

American Lung Association   www.lungusa.org/index.htm
American Thoracic Society   www.thoracic.org
National Asthma Education and Prevention Program Expert Panel Report 2: Guidelines for the Diagnosis and Management of Asthma   www.nhlbi.nih.gov/guidelines/asthma/asthgdln.htm

References

1. Chestnut M.S., Prendergast T.J. (2001). Lung. In Tierney L.M., McPhee S.J., Papadakis M.A. (Eds.), *Current medical diagnosis and treatment* (40th ed., pp. 283–287, 339–344). New York: Lange Medical Books/McGraw-Hill.

2. Romero S. (2000). Nontraumatic chylothorax. *Current Opinion in Pulmonary Medicine* 6, 287–291.

3. Guenther C.A., Welch M.H. (1982). *Pulmonary medicine* (2nd ed., 524–526). Philadelphia: J.B. Lippincott.

4. Sahn S.A., Heffner J.E. (2000). Spontaneous pneumothorax. *New England Journal of Medicine* 342, 868–874.

5. Light R.W. (1995). Diseases of the pleura, mediastinum, chest wall, and diaphragm. In George R.B., Light R.W., Matthay M.A., Matthay R.A. (Eds.), *Chest medicine* (3rd ed., pp. 501–520). Baltimore: Williams & Wilkins.

6. American Lung Association. (2000). *Asthma statistics*. [On-line.] Available: http://lungusa.org/data.

7. Buist A.S., Vollmer W.M. (1994). Preventing death from asthma. *New England Journal of Medicine* 331, 1584–1585.

8. National Asthma Education and Prevention Program. (1997). *Expert Panel report 2: Guidelines for the diagnosis and management of bronchial asthma*. Bethesda, MD: National Institutes of Health, National Heart, Lung, and Blood Institute.

9. Cotran R.S., Kumar V., Collins T. (1999). *Pathologic basis of disease* (6th ed., p. 713). Philadelphia: W.B. Saunders.

10. McFadden E.R., Gilbert I.A. (1994). Exercise-induced asthma. *New England Journal of Medicine* 330, 1362–1366.

11. Roberts J.A. (1988). Exercise-induced asthma in athletes. *Sports Medicine* 6, 193–195.

12. Young S., LeSouef P.N., Geelhoed G.C., Sticks M., Turner K.T., Landau, L.I. (1991). The influence of a family history of asthma and parental smoking on airway responsiveness in early infancy. *New England Journal of Medicine* 324, 1168–1173.

13. Chan-Yeung M., Malo J. (1995). Occupational asthma. *New England Journal of Medicine* 333, 107–112.

14. Babu K.S., Salvi S.S. (2000). Aspirin and asthma. *Chest* 118, 1470–1476.

15. Szczeklik A., Nizankowska E. (2000). Clinical features and diagnosis of aspirin induced asthma. *Thorax* 55 (Suppl. 2), S42–S44.

16. Tan K.S., McFarlane L.C., Lipworth B.J. (1997). Loss of normal cyclical B2 adrenoreceptor regulation and increased premenstrual responsiveness to adenosine monophosphate in stable female asthmatic patients. *Thorax* 52, 608–611.

17. Dubuske D.M. (1994). Asthma: Diagnosis and management of nocturnal symptoms. *Comprehensive Therapy* 20, 628–639.

18. Drazen J.M., Israel E., O'Bryne P.M. (1999). Treatment of asthma with drugs modifying the leukotriene pathway. *New England Journal of Medicine* 340, 197–204.

19. Benatar S.R. (1986). Fatal asthma. *New England Journal of Medicine* 314, 423–428.

20. Macklem P. (1996). Fatal asthma. *Annual Review of Medicine* 47, 161–168.

21. Barnes P.J. (1994). Blunted perception and death from asthma. *New England Journal of Medicine* 330, 1383–1384.

22. Behrman R.E., Kliegman R.M., Jensen H.B. (2000). *Nelson textbook of pediatrics* (16th ed., pp. 664–685). Philadelphia: W.B. Saunders.

23. Gilliland F.D., Berhane K., McConnell R., Gauderman W.J., Vora H., Rappaport E.B., Avol E., Peters J.M. (2000). Maternal smoking during pregnancy, environmental tobacco smoke exposure and childhood lung function. *Thorax* 55, 271–276.

24. Stein R.T., Holberg C.J., Sherrill D., Wright A.L., Morgan W.J., Taussig L., Martinez F.D. (1999). Influence of parental smoking on respiratory symptoms during the first decade of life: The Tucson Children's Respiratory Study. *American Journal of Epidemiology* 149, 1030–1037.

25. American Thoracic Society. (1995). Standards for the diagnosis and care of patients with chronic obstructive pulmonary disease. *American Journal of Respiratory Critical Care Medicine* 152, S77–S120.

26. Mannino D.M., Gagnon R.C., Petty T.L., Lydick E. (2000). Obstructive lung disease and low lung function in adults in the United States. *Archives of Internal Medicine* 160, 1683–1689.

27. Barnes P.J. (2000). Medical progress: Chronic obstructive pulmonary disease. *New England Journal of Medicine* 343, 269–280.

28. Silverman E.K., Chapman H.A., Drazen J.M., Weiss S.T., Rosner B., Campbell E.J., O'Donnell W.J., Reilly L.G., Mentzer S., Wain J., Speizer F.E. (1998). Genetic epidemiology of severe, early-onset chronic obstructive pulmonary disease. *American Journal of Critical Care Medicine* 157, 1770–1778.

29. Travis W.D., Farber J.L., Rubin E. (1999). The respiratory system. In Rubin E., Farber J.L. (Eds.), *Pathology* (3nd ed., pp. 600–601, 623–630). Philadelphia: Lippincott Williams & Wilkins.

30. Stoller J.K., Aboussouan L.S. (1995). Chronic obstructive lung diseases: Emphysema, chronic bronchitis, bronchiectasis, and cystic fibrosis. In George R.B., Light R.W., Matthay M.A., Matthay R.A. (Eds.), *Chest medicine* (3rd ed., pp. 201–246). Baltimore: Williams & Wilkins.

31. Ferguson G.T., Cherniack R.M. (1993). Management of chronic obstructive pulmonary disease. *New England Journal of Medicine* 328, 1017–1022.

32. Tarpy S.P., Celli B.R. (1995). Long-term oxygen therapy. *New England Journal of Medicine* 333, 710–714.

33. McGraw L.R. (1996). Lung volume reduction surgery: An overview. *Heart and Lung* 26, 131–138.

34. Rogers R.M., Sciurba F.C., Keenan R.J. (1996). Lung reduction surgery in chronic obstructive lung disease. *Medical Clinics of North America* 80, 623–643.

35. Mysliwiec V., Pina J.S. (1999). Bronchiectasis: The "other" obstructive lung disease. *Postgraduate Medicine* 106, 123–131.

36. Cystic Fibrosis Foundation. (2000). *Facts about cystic fibrosis*. [On-line.] Available: http://www.cff.org/facts.htm.

37. Rubin E., Farber J.L. (1999). Developmental and genetic diseases. In Rubin E., Farber J.L. (Eds.), *Pathology* (3rd ed., pp. 246–249). Philadelphia: Lippincott Williams & Wilkins.

38. Welsh M.J., Smith A.E. (1995). Cystic fibrosis. *Scientific American* 73 (6), 52–59.

39. Tsui G., Durie P. (1997). Genotype and phenotype in cystic fibrosis. *Hospital Practice* 32 (6), 115–142.

40. Stern R.C. (1997). The diagnosis of cystic fibrosis. *New England Journal of Medicine* 336, 487–491.

41. Boat T.F. (2000). Cystic fibrosis. In Behrman R.E., Kliegman R.M., Jensen H.B. (Eds.), *Nelson textbook of pediatrics* (16th ed., pp. 664–685). Philadelphia: W.B. Saunders.

42. Reynolds H.V., Matthay R.A. (1995). Diffuse interstitial and alveolar inflammatory diseases. In George R.B., Light R.W., Matthay M.A., Matthay R.A. (Eds.), *Chest medicine* (3rd ed., pp. 303–323). Baltimore: Williams & Wilkins.

43. Kobzik L. (1999). The lung. In Cotran R.S., Kumar V., Collins T. (Eds.), *Robbins pathologic basis of disease* (6th ed., pp. 697–755). Philadelphia: W.B. Saunders Co.

44. Newman L.S., Rose C.S., Maier L.A. (1997). Sarcoidosis. *New England Journal of Medicine* 336, 1224–1233.

45. Belfer M.H., Stevens R.W. (1998). Sarcoidosis: A primary care review. *American Family Physician* 58 (9), 2041–2050.

46. Goldhaber S.Z. (1998). Pulmonary embolism. *New England Journal of Medicine* 339, 93–104.

47. Perrier A. (1998). Noninvasive diagnosis of pulmonary embolism. *Hospital Practice* 33 (9), 47–55.

48. Richardi M.J., Rubenfire M. (1999). How to manage secondary pulmonary hypertension. *Postgraduate Medicine* 105 (2), 183–190.

49. Rubin L.J. (1997). Primary pulmonary hypertension. *New England Journal of Medicine* 336, 111–117.

50. Richardi M.J., Rubenfire M. (1999). How to manage primary pulmonary hypertension. *Postgraduate Medicine* 105 (2), 45–56.

51. Kollef M.H., Schuster D.P. (1995). The acute respiratory distress syndrome. *New England Journal of Medicine* 332, 27–36.

52. Ware L.B., Matthay M.A. (2000). The acute respiratory distress syndrome. *New England Journal of Medicine* 342, 1334–1348.

53. Fulkerson W.J., MacIntyre N., Stamler J., Crapo J.D. (1996). Pathogenesis and treatment of adult respiratory distress syndrome. *Archives of Internal Medicine* 156, 29–38.

54. West J.B. (1997). Pulmonary pathophysiology: The essentials (5th ed., pp. 18–40, 132–142, 151). Philadelphia: Lippincott-Raven.

55. Katzung B.G. (2001). *Basic and clinical pharmacology* (8th ed., p. 186). New York: Lange Medical Books/McGraw-Hill.

56. White K.M., Winslow E.H., Clark A., Tyler D.O. (1990). The physiologic basis for continuous mixed oxygen saturation. *Heart and Lung* 19, 548–551.

57. Rueden K.T. (1990). Noninvasive assessment of gas exchange in the critically ill patient. *AACN Clinical Issues in Critical Care Nursing* 1, 239–247.

58. St. John R.E., Thomson P.D. (1999). Noninvasive respiratory monitoring. *Critical Care Nursing Clinics of North America* 11, 423–434.

59. Guyton A.C., Hall J.E. (2000). *Textbook of medical physiology* (10th ed., pp. 477–478, 491, 804). Philadelphia: W.B. Saunders.

60. Weinberger S.E., Schwartzstein R.M., Weiss J.W. (1989). Hypercapnia. *New England Journal of Medicine* 321, 1223–1230.

61. St. John R.E., Eisenberg P. (1991). Nutrition and use of metabolic assessment in the ventilator-dependent patient. *AACN Clinical Issues in Critical Care Nursing* 2, 453–462.

62. Hudak C.M., Gallo B.M., Morton P.G. (1998). *Critical care nursing* (7th ed., pp. 476–489). Philadelphia: Lippincott Williams & Wilkins.

63. Hillberg R.E., Johnson D.C. (1997). Current concepts: Noninvasive ventilation. *New England Journal of Medicine* 337, 1746–1752.

64. Knebel A., Allen M., McNemar A., Peterson A., Feigenbaum K. (1997). A guide to noninvasive intermittent ventilatory support. *Heart and Lung* 26, 307–316.

65. Evans R.W. (1995). Neurologic aspects of hyperventilation syndrome. *Seminars in Neurology* 15, 115–125.

66. Gardner W.N. (1996). The pathophysiology of hyperventilation disorders. *Chest* 109, 516–534.

67. Cowley D.S., Roy-Byrne P.P. (1987). Hyperventilation and panic disorder. *American Journal of Medicine* 83, 929–937.

68. Tavel M.E. (1990). Hyperventilation syndrome: Hiding behind pseudonyms. *Chest* 97, 1285–1288.

Renal Function and Fluid and Electrolytes

Throughout the earlier part of the Middle Ages, one of the major concerns of the physician was examination of the urine. Many physicians of this time thought that most diseases could be diagnosed by careful examination of the urine. Numerous illustrations taken from this period show early physicians holding up flasks of urine to study its color, cloudiness, and other properties. It was thought that if the cloudiness was at the top of the urine, the problem was in the head, and if it was at the bottom, the problem was in the legs.

From the 16th century on, anatomists began to acquire a fairly good understanding of the gross structure of the kidney, ureters, and bladder. The first great discovery of the minute structures of the kidney was made by Marcello Malphigi (1628–1694), one of the earliest microscopists, who described the ball-shaped structure of the glomerulus. The work of Malphigi was followed by that of Sir William Bowman (1816–1892), who described the urine collecting capsule of the nephron, Bowman's capsule. Bowman also described the relationship between the glomerulus and the tubules. German pathologist Friedrich Henle (1809–1885) described the long U-shaped loop, called the loop of Henle, that contributes to the concentrating abilities of the kidney. Once this structure of the kidney was established, other scientists began to focus on the chemical composition of urine and on the function of the kidney in the regulation of blood pressure.

Control of Renal Function

It is no exaggeration to say that the composition of the blood is determined not so much by what the mouth takes in as by what the kidneys keep.

—Homer Smith, *From Fish to Philosopher*

The kidneys are remarkable organs. Each is smaller than a person's fist, but in a single day the two organs process approximately 1700 L of blood and combine its waste products into approximately 1.5 L of urine. As part of their function, the kidneys filter physiologically essential substances, such as sodium and potassium ions, from the blood and selectively reabsorb those substances that are needed to maintain the normal composition of internal body fluids. Substances that are not needed for this purpose or are in excess pass into the urine. In regulating the volume and composition of body fluids, the kidneys perform excretory and endocrine functions. The renin-angiotensin mechanism participates in the regulation of blood pressure and the maintenance of circulating blood volume, and erythropoietin stimulates red blood cell production. The discussion in this chapter focuses on the structure and function of the kidneys, tests of renal function, and the physiologic action of diuretics.

Kidney Structure and Function

After you have completed this section of the chapter, you should be able to meet the following objectives:

+ Describe the location and gross structure of the kidney
+ Describe the kidney blood supply and mechanisms for regulating blood flow
+ Explain the structure and function of the glomerulus and tubular components of the nephron
+ Explain the function of sodium in terms of tubular transport mechanisms
+ Describe how the kidney produces a concentrated or dilute urine
+ Describe the elimination functions of the kidney
+ Characterize the function of the juxtaglomerular complex
+ Explain the endocrine functions of the kidney

GROSS STRUCTURE AND LOCATION

The kidneys are paired, bean-shaped organs that lie outside the peritoneal cavity in the back of the upper abdomen, one on each side of the vertebral column at the level of the 12th thoracic to 3rd lumbar vertebrae (Fig. 30-1). The right kidney normally is situated lower than the left, presumably because of the position of the liver. In the adult, each kidney is approximately 10 to 12 cm long, 5 to 6 cm wide, and 2.5 cm deep and weighs approximately 113 to 170 g. The medial border of the kidney is indented by a deep fissure called the *hilus*. It is here that blood vessels and nerves enter and leave the kidney. The ureters, which connect the kidneys with the bladder, also enter the kidney at the hilus.

The kidney is a multilobular structure, composed of up to 18 lobes. Each lobule is composed of nephrons, which are the functional units of the kidney. Each nephron has a glomerulus that filters the blood and a system of tubular structures that selectively reabsorb material from the filtrate back into the blood and secrete materials from the blood into the filtrate as urine is being formed.

On longitudinal section, a kidney can be divided into an outer cortex and an inner medulla (Fig. 30-2). The cortex, which is reddish-brown, contains the glomeruli and convoluted tubules of the nephron and blood vessels. The medulla consists of light-colored, cone-shaped masses—the renal pyramids—that are divided by the columns of the cortex (*i.e.*, columns of Bertin) that extend into the medulla. Each pyramid, topped by a region of cortex, forms a lobe of the kidney. The apices of the pyramids form the papillae (*i.e.*, 8 to 18 per kidney, corresponding to the number of lobes), which are perforated by the openings of the collecting ducts. The renal pelvis is a wide, funnel-shaped structure at the upper end of the ureter. It is made up of the calyces or cuplike structures that drain the upper and lower halves of the kidney.

The kidney is ensheathed in a fibrous external capsule and surrounded by a mass of fatty connective tissue, especially at its ends and borders. The adipose tissue protects

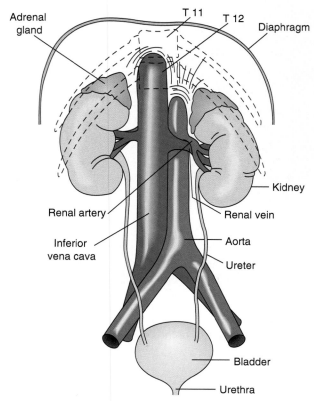

FIGURE 30-1 Kidneys, ureters, and bladder. (The right kidney is usually lower than the left.)

the kidney from mechanical blows and assists, together with the attached blood vessels and fascia, in holding the kidney in place. Although the kidneys are relatively well protected, they may be bruised by blows to the loin or by compression between the lower ribs and the ilium. Because the kidneys are outside the peritoneal cavity, injury and

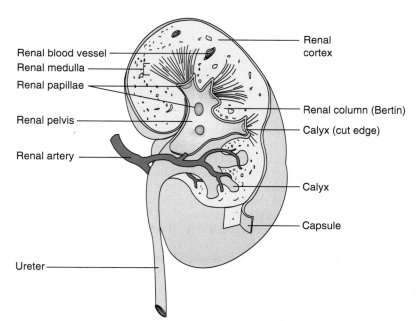

FIGURE 30-2 Internal structure of the kidney. (Chaffee E.E., Lytle I.M. [1980]. *Basic physiology and anatomy* [4th ed.]. Philadelphia: J.B. Lippincott)

rupture do not produce the same threat of peritoneal involvement as rupture of organs such as the liver or spleen.

RENAL BLOOD SUPPLY

Each kidney is supplied by a single renal artery that arises on either side of the aorta. As the renal artery approaches the kidney, it divides into five segmental arteries that enter the hilus of the kidney. In the kidney, each segmental artery branches into several lobular arteries that supply the upper, middle, and lower parts of the kidney. The lobar arteries further subdivide to form the interlobular arteries at the level of the cortical medullary junction (Fig. 30-3). These arteries give off branches, called the arcuate arteries, that arch across the top of the pyramids. Small intralobular arteries radiate from the arcuate arteries to supply the cortex of the kidney. The afferent arterioles that supply the glomeruli arise from the intralobular arteries.

The nephron is supplied by two capillary systems, the glomerulus and the peritubular capillary network (Fig. 30-4).

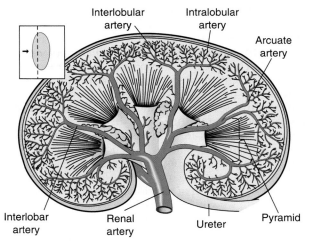

FIGURE 30-3 Simplified illustration of the arterial supply of the kidney. (Cormack D.H. [1987]. *Ham's histology* [9th ed.]. Philadelphia: J.B. Lippincott)

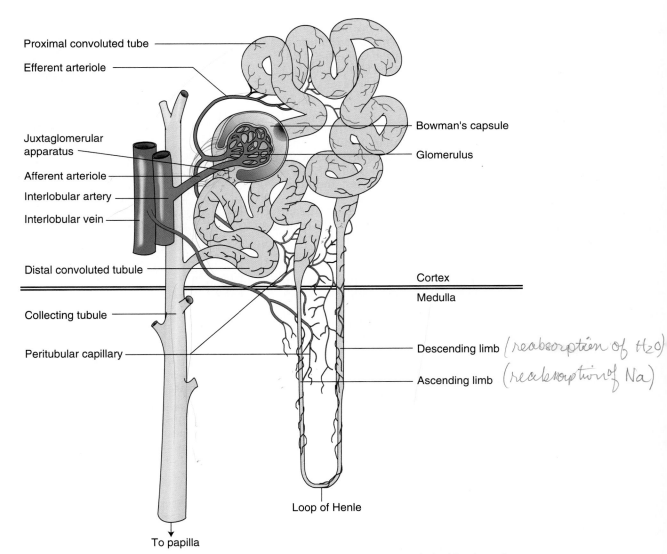

FIGURE 30-4 Nephron, showing the glomerular and tubular structures along with the blood supply. (Chaffee E.E., Lytle I.M. [1980]. *Basic physiology and anatomy* [4th ed.]. Philadelphia: J.B. Lippincott)

The glomerulus is a unique, high-pressure capillary filtration system located between two arterioles—the afferent and the efferent arterioles—that selectively dilate or constrict to regulate glomerular capillary pressure. The peritubular capillary network is a low-pressure reabsorptive system that originates from the efferent arteriole. These capillaries surround all portions of the tubules, an arrangement that permits rapid movement of solutes and water between the fluid in the tubular lumen and the blood in the capillaries. The medullary nephrons are supplied with two types of capillaries: the peritubular capillaries, which are similar to those in the cortex, and the vasa recta, which are long, straight capillaries. The vasa recta accompany the long loops of Henle in the medullary portion of the kidney to assist in exchange of substances flowing in and out of that portion of the kidney. The peritubular capillaries rejoin to form the venous channels by which blood leaves the kidneys and empties into the inferior vena cava.

Although nearly all the blood flow to the kidneys passes through the cortex, less than 10% is directed to the medulla and only approximately 1% goes to the papillae. Under conditions of decreased perfusion or increased sympathetic nervous system stimulation, blood flow is redistributed away from the cortex toward the medulla. This redistribution of blood flow decreases glomerular filtration while maintaining the urine concentrating ability of the kidneys, a factor that is important during conditions such as shock.

THE NEPHRON

Each kidney is composed of more than 1 million tiny, closely packed functional units called *nephrons*. Each nephron consists of a glomerulus, where blood is filtered, and a tubular component. Here, water, electrolytes, and other substances needed to maintain the constancy of the internal environment are reabsorbed into the bloodstream while other unneeded materials are secreted into the tubular filtrate for elimination (see Fig. 30-4).

The Glomerulus

The glomerulus consists of a compact tuft of capillaries encased in a thin, double-walled capsule, called *Bowman's capsule*. Blood flows into the glomerular capillaries from the afferent arteriole and flows out of the glomerular capillaries into the efferent arteriole, which leads into the peritubular capillaries. Fluid and particles from the blood are filtered through the capillary membrane into a fluid-filled space in Bowman's capsule, called *Bowman's space*. The portion of the blood that is filtered into the capsule space is called the *filtrate*. The mass of capillaries and its surrounding epithelial capsule are collectively referred to as the *renal corpuscle* (Fig. 30-5A).

The glomerular capillary membrane is composed of three layers: the capillary endothelial layer, the basement membrane, and the single-celled capsular epithelial layer (see Fig. 30-5). The endothelial layer lines the glomerulus and interfaces with blood as it moves through the capillary. This layer contains many small perforations, called *fenestrations*.

The epithelial layer that covers the glomerulus is continuous with the epithelium that lines Bowman's capsule.

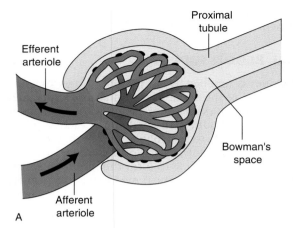

A

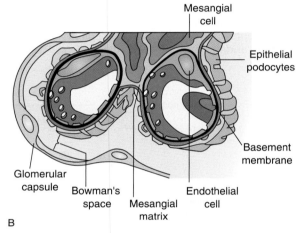

B

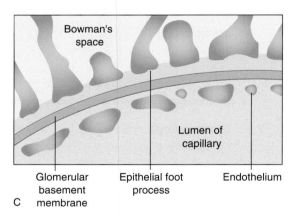

C

FIGURE 30-5 Renal corpuscle. (**A**) Structures of the glomerulus. (**B**) Position of the mesangial cells in relation to the capillary loops and Bowman's capsule. (**C**) Cross-section of the glomerular membrane, showing the position of the endothelium, basement membrane, and epithelial foot processes.

The cells of the epithelial layer have unusual octopus-like structures that possess a large number of extensions, or *foot processes* (i.e., *podocytes*), which are embedded in the basement membrane (Fig. 30-6). These foot processes form *slit pores* through which the glomerular filtrate passes. The

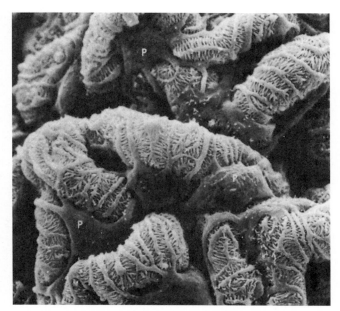

FIGURE 30-6 Scanning electron micrograph of a glomerulus from the kidney of a normal rat. The visceral epithelial cells, or podocytes (P), extend multiple processes outward from the main cell body to wrap around individual capillary loops. Immediately adjacent pedicels, or foot processes, arise from different podocytes (original magnification 2 × 4800). (Brenner B.M., Rector F.C. [1981]. *The kidney.* Philadelphia: W.B. Saunders)

basement membrane consists of a homogeneous acellular meshwork of collagen fibers, glycoproteins, and mucopolysaccharides (see Fig. 30-5C). Because the endothelial and the epithelial layers of the glomerular capillary have porous structures, the basement membrane determines the permeability of the glomerular capillary membrane. The spaces between the fibers that make up the basement membrane represent the pores of a filter and determine the size-dependent permeability barrier of the glomerulus. The size of the pores in the basement membrane normally prevents red blood cells and plasma proteins from passing through the glomerular membrane into the filtrate. There is evidence that the epithelium plays a major role in producing the basement membrane components, and it is probable that the epithelial cells are active in forming new basement membrane material throughout life. Alterations in the structure and function of the glomerular basement membrane are responsible for the leakage of proteins and blood cells into the filtrate that occurs in many forms of glomerular disease.

Another important component of the glomerulus is the *mesangium.* In some areas, the capillary endothelium and the basement membrane do not completely surround each capillary. Instead, the mesangial cells, which lie between the capillary tufts, provide support for the glomerulus in these areas (see Fig. 30-5B). The mesangial cells produce an intercellular substance similar to that of the basement membrane. This substance covers the endothelial cells where they are not covered by basement membrane. The mesangial cells possess (or can develop) phagocytic properties

and remove macromolecular materials that enter the intercapillary spaces. Mesangial cells also exhibit contractile properties in response to neurohumoral substances and are thought to contribute to the regulation of blood flow through the glomerulus. In normal glomeruli, the mesangial area is narrow and contains only a small number of cells. Mesangial hyperplasia and increased mesangial matrix occur in a number of glomerular diseases.

Tubular Components of the Nephron

The nephron tubule is divided into four segments: a highly coiled segment called the *proximal convoluted tubule,* which drains Bowman's capsule; a thin, looped structure called the *loop of Henle*; a distal coiled portion called the *distal convoluted tubule*; and the final segment called the *collecting tubule,* which joins with several tubules to collect the filtrate. The filtrate passes through each of these segments before reaching the pelvis of the kidney.

Nephrons can be roughly grouped into two categories. Approximately 85% of the nephrons originate in the superficial part of the cortex and are called *cortical nephrons.* They have short, thick loops of Henle that penetrate only a short distance into the medulla. The remaining 15% are called *juxtamedullary nephrons.* They originate deeper in the cortex and have longer and thinner loops of Henle that penetrate the entire length of the medulla. The juxtamedullary nephrons are largely concerned with urine concentration.

The proximal tubule is a highly coiled structure that dips toward the renal pelvis to become the descending limb of the loop of Henle. The ascending loop of Henle returns to the region of the renal corpuscle, where it becomes the distal tubule. The distal convoluted tubule, which begins at the juxtaglomerular complex, is divided into two segments:

The Nephron and Glomerular Filtration Rate

➤ The nephron is the functional unit of the kidney and is composed of a glomerulus and a tubule.

➤ Arterial blood enters the nephron through the afferent arteriole; approximately 20% is filtered from the capillaries of the glomerulus into Bowman's capsule (urine filtrate). The remainder leaves the nephron through the efferent arteriole and into the peritubular capillaries.

➤ The rate at which the blood is filtered into Bowman's capsule (glomerular filtration rate) is determined by glomerular capillary hydrostatic pressure, glomerular capillary osmotic pressure, and the hydrostatic and osmotic pressures in Bowman's capsule.

➤ The glomerular capillary serves as a filtration barrier, such that the urine filtrate is free of red blood cells and plasma proteins.

the *diluting segment* and the *late distal tubule*. The late distal tubule fuses with the collecting tubule. Like the distal tubule, the collecting duct is divided into two segments: the *cortical collecting tubule* and the *inner medullary collecting tubule*.

Throughout its course, the tubule is composed of a single layer of epithelial cells resting on a basement membrane. The structure of the epithelial cells varies with tubular function. The cells of the proximal tubule have a fine villous structure that increases the surface area for reabsorption; they also are rich in mitochondria, which support active transport processes. The epithelial layer of the thin segment of the loop of Henle has few mitochondria, indicating minimal metabolic activity and passive reabsorptive function.

URINE FORMATION

Urine formation involves the filtration of blood by the glomerulus to form an *ultrafiltrate of urine* and the tubular reabsorption of electrolytes and nutrients needed to maintain the constancy of the internal environment while eliminating waste materials.

Glomerular Filtration
Urine formation begins with the filtration of essentially protein-free plasma through the glomerular capillaries into Bowman's space. The movement of fluid through the glomerular capillaries is determined by the same factors (*i.e.,* capillary filtration pressure, colloidal osmotic pressure, and capillary permeability) that affect fluid movement through other capillaries in the body (see Chapter 21). The glomerular filtrate has a chemical composition similar to plasma, but it contains almost no proteins because large molecules do not readily cross the glomerular wall. Approximately 125 mL of filtrate is formed each minute. This is called the *glomerular filtration rate (GFR)*. This rate can vary from a few milliliters per minute to as high as 200 mL/minute.

The location of the glomerulus between two arterioles allows for maintenance of a high-pressure filtration system. The capillary filtration pressure (approximately 60 mm Hg) in the glomerulus is approximately two to three times higher than that of other capillary beds in the body. The filtration pressure and the GFR are regulated by the constriction and relaxation of the afferent and efferent arterioles. Constriction of the efferent arteriole increases resistance to outflow from the glomeruli and increases the glomerular pressure and the GFR. Constriction of the afferent arteriole causes a reduction in the renal blood flow, glomerular filtration pressure, and GFR. The afferent and the efferent arterioles are innervated by the sympathetic nervous system and are sensitive to vasoactive hormones, such as angiotensin II, as well. During periods of strong sympathetic stimulation, as occurs during shock, constriction of the afferent arteriole causes a marked decrease in renal blood flow and thus glomerular filtration pressure. Consequently, urine output can fall almost to zero.

Tubular Reabsorption and Secretion
From Bowman's capsule, the glomerular filtrate moves into the tubular segments of the nephron. In its movement through the lumen of the tubular segments, the glomerular filtrate is changed considerably by the tubular transport of water and solutes. Tubular transport can result in reabsorption of substances from the tubular fluid into the blood or secretion of substances into the tubular fluid from the blood (Fig. 30-7).

The basic mechanisms of transport across the tubular epithelial cell membrane are similar to those of other cell membranes in the body and include active and passive transport mechanisms. Water and urea are passively absorbed along concentration gradients. Sodium, potassium, chloride, calcium, and phosphate ions, as well as urate, glucose, and amino acids are reabsorbed using primary or secondary active transport mechanisms to move across the tubular membrane. Some substances, such as hydrogen, potassium, and urate ions, are secreted into the tubular fluids. Under normal conditions, only approximately 1 mL of the 125 mL of glomerular filtrate that is formed each minute is excreted in the urine. The other 124 mL is reabsorbed in the tubules. This means that the average output of urine is approximately 60 mL/hour.

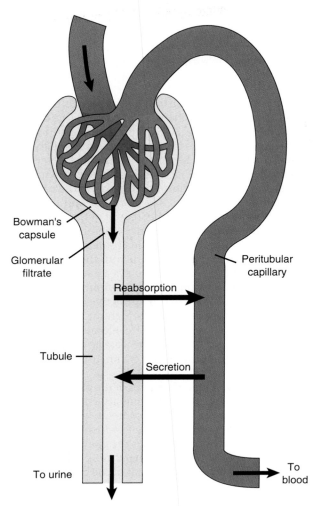

FIGURE 30-7 Reabsorption and secretion of substances between the renal tubules and peritubular capillaries.

Renal tubular cells have two membrane surfaces through which substances must pass as they are reabsorbed from the tubular fluid. The side of the cell that is in contact with the tubular lumen and tubular filtrate is called the *luminal membrane*. The outside membrane that lies adjacent to the interstitial fluid is called the *basolateral membrane*. In most cases, substances move from the tubular filtrate into the tubular cell along a concentration gradient, but they require facilitated transport or carrier systems to move across the basolateral membrane into the interstitial fluid, where they are absorbed into the peritubular capillaries.

The bulk of energy used by the kidney is for active sodium transport mechanisms that facilitate sodium reabsorption and cotransport of other electrolytes and substances such as glucose and amino acids. This is called *secondary active transport* or *cotransport* (Fig. 30-8). Secondary active transport depends on the energy-dependent sodium-potassium adenosine triphosphatase (ATPase) pump on the basolateral side of renal tubular cells. The pump maintains a low intracellular sodium concentration that facilitates the downhill (*i.e.*, from a higher to lower concentration) movement of sodium from the filtrate across the luminal membrane. Cotransport uses a carrier system in which the downhill movement of one substance such as sodium is coupled to the uphill movement (*i.e.*, from a lower to higher concentration) of another substance such as glucose or an amino acid. A few substances, such as hydrogen, are secreted into the tubule using countertransport, in which the movement of one substance, such as sodium, enables the movement of a second substance in the opposite direction.

Proximal Tubule. Approximately 65% of all reabsorptive and secretory processes that occur in the tubular system take place in the proximal tubule. There is almost complete reabsorption of nutritionally important substances, such as glucose, amino acids, lactate, and water-soluble vitamins. Electrolytes, such as sodium, potassium, chloride, and bicarbonate, are 65% to 80% reabsorbed. As these solutes move into the tubular cells, their concentration in the tubular lumen decreases, providing a concentration gradient for the osmotic reabsorption of water and urea. The proximal tubule is highly permeable to water, and the osmotic movement of water occurs so rapidly that the concentration difference of solutes on either side of the membrane seldom is more than a few milliosmoles.

Many substances, such as glucose, are freely filtered in the glomerulus and reabsorbed by energy-dependent cotransport carrier mechanisms. The maximum amount of substance that these transport systems can reabsorb per unit time is called the *transport maximum*. The transport maximum is related to the number of carrier proteins that are available for transport and usually is sufficient to ensure that all of a filtered substance such as glucose can be reabsorbed rather than being eliminated in the urine. The plasma level at which the substance appears in the urine is called the *renal threshold* (Fig. 30-9). Under some circumstances, the amount of substance filtered in the glomerulus exceeds the transport maximum. For example, when the blood glucose level is elevated in uncontrolled diabetes mellitus, the amount that is filtered in the glomerulus often exceeds the transport maximum (approximately 320 mg/minute), and glucose spills into the urine.

The Loop of Henle. The loop of Henle is divided into three segments: the thin descending segment, the thin ascending

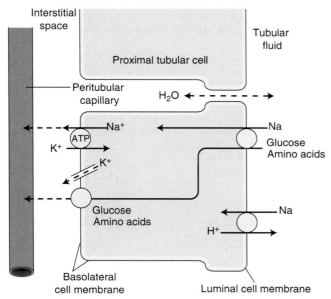

FIGURE 30-8 Mechanism for secondary active transport or cotransport of glucose and amino acids in the proximal tubule. The energy-dependent sodium-potassium pump on the basal lateral surface of the cell maintains a low intracellular gradient that facilitates the downhill movement of sodium and glucose or amino acids (cotransport) from the tubular lumen into the tubular cell and then into the peritubular capillary.

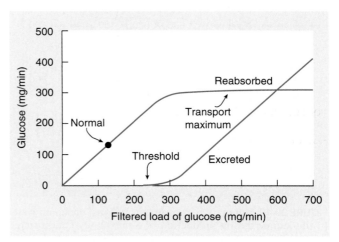

FIGURE 30-9 Relations among the filtered load (plasma concentration of glucose × GFR) of glucose, the rate of glucose reabsorption by the renal tubules, and the rate of glucose excretion in the urine. The *transport maximum* is the maximum rate at which glucose can be reabsorbed from the tubules. The *threshold* for glucose refers to the filtered load of glucose at which glucose first begins to appear in the urine. (Guyton A., Hall J.E. [1996]. *Textbook of medical physiology* [9th ed., p. 335]. Philadelphia: W.B. Saunders)

segment, and thick ascending segment. Each of these segments has special structural and functional properties.

Fluid that enters the loop of Henle is iso-osmotic to plasma, but it becomes hypo-osmotic as it moves through the loop. The thin descending limb is highly permeable to water and moderately permeable to urea, sodium, and other ions. The ascending limb, in contrast to the descending limb, is impermeable to water. As fluid moves down the descending limb, water is reabsorbed until the osmolality of the tubular fluid reaches an equilibrium with the interstitial fluid, which is more hypertonic. In the ascending limb, which is impermeable to water, solutes are reabsorbed, but water cannot follow; as a result, the tubular fluid becomes more and more dilute, often reaching an osmolality of 100 mOsm/kg of H_2O as it enters the distal convoluted tubule, compared with the 285 mOsm/kg of H_2O in plasma (Fig. 30-10).

The thick segment of the loop of Henle begins in the ascending limb where the epithelial cells become thickened. As with the thin ascending limb, this segment is impermeable to water. The thick segment contains a Na^+–K^+–$2Cl^-$

cotransport system. This system involves the cotransport of a positively charged sodium and positively charged potassium ion accompanied by two negatively charged chloride ions (Fig. 30-11). The gradient for the operation of this cotransport system is provided by the basolateral sodium-potassium pump, which maintains a low intracellular sodium concentration. The repetitive reabsorption of sodium chloride from the thick ascending limb of Henle and continued inflow of new sodium chloride from the proximal tubule into the loop of Henle serve to trap solutes in the medullary interstitium, contributing to the high osmolality in this part of the nephron. Approximately 20% to 25% of the filtered load of sodium, potassium, and chloride is reabsorbed in the thick loop of Henle. Movement of these ions out of the tubule leads to the development of a transmembrane potential that favors the passive reabsorption of small divalent cations such as calcium and magnesium. Inhibition of sodium transport in the thick loop of Henle by loop diuretics causes an increase in urinary excretion of these divalent ions in addition to sodium and chloride.

In approximately one fifth of the juxtamedullary nephrons, the loops of Henle and special hairpin-shaped capillaries called the *vasa recta* descend into the medullary portion of the kidney. A countercurrent mechanism controls water and solute movement so that water is kept out of the peritubular area and sodium and urea are retained (see Fig. 30-10). The term *countercurrent* refers to a flow of fluids in opposite directions in adjacent structures. There is an exchange of solutes between the adjacent descending and ascending loops of Henle and between the ascending and descending sections of the vasa recta. Because of these exchange processes, a high concentration of osmotically active particles (approximately 1200 mOsm/kg of H_2O) collects in the interstitium of the kidney medulla. The presence of these osmotically active particles in the interstitium surrounding the medullary collecting tubules facil-

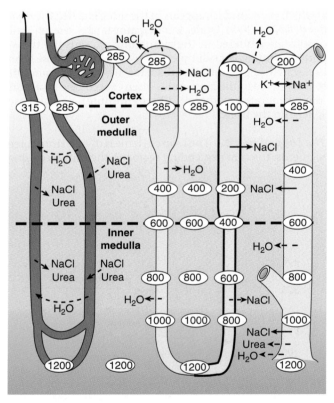

FIGURE 30-10 Summary of movements of ions, urea, and water in the kidney during production of a maximally concentrated urine (1200 mOsm/kg H_2O). Numbers in ovals give osmolality of the urine filtrate and medullary interstitium in mOsm/kg H_2O. Solid arrows indicate active transport; dashed arrows indicate passive transport. The heavy outlining along the ascending limb of Henle's loop indicates a decreased water permeability in that tubule segment. Note the osmotic gradient in the medulla from the outer to the inner medulla. (Rhoades R.A., Tanner G.A. [1996]. *Medical physiology* [p. 441]. Boston: Little, Brown)

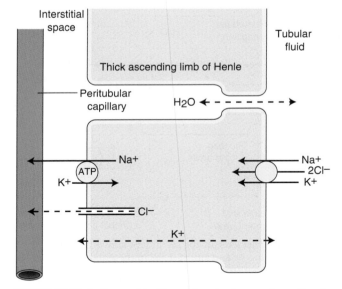

FIGURE 30-11 Sodium, chloride, and potassium reabsorption in the thick segment of the loop of Henle.

itates the antidiuretic hormone (ADH)–mediated reabsorption of water (see following discussion).

Distal Convoluted Tubule.

Like the thick ascending loop of Henle, the distal convoluted tubule is relatively impermeable to water, and reabsorption of sodium chloride from this segment further dilutes the tubular fluid (see Fig. 30-10). Sodium reabsorption occurs through a sodium and chloride cotransport mechanism. Approximately 10% of filtered sodium chloride is reabsorbed in this section of the tubule. Unlike the thick ascending loop of Henle, neither calcium nor magnesium are passively absorbed in this segment of the tubule. Instead, calcium ions are actively reabsorbed in a process that is largely regulated by parathyroid hormone and possibly by vitamin D.

The thick ascending loop of Henle, the distal tubule, and cortical collecting tubule are often referred to as the *diluting segment* of the tubule. As solutes are reabsorbed from these segments, the urine becomes more and more dilute, often reaching an osmolar concentration that is equal to or less than that of plasma. This allows excretion of free water from the body.

Late Distal Tubule and Cortical Collecting Tubule.

The late distal tubule and the cortical collecting tubule constitute the site where aldosterone exerts its action on sodium and potassium reabsorption. Although responsible for only 2% to 5% of sodium chloride reabsorption, this site is largely responsible for determining the final sodium concentration of the urine. The late distal tubule with the cortical collecting tubule also is the major site for regulation of potassium excretion by the kidney. When the body is confronted with a potassium excess, as occurs with a diet high in potassium content, the amount of potassium secreted at this site may exceed the amount filtered in the glomerulus.

The mechanism for sodium reabsorption and potassium secretion by this section of the kidney is distinct from other tubular segments. This tubular segment is composed of two types of cells, the *principal cells* and the *intercalated cells*. The principal cells reabsorb sodium and water from the lumen filtrate and secrete potassium into the lumen. The intercalated cells reabsorb potassium and secrete hydrogen ions into the lumen. The principal cells use separate channels for transport of sodium and potassium rather than cotransport mechanisms (Fig. 30-12). Aldosterone is thought to exert its effect on sodium and potassium excretion by increasing the number of ion channels and the function of the basolateral sodium-potassium pump.

Medullary Collecting Duct.

The epithelium of the inner medullary collecting duct is well designed to resist extreme changes in the osmotic or pH characteristics of tubular fluid, and it is here that the urine becomes highly concentrated, highly diluted, highly alkaline, or highly acidic. During periods of water excess or dehydration, the kidneys play a major role in maintaining water balance.

ADH exerts its effect in the medullary collecting duct. ADH maintains extracellular volume by returning water to the vascular compartment and leads to the production of a concentrated urine by removing water from the tubular filtrate. Osmoreceptors in the hypothalamus sense the in-

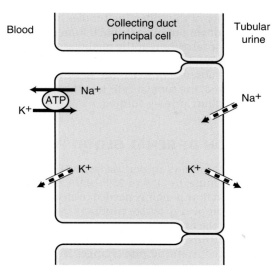

FIGURE 30-12 Model for ion transport of sodium and potassium by collecting duct principal cells. (Rhoades R.A., Tanner G.A. [1996]. *Medical physiology* [p. 438]. Boston: Little, Brown)

crease in osmolality of extracellular fluids and stimulate the release of ADH from the posterior pituitary gland (see Chapter 31). The permeability of the collecting ducts to water is determined mainly by the concentration of ADH. In exerting its effect, ADH, also known as *vasopressin*, binds to vasopressin receptors on the blood side of the tubular cells (Fig. 30-13). Binding of ADH to the vasopressin receptors causes insertion of water channels into the cell membrane on the luminal side of the tubular cells, producing a marked increase in water permeability. After

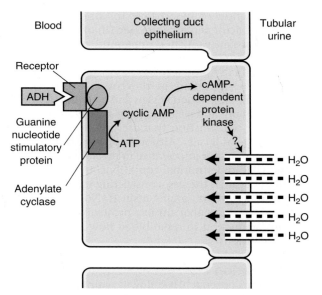

FIGURE 30-13 Model for the action of antidiuretic hormone (ADH) on the epithelium of the collecting duct. The ADH receptor is on the basolateral side, but the water permeability increase occurs on the luminal side. (Rhoades R.A., Tanner G.A. [1996]. *Medical physiology* [p. 439]. Boston: Little, Brown)

the permeability of the collecting tubules has been established, water moves out of the tubular lumen and into the hyperosmotic interstitium of the medullary area, where it enters the peritubular capillaries for return to the vascular system. In the absence of ADH, the inserted water channels are removed, the tubular cells lose their water permeability, and a dilute urine is formed.

REGULATION OF RENAL BLOOD FLOW

In the adult, the kidneys are perfused with 1000 to 1300 mL of blood per minute, or 20% to 25% of the cardiac output. This large blood flow is mainly needed to ensure a sufficient GFR for the removal of waste products from the blood, rather than for the metabolic needs of the kidney. Feedback mechanisms intrinsic to the kidney normally keep blood flow and GFR constant despite changes in arterial blood pressure.

Neural and Humoral Control Mechanisms

The kidney is richly innervated by the sympathetic nervous system. Increased sympathetic activity causes constriction of the afferent and efferent arterioles and thus a decrease in renal blood flow. Intense sympathetic stimulation such as occurs in shock and trauma can produce marked decreases in renal blood flow and GFR, even to the extent of causing blood flow to cease altogether.

Several humoral substances, including angiotensin II, ADH, and endothelins, cause vasoconstriction of renal vessels. The endothelins are a group of peptides released from damaged endothelial cells in the kidney and other tissues. Although not thought to be important regulators of renal blood flow during everyday activities, endothelin I, which is released by renal endothelial cells, may play a role in reduction of blood flow in conditions such as postischemic acute renal failure (see Chapter 34).

Other substances such as dopamine, nitric oxide, and prostaglandins (*i.e.*, E_2 and I_2) produce vasodilation. Nitric oxide, a vasodilator produced by the vascular endothelium, appears to be important in preventing excessive vasoconstriction of renal blood vessels and allowing normal excretion of sodium and water. Prostaglandins are a group of mediators of cell function that are produced locally and exert their effects locally. Although prostaglandins do not appear to be of major importance in regulating renal blood flow and GFR under normal conditions, they may protect the kidneys against the vasoconstricting effects of sympathetic stimulation and angiotensin II. Nonsteroidal antiinflammatory drugs that inhibit prostaglandin synthesis may cause reduction in renal blood flow and GFR under certain conditions.

Autoregulation

The constancy of renal blood flow is maintained by a process called *autoregulation* (see Chapter 21). Normally, autoregulation of blood flow is designed to maintain blood flow at a level consistent with the metabolic needs of the tissues. In the kidney, autoregulation of blood flow also must allow for precise regulation of renal excretion of water and solutes.

For autoregulation to occur, the resistance to blood flow through the kidneys must be varied in direct proportion to the arterial pressure. The exact mechanisms responsible for the intrarenal regulation of blood flow are unclear. One of the proposed mechanisms is a direct effect on vascular smooth muscle that causes the blood vessels to relax when there is an increase in blood pressure, and to constrict when there is a decrease in pressure. A second proposed mechanism is the juxtaglomerular complex.

The Juxtaglomerular Complex. The juxtaglomerular complex is thought to represent a feedback control system that links changes in the GFR with renal blood flow. The juxtaglomerular complex is located at the site where the distal tubule extends back to the glomerulus and then passes between the afferent and efferent arteriole (Fig. 30-14). The distal tubular site that is nearest the glomerulus is characterized by densely nucleated cells called the *macula densa*.

In the adjacent afferent arteriole, the smooth muscle cells of the media are modified as special secretory cells called *juxtaglomerular cells*. These cells contain granules of inactive renin, an enzyme that functions in the conversion of angiotensinogen to angiotensin. Renin functions by means of angiotensin II to produce vasoconstriction of the efferent arteriole as a means of preventing serious decreases in glomerular filtration rate. Angiotensin II also increases sodium reabsorption indirectly by stimulating aldosterone secretion from the adrenal gland and directly by increasing sodium reabsorption by the proximal tubule cells.

Because of its location between the afferent and efferent arteriole, the juxtaglomerular complex is thought to play an essential feedback role in linking the level of arterial blood pressure and renal blood flow to the GFR and the composition of the distal tubular fluid. The juxtaglomerular complex monitors the systemic blood pressure by sensing the stretch of the afferent arteriole, and it monitors the

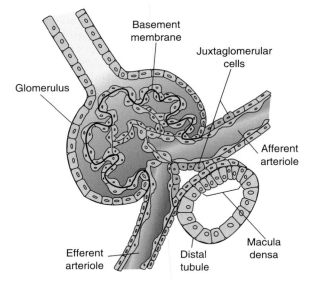

FIGURE 30-14 Juxtaglomerular apparatus, showing the close contact of the distal tubule with the afferent arteriole, the macula densa, and the juxtaglomerular cells.

concentration of sodium chloride in the tubular filtrate as it passes through the macula densa. This information is then used in determining how much renin should be released to keep the arterial blood pressure in its normal range and maintain a relatively constant GFR.

Effect of Increased Protein and Glucose Load. Although renal blood flow and glomerular filtration are relatively stable under most conditions, two conditions can increase renal blood flow and glomerular filtration. These are an increased amount of protein in the diet and an increase in blood glucose. With ingestion of a high-protein diet, renal blood flow increases 20% to 30% within 1 to 2 hours. Although the exact mechanism for this increase is uncertain, it is thought to be related to the fact that amino acids and sodium are absorbed together in the proximal tubule (secondary active transport). As a result, delivery of sodium to the macula densa is decreased, which elicits an increase in renal blood flow through the juxtaglomerular complex feedback mechanism. The resultant increase in blood flow and GFR allows sodium excretion to be maintained at a near-normal level while increasing the excretion of the waste products of protein metabolism, such as urea. The same mechanism is thought to explain the large increases in renal blood flow and GFR that occur with high blood glucose levels in persons with uncontrolled diabetes mellitus.

ELIMINATION FUNCTIONS OF THE KIDNEY

Renal Clearance

Renal clearance is the volume of plasma that is completely cleared each minute of any substance that finds its way into the urine. It is determined by the ability of the substance to be filtered in the glomeruli and the capacity of the renal tubules to reabsorb or secrete the substance. Every substance has its own clearance rate, the units of which are always volume of plasma per unit time. It can be determined by measuring the amount of a substance that is excreted in the urine (*i.e.,* urine concentration × urine flow rate in milliliters per minute) and dividing by its plasma concentration. Inulin, a large polysaccharide, is freely filtered in the glomeruli and neither reabsorbed nor secreted by the tubular cells. After intravenous injection, the amount that appears in the urine is equal to the amount that is filtered in the glomeruli (*i.e.,* the clearance rate is equal to the GFR). Because of these properties, inulin can be used as a laboratory measure of the GFR. Some substances, such as urea, are freely filtered in the glomeruli, but the volume that is cleared from the plasma is less than the GFR, indicating that at least some of the substance is being reabsorbed. At normal plasma levels, glucose has a clearance of zero because it is reabsorbed in the tubules and none appears in the urine.

Regulation of Sodium and Potassium Elimination

Elimination of sodium and potassium is regulated by the GFR and by humoral agents that control reabsorption. Aldosterone functions in the regulation of sodium and potassium elimination. Atrial natriuretic peptide (ANP) contributes to the regulation of sodium elimination.

Tubular Function

➤ The urine filtrate flows through the tubular component of the nephron, which is divided into four major segments. The tubules are composed of epithelial cells supported by a basement membrane and surrounded by peritubular capillaries. The structure of the epithelial cell varies among segments, depending on reabsorptive or secretory function.

➤ As the filtrate flows through the tubule, the concentration of water and electrolytes in the filtrate changes because of reabsorption of water and solutes by tubular cells into the peritubular capillary blood and secretion from the blood into the tubular lumen.

➤ Reabsorption and secretion of substances across the tubular epithelial cell are accomplished through both active and passive transport processes. Most of the reabsorption and secretion occurs in the proximal tubule.

➤ The reabsorption of most substances (*i.e.,* water, chloride, bicarbonate, glucose, amino acids) depends on the maintenance of a low epithelial intracellular concentration of sodium by the basolateral membrane Na^+-K^+ ATPase pump. Sodium moves into the cell down its concentration gradient and other substances are reabsorbed by cotransport processes, or by the osmotic or electrical gradients created by the movement of sodium out of the lumen. Other substances such as hydrogen are secreted into the lumen by countertransport pumps.

➤ The kidney is able to concentrate urine because of the creation of a hyperosmotic medullary interstitium and the presence of receptors on the collecting ducts for antidiuretic hormone (ADH). In the presence of ADH, there is an increase in the number of protein water channels expressed on the luminal membrane, and water moves into the cell down its concentration gradient.

Aldosterone. Sodium reabsorption in the distal tubule and collecting duct is highly variable and depends on the presence of aldosterone, a hormone secreted by the adrenal gland. In the presence of aldosterone, almost all the sodium in the distal tubular fluid is reabsorbed, and the urine essentially becomes sodium free. In the absence of aldosterone, virtually no sodium is reabsorbed from the distal tubule. The remarkable ability of the distal tubular and collecting duct cells to alter sodium reabsorption in relation to changes in aldosterone allows the kidneys to excrete urine with sodium levels that range from a few tenths of a gram to 40 g per day.

Like sodium, potassium is freely filtered in the glomerulus, but unlike sodium, potassium is reabsorbed from and secreted into the tubular fluid. The secretion of potassium into the tubular fluid occurs in the distal tubule and, like that of sodium, is regulated by aldosterone. Only approximately 70 mEq of potassium is delivered to the distal tubule each day, but the average person consumes this much and more potassium in the diet. Excess potassium that is not filtered in the glomerulus and delivered to the collecting tubule therefore must be secreted (*i.e.*, transported from the blood) into the tubular fluid for elimination from the body. In the absence of aldosterone (as in Addison's disease; see Chapter 40), potassium secretion becomes minimal. In these circumstances, potassium reabsorption exceeds secretion, and blood levels of potassium increase.

Atrial Natriuretic Peptide.   Atrial natriuretic peptide, discovered in 1981, is a hormone believed to have an important role in salt and water excretion by the kidney. It is synthesized in muscle cells of the atria of the heart and released when the atria are stretched. The actions of ANP include vasodilation of the afferent and efferent arterioles, which results in an increase in renal blood flow and glomerular filtration rate. ANP inhibits aldosterone secretion by the adrenal gland and sodium reabsorption from the collecting tubules through its action on aldosterone and through direct action on the tubular cells. It also inhibits ADH release from the posterior pituitary gland, thereby increasing excretion of water by the kidneys. ANP also has vasodilator properties. Whether these effects are sufficient to produce long-term changes in blood pressure is uncertain.

Regulation of pH

The kidneys regulate body pH by conserving base bicarbonate and eliminating hydrogen ions (H^+). Neither the blood buffer systems nor the respiratory control mechanisms for carbon dioxide elimination can eliminate hydrogen ions from the body. This is accomplished by the kidneys. The average North American diet results in the liberation of 40 to 80 mmol of hydrogen ions each day. Virtually all the hydrogen ions excreted in the urine are secreted into the tubular fluid by means of tubular secretory mechanisms. The lowest tubular fluid pH that can be achieved is 4.4 to 4.5. The ability of the kidneys to excrete hydrogen ions depends on buffers in the urine that combine with the hydrogen ion. The three major urine buffers are bicarbonate (HCO_3^-), phosphate (HPO_4^-), and ammonia (NH_3). Bicarbonate ions, which are present in the urine filtrate, combine with hydrogen ions that have been secreted into the tubular fluid; this results in the formation of carbon dioxide and water. The carbon dioxide is then absorbed into the tubular cells and bicarbonate is regenerated. The phosphate ion is a metabolic end product that is filtered into the tubular fluid; it combines with a secreted hydrogen ion and is not reabsorbed. Ammonia is synthesized in tubular cells by deamination of the amino acid glutamine; it diffuses into the tubular fluid and combines with the hydrogen ion. An important aspect of this buffer system is that the deamination process increases whenever the body's hydrogen ion concentration remains elevated for 1 to 2 days. These mechanisms for pH regulation are described more fully in Chapter 32.

pH-Dependent Elimination of Organic Ions

The proximal tubule actively secretes large amounts of different organic anions. Foreign anions (*e.g.*, salicylates, penicillin) and endogenously produced anions (*e.g.*, bile acids, uric acid) are actively secreted into the tubular fluid. Most of the anions that are secreted use the same transport system, allowing the kidneys to rid the body of many different drugs and environmental agents. Because the same transport system is shared by different anions, there is competition for transport such that elevated levels of one substance tend to inhibit the secretion of other anions. The proximal tubules also possess an active transport system for organic cations that is analogous to that for organic ions.

Uric Acid Elimination

Uric acid is a product of purine metabolism (see Chapter 59). Excessively high blood levels (*i.e.*, hyperuricemia) can cause gout, and excessive levels in the urine can cause kidney stones. Uric acid is freely filtered in the glomerulus and is reabsorbed and secreted into the proximal tubules. Uric acid is one of the anions that uses the previously described anion transport system in the proximal tubule. Tubular reabsorption normally exceeds secretion, and the net effect is removal of uric acid from the filtrate. Although the rate of reabsorption exceeds secretion, the secretory process is homeostatically controlled to maintain a constant plasma level. Many persons with elevated uric acid levels secrete less uric acid than do persons with normal uric acid levels.

Uric acid uses the same transport systems as other anions, such as aspirin, sulfinpyrazone, and probenecid. Small doses of aspirin compete with uric acid for secretion into the tubular fluid and reduce uric acid secretion, and large doses compete with uric acid for reabsorption and increase uric acid excretion in the urine. Because of its effect on uric acid secretion, aspirin is not recommended for treatment of gouty arthritis. Thiazide and loop diuretics (*i.e.*, furosemide and ethacrynic acid) also can cause hyperuricemia and gouty arthritis, presumably through a decrease in extracellular fluid volume and enhanced uric acid reabsorption.

Urea Elimination

Urea is an end product of protein metabolism. The normal adult produces 25 to 30 g/day; the quantity rises when a high-protein diet is consumed, when there is excessive tissue breakdown, or in the presence of gastrointestinal bleeding. With gastrointestinal bleeding, the blood proteins are broken down to form ammonia in the intestine; the ammonia is then absorbed into the portal circulation and converted to urea by the liver before being released into the bloodstream. The kidneys, in their role as regulators of blood urea nitrogen (BUN) levels, filter urea in the glomeruli and then reabsorb it in the tubules. This enables maintenance of a normal BUN, which is in the range of 8 to 25 mg/dL (2.9 to 8.9 mmol/L). During periods of dehydration, the blood volume and GFR drop, and BUN levels increase. The renal tubules are permeable to urea, which means that the longer the tubular fluid remains in the kidneys, the greater is the reabsorption of urea into the blood. Only small amounts of urea are reabsorbed into the blood when the GFR is high, but relatively large amounts of urea are returned to the blood when the GFR is reduced.

DRUG ELIMINATION

Many drugs are eliminated in the urine. These drugs are selectively filtered in the glomerulus and reabsorbed or secreted into the tubular fluid. Only drugs that are not bound to plasma proteins are filtered in the glomerulus and therefore able to be eliminated by the kidneys.

Many drugs are weak acids or weak bases and are present in the renal tubular fluid partly as water-soluble ions and partly as nonionized lipid-soluble molecules. The nonionized lipid-soluble form of a drug diffuses more readily through the lipid membrane of the tubule and then back into the bloodstream. The water-soluble ionized form remains in the urine filtrate. The ratio of ionized to nonionized drug depends on the pH of the urine. For example, aspirin is highly ionized in alkaline urine and in this form is rapidly excreted in the urine. Aspirin is largely nonionized in acid urine and is reabsorbed rather than excreted. Alkaline or acid diuresis may be used to increase elimination of drugs in the urine, particularly in situations of drug overdose.

ENDOCRINE FUNCTIONS OF THE KIDNEY

In addition to their function in regulating body fluids and electrolytes, the kidneys function as an endocrine organ in that they produce chemical mediators that travel through the blood to distant sites where they exert their actions. The kidneys participate in control of blood pressure by way of the renin-angiotensin mechanism, in calcium metabolism by activating vitamin D, and in regulating red blood cell production through the synthesis of erythropoietin.

The Renin-Angiotensin-Aldosterone Mechanism

The renin-angiotensin-aldosterone mechanism plays an important part in short-term and long-term regulation of blood pressure (see Chapter 21). Renin is synthesized and stored in the juxtaglomerular cells of the kidney. This enzyme is thought to be released in response to a decrease in renal blood flow or a change in the composition of the distal tubular fluid, or as the result of sympathetic nervous system stimulation. Renin itself has no direct effect on blood pressure. Rather, it acts enzymatically to convert a circulating plasma protein called *angiotensinogen* to angiotensin I. Angiotensin I, which has few vasoconstrictor properties, leaves the kidneys and enters the circulation; as it is circulated through the lungs, *angiotensin-converting enzyme* catalyzes the conversion of angiotensin I to angiotensin II. Angiotensin II is a potent vasoconstrictor, and it acts directly on the kidneys to decrease salt and water excretion. Both mechanisms have relatively short periods of action. Angiotensin II also stimulates aldosterone secretion by the adrenal gland. Aldosterone acts on the distal tubule to increase sodium reabsorption and exerts a longer-term effect on the maintenance of blood pressure. Renin also functions by means of angiotensin II to produce constriction of the efferent arteriole as a means of preventing a serious decrease in glomerular filtration pressure.

Erythropoietin

Erythropoietin is a polypeptide hormone that regulates the differentiation of red blood cells in the bone marrow (see Chapter 15). Between 89% and 95% of erythropoietin is formed in the kidneys. The synthesis of erythropoietin is stimulated by tissue hypoxia, which may be brought about by anemia, residence at high altitudes, or impaired oxygenation of tissues due to cardiac or pulmonary disease. Persons with end-stage kidney disease often are anemic because of an inability of the kidneys to produce erythropoietin. This anemia usually is managed by the administration of epoetin-alfa, a synthetic form of erythropoietin produced through DNA technology, to stimulate erythropoiesis.

Vitamin D

Activation of vitamin D occurs in the kidneys. Vitamin D increases calcium absorption from the gastrointestinal tract and helps to regulate calcium deposition in bone. It also has a weak stimulatory effect on renal calcium absorption. Although vitamin D is not synthesized and released from an endocrine gland, it often is considered as a hormone because of its pathway of molecular activation and mechanism of action.

It exists in several forms: natural vitamin D (cholecalciferol), which results from ultraviolet irradiation of the skin, and synthetic vitamin D (ergocalciferol), which is derived from irradiation of ergosterol. The active form of vitamin D is 1,25-dihydroxycholecalciferol. Cholecalciferol and ergocalciferol must undergo chemical transformation to become active: first to 25-hydroxycholecalciferol in the liver and then to 1,25-dihydroxycholecalciferol in the kidneys. Persons with end-stage renal disease are unable to transform vitamin D to its active form and must rely on pharmacologic preparations of the active vitamin (calcitriol) for maintaining mineralization of their bones.

In summary, the kidneys perform excretory and endocrine functions. In the process of excreting wastes, the kidneys filter the blood and then selectively reabsorb those materials that are needed to maintain a stable internal environment. The kidneys rid the body of metabolic wastes, regulate fluid volume, regulate the concentration of electrolytes, assist in maintaining acid-base balance, aid in regulation of blood pressure through the renin-angiotensin-aldosterone mechanism and control of extracellular fluid volume, regulate red blood cell production through erythropoietin, and aid in calcium metabolism by activating vitamin D.

The nephron is the functional unit of the kidney. It is composed of a glomerulus, which filters the blood, and a tubular component, where electrolytes and other substances needed to maintain the constancy of

TABLE 30-1 ✦ Normal Values for Routine Urinalysis		
General Characteristics and Measurements	**Chemical Determinations**	**Microscopic Examination of Sediment**
Color: yellow-amber—indicates a high specific gravity and small output of urine Turbidity: clear to slightly hazy Specific gravity: 1.010–1.025 with a normal fluid intake pH: 4.6–4.8—average person has a pH of about 6 (acid)	Glucose: negative Ketones: negative Blood: negative Protein: negative Bilirubin: negative Urobilinogen: 0.1–1 Nitrate for bacteria: negative Leukocyte esterase: negative	Casts negative: occasional hyaline casts Red blood cells: negative or rare Crystals: negative White blood cells; negative or rare Epithelial cells: few

(From Fischbach F. [1992]. *A manual of laboratory diagnostic tests* [p. 148]. Philadelphia: J.B. Lippincott)

the internal environment are reabsorbed into the bloodstream while unneeded materials are secreted into the tubular filtrate for elimination. Urine concentration occurs in the collecting tubules under the influence of ADH. ADH maintains extracellular volume by returning water to the vascular compartment, producing a concentrated urine by removing water from the tubular filtrate.

The GFR is the amount of filtrate that is formed each minute as blood moves through the glomeruli. It is regulated by the arterial blood pressure and renal blood flow in the normally functioning kidney. The juxtaglomerular complex is thought to represent a feedback control system that links changes in the GFR with renal blood flow. Renal clearance is the volume of plasma that is completely cleared each minute of any substance that finds its way into the urine. It is determined by the ability of the substance to be filtered in the glomeruli and the capacity of the renal tubules to reabsorb or secrete the substance.

 Other Functions of the Kidney

➤ Long-term regulation of arterial pressure through regulation of sodium and water balance

➤ Synthesis and release of the enzyme renin, which is the first step in the biochemical synthesis of angiotensin II, a vasoconstrictor hormone that also increases sodium reabsorption by the proximal tubule

➤ Activation of vitamin D, which is important for intestinal absorption of calcium

➤ Production of erythropoietin, which stimulates bone marrow production of red blood cells

➤ pH regulation through bicarbonate reabsorption and hydrogen ion excretion

Tests of Renal Function

After you have completed this section of the chapter, you should be able to meet the following objectives:

✦ Describe the characteristics of normal urine
✦ Explain the significance of casts in the urine
✦ Explain the value of urine specific gravity in evaluating renal function
✦ Explain the concept of the glomerular filtration rate
✦ Explain the value of serum creatinine levels in evaluating renal function
✦ Describe the methods used in cystoscopic examination of the urinary tract, ultrasound studies of the urinary tract, computed tomographic scans, magnetic resonance imaging studies, excretory urography, and renal angiography

The function of the kidneys is to filter the blood, selectively reabsorb those substances that are needed to maintain the constancy of body fluid, and excrete metabolic wastes. The composition of urine and blood provides valuable information about the adequacy of renal function. Radiologic tests, endoscopy, and renal biopsy afford means for viewing the gross and microscopic structures of the kidneys and urinary system.

URINALYSIS

Urine is a clear, amber-colored fluid that is approximately 95% water and 5% dissolved solids. The kidneys normally produce approximately 1.5 L of urine each day. Normal urine contains metabolic wastes and few or no plasma proteins, blood cells, or glucose molecules.

Urine tests can be performed on a single urine specimen or on a 24-hour urine specimen. First-voided morning specimens are useful for qualitative protein and specific gravity testing. A freshly voided specimen is most reliable. Urine specimens that have been left standing may contain lysed red blood cells, disintegrating *casts*, and rapidly multiplying bacteria. Table 30-1 describes urinalysis values for normal urine.

Casts are molds of the distal nephron lumen. A gel-like substance called *Tamm-Horsfall mucoprotein*, which is formed in the tubular epithelium, is the major protein constituent of urinary casts. Casts composed of this gel but devoid of cells are called *hyaline casts*. These casts develop when the protein concentration of the urine is high (as in nephrotic syndrome), urine osmolality is high, and urine pH is low. The inclusion of granules or cells in the matrix of the protein gel leads to the formation of various other types of casts.

Because of the glomerular capillary filtration barrier, less than 150 mg of protein is excreted in the urine over 24 hours in a healthy person. Qualitative and quantitative tests to determine urinary protein content are important tools to assess the extent of glomerular disease. pH-sensitive reagent strips are used to test for the presence of proteins, whereas immunoassay methods are used to test for microalbuminuria (30 to 300 mg albumin/24 hours).

The *specific gravity* (or osmolality) of urine varies with its concentration of solutes. Urine specific gravity provides a valuable index of the hydration status and functional ability of the kidneys. Although there are more sophisticated methods for measuring specific gravity, it can be measured easily using an inexpensive piece of equipment called a *urinometer*. Healthy kidneys can produce a concentrated urine with a specific gravity of 1.030 to 1.040. During periods of marked hydration, the specific gravity can approach 1.000. With diminished renal function, there is a loss of renal concentrating ability, and the urine specific gravity may fall to levels of 1.006 to 1.010 (usual range is 1.010 to 1.025 with normal fluid intake). These low levels are particularly significant if they occur during periods that follow a decrease in water intake (*e.g.*, during the first urine specimen on arising in the morning).

GLOMERULAR FILTRATION RATE

The GFR provides a gauge of renal function. It can be measured clinically by collecting timed samples of blood and urine. *Creatinine*, a product of creatine metabolism by the muscle, is filtered by the kidneys but not reabsorbed in the renal tubule. Creatinine levels in the blood and urine can be used to measure GFR. The clearance rate for creatinine is the amount that is completely cleared by the kidneys in 1 minute. The formula is expressed as $C = UV/P$, in which C is the clearance rate (mL/minute), U is the urine concentration (mg/dL), V is the urine volume excreted (mL/minute or 24 hours), and P is plasma concentration (mg/dL).

Normal creatinine clearance is 115 to 125 mL/minute. This value is corrected for body surface area, which reflects the muscle mass where creatinine metabolism takes place. The test may be done on a 24-hour basis, with blood being drawn when the urine collection is completed. In another method, two 1-hour urine specimens are collected, and a blood sample is drawn in between.

BLOOD TESTS

Blood tests can provide valuable information about the kidneys' ability to remove metabolic wastes from the blood and maintain normal electrolyte and pH composition of the blood. Normal blood values are listed in Table 30-2. Serum levels of potassium, phosphate, BUN, and creatinine increase in renal failure. Serum pH, calcium, and bicarbonate levels decrease in renal failure. The effect of renal failure on the concentration of serum electrolytes and metabolic end products is discussed in Chapter 34.

Serum Creatinine

Serum creatinine levels reflect the glomerular filtration rate. Because these measurements are easily obtained and relatively inexpensive, they often are used as a screening measure of renal function. Creatinine is a product of creatine metabolism in muscles; its formation and release are relatively constant and proportional to the amount of muscle mass present. Creatinine is freely filtered in the glomeruli, is not reabsorbed from the tubules into the blood, and is only minimally secreted into the tubules from the blood; therefore, its blood values depend closely on the GFR.

The normal creatinine value is approximately 0.7 mg/dL of blood for a woman with a small frame, approximately 1.0 mg/dL of blood for a normal adult man, and approximately 1.5 mg/dL of blood (60 to 130 mmol/L) for a muscular man. There is an age-related decline in creatinine clearance in many elderly persons because muscle mass and the GFR decline with age (see Chapter 34). A normal serum creatinine level usually indicates normal renal function. In addition to its use in calculating the GFR, the serum creatinine level is used in estimating the functional capacity of the kidneys (Fig. 30-15). If the value doubles, the GFR—and renal function—probably has fallen to one half of its normal state. A rise in the serum creatinine level to three times its normal value suggests that there is a 75% loss of renal function, and with creatinine values of 10 mg/dL or more, it can be assumed that approximately 90% of renal function has been lost.

Recently it has been proposed that another serum protein, *cystatin-C* (a cysteine protease inhibitor), could be useful as a marker of GFR because it has a stable production rate, is freely filtered at the glomerulus, and in several studies to date has shown a greater sensitivity in detecting a decreased GFR. Further clinical studies are needed to de-

TABLE 30-2 ✦ **Normal Blood Chemistry Levels**	
Substance	**Normal Value***
Blood urea nitrogen	8.0–20.0 mg/dL (2.9–7.1 mmol/L)
Creatinine	0.7–1.5 mg/dL (60–130 µmol/L)
Sodium	135–145 mEq/L (135–148 mmol/L)
Chloride	98–106 mEq/L (98–106 mmol/L)
Potassium	3.5–5 mEq/L (3.5–5 mmol/L)
Carbon dioxide (CO_2 content)	24–29 mEq/L (24–29 mmol/L)
Calcium	8.5–10.5 mg/dL (2.1–2.6 mmol/L)
Phosphate	2.5–4.5 mg/dL (1–1.5 mmol/L)
Uric acid	1.4–7.4 mg/dL (0.154–0.42 mmol/L)
pH	7.35–7.45

*Values may vary among laboratories, depending on the method of analysis used.

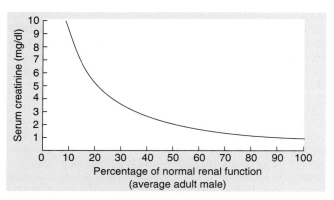

FIGURE 30-15 Relation between the percentage of renal function and serum creatinine levels.

termine the clinical efficacy of cystatin-C as a marker and to determine whether there is an advantage in its use compared with creatinine.

Blood Urea Nitrogen

Urea is formed in the liver as a byproduct of protein metabolism and is eliminated entirely by the kidneys. BUN therefore is related to the GFR but, unlike creatinine, also is influenced by protein intake, gastrointestinal bleeding, and hydration status. Increased protein intake and gastrointestinal bleeding increase urea by means of protein metabolism. In gastrointestinal bleeding, the blood is broken down by the intestinal flora, and the nitrogenous waste is absorbed into the portal vein and transported to the liver, where it is converted to urea. During dehydration, elevated BUN levels result from increased concentration. Approximately two thirds of renal function must be lost before a significant rise in the BUN level occurs.

The BUN is less specific for renal insufficiency than creatinine, but the *BUN–creatinine ratio* may provide useful diagnostic information. The ratio normally is approximately 10:1. Ratios greater than 15:1 represent prerenal conditions, such as congestive heart failure and upper gastrointestinal tract bleeding, that produce an increase in BUN but not in creatinine. A ratio of less than 10:1 occurs in persons with liver disease and in those who receive a low-protein diet or chronic dialysis, because BUN is more readily dialyzable than creatinine.

CYSTOSCOPY

Cystoscopy provides a means for direct visualization of the urethra, bladder, and ureteral orifices. It relies on the use of a cystoscope, an instrument with a lighted lens. The cystoscope is inserted through the urethra into the bladder. Biopsy specimens, lesions, small stones, and foreign bodies can be removed from the bladder. Urethroscopy may be used to remove stones from the ureter and aid in the treatment of ureteral disorders such as ureteral strictures.

ULTRASONOGRAPHY

Ultrasound studies use the reflection of ultrasonic (high-frequency) waves to visualize the deep structures of the

body. The procedure is painless and noninvasive and requires no patient preparation. Ultrasonography is used to visualize the structures of the kidneys and has proved useful in the diagnosis of many urinary tract disorders, including congenital anomalies, renal abscesses, hydronephrosis, and kidney stones. It can differentiate a renal cyst from a renal tumor. The use of ultrasonography also enables accurate placement of needles for renal biopsy and catheters for percutaneous nephrostomy.

RADIOLOGIC AND OTHER IMAGING STUDIES

Radiologic studies include a simple flat plate (radiograph) of the kidneys, ureters, and bladder that can be used to determine the size, shape, and position of the kidneys and observe any radiopaque stones that may be in the kidney pelvis or ureters. In excretory urography, or *intravenous pyelography*, a radiopaque dye is injected into a peripheral vein; the dye is then filtered by the glomerulus and excreted into the urine, and x-ray films are taken as it moves through the kidneys and ureters.

Urography is used to detect space-occupying lesions of the kidneys, pyelonephritis, hydronephrosis, vesicoureteral reflux, and kidney stones. Some persons are allergic to the dye used for urography and may have an anaphylactic reaction after its administration. Every person undergoing urography studies should be questioned about previous reactions to the dye or to similar dyes. If the test is considered essential in such persons, premedication with antihistamines and corticosteroids may be used. The dye also reduces renal blood flow; acute renal failure can occur, particularly in persons with vascular disease or preexisting renal insufficiency.

Other diagnostic tests include computed tomographic (CT) scans, magnetic resonance imaging (MRI), radionuclide imaging, and renal angiography. CT scans may be used to outline the kidneys and detect renal masses and tumors. MRI is becoming readily available and is used in imaging the kidneys, retroperitoneum, and urinary bladder. It is particularly useful in evaluating vascular abnormalities in and around the kidneys. Radionuclide imaging involves the injection of a radioactive material that subsequently is detected externally by a scintillation camera, which detects the radioactive emissions. Radionuclide imaging is used to evaluate renal function and structures, as well as the ureters and bladder. It is particularly useful in evaluating the function of kidney transplants. Renal angiography provides x-ray pictures of the blood vessels that supply the kidneys. It involves the injection of a radiopaque dye directly into the renal artery. A catheter usually is introduced through the femoral artery and advanced under fluoroscopic view into the abdominal aorta. The catheter tip then is maneuvered into the renal artery, and the dye is injected. This test is used to evaluate persons suspected of having renal artery stenosis, abnormalities of renal blood vessels, or vascular damage to the renal arteries after trauma.

In summary, urinalysis and blood tests that measure levels of byproducts of metabolism and electrolytes provide information about renal function. Cystoscopic examinations can be used for direct visualization of the urethra, bladder, and ureters. Ultrasonography can be used to determine kidney size, and renal radionuclide imaging can be used to evaluate the kidney structures. Radiologic methods such as excretory urography provide a means by which kidney structures such as the renal calyces, pelvis, ureters, and bladder can be outlined.

Physiologic Action of Diuretics

After you have completed this section of the chapter, you should be able to meet the following objectives:

- ✦ Describe the physiologic action of diuretics
- ✦ Contrast and compare the actions of osmotic diuretics, loop diuretics, thiazide diuretics, aldosterone antagonists, and carbonic anhydrase inhibitors

Diuresis is the rapid passage of urine through the kidneys. In some disease states, it is desirable to increase urine output through the use of diuretics. Water reabsorption in the kidneys is largely passive and depends on sodium reabsorption. Most diuretics exert their action by interfering with sodium reabsorption. Approximately 60% to 65% of sodium reabsorption takes place in the proximal tubule, 20% to 25% in the loop of Henle, 10% in the distal convoluted tubule, and 2% to 5% in the late distal and cortical tubules (Fig. 30-16). The effectiveness of a diuretic in promoting salt and water excretion depends on the tubular site of action. There are four types of diuretics: *osmotic diuretics, inhibitors of sodium transport, aldosterone antagonists,* and *inhibitors of urine acidification.*

OSMOTIC DIURETICS

Osmotic diuretics, such as mannitol, are filtered in the glomerulus but not reabsorbed in the tubules. The proximal tubule and descending limb are freely permeable to water. Because these substances are poorly reabsorbed, they increase the osmolality of the tubular filtrate and cause water diuresis. Because these agents are poorly absorbed, they must be given intravenously rather than orally. The osmotic diuretics increase water elimination in preference to sodium; therefore, they reduce total body water more than cation content and reduce intracellular volume. This effect is used to reduce intracranial pressure in persons with neurologic conditions or intraocular pressure before eye surgery. They also are used to maintain a high urine volume after a hemolytic reaction or the ingestion of toxic substances, such as salicylates or barbiturates, which are excreted in the urine.

INHIBITORS OF SODIUM TRANSPORT

Sodium reabsorption occurs in the proximal tubule, the thick ascending loop of Henle, and the distal tubule, where aldosterone regulates sodium and potassium exchange. Diuretics that alter sodium transport can act at any of these

levels. Approximately 25% to 30% of sodium is reabsorbed in the thick ascending loop of Henle, approximately 10% in the distal convoluted tubule, and 2% to 5% is reabsorbed in the late distal and cortical collecting tubule. The effectiveness of a diuretic is determined by its site of action.

Loop Diuretics

Loop diuretics exert their effect in the thick ascending loop of Henle. Because of their site of action, these drugs are the most effective diuretic agents available. These drugs inhibit the coupled Na^+–K^+–$2Cl^-$ transport system on the luminal side of the ascending limb of Henle. By inhibiting this transport system, they reduce the reabsorption of NaCl, decrease potassium reabsorption, and increase calcium and magnesium elimination. Prolonged use can cause significant loss of magnesium in some persons. Because calcium is actively reabsorbed in the distal convoluted tubule, loop diuretics usually do not cause hypocalcemia. Impairment of sodium reabsorption in the loop of Henle causes a decrease in the osmolarity of the interstitial fluid surrounding the collecting ducts and further impedes the kidneys' ability to concentrate urine. The loop diuretics may increase uric acid retention and impair glucose tolerance. These drugs also can cause hypovolemia.

Thiazide Diuretics

Thiazide diuretics act by preventing the reabsorption of NaCl in the distal convoluted tubule. Because of their site of action, the thiazide diuretics are less effective than loop diuretics in terms of effecting diuresis. The thiazides produce increased losses of potassium in the urine, uric acid retention, and some impairment in glucose tolerance. Thiazide diuretics also reduce peripheral vascular resistance, and therefore often are prescribed as a first-line antihypertensive treatment.

ALDOSTERONE ANTAGONISTS

The aldosterone antagonists, also called *potassium-sparing diuretics,* reduce sodium reabsorption and increase potassium secretion in the late distal tubule and cortical collecting tubule site regulated by aldosterone. Because of their site of action, the aldosterone antagonists have the least effect on diuresis compared with the loop diuretics and the thiazide diuretics. They have the advantage of increasing potassium reabsorption and thereby eliminating the risk of hypokalemia. These agents also tend to interfere with secretion of hydrogen ions in the collecting duct, explaining in part the metabolic acidosis sometimes seen with the use of these agents.

There are two types of potassium-sparing diuretics: those that act as direct aldosterone antagonists and those that act independently of aldosterone. The first type (*e.g.,* spironolactone) binds to the mineralocorticoid receptor in the tubule, preventing aldosterone from binding and exerting its effects. The second type (*e.g.,* triamterene, amiloride) does not bind to the receptor, but instead directly interferes with sodium entry through the sodium-selective ion channel. Because potassium secretion is coupled with sodium reabsorption in this segment of the tubule, these agents

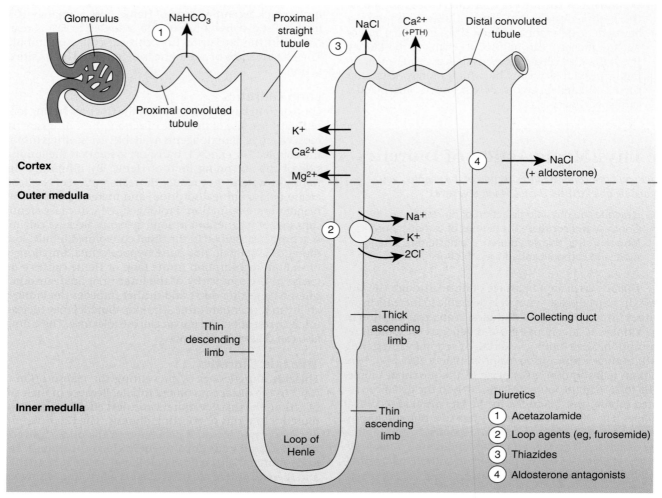

FIGURE 30-16 Sites of action of diuretics.

are effective potassium-sparing diuretics. These diuretics are used during states of mineralocorticoid excess and because of their effects on potassium excretion. Because the thiazide and aldosterone antagonists affect sodium reabsorption at different tubule sites, combination products of the two agents (*i.e.,* hydrochlorothiazide with triamterene [Dyazide], hydrochlorothiazide with amiloride [Moduretic], hydrochlorothiazide with spironolactone [Aldactazide]) are available. Because of their mechanism of action, these diuretics may cause severe hyperkalemia.

INHIBITORS OF URINE ACIDIFICATION

Acetazolamide, a carbonic anhydrase inhibitor, impairs the reaction that converts carbon dioxide and water to bicarbonate and hydrogen ions. Bicarbonate is poorly absorbed in the renal tubules; instead, it combines with hydrogen that is secreted into the tubule to form carbon dioxide and water. The carbon dioxide is then reabsorbed into the tubular cells, where it combines with water in a carbonic

anhydrase–catalyzed reaction to form bicarbonate and hydrogen ions. When hydrogen ion secretion is blocked by the action of acetazolamide, the bicarbonate ion and the sodium ion that accompany it are lost in the urine. The loss of bicarbonate results in a mild systemic acidosis. As this occurs, the kidneys resume the secretion of hydrogen ions, overcoming the effect of the carbonic anhydrase inhibition.

The duration of action of acetazolamide is short. This drug has been largely replaced by more effective diuretics, such as the thiazides. Acetazolamide also decreases the formation of aqueous humor and cerebrospinal fluid and continues to be used for that purpose. The drug also is used for prophylaxis and treatment of the symptoms of acute mountain sickness, which are related to hypoxia-induced hyperventilation and respiratory alkalosis.

In summary, diuretics are drugs that increase urine output. With the exception of osmotic diuretics, they exert their action by altering sodium transport. Osmotic diuretics are filtered in the glomerulus and reabsorbed in the tubules. They act by increasing the osmolarity of tubular fluid. Inhibitors of urine acidification, such as acetazolamide, prevent bicarbonate reabsorption and the accompanying sodium reabsorption. Loop diuretics block sodium reabsorption in the thick ascending loop of Henle, and thiazide diuretics function in the section of the tubule between the thick ascending loop of Henle and the distal tubule. The potassium-sparing diuretics decrease sodium reabsorption while causing potassium retention.

Bibliography

Brater D.C. (2000). Pharmacology of diuretics. *American Journal of Medical Sciences* 319, 38–50.

Cormack D.H. (1993). *Essential histology* (pp. 322–333). Philadelphia: J.B. Lippincott.

Guyton A.C., Hall J.E. (2000). *Textbook of medical physiology* (10th ed., pp. 279–311). Philadelphia: W.B. Saunders.

Koeppen B.M., Stanton B.A. (1997). *Renal physiology* (2nd ed.). St. Louis: Mosby.

Price C.P., Finney H. (2000). Developments in the assessment of glomerular filtration rate. *Clinica Chimica Acta* 297, 55–66.

Rahn K.H., Heidenreich S., Bruckner D. (1999). How to assess glomerular function and damage in humans. *Journal of Hypertension* 17, 309–317.

Rhoades R.A., Tanner G.A. (1996). *Medical physiology* (pp. 417–445). Boston: Little, Brown.

Smith H. (1953). *From fish to philosopher* (p. 4). Boston: Little, Brown.

Vander A.J. (1995). *Renal physiology* (5th ed.). New York: McGraw-Hill.

Alterations in Fluids and Electrolytes

Fluids and electrolytes are present in body cells, in the tissue spaces between the cells, and in the blood that fills the vascular compartment. Fluids transport gases, nutrients, and wastes; help generate the electrical activity needed to power body functions; take part in the transforming of food into energy; and otherwise maintain the overall function of the body. Although fluid volume and composition remain relatively constant in the presence of a wide range of changes in intake and output, conditions such as environmental stresses and disease can increase fluid loss, impair its intake, and otherwise interfere with mechanisms that regulate fluid volume, composition, and distribution.

This chapter is divided into four sections: (1) Composition and Compartmental Distribution of Body Fluids, (2) Sodium and Water Balance, (3) Potassium Balance, and (4) Calcium, Phosphate, and Magnesium Balance.

The mechanisms of edema formation are discussed in the section on composition and compartmentalization of body fluids.

Composition and Compartmental Distribution of Body Fluids

After you have completed this section of the chapter, you should be able to meet the following objectives:

✦ Define *electrolyte*, *ion*, and *nonelectrolyte*
✦ Differentiate intracellular from extracellular compartments in terms of distribution and composition of water, electrolytes, and other osmotically active solutes
✦ Cite the rationale for the use of concentration rather than absolute values in describing electrolyte content of body fluids
✦ Relate the concept of a concentration gradient to the processes of diffusion and osmosis
✦ Differentiate between effective and ineffective osmoles in determining the tonicity of a solution

+ Describe the control of cell volume and the effect of isotonic, hypotonic, and hypertonic solutions on cell size
+ Describe factors that control fluid exchange between the vascular and interstitial fluid compartments and relate them to the development of edema and third spacing of extracellular fluids
+ Describe the manifestations and treatment of edema

Body fluids are distributed between the intracellular and extracellular fluid compartments. The intracellular compartment consists of fluid contained within all of the billions of cells in the body. It is the larger of the two compartments, with approximately two thirds of the body water in healthy adults. The remaining one third of body water is in the extracellular compartment, which contains all the fluids outside the cells, including that in the interstitial or tissue spaces and blood vessels (Fig. 31-1). The extracellular fluids, including the plasma and interstitial fluids, contain large amounts of sodium and chloride, moderate amounts of bicarbonate, but only small quantities of potassium, magnesium, calcium, and phosphate. In contrast to the extracellular fluid, the intracellular fluid contains almost no calcium; small amounts of sodium, chloride, bicarbonate, and phosphate; moderate amounts of magnesium; and large amounts of potassium (Table 31-1). It is the extracellular levels of electrolytes in the blood or blood serum that are measured clinically. Although blood levels usually are representative of the total body levels of an electrolyte, this is not always the case, particularly with potassium, which is approximately 28 times more concentrated inside the cell than outside.

The cell membrane serves as the primary barrier to the movement of substances between the extracellular and intracellular compartments. Lipid-soluble substances such as gases (*i.e.*, oxygen and carbon dioxide), which dissolve in

TABLE 31-1 ✦ Concentrations of Extracellular and Intracellular Electrolytes in Adults		
Electrolyte	Extracellular Concentration*	Intracellular Concentration*
Sodium	135–145 mEq/L	10–14 mEq/L
Potassium	3.5–5.0 mEq/L	140–150 mEq/L
Chloride	98–106 mEq/L	3–4 mEq/L
Bicarbonate	24–31 mEq/L	7–10 mEq/L
Calcium	8.5–10.5 mg/dL	<1 mEq/L
Phosphate/ phosphorus	2.5–4.5 mg/dL	4 mEq/kg†
Magnesium	1.8–3.0 mg/dL	40 mEq/kg†

* Values may vary among laboratories, depending on the method of analysis used.
† Values vary among various tissues and with nutritional status.

the lipid bilayer of the cell membrane, pass directly through the membrane. Many ions, such as sodium (Na^+) and potassium (K^+) ions, rely on transport mechanisms such as the Na^+/K^+ pump that is located in the cell membrane for movement across the membrane (see Chapter 4). Because the Na^+/K^+ pump relies on adenosine triphosphate (ATP) and the enzyme ATPase for energy, it is often referred to as the Na^+/K^+-ATPase membrane pump. Water crosses the cell membrane by osmosis using special protein channels.

INTRODUCTORY CONCEPTS

Dissociation of Electrolytes

Body fluids contain water and electrolytes. Electrolytes are substances that dissociate in solution to form charged particles, or *ions*. For example, a sodium chloride (NaCl) molecule dissociates to form a positively charged sodium ion (Na^+) and a negatively charged chloride ion (Cl^-). Particles that do not dissociate into ions such as glucose and urea are called *nonelectrolytes*. Positively charged ions are called *cations* because they are attracted to the cathode of a wet electric cell, and negatively charged ions are called *anions* because they are attracted to the anode. The ions found in body fluids carry one charge (*i.e.*, monovalent ion) or two charges (*i.e.*, divalent ion). Because of their attraction forces, positively charged cations are always accompanied by negatively charged anions. The distribution of electrolytes between body compartments is influenced by their electrical charge. However, one cation may be exchanged for another, providing it carries the same charge. For example, a positively charged hydrogen ion may be exchanged for a positively charged potassium ion and a negatively charged bicarbonate ion may be exchanged for another negatively charged chloride anion.

Diffusion and Osmosis

Diffusion. *Diffusion* is the movement of charged or uncharged particles along a concentration gradient. All molecules and ions, including water and dissolved molecules,

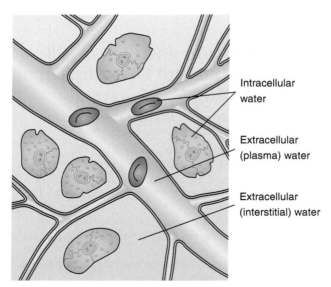

FIGURE 31-1 Distribution of body water. The extracellular space includes the vascular compartment and the interstitial spaces.

Intracellular water

Extracellular (plasma) water

Extracellular (interstitial) water

Measurement Units

The amount of electrolytes and solutes in body fluids is expressed as a concentration or amount of solute in a given volume of fluid, such as milligrams per deciliter (mg/dL), milliequivalents per liter (mEq/L), or millimoles per liter (mmol/L). The *milligrams per deciliter* measurement unit expresses the weight of the solute in one tenth of a liter (dL) or 100 mL of solution. The concentration of electrolytes, such as calcium, phosphate, and magnesium, is often expressed in mg/dL.

The *milliequivalent* is used to express the charge equivalency for a given weight of an electrolyte. Electroneutrality requires that the total number of cations in the body equals the total number of anions. When cations and anions combine, they do so according to their ionic charge, not according to their atomic weight. Thus, 1 mEq of sodium has the same number of charges as 1 mEq of chloride, regardless of molecular weight (although sodium is positive and chloride is negative). The number of milliequivalents of an electrolyte in a liter of solution can be derived from the following equation:

$$mEq = \frac{mg/100\,mL \times 10 \times valence}{atomic\ weight}$$

The Système Internationale (SI) units express electrolyte content of body fluids in *millimoles per liter* (mmol/L). A millimole is one thousandth of a mole, or the molecular weight of a substance expressed in milligrams. The number of millimoles of an electrolyte in a liter of solution can be calculated using the following equation:

$$mmol/L = \frac{mEq/L}{valence}$$

For monovalent electrolytes such as sodium and potassium, the mmol and mEq values are identical. For example 140 mEq is equal to 140 mmol of sodium.

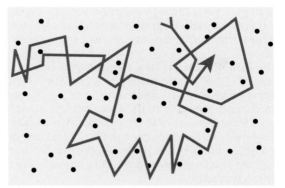

FIGURE 31-2 Diffusion of a fluid molecule during a billionth of a second. (Used with permission from Guyton A.C., Hall J.E. [1996]. *Textbook of medical physiology* [9th ed., p. 45]. Philadelphia: W.B. Saunders)

sure (measured in millimeters of mercury [mm Hg]) needed to oppose the movement of water across the membrane.

The osmotic activity that nondiffusible particles exert in pulling water from one side of the semipermeable membrane to the other is measured by a unit called an *osmole*. The osmole is derived from the gram molecular weight of a substance (*i.e.*, 1 gram molecular weight of a nondiffusible and nonionizable substance is equal to 1 osmole). In the clinical setting, osmotic activity usually is expressed in milliosmoles (one thousandth of an osmole) per liter. Each nondiffusible particle, large or small, is equally effective in its

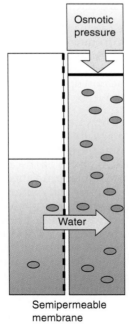

FIGURE 31-3 Movement of water across a semipermeable membrane. Water moves from the side that has fewer nondiffusible particles to the side that has more. The osmotic pressure is equal to the hydrostatic pressure needed to oppose water movement across the membrane.

are in constant random motion. It is the motion of these particles, each colliding with one another, that supplies the energy for diffusion. Because there are more molecules in constant motion in a concentrated solution, particles move from an area of higher concentration to one of lower concentration (Fig. 31-2).

Osmosis. *Osmosis* is the movement of water across a semipermeable membrane (*i.e.*, one that is permeable to water but impermeable to most solutes). As with particles, water diffuses down its concentration gradient, moving from the side of the membrane with the lesser number of particles and greater concentration of water to the side with the greater number of particles and lesser concentration of water (Fig. 31-3). As water moves across the semipermeable membrane, it generates a pressure, called the *osmotic pressure*. The osmotic pressure represents the pres-

ability to pull water through a semipermeable membrane. Thus, it is the number, rather than the size, of the non-diffusible particles that determines the osmotic activity of a solution.

The osmotic activity of a solution may be expressed in terms of either its osmolarity or osmolality. *Osmolarity* refers to the osmolar concentration in 1 L of solution (mOsm/L) and *osmolality* to the osmolar concentration in 1 kg of water (mOsm/kg of H_2O). Osmolarity is usually used when referring to fluids outside the body and osmolality for describing fluids inside the body. Because 1 L of water weighs 1 kg, the terms *osmolarity* and *osmolality* are often used interchangeably.

The predominant osmotically active particles in the extracellular fluid are Na^+ and its attendant anions (Cl^- and HCO_3^-), which together account for 90% to 95% of the osmotic pressure. Blood urea nitrogen (BUN) and glucose, which also are osmotically active, account for less than 5% of the total osmotic pressure in the extracellular compartment. This can change, however, as when blood glucose levels are elevated in persons with diabetes mellitus or when BUN levels change rapidly in persons with renal failure. Serum osmolality, which normally ranges between 275 and 295 mOsm/kg, can be calculated using the following equation:

$$\text{Osmolality (mOsm/kg)} = 2[Na^+(mmol/L)] +$$

$$\frac{\text{glucose (mg/dL)}^*}{18} + \frac{\text{BUN (mg/dL)}^*}{2.8}$$

* 1 mOsm of glucose equals 180 mg/L, and 1 mOsm of urea equals 28 mg/L

Ordinarily, the calculated and measured osmolality are within 10 mOsm of one another. The difference between the calculated and measured osmolality is called the *osmolar gap*. An osmolar gap larger than 10 mOsm suggests the presence of an unmeasured, osmotically active substance such as alcohol, acetone, or mannitol.

Tonicity. A change in water content causes cells to swell or shrink. The term *tonicity* refers to the tension or effect that the effective osmotic pressure of a solution with impermeable solutes exerts on cell size because of water movement across the cell membrane. An effective osmole is one that exerts an osmotic force and cannot permeate the cell membrane, whereas an ineffective osmole is one that exerts an osmotic force but crosses the cell membrane. Tonicity is determined solely by effective solutes such as glucose that cannot penetrate the cell membrane, thereby producing an osmotic force that pulls water into or out of the cell and causing it to change size. In contrast, urea, which is osmotically active but lipid soluble, tends to distribute equally across the cell membrane. Therefore, when extracellular levels of urea are elevated, intracellular levels also are elevated. Urea is therefore considered to be an ineffective osmole. It is only when extracellular levels of urea change rapidly, as during hemodialysis treatment, that urea affects tonicity.

Solutions to which body cells are exposed can be classified as isotonic, hypotonic, or hypertonic depending on

---

whether they cause cells to swell or shrink (Fig. 31-4). Cells placed in an isotonic solution, which has the same effective osmolality as intracellular fluids (*i.e.*, 280 mOsm/L), neither shrink nor swell. An example of an isotonic solution is 0.9% sodium chloride. When cells are placed in a hypotonic solution, which has a lower effective osmolality than intracellular fluids, they swell as water moves into the cell, and when they are placed in a hypertonic solution, which has a greater effective osmolality than intracellular fluid, they shrink as water is pulled out of the cell. How-

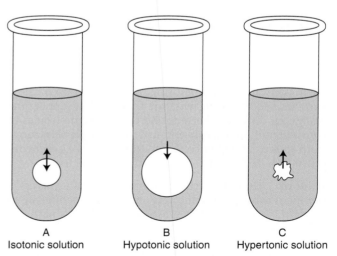

A	B	C
Isotonic solution	Hypotonic solution	Hypertonic solution

FIGURE 31-4 Osmosis. Red cells undergo no change in size in isotonic solutions (**A**). They increase in size in hypotonic solutions (**B**) and decrease in size in hypertonic solutions (**C**). (Chaffee E.E., Lytle I.M. [1980]. *Basic physiology and anatomy* [4th ed.]. Philadelphia: J.B. Lippincott)

ever, an iso-osmotic solution is not necessarily isotonic. For example, the intravenous administration of a solution of 5% dextrose in water, which is iso-osmotic, is equivalent to the infusion of a hypotonic solution of distilled water because the glucose is rapidly metabolized to carbon dioxide and water.

COMPARTMENTAL DISTRIBUTION OF BODY FLUIDS

Body water is distributed between the intracellular and extracellular compartments. In the adult, the fluid in the intracellular compartment constitutes approximately 40% of body weight.[1] The fluid in the extracellular compartment is further divided into two major subdivisions: the plasma compartment, which constitutes approximately 4% of body weight, and the interstitial fluid compartment, which constitutes approximately 15% of body weight (Fig. 31-5).

A third, usually minor, subdivision of the extracellular fluid compartment is the transcellular compartment, which is defined as being separated by a layer of epithelium. It includes the cerebrospinal fluid and fluid contained in the various body spaces, such as the peritoneal, pleural, and pericardial cavities; the joint spaces; and the gastrointestinal tract. Normally, only approximately 1% of extracellular fluid is in the transcellular space. This amount can increase considerably in conditions such as ascites, in which large amounts of fluid are sequestered in the peritoneal cavity. When the transcellular fluid compartment becomes considerably enlarged, it is referred to as a *third space*, because this fluid is not readily available for exchange with the rest of the extracellular fluid.

Intracellular Fluid Volume

Most cells are freely permeable to water. Intracellular volume is regulated by large numbers of osmotically active proteins and other organic compounds that cannot escape through the cell membrane and by solutes such as sodium, potassium, and glucose that pass through the cell membrane. Many of the intracellular proteins are negatively charged and attract positively charged ions such as potassium. The Na^+ ion, which has a greater concentration in the extracellular fluid, tends to enter the cell by diffusion. The Na^+ ion is osmotically active and its entry would, if left unchecked, pull water into the cell until it ruptured. The reason this does not occur is because the Na^+/K^+-ATPase membrane pump continuously removes three Na^+ ions from the cell for every two K^+ ions that are moved back into the cell (see Chapter 4). Situations that impair the function of the Na^+/K^+-ATPase pump, such as hypoxia, cause cells to swell because of an accumulation of Na^+ ions. Other ions, such as Ca^{2+} and H^+, are exchanged by similar transport systems.

Extracellular Fluid Volume

Extracellular fluid is divided between the vascular and interstitial fluid compartments. The vascular compartment contains blood, which is essential to the transport of substances such as electrolytes, gases, nutrients, and waste products throughout the body. Interstitial fluid acts as a transport vehicle for gases, nutrients, wastes, and other materials that move between the vascular compartment and body cells. Interstitial fluid also provides a reservoir from which vascular volume can be maintained during periods of hemorrhage or loss of vascular volume. A tissue gel, which is a spongelike material composed of large quantities of mucopolysaccharides, fills the tissue spaces and aids in even distribution of interstitial fluid. Normally, most of the fluid in the interstitium is in gel form. The tissue gel is supported by collagen fibers that hold the gel in place. The tissue gel, which has a firmer consistency than water, opposes the outflow of water from the capillaries and prevents the accumulation of free water in the interstitial spaces.

CAPILLARY/INTERSTITIAL FLUID EXCHANGE

The transfer of water between the vascular and interstitial compartments occurs at the capillary level and is governed by the Starling forces described in Chapter 21. Four forces control the movement of water between the capillary and interstitial spaces (Fig. 31-6): (1) the capillary filtration pressure, which pushes water out of the capillary into the interstitial spaces; (2) the capillary colloidal osmotic pressure, which pulls water back into the capillary; (3) the interstitial fluid pressure, which opposes the movement of water out of the capillary; and (4) the tissue colloidal osmotic pressure, which pulls water out of the capillary into the interstitial spaces.

Normally, the combination of these four forces is such that only a small excess of fluid remains in the interstitial compartment. This excess fluid is removed from the interstitium by the lymphatic system and returned to the systemic circulation.

Capillary filtration refers to the movement of water through capillary pores because of a mechanical rather than an osmotic force. The capillary filtration pressure, sometimes called the *capillary hydrostatic pressure*, is the pressure pushing water out of the capillary into the interstitial spaces. It reflects the arterial and venous pressures, the precapillary (arterioles) and postcapillary (venules) resistances, and the

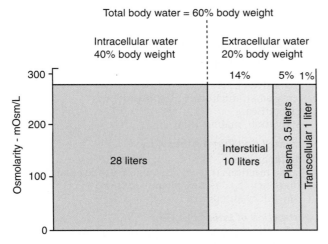

FIGURE 31-5 Approximate size of body compartments in a 70-kg adult.

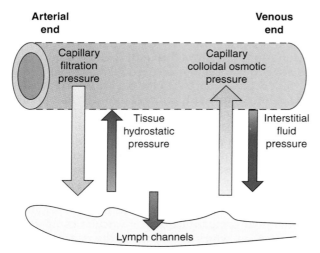

Arterial end

Venous end

Capillary filtration pressure

Capillary colloidal osmotic pressure

Tissue hydrostatic pressure

Interstitial fluid pressure

Lymph channels

FIGURE 31-6 Exchange of fluid at the capillary level.

force of gravity.[2] A rise in arterial or venous pressure increases capillary pressure. A decrease in arterial resistance or increase in venous resistance increases capillary pressure, and an increase in arterial resistance or decrease in venous resistance decreases capillary pressure. The force of gravity increases capillary pressure in the dependent parts of the body. In a person who is standing absolutely still, the weight of blood in the vascular column causes an increase of 1 mm Hg in pressure for every 13.6 mm of distance from the heart.[2] This pressure results from the weight of water and is therefore called *hydrostatic pressure*. For example, the hydrostatic pressure in the veins of an adult man can reach 90 mm Hg. This pressure is then transmitted to the capillaries.

The capillary colloidal osmotic pressure is the osmotic pressure generated by the plasma proteins that are too large to pass through the pores of the capillary wall. The term *colloidal osmotic pressure* differentiates this type of osmotic pressure from the osmotic pressure that develops at the cell membrane from the presence of electrolytes and non-electrolytes. Because plasma proteins do not normally penetrate the capillary pores and because their concentration is greater in the plasma than in the interstitial fluids, it is capillary colloidal osmotic pressure that pulls fluids back into the capillary.

The interstitial fluid pressure and the tissue colloidal osmotic pressure contribute to movement of water into and out of the interstitial spaces. The interstitial fluid pressure opposes the outward movement of water from the capillary into the interstitial spaces. The tissue colloidal osmotic pressure pulls water out of the capillary into the tissue spaces. It reflects the small amount of plasma proteins that normally escape from the capillary to enter the interstitial spaces.

Edema

Edema can be defined as palpable swelling produced by expansion of the interstitial fluid volume. Edema does not become evident until the interstitial volume has been increased by 2.5 to 3 L.[3]

Causes. The physiologic mechanisms that contribute to edema formation include factors that increase the capillary filtration pressure, decrease the capillary colloidal osmotic pressure, increase capillary permeability, or produce obstruction to lymph flow. The causes of edema are summarized in Chart 31-1.

Increased Capillary Filtration Pressure. As the capillary filtration pressure rises, the movement of vascular fluid into the interstitial spaces increases. Among the factors that increase capillary pressure are increased arterial pressure or decreased resistance to flow through the precapillary sphincters, increased venous pressure or increased resistance to outflow at the postcapillary sphincter, and capillary distention due to increased vascular volume.

Edema can be either localized or generalized. The localized edema that occurs with urticaria (*i.e.*, hives) or other allergic or inflammatory conditions results from the release of histamine and other inflammatory mediators that cause dilation of the precapillary sphincters and arterioles that supply the swollen lesions. Thrombophlebitis obstructs venous flow, producing an elevation of venous pressure and edema of the affected part, usually one of the lower extremities.

CHART 31-1

Causes of Edema

Increased Capillary Pressure

Increased vascular volume
   Heart failure
   Kidney disease
   Premenstrual sodium retention
   Pregnancy
   Environmental heat stress
Venous obstruction
   Liver disease with portal vein obstruction
   Acute pulmonary edema
   Venous thrombosis (thrombophlebitis)
Decreased arteriolar resistance
   Calcium channel–blocking drug responses

Decreased Colloidal Osmotic Pressure

Increased loss of plasma proteins
   Protein-losing kidney diseases
   Extensive burns
Decreased production of plasma proteins
   Liver disease
   Starvation, malnutrition

Increased Capillary Permeability

Inflammation
Allergic reactions (*e.g.*, hives, angioneurotic edema)
Malignancy (*e.g.*, ascites, pleural effusion)
Tissue injury and burns

Obstruction of Lymphatic Flow

Malignant obstruction of lymphatic structures
Surgical removal of lymph nodes

Generalized edema is common in conditions such as congestive heart failure that produce fluid retention and venous congestion. In right-sided heart failure, blood dams up throughout the entire venous system, causing organ congestion and edema of the dependent extremities. Decreased sodium and water excretion by the kidneys leads to an increase in extracellular volume with an increase in capillary volume and pressure with subsequent movement of fluid into the tissue spaces. The swelling of hands and feet that occurs in healthy persons during hot weather results from vasodilation of superficial blood vessels along with sodium and water retention.

Because of the effects of gravity, edema resulting from increased capillary pressure commonly causes fluid to accumulate in the dependent parts of the body, a condition referred to as *dependent edema*. For example, edema of the ankles and feet becomes more pronounced during prolonged periods of standing.

Decreased Capillary Colloidal Osmotic Pressure. Plasma proteins exert the osmotic force needed to pull fluid back into the capillary from the tissue spaces. The plasma proteins constitute a mixture of proteins, including albumin, globulins, and fibrinogen. Albumin, the smallest of the plasma proteins, has a molecular weight of 69,000; globulins have molecular weights of approximately 140,000; and fibrinogen has a molecular weight of 400,000.[2] Because of its lower molecular weight, 1 g of albumin has approximately twice as many osmotically active molecules as 1 g of globulin and almost six times as many osmotically active molecules as 1 g of fibrinogen. Also, the concentration of albumin (approximately 4.5 g/dL) is greater than that of the globulins (2.5 g/dL) and fibrinogen (0.3 mg/dL).

Edema due to decreased capillary colloidal osmotic pressure usually is the result of inadequate production or abnormal loss of plasma proteins, mainly albumin. The plasma proteins are synthesized in the liver. In persons with severe liver failure, impaired synthesis of albumin results in a decrease in colloidal osmotic pressure. In starvation and malnutrition, edema develops because there is a lack of amino acids needed in plasma protein synthesis.

The most common site of plasma protein loss is the kidney. In kidney diseases such as nephrosis, the glomerular capillaries become permeable to the plasma proteins, particularly albumin, which is the smallest of the proteins. When this happens, large amounts of albumin are filtered out of the blood and lost in the urine. An excessive loss of plasma proteins also occurs when large areas of skin are injured or destroyed. Edema is a common problem during the early stages of a burn, resulting from capillary injury and loss of plasma proteins.

Because the plasma proteins are evenly distributed throughout the body and are not affected by the force of gravity, edema due to a decrease in capillary colloidal osmotic pressure tends to affect tissues in nondependent as well as dependent parts of the body. There is swelling of the face as well as the legs and feet.

Increased Capillary Permeability. When the capillary pores become enlarged or the integrity of the capillary wall is damaged, capillary permeability is increased. When this happens, plasma proteins and other osmotically active particles leak into the interstitial spaces, increasing the tissue colloidal osmotic pressure and thereby contributing to the accumulation of interstitial fluid. Among the conditions that increase capillary permeability are burn injury, capillary congestion, inflammation, and immune responses.

Obstruction of Lymph Flow. Osmotically active plasma proteins and other large particles that cannot be reabsorbed through the pores in the capillary membrane rely on the lymphatic system for movement back into the circulatory system. Edema due to impaired lymph flow is commonly referred to as *lymphedema*. Malignant involvement of lymph structures and removal of lymph nodes at the time of cancer surgery are common causes of lymphedema. Another cause of lymphedema is infection involving the lymphatic channels and lymph nodes.

Manifestations. The effects of edema are determined largely by its location. Edema of the brain, larynx, or lungs is an acute, life-threatening condition. Although not life threatening, edema may interfere with movement, limiting joint motion. Swelling of the ankles and feet often is insidious in onset and may or may not be associated with disease. At the tissue level, edema increases the distance for diffusion of oxygen, nutrients, and wastes. Edematous tissues usually are more susceptible to injury and development of ischemic tissue damage, including pressure ulcers. Edema can also compress blood vessels. The skin of a severely swollen finger can act as a tourniquet, shutting off the blood flow to the finger. Edema can also be disfiguring, causing psychological effects and disturbances in self-concept. Edema often causes a distortion of body features and creates problems in obtaining proper-fitting clothing and shoes.

Pitting edema occurs when the accumulation of interstitial fluid exceeds the absorptive capacity of the tissue gel. In this form of edema, the tissue water becomes mobile and can be translocated with pressure exerted by a finger. Nonpitting edema usually reflects a condition in which serum proteins have accumulated in the tissue spaces and coagulated. The area often is firm and discolored. Brawny edema is a type of nonpitting edema in which the skin thickens and hardens. Nonpitting edema most frequently is seen after local infection or trauma.

Assessment and Treatment. Methods for assessing edema include daily weight, visual assessment, measurement of the affected part, and application of finger pressure to assess for pitting edema. Daily weight performed at the same time each day with the same amount of clothing provides a useful index of water gain (1 L of water weighs 2.2 pounds) due to edema. Visual inspection and measurement of the circumference of an extremity can also be used to assess the degree of swelling. This is particularly useful when swelling is due to thrombophlebitis. Finger pressure can be used to assess the degree of pitting edema. If an indentation remains after the finger has been removed, pitting edema is identified. It is evaluated on a scale of +1 (minimal) to +4 (severe) (Fig. 31-7).

Treatment of edema usually is directed toward maintaining life when the swelling involves vital structures, correcting or controlling the cause, and preventing tissue

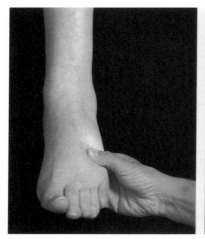
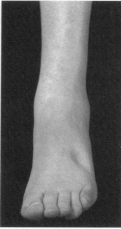

FIGURE 31-7 3 + pitting edema of the left foot. (Used with permission from Bates B. [1995]. *Bates' guide to physical examination and history taking* [6th ed., p. 438]. Philadelphia: Lippincott Williams & Wilkins)

injury. Diuretic therapy commonly is used to treat edema. Edema of the lower extremities may respond to simple measures such as elevating the feet.

Elastic support stockings and sleeves increase interstitial fluid pressure and resistance to outward movement of fluid from the capillary into the tissue spaces. These support devices typically are prescribed for patients with conditions such as lymphatic or venous obstruction and are most efficient if applied before the tissue spaces have filled with fluid—in the morning, for example, before the effects of gravity have caused fluid to move into the ankles.

Serum albumin levels can be measured, as can the colloidal osmotic pressure of the plasma (normally approximately 25.4 mm Hg). Albumin can be administered intravenously to raise the plasma colloidal osmotic pressure when edema is caused by hypoalbuminemia.

Third-Space Accumulation

Third spacing represents the loss or trapping of extracellular fluid into the transcellular space. The serous cavities are part of the transcellular compartment (*i.e.*, third-space) located in strategic body areas where there is continual movement of body structures—the pericardial sac, the peritoneal cavity, and the pleural cavity. The exchange of extracellular fluid between the capillaries, the interstitial spaces, and the transcellular space of the serous cavity uses the same mechanisms as capillaries elsewhere in the body. The serous cavities are closely linked with lymphatic drainage systems. The milking action of the moving structures, such as the lungs, continually forces fluid and plasma proteins back into the circulation, keeping these cavities empty. Any obstruction to lymph flow causes fluid accumulation in the serous cavities. As with edema fluid, third-space fluids represent an accumulation or trapping of body fluids that contribute to body weight but not to fluid reserve or function.

The prefix *hydro-* may be used to indicate the presence of excessive fluid, as in *hydrothorax*, which means excessive fluid in the pleural cavity. The accumulation of fluid in the peritoneal cavity is called *ascites*. The transudation of fluid into the serous cavities is also referred to as *effusion*. Effusion can contain blood, plasma proteins, inflammatory cells (*i.e.*, pus), and extracellular fluid.

> In summary, body fluids are distributed between the intracellular and extracellular compartments of the body. Two thirds of body fluids are contained in the body cells of the intracellular compartment and one third is contained in the vascular compartment, interstitial spaces, and third space areas of the extracellular compartment. Body fluids contain water, charged particles called *electrolytes*, and noncharged particles called *nonelectrolytes*. Intracellular fluids have higher concentrations of potassium, calcium, phosphates, and magnesium, and extracellular fluids have high concentrations of sodium, chloride, and bicarbonate. Electrolytes and nonelectrolytes move by diffusion across cell membranes that separate the intracellular and extracellular fluid compartments. Water moves by osmosis across semipermeable membranes, moving from the side of the membrane that has the lesser number of particles and greater concentration of water to the side that has the greater number of particles and lesser concentration of water. The osmotic tension or effect that a solution exerts on cell volume in terms of causing the cell to swell or shrink is called *tonicity*.
>
> Intracellular volume is regulated by the large numbers of proteins and other inorganic solutes that cannot cross the cell's membrane and the Na^+/K^+-ATPase membrane pump, which continually removes three sodium ions for every two potassium ions that are moved back into the cell. Extracellular fluid volume, which is distributed between the vascular and interstitial compartments, is regulated by the elimination of sodium and water by the kidney.
>
> Edema represents an increase in interstitial fluid volume. The physiologic mechanisms that predispose to edema formation are increased capillary filtration pressure, decreased capillary colloidal osmotic pressure, increased capillary permeability, and obstruction of lymphatic flow. The effect that edema exerts on body function is determined by its location; cerebral edema can be a life-threatening situation, but swollen feet can be a normal discomfort that accompanies hot weather. Fluid can also accumulate in the transcellular compartment—the joint spaces, pericardial sac, the peritoneal cavity, and the pleural cavity. Because this fluid is not easily exchanged with the rest of the extracellular fluid, it is often referred to as third-space fluid.

Sodium and Water Balance

After you have completed this section of the chapter, you should be able to meet the following objectives:

✦ State the functions and physiologic mechanisms controlling body water levels and sodium concentration

✦ Describe the relationship between body water and the extracellular sodium concentration

✦ Describe measures that can be used in assessing sodium concentration and body fluid levels

✦ Compare and contrast the causes, manifestations, and treatment of isotonic fluid volume deficit, isotonic fluid volume excess, hyponatremia with water excess, and hypernatremia with water deficit

✦ Describe the causes, manifestations, and treatment of psychogenic polydipsia

✦ Compare the pathology, manifestations, and treatment of diabetes insipidus and the syndrome of inappropriate antidiuretic hormone

The movement of body fluids between the intracellular and extracellular compartments occurs at the cell membrane and depends on regulation of extracellular water and sodium. Water provides approximately 90% to 93% of the volume of body fluids and sodium salts approximately 90% to 95% of extracellular solutes. Normally, equivalent changes in sodium and water are such that the volume and osmolality of extracellular fluids are maintained within a normal range. Because it is the concentration of sodium (in milligrams per liter) that controls extracellular fluid osmolality, changes in sodium are usually accompanied by proportionate changes in water volume.

Protection of the circulatory volume can be viewed as the single most important characteristic of body fluid homeostasis. In situations in which multiple physiologic variables are threatened simultaneously, the homeostatic response protects the vascular volume even at the expense of aggravating another electrolyte disorder.[4] For example, a volume-depleted person who is given water but no sodium retains water and becomes hyponatremic as a means of avoiding circulatory collapse. Two mechanisms protect extracellular fluid (and vascular) volume: (1) alterations in hemodynamic variables such as vasoconstriction and an increase in heart rate, and (2) alterations in sodium and water balance. Both mechanisms serve to maintain filling of the vascular compartment. Tachycardia, peripheral arterial vasoconstriction, and venoconstriction occur within minutes of external fluid losses, whereas salt and water retention take hours to become effective.

Alterations of sodium and water balance can be divided into two main categories: (1) isotonic contraction or expansion of extracellular fluid volume, and (2) hypotonic dilution (dilutional hyponatremia) or hypertonic concentration (hypernatremia) of extracellular sodium brought about by changes in extracellular water. Isotonic disorders usually are confined to the extracellular fluid compartment (*i.e.*, extracellular fluid volume deficit or excess), whereas disorders of sodium concentration arise with the addition or removal of fluid from the intracellular compartment (Fig. 31-8).

REGULATION OF SODIUM BALANCE

Sodium is the most abundant cation in the body, averaging approximately 60 mEq/kg of body weight.[5] Most of the body's sodium is in the extracellular fluid compartment (135 to 145 mEq/L), with only a small amount (10 to 14 mEq/L) located in the intracellular compartment. The resting cell membrane is relatively impermeable to sodium. Sodium that enters the cell is transported out of the cell against an electrochemical gradient by the energy-dependent Na^+/K^+-ATPase membrane pump.

Sodium functions mainly in regulating extracellular and vascular volume. As the major cation in the extracellular compartment, Na^+ and its attendant anions (Cl^- and HCO_3^-) account for approximately 90% to 95% of the osmotic activity in the extracellular fluid. Because sodium is part of the sodium bicarbonate molecule, it is important in regulating acid-base balance. As a current-carrying ion, sodium contributes to the function of the nervous system and other excitable tissue.

Gains and Losses

Sodium normally enters the body through the gastrointestinal tract and is eliminated by the kidneys or lost from the gastrointestinal tract or skin. Sodium intake normally is derived from dietary sources. Body needs for sodium usually can be met by as little as 500 mg/day. In the United States, the average salt intake is approximately 6 to 15 g/day, or 12 to 30 times the daily requirement. Dietary intake, which frequently exceeds the amount needed by the body, is often influenced by culture and food preferences rather than need. As package labels indicate, many commercially prepared foods and soft drinks contain considerable amounts of sodium. Other sources of sodium are intravenous saline infusions and medications that contain sodium. An often-forgotten source of sodium is the sodium bicarbonate or other sodium-containing home remedies or over-the-counter medications used to treat upset stomach or other ailments.

Water Balance

➤ Protection of blood volume and filling of the vascular compartment can be viewed as the single most important characteristic of body fluid homeostasis.

➤ Two homeostatic mechanisms protect the vascular volume component of the extracellular fluid compartment: (1) the immediate recruitment of hemodynamic responses such as increased heart rate and vasoconstriction that function to maintain blood flow to vital organs, and (2) more long-term alterations in sodium and water balance that function to restore extracellular fluid volume.

➤ In situations where multiple physiologic functions are threatened simultaneously, homeostatic mechanisms strive to protect the volume of the vascular compartment at the expense of aggravating other electrolyte disorders.

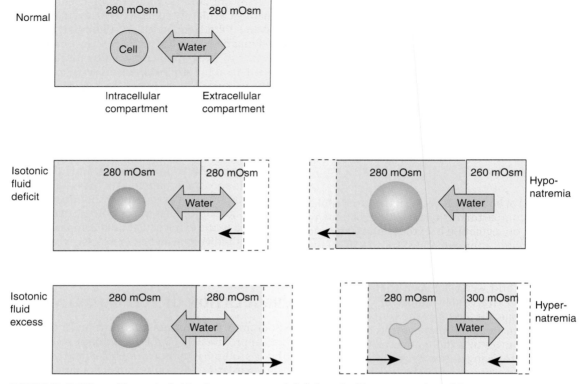

FIGURE 31-8 Effect of isotonic fluid volume excess and deficit and of hyponatremia and hypernatremia on extracellular and intracellular fluid volume.

Most sodium losses occur through the kidney. The kidneys are extremely efficient in regulating sodium output, and when sodium intake is limited or conservation of sodium is needed, the kidneys are able to reabsorb almost all the sodium that has been filtered by the glomerulus.

🔑 Sodium Balance

➤ Water provides about 90% to 93% of the volume of body fluids and sodium salts approximately 90% to 95% of the solutes in the extracellular compartment. Together they serve to regulate the distribution of fluid between the intracellular and extracellular compartments.

➤ All gains or losses of sodium and water occur through the extracellular fluid compartment.

➤ Isotonic changes in body fluids that result from proportionate gains or losses of sodium and water are largely confined to the extracellular compartment.

➤ In contrast, changes in the tonicity of extracellular fluid brought about by disproportionate losses or gains of sodium or water are transmitted to the intracellular compartment, causing water to move in or out of body cells.

This results in an essentially sodium-free urine. Conversely, urinary losses of sodium increase as intake increases.

Usually less than 10% of sodium intake is lost through the gastrointestinal tract and skin. Although the sodium concentration of fluids in the upper part of the gastrointestinal tract approaches that of the extracellular fluid, sodium is reabsorbed as the fluids move through the lower part of the bowel, so that the concentration of sodium in the stool is only approximately 40 mEq/L. Sodium losses increase with conditions such as vomiting, diarrhea, fistula drainage, and gastrointestinal suction that remove sodium from the upper gastrointestinal tract. Irrigation of gastrointestinal tubes with distilled water removes sodium from the gastrointestinal tract, as do repeated tap water enemas.

Excessive amounts of sodium can also be lost through the skin. Sweat losses, which usually are negligible, can increase greatly during exercise and periods of exposure to a hot environment. A person who sweats profusely can lose as much as 15 to 30 g of sodium per day. Fortunately, this amount decreases to as little as 3 to 5 g/day with acclimatization to the heat.[2] Loss of skin integrity, such as occurs in extensive burns, also leads to excessive skin losses of sodium.

Mechanisms of Regulation

The kidney is the main regulator of sodium. The kidney monitors arterial pressure and retains sodium when arterial pressure is decreased and eliminates it when arterial pressure is increased. The rate at which the kidney excretes or conserves sodium is coordinated by the sympathetic nervous system and the renin-angiotensin-aldosterone mechanism. Another possible regulator of sodium excretion by the kidney is atrial natriuretic peptide (ANP), which is released from cells in the atria of the heart. ANP, which is released in response to atrial stretch and overfilling, increases sodium excretion by the kidney (see Chapter 30). Although ANP acts at several sites in the kidney to increase sodium excretion, its role in regulating sodium balance remains uncertain.[3]

The Sympathetic Nervous System. The sympathetic nervous system responds to changes in arterial pressure and blood volume by adjusting the glomerular filtration rate and thus the rate at which sodium is filtered from the blood. Sympathetic activity also regulates tubular reabsorption of sodium and renin release.

The Renin-Angiotensin-Aldosterone Mechanism. The renin-angiotensin-aldosterone system exerts its action through angiotensin II and aldosterone (see Chapter 21). Renin is a small protein enzyme that is released by the kidney in response to changes in arterial pressure, the glomerular filtration rate, and the amount of sodium in the tubular fluid. Most of the renin that is released leaves the kidney and enters the bloodstream, where it interacts enzymatically to convert a circulating plasma protein called *angiotensinogen* to angiotensin I. Angiotensin I is rapidly converted to angiotensin II by the angiotensin-converting enzyme in the small blood vessels of the lung. Angiotensin II acts directly on the renal tubules to increase sodium reabsorption. It also acts to constrict renal blood vessels, thereby decreasing the glomerular filtration rate and slowing renal blood flow so that less sodium is filtered and more is reabsorbed. Angiotensin II is also a powerful regulator of aldosterone, a hormone secreted by the adrenal cortex. Aldosterone acts at the level of the cortical collecting tubules of the kidneys to increase sodium reabsorption while increasing potassium elimination (see Chapter 30).

The sodium-retaining action of aldosterone can be inhibited by blocking the actions of aldosterone with potassium-sparing diuretics (*e.g.*, spironolactone, amiloride, and triamterene), by suppressing renin release (*e.g.*, β-adrenergic blocking drugs), or by inhibiting the conversion of angiotensin I to angiotensin II (*e.g.*, angiotensin-converting enzyme inhibitors).

REGULATION OF WATER BALANCE

Total body water (TBW) varies with sex and weight. These differences can be explained by differences in body fat, which is essentially water free. In men, body water approximates 60% of body weight during young adulthood and decreases to approximately 50% in old age; in young women it is approximately 50% and in elderly women approximately 40%.[6] Obesity produces further decreases in body water, sometimes reducing these levels to values as low as 30% to 40% of body weight in adults (Fig. 31-9).

Infants have a high water content. TBW constitutes approximately 75% to 80% of body weight in full-term infants and is even greater in premature infants. In addition to having proportionately more body water than adults have, infants have relatively more water in their extracellular compartment. Infants have more than half of their TBW in

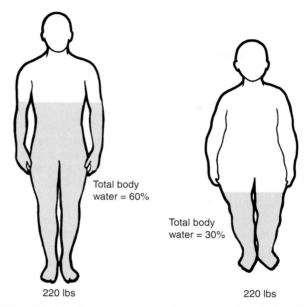

FIGURE 31-9 Body composition of a lean and an obese individual. (Adapted with permission from Statland H. [1963]. *Fluids and electrolytes in practice.* [3rd ed.]. Philadelphia: J.B. Lippincott)

Total body water = 60%

Total body water = 30%

220 lbs   220 lbs

the extracellular compartment, whereas adults have only approximately a third.[7] The greater extracellular water content of an infant can be explained in terms of its higher metabolic rate, larger surface area in relation to its body mass, and its inability to concentrate its urine because of immature kidney structures. Because extracellular fluids are more readily lost from the body, infants are more vulnerable to fluid deficit than are older children and adults. As an infant grows older, TBW decreases, and by the second year of life, the percentages and distribution of body water approach those of an adult.[7]

Gains and Losses

Regardless of age, all healthy persons require approximately 100 mL of water per 100 calories metabolized for dissolving and eliminating metabolic wastes. This means that a person who expends 1800 calories for energy requires approximately 1800 mL of water for metabolic purposes. The metabolic rate increases with fever; it rises approximately 12% for every 1°C (7% for every 1°F) increase in body temperature.[2] Fever also increases the respiratory rate, resulting in additional loss of water vapor through the lungs.

The main source of water gain is through oral intake and metabolism of nutrients. Water, including that obtained from liquids and solid foods, is absorbed from the gastrointestinal tract. Tube feedings and parenterally administered fluids are also a source of water gain. Metabolic processes also generate a small amount of water. The amount of water gained from these processes varies from 150 to 300 mL/day, depending on metabolic rate.

Normally, the largest loss of water occurs through the kidneys, with lesser amounts being lost through the skin, lungs, and gastrointestinal tract. Even when oral or parenteral fluids are withheld, the kidneys continue to produce urine as a means of ridding the body of metabolic wastes. The urine output that is required to eliminate these wastes is called the *obligatory urine output*. The obligatory urine loss is approximately 300 to 500 mL/day. Water losses that occur through the skin and lungs are referred to as *insensible water losses* because they occur without a person's awareness. The gains and losses of body water are summarized in Table 31-2.

Mechanisms of Regulation

There are two main physiologic mechanisms that assist in regulating body water: thirst and antidiuretic hormone (ADH). Thirst is primarily a regulator of water intake and ADH a regulator of water output. Both mechanisms respond to changes in extracellular osmolality and volume (Fig. 31-10).

Thirst.   Like appetite and eating, thirst and drinking behavior are two separate entities.[8] Thirst is a conscious sensation of the need to obtain and drink fluids high in water content. Drinking of water or other fluids often occurs as the result of habit or for reasons other than those related to thirst. Most persons drink without being thirsty, and water is consumed before it is needed. As a result, thirst is basically an emergency response. It usually occurs only when the need for water has not been anticipated.

Thirst is controlled by the thirst center in the hypothalamus. There are two stimuli for true thirst based on water need: cellular dehydration caused by an increase in extracellular osmolality, and a decrease in blood volume, which may or may not be associated with a decrease in serum osmolality. Sensory neurons, called *osmoreceptors*, which are located in or near the thirst center in the hypothalamus, respond to changes in extracellular osmolality by swelling or shrinking (Fig. 31-11). Thirst normally develops when there is as little as a 1% to 2% change in serum osmolality.[9] Blood pressure and blood volume are sensed by stretch receptors that are sensitive to changes in blood pressure (high-pressure baroreceptors located in the carotid sinus and aorta) and central blood volume (low-pressure baroreceptors located in the left atrium and major thoracic veins). Thirst is one of the earliest symptoms of hemorrhage and is often present before other signs of blood loss appear.

Dryness of the mouth, such as the thirst a lecturer experiences during speaking, produces a sensation of thirst that is not necessarily associated with the body's hydration status. Thirst sensation also occurs in those who breathe

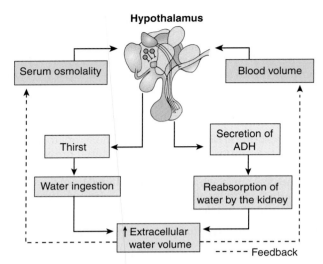

FIGURE 31-10 Pathways for regulation of extracellular water volume by thirst and antidiuretic hormone.

through their mouths, such as smokers and persons with chronic respiratory disease or hyperventilation syndrome.

The renin-angiotensin mechanism contributes to nonosmotic thirst. This system is considered a backup system for thirst should other systems fail. Because it is a backup system, it probably does not contribute to the regulation of

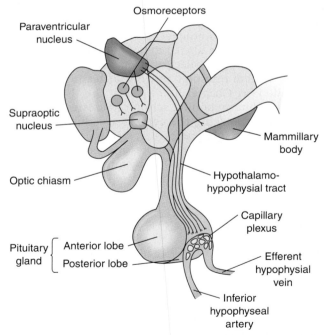

FIGURE 31-11 Sagittal section through the pituitary and anterior hypothalamus. Antidiuretic hormone (ADH) is formed primarily in the supraoptic nucleus and to a lesser extent in the paraventricular nucleus of the hypothalamus. It is then transported down the hypothalamohypophysial tract and stored in secretory granules in the posterior pituitary, where it can be released into the blood. (Adapted from Rhoades R.A., Tanner G.A. [1996]. *Medical physiology* [p. 449]. Boston: Little, Brown)

TABLE 31-2 ✦ Sources of Body Water Gains and Losses in the Adult			
Gains		**Losses**	
Oral intake		Urine	1500 mL
As water	1000 mL	Insensible losses	
In food	1300 mL	Lungs	300 mL
Water of	200 mL	Skin	500 mL
oxidation		Feces	200 mL
Total	**2500 mL**	**Total**	**2500 mL**

normal thirst. However, elevated levels of angiotensin II may lead to thirst in conditions such as chronic renal failure and congestive heart failure, in which renin levels may be elevated. Thirst and elevated renin levels are also found in persons with primary hyperaldosteronism and in those with secondary hyperaldosteronism accompanying anorexia nervosa, hemorrhage, and sodium depletion.

Hypodipsia. Hypodipsia represents a decrease in the ability to sense thirst. There is evidence that thirst is decreased and water intake reduced in elderly persons, despite higher serum sodium and osmolality levels.[10–12] The inability to perceive and respond to thirst is compounded in elderly persons who have had a stroke and may be further influenced by confusion and sensory disturbances.

Polydipsia. Polydipsia, or excessive thirst, is normal when it accompanies conditions of water deficit. Increased thirst and drinking behavior can be classified into three categories: symptomatic or true thirst, inappropriate or false thirst that occurs despite normal levels of body water and serum osmolality, and compulsive water drinking. Symptomatic thirst develops when there is a loss of body water and resolves after the loss has been replaced. Among the most common causes of symptomatic thirst are water losses associated with diarrhea, vomiting, diabetes mellitus, and diabetes insipidus. Inappropriate or excessive thirst may persist despite adequate hydration. It is a common complaint in persons with renal failure and congestive heart failure. Although the cause of thirst in these persons is unclear, it may result from increased angiotensin levels. Thirst is also a common complaint in persons with dry mouth caused by decreased salivary function or treatment with drugs with an anticholinergic action (*e.g.*, antihistamines, atropine) that lead to decreased salivary flow.

Psychogenic polydipsia involves compulsive water drinking and is usually seen in persons with psychiatric disorders, most commonly schizophrenia. Persons with the disorder drink large amounts of water and excrete large amounts of urine. The cause of excessive water drinking in these persons is uncertain. It has been suggested that the compulsive water drinking may share the same pathology as the psychosis because persons with the disorder often increase their water drinking during periods of exacerbation of their psychotic symptoms.[13] The condition may be compounded by antipsychotic medications that increase ADH levels and interfere with water excretion by the kidneys. Cigarette smoking, which is common among persons with psychiatric disorders, also stimulates ADH secretion.

Excessive water ingestion coupled with impaired water excretion (or rapid ingestion at a rate that exceeds renal excretion) in persons with psychogenic polydipsia can lead to water intoxication (see Hyponatremia).

Treatment usually consists of water restriction and behavioral measures aimed at decreasing water consumption. Measurements of body weight can be used to provide an estimate of water consumption.[14]

Antidiuretic Hormone. The reabsorption of water by the kidneys is regulated by ADH, also known as *vasopressin*. ADH is synthesized by cells in the supraoptic and paraventricular nuclei of the hypothalamus (see Fig. 31-11). ADH from neurons in the supraoptic and paraventricular nuclei is transported along a neural pathway (*i.e.*, hypothalamohypophysial tract) to the neurohypophysis (*i.e.*, posterior pituitary) and then stored for future release

ADH exerts its effects through two types of vasopressin (V) receptors—V_1 and V_2 receptors. The V_2 receptors, located on the tubular cells of the cortical collecting duct, control water reabsorption by the kidney (see Chapter 30). Binding of ADH to the V_2 receptors increases water reabsorption by increasing the permeability of the collecting duct to water (*i.e.*, the antidiuretic effect). In the absence of ADH, the permeability of the collecting duct to water is very low, and reabsorption of water decreases, leading to polyuria. V_1 receptors, which are located in vascular smooth muscle, cause vasoconstriction—hence the name *vasopressin*. Although ADH can increase blood pressure through V_1 receptors, this response occurs only when ADH levels are very high.

As with thirst, ADH levels are controlled by extracellular volume and osmolality. Osmoreceptors in the hypothalamus sense changes in extracellular osmolality and stimulate the production and release of ADH. A small increase in serum osmolality of 1% is sufficient to cause ADH release.[15] Likewise, stretch receptors that are sensitive to changes in blood pressure and central blood volume aid in the regulation of ADH release. A blood volume decrease of 5% to 10% produces a maximal increase in ADH levels.[15] As with many other homeostatic mechanisms, acute conditions produce greater changes in ADH levels than do chronic conditions; long-term changes in blood volume or blood pressure may exist without affecting ADH levels.

The effect of changes in glucose concentration on ADH secretion depends on the presence or absence of insulin. In nondiabetic persons, insulin facilitates glucose entry into the osmoreceptors, rendering it an ineffective osmole. In contrast, glucose stimulates ADH secretion in persons with diabetes, presumably because insulin is required for glucose uptake by the osmoreceptors.[5]

Responsiveness to ADH increases with age, with older persons being more responsive to changes in serum osmolality.[6] Osmoregulation is also altered in normal pregnancy and the menstrual cycle. Serum sodium concentration normally falls by an average of 5 mEq/L and serum osmolality by 10 mOsm/kg within 5 to 8 weeks of conception, and then remains stable for the duration of pregnancy.[5] This change represents a resetting of the osmotic threshold for ADH and an increase in the extracellular fluid volume that accompanies pregnancy. A decrease in plasma osmolality of 2 to 3 mOsm/kg occurs during the ovulatory luteal phase of the menstrual cycle in healthy young women.[5]

The abnormal synthesis and release of ADH occurs in a number of stress situations. Severe pain, nausea, trauma, surgery, certain anesthetic agents, and some analgesic drugs increase ADH levels. Nausea is a potent stimulus of ADH secretion; it can increase ADH levels 10 to 1000 times those required for maximal diuresis.[16] The stimulus is mediated by the chemoreceptor trigger zone in the medulla oblongata, which then relays the impulse to the supraoptic and paraventricular nuclei in the hypothalamus. Afferent input from the gastrointestinal tract also may be important in some circumstances. Among the drugs that affect ADH are nicotine, which stimulates its release, and alcohol, which inhibits it (Table 31-3). Two important conditions alter ADH levels: diabetes insipidus and inappropriate secretion of ADH.

Diabetes Insipidus. Diabetes insipidus, which means "tasteless diabetes," as opposed to diabetes mellitus, or "sweet diabetes," is caused by a deficiency of or a decreased response to ADH. Diabetes insipidus is characterized by excessive urination of a dilute urine (polyuria) and polydipsia.

There are two types of diabetes insipidus: central or neurogenic diabetes insipidus, which occurs because of a defect in the synthesis or release of ADH, and nephrogenic diabetes insipidus, which occurs because the kidneys do not respond to ADH.[17–20] In neurogenic diabetes insipidus, loss of 75% to 80% of ADH-secretory neurons is necessary before polyuria becomes evident. Most persons with neurogenic diabetes insipidus have an incomplete form of the disorder and retain some ability to concentrate their urine. Temporary neurogenic diabetes insipidus may follow head injury or surgery near the hypothalamohypophysial tract. Nephrogenic diabetes insipidus is characterized by impairment of urine-concentrating ability and free-water conservation. It may occur as a genetic trait that affects the V_2 receptor that binds ADH or the protein that forms the water channels in the collecting tubules. Other acquired causes of nephrogenic diabetes insipidus are drugs such as lithium[21] and electrolyte disorders such as potassium depletion or chronic hypercalcemia. Lithium and the electrolyte disorders are thought to interfere with the postreceptor actions of ADH on the permeability of the collecting ducts.

Persons with diabetes insipidus are unable to concentrate their urine during periods of water restriction; they excrete large volumes of urine, usually 3 to 20 L/day, depending on the degree of ADH deficiency or renal insensitivity to ADH. This large urine output is accompanied by excessive thirst. As long as the thirst mechanism is normal and fluid is readily available, there is little or no alteration in the fluid levels in persons with diabetes insipidus. The danger arises when the condition develops in someone who is unable to communicate the need for water or is unable to secure the needed water. In such cases, inadequate fluid intake rapidly leads to hypertonic dehydration and increased serum osmolality.

Diagnosis of diabetes insipidus is based on measurement of ADH levels along with plasma and urine osmolality before and after a period of fluid deprivation or hypertonic saline infusion. Persons with neurogenic diabetes insipidus do not increase their ADH levels in response to increased plasma osmolality. Another diagnostic approach is to conduct a carefully monitored trial of a pharmacologic form of ADH. Persons with nephrogenic diabetes insipidus do not respond to pharmacologic preparations of the hormone. When central diabetes insipidus is suspected, diagnostic methods such as skull x-ray studies and magnetic resonance imaging (MRI) of the pituitary-hypothalamic area are used to determine the cause of the disorder.

The management of central diabetes insipidus depends on the cause and severity of the disorder. Many persons with incomplete neurogenic diabetes insipidus maintain near-normal water balance when permitted to ingest water in response to thirst. Pharmacologic preparations of ADH are available for persons who cannot be managed by conservative measures. The preferred drug for treating chronic diabetes insipidus is desmopressin acetate (DDAVP). It usually is given nasally, but is available in parenteral and oral forms. The oral antidiabetic agent chlorpropamide may be used to stimulate ADH release in neurogenic diabetes insipidus. It usually is reserved for special cases because of its ability to cause hypoglycemia. Both neurogenic and nephrogenic forms of the disorder respond partially to the thiazide diuretics (*e.g.*, hydrochlorothiazide). These diuretics are thought to act by increasing sodium excretion by the kidneys, which lowers the glomerular filtration rate and increases reabsorption of water in the proximal tubule.

Syndrome of Inappropriate Antidiuretic Hormone. The syndrome of inappropriate ADH (SIADH) results from a failure of the negative feedback system that regulates the release and inhibition of ADH.[22] In persons with this syndrome, ADH secretion continues even when serum osmolality is decreased; this causes marked retention of water in excess of sodium and dilutional hyponatremia (see Hyponatremia). An increase in the glomerular filtration rate resulting from an increased plasma volume causes further increases in sodium loss by suppressing the renin-angiotensin mechanism. Urine osmolality is high and serum osmolality is low. Urine output decreases despite adequate or increased fluid intake. Hematocrit and the serum sodium and BUN levels are all decreased because of the expansion of the extracellular fluid volume.

TABLE 31-3 ✦ Drugs That Affect Antidiuretic Hormone Levels*	
Drugs That Decrease ADH Levels/Action	**Drugs That Increase ADH Levels/Action**
Amphotericin B	Anticancer drugs (vincristine and cyclophosphamide)
Demeclocycline	Carbamazepine
Ethanol	Chlorpropamide
Foscarnet	Clofibrate
Lithium	General anesthetics (most)
Morphine antagonists	Narcotics (morphine and meperidine)
	Nicotine
	Nonsteroidal anti-inflammatory drugs
	Phenothiazine antipsychotic drugs
	Selective serotonin reuptake inhibitors
	Thiazide diuretics (chlorothiazide)
	Thiothixene (antipsychotic drug)
	Tricyclic antidepressants

ADH, antidiuretic hormone
* List not inclusive.

SIADH can be caused by a number of conditions, including lung tumors, chest lesions, and central nervous system (CNS) disorders, and by various pharmacologic agents. Tumors, particularly bronchogenic carcinomas and cancers of the lymphoid tissue, prostate, and pancreas, are known to produce and release ADH independent of normal hypothalamic control mechanisms. Other intrathoracic conditions, such as advanced tuberculosis, severe pneumonia, and positive-pressure breathing, also cause SIADH. The suggested mechanism for SIADH in positive-pressure ventilation is activation of baroreceptors (*e.g.*, aortic baroreceptors, cardiopulmonary receptors) that respond to marked changes in intrathoracic pressure. Disease and injury to the CNS can cause direct pressure on or direct involvement of the hypothalamic–posterior pituitary structures. Examples include brain tumors, hydrocephalus, head injury, meningitis, and encephalitis. Other stimuli, such as surgery, pain, stress, and temperature changes, are capable of stimulating ADH release through the limbic system. Human immunodeficiency virus infection is emerging as a new cause of SIADH. It has been reported that up to 35% of persons with acquired immunodeficiency syndrome who are admitted to the acute care setting have SIADH related to *Pneumocystis carinii* pneumonia, CNS infections, or malignancies.[23]

Drugs induce SIADH in different ways; some drugs are thought to increase hypothalamic production and release, and others are believed to act directly on the renal tubules to enhance the action of ADH.

SIADH may occur as a transient condition, as in a stress situation, or as a chronic condition, resulting from disorders such as lung tumors. The manifestations of SIADH are those of dilutional hyponatremia. The severity of symptoms usually is proportional to the extent of sodium depletion and water intoxication.

The treatment of SIADH depends on its severity. In mild cases, treatment consists of fluid restriction. If fluid restriction is not sufficient, diuretics such as mannitol and furosemide (Lasix) may be given to promote diuresis and free-water clearance. Lithium and the antibiotic demeclocycline inhibit the action of ADH on the renal collecting ducts and sometimes are used in treating the disorder. In cases of severe water intoxication, a hypertonic (*e.g.*, 3%) sodium chloride solution may be administered intravenously.

ALTERATIONS IN FLUID VOLUME

Alterations in fluid volume represent an isotonic contraction or expansion of extracellular fluids. The kidneys regulate the volume and solute concentration of extracellular fluid, promoting diuresis in conditions of fluid excess and conserving water when extracellular fluid volume is decreased. As a rule of thumb, water follows sodium reabsorption; conditions that increase sodium loss or gain produce proportionate losses or gains in water.

Fluid Volume Deficit

Fluid volume deficit is characterized by a decrease in extracellular fluid, including circulating blood volume. The term *isotonic fluid volume deficit* is used to differentiate the type of fluid deficit in which there are proportionate losses in sodium and water from water deficit and the hyperosmolar state associated with hypernatremia. Unless other fluid and electrolyte imbalances are present, the concentration of serum electrolytes remains essentially unchanged.

Causes. Isotonic fluid volume deficit can result from impaired intake or excessive losses of body fluids (Table 31-4). Fluid intake may be reduced because of a lack of access to fluids, impaired thirst, unconsciousness, oral trauma, impaired swallowing, or neuromuscular problems that prevent fluid access. Although access to fluids is taken for granted, for someone with impaired mobility, fluid availability may become a problem. Fluid volume deficit can also result from loss of gastrointestinal fluids, polyuria, sweating due to fever and exercise, and third-space losses. When the effective circulating blood volume is compromised, the condition is often referred to as *hypovolemia*.

In a single day, 8 to 10 L of extracellular fluid is secreted into the gastrointestinal tract. Most of it is reabsorbed in the ileum and proximal colon, and only approximately 150 to 200 mL/day is eliminated in the feces. Vomiting and diarrhea interrupt the reabsorption process and, in some situations, lead to increased secretion of fluid into the intestinal tract. In Asiatic cholera, death can occur within a matter of hours as the cholera organism causes excessive amounts of fluid to be secreted into the bowel. These fluids are then lost as vomitus or excreted as diarrheal fluid. Gastrointestinal suction, fistulas, and drainage tubes can remove large amounts of fluid from the gastrointestinal tract.

Excess sodium and water losses also can occur through the kidney. Certain forms of kidney disease are characterized by salt wasting due to impaired sodium reabsorption. Fluid volume deficit also can result from osmotic diuresis or injudicious use of diuretic therapy. Glucose in the urine filtrate prevents reabsorption of water by the renal tubules, causing a loss of sodium and water. In Addison's disease, a condition of chronic adrenocortical insufficiency, there is unregulated loss of sodium in the urine with a resultant loss of extracellular fluid (see Chapter 40). This is accompanied by increased potassium retention. The loss of extracellular fluid and low blood volume can lead to circulatory collapse.

The skin acts as an exchange surface for heat and as a vapor barrier to prevent water from leaving the body. Body surface losses of sodium and water increase when there is excessive sweating or when large areas of skin have been damaged. Hot weather and fever increase sweating. In hot weather, water losses through sweating may be increased by as much as 1 to 3 L/hour, depending on acclimatization.[2] The respiratory rate and sweating usually are increased as body temperature rises. As much as 3 L of water may be lost in a single day as a result of fever. Burns are another cause of excess fluid loss. Evaporative losses can increase 10-fold with severe burns, to 3 to 5 L/day.[2]

Third-space losses cause sequestering of extracellular fluids in the serous cavities, extracellular spaces in injured tissues, or lumen of the gut. Because the fluid remains in the body, fluid volume deficit caused by third spacing does not usually cause weight loss.

TABLE 31-4 ✦ Causes and Manifestations of Fluid Volume Deficit

Causes	Manifestations
Inadequate Fluid Intake	**Acute Weight Loss**
Oral trauma or inability to swallow	Mild fluid volume deficit: 2%
Inability to obtain fluids (*e.g.*, impaired mobility)	Moderate fluid volume deficit: 2%–5%
Impaired thirst mechanism	Severe fluid deficit: 8% or greater
Therapeutic withholding of fluids	
Unconsciousness or inability to express thirst	**Compensatory Increase in Antidiuretic Hormone**
	Decreased urine output
Excessive Gastrointestinal Fluid Losses	Increased osmolality and specific gravity
Vomiting	
Diarrhea	**Increased Serum Osmolality**
Gastrointestinal suction	Thirst
Draining gastrointestinal fistula	Increased hematocrit and blood urea nitrogen
Excessive Renal Losses	
Diuretic therapy	**Decreased Vascular Volume**
Osmotic diuresis (hyperglycemia)	Postural hypotension
Adrenal insufficiency (Addison's disease)	Tachycardia, weak and thready pulse
Salt-wasting kidney disease	Decreased vein filling and increased vein refill time
	Hypotension and shock
Excessive Skin Losses	
Fever	**Decreased Extracellular Fluid Volume**
Exposure to hot environment	Depressed fontanel in an infant
Burns and wounds that remove skin	Sunken eyes and soft eyeballs
Third-Space Losses	**Impaired Temperature Regulation**
Intestinal obstruction	Elevated body temperature
Edema	
Ascites	
Burns (first several days)	

Manifestations. The manifestations of fluid volume deficit reflect a decrease in extracellular fluid volume. They include thirst, loss of body weight, signs of water conservation by the kidney, impaired temperature regulation, and signs of reduced interstitial and vascular volume (see Table 31-4).

A loss in fluid volume is accompanied by a decrease in body weight. One liter of water weighs 1 kg (2.2 lb). A mild extracellular fluid deficit exists when weight loss equals 2% of body weight. In a person who weighs 68 kg (150 lb), this percentage of weight loss equals 1.4 L of water. A moderate deficit equates to a 5% loss in weight and a severe deficit to an 8% or greater loss in weight.[7] To be accurate, weight must be measured at the same time each day with the person wearing the same amount of clothing. Because extracellular fluid is trapped in the body in persons with third-space losses, their body weight may not decrease.

Thirst is a common symptom of fluid deficit, although it is not always present in early stages of isotonic fluid deficit. It develops as the effective circulating volume decreases to a point sufficient to stimulate the thirst mechanism. Urine output decreases and urine osmolality and specific gravity increase as ADH levels rise because of a decrease in vascular volume. Although there is an isotonic loss of fluid from the vascular compartment, blood components such as red blood cells and urea become more concentrated.

The fluid content of body tissues decreases as fluid is removed from the interstitial spaces. The eyes assume a sunken appearance and feel softer than normal as the fluid content in the anterior chamber of the eye is decreased. Fluids add resiliency to the skin and underlying tissues that is referred to as *skin* or *tissue turgor*. Tissue turgor is assessed by pinching a fold of skin between the thumb and forefinger. The skin should immediately return to its original configuration when the fingers are released. A loss of 3% to 5% of body water in children causes the resiliency of the skin to be lost, and the tissue remains raised for several seconds. Decreased tissue turgor is less predictive of fluid deficit in older persons (>65 years) because of the loss of tissue elasticity. In infants, fluid deficit may be evidenced by depression of the anterior fontanel due to a decrease in cerebrospinal fluid. There may be a rise in body temperature that accompanies fluid volume deficit. Interstitial fluids insulate the body against changes in the external temperature and vascular fluids transport heat from the inner core of the body to the periphery, where it can be released into the external environment.

Arterial and venous volumes decline during periods of fluid deficit, as does filling of the capillary circulation. As the volume in the arterial system declines, the blood pressure decreases and heart rate increases, and the pulse becomes weak and thready. Postural hypotension is an early sign of fluid deficit, characterized by a blood pressure that is at least 10 mm Hg lower when the patient is sitting or standing than when the patient is lying down. When volume depletion becomes severe, signs of hypovolemic shock and vascular collapse appear (see Chapter 26). On the venous side of the circulation, the veins become less prominent, and venous refill time increases.

Diagnosis and Treatment. Diagnosis of fluid volume deficit is based on a history of conditions that predispose to sodium and water losses, weight loss, and observations of altered physiologic function indicative of decreased fluid volume. Intake and output measurements afford a means for assessing fluid balance. Although these measurements provide insight into the causes of fluid imbalance, they often are inadequate in measuring actual losses and gains, because accurate measurements of intake and output often are difficult to obtain and insensible losses are difficult to estimate.

Measurement of heart rate and blood pressure provides useful information about vascular volume. A simple test to determine venous refill time consists of compressing the distal end of a vein on the dorsal aspect of the hand when it is not in the dependent position. The vein is then emptied by "milking" the blood toward the heart. The vein should refill almost immediately when the occluding finger is removed. When venous volume is decreased, as occurs in fluid deficit, venous refill time increases. Capillary refill time is

also increased. Capillary refill can be assessed by applying pressure to a fingernail for 5 seconds and then releasing the pressure and observing the time (normally 1 to 2 seconds) that it takes for the color to return to normal.[7]

Treatment of fluid volume deficit consists of fluid replacement and measures to correct the underlying cause. Usually, isotonic electrolyte solutions are used for fluid replacement. Acute hypovolemia and hypovolemic shock can cause renal damage; therefore, prompt assessment of the degree of fluid deficit and adequate measures to resolve the deficit and treat the underlying cause are essential (see Chapter 26).

Fluid Volume Excess

Fluid volume excess represents an isotonic expansion of the extracellular fluid compartment. It occurs secondary to an increase in total body sodium, which in turn leads to an increase in body water. Fluid volume excess involves an increase in interstitial and vascular volumes. Although increased fluid volume is usually the result of a disease condition, this is not always true. For example, a compensatory isotonic expansion of body fluids can occur in healthy persons during hot weather as a mechanism for increasing body heat loss.

Causes. Although fluid volume excess can occur as the result of increased sodium intake, it is most commonly caused by a decrease in sodium and water elimination by the kidney. Among the causes of decreased sodium and water elimination are decreased renal function, heart failure, liver failure, and corticosteroid excess (Table 31-5).

TABLE 31-5 ◆ Causes and Manifestations of Fluid Volume Excess

Causes	Manifestations
Inadequate Sodium and Water Elimination	**Acute Weight Gain**
Congestive heart failure	Mild fluid volume excess: 2%
Renal failure	Moderate fluid volume excess: 5%
Increased corticosteroid levels	Severe fluid volume excess: 8% or greater
Hyperaldosteronism	
Cushing's disease	**Increased Interstitial Fluid Volume**
Liver failure (*e.g.*, cirrhosis)	Dependent and generalized edema
Excessive Sodium Intake in Relation to Output	**Increased Vascular Volume**
Excessive dietary intake	Full and bounding pulse
Excessive ingestion of sodium-containing	Venous distention
medications or home remedies	Pulmonary edema
Excessive administration of sodium-containing	Shortness of breath
parenteral fluids	Crackles
Excessive Fluid Intake in Relation to Output	Dyspnea
Ingestion of fluid in excess of elimination	Cough
Administration of parenteral fluids or blood at	
an excessive rate	

Heart failure produces a decrease in renal blood flow and a compensatory increase in sodium and water retention (see Chapter 26). Persons with severe congestive heart failure maintain a precarious balance between sodium and water intake and output. Even small increases in sodium intake can precipitate a state of fluid volume excess and a worsening of heart failure. A condition called *circulatory overload* results from an increase in intravascular blood volume; it can occur during infusion of intravenous fluids or transfusion of blood if the amount or rate of administration is excessive. Elderly persons and those with heart disease require careful observation because even small amounts of intravenous fluid or blood may overload the circulatory system. Liver failure (*e.g.*, cirrhosis of the liver) impairs aldosterone metabolism and alters renal perfusion, leading to increased salt and water retention.

Cushing's syndrome is a condition of glucocorticoid excess (see Chapter 40). Because cortisol, the most active of the glucocorticoids, has weak mineralocorticoid activity, Cushing's syndrome predisposes to increased sodium retention. The fact that cortisol increases salt and water retention also helps to explain why edema and hypertension may develop in persons who are being treated with corticosteroid drugs.

Manifestations. Isotonic fluid volume excess is manifested by an increase in interstitial and vascular fluids. It is characterized by weight gain over a short period of time. A mild fluid volume excess represents a 2% gain in weight; moderate fluid volume excess, a 5% gain in weight; and severe fluid volume excess, a gain of 8% or more in weight[7] (see Table 31-5). Edema is characteristic of isotonic fluid excess. When the fluid excess accumulates gradually, as often happens in debilitating diseases and starvation, edema fluid may mask the loss of tissue mass. The edema associated with extracellular fluid excess may be generalized or it may be confined to dependent areas of the body, such as the legs and feet. The eyelids often are puffy when the person awakens. There may be a decrease in BUN and hematocrit as a result of dilution due to expansion of the plasma volume. An increase in vascular volume may be evidenced by distended neck veins, slow-emptying peripheral veins, a full and bounding pulse, and an increase in central venous pressure. When excess fluid accumulates in the lungs (*i.e.*, pulmonary edema), there are complaints of shortness of breath and difficult breathing, respiratory crackles, and a productive cough (see Chapter 26).

Diagnosis and Treatment. Diagnosis of fluid volume excess is usually based on a history of factors that predispose to sodium and water retention, weight gain, and manifestations such as edema and cardiovascular symptoms indicative of an expanded extracellular fluid volume.

The treatment of fluid volume excess focuses on providing a more favorable balance between sodium and water intake and output. A sodium-restricted diet is often prescribed as a means of decreasing extracellular sodium and water levels. Diuretic therapy is commonly used to increase sodium elimination. When there is need for intravenous fluid administration or transfusion of blood components, the procedure requires careful monitoring to prevent fluid overload.

ALTERATIONS IN SODIUM CONCENTRATION

The normal serum concentration of sodium ranges from 135 to 145 mEq/L (135 to 145 mmol/L). Serum sodium values reflect the sodium concentration (or dilution of sodium by extracellular water) expressed in milliequivalents or millimoles per liter, rather than an absolute amount. Sodium dilution occurs when excess water is added to extracellular fluid, reducing its sodium concentration. This can occur because of water retention or because of redistribution of intracellular water to the extracellular fluid. Dehydration increases sodium concentration by decreasing its dilution. This occurs when water is lost from the extracellular compartment in excess of sodium. Because sodium and its attendant anions account for 90% to 95% of the osmolality of extracellular fluids, serum osmolality (normal range, 275 to 295 mOsm/kg) usually changes with changes in serum sodium concentration.

Hyponatremia

Hyponatremia represents a decrease in serum sodium concentration below 135 mEq/L (135 mmol/L). Unlike hypernatremia, which is always associated with hypertonicity, hyponatremia may be associated with high, normal, or low tonicity.[23–27]

Hypertonic (translocational) hyponatremia results from a shift of water from cells to the extracellular fluid that is driven by solutes confined to the extracellular fluids, such as occurs with hyperglycemia. Because sodium is largely an extracellular cation, it becomes diluted as water moves out of cells in response to the osmotic effects of the elevated blood glucose level. There is approximately a 1.7 mEq/L decrease in serum sodium for every 100 mg/dL rise in serum glucose above the normal level (100 mg/dL).[25] A normotonic hyponatremia, termed *pseudohyponatremia*, can be detected in serum samples from persons with hyperlipidemia and hyperproteinemia because of laboratory methods. This disturbance is caused by laboratory methods that include excess lipids or proteins in the water volume of the sample, causing an artifactual dilution of sodium. The increased availability of direct measurement of serum sodium by ion-specific electrodes has helped to eliminate this laboratory artifact. Hypotonic (dilutional) hyponatremia, which is caused by water retention and is characterized by a serum osmolality of less than 280 mOsm/kg, is by far the most common form of hyponatremia.

Dilutional hyponatremia can present as a hypervolemic, euvolemic, or hypovolemic condition. Hypervolemic hyponatremia involves an increase in extracellular fluid volume and is seen when hyponatremic conditions are accompanied by edema-forming disorders such as congestive heart failure, cirrhosis, and advanced kidney disease. Euvolemic hyponatremia represents a retention of water with dilution of sodium while extracellular volume is maintained within a normal range. It usually is the result of inappropriate thirst or SIADH. Hypovolemic hyponatremia occurs when water is lost along with sodium, but to a lesser extent. It occurs with diuretic use, excessive sweating in hot weather, and vomiting and diarrhea.

Causes. Dilutional, or hypotonic, hyponatremia represents a decreased sodium concentration and tonicity of the extracellular fluids (Table 31-6). The most common causes of acute dilutional hyponatremia in adults are diuretic therapy, inappropriate fluid replacement during heat exposure or after heavy exercise, the postoperative state, SIADH, and polydipsia in persons with psychotic disorders. Gastrointestinal fluid loss and ingestion of excessively diluted formula are common causes of acute hyponatremia in infants and children. Adrenal insufficiency is characterized by reduced levels of aldosterone and a resultant decrease in sodium reabsorption by the kidney.

Diuretic-induced hyponatremia is primarily a complication of thiazide diuretics. These agents block the reabsorption of sodium in the cortical diluting segment of the nephron, preventing the generation of maximally dilute urine. In this situation, urine sodium losses exceed water losses. Loop diuretics do not pose the same risk of hyponatremia because they simultaneously block the urine concentrating ability of the kidney, so both sodium and water are lost in the urine.

Excessive sweating in hot weather, particularly during heavy exercise, leads to loss of sodium and water. Hyponatremia develops when water rather than electrolyte-containing liquids is used to replace fluids lost in sweating. Iso-osmotic fluid loss, as in vomiting or diarrhea, does not usually lower the serum sodium concentration unless these losses are replaced with disproportionate amounts of orally ingested or parenterally administered water. Another potential cause of sodium loss from the gastrointestinal tract is repeated tap water enemas or frequent gastrointestinal irrigations with distilled water. Massive absorption of irrigating solutions that do not contain sodium during transurethral prostatectomy is another cause of dilutional hyponatremia. During prostatectomy, the surgeon irrigates the operative site for better visibility. Because electrocautery is used, the irrigating solution must be nonconductive (electrolyte free).

There is also risk of hyponatremia during the postoperative period. During this time, ADH levels are often high, producing an increase in water reabsorption by the kidney (see section on SIADH). Although these elevated levels usually resolve in approximately 72 hours, they can persist for up to 5 days. The hyponatremia becomes exaggerated when electrolyte-free fluids, such as glucose, are used for fluid replacement. Excessive water drinking during this period can also increase the risk of hyponatremia.

TABLE 31-6 ✦ Causes and Manifestations of Hyponatremia

Causes	Manifestations
Excessive Sodium Losses and Replacement With Tap Water or Sodium-Free Losses	**Laboratory Values**
Exercise- or heat-induced sweating and replacement with sodium-free fluids	Serum sodium level below 135 mEq/L (135 mmol/L)
Gastrointestinal losses	Decreased serum osmolality
Vomiting	Dilution of blood components, including
Diarrhea	hematocrit, blood urea nitrogen
Diuresis	
	Signs Related to Hypo-osmolality of Extracellular Fluids and Movement of Water Into Brain Cells and Neuromuscular Tissue
Excessive Water Intake in Relation to Output	
Excessively diluted infant formula	Muscle cramps
Excessive administration of sodium-free parenteral solutions	Weakness
	Headache
Repeated irrigation of body cavities with sodium-free solutions	Depression
Irrigation of gastrointestinal tube with distilled water	Apprehension, feeling of impending doom
	Personality changes
Tap water enemas	Lethargy
Use of nonelectrolyte irrigating solutions during prostate surgery	Stupor, coma
Kidney disorders that impair water elimination	**Gastrointestinal Manifestations**
Increased ADH levels	Anorexia, nausea, vomiting
Trauma, stress, pain	Abdominal cramps, diarrhea
Syndrome of inappropriate ADH	
Use of medications that increase ADH	**Increased Intracellular Fluid**
Psychogenic polydipsia	Fingerprint edema

ADH, antidiuretic hormone

Manifestations. The manifestations of hypotonic hyponatremia are largely related to sodium dilution (see Table 31-6). Serum osmolality is decreased and cellular swelling occurs owing to the movement of water from the extracellular to the intracellular compartment. The manifestations of hyponatremia depend on the rapidity of onset and the severity of the sodium dilution. The signs and symptoms may be acute, as in severe water intoxication, or more insidious in onset and less severe as in chronic hyponatremia. Because of water movement, hyponatremia causes intracellular hypo-osmolality, which is responsible for many of the clinical manifestations of the disorder.[27]

Fingerprint edema is a sign of excess intracellular water. This phenomenon is demonstrated by pressing the finger firmly over the bony surface of the sternum for 15 to 30 seconds. When excess intracellular water is present, a fingerprint similar to that observed when pressing on a piece of modeling clay is seen.

Muscle cramps, weakness, and fatigue reflect the hypo-osmolality of skeletal muscle cells and are often early signs of hyponatremia. These effects commonly are observed in persons with hyponatremia that occurs during heavy exercise in hot weather. Gastrointestinal manifestations such as nausea and vomiting, abdominal cramps, and diarrhea may develop. The brain and nervous system are the most seriously affected by increases in intracellular water. Symptoms include apathy, lethargy, and headache, which can progress to disorientation, confusion, gross motor weakness, and depression of deep tendon reflexes. Seizures and coma occur when serum sodium levels reach extremely low levels. These severe effects, which are caused by brain swelling, may be irreversible.[27] If the condition develops slowly, signs and symptoms do not develop until serum sodium levels approach 125 mEq/L. Progressive neurologic symptoms occur when the serum sodium falls below this level. The term *water intoxication* is often used to describe the neurologic effects of acute hypotonic hyponatremia.

Diagnosis and Treatment. Diagnosis of hyponatremia is based on laboratory reports of decreased sodium concentration, the presence of conditions that predispose to sodium loss or water retention, and signs and symptoms indicative of the disorder.

The treatment of hyponatremia with water excess focuses on the underlying cause. When hyponatremia is caused by water intoxication, limiting water intake or discontinuing medications that contribute to SIADH may be sufficient. The administration of a saline solution orally or intravenously may be needed when hyponatremia is caused by sodium deficiency. Symptomatic hyponatremia (*i.e.*, neurologic manifestations) is often treated with hypertonic saline solution and a loop diuretic, such as furosemide, to increase water elimination. This combination allows for correction of serum sodium levels while ridding the body of excess water.

There is concern about the rapidity with which serum sodium levels are corrected, particularly in persons with chronic symptomatic hyponatremia. Cells, particularly those in the brain, tend to defend against changes in cell volume caused by increased extracellular osmolality by synthesizing amino acids and other osmotically active organic solutes.[28] Because these solutes cannot cross the cell membrane, they confine their osmotic activity to the intracellular compartment. In contrast to electrolytes and other solutes that disturb cell function and harm cells by altering the resting membrane potential or disrupting metabolic processes when they are present in large amounts, these organic osmoles have unique biochemical properties that allow them to accumulate in high concentrations without disrupting cell structure or function. In the case of prolonged water intoxication, brain cells reduce their concentration of organic osmoles as a means of preventing an increase in cell volume. It takes several days for brain cells to restore the organic osmoles lost during hyponatremia.[29] Rapid changes in serum osmolality when brain cells have already undergone volume regulation may cause a dramatic change in brain cell volume. One of the reported effects of rapid treatment of hyponatremia is an osmotic demyelinating condition called *central pontine myelosis*, which produces serious neurologic sequelae and sometimes causes death.[30]

Hypernatremia

Hypernatremia implies a serum sodium level above 145 mEq/L and a serum osmolality greater than 295 mOsm/kg. Because sodium is functionally an impermeable solute, it contributes to tonicity and induces movement of water across cell membranes. Hypernatremia is characterized by hypertonicity of extracellular fluids and almost always causes cellular dehydration.[31]

Causes. Hypernatremia represents a deficit of water in relation to the body's sodium stores. It can be caused by net loss of water or sodium gain. Net water loss can occur through the urine, gastrointestinal tract, lungs, or skin. A defect in thirst or inability to obtain or drink water can interfere with water replacement. Rapid ingestion or infusion of sodium with insufficient time or opportunity for water ingestion can produce a disproportionate gain in sodium (Table 31-7). Hypernatremia almost always follows a loss of body fluids that have a lower than normal concentration of sodium, so that water is lost in excess of sodium. This can result from increased losses from the respiratory tract during fever or strenuous exercise, from watery diarrhea, or when osmotically active tube feedings are given with inadequate amounts of water. With pure water loss, each body fluid compartment loses an equal percentage of its volume. Because approximately one third of the water is in the extracellular compartment, compared with the two thirds in the intracellular compartment, more actual water volume is lost from the intracellular than the extracellular compartment.[6]

Normally, water deficit stimulates thirst and increases water intake. Therefore, hypernatremia is more likely to occur in infants and in persons who cannot express their thirst or obtain water to drink. With hypodipsia, or impaired thirst, the need for fluid intake does not activate the thirst response. Hypodipsia is particularly prevalent among the elderly. In persons with diabetes insipidus, hypernatremia can develop when thirst is impaired or access to water is impeded. The therapeutic administration of

TABLE 31-7 ✦ Causes and Manifestations of Hypernatremia

Causes	Manifestations
Excessive Water Losses	**Laboratory Values**
Watery diarrhea	Serum sodium level above 145 mEq/L
Excessive sweating	(145 mmol/L)
Increased respirations due to conditions such	Increased serum osmolality
as tracheobronchitis	Increased hematocrit and blood urea
Hypertonic tube feedings	nitrogen
Diabetes insipidus	
	Thirst and Signs of Increased ADH Levels
Decreased Water Intake	Polydipsia
Unavailability of water	Oliguria or anuria
Oral trauma or inability to swallow	High urine specific gravity
Impaired thirst sensation	
Withholding water for therapeutic reasons	**Intracellular Dehydration**
Unconsciousness or inability to express thirst	Dry skin and mucous membranes
	Decreased tissue turgor
Excessive Sodium Intake	Tongue rough and fissured
Rapid or excessive administration of sodium-	Decreased salivation and lacrimation
containing parenteral solutions	
Near-drowning in salt water	**Signs Related to Hyperosmolality of**
	Extracellular Fluids and Movement of
	Water Out of Brain Cells
	Headache
	Agitation and restlessness
	Decreased reflexes
	Seizures and coma
	Extracellular Dehydration and Decreased
	Vascular Volume
	Tachycardia
	Weak and thready pulse
	Decreased blood pressure
	Vascular collapse

sodium-containing solutions may also cause hypernatremia. For example, the administration of sodium bicarbonate during cardiopulmonary resuscitation increases body sodium levels because the sodium concentration of each 50-mL ampule of 7.5% sodium bicarbonate contains 892 mEq of sodium.[5] Hypertonic saline solution intended for intra-amniotic instillation for therapeutic abortion may inadvertently be injected intravenously, causing hypernatremia. Rarely, salt intake occurs rapidly, as in taking excess salt tablets or during near-drowning in salt water.

Manifestations. The clinical manifestations of hyper-natremia caused by water loss are largely those of water loss and cellular dehydration (see Table 31-7). The severity of signs and symptoms is greatest when the increase in serum sodium is large and occurs rapidly. Body weight is decreased in proportion to the amount of water that has been lost. Because blood plasma is roughly 90% to 93% water, the concentrations of blood cells and other blood components increase as extracellular water decreases.

Thirst is an early symptom of water deficit, occurring when water losses are equal to 0.5% of body water. Urine output is decreased and urine osmolality increased because of renal water-conserving mechanisms. Body temperature frequently is elevated, and the skin becomes warm and flushed. The vascular volume decreases, the pulse becomes rapid and thready, and the blood pressure drops. Hyperna-tremia produces an increase in serum osmolality and results in water being pulled out of body cells. As a result, the skin and mucous membranes become dry, and salivation and lacrimation are decreased. The mouth becomes dry and sticky, and the tongue becomes rough and fissured. Swallowing is difficult. The subcutaneous tissues assume a firm, rubbery texture. Most significantly, water is pulled out of the cells in the CNS, causing decreased reflexes, agitation, headache, and restlessness. Coma and seizures may develop as hypernatremia progresses.

Diagnosis and Treatment. The diagnosis of hyper-natremia is based on history, physical examination findings indicative of dehydration, and results of laboratory tests. The treatment of hypernatremia includes measures to treat the underlying cause of the disorder and fluid replacement therapy to treat the accompanying dehydration. Replacement fluids can be given orally or intravenously. The oral route is preferable. Oral glucose–electrolyte replacement solutions are available for the treatment of infants with diarrhea.[32–34] Until recently, these solutions were used only early in diarrheal illness or as a first step in reestablishing oral intake after parenteral replacement therapy. These solutions are now widely available in grocery stores and pharmacies for use in the treatment of diarrhea and other dehydrating disorders in infants and young children. They are particularly important in developing countries, where the availability of intravenous fluids is limited and diarrhea is a leading cause of death among children.

The composition of the oral rehydration solution recommended by the Diarrheal Disease Control Center of the World Health Organization (WHO) contains glucose (2.0 g/L), sodium (90 mEq/L), potassium (20 mEq/L), chloride (80 mEq/L), and bicarbonate (30 mEq/L).[33] It is recommended that ingredients be supplied in preweighed packets. Using teaspoons or other household items for measuring the ingredients often is inaccurate and is not recommended. Glucose is preferred to sucrose (*i.e.*, table sugar), which is a disaccharide and must be broken down before it can be absorbed. Commercially available preparations usually contain less sodium and chloride (*e.g.*, 45 to 50 mEq/L of sodium, 35 to 45 mEq/L of chloride) than the WHO formulation, with citrate being substituted for bicarbonate. Although cola drinks commonly are recommended as a remedy for dehydration caused by acute diarrhea, their electrolyte content often is inadequate for replacement purposes, and their high sugar content may complicate the situation by inducing an osmotic diarrhea.[33,35] Sport drinks usually contain more sodium and sugar than the oral rehydration solutions. Intravenous replacement solutions continue to be the treatment of choice for severe fluid deficit.

One of the serious aspects of fluid volume deficit is dehydration of brain and nerve cells. Serum osmolality should be corrected slowly in cases of chronic hypernatremia. This is because brain cells synthesize osmotically active organic solutes to protect against volume changes. These organic solutes serve to produce a gradual increase in intracellular osmolality, allowing osmotic flow of water back into the cell and restoring cell volume. This response begins within 4 to 6 hours of increased serum osmolality and takes several days to become fully effective.[5] Changes in brain water content are greatest during acute hypernatremia but only slightly reduced in chronic hypernatremia. If hypernatremia is corrected too rapidly before the organic osmoles have had a chance to dissipate, the plasma may become relatively hypotonic in relation to brain cell osmolality. When this occurs, water moves into the brain cells, causing cerebral edema and potentially severe neurologic impairment.

In summary, body fluids are distributed between the intracellular and extracellular compartments. Regulation of fluid volume, solute concentration, and distribution between the two compartments depends on water and sodium balance. Water provides approxi-

mately 90% to 93% of fluid volume and sodium salts, approximately 90% to 95% of extracellular solutes. Body water is regulated by thirst, which controls water intake, and by ADH, which controls urine concentration and renal output. Sodium is largely regulated by the kidney under the influence of the sympathetic nervous system and the renin-angiotensin-aldosterone mechanism.

Alterations of salt and water balance can be divided into two main categories: (1) isotonic contraction or expansion of extracellular fluid volume brought about by proportionate losses of sodium and water, and (2) hypotonic dilution (dilutional hyponatremia) or hypertonic concentration (hypernatremia) of extracellular sodium brought about by disproportionate increases or decreases in extracellular water.

Isotonic fluid volume deficit is characterized by a reduction in extracellular fluids. It causes thirst, decreased vascular volume and circulatory function, decreased urine output, and increased urine specific gravity. Isotonic fluid volume excess is characterized by an increase in extracellular fluids. It is manifested by signs of increased vascular volume and edema.

Alterations in extracellular sodium concentration are brought about by a disproportionate gain (hyponatremia) or loss (hypernatremia) of water. As the major cation in the extracellular fluid compartment, sodium concentration controls the osmolality of extracellular fluids and their effect on cell volume. Many of the manifestations of altered sodium concentration are caused by swelling (hyponatremia) or shrinking (hypernatremia) of body cells, including those of the CNS.

Potassium Balance

After you have completed this section of the chapter, you should be able to meet the following objectives:

✦ Characterize the distribution of potassium in the body and explain how extracellular potassium levels are regulated in relation to body gains and losses
✦ State the causes of hypokalemia and hyperkalemia in terms of altered intake, output, and transcellular shifts
✦ Relate the functions of potassium to the manifestations of hypokalemia and hyperkalemia
✦ Describe methods of diagnosis and treatment of hypokalemia and hyperkalemia

REGULATION OF POTASSIUM BALANCE

Potassium is the second most abundant cation in the body and the major cation in the intracellular compartment. All but approximately 2% of body potassium is contained within body cells, with an intracellular concentration of 140 to 150 mEq/L.[36] The potassium content of extracellular fluid (3.5 to 5.0 mEq/L) is considerably less. Because potassium is an intracellular ion, total body stores of potassium are related to body size and muscle mass. In adults, total body potassium ranges from 50 to 55 mmol/kg of body weight.[37,38]

Approximately 65% to 75% of potassium is in muscle.[39] Thus, potassium content declines with age, mainly as a result of a decrease in muscle mass.

Gains and Losses

Potassium intake is normally derived from dietary sources. In healthy persons, potassium balance usually can be maintained by a daily dietary intake of 50 to 100 mEq. Additional amounts of potassium are needed during periods of trauma and stress. The kidneys are the main source of potassium loss. Approximately 80% to 90% of potassium losses occur in the urine, with the remainder being lost in stools or sweat.

Mechanisms of Regulation

Potassium regulation must be extremely efficient, because even a 1% to 2% addition of potassium to the extracellular compartment can elevate serum levels to dangerously high levels. Serum potassium is largely regulated through two mechanisms: (1) renal mechanisms that conserve or eliminate potassium, and (2) a transcellular shift between the intracellular and extracellular compartments. Normally, it takes 6 to 8 hours to eliminate 50% of potassium intake.[5] To avoid an increase in extracellular potassium during this time, excess potassium is temporarily shifted in cells such as those of muscle, liver, red blood cells, and bone.

Renal Regulation.   The major route for potassium elimination is the kidney. Unlike other electrolytes, the regulation of potassium elimination is controlled by secretion from the blood into the tubular filtrate rather than through reabsorption from the tubular filtrate into the blood. Potassium is filtered in the glomerulus, reabsorbed along with sodium and water in the proximal tubule and with sodium and chloride in the thick ascending loop of Henle, and then secreted into the late distal and cortical collecting tubules for elimination in the urine. The latter mechanism serves to "fine-tune" the concentration of potassium in the extracellular fluid.

Aldosterone plays an essential role in regulating potassium elimination by the kidney. The effects of aldosterone on potassium elimination are mediated through a sodium-potassium exchange system located in the late distal and cortical collecting tubules of the kidney (see Chapter 30). In the presence of aldosterone, sodium is transported back into the blood and potassium is secreted in the tubular filtrate for elimination in the urine. The rate of aldosterone secretion by the adrenal gland is strongly controlled by serum potassium levels. For example, an increase of less than 1 mEq/L of potassium causes aldosterone levels to triple.[2] The effect of serum potassium on aldosterone secretion is an example of the powerful feedback regulation of potassium elimination. In the absence of aldosterone, as occurs in persons with Addison's disease, renal elimination of potassium is impaired, causing serum potassium levels to rise to dangerously high levels. Aldosterone is often referred to as a *mineralocorticoid hormone* because of its effect on sodium and potassium. The term *mineralocorticoid activity* is used to describe the aldosterone-like actions of other adrenocortical hormones such as cortisol.

There is also a potassium-hydrogen ion exchange mechanism in the cortical collecting tubules of the kidney (see Chapter 30). When serum potassium levels are increased, K^+ ions are secreted into the urine and H^+ ions are reabsorbed into the blood, producing a decrease in pH and metabolic acidosis. Conversely, when potassium levels are low, K^+ ions are reabsorbed and H^+ ions secreted in the urine, leading to metabolic alkalosis.

Intracellular-Extracellular Shifts.   The transcellular shift of potassium between the extracellular and intracellular compartments is controlled by the function of the Na^+/K^+-ATPase membrane pump and the permeability of ion channels in the cell membrane.

Both insulin and β-adrenergic catecholamines (*e.g.*, epinephrine) increase cellular uptake of potassium by increasing the activity of the Na^+/K^+-ATPase membrane pump (Fig. 31-12). Studies indicate that insulin deficiency impedes cellular uptake of potassium and insulin excess increases uptake. The serum potassium concentration directly affects insulin release from beta cells in the pancreas. Increased potassium stimulates insulin release and a low potassium level inhibits release, suggesting a potassium-insulin regulatory feedback mechanism.[39,40] The catecholamines, particularly epinephrine, facilitate the movement of potassium into muscle tissue. The action of epinephrine on potassium transport is additive to that of insulin.

Extracellular osmolality and pH also influence transcellular potassium exchange by means of either the Na^+/K^+-ATPase pump or ion channels in the cell membrane. Acute

Potassium Balance

➤ Potassium is mainly an intracellular ion with only a small, but vital, amount being present in the extracellular fluids.

➤ The distribution of potassium between the intracellular and extracellular compartments regulates electrical membrane potentials controlling the excitability of nerve and muscle cells as well as contractility of skeletal, cardiac, and smooth muscle tissue.

➤ Because of its vital role in regulating neuromuscular excitability, potassium regulation must be extremely efficient. Even a 1% to 2% addition of potassium to the extracellular fluid compartment can elevate serum levels to dangerously high levels.

➤ Two major mechanisms function in the control of serum potassium: (1) renal mechanisms that conserve or eliminate potassium, and (2) transcellular buffer systems that remove potassium from and release it into the serum as needed. Conditions that disrupt the function of either mechanism can result in serious alteration in serum potassium levels.

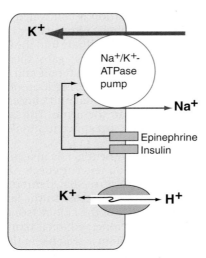

FIGURE 31-12 Mechanisms regulating transcellular shifts in potassium.

increases in serum osmolality cause potassium to move out of cells. When serum osmolality increases because of the presence of impermeable extracellular solutes such as mannitol or glucose (without insulin), water leaves the cell. The loss of cell water produces an increase in intracellular potassium concentration, causing potassium to diffuse out of the cell. A 1.0 to 1.5 mEq/L rise in serum potassium occurs in response to an acute 10% increase in serum osmolality.[5] A hyperosmolality-induced increase in serum potassium is usually counteracted by the opposing actions of insulin and epinephrine. The reverse condition, hypo-osmolality, usually occurs more slowly and does not affect serum potassium levels.

The H^+ ion concentration (pH) of extracellular fluids contributes to the transcellular shift of potassium. In acidosis, H^+ ions move into the cell as a means of preventing large changes in extracellular pH changes. As H^+ ions move into the cell, other positively charged ions, such as K^+, must move out as a means of maintaining electrical neutrality. The serum potassium concentration rises 0.7 mEq/L for each 0.1-unit fall in serum pH.[5] The pH-related shifts in intracellular-extracellular potassium are more pronounced when changes in pH are caused by nonorganic acids (*i.e.*, hyperchloremic acidosis associated with diarrhea and renal failure), in which the companion anion, chloride, cannot permeate the cell membrane and remains outside the cell as a companion for the potassium ion. In contrast, acidosis due to accumulation of organic acids (*i.e.*, lactic acidosis and ketoacidosis) has little effect on potassium because the companion anion is able to enter the cell. Although there is increased movement of potassium out of the cell in diabetic ketoacidosis, it is more likely related to the effects of insulin deficiency and the hyperosmolality of the extracellular fluids. Respiratory acidosis and alkalosis cause little change in serum potassium concentration. Metabolic alkalosis tends to have a smaller opposite effect—H^+ ions move out of the cell as K^+ ions move in. Serum potassium concentration falls by approximately 0.3 mEq/L for each 0.1-unit increase in serum pH.[5]

Exercise also produces compartmental shifts in potassium. Repeated muscle contraction releases potassium into the extracellular fluids. Although the increase usually is small with modest exercise, it can be considerable during exhaustive exercise. Even the repeated clenching and unclenching of the fist during a blood draw can cause potassium to move out of cells and artificially elevate serum potassium levels.

ALTERATIONS IN POTASSIUM BALANCE

As the major intracellular cation, potassium is critical to many body functions. It is involved in a wide range of body functions, including the maintenance of the osmotic integrity of cells, acid-base balance, and the kidney's ability to concentrate urine. Potassium is necessary for growth and it contributes to the intricate chemical reactions that transform carbohydrates into energy, change glucose into glycogen, and convert amino acids to proteins. The difference between the intracellular and extracellular potassium concentrations maintains the normal resting membrane potential for excitable tissues and is essential to skeletal, cardiac, and smooth muscle function (see Chapter 4).

Hypokalemia

Hypokalemia refers to a decrease in serum potassium levels below 3.5 mEq/L (3.5 mmol/L). Because of transcellular shifts, temporary changes in serum potassium may occur as the result of movement between the intracellular and extracellular compartments.

Causes. The causes of potassium deficit can be grouped into three categories: (1) inadequate intake; (2) excessive gastrointestinal, renal, and skin losses; and (3) redistribution between the intracellular and extracellular compartments (Table 31-8).

Inadequate Intake. Inadequate intake is a frequent cause of hypokalemia. A potassium intake of at least 10 to 30 mEq/day is needed to compensate for obligatory urine losses.[5,39] A person on a potassium-free diet continues to lose approximately 5 to 15 mEq of potassium daily. Insufficient dietary intake may result from the inability to obtain or ingest food or from a diet that is low in potassium-containing foods. Potassium intake is often inadequate in persons on fad diets and those who have eating disorders. Elderly persons are particularly likely to have potassium deficits. Many have poor eating habits as a consequence of living alone; they may have limited income, which makes buying foods high in potassium difficult; they may have difficulty chewing many foods that have a high potassium content because of poorly fitting dentures; or they may have problems with swallowing. Also, many medical problems in elderly persons require treatment with drugs, such as diuretics, that increase potassium losses.

Excessive Renal Losses. The kidneys are the main source of potassium loss. Approximately 80% to 90% of potassium losses occur in the urine, with the remaining losses occurring in the stool and sweat. The kidneys do not have the homeostatic mechanisms needed to conserve potas-

TABLE 31-8 ✦ Causes and Manifestations of Hypokalemia	
Causes	**Manifestations**
Inadequate Intake	**Laboratory Values**
Diet deficient in potassium	Serum potassium less than 3.5 mEq/L
Inability to eat	(3.5 mmol/L)
Administration of potassium-free parenteral solutions	**Impaired Ability to Concentrate Urine**
	Polyuria
Excessive Renal Losses	Urine with low osmolality and specific gravity
Diuretic therapy (except potassium-sparing diuretics)	Polydipsia
Diuretic phase of renal failure	**Gastrointestinal Manifestations**
Increased mineralocorticoid levels	Anorexia, nausea, vomiting
Primary hyperaldosteronism	Abdominal distention
Treatment with corticosteroid drugs	Paralytic ileus
Excessive Gastrointestinal Losses	**Neuromuscular Manifestations**
Vomiting	Muscle flabbiness, weakness, and fatigue
Diarrhea	Muscle cramps and tenderness
Gastrointestinal suction	Paresthesias
Draining gastrointestinal fistula	Paralysis
Transcompartmental Shift	**Cardiovascular Manifestations**
Administration of β-adrenergic agonist (*e.g.*, albuterol)	Postural hypotension
Administration of insulin for treatment of diabetic ketoacidosis	Increased sensitivity to digitalis toxicity
Alkalosis, metabolic or respiratory	Changes in electrocardiogram
	Cardiac dysrhythmias
	Central Nervous System Manifestations
	Confusion
	Depression
	Acid–Base Disorders
	Metabolic alkalosis

sium during periods of insufficient intake. After trauma and in stress situations, urinary losses of potassium are greatly increased, sometimes approaching levels of 150 to 200 mEq/L.[40] This means that a potassium deficit can develop rather quickly if intake is inadequate. Renal losses also can be increased by medications, metabolic alkalosis, magnesium depletion, and increased levels of aldosterone. Some antibiotics, particularly amphotericin B and gentamicin, are impermeable anions that require the presence of positively charged cations for elimination in the urine; this causes potassium wasting.

Diuretic therapy, with the exception of potassium-sparing diuretics, is the most common cause of hypokalemia. Both thiazide and loop diuretics increase the loss of potassium in the urine. The degree of hypokalemia is directly related to diuretic dose and is greater when sodium intake is higher.[39] Magnesium depletion causes renal potassium wasting. Magnesium deficiency often coexists with potassium depletion due to diuretic therapy or disease processes such as diarrhea. Importantly, the ability to correct potassium deficiency is impaired when magnesium deficiency is present.

Renal losses of potassium are accentuated by aldosterone and cortisol. Increased potassium losses occur in situations such as trauma and surgery that produce a stress-related increase in these hormones. Primary aldosteronism is caused by a tumor in the cells of the adrenal cortex (in the zona glomerulosa) that secrete aldosterone. Excess secretion of aldosterone by the tumor cells causes severe potassium losses and a decrease in serum potassium levels. Licorice-induced hypokalemia results from inhibition of the enzyme that inactivates cortisol. Cortisol binds to aldosterone receptors and exerts aldosterone-like effects on potassium elimination.

Excessive Nonrenal Losses.   Although potassium losses from the skin and the gastrointestinal tract usually are minimal, these losses can become excessive under certain conditions. For example, burns increase surface losses of potassium. Losses due to sweating increase in persons who are acclimated to a hot climate, partly because increased secretion of aldosterone during heat acclimatization increases the loss of potassium in urine and sweat. Gastrointestinal losses also can become excessive; this occurs with vomiting and diarrhea and when gastrointestinal suction is being used. The potassium content of liquid stools, for example, is approximately 40 to 60 mEq/L.[37]

Transcellular Shifts.   Because of the high ratio of intracellular to extracellular potassium, a redistribution of potassium from the extracellular to the intracellular compartment can produce a marked decrease in the serum concentration (see Fig. 31-12). One cause of potassium redistribution is insulin. After insulin administration, there is increased movement of glucose and potassium into cells. This is one of the reasons that potassium deficit often develops during treatment of diabetic ketoacidosis. β-adrenergic agonist drugs, such as pseudoephedrine and albuterol, have a similar effect on potassium distribution. For example, a standard dose of nebulized albuterol (a bronchodilator) reduces serum potassium by 0.2 to 0.4 mEq/L, and a second dose taken within 1 hour reduces it by almost 1 mEq/L.[39] Ingestion of excess doses of pseudoephedrine, an over-the-counter decongestant, can cause severe hypokalemia. Theophylline and caffeine, although not catecholamines, may increase Na+/K+-ATPase membrane pump activity by inhibiting phospho-diesterase. Severe hypokalemia is a common manifestation of theophylline toxicity.[39]

Manifestations.   The manifestations of hypokalemia include alterations in renal, gastrointestinal, cardiovascular, and skeletal muscle function (see Table 31-8). These manifestations reflect both the intracellular functions of potassium as well as the body's attempt to regulate serum potassium levels within the very narrow range needed to maintain the normal electrical activity of excitable tissues such as nerve and muscle cells. The signs and symptoms of potassium deficit seldom develop until the serum potassium level has fallen below 3.0 mEq/L. They are typically gradual in onset, and therefore the disorder may go undetected for some time.

The renal processes that conserve potassium during hypokalemia interfere with the kidney's ability to concentrate urine. Urine output and serum osmolality are increased, urine specific gravity is decreased, and complaints of polyuria, nocturia, and thirst are common. Metabolic alkalosis and renal chloride wasting are signs of severe hypokalemia.

There are numerous signs and symptoms associated with gastrointestinal function, including anorexia, nausea, and vomiting. Atony of the gastrointestinal smooth muscle can cause constipation, abdominal distention, and, in severe hypokalemia, paralytic ileus. When gastrointestinal symptoms occur gradually and are not severe, they often impair potassium intake and exaggerate the condition.

The most serious effects of hypokalemia are those affecting cardiovascular function. Postural hypotension is common. Digitalis toxicity can be provoked in persons treated with this drug and there is an increased risk of ventricular dysrhythmias, particularly in persons with underlying heart disease. Potassium and digitalis compounds compete for binding to sites on the Na+/K+-ATPase membrane pump. In hypokalemia, more sites are available for digitalis to bind to and exert its action. The dangers associated with digitalis toxicity are compounded in persons who are receiving diuretics that increase urinary losses of potassium.

Most persons with a serum potassium below 3.0 mEq/L demonstrate electrocardiographic (ECG) changes typical of hypokalemia. These changes include prolongation of the PR interval, depression of the ST segment, flattening of the T wave, and appearance of a prominent U wave (Fig. 31-13). Normally, potassium leaves the cell during the repolarization phase of the action potential, returning the membrane potential to its normal resting value. Hypokalemia produces a decrease in potassium efflux that prolongs the rate of repolarization and lengthens the relative refractory period. The U wave normally may be present on the ECG but should be of lower amplitude than the T wave. With hypokalemia, the amplitude of the T wave decreases as the U-wave amplitude increases. Although these ECG changes usually are not serious, they may predispose to sinus bradycardia and ectopic ventricular dysrhythmias. The reader is referred to Chapter 25 for additional information on the ECG and cardiac dysrhythmias.

Complaints of weakness, fatigue, and muscle cramps, particularly during exercise, are common in moderate hypokalemia (serum potassium 3.0 to 2.5 mEq/L). Muscle paralysis with life-threatening respiratory insufficiency can occur with severe hypokalemia (serum potassium <2.5 mEq/L). Leg muscles, particularly the quadriceps, are most prominently affected. Some persons complain of muscle tenderness and paresthesias rather than weakness. In chronic potassium deficiency, muscle atrophy may contribute to muscle weakness. At least three defects in skeletal muscle function occur with potassium deficiency: alterations in the resting membrane potential, alterations in glycogen synthesis and storage, and impaired ability to increase blood flow during strenuous exercise.[41] In hypokalemia, the rest-

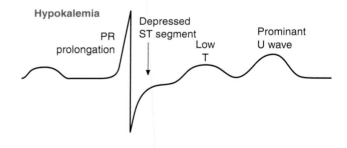

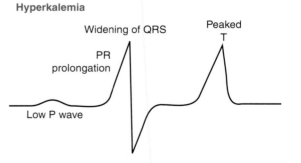

FIGURE 31-13 Electrocardiographic changes with hyperkalemia and hypokalemia.

ing membrane potential becomes more negative, resulting in a decrease in neuromuscular excitability (see Chapter 4). Normal concentrations of intracellular potassium are necessary for glycogen synthesis in muscle cells. Therefore, hypokalemia can interfere with muscle metabolism, especially under exercise conditions that rely heavily on anaerobic pathways that use glycogen as fuel. Potassium released from muscle normally contributes to the autoregulation of blood flow during exercise. Thus, potassium deficiency is thought to lead to impaired blood flow with increased risk of ischemic injury to muscle cells during intense physical exercise.[41]

In a rare condition called *hypokalemic familial periodic paralysis*, episodes of hypokalemia cause attacks of flaccid paralysis that last 6 to 48 hours if untreated.[3] The paralysis may be precipitated by situations that cause severe hypokalemia by producing an intracellular shift in potassium, such as ingestion of a high-carbohydrate meal or administration of insulin, epinephrine, or glucocorticoid drugs. The paralysis often can be reversed by potassium replacement therapy.

Treatment.   When possible, hypokalemia caused by potassium deficit is treated by increasing the intake of foods high in potassium content—meats, dried fruits, fruit juices (particularly orange juice), and bananas. Oral potassium supplements are prescribed for persons whose intake of potassium is insufficient in relation to losses. This is particularly true of persons who are receiving diuretic therapy and those who are taking digitalis.

Potassium may be given intravenously when the oral route is not tolerated or when rapid replacement is needed. Magnesium deficiency may impair potassium correction; in such cases, magnesium replacement is indicated.[42] The rapid infusion of a concentrated potassium solution can cause death from cardiac arrest. Health personnel who assume responsibility for administering intravenous solutions that contain potassium should be fully aware of all the precautions pertaining to their dilution and flow rate.

Hyperkalemia

Hyperkalemia refers to an increase in serum levels of potassium in excess of 5.0 mEq/L (5.0 mmol/L). It seldom occurs in healthy persons because the body is extremely effective in preventing excess potassium accumulation in the extracellular fluid.

Causes.   The three major causes of potassium excess are decreased renal elimination, excessively rapid administration, and movement of potassium from the intracellular to extracellular compartment (Table 31-9). A pseudohyperkalemia can occur secondary to release of potassium from intracellular stores after a blood sample has been collected, hemolysis of red blood cells from excessive agitation of a blood sample, traumatic venipuncture, or prolonged application of a tourniquet during venipuncture.[43]

The most common cause of hyperkalemia is decreased renal function. Chronic hyperkalemia is almost always associated with renal failure. Usually, the glomerular filtration rate must decline to less than 10 mL/minute before hyperkalemia develops. Some renal disorders, such as sickle cell nephropathy, lead nephropathy, and systemic lupus nephritis, can selectively impair tubular secretion of potassium without causing renal failure. As discussed previously, acidosis diminishes potassium elimination by the kidney. Persons with acute renal failure accompanied by lactic acidosis or ketoacidosis are at increased risk for development of hyperkalemia. Correcting the acidosis usually helps to correct the hyperkalemia.[43]

Aldosterone acts at the level of the distal tubular sodium/potassium exchange system to increase potassium excretion while facilitating sodium reabsorption. A decrease

---

TABLE 31-9 ✦ Causes and Manifestations of Hyperkalemia

Causes	Manifestations
Excessive Intake	**Laboratory Values**
Excessive oral intake	Serum potassium above 5.0 mEq/L
Treatment with oral potassium supplements	(5.0 mmol/L)
Excessive or rapid infusion of potassium-containing parenteral fluids	**Gastrointestinal Manifestations**
Release From Intracellular Compartment	Nausea and vomiting
	Intestinal cramps
Tissue trauma	Diarrhea
Burns	
Crushing injuries	**Neuromuscular Manifestations**
Extreme exercise or seizures	Paresthesias
	Weakness, dizziness
Inadequate Elimination by Kidneys	Muscle cramps
Renal failure	
Adrenal insufficiency (Addison's disease)	**Cardiovascular Manifestations**
Treatment with potassium-sparing diuretics	Changes in electrocardiogram
Treatment with angiotensin-converting enzyme inhibitors	Risk of cardiac arrest with severe excess

in aldosterone-mediated potassium elimination can result from adrenal insufficiency (*i.e.*, Addison's disease), depression of aldosterone release due to a decrease in renin or angiotensin II, or impaired ability of the kidneys to respond to aldosterone. Potassium-sparing diuretics (*e.g.*, spironolactone, amiloride, triamterene) can produce hyperkalemia by means of the latter mechanism. Because of their ability to decrease aldosterone levels, angiotensin-converting enzyme inhibitors also can produce an increase in serum potassium levels.

Potassium excess can result from excessive oral ingestion or intravenous administration of potassium. It is difficult to increase potassium intake to the point of causing hyperkalemia when renal function is adequate and the aldosterone sodium/potassium exchange system is functioning. An exception to this rule is the intravenous route of administration. In some cases, severe and fatal incidents of hyperkalemia have occurred when intravenous potassium solutions were infused too rapidly. Because the kidneys control potassium elimination, intravenous solutions that contain potassium should never be started until urine output has been assessed and renal function has been deemed to be adequate.

The movement of potassium out of body cells into the extracellular fluids also can lead to elevated serum potassium levels. Tissue injury causes release of intracellular potassium into the extracellular fluid compartment. For example, burns and crushing injuries cause cell death and release of potassium into the extracellular fluids. The same injuries often diminish renal function, which contributes to the development of hyperkalemia. Transient hyperkalemia may be induced during extreme exercise or seizures, when muscle cells are permeable to potassium. In a rare autosomal dominant disorder called *hyperkalemic periodic paralysis*, hyperkalemia may cause transient periods of muscle weakness and paralysis after exercise, cold exposure, or other situations that cause potassium to move out of the cells. In contrast to hypokalemic periodic paralysis, the episodes are mild, lasting less than 2 hours.[3]

Manifestations.   The signs and symptoms of potassium excess are closely related to the alterations in neuromuscular excitability (see Table 31-9). The effect that potassium has on membrane excitability is determined by the ratio of K^+ ions inside the cell membrane to those outside the cell membrane. As the extracellular potassium concentration rises, there is a decrease in the potassium ratio. This change produces an initial increase in membrane excitability because it brings the resting membrane potential closer to the threshold potential, such that a lesser stimulus is needed for depolarization (see Chapter 4). However, with persistent depolarization, as occurs with severe hyperkalemia, the Na^+ channels become inactivated, producing a net decrease in excitability. The neuromuscular manifestations of potassium excess usually are absent until the serum concentration exceeds 6 mEq/L. The first symptom associated with hyperkalemia typically is paresthesia. There may be complaints of generalized muscle weakness or dyspnea secondary to respiratory muscle weakness.

The most serious effect of hyperkalemia is on the heart. As potassium levels increase, disturbances in cardiac conduction occur. The earliest changes are peaked, narrow T waves and widening of the QRS complex. If serum levels continue to rise, the PR interval becomes prolonged and is followed by disappearance of P waves (see Fig. 31-13). The heart rate may be slow. Ventricular fibrillation and cardiac arrest are terminal events. Detrimental effects of hyperkalemia on the heart are most pronounced when the serum potassium level rises rapidly.

Diagnosis and Treatment.   Diagnosis of hyperkalemia is based on complete history, physical examination to detect muscle weakness and signs of volume depletion, serum potassium levels, and ECG findings. The history should include questions about dietary intake, use of potassium-sparing diuretics, history of kidney disease, and recurrent episodes of muscle weakness.

The treatment of potassium excess varies with the severity of the disturbance and focuses on decreasing or curtailing intake or absorption, increasing renal excretion, and increasing cellular uptake. Decreased intake can be achieved by restricting dietary sources of potassium. The major ingredient in most salt substitutes is potassium chloride, and such substitutes should not be given to patients with renal problems. Increasing potassium output often is more difficult. Patients with renal failure may require hemodialysis or peritoneal dialysis to reduce serum potassium levels. Sodium polystyrene sulfonate, a cation exchange resin, also may be used to remove potassium ions from the colon. The sodium ions in the resin are exchanged for potassium ions, and then the potassium-containing resin is eliminated in the stool.

Most emergency methods focus on measures that cause serum potassium to move into the intracellular compartment. Sometimes the intravenous infusion of insulin and glucose is used for this purpose.

In summary, potassium is the major intracellular cation. It contributes to the maintenance of intracellular osmolality, is necessary for normal neuromuscular function, and influences acid-base balance. Potassium is ingested in the diet and eliminated through the kidney. Because potassium is poorly conserved by the kidney, an adequate daily intake is needed. A transcellular shift can produce a redistribution of potassium between the extracellular and intracellular compartments, causing blood levels to increase or decrease.

Hypokalemia represents a decrease in serum potassium levels below 3.5 mEq/L. It can result from inadequate intake, excessive losses, or redistribution between the intracellular and extracellular fluid compartments. The manifestations of potassium deficit include alterations in renal, skeletal muscle, gastrointestinal, and cardiovascular function, reflecting the crucial role of potassium in cell metabolism and neuromuscular function.

Hyperkalemia represents an increase in serum potassium greater than 5.0 mEq/L. It seldom occurs in healthy persons because the body is extremely effective in preventing excess potassium accumulation in the extracellular fluid. The major causes of potassium excess are decreased renal elimination of potassium, excessively rapid intravenous administration of potassium, and a transcellular shift of potassium out of the cell to the extracellular compartment. The most serious effect of hyperkalemia is cardiac arrest.

Calcium, Phosphate, and Magnesium Balance

After you have completed this section of the chapter, you should be able to meet the following objectives:

+ Describe the associations among intestinal absorption, renal elimination, bone stores, and the functions of vitamin D and parathyroid hormone in regulating calcium, phosphate, and magnesium levels
+ State the difference between ionized and bound or chelated forms of calcium in terms of physiologic function
+ Describe the mechanisms of calcium gain and loss and relate them to the causes of hypocalcemia and hypercalcemia
+ Relate the functions of calcium to the manifestations of hypocalcemia and hypercalcemia
+ Describe the mechanisms of phosphate gain and loss and relate them to causes of hypophosphatemia and hyperphosphatemia
+ Relate the functions of phosphate to the manifestations of hypophosphatemia and hyperphosphatemia
+ Describe the mechanisms of magnesium gain and loss and relate them to the causes of hypomagnesemia and hypermagnesemia
+ Relate the functions of magnesium to the manifestations of hypomagnesemia and hypermagnesemia

MECHANISMS REGULATING CALCIUM, PHOSPHATE, AND MAGNESIUM BALANCE

Calcium, phosphate, and magnesium are the major divalent cations in the body. They are ingested in the diet, absorbed from the intestine, filtered in the glomerulus of the kidney, reabsorbed in the renal tubules, and eliminated in the urine. Approximately 99% of calcium, 85% of phosphate, and 50% to 60% of magnesium are found in bone. Most of the remaining calcium (approximately 1%), phosphate (approximately 14%), and magnesium (approximately 40% to 50%) is located inside cells. Only a small amount of these three ions is present in extracellular fluid. This small, but vital, amount of extracellular calcium, phosphate, and magnesium is directly or indirectly regulated by vitamin D and parathyroid hormone (PTH). Calcitonin, a hormone produced by C cells in the thyroid, is thought to act on the kidney and bone to remove calcium from the extracellular circulation. The role of vitamin D, PTH, and calcitonin on skeletal function is discussed further in Chapters 56 and 58.

Vitamin D

Although classified as a vitamin, vitamin D functions as a hormone. It acts to sustain normal serum levels of calcium and phosphate by increasing their absorption from the intestine, and it also is necessary for normal bone formation. Vitamin D is synthesized by ultraviolet irradiation of 7-dehydrocholesterol, which is present in the skin or obtained from foods in the diet, many of which are fortified with vitamin D. The synthesized or ingested forms of vitamin D are essentially prohormones that lack biologic activity and must undergo metabolic transformation to achieve potency. Once vitamin D enters the circulation from the skin or intestine, it is concentrated in the liver. There it is hydroxylated to form 25-hydroxyvitamin D [25-$(OH)D_3$]. It is then transported to the kidney, where it is transformed into active 1,25-$(OH)_2D_3$. The major action of the activated form of vitamin D, also called *calcitriol*, is to increase the absorption of calcium from the intestine. 1,25-$(OH)_2D_3$ also increases intestinal reabsorption of calcium and sensitizes bone to the resorptive actions of PTH. There is also recent evidence that vitamin D controls parathyroid gland growth and suppresses the synthesis and secretion of PTH.[44] The formation of 1,25-$(OH)_2D_3$ in the kidneys is regulated in feedback fashion by serum calcium and phosphate levels. Low calcium levels lead to an increase in PTH, which then increases vitamin D activation. A lowering of serum phosphate also augments vitamin D activation. Additional control of renal activation of vitamin D is exerted by a negative feedback loop that monitors 1,25-$(OH)_2D_3$ levels.

Parathyroid Hormone

Parathyroid hormone, a major regulator of serum calcium and phosphate, is secreted by the parathyroid glands. There are four parathyroid glands located on the dorsal surface of the thyroid gland. The dominant regulator of PTH is a decrease in serum calcium concentration. A unique calcium receptor on the parathyroid cell membrane responds rapidly to changes in serum calcium levels. The response to a decrease in serum calcium is prompt, occurring within seconds. Phosphate does not exert a direct effect on PTH secretion. Instead, it acts indirectly by complexing with calcium and decreasing serum calcium concentration.

The secretion, synthesis, and action of PTH are also influenced by magnesium. Magnesium serves as a cofactor in the generation of cellular energy and is important in the function of second messenger systems. Magnesium's effects on the synthesis and release of PTH are thought to be mediated through these mechanisms.[45] Because of its function in regulating PTH release, severe and prolonged hypomagnesemia can markedly inhibit PTH levels.

The main function of PTH is to maintain the calcium concentration of the extracellular fluids. It performs this function by promoting the release of calcium from bone, increasing the activation of vitamin D as a means of enhancing intestinal absorption of calcium, and stimulating calcium conservation by the kidney while increasing phosphate excretion (Fig. 31-14).

Parathyroid hormone acts on bone to accelerate the mobilization and transfer of calcium to the extracellular fluid. The skeletal response to PTH is a two-step process.

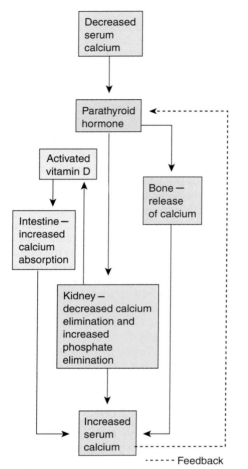

FIGURE 31-14 Regulation of serum calcium concentration by parathyroid hormone.

There is an immediate response in which calcium that is present in bone fluid is released into the extracellular fluid, and a second, more slowly developing response in which completely mineralized bone is resorbed, resulting in the release of both calcium and phosphate. The actions of PTH in terms of bone resorption require normal levels of both vitamin D and magnesium. The activation of vitamin D by the kidney is enhanced by the presence of PTH; it is through the activation of vitamin D that PTH increases intestinal absorption of calcium and phosphate. PTH acts directly on the kidney to increase tubular reabsorption of calcium and magnesium while increasing phosphate elimination. The accompanying increase in phosphate elimination ensures that calcium released from bone does not produce hyperphosphatemia and increase the risk of soft tissue deposition of calcium-phosphate crystals.

Hypoparathyroidism. Hypoparathyroidism reflects deficient PTH secretion, resulting in hypocalcemia. PTH deficiency may be caused by a congenital absence of all of the parathyroid glands, as in DiGeorge syndrome. An acquired deficiency of PTH may occur after neck surgery, particularly if the surgery involves removal of a parathyroid adenoma,

thyroidectomy, or bilateral neck resection for cancer. A transient form of PTH deficiency, occurring within 1 to 2 days and lasting up to 5 days, may occur after thyroid surgery owing to parathyroid gland suppression.[7] Hypoparathyroidism also may have an autoimmune origin. Antiparathyroid antibodies have been detected in some persons with hypoparathyroidism, particularly those with multiple endocrine disorders. Other causes of hypoparathyroidism include heavy metal damage such as occurs with Wilson's disease, metastatic tumors, and infection. Functional impairment of parathyroid function occurs with magnesium deficiency. Correction of the hypomagnesemia results in rapid disappearance of the condition.

Manifestations of acute hypoparathyroidism, which result from a decrease in serum calcium, include tetany with muscle cramps, carpopedal spasm, and convulsions (see Hypocalcemia). Paresthesias, such as tingling of the circumoral area and in the hands and feet, are almost always present. Low calcium levels may cause prolongation of the QT interval, resistance to digitalis, hypotension, and refractory heart failure. Symptoms of chronic PTH deficiency include lethargy, anxiety state, and personality changes. There may be blurring of vision because of cataracts, which develop over a number of years. Extrapyramidal signs, such as those seen with Parkinson's disease, may occur because of calcification of the basal ganglia. Successful treatment of the hypocalcemia may improve the disorder and is sometimes associated with decreases in basal ganglia calcification on x-ray. Teeth may be defective if the disorder occurs during childhood.

Diagnosis of hypoparathyroidism is based on low serum calcium levels, high serum phosphate levels, and low serum PTH levels. Serum magnesium levels usually are measured to rule out hypomagnesemia as a cause of the disorder.

Acute hypoparathyroid tetany is treated with intravenous calcium gluconate followed by oral administration of calcium salts and vitamin D. Magnesium supplementation is used when the disorder is caused by magnesium deficiency. Persons with chronic hypoparathyroidism are treated with oral calcium and vitamin D. Serum calcium levels are monitored at regular intervals (at least every 3 months) as a means of maintaining serum calcium within a slightly low but asymptomatic range. Maintaining serum calcium within this range helps to prevent hypercalciuria and kidney damage.

Pseudohypoparathyroidism is a rare familial disorder characterized by target tissue resistance to PTH. It is characterized by hypocalcemia, increased parathyroid function, and a variety of congenital defects in the growth and development of the skeleton, including short stature and short metacarpal and metatarsal bones. There are variants in the disorder, with some persons having the pseudohypoparathyroidism with the congenital defects and others having the congenital defects with normal calcium and phosphate levels. The manifestations of the disorder are due primarily to chronic hypocalcemia. Treatment is similar to that for hypoparathyroidism.

Hyperparathyroidism. Hyperparathyroidism is caused by hypersecretion of parathyroid hormone. Hyperparathyroidism can manifest as a primary disorder caused by hyperplasia, an adenoma, or carcinoma of the parathyroid glands or as a secondary disorder seen in persons with renal failure.

Primary hyperparathyroidism is seen more commonly after 50 years of age and is more common in women than men. Primary hyperparathyroidism causes hypercalcemia and an increase in calcium in the urine filtrate, resulting in hypercalciuria and the potential for development of kidney stones. Chronic bone resorption may produce diffuse demineralization, pathologic fractures, and cystic bone lesions. Signs and symptoms of the disorder are related to skeletal abnormalities, exposure of the kidney to high calcium levels, and elevated serum calcium levels (see Hypercalcemia). Diagnostic procedures include serum calcium and parathyroid hormone levels. Imaging studies of the parathyroid area may be used to identify a parathyroid adenoma.

Secondary hyperparathyroidism involves hyperplasia of the parathyroid glands and occurs primarily in persons with renal failure (see Chapter 34). In early renal failure, an increase in PTH results from decreased serum calcium and activated vitamin D levels. As the disease progresses, there is a decrease in vitamin D and calcium receptors, making the parathyroid glands more resistant to vitamin D and calcium.[46,47] At this point, elevated phosphate levels induce hyperplasia of the parathyroid glands independent of calcium and activated vitamin D.

The bone disease seen in persons with secondary hyperparathyroidism due to renal failure is known as *renal osteodystrophy*. Treatment includes resolving the hypercalcemia with large fluid intake. Persons with mild disease are advised to keep active and drink adequate fluids. They also are advised to avoid calcium-containing antacids, vitamin D, and thiazide diuretics, which increase reabsorption of calcium by the kidney. Bisphosphonates (*e.g.,* pamidronate and alendronate), which are potent inhibitors of bone resorption, may be used temporarily to treat the hypercalcemia of hyperparathyroidism. Parathyroidectomy may be indicated in persons with symptomatic hyperthyroidism, kidney stones, or bone disease. Avoiding hyperphosphatemia may prevent renal osteodystrophies caused by secondary hyperthyroidism in renal failure. Calcium acetate or a newer calcium-free agent (sevelamer HCl [Renagel]) can be given with meals to bind phosphate. Calcitriol, the activated form of vitamin D, may be used to control parathyroid growth and suppress the synthesis and secretion of PTH. However, because of its potent effect on intestinal absorption and bone mobilization, calcitriol can cause hypercalcemia. Newer analogs of activated vitamin D (*e.g.,* paracalcitriol) are being developed that retain the ability to suppress parathyroid function while having minimal effects on calcium or phosphate reabsorption.[44]

ALTERATIONS IN CALCIUM BALANCE

Calcium enters the body through the gastrointestinal tract, is absorbed from the intestine under the influence of vitamin D, is stored in bone, and is excreted by the kidney. Approximately 99% of body calcium is found in bone,

where it provides the strength and stability for the skeletal system and serves as an exchangeable source to maintain extracellular calcium levels. Only approximately 0.1% (approximately 8.5 to 10.5 mg/dL) of the remaining calcium is present in the extracellular fluid. The extracellular concentrations of calcium and phosphate are reciprocally regulated such that calcium levels fall when phosphate levels are high, and vice versa. Normal serum levels of calcium (8.5 to 10.5 mg/dL in adults) and phosphate (2.5 to 4.5 mg/dL in adults) are regulated so that the product of the two concentrations ($[Ca^{2+}] \times [PO_4^{2-}]$) is normally maintained below 70.[46] Maintenance of the calcium-phosphate product within this range is important in preventing the deposition of $CaPO_4$ salts in soft tissue, damaging the kidneys, blood vessels, and lungs.

Ionized calcium serves a number of functions. It participates in many enzyme reactions; exerts an important effect on membrane potentials and neuronal excitability; is necessary for contraction in skeletal, cardiac, and smooth muscle; participates in the release of hormones, neurotransmitters, and other chemical messengers; influences cardiac contractility and automaticity by way of slow calcium channels; and is essential for blood clotting. The use of calcium channel–blocking drugs in circulatory disorders demonstrates the importance of the calcium ion in the normal function of the heart and blood vessels. Calcium is required for all but the first two steps of the intrinsic pathway for blood coagulation. Because of its ability to bind calcium, citrate often is used to prevent clotting in blood that is to be used for transfusions.

Gains and Losses

The major sources of calcium are milk and milk products. Only 30% to 50% of dietary calcium is absorbed from the duodenum and upper jejunum; the remainder is eliminated in the stool. There is a calcium influx of approximately 150 mg/day into the intestine from the blood. Net absorption of calcium is equal to the amount that is absorbed from the intestine less the amount that moves into the intestine. Calcium balance can become negative when dietary intake (and calcium absorption) is less than intestinal secretion. A dietary intake of less than 400 mg/day can be associated with negative calcium balance.[5]

 Calcium Balance

➤ Extracellular calcium levels are made up of free, complexed, and protein-bound fractions. Only the free, or ionized, calcium functions in the regulation of physiologic functions.

➤ Extracellular calcium ions play an essential role in neuromuscular and cardiac excitability. A decrease in ionized calcium leads to increased excitability and an increase to decreased excitability.

Calcium is stored in bone and excreted by the kidney. Approximately 60% to 65% of filtered calcium is passively reabsorbed in the proximal tubule, driven by the reabsorption of sodium chloride; 15% to 20% is reabsorbed in the thick ascending loop of Henle, driven by the $Na^+/K^+/2Cl^-$ cotransport system; and 5% to 10% is reabsorbed in the distal convoluted tubule (see Chapter 30). The distal convoluted tubule is an important regulatory site for controlling the amount of calcium that enters the urine. PTH and possibly vitamin D stimulate calcium reabsorption in this segment of the nephron. Other factors that may influence calcium reabsorption in the distal convoluted tubule are phosphate levels and glucose and insulin levels. Thiazide diuretics, which exert their effects in the distal convoluted tubule, enhance calcium reabsorption.

Serum calcium exists in three forms: (1) protein bound, (2) complexed, and (3) ionized. Approximately 40% of serum calcium is bound to plasma proteins, mostly albumin, and cannot diffuse or pass through the capillary wall to leave the vascular compartment (Fig. 31-15). Another 10% is complexed (*i.e.*, chelated) with substances such as citrate, phosphate, and sulfate. This form is not ionized. The remaining 50% of serum calcium is present in the ionized form. It is the ionized form of calcium that is free to leave the vascular compartment and participate in cellular functions. The total serum calcium level fluctuates with changes in serum albumin and pH. As a rule, the total serum calcium level is decreased 0.75 to 1.0 mg/dL for every 1-g/dL decrease from normal in the serum albumin level, and by 0.16 mg/dL for each 0.1-unit rise in pH.[5]

Hypocalcemia

Hypocalcemia represents a serum calcium level of less than 8.5 mg/dL. Hypocalcemia occurs in many forms of critical illness and has affected as many as 70% to 90% of patients in intensive care units.[48]

Causes. The causes of hypocalcemia can be divided into four categories: (1) impaired ability to mobilize calcium bone stores, (2) abnormal losses of calcium from the kidney, (3) increased protein binding or chelation such that greater proportions of calcium are in the nonionized form, and (4) soft tissue sequestration (Table 31-10). A pseudohypocalcemia is caused by hypoalbuminemia. It results in a decrease in protein-bound, rather than ionized, calcium and usually is asymptomatic.[49,50]

Serum calcium exists in a dynamic equilibrium with calcium in bone. The ability to mobilize calcium from bone depends on adequate levels of PTH. Decreased levels of PTH may result from primary or secondary forms of hypoparathyroidism. Suppression of PTH release may also occur when vitamin D levels are elevated. The activated form of vitamin D (calcitriol) can be used to suppress the secondary hyperparathyroidism that occurs in persons with kidney failure. Magnesium deficiency inhibits PTH release and impairs the action of PTH on bone resorption. This form of hypocalcemia is difficult to treat with calcium supplementation alone and requires correction of the magnesium deficiency.

There is an inverse relation between calcium and phosphate excretion by the kidneys. Phosphate elimination is impaired in renal failure, causing serum calcium levels to decrease. Hypocalcemia and hyperphosphatemia occur when the glomerular filtration rate falls below 25 to 30 mL/minute (normal is 100 to 120 mL/minute).

Only the ionized form of calcium is able to leave the capillary and participate in body functions. A change in pH alters the proportion of calcium that is in the bound and ionized forms. An acid pH decreases binding of calcium to protein, causing a proportionate increase in ionized calcium, whereas total serum calcium remains unchanged. An alkaline pH has the opposite effect. As an example, hyperventilation sufficient to cause respiratory alkalosis can produce tetany because of increased protein binding of calcium. Free fatty acids increase binding of calcium to albumin, causing a reduction in ionized calcium. Elevations in free fatty acids sufficient to alter calcium binding may occur during stressful situations that cause elevations of epinephrine, glucagon, growth hormone, and adrenocorticotropic hormone levels. Heparin, β-adrenergic drugs (*i.e.*, epinephrine, isoproterenol, and norepinephrine), and alcohol can also produce elevations in free fatty acids levels sufficient to increase calcium binding.

Citrate, which is often used as an anticoagulant in blood transfusions, complexes with calcium. Theoretically, excess citrate in donor blood could combine with the calcium in a recipient's blood, producing a sharp drop in ionized calcium. This normally does not occur because the liver removes the citrate within a matter of minutes. When blood transfusions are administered at a slow rate, there is little danger of hypocalcemia caused by citrate binding.[2]

Hypocalcemia is a common finding in a patient with acute pancreatitis. Inflammation of the pancreas causes release of proteolytic and lipolytic enzymes. It is thought that the calcium ion combines with free fatty acids released by

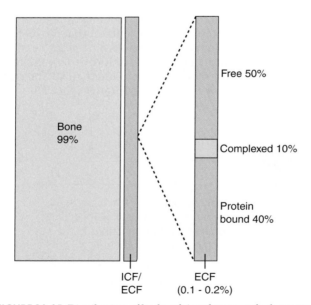

FIGURE 31-15 Distribution of body calcium between the bone and the intracellular and extracellular fluids. The percentages of free, complexed, and protein-bound calcium in extracellular fluids are indicated.

TABLE 31-10 ◆ Causes and Manifestations of Hypocalcemia	
Causes	**Manifestations**

Impaired Ability to Mobilize Calcium From Bone
 	
Hypoparathyroidism
Resistance to the actions of parathyroid hormone
Hypomagnesemia
 	
Decreased Intake or Absorption
 	
Malabsorption
Vitamin D deficiency
  Failure to activate
    Liver disease
    Kidney disease
    Medications that impair activation of vitamin D (*e.g.,* phenytoin)
 	
Abnormal Renal Losses
 	
Renal failure and hyperphosphatemia
 	
Increased Protein Binding or Chelation
 	
Increased pH
Increased fatty acids
Rapid transfusion of citrated blood
 	
Increased Sequestration
 	
Acute pancreatitis
	Laboratory Values
	
	Serum calcium level below 8.5 mg/dL
	
	Neuromuscular Manifestations (Increased Neuromuscular Excitability)
	
	Paresthesias, especially numbness and tingling
	Skeletal muscle cramps
	Abdominal spasms and cramps
	Hyperactive reflexes
	Carpopedal spasm
	Tetany
	Laryngeal spasm
	Positive Chvostek's and Trousseau's signs
	
	Cardiovascular Manifestations
	
	Hypotension
	Signs of cardiac insufficiency
	Failure to respond to drugs that act by calcium-mediated mechanisms
	Prolongation of QT interval predisposes to ventricular dysrhythmias
	
	Skeletal Manifestations (Chronic Deficiency)
	
	Osteomalacia
	Bone pain, deformities, fracture

lipolysis in the pancreas, forming soaps and removing calcium from the circulation.

Calcium deficit due to dietary deficiency exerts its effects on bone stores rather than extracellular calcium levels. A dietary deficiency of vitamin D is seldom seen today because many foods are fortified with vitamin D. Vitamin D deficiency is more likely to occur in malabsorption states, such as biliary obstruction, pancreatic insufficiency, and celiac disease, in which the ability to absorb fat and fat-soluble vitamins is impaired. Failure to activate vitamin D is another cause of hypocalcemia. Anticonvulsant medications, particularly phenytoin, can impair initial activation of vitamin D in the liver. The final step in activation of vitamin D is impaired in persons with renal failure (see Chapter 34). Fortunately, the activated form of vitamin D, calcitriol, has been synthesized and is available for use in the treatment of calcium deficit in persons with renal failure.

Manifestations. Hypocalcemia can manifest as an acute or chronic condition. The manifestations of acute hypocalcemia reflect the increased neuromuscular excitability and cardiovascular effects of a decrease in ionized calcium (see Table 31-10). Ionized calcium stabilizes neuromuscular excitability, thereby making nerve cells less sensitive to stimuli. Nerves exposed to low ionized calcium levels show decreased thresholds for excitation, repetitive responses

to a single stimulus, and, in extreme cases, continuous activity. The severity of the manifestations depends on the underlying cause, rapidity of onset, accompanying electrolyte disorders, and extracellular pH. Increased neuromuscular excitability can manifest as paresthesias (*i.e.,* tingling around the mouth and in the hands and feet) and tetany (*i.e.,* muscle spasms of the muscles of the face, hands, and feet). Severe hypocalcemia can lead to laryngeal spasm, seizures, and even death.

Cardiovascular effects of acute hypocalcemia include hypotension, cardiac insufficiency, cardiac dysrhythmias (particularly heart block and ventricular fibrillation), and failure to respond to drugs such as digitalis, norepinephrine, and dopamine that act through calcium-mediated mechanisms.

Chronic hypocalcemia is often accompanied by skeletal manifestations and skin changes. There may be bone pain, fragility, deformities, and fractures. The skin may be dry and scaling, the nails brittle, and hair dry. Development of cataracts is common. A person with chronic hypocalcemia may also present with mild diffuse brain disease mimicking depression, dementia, or psychoses.

Chvostek's and Trousseau's tests can be used to assess for an increase in neuromuscular excitability and tetany.[7] Chvostek's sign is elicited by tapping the face just below the temple at the point where the facial nerve emerges. Tapping the face over the facial nerve causes spasm of the lip, nose, or face when the test result is positive. An inflated blood pressure cuff is used to test for Trousseau's sign. The cuff is inflated above systolic blood pressure for 3 minutes. Contraction of the fingers and hands (*i.e.*, carpopedal spasm) indicates the presence of tetany.

Treatment. Acute hypocalcemia is an emergency situation, requiring prompt treatment. An intravenous infusion containing calcium (*e.g.*, calcium gluconate, calcium gluceptate, calcium chloride) is used when tetany or acute symptoms are present or anticipated because of a decrease in the serum calcium level.

Chronic hypocalcemia is treated with oral intake of calcium. One glass of milk contains approximately 300 mg of calcium. Oral calcium supplements of carbonate, gluconate, or lactate salts may be used. In some cases, long-term treatment may require the use of vitamin D preparations. The active form of vitamin D is administered when the liver or kidney mechanisms needed for hormone activation are impaired.

Hypercalcemia

Hypercalcemia represents a total serum calcium concentration greater than 10.5 mg/dL. Falsely elevated levels of calcium can result from prolonged drawing of blood with an excessively tight tourniquet. Increased plasma proteins (*e.g.*, hyperalbuminemia, hyperglobulinemia) may elevate the total serum calcium but not affect the ionized calcium concentration.

Causes. A serum calcium excess (*i.e.*, hypercalcemia) results when calcium movement into the circulation overwhelms the calcium regulatory hormones or the ability of the kidney to remove excess calcium ions (Table 31-11). The most common causes of hypercalcemia are increased bone resorption due to neoplasms or hyperparathyroidism.[51–53] Hypercalcemia is a common complication of malignancy, occurring in approximately 10% to 20% of persons with advanced disease.[52] A number of malignant tumors, including carcinoma of the lungs, have been associated with hypercalcemia. Some tumors destroy the bone, but others produce humoral agents that stimulate osteoclastic activity, increase bone resorption, or inhibit bone formation.

Less frequent causes of hypercalcemia are prolonged immobilization, increased intestinal absorption of calcium, excessive doses of vitamin D, and the effects of drugs such as lithium and thiazide diuretics. Prolonged immobilization and lack of weight bearing cause demineralization of bone

---

TABLE 31-11 ✦ Causes and Manifestations of Hypercalcemia

Causes	Manifestations
Increased Intestinal Absorption	**Laboratory Values**
Excessive vitamin D	Serum calcium level above 10.5 mg/dL
Excessive calcium in the diet	
Milk-alkali syndrome	**Impaired Ability to Concentrate Urine and Exposure of Kidney to Increased Concentration of Calcium**
Increased Bone Resorption	
Increased levels of parathyroid hormone	Polyuria
Malignant neoplasms	Polydipsia
Prolonged immobilization	Flank pain
	Signs of acute renal insufficiency
Decreased Elimination	Signs of kidney stones
Thiazide diuretics	**Gastrointestinal Manifestations**
Lithium therapy	
	Anorexia
	Nausea, vomiting
	Constipation
	Neuromuscular Manifestations (Decreased Neuromuscular Excitability)
	Muscle weakness and atrophy
	Ataxia, loss of muscle tone
	Central Nervous System Manifestations
	Lethargy
	Personality and behavioral changes
	Stupor and coma
	Cardiovascular Manifestations
	Hypertension
	Shortening of the QT interval
	Atrioventricular block on electrocardiogram

and release of calcium into the bloodstream. Intestinal absorption of calcium can be increased by excessive doses of vitamin D or as a result of a condition called the *milk-alkali syndrome*. The milk-alkali syndrome is caused by excessive ingestion of calcium (often in the form of milk) and absorbable antacids. Because of the advent of nonabsorbable antacids, the condition is seen less frequently than in the past, but it may occur in women who are overzealous in taking calcium preparations for osteoporosis prevention. The condition is thought to be initiated by mild hypercalcemia leading to increased sodium excretion along with a decrease in extracellular fluid volume and glomerular filtration rate. The decreased glomerular filtration rate leads to alkalosis and increased calcium reabsorption by the kidney. Discontinuance of the antacid repairs the alkalosis and increases calcium elimination.

A variety of drugs elevate calcium levels. The use of lithium to treat bipolar disorders has caused hypercalcemia and hyperparathyroidism. The thiazide diuretics increase calcium reabsorption in the distal convoluted tubule of the kidney. Although the thiazide diuretics seldom cause hypercalcemia, they can unmask hypercalcemia from other causes such as underlying bone disorders and conditions that increase bone resorption.

Manifestations. The signs and symptoms associated with calcium excess originate from three sources: changes in neural excitability and smooth and cardiac muscle function and exposure of the kidneys to high concentrations of calcium (see Table 31-11).

Neural excitability is decreased in patients with hypercalcemia. There may be a dulling of consciousness, stupor, weakness, and muscle flaccidity. Behavioral changes may range from subtle alterations in personality to acute psychoses.

The heart responds to elevated levels of calcium with increased contractility and ventricular dysrhythmias. Digitalis accentuates these responses. Gastrointestinal symptoms reflect a decrease in smooth muscle activity and include constipation, anorexia, nausea, and vomiting. Pancreatitis is another potential complication of hypercalcemia and is probably related to stones in the pancreatic ducts.

High calcium concentrations in the urine impair the ability of the kidneys to concentrate urine by interfering with the action of ADH. This causes salt and water diuresis and an increased sensation of thirst. Hypercalciuria also predisposes to the development of renal calculi.

Hypercalcemic crisis describes an acute increase in the serum calcium level.[54] Malignant disease and hyperparathyroidism are major causes of hypercalcemic crisis. In hypercalcemic crisis, polyuria, excessive thirst, volume depletion, fever, altered levels of consciousness, azotemia (*i.e.*, nitrogenous wastes in the blood), and a disturbed mental state accompany other signs of calcium excess. Symptomatic hypercalcemia is associated with a high mortality rate; death often is caused by cardiac arrest.

Treatment. The treatment of calcium excess usually is directed toward rehydration and measures to increase urinary excretion of calcium and inhibit release of calcium from bone.[54] Fluid replacement is needed in situations of volume depletion. The excretion of sodium is accompanied by calcium excretion. Diuretics and sodium chloride can be administered to increase urinary elimination of calcium after the extracellular fluid volume has been restored. Loop diuretics commonly are used rather than thiazide diuretics, which increase calcium reabsorption.

Initial lowering of calcium levels is followed by measures to inhibit bone reabsorption. Drugs that are used to inhibit calcium mobilization include bisphosphonates, calcitonin, plicamycin, glucocorticosteroids, and gallium nitrate. The bisphosphonates are a relatively new group of drugs that act mainly by inhibiting osteoclastic activity. These agents provide a significant reduction in calcium levels with relatively few side effects. Calcitonin inhibits osteoclastic activity, thereby decreasing resorption. The corticosteroids and plicamycin (mithramycin) inhibit bone resorption and are used to treat hypercalcemia associated with cancer. The long-term use of plicamycin, an antineoplastic drug, is limited because of its potential for nephrotoxicity and hepatotoxicity. Gallium nitrate is also used in the treatment of severe hypercalcemia associated with malignancy. It is a chemical compound that inhibits bone resorption, although the precise mechanism of action is unclear.

ALTERATIONS IN PHOSPHATE BALANCE

Phosphorus is mainly an intracellular anion. It is the fourth most abundant element in the body after carbon, nitrogen, and calcium. Phosphate is essential to many bodily functions. It plays a major role in bone formation; is essential to certain metabolic processes, including the formation of ATP and the enzymes needed for metabolism of glucose, fat, and protein; is a necessary component of several vital parts of the cell, being incorporated into the nucleic acids of DNA and RNA and the phospholipids of the cell membrane; and serves as an acid-base buffer in the extracellular fluid and in the renal excretion of hydrogen ions. Delivery of oxygen by the red blood cell depends on organic phosphates in ATP and 2,3-diphosphoglycerate. Phosphate is also needed for normal function of other blood cells, including the white blood cells and platelets.

Approximately 85% of phosphate is contained in bone, and most of the remainder (14%) is located in cells. Only approximately 1% is in the extracellular compartment, and of that, only a minute proportion is in the plasma. Extracellular phosphorus exists mainly as phosphate, although laboratory measurements are often reported as elemental phosphorus.[55,56] Most of the intracellular phosphorus (approximately 90%) is in the organic form (*e.g.*, nucleic acids, phosphoproteins, ATP). Entry of phosphate into cells is enhanced after glucose uptake, because phosphorus is incorporated into the phosphorylated intermediates of glucose metabolism. Cell injury or atrophy leads to a loss of cell components that contain organic phosphate; regeneration of these cellular components results in withdrawal of inorganic phosphate from the extracellular compartment.

In the adult, the normal serum phosphate level ranges from 2.5 to 4.5 mg/dL. These values are slightly higher in infants (3.7 to 8.5 mg/dL) and children (4.0 to 5.4 mg/dL), probably because of increased growth hormone and decreased gonadal hormones. Changing the serum phosphate levels to as high as three to four times the normal value does not seem to have an immediate effect on body function.

Gains and Losses

Phosphate is ingested in the diet and eliminated in the urine. Phosphate is derived from many dietary sources, including milk and meats. Approximately 80% of ingested phosphate is absorbed in the intestine, primarily in the jejunum. Absorption is diminished by concurrent ingestion of substances that bind phosphate, including calcium, magnesium, and aluminum.

The overall elimination of phosphate by the kidney involves glomerular filtration and tubular reabsorption. Essentially all of the phosphate that is present in the plasma is filtered in the glomerulus. Renal elimination of phosphate is then regulated by an overflow mechanism in which the amount of phosphate lost in the urine is directly related to phosphate concentrations in the blood. Essentially all the filtered phosphate is reabsorbed when phosphate levels are low. When serum phosphate levels rise above a critical level, the rate of phosphate loss in the urine reflects the excess serum phosphate levels. Parathyroid hormone also plays a significant role in regulating phosphate concentration. It does this by promoting bone resorption, which dumps large amounts of phosphate into the extracellular fluid, and it increases the renal threshold for phosphate reabsorption. Thus, whenever PTH is increased, tubular phosphate reabsorption is decreased and more phosphate is lost in the urine.

Hypophosphatemia

Hypophosphatemia is commonly defined by a serum phosphorus level of less than 2.5 mg/dL in adults; it is considered

---

Phosphate Balance

➤ Approximately 85% of the phosphorus is contained in bone. Most of the remaining phosphorus is incorporated into organic compounds such as nucleic acids, high-energy compounds (*e.g.*, ATP), and coenzymes which are critically important for cell function.

➤ Many of the manifestations of hypophosphatemia are related to a decrease in cell energy due to ATP depletion.

➤ Serum phosphate levels are regulated by the kidneys, which eliminate or conserve phosphate as serum levels change. Serum levels of calcium and phosphate are reciprocally regulated to prevent the damaging deposition of calcium phosphate crystals in the soft tissues of the body. Many of the manifestations of hyperphosphatemia reflect a decrease in serum calcium levels.

---

severe at concentration of less than 1.0 mEq/L.[56] Hypophosphatemia may occur despite normal body phosphate stores as a result of movement into the intracellular compartment. Serious depletion of phosphate may exist with low, normal, or high serum concentrations.

Causes.   The most common causes of hypophosphatemia are depletion of phosphate because of insufficient intestinal absorption, transcompartmental shifts, and increased renal losses (Table 31-12). Often, more than one of these mechanisms is active. Unless food intake is severely restricted, dietary intake and intestinal absorption of phosphorus is usually adequate. Intestinal absorption may be inhibited by administration of glucocorticoids, high dietary levels of magnesium, and hypothyroidism. Prolonged ingestion of antacids may also interfere with intestinal absorption. Antacids that contain aluminum hydroxide, aluminum carbonate, and calcium carbonate bind with phosphate, causing increased phosphate losses in the stool. Because of their ability to bind phosphate, calcium-based antacids are sometimes used therapeutically to decrease phosphate levels in persons with chronic renal failure.

Alcoholism is a common cause of hypophosphatemia. The mechanisms underlying hypophosphatemia in the person addicted to alcohol may be related to malnutrition, increased renal excretion rates, or hypomagnesemia. Malnutrition and diabetic ketoacidosis increase phosphate excretion and phosphate loss from the body. Refeeding of malnourished patients increases the incorporation of phosphate into nucleic acids and phosphorylated compounds in the cell. The same thing happens when diabetic ketoacidosis is reversed with insulin therapy. Urinary losses of phosphate may be caused by drugs, such as theophylline, corticosteroids, and loop diuretics, that increase renal excretion.

Hypophosphatemia can occur during prolonged courses of glucose administration or hyperalimentation. Glucose administration causes insulin release, with transport of glucose and phosphorus into the cell. The catabolic events that occur with diabetic ketoacidosis also deplete phosphate stores. However, hypophosphatemia does not become apparent until insulin and fluid replacement have reversed dehydration and glucose has started to move back into the cell. Administration of hyperalimentation solutions without adequate phosphorus can cause a rapid influx of phosphorus into the body's muscle mass, particularly if treatment is initiated after a period of tissue catabolism. Because only a small amount of total body phosphorus is in the extracellular compartment, even a small redistribution between the extracellular and intracellular compartments can cause hypophosphatemia, even though total phosphate levels have not changed.

Respiratory alkalosis due to prolonged hyperventilation can produce hypophosphatemia through decreased levels of ionized calcium from increased protein binding, increased PTH release, and increased phosphate excretion. Clinical conditions associated with hyperventilation include gram-negative septicemia, alcohol withdrawal, heat stroke, and primary hyperventilation.[56,57]

Manifestations.   Many of the manifestations of phosphorus deficiency result from a decrease in cellular energy stores

TABLE 31-12 ✦ Causes and Manifestations of Hypophosphatemia

Causes	Manifestations
Decreased Intestinal Absorption	**Laboratory Values**
Antacids (aluminum and calcium)	Serum levels below 2.5 mg/dL in adults and
Severe diarrhea	4.0 mg/dL in children
Lack of vitamin D	**Neural Manifestations**
Increased Renal Elimination	Intention tremor
Alkalosis	Ataxia
Hyperparathyroidism	Paresthesias
Diabetic ketoacidosis	Confusion, stupor, coma
Renal tubular absorption defects	Seizures
Malnutrition and Intracellular Shifts	**Musculoskeletal Manifestations**
Alcoholism	Muscle weakness
Total parenteral hyperalimentation	Joint stiffness
Recovery from malnutrition	Bone pain
Administration of insulin and recovery from	Osteomalacia
diabetic ketoacidosis	**Blood Disorders**
	Hemolytic anemia
	Platelet dysfunction with bleeding disorders
	Impaired white blood cell function

due to deficiency in ATP and impaired oxygen transport due to a decrease in red blood cell 2,3-diphosphoglycerate (see Chapter 15). Hypophosphatemia results in altered neural function, disturbed musculoskeletal function, and hematologic disorders (see Table 31-12).

Red blood cell metabolism is impaired by phosphate deficiency; the cells become rigid, undergo increased hemolysis, and have diminished ATP and 2,3-diphosphoglycerate levels. Chemotaxis and phagocytosis by white blood cells are impaired. Platelet function also is disturbed. Respiratory insufficiency resulting from impaired function of the respiratory muscles can develop in patients with severe hypophosphatemia.

Neural manifestations include intention tremors, paresthesia, hyporeflexia, stupor, coma, and seizures. Anorexia and dysphagia can occur. Muscle weakness, which is common in hypophosphatemia, is related to a reduction in 2,3-diphosphoglycerate. Chronic phosphate depletion interferes with mineralization of newly formed bone matrix. In growing children, this process causes abnormal endochondral growth and clinical manifestations of rickets. In adults, the condition leads to joint stiffness, bone pain, and skeletal deformities consistent with osteomalacia (see Chapter 58).

Treatment.   The treatment of hypophosphatemia is replacement therapy. This may be accomplished with dietary sources high in phosphate (one glassful of milk contains approximately 250 mg of phosphate) or with oral or intravenous replacement solutions. Phosphate supplements usually are contraindicated in hypercalcemia and renal failure because of increased risk of extracellular calcifications that occur when the calcium × phosphate product exceeds that needed for precipitation of calcium phosphate.

Hyperphosphatemia

Hyperphosphatemia represents a serum phosphorus concentration in excess of 4.5 mg/dL in adults. Growing children normally have serum phosphate levels higher than those of adults.

Causes.   Hyperphosphatemia results from failure of the kidneys to excrete excess phosphate, rapid redistribution of intracellular phosphate to the extracellular compartment, and excessive intake of phosphate.[57] The most common cause of hyperphosphatemia is impaired renal function (Table 31-13).

Hyperphosphatemia is a common electrolyte disorder in persons with chronic renal failure. A reduction in glomerular filtration rate to less than 30 to 50 mL/minute results in a reduction of phosphate elimination. The increase in phosphate levels in persons with end-stage renal disease occurs despite compensatory increases in PTH. A recent study has shown an increase in soft tissue calcification and mortality among patients with end-stage renal disease with hyperphosphatemia.[46] Release of intracellular phosphate can result from conditions such as massive tissue injury, heat stroke, potassium deficiency, and seizures. Chemotherapy can raise serum phosphate levels because of the rapid destruction of tumor cells.

The administration of excess phosphate-containing antacids, laxatives, or enemas can be another cause of hyperphosphatemia, especially when there is a decrease in vascular volume and a reduced glomerular filtration rate. Phosphate-containing laxatives and enemas predispose to hypovolemia and a decreased glomerular filtration rate by inducing diarrhea, thereby increasing the risk of hypophosphatemia. Serious and even fatal hyperphosphatemia has

TABLE 31-13 ◆ Causes and Manifestations of Hyperphosphatemia	
Causes	**Manifestations**
Acute Phosphate Overload	**Laboratory Values**
Laxatives and enemas containing phosphate	Serum levels above 4.5 mg/dL in adults and
Intravenous phosphate supplementation	5.4 mg/dL in children
	Ectopic calcification when Ca × PO₄ > 60
Intracellular-to-Extracellular Shift	
Massive trauma	**Neuromuscular Manifestations**
Heat stroke	**(Reciprocal Decrease in Serum Calcium)**
Seizures	
Tumor lysis syndrome	Paresthesias
Potassium deficiency	Tetany
Impaired Elimination	**Cardiovascular Manifestations**
Kidney failure	Hypotension
Hypoparathyroidism	Cardiac dysrhythmias

resulted from administration of Fleet Phospho-Soda enterally[58] or as an enema.

Manifestations. Hyperphosphatemia is accompanied by a decrease in serum calcium. Many of the signs and symptoms of a phosphate excess are related to a calcium deficit (see Table 31-13). Ectopic calcifications may develop when the calcium × phosphate concentration product exceeds 60.

Treatment. The treatment of hyperphosphatemia is directed at the cause of the disorder. Dietary restriction of foods that are high in phosphate may be used. Calcium-based phosphate binders are useful in chronic hyperphosphatemia. Hemodialysis is used to reduce phosphate levels in persons with end-stage renal disease.

ALTERATIONS IN MAGNESIUM BALANCE

Magnesium is the second most abundant intracellular cation. The average adult has approximately 24 g of magnesium distributed throughout the body.[59] Of the total magnesium content, approximately 50% to 60% is stored in bone, 39% to 49% is contained in the body cells, and the remaining 1% is dispersed in the extracellular fluids.[60–62] Approximately 20% to 30% of the extracellular magnesium is protein bound, and only a small fraction of intracellular magnesium (15% to 30%) is exchangeable with the extracellular fluid. The normal serum concentration of magnesium is 1.8 to 2.7 mg/dL.

Only recently has the importance of magnesium to the overall function of the body been recognized. Magnesium acts as a cofactor in many intracellular enzyme reactions, including those related to transfer of phosphate groups. It is essential to all reactions that require ATP, for every step related to replication and transcription of DNA, and for the translation of messenger RNA. It is required for cellular energy metabolism, functioning of the sodium-potassium membrane pump, membrane stabilization, nerve conduction, ion transport, and calcium channel activity. Magnesium binds to calcium receptors, and it has been suggested

that alterations in magnesium levels may exert their effects through calcium-mediated mechanisms. Magnesium may bind competitively to calcium binding sites, producing the appropriate response; it may compete with calcium for a binding site but not exert an effect; or it may alter the distribution of calcium by interfering with its movement across the cell membrane.

Gains and Losses

Magnesium is ingested in the diet, absorbed from the intestine, and excreted by the kidneys. Intestinal absorption is not closely regulated, and approximately 25% to 65% of dietary magnesium is absorbed. Magnesium is contained in

  Magnesium Balance

➤ Most of the body's magnesium is located within cells, where it functions in regulation of enzyme activity, generation of ATP, and calcium transport. Magnesium is necessary for parathyroid hormone function and hypomagnesemia is a common cause of hypocalcemia.

➤ Elimination of magnesium occurs mainly through the kidney, which adjusts urinary excretion as a means of maintaining serum magnesium levels. Diuretics tend to disrupt renal regulatory mechanisms and increase urinary losses of magnesium.

➤ There is an interdependency between intracellular concentrations of magnesium and potassium such that a decrease in one is accompanied by a decrease in the other. Magnesium deficiency contributes to cardiac dysrhythmias that occur with hypokalemia.

all green vegetables, grains, nuts, meats, and seafood. Magnesium is also present in much of the groundwater in North America.

The kidney is the principal organ of magnesium regulation. Magnesium is a unique electrolyte in that only approximately 30% to 40% of the filtered amount is reabsorbed in the proximal tubule. The greatest quantity, approximately 50% to 70%, is reabsorbed in the thick ascending loop of Henle. The distal tubule, which reabsorbs a small amount of magnesium, is the major site of magnesium regulation. Magnesium reabsorption is decreased in the presence of increased serum levels, stimulated by PTH, and inhibited by increased calcium levels. The major driving force for magnesium absorption in the thick ascending loop of Henle is the $Na^+/K^+/2Cl^-$ cotransport system (see Chapter 30). Inhibition of this transport system by loop diuretics lowers magnesium reabsorption.

Hypomagnesemia

Hypomagnesemia represents a serum magnesium concentration of less than 1.8 mg/dL.[63] It is seen in conditions that limit intake or increase intestinal or renal losses, and it is a common finding in emergency departments and critical care patients.

Causes. Magnesium deficiency can result from insufficient intake, excessive losses, or movement between the extracellular and intracellular compartments (Table 31-14). It can result from conditions that directly limit intake, such as malnutrition, starvation, or prolonged maintenance of magnesium-free parenteral nutrition. Other conditions, such as diarrhea, malabsorption syndromes, prolonged nasogastric suction, or laxative abuse, decrease intestinal absorption. Excessive calcium intake impairs intestinal absorption of magnesium by competing for the same transport site. Another common cause of magnesium deficiency is chronic alcoholism. Many factors contribute to hypomagnesemia in alcoholism, including low intake and gastrointestinal losses from diarrhea. The effects of hypomagnesemia are exaggerated by other electrolyte disorders, such as hypokalemia, hypocalcemia, and metabolic acidosis. There also is evidence that alcohol inhibits reabsorption of magnesium by the kidney.[59]

Although the kidneys are able to defend against hypermagnesemia, they are less able to conserve magnesium and prevent hypomagnesemia. Urine losses are increased in diabetic ketoacidosis, hyperparathyroidism, and hyperaldosteronism. Some drugs increase renal losses of magnesium, including diuretics (particularly loop diuretics) and nephrotoxic drugs such as aminoglycoside antibiotics, cyclosporine, cisplatin, and amphotericin B.

Relative hypomagnesemia may also develop in conditions that promote movement of magnesium between the extracellular and intracellular compartments, including rapid administration of glucose, insulin-containing parenteral solutions, and alkalosis. Although transient, these conditions can cause serious alterations in body function.

Manifestations. Magnesium deficiency usually occurs in conjunction with hypocalcemia and hypokalemia, producing a number of related neurologic and cardiovascular manifestations (see Table 31-14). Hypocalcemia is typical of severe hypomagnesemia. Most persons with hypomagnesemia-related hypocalcemia have decreased PTH levels, probably as a result of impaired magnesium-dependent mechanisms that control PTH release and synthesis. There is also evidence that hypomagnesemia decreases both the PTH-dependent and PTH-independent release of calcium from bone. In hypomagnesemia, magnesium ions are released from bone in exchange for increased uptake of calcium from the serum.

Hypokalemia also is a typical feature of hypomagnesemia. It leads to a reduction in intracellular potassium and impairs the ability of the kidney to conserve potassium. When hypomagnesemia is present, hypokalemia is unresponsive to potassium replacement therapy.

TABLE 31-14 ✦ Causes and Manifestations of Hypomagnesemia

Causes	Manifestations
Impaired Intake or Absorption	**Laboratory Values**
Alcoholism	Serum magnesium level less than 1.8 mg/dL
Malnutrition or starvation	
Malabsorption	**Neuromuscular Manifestations**
Small bowel bypass surgery	Personality change
Parenteral hyperalimentation with inadequate amounts of magnesium	Athetoid or choreiform movements
High dietary intake of calcium without concomitant amounts of magnesium	Nystagmus
	Tetany
	Positive Babinski's, Chvostek's, Trousseau's signs
Increased Losses	
Diuretic therapy	**Cardiovascular Manifestations**
Hyperparathyroidism	
Hyperaldosteronism	Tachycardia
Diabetic ketoacidosis	Hypertension
Magnesium-wasting kidney disease	Cardiac dysrhythmias

Magnesium is vital to carbohydrate metabolism and the generation of both aerobic and anaerobic metabolisms. Many of the manifestations of magnesium deficit are due to related electrolyte disorders such as hypokalemia and hypocalcemia. Hypocalcemia may be evidenced by personality changes and neuromuscular irritability along with tremors, athetoid or choreiform movements, and positive Chvostek's or Trousseau's signs. Cardiovascular manifestations include tachycardia, hypertension, and ventricular dysrhythmias. There may be ECG changes such as widening of the QRS complex, appearance of peak T waves, and prolongation of PR interval, T-wave inversion, and appearance of U waves. Ventricular dysrhythmias, particularly in the presence of digitalis, may be difficult to treat unless magnesium levels are normalized.

Persistent magnesium deficiency has been implicated as a risk factor for osteoporosis and osteomalacia, particularly in persons with chronic alcoholism, diabetes mellitus, and malabsorption syndrome.

Treatment.   Hypomagnesemia is treated with magnesium replacement. The route of administration depends on the severity of the condition. Symptomatic, moderate to severe magnesium deficiency is treated by parenteral administration. Treatment must be continued for several days to replace stored and serum levels. In conditions of chronic intestinal or renal loss, maintenance support with oral magnesium may be required. Patients with any degree of renal failure must be carefully monitored to prevent magnesium excess. Magnesium often is used therapeutically to treat cardiac arrhythmia, myocardial infarct, angina, and pregnancy complicated by preeclampsia or eclampsia. Caution to prevent hypermagnesemia is essential.

Hypermagnesemia

Hypermagnesemia represents a serum magnesium concentration in excess of 2.7 mg/dL. Because of the ability of the normal kidney to excrete magnesium, hypermagnesemia is rare.

Causes.   When hypermagnesemia does occur, it usually is related to renal insufficiency and the injudicious use of magnesium-containing medications such as antacids, mineral supplements, or laxatives (Table 31-15). The elderly are particularly at risk because they have age-related reductions in renal function and tend to consume more magnesium-containing medications. Magnesium sulfate is used to treat toxemia of pregnancy and premature labor; in these cases, careful monitoring for signs of hypermagnesemia is essential

Manifestations.   Hypermagnesemia affects neuromuscular and cardiovascular function (see Table 31-15). Because magnesium tends to suppress PTH secretion, hypocalcemia may accompany hypermagnesemia. The signs and symptoms occur only when serum magnesium levels exceed 4.9 mg/dL (2 mmol/L). Deep tendon reflexes begin to decrease as magnesium serum levels exceed 4 mEq/L.[64]

Hypermagnesemia diminishes neuromuscular function, causing hyporeflexia, muscle weakness, and confusion. Magnesium decreases acetylcholine release at the myoneural junction and may cause neuromuscular blockade and respiratory paralysis. Cardiovascular effects are related to the calcium channel–blocking effects of magnesium. Blood pressure is decreased, and the ECG shows an increase in the PR interval, a shortening of the QT interval, T-wave abnormalities, and prolongation of the QRS and PR intervals. Hypotension due to vasodilation and cardiac dysrhythmias can occur with moderate hypermagnesemia (<10 mg/dL), and confusion and coma can occur with severe hypermagnesemia (≥10 mg/dL). Very severe hypermagnesemia (>15 mg/dL) may cause cardiac arrest.

Treatment.   The treatment of hypermagnesemia includes cessation of magnesium administration. Calcium is a direct antagonist of magnesium, and intravenous administration of calcium may be used. Peritoneal dialysis or hemodialysis may be required.

TABLE 31-15 ✦ Causes and Manifestations of Hypermagnesemia

Causes	Manifestations
Excessive Intake	**Laboratory Values**
Intravenous administration of magnesium for treatment of preeclampsia	Serum values in excess of 2.7 mg/dL
Excessive use of oral magnesium-containing medications	**Neuromuscular Manifestations**
Decreased Excretion	Lethargy
	Hyporeflexia
Kidney disease	Confusion
Glomerulonephritis	Coma
Tubulointerstitial kidney disease	
Acute renal failure	**Cardiovascular Manifestations**
	Hypotension
	Cardiac dysrhythmias
	Cardiac arrest

In summary, calcium, phosphate, and magnesium are major divalent ions in the body. Calcium is a major divalent cation. Approximately 99% of body calcium is found in bone; less than 1% is found in the extracellular fluid compartment. The calcium in bone is in dynamic equilibrium with extracellular calcium. Of the three forms of extracellular calcium (*i.e.*, protein bound, complexed, and ionized), only the ionized form can cross the cell membrane and contribute to cellular function. Ionized calcium has a number of functions. It contributes to neuromuscular function, plays a vital role in the blood clotting process, and participates in a number of enzyme reactions. Alterations in ionized calcium levels produce neural effects; neural excitability is increased in hypocalcemia and decreased in hypercalcemia.

Phosphate is largely an intracellular anion. It is incorporated into the nucleic acids and ATP. The most common causes of altered levels of serum phosphate are alterations in intestinal absorption, transcompartmental shifts, and disorders of renal elimination. Phosphate deficit causes signs and symptoms of neural dysfunction, disturbed musculoskeletal function, and hematologic disorders. Most of these manifestations result from a decrease in cellular energy stores from a deficiency in ATP and oxygen transport by 2,3-diphosphoglycerate in the red blood cell. Phosphate excess occurs with renal failure and PTH deficit; it is associated with decreased serum calcium levels.

Magnesium is the second most abundant intracellular cation. It acts as a cofactor in many enzyme reactions and affects neuromuscular function in the same manner as the calcium ion. Magnesium deficiency can result from insufficient intake, excessive losses, or movement between the extracellular and intracellular compartments. Hypomagnesemia impairs PTH release and the actions of PTH; it leads to a reduction in intracellular potassium and impairs the ability of the kidney to conserve potassium. The signs and symptoms of hypomagnesemia are therefore similar to those of hypocalcemia. Hypermagnesemia usually is related to renal insufficiency and the injudicious use of magnesium-containing medications such as antacids, mineral supplements, or laxatives. It can cause neuromuscular dysfunction with hyporeflexia, muscle weakness, and confusion. Magnesium decreases acetylcholine release at the myoneural junction and may cause neuromuscular blockade and respiratory paralysis.

Related Web Sites

Diarrhea/Rehydration Information   www.rehydrate.org/html/deh.htm

Merck Manual of Geriatrics (fluid and electrolytes in the elderly)   www.merck.com/pubs/mm_geriatrics/3×.htm

National Diabetes Insipidus Foundation   www.ndif.org/index.html

World Health Organization (site contains information on diarrhea in children, cholera, rehydration)   www.who.int

References

1. Krieger J.N., Sherrad D.J. (1991). *Practical fluid and electrolytes* (pp. 104–105). Norwalk, CT: Appleton & Lange.
2. Guyton A., Hall J.E. (2001). *Textbook of medical physiology* (10th ed., pp. 158–171, 264–278, 322–345, 820–826). Philadelphia: W. B. Saunders.
3. Rose B.D., Post T.W. (2001). *Clinical physiology of acid-base and electrolyte disorders* (5th ed., pp. 187–190, 478–479, 547, 841–842, 896–897). New York: McGraw-Hill.
4. Kokko J.P. (1996). Disorders of fluid volume, electrolyte, and acid-base balance. In Bennett J.C., Plum F. (Eds.), *Cecil textbook of medicine* (20th ed., p. 525–543). Philadelphia: W.B. Saunders.
5. Cogan M.G. (1991). *Fluid and electrolytes* (pp. 43, 112–123, 80–84, 1, 100–111, 125–130, 242–245). Norwalk, CT: Appleton & Lange.
6. Stearns R.H., Spital A., Clark E. C. (1996). Disorders of water balance. In Kokko J., Tannen R.L. (Eds.), *Fluids and electrolytes* (3rd ed., pp. 65, 69, 95). Philadelphia: W.B. Saunders.
7. Metheney N.M. (2000). *Fluid and electrolyte balance* (4th ed., pp. 3, 18, 47, 56, 256). Philadelphia: Lippincott Williams & Wilkins.
8. Porth C.J.M., Erickson M. (1992). Physiology of thirst and drinking: Implications for nursing practice. *Heart and Lung* 21, 273–284.
9. Ayus J.C., Arieff A.I. (1996). Abnormalities of water metabolism in the elderly. *Seminars in Nephrology* 16 (4), 277–288.
10. Rolls B., Phillips P.A. (1990). Aging and disturbances of thirst and fluid balance. *Nutrition Reviews* 48 (3), 137–143.
11. Phillips P.A., Johnson C.L., Gray L. (1993). Disturbed fluid and electrolyte homeostasis following dehydration in elderly people. *Age and Ageing* 22, S26–S33.
12. Kugler J.P., Hustead T. (2000). Hyponatremia and hypernatremia in the elderly. *American Family Physician* 61, 3623–3630.
13. Illowsky B.P., Kirch D.G. (1988). Polydipsia and hyponatremia in psychiatric patients. *American Journal of Psychiatry* 145, 675–683.
14. Vieweg W.V.R. (1994). Treatment strategies for polydipsia-hyponatremia syndrome. *Journal of Clinical Psychiatry* 55 (4), 154–159.
15. Berne R.M., Levy M. (2000). *Principles of physiology* (3rd ed., p. 438). St Louis: Mosby.
16. Robertson G.L. (1983). Thirst and vasopressin function in normal and disordered states of water balance. *Journal of Laboratory and Clinical Medicine* 101, 351–371.
17. Robertson G.L. (1995). Diabetes insipidus. *Endocrinology and Metabolic Clinics of North America* 24, 549–571.
18. Holzman E.J., Ausiello D.A. (1994). Nephrogenic diabetes insipidus: Causes revealed. *Hospital Practice* 29 (3), 89–104.
19. Miller K.L (1996). Diabetes insipidus. *ANNA Journal* 23 (3), 285–293.
20. Singer I., Oster J.R., Fishman L.M. (1997). The management of diabetes insipidus in adults. *Archives of Internal Medicine* 157, 1293–1301.
21. Bendz H., Aurell M. (1999). Drug-induced diabetes insipidus. *Drug Safety* 21, 449–456.
22. Batchell J. (1994). Syndrome of inappropriate antidiuretic hormone. *Critical Care Clinics of North America* 69, 687–691.
23. Kumar S., Beri T. (1998). Sodium. *Lancet* 352, 220–228.
24. Fried L.F., Palevsky P.M. (1997). Hyponatremia and Hypernatremia. *Medical Clinics of North America* 81, 585–606.
25. Androgue H.J., Madias N.E. (2000). Hyponatremia. *New England Journal of Medicine* 343, 1581–1589.

26. Schreir R.W., Briner V.A. (1994). The differential diagnosis of hyponatremia. *Hospital Practice* 29 (9), 29–37.

27. Oh M.S., Carroll H.J. (1992). Disorders of sodium metabolism: Hypernatremia and hyponatremia. *Critical Care Medicine* 20, 94–103.

28. McManus M.L., Churchwell K.B., Strange K. (1995). Regulation of cell volume in health and disease. *New England Journal of Medicine* 333, 1260–1266.

29. Sterns R.H. (1994). Treating hyponatremia. *Southern Medical Journal* 87, 1283–1287.

30. Oh M.S. (1995). Recommendations for treatment of symptomatic hyponatremia. *Nephron* 70, 143–150.

31. Androgue H.J. (2000). Hypernatremia. *New England Journal of Medicine* 342, 1493–1499.

32. Casteel H.B., Fiedorek S. C. (1990). Oral rehydration therapy. *Pediatric Clinics of North America* 37, 295–311.

33. Behrman R.E., Kliegman R.M., Jenson H.B. (2000). *Nelson textbook of pediatrics* (16th ed., pp. 215–218). Philadelphia: W.B Saunders.

34. Meyers A. (1995). Modern management of acute diarrhea and dehydration in children. *American Family Physician* 51 (5), 1103–1118.

35. Weisman Z. (1986). Cola drinks and rehydration in acute diarrhea [Letter]. *New England Journal of Medicine* 315, 768.

36. Bräxmeyer D.L., Keyes J.L. (1996). The pathophysiology of potassium balance. *Critical Care Nurse* 16 (5), 59–71.

37. Knochel J.F. (1987). Etiology and management of potassium deficiency. *Hospital Practice* 22 (1), 153–160.

38. Mandel A.K. (1997). Hypokalemia and hyperkalemia. *Medical Clinics of North America* 81, 611–639.

39. Gennari F.J. (1998). Hypokalemia. *New England Journal of Medicine* 339, 451–458.

40. Tannen R.L (1996). Potassium disorders. In Kokko J., Tannen R.L. (Eds.). *Fluids and electrolytes* (3rd ed., pp. 116–118). Philadelphia: W. B. Saunders.

41. Knochel J.P. (1982). Neuromuscular manifestations of electrolyte disorders. *American Journal of Medicine* 72 (3), 521–535.

42. Whang G., Whang G.G., Ryan M.P. (1992). Refractory potassium repletion: A consequence of magnesium deficiency. *Archives of Internal Medicine* 152 (1), 40–45.

43. Clark B.A., Brown R.S. (1995). Potassium homeostasis and hyperkalemic syndromes. *Endocrinology and Metabolic Clinics of North America* 24, 573–590.

44. Slatopolsky E., Dusso A., Brown A. (1999). New analogs of vitamin D3. *Kidney International* 56 (Suppl. 73), S46–S51.

45. Korbin S.M., Goldfarb S. (1990). Magnesium deficiency. *Seminars in Nephrology* 10, 525–535.

46. Llach F. (1999). Hyperphosphemia in end-stage renal disease patients: Pathological consequences. *Kidney International* 56 (Suppl. 73), S31–S37.

47. Slaptopolsky E., Brown A., Dusso A. (1999). Pathogenesis of secondary hyperthyroidism. *Kidney International* 56 (Suppl. 73), S14–S19.

48. Zaloga G.F. (1992). Hypocalcemia in critically ill patients. *Critical Care Medicine* 20, 251–262.

49. Yucha C.B., Toto K.H. (1994). Calcium and phosphorous derangements. *Critical Care Clinics of North America* 6, 747–765.

50. Reber R.M., Heath H. (1995). Hypocalcemic emergencies. *Medical Clinics of North America* 79, 93–165.

51. Marx S.J. (1996). Diseases of bone and bone metabolism. In Bennett J.C., Plum F. (Eds.), *Cecil textbook of medicine* (20th ed., pp. 1363–1373). Philadelphia: W.B. Saunders.

52. Kaplan M. (1994). Hypercalcemia of malignancy. *Oncology Nursing Forum* 21 (6), 1039–1046.

53. Barnett M.L. (1999). Hypercalcemia. *Seminars in Oncology Nursing* 15, 190–201.

54. Edelson G.W., Kleerekoper M. (1995). Hypercalcemic crisis. *Medical Clinics of North America* 79, 79–92.

55. Dennis V.W. (1996). Phosphate disorders. In Kokko J., Tannen R.L. (Eds.), *Fluids and electrolytes* (3rd ed., pp. 359–382). Philadelphia: W.B. Saunders.

56. Hodgson S.F., Hurley D. (1993). Acquired hypophosphatemia. *Endocrinology and Metabolism Clinics of North America* 22, 397–409.

57. Weisinger J., Bellorin-Font E. (1998). Magnesium and phosphate. *Lancet* 352, 391–396.

58. Fass R., Do S., Hixson L.J. (1993). Fatal hyperphosphatemia following Fleet Phospho-Soda in patient with colonic ileus. *American Journal of Gastroenterology* 88 (6), 929–932.

59. Workman L. (1992). Magnesium and phosphorus: The neglected electrolytes. *ACCN Clinical Issues* 3, 655–663.

60. Swain R., Kaplan-Machlis B. (1999). Magnesium for the next millennium. *Southern Medical Journal* 92, 1040–1046.

61. Nadler J.L., Rude R.K. (1995). Disorders of magnesium metabolism. *Endocrinology and Metabolism Clinics of North America* 24, 623–639.

62. Rude R.K. (1998). Magnesium deficiency: A cause for heterogenous disease in humans. *Journal of Bone and Mineral Metabolism* 13, 749–755.

63. Toto K., Yucha C.B. (1994). Magnesium: Homeostasis, imbalances, and therapeutic uses. *Critical Care Nursing Clinics of North America* 6, 767–778.

64. Matz R. (1993). Magnesium deficiencies and therapeutic uses. *Hospital Practice* 28 (4), 79–92.

Alterations in Acid-Base Balance

Metabolic activities of the body require the precise regulation of acid-base balance, which is reflected by the pH of extracellular fluid. Membrane excitability, enzyme systems, and chemical reactions depend on pH being regulated within a narrow physiologic range to function in an optimal way. Many conditions, pathologic or otherwise, can alter body pH. This chapter has been organized into two sections: Mechanisms of Acid-Base Balance and Alterations in Acid-Base Balance.

Mechanisms of Acid-Base Balance

After you have completed this section of the chapter, you should be able to meet the following objectives:

✦ Characterize an acid and a base
✦ Cite the source of metabolic acids
✦ Describe the three forms of carbon dioxide transport and their contribution to acid-base balance
✦ Use the Henderson-Hasselbalch equation to calculate pH and compare compensatory mechanisms for regulating pH

✦ Describe the intracellular and extracellular mechanisms for buffering changes in body pH
✦ Compare the role of the kidneys and respiratory system in regulation of acid-base balance
✦ Explain how potassium and hydrogen ions and how bicarbonate and chloride ions interact in pH regulation

Normally, the concentration of body acids and bases is regulated so that the pH of extracellular body fluids is maintained within a very narrow range of 7.35 to 7.45. This balance is maintained through mechanisms that generate, buffer, and eliminate acids and bases. This section focuses on acid-base chemistry, the production and regulation of metabolic acids and bicarbonate, and calculation of pH.

ACID-BASE CHEMISTRY

An *acid* is a molecule that can release a hydrogen ion (H^+), and a *base* is a molecule that can accept or combine with an H^+ ion. When an acid (HA) is added to water, it dissociates reversibly to form H^+ and anions (*e.g.*, HA $\rightleftharpoons$ H^+ + A^- [A = anion]). The degree to which an acid dissociates and acts as a H^+ ion donor determines whether it is a strong or weak acid. *Strong acids*, such as sulfuric acid, dissociate completely; *weak acids*, such as acetic acid, dissociate only to a limited extent. The same is true of a base and its ability to dissociate and accept an H+ ion. Most of the body's acids and bases are weak acids and bases; the most important are *carbonic acid*, which is a weak acid derived from carbon dioxide, and *bicarbonate*, which is a weak base.

The concentration of the H+ ion in body fluids is low compared with other ions. For example, the sodium ion (Na+) is present at a concentration approximately 1 million times that of the H+ ion. Because of its low concentration in body fluids, the H+ ion is commonly expressed in terms of pH. Specifically, *pH* represents the negative logarithm (p) of the H+ ion concentration in milliequivalents per liter; a pH value of 7.0 implies a hydrogen ion concentration of 10^{-7} (0.0000001) equivalents per liter (mEq/L). The pH is inversely related to the H+ ion concentration; a low pH indicates a high concentration of H+ ions and a high pH a low concentration of H+ ions.

The *dissociation constant* (K) is used to describe the degree to which an acid or base dissociates. The symbol pK_a

refers to the negative logarithm of the dissociation constant for an acid and represents the pH at which the acid is 50% dissociated. The use of a negative logarithm for the dissociation constant allows pH to be expressed as a positive value. Each acid in an aqueous solution has a characteristic pK_a that varies slightly with temperature and pH. At normal body temperature, the pK_a for the bicarbonate buffer system of the extracellular fluid compartment is 6.1.

METABOLIC ACID AND BICARBONATE PRODUCTION

Acids are continuously generated as byproducts of metabolic processes. Physiologically, these acids fall into two groups: the volatile acid carbonic acid (H_2CO_3) and all other nonvolatile or fixed acids.

The difference between the two types of acids arises because H_2CO_3 is in equilibrium with the volatile carbon dioxide gas (CO_2), which leaves the body by way of the lungs (Fig. 32-1). The concentration of H_2CO_3 is therefore

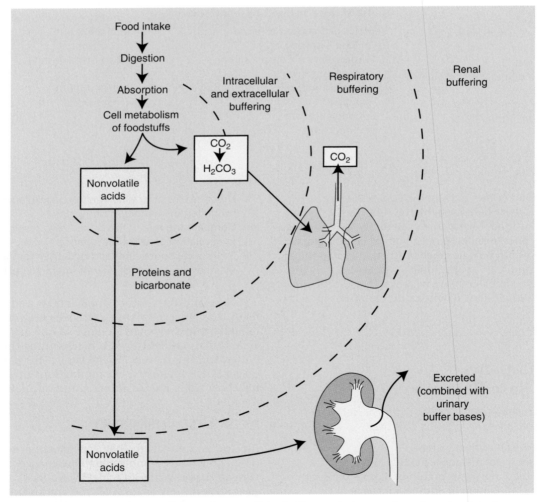

FIGURE 32-1 The role of intracellular and extracellular buffer, respiratory, and renal mechanisms in maintaining normal blood pH. (Rhoades R.A., Tanner G.A. [1996]. *Medical physiology* [p. 468]. Boston: Little, Brown)

determined by the lungs and their respiratory capacity. The *noncarbonic acids* (*e.g.*, sulfuric, hydrochloric, phosphoric) are *nonvolatile* and are not eliminated by the lungs. Instead, they are buffered by body proteins or extracellular buffers, such as bicarbonate, and then excreted by the kidney.

Carbon Dioxide and Bicarbonate Production

Body metabolism results in the production of approximately 15,000 mmol of CO_2 each day.[1] Carbon dioxide is transported in the circulation in three forms: attached to hemoglobin, dissolved (in the serum) CO_2, and as bicarbonate (Fig. 32-2). Collectively, dissolved CO_2 and bicarbonate constitute approximately 77% of the CO_2 that is transported in the extracellular fluid; the remaining CO_2 travels attached to hemoglobin. Although CO_2 is not an acid, a small percentage of the gas combines with water in the bloodstream to form carbonic acid (H_2CO_3):

$$CO_2 + H_2O \rightleftharpoons H_2CO_3 \rightleftharpoons H^+ + HCO_3^-$$

The reaction between CO_2 and water is catalyzed by an enzyme called *carbonic anhydrase*, which is present in large quantities in red blood cells, renal tubular cells, and other tissues in the body. The rate of the reaction between CO_2 and water is increased approximately 5000 times by the presence of carbonic anhydrase. Were it not for this enzyme, the reaction would occur too slowly to be of any significance.

Because it is almost impossible to measure H_2CO_3, dissolved CO_2 measurements are commonly substituted when calculating pH. The H_2CO_3 content of the blood can be calculated by multiplying the partial pressure of CO_2 (PCO_2) by its solubility coefficient, which is 0.03. This means that the concentration of H_2CO_3 in venous blood, which normally has a PCO_2 of approximately 45 mm Hg, is 1.35 mEq/L ($45 \times 0.03 = 1.35$).

Production of Metabolic Acids

The metabolism of dietary proteins is the major source of strong *inorganic acids*—sulfuric acid, hydrochloric acid, and phosphoric acid.[2] Oxidation of the sulfur-containing amino acids (*e.g.*, methionine, cysteine, cystine) results in the production of sulfuric acid. Oxidation of arginine and lysine produces hydrochloric acid, and oxidation of phosphorus-containing nucleic acids yields phosphoric acid. Incomplete oxidation of glucose results in the formation of lactic acid, and incomplete oxidation of fats results in the production of ketoacids. The major source of base is the metabolism of amino acids such as aspartate and glutamate and the metabolism of certain organic anions (*e.g.*, citrate, lactate, acetate). Acid production normally exceeds base production, with the net effect being the addition of approximately 1 mmol/kg body weight of nonvolatile acid to the body each day.[2] A vegetarian diet, which contains large amounts of organic anions, results in the net production of base.

CALCULATION OF pH

The serum pH can be calculated using an equation called the *Henderson-Hasselbalch equation* (Fig. 32-3). This equation uses the negative logarithm of the dissociation constant and the logarithm of the bicarbonate to carbon dioxide (HCO_3^-/CO_2) ratio to calculate pH:

$$pH = pK_a + \log \frac{[HCO_3^-]}{[CO_2]}$$

It is the ratio rather than the absolute values for bicarbonate and dissolved CO_2 that determines pH (*e.g.*, when the ratio is 20:1, pH = 7.4). Let us consider two examples to emphasize this point. The first situation uses normal serum values (HCO_3 = 24 mEq/L, PCO_2 = 40 mm Hg [1.2 mEq/L H_2CO_3])

Situation 1
$$pH = 7.4 = 6.1 + \log \frac{24 \text{ mEq/L } (HCO_3^-)}{1.2 \text{ mEq/L } (H_2CO_3)}$$

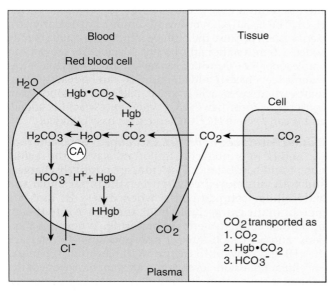

FIGURE 32-2 Mechanisms of carbon dioxide transport. (Adapted from Guyton A.C., Hall J.E. [1996]. *Textbook of medical physiology* [9th ed.]. Philadelphia: W.B. Saunders)

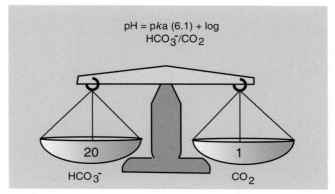

FIGURE 32-3 The Henderson-Hasselbalch equation expressed as a simple scale.

The second situation uses increased serum values (HCO_3 = 48 mEq/L, PCO_2 = 80 mm Hg [2.4 mEq/L H_2CO_3])

Situation 2

$$pH = 7.4 = 6.1 + \log \frac{48 \text{ mEq/L } (HCO_3^-)}{2.4 \text{ mEq/L } (H_2CO_3)}$$

These examples demonstrate that pH remains relatively stable over a wide range of changes in bicarbonate and dissolved CO_2 concentrations, provided the two concentrations approach a ratio of 20:1 (Fig. 32-4). Plasma pH decreases when the ratio is less than 20:1, and it increases when the ratio is greater than 20:1.

The Henderson-Hasselbalch equation provides the mechanism for calculating pH, and it provides an insight into the physiologic control of acid-base balance. The bicarbonate part of the equation is controlled by the generation of metabolic acids and the availability of bicarbonate to buffer these acids. The H_2CO_3 part of the equation is regulated by respiration. The equation could be represented as:

$$pH = pK_a + \log \frac{[HCO_3^-] \text{ (controlled by metabolism)}}{[CO_2] \text{ (controlled by respiration)}}$$

The kidney functions in the generation and reabsorption of bicarbonate and contributes to control of the metabolic part of the equation.

REGULATION OF pH

The pH of body fluids is regulated by intracellular and extracellular buffering systems that prevent large changes in the extracellular pH from occurring through respiratory mechanisms that eliminate CO_2 and by renal mechanisms that conserve bicarbonate and eliminate H^+ ions. The pH

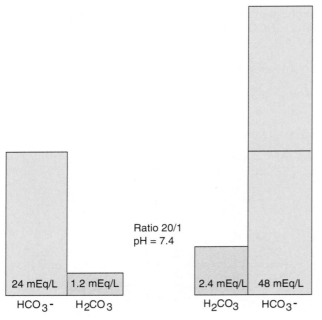

FIGURE 32-4 It is the ratio of HCO_3^- to H_2CO_3 that determines pH, not the concentration.

is further influenced by the electrolyte composition of the intracellular and extracellular compartments.

Intracellular and Extracellular Buffer Systems

The moment-by-moment regulation of pH depends on intracellular and extracellular buffer systems. A *buffer system* consists of a weak acid and the base salt of that acid or of a weak base and its acid salt. In the process of preventing large changes in pH, the system trades a strong acid for a weak acid or a strong base for a weak base.

The two major buffer systems that protect the pH of body fluids are proteins and the bicarbonate buffer system. These buffer systems are immediately available to combine with excess acids or bases and prevent large changes in pH from occurring during the time it takes for respiratory and renal mechanisms to become effective. Bone also represents an important site for buffering of acids and bases. Although it is difficult to measure, it has been estimated that 40% of acute acid-base buffering occurs in bone.[1] The role of bone buffers is even higher in chronic acid-base disorders. One consequence of bone buffering is the release of calcium from bone and increased renal excretion of calcium. In addition to causing demineralization of bone, it also predisposes to kidney stones.

Protein Buffer Systems.   Proteins are the largest buffer system in the body. Proteins are amphoteric, meaning that they can function as acids or bases. They contain many ionizable groups that can release or bind H^+. The protein buffers are largely located in cells, and H^+ ions and CO_2 diffuse across cell membranes for buffering by intracellular proteins. Albumin and plasma globulins are the major protein buffers in the vascular compartment.

Bicarbonate Buffer System.   The bicarbonate buffer system uses carbonic acid as its weak acid and bicarbonate as its weak base. It substitutes the weak carbonic acid for a strong acid such as hydrochloric acid ($HCl + NaHCO_3 \rightleftharpoons H_2CO_3 + NaCl$) or the weak bicarbonate base for a strong base such as sodium hydroxide ($NaOH + H_2CO_3 \rightleftharpoons NaHCO_3 + H_2O$). The HCO_3^-/CO_2 buffer system is a particularly efficient system because the buffer components can be readily added or removed from the body.[2,3] Metabolism provides an ample supply of CO_2, which can replace any H_2CO_3 that is lost when excess base is added, and CO_2 can be readily eliminated when excess acid is added. Likewise, the kidney can conserve or form new HCO_3^- when excess acid is added, and it can excrete HCO_3^- when excess base is added.

Plasma Potassium-Hydrogen Exchange.   Potassium ions (K^+) and H^+ ions interact in important ways in the regulation of acid-base balance. Both ions are positively charged, and both ions move freely between the intracellular and extracellular compartments; when excess H^+ ions are present in the extracellular fluid, they move into the intracellular compartment for buffering. When this happens, another cation—in this case, potassium—must leave the cell and move into the extracellular fluid. When extracellular potassium levels fall, potassium moves out of the cell and is replaced by H^+ ions. Thus, alterations in potassium levels can affect acid-base balance, and changes in acid-base balance can influence potassium levels. Potassium shifts tend to be more pronounced in acidemia than alkalemia and are greater in metabolic acidosis than respiratory acidosis.[3,4] Metabolic acidosis caused by an accumulation of non-organic acids (*e.g.*, hydrochloric acid that occurs in diarrhea, phosphoric acid that occurs in renal failure) produces a greater increase in potassium than does acidosis caused by an accumulation of organic acids (*e.g.*, lactic acid, ketoacids).

An important implication of the potassium and hydrogen transmembrane exchange is its effect on the resting membrane potential of neurons and other excitable tissue. In acidosis, increased levels of extracellular potassium cause the resting membrane potential to become less negative or depolarized such that a smaller stimulus is needed for excitation (see Chapter 31). In alkalosis, decreased levels of extracellular potassium cause the resting membrane potential to become more negative or hyperpolarized so that neurons become less excitable. Changes in neural excitability are further influenced by alterations in ionized calcium. In acidosis, the ionized portion of the extracellular calcium is increased, making neurons less excitable, and in alkalosis, the amount of ionized calcium is reduced, making neurons more excitable.

Respiratory Control Mechanisms

The respiratory system provides for the elimination of CO_2 into the air and plays a major role in acid-base regulation. An elevated PCO_2 is a powerful stimulus for ventilation. CO_2 readily crosses the blood-brain barrier and in the process reacts with water to form carbonic acid, which dissociates into H^+ and HCO_3^- ions. It is the H^+ ion that stimulates the respiratory center, causing an increase or decrease in ventilation. The respiratory control of pH is rapid, occurring within minutes, and is maximal within 12 to 24 hours.[1] Although the respiratory response is rapid, it does not completely return the pH to normal. Although CO_2 readily crosses the blood-brain barrier, there is a lag for entry of the HCO_3^- ion. Thus, blood pH and bicarbonate levels drop more rapidly than cerebrospinal fluid (CSF) levels. In metabolic acidosis, for example, there is often a 12- to 32-hour delay in maximal respiratory response.[2] Likewise, when metabolic acid-base disorders are corrected rapidly, the respiratory response may persist because of a delay in CSF adjustments.

In severe ketoacidosis and other forms of metabolic acidosis, the peripheral arterial chemoreceptors in the aortic and carotid bodies, rather than the medullary chemoreceptors in the brain, provide the major stimulus for ventilation. In this case, rapid correction of acidosis by administration of sodium bicarbonate may decrease the respiratory stimulus for ventilation. Because of the delay in HCO_3^- ion entry into the CSF, there may be a drop in the pH of the CSF that occurs simultaneously with a rise in blood pH.

Renal Control Mechanisms

The kidneys regulate acid-base balance by excreting an acidic or an alkaline urine. Excreting an acidic urine reduces the amount of acid in the extracellular fluid, and excreting an alkaline urine removes base from the extracellular fluid. The renal mechanisms for regulating acid-base balance cannot adjust the pH within minutes, as respiratory mechanisms can, but they continue to function for days until the pH has returned to normal or near-normal range.

Hydrogen Ion Elimination and Bicarbonate Conservation. The average diet contains acid-generating foods. The strong acids produced by metabolism of these foods combine with buffers, particularly bicarbonate. The kidney must then secrete the excess H^+ ions and restore the HCO_3^- ions. Bicarbonate is freely filtered in the glomerulus (approximately 4500 mEq/day).[3] Loss of even small amounts of bicarbonate impairs the body's ability to buffer its daily load of metabolic acids.

Most of the H^+ ion secretion and reabsorption of bicarbonate ions takes place in the proximal tubule. The process begins with a coupled Na^+/H^+ transport system in which a H^+ ion is secreted into the tubular fluid and a Na^+ ion is reabsorbed into the tubular cell (Fig. 32-5). The secreted H^+ ion combines with a filtered HCO_3^- ion to yield CO_2 and H_2O. The water is eliminated in the urine, and the CO_2 diffuses into the tubular cell, where it combines with water, in a carbonic anhydrase–mediated reaction to form a HCO_3^- ion and a H^+ ion. The HCO_3^- ion is reabsorbed into the blood along with the Na^+ ion; the newly generated H^+ ion is secreted into the tubular fluid to begin another cycle. Normally, only a few of the secreted H^+ ions remain in the tubular fluid because the secretion of H^+ ions is roughly equivalent to the number of HCO_3^- ions that are filtered in the glomerulus.

Tubular Buffering Systems. Because an extremely acidic urine would be damaging to structures in the urinary tract, the pH of the urine is maintained within a range from 4.5 to 8.0. This limits the number of unbuffered H^+ ions that can be excreted by the kidney. When the number of free H^+ ions secreted into the tubular fluid threatens to cause the pH of the urine to become too acidic, they must be carried in some other form. This is accomplished by combining H^+ ions with intratubular buffers before they are excreted in

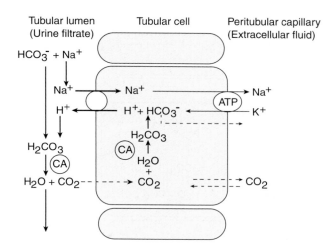

FIGURE 32-5 Hydrogen ion (H^+) secretion and bicarbonate ion (HCO_3^-) reabsorption in a renal tubular cell. Carbon dioxide (CO_2) diffuses from the blood or urine filtrate into the tubular cell, where it combines with water in a carbonic anhydrase-catalyzed reaction that yields carbonic acid (H_2CO_3). The H_2CO_3 dissociates to form H^+ and HCO_3^-. The H^+ is secreted into the tubular fluid in exchange for Na^+. The Na^+ and HCO_3^- enter the extracellular fluid.

the urine. There are two important intratubular buffer systems: the phosphate buffer system and the ammonia buffer system.

The *phosphate buffer system* uses HPO_4^{2-} and $H_2PO_4^-$ that are present in the tubular filtrate. The combination of H^+ with HPO_4^{2-} to form $H_2PO_4^-$ allows the kidneys to increase their secretion of H^+ ions (Fig. 32-6). Because they are poorly reabsorbed, the phosphates become more concentrated as they move through the tubules. This system works best when the renal tubular fluid contains a high concentration of H^+ ions.

Another important but more complex buffer system is the *ammonia buffer system*. Renal tubular cells are able to use the amino acid glutamine to synthesize ammonia (NH_3) and secrete it into the tubular fluid (Fig. 32-7). The H^+ ions then combine with the NH_3 to form an ammonium ion (NH_4^+). The NH_4^+ ions combine with chloride ions (Cl^-), which are present in the tubular fluid, to form ammonium chloride (NH_4Cl), which is then excreted in the urine. The ammonia buffer system allows for elimination of Cl^- and H^+ ions without effecting a change in urine pH. Although most of the negative ions in the tubular fluid are Cl^- ions, only a few Cl^- ions can be transported in direct combination with H^+ because the generation of hydrochloric acid would cause a sharp drop in urine pH. The ammonia buffer system requires large amounts of an enzyme that deaminates the glutamine that is used in ammonia synthesis; it takes 2 or 3 days for the tubular cells to increase enzyme synthesis and for this buffer system to become efficient.

The kidney also participates in gluconeogenesis (*i.e.*, generation of new glucose from sources such as amino acids). The use of glutamine for buffering metabolic acids enables the kidney to increase its production of glucose. This can be particularly effective in situations of starvation and calorie deprivation, when excess ketoacids are formed as

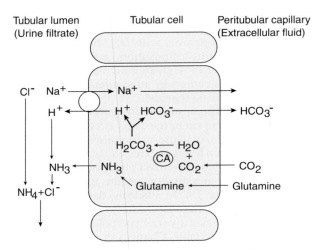

FIGURE 32-7 The ammonia buffer system in a renal tubular cell. The tubular cell synthesizes ammonia (NH_3) from glutamine. The NH_3 is secreted into the tubular fluid, where it combines with an H^+ to form an ammonium ion (NH_4^+). The ammonium ion combines with chloride for excretion in the urine. The HCO_3^- moves into the extracellular fluid along with the Na^+ that was exchanged during secretion of the H^+.

the body reverts to using body fats and proteins as fuel sources. In this case, the kidney uses glutamine for generating the ammonia needed for buffering excess metabolic acids and as a substrate for gluconeogenesis and maintenance of blood glucose levels.

Hydrogen and Potassium Ions Compete for Elimination in the Urine. Plasma potassium levels influence renal elimination of H^+ ions and vice versa. When plasma potassium levels fall, there is movement of K^+ ions from body cells into the plasma and a reciprocal movement of H^+ ions from the plasma into body cells. In the kidney, these movements lower the intracellular pH of tubular cells, causing an increase in H^+ secretion. Potassium depletion also stimulates ammonia synthesis by the kidney as a means of buffering the secreted H^+ ions. The result is increased reabsorption of the filtered bicarbonate and development of metabolic alkalosis. An elevation in plasma potassium has the opposite effect. Because of the K^+/H^+ ion exchange that occurs in the kidney, acidosis tends to increase H^+ ion elimination and decrease K^+ ion elimination, with a resultant increase in serum potassium levels. Alkalosis has the opposite effect; it tends to increase K^+ elimination, producing a decrease in serum potassium levels.

Aldosterone also influences H^+ ion elimination by the kidney. It acts in the collecting duct to indirectly stimulate H^+ ion secretion, while increasing Na^+ ion reabsorption and K^+ secretion. Hyperaldosteronism tends to lead to a decrease in serum potassium levels and increased pH and alkalosis because of increased H^+ ion secretion. Hypoaldosteronism has the opposite effect. It leads to increased potassium levels, decreased H^+ ion secretion, and acidosis.

Influence of Sodium Chloride–Bicarbonate Exchange on pH. Body sodium levels can indirectly influence acid-

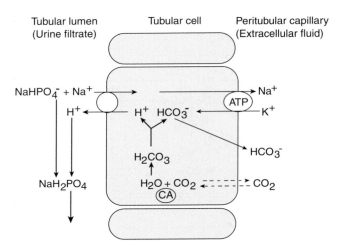

FIGURE 32-6 The renal phosphate buffer system. The mono–hydrogen phosphate ion (HPO_4^{2-}) enters the renal tubular fluid in the glomerulus. A H^+ combines with the HPO_4^{2-} to form $H_2PO_4^-$ and is then excreted into the urine in combination with Na^+. The HCO_3^- moves into the extracellular fluid along with the Na^+ that was exchanged during secretion of the H^+.

base balance by way of the chloride–bicarbonate exchange system. Sodium reabsorption in the kidneys requires the reabsorption of an accompanying anion. The two major anions in the extracellular fluid are Cl^- and HCO_3^-.

One of the mechanisms that the kidneys use in regulating the pH of the extracellular fluids is to conserve or eliminate HCO_3^- ions; in the process, it often is necessary to shuffle anions. Chloride is the most abundant anion in the extracellular fluid and can substitute for bicarbonate when an anion shift is needed. As an example, serum HCO_3^- levels normally increase as hydrochloric acid is secreted into the stomach after a heavy meal, causing what is called the *postprandial alkaline tide*. Later, as the Cl^- is reabsorbed in the small intestine, the pH returns to normal. *Hypochloremic alkalosis* refers to an increase in pH that is induced by a decrease in serum Cl^- levels. *Hyperchloremic acidosis* occurs when excess levels of Cl^- are present.

Mechanisms of Acid-Base Balance

➤ The pH of the extracellular fluid must be maintained within the narrow range of 7.35 to 7.45 for the optimal functioning of body cells.

➤ pH is determined by the ratio of the bicarbonate (HCO_3^-) base to the volatile carbonic acid ($H_2CO_3 \rightleftharpoons H^+ + HCO_3^-$). At a pH of 7.4, the ratio is normally 20 to 1.

➤ The concentration of metabolic acids and bicarbonate base is regulated by the kidney. The concentration of CO_2 is regulated by the respiratory system.

➤ Extracellular (carbonic acid/bicarbonate) and intracellular (proteins) systems buffer the changes in pH that would otherwise occur because of the metabolic production of volatile (CO_2) and non-volatile acids (*i.e.*, sulfuric, phosphoric).

➤ The respiratory system regulates the concentration of the volatile carbonic acid ($CO_2 + H_2O \rightleftharpoons H_2CO_3 \rightleftharpoons H^+ + HCO_3^-$) by changing the rate and depth of respiration.

➤ The kidneys regulate the plasma concentration of HCO_3^- by two processes: reabsorption of the filtered bicarbonate and generation of new bicarbonate. The latter is accomplished by excretion of nonvolatile acids and is an important means by which the body replaces bicarbonate consumed in the process of buffering acids produced by metabolism. The excreted H^+ ions are buffered by tubular buffer systems (phosphate and ammonia) to maintain a luminal pH of at least 4.5.

LABORATORY TESTS

Laboratory tests that are used in assessing acid-base balance include those for arterial blood gases and pH, carbon dioxide content and bicarbonate levels, base excess or deficit, and the anion gap. Although useful in determining whether acidosis or alkalosis is present, the pH of the blood as measured by a pH meter or electrode provides little information about the cause of an acid-base disorder.

Carbon Dioxide and Bicarbonate Levels

Arterial blood gases provide a means of assessing the respiratory component of acid-base balance. Arterial blood gases are used, because venous blood gases are highly variable, depending on metabolic demands of the various tissues that empty into the vein from where the sample is being drawn. The dissolved CO_2 levels can be determined from arterial blood gas measurements using the PCO_2 and the solubility coefficient for CO_2 (normal arterial PCO_2 is 38 to 42 mm Hg). Arterial blood gases also provide a measure of blood oxygen (PO_2) levels. This can be important in assessing respiratory acid-base disorders. Laboratory measurements of electrolytes include the CO_2 content and bicarbonate levels. However, the CO_2 content that is included in these measurements does not refer to arterial blood gases. Instead, it refers to the total CO_2 content of blood, including that contained in bicarbonate. More than 70% of the CO_2 in the blood is in the form of bicarbonate. The CO_2 content is determined by adding a strong acid to a plasma sample and measuring the amount of CO_2 generated. The serum bicarbonate concentration is then determined from the total CO_2 content of the blood. The normal range of values for venous bicarbonate concentration is 24 to 29 mEq/L (24 to 29 mmol/L).

Base Excess or Deficit

Base excess or deficit measures the level of all the buffer systems of the blood—hemoglobin, protein, phosphate, and bicarbonate. The base excess or deficit describes the amount of a fixed acid or base that must be added to a blood sample to achieve a pH of 7.4 (normal ± 3.0 mEq/L).[1] For practical purposes, base excess or deficit is a measurement of bicarbonate excess or deficit. A base excess indicates metabolic alkalosis, and a base deficit indicates metabolic acidosis.

Anion Gap

The anion gap describes the difference between the plasma concentration of the major measured cation (Na^+) and the sum of the measured anions (Cl^- and HCO_3^-). This difference represents the concentration of unmeasured anions, such as phosphates, sulfates, organic acids, and proteins (Fig. 32-8). Normally, the anion gap ranges between 8 and 12 mEq/L (a value of 16 mEq/L is normal if sodium and potassium concentrations are used in the calculation). The anion gap is increased in conditions such as lactic acidosis and ketoacidosis that result from elevated levels of metabolic acids. A low anion gap is found in conditions that produce a fall in unmeasured anions (primarily albumin) or rise in unmeasured cations. The latter can occur in hyperkalemia, hypercalcemia, hypermagnesemia, lithium intoxication, or multiple myeloma, in which an abnormal immunoglobulin is produced.[2]

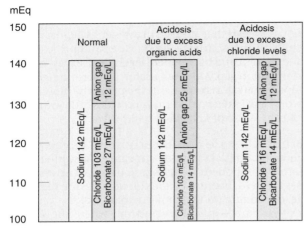

FIGURE 32-8 The anion gap in acidosis due to excess metabolic acids and excess serum chloride levels. Unmeasured anions such as phosphates, sulfates, and organic acids increase the anion gap because they replace bicarbonate. This assumes there is no change in sodium content.

The anion gap of urine can also be measured. It uses values for the measurable cations (Na^+ and K^+) and measurable anion (Cl^-) to provide an estimate of ammonium (NH_4^+) excretion. Because ammonium is a cation, the value of the anion gap becomes more negative as the ammonium level increases. In normal persons secreting 20 to 40 mmol of ammonium per liter, the urine anion gap is close to zero. In metabolic acidosis, the amount of unmeasurable NH_4^+ should increase if renal excretion of H^+ is intact; as a result, the urine anion gap should become more negative.

In summary, normal body function depends on the precise regulation of acid-base balance. The pH of the extracellular fluid is normally maintained within the narrow physiologic range of 7.35 to 7.45. Metabolic processes produce volatile and nonvolatile metabolic acids that must be buffered and eliminated from the body. The volatile acid, H_2CO_3, is in equilibrium with dissolved CO_2, which is eliminated through the lungs. The nonvolatile metabolic acids, most of which are excreted by the kidneys, are derived mainly from protein metabolism and incomplete carbohydrate and fat metabolism. It is the ratio of the bicarbonate ion concentration to dissolved CO_2 (carbonic acid concentration) that determines body pH. When this ratio is 20:1, the pH is 7.4.

The ability of the body to maintain pH within the normal physiologic range depends on respiratory and renal mechanisms and on intracellular and extracellular buffers; the most important of these is the bicarbonate buffer system. The kidney aids in regulation of pH by eliminating H^+ ions or conserving HCO_3^- ions. In the process of eliminating H^+ ions, it uses the phosphate and ammonia buffer systems. Body pH is also affected by the distribution of exchangeable cations (K^+ and H^+) and anions (Cl^- and HCO_3^-).

Laboratory tests that are used in assessing acid-base balance include arterial blood gas measurements, carbon dioxide content and bicarbonate levels, base excess or deficit, and the anion gap. The base excess or deficit describes the amount of a fixed acid or base that must be added to a blood sample to achieve a pH of 7.4. The anion gap describes the difference between the plasma concentration of the major measured cation (Na^+) and the sum of the measured anions (Cl^- and HCO_3^-). This difference represents the concentration of unmeasured anions, such as phosphates, sulfates, organic acids, and proteins, that are present.

Alterations in Acid-Base Balance

After you have completed this section of the chapter, you should be able to meet the following objectives:

+ Differentiate the terms *acidemia, alkalemia, acidosis,* and *alkalosis*
+ Describe a clinical situation involving an acid-base disorder in which primary and compensatory mechanisms might be active
+ Define metabolic acidosis, metabolic alkalosis, respiratory acidosis, and respiratory alkalosis
+ Explain the use of the plasma anion gap in differentiating types of metabolic acidosis
+ List common causes of metabolic and respiratory acidosis and metabolic and respiratory alkalosis
+ Contrast and compare the clinical manifestations and treatment of metabolic and respiratory acidosis and of metabolic and respiratory alkalosis

The terms *acidosis* and *alkalosis* describe the clinical conditions that arise as a result of changes in dissolved CO_2 and HCO_3^- concentration. An alkali represents a combination of one or more alkali metals such as sodium or potassium with a highly basic ion such as a hydroxyl ion (OH^-). Sodium bicarbonate ($NaHCO_3$) is the main alkali in the extracellular fluid. Although the definitions differ somewhat, the terms *alkali* and *base* are often used interchangeably. Hence, the term *alkalosis* has come to mean the opposite of *acidosis*.

METABOLIC VERSUS RESPIRATORY ACID-BASE DISORDERS

There are two types of acid-base disorders: metabolic and respiratory (Table 32-1). *Metabolic disorders* produce an alteration in bicarbonate concentration and result from addition or loss of nonvolatile acid or alkali to or from the extracellular fluid. A decrease in pH due to a reduced bicarbonate is called *metabolic acidosis*, and an elevated pH due to increased bicarbonate levels is called *metabolic alkalosis*. *Respiratory disorders* involve a disorder in the PCO_2, reflecting an increase or decrease in alveolar ventilation. *Respiratory acidosis* is characterized by a decrease in pH, reflecting a decrease in ventilation and an increase in PCO_2. *Respiratory alkalosis* involves an increase in pH, resulting from an increase in alveolar ventilation and a decrease in PCO_2.

TABLE 32-1 ✦ Summary of Acid-Base Imbalances

Acid-Base Imbalance	Primary Disturbance	Respiratory Compensation	Renal Compensation
Metabolic acidosis	Decrease in bicarbonate	Hyperventilation to decrease PCO_2	If no renal disease, increased H^+ excretion and increased HCO_3^- reabsorption
Metabolic alkalosis	Increase in bicarbonate	Hypoventilation to increase PCO_2	If no renal disease, decreased H^+ excretion and decreased HCO_3^- reabsorption
Respiratory acidosis	Increase in PCO_2	None	Increased H^+ excretion and increased HCO_3^- reabsorption
Respiratory alkalosis	Decrease in PCO_2	None	Decreased H^+ excretion and decreased HCO_3^- reabsorption

PRIMARY VERSUS COMPENSATORY MECHANISMS

Acidosis and alkalosis typically involve a *primary* or *initiating event* and a *compensatory state* that results from homeostatic mechanisms that attempt to correct or prevent large changes in pH. For example, a person may have a primary metabolic acidosis as a result of overproduction of ketoacids and respiratory alkalosis because of a compensatory increase in ventilation (see Table 32-1). *Compensatory mechanisms* adjust the pH toward a more normal level without correcting the underlying cause of the disorder. The respiratory mechanisms, which compensate by increasing or decreasing ventilation, are rapid but seldom able to return the pH to normal because, as the pH returns toward normal, the respiratory stimulus is lost. The kidneys compensate by conserving HCO_3^- or H^+ ions. It normally takes longer to recruit renal compensatory mechanisms than it does respiratory compensatory mechanisms. Renal mechanisms are more efficient, however, because they continue to operate until the pH has returned to a normal or near-normal value.

Compensatory mechanisms provide a means to control pH when correction is impossible or cannot be immediately achieved. Often, compensatory mechanisms are interim measures that permit survival while the body attempts to correct the primary disorder. Compensation requires the use of mechanisms that are different from those that caused the primary disorder. In other words, the lungs cannot compensate for respiratory acidosis that is caused by lung disease, nor can the kidneys compensate for metabolic acidosis that occurs because of renal failure. The body can, however, use renal mechanisms to compensate for respiratory-induced changes in pH, and it can use respiratory mechanisms to compensate for metabolically induced changes in acid-base balance. Compensatory mechanisms often become more effective with time, and there are differences between the level of pH change that occurs with acute and chronic acid-base disorders.

Most of the manifestations of acid-base disorders fall into three categories: those associated with the primary disorder that caused the pH disturbance, those related to the altered pH, and those that occur because of the body's attempt to compensate for the altered pH.

METABOLIC ACIDOSIS

Metabolic acidosis involves a primary deficit in base bicarbonate along with a decrease in plasma pH. Metabolic acidosis can result from a decrease in bicarbonate with an increase in the anion gap or from replacement of bicarbonate with chloride ions in which the anion gap remains within the normal range.[5] In metabolic acidosis, the body compensates for the decrease in pH by increasing the respiratory rate in an effort to decrease CO_2 and H_2CO_3 levels.

Causes

Metabolic acidosis can be caused by one of four mechanisms: increased production of nonvolatile metabolic acids, decreased acid secretion by the kidney, excessive loss of bicarbonate, or an increase in chloride. The causes of metabolic acidosis are summarized in Table 32-2.

Metabolic acids increase when there is an accumulation of lactic acid, overproduction of ketoacids, drug and chemical anion ingestion, or an inability of the kidneys to excrete metabolic acids or conserve bicarbonate. The anion gap is often useful in determining the cause of the metabolic acidosis (Chart 32-1). The presence of excess metabolic acids produces an increase in the anion gap as sodium bicarbonate is replaced by the sodium salt of the offending acid (*e.g.*, sodium lactate). When acidosis results from increased chloride levels (*e.g.*, hyperchloremic acidosis), the anion gap remains within normal levels.

Lactic Acidosis.   Acute lactic acidosis is one of the most common types of metabolic acidosis. Lactic acidosis develops when there is excess production of lactic acid or diminished lactic acid removal from the blood. Lactic acid is produced by the anaerobic metabolism of glucose. Virtually all tissues can produce lactic acid under appropriate circumstances. Tissues such as red blood cells, intestine, and skeletal muscle do so under normal conditions. The liver and, to a lesser extent, the kidney normally remove lactic acid from the blood and use it for energy or convert it back to glucose.

Most cases of lactic acidosis are caused by inadequate oxygen delivery, as in shock or cardiac arrest.[6] These conditions increase lactic acid production, and they impair lactic

TABLE 32-2 ✦ Metabolic Acidosis	
Causes	**Manifestations**
Excess Metabolic Acids (Increased Anion Gap)	**Blood pH, HCO₃⁻, CO₂**
Excessive production of metabolic acids	pH decreased
Lactic acidosis	HCO₃⁻ (primary) decreased
Diabetic ketoacidosis	PCO₂ (compensatory) decreased
Alcoholic ketoacidosis	
Fasting and starvation	**Gastrointestinal Function**
Poisoning (*e.g.*, salicylate, methanol, ethylene glycol)	Anorexia
Impaired elimination of metabolic acids	Nausea and vomiting
Kidney failure or dysfunction	Abdominal pain
	Neural Function
Excessive Bicarbonate Loss (Normal Anion Gap)	Weakness
Loss of intestinal secretions	Lethargy
Diarrhea	General malaise
Intestinal suction	Confusion
Intestinal or biliary fistula	Stupor
Increased renal losses	Coma
Renal tubular acidosis	Depression of vital functions
Treatment with carbonic anhydrase inhibitors	
Hyperaldosteronism	**Cardiovascular Function**
	Peripheral vasodilation
Increased Chloride Levels (Normal Anion Gap)	Decreased heart rate
Excessive reabsorption of chloride by the kidney	Cardiac dysrhythmias
Sodium chloride infusions	
Treatment with ammonium chloride	**Skin**
Parenteral hyperalimentation	Warm and flushed
	Skeletal System
	Bone disease (*e.g.*, chronic acidosis)
	Signs of Compensation
	Increased rate and depth of respiration (*i.e.*, Kussmaul breathing)
	Hyperkalemia
	Acid urine
	Increased ammonia in urine

acid clearance because of poor liver perfusion. Mortality rates are high for persons with lactic acidosis because of shock and tissue hypoxia. Excess lactate also is produced with vigorous exercise or grand mal seizures (*i.e.*, convulsions), during which there is a local disproportion between oxygen supply and demand in the contracting muscles.

Lactic acidosis is also associated with disorders in which tissue hypoxia does not appear to be present. It has been reported in patients with leukemia, lymphomas, and other cancers; those with poorly controlled diabetes; and patients with severe liver failure. Mechanisms causing lactic acidosis in these conditions are poorly understood. Some conditions such as neoplasms may produce local increases in tissue metabolism and lactate production or may interfere with blood flow delivery to noncancerous cells. Ethanol produces a slight elevation in lactic acid, but clinically significant lactic acidosis does not occur in alcohol intoxication unless other problems such as liver failure are present. Lactic acidosis may also complicate the severe acidosis that occurs in salicylate poisoning.

Lactic acidosis also occurs in genetic mitochondrial disorders that impair lactate metabolism.[7,8] One of these disorders, referred to by the acronym MELAS, involves mitochondrial encephalopathy (ME), lactic acidosis (LA), and strokelike episodes (S). Children with the disorder are normal for the first few years of life and then begin to display impaired motor and cognitive development. The mitochondrial defect also leads to short stature, seizure disorders, and multiple strokes. Lowering the serum lactate level of children with severe lactic acidosis may result in marked clinical improvement.

A unique form of lactic acidosis, called D-lactic acidosis, can occur in persons with intestinal disorders that involve the generation and absorption of D-lactic acid (L-lactic acid is the usual cause of lactic acidosis). D-lactic acidosis can occur in persons with jejunoileal bypass, small bowel resection, or short bowel syndrome, in which there is impaired reabsorption of carbohydrate in the small intestine.[9] In these cases, the unabsorbed carbohydrate is delivered to the colon, where it is converted to D-lactic acid by an overgrowth of

The Anion Gap in Differential Diagnosis of Metabolic Acidosis

Decreased Anion Gap (<8 mEq/L)

Hypoalbuminemia (decrease in unmeasured anions)
Multiple myeloma (increase in unmeasured cationic IgG paraproteins)
Increased unmeasured cations (hyperkalemia, hypercalcemia, hypermagnesemia, lithium intoxication)

Increased Anion Gap (>12 mEq/L)

Presence of unmeasured metabolic anion
    Diabetic ketoacidosis
    Alcoholic ketoacidosis
    Lactic acidosis
    Starvation
    Renal insufficiency
Presence of drug or chemical anion
    Salicylate poisoning
    Methanol poisoning
    Ethylene glycol poisoning

Normal Anion Gap (8–12 mEq/L)

Loss of bicarbonate
    Diarrhea
    Pancreatic fluid loss
    Ileostomy (unadapted)
Chloride retention
    Renal tubular acidosis
    Ileal loop bladder
    Parenteral nutrition (arginine and lysine)

gram-positive anaerobes. Persons with D-lactic acidosis experience episodic periods of metabolic acidosis often brought on by eating a meal high in carbohydrates. Manifestations include confusion, cerebellar ataxia, slurred speech, and loss of memory. They may complain of feeling (or appear) intoxicated. Treatment includes use of antimicrobial agents to decrease the number of D-lactic acid–producing microorganisms in the bowel along with a low-carbohydrate diet.

Ketoacidosis. Ketoacids (*i.e.*, acetoacetic and β-hydroxybutyric acid), produced in the liver from fatty acids, are the source of fuel for many body tissues. An overproduction of ketoacids occurs when carbohydrate stores are inadequate or when the body cannot use available carbohydrates as a fuel. Under these conditions, fatty acids are mobilized from adipose tissue and delivered to the liver, where they are converted to ketones. Ketoacidosis develops when ketone production exceeds tissue use.

The most common cause of ketoacidosis is uncontrolled diabetes mellitus, in which an insulin deficiency leads to the release of fatty acids from adipose cells with subsequent production of excess ketoacids (see Chapter 41). Ketoacidosis may also develop as the result of fasting or food deprivation, during which the lack of carbohydrates produces a self-limited state of ketoacidosis. The self-limited nature of

ketoacidosis results from a decrease in insulin, which further suppresses the release of fatty acids from fat cells. A ketogenic diet is one that is low in carbohydrate and favors ketoacid production. Over the years, various ketogenic diets have been used for weight reduction; part of the success of these diets derives from symptoms such as anorexia that occur as a consequence of the metabolic acidosis caused by many of these diets.

Ketones are also formed during the oxidation of alcohol, a process that occurs in the liver. A condition called *alcoholic ketoacidosis* can develop in persons who engage in excess alcohol consumption.[10] It usually follows prolonged alcohol ingestion, particularly if accompanied by decreased food intake and vomiting that results in using fatty acids as an energy source. The ketoacids responsible for alcoholic ketoacidosis are formed in part as a result of alcohol metabolism. Extracellular fluid volume depletion caused by vomiting and decreased fluid intake, along with alcohol-induced inhibition of antidiuretic hormone (see Chapter 31), often contribute to the acidosis. Ketone formation may be further enhanced by the hypoglycemia that results from alcohol-induced inhibition of glucose synthesis (*i.e.*, gluconeogenesis) by the liver and impaired ketone elimination by the kidneys because of dehydration. Numerous other factors, such as elevations in cortisol, growth hormone, glucagon, and catecholamines, mediate free fatty acid release and thereby contribute to the development of alcoholic ketoacidosis.

Salicylate Toxicity. Aspirin (acetylsalicylic acid) is rapidly converted to salicylic acid in the body. Salicylate overdose produces serious toxic effects, including death. A fatal overdose can occur with as little as 10 to 30 g in adults and 3 g in children.[1,2] The diagnosis can be made with certainty only by measurement of serum salicylate concentration. Although aspirin is the most common cause of salicylate toxicity, other salicylate preparations such as methyl salicylate, sodium salicylate, and salicylic acid may be involved.

Increasing doses of aspirin cause a progressively greater risk of toxicity because of the saturation of normal protective mechanisms. At therapeutic levels, much of salicylate is protein bound so that it remains in the vascular compartment; the drug is partially changed in the liver to salicyluric acid, which is less toxic and more rapidly excreted by the kidney than salicylate. With salicylate toxicity, these mechanisms become saturated, and renal elimination is decreased and more salicylate is able to reach the tissues and exert its toxic effects.

A variety of acid-base disturbances occur with salicylate toxicity. The salicylates cross the blood-brain barrier and directly stimulate the respiratory center, causing hyperventilation and respiratory alkalosis. The kidneys compensate by secreting increased amounts of bicarbonate, potassium, and sodium, thereby contributing to the development of metabolic acidosis. Salicylates also interfere with carbohydrate metabolism, which results in increased production of metabolic acids.

One of the treatments for salicylate toxicity is *alkalinization* of the plasma. Salicylic acid, which is a weak acid, exists in equilibrium with the alkaline salicylate anion. It is the salicylic acid that is toxic because of its ability to cross cell membranes and enter brain cells. The salicylate anion crosses membranes poorly and is less toxic. With alkalinization of the extracellular fluids, the ratio of salicylic acid to salicylate is greatly reduced. This allows cellular salicylic acid to move out of cells into the extracellular fluid along a concentration gradient. The renal elimination of salicylates follows a similar pattern when the urine is alkalinized.

Methanol and Ethylene Glycol Toxicity. Ingestion of methanol and ethylene glycol results in the production of metabolic acids and causes metabolic acidosis. Both produce an osmolar gap because of their small size and osmotic properties. Methanol (wood alcohol) is a component of shellac, varnish, deicing solutions, sterno, and other commercial products. Methanol can be absorbed through the skin or gastrointestinal tract or inhaled through the lungs. A dose as small as 30 mL can be fatal.[11] In addition to metabolic acidosis, methanol produces severe optic nerve and central nervous system toxicity. Organ system damage occurs after a 24-hour period in which methanol is converted to formaldehyde and formic acid.

Ethylene glycol is a component of antifreeze and solvents. It tastes sweet and is intoxicating, factors that contribute to its abuse potential. A lethal dose is approximately 100 mL. Acidosis occurs as ethylene glycol is converted to oxalic and lactic acid. Manifestations of ethylene glycol toxicity occur in three stages: neurologic symptoms ranging from drunkenness to coma, which appear during the first 12 hours; cardiorespiratory disorders such as tachycardia and pulmonary edema; and flank pain and renal failure caused by plugging of the tubules with oxalate crystals (from excess oxalic acid production).[12]

The enzyme *alcohol dehydrogenase* metabolizes methanol and ethylene glycol into toxic metabolites. This is the same enzyme that is used in the metabolism of ethanol. Because alcohol dehydrogenase has an affinity for ethanol 10 times its affinity for methanol or ethylene glycol, intravenous or oral ethanol is used as an antidote for methanol and ethylene glycol poisoning.[1] Extracellular volume expansion and hemodialysis are also used.

Decreased Renal Function. Renal disease is the most common cause of chronic metabolic acidosis. The kidneys normally conserve HCO_3^- and secrete H^+ ions into the urine as a means of regulating acid-base balance. In renal failure, there is loss of glomerular and tubular function, with retention of nitrogenous wastes and metabolic acids. In a condition called *renal tubular acidosis*, glomerular function is normal, but the tubular secretion of H^+ or reabsorption of HCO_3^- is abnormal. Renal tubular acidosis is discussed in Chapter 33.

Increased Bicarbonate Losses. Increased HCO_3^- losses occur with the loss of bicarbonate-rich body fluids or with impaired conservation of HCO_3^- by the kidney. Intestinal secretions have a high HCO_3^- concentration. Consequently, excessive losses of HCO_3^- ions occur with severe diarrhea; small bowel, pancreatic, or biliary fistula drainage; ileostomy drainage; and intestinal suction. In diarrhea of microbial origin, HCO_3^- is secreted into the bowel to neutralize the metabolic acids produced by the microorganisms causing the diarrhea. Creation of an ileal bladder, which is done for conditions such as neurogenic bladder or surgical removal of the bladder because of cancer, involves the implantation of the ureters into a short, isolated loop of ileum that serves as a conduit for urine collection. With this procedure, contact time between the urine and ileal bladder is normally too short for significant anion exchange, and HCO_3^- is lost in the urine.[1]

Hyperchloremic Acidosis. Hyperchloremic acidosis occurs when Cl^- ion levels are increased. Because Cl^- and HCO_3^- are anions, the HCO_3^- ion concentration decreases when there is an increase in Cl^- ions. Hyperchloremic acidosis can occur as the result of abnormal absorption of chloride by the kidneys or as a result of treatment with chloride-containing medications (*i.e.*, sodium chloride, amino acid–chloride hyperalimentation solutions, and ammonium chloride). Ammonium chloride is broken down into NH_4^+ and Cl^-. The ammonium ion is converted to urea in the liver, leaving the chloride ion free to react with hydrogen to form hydrochloric acid. The administration of intravenous sodium chloride or parenteral hyperalimentation solutions that contain an amino acid–chloride combination can cause acidosis in a similar manner.[13] With hyperchloremic acidosis, the anion gap is within the normal range, but the chloride levels are increased and bicarbonate levels are decreased.

Manifestations

Metabolic acidosis is characterized by a decrease in pH (<7.35) because of an increase in extracellular H^+ ion concentration and a decrease in HCO_3^- levels (<24 mEq/L). Acidosis typically produces a compensatory increase in respiratory rate with a decrease in PCO_2 and H_2CO_3.

The manifestations of metabolic acidosis fall into three categories: signs and symptoms of the disorder causing the acidosis, alterations in function resulting from the decreased pH, and changes in body function related to recruitment of compensatory mechanisms (see Table 32-2). The signs and symptoms of metabolic acidosis usually begin to appear when the plasma HCO_3^- concentration falls to 20 mEq/L or less. Metabolic acidosis is seldom a primary disorder; it usually develops during the course of another disease. The manifestations of metabolic acidosis frequently are superimposed on the symptoms of the contributing health problem. With diabetic ketoacidosis, which is a common cause of metabolic acidosis, there is an increase in blood and urine glucose and a characteristic smell of ketones to the breath. In metabolic acidosis that accompanies renal failure, blood urea nitrogen levels are elevated, and tests of renal function yield abnormal results.

Changes in pH have a direct effect on body function that can produce signs and symptoms common to most types of metabolic acidosis, regardless of cause. A person with metabolic acidosis often complains of weakness, fatigue, general malaise, and a dull headache. The patient also may have anorexia, nausea, vomiting, and abdominal pain. Tissue turgor is impaired, and the skin is dry when fluid deficit accompanies acidosis. In persons with undiagnosed diabetes mellitus, the nausea, vomiting, and abdominal symptoms may be misinterpreted as being caused by gastrointestinal flu or other abdominal disease, such as appendicitis. Neural activity becomes depressed as body pH declines. Acidosis directly depresses membrane excitability, and it decreases binding of calcium to plasma proteins so that more free calcium is available to decrease neural activity. As acidosis progresses, the level of consciousness declines, and stupor and coma develop. The skin is often warm and flushed because skin vessels become less responsive to sympathetic stimulation and lose tone.

When the pH falls to 7.0, cardiac contractility and cardiac output decreases, the heart becomes less responsive to catecholamines (*i.e.*, epinephrine and norepinephrine), and dysrhythmias, including fatal ventricular dysrhythmias, can develop. A decrease in ventricular function may be particularly important in perpetuating shock-induced lactic acidosis, and partial correction of the acidemia may be necessary before tissue perfusion can be restored.[1]

Metabolic acidosis also is accompanied by signs and symptoms related to the recruitment of compensatory mechanisms. In situations of acute metabolic acidosis, the respiratory system compensates for a decrease in pH by increasing ventilation to reduce PCO_2; this is accomplished through deep and rapid respirations. In diabetic ketoacidosis, this breathing pattern is referred to as *Kussmaul breathing*. For descriptive purposes, it can be said that Kussmaul breathing resembles the hyperpnea of exercise—the person breathes as though he or she had been running. There may be complaints of difficult breathing or dyspnea with exertion; with severe acidosis, dyspnea may be present even at rest. Respiratory compensation for acute acidosis tends to be somewhat greater than for chronic metabolic alkalosis.

When kidney function is normal, net acid excretion increases promptly in response to acidosis, and the urine becomes more acid. Net acid excretion may increase 5 to 10 times above normal. Most of the initial acid secretion into the urine is facilitated through use of the phosphate buffer system. Over several days, ammonia production by the kidney increases and becomes the most important mechanism for excreting excess H^+ ions.

Chronic acidemia, as in renal failure, can lead to a variety of skeletal problems, some of which result from the release of calcium and phosphate during bone buffering of excess H^+ ions.[14] Of particular importance is impaired growth in children. In infants and children, acidemia may be associated with a variety of nonspecific symptoms such as anorexia, weight loss, muscle weakness, and listlessness.[1,14] Muscle weakness and listlessness may result from alterations in muscle metabolism.

Treatment

The treatment of metabolic acidosis focuses on correcting the condition that caused the disorder and restoring the fluids and electrolytes that have been lost from the body. The treatment of diabetic ketoacidosis is discussed in Chapter 41.

The use of supplemental sodium bicarbonate may be indicated in the treatment of some forms of normal anion gap acidosis. However, its use in treatment of metabolic acidosis with an increased anion gap is controversial, particularly in cases of lactic acidosis. In most patients with cardiac arrest, shock, or sepsis, impaired oxygen delivery is the primary cause of lactic acidosis. In these situations, the administration of large amounts of sodium bicarbonate does not improve oxygen delivery and may produce hypernatremia, hyperosmolality, and decreased oxygen release by hemoglobin because of a shift in the oxygen dissociation curve.[6]

METABOLIC ALKALOSIS

Metabolic alkalosis involves a primary excess of base bicarbonate along with an increased plasma pH. It can be caused by a gain in HCO_3^- or loss of H^+ ions. The body compensates for the increase in pH by decreasing the respiratory rate as a means of increasing PCO_2 and H_2CO_3 levels.

Causes

The causes of metabolic alkalosis can be divided into two major groups: those that are associated with a combination of large losses of extracellular volume and potassium and those that are associated with an increase in potassium excretion and thus hypokalemia due to a primary excess in mineralocorticoid activity.[2] The first group accounts for approximately 95% of all cases of metabolic alkalosis. Specifically, metabolic alkalosis may occur because of ingestion or administration of excess bicarbonate or other alkali (*e.g.*, carbonate, citrate, acetate), increased gastrointestinal or renal loss of H^+ ions, or volume contraction of the extracellular fluid compartment (Table 32-3).

Most of the body's serum bicarbonate is obtained from CO_2 that is produced during metabolic processes, from reabsorption of filtered bicarbonate, or generation of new bicarbonate by the kidney. Usually, bicarbonate production and renal reabsorption are balanced in a manner that prevents alkalosis from occurring. The proximal tubule reabsorbs 99.9% of the filtered bicarbonate, but if plasma levels of bicarbonate rise above the renal reabsorptive threshold, the reabsorption of filtered bicarbonate is reduced and the excess is excreted in the urine. However, many conditions that increase plasma bicarbonate levels also raise the renal threshold for bicarbonate reabsorption. Thus, the metabolic alkalosis not only is generated but is maintained.

Excess Bicarbonate Intake. Excessive alkali ingestion, as in the use of bicarbonate-containing antacids (*e.g.*, Alka-Seltzer) or sodium bicarbonate administration during cardiopulmonary resuscitation, can cause metabolic alkalosis. Other sources of alkali intake are acetate in hyperalimentation solutions, lactate in parenteral solutions such as Ringer's lactate, and citrate used in blood transfusions. A condition called the *milk-alkali syndrome* may develop in persons who consume excessive amounts of milk (calcium source) along with alkaline antacids. In this case, metabolic alkalosis develops as a consequence of vomiting (volume depletion and hypokalemia), hypercalcemia (increased bicarbonate reabsorption), and reduced glomerular filtration rate (increased bicarbonate reabsorption).[2,15]

Hydrogen, Chloride, and Potassium Ion Loss Associated With Bicarbonate Ion Retention. Vomiting, removal of gastric secretions through use of nasogastric suction, and

TABLE 32-3 ✦ Metabolic Alkalosis	
Causes	**Manifestations**
Excessive Gain of Bicarbonate or Alkali	**Blood pH, HCO_3^-, CO_2**
Ingestion or administration of sodium bicarbonate	pH increased
Administration of hyperalimentation solutions containing acetate	HCO_3^- (primary) increased
Administration of parenteral solutions containing lactate	PCO_2 (compensatory) increased
Administration of citrate-containing blood transfusions	
	Neural Function
Excessive Loss of Hydrogen Ions	Confusion
Vomiting	Hyperactive reflexes
Gastric suction	Tetany
Binge-purge syndrome	Convulsions
Potassium deficit	
Diuretic therapy	**Cardiovascular Function**
Hyperaldosteronism	Hypotension
Milk-alkali syndrome	Dysrhythmias
Increased Bicarbonate Retention	**Respiratory Function**
Loss of chloride with bicarbonate retention	Respiratory acidosis due to decreased respiratory rate
Volume Contraction	**Signs of Compensation**
Loss of body fluids	Decreased rate and depth of respiration
Diuretic therapy	Increased urine pH

low potassium levels resulting from diuretic therapy are the most common causes of metabolic alkalosis in hospitalized patients. The binge-purge syndrome, or self-induced vomiting, often is associated with metabolic alkalosis.[15] Gastric secretions contain high concentrations of hydrochloric acid and lesser concentrations of potassium chloride. As chloride is taken from the blood and secreted into the stomach with the H^+ ion, it is replaced by bicarbonate. Under normal conditions, each 1 mEq of H^+ ion that is secreted into the stomach generates 1 mEq of serum HCO_3^-.[15] Normally, the increase in serum HCO_3^- concentration is transient only, because the entry of acid into the duodenum stimulates an equal amount of pancreatic HCO_3^- secretion. However, loss of H^+ and Cl^- ions from the stomach due to vomiting or gastric suction stimulates continued production of gastric acid and thus the addition of more bicarbonate into the blood.

Maintenance of Metabolic Alkalosis by Volume Contraction, Hypokalemia, and Hypochloremia. Vomiting also results in the loss of water, sodium, and potassium (Fig. 32-9). The resultant volume depletion and hypokalemia maintain the generated metabolic alkalosis by increasing the renal reabsorption of bicarbonate. The details of the mechanisms by which volume depletion and hypokalemia stimulate the increased reabsorption of bicarbonate are not fully understood; however, volume depletion activates the renin-angiotensin-aldosterone system, which increases Na^+ reabsorption to maintain fluid volume. Na^+ reabsorption requires concomitant anion reabsorption. Because there is a Cl^- deficit, HCO_3^- is reab-

sorbed along with Na^+, leading to metabolic alkalosis. Angiotensin II also increases the activity of the proximal tubule Na^+/H^+ antiport transporter, which increases hydrogen ion excretion and bicarbonate reabsorption.

It has been proposed recently that the reduced delivery of chloride to the distal tubule of the kidney due to hypochloremia is responsible for maintaining metabolic alkalosis, rather than volume depletion per se. The low luminal chloride is interpreted as a sign of low tubular flow by the macula densa, and thus the renin-angiotensin-aldosterone system is stimulated. Low luminal concentrations of chloride also reduce the driving force for bicarbonate reabsorption. Diuretics that block chloride reabsorption in the kidney (*i.e.*, loop and thiazide diuretics) produce a bicarbonate retention through volume contraction and loss of Cl^- ions.[15]

The possible mechanisms by which hypokalemia increases bicarbonate reabsorption include an increased driving force for HCO_3^- reabsorption due to a decreased intracellular bicarbonate concentration in the tubular cells of the kidney. The decreased intracellular concentration results from increased movement of HCO_3^- as it accompanies K^+ moving from the renal tubular cells into the blood owing to the concentration gradient that exists because of low serum K^+ levels. Hypokalemia may also produce an up-regulation of H^+/K^+ luminal antiport transporters, thereby increasing K^+ reabsorption and H^+ secretion and simultaneously increasing HCO_3^- reabsorption.[2]

Metabolic alkalosis also is associated with low potassium levels caused by certain diuretics (*e.g.*, thiazides, furosemide) and excessive adrenocorticosteroid hormones (*e.g.*,

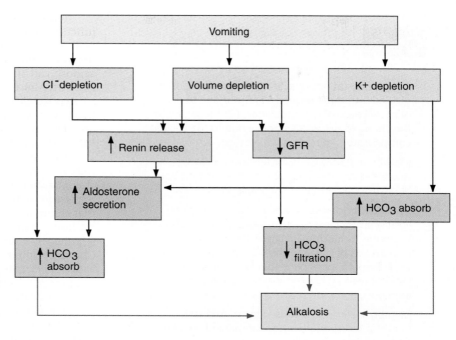

FIGURE 32-9 The mechanisms by which vomiting maintains metabolic alkalosis. See text for explanation. (Adapted from Galla J.H., Luke R.G. [1987]. Pathophysiology of metabolic alkalosis. *Hospital Practice* 22 (10), 130)

hyperaldosteronism, Cushing's syndrome). In situations of low potassium levels, renal excretion of H^+ ions is increased as the kidneys focus on conserving potassium. The hormone aldosterone increases H^+ ion secretion as it increases Na^+ and HCO_3^- ion reabsorption. In hyperaldosteronism, the concurrent loss of K^+ in the urine serves to perpetuate the alkalosis.

Chronic respiratory acidosis produces a compensatory loss of H^+ and Cl^- ions in the urine along with HCO_3^- retention. When respiratory acidosis is corrected abruptly, as with mechanical ventilation, a "posthypercapneic" metabolic alkalosis may develop because of a rapid drop in PCO_2, but the concentration of HCO_3^- ions, which are eliminated renally, remains elevated.

Manifestations

Metabolic alkalosis is characterized by a plasma pH above 7.45, plasma HCO_3^- level above 29 mEq/L (29 mmol/L), and base excess above 3.0 mEq/L (3 mmol/L). Persons with metabolic alkalosis often are asymptomatic or have signs related to volume depletion or hypokalemia. The neurologic signs (*e.g.*, hyperexcitability) occur less frequently with metabolic alkalosis than with other acid-base disorders because the HCO_3^- ion enters the CSF more slowly than CO_2. When neurologic manifestations do occur, as in acute and severe metabolic alkalosis, they include mental confusion, hyperactive reflexes, tetany, and carpopedal spasm. Metabolic alkalosis also leads to a compensatory hypoventilation with development of various degrees of hypoxemia and respiratory acidosis. Significant morbidity occurs with severe metabolic alkalosis (pH >7.55), including respiratory failure, dysrhythmias, seizures, and coma.

Treatment

The treatment of metabolic alkalosis usually is directed toward correcting the cause of the condition. A chloride deficit requires correction. Potassium chloride usually is the treatment of choice for metabolic alkalosis when there is an accompanying potassium deficit. When potassium chloride is used as a therapy, the chloride anion replaces the bicarbonate anion, and the administration of potassium corrects the potassium deficit and allows the kidneys to conserve H^+ ions while eliminating the K^+ ions. Fluid replacement with normal saline or one-half normal saline often is used in the treatment of patients with volume contraction alkalosis.

RESPIRATORY ACIDOSIS

Respiratory acidosis involves an increase in PCO_2 and H_2CO_3 along with a decrease in pH. Acute respiratory failure is associated with severe acidosis and only a small change in serum bicarbonate levels. Within 1 day, renal compensatory mechanisms become effective in generating more HCO_3^- ions, and the bicarbonate levels rise. In chronic respiratory acidosis, there is a compensatory increase in bicarbonate levels.[16]

Causes

Respiratory acidosis occurs in conditions that impair alveolar ventilation and cause an accumulation of PCO_2 (Table 32-4). It can occur as an acute or chronic disorder. Because renal compensatory mechanisms take time to exert their effects, blood pH can drop sharply in persons with acute respiratory acidosis.

Metabolic Acid-Base Imbalance

➤ The manifestations of acid-base disorders can be divided into three groups: (1) those due to the primary cause of the imbalance, (2) those due to the changed pH, and (3) those due to the elicited compensatory mechanisms.

➤ Metabolic acid-base disorders are the consequence of primary changes in the concentration of bicarbonate in the extracellular fluid.

➤ Metabolic acidosis is caused by an excess of nonvolatile acids or loss of bicarbonate. Compensatory responses include an increased respiratory rate (elimination of CO_2 and therefore H^+), reabsorption of all filtered bicarbonate, tubular secretion of H^+ ions buffered by intraluminal phosphates and ammonia, and production of acidic urine.

➤ Metabolic alkalosis is caused by an excessive intake of bicarbonate ion accompanied by an impaired ability of the kidney to excrete bicarbonate ion or by gastrointestinal or renal losses of H^+ ion. Compensatory responses include a decreased respiratory rate (retention of CO_2 and therefore H^+), increased excretion of bicarbonate (unless the primary problem is renal), and the production of an alkaline urine.

Acute respiratory acidosis can be caused by impaired function of the respiratory center in the medulla (as in narcotic overdose), lung disease, chest injury, weakness of the respiratory muscles, or airway obstruction. Acute respiratory acidosis can also result from breathing air with a high CO_2 content. Almost all persons with acute respiratory acidosis are hypoxemic if they are breathing room air. In many cases, signs of hypoxemia develop before those of respiratory acidosis because CO_2 diffuses across the alveolar capillary membrane 20 times more rapidly than oxygen.[1,2]

In many lung disorders, there are some areas of the lung that are more severely compromised in terms of gas exchange function than others. In these circumstances, the respiratory acidosis or hypoxemia stimulates ventilation so that elimination of CO_2 from the relatively normal areas of the lung is increased, but oxygen uptake from the same area is limited by a hemoglobin saturation that approaches 100%. Chronic respiratory acidosis is a relatively common disturbance in patients with chronic obstructive lung disease (see Chapter 29). In these persons, the persistent elevation of PCO_2 stimulates renal H^+ ion secretion and HCO_3^- reabsorption. The effectiveness of these compensatory mechanisms can often return the pH to near-normal values as long as oxygen levels are maintained within a range that does not unduly suppress chemoreceptor control of respirations.

An acute episode of respiratory acidosis can develop in patients with chronic lung disease who have chronically elevated PCO_2 levels. This is sometimes called *carbon dioxide narcosis*. In these persons, the medullary respiratory center has become adapted to the elevated levels of CO_2 and no longer responds to increases in PCO_2. Instead, the oxygen content of their blood becomes the major stimu-

---

TABLE 32-4 ✦ Causes and Manifestations of Respiratory Acidosis

Causes	Manifestations
Depression of Respiratory Center	**Blood pH, CO_2, HCO_3^-**
Drug overdose	pH decreased
Head injury	PCO_2 (primary) increased
	HCO_3^- (compensatory) increased
Lung Disease	
Bronchial asthma	**Neural Function**
Emphysema	Dilation of cerebral vessels and depression of neural function
Chronic bronchitis	Headache
Pneumonia	Weakness
Pulmonary edema	Behavior changes
Respiratory distress syndrome	Confusion
	Depression
Airway Obstruction, Disorders of Chest	Paranoia
Wall and Respiratory Muscles	Hallucinations
Paralysis of respiratory muscles	Tremors
Chest injuries	Paralysis
Kyphoscoliosis	Stupor and coma
Extreme obesity	
Treatment with paralytic drugs	**Skin**
	Skin warm and flushed
Breathing Air With High CO_2 Content	
	Signs of Compensation
	Acid urine

lus for respiration. If oxygen is administered at a flow rate that is sufficient to suppress this stimulus, the rate and depth of respiration decrease, and the CO_2 content of the blood increases.

Manifestations

Respiratory acidosis is associated with a plasma pH below 7.35 and an arterial PCO_2 above 50 mm Hg. The signs and symptoms of respiratory acidosis depend on the rapidity of onset and whether the condition is acute or chronic. Because respiratory acidosis often is accompanied by hypoxemia, the manifestations of respiratory acidosis often are intermixed with those of oxygen deficit. Carbon dioxide readily crosses the blood-brain barrier, exerting its effects by changing the pH of brain fluids. Elevated levels of CO_2 produce vasodilation of cerebral blood vessels. Headache, blurred vision, irritability, muscle twitching, and psychological disturbances can occur with acute respiratory acidosis. If the condition is severe and prolonged, it can cause an increase in CSF pressure and papilledema. Impaired consciousness, ranging from lethargy to coma, develops as the PCO_2 rises. Paralysis of extremities may occur, and there may be respiratory depression. Less severe forms of acidosis often are accompanied by warm and flushed skin, weakness, and tachycardia.

Treatment

The treatment of acute and chronic respiratory acidosis is directed toward improving ventilation. In severe cases, mechanical ventilation may be necessary. The treatment of respiratory acidosis due to respiratory failure is discussed in Chapter 29.

RESPIRATORY ALKALOSIS

Respiratory alkalosis involves a decrease in PCO_2 and a primary deficit in carbonic acid (H_2CO_3) along with an increase in pH. Because respiratory alkalosis can occur suddenly, a compensatory decrease in bicarbonate level may not occur before respiratory correction has been accomplished. The increase in pH is less in chronic compensated respiratory alkalosis, and the fall in bicarbonate concentration is greater.

Causes

Respiratory alkalosis is caused by hyperventilation or a respiratory rate in excess of that needed to maintain normal PCO_2 levels (Table 32-5). One of the most common causes of respiratory alkalosis is the hyperventilation syndrome, which is characterized by recurring episodes of overbreathing often associated with anxiety (see Chapter 29). Persons experiencing panic attacks frequently present in the emergency room with acute respiratory alkalosis. Other causes of hyperventilation are fever, oxygen deficiency, early salicylate toxicity, and encephalitis. Hypoxemia exerts its effect through the peripheral chemoreceptors. Salicylate toxicity and encephalitis produce hyperventilation by directly stimulating the medullary respiratory center. Hyperventilation can also occur during anesthesia or with use of mechanical ventilatory devices.

Manifestations

Respiratory alkalosis manifests with a decrease in PCO_2 and a deficit in H_2CO_3. In respiratory alkalosis, the pH is above 7.45, arterial PCO_2 is below 35 mm Hg, and serum HCO_3^- levels usually are below 24 mEq/L (24 mmol/L). The signs and symptoms of respiratory alkalosis are associated with hyperexcitability of the nervous system and a decrease in cerebral blood flow. Alkalosis increases protein binding of extracellular calcium. This reduces ionized calcium levels, causing an increase in neuromuscular excitability. A decrease in the CO_2 content of the blood causes constriction of cerebral blood vessels. CO_2 crosses the blood-brain barrier rather quickly; therefore, manifestations of acute respiratory alkalosis often are of sudden onset. The patient often experiences light-headedness, dizziness, tingling, and numbness of the fingers and toes. These manifestations may be accompanied by sweating, palpitations, panic, air hunger, and dyspnea. Chvostek's and Trousseau's signs may be positive

TABLE 32-5 ✦ Causes and Manifestations of Respiratory Alkalosis

Causes	Manifestations
Excessive Ventilation	**Blood pH, CO_2, HCO_3^-**
Anxiety and psychogenic hyperventilation	pH increased
Hypoxia and reflex stimulation of ventilation	PCO_2 (primary) decreased
Lung disease that reflexly stimulates ventilation	HCO_3^- (compensatory) decreased
Stimulation of respiratory center	**Neural Function**
Elevated blood ammonia level	Constriction of cerebral vessels and increased neuronal excitability
Salicylate toxicity	Dizziness, panic, light-headedness
Encephalitis	Tetany
Fever	Numbness and tingling of fingers and toes
Mechanical ventilation	Positive Chvostek's and Trousseau's signs
	Seizures
	Cardiovascular Function
	Cardiac dysrhythmias

(see Chapter 31), and tetany and convulsions may occur. Because CO_2 provides the stimulus for short-term regulation of respiration, short periods of apnea may occur in persons with acute episodes of hyperventilation.

Treatment

The treatment of respiratory alkalosis focuses on measures to increase the PCO_2. Attention is directed toward correcting the disorder that caused the overbreathing. Rebreathing of small amounts of expired air (breathing into a paper bag) may prove useful in restoring PCO_2 levels in persons with anxiety-produced respiratory alkalosis.

In summary, acidosis describes a decrease in pH, and alkalosis describes an increase in pH. Acid-base disorders may be caused by alterations in the body's volatile acids (*i.e.*, respiratory acidosis or respiratory alkalosis) or nonvolatile acids (*i.e.*, metabolic acidosis or metabolic alkalosis).

Metabolic acidosis is defined as a decrease in bicarbonate, and metabolic alkalosis is defined as an increase in bicarbonate. Metabolic acidosis is caused by an excessive production and accumulation of metabolic acids or an excessive loss of bicarbonate. Metabolic alkalosis is caused by an increase in bicarbonate or a decrease in H^+ or Cl^- ion levels. Respiratory acidosis reflects an increase in CO_2 levels and is caused by conditions that produce hypoventilation. Respiratory alkalosis is caused by conditions that cause hyperventilation and a reduction in CO_2 levels.

The signs and symptoms of acidosis and alkalosis reflect alterations in body function associated with the disorder causing the acid-base disturbance, the effect of the change of pH on body function, and the body's attempt to correct and maintain the pH within a normal physiologic range. In general, neuromuscular excitability is decreased in acidosis and increased in alkalosis.

Related Web Sites

Acid-Base Tutorial   www.tmc.tulane.edu/anes/acid
Fundamentals of Acid-Base Balance   www.gasnet.org/education/acid-base
Acid-Base Balance Continuing Education Course   www.nursingceu.com/NCEU/courses/acidbase2
Acid-Base Balance: Clinical Considerations   www1.omi.tulane.edu/anes/acid/practical.html

References

1. Rose B.D. (1994). *Clinical physiology of acid-base and electrolyte disorders* (3rd ed., pp. 288, 485, 520–527, 540–557, 565). New York: McGraw-Hill.
2. Abelow B. (1998). *Understanding acid-base* (pp. 43–49, 83–93, 139–169, 171–188, 189–198, 224–230). Baltimore: Williams & Wilkins.
3. Rhoades R.A., Tanner G.A. (1996). *Medical physiology* (pp. 465–483). Boston: Little, Brown.
4. Metheny N.M. (1996). *Fluid and electrolyte balance* (3rd ed., p. 162). Philadelphia: J.B. Lippincott.
5. Adrogue H.J., Madias N.E. (1998). Management of life-threatening acid-base disorders: First of two parts. *New England Journal of Medicine* 338, 26–34.
6. Forsythe S.M., Schmidt G.A. (2000). Sodium bicarbonate for the treatment of lactic acidosis. *Chest* 117, 260–267.
7. Rothman S.M. (1999). Mutations of the mitochondrial genome: Clinical overview and possible pathophysiology of cell damage. *Biochemical Society Symposia* 66, 111–122.
8. Howell N. (1999). Human mitochondrial diseases: Answering questions and questioning answers. *International Review of Cytology* 186, 49–116.
9. Uribarri J., Oh M.S., Carroll H.J. (1998). D-Lactic acidosis: A review of clinical presentation, biochemical features and pathophysiological mechanisms. *Medicine (Baltimore)* 77 (2), 73–82.
10. Umpierrez G.E., DiGirolamo M., Tuvlin J.A., Isaacs S.D., Bhoola S.M., Kokko J.P. (2000). Differences in metabolic and hormonal milieu in diabetic and alcohol-induced ketoacidosis. *Journal of Critical Care* 15 (2), 52–59.
11. Meyer R.J., Beard M.E., Ardagh M.W., Henderson S. (2000). Methanol poisoning. *New Zealand Medical Journal* 113 (1102), 3–11.
12. Egbert P.A., Abraham K. (1999). Ethylene glycol intoxication: Pathophysiology, diagnosis, and emergency management. *ANNA Journal* 26, 295–300.
13. Powers F. (1999). The role of chloride in acid-base balance. *Journal of Intravenous Nursing* 22, 286–291.
14. Alpern R.J., Sakhaee K. (1997). The clinical spectrum of chronic metabolic acidosis: Homeostatic mechanisms produce significant morbidity. *American Journal of Kidney Diseases* 29, 291–302.
15. Galla J.H. (2000). Metabolic alkalosis. *Journal of the American Society of Nephrology* 11, 369–375.
16. Adrogue H.J., Madias N.E. (1998). Management of life-threatening acid-base disorders. *New England Journal of Medicine* 338, 107–111.

Respiratory Acid-Base Imbalance

➤ Respiratory acid-base imbalances are due to a primary disturbance in PCO_2 reflecting an increase or decrease in ventilation.

➤ Respiratory acidosis is caused by a decrease in ventilation such that PCO_2 increases above normal. Compensatory mechanisms include the renal reabsorption of all filtered bicarbonate, the secretion of acid buffered by phosphate and ammonia, and the excretion of an acid urine.

➤ Respiratory alkalosis is caused by an increase in ventilation such that PCO_2 decreases below normal. Compensatory mechanisms include decreased renal bicarbonate reabsorption and excretion of nonvolatile acids.

Alterations in Renal Function

Mﾠore than 20 million North Americans have diseases of the kidneys and urinary tract. Each year, over 8 million people are diagnosed with acute urinary tract disorders, and approximately 50,000 die because of these diseases.[1]

The kidneys are subject to many of the same types of disorders that affect other body structures, including developmental defects, infections, altered immune responses, and neoplasms. The kidneys filter blood from all parts of the body, and although many forms of kidney disease originate in the kidneys, others develop secondary to disorders such as hypertension, diabetes mellitus, and systemic lupus erythematosus (SLE). The content in this chapter focuses on congenital disorders of the kidneys, obstructive disorders, urinary tract infections (UTIs), disorders of glomerular function, tubulointerstitial disorders, and neoplasms of the kidneys. Acute and chronic renal failure are discussed in Chapter 34, and the effects of other disease conditions, such as hypertension, shock, and diabetes mellitus, are discussed in other sections of the book.

Congenital Disorders of the Kidneys

After you have completed this section of the chapter, you should be able to meet the following objectives:

- Define the terms *agenesis, dysgenesis,* and *hypoplasia* as they refer to the development of the kidney
- Cite the effect of urinary obstruction in the fetus
- Describe the genetic basis for renal cystic disease, the pathology of the disorder, and its signs and symptoms

Some abnormality of the kidneys and ureters occur in approximately 3% to 4% of newborn infants.[2] Anomalies in shape and position are the most common. Less common are disorders involving a decrease in renal mass (*e.g.,* agenesis, hypogenesis) or a change in renal structure (*e.g.,* renal cysts). Many fetal anomalies can be detected before birth by ultrasonography. In the normal fetus, the kidneys can be visualized as early as 12 weeks.

AGENESIS AND HYPOPLASIA

The kidneys begin to develop early in the fifth week of gestation and start to function approximately 3 weeks later. Formation of urine is thought to begin in the 9th to 12th weeks of gestation; by the 32nd week, fetal production of urine reaches approximately 28 mL/hour.[3] Urine is the main constituent of amniotic fluid. The relative amount of amniotic fluid can provide information about the status of fetal renal function.

The term *dysgenesis* refers to a failure of an organ to develop normally. *Agenesis* is the complete failure of an organ to develop. Total agenesis of both kidneys is incompatible with extrauterine life. Infants are stillborn or die shortly after birth of pulmonary hypoplasia. Newborns with renal agenesis often have characteristic facial features, termed *Potter's syndrome*.[4] The eyes are widely separated and have epicanthic folds, the ears are low set, the nose is broad and flat, the chin is receding, and limb defects often are present.[4,5] Other causes of neonatal renal failure with the Potter phenotype include cystic renal dysplasia, obstructive uropathy, and autosomal recessive polycystic disease. Unilateral agenesis is an uncommon anomaly that is compatible with life if no other abnormality is present. The opposite kidney usually is enlarged as a result of compensatory hypertrophy.

In *renal hypoplasia*, the kidneys do not develop to normal size. Like agenesis, hypoplasia more commonly affects only one kidney. When both kidneys are affected, there is progressive development of renal failure. It has been suggested that true hypoplasia is extremely rare; most cases probably represent acquired scarring due to vascular, infectious, or other kidney diseases rather than an underlying developmental failure.[5,6]

In pregnancies that involve infants with nonfunctional kidneys or outflow obstruction of the kidneys, the amount of amniotic fluid is small—a condition called *oligohydramnios*. The cause of fetal death in these infants is thought to be cord compression due to the oligohydramnios.[2]

ALTERATIONS IN KIDNEY POSITION AND FORM

The development of the kidneys during embryonic life can result in kidneys that lie outside their normal position, usually just above the pelvic brim or within the pelvis. Because of the abnormal position, kinking of the ureters and obstruction of urine flow may occur.

One of the most common alterations in kidney form is an abnormality called a *horseshoe kidney*. This abnormality occurs in approximately 1 of every 500 to 1000 persons.[4,5]

In this disorder, the upper or lower poles of the two kidneys are fused, producing a horseshoe-shaped structure that is continuous along the midline of the body anterior to the great vessels. Most horseshoe kidneys are fused at the lower pole[6] (Fig. 33-1). The condition usually does not cause problems unless there is an associated defect in the renal pelvis or other urinary structures that obstructs urine flow.

CYSTIC DISEASE OF THE KIDNEY

Renal cysts are fluid-filled sacs or segments of a dilated nephron. The cysts may be single or multiple and can vary in size from microscopic to several centimeters in diameter. There are four basic types of renal cystic disease: polycystic kidney disease, medullary sponge kidney, acquired cystic disease, and simple kidney cysts (Fig. 33-2). Although some types of cysts are not congenital, they are included in this section.

Renal cystic disease is thought to result from tubular obstructions that increase intratubular pressure or from changes in the basement membrane of the renal tubules that predispose to cystic dilatation. After a cyst begins to form, continued fluid accumulation contributes to its persistent growth. Renal cystic diseases probably exert their effects by compressing renal blood vessels, producing degeneration of functional renal tissue and obstructing tubular flow.

Simple and Acquired Renal Cysts

Simple cysts are a common disorder of the kidney. The cysts may be single or multiple, unilateral or bilateral, and usu-

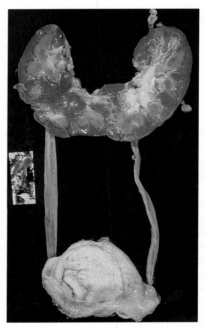

FIGURE 33-1 Horseshoe kidney. The kidneys are fused at the lower poles. (Rubin E., Farber J.L. [1999]. *Pathology* [3rd ed., p. 865]. Philadelphia: Lippincott Williams & Wilkins)

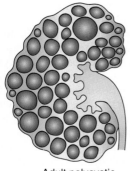
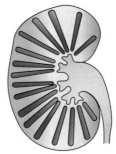

Adult polycystic
disease

Infantile polycystic
disease

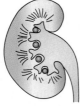
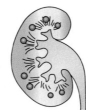

Medullary
sponge kidney

Medullary cystic
disease complex

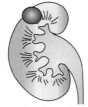

Simple cyst

FIGURE 33-2 Cystic diseases of the kidney. (Rubin E., Farber J.L. [1999]. *Pathology* [3rd ed., p. 866]. Philadelphia: Lippincott Williams & Wilkins.) (Courtesy of Dmitri Kartenikov, artist)

ally are less than 1 cm in diameter, although they may grow larger. Most simple cysts do not produce signs or symptoms or compromise renal function. When symptomatic, they may cause flank pain, hematuria, infection, and hypertension related to ischemia-produced stimulation of the renin-angiotensin system. They are most common in older persons. Although the cysts are benign, they may be confused clinically with renal cell carcinoma.

An acquired form of renal cystic disease occurs in persons with end-stage renal failure who have undergone prolonged dialysis treatment. The cysts, which measure 0.2 to 2 cm in diameter, probably develop as a result of tubular obstruction.[5] Although the condition is largely asymptomatic, the cysts may bleed, causing hematuria. Tumors, usually adenomas but occasionally adenosarcomas, may develop in the walls of these cysts.

Medullary Cystic Disease

There are two major types of cystic disease that involve the medullary portion of the kidney—medullary sponge kidney and nephronophthisis–medullary cystic disease complex.[5,6]

Medullary sponge kidney is characterized by small (<5 mm in diameter), multiple cystic dilations of the collecting ducts of the medulla. The disorder does not cause progressive renal failure; it does, however, produce urinary stasis and predisposes to kidney infections and kidney stones. The disease usually is asymptomatic in young adults. Symptomatic disease usually develops between the ages of 30 and 60 years, when affected persons begin to have flank pain, dysuria, hematuria, and "gravel" in the urine as a result of stone formation in the cysts.[6]

Nephronophthisis–medullary cystic disease complex is a group of related diseases characterized by renal medullary cysts, sclerotic kidneys, and renal failure. Approximately 85% of cases have a hereditary basis. Symptoms usually develop during childhood, and the disorder accounts for 10% to 20% of renal failure in children. Polyuria, polydipsia, and enuresis (bed-wetting), which are early manifestations of the disorder, reflect impaired ability of the kidneys to concentrate urine.[5,6]

Polycystic Kidney Disease

The most common form of renal cystic disease is polycystic kidney disease, which is the result of a hereditary trait. It is one of the most common hereditary diseases in the United States, affecting more than 600,000 Americans.[1] There are two types of inherited polycystic disease: autosomal recessive and autosomal dominant.

Autosomal Recessive Polycystic Kidney Disease. Autosomal recessive polycystic kidney disease, which is present at birth, is rare compared with the adult variety.[5,6] The disorder is inherited as a recessive trait, meaning that both parents are carriers of the gene and that there is a one in four chance of the parents having another child with the disorder. Because the condition is present at birth, it formerly was called *infantile* or *childhood polycystic disease*. The condition is bilateral, and significant renal dysfunction usually is present, accompanied by variable degrees of liver fibrosis and portal hypertension. The disorder can be diagnosed by ultrasonography.

There is no known treatment for the disease. Approximately 75% of infants die in the perinatal period, often because the large kidneys compromise expansion of the lungs.[6] Some children may present with less severe kidney problems and more severe liver disease.

Autosomal Dominant Polycystic Kidney Disease. Autosomal dominant polycystic kidney disease, also called *adult polycystic kidney disease,* affects children and adults in the prime of life and accounts for 10% of persons who require treatment for end-stage renal disease. This disorder is transmitted as an autosomal dominant trait. There is considerable variability in gene expression, and many affected persons do not have clinical symptoms, or if they do, the symptoms occur later in life.

Three mutant genes have been implicated in the disorder.[5–7] A polycystic kidney disease gene called *PKD1*, located on chromosome 16, is responsible for approximately 85% of cases. It encodes a large membrane protein called *polycystin 1* that has domains similar to proteins involved in cell-to-cell and cell-extracellular matrix interactions.[5,7] A second gene, called *PKD2*, which is located on chromosome 4, is responsible for a milder form of the disease. It encodes for a product called *polycystin 2*, which is an integral membrane protein that is similar to certain calcium and sodium channel proteins as well as to a portion of polycystin 1. A third gene, *PKD3*, is responsible for a minority of cases and has yet to be mapped.

How the genetic defects in the polycystin proteins cause cyst formation is largely speculative. It is thought that the membrane proteins may play a role in extracellular matrix interactions that are important in tubular epithelial cell growth and differentiation. Accordingly, it is hypothesized that cysts develop as a result of an abnormality in cell differentiation, increased transepithelial fluid secretion, and formation of an abnormal extracellular matrix that allows the cyst to separate from adjacent tubules. In addition, cyst fluids have been shown to harbor mediators that enhance fluid secretion and induce inflammation, resulting in further enlargement of the cysts and the interstitial fibrosis that is characteristic of progressive polycystic kidney disease.

The disease is characterized by tubular dilatation with cyst formation interspersed between normally functioning nephrons. Fluid collects in the cyst while it is still part of the tubular lumen, or it is secreted into the cyst after it has separated from the tubule. As the fluid accumulates, the cysts gradually increase in size, with some becoming as large as 5 cm in diameter. The kidneys of persons with polycystic kidney disease eventually become enlarged because of the presence of multiple cysts (Fig. 33-3). Cysts also may be found in the liver and, less commonly, the pancreas and spleen. Mitral valve prolapse and other valvular heart diseases occur in 20% to 25% of persons, but are largely asymptomatic. Most persons with polycystic disease also have colonic diverticula. One of the most devastating extrarenal manifestations is a weakness in the walls of the cerebral arteries that can lead to aneurysm formation. Approximately 20% of persons with polycystic kidney disease

have an associated aneurysm, and subarachnoid hemorrhage is a frequent cause of death.[6]

The manifestations of polycystic kidney disease include pain from the enlarging cysts that may reach debilitating levels, episodes of gross hematuria from bleeding into a cyst, infected cysts from ascending UTI, and hypertension resulting from compression of intrarenal blood vessels with activation of the renin-angiotensin mechanism.[8,9] Persons with polycystic kidney disease also are at risk for development of renal cell carcinoma. The progress of the disease is slow, and end-stage renal failure is uncommon before 40 years of age.

The diagnosis of autosomal polycystic kidney disease can be made by radiologic studies, such as excretory urography, and by ultrasonography or computed tomography (CT). Ultrasonography and CT have largely replaced excretory urography because they are better able to detect small cysts. Ultrasonography is particularly useful as a screening test for the disease.

The treatment of polycystic kidney disease is largely supportive. Control of hypertension and prevention of ascending UTIs are important. The cysts may be surgically decompressed in persons with severe, disabling pain.[8,9] The procedure permits removal of fluid from the cyst. Although affording pain relief, the procedure does not appear to alter the course of the disease.[8] Dialysis and kidney transplantation are reserved for those who progress to end-stage renal disease.

In summary, approximately 10% of infants are born with potentially significant malformations of the urinary system. These abnormalities can range from bilateral renal agenesis, which is incompatible with life, to hypogenesis of one kidney, which usually causes no problems unless the function of the remaining kidney is impaired. The developmental process can result in kidneys that lie outside their normal position. Because of the abnormal position, kinking of the ureters and obstruction of urine flow can occur.

Renal cystic disease is a condition in which there is dilatation of tubular structures with cyst formation. Cysts may be single or multiple. Polycystic kidney disease is an inherited form of renal cystic disease; it can be inherited as an autosomal recessive or an autosomal dominant trait. Autosomal recessive polycystic kidney disease is rare and usually presents as severe renal dysfunction during infancy. Autosomal dominant polycystic disease usually does not become symptomatic until later in life, often after 40 years of age.

Obstructive Disorders

After you have completed this section of the chapter, you should be able to meet the following objectives:

✦ List common causes of urinary tract obstruction
✦ Describe the effects of urinary tract obstruction on renal structure and function
✦ Cite three theories that are used to explain the formation of kidney stones

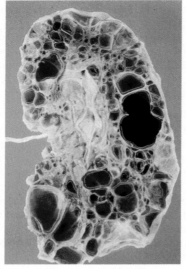

FIGURE 33-3 Adult polycystic disease. The kidney is enlarged, and the parenchyma is almost entirely replaced by cysts of varying size. (Rubin E., Farber J.L. [1999]. *Pathology* [3rd ed., p. 867]. Philadelphia: Lippincott Williams & Wilkins)

+ Explain the mechanisms of pain and infection that occur with kidney stones
+ Describe methods used in diagnosis and treatment of kidney stones

Urinary obstruction can occur in persons of any age and can involve any level of the urinary tract from the urethra to the renal pelvis (Fig. 33-4). The conditions that cause urinary tract obstruction include developmental defects, calculi (*i.e.*, stones), pregnancy, benign prostatic hyperplasia, scar tissue resulting from infection and inflammation, tumors, and neurologic disorders such as spinal cord injury. The causes of urinary tract obstructions are summarized in Table 33-1.

MECHANISMS OF RENAL DAMAGE

The destructive effects of urinary obstruction on kidney structures are determined by the degree (*i.e.*, partial vs. complete, unilateral vs. bilateral) and the duration of the obstruction. The two most damaging effects of urinary obstruction are stasis of urine, which predisposes to infection and stone formation, and development of backpressure, which interferes with renal blood flow and destroys kidney tissue.

A common complication of urinary tract obstruction is infection. Stagnation of urine predisposes to infection, which may spread throughout the urinary tract. When present, urinary calculi serve as foreign bodies and contribute to the infection. Once established, the infection is difficult to treat. It often is caused by urea-splitting organisms (*e.g.*,

TABLE 33-1 ◆ **Causes of Urinary Tract Obstruction**	
Level of Obstruction	**Cause**
Renal pelvis	Renal calculi
	Papillary necrosis
Ureter	Renal calculi
	Pregnancy
	Tumors that compress the ureter
	Ureteral stricture
	Congenital disorders of the ureterovesical junction and ureteropelvic junction strictures
Bladder and urethra	Bladder cancer
	Neurogenic bladder
	Bladder stones
	Prostatic hyperplasia or cancer
	Urethral strictures
	Congenital urethral defects

Proteus, staphylococci) that increase ammonia production and cause the urine to become alkaline.[10] Calcium salts precipitate more readily in stagnant alkaline urine; thus, urinary tract obstructions also predispose to stone formation.

In situations of marked or complete obstruction, backpressure develops because of a combination of continued glomerular filtration and impedance to urinary flow. Prolonged or severe partial obstruction causes irreversible kidney damage. Depending on the degree of obstruction, pressure builds up, beginning at the site of obstruction and moving backward from the ureter or renal pelvis into the calices and collecting tubules. Typically, the most severe effects occur at the level of the papillae because these structures are subjected to the greatest pressure. Damage to the nephrons and other functional components of the kidney is caused by compression from increased intrapelvic pressure and ischemia from disturbances in blood flow. Experiments have shown recovery of renal function after release of complete obstruction of up to 4 weeks' duration.[10] Irreversible damage, however, can begin as early as 7 days.[10]

Dilatation of the ureters and renal pelves occurs with prolonged urinary tract obstruction. When the obstruction is in the distal ureter, the increased pressure dilates the proximal ureter, a condition called *hydroureter* (Fig. 33-5). Hydroureter also is a complication of bladder outflow obstruction due to prostatic hyperplasia (see Chapter 43). With increasing pressure, the ureteral wall becomes severely stretched and loses its ability to undergo peristaltic contractions. In extreme cases, the ureter may become so dilated that it resembles a loop of bowel. *Hydronephrosis* refers to urine-filled dilatation of the renal pelvis and calices. The degree of hydronephrosis depends on the duration, degree, and site of obstruction. Bilateral hydronephrosis occurs only when the obstruction is below the level of the ureters. If the obstruction occurs at the level of the ureters or above, hydronephrosis is unilateral. The kidney eventually is destroyed and appears as a thin-walled shell that is filled with fluid (Fig. 33-6).

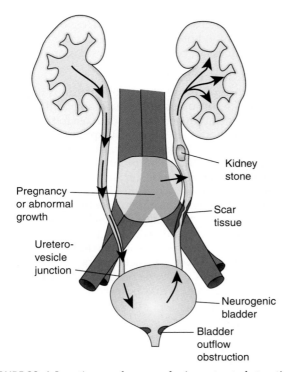

Kidney stone

Pregnancy or abnormal growth

Uretero-vesicle junction

Scar tissue

Neurogenic bladder

Bladder outflow obstruction

FIGURE 33-4 Locations and causes of urinary tract obstruction.

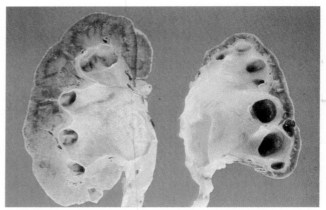

FIGURE 33-6 Hydronephrosis. Bilateral urinary tract obstruction has led to conspicuous dilatation of the ureters, pelves, and calyces. The kidney on the right shows severe cortical atrophy. (Rubin E., Farber J.L. [1999]. *Pathology* [3rd ed., p. 910]. Philadelphia: Lippincott Williams & Wilkins)

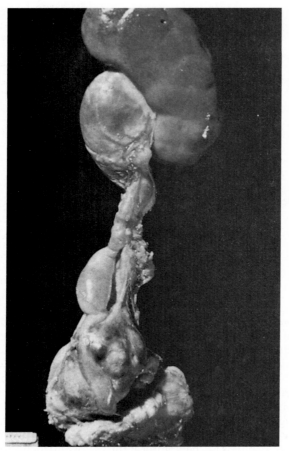

FIGURE 33-5 Hydroureter caused by ureteral obstruction in a woman with cancer of the uterus.

Manifestations

The manifestations of urinary obstruction depend on the site of obstruction, the cause, and the rapidity with which the condition developed. Most commonly, the person has pain, signs and symptoms of UTI, and manifestations of renal dysfunction, such as an impaired ability to concentrate urine. Changes in urine output may be misleading because output may be normal or even high in cases of partial obstruction.

Pain, which often is the factor that causes a person to seek medical attention, is the result of distention of the bladder, collecting system, or renal capsule. Its severity is related most closely to the rate rather than the degree of distention. Pain most often occurs with acute obstruction, in which the distention of urinary structures is rapid. This contrasts with chronic obstruction, in which distention is gradual and may not cause pain. Instead, gradual obstruction may produce only vague abdominal or back discomfort. When pain occurs, it is related to the site of obstruction. Obstruction of the renal pelvis or upper ureter causes pain and tenderness over the flank area. With lower levels of obstruction, the pain may radiate to the testes in the male or the labia in the female. With partial obstruction, particularly of the ureteropelvic junction, pain may occur during periods of high fluid

intake, when a high rate of urine flow causes an acute distention of the renal pelvis. Because of its visceral innervation, ureteral obstruction may produce reflex impairment of gastrointestinal tract peristalsis and motility with abdominal distention and, in severe cases, paralytic ileus.

Hypertension is an occasional complication of urinary tract obstruction. It is more common in cases of unilateral obstruction in which renin secretion is enhanced, probably secondary to impaired renal blood flow. In these circumstances, removal of the obstruction often leads to a reduction in blood pressure. When hypertension accompanies bilateral obstruction, renin levels usually are normal, and the elevated blood pressure probably is volume related. The relief of bilateral obstruction leads to a loss of volume and a decrease in blood pressure. In some cases, relieving the obstruction does not correct the hypertension.

Diagnosis and Treatment

Early diagnosis of urinary tract obstruction is important because the condition usually is treatable and a delay in therapy may result in permanent damage to the kidneys. Diagnostic methods vary with the symptoms. For example, a distended bladder suggests prostatic hyperplasia in the male. Radiologic methods commonly are used. The opaque kidney stones often are visible on x-ray films. CT scans and intravenous urography may be used. Ultrasonography has proved to be the single most useful noninvasive diagnostic modality for urinary obstruction. Other diagnostic methods, such as urinalysis, are used to determine the extent of renal involvement and the presence of infection.

Treatment of urinary obstruction depends on the cause. Urinary stone removal may be necessary, or surgical treatment of structural defects may be indicated.

RENAL CALCULI

The term *nephrolithiasis* refers to kidney stones. The most common cause of upper urinary tract obstruction is urinary calculi. Although stones can form in any part of the urinary

Kidney Stones

> ► Kidney stones are crystalline structures that form from components of the urine.

> ► Stones require a nidus to form and a urinary environment that supports continued crystalization of stone components.

> ► Stone formation is influenced by the concentration of stone components in the urine, the ability of the stone components to complex and form stones, and the presence of substances that inhibit stone formation.

tract, most develop in the kidneys. Approximately 1 million North Americans are hospitalized each year with kidney stones, and an equal number are treated for stones without hospitalization.[1] Men are more frequently affected than women, with a ratio of 4:1.[11]

Kidney stones are crystalline structures made up of materials that the kidneys normally excrete in the urine. The etiology of urinary stone formation is complex and not all aspects are well understood. It is thought to encompass a number of factors, including increases in blood and urinary levels of stone components and interactions among the components; anatomic changes in urinary tract structures; metabolic and endocrine influences; dietary and intestinal absorption factors; and UTI. To add to the mystery of stone formation is the fact that although both kidneys are exposed to the same urinary constituents, kidney stones tend to form in only one kidney. Three major theories are used to explain stone formation: the saturation theory, the matrix theory, and the inhibitor deficiency theory.[12–14] One or more of these theories may apply to stone formation in the same person.

Kidney stones require a nidus, or nucleus, to form and a urinary environment that supports continued precipitation of stone components to grow. The *saturation theory* states that the risk of stone formation is increased when the urine is supersaturated with stone components (*e.g.*, calcium salts, uric acid, magnesium ammonium phosphate, cystine). Supersaturation depends on urinary pH, solute concentration, ionic strength, and complexation. The greater the concentration of two ions, the more likely they are to precipitate. Complexation influences the availability of specific ions. For example, sodium complexes with oxalate and decreases its free ionic form.

The *matrix theory* proposes that organic materials, such as mucopolysaccharides derived from the epithelial cells that line the tubules, act as a nidus for stone formation. This theory is based on the observation that organic matrix materials can be found in all layers of kidney stones. It is not known whether the matrix material contributes to the initiation of stone formation or the material is merely entrapped as the stone forms.

Kidney proteins inhibit all phases of crystallization. The *inhibitor theory* suggests that persons who have a deficiency of proteins that inhibit stone formation in their urine are at increased risk for stone formation. Kidney cells produce at least three proteins that are thought to slow the rate of calcium oxalate crystallization: nephrocalcin, Tamm-Horsfall mucoprotein, and uropontin.[12,15] Nephrocalcin inhibits nucleation, aggregation, and growth of calcium oxalate stones. *Tamm-Horsfall mucoprotein* is thought to exert a minor effect on crystal aggregation. Uropontin inhibits the growth of calcium oxalate crystals. Much of the information about the function of organic inhibitors in terms of stone formation is still experimental. Nonorganic substances also can act as inhibitors of stone formation. For example, citrate is a key factor affecting development of calcium stones. It complexes with calcium, thereby decreasing the concentration of ionic calcium. Citrate is a normal byproduct of the citric acid cycle in renal cells; metabolic stimuli that consume this product (as with metabolic acidosis due to fasting, hypokalemia, or hypomagnesemia) reduce the urinary excretion of citrate. Citrate supplementation (potassium citrate) may be used in the treatment of some forms of hypocitraturic kidney stones.[10,11,14]

Types of Stones

There are four basic types of kidney stones: calcium stones (*i.e.*, oxalate or phosphate), magnesium ammonium phosphate stones, uric acid stones, and cystine stones. The causes and treatment measures for each of these types of renal stones are described in Table 33-2.

Most kidney stones (70% to 80%) are calcium stones—calcium oxalate, calcium phosphate, or a combination of the two materials. Calcium stones usually are associated with increased concentrations of calcium in the blood and urine. Excessive bone resorption caused by immobility, bone disease, hyperparathyroidism, and renal tubular acidosis all are contributing conditions. High oxalate concentrations in the blood and urine predispose to formation of calcium oxalate stones. A recent addition to the spectrum of kidney stones are those seen in persons with human immunodeficiency virus (HIV) infection who are being treated with indinavir, a protease inhibitor. The calcium-containing calculi develop in up to 6% of persons treated with the drug.[10]

Magnesium ammonium phosphate stones, also called *struvite stones*, form only in alkaline urine and in the presence of bacteria that possess an enzyme called *urease*, which splits the urea in the urine into ammonia and carbon dioxide. The ammonia that is formed takes up a hydrogen ion to become an ammonium ion, increasing the pH of the urine so that it becomes more alkaline. Because phosphate levels are increased in alkaline urine and because magnesium always is present in the urine, struvite stones form. These stones enlarge as the bacterial count grows, and they can increase in size until they fill an entire renal pelvis (Fig. 33-7). Because of their shape, they often are called *staghorn stones*. Staghorn stones almost always are associated with UTIs and persistently alkaline urine. Because these stones act as a foreign body, treatment of the infection often is difficult. Struvite stones usually are too large to be passed and require lithotripsy or surgical removal.

TABLE 33-2 ◆ Composition, Contributing Factors, and Treatment of Kidney Stones

Type of Stone	Contributing Factors	Treatment
Calcium (oxalate and phosphate)	Hypercalcemia and hypercalciuria Immobilization	Treatment of underlying conditions Increased fluid intake Thiazide diuretics
	Hyperparathyroidism Vitamin D intoxication Diffuse bone disease Milk-alkali syndrome Renal tubular acidosis Hyperoxaluria Intestinal bypass surgery	Dietary restriction of foods high in oxalate
Magnesium ammonium phosphate (struvite)	Urea-splitting urinary tract infections	Treatment of urinary tract infection Acidification of the urine Increased fluid intake
Uric acid (urate)	Formed in acid urine with pH of approximately 5.5 Gout High-purine diet	Increased fluid intake Allopurinol for hyperuricuria Alkalinization of urine
Cystine	Cystinuria (inherited disorder of amino acid metabolism)	Increased fluid intake Alkalinization of urine

Uric acid stones develop in conditions of gout and high concentrations of uric acid in the urine. Hyperuricosuria also may contribute to calcium stone formation by acting as a nucleus for calcium oxalate stone formation. Unlike radiopaque calcium stones, uric acid stones are not visible on x-ray films. Uric acid stones form most readily in urine with a pH of 5.1 to 5.9.[12] Thus, these stones can be treated by raising the urinary pH to 6 to 6.5 with potassium alkali salts.

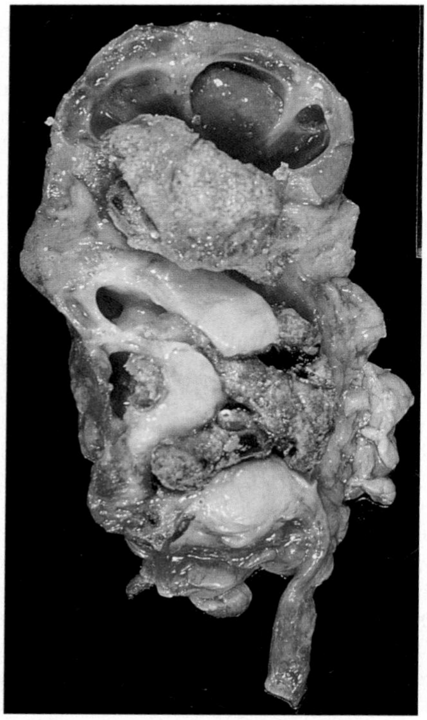

Cystine stones are rare. They are seen in cystinuria, which results from a genetic defect in renal transport of cystine. These stones resemble struvite stones except that infection is unlikely to be present.

Manifestations

One of the major manifestations of kidney stones is pain. Depending on location, there are two types of pain associated with kidney stones: renal colic and noncolicky renal pain.[10] *Renal colic* is the term used to describe the colicky pain that accompanies stretching of the collecting system or ureter. The symptoms of renal colic are caused by stones 1 to 5 mm in diameter that can move into the ureter and obstruct flow. Classic ureteral colic is manifested by acute, intermittent, and excruciating pain in the flank and upper outer quadrant of the abdomen on the affected side. The pain may radiate to the lower abdominal quadrant, bladder area, perineum, or scrotum in the male. The skin may be cool and clammy, and nausea and vomiting are common. Noncolicky pain is caused by stones that produce distention of the renal calices or renal pelvis. The pain usually is a dull, deep ache in flank or back that can vary in intensity from mild to severe. The pain may be exaggerated by drinking large amounts of fluid.[10]

Diagnosis and Treatment

Patients with kidney stones often present with acute renal colic, and the diagnosis is based on symptomatology and diagnostic tests, which include urinalysis, abdominal radiographs, and excretory urography. Urinalysis provides infor-

FIGURE 33-7 Staghorn calculi. The kidney shows hydronephrosis and stones that are casts of the dilated calyces. (Rubin E., Farber J.L. [1999]. *Pathology* [3rd ed., p. 909]. Philadelphia: Lippincott Williams & Wilkins)

mation related to hematuria, infection, the presence of stone-forming crystals, and urine pH. At least 90% of stones are radiopaque and readily visible on a plain radiograph of the abdomen. Excretory urography uses an intravenously injected contrast medium that is filtered in the glomeruli to visualize the collecting system and the ureters of the kidneys. Retrograde urography, ultrasonography, and CT scanning also may be used. A new imaging technique called *nuclear scintigraphy* uses bisphosphonate markers as a means of imaging stones.[10] The method has been credited with identifying stones that are too small to be detected by other methods.

Treatment of acute renal colic usually is supportive. Pain relief may be needed during acute phases of obstruction, and antibiotic therapy may be necessary to treat urinary infections. Most stones that are less than 5 mm in diameter pass spontaneously. All urine should be strained during an attack in the hope of retrieving the stone for chemical analysis and determination of type. This information, along with a careful history and laboratory tests, provides the basis for long-term preventive measures.

A major goal of treatment in persons who have passed kidney stones or have had them removed is to prevent their recurrence. Prevention requires investigation into the cause of stone formation using urine tests, blood chemistries, and stone analysis. Underlying disease conditions, such as hyperparathyroidism, are treated. Adequate fluid intake reduces the concentration of stone-forming crystals in the urine and needs to be encouraged. Depending on the type of stone that is formed, dietary changes, medications, or both may be used to alter the concentration of stone-forming elements in the urine. For example, persons who form calcium oxalate stones may need to decrease their intake of foods that are high in oxalate (*e.g.*, spinach, Swiss chard, cocoa, chocolate, pecans, peanuts). Calcium supplementation with calcium salts such calcium carbonate and calcium phosphate also may be used to bind oxalate in the intestine and decrease its absorption.[10] Thiazide diuretics lower urinary calcium by increasing tubular reabsorption so that less remains in the urine. Drugs that bind calcium in the gut (*e.g.*, cellulose phosphate) may be used to inhibit calcium absorption and urinary excretion.

Measures to change the pH of the urine also can influence kidney stone formation. In persons who lose the ability to lower the pH of (or acidify) their urine, there is an increase in the divalent and trivalent forms of urine phosphate that combine with calcium to form calcium phosphate stones. The formation of uric acid stones is increased in acid urine; stone formation can be reduced by raising the pH of urine to 6.0 to 6.5 with potassium alkali (*e.g.*, potassium citrate) salts. Table 33-2 summarizes measures for preventing the recurrence of different types of kidney stones.

In some cases, stone removal may be necessary. Several methods are available for removing kidney stones: ureteroscopic removal, percutaneous removal, and extracorporeal lithotripsy. All these procedures eliminate the need for an open surgical procedure, which is another form of treatment. Open stone surgery may be required to remove large calculi or those that are resistant to other forms of removal.

Ureteroscopic removal involves the passage of an instrument through the urethra into the bladder and then into the ureter. The development of high-quality optics has improved the ease with which this procedure is performed and its outcome. The procedure, which is performed under fluoroscopic guidance, involves the use of various instruments for dilating the ureter and for grasping, fragmenting, and removing the stone. Preprocedure radiologic studies using a contrast medium (*i.e.*, excretory urography) are done to determine the position of the stone and direct the placement of the ureteroscope.

Percutaneous nephrolithotomy is the treatment of choice for removal of renal or proximal ureteral calculi. It involves the insertion through the flank of a small-gauge needle into the collecting system of the kidney; the needle tract is then dilated, and an instrument called a *nephroscope* is inserted into the renal pelvis. The procedure is performed under fluoroscopic guidance. Preprocedure radiologic and ultrasonographic examinations of the kidney and ureter are used in determining the placement of the nephroscope. Stones up to 1 cm in diameter can be removed through this method. Larger stones must be broken up with an electrohydraulic or ultrasonic lithotriptor (*i.e.*, stone breaker).

A nonsurgical treatment called *extracorporeal shock-wave lithotripsy*, introduced in Germany in 1980, received U.S. Food and Drug Administration approval in 1984 for treatment of stones primarily in the renal calix and pelvis and the upper third of the ureter. The procedure uses acoustic shock waves to fragment calculi into sandlike particles that are passed in the urine over the next few days. Because of the large amount of stone particles that are generated during the procedure, a ureteral stent (*i.e.*, tubelike device used to hold the ureter open) may be inserted to ensure adequate urine drainage.

In summary, obstruction of urine flow can occur at any level of the urinary tract. Among the causes of urinary tract obstruction are developmental defects, pregnancy, infection and inflammation, kidney stones, neurologic defects, and prostatic hypertrophy. Obstructive disorders produce stasis of urine, increasing the risk of infection and calculi formation and resulting in back pressure that is damaging to kidney structures.

Kidney stones are a major cause of upper urinary tract obstruction. There are four types of kidney stones: calcium (*i.e.*, oxalate and phosphate) stones, which are associated with increased serum calcium levels; magnesium ammonium phosphate (*i.e.*, struvite) stones, which are associated with UTIs; uric acid stones, which are related to elevated uric acid levels; and cystine stones, which are seen in cystinuria. A major goal of treatment for persons who have passed kidney stones or have had them removed is to identify stone composition and prevent their recurrence. Treatment measures depend on stone type and include adequate fluid intake to prevent urine saturation, dietary modification to decrease intake of stone-forming constituents, treatment of UTI, measures to change urine pH, and the use of diuretics that decrease the calcium concentration of urine.

Urinary Tract Infections

After you have completed this section of the chapter, you should be able to meet the following objectives:

✦ Cite the organisms most responsible for UTIs and state why urinary catheters, obstruction, and reflux predispose to infections

✦ List three physiologic mechanisms that protect against UTIs

✦ Compare the signs and symptoms of upper and lower UTIs

✦ Describe factors that predispose to UTIs in children, sexually active women, pregnant women, and older adults

✦ Compare the manifestations of UTIs in different age groups, including infants, toddlers, adolescents, adults, and older adults

✦ Cite measures used in the diagnosis and treatment of UTIs

Urinary tract infections are the second most common type of bacterial infections seen by health care providers (respiratory tract infections are first). Each year, over 8 million people are diagnosed with UTIs. In 1997, UTIs accounted for 8.3 million physician visits and 1.68 million hospitalizations.[1] UTIs can include several distinct entities, including asymptomatic bacteriuria, symptomatic infections, lower UTIs such as cystitis, and upper UTIs such as pyelonephritis. Because of their ability to cause renal damage, upper UTIs are considered more serious than lower UTIs.

ETIOLOGIC FACTORS

Most UTIs are caused by *Escherichia coli.* Other common pathogens include *Staphylococcus saprophyticus, Proteus mirabilis, Klebsiella pneumoniae,* and *Enterococcus* species.[16–18] Bacteria can enter the kidneys either through the bloodstream or as an ascending infection from the lower urinary tract. Most infections are of the ascending type. Although the distal portion of the urethra often contains pathogens, the urine formed in the kidneys and found in the bladder normally is sterile or free of bacteria. This is because of the *washout phenomenon,* in which urine from the bladder normally washes bacteria out of the urethra. When a UTI occurs, the bacteria that have colonized the urethra, vagina, or perineal area often are responsible.

There is an increased risk of UTI in persons with urinary obstruction and reflux; in people with neurogenic disorders that impair bladder emptying; in women who are sexually active, especially if they use a diaphragm or spermicide for contraception; in postmenopausal women; in men with diseases of the prostate; and in elderly persons. Instrumentation and urinary catheterization are the most common predisposing factors for nosocomial UTIs.

Because certain people tend to be predisposed to development of UTIs, considerable interest has been focused on host-agent interactions and factors that increase the risk of UTI.

Host Defenses

In the development of a UTI, host defenses are matched against the virulence of the pathogen. The host defenses of the bladder have several components, including the washout phenomenon, in which bacteria are removed from the bladder and urethra during voiding; the protective mucin layer that lines the bladder and protects against bacterial invasion; and local immune responses. In the ureters, peristaltic movements facilitate the movement of urine from the renal pelvis through the ureters and into the bladder. Immune mechanisms, particularly secretory immunoglobulin A (IgA), appear to provide an important antibacterial defense. Phagocytic blood cells further assist in the removal of bacteria from the urinary tract.

There has been a growing appreciation of the protective function of the bladder's mucin layer.[19] It is thought that the epithelial cells that line the bladder synthesize protective substances that subsequently become incorporated into the mucin layer that adheres to the bladder wall. One theory proposes that the mucin layer acts by binding water, which then constitutes a protective barrier between the bacteria and the bladder epithelium. Elderly and postmenopausal women produce less mucin than younger women, suggesting that estrogen may play a role in mucin production in women.

Pathogen Virulence

Investigations are focusing on the adherence properties of the bacteria that infect the urinary tract. These bacteria have fine protein filaments that help them adhere to receptors on the lining of urinary tract structures.[19,20] These filaments are called *fimbriae* or *pili.* Among the factors that contribute to bacterial virulence, the type of fimbriae that the bacteria possess may be the most important. Bacteria with certain types of fimbriae are associated primarily with cystitis, and those with other types are associated with a high incidence of pyelonephritis. The bacteria associated with pyelonephritis are thought to have fimbriae that bind to carbohydrates that are specific to the surfaces of epithelial cells in this part of the urinary tract.

Urinary Tract Infections

➤ Urinary tract infections involve both the lower and upper urinary tract structures.

➤ In lower urinary tract infections, the infecting pathogens tend to propagate in the urine and cause irritative voiding symptoms, often with minimal systemic signs of infection.

➤ Upper urinary tract infections tend to invade the tissues of the kidney pelvis, inciting an acute inflammatory response with marked systemic manifestations of infection.

Obstruction and Reflux

Obstruction and reflux are important contributing factors in the development of UTIs. Any microorganisms that enter the bladder normally are washed out during voiding. When outflow is obstructed, urine remains in the bladder and acts as a medium for microbial growth; the microorganisms in the contaminated urine can then ascend along the ureters to infect the kidneys. The presence of residual urine correlates closely with bacteriuria and with its recurrence after treatment. Another aspect of bladder outflow obstruction and bladder distention is increased intravesicular pressure, which compresses blood vessels in the bladder wall, leading to a decrease in the mucosal defenses of the bladder.

In UTIs associated with stasis of urine flow, the obstruction may be anatomic or functional. Anatomic obstructions include urinary tract stones, prostatic hyperplasia, pregnancy, and malformations of the ureterovesical junction. Functional obstructions include neurogenic bladder, infrequent voiding, detrusor (bladder) muscle instability, and constipation.

Reflux occurs when urine from the urethra moves into the bladder (*i.e.*, urethrovesical reflux) or from the bladder into the ureters (*i.e.*, vesicoureteral reflux). In women, *urethrovesical reflux* can occur during activities such as coughing or squatting, in which an increase in intra-abdominal pressure causes the urine to be squeezed into the urethra and then to flow back into the bladder as the pressure decreases. This also can happen when voiding is abruptly interrupted. Because the urethral orifice frequently is contaminated with bacteria, the reflux mechanism may cause bacteria to be drawn back into the bladder.

A second type of reflux mechanism, *vesicoureteral reflux*, occurs at the level of the bladder and ureter. Normally, the distal portion of the ureter courses between the muscle layer and the mucosal surface of the bladder wall, forming a flap. The flap is compressed against the bladder wall during micturition, preventing urine from being forced into the ureter (Fig. 33-8). In persons with vesicoureteral reflux, the ureter enters the bladder at an approximate right angle such that urine is forced into the ureter during micturition. It is seen most commonly in children with UTIs and is believed to result from congenital defects in length, diameter, muscle structure, or innervation of the submucosal segment of the ureter. Vesicoureteral reflux also is seen in adults with obstruction to bladder outflow, primarily due to increased bladder volume and pressure.

Catheter-Induced Infection

Urinary catheters are tubes made of latex or plastic. They are inserted through the urethra into the bladder for the purpose of draining urine. They are a source of urethral irritation and provide a means for entry of microorganisms into the urinary tract.

Catheter-associated bacteriuria remains the most frequent cause of gram-negative septicemia in hospitalized patients. Studies have shown that bacteria adhere to the surface of the catheter and initiate the growth of a biofilm that then covers the surface of the catheter.[16] The biofilm tends to protect the bacteria from the action of antibiotics and

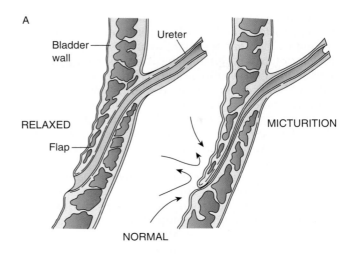

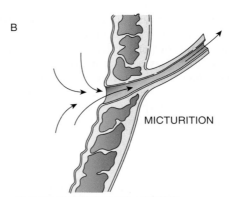

FIGURE 33-8 Anatomic features of the bladder and kidney in pyelonephritis caused by vesicoureteral reflux. Bladder. (**A**) In the normal bladder, the distal portion of the intravesical ureter courses between the mucosa and the muscularis of the bladder. A mucosal flap is thus formed. On micturition, the elevated intravesicular pressure compresses the flap against the bladder wall, thereby occluding the lumen. (**B**) Persons with a congenitally short intravesical ureter have no mucosal flap, because the entry of the ureter into the bladder approaches a right angle. Thus, micturition forces urine into the ureter. (Rubin E., Farber J.L. [1999]. *Pathology* [3rd ed., p. 903]. Philadelphia: Lippincott Williams & Wilkins.) (Courtesy of Dmitri Karetnikov, artist)

makes treatment difficult. A closed drainage system (*i.e.*, closed to air and other sources of contamination) and careful attention to perineal hygiene (*i.e.*, cleaning the area around the urethral meatus) help to prevent infections in persons who require an indwelling catheter. Careful hand washing and early detection and treatment of UTIs also are essential.

MANIFESTATIONS

The manifestations of UTI depend on whether the infection involves the lower or upper urinary tract. An acute episode of cystitis (bladder infection) or lower UTI is characterized by frequency of urination (sometimes as often as every 20 minutes), lower abdominal or back discomfort, and burning and pain on urination (*i.e.*, dysuria). Occasionally the urine is cloudy and foul smelling. In adults, fever and other signs of infection usually are absent. If there are no complications, the symptoms disappear within 48 hours of treatment. This type of UTI is common in younger women. The symptoms of cystitis also may represent urethritis caused by *Chlamydia trachomatis*, *Neisseria gonorrhoeae*, or herpes simplex virus, or vaginitis attributable to *Trichomonas vaginalis* or *Candida* species.

Upper UTIs affect the parenchyma and pelvis of the kidney (pyelonephritis). They tend to produce more systemic signs of infection than lower UTIs because of closer proximity to the vascular compartment and blood cells (*e.g.*, neutrophils) that incite the inflammatory response. Acute pyelonephritis tends to present with an abrupt onset of shaking chills, moderate to high fever, and constant ache in the loin area of the back that is unilateral or bilateral.[19,20] Lower urinary tract symptoms, including dysuria, frequency, and urgency, also are common. There may be significant malaise, and the person usually looks and feels ill. Nausea and vomiting may occur along with abdominal pain. Palpation or percussion over the costovertebral angle on the affected side usually causes pain. Pyelonephritis occurs more frequently in children and adults with urinary tract obstructions or other predisposing conditions.

DIAGNOSIS

The diagnosis of UTI usually is based on symptoms and on examination of the urine for the presence of microorganisms. When necessary, x-ray films, ultrasonography, and CT and renal scans are used to identify contributing factors, such as obstruction.

Microscopic urine tests are used establish the presence of bacteria and blood cells in the urine.[10] A commonly accepted criterion for diagnosis of a UTI is the presence of 10^5 or more bacteria per milliliter of urine.[10] Colonization usually is defined as the multiplication of microorganisms in or on a host without apparent evidence of invasiveness or tissue injury. Pyuria (the presence of less than five to eight leukocytes per high-power field) indicates a host response to infection rather than asymptomatic bacterial colonization. A Gram stain may be done to determine the type of organism that is present (gram positive or gram negative).

Chemical screening (urine dipstick) for markers of infection may provide useful information but is less sensitive than microscopic analysis. Bacteria reduce nitrates in the urine to nitrites, providing a means for chemical analysis. Similarly, activated leukocytes secrete leukocyte esterase, which can be detected chemically. These two chemical tests have sensitivities ranging from 56% to 92% and rarely are positive in the absence of infection.[10] Therefore, they are commonly used as a screening tool in persons with symptoms of UTI. The tests are relatively inexpensive, easy to perform, and can be done in the clinic setting or even in the home.

A urine culture confirms the presence of pathogenic bacteria in urine specimens, allows for their identification, and permits the determination of their sensitivity to specific antibiotics. Urine culture requires collection of urine in a sterile container, and efforts are made to prevent contamination of the specimen. Specimens that are kept for longer than 1 hour must be refrigerated to prevent the contaminating organisms from multiplying. The use of catheterized urine specimens, once common, has largely been replaced with clean-voided specimens. To obtain a clean-voided specimen, the area around the urethra is carefully cleansed and a midstream specimen is obtained by having the person void directly into a sterile container. This method usually is adequate and eliminates the risk of introducing microorganisms into the bladder during insertion of a catheter. In infants and sometimes in other age groups, suprapubic aspiration may be done to obtain a sample of bladder urine.

TREATMENT

The treatment of UTI is based on the type of infection that is present (lower or upper UTI), the pathogen causing the infection, and the presence of contributing host-agent factors. Other considerations include whether the infection is acute, recurrent, or chronic.

Acute Urinary Tract Infections

Most acute lower UTIs are treated successfully with antimicrobial therapy and increased fluid intake. Acute cystitis commonly is treated with a 3-day course of antibiotics, although a longer course of treatment may be needed. Forcing fluids may relieve signs and symptoms, and this approach is used as an adjunct to antibiotic treatment.

Because there is risk of permanent kidney damage with pyelonephritis, these infections are treated more aggressively. Treatment with an appropriate antimicrobial agent usually is continued for 10 to 14 days. Hospitalization may be recommended during the early stages of infection until a response to treatment is observed.[21]

Recurrent Urinary Tract Infections

Recurrent lower UTIs are those that recur after treatment. They are due either to bacterial persistence or reinfection. Bacterial persistence usually is curable by removal of the infectious source (*e.g.*, urinary catheter or infected bladder stones). Reinfection is managed principally through education regarding pathogen transmission and prevention measures. Cranberry juice or blueberry juice has been suggested as a preventive measure for persons with frequent UTIs. Studies suggest that these juices reduce bacterial adherence to the epithelial lining of the urinary tract.[22,23] Because of their mechanism of action, these juices are used more appropriately in prevention rather than treatment of an established UTI.

Chronic Urinary Tract Infections

Chronic UTIs are more difficult to treat. Because they often are associated with obstructive uropathy or reflux flow of urine, diagnostic tests usually are performed to detect such abnormalities. When possible, the condition causing the reflux flow or obstruction is corrected. Most persons with recurrent UTIs are treated with antibiotics for 10 to 14 days in doses sufficient to maintain high urine levels of the drug, and they are examined for obstruction or other causes of infection. Men in particular should be investigated for obstructive disorders or a prostatic focus of infection.

INFECTIONS IN SPECIAL POPULATIONS

Urinary tract infections affect persons of all ages. In infants, they occur more often in boys than in girls. After the first year of life, however, UTIs are more frequent in females because of the shorter length of the urethra and because the vaginal vestibule can be easily contaminated with fecal flora. Approximately 20% of all adult women have at least one UTI during their lifetime. In men, the longer length of the urethra and the antibacterial properties of the prostatic fluid provide some protection from ascending UTIs until approximately 50 years of age. After this age, prostatic hypertrophy becomes more common, and with it may come obstruction and increased risk of UTI (see Chapter 43).

Urinary Tract Infections in Women

In women, the urethra is short and close to the vagina and rectum, offering little protection against entry of microorganisms into the bladder. There is a peak incidence of these infections in the 15- to 24-year-old age group, suggesting that hormonal and anatomic changes associated with puberty and sexual activity contribute to UTIs.

The role of sexual activity in the development of urethritis and cystitis is controversial. The well-documented "honeymoon cystitis" suggests that sexual activity may contribute to such infections in susceptible women. The anterior urethra usually is colonized with bacteria; urethral massage or sexual intercourse can force these bacteria back into the bladder. Using a diaphragm and spermicide enhances the susceptibility to infection.[24] A nonpharmacologic approach to the treatment of frequent UTIs associated with sexual intercourse is to increase fluid intake before intercourse and to void soon after intercourse. This procedure uses the washout phenomenon to remove bacteria from the bladder.

Pregnant women are at increased risk for UTIs. Normal changes in the functioning of the urinary tract that occur during pregnancy predispose to UTIs.[25] These changes involve the collecting system of the kidneys and include dilatation of the renal calices, pelves, and ureters that begins during the first trimester and becomes most pronounced during the third trimester. This dilatation of the upper urinary system is accompanied by a reduction in the peristaltic activity of the ureters that is thought to result from the muscle-relaxing effects of progesterone-like hormones and mechanical obstruction from the enlarging uterus. In addition to the changes in the kidneys and ureters, the bladder becomes displaced from its pelvic position to a more abdominal position, producing further changes in ureteral position.

Asymptomatic UTIs are common, with a prevalence rate of 10% in pregnant women. The complications of asymptomatic UTIs during pregnancy include persistent bacteriuria, acute and chronic pyelonephritis, toxemia of pregnancy, and premature delivery. Evidence suggests that few women become bacteriuric during pregnancy. Rather, it appears that symptomatic UTIs during pregnancy reflect preexisting asymptomatic bacteriuria, and that changes occurring during pregnancy simply permit the prior urinary colonization to lead to symptomatic infection and invasion of the kidneys.[26] Untreated asymptomatic bacteriuria leads to symptomatic cystitis in approximately 30% of pregnant women.[25] Because bacteriuria may occur as an asymptomatic condition in pregnant women, the American College of Obstetrics and Gynecology recommends that a urine culture be obtained at the first prenatal visit.[25,27] A repeat culture should be obtained during the third trimester. Women with bacteriuria should be followed closely, and infections should be properly treated to prevent complications. The choice of antimicrobial agent should address the common infecting organisms and should be safe for the mother and fetus.

Urinary Tract Infections in Children

Urinary tract infections occur in as many as 3% to 5% of female and 1% of male children.[4] In girls, the average age at first diagnosis is 3 years, which coincides with onset of toilet training. In boys, most UTIs occur during the first year of life; they are more common in uncircumcised than in circumcised boys. Children who are at increased risk for bacteriuria or symptomatic UTIs are premature infants discharged from neonatal intensive care units; children with systemic or immunologic disease or urinary tract abnormalities such as neurogenic bladder or vesicoureteral reflux; those with a family history of UTI or urinary tract anomalies with reflux; and girls younger than 5 years of age with a history of UTI.[28]

UTIs in children frequently involve the upper urinary tract (pyelonephritis). In children in whom renal development is not complete, pyelonephritis can lead to renal scarring and permanent kidney damage. It has been reported that more than 75% of children younger than 5 years of age with febrile UTIs have pyelonephritis, and that renal scarring occurs in 27% to 64% of children with pyelonephritis.[29] Most UTIs that lead to scarring and diminished kidney growth occur in children younger than 4 years, especially infants younger than 1 year of age. The incidence of scarring is greatest in children with gross vesicoureteral reflux or obstruction, in children with recurrent UTIs, and those with a delay in treatment.

Unlike adults, children frequently do not present with the typical signs of a UTI.[29,30] Many neonates with UTIs have bacteremia and may show signs and symptoms of septicemia, including fever, hypothermia, apneic spells, poor skin perfusion, abdominal distention, diarrhea, vomiting, lethargy, and irritability. Older infants may present with feeding problems, failure to thrive, diarrhea, vomiting, fever, and foul-smelling urine. Toddlers often present with abdominal pain, vomiting, diarrhea, abnormal voiding patterns, foul-smelling urine, fever, and poor growth. In older children with lower UTIs, the classic features—enuresis, frequency, dysuria, and suprapubic discomfort—are more common. Fever is a common sign of UTI in children, and the possibility of UTI should be considered in children with unexplained fever.

Diagnosis is based on a careful history of voiding patterns and symptomatology; physical examination to determine fever, hypertension, abdominal or suprapubic tenderness, and other manifestations of UTI; and urinalysis to determine bacteriuria, pyuria, proteinuria, and hematuria. A positive urine culture that is obtained correctly is essential for the diagnosis. Additional diagnostic methods may be needed to determine the cause of the disorder. Vesicoureteral reflux is the most commonly associated abnormality in UTIs, and reflux nephropathy is an important cause of end-stage renal disease in children and adolescents. Children with a relatively uncomplicated first UTI may turn out to have significant reflux. Therefore, even a single documented UTI in a child requires careful diagnosis. Urinary symptoms in the absence of bacteriuria suggest vaginitis, urethritis, sexual molestation, the use of irritating bubble baths, pinworms, or viral cystitis. In adolescent girls, a history of dysuria and vaginal discharge makes vaginitis or vulvitis a consideration.

The approach to treatment is based on the clinical severity of the infection, the site of infection (*i.e.*, lower vs. upper urinary tract), the risk of sepsis, and the presence of structural abnormalities. The immediate treatment of infants and young children is essential. Most infants with symptomatic UTIs and many children with clinical evidence of acute upper UTIs require hospitalization and intravenous antibiotic therapy. Follow-up is essential for children with febrile UTIs to ensure resolution of the infection. Follow-up urine cultures often are done at the end of treatment. Imaging studies often are recommended for all children after first UTIs to detect renal scarring, vesicoureteral reflux, or other abnormalities.[29,31]

Urinary Tract Infections in the Elderly

Urinary tract infections are relatively common in elderly persons. It has been reported that 5% to 20% of the elderly living at home have bacteriuria. These numbers increase to 15% to 25% for the elderly living in nursing homes or extended-care facilities.[32]

Most of these infections follow invasion of the urinary tract by the ascending route. Several factors predispose elderly persons to UTIs: immobility resulting in poor bladder emptying, bladder outflow obstruction caused by prostatic hyperplasia or kidney stones, bladder ischemia caused by urine retention, senile vaginitis, constipation, and diminished bactericidal activity of urine and prostatic secretions. Added to these risks are other health problems that necessitate instrumentation of the urinary tract. UTIs develop in 1% of ambulatory patients after a single catheterization and within 3 to 4 days in essentially all patients with indwelling catheters.[33]

Elderly persons with bacteriuria have varying symptoms, ranging from the absence of symptoms to the presence of typical UTI symptoms. Even when symptoms of lower UTIs are present, they may be difficult to interpret because elderly persons without UTIs commonly experience urgency, frequency, and incontinence. Alternatively, elderly persons may have vague symptoms such as anorexia, fatigue, weakness, or change in mental status. Even with more serious upper UTIs (*e.g.*, pyelonephritis), the classic signs of infection such as fever, chills, flank pain, and tenderness may be altered or absent in elderly persons.[32] Sometimes, no symptoms occur until the infection is far advanced.

In summary, UTI is the second most common type of bacterial infection seen by health care professionals. Infections can range from simple bacteriuria to severe kidney infections that cause irreversible kidney damage. Predisposition to infection is determined by host defenses and pathogen virulence. Host defenses include the washout phenomenon associated with voiding, the protective mucin lining of the bladder, and local immune defenses. Pathogen virulence is enhanced by the presence of fimbriae that facilitate adherence to structures in the urinary tract.

Most UTIs ascend from the urethra and bladder. A number of factors interact in determining the predisposition to development of UTIs, including urinary tract obstruction, urine stasis and reflux, pregnancy-induced changes in urinary tract function, age-related changes in the urinary tract, changes in the protective mechanisms of the bladder and ureters, impaired immune function, and virulence of the pathogen. Urinary tract catheters and urinary instrumentation contribute to the incidence of UTIs. Early diagnosis and treatment of UTI are essential to preventing permanent kidney damage.

Disorders of Glomerular Function

After you have completed this section of the chapter, you should be able to meet the following objectives:

+ Describe the two types of immune mechanisms involved in glomerular disorders
+ Use the terms *proliferation, sclerosis, membranous, diffuse, focal, segmental,* and *mesangial* to explain changes in glomerular structure that occur with glomerulonephritis
+ Relate the proteinuria, hematuria, pyuria, oliguria, edema, hypertension, and azotemia that occur with glomerulonephritis to changes in glomerular structure
+ Differentiate the pathology and manifestations of the nephrotic syndrome from those of the nephritic syndrome

The glomeruli are tufts of capillaries that lie between the afferent and efferent arterioles. The capillaries of the glomeruli are arranged in lobules and supported by a stalk consisting of mesangial cells and a basement membrane-like extracellular matrix (Fig. 33-9). The glomerular membrane is composed of three layers: an endothelial layer lining the capillary, a basement membrane, and a layer of epithelial cells forming the outer surface of the capillary and lining Bowman's capsule (see Fig. 30-5, Chapter 30). The epithelial

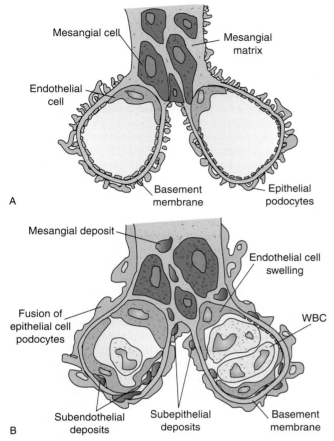

A

B

FIGURE 33-9 Schematic representation of glomerulus. (**A**) Normal; (**B**) localization of immune deposits (mesangial, subendothelial, subepithelial) and changes in glomerular architecture associated with injury. (Whitley K., Keane W.F., & Vernier R.L. [1984]. Acute glomerulonephritis: A clinical overview. *Medical Clinics of North America* 68 [2], 263)

cells are attached to the basement membrane by discrete cytoplasmic extensions, the foot processes (*i.e.*, podocytes). In the glomeruli, blood is filtered, and the urine filtrate formed. The capillary membrane is selectively permeable: it allows water, electrolytes, and dissolved particles, such as glucose and amino acids, to leave the capillary and enter Bowman's space and prevents larger particles, such as plasma proteins and blood cells, from leaving the blood.

MECHANISMS OF GLOMERULAR INJURY

Glomerulonephritis, an inflammatory process that involves glomerular structures, is the leading cause of chronic renal failure in the United States, accounting for one half of persons with end-stage renal disease.[34] There are many causes of glomerular disease. The disease may occur as a primary condition in which the glomerular abnormality is the only disease present, or it may occur as a secondary condition in which the glomerular abnormality results from another disease, such as diabetes mellitus or SLE. An understanding of the various forms of glomerular disease has emerged only recently. Much of this knowledge can be attributed to advances in immunobiology and electron microscopy, development of animal models, and increased use of renal biopsy during the early stages of glomerular disease.

Glomerulonephritis is characterized by hematuria with red cell casts, a diminished glomerular filtration rate (GFR), azotemia (presence of nitrogenous wastes in the blood), oliguria, and hypertension. It is caused by diseases that provoke a proliferative inflammatory response of the endothelial, mesangial, or epithelial cells of the glomeruli. The inflammatory process damages the capillary wall, permitting red blood cells to escape into the urine and producing hemodynamic changes that decrease the GFR.

Although little is known about the causative agents or triggering events that produce glomerular disease, most cases of primary and many cases of secondary glomerular disease probably have an immune origin.[5,6,34,35] Two types of immune mechanisms have been implicated in the development of glomerular disease: injury resulting from antibodies reacting with fixed glomerular antigens, and injury resulting from circulating antigen-antibody complexes that become trapped in the glomerular membrane (Fig. 33-10). Antigens responsible for development of the immune response may be of endogenous origin, such as DNA in SLE, or they may be of exogenous origin, such as streptococcal membrane antigens in poststreptococcal glomerulonephritis. Frequently, the source of the antigen is unknown.

FIGURE 33-10 Immune mechanisms of glomerular disease. (**A**) Antiglomerular antibodies leave the circulation and interact with antigens that are present in the basement membrane of the glomerulus. (**B**) Antigen-antibody complexes circulating in the blood become trapped as they are filtered in the glomerulus.

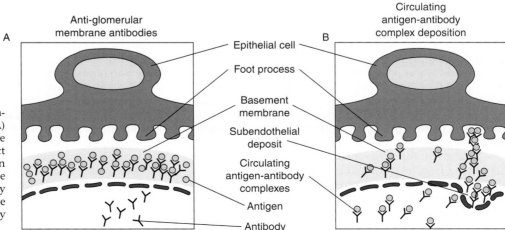

SPECIFIC TYPES OF GLOMERULAR DISEASE

The cellular changes that occur with glomerular disease include proliferative, sclerotic, and membranous changes. The term *proliferative* refers to an increase in the cellular components of the glomerulus, regardless of origin; *sclerotic* to an increase in the noncellular components of the glomerulus, primarily collagen; and *membranous* to an increase in the thickness of the glomerular capillary wall, often caused by immune complex deposition. Glomerular changes can be *diffuse*, involving all glomeruli and all parts of the glomeruli; *focal*, in which only some glomeruli are affected and others are essentially normal; *segmental*, involving only a certain segment of each glomeruli; or *mesangial*, affecting only the mesangial cell. Figure 33-9 shows changes associated with various types of glomerular disease.

Among the different types of glomerular diseases are acute proliferative glomerulonephritis, rapidly progressive glomerulonephritis, nephrotic syndrome, membranous glomerulonephritis, minimal change disease (lipoid nephrosis), focal segmental glomerulosclerosis, and IgA nephropathy, and chronic glomerulonephritis.

Acute Proliferative Glomerulonephritis

The most commonly recognized form of acute glomerulonephritis is diffuse proliferative glomerulonephritis, which follows infections caused by strains of group A β-hemolytic streptococci. Diffuse proliferative glomerulonephritis also may occur after infections by other organisms, including staphylococci and a number of viral agents, such as those responsible for mumps, measles, and chickenpox. With this type of nephritis, the inflammatory response is caused by an immune reaction that occurs when circulating immune complexes become entrapped in the glomerular membrane. Proliferation of the endothelial cells lining the glomerular capillary (*i.e.*, endocapillary form of the disease) and the mesangial cells lying between the endothelium and the epithelium follows (see Fig. 33-9). The capillary membrane swells and becomes permeable to plasma proteins and blood cells. Although the disease is seen primarily in children, adults of any age also can be affected.

The classic case of poststreptococcal glomerulonephritis follows a streptococcal infection by approximately 7 to 12 days—the time needed for the development of antibodies.[34] Oliguria, which develops as the GFR decreases, is one of the first symptoms. Proteinuria and hematuria follow because of increased glomerular capillary wall permeability. The blood is degraded by materials in the urine, and a cola-colored urine may be the first sign of the disorder. Sodium and water retention gives rise to edema, particularly of the face and hands, and hypertension. Important laboratory findings include an elevated streptococcal exoenzyme (antistreptolysin O) titer, a decline in C3 complement (see Chapter 18), and cryoglobulins (*i.e.*, large immune complexes) in the serum.

Treatment for acute poststreptococcal glomerulonephritis is largely symptomatic. The acute symptoms usually begin to subside in approximately 10 days to 2 weeks, although in some children the proteinuria may persist for several months. The immediate prognosis is favorable and approximately 95% of children recover spontaneously.[5] The outlook for adults is less favorable; approximately 60% recover completely. In the remainder of cases, the lesions eventually resolve, but there may be permanent kidney damage.

Rapidly Progressive Glomerulonephritis

Rapidly progressive glomerulonephritis is a clinical syndrome characterized by signs of severe glomerular injury that does not have a specific cause. As its name indicates, this type of glomerulonephritis is rapidly progressive, often within a matter of months. The disorder involves focal and segmental proliferation of glomerular cells and recruitment of monocytes (macrophages) with formation of crescent-shaped structures that obliterate Bowman's space.[5] Rapidly proliferative glomerulonephritis may be caused by a number of immunologic disorders, some systemic and others restricted to the kidney. Among the diseases associated with this form of glomerulonephritis are immune complex disorders such as SLE, the small vessel vasculitides (*e.g.*, microscopic polyangiitis), and an immune disorder condition called *Goodpasture's syndrome*.

Goodpasture's syndrome, which is caused by antibodies to the glomerular basement membrane (GBM), accounts for approximately 5% of cases of rapidly progressive glomerulonephritis. It is a rare disease and is associated with a triad of pulmonary hemorrhage, iron-deficiency anemia, and glomerulonephritis. All of these manifestations result from anti-GBM antibody deposition in the lungs and glomeruli. The cause of the disorder is unknown, although influenza infection and exposure to hydrocarbon solvent (found in paints and dyes) have been implicated in some persons, as have various drugs and cancers. There is a high prevalence of certain human leukocyte antigen subtypes (*e.g.*, HLA-DRB1), suggesting a genetic predisposition.[5] Treatment includes plasmapheresis to remove circulating anti-GBM antibodies and immunosuppressive therapy (*i.e.*, corticosteroids and cyclophosphamide) to inhibit antibody production.

NEPHROTIC SYNDROME

Nephrotic syndrome is not a specific glomerular disease but a constellation of clinical findings that result from increased glomerular permeability to the plasma proteins (Fig. 33-11). The glomerular derangements that occur with nephrosis can develop as a primary disorder or secondary to changes caused by systemic diseases such as diabetes mellitus, amyloidosis, and SLE. Among the primary glomerular lesions leading to nephrotic syndrome are minimal change disease (lipoid nephrosis), focal segmental glomerulosclerosis, and membranous glomerulonephritis. The relative frequency of these causes varies with age. In children younger than 15 years of age, nephrotic syndrome almost always is caused by primary glomerular disease, whereas in adults it often is a secondary disorder.[5]

The nephrotic syndrome is characterized by massive proteinuria (>3.5 g/day) and lipiduria (*e.g.*, free fat, oval bodies, fatty casts), along with an associated hypoalbuminemia (<3 g/dL), generalized edema, and hyperlipidemia

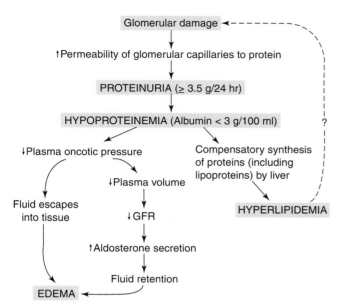

FIGURE 33-11 Pathophysiology of the nephrotic syndrome. The relationship between hyperlipidemia and glomerular damage (*dashed line*) has been demonstrated in experimental models of certain diseases associated with nephrotic range proteinuria (*e.g.,* focal segmental glomerulosclerosis), but its significance in human renal disease is still somewhat unknown. (GFR, glomerular filtration rate.) (Rubin E., Farber J.L. [1999]. *Pathology* [3rd ed., p. 869]. Philadelphia: Lippincott Williams & Wilkins)

(cholesterol >300 mg/dL).[6,36,37,38] The initiating event in the development of nephrosis is a derangement in the glomerular membrane that causes increased permeability to plasma proteins. The glomerular membrane acts as a size and charge barrier through which the glomerular filtrate must pass. Any increased permeability allows protein to escape from the plasma into the glomerular filtrate.

Generalized edema, which is a hallmark of nephrosis, results from salt and water retention and a loss of serum albumin below that needed to maintain the colloid osmotic pressure of the vascular compartment.[5] The sodium and water retention appears to be due to several factors, including a compensatory increase in aldosterone, stimulation of the sympathetic nervous system, and a reduction in secretion of natriuretic factors. Initially, the edema presents in dependent parts of the body such as the lower extremities, but becomes more generalized as the disease progresses. Dyspnea due to pulmonary edema, pleural effusions, and diaphragmatic compromise due to ascites can develop in persons with nephrotic syndrome.[20]

Although the largest proportion of plasma protein loss is in albumin, globulins also are lost. As a result, persons with nephrosis are particularly vulnerable to infections, particularly those caused by staphylococci and pneumococci.[5] This decreased resistance to infection probably is related to loss of both immunoglobulins and low–molecular-weight complement components in the urine. Many binding proteins also are lost in the urine. Consequently, the plasma levels of many ions (iron, copper, zinc), hormones (thyroid and sex hormones), and drugs may be low because of decreased binding proteins. Many drugs require protein binding for transport. Hypoalbuminemia reduces the number of available protein binding sites, thereby producing a potential increase in the amount free (active) drug that is available.[36]

Thrombotic complications also have evolved as a risk in persons with nephrotic syndrome. These disorders are thought to be related to a disruption in the function of the coagulation system brought about by a loss of coagulation and anticoagulation factors.[20,36] Renal vein thrombosis, once thought to be a cause of the disorder, is more likely a consequence of the hypercoagulable state.[5] Other thrombotic complications include deep vein thrombosis and pulmonary emboli.

The hyperlipidemia that occurs in persons with nephrosis is characterized by elevated levels of triglycerides and low-density lipoproteins (LDL). Levels of high-density lipoproteins (HDL) usually are normal. These abnormalities are thought to be related, in part, to increased synthesis of lipoproteins in the liver secondary to a compensatory increase in albumin production. Because of the elevated LDL levels, persons with nephrotic syndrome are at increased risk for development of atherosclerosis.

Membranous Glomerulonephritis
Membranous glomerulonephritis is the most common cause of primary nephrosis in adults, most commonly in their sixth or seventh decade. The disorders are caused by diffuse thickening of the GBM due to deposition of immune complexes. The disorder may be idiopathic or associated with a number of disorders, including autoimmune diseases such as SLE, infections such as chronic hepatitis B, metabolic disorders such as diabetes mellitus and thyroiditis, and use of certain drugs such as gold, penicillamine, and captopril.[5] Because of the presence of immunoglobulins and complement in the subendothelial deposits, it is thought that the disease represents a chronic antigen-antibody complex–mediated disorder.

The disorder is treated with corticosteroids. Cytotoxic drugs may be added to the treatment regimen. The progress of the disease is variable; approximately one half of persons sustain a slow but progressive loss of renal function.

Minimal Change Disease (Lipoid Nephrosis)
Minimal change disease is characterized by diffuse loss (through fusion) of the foot processes from the epithelial layer of the glomerular membrane. The peak incidence is between 2 and 6 years of age. The cause of minimal change nephrosis is unknown; however, children in whom the disease develops often have a history of recent upper respiratory infections or of receiving routine immunizations.[5] Although minimal change disease does not progress to renal failure, it can cause significant complications, including predisposition to infection with gram-positive organisms, a tendency toward thromboembolic events, hyperlipidemia, and protein malnutrition. There usually is a dramatic response to corticosteroid therapy.[5]

Focal Segmental Glomerulosclerosis
Focal segmental glomerulosclerosis is characterized by sclerosis (*i.e.,* increased collagen deposition) of some but not all

glomeruli, and in the affected glomeruli, only a portion of the glomerular tuft is involved. Although focal segmental sclerosis often is an idiopathic syndrome, it may be associated with reduced oxygen in the blood (*e.g.*, sickle cell disease and cyanotic congenital heart disease), HIV infection, or intravenous drug abuse, or it may be a secondary event reflecting glomerular scarring due to other forms of glomerulonephritis or reflux nephropathy.[5,6] The presence of hypertension and decreased renal function distinguishes focal sclerosis from minimal change disease. The disorder usually is treated with corticosteroids. Most persons with the disorder progress to end-stage renal disease within 5 to 10 years.

Immunoglobulin A Nephropathy

Immunoglobulin A nephropathy (*i.e.*, Buerger's disease) is a primary type of glomerulonephritis. Most persons are between 16 and 35 years of age at the time of diagnosis. The disease occurs more commonly in males than females and is the most common cause of glomerular nephritis in Asians.[20] The disorder is characterized by the deposition of IgA and occasionally IgG with complement and fibrin-associated antigens in the mesangium of the glomerulus. Serum IgA levels are elevated and may be helpful in the diagnosis of the disorder. The disorder tends to present with hematuria and often is preceded by upper respiratory tract infection, gastrointestinal tract symptoms, or a flulike illness. The association with respiratory and gastrointestinal disorders suggests a genetic or acquired abnormality in immune regulation leading to increased mucosal IgA synthesis in response to antigen exposure.

Gross hematuria usually lasts for 2 to 6 days. Approximately one half of the persons with gross hematuria have a single episode; the remainder have gradual progression of glomerular disease with recurrent episodes of hematuria and mild proteinuria. Progression usually is slow, extending over several decades. There is no satisfactory treatment for IgA nephropathy. The role of immunosuppressive drugs such as steroids and cytotoxic drugs is not clear. There has been recent interest the use of omega-3 fatty acids (fish oil) in delaying the progression of the disease. Evidence suggests that the daily use of fish oil in the diet may retard the progress of the disease, particularly in persons with mildly impaired renal function.[39]

CHRONIC GLOMERULONEPHRITIS

Chronic glomerulonephritis represents the chronic phase of a number of specific types of glomerulonephritis.[5] Some forms of glomerulonephritis (*e.g.*, poststreptococcal glomerulonephritis) undergo complete resolution, whereas others progress at variable rates to chronic glomerulonephritis. Some persons who present with chronic glomerulonephritis have no history of glomerular disease. These cases may represent the end result of relatively asymptomatic forms of glomerulonephritis. Histologically, the condition is characterized by small kidneys with sclerosed glomeruli. In most cases, chronic glomerulonephritis develops insidiously and

slowly progresses to end-stage renal disease over a period of years (see Chapter 34).

GLOMERULAR LESIONS ASSOCIATED WITH SYSTEMIC DISEASE

Many immunologic, metabolic, or hereditary systemic diseases are associated with glomerular injury. In some diseases, such as SLE and diabetes mellitus, the glomerular involvement may be a major clinical manifestation. The glomerular lesions associated with diabetes mellitus and hypertension are discussed in this chapter.

Diabetic Glomerulosclerosis

Diabetic nephropathy, or kidney disease, is a major complication of diabetes mellitus. It affects approximately 30% of persons with type 1 diabetes and accounts for 20% of deaths in diabetic patients younger than 40 years of age.[5]

The glomerulus is the most commonly affected structure in diabetic nephropathy, evidenced by three glomerular syndromes: non-nephrotic proteinuria, nephrotic syndrome, and renal failure. Widespread thickening of the glomerular capillary basement membrane occurs in almost all persons with diabetes and can occur without evidence of proteinuria.[5] This is followed by a diffuse increase in mesangial matrix, with mild proliferation of mesangial cells. As the disease progresses, the mesangial cells impinge on the capillary lumen, drastically reducing the surface area for glomerular filtration.[40] In nodular glomerulosclerosis, also known as *Kimmelstiel-Wilson syndrome*, there is nodular deposition of hyaline in the mesangial portion of the glomerulus. As the sclerotic process progresses in the diffuse and nodular forms of glomerulosclerosis, there is complete obliteration of the glomerulus, with impairment of renal function.

Although the mechanisms of glomerular change in diabetes are uncertain, they are thought to represent enhanced or defective synthesis of the GBM and mesangial matrix with an inappropriate incorporation of glucose into the noncellular components of these glomerular structures. Alternatively, hemodynamic changes that occur secondary to elevated blood glucose levels may contribute to the initiation and progression of diabetic glomerulosclerosis. It has been hypothesized that elevations in blood glucose produce an increase in GFR and glomerular intracapillary pressure that leads to an enlargement of glomerular capillary pores by a mechanism that is at least partly mediated by angiotensin II. This enlargement impairs the size-selective function of the membrane so that the protein content of the glomerular filtrate increases, which in turn requires increased endocytosis of protein by the tubular endothelial cells, a process that ultimately leads to nephron destruction and progressive deterioration of renal function.[41,42]

The clinical manifestations of diabetic glomerulosclerosis are closely linked to those of diabetes. The increased GFR that occurs in persons with early alterations in renal function is associated with *microalbuminuria*, defined as urinary albumin excretion greater than 30 mg/24 hours and no more than 300 mg/24 hours.[42] Microalbuminuria is an important predictor of future diabetic nephropathies.[5,42] In many cases, these early changes in glomerular function can be reversed by careful control of blood glucose levels (see Chapter 41).[40,42] Inhibition of angiotensin by angiotensin-converting enzyme inhibitors (*e.g.*, captopril) has been shown to have a beneficial effect, possibly by reversing increased glomerular pressure.[6,40,42] Hypertension and cigarette smoking have been implicated in the progression of diabetic nephropathy. Thus, control of high blood pressure and smoking cessation are recommended as primary and secondary prevention strategies in persons with diabetes.

Hypertensive Glomerular Disease

Hypertension can be viewed as both a cause and an effect of kidney disease. Most persons with advanced kidney disease have hypertension, and many persons with long-standing hypertension eventually sustain changes in kidney function. Renal failure and azotemia occur in 1% to 5% of persons with long-standing hypertension (see Chapter 23). Hypertension is associated with a number of changes in glomerular structures, including sclerotic changes. As the glomerular vascular structures thicken and perfusion diminishes, the blood supply to the nephron decreases, causing the kidneys to lose some of their ability to concentrate the urine. This may be evidenced by nocturia. Blood urea nitrogen levels also may become elevated, particularly during periods of water deprivation. Proteinuria may occur as a result of changes in glomerular structure.

In summary, diseases of the glomerulus disrupt glomerular filtration and alter the permeability of glomerular capillary membrane to plasma proteins and blood cells. *Glomerulonephritis* is a term used to describe a group of diseases that result in inflammation and injury of the glomerulus. These diseases disrupt the capillary membrane and cause proteinuria, hematuria, pyuria, oliguria, edema, hypertension, and azotemia. Almost all types of glomerulonephritis are caused by immune mechanisms.

Glomerular diseases have been grouped into two categories: the nephritic and the nephrotic syndromes. The nephritic syndrome evokes an inflammatory response in the glomeruli and is characterized by hematuria with red cell casts in the urine, a diminished GFR, azotemia, oliguria, and hypertension. The nephrotic syndrome affects the integrity of the glomerular capillary membrane and is characterized by massive proteinuria, hypoalbuminemia, generalized edema, lipiduria, and hyperlipidemia. Both conditions can lead to progressive loss of glomerular function and eventual development of end-stage renal disease. Among the secondary causes of glomerular kidney disease are diabetes and hypertension. Kidney disease is a major complication of diabetes mellitus and is thought to be related to hemodynamic changes associated and defective synthesis of glomerular structures associated with increased blood glucose levels. Hypertension is closely linked with kidney disease, and kidney disease can be a cause or effect of elevated blood pressure.

Tubulointerstitial Disorders

After you have completed this section of the chapter, you should be able to meet the following objectives:

✦ Cite a definition of tubulointerstitial kidney disease
✦ Differentiate between the defects in tubular function that occur in proximal and distal tubular acidosis
✦ Explain the pathogenesis of kidney damage in pyelonephritis
✦ Explain the vulnerability of the kidneys to injury caused by drugs and toxins

Several disorders affect renal tubular structures, including the proximal and distal tubules. Most of these disorders also affect the interstitial tissue that surrounds the tubules. These disorders, which sometimes are referred to as *tubulointerstitial disorders*, include acute tubular necrosis (see Chapter 34), renal tubular acidosis, pyelonephritis, and the effects of drugs and toxins.

Tubulointerstitial renal diseases may be divided into acute and chronic disorders. The acute disorders are characterized by their sudden onset and by signs and symptoms of interstitial edema; they include acute pyelonephritis and acute hypersensitivity reaction to drugs. The chronic disorders produce interstitial fibrosis, atrophy, and mononuclear infiltrates; most persons are asymptomatic until late in the course of the disease. In the early stages, tubulointerstitial diseases commonly are manifested by fluid and electrolyte imbalances that reflect subtle changes in tubular function. These manifestations can include inability to concentrate urine, as evidenced by polyuria and nocturia; interference with acidification of urine, resulting in metabolic acidosis; and diminished tubular reabsorption of sodium and other substances.[5]

RENAL TUBULAR ACIDOSIS

Renal tubular acidosis refers to a group of tubular disorders that result in acidosis and its subsequent complications, including metabolic bone disease, kidney stones, and growth failure in children. There are two main types of renal tubular acidosis: proximal tubular disorders that affect bicarbonate reabsorption and distal tubular defects that affect the secretion of fixed metabolic acids.[43,44]

The proximal tubule is the site where 90% to 95% of filtered bicarbonate is reabsorbed. With the onset of impaired tubular bicarbonate absorption, there is a loss of bicarbonate in the urine that reduces plasma bicarbonate levels. The concomitant loss of sodium in the urine that accompanies the bicarbonate loss leads to contraction of the extracellular fluid volume with increased aldosterone secretion and a resultant decrease in serum potassium levels (see Chapter 31). With proximal tubular defects in acid-base regulation, the distal tubular sites for secretion of the fixed acids into the urine continue to function, and the reabsorption of bicarbonate by the proximal cells eventually resumes, albeit at a lower level of serum bicarbonate. Whenever serum levels rise above this decreased level, bicarbonate is lost in the urine. The proximal tubular defect in bicarbonate reabsorption can extend to other substances, such as glucose, amino acids, and phosphate. Defects in calcium and phosphate reabsorption may accentuate bicarbonate losses.

The most common type of distal tubular acidosis usually is a defect in the secretion of hydrogen ions with failure to acidify the urine. Because the secretion of hydrogen ions in the distal tubules is linked to sodium reabsorption, failure to secrete hydrogen ions results in a net loss of sodium bicarbonate in the urine. There is a resultant contraction of fluids in the extracellular fluid compartment, a compensatory increase in aldosterone levels, and development of hypokalemia. The persistent acidosis, which requires buffering by the skeletal system, causes calcium to be released from bone. Increased losses of calcium in the urine lead to increased levels of parathyroid hormone, osteomalacia, bone pain, impaired growth in children, and development of kidney stones.

The treatment of renal tubular acidosis depends on the defect and may require administration of bicarbonate and potassium. The selective use of diuretics also may be indicated.

PYELONEPHRITIS

Pyelonephritis refers to an infection of the kidneys and renal pelves. In its earliest stages, it is characterized by inflammatory foci that are interspersed throughout the renal interstitium. Small abscesses may form on the surface of the kidneys. In time, the lesions are replaced by scar tissue. There are two forms of pyelonephritis: acute and chronic. Because pyelonephritis affects the tubules and interstitium of the kidneys, it is classified as a tubulointerstitial kidney disease.

Acute pyelonephritis represents an acute suppurative inflammation of renal tubulointerstitial tissues caused by bacterial infection (see previous discussion of UTIs). Infection may occur through the bloodstream or ascend from the bladder. Factors that contribute to the development of acute pyelonephritis are catheterization and urinary tract instrumentation, vesicoureteral reflux, pregnancy, increased susceptibility to infection, and neurogenic bladder.

The onset of acute pyelonephritis typically is abrupt, with chills, fever, headache, back pain, tenderness over the costovertebral angle, and general malaise. It usually is accompanied by symptoms of bladder irritation, such as dysuria, frequency, and urgency. Pyuria occurs but is not diagnostic because it also occurs in lower UTIs. It is possible to determine whether an infection involves the upper or lower urinary tract through detection of the antibody coating on the bacteria. The finding of leukocyte casts in the urine also indicates that the infection is in the kidneys rather than the lower urinary tract.

Acute pyelonephritis is treated with appropriate antimicrobial drugs. Unless obstruction or other complications occur, the symptoms usually disappear within several days. Hospitalization during initial treatment may be necessary. Depending on the cause, recurrent infections are possible.

Chronic pyelonephritis represents a progressive process. There is scarring and deformation of the renal calices and pelvis[6] (Fig. 33-12). The disorder appears to involve a bacterial infection superimposed on obstructive abnormalities or vesicoureteral reflux. Although the mechanisms by which the urinary obstruction interacts to produce kidney damage in chronic pyelonephritis are unknown, observations sug-

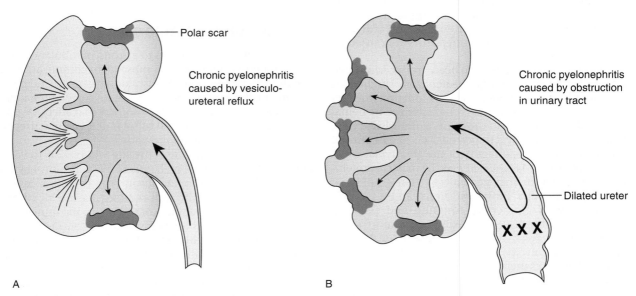

A   B

FIGURE 33-12 The two major types of chronic pyelonephritis. (**A**) Vesicoureteral reflux causes infection of the peripheral compound papillae and, therefore, scars in the poles of the kidney. (**B**) Obstruction of the urinary tract leads to high-pressure backflow of urine that causes infection of all papillae and diffuse scarring of the kidney and thinning of the cortex. (Rubin E., Farber J.L. [1999]. *Pathology* [3rd ed., p. 905]. Philadelphia: Lippincott Williams & Wilkins.) (Courtesy of Dmitri Karetnikov, artist)

gest that some component of the urine may serve as an antigenic determinant to induce an immune response. Among the suspected urinary components are Tamm-Horsfall proteins, which are synthesized in the tubular epithelial cells of the thick ascending loop of Henle and the distal convoluted tubules.[45]

Chronic pyelonephritis may cause many of the same symptoms as acute pyelonephritis, or its onset may be insidious. Loss of tubular function and of the ability to concentrate urine give rise to polyuria and nocturia, and mild proteinuria is common. Severe hypertension often is a contributing factor in the progress of the disease. Chronic pyelonephritis is a significant cause of renal failure. It is thought to be responsible for 11% to 20% of all cases of end-stage renal disease.[5]

DRUG-RELATED NEPHROPATHIES

Drug-related nephropathies involve functional or structural changes in the kidneys that occur after exposure to a drug. The kidneys are exposed to a high rate of delivery of any substance in the blood because of their large blood flow and high filtration pressure. The kidneys also are active in the metabolic transformation of drugs and therefore are exposed to a number of toxic metabolites. Some drugs and toxic substances damage the kidneys by causing a decrease in blood flow; others directly damage tubulointerstitial structures; and still others cause damage by producing hypersensitivity reactions.

The tolerance to drugs varies with age and depends on renal function, state of hydration, blood pressure, and the pH of the urine. Because of a decrease in physiologic function, elderly persons are particularly susceptible to kidney damage caused by drugs and toxins. The dangers of nephrotoxicity are increased when two or more drugs capable of producing kidney damage are given at the same time.

Acute drug-related hypersensitivity reactions produce tubulointerstitial nephritis, with damage to the tubules and interstitium. This condition was observed initially in persons who were sensitive to the sulfonamide drugs; currently, it is observed most often with the use of methicillin and other synthetic antibiotics, and with the use of furosemide and the thiazide diuretics in persons sensitive to these drugs. The condition begins approximately 15 days (range, 2 to 40 days) after exposure to the drug.[5,6] At the onset, there is fever, eosinophilia, hematuria, mild proteinuria, and in approximately one fourth of cases, a rash. In approximately 50% of cases, signs and symptoms of acute renal failure develop. Withdrawal of the drug commonly is followed by complete recovery, but there may be permanent damage in some persons, usually in older persons. Drug nephritis may not be recognized in its early stage because it is uncommon.

Chronic analgesic nephritis, which is associated with analgesic abuse, causes interstitial nephritis with renal papillary necrosis. When first observed, it was attributed to phenacetin, a then-common ingredient of over-the-counter medications containing aspirin, phenacetin, and caffeine. Although phenacetin is no longer contained in these preparations, it has been suggested that other ingredients, such as aspirin and acetaminophen, also may contribute to the

disorder. How much analgesic it takes to produce papillary necrosis is unknown.

Nonsteroidal anti-inflammatory drugs (NSAIDs) also have the potential for damaging renal structures, including medullary interstitial cells. Prostaglandins (particularly PGI_2 and PGE_2) contribute to regulation of tubular blood flow.[46] The deleterious effects of NSAIDs on the kidney are thought to result from their ability to inhibit prostaglandin synthesis. Persons who are particularly at risk are the elderly because of age-related changes in renal function, persons who are dehydrated or have a decrease in blood volume, and persons with preexisting kidney disease or renal insufficiency.

> In summary, tubulointerstitial diseases affect the tubules and the surrounding interstitium of the kidneys. These disorders include renal tubular acidosis, chronic pyelonephritis, and the effects of drugs and toxins. Renal tubular acidosis describes a form of systemic acidosis that results from tubular defects in bicarbonate reabsorption or hydrogen ion secretion. Pyelonephritis, or infection of the kidney and kidney pelvis, can occur as an acute or a chronic condition. Acute pyelonephritis typically is caused by ascending bladder infections or infections that come from the bloodstream; it usually is successfully treated with appropriate antimicrobial drugs. Chronic pyelonephritis is a progressive disease that produces scarring and deformation of the renal calices and pelvis. Drug-induced impairment of tubulointerstitial structure and function usually is the result of direct toxic injury, decreased blood flow, or hypersensitivity reactions.

■ Neoplasms

After you have completed this section of the chapter, you should be able to meet the following objectives:

✦ Characterize Wilms' tumor in terms of age of onset, possible oncogenic origin, manifestations, and treatment

✦ Cite the risk factors for renal cell carcinoma, describe the manifestations, and explain why the 5-year survival rate has been so low

There are two major groups of renal neoplasms: embryonic kidney tumors (*i.e.*, Wilms' tumor), which occur during childhood, and adult kidney cancers.

WILMS' TUMOR

Wilms' tumor (*i.e.*, nephroblastoma) is one of the most common primary neoplasms of young children. The median age at time of diagnosis of unilateral Wilms' tumor is approximately 3 years.[47] It is a mixed tumor, composed of epithelial and mesenchymal embryonic tissue elements.[5] An important feature of Wilms' tumor is its association with congenital anomalies, the most frequent being those affecting genitourinary structures.[47] Deletions involving at least two loci on chromosome 11 have been found in approximately 30% of children with Wilms' tumors. Some familial cases of Wilms' tumor are not associated with identifiable chromosomal deletions or mutations, suggesting a third locus may be involved.

Wilms' tumor usually is a solitary mass that occurs in any part of the kidney. It usually is sharply demarcated and variably encapsulated.[6] The tumors grow to a large size, distorting kidney structure. The tumors usually are staged using the Wilms' Tumor Study Group classification.[47] Stage I tumors are limited to the kidney and can be excised with the capsular surface intact. Stage II tumors extend into the kidney but can be excised. In stage III, extension of the tumor is confined to the abdomen, and in stage IV, hematogenous metastasis most commonly involves the lung. Bilateral kidney involvement occurs in 5% to 10% of cases.

The common presenting signs are a large asymptomatic abdominal mass and hypertension. Approximately 50% of children have abdominal pain, vomiting, or both.[47] Microscopic and gross hematuria are present in 10% to 25% of children. CT scans are used to confirm the diagnosis.

Treatment involves surgery, chemotherapy, and sometimes radiation therapy. Long-term survival rates have increased to approximately 90% with an aggressive treatment plan.[47]

ADULT KIDNEY CANCER

Adult kidney cancer accounts for 2% of all cancer incidence and mortality in the United States, with nearly 30,000 new cases and 12,000 deaths estimated for 1998.[48] The increased use of imaging procedures such as ultrasonography, CT scanning, and magnetic resonance imaging (MRI) has contributed significantly to earlier diagnosis and more accurate staging of kidney cancers.[48,49]

Renal cell carcinoma originates in the renal cortex and accounts for approximately 80% to 85% of kidney tumors, with transitional or squamous cell cancers of the renal pelvis accounting for most of the remaining cancers.[50] The cause of renal cell carcinoma remains unclear. It occurs most often in older persons in the sixth to seventh decade. Men are affected twice as frequently as women. Some of these tumors may occur as a result of chronic irritation associated with kidney stones. Epidemiologic evidence suggests a correlation between smoking and kidney cancer. Obesity also is a risk factor, particularly in women.[50] Additional risk factors include occupational exposure to petroleum products, heavy metals, and asbestos. The risk of renal cell carcinoma also is increased in persons with acquired cystic kidney disease associated with chronic renal insufficiency.[50,51] Most cases of renal cell carcinoma occur without a recognizable hereditary pattern. However, there are several rare forms of renal cell cancer that are characterized by an autosomal dominant pattern of inheritance, young age at onset (third and fourth decade), and bilateral or multifocal tumors.[50,51]

Kidney cancer is largely a silent disorder during its early stages, and symptoms usually denote advanced disease. Presenting features include hematuria, costovertebral pain, presence of a palpable flank mass, polycythemia, and fever. Hematuria, which occurs in 70% to 90% of cases, is the most

reliable sign. It is, however, intermittent and may be microscopic; as a result, the tumor may reach considerable size before it is detected. In approximately one third of cases, metastases are present at the time of diagnosis.

Kidney cancer is suspected when there are findings of hematuria and a renal mass. Ultrasonography, CT scanning, excretory urography, and renal angiography are used to confirm the diagnosis. MRI with intravenous gadolinium may be used when involvement of the inferior vena cava is suspected.

Surgery (radical nephrectomy with lymph node dissection) is the treatment of choice for all resectable tumors. Nephron-sparing surgery may be done when both kidneys are involved or when the contralateral kidney is threatened by an associated disease such as hypertension or diabetes mellitus. Single-agent and combination chemotherapy have been used with limited success. Immunotherapy involving interferon-alfa and interleukin-2 has been used with some success.[51] The 5-year survival rate for stage I disease ranges from 65% to 85%; 45% to 80% for stage II disease; 15% to 35% for stage III disease; and 0% to 10% for stage IV disease.[50]

> In summary, there are two major groups of renal neoplasms: embryonic kidney tumors (*i.e.*, Wilms' tumor) that occur during childhood and adult renal cell carcinomas. Wilms' tumor is the most common malignant tumor of children. The most common presenting signs are a large abdominal mass and hypertension. Treatment is surgery, chemotherapy, and sometimes radiation therapy. The long-term survival rate for children with Wilms' tumor is approximately 90% with an aggressive plan of treatment.
>
> Adult kidney cancers account for 2% of all cancers. Renal cell carcinoma is the most frequent type of kidney cancer. These tumors are characterized by a lack of early warning signs, diverse clinical manifestations, and resistance to chemotherapy and radiation therapy. Because of the lack of early warning signs, the tumors often are far advanced at the time of diagnosis. Diagnostic methods include ultrasonography and CT scans. The treatment of choice is surgical resection. Prognosis depends on the stage of the cancer; the 5-year survival rate for stage I tumors is 65% to 85%, and for stage IV tumors, it is 0% to 10%.

References

1. National Kidney Foundation. (2000). *Facts about transplantation and kidney and urologic diseases.* [On-line]. Available: http://www.kidney.org.
2. Moore K.L., Persaud T.V.N. (1988). *The developing human: Clinically oriented embryology* (6th ed., pp. 305–315). Philadelphia: W.B. Saunders.
3. Stewart C.L., Jose P.A. (1991). Transitional nephrology. *Urologic Clinics of North America* 18, 143–149.
4. Elder J.S. (2000). Urologic disorders in infants and children. In Behrman R.E., Kliegman R.M., Jenson H.B. (Eds.), *Nelson textbook of pediatrics* (16th ed., pp. 619–623, 1621–1623). Philadelphia: W.B. Saunders.

5. Cotran R.S., Kumar V., Collins T. (1999). *Robbins pathologic basis of disease* (6th ed., pp. 936–965, 971–979). Philadelphia: W.B. Saunders.

6. Jennette J.C., Spargo B.H. (1999). The kidney. In Rubin E., Farber J.L. (Eds.), *Pathology* (3rd ed., pp. 865–893, 902–907, 913–917). Philadelphia: Lippincott Williams & Wilkins.

7. Germino G.G. (1997). Autosomal dominant polycystic kidney disease: A two-hit model. *Hospital Practice* 32 (3), 81–92.

8. Gabow P.A. (1993). Autosomal dominant polycystic kidney disease. *New England Journal of Medicine* 329, 332–342.

9. Grantham J.J. (1992). Polycystic kidney disease: I. Etiology and pathogenesis. *Hospital Practice* 27 (3A), 51–59.

10. Tanagho E.A. (2000). Urinary obstruction and stasis. In Tanagho E.A., McAninch J.W. (Eds.), *Smith's general urology* (15th ed., pp. 208–219, 291–320). New York: Lange Medical Books/McGraw-Hill.

11. Stoller M.L., Presti J.C., Carroll P.R. (2001). Urology. In Tierney L.M., McPhee S.J., Papadakis M.A. (Eds.), *Current medical diagnosis and treatment* (40th ed., pp. 939–943). New York: Lange Medical Books/McGraw-Hill.

12. Coe F.L., Parks J.H., Asplin J.R. (1992). The pathogenesis and treatment of kidney stones. *New England Journal of Medicine* 327, 1141–1152.

13. Mandel N. (1996). Mechanisms of stone formation. *Seminars in Nephrology* 16, 364–374.

14. Scheinman S.J. (2000). New insights into causes and treatments of kidney stones. *Hospital Practice* 35 (3), 49–56, 67–68.

15. Worchester E.M. (1996). Inhibitors of stone formation. *Seminars in Nephrology* 16, 474–486.

16. Stamm W.E., Hooton T.M. (1993). Management of urinary tract infections in adults. *New England Journal of Medicine* 329, 1328–1334.

17. Orenstein R., Wong E.S. (1999). Urinary tract infections in adults. *American Family Physician* 59 (5), 1225–1237.

18. Hooton T.M. (1995). A simplified approach to urinary tract infection. *Hospital Practice* 28 (2), 15, 23–30.

19. McRae S.N., Shortliffe L.M. (2000). Bacterial infections of the genitourinary tract. In Tanagho E.A., McAninch J.W. (Eds.), *Smith's general urology* (15th ed., pp. 237–264). New York: Lange Medical Books/McGraw-Hill.

20. Watnick S., Morrison G. (2001). Kidney. In Tierney L.M., McPhee S.J., Papadakis M.A. (Eds.), *Current medical diagnosis and treatment* (40th ed., pp. 912–923, 932–936). New York: Lange Medical Books/McGraw-Hill

21. Roberts J.A. (1999). Management of pyelonephritis and upper urinary tract infections. *Urologic Clinics of North America* 26, 753–763.

22. Ofek I., Goldhar J., Zafriri D., Lis H., Adar R., Sharon N. (1991). Anti-*Escherichia coli* adhesin activity of cranberry and blueberry juices. *New England Journal of Medicine* 324, 1599.

23. Lowe F.C., Fagelman E. (2001). Cranberry juice and urinary tract infections: What is the evidence? *Urology* 57, 407–413.

24. Hooton T.M., Scholes D., Hughes J.P., Winter C., Roberts P.L., Stapleton A.E., Stergachis A., Stamm W.E. (1996). A prospective study of risk factors for symptomatic urinary tract infections in young women. *New England Journal of Medicine* 335, 468–474.

25. Delzell J.E., Lefevre M.L. (2000). Urinary tract infections during pregnancy. *American Family Physician* 61, 713–721.

26. Andriole V.T., Patterson T.F. (1991). Epidemiology, natural history, and management of urinary tract infections during pregnancy. *Medical Clinics of North America* 75, 359–373.

27. American College of Obstetricians and Gynecologists. (1998). *Antimicrobial therapy for obstetric patients* (pp. 8–10). ACOG Educational Bulletin no. 245. Washington, DC: Author.

28. Zelikovic I., Adelman R.D., Nancarrow R.A. (1992). Urinary tract infections in children: An update. *Western Journal of Medicine* 157, 554–556.

29. Shaw K.N., Gorelick M.H. (1999). Urinary tract infections in children. *Pediatric Clinics of North America* 46, 1111–1122.

30. Bartkowski D.P. (2001). Recognizing UTIs in infants and children. *Postgraduate Medicine* 109, 171–181.

31. Johnson C.E. (1999). New advances in childhood urinary tract infections. *Pediatrics in Review* 20, 335–342.

32. Yoshikawa T.T. (1993). Chronic urinary tract infections in elderly patients. *Hospital Practice* 28(6), 103–118.

33. Mouton C.P., Pierce B., Espino D.V. (2001). Common infections in older adults. *American Family Physician* 63, 257–268.

34. Hricik D.E., Chung-Park M., Sedor J.R. (1998). Glomerulonephritis. *New England Journal of Medicine* 339, 888–899.

35. Couser W.O. (1999). Glomerulonephritis. *Lancet* 35, 1509–1515.

36. Vincenti F.G., Amend W.J.C. (2000). Diagnosis of medical renal diseases. In Tanagho E.A., McAninch J.W. (Eds.), *Smith's general urology* (15th ed., pp. 594–599). New York: Lange Medical Books/McGraw-Hill.

37. Orth S.R., Ritz E. (1998). The nephrotic syndrome. *New England Journal of Medicine* 339, 1202–1211.

38. Jennette J.C., Falk R.J. (1997). Diagnosis and management of glomerular disease. *Medical Clinics of North America* 81(3), 653–675.

39. Donadio J.V., Bergstralh E.J., Offord K.P., Spencer D.C., Holley K.E. (1994). A controlled trial of fish oil in IgA nephropathy. *New England Journal of Medicine* 331, 1194–1199.

40. Dunfee T.P. (1995). The changing management of diabetic nephropathy. *Hospital Practice* 30 (5), 45–55.

41. Remuzzi G., Bertani T. (1998). Pathophysiology of progressive nephropathies. *New England Journal of Medicine* 339, 1448–1455.

42. Parving H.-H., Østerby R., Ritz E. (2000). Diabetic nephropathy. In Brenner B.M. (Ed.), *Brenner and Rector's The kidney* (6th ed., pp. 1731–1753). Philadelphia: W.B. Saunders.

43. Davidman M., Schmitz P. (1988). Renal tubular acidosis: A pathophysiologic approach. *Hospital Practice* 23 (1), 77–96.

44. Arruda J.A.L., Cowell G. (1994). Distal renal tubular acidosis: Molecular and clinical aspects. *Hospital Practice* 29 (1), 75–88.

45. Andriole V.T. (1985). The role of Tamm-Horsfall protein in the pathogenesis of reflux nephropathy and chronic pyelonephritis. *Yale Journal of Biology and Medicine* 58, 91–100.

46. Palmer B., Hendrich W.L. (1995). Clinical acute renal failure with nonsteroidal anti-inflammatory drugs. *Seminars in Nephrology* 15, 214–227.

47. Anderson P.M. (2000). Neoplasms of the kidney. In Behrman R.E., Kiegman R.M., Jenson H.B. (Eds.), *Nelson textbook of pediatrics* (16th ed., pp. 1554–1556). Philadelphia: W.B. Saunders.

48. Schofield D., Cotran R.S. (1999). Diseases of infancy and childhood. In Cotran R.S., Kumar V., Collins T. (Eds.), *Robbins pathologic basis of disease* (6th ed., pp. 487–489). Philadelphia: W.B. Saunders.

49. Chow W.-H., Devesa S.S., Warren J.L., Fraumeni J.F. (1999). Rising incidence of renal cell cancer in the United States. *Journal of the American Medical Association* 281, 1628–1631.

50. Motzer R.J., Bander N.H., Nanus D.M. (1997). Medical progress: Renal-cell carcinoma. *New England Journal of Medicine* 335, 865–875.

51. Dreicer R., Williams R.D. (2000). Renal parenchymal neoplasms. In Tanagho E.A., McAninch J.W. (Eds.), *Smith's general urology* (15th ed., pp. 378–394). New York: Lange Medical Books/McGraw-Hill.

Renal Failure

Renal failure is a condition in which the kidneys fail to remove metabolic end products from the blood and regulate the fluid, electrolyte, and pH balance of the extracellular fluids. The underlying cause may be renal disease, systemic disease, or urologic defects of nonrenal origin. Renal failure can occur as an acute or a chronic disorder. Acute renal failure is abrupt in onset and often is reversible if recognized early and treated appropriately. In contrast, chronic renal failure is the end result of irreparable damage to the kidneys. It develops slowly, usually over the course of a number of years.

Acute Renal Failure

After you have completed this section of the chapter, you should be able to meet the following objectives:

✦ Distinguish between acute and chronic renal failure in terms of causes, treatment, and outcome
✦ Differentiate the prerenal, intrinsic, and extrarenal forms of acute renal failure in terms of the mechanisms of development and manifestations
✦ Cite the two most common causes of acute tubular necrosis and describe the course of the disease in terms of the initiation, maintenance, and recovery phases

Acute renal failure represents a rapid decline in renal function sufficient to increase blood levels of nitrogenous wastes and impair fluid and electrolyte balance. Unlike chronic renal failure, acute renal failure is potentially reversible if the precipitating factors can be corrected or removed before permanent kidney damage has occurred.

Acute renal failure is a common threat to seriously ill persons in intensive care units, with a mortality rate ranging from 42% to 88%.[1] Although treatment methods such as dialysis and renal replacement methods are effective in correcting life-threatening fluid and electrolyte disorders, the mortality rate from acute renal failure has not changed substantially since the 1960s.[2,3] This probably is because acute renal failure is seen more often in older persons than before, and because it frequently is superimposed on other life-threatening conditions such as trauma, shock, and sepsis.

The most common indicator of acute renal failure is *azotemia*, an accumulation of nitrogenous wastes (urea nitrogen, uric acid, and creatinine) in the blood. In acute renal failure the glomerular filtration rate (GFR) is decreased. As a result, excretion of nitrogenous wastes is reduced and fluid and electrolyte balance cannot be maintained. Persons with acute renal failure often are asymptomatic, and the condition is diagnosed by observation of elevations in blood urea nitrogen (BUN) and creatinine.

TYPES OF ACUTE RENAL FAILURE

Acute renal failure can be caused by several types of conditions, including a decrease in blood flow without ischemic injury; ischemic, toxic, or obstructive tubular injury; and obstruction of urinary tract outflow. The causes of acute renal failure commonly are categorized as prerenal (55% to 60%), intrinsic (35% to 40%), and postrenal (<5%).[3] Causes of renal failure within these categories are summarized in Chart 34-1.

Prerenal Failure

Prerenal failure, the most common form of acute renal failure, is characterized by a marked decrease in renal blood flow. It is reversible if the cause of the decreased renal blood flow can be identified and corrected before kidney damage occurs. Causes of prerenal failure include profound depletion of vascular volume (*e.g.*, hemorrhage, loss of extracellular fluid volume), impaired perfusion due to heart failure and cardiogenic shock, and decreased vascular filling because of increased vascular capacity (*e.g.*, anaphylaxis or sepsis). Elderly persons are particularly at risk because of their predisposition to hypovolemia and their high prevalence of renal vascular disorders.

Some vasoactive mediators, drugs, and diagnostic agents stimulate intense intrarenal vasoconstriction and induce glomerular hypoperfusion and prerenal failure.[3–5] Examples include hypercalcemia, endotoxins, radiocontrast

Acute Renal Failure

➤ Acute renal failure is caused by conditions that produce an acute shutdown in renal function.

➤ It can result from decreased blood flow to the kidney (prerenal failure), disorders that disrupt the structures in the kidney (intrinsic or intrarenal failure), or disorders that interfere with the elimination of urine from the kidney (postrenal failure).

➤ Acute renal failure, although it causes an accumulation of products normally cleared by the kidney, is a reversible process if the factors causing the condition can be corrected.

---

agents such as those used for cardiac catheterization, cyclosporine (an immunosuppressant drug that is used to prevent transplant rejection), amphotericin B (an antifungal agent), epinephrine, and high doses of dopamine.[3] Many of these drugs also cause acute tubular necrosis (discussed later). In addition, several commonly used classes of drugs impair renal adaptive mechanisms and can convert compensated renal hypoperfusion into prerenal failure. Angiotensin-converting enzyme inhibitors reduce the effects of renin on renal blood flow; when combined with diuretics, they may cause prerenal failure in persons with decreased blood flow due to large-vessel or small-vessel renal vascular disease. Prostaglandins have a vasodilatory effect on renal blood vessels. Nonsteroidal anti-inflammatory drugs (NSAIDs) reduce renal blood flow through inhibition of prostaglandin synthesis. In some persons with diminished renal perfusion, NSAIDs can precipitate prerenal failure.

Normally, the kidneys receive 20% to 25% of the cardiac output.[6] This large blood supply is required to remove metabolic wastes and regulate body fluids and electrolytes. Fortunately, the normal kidney can tolerate relatively large reductions in blood flow before renal damage occurs. As renal blood flow is reduced, the GFR drops, the amount of sodium and other substances that is filtered by the glomeruli is reduced, and the need for energy-dependent mechanisms to reabsorb these substance is reduced (see Chapter 30). As the GFR and urine output approach zero, oxygen consumption by the kidney approximates that required to keep renal tubular cells alive.[6] When blood flow falls below this level, which is about 20% of normal, ischemic changes occur. Because of their high metabolic rate, the tubular epithelial cells are most vulnerable to ischemic injury. Improperly treated, prolonged renal hypoperfusion can lead to ischemic tubular necrosis with significant morbidity and mortality.

Acute renal failure is manifested by a sharp decrease in urine output and a disproportionate elevation of BUN in relation to serum creatinine levels. The kidney normally responds to a decrease in the GFR with a decrease in urine

---

CHART 34-1

Causes of Acute Renal Failure

Prerenal
Hypovolemia
  Hemorrhage
  Dehydration
  Excessive loss of gastrointestinal tract fluids
  Excessive loss of fluid due to burn injury
Decreased vascular filling
  Anaphylactic shock
  Septic shock
Heart failure and cardiogenic shock
Decreased renal perfusion due to vasoactive mediators, drugs, diagnostic agents

Intrinsic or intrarenal
Acute tubular necrosis
  Prolonged renal ischemia
  Exposure to nephrotoxic drugs, heavy metals, and organic solvents
  Intratubular obstruction resulting from hemoglobinuria, myoglobinuria, myeloma light chains, or uric acid casts
  Acute renal disease (acute glomerulonephritis, pyelonephritis)

Postrenal
Bilateral ureteral obstruction
Bladder outlet obstruction

output. An early sign of prerenal failure is a sharp decrease in urine output. A low fractional excretion of sodium (<1%) suggests that oliguria is due to decreased renal perfusion and that the nephrons are responding appropriately by decreasing the excretion of filtered sodium in an attempt to preserve vascular volume.[4] BUN levels also depend on the GFR. A low GFR allows more time for small particles such as urea to be reabsorbed into the blood. Creatinine, which is larger and nondiffusible, remains in the tubular fluid, and the total amount of creatinine that is filtered, although small, is excreted in the urine. Thus, there also is a disproportionate elevation in the ratio of BUN to serum creatinine to greater than 20:1 (normal, approximately 10:1).[4]

Postrenal Failure

Postrenal failure results from obstruction of urine outflow from the kidneys. The obstruction can occur in the ureter (*i.e.*, calculi and strictures), bladder (*i.e.*, tumors or neurogenic bladder), or urethra (*i.e.*, prostatic hypertrophy). Prostatic hyperplasia is the most common underlying problem. Because both ureters must be occluded to produce renal failure, obstruction of the bladder rarely causes acute renal failure unless one of the kidneys already is damaged or a person has only one kidney. The treatment of acute postrenal failure consists of treating the underlying cause of obstruction so that urine flow can be reestablished before permanent nephron damage occurs.

Intrinsic Renal Failure

Intrinsic or intrarenal renal failure results from conditions that cause damage to structures within the kidney—glomerular, tubular, or interstitial. Injury to the tubules is most common and often is ischemic or toxic in origin. The major causes of intrarenal failure are ischemia associated with prerenal failure, toxic insult to the tubular structures of the nephron, and intratubular obstruction. Acute glomerulonephritis and acute pyelonephritis also are intrarenal causes of acute renal failure.

ACUTE TUBULAR NECROSIS

Acute tubular necrosis (ATN) is characterized by destruction of tubular epithelial cells with acute suppression of renal function.[3,7] It is the most common cause of intrinsic renal failure. ATN can be caused by a variety of conditions, including acute tubular damage due to ischemia, the nephrotoxic effects of drugs, tubular obstruction, and toxins from a massive infection. Tubular epithelial cells are particularly sensitive to ischemia and also are vulnerable to toxins; ischemia and toxins account for most cases of ATN. The tubular injury that occurs in ATN frequently is reversible. The process depends on the recovery of the injured cells, removal of the necrotic cells and intratubular casts, and regeneration of renal cells to restore the normal continuity of the tubular epithelium. If, however, the ischemia is severe enough to cause cortical necrosis, irreversible renal failure occurs.

Ischemic ATN occurs most frequently in persons who have major surgery, severe hypovolemia, overwhelming sepsis, trauma, and burns.[3] Sepsis produces ischemia by provoking a combination of systemic vasodilation and intrarenal hypoperfusion. In addition, sepsis results in the generation of toxins that sensitize renal tubular cells to the damaging effects of ischemia. ATN complicating trauma and burns frequently is multifactorial in origin and due to the combined effects of hypovolemia and myoglobin or other toxins released from damaged tissue. In contrast to prerenal failure, the GFR does not improve with the restoration of renal blood flow in acute renal failure caused by ischemic ATN.

Nephrotoxic ATN complicates the administration of or exposure to many structurally diverse drugs and other toxic agents. Nephrotoxic agents cause renal injury by inducing varying combinations of renal vasoconstriction, direct tubular damage, or intratubular obstruction. The kidney is particularly vulnerable to nephrotic injury because of its rich blood supply and ability to concentrate toxins to high levels in the medullary portion of the kidney. In addition, the kidney is an important site for metabolic processes that transform relatively harmless agents into toxic metabolites. Pharmacologic agents that are directly toxic to the renal tubule include antimicrobials such as the aminoglycosides, chemotherapeutic agents such cisplatin and ifosfamide, and the radiocontrast agents.[7,8,9] Several factors contribute to aminoglycoside nephrotoxicity, including a decrease in the GFR, preexisting renal disease, hypovolemia, and concurrent administration of other drugs that have a nephrotoxic effect.[3] Nonoliguric ATN occurs in 10% to 30% of courses of aminoglycoside therapy, even when the blood levels of the drug are within therapeutic range.[3] Cisplatin accumulates in proximal tubule cells, inducing mitochondrial injury and inhibition of adenosine triphosphatase (ATP) activity and solute transport. ATN complicates up to 70% of courses of cisplatin therapy. Radio contrast media–induced nephrotoxicity is thought to result from direct tubular toxicity and renal ischemia.[10] The risk of renal damage caused by radio contrast media is greatest in elderly persons, in persons with diabetes mellitus, and in persons who, for various reasons, are susceptible to kidney disease.[3] Heavy metals (*e.g.*, lead, mercury) and organic solvents (*e.g.*, carbon tetrachloride, ethylene glycol) are other nephrotoxic agents.

Myoglobin, hemoglobin, uric acid, and myeloma light chains are the most frequent cause of ATN due to intratubular obstruction. Both myeloma cast nephropathy and acute urate nephropathy usually are seen in the setting of widespread malignancy or massive tumor destruction by therapeutic agents.[3] Hemoglobinuria results from blood transfusion reactions and other hemolytic crises. Skeletal and cardiac muscles contain myoglobin, which accounts for their rubiginous color. Myoglobin corresponds to hemoglobin in function, serving as an oxygen reservoir in the muscle fibers. Myoglobin normally is not found in the serum or urine. It has a low molecular weight of 17,000 daltons; if it escapes into the circulation, it is rapidly filtered in the glomerulus. Myoglobinuria most commonly results from muscle trauma, but may result from extreme exertion, hyperthermia, sepsis, prolonged seizures, potassium or phosphate depletion, and alcoholism or drug abuse. Both myoglobin and hemoglobin discolor the urine, which may range from the color of tea to red, brown, or black.

The course of ATN can be divided into three phases: the onset or initiating phase, the maintenance phase, and the recovery or convalescent phase.[3,4] The *onset* or *initiating phase*, which lasts hours or days, is the time from the onset of the precipitating event (*e.g.,* ischemic phase of prerenal failure or toxin exposure) until tubular injury occurs.

The *maintenance phase* of ATN is characterized by a marked decrease in the GFR, causing sudden retention of endogenous metabolites such as urea, potassium, sulfate, and creatinine that normally are cleared by the kidneys. The urine output usually is lowest at this point. Fluid retention gives rise to edema, water intoxication, and pulmonary congestion. If the period of oliguria is prolonged, hypertension frequently develops and with it signs of uremia. When untreated, the neurologic manifestations of uremia progress from neuromuscular irritability to seizures, somnolence, coma, and death. Hyperkalemia usually is asymptomatic until serum levels of potassium rise above 6.0 to 6.5 mEq/L, at which point characteristic electrocardiographic changes and symptoms of muscle weakness are seen.

Formerly, most patients with ATN were oliguric. During the past several decades, a nonoliguric form of ATN has become increasingly prevalent. Persons with nonoliguric failure have higher levels of glomerular filtration and excrete more nitrogenous waste, water, and electrolytes in their urine than persons with acute oliguric renal failure. Abnormalities in blood chemistry levels usually are milder and cause fewer complications. The decrease in oliguric ATN probably reflects new approaches to the treatment of poor cardiac performance and circulatory failure that focus on vigorous plasma volume expansion and the selective use of dopamine and other drugs to improve renal blood flow. Dopamine has renal vasodilator properties and inhibits sodium reabsorption in the proximal tubule, thereby decreasing the work demands of the nephron.

The *recovery phase* is the period during which repair of renal tissue takes place. Its onset usually is heralded by a gradual increase in urine output and a fall in serum creatinine, indicating that the nephrons have recovered to the point where urine excretion is possible. Diuresis often occurs before renal function has fully returned to normal. Consequently, BUN and serum creatinine, potassium, and phosphate levels may remain elevated or continue to rise even though urine output is increased. In some cases, the diuresis may result from impaired nephron function and may cause excessive loss of water and electrolytes. Eventually, renal tubular function is restored with improvement in concentrating ability. At about the same time, the BUN and creatinine begin to return to normal. In some cases, mild to moderate kidney damage persists.

DIAGNOSIS AND TREATMENT

Given the high morbidity and mortality rates associated with acute renal failure, attention should be focused on prevention and early diagnosis. This includes assessment measures to identify persons at risk for development of acute renal failure, including those with preexisting renal insufficiency and diabetes. These persons are particularly at risk for development of acute renal failure due to nephrotoxic

drugs such as aminoglycosides and contrast agents, or to drugs such as the NSAIDs that alter intrarenal hemodynamics. Elderly persons are susceptible to all forms of acute renal failure because of the effects of aging on renal reserve.

Careful observation of urine output is essential for persons at risk for development of acute renal failure. Urine tests that measure urine osmolality, urinary sodium concentration, and fractional excretion of sodium help differentiate prerenal azotemia, in which the reabsorptive capacity of the tubular cells is maintained, from tubular necrosis, in which these functions are lost. One of the earliest manifestations of tubular damage is the inability to concentrate the urine.

Further diagnostic information that can be obtained from the urinalysis includes evidence of proteinuria, hemoglobinuria, and casts or crystals in the urine. Blood tests for BUN and creatinine provide information regarding the ability to remove nitrogenous wastes from the blood. It also is important to exclude urinary obstruction.

A major concern in the treatment of acute renal failure is identifying and correcting the cause (*e.g.,* improving renal perfusion, discontinuing nephrotoxic drugs). Fluids are carefully regulated in an effort to maintain normal fluid volume and electrolyte concentrations. Adequate caloric intake is needed to prevent the breakdown of body proteins, which increases nitrogenous wastes. Parenteral hyperalimentation may be used for this purpose. Because secondary infections are a major cause of death in persons with acute renal failure, constant effort is needed to prevent and treat such infections.

Dialysis or continuous renal replacement therapy (CRRT) may be indicated when nitrogenous wastes and the water and electrolyte balance cannot be kept under control by other means. Venovenous or arteriovenous CRRT has emerged as a method for treating acute renal failure in patients too hemodynamically unstable to tolerate hemodialysis.[11] An associated advantage of the continuous renal replacement therapies is the ability to administer nutritional support. The disadvantages are the need for prolonged anticoagulation and continuous sophisticated monitoring.

In summary, acute renal failure is an acute, reversible suppression of kidney function. It is a common threat to seriously ill persons in intensive care units, with a mortality rate of 42% to 88%. Acute renal failure is characterized by an accumulation of nitrogenous wastes in the blood (*i.e.,* azotemia) and alterations in body fluids and electrolytes. Acute renal failure is classified as prerenal, intrinsic or intrarenal, or postrenal in origin. Prerenal failure is caused by decreased blood flow to the kidneys; postrenal failure by obstruction to urine output; and intrinsic renal failure by disorders in the kidney itself. ATN, due to ischemia or nephrotoxic agents, is a common cause of acute intrinsic renal failure. ATN typically progresses through three phases: the initiation phase, during which tubular injury is induced; the maintenance phase, during which the GFR falls, nitrogenous wastes accumulate, and urine output decreases;

and the recovery or reparative phase, during which the GFR, urine output, and blood levels of nitrogenous wastes return to normal.

Because of the high morbidity and mortality rates associated with acute renal failure, identification of persons at risk is important to clinical decision making. Acute renal failure often is reversible, making early identification and correction of the underlying cause (*e.g.*, improving renal perfusion, discontinuing nephrotoxic drugs) important. Treatment includes the judicious administration of fluids and dialysis or CRRT.

Chronic Renal Failure

After you have completed this section of the chapter, you should be able to meet the following objectives:

✦ State the definitions of renal impairment, renal insufficiency, renal failure, and end-stage renal disease
✦ List the common problems associated with end-stage renal disease, including alterations in fluid and electrolyte balance and disorders of skeletal, hematologic, cardiovascular, immune, neurologic, skin, and sexual function, and explain their physiologic significance
✦ State the basis for adverse drug reactions in patients with end-stage renal disease
✦ Describe the scientific principles underlying dialysis treatment, and compare hemodialysis with peritoneal dialysis
✦ Cite the complications of kidney transplantation
✦ State the goals for dietary management of persons with end-stage renal disease.

Unlike acute renal failure, chronic renal failure represents progressive and irreversible destruction of kidney structures. As recently as 1965, many patients with chronic renal failure progressed to the final stages of the disease and then died. The high mortality rate was associated with limitations in the treatment of renal disease and with the tremendous cost of ongoing treatment. In 1972, federal support began for dialysis and transplantation through a Medicare entitlement program.[12] Technologic advances in renal replacement therapy (*i.e.*, dialysis therapy and transplantation) have improved the outcomes for persons with renal failure. In the United States, there are approximately 400,000 persons with end-stage renal disease (ESRD) who are living today, a product of continued research and advances in treatment methods.[13] In 1998, almost 246,000 of these people were receiving dialysis treatment and 13,300 received a kidney transplant.

Chronic renal failure can result from a number of conditions that cause permanent loss of nephrons, including diabetes, hypertension, glomerulonephritis, and polycystic kidney disease. Typically, the signs and symptoms of renal failure occur gradually and do not become evident until the disease is far advanced. This is because of the amazing compensatory ability of the kidneys. As kidney structures are destroyed, the remaining nephrons undergo structural and functional hypertrophy, each increasing its func-

tion as a means of compensating for those that have been lost (Fig. 34-1). It is only when the few remaining nephrons are destroyed that the manifestations of renal failure become evident.

STAGES OF PROGRESSION

Regardless of cause, chronic renal failure results in progressive deterioration of glomerular filtration, tubular reabsorptive capacity, and endocrine functions of the kidneys. All forms of renal failure are characterized by a reduction in the GFR, reflecting a corresponding reduction in the number of functional nephrons. The rate of nephron destruction differs from case to case, ranging from several months to many years. The progression of chronic renal failure usually occurs in four stages: diminished renal reserve, renal insufficiency, renal failure, and ESRD.[7]

Diminished Renal Reserve
Diminished renal reserve occurs when the GFR drops to approximately 50% of normal. At this point, the serum BUN and creatinine levels still are normal, and no symptoms of

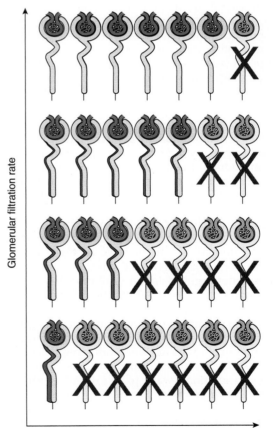

Glomerular filtration rate

Number of functioning nephrons

FIGURE 34-1 Relation of renal function and nephron mass. Each kidney contains 1 million tiny nephrons. A proportional relation exists between the number of nephrons affected by disease and the resulting glomerular filtration rate.

Chronic Renal Failure

➤ Chronic renal failure represents the end result of conditions that greatly reduce renal function by destroying renal nephrons and producing a marked decrease in the glomerular filtration rate (GFR).

➤ Because of the remarkable ability of the kidneys to adapt, signs of renal failure do not appear until 50% or more of the renal functional tissue has been destroyed. After this, signs of renal failure begin to appear as renal function moves from renal insufficiency (GFR 50% to 20% normal), to renal failure (20% to 5% normal), to end-stage renal disease (<5% normal). When the GFR decreases to less than 5% of normal, dialysis or kidney transplantation is necessary for survival.

➤ The manifestations of chronic renal failure represent the inability of the kidney to perform its normal functions in terms of regulating fluid and electrolyte balance, controlling blood pressure through fluid volume and the renin-angiotensin system, eliminating nitrogenous and other waste products, governing the red blood cell count through erythropoietin synthesis, and directing parathyroid and skeletal function through phosphate elimination and activation of vitamin D.

impaired renal function are evident. This is supported by the fact that many persons survive an entire lifetime with only one kidney. Because of the diminished reserve, the risk for development of azotemia increases with an additional renal insult, such as that due to nephrotoxic drugs.

Renal Insufficiency

Renal insufficiency represents a reduction in the GFR to 20% to 50% of normal. During this stage, azotemia, anemia, and hypertension appear. Signs and symptoms of renal insufficiency do not begin to appear until more than 50% of the function in both kidneys is lost. The kidneys initially have tremendous adaptive capabilities. As nephrons are destroyed, the remaining nephrons undergo changes to compensate for those that are lost. In the process, each of the remaining nephrons must filter more solute particles from the blood. Because the solute particles are osmotically active, they cause additional water to be lost in the urine. One of the earliest symptoms of renal insufficiency is *isosthenuria*, or polyuria with urine that is almost isotonic with plasma.[6]

Conservative treatment during this stage includes measures to retard deterioration of renal function and assist the body in managing the effects of impaired function. Because the kidneys have difficulty eliminating the waste products of protein metabolism, a restricted-protein diet usually produces fewer uremic symptoms and slows progression of renal failure. The few remaining nephrons that constitute

the functional reserve of the kidneys can be easily disrupted; at that point, renal failure progresses rapidly.

Renal Failure

Renal failure develops when the GFR is less than 20% of normal. At this point, the kidneys cannot regulate volume and solute composition, and edema, metabolic acidosis, and hypercalcemia develop. Overt uremia may ensue with neurologic, gastrointestinal, and cardiovascular manifestations.

End-Stage Renal Disease

End-stage renal disease occurs when the GFR is less than 5% of normal. Histologic findings of an end-stage kidney include a reduction in renal capillaries and scarring in the glomeruli. Atrophy and fibrosis are evident in the tubules. The mass of the kidneys usually is reduced. At this final phase of renal failure, treatment with dialysis or transplantation is necessary for survival.

CLINICAL MANIFESTATIONS

The manifestations of renal failure include an accumulation of nitrogenous wastes; alterations in water, electrolyte and acid-base balance; mineral and skeletal disorders; anemia and coagulation disorders; hypertension and alterations in cardiovascular function; gastrointestinal disorders; neurologic complications; disorders of skin integrity; and immunologic disorders (Table 34-1). There currently are four target populations that comprise the entire population of persons with chronic renal failure: persons with chronic renal insufficiency, those with ESRD being treated with hemodialysis, those being treated with peritoneal dialysis, and renal transplant recipients. The manifestations of renal failure are determined largely by the extent of renal function that is present (*e.g.*, renal insufficiency, ESRD), coexisting disease conditions, and the type of renal replacement therapy that the person is receiving.

Accumulation of Nitrogenous Wastes

The accumulation of nitrogenous wastes is an early sign of renal failure, usually occurring before other symptoms become evident. Urea is one of the first nitrogenous wastes to accumulate in the blood, and the BUN level becomes increasingly elevated as renal failure progresses. The normal concentration of urea in the plasma is approximately 20 mg/dL. In renal failure, this level may rise to as high as 800 mg/dL. Creatinine, a byproduct of muscle metabolism, is freely filtered in the glomerulus and is not reabsorbed in the renal tubules. Creatinine is produced at a relatively constant rate and any creatinine that is filtered in the glomerulus is lost in the urine rather than being reabsorbed into the blood. Thus, serum creatinine can be used as an indirect method for assessing the GFR and the extent of renal damage that has occurred in renal failure (see Chapter 30).

Uremia, which literally means "urine in the blood," is the term used to describe the clinical manifestations of ESRD. Few symptoms of uremia appear until at least two thirds of the nephrons have been destroyed. Uremia differs from azotemia, which merely indicates the accumulation of nitrogenous wastes in the blood and can occur without symptoms. The uremic state includes signs and symptoms

TABLE 34-1 ✦ Alterations in Body Function That Occur With Chronic Renal Failure

Body System	Change in Function	Manifestation
Body fluids	Compensatory changes in tubular functions	Fixed specific gravity of urine; polyuria and nocturia
	Decreased ability to synthesize ammonia and conserve bicarbonate	Metabolic acidosis
	Inability to excrete potassium	Hyperkalemia
	Inability to regulate sodium excretion	Salt wasting or sodium retention
	Impaired ability to excrete phosphate	Hyperphosphatemia
	Hyperphosphatemia and inability to activate vitamin D	Hypocalcemia and increased levels of parathyroid hormone
Hematologic	Impaired synthesis of erythropoietin and effects of uremia	Anemia
	Impaired platelet function	Bleeding tendencies
Cardiovascular	Activation of renin-angiotensin mechanism, increased vascular volume, and failure to produce vasopressor substances	Hypertension
	Fluid retention and hypoalbuminemia	Edema
	Excess extracellular fluid volume, left ventricular hypertrophy, and anemia	Congestive heart failure; pulmonary edema
	Increased metabolic wastes in blood	Uremic pericarditis
Gastrointestinal	Increased metabolic wastes	Anorexia, nausea, vomiting
	Decreased platelet function and increased gastric acid secretion due to hyperparathyroidism	Gastrointestinal bleeding
Neurologic	Fluid and electrolyte imbalance	Headache
	Increase in blood levels of metabolic acids and other small, diffusible particles, such as urea	Signs of uremic encephalopathy: lethargy, decreased alertness, loss of recent memory, delirium, coma, seizures, asterixis, muscle twitching, and tremulousness
		Signs of neuropathy: restless leg syndrome, paresthesias, muscle weakness, and paralysis
Osteodystrophy	High bone turnover (osteitis fibrosa)	Muscle weakness
	Low bone turnover (Osteomalacia and adynamic osteodystrophy)	Bone pain and tenderness
		Spontaneous fractures
Skin	Anemia	Pale, sallow complexion
	Hyperparathyroidism	Pruritus
	High concentration of metabolic end products in body fluids	Uremic frost and odor of urine on skin and breath
Genitourinary	Impaired general health	
	Decreased testosterone	Impotence and loss of libido
	Decreased estrogen	Amenorrhea and loss of libido

of altered fluid, electrolyte, and acid-base balance; alterations in regulatory functions (*e.g.*, hypertension, anemia, osteodystrophy); and the effects of uremia on body function (*e.g.*, uremic encephalopathy, peripheral neuropathy, pruritus). At this stage, virtually every organ and structure in the body is affected. The symptoms at the onset of uremia (*e.g.*, weakness, fatigue, nausea, apathy) often are subtle. More severe symptoms include extreme weakness, frequent vomiting, lethargy, and confusion. Without treatment, coma and death follow.

Disorders of Water, Electrolyte, and Acid-Base Balance

Sodium and Water Balance. The kidneys function in the regulation of extracellular fluid volume. They do this by either eliminating or conserving sodium and water.

Chronic renal failure can produce dehydration or fluid overload, depending on the pathology of the renal disease. In addition to volume regulation, the ability of the kidneys to concentrate the urine is diminished. In renal failure, the specific gravity of the urine becomes fixed (1.008 to 1.012) and varies little from voiding to voiding. Polyuria and nocturia are common.

As renal function declines further, the ability to regulate sodium excretion is reduced. The kidneys normally tolerate large variations in sodium intake while maintaining normal serum sodium levels. In chronic renal failure, they lose the ability to regulate sodium excretion. There is impaired ability to adjust to a sudden reduction in sodium intake and poor tolerance of an acute sodium overload. Volume depletion with an accompanying decrease in the GFR can occur with a restricted sodium intake or excess sodium loss caused by diarrhea or vomiting. Salt wasting is a common problem in advanced renal failure because of impaired tubular re-absorption of sodium. Increasing sodium intake in persons with chronic renal failure often improves the GFR and whatever renal function remains. In patients with associated hypertension, the possibility of increasing blood pressure or production of congestive heart failure often excludes supplemental sodium intake.

Potassium Balance. Approximately 90% of potassium excretion is through the kidneys. In renal failure, potassium excretion by each nephron increases as the kidneys adapt to a decrease in the GFR. As a result, hyperkalemia usually does not develop until renal function is severely compromised. Because of this adaptive mechanism, it usually is not necessary to restrict potassium intake in patients with chronic renal failure until the GFR has dropped below 5 mL/minute. In patients with chronic renal failure, hyperkalemia often results from failure to follow dietary potassium restrictions and ingestion of medications that contain potassium, or from an endogenous release of potassium, as in trauma or infection.

Acid-Base Balance. The kidneys normally regulate blood pH by eliminating hydrogen ions produced in metabolic processes and regenerating bicarbonate. This is achieved through hydrogen ion secretion, sodium and bicarbonate reabsorption, and the production of ammonia, which acts as a buffer for titratable acids (see Chapter 32). With a decline in renal function, these mechanisms become impaired, and metabolic acidosis results. In chronic renal failure, acidosis seems to stabilize as the disease progresses, probably as a result of the tremendous buffering capacity of bone. However, this buffering action is thought to increase bone resorption and contribute to the skeletal defects present in chronic renal failure.

Mineral and Bone Disorders

Abnormalities of calcium, phosphate, and vitamin D metabolism occur early in the course of chronic renal failure.[14] The regulation of serum phosphate levels requires a daily urinary excretion of an amount equal to that ingested in the diet. With deteriorating renal function, phosphate excretion is impaired, and as a result, serum phosphate levels rise. At the same time, serum calcium levels, which are inversely regulated in relation to serum phosphate levels, fall (see Chapter 31). In turn, the drop in serum calcium stimulates parathyroid hormone release, with a resultant increase in calcium resorption from bone. Most persons with ESRD acquire secondary hyperparathyroidism, the result of chronic stimulation of the parathyroid glands. Although serum calcium levels are maintained through increased parathyroid hormone function, this adjustment is accomplished at the expense of the skeletal system and other body organs.

Vitamin D synthesis also is impaired in renal failure. The kidneys regulate vitamin D activity by converting the inactive form of vitamin D [25(OH) vitamin D_3] to its active form (1,25-OH$_2$ vitamin D_3). Decreased levels of active vitamin D lead to a decrease in intestinal absorption of calcium with a resultant increase in parathyroid hormone levels.

Vitamin D also regulates osteoblast differentiation, thereby affecting bone matrix formation and mineralization.

Skeletal Disorders. The term *renal osteodystrophy* is used to describe the skeletal complications of ESRD.[14,15] Several factors are thought to contribute to the development of renal osteodystrophy, including elevated serum phosphate levels, decreased serum calcium levels, impaired renal activation of vitamin D, and hyperparathyroidism. The skeletal changes that occur with renal failure have been divided into two major types of disorders: high-turnover and low-turnover osteodystrophy.[7] Inherent to both of these conditions is abnormal reabsorption and defective remodeling of bone (see Chapter 58).

High–bone-turnover osteodystrophy, sometimes referred to as *osteitis fibrosa*,[15] is characterized by increased bone resorption and formation, with bone resorption predominating. The disorder is associated with secondary hyperparathyroidism; altered vitamin D metabolism along with resistance to the action of vitamin D; and impaired regulation of locally produced growth factors and inhibitors. There is an increase in both osteoblast and osteoclast numbers and activity. Although the osteoblasts produce excessive amounts of bone matrix, mineralization fails to keep pace, and there is a decrease in bone density and formation of porous and coarse-fibered bone. Cortical bone is affected more severely than cancellous bone. Marrow fibrosis is another component of osteitis fibrosa; it occurs in areas of increased bone cell activity. In advanced stages of the disorder, cysts may develop in the bone, a condition called *osteitis fibrosa cystica*.[15]

Low–bone-turnover osteodystrophy is characterized by decreased numbers of osteoblasts and low or reduced numbers of osteoclasts, a low rate of bone turnover, and an accumulation of unmineralized bone matrix.[16] There are two forms of low-turnover osteodystrophy: osteomalacia and adynamic osteodystrophy. *Osteomalacia* is characterized by a slow rate of bone formation and defects in bone mineralization. Several factors are thought to contribute to the development of osteomalacia in ESRD including decreased levels of 25(OH) vitamin D_3, the precursor of activated 1,25-OH$_2$ vitamin D_3, and metabolic acidosis. It is thought that 25(OH) vitamin D_3 deficiency is a major risk factor for defective bone mineralization, completely independent of 1,25-OH$_2$ vitamin D_3 levels.[17] Metabolic acidosis is thought to have a direct effect on both osteoblastic and osteoclastic activity, as well as on the mineralization process by decreasing the availability of trivalent phosphate.[16] Until the 1980s, osteomalacia in ESRD resulted mainly from aluminum intoxication. Aluminum intoxication causes decreased and defective mineralization of bone by existing osteoblasts and more long-term inhibition of osteoblast differentiation. During the 1970s and 1980s, it was discovered that accumulation of aluminum from water used in dialysis and aluminum salts used as phosphate binders caused osteomalacia and adynamic bone disease.[18] This discovery led to a change in the composition of dialysis solutions and substitution of calcium carbonate for aluminum salts as phosphate binders. As a result, the prevalence of osteomalacia in persons with ESRD is declining.

The second type of low-turnover osteodystrophy, *adynamic osteodystrophy*, is characterized by a low number of osteoblasts, the osteoclast number being normal or reduced.[16] In persons with adynamic bone disease, bone remodeling is greatly reduced, and the bone surfaces become hypocellular. Adynamic bone disease is associated with an increased fracture rate. The disease is associated with a "relative hypothyroidism." It has been suggested that hypersecretion of parathyroid hormone may be necessary to maintain normal rates of bone formation in persons with ESRD. Thus, this form of renal osteodystrophy is seen more commonly in persons with ESRD who do not have secondary hyperparathyroidism (*i.e.*, those who have been treated with parathyroidectomy) or have been overtreated with calcium and vitamin D.

The symptoms of renal osteodystrophy, which occur late in the disease, include bone tenderness and muscle weakness. Proximal muscle weakness in the lower extremities is common, making it difficult to get out of a chair or climb stairs.[15] Fractures are more common with low-turnover osteomalacia and adynamic renal bone disease.

Early treatment of hyperphosphatemia and hypocalcemia is important to prevent or slow long-term skeletal complications.[19] Milk products and other foods high in phosphorus content are restricted in the diet. Phosphate-binding antacids (aluminum salts, calcium carbonate, or calcium acetate) may be prescribed to decrease absorption of phosphate from the gastrointestinal tract. Calcium-containing phosphate binders can lead to hypercalcemia, thus worsening soft tissue calcification, especially in persons on vitamin D therapy. Aluminum-containing antacids can contribute to the development of osteodystrophy. To avoid these side effects, a new, well-tolerated aluminum- and calcium-free binder (RenaGel) has been developed. RenaGel is a hydrogel that is resistant to digestive degradation and not absorbed.

Activated forms of vitamin D (calcitriol or alfacalcidol) and calcium supplements often are used to facilitate intestinal absorption of calcium, increase serum calcium levels, and reduce parathyroid hormone levels. Because excessive vitamin D can lead to hypercalcemia and more rapid progression of renal failure, there has been recent concern over using lower doses of vitamin D to reduce parathyroid hormone levels and correct skeletal abnormalities.[17]

Hematologic Disorders

Anemia. Chronic anemia is the most profound hematologic alteration that accompanies renal failure. Anemia first appears when the GFR falls below 40 mL/minute, and is present in most persons with ESRD.[20] Nephrologists have defined clinically significant anemia as a hemoglobin level less than 10 g/dL and a hematocrit less than 30%, in the absence of erythropoietin therapy.[21] An analysis of patients beginning dialysis in the United States found that 67% had a hematocrit less than 30%, and 51% had a hematocrit less than 28%.[22]

The kidneys are the primary site for the production of the hormone *erythropoietin*, which controls red blood cell production. In renal failure, erythropoietin production usu-

ally is insufficient to stimulate adequate red blood cell production by the bone marrow. The accumulation of uremic toxins further suppresses red cell production in the bone marrow, and the cells that are produced have a shortened life span. Iron is essential for erythropoiesis. Many persons on maintenance hemodialysis also are iron deficient because of blood sampling and accidental loss of blood during dialysis. Other causes of iron deficiency include factors such as anorexia and dietary restrictions that limit intake.

When untreated, anemia causes or contributes to weakness, fatigue, depression, insomnia, and decreased cognitive function. There is increasing concern regarding the physiologic effects of anemia on cardiovascular function. The anemia of renal failure produces a decrease in blood viscosity and a compensatory increase in heart rate. The decreased blood viscosity also exacerbates peripheral vasodilatation and contributes to decreased vascular resistance. Cardiac output increases in a compensatory fashion to maintain tissue perfusion. Echocardiographic studies after initiation of chronic dialysis have shown ventricular dilatation with compensatory left ventricular hypertrophy.[20] Anemia also limits myocardial oxygen supply, particularly in persons with coronary heart disease, leading to angina pectoris and other ischemic events.[21] Thus, anemia, when coupled with hypertension, may be a major contributing factor to the development of left ventricular dysfunction and congestive heart failure in persons with ESRD.

A remarkable advance in medical management of ESRD occurred with the availability of recombinant human erythropoietin (rhEPO). Since its approval by the U.S. Food and Drug Administration in June 1989, rhEPO therapy has been used to maintain hematocrit levels in the range of 28% to 33%, with an upper limit of 36%. It currently is recommended that the hematocrit be maintained at the higher target range of 33% to 36% (hemoglobin 11 to 12 g/dL).[23,24] Secondary benefits of treating anemia with rhEPO, previously attributed to the correction of uremia, include improvement in appetite, energy level, sexual function, skin color, and hair and nail growth, and reduced cold intolerance. Frequent measurements of hematocrit are necessary. Worsening hypertension and seizures have occurred when the hematocrit was raised too suddenly.

Because iron deficiency is common among persons with chronic renal failure, iron supplementation often is needed. Iron can be given orally or intravenously. Intravenous iron (iron dextran and ferric sodium gluconate) is used for treatment of persons who are not able to maintain adequate iron status with oral iron. Because intravenously administered iron may cause serious immediate and delayed hypersensitivity reactions, including life-threatening anaphylactic reactions, care is required when prescribing and administering these drugs.[23,24]

Coagulopathies. Bleeding disorders are manifested by epistaxis, menorrhagia, gastrointestinal bleeding, and bruising of the skin and subcutaneous tissues. Although platelet production often is normal in ESRD, platelet function is impaired. Coagulative function improves with dialysis but does not completely normalize, suggesting that uremia contributes to the problem. Anemia may accentuate the problem by changing the position of the platelets with respect to the vessel wall. Normally the red cells occupy the center of the bloodstream and the platelets are in the skimming layer along the endothelial surface. In anemia, the platelets become dispersed, impairing the platelet–endothelial cell adherence needed to initiate hemostasis.[25]

Cardiovascular Disorders

Cardiovascular disease is the major cause of death in patients with ESRD. The overall mortality rate from cardiovascular disease for people with renal failure is 30 times that of the general population. Even after stratification for age, the incidence of cardiovascular disease remains 10 to 20 times higher in persons with ESRD than in the general population.[26]

Hypertension. Hypertension commonly is an early manifestation of chronic renal failure. The mechanisms that produce hypertension in ESRD are multifactorial; they include an increased vascular volume, elevation of peripheral vascular resistance, decreased levels of renal vasodilator prostaglandins, and increased activity of the renin-angiotensin system.[27]

Early identification and aggressive treatment of hypertension has been shown to slow the rate of renal impairment in many types of renal disease. Treatment involves salt and water restriction and the use antihypertensive medications to control blood pressure. Many persons with renal insufficiency need to take several antihypertensive medications to control blood pressure (see Chapter 23).

Heart Disease. The spectrum of cardiovascular disease includes left ventricular hypertrophy and ischemic heart disease. Congestive heart failure and pulmonary edema tend to occur in the late stages of renal failure. Coexisting conditions that have been identified as contributing to the burden of cardiovascular disease include hypertension, anemia, diabetes mellitus, dyslipidemia, and coagulopathies. Anemia, in particular, has been correlated with the presence of left ventricular hypertrophy. Parathyroid hormone also may play a role in the pathogenesis of cardiomyopathy in renal failure.

People with ESRD tend to have an increased prevalence of left ventricular dysfunction, both with a depressed left ventricular ejection fraction, as in systolic dysfunction, as well as impaired ventricular filling, as in diastolic failure (see Chapter 26).[28,29] There are multiple factors that lead to development of left ventricular dysfunction, including extracellular fluid overload, shunting of blood through an arteriovenous fistula for dialysis, and anemia. These abnormalities, coupled with the hypertension that often is present, cause increased myocardial work and oxygen demand, with eventual development of heart failure.

Pericarditis. Pericarditis occurs in approximately 20% of persons receiving chronic dialysis.[30] It can result from metabolic toxins associated with the uremic state or from dialysis. The manifestations of uremic pericarditis resemble those of viral pericarditis, with all its complications, including cardiac tamponade (see Chapter 24).

The presenting signs include mild to severe chest pain with respiratory accentuation and a pericardial friction rub.

Fever is variable in the absence of infection, and is more common in dialysis than uremic pericarditis.

Gastrointestinal Disorders

Anorexia, nausea, and vomiting are common in patients with uremia, along with a metallic taste in the mouth that further depresses the appetite. Early-morning nausea is common. Ulceration and bleeding of the gastrointestinal mucosa may develop, and hiccups are common. A possible cause of nausea and vomiting is the decomposition of urea by intestinal flora, resulting in a high concentration of ammonia. Parathyroid hormone increases gastric acid secretion and contributes to gastrointestinal problems. Nausea and vomiting often improve with restriction of dietary protein and after initiation of dialysis, and disappear after kidney transplantation.

Disorders of Neural Function

Many persons with chronic renal failure have alterations in peripheral and central nervous system function. Peripheral neuropathy, or involvement of the peripheral nerves, affects the lower limbs more frequently than the upper limbs. It is symmetric and affects both sensory and motor function. Neuropathy is caused by atrophy and demyelination of nerve fibers, possibly caused by uremic toxins. Restless legs syndrome is a manifestation of peripheral nerve involvement and can be seen in as many as two thirds of patients on dialysis. This syndrome is characterized by creeping, prickling, and itching sensations that typically are more intense at rest. Temporary relief is obtained by moving the legs. A burning sensation of the feet, which may be followed by muscle weakness and atrophy, is a manifestation of uremia.

The central nervous system disturbances in uremia are similar to those caused by other metabolic and toxic disorders. Sometimes referred to as *uremic encephalopathy*, the condition is poorly understood and may result, at least in part, from an excess of toxic organic acids that alter neural function. Electrolyte abnormalities, such as sodium shifts, also may contribute. The manifestations are more closely related to the progress of the uremic disorder than to the level of the metabolic end products. Reductions in alertness and awareness are the earliest and most significant indications of uremic encephalopathy. This often is followed by an inability to fix attention, loss of recent memory, and perceptual errors in identifying persons and objects. Delirium and coma occur late in the course; seizures are the preterminal event.

Disorders of motor function commonly accompany the neurologic manifestations of uremic encephalopathy. During the early stages, there often is difficulty in performing fine movements of the extremities; the gait becomes unsteady and clumsy with tremulousness of movement. Asterixis (dorsiflexion movements of the hands and feet) typically occurs as the disease progresses. It can be elicited by having the person hyperextend his or her arms at the elbow and wrist with the fingers spread apart. If asterixis is present, this position causes side-to-side flapping movements of the fingers.

Altered Immune Function

Infection is a common complication and cause of hospitalization and death of patients with chronic renal failure. Immunologic abnormalities decrease the efficiency of the immune response to infection. All aspects of inflammation and immune function may be affected adversely by the high levels of urea and metabolic wastes, including a decrease in granulocyte count, impaired humoral and cell-mediated immunity, and defective phagocyte function. The acute inflammatory response and delayed-type hypersensitivity response are impaired. Although persons with ESRD have normal humoral responses to vaccines, a more aggressive immunization program may be needed. Skin and mucosal barriers to infection also may be defective. In persons who are maintained on dialysis, vascular access devices are common portals of entry for pathogens. Many persons with ESRD fail to mount a fever with infection, making the diagnosis more difficult.

Disorders of Skin Integrity

Skin manifestations are common in persons with renal failure. The skin often is pale owing to anemia and may have a sallow, yellow-brown hue. The skin and mucous membranes often are dry, and subcutaneous bruising is common. Skin dryness is caused by a reduction in perspiration owing to the decreased size of sweat glands and the diminished activity of oil glands. Pruritus is common; it results from the high serum phosphate levels and the development of phosphate crystals that occur with hyperparathyroidism. Severe scratching and repeated needlesticks, especially with hemodialysis, break the skin integrity and increase the risk for infection. In the advanced stages of untreated renal failure, urea crystals may precipitate on the skin as a result of the high urea concentration in body fluids. The fingernails may become thin and brittle, with a dark band just behind the leading edge of the nail, followed by a white band. This appearance is known as *Terry's nails*.

Sexual Dysfunction

The cause of sexual dysfunction in men and women with chronic renal failure is unclear. The cause probably is multifactorial and may result from high levels of uremic toxins, neuropathy, altered endocrine function, psychological factors, and medications (*e.g.*, antihypertensive drugs). Alterations in physiologic sexual responses, reproductive ability, and libido are common.

Impotence occurs in as many as 56% of male patients on dialysis.[31] Derangements of the pituitary and gonadal hormones, such as decreases in testosterone levels and increases in prolactin and luteinizing hormone levels, are common and cause erectile difficulties and decreased spermatocyte counts. Loss of libido may result from chronic anemia and decreased testosterone levels. Several drugs, such as exogenous testosterone and bromocriptine, have been used in an attempt to return hormone levels to normal.

Impaired sexual function in women is manifested by abnormal levels of progesterone, luteinizing hormone, and prolactin. Hypofertility, menstrual abnormalities, decreased vaginal lubrication, and various orgasmic problems have been described.[32] Amenorrhea is common among women who are on dialysis therapy.

Elimination of Drugs

The kidneys are responsible for the elimination of many drugs and their metabolites.[9] Renal failure and its treatment can interfere with the absorption, distribution, and elimination of drugs. The administration of large quantities of phosphate-binding antacids to control hyperphosphatemia and hypocalcemia in patients with advanced renal failure interferes with the absorption of some drugs. Many drugs are bound to plasma proteins, such as albumin, for transport in the body; the unbound portion of the drug is available to act at the various receptor sites and is free to be metabolized. A decrease in plasma proteins, particularly albumin, that occurs in many persons with ESRD results in less protein-bound drug and greater amounts of free drug.

In the process of metabolism, some drugs form intermediate metabolites that are toxic if not eliminated. This is true of meperidine (Demerol); it is metabolized to the toxic intermediate normeperidine, which causes excessive sedation, nausea, and vomiting. Some pathways of drug metabolism, such as hydrolysis, are slowed with uremia. In persons with diabetes, for example, insulin requirements may be reduced as renal function deteriorates. Decreased elimination by the kidneys allows drugs or their metabolites to accumulate in the body and requires that drug dosages be adjusted accordingly. Some drugs contain unwanted nitrogen, sodium, potassium, and magnesium and must be avoided in patients with renal failure. Penicillin, for example, contains potassium. Nitrofurantoin and ammonium chloride add to the body's nitrogen pool. Many antacids contain magnesium. Because of problems with drug dosing and elimination, persons with renal failure should be cautioned against the use of over-the-counter remedies.

TREATMENT

During the past several decades, an increasing number of persons have required renal replacement therapy with dialysis or transplantation. The growing volume is largely attributable to the improvement in treatment and more liberal policies regarding who is treated. Between 1980 and 1992, there was a twofold reported increase in treatment for ESRD.[33] In 1998, almost 245,910 persons were maintained by dialysis therapy in the United States, and another 13,272 underwent kidney transplantation.[34]

Medical Management

Chronic renal failure can treated by conservative management of renal insufficiency and by renal replacement therapy with dialysis or transplantation. Conservative treatment consists of measures to prevent or retard deterioration in remaining renal function and to assist the body in compensating for the existing impairment. Interventions that have been shown to significantly retard the progression of chronic renal insufficiency include dietary protein restriction and blood pressure normalization. Various interventions are used to compensate for reduced renal function and correct the resulting anemia, hypocalcemia, and acidosis. These interventions often are used in conjunction with dialysis therapy for patients with ESRD.

Dialysis and Transplantation

Dialysis or renal replacement therapy is indicated when advanced uremia or serious electrolyte imbalances are present. The choice between dialysis and transplantation is dictated by age, related health problems, donor availability, and personal preference. Although transplantation often is the treatment preference, dialysis plays a critical role as a treatment method for ESRD. It is life sustaining for persons who are not candidates for transplantation or who are awaiting transplantation. There are two broad categories of dialysis: hemodialysis and peritoneal dialysis.

Hemodialysis. The basic principles of hemodialysis have remained unchanged over the years, although new technology has improved the efficiency and speed of dialysis.[35,36] A hemodialysis system, or artificial kidney, consists of three parts: a blood compartment, a dialysis fluid compartment, and a cellophane membrane that separates the two compartments. There are several types of dialyzers; all incorporate these parts, and all function in a similar manner.

The cellophane membrane is semipermeable, permitting all molecules except blood cells and plasma proteins to move freely in both directions—from the blood into the dialyzing solution and from the dialyzing solution into the blood. The direction of flow is determined by the concentration of the substances contained in the two solutions. The waste products and excess electrolytes in the blood normally diffuse into the dialyzing solution. If there is a need to replace or add substances, such as bicarbonate, to the blood, these can be added to the dialyzing solution (Fig. 34-2).

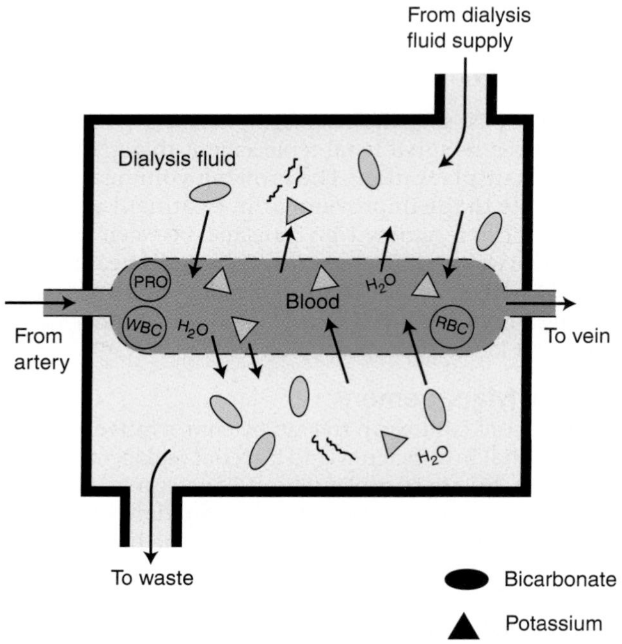

During dialysis, blood moves from an artery through the tubing and blood chamber in the dialysis machine and then back into the body through a vein. Access to the vascular system is accomplished through an external arteriovenous shunt (*i.e.,* tubing implanted into an artery and a vein) or, more commonly, through an internal arteriovenous fistula (*i.e.,* anastomosis of a vein to an artery, usually in the forearm). Heparin is used to prevent clotting during the dialysis treatment; it can be administered continuously or intermittently. Problems that may occur during dialysis, depending on the rates of blood flow and solute removal, include hypotension, nausea, vomiting, muscle cramps, headache, chest pain, and disequilibrium syndrome.

Most persons are dialyzed three times each week for 3 to 4 hours; treatment is determined by kinetic profiles, referred to as Kt/V values, which consider dialyzer size, dialysate, flow rate, time of dialysis, and body size. The adequacy of dialysis is a significant predictor of mortality; the clinical standard for hemodialysis is a Kt/V of 1.2.[37] Many dialysis centers provide the option for patients to learn how to perform hemodialysis at home.

Peritoneal Dialysis. Peritoneal dialysis was introduced in the mid-1970s. Improvements in technology and the ability to deliver adequate dialysis resulted in improved outcomes and the acceptance of peritoneal dialysis as a renal replacement therapy.

The same principles of diffusion, osmosis, and ultrafiltration that apply to hemodialysis apply to peritoneal dialysis. The thin serous membrane of the peritoneal cavity serves as the dialyzing membrane. A Silastic catheter is surgically implanted in the peritoneal cavity below the umbilicus to provide access. The catheter is tunneled through subcutaneous tissue and exits on the side of the abdomen (Fig. 34-3). The dialysis process involves instilling a sterile

FIGURE 34-2 Schematic diagram of a hemodialysis system. The blood compartment and dialysis solution compartment are separated by a cellophane membrane. This membrane is porous enough to allow all the constituents, except the plasma proteins and blood cells, to diffuse between the two compartments.

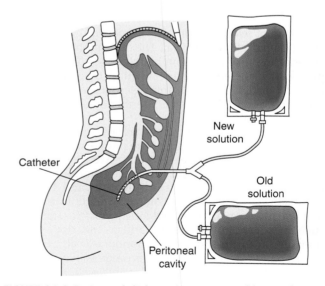

FIGURE 34-3 Peritoneal dialysis. A semipermeable membrane, richly supplied with small blood vessels, lines the peritoneal cavity. With dialysate dwelling in the peritoneal cavity, waste products diffuse from the network of blood cells into the dialysate.

dialyzing solution (usually 2 L) through the catheter over a period of approximately 10 minutes. The solution then is allowed to remain, or dwell, in the peritoneal cavity for a prescribed amount of time, during which the metabolic end products and extracellular fluid diffuse into the dialysis solution. At the end of the dwell time, the dialysis fluid is drained out of the peritoneal cavity by gravity into a sterile bag. Glucose in the dialysis solution accounts for water removal. Commercial dialysis solution is available in 1.5%, 2.5%, and 4.25% dextrose concentrations. Solutions with higher dextrose levels increase osmosis, causing more fluid to be removed. As with hemodialysis, Kt/V values are used to evaluate adequacy of peritoneal analysis. A Kt/V of at least 2.0 is recommended for continuous ambulatory peritoneal dialysis (CAPD).

Peritoneal dialysis can be performed at home or in a center, by an automated or manual system, and on an intermittent or continuous basis—all with variations in the number of exchanges and in dwell time. Individual preference, manual ability, lifestyle, knowledge of the procedure, and physiologic response to treatment influence the dialysis schedule. The most common method is CAPD, a self-care procedure in which the person manages the dialysis procedure and the type of solution (*i.e.*, dextrose concentration) used at home. CAPD involves instilling dialysate into the peritoneal cavity and rolling up the bag and tubing and securing them under clothing during the dwell. After the dwell time is completed (4 to 6 hours during the day), the bag is unrolled and lowered, allowing the waste-containing dialysis solution to drain from the peritoneal cavity into the bag. Each exchange, which involves draining the solution and infusing a new solution, requires approximately 30 to 45 minutes. Four exchanges usually are performed each day. The continuous rather than intermittent nature of CAPD ensures that the rapid fluctuations in extracellular fluid volume associated with hemodialysis are avoided, and dietary restrictions can be liberalized somewhat.

Potential problems with peritoneal dialysis include infection, catheter malfunction, dehydration caused by excessive fluid removal, hyperglycemia, and hernia. The most serious complication is infection, which can occur at the catheter exit site, in the subcutaneous tunnel, or in the peritoneal cavity (*i.e.*, peritonitis).

Transplantation. Greatly improved success rates have made kidney transplantation the treatment of choice for many patients with chronic renal failure. The availability of donor organs continues to limit the number of transplantations performed each year. Donor organs are obtained from cadavers and living related donors (e.g., parent, sibling). Transplants from living nonrelated donors (e.g., spouse) have been used in cases of suitable ABO and tissue compatibility. Of the transplantations performed in 1998, 8752 were from cadaver donors, 3453 were from living related donors, and 1067 were from living unrelated donors.[34] The 1-year graft survival rates for cadaver transplants were 87.7%, and for living related donors, 92.1%.[34]

The success of transplantation depends primarily on the degree of histocompatibility, adequate organ preservation, and immunologic management.[38] Maintenance immuno-suppressive therapy typically consists of corticosteroids, azathioprine, and cyclosporine (or tacrolimus [FK506] or sirolimus). Interleukin-2, a cytokine, plays an essential role in T- and B-cell activation (see Chapter 18). Cyclosporine and tacrolimus inhibit interleukin-2 synthesis, and sirolimus inhibits the T-cell response to interleukin. Genetically engineered antibodies that selectively target interleukin receptors also are available. Monoclonal antibodies such as OKT-3 (directed against the CD3 T-cell receptor) and antilymphocyte antibodies may be used as induction therapy. Because of the increased number of effective immunosuppressive agents that have become available, lower corticosteroid doses are used, resulting in reduced cushingoid effects after transplantation.

Rejection, which is categorized as acute and chronic, can occur at any time. Acute rejection most commonly occurs during the first several months after transplantation and involves a cellular response with the proliferation of T lymphocytes. Chronic rejection can occur months to years after transplantation. Because chronic rejection is caused by both cellular and humoral immunity, it does not respond to increased immunosuppressive therapy.

Maintenance immunosuppressive therapy and increased use of immunosuppression to treat rejection predispose the person to a spectrum of infectious complications. Prophylactic antimicrobials may be prescribed to decrease the incidence of common infections, such as candidiasis, herpesvirus infections, and *Pneumocystis carinii* pneumonia. Other infections, such as cytomegalovirus infection and aspergillosis, are seen with chronic immunosuppression.

Dietary Management

A major component in the treatment of chronic renal failure is dietary management. The goal of dietary treatment is to provide optimum nutrition while maintaining tolerable levels of metabolic wastes. The specific diet prescription depends on the type and severity of renal disease and on the dialysis modality. Because of the severe restrictions placed on food and fluid intake, these diets may be complicated and unappetizing. After kidney transplantation, some dietary restrictions still may be necessary, even when renal function is normal, to control the adverse effects from immunosuppressive medication.

Protein. Restriction of dietary proteins may decrease the progress of renal impairment in persons with advanced renal disease. Proteins are broken down to form nitrogenous wastes, and reducing the amount of protein in the diet lowers the BUN and reduces symptoms. Moreover, a high-protein diet is high in phosphates and inorganic acids. The Modification of Diet in Renal Disease (MDRD) Study, which was conducted in 15 university hospital outpatient nephrology clinics and included 255 patients between the ages of 18 and 70 years, demonstrated a slower decline in GFR among patients randomized to the very–low-protein diet compared with patients on a low-protein diet.[39]

Considerable controversy exists over the degree of restriction needed. If the diet is too low in protein, protein malnutrition can occur, with a loss of strength, muscle mass, and body weight. Results of the MDRD Study indicate that protein requirements can be met by providing 0.6 g of protein per kilogram of body weight per day (g/kg/day).[40] The maintenance dietary protein intake for persons on hemodialysis is 1.2 g/kg/day. Persons on hemodialysis experience protein and energy malnutrition due to anorexia from uremia itself, the dialysis procedure, intercurrent illness, and acidemia. Persons on peritoneal dialysis have significant protein losses, ranging from 5 to 15 g/day, through dialysis and require a dietary protein intake of 1.2 to 1.3 g/kg/day.[41] At least 50% of the protein intake should consist of proteins of high biologic value, such as those in eggs, lean meat, and milk, which are rich in essential amino acids. Proteins with a high biologic value are believed to promote the reuse of endogenous nitrogen, decreasing the amount of nitrogenous wastes that are produced and ameliorating the symptoms of uremia. In reusing nitrogen, the proteins ingested in the diet are broken down into their constituent amino acids and recycled in the synthesis of protein required by the body. In contrast to proteins with a high biologic value, fewer than half of the amino acids in cereal proteins are reused. Amino acids that are not reused to build body proteins are broken down and form the end products of protein metabolism, such as urea.

Carbohydrates, Fat, and Calories. With renal failure, adequate calories in the form of carbohydrates and fat are required to meet energy needs. This is particularly important when the protein content of the diet is severely restricted. If sufficient calories are not available, the limited protein in the diet goes into energy production, or body tissue itself is used for energy purposes. Caloric intake for persons on CAPD includes food intake and calories absorbed from the dialysis solution. A 2-L bag of 1.5% dialysate solution equals 105 calories, and a 4.25% solution delivers 289 calories.

Potassium. When the GFR falls to extremely low levels in ESRD or when undergoing hemodialysis therapy, dietary restriction of potassium becomes mandatory. Using salt substitutes that contain potassium, or ingesting fruits, fruit juice, chocolate, potatoes, or other high-potassium foods can cause hyperkalemia. Most persons on CAPD do not need to limit potassium intake and often may even need to increase intake.

Sodium and Fluid Intake. The sodium and fluid restrictions depend on the kidneys' ability to excrete sodium and water and must be individually determined. Renal disease of glomerular origin is more likely to contribute to sodium retention, whereas tubular dysfunction causes salt wasting. Fluid intake in excess of what the kidneys can excrete causes circulatory overload, edema, and water intoxication. Thirst is a common problem among patients on hemodialysis, often resulting in large weight gains between treatments. Increased thirst appears to be related to elevated renin levels and the production of angiotensin II.[42] Inadequate intake, on the other hand, causes volume depletion and hypotension and can cause further decreases in the already compromised GFR. It is common practice to allow a daily fluid intake of 500 to 800 mL, which is equal to insensible water loss plus a quantity equal to the 24-hour urine output.

In summary, chronic renal failure results from the destructive effects of many forms of renal disease. Regardless of the cause, the consequences of nephron destruction in ESRD are alterations in the filtration, reabsorption, and endocrine functions of the kidneys. The progression of chronic renal failure usually occurs in four stages: diminished renal reserve, renal insufficiency, renal failure, and ESRD. Renal insufficiency represents a reduction in the GFR to approximately 20% to 50% of normal; renal failure, a reduction to less than 20% to 25% of normal; and ESRD, a decrease in GFR to less than 5% of normal.

End-stage renal disease affects almost every body system. It causes an accumulation of nitrogenous wastes (*i.e.,* azotemia), alters sodium and water excretion, and alters regulation of body levels of potassium, phosphate, calcium, and magnesium. It also causes skeletal disorders, anemia, alterations in cardiovascular function, neurologic disturbances, gastrointestinal dysfunction, and discomforting skin changes.

The treatment of ESRD can be divided into two types: conservative management of renal insufficiency and renal replacement therapy with dialysis or transplantation. Conservative treatment consists of measures to prevent or retard deterioration in remaining renal function and to assist the body in compensating for the existing impairment. Interventions that have been shown significantly to retard the progression of chronic renal insufficiency include dietary protein restriction and blood pressure normalization. Activated vitamin D can be used to increase calcium absorption and control secondary hyperparathyroidism. Recombinant human erythropoietin is used to treat the profound anemia that occurs in persons with ESRD.

Renal Failure in Children and Elderly Persons

After you have completed this section of the chapter, you should be able to meet the following objectives:

✦ List the causes of renal failure in children and describe the special problems of children with ESRD
✦ State why renal failure is so common in the elderly and describe measures to prevent or delay the onset of ESRD in this population
✦ Describe the treatment of ESRD in children and the elderly

Although the spectrum of renal disease among children and elderly persons is similar to that of adults, several unique issues affecting these groups warrant further discussion.

CHRONIC RENAL FAILURE IN CHILDREN

The true incidence of chronic renal failure in infants and children is unknown. The data indicate that 2500 people in the United States who are younger than 20 years of age begin treatment for chronic renal failure each year; 100 of these children are younger than 2 years of age.[42] The most common cause of chronic renal failure in children is glomerulonephritis and congenital malformations, such as renal hypoplasia or dysplasia, obstructive uropathy, and reflux nephropathy.[43]

Features of renal disease that are marked during childhood include severe growth impairment, developmental delay, delay in sexual maturation, bone abnormalities, and development of psychosocial problems. Critical growth periods occur during the first 2 years of life and during adolescence. Physical growth and cognitive development occur at a slower rate as consequences of renal disease, especially among children with congenital renal disease. Puberty usually occurs at a later age in children with renal failure, partly because of endocrine abnormalities. Renal osteodystrophy is more common and extensive in children than in adults because of the presence of open epiphyses. As a result, metaphyseal fractures, bone pain, impaired bone growth, short stature, and osteitis fibrosa cystica occur with greater frequency. Some hereditary renal diseases, such as medullary cystic disease, have patterns of skeletal involvement that further complicate the problems of renal osteodystrophy. Factors related to impaired growth include deficient nutrition, anemia, renal osteodystrophy, chronic acidosis, and cases of nephrotic syndrome that require high-dose corticosteroid therapy.

Success of treatment depends on the level of bone maturation at the initiation of therapy. Nutrition is believed to be the most important determinant during infancy.[44] During childhood, growth hormone is important, and gonadotropic hormones become important during puberty.[44] Parental heights provide a means of assessing growth potential. For many children, catch-up growth is important because a growth deficit frequently is established during the first months of life. Recombinant human growth hormone therapy has been used to improve growth in children with ESRD.[44,45] Success of treatment depends on the level of bone maturation at the initiation of therapy.

All forms of renal replacement therapy can be safely and reliably used for children. Children typically are treated with CAPD or transplantation to optimize growth and development.[43] An alternative to CAPD is continuous cyclic peritoneal dialysis. The procedure reverses the schedule of CAPD by providing the exchanges at night rather than during the day. The exchanges are performed automatically during sleep by a simple cycler machine. Renal transplantation is considered the best alternative for children.[42,44,46,47] Early transplantation in young children is regarded as the best way to promote physical growth, improve cognitive function, and foster psychosocial development.[46–48] Immunosuppressive therapy in children is similar to that used in adults. All of these immunosuppressive agents have side effects, including increased risk of infection. Corticosteroids, which have been the mainstay of chronic immunosuppressive therapy for decades, carry the risk of hypertension, orthopedic complications (especially aseptic necrosis), cataracts, and growth retardation.

CHRONIC RENAL FAILURE IN ELDERLY PERSONS

Since the mid-1980s, there have been increasing numbers of elderly persons accepted to ESRD programs. In 1998, 20.6% of persons being treated for ESRD were 65 to 74 years of age, and 12.9% were older than 75 years of age.[49] Among elderly persons, the presentation and course of renal failure may be altered because of age-related changes in the kidneys and concurrent medical conditions.

Normal aging is associated with a decline in the GFR and subsequently with reduced homeostatic regulation under stressful conditions.[50] This reduction in GFR makes elderly persons more susceptible to the detrimental effects of nephrotoxic drugs, such as radiographic contrast compounds. The reduction in GFR related to aging is not accompanied by a parallel rise in the serum creatinine level because the serum creatinine level, which results from muscle metabolism, is significantly reduced in elderly persons because of diminished muscle mass and other age-related changes. Evaluation of renal function in elderly persons should include a measurement of creatinine clearance along with the serum creatinine level. The Cockroft and Gault equation can be used to provide an estimate of GFR and of renal function with allowance for age.

The prevalence of chronic disease affecting the cerebrovascular, cardiovascular, and skeletal systems is higher in this age group. Because of concurrent disease, the presenting symptoms of renal disease in elderly persons may be less typical than those observed in younger adults. For example, congestive heart failure and hypertension may be the dominant clinical features with the onset of acute glomerulonephritis, whereas oliguria and discolored urine more often are the first signs in younger adults. The course of renal failure may be more complicated in older patients with numerous chronic diseases.

Treatment options for chronic renal failure in elderly patients include hemodialysis, peritoneal dialysis, transplantation, and acceptance of death from uremia. Neither hemodialysis nor peritoneal dialysis has proven to be superior in the elderly. The mode of renal replacement therapy

---

*Prediction of Creatinine Clearance Using Serum Clearance**

$$\text{Creatinine clearance (mL/minute)} = \frac{(140 - \text{age}) \times (\text{body weight in kg})}{72 \times \text{serum creatinine in mg/dL}}$$

*The equation result should be multiplied by a factor of 0.85 for women.

(From Cockroft D.W., Gault M.H. [1976]. Prediction of creatinine clearance from serum creatinine. *Nephron 16*, 31.)

should be individualized, taking into account underlying medical and psychosocial factors. Age alone should not preclude renal transplantation.[50] With increasing experience, many transplantation centers have increased the age for acceptance on transplant waiting lists. Reluctance to provide transplantation as an alternative may have been due, at least in part, to the scarcity of available organs and the view that younger persons are more likely to benefit for a longer time.[51] The general reduction in T-cell function that occurs with aging has been suggested as a beneficial effect that increases transplant graft survival.

In summary, there is approximately a 2% per year incidence of renal failure in children, most frequently resulting from congenital malformations and glomerulonephritis. Problems associated with renal failure in children include growth impairment, delay in sexual maturation, and more extensive bone abnormalities than in adults. Although all forms of renal replacement therapy can be safely and reliably used for children, CAPD or transplantation optimize growth and development.

Adults 65 years of age and older account for close to one half of the new cases of ESRD each year. Normal aging is associated with a decline in the GFR, which makes elderly persons more susceptible to the detrimental effects of nephrotoxic drugs and other conditions that compromise renal function. Treatment options for chronic renal failure in elderly patients are similar to those for younger persons.

References

1. Levy E.M., Viscose C.M., Horwitz R.I. (1996). The effect of acute renal failure on mortality: A cohort analysis. *Journal of the American Medical Association* 275, 1489–1494.
2. Thadhani R., Pascual M., Bonventre J.V. (1996). Acute renal failure. *New England Journal of Medicine* 334, 1448–1460.
3. Brady H.R., Brenner B.M., Clarkson M.R., Liebman W. (2000). Acute renal failure. In Brenner B.M. (Ed.), *Brenner and Rector's The kidney* (6th ed., pp. 1201–1247). Philadelphia: W.B Saunders.
4. Agrawal M., Schwartz R. (2000). Acute renal failure. *American Family Physician* 61, 2077–2088.
5. Albright R.C. (2001). Acute renal failure: A practical update. *Mayo Clinic Proceedings* 76, 67–74.
6. Guyton A., Hall J.E. (2000). *Textbook of medical physiology* (10th ed., pp. 369–371, 373–378). Philadelphia: W.B. Saunders.
7. Cotran R.S., Kumar V., Collins T. (1999). *Robbins pathologic basis of disease* (6th ed., pp. 932–933, 969–971, 1229). Philadelphia: W.B. Saunders.
8. Garella S. (1993). Drug-induced renal disease. *Hospital Practice* 28(4), 129–140.
9. Bailie G.R. (1996). Acute renal failure. In Young L.Y., Koda-Kimble M.A. (Eds.), *Applied therapeutics: The clinical use of drugs* (6th ed., pp. 29-6–29-17). Vancouver, WA: Applied Therapeutics.
10. Gerlach A.T., Pickworth K.K. (2000). Contrast medium-induced nephrotoxicity: Pathophysiology and prevention. *Pharmacotherapy* 20, 540–548.
11. Forni L.G., Hilton P.J. (1997). Continuous hemodilution in the treatment of acute renal failure. *New England Journal of Medicine* 336, 1303–1309.
12. Rettig R.A. (1996). The social contract and the treatment of permanent renal failure. *Journal of the American Medical Association* 274, 1123–1126.
13. National Kidney and Urological Information Center. (2001). *Kidney and urologic disease statistics for the United States.* [On-line]. Available: http://www.niddk.nih.gov/health/kidney/pubs/kstats/kstats.htm.
14. Llach F., Bover J. (2000). Renal osteodystrophies. In Brenner B.M. (Ed.), *Brenner and Rector's The kidney* (6th ed., pp. 2103–2135). Philadelphia: W.B Saunders.
15. Hrusks K.A., Teitelbaum S.L. (1995). Renal osteodystrophy. *New England Journal of Medicine* 333, 166–174.
16. Couttenye M.M., D'Haese P.C., Verschoren W.J., Behets G.J., Schrooten I., Broe M.E. (1999). Low bone turnover in patients with renal failure. *Kidney International* 56 (7 Suppl. 73), S70–S76.
17. Brenner B.M., Lazarus J.M. (1991). Chronic renal failure. In Wilson J.D., Braunwald E., Isselbacher K.J., et al. (Eds.), *Harrison's principles of internal medicine* (12th ed., pp. 1150–1156). New York: McGraw-Hill.
18. Slatopolsky E., Brown A., Dusso A. (2000). Role of phosphorus in pathogenesis of secondary hyperparathyroidism. *American Journal of Kidney Diseases* 37 (1 Suppl. 2), S54–S57.
19. Drüeke T.B. (2001). Control of secondary hyperthyroidism by vitamin D derivatives. *American Journal of Kidney Diseases* 37 (1 Suppl. 2), S58–S61.
20. Tong E.M., Nissenson A.R. (2001). Erythropoietin and anemia. *Seminars in Nephrology* 21, 190–203.
21. Besarab A., Levin A. (2000). Defining a renal anemia management period. *American Journal of Kidney Diseases* 36 (6 Suppl. 3), S13–S23.
22. Obrador G.T., Ruthazer R., Aora P., Kausz A.T., Pereira B.J. (1999). Prevalence of and factors associated with suboptimal care before initiation of dialysis in the United States. *Journal of the American Society of Nephrologists* 10, 1793–1800.
23. Kautz A.T., Obrader G.T., Pereira B.J.G. (2000). Anemia management in patients with chronic renal failure. *American Journal of Kidney Diseases* 36(6 Suppl. 3), S39–S49.
24. National Kidney Foundation. (2001). NKF-KDOQ Clinical practice guidelines for anemia in chronic renal failure. Target hemoglobin/hematocrit. *American Journal of Kidney Diseases* 37 (1 Suppl. 1), S182–238.
25. Eberst M.E., Berkowitz L.R. (1993). Hemostasis in renal disease: Pathophysiology and management. *American Journal of Medicine* 96, 168–179.
26. National Kidney Foundation Task Force on Cardiovascular Disease. (1998). Controlling the epidemic of cardiovascular disease in chronic renal disease. *American Journal of Kidney Diseases* 32, 853–906.
27. Preston R.A., Singer I., Epstein M. (1996). Renal parenchymal hypertension. *Archives of Internal Medicine* 156, 602–611.
28. Levin A., Foley R.N. (2000). Cardiovascular disease in chronic renal failure. *American Journal of Kidney Diseases* 36 (6 Suppl. 3), S24–S30.
29. Al-Ahmad A., Sarnak M.J., Salem D.N., Konstam M.A. (2001). Cause and management of heart failure in patients with chronic renal disease. *Seminars in Nephrology* 21, 3–12.
30. Gunukula S., Spodick D.H. (2001). Pericardial disease in renal failure. *Seminars in Nephrology* 21, 52–56.
31. Rickus M.A. (1987). Sexual dysfunction in the female ESRD patient. *American Nephrology Nurses' Association Journal* 14, 185–186.
32. Foulks C.J., Cushner H.M. (1986). Sexual dysfunction in the male dialysis patient: Pathogenesis, evaluation, and therapy. *American Journal of Kidney Diseases* 8, 211–212.

33. Agodaoa L.Y., Eggers P.W. (1995). Renal replacement therapy in the United States: Data from the United States Renal Data System. *American Journal of Kidney Diseases* 25, 119–133.
34. National Kidney and Urologic Diseases Information Clearinghouse. (2001). *Kidney and urologic diseases statistics in the United States.* [On-line]. Available: http://www.niddk.gov/health/kidney/pubs/kustats/kustats.htm.
35. Ifudu O. (1998). Care of patients undergoing hemodialysis. *New England Journal of Medicine* 339, 1054–1062.
36. Daelemans R.A., D'Haese P.C., BeBroe M.E. (2001). Dialysis. *Seminars in Nephrology* 21, 204–212.
37. Renal Physicians' Association, Working Committee on Clinical Practice Guidelines. (1993). *Clinical practice guidelines on adequacy of hemodialysis.* Washington, DC: Author.
38. Ramanathan V., Goral S., Helderman J.H. (2001). Renal transplantation. *Seminars in Nephrology* 21, 213–219.
39. Levey A.S., Adler S., Caggiula A.W., England B.K., Greene T., Hunsicker H.G., et al. (1996). Effects of dietary protein restriction on the progression of advanced renal disease in the modification of diet in renal disease study. *American Journal of Kidney Diseases* 27, 652–663.
40. National Kidney Foundation. (2000). *Clinical practice guidelines for nutrition in chronic renal failure.* [On-line]. Available: http://kidney.org/professionals/doqi/doqi/doqi_nut.html.
41. Porth C.M., Erickson M. (1992). Physiology of thirst and drinking: Implication for nursing practice. *Heart and Lung* 21, 275.
42. Hanna J.D., Krieg R.J., Scheinman J.I., Chan J.C.M. (1996). Effects of uremia on growth in children. *Seminars in Nephrology* 16, 230–241.
43. Bergstein J.M. (2000). Renal failure. In Behrman R.E., Kliegman R.M., Jensen H.B. (Eds.), *Nelson textbook of pediatrics* (16th ed., pp. 1605–1617). Philadelphia: W.B. Saunders.
44. Abitbol C., Chan J.C.M., Trachtman H., Strauss J., Greifer I. (1996). Growth in children with moderate renal insufficiency: Measurement, evaluation, and treatment. *Journal of Pediatrics* 129, S3–S7.
45. Haffner D., Schaffer F., Nissel R., Wühl E., Tönshoff B., Mehls O. (Study Group for Growth Hormone Treatment in Chronic Renal Failure). (2000). Effect of growth hormone treatment on the adult height of children with chronic renal failure. *New England Journal of Medicine* 343, 923–930.
46. Bereket G., Fine R.N. (1995). Pediatric renal transplantation. *Pediatric Clinics of North America* 42, 1603–1627.
47. Urizar R.E. (2000). Renal transplantation. In Behrman R.E., Kliegman R.M., Jensen H.B. (Eds.), *Nelson textbook of pediatrics* (16th ed., pp. 1612–1617). Philadelphia: W.B. Saunders.
48. Fennell R.S., Ruley E.J., Vehaskari M. (1996). Psychosocial aspects of care of the child with moderate renal failure. *Journal of Pediatrics* 129, S8–S12.
49. National Kidney Foundation. (2000). *End stage renal disease.* [On-line]. Available: http://www.kidney.org/general/news/esrd/cfm.
50. Choudhury D., Raj D.S.D., Palmer B., Levi M. (2000). Effect of aging on renal function and disease. In Brenner B.M. (Ed.), *Brenner and Rector's The kidney* (6th ed., pp. 2187–2210). Philadelphia: W.B Saunders.
51. Davison A.M. (1998). Renal disease in the elderly. *Nephron* 80, 6–16.

Alterations in Urine Elimination

Although the kidneys control the formation of urine and regulate the composition of body fluids, it is the bladder that stores urine and controls its elimination from the body. Alterations in the storage and expulsion functions of the bladder can result in incontinence, with its accompanying social and hygienic problems, or obstruction of urinary flow, which has deleterious effects on ureteral and, ultimately, renal function. The discussion in this chapter focuses on normal control of urine elimination, urinary obstruction and stasis, neurogenic bladder, incontinence, and bladder cancer. Urinary tract infections are discussed in Chapter 33.

Control of Urine Elimination

After you have completed this section of the chapter, you should be able to meet the following objectives:

- ✦ Trace the innervation of the bladder and control of micturition from the detrusor muscle and external sphincter, the micturition centers in the sacral and thoracolumbar cord, the pontine micturition center, and the cerebral cortex
- ✦ Explain the mechanism of low-pressure urine storage in the bladder

- ✦ List at least three classes of autonomic drugs and explain their potential effect on bladder function
- ✦ Describe at least three urodynamic studies that can be used to assess bladder function

The bladder, also known as the *urinary vesicle*, is a freely movable organ located behind the pelvic bone in the male and in front of the vagina in the female. It consists of two parts: the fundus, or body, and the neck, or posterior urethra. In the man, the urethra continues anteriorly through the penis. Urine passes from the kidneys to the bladder through the ureters, which are 4 to 5 mm in diameter and approximately 30 cm long. The ureters enter the bladder bilaterally at a location toward its base and close to the urethra Fig. 35-1). The triangular area that is bounded by the ureters and the urethra is called the *trigone*. There are no valves at the ureteral openings, but as the pressure of the urine in the bladder rises, the ends of the ureters are compressed against the bladder wall to prevent the backflow of urine.

BLADDER STRUCTURE

The bladder is composed of four layers. The first is an outer serosal layer, which covers the upper surface and is continuous with the peritoneum. The second is a network

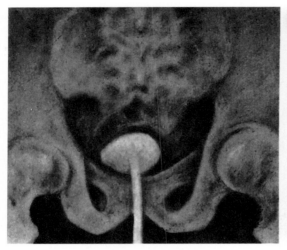
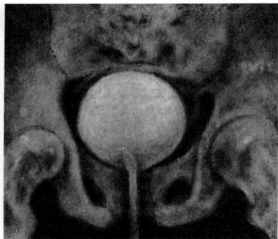

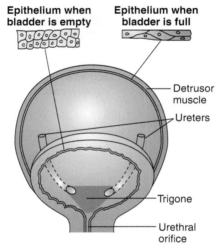

Epithelium when bladder is empty

Epithelium when bladder is full

Detrusor muscle

Ureters

Trigone

Urethral orifice

FIGURE 35-1 (**Top**) Cystogram of male bladder, showing position and filling. (**Bottom**) Diagram of the bladder, showing the detrusor muscle, ureters, trigone area, and urethral orifice. Note the flattening of epithelial cells when the bladder is full and the wall is stretched. (Chaffee E.E., Lytle I.M. [1980]. *Basic physiology and anatomy.* Philadelphia: J.B. Lippincott)

of smooth muscle fibers called the *detrusor muscle.* The third is a submucosal layer of loose connective tissue, and the fourth is an inner mucosal lining of transitional epithelium.

The tonicity of the urine often is quite different from that of the blood, and the transitional epithelial lining of the bladder acts as an effective barrier to prevent the passage of water between the bladder contents and the blood. The inner elements of the bladder form smooth folds, or rugae. As the bladder expands during filling, these rugae spread out to form a single layer without disrupting the integrity of the epithelial lining.

The detrusor muscle is the muscle of micturition (passage of urine). When it contracts, urine is expelled from the bladder. The abdominal muscles play a secondary role in micturition. Their contraction increases intra-abdominal pressure, which further increases intravesicular pressure.

Muscles in the bladder neck, sometimes referred to as the *internal sphincter,* are a continuation of the detrusor muscle. They run down obliquely behind the proximal urethra, forming the posterior urethra in males and the entire urethra in females. When the bladder is relaxed, these circular muscle fibers are closed and act as a sphincter. When the detrusor muscle contracts, the sphincter is pulled open by the changes that occur in bladder shape. In the female, the urethra (2.5 to 3.5 cm) is shorter than in the male (16.5 to 18.5 cm), and usually affords less resistance to urine outflow.

Another muscle important to bladder function is the *external sphincter,* a circular muscle composed of striated muscle fibers that surrounds the urethra distal to the base of the bladder. The external sphincter operates as a reserve mechanism to stop micturition when it is occurring and to maintain continence in the face of unusually high blad-

Bladder Function

> ➤ The functions of the bladder are storage and emptying of urine.

> ➤ The control of the storage and emptying functions of the bladder involves both involuntary (autonomic nervous system) and voluntary (somatic nervous system) control.

> ➤ The parasympathetic nervous system promotes bladder emptying. It produces contraction of the smooth muscle of the bladder wall and relaxation of the internal sphincter.

> ➤ The sympathetic nervous system promotes bladder filling. It produces relaxation of the smooth muscle of the bladder wall and contraction of the internal sphincter.

> ➤ The striated muscles in the external sphincter and pelvic floor, which are innervated by the somatic nervous system, provide for the voluntary control of urination and maintenance of continence.

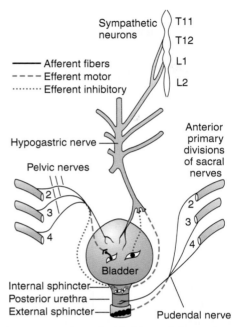

FIGURE 35-2 Nerve supply to the bladder and the urethra. (Chaffee E.E., Lytle I.M. [1980]. *Basic physiology and anatomy*. Philadelphia: J.B. Lippincott)

der pressure. The skeletal muscle of the pelvic floor also contributes to the support of the bladder and the maintenance of continence.

NEURAL CONTROL OF BLADDER FUNCTION

The control of bladder emptying is unique in that it involves both involuntary autonomic nervous system (ANS) reflexes and some voluntary control. The excitatory input to the bladder that causes bladder emptying is controlled by the parasympathetic nervous system. The sympathetic nervous system relaxes the bladder smooth muscle. There are three main levels of neurologic control for bladder function: the spinal cord reflex centers, the micturition center in the pons, and the cortical and subcortical centers.

Spinal Cord Centers

The centers for reflex control of micturition are located in the sacral (S2 through S4) and thoracolumbar (T11 through L1) segments of the spinal cord (Fig. 35-2). The parasympathetic lower motor neurons (LMNs) for the detrusor muscle of the bladder are located in the sacral segments of the spinal cord; their axons travel to the bladder by way of the *pelvic nerve*. LMNs for the external sphincter also are located in the sacral segments of the spinal cord. These LMNs receive their control from the motor cortex by way of the corticospinal tract and send impulses to the external sphincter through the *pudendal nerve*. The bladder neck and trigone area of the bladder, because of their different embryonic origin, receive their innervation from sympathetic outflow from the thoracolumbar (T11 to L2) segments of the spinal cord. The seminal vesicles, ampulla

of the vas, and vas deferens also receive sympathetic innervation from the thoracolumbar segments of the cord.

The afferent input from the bladder and urethra is carried to the central nervous system (CNS) by means of fibers that travel with the parasympathetic (pelvic), somatic (pudendal), and sympathetic (hypogastric) nerves. The pelvic nerve carries sensory fibers from the stretch receptors in the bladder wall; the pudendal nerve carries sensory fibers from the external sphincter and pelvic muscles; and the hypogastric nerve carries sensory fibers from the trigone area.

Pontine Micturition Center

The immediate coordination of the normal micturition reflex occurs in the micturition center in the pons, facilitated by descending input from the forebrain and ascending input from the reflex centers in the spinal cord[1,2] (Fig. 35-3). This center is thought to coordinate the activity of the detrusor muscle and the external sphincter. As bladder filling occurs, ascending spinal afferents relay this information to the micturition center, which also receives important descending information from the forebrain concerning behavioral cues for bladder emptying. Descending pathways from the pontine micturition center produce coordinated inhibition of somatic systems, relaxing both sphincters. The onset of urinary flow through the urethra causes reflex contraction of the bladder.

Cortical and Subcortical Centers

Cortical brain centers enable inhibition of the micturition center in the pons and conscious control of urination. Neural influences from the subcortical centers in the basal

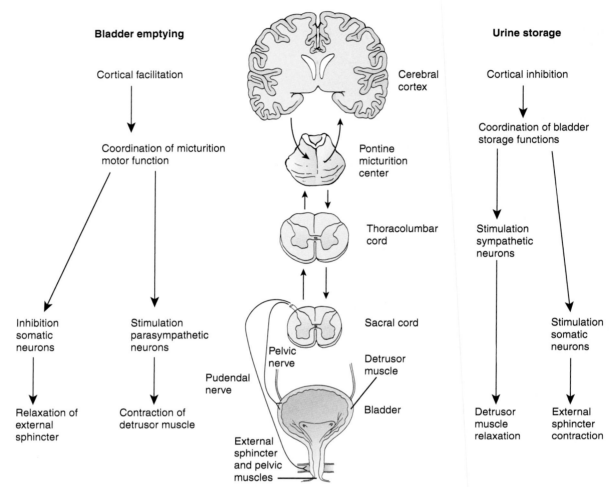

Bladder emptying

Cortical facilitation

Coordination of micturition motor function

Inhibition somatic neurons

Stimulation parasympathetic neurons

Relaxation of external sphincter

Contraction of detrusor muscle

Cerebral cortex

Pontine micturition center

Thoracolumbar cord

Sacral cord

Pelvic nerve

Pudendal nerve

Detrusor muscle

Bladder

External sphincter and pelvic muscles

Urine storage

Cortical inhibition

Coordination of bladder storage functions

Stimulation sympathetic neurons

Stimulation somatic neurons

Detrusor muscle relaxation

External sphincter contraction

FIGURE 35-3 Pathways and central nervous system centers involved in control of bladder function. Efferent pathways for micturition (**left**) and urine storage (**right**).

ganglia, which are conveyed by extrapyramidal pathways, modulate the contractile response. They modify and delay the detrusor contractile response during filling and then modulate the expulsive activity of the bladder to facilitate complete emptying.

Micturition

When the bladder is distended to 150 to 300 mL, the sensation of fullness is transmitted to the spinal cord and then to the cerebral cortex, allowing for conscious inhibition of the micturition reflex. During the act of micturition, the detrusor muscle of the bladder fundus and bladder neck contract down on the urine in the fundus of the bladder; the ureteral orifices are forced shut; the bladder neck is widened and shortened as it is pulled up by the globular muscles in the bladder fundus; the resistance of the internal sphincter in the bladder neck is decreased; and the external sphincter relaxes as urine moves out of the bladder.

In infants and young children, micturition is an involuntary act that is triggered by a spinal cord reflex; when the bladder fills to a given capacity, the detrusor muscle

contracts and the external sphincter relaxes. As the bladder grows and increases in capacity, the tone of the external sphincter muscle increases. At 2 to 3 years of age, the child becomes conscious of the need to urinate and can learn to contract the pelvic muscles to maintain closure of the sphincter and delay urination. As the nervous system continues to mature, inhibition of involuntary detrusor muscle activity takes place. After the child achieves continence, micturition becomes voluntary.

To maintain continence, or retention of urine, the bladder must function as a low-pressure storage system; the pressure in the bladder must remain lower than urethral pressure. To ensure that this condition is met, the increase in intravesicular pressure that accompanies bladder filling is almost imperceptible. An increase in bladder volume from 10 to 400 mL may be accompanied by only a 5 cm H_2O increase in pressure.[3] Sustained elevations in intravesicular pressures (>40 to 50 cm H_2O) often are associated with vesicoureteral reflux (*i.e.*, backward movement of urine from the bladder into the ureter) and the development of ureteral dilatation. Although the pressure in the bladder is maintained at low levels, sphincter pressure remains high (45 to 65 cm H_2O) as a means of preventing loss of urine as the bladder fills.

Pharmacology of Micturition

The ANS and its neuromediators play a central role in micturition. Parasympathetic innervation of the bladder is mediated by the neurotransmitter acetylcholine. Two types of cholinergic receptors affect various aspects of micturition: nicotinic and muscarinic. *Nicotinic* (N) receptors are found in the synapses between the preganglionic and postganglionic neurons of the sympathetic and the parasympathetic system, as well as in the neuromuscular end plates of the striated muscle fibers of the external sphincter and pelvic muscles. *Muscarinic* (M) receptors are found in the postganglionic parasympathetic endings of the detrusor muscle. Several subtypes of M receptors have been identified. The M_2 and M_3 receptors appear predominantly to mediate detrusor contraction and internal sphincter contraction. The M_3 receptor also mediates salivary secretion and bowel activity.[4] The identification of receptor subtypes has facilitated the development of medications that selectively target bladder structures while minimizing other, undesired effects.

Although sympathetic innervation is not essential to the act of micturition, it allows the bladder to store a large volume without the involuntary escape of urine—a mechanism that is consistent with the fight-or-flight function subserved by the sympathetic nervous system. The bladder is supplied with α_1- and β_2-adrenergic receptors. The β_2-adrenergic receptors are found in the detrusor muscle; they produce relaxation of the detrusor muscle, increasing the bladder volume at which the micturition reflex is triggered. The α_1-adrenergic receptors are found in the trigone area, including the intramural ureteral musculature, bladder neck, and internal sphincter. The activation of α_1 receptors produces contraction of these muscles. Sympathetic activity ceases when the micturition reflex is activated. During male ejaculation, which is mediated by the sympathetic nervous system, the musculature of the trigone area and that of the bladder neck and prostatic urethra contracts and prevents the backflow of seminal fluid into the bladder.

Because of their effects on bladder function, drugs that selectively activate or block ANS outflow or receptor activity can alter urine elimination. Table 35-1 describes the action of drug groups that can impair bladder function or can be used in the treatment of micturition disorders. Many of the nonprescription cold preparations contain α-adrenergic agonists and antihistamine agents that have anticholinergic properties. These drugs can cause urinary retention. Many of the antidepressant and antipsychotic drugs also have anticholinergic actions that influence urination.

DIAGNOSTIC METHODS OF EVALUATING BLADDER FUNCTION

Bladder structure and function can be assessed by a number of methods.[5] Reports or observations of frequency, hesitancy, straining to void, and a weak or interrupted stream are suggestive of outflow obstruction. Palpation and percussion provide information about bladder distention.

TABLE 35-1 ✦ Action of Drug Groups on Bladder Function

Function	Drug Groups	Mechanism of Action
Detrusor Muscle		
Increased tone and contraction	Cholinergic drugs	Stimulate parasympathetic receptors that cause detrusor contraction
Inhibition of detrusor muscle relaxation during filling	β_2-Adrenergic–blocking drugs	Block β_2 receptors that produce detrusor muscle relaxation
Decreased tone	Anticholinergic drugs and drugs with an anticholinergic action	Block the muscarinic receptors that cause detrusor muscle contraction
	Calcium channel–blocking drugs	May interfere with influx of calcium to support contraction of detrusor smooth muscle
Internal Bladder Sphincter		
Increased tone	α_1-Adrenergic agonists	Activate α_1 receptors that produce contraction of the smooth muscle of the internal sphincter
Decreased tone	α_1-Adrenergic–blocking drugs	Block contraction of the smooth muscle of the internal sphincter
External Sphincter		
Decreased tone	Skeletal muscle relaxants	Decrease the tone of the external sphincter by acting at the level of the spinal cord or by interfering with release of calcium in muscle fiber

Physical Examination

Postvoided residual (PVR) urine volume provides information about bladder emptying. It can be estimated by abdominal palpation and percussion. Catheterization and ultrasonography can be used to obtain specific measurements of PVR. A PVR value of less than 50 mL is considered adequate bladder emptying, and more than 200 mL indicates inadequate bladder emptying.[6]

Pelvic examination is used in women to assess perineal skin condition, perivaginal muscle tone, genital atrophy, pelvic prolapse (*e.g.*, cystocele, rectocele, uterine prolapse), pelvic mass, or other conditions that may impair bladder function. Bimanual examination (*i.e.*, pelvic and abdominal palpation) can be used to assess PVR volume. Rectal examination is used to test for perineal sensation, sphincter tone, fecal impaction, and rectal mass. It is used to assess the contour of the prostate in men.

Laboratory and Radiologic Studies

Urine tests provide information about kidney function and urinary tract infections. The presence of bacteriuria or pyuria suggests urinary tract infection and the possibility of urinary tract obstruction. Blood tests (*i.e.*, blood urea nitrogen and creatinine) provide information about renal function.

Bladder structures can be visualized indirectly by taking x-ray films of the abdomen and by using excretory urography (which involves the use of a radiopaque dye [see Fig. 35-1]), computed tomographic (CT) scanning, magnetic resonance imaging (MRI), or ultrasonography. Cystoscopy enables direct visualization of the urethra, bladder, and ureteral orifices.

Urodynamic Studies

Urodynamic studies are used to study bladder function and voiding problems. Three aspects of bladder function can be assessed by urodynamic studies: bladder, urethral, and intra-abdominal pressure changes; characteristics of urine flow; and the activity of the striated muscles of the external sphincter and pelvic floor. Specific urodynamic tests include uroflowmetry, cystometry, urethral pressure profile, sphincter electromyography (EMG), and uroflow studies. It often is advantageous to evaluate several components of bladder function simultaneously.

Uroflowmetry. Uroflowmetry measures the flow rate (milliliters per minute) during urination. It commonly is done using a weight-recording device located at the bottom of a commode receptacle unit. As the person being tested voids, the weight of the commode receptacle unit increases. This weight change is electronically recorded and then analyzed using weight (converted to milliliters) and time.

Cystometry. Cystometry is used to measure bladder pressure during filling and voiding. It provides valuable information about total bladder capacity, intravesicular pressures during bladder filling, the ability to perceive bladder fullness and the desire to urinate, the ability of the bladder to contract and sustain a contraction, uninhibited bladder contractions, and the ability to inhibit urination. The test can be done by allowing physiologic filling of the bladder with urine and recording intravesicular pressure throughout a voiding cycle, or by filling the bladder with water and measuring intravesicular pressure against the volume of water instilled into the bladder.[5]

In a normally functioning bladder, the sensation of bladder fullness is first perceived when the bladder contains 100 to 200 mL of urine while bladder pressure remains constant at approximately 8 to 15 cm H_2O. The desire to void occurs when the bladder is full (normal capacity is approximately 400 to 500 mL). At this point, a definite sensation of fullness occurs, the pressure rises sharply to 40 to 100 cm H_2O, and voiding occurs around the catheter. Urinary continence requires that urethral pressure exceed bladder pressure. Bladder pressure usually rises 30 to 40 cm H_2O during voiding. If the urethral resistance is high because of obstruction, greater pressure is required, a condition that can be detected by cystometry.

Urethral Pressure Profile. The urethral pressure profile is used to evaluate the intraluminal pressure changes along the length of the urethra with the bladder at rest.[5] It provides information about smooth muscle activity along the length of the urethra. This test can be done using the infusion method (most commonly used), the membrane catheter method, or the microtip transducer. The infusion method involves the insertion of a small double-lumen urethral catheter, then infusing water into the bladder and measuring the changes in urethral pressure as the catheter is slowly withdrawn.

Sphincter Electromyography. Sphincter EMG allows the activity of the striated (voluntary) muscles of the perineal area to be studied. Activity is recorded using an anal plug electrode, a catheter electrode, adhesive skin electrodes, or needle electrodes. Electrode placement is based on the muscle groups that need to be tested. The test usually is done along with urodynamic tests such as the cystometrogram and uroflow studies.

Ultrasound Bladder Scan. The ultrasound bladder scan provides a noninvasive method for estimating bladder volume. The device measures ultrasonic reflections to differentiate the urinary bladder from the surrounding tissue. A computer system calculates and displays bladder volume. The device can be used to determine the need for catheterization, for evaluation and diagnosis of urinary retention, to measure PVR volumes, and for facilitating volume-dependent or time-dependent catheterization or toileting programs.

In summary, although the kidneys function in the formation of urine and the regulation of body fluids, it is the bladder that stores and controls the elimination of urine. Micturition is a function of the peripheral ANS, subject to facilitation or inhibition from higher neurologic centers. The parasympathetic nervous system controls the motor function of the bladder detrusor muscle and the tone of the internal sphincter; its cell bodies are located in the sacral spinal cord and communicate with the bladder through the pelvic nerve. Efferent sympathetic control originates at the level of segments T11 through L1 of the spinal cord and produces relaxation of the detrusor muscle and contraction of the internal sphincter. Skeletal muscle found in the external sphincter and the pelvic muscles that support the bladder are supplied by the pudendal nerve, which exits the spinal cord at the level of segments S2 through S4. The micturition center in the brain stem coordinates the action of the detrusor muscle and the external sphincter, whereas cortical centers permit conscious control of micturition.

Bladder function can be evaluated using urodynamic studies that measure bladder, urethral, and abdominal pressures; urine flow characteristics; and skeletal muscle activity of the external sphincter.

Alterations in Bladder Function

After you have completed this section of the chapter, you should be able to meet the following objectives:

✦ Describe the causes of and compensatory changes that occur with urinary tract obstruction

✦ Differentiate lesions that produce storage dysfunction associated with spastic bladder from those that produce emptying dysfunction associated with flaccid bladder in terms of the level of the lesions and their effects on bladder function

✦ Cite the pathology and causes of nonrelaxing external sphincter

✦ Describe methods used in treatment of neurogenic bladder

✦ Define *incontinence* and list the categories of this condition

✦ Describe behavioral, pharmacologic, and surgical methods used in treatment of incontinence

Alterations in bladder function include urinary obstruction with retention or stasis of urine and urinary incontinence with involuntary loss of urine. Although the two conditions have almost opposite effects on urination, they can have similar causes. Both can result from structural changes in the bladder, urethra, or surrounding organs or from impairment of neurologic control of bladder function.

URINARY OBSTRUCTION AND STASIS

In lower urinary tract obstruction and stasis, urine is produced normally by the kidneys but is retained in the bladder. Obstructions are classified according to cause (congenital or acquired), degree (partial or complete), duration (acute or chronic), and level (upper or lower urinary tract).[7] Because it has the potential to produce vesicoureteral reflux and cause kidney damage, urinary obstruction and stasis is a serious disorder.

Congenital narrowing of the external meatus (*i.e.,* meatal stenosis) is more common in boys, and obstructive disorders of the posterior urethra are more common in girls. Another common cause of congenital obstruction is the damage to sacral nerves that occurs in spina bifida and meningomyelocele.

The acquired causes of lower urinary tract obstruction and stasis are numerous. In males, the most important cause of urinary obstruction is external compression of the urethra caused by the enlargement of the prostate gland. Gonorrhea and other sexually transmitted diseases contribute to the incidence of infection-produced urethral strictures. Bladder tumors and secondary invasion of the bladder by tumors arising in structures that surround the bladder and urethra can compress the bladder neck or urethra and cause obstruction. Constipation and fecal impaction can compress the urethra and produce urethral obstruction. This can be a particular problem in elderly persons.

Compensatory Changes

The body compensates for the obstruction of urine outflow with mechanisms designed to prevent urine retention. These mechanisms can be divided into two stages: a compensatory stage and a decompensatory stage.[7] The degree to which these changes occur and their effect on bladder structure and urinary function depend on the extent of the obstruction, the rapidity with which it occurs, and the presence of other contributing factors, such as neurologic impairment and infection.

During the early stage of obstruction, the bladder begins to hypertrophy and becomes hypersensitive to afferent stimuli arising from bladder filling. The ability to suppress urination is diminished, and bladder contraction can become so strong that it virtually produces bladder spasm. There is urgency, sometimes to the point of incontinence, and frequency during the day and at night.

With continuation and progression of the obstruction, compensatory changes begin to occur. There is further hypertrophy of the bladder muscle, the thickness of the bladder wall may double, and the pressure generated by detrusor contraction can increase from a normal 20 to 40 cm H_2O to 50 to 100 cm H_2O to overcome the resistance from the obstruction. As the force needed to expel urine from the bladder increases, compensatory mechanisms may become ineffective, causing muscle fatigue before complete emptying can be accomplished. After a few minutes, voiding can again be initiated and completed, accounting for the frequency of urination.

The inner bladder surface forms smooth folds. With continued outflow obstruction, this smooth surface is replaced with coarsely woven structures (*i.e.,* hypertrophied smooth muscle fibers) called *trabeculae*. Small pockets of mucosal tissue, called *cellules*, commonly develop between the trabecular ridges. These pockets form diverticula when they extend between the actual fibers of the bladder muscle (Fig. 35-4). Because the diverticula have no muscle, they are unable to contract and expel their urine into the bladder, and secondary infections caused by stasis are common.

Along with hypertrophy of the bladder wall, there is hypertrophy of the trigone area and the interureteric ridge,

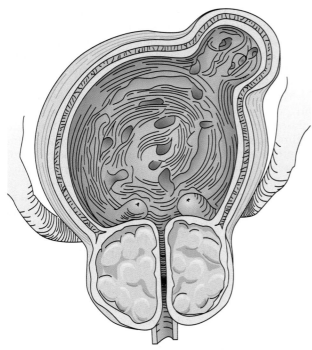

FIGURE 35-4 Destructive changes of the bladder wall with development of diverticula caused by benign prostatic hypertrophy.

which is located between the two ureters. This causes backpressure on the ureters, the development of hydroureters (*i.e.*, dilated, urine-filled ureters), and eventually, kidney damage. Stasis of urine predisposes to urinary tract infections.

When compensatory mechanisms no longer are effective, signs of decompensation begin to occur. The period of detrusor muscle contraction becomes too short to completely expel the urine, and residual urine remains in the bladder. At this point, the symptoms of obstruction—frequency of urination, hesitancy, a need to strain to initiate urination, a weak and small stream, and termination of the stream before the bladder is completely emptied—become pronounced. The amount of residual urine may increase up to 1000 to 3000 mL, and overflow incontinence occurs. There also may be acute retention of urine. The signs of urine retention are summarized in Chart 35-1.

CHART 35-1

Signs of Outflow Obstruction and Urine Retention

Bladder distention
Hesitancy
Straining when initiating urination
Small and weak stream
Frequency
Feeling of incomplete bladder emptying
Overflow incontinence

Treatment

The immediate treatment of lower urinary obstruction and stasis is directed toward relief of bladder distention. This usually is accomplished through urinary catheterization (discussed later in this chapter). Constipation or fecal impaction should be corrected. Long-term treatment is directed toward correcting the problem causing the obstruction.

NEUROGENIC BLADDER DISORDERS

The urinary bladder is unique in that it is probably the only autonomically innervated visceral organ that is under CNS control. The neural control of bladder function can be interrupted at any level. It can be interrupted at the level of the peripheral nerves that connect the bladder to the micturition center to the sacral cord, the ascending and descending tracts in the spinal cord, the pontine micturition center, or the cortical centers that are involved in voluntary control of micturition.[8,9] Neurogenic disorders of bladder function commonly are manifested in one of two ways: failure to store urine (spastic bladder dysfunction) or failure to empty (flaccid bladder dysfunction). Spastic bladder dysfunction usually results from neurologic lesions located above the level of the sacral micturition reflexes, whereas flaccid bladder dysfunction results from lesions at the level of sacral reflexes or the peripheral nerves that innervate the bladder. In addition to disorders of detrusor muscle function, disruption of micturition occurs when the neurologic control of external sphincter function is disrupted. Some disorders, such as stroke and Parkinson's disease, may affect both the storage and emptying functions of the bladder. Table 35-2 describes the characteristics of neurogenic bladder according to the level of the lesion.

Spastic Bladder: Failure to Store Urine

Failure to store urine results from conditions that cause reflex bladder spasm and a decrease in bladder volume. It commonly is caused by conditions that produce partial or extensive neural damage above the micturition reflex center in the sacral cord. As a result, bladder function is regulated by segmental reflexes, without control from higher brain centers. The degree of bladder spasticity and dysfunction depends on the level and extent of neurologic dysfunction. Usually both the ANS neurons controlling bladder function and the somatic neurons controlling the function of the striated muscles in the external sphincter are affected. In some cases, there is a detrusor-sphincter dyssynergia with uncoordinated contraction and relaxation of the detrusor and external sphincter muscles. The most common causes of spastic bladder dysfunction are spinal cord lesions such as spinal cord injury, herniated intervertebral disk, vascular lesions, tumors, and myelitis. Other neurologic conditions that affect voiding are stroke, multiple sclerosis, and brain tumors.

Bladder Dysfunction Caused by Spinal Cord Injury.
One of the most common types of spinal cord lesions is spinal cord injury (see Chapter 49). The immediate and early effects of spinal cord injury on bladder function are

TABLE 35-2 ✦ Types and Characteristics of Neurogenic Bladder

Level of Lesion	Change in Bladder Function	Common Causes
Sensory cortex, motor cortex, or corticospinal tract	Loss of ability to perceive bladder filling; low-volume, physiologically normal micturition that occurs suddenly and is difficult to inhibit	Stroke and advanced age
Basal ganglia or extrapyramidal tract	Detrusor contractions are elicited suddenly without warning and are difficult to control; bladder contraction is shorter than normal and does not produce full bladder emptying	Parkinson's disease
Pontine micturition center or communicating tracts in the spinal cord	Storage reflexes are provoked during filling, and external sphincter responses are heightened; uninhibited bladder contractions occur at a lower volume than normal and do not continue until the bladder is emptied; antagonistic activity occurs between the detrusor muscle and the external sphincter	Spinal cord injury
Sacral cord or nerve roots	Areflexic bladder fills but does not contract; loss of external sphincter tone occurs when the lesion affects the α-adrenergic motor neurons or pudendal nerve	Injury to sacral cord or spinal roots
Pelvic nerve	Increased filling and impaired sphincter control cause increased intravesicular pressure	Radical pelvic surgery
Autonomic peripheral sensory pathways	Bladder overfilling occurs owing to a loss of ability to perceive bladder filling	Diabetic neuropathies, multiple sclerosis

quite different from those that follow recovery from the initial injury. During the period immediately after spinal cord injury, a state of spinal shock develops, during which all the reflexes, including the micturition reflex, are depressed. During this stage, the bladder becomes atonic and cannot contract. Catheterization is necessary to prevent injury to urinary structures associated with overdistention of the bladder. Aseptic intermittent catheterization is the preferred method of catheterization. Depression of reflexes lasts from a few weeks to 6 months (usually 2 to 3 months), after which the spinal reflexes return and become hyperactive.[9]

After the acute stage of spinal cord injury, the micturition response changes from a long-tract reflex to a segmental reflex. Because the sacral reflex arc remains intact, stimuli generated by bladder stretch receptors during filling produce frequent spontaneous contractions of the detrusor muscle. This creates a small, hyperactive bladder subject to high-pressure and short-duration uninhibited bladder contractions. Voiding is interrupted, involuntary, or incomplete. Dilation of the internal sphincter and spasticity of the external sphincter and perineal muscles innervated by upper motoneurons occur, producing resistance to bladder emptying. Hypertrophy of the trigone develops, often leading to vesicoureteral reflux and renal damage.

Uninhibited Neurogenic Bladder.   A mild form of reflex neurogenic bladder, sometimes called *uninhibited bladder,* can develop after a stroke, during the early stages of multiple sclerosis, or as a result of lesions located in the inhibitory centers of the cortex or the pyramidal tract. With this type of disorder, the sacral reflex arc and sensation are retained, the urine stream is normal, and there is no residual urine. Bladder capacity is diminished, however, because of increased detrusor muscle tone and spasticity.

Detrusor-Sphincter Dyssynergia.   Depending on the level of the lesion, the coordinated activity of the detrusor muscle and the external sphincter may be affected. Lesions that affect the micturition center in the pons or impair

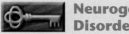

Neurogenic Bladder Disorders

➤ Neurogenic disorders of the bladder commonly are manifested by a spastic bladder dysfunction, in which there is failure to store urine, or as flaccid bladder dysfunction, in which bladder emptying is impaired.

➤ Spastic bladder dysfunction results from neurologic lesions above the level of the sacral cord that allow neurons in the micturition center to function reflexively without control from higher central nervous system centers.

➤ Flaccid bladder dysfunction results from neurologic disorders affecting the motor neurons in the sacral cord or peripheral nerves that control detrusor muscle contraction and bladder emptying.

communication between this center and spinal cord centers interrupt the coordinated activity of the detrusor muscle and the external sphincter. This is called *detrusor-sphincter dyssynergia*. Instead of relaxing during micturition, the external sphincter becomes more constricted. This condition can lead to elevated intravesicular pressures, vesicoureteral reflux, and kidney damage.

Treatment. Among the methods used to treat spastic bladder and detrusor-sphincter dyssynergia are the use of anticholinergic medications to decrease bladder hyperactivity and urinary catheterization to produce bladder emptying (discussed later). A sphincterotomy (surgical resection of the external sphincter) or implantable urethral stent may be used to decrease outflow resistance in a person who cannot be managed with medications and catheterization procedures. An alternative to surgical resection of the external sphincter is the injection of botulinum-A toxin to produce paralysis of the striated muscles in the external sphincter. The effects of the injection last from 3 to 9 months, after which the injection must be repeated.[8]

Flaccid Bladder: Failure to Empty Urine

Failure to empty the bladder can be due to flaccid bladder dysfunction, peripheral neuropathies that interrupt afferent or efferent communication between the bladder and the spinal cord, or conditions that prevent relaxation of the external sphincter.

Flaccid Bladder Dysfunction. Detrusor muscle areflexia, or flaccid neurogenic bladder, occurs when there is injury to the micturition center of the sacral cord, the cauda equina, or the sacral roots that supply the bladder.[9] Atony of the detrusor muscle and loss of the perception of bladder fullness permit the overstretching of the detrusor muscle that contributes to weak and ineffective bladder contractions. External sphincter tone and perineal muscle tone are diminished. Voluntary urination does not occur, but fairly efficient emptying usually can be achieved by increased intra-abdominal pressure or manual suprapubic pressure. Among the causes of flaccid neurogenic bladder are spina bifida and meningomyelocele.

Bladder Dysfunction Caused by Peripheral Neuropathies. In addition to CNS lesions and conditions that disrupt bladder function, disorders of the peripheral (pelvic, pudendal, and hypogastric) neurons that supply the bladder can occur. These neuropathies can selectively interrupt sensory or motor pathways for the bladder or involve both pathways.

Bladder atony and dysfunction is a frequent complication of diabetes mellitus.[10] The disorder initially affects the sensory axons of the urinary bladder without involvement of the pudendal nerve. This leads to large residual volumes after micturition, sometimes complicated by infection.[11] There frequently is a need for straining, accompanied by hesitation, weakness of the stream, dribbling, and a sensation of incomplete bladder emptying.[12] The chief complications are vesicoureteral reflux and ascending urinary tract infection. Because persons with diabetes are already at risk for development of glomerular disease

(see Chapter 33), reflux can have serious effects on kidney function. Treatment consists of client education, including the need for frequent voidings (*e.g.*, every 3 to 4 hours while awake), use of abdominal compression to effect more complete bladder emptying, and intermittent catheterization when necessary.[12]

Nonrelaxing External Sphincter

Another condition that affects micturition and bladder function is the nonrelaxing external sphincter.[13] This condition usually is related to a delay in maturation, developmental regression, psychomotor disorders, or locally irritative lesions. Inadequate relaxation of the external sphincter can be the result of anxiety or depression. Any local irritation can produce spasms of the sphincter by means of afferent sensory input from the pudendal nerve; included are vaginitis, perineal inflammation, and inflammation or irritation of the urethra. In men, chronic prostatitis contributes to the impaired relaxation of the external sphincter.

Treatment

The goals of treatment for neurogenic bladder disorders focus on preventing bladder overdistention, urinary tract infections, and potentially life-threatening renal damage, and reducing the undesirable social and psychological effects of the disorder. The methods used in treatment of neurogenic bladder disorders are individualized based on the type of neurologic lesion that is involved; information obtained through the health history, including fluid intake; report or observation of voiding patterns; presence of other health problems; urodynamic studies when indicated; and the ability of the person to participate in the treatment. Treatment methods include catheterization, bladder training, pharmacologic manipulation of bladder function, and surgery.

Catheterization. Catheterization involves the insertion of a small-diameter latex or silicone tube into the bladder through the urethra.[14] The catheter may be inserted on a one-time basis to relieve temporary bladder distention, left indwelling (*i.e.*, retention catheter), or inserted intermittently. With acute overdistention of the bladder, usually no more than 1000 mL of urine is removed from the bladder at one time. The theory behind this limitation is that removing more than this amount at one time releases pressure on the pelvic blood vessels and predisposes to alterations in circulatory function.

Permanent indwelling catheters sometimes are used when there is urine retention or incontinence in persons who are ill or debilitated or when conservative or surgical methods for the correction of incontinence are not feasible. The use of permanent indwelling bladder catheters in patients with spinal cord injury has been shown to produce a number of complications, including urinary tract infections, urethral irritation and injury, epididymoorchitis, pyelonephritis, and kidney stones.

Intermittent catheterization is used to treat urine retention or incomplete emptying secondary to various neurologic or obstructive disorders. Properly used, it prevents bladder overdistention and urethral irritation, allows more freedom of activity, and provides periodic distention of the bladder to prevent muscle atony. It often is used with pharmacologic manipulation to achieve continence; when possible, it is learned and managed as a self-care procedure (*i.e.*, intermittent self-catheterization). It may be carried out as an aseptic (sterile) or a clean procedure. Aseptic intermittent catheterization is used in persons with spinal shock and in those who need short-term catheterization.

The clean procedure typically is used for self-catheterization. It is performed at 3- to 4-hour intervals to prevent overdistention of the bladder. The best results are obtained if only 300 to 400 mL is allowed to collect in the bladder between catheterizations. The use of the clean instead of the sterile procedure has been defended on the basis that most urinary tract infections are caused by some underlying abnormality of the urinary tract that leads to impaired mucosal resistance to bacterial infection, the most common cause of which is decreased blood flow because of bladder overdistention.[15]

Bladder Retraining. Bladder retraining differs with the type of disorder. Methods used to supplement bladder retraining include monitoring fluid intake to prevent urinary tract infections and control urine volume and osmolality, developing scheduled times for urination, and using body positions that facilitate micturition.

Among the considerations when monitoring fluid intake is the need to ensure adequate fluid intake to prevent unduly concentrated urine, which may serve to stimulate afferent neurons of the micturition reflex. In hyperreflexive bladder or detrusor-sphincter dyssynergia, the stimulation of afferent nerve endings by irritating urinary constituents results in increased vesicular pressures, vesicoureteral reflux, and overflow incontinence. Fluid intake must be balanced to prevent bladder overdistention from occurring during the night. Adequate fluid intake also is needed to prevent urinary tract infections, the irritating effects of which increase bladder irritability and the risk of urinary incontinence and renal damage. Developing scheduled times for urinating prevents overdistention of the bladder.

The methods used for bladder retraining depend on the type of lesion causing the disorder. In spastic neurogenic bladder, methods designed to trigger the sacral micturition reflex are used; in flaccid neurogenic bladder, manual methods that increase intravesicular pressure are used. Trigger voiding methods include manual stimulation of the afferent loop of the micturition reflex through such maneuvers as tapping the suprapubic area, pulling on the pubic hairs, stroking the glans penis, or rubbing the thighs. Credé's method, which is done with the person in a sitting position, consists of applying pressure with four fingers of one hand or both hands to the suprapubic area as a means of increasing intravesicular pressure. The use of Valsalva's maneuver (*i.e.*, bearing down by exhaling against a closed glottis) increases intra-abdominal pressure and aids in bladder emptying. This maneuver is repeated until the bladder is empty. For the best results, the patient must cooperate fully with the procedures and, if possible, learn to perform them independently.

Biofeedback methods have been useful for teaching some aspects of bladder control. They involve the use of EMG or cystometry as a feedback signal for training a person to control the function of the external sphincter or raise intravesicular pressure enough to overcome outflow resistance.

Pharmacologic Manipulation. Pharmacologic manipulation includes the use of drugs to alter the contractile properties of the bladder, decrease the outflow resistance of the internal sphincter, and relax the external sphincter. The usefulness of drug therapy often is evaluated during cystometric studies. Anticholinergic drugs, such as tolterodine (Detrol), oxybutynin (Ditropan), and propantheline (generic; Pro-Banthine), decrease detrusor muscle tone and increase bladder capacity in persons with spastic bladder dysfunction. Cholinergic drugs that stimulate parasympathetic receptors, such as bethanechol chloride (generic; Urecholine), provide increased bladder tonus and may prove helpful in the symptomatic treatment of milder forms of flaccid neurogenic bladder. Muscle relaxants, such as diazepam (Valium) and baclofen (Lioresal), may be used to decrease the tone of the external sphincter. A nasal spray preparation of desmopressin (DDAVP), a synthetic antidiuretic hormone, can be used to treat persons with nighttime frequency due to spastic bladder symptoms.[2]

Surgical Procedures. Among the surgical procedures used in the management of neurogenic bladder are sphincterectomy, reconstruction of the sphincter, nerve resection of the sacral reflex nerves that cause spasticity or the pudendal nerve that controls the external sphincter, and urinary diversion. Urinary diversion can be done by creating an ileal or a colon loop into which the ureters are anastomosed; the distal end of the loop is brought out and attached to the abdominal wall. Other procedures include the attachment of the ureters to the skin of the abdominal wall or the attachment of the ureters to the sigmoid colon, with the rectum serving as a receptacle for the urine.

Extensive research is being conducted on methods of restoring voluntary control of the storage and evacuation functions of the bladder through the use of implanted electrodes. Single and multiple electrodes can be placed on selected nerves and then coupled to a subcutaneous receiver.

URINARY INCONTINENCE

The Urinary Incontinence Guideline Panel defines urinary incontinence as an involuntary loss of urine that is sufficient to be a problem.[16] This panel was convened by the Agency for Health Care Policy and Research in 1992 and again in 1996 for the purpose of developing specific guidelines to improve the care of persons with urinary incontinence.[6]

Urinary incontinence affects approximately 13 million Americans. Many body functions decline with age, and incontinence, although not a normal accompaniment of the aging process, is seen with increased frequency in elderly persons. For noninstitutionalized persons older than 60 years of age, the prevalence of urinary incontinence ranges from 15% to 35%, with women affected twice as often as men.[6] The increase in health problems often seen in elderly persons probably contributes to the greater

Incontinence

> ➤ Incontinence represents the involuntary loss of urine due to increased bladder pressures (overactive bladder with urge incontinence or overflow incontinence) or decreased ability of the vesicourethral sphincter to prevent the escape of urine (stress incontinence).
>
> ➤ Overactive bladder with urge incontinence is caused by neurogenic or myogenic disorders that result in hyperactive bladder contractions.
>
> ➤ Overflow incontinence results from overfilling of the bladder with escape of urine.
>
> ➤ Stress incontinence is caused by the decreased ability of the vesicourethral sphincter to prevent the escape of urine during activities, such as lifting and coughing, that raise bladder pressure above the sphincter closing pressure.

frequency of incontinence. Despite the prevalence of incontinence, most affected persons do not seek help for it, primarily because of embarrassment or because they are not aware that help is available.

Incontinence can be caused by a number of conditions. It can occur without the person's knowledge; at other times, the person may be aware of the condition but be unable to prevent it. The Urinary Incontinence Guideline Panel has identified four main types of incontinence: stress incontinence, urge incontinence, overflow incontinence, and mixed incontinence, which is a combination of stress and urge incontinence.[6] Recently, the term *overactive bladder* has been designated as a term to replace *urge incontinence*.[17] Table 35-3 summarizes the characteristics of

TABLE 35-3 ✦ Types and Characteristics of Urinary Incontinence	
Type	**Characteristics**
Stress	Involuntary loss of urine associated with activities, such as coughing, that increase intra-abdominal pressure
Overactive bladder/ urge incontinence	Urgency and frequency associated with hyperactivity of the detrusor muscle; may or may not involve involuntary loss of urine
Overflow	Involuntary loss of urine when intra-vesicular pressure exceeds maximal urethral pressure in the absence of detrusor activity

stress, urge incontinence/overactive bladder, and overflow incontinence.

Incontinence may occur as a transient and correctable phenomenon, or it may not be totally correctable and occur with various degrees of frequency. Among the transient causes of urinary incontinence are confusional states; medications that alter bladder function or perception of bladder filling and the need to urinate; diuretics and conditions that increase bladder filling; restricted mobility; and stool impaction.[18]

Stress Incontinence

Stress incontinence is the involuntary loss of urine during coughing, laughing, sneezing, or lifting that increases intra-abdominal pressure. The most common cause is hypermobility and significant displacement of the urethra during exertion.

In women, the angle between the bladder and the posterior proximal urethra (*i.e.*, urethrovesical junction) is important to continence. This angle normally is 90 to 100 degrees, with at least one third of the bladder base contributing to the angle when not voiding[19] (Fig. 35-5). During the first stage of voiding, this angle is lost as the bladder

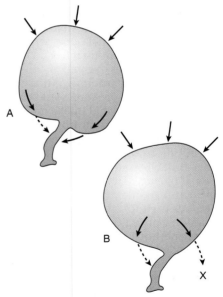

FIGURE 35-5 Importance of the posterior urethrovesical (PU-V) angle to the continence mechanism. (**A**) In the presence of the normal PU-V angle, sudden changes in intra-abdominal pressure are transmitted optimally (indicated by the *arrows* with dotted lines) to all sides of the proximal urethra. In this way, intra-urethral pressure is maintained higher than the simultaneously elevated intravesicular pressure. This prevents loss of urine with sudden stress. (**B**) Loss of the PU-V angle results in displacement of the vesicle neck to the most dependent portion of the bladder, preventing the equal transmission of sudden increases in intra-abdominal pressure to the lumen of the proximal urethra. Thus, the pressure in the region of the vesicle neck rises considerably more than the intraurethral pressure just beyond it, and stress incontinence occurs. (Green J.T., Jr. [1968]. *Obstetrical and Gynecological Survey* 23, 603. Reprinted with permission)

descends. In women, diminution of muscle tone associated with normal aging, childbirth, or surgical procedures can cause weakness of the pelvic floor muscles and result in stress incontinence by obliterating the critical posterior urethrovesical angle. In these women, loss of the posterior urethrovesical angle, descent and funneling of the bladder neck, and backward and downward rotation of the bladder occur, so that the bladder and urethra are already in an anatomic position for the first stage of voiding. Any activity that causes downward pressure on the bladder is sufficient to allow the urine to escape involuntarily.

Another cause of stress incontinence is intrinsic urethral deficiency, which may result from congenital sphincter weakness, as occurs with meningomyelocele. It also may be acquired as a result of trauma, irradiation, or sacral cord lesion. Stress incontinence in men may result from a congenital defect or from trauma or surgery to the bladder outlet, as occurs with prostatectomy. Neurologic dysfunction, as occurs with impaired sympathetic innervation of the bladder neck, impaired pelvic nerve innervation to the intrinsic sphincter, or impaired pudendal nerve innervation to the external sphincter, may be a contributing factor.

Urge Incontinence/Overactive Bladder

The Urinary Incontinence Guideline Panel has defined urge incontinence as the involuntary loss of urine associated with a strong desire to void (urgency).[6] To expand the number and types of patients eligible for clinical trials, the U.S. Food and Drug Administration adopted the term *overactive bladder* to describe the clinical syndrome that describes not only urge incontinence, but urgency, frequency, dysuria, and nocturia.[17] Although overactive bladder often is associated with urge incontinence, it can occur without incontinence.[20]

Although some cases of overactive bladder result from specific conditions such as acute or chronic urinary tract infections, in many cases the cause is unknown. Regardless of the primary cause of overactive bladder, two types of mechanisms are thought to contribute to its symptomatology: those involving CNS control of bladder sensation and emptying (neurogenic), and those involving the smooth muscle of the bladder itself (myogenic).[20]

The CNS functions as an on-off switching circuit for voluntary control of bladder function. Therefore, neurologic damage to central inhibitory pathways or sensitization of peripheral afferent terminals in the bladder may trigger bladder overactivity owing to uncontrolled voiding reflexes. Neurogenic causes of overactive bladder include stroke, Parkinson's disease, and multiple sclerosis. Other neurogenic causes of overactive bladder include increased peripheral afferent activity or increased peripheral sensitivity to efferent impulses.

Myogenic causes of overactive bladder are thought to be caused by spontaneous elevations in bladder pressure arising from changes in the properties of the smooth muscle of the bladder itself. One example is overactive bladder associated with bladder outlet obstruction. It is hypothesized that the sustained increase in intravesicular pressure that occurs with the outlet obstruction causes a partial destruction of the efferent nerve endings that control bladder excitability.[20] The result is urgency and frequency of urination due to spontaneous bladder contractions resulting from detrusor muscle hyperexcitability. Disorders of detrusor muscle structure and excitability also can occur as the result of the aging process or disease conditions such as diabetes mellitus. Overactive bladder symptoms usually are exaggerated by incomplete bladder emptying.

In persons with overactive bladder, urge incontinence may occur because the interval between knowing the bladder needs to be emptied and being able to stop it from emptying may be less than the time needed to reach the lavatory. Musculoskeletal disorders, such as arthritis and joint instability, also may prevent an otherwise continent person from reaching the toilet in time. Drugs such as hypnotics, tranquilizers, and sedatives can interfere with the conscious inhibition of voiding, leading to urge incontinence. Diuretics, particularly in elderly persons, increase the flow of urine and may contribute to incontinence, particularly in persons with diminished bladder capacity and in those who have difficulty reaching the toilet.

Treatment methods for overactive bladder include the use of behavioral methods and pharmacologic agents. Behavioral methods include fluid management, modification of voiding frequency, and bladder retraining.[21] Bladder retraining and biofeedback techniques seek to reestablish cortical control over bladder function by having the person ignore urgency and respond only to cortical signals during waking hours. Two newer anticholinergic medications, tolterodine (Detrol) and extended-release oxybutynin (Ditropan XL), may be used to inhibit detrusor muscle hyperactivity and thereby increase overall bladder capacity.[21,22]

Overflow Incontinence

Overflow incontinence is an involuntary loss of urine that occurs when intravesicular pressure exceeds the maximal urethral pressure because of bladder distention in the absence of detrusor activity. It can occur with retention of urine owing to nervous system lesions or obstruction of the bladder neck. With this type of incontinence, the bladder is distended and small amounts of urine are passed, particularly at night. In males, one of the most common causes of obstructive incontinence is enlargement of the prostate gland. Another cause that commonly is overlooked is fecal impaction (*i.e.*, dry, hard feces in the rectum). When a large bolus of stool forms in the rectum, it can push against the urethra and block the flow of urine.

Other Causes of Incontinence

Another cause of incontinence is decreased bladder compliance or distensibility. This abnormal bladder condition may result from radiation therapy, radical pelvic surgery, or interstitial cystitis. Many persons with this disorder have severe urgency related to bladder hypersensitivity that results in loss of bladder elasticity, such that any small increase in bladder volume or detrusor function causes a sharp rise in bladder pressure and severe urgency.

Incontinence also may be caused by factors outside the lower urinary tract, such as the inability to locate, reach, or receive assistance in reaching an appropriate place to void.[14]

This may be a particular problem for elderly persons, who may have problems with mobility and manual dexterity or find themselves in unfamiliar surroundings. It occurs when a person cannot find or reach the bathroom or manipulate clothing quickly enough. Failing vision may contribute to the problem. Embarrassment in front of other persons at having to use the bathroom, particularly if the timing seems inappropriate, may cause a person to delay emptying the bladder and may lead to incontinence.

Treatment with drugs such as diuretics may cause the bladder to fill more rapidly than usual, making it difficult to reach the bathroom in time if there are problems with mobility or if a bathroom is not readily available. Night sedation may cause a person to sleep through the signal that normally would waken a person so he or she could get up and empty the bladder and avoid wetting the bed.

Diagnosis and Treatment

Urinary incontinence is a frequent and major health problem. It increases social isolation, frequently leads to institutionalization of elderly persons, and predisposes to infections and skin breakdown.

Urinary incontinence is not a single disease but a symptom with many possible causes. As a symptom, it requires full investigation to establish its cause. This usually is accomplished through a careful history, physical examination, blood tests, and urinalysis. A voiding record (*i.e.*, diary) may be used to determine the frequency, timing, amount of voiding, and other factors associated with the incontinence.[16,17] Because many drugs affect bladder function, a full drug history is essential. Estimation of PVR volume is recommended for all persons with incontinence. Provocative stress testing is done when stress incontinence is suspected. This test is done by having the person relax and then cough vigorously while the examiner observes for urine loss. The test usually is done in the lithotomy position; if no leakage is observed, it is repeated in the standing position.[16] Urodynamic studies may be needed to provide information about urinary pressures and urine flow rates.

Treatment or management depends on the type of incontinence, accompanying health problems, and the person's age. Exercises to strengthen the pelvic muscles and surgical correction of pelvic relaxation disorders often are used for women with stress incontinence. Noncatheter devices to obstruct urine flow or collect urine as it is passed may be used when urine flow cannot be controlled. Indwelling catheters (discussed earlier in the chapter), although a solution to the problem of urinary incontinence, usually are considered only after all other treatment methods have failed. In some types of incontinence, such as that associated with spinal cord injury or meningomyelocele, self-catheterization provides the means for controlling urine elimination.

Treatment of Stress Incontinence.   Stress incontinence can be treated by physiotherapeutic measures, surgery, or a combination of the two. Surgical correction of cystocele and pelvic relaxation disorders may be needed for women.

Active muscle-tensing exercises of the pelvic muscles may prove effective.[23] These exercises were first advocated by Kegel, and they commonly are called *Kegel's exercises*.[24]

Two groups of muscles are strengthened: those of the back part of the pelvic floor (*i.e.*, muscles used to contract the anus and control the passing of stool) and the front muscles of the pelvic floor (*i.e.*, muscles used to stop the flow of urine during voiding). In learning the exercises, a woman concentrates on identifying the muscle groups and learning how to control contraction. After this has been accomplished, she can start an exercise program that consists of slowly contracting the muscles, beginning at the front and working to the back while counting to four and then releasing. The exercises can be done while sitting or standing and usually are performed in repetitions of 10, 3 times each day. A vaginal cone, a tampon-like device, may be used to enhance the benefits of the exercise. The cone is placed in the vagina, and the woman instructed to hold it in place by contracting the proper inner muscles.[25]

The α-adrenergic agonist drugs, such as pseudoephedrine, increase sympathetic relaxation of the detrusor muscle and internal sphincter tone and may be used in treating stress incontinence.[6,17] Imipramine, a tricyclic antidepressant agent that has α-adrenergic and anticholinergic properties, has proved useful in some women. Estrogen therapy (oral or vaginal) may be considered as an adjunctive pharmacologic agent for postmenopausal women.

Surgical intervention may be considered when other treatment methods have proved ineffective. Three types of surgical procedures are used: procedures that increase outlet resistance, surgeries that decrease detrusor muscle instability, and operations that remove outflow obstruction to reduce overflow incontinence and detrusor muscle instability.[6] A new development for the treatment of stress incontinence is the tension-free vaginal tape procedure. The procedure, which is minimally invasive and performed under local anesthesia, involves recreating suburethral support with a polypropylene mesh, without repositioning the bladder or urethra. Initial results from the procedure appear to be promising, with one study reporting a 90% cure rate.[26]

Another minimally invasive procedure for the treatment of stress incontinence is periurethral injection of a bulking agent (glutaraldehyde cross-linked bovine collagen or carbon-coated beads). Both of these agents typically require multiple treatment sessions to achieve cure.[17]

Noncatheter Devices.   Two types of noncatheter devices commonly are used in the management of urinary incontinence: one obstructs flow, and the other collects urine as it is passed. Obstruction of urine flow is achieved by compressing the urethra or stimulating contraction of the pelvic floor muscles. Penile clamps are available that occlude the urethra without obstructing blood circulation to the penis. Clamps must be removed at 3-hour intervals to empty the bladder. Complications such as penile and urethral erosion can occur if clamps are used incorrectly. In females, compression of the urethra usually is accomplished by intravaginal devices.

Surgically implanted artificial sphincters are available for use in males and females. These devices consist of an inflatable cuff that surrounds the proximal urethra. The cuff is connected by tubing to an implanted fluid reservoir and an inflation bulb. Pressing the bulb, which is placed in the scrotum in males, inflates the cuff. It is emptied in a similar manner.

When urinary incontinence cannot be prevented, various types of urine collection devices or protective pads are used. Men can be fitted with collection devices (*i.e.*, condom or sheath urinals) that are worn over the penis and attached to a container at the bedside or fastened to the body. There are no effective external collection devices for women. Pants and pads usually are used. Dribbling bags (males) and pads (females) in which the urine changes to a nonpourable gel are available for occasional dribbling, but are unsuitable for considerable wetting.

Special Needs of Elderly Persons

Urinary incontinence is a common problem in elderly persons. An estimated 15% to 35% of community-dwelling elders and 50% of institutionalized elders have severe urinary incontinence.[27,28] Many factors contribute to incontinence in elderly persons, a number of which can be altered.

Physiologically, detrusor muscle function tends to decline with aging so there is a trend toward a reduction in the strength of bladder contraction and impairment in emptying that leads to larger PVR volumes.[2] It has been proposed that many of these changes are due to degenerative detrusor muscle changes rather than neurologic changes, as was once thought. The combination of involuntary detrusor contraction (detrusor hyperactivity) leading to urge incontinence along with impaired contractile function leads to incomplete bladder emptying.

Pelvic relaxation disorders are more frequent in older than in younger women, and prostatic hypertrophy is more common in older than in younger men. Many elderly persons have difficulty getting to the toilet in time. This can be caused by arthritis that makes walking or removing clothing difficult or by failing vision that makes trips to the bathroom precarious, especially in new and unfamiliar surroundings.

Medication prescribed for other health problems may prevent a healthy bladder from functioning normally. Potent, fast-acting diuretics are known for their ability to cause urge incontinence. Psychoactive drugs, such as tranquilizers and sedatives, may diminish normal attention to bladder clues. Impaired thirst or limited access to fluids predisposes to constipation with urethral obstruction and overflow incontinence and to concentrated and infected urine, which increases bladder excitability.

According to Stanton, "there are two guiding principles in management of incontinence in the elderly. First, growing old does not imply becoming incontinent, and second, incontinence should not be left untreated just because the patient is old."[29] Treatment may involve changes in the physical environment so that the older person can reach the bathroom more easily or remove clothing more quickly. Habit training with regularly scheduled toileting— usually every 2 to 4 hours—often is effective. Many elderly persons who void on a regular schedule can gradually increase the interval between toileting while improving their ability to suppress bladder instability. The treatment plan may require dietary changes to prevent constipation or a plan to promote adequate fluid intake to ensure adequate

bladder filling and prevent urinary stasis and symptomatic urinary tract infections.

> In summary, alterations in bladder function include urinary obstruction with retention of urine, neurogenic bladder, and urinary incontinence with involuntary loss of urine. Urine retention occurs when the outflow of urine from the bladder is obstructed because of urethral obstruction or impaired bladder innervation. Urethral obstruction causes bladder irritability, detrusor muscle hypertrophy, trabeculation and the formation of diverticula, development of hydroureters, and, eventually, renal failure.
>
> Neurogenic bladder is caused by interruption in the innervation of the bladder. It can result in spastic bladder dysfunction caused by failure of the bladder to fill or flaccid bladder dysfunction caused by failure of the bladder to empty. Spastic bladder dysfunction usually results from neurologic lesions that are above the level of the sacral micturition reflex center; flaccid bladder dysfunction results from lesions at the level of the sacral micturition reflexes or peripheral innervation of the bladder. A third type of neurogenic disorder involves a nonrelaxing external sphincter.
>
> Urinary incontinence is the involuntary loss of urine in amounts sufficient to be a problem. It may manifest as stress incontinence, in which the loss of urine occurs as a result of coughing, sneezing, laughing, or lifting; overactive bladder, characterized by frequency and urgency associated with hyperactive bladder contractions; or overflow incontinence, which results when intravesicular pressure exceeds the maximal urethral pressure because of bladder distention. Other causes of incontinence include a small, contracted bladder or external environmental conditions that make it difficult to access proper toileting facilities.
>
> The treatment of urinary obstruction, neurogenic bladder, and incontinence requires careful diagnosis to determine the cause and contributing factors. Treatment methods include correction of the underlying cause, such as obstruction due to prostatic hyperplasia; pharmacologic methods to improve bladder and external sphincter tone; behavior methods that focus on bladder and habit training; exercises to improve pelvic floor function; and the use of catheters and urine collection devices.

Cancer of the Bladder

After you have completed this section of the chapter, you should be able to meet the following objectives:

✦ Discuss the difference between superficial and invasive bladder cancer in terms of bladder involvement, extension of the disease, and prognosis

✦ State the most common sign of bladder cancer

Bladder cancer is the most frequent form of urinary tract cancer in the United States, accounting for over

53,000 new cases and 12,000 deaths each year.[30,31] Whites are twice as likely to have bladder cancer as African Americans.[30] It occurs most commonly in people in their late seventh decade.[30] When detected and treated early, the chances for survival are very good. The 5-year survival rate for early noninvasive bladder cancers is approximately 94%.

Approximately 90% of bladder cancers are derived from the transitional (urothelial) cells that line the bladder.[32] The gross patterns of urothelial cell tumors vary from papillary to nodular or flat to mixed papillary and nodular tumors. These tumors can range from low-grade noninvasive tumors to high-grade tumors that invade the bladder wall and metastasize frequently. The low-grade tumors are papillary noninvasive lesions. These tumors, which may recur after resection, have an excellent prognosis, with only a small number (2% to 10%) progressing to higher-grade tumors.[32] The high-grade tumors may be papillary, nodular, or both. They tend to have greater invasive and metastatic potential and are potentially fatal in approximately 60% of cases within 10 years of diagnosis.[32]

Although the cause of bladder cancer is unknown, evidence suggests that its origin is related to local influences, such as carcinogens that are excreted in the urine and stored in the bladder. These include the breakdown products of aniline dyes used in the rubber and cable industries. Smoking also deserves attention. Fifty percent to 80% of all bladder cancers in men are associated with cigarette smoking. Chronic bladder infections and bladder stones also increase the risk of bladder cancer. Bladder cancer is more frequent among persons harboring the parasite *Schistosoma haematocium* in their bladders. The parasite is endemic in Egypt and Sudan. It is not known whether the parasite excretes a carcinogen or produces its effects through irritation of the bladder.

DIAGNOSIS AND TREATMENT

The most common sign of bladder cancer is painless hematuria.[32–35] Gross hematuria is a presenting sign in 75% of persons with the disease, and microscopic hematuria is present in most others. Frequency, urgency, and dysuria occasionally accompany the hematuria. Because hematuria often is intermittent, the diagnosis may be delayed. Periodic urine cytology is recommended for all persons who are at high risk for the development of bladder cancer because of exposure to urinary tract carcinogens. Ureteral invasion leading to bacterial and obstructive renal disease and dissemination of the cancer are potential complications and ultimate causes of death. The prognosis depends on the histologic grade of the cancer and the stage of the disease at the time of diagnosis.

Diagnostic methods include cytologic studies, excretory urography, cystoscopy, and biopsy. Ultrasonography, CT scans, and MRI are used as aids for staging the tumor. Cytologic studies performed on biopsy tissues or cells obtained from bladder washings may be used to detect the presence of malignant cells. A technique called *flow cytom-etry* is helpful in screening persons at high risk for the disease and for monitoring the results of therapy. In flow cytometry, the interaction between fluorochromes or dyes with DNA causes the emission of high-intensity light similar to that produced by a laser.[33] Flow cytometry can be carried out on biopsy specimens, bladder washings, or cytologic preparations. There appears to be a correlation between the DNA content (*i.e.*, ploidy) of the cancer cells and the level of differentiation (*i.e.*, grade), depth of invasion (*i.e.*, stage), and response to treatment. The expression of blood group antigens on the surface of bladder cancer cells has proved to be a useful prognostic determinant. Tumors that express the A, B, or H antigens have a better prognosis than tumors that do not express these antigens.[33] However, the secretory status of the person being tested must be considered because approximately 20% of persons normally are nonsecretors of blood antigens. Other urine markers that can be used for the detection and follow-up of bladder cancer are being investigated.

The treatment of bladder cancer depends on the extent of the lesion and the health of the patient. Endoscopic resection usually is done for diagnostic purposes and may be used as a treatment for superficial lesions. Diathermy (*i.e.*, electrocautery) may be used to remove the tumors. Segmental surgical resection may be used for removing a large single lesion. When the tumor is invasive, cystectomy with resection of the pelvic lymph nodes frequently is the treatment of choice. In males, the prostate and seminal vesicles often are removed as well. Until the 1980s, most men who underwent radical cystectomy became impotent. Newer surgical approaches designed to preserve erectile function now are being used. Cystectomy requires urinary diversion, an alternative reservoir, usually created from the ileum (*e.g.*, an ileal loop), that is designed to collect the urine. Traditionally, the ileostomy reservoir drains urine continuously into an external collecting device. Methods of urinary diversion have been developed that provide continence and eliminate the need to wear an external collection bag.[33]

External beam radiation is an alternative to radical cystectomy in some persons with deeply infiltrating bladder cancers. The treatment usually is well tolerated, but approximately 15% of persons experience significant bowel, bladder, and rectal complications.

Although a number of chemotherapeutic drugs have been used in the treatment of bladder cancer, no chemotherapeutic regimens for the disease have been established. Perhaps of more importance is the increasing use of intravesicular chemotherapy, in which the cytotoxic drug is instilled directly into the bladder.[33–35] These drugs can be instilled prophylactically after surgical resection of all demonstrable tumor or therapeutically in the presence of residual disease. Among the chemotherapeutic drugs that have been used for this purpose are thiotepa, mitomycin C, and doxorubicin (Adriamycin). The intervesicular administration of bacillus Calmette-Guérin (BCG) vaccine, made from a strain of *Mycobacterium bovis* that formerly was used to protect against tuberculosis, causes a significant reduction in the rate of relapse and prolongs relapse-free interval in persons with cancer in situ. The vaccine is thought to act as a nonspecific stimulator of cell-mediated immunity. It is not known whether the effects of BCG are immunologic or include a component of direct toxicity. Several strains of this agent exist, and it is not known which is the most active and least toxic. The intravesicular instillation of immunomodulators such as interferon alfa are being investigated.

> In summary, cancer of the bladder is the most common cause of urinary tract cancer in the United States, accounting for over 53,000 new cases and 12,000 deaths each year. Bladder cancers fall into two major groups: low-grade noninvasive tumors and high-grade invasive tumors that are associated with metastasis and a worse prognosis. Although the cause of cancer of the bladder is unknown, evidence suggests that carcinogens excreted in the urine may play a role. Microscopic and gross, painless hematuria are the most frequent presenting signs of bladder cancer. The methods used in treatment of bladder cancer depend on the cytologic grade of the tumor and the lesion's degree of invasiveness. The methods include surgical removal of the tumor, radiation therapy, and chemotherapy. In many cases, immunotherapeutic and chemotherapeutic agents can be instilled directly into the bladder through a catheter, thereby avoiding the side effects of systemic therapy.

Related Web Sites

American Cancer Society Cancer Resource Center—information on bladder cancer   www3.cancer.org/cancerinfo/load_cont.asp

American Foundation for Urologic Disease   www.afud.org

Medline Plus Health Information—Bladder Diseases   medlineplus.nlm.nih.gov/medlineplus/bladderdiseases.html#picturesdiagrams

National Cancer Institute Cancernet—information on bladder cancer   cancernet.nci.nih.gov/cancer_types/bladder_cancer.shtml

Urology Channel—Conditions: Interstitial Cystitis   www.urogynecology.com/interstitialcystitis/index.shtml

References

1. Kandel E.R., Schwartz J.H., Jessel T.M. (2000). *Principles of neural science* (4th ed.). New York: McGraw-Hill.
2. Fowler C.J. (1999). Neurological disorders of micturition and their treatment. *Brain* 122, 1213–1231.
3. Berne R.M., Levy M.N. (1993). *Physiology* (3rd ed., p. 726). St. Louis: C.V. Mosby.
4. Dmochowski R.R., Appell R.A. (2000). Advances in pharmacologic management of overactive bladder. *Urology* 56 (Suppl. 6A), 41–49.
5. Tanagho E.A. (2000). Urodynamic studies. In Tanagho E.A., McAninch J.W. (Eds.), *Smith's general urology* (15th ed., pp. 516–537). New York: Lange Medical Books/McGraw-Hill.
6. Fantl J.A., Newman D.K., Colling J., et al., for the Public Health Service, Agency for Health Care Policy and Research. (1996). *Urinary incontinence in adults: Acute and chronic management.* Clinical Practice Guideline no. 2, 1996 update. AHCPR publication no. 96-0682. Rockville, MD: U.S. Department of Health and Human Services.
7. Tanagho E.A. (2000). Urinary obstruction and stasis. In Tanagho E.A., McAninch J.W. (Eds.), *Smith's general urology* (15th ed., pp. 208–220). New York: Lange Medical Books/McGraw-Hill.
8. Elliott D.S., Boone T.B. (2000). Recent advances in management of neurogenic bladder. *Urology* 56 (Suppl. 6A), 76–81.
9. Tanagho E.A., Lue T.F. (2000). Neuropathic bladder disorders. In Tanagho E.A., McAninch J.W. (Eds.), *Smith's general urology* (15th ed., pp. 498–515). New York: Lange Medical Books/McGraw-Hill.
10. Frimodt-Møller C. (1980). Diabetic cystopathy: Epidemiology and related disorders. *Annals of Internal Medicine* 92, 318–321.
11. Said G. (1996). Diabetic neuropathy. *Journal of Neurology* 243, 431–440.
12. Bays H.E., Pfiefer M.A. (1988). Peripheral diabetic neuropathy. *Medical Clinics of North America* 72, 1439–1464.
13. Thon W., Altwein J.E. (1984). Voiding dysfunction. *Urology* 23, 323.
14. Cravens D.D., Zwieg S. (2000). Urinary catheter management. *American Family Physician* 61, 369–376.
15. Lapides J., Diokno A.C., Silber S.J. (1971). Clean, intermittent self-catheterization in treatment of urinary tract disease. *Transactions of the American Association of Genitourinary Surgeons* 63, 92.
16. Urinary Incontinence Guideline Panel. (1992). *Urinary incontinence in adults: Clinical practice guidelines.* AHCPR publication no. 92-0038. Rockville, MD: Agency for Health Care Policy and Research, Public Health Service, U.S. Department of Health and Human Services.
17. Culligan P.J., Heit M. (2000). Urinary incontinence in women: Evaluation and management. *American Family Physician* 62, 2433–2452.
18. Gray M., Burns S.M. (1996). Continence management. *Critical Care Clinics of North America* 8, 29–38.
19. Green T.H. (1975). Urinary stress incontinence: Differential diagnosis, pathophysiology, and management. *American Journal of Obstetrics and Gynecology* 122, 368–382.
20. Dmochowski R.R., Appell R.A. (2000). Advancements in pharmacologic management of overactive bladder. *Urology* 56 (Suppl. 6A), 41–49.
21. Wein A.J. (2001). Putting overactive bladder into clinical perspective. *Patient Care for the Nurse Practitioner* (Spring Suppl.), 1–5.
22. Roberts R.R. (2001). Current management strategies for overactive bladder. *Patient Care for the Nurse Practitioner* (Spring Suppl.), 22–30.
23. Wells T.J., Brink C.A., Kiokno A.C, Wolfe R., Gillis G.L. (1991). Pelvic muscle exercise for stress urinary incontinence in elderly women. *Journal of the American Geriatrics Society* 39, 785–791.
24. Kegel A.H. (1948). Progressive resistance exercises in the functional restoration of the perineal muscles. *American Journal of Obstetrics and Gynecology* 56, 238–248.
25. Boourcier A.P., Jurat J.C. (1995). Nonsurgical therapy for stress incontinence. *Urologic Clinics of North America* 22, 613–627.
26. Carlin B.I., Klutke J.J., Klutke C.G. (2000). The tension-free vaginal tape procedure for treatment of stress incontinence in the female patient. *Urology* 56 (Suppl. 6A), 28–31.

27. Lee S.Y., Phanumus D., Fields S.D. (2000). Urinary incontinence: A primary guide to managing acute and chronic symptoms in older adults. *Geriatrics* 55(11), 65–71.

28. Weiss B.D. (1998). Diagnostic evaluation of urinary incontinence in geriatric patients. *American Family Physician* 57, 2675–2684, 2688–2690.

29. Stanton S.L. (1984). Surgical management of female incontinence. In Brocklehurst J.C. (Ed.), *Urology in the elderly* (p. 93). New York: Churchill Livingstone.

30. American Cancer Society (2000). *Bladder cancer: Overview*. [On-line]. Available: http://www3.cancer.org/cancerinfo.

31. Lee R., Droller M.J. (2000). The natural history of bladder cancer. *Urologic Clinics of North America* 27(1), 1–13.

32. Cotran R.S., Kumar V., Collins T. (1999). *Robbins pathologic basis of disease* (6th ed., pp. 1003–1008). Philadelphia: W.B. Saunders.

33. Carroll P. (2000). Urothelial carcinoma: Cancers of the bladder, ureter, and renal pelvis. In Tanagho E.A., McAninch J.W. (Eds.), *Smith's general urology* (15th ed., pp. 355–376). New York: Lange Medical Books/ McGraw-Hill.

34. Kelly L.P., Miaskowski C. (1996). An overview of bladder cancer: Treatment and nursing implications. *Oncology Nursing Forum* 23, 459–467.

35. Badalament R.A., Schervish E.W. (1996). Bladder cancer. *Postgraduate Medicine* 100, 217–224.

Gastrointestinal Function

The study of the gastrointestinal system aroused none of the philosophical interest that surrounded the elements, humors, and pneuma of Galen's time. During ancient times, the gut was thought merely to provide the chyle that was turned into blood by the liver. Although the structures of the gut had been fairly well described, perhaps owing to observations made during the slaughtering of animals, it was not until the 18th and 19th centuries that the function of the gastrointestinal tract began to unfold.

One of the breakthroughs in gastrointestinal physiology came as the result of an accident. In 1822, William Beaumont (1785–1853), a self-trained surgeon in the United States Army, was called upon to render aid to Alexis St. Martin, a Canadian traveler who had suffered a large gunshot wound to the chest and abdomen. Although not expected to live, young St. Martin rallied and his wounds healed; however, he was left with a permanent fistula that opened to his stomach. Beaumont became intrigued with this patient's unique defect, using this living laboratory to study the process of digestion. He would have St. Martin swallow different types of food and then collect the stomach contents by means of a tube passed into the fistula. Beaumont described the movement of the stomach, and he confirmed the presence of hydrochloric acid and a ferment, later shown to be the result of the protein-breaking enzyme pepsin. Because of an unfortunate accident, both Beaumont and St. Martin gained a place in the history of gastrointestinal physiology.

Control of Gastrointestinal Function

The digestive system is an amazing structure. In this system, enzymes and hormones are produced, vitamins are synthesized and stored, and food is dismantled and then reassembled. Nutrients, vitamins, minerals, electrolytes, and water enter the body through the gastrointestinal tract. Wastes are collected and eliminated efficiently.

Structurally, the gastrointestinal tract is a long, hollow tube with its lumen inside the body and its wall acting as an interface between the internal and external environments. The wall does not normally allow harmful agents to enter the body, nor does it permit body fluids and other materials to escape. The process of digestion and absorption of nutrients requires an intact and healthy gastrointestinal tract epithelial lining that can resist the effects of its own digestive secretions. The process also involves movement of materials through the gastrointestinal tract at a rate that facilitates absorption, and it requires the presence of enzymes for the digestion and absorption of nutrients.

Although this chapter cannot cover gastrointestinal function in its entirety, it is designed to provide the reader with an overview essential to an understanding of subsequent chapters. As a matter of semantics, the gastrointestinal tract also is referred to as the *digestive tract*, the *alimentary canal*, and, at times, the *gut*. The intestinal portion also may be called the *bowel*. For the purposes of this text, the salivary glands, the liver, and the pancreas, which produce secretions that aid in digestion, are considered *accessory organs*.

Structure and Organization of the Gastrointestinal Tract

After you have completed this section of the chapter, you should be able to meet the following objectives:

✦ Describe the physiologic function of the four parts of the digestive system
✦ List the five layers of the digestive tract and describe their function
✦ Characterize the function of the intramural neural plexuses in control of gastrointestinal function

In the digestive tract, food and other materials move slowly along its length as they are systematically broken down into ions and molecules that can be absorbed into the body. In the large intestine, unabsorbed nutrients and wastes are collected for later elimination. Although the gastrointestinal tract is located inside the body, it is a long, hollow tube, the lumen (*i.e.*, hollow center) of which is an extension of the external environment. Nutrients do not become part of the internal environment until they have passed through the intestinal wall and have entered the blood or lymph channels.

For simplicity and understanding, the digestive system can be divided into four parts (Fig. 36-1). The upper part—the mouth, esophagus, and stomach—acts as an intake source and receptacle through which food passes and in

Structure and Function of the Gastrointestinal Tract

➤ The gastrointestinal tract is a long, hollow tube that extends from the mouth to the anus; food and fluids that enter the gastrointestinal tract do not become part of the internal environment until they have been broken down and absorbed into the blood or lymph channels.

➤ The wall of the gastrointestinal tract is essentially a five-layered tube: an inner mucosal layer; a supporting submucosal layer of connective tissue; a fourth and fifth layer of circular and longitudinal smooth muscle that functions to propel its contents in a proximal-to-distal direction; and an outer, two-layered peritoneum that encloses and prevents friction between the continuously moving segments of the intestine.

➤ The nutrients contained in ingested foods and fluids must be broken down into molecules that can be absorbed across the wall of the intestine. Gastric acids and pepsin from the stomach begin the digestive process: bile from the liver, digestive enzymes from the pancreas, and brush border enzymes break carbohydrates, fats, and proteins into molecules that can be absorbed from the intestine.

which initial digestive processes take place. The middle portion consists of the small intestine—the duodenum, jejunum, and ileum. Most digestive and absorptive processes occur in the small intestine. The lower segment—the cecum, colon, and rectum—serves as a storage channel for the efficient elimination of waste. The fourth part consists of the accessory organs—the salivary glands, liver, and pancreas. These structures produce digestive secretions that help dismantle foods and regulate the use and storage of nutrients. The discussion in this chapter focuses on the first three parts of the gastrointestinal tract. The liver and pancreas are discussed in Chapter 38.

UPPER GASTROINTESTINAL TRACT

The mouth forms the entryway into the gastrointestinal tract for food; it contains the teeth, used in the mastication of food, and the tongue and other structures needed to direct food toward the pharyngeal structures and the esophagus.

The esophagus begins at the lower end of the pharynx. It receives food from the pharynx, and in the process of swallowing, a series of peristaltic contractions moves the food into the stomach. The esophagus is a muscular, collapsible tube, approximately 25 cm (10 in) long, that lies behind the trachea. The muscular walls of the upper third

of the esophagus are skeletal-type striated muscle; these muscle fibers are gradually replaced by smooth muscle fibers until, at the lower third of the esophagus, the muscle layer is entirely smooth muscle.

The upper and lower ends of the esophagus act as sphincters. The upper sphincter is formed by a thickening of the striated muscle; it prevents air from entering the esophagus during respiration. The lower sphincter, which is not identifiable anatomically, occurs at a point 1 to 2 cm (0.4 to 0.8 in) from where the esophagus joins the stomach. The lower sphincter prevents gastric reflux into the esophagus.

The stomach is a pouchlike structure that lies in the upper part of the abdomen and serves as a food storage reservoir during the early stages of digestion. Although the residual volume of the stomach is only approximately 50 mL, it can increase to almost 1000 mL before the intraluminal pressure begins to rise. The esophagus opens into the stomach through an opening called the *cardiac orifice*, so named because of its proximity to the heart. The part of the stomach that lies above and to the left of the cardiac orifice is called the *fundus*, the central portion is called the *body*, the orifice encircled by a ringlike muscle that opens into the small intestine is called the *pylorus*, and the portion between the body and pylorus is called the *antrum* (Fig. 36-2). The presence of a true pyloric sphincter is controversial. Regardless of whether an actual sphincter exists, contractions of the smooth muscle in the pyloric area control the rate of gastric emptying.

MIDDLE GASTROINTESTINAL TRACT

The small intestine, which forms the middle portion of the digestive tract, consists of three subdivisions: the duodenum, the jejunum, and the ileum. The duodenum, which is approximately 22 cm (10 in) long, connects the stomach to the jejunum and contains the opening for the common bile duct and the main pancreatic duct. Bile and pancreatic juices enter the intestine through these ducts. It is in the jejunum and ileum, which together are approximately 7 m (23 ft) long and must be folded onto themselves to fit into the abdominal cavity, that food is digested and absorbed.

LOWER GASTROINTESTINAL TRACT

The large intestine, which forms the lower gastrointestinal tract, is approximately 1.5 m (4.5 to 5 ft) long and 6 to 7 cm (2.4 to 2.7 in) in diameter. It is divided into the cecum, colon, rectum, and anal canal. The cecum is a blind pouch that projects down at the junction of the ileum and the colon. The ileocecal valve lies at the upper border of the cecum and prevents the return of feces from the cecum into the small intestine. The appendix arises from the cecum approximately 2.5 cm (1 in) from the ileocecal valve. The colon is further divided into ascending, transverse, descending, and sigmoid portions. The ascending colon extends from the cecum to the undersurface of the liver, where it turns abruptly to form the right colic (hepatic) flexure. The transverse colon crosses the upper half of the abdominal cavity from right to left and then curves sharply downward

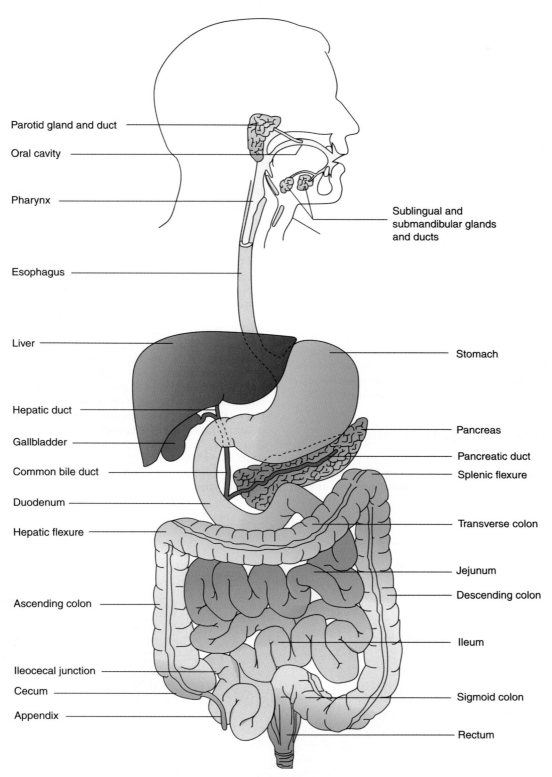

FIGURE 36-1 The digestive system. (Chaffee E.E., Lytle I.M. [1980]. *Basic physiology and anatomy* [4th ed.]. Philadelphia: J.B. Lippincott)

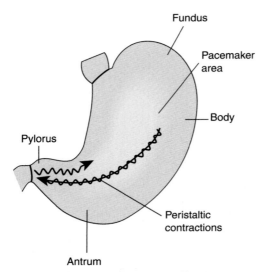

FIGURE 36-2 Structures of the stomach, showing the pacemaker area and the direction of chyme movement resulting from peristaltic contractions.

beneath the lower end of the spleen, forming the left colic (splenic) flexure. The descending colon extends from the colic flexure to the rectum. The rectum extends from the sigmoid colon to the anus. The anal canal passes between the two medial borders of the levator ani muscles. Powerful sphincter muscles guard against fecal incontinence.

GASTROINTESTINAL WALL STRUCTURE

The digestive tract, below the upper third of the esophagus, is essentially a five-layered tube (Fig. 36-3). The inner luminal layer, or *mucosal layer*, is so named because its cells produce mucus that lubricates and protects the inner surface of the alimentary canal. The epithelial cells in this layer have a rapid turnover rate and are replaced every 4 to 5 days. Approximately 250 g of these cells are shed each day in the stool. Because of the regenerative capabilities of the mucosal layer, injury to this layer of tissue heals rapidly without leaving scar tissue. The *submucosal layer* consists of connective tissue. This layer contains blood vessels, nerves, and structures responsible for secreting digestive enzymes. The third and fourth layers, the *circular* and *longitudinal muscle layers*, facilitate movement of the contents of the gastrointestinal tract. The outer layer, the *peritoneum*, is loosely attached to the outer wall of the intestine.

The peritoneum is the largest serous membrane in the body, having a surface area approximately equal to that of the skin. The peritoneal membrane is composed of two layers, a thin layer of simple squamous epithelial cells resting on a layer of connective tissue. If the epithelial layer is injured because of surgery or inflammation, there is danger that adhesions (*i.e.*, fibrous scar tissue bands) may form, causing sections of the viscera to heal together. Adhesions can alter the position and movement of the abdominal viscera.

The peritoneal cavity is a potential space formed between what is called the *parietal peritoneum* and the *visceral peritoneum*. The parietal peritoneum comes in contact with and is loosely attached to the abdominal wall, whereas the abdominal organs are in contact with the visceral peritoneum. The two layers of the peritoneum can be compared with a deflated balloon. If one makes a fist into the balloon, the outer surface can be equated with the parietal peritoneum, and the fist interfaces with the visceral peritoneum (Fig. 36-4). In this case, the area within the balloon represents the peritoneal cavity. The connective tissue layer of the peritoneum forms the parietal and the visceral peritoneum, and the smooth, epithelial cell layer of the mem-

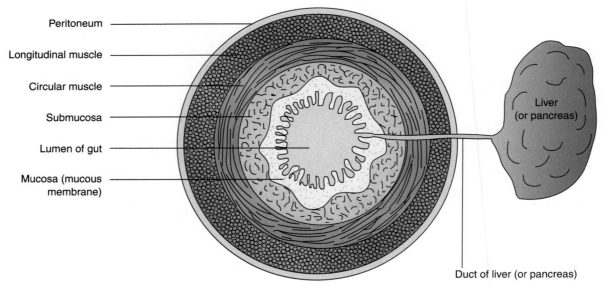

FIGURE 36-3 Transverse section of the digestive system. (Thomson J.S. [1977]. *Core textbook of anatomy.* Philadelphia: J.B. Lippincott)

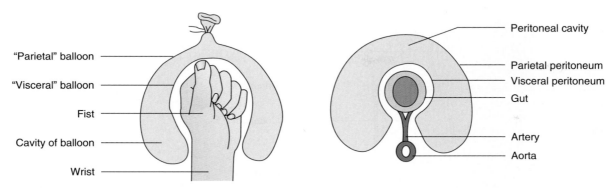

FIGURE 36-4 Comparison of the peritoneal cavity with a balloon. (Thomson J.S. [1977]. *Core textbook of anatomy*. Philadelphia: J.B. Lippincott)

brane lines the cavity. The adjacent membrane layers in the peritoneal cavity are separated by a thin layer of serous fluid. This fluid forms a moist and slippery surface that prevents friction between the continuously moving abdominal structures. In certain pathologic states, the amount of fluid in the potential space of the peritoneal cavity is increased, causing a condition called *ascites*.

The jejunum and ileum are suspended by a double-layered fold of peritoneum called the *mesentery* (Fig. 36-5). The mesentery contains the blood vessels, nerves, and lymphatic vessels that supply the intestinal wall. The mesentery is gathered in folds that attach to the dorsal abdominal wall along a short line of insertion, giving a fan-shaped appearance, with the intestines at the edge. A filmy, double fold of peritoneal membrane called the *greater omentum* extends from the stomach to cover the transverse colon and

folds of the intestine (Fig. 36-6). The greater omentum protects the intestines from cold. It always contains some fat, which in obese persons can be a considerable amount. The omentum also controls the spread of infection from gastrointestinal contents. In the case of infection, the omentum adheres to the inflamed area so that the infection is less likely to enter the peritoneal cavity. The lesser omentum extends between the transverse fissure of the liver and the lesser curvature of the stomach.

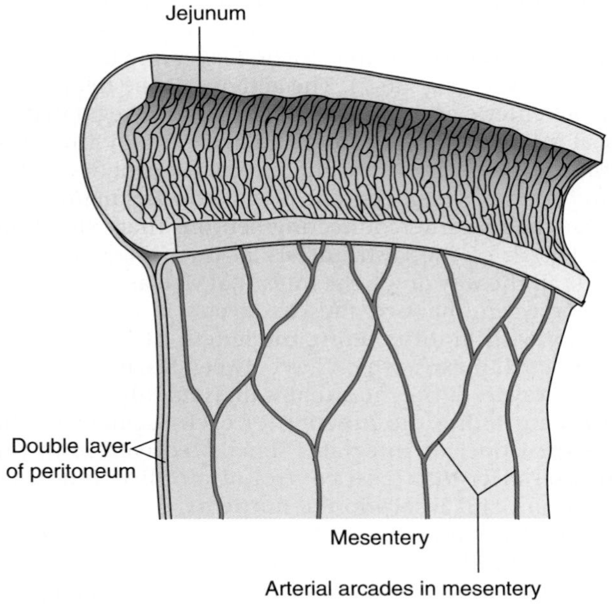

> In summary, the gastrointestinal tract is a long, hollow tube, the lumen of which is an extension of the external environment. The digestive tract can be divided into four parts: an upper part, consisting of the mouth, esophagus, and stomach; a middle part, consisting of the small intestine; a lower part, consisting of the cecum, colon, and rectum; and the accessory organs, consisting of the salivary glands, the liver, and the pancreas. Throughout its length, except for the mouth, throat, and upper esophagus, the gastrointestinal tract is composed of five layers: an inner mucosal layer, a submucosal layer, a layer of circular smooth muscle fibers, a layer of longitudinal smooth muscle fibers, and an outer serosal layer that forms the peritoneum and is continuous with the mesentery.

FIGURE 36-5 The attachment of the mesentery to the small bowel. (Thomson J.S. [1977]. *Core textbook of anatomy*. Philadelphia: J.B. Lippincott)

Motility

After you have completed this section of the chapter, you should be able to meet the following objectives:

✦ Compare the effects of parasympathetic and sympathetic activity on the motility and secretory function of the gastrointestinal tract
✦ Differentiate tonic and peristaltic movements in the gastrointestinal tract
✦ Trace a bolus of food through the stages of swallowing
✦ Describe the action of the internal and external sphincters in the control of defecation

The motility of the gastrointestinal tract propels food products and fluids along its length, from mouth to anus,

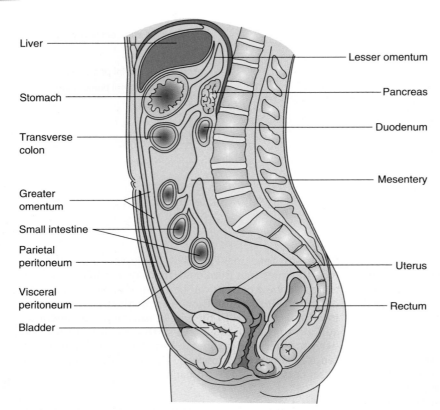

Liver

Stomach

Transverse colon

Greater omentum

Small intestine

Parietal peritoneum

Visceral peritoneum

Bladder

Lesser omentum

Pancreas

Duodenum

Mesentery

Uterus

Rectum

FIGURE 36-6 Reflections of the peritoneum as seen in sagittal section. (Chaffee E.E., Lytle I.M. [1980]. *Basic physiology and anatomy* [4th ed.]. Philadelphia: J.B. Lippincott)

in a manner that facilitates digestion and absorption. Except in the pharynx and upper third of the esophagus, smooth muscle provides the contractile force for gastrointestinal motility (the actions of smooth muscle are discussed in Chapter 4). The rhythmic movements of the digestive tract are self-perpetuating, much like the activity of the heart, and are influenced by local, humoral (*i.e.,* blood-borne), and neural influences. The ability to initiate impulses is a property of the smooth muscle itself. Impulses are conducted from one muscle fiber to another.

The movements of the gastrointestinal tract are tonic and rhythmic. The tonic movements are continuous movements that last for minutes or even hours. Tonic contractions occur at sphincters. The rhythmic movements consist of intermittent contractions that are responsible for mixing and moving food along the digestive tract. Peristaltic movements are rhythmic propulsive movements that occur when the smooth muscle layer constricts, forming a contractile band that forces the intraluminal contents forward. During peristalsis, the segment that lies distal to, or ahead of, the contracted portion relaxes, and the contents move forward with ease. Normal peristalsis always moves in the direction from the mouth toward the anus.

NEURAL CONTROL MECHANISMS

Gastrointestinal function is controlled by the *enteric nervous system,* which lies entirely within the wall of the gastrointestinal tract, and by the parasympathetic and sympathetic divisions of the autonomic nervous system (ANS). The

intramural neurons (*i.e.,* those contained within the wall of the gastrointestinal tract) consist of two networks, the myenteric and submucosal plexuses. Both plexuses are aggregates of ganglionic cells that extend along the length of the gastrointestinal wall. The myenteric (Auerbach's) plexus is located between the circular muscle and longitudinal muscle layers, and the submucosal (Meissner's) plexus between the mucosal layer and the circular muscle layers (Fig. 36-7). The activity of the neurons in the myenteric and submucosal plexuses is regulated by local influences, input from the ANS, and by interconnecting fibers that transmit information between the two plexuses. The myenteric plexus consists mainly of a linear chain of interconnecting neurons that extend the full length of the gastrointestinal tract. Because it extends all the way down the intestinal wall and because it lies between the two muscle layers, it is concerned mainly with motility along the length of the gut. The submucosal plexus, which lies between the mucosal and muscle layers of the intestinal wall, is mainly concerned with controlling the function of each segment of the intestinal tract. It integrates signals received from the mucosal layer into local control of motility, intestinal secretions, and absorption of nutrients.

The digestive tract contains two types of afferent fibers: those with cell bodies located in the nervous system and those with cell bodies located in the intramural plexuses. The first group has receptors in the mucosal epithelium and in the muscle layers; their fibers pass centrally in vagal and sympathetic fibers. The second group is lo-

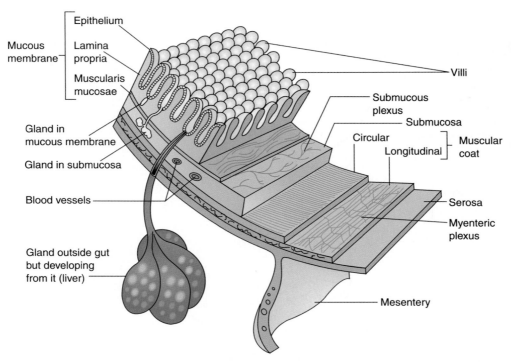

FIGURE 36-7 Diagram of the four main layers of the wall of the digestive tube: mucosa, submucosa, muscular, and serosa (below the diaphragm). (Chaffee E.E., Lytle I.M. [1980]. *Basic physiology and anatomy* [4th ed.]. Philadelphia: J.B. Lippincott)

cated in the intramural plexus and exerts local control over motility.

Efferent parasympathetic innervation to the stomach, small intestine, cecum, ascending colon, and transverse colon occurs by way of the vagus nerve (Fig. 36-8). The remainder of the colon is innervated by parasympathetic fibers that exit the sacral segments of the spinal cord by way of the pelvic nerve. Preganglionic parasympathetic fibers can synapse with intramural plexus neurons, or they can act directly on intestinal smooth muscle. Most parasympathetic fibers are excitatory. Numerous vagovagal reflexes influence motility and secretions of the digestive tract.

Efferent sympathetic innervation of the gastrointestinal tract occurs through the thoracic chain of sympathetic ganglia and the celiac, superior mesenteric, and inferior mesenteric ganglia. The sympathetic nervous system exerts several effects on gastrointestinal function. It controls the extent of mucus secretion by the mucosal glands, reduces motility by inhibiting the activity of intramural plexus neurons, enhances sphincter function, and increases the vascular smooth muscle tone of the blood vessels that supply the gastrointestinal tract. The effect of the sympathetic stimulation is to block the release of the excitatory neuromediators in the intramural plexuses, inhibiting gastrointestinal motility. Sympathetic control of gastrointestinal function is largely mediated by activity in the intramural plexuses. For example, when gastric motility is enhanced because of increased vagal activity, stimulation of sympathetic centers in the hypothalamus promptly and often completely inhibits motility. The sympathetic fibers that supply the lower

esophageal, pyloric, and internal and external anal sphincters are largely excitatory, but their role in controlling these sphincters is poorly understood.

Intramural plexus neurons also communicate with receptors in the mucosal and muscle layers. Mechanoreceptors monitor the stretch and distention of the gastrointestinal tract wall, and chemoreceptors monitor the chemical composition (*i.e.,* osmolality, pH, and digestive products of protein and fat metabolism) of its contents. These receptors can communicate directly with ganglionic cells in the intramural plexuses or with visceral afferent fibers that influence ANS control of gastrointestinal function.

CHEWING AND SWALLOWING

Chewing begins the digestive process; it breaks the food into particles of a size that can be swallowed, lubricates it by mixing it with saliva, and mixes starch-containing food with salivary amylase. Although chewing usually is considered a voluntary act, it can be carried out involuntarily by a person who has lost the function of the cerebral cortex.

The swallowing reflex is a rigidly ordered sequence of events that results in the propulsion of food from the mouth to the stomach through the esophagus. Although swallowing is initiated as a voluntary activity, it becomes involuntary as food or fluid reaches the pharynx. Sensory impulses for the reflex begin at tactile receptors in the pharynx and esophagus and are integrated with the motor components of the response in an area of the reticular formation of the medulla and lower pons called the *swallowing center*. The

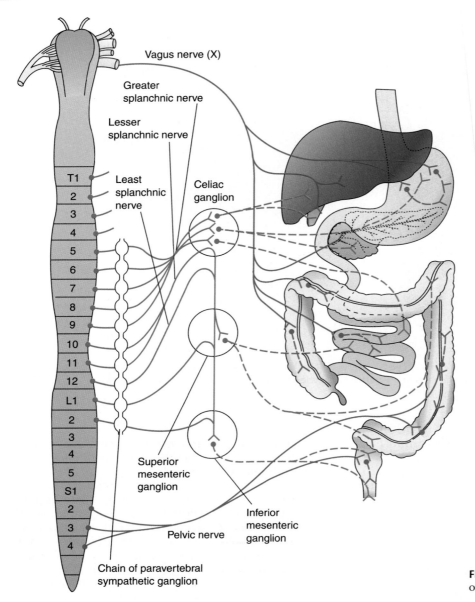

FIGURE 36-8 The autonomic innervation of the gastrointestinal tract.

motor impulses for the oral and pharyngeal phases of swallowing are carried in the trigeminal (V), glossopharyngeal (IX), vagus (X), and hypoglossal (XII) cranial nerves, and impulses for the esophageal phase are carried by the vagus nerve. Diseases that disrupt these brain centers or their cranial nerves disrupt the coordination of swallowing and predispose an individual to food and fluid lodging in the trachea and bronchi, leading to risk of asphyxiation or aspiration pneumonia.

Swallowing consists of three phases: an oral, or voluntary phase; a pharyngeal phase; and an esophageal phase. During the *oral phase*, the bolus is collected at the back of the mouth so the tongue can lift the food upward until it touches the posterior wall of the pharynx. At this point, the *pharyngeal phase* of swallowing is initiated. The soft palate is pulled upward, the palatopharyngeal folds are pulled to-

gether so that food does not enter the nasopharynx, the vocal cords are pulled together, and the epiglottis is moved so that it covers the larynx. Respiration is inhibited, and the bolus is moved backward into the esophagus by constrictive movements of the pharynx. Although the striated muscles of the pharynx are involved in the second stage of swallowing, it is an involuntary stage.

The third phase of swallowing is the *esophageal stage*. As food enters the esophagus and stretches its walls, local and central nervous system reflexes that initiate peristalsis are triggered. There are two types of peristalsis—primary and secondary. Primary peristalsis is controlled by the swallowing center in the brain stem and begins when food enters the esophagus. Secondary peristalsis is partially mediated by smooth muscle fibers in the esophagus and occurs when primary peristalsis is inadequate to move food through the esophagus. Peristalsis begins at the site of distention and moves downward. Before the peristaltic wave reaches the stomach, the lower esophageal sphincter relaxes to allow the bolus of food to enter the stomach. The pressure in the lower esophageal sphincter normally is greater than that in the stomach, an important factor in preventing the reflux of gastric contents. The lower esophageal sphincter is innervated by the vagus nerve. Increased levels of parasympathetic stimulation increase the constriction of the sphincter. The hormone gastrin also increases constriction of the sphincter. Gastrin provides the major stimulus for gastric acid production, and its action on the lower esophageal sphincter protects the esophageal mucosa when gastric acid levels are elevated.

GASTRIC MOTILITY

The stomach serves as a reservoir for ingested solids and liquids. Motility of the stomach results in the churning and grinding of solid foods and regulates the emptying of the gastric contents, or chyme, into the duodenum. Peristaltic mixing and churning contractions begin in a pacemaker area in the middle of the stomach and move toward the antrum (see Fig. 36-2). They occur at a frequency of three to five contractions per minute, each with a duration of 2 to 20 seconds. As the peristaltic wave approaches the antrum, it speeds up, and the entire terminal 5 to 10 cm of the antrum contracts, occluding the pyloric opening. Contraction of the antrum reverses the movement of the chyme, returning the larger particles to the body of the stomach for further churning and kneading. Because the pylorus is contracted during antral contraction, the gastric contents are emptied into the duodenum between contractions.

Although the pylorus does not contain a true anatomic sphincter, it does function as a physiologic sphincter to prevent the backflow of gastric contents and allow them to flow into the duodenum at a rate commensurate with the ability of the duodenum to accept them. This is important because the regurgitation of bile salts and duodenal contents can damage the mucosal surface of the antrum and lead to gastric ulcers. Likewise, the duodenal mucosa can be damaged by the rapid influx of highly acid gastric contents.

Like other parts of the gastrointestinal tract, the stomach is richly innervated by the enteric nervous system and its connections with the sympathetic and parasympathetic nervous systems. Axons from the intramural plexuses innervate the smooth muscles and glands of the stomach. Parasympathetic innervation is provided by the vagus nerve and sympathetic innervation by the celiac ganglia. The emptying of the stomach is regulated by hormonal and neural mechanisms. The hormones cholecystokinin (CCK) and gastric inhibitory peptide, which are thought to control gastric emptying, are released in response to the pH and the osmolar and fatty acid composition of the chyme. Local and central circuitry are involved in the neural control of gastric emptying. Afferent receptor fibers synapse with the neurons in the intramural plexus or trigger intrinsic reflexes by means of vagal or sympathetic pathways that participate in extrinsic reflexes.

Disorders of gastric motility can occur when the rate is too slow or too fast (see Chapter 37). A rate that is too slow leads to gastric retention. It can be caused by obstruction or gastric atony. Obstruction can result from the formation of scar tissue in the pyloric area after a peptic ulcer. Another example of obstruction is hypertrophic pyloric stenosis, which can occur in infants with an abnormally thick muscularis layer in the terminal pylorus. Myotomy, or surgical incision of the muscular ring, may be done to relieve the obstruction. Gastric atony can occur as a complication of visceral neuropathies in diabetes mellitus. Surgical procedures that disrupt vagal activity also can result in gastric atony. Abnormally fast emptying occurs in the dumping syndrome, which is a consequence of certain types of gastric operations. This condition is characterized by the rapid dumping of highly acidic and hyperosmotic gastric secretions into the duodenum and jejunum.

SMALL INTESTINE MOTILITY

The small intestine is the major site for the digestion and absorption of food; its movements are mixing and propulsive. Regular peristaltic movements begin in the duodenum near the entry sites of the common duct and the main hepatic duct. A series of local pacemakers maintains the frequency of intestinal contraction. The peristaltic movements (approximately 12 per minute in the jejunum) become less frequent as they move further from the pylorus, becoming approximately 9 per minute in the ileum.

The peristaltic contractions produce segmentation waves and propulsive movements through the muscles of the small intestine. With segmentation waves, slow contractions of circular muscle occlude the lumen and drive the contents forward and backward. Most of the contractions that produce segmentation waves are local events involving only 1 to 4 cm at a time. They function mainly to mix the chyme with the digestive enzymes from the pancreas and to ensure adequate exposure of all parts of the chyme to the mucosal surface of the intestine, where absorption takes place. The frequency of segmenting activity increases after a meal. Presumably, it is stimulated by receptors in the stomach and intestine.

Propulsive movements occur with synchronized activity in a section 10 to 20 cm long. They are accomplished by contraction of the proximal, or orad, portion of the intestine with the sequential relaxation of its distal, or anal, portion. After material has been propelled to the ileocecal junction by peristaltic movement, stretching of the distal ileum produces a local reflex that relaxes the sphincter and allows fluid to squirt into the cecum.

Motility disturbances of the small bowel are common, and auscultation of the abdomen can be used to assess bowel activity. Inflammatory changes increase motility. In many instances, it is not certain whether changes in motility occur because of inflammation or occur secondary to toxins and unabsorbed materials. Delayed passage of materials in the small intestine also can be a problem. Transient interruption of intestinal motility often occurs after gastrointestinal surgery. Intubation with suction often is required to remove the accumulating intestinal contents and gases until activity is resumed.

COLONIC MOTILITY

The storage function of the colon dictates that movements in this section of the gut are different from those in the small intestine. Movements in the colon are of two types. First are the segmental mixing movements, called *haustrations*, so named because they occur within sacculations called *haustra*. These movements produce a local digging-type action, which ensures that all portions of the fecal mass are exposed to the intestinal surface. Second are the propulsive mass movements, in which a large segment of the colon (≥20 cm) contracts as a unit, moving the fecal contents forward as a unit. Mass movements last approximately 30 seconds, followed by a 2- to 3-minute period of relaxation, after which another contraction occurs. A series of mass movements lasts only for 10 to 30 minutes and may occur only several times a day. Defecation normally is initiated by the mass movements.

DEFECATION

Defecation is controlled by the action of two sphincters, the internal and external anal sphincters (Fig. 36-9). The internal sphincter is a several-centimeters long circular thickening of smooth muscle that lies inside the anus. The external sphincter, which is composed of striated voluntary muscle, surrounds the internal sphincter. The external

sphincter is controlled by nerve fibers in the pudendal nerve, which is part of the somatic nervous system and therefore under voluntary control. Defecation is controlled by defecation reflexes. One of these reflexes is the intrinsic myenteric reflex mediated by the local enteric nervous system. It is initiated by distention of the rectal wall, with initiation of reflex peristaltic waves that spread through the descending colon, sigmoid colon, and rectum. A second defecation reflex, the parasympathetic reflex, is integrated at the level of the sacral cord. When the nerve endings in the rectum are stimulated, signals are transmitted first to the sacral cord and then reflexly back to the descending colon, sigmoid colon, rectum, and anus by way of the pelvic nerves (Fig. 36-8). These impulses greatly increase peristaltic movements as well as relax the internal sphincter.

To prevent involuntary defecation from occurring, the external anal sphincter is under the conscious control of the cortex. As afferent impulses arrive at the sacral cord, signaling the presence of a distended rectum, messages are transmitted to the cortex. If defecation is inappropriate, the cortex initiates impulses that constrict the external sphincter and inhibit efferent parasympathetic activity. Normally, the afferent impulses in this reflex loop fatigue easily, and the urge to defecate soon ceases. At a more convenient time, contraction of the abdominal muscles compresses the contents in the large bowel, reinitiating afferent impulses to the cord.

> In summary, motility of the gastrointestinal tract propels food products and fluids along its length from mouth to anus. Although the activity of gastrointestinal smooth muscle is self-propagating and can continue without input from the nervous system, its rate and strength of contractions are regulated by a network of intramural neurons that receive input from the ANS and local receptors that monitor wall stretch and the chemical composition of luminal contents. Parasympathetic innervation occurs by means of the vagus nerve and nerve fibers from sacral segments of the spinal cord; it increases gastrointestinal motility. Sympathetic activity occurs by way of thoracolumbar output from the spinal cord, its paravertebral ganglia, and celiac, superior mesenteric, and inferior mesenteric ganglia. Sympathetic stimulation enhances sphincter function and reduces motility by inhibiting the activity of intramural plexus neurons.

Secretory Function

After you have completed this section of the chapter, you should be able to meet the following objectives:

✦ State the source of water and electrolytes in digestive secretions
✦ Explain the protective function of saliva
✦ Describe the function of the gastric secretions in the process of digestion
✦ List three major gastrointestinal hormones and cite their function

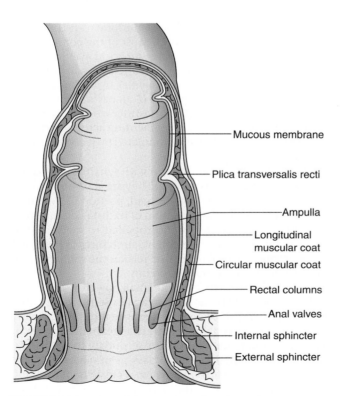

Mucous membrane

Plica transversalis recti

Ampulla

Longitudinal muscular coat

Circular muscular coat

Rectal columns

Anal valves

Internal sphincter

External sphincter

FIGURE 36-9 Interior of the rectum and anal canal.

✦ Describe the site of gastric acid and pepsin production and secretion in the stomach
✦ Describe the function of the gastric mucosal barrier
✦ Name the secretions of the small and the large intestine

Each day, approximately 7000 mL of fluid is secreted into the gastrointestinal tract (Table 36-1). Approximately 50 to 200 mL of this fluid leaves the body in the stool; the remainder is reabsorbed in the small and large intestines. These secretions are mainly water and have sodium and potassium concentrations similar to those of extracellular fluid. Because water and electrolytes for digestive tract secretions are derived from the extracellular fluid compartment, excessive secretion or impaired absorption can lead to extracellular fluid deficit.

CONTROL OF SECRETORY FUNCTION

The secretory activity of the gut is influenced by local, humoral, and neural influences. Neural control of gastrointestinal secretory activity is mediated through the ANS. Secretory activity, like motility, is increased with parasympathetic stimulation and inhibited with sympathetic activity. Many of the local influences, including pH, osmolality, and chyme, consistently act as stimuli for neural and humoral mechanisms.

GASTROINTESTINAL HORMONES

The gastrointestinal tract is the largest endocrine organ in the body. It produces hormones that pass from the portal circulation into the general circulation and then back to the digestive tract, where they exert their actions. Among the hormones produced by the gastrointestinal tract are gastrin, secretin, and CCK. These hormones influence motility and the secretion of electrolytes, enzymes, and other hormones. The gastrointestinal tract hormones and their functions are summarized in Table 36-2.

The primary function of gastrin is the stimulation of gastric acid secretion. Gastrin also has a trophic, or growth-producing, effect on the mucosa of the small intestine, colon, and oxyntic (acid-secreting) gland area of the stomach. Removal of the tissue that produces gastrin results in atrophy of these structures. This atrophy can be reversed by the administration of exogenous gastrin.

Secretin is secreted by S cells in the mucosa of the duodenum and jejunum in an inactive form called *prosecretin*. When an acid chyme with a pH of less than 4.5 to 5.0 enters the intestine, secretin is activated and absorbed into the blood. *Secretin* causes the pancreas to secrete large quantities of fluid with a high bicarbonate concentration and low chloride concentration.

The primary function of *cholecystokinin* is stimulation of pancreatic enzyme secretion. CCK also regulates gallbladder contraction and gastric emptying. CCK potentiates the action of secretin, increasing the pancreatic bicarbonate response to low circulating levels of secretin. In addition to its effects on the pancreas, CCK secretion stimulates biliary secretion of fluid and bicarbonate.

Two other hormones that contribute to gastrointestinal function are gastric inhibitory peptide and motilin. *Gastric inhibitory peptide*, which is released from the intestinal mucosa in response to increased concentration of glucose and fats, inhibits gastric acid secretion, gastric motility, and gastric emptying. *Motilin*, which stimulates intestinal motility and contributes to the control of the interdigestive actions of the intestinal neurons, is released from the upper small intestine.

TABLE 36-1 ✦ Secretions of the Gastrointestinal Tract

Secretions	Amount Daily (mL)
Salivary	1200
Gastric	2000
Pancreatic	1200
Biliary	700
Intestinal	2000
Total	7100

TABLE 36-2 ✦ Major Gastrointestinal Hormones and Their Actions

Hormone	Site of Secretion	Stimulus for Secretion	Action
Cholecystokinin	Duodenum, jejunum	Amino acids	Stimulates contraction of the gallbladder; stimulates secretion of pancreatic enzymes; slows gastric emptying
Gastrin	Antrum of the stomach, duodenum	Vagal stimulation; epinephrine; neutral amino acids; calcium-containing fluids such as milk; and alcohol. Secretion is inhibited by acid contents in the antrum of the stomach (below pH 2.5)	Stimulates secretion of gastric acid and pepsinogen; increases gastric blood flow; stimulates gastric smooth muscle contraction; stimulates growth of gastric, small intestine, and colon mucosa
Secretin	Duodenum	Acid pH or chyme entering duodenum (below pH 3.0)	Stimulates secretion of bicarbonate-containing solution by pancreas and liver

Other neural peptides are found in the neurons of the gut. These include *vasoactive intestinal peptide* (VIP), *gastrin-releasing peptide* (GRP), and the *enkephalins*. Gastrointestinal muscle is innervated by VIP-containing neurons. VIP mediates relaxation of gastrointestinal smooth muscle and is thought also to cause relaxation of vascular smooth muscle. GRP-containing neurons are located in the gastric mucosa and function in the release of gastrin. The action of the enkephalins, which exert their function through opioid receptors (see Chapter 48), is to slow the transit of material through the gut and inhibit intestinal secretions. The combination of these actions probably accounts for the effectiveness of selected opioid drugs in treating diarrhea.

Histamine and somatostatin are paracrine agents that act at receptors close to the site of release. *Somatostatin* inhibits gastrin release and gastric acid secretion. *Histamine*, which is released in response to gastrin, stimulates gastric acid secretion by the parietal cells. Histamine also potentiates the action of gastrin and acetylcholine on gastric acid secretion. Histamine type 2 (H_2) antagonists reduce gastric acid secretion by blocking H_2 receptors.

SALIVARY SECRETIONS

Saliva is secreted by the salivary glands. The salivary glands consist of the parotid, submaxillary, sublingual, and buccal glands. Saliva has three functions. The first is protection and lubrication. Saliva is rich in mucus, which protects the oral mucosa and coats the food as it passes through the mouth, pharynx, and esophagus. The sublingual and buccal glands produce only mucus-type secretions. The second function of saliva is its protective antimicrobial action. The saliva cleans the mouth and contains the enzyme lyso-

zyme, which has an antibacterial action. Third, saliva contains ptyalin and amylase, which initiate the digestion of dietary starches. Secretions from the salivary glands are primarily regulated by the ANS. Parasympathetic stimulation increases flow and sympathetic stimulation decreases flow. The dry mouth that accompanies anxiety attests to the effects of sympathetic activity on salivary secretions.

Mumps, or parotitis, is an infection of the parotid glands. Although most of us associate mumps with the contagious viral form of the disease, inflammation of the parotid glands can occur in the seriously ill person who does not receive adequate oral hygiene and who is unable to take fluids orally. Potassium iodide increases the secretory activity of the salivary glands, including the parotid glands. In a small percentage of persons, parotid swelling may occur in the course of treatment with this drug.

GASTRIC SECRETIONS

In addition to mucus-secreting cells that line the entire surface of the stomach, the stomach mucosa has two types of glands: oxyntic (or gastric) glands and pyloric glands. The *oxyntic glands* are located in the proximal 80% (body and fundus) of the stomach. They secrete hydrochloric acid, pepsinogen, intrinsic factor, and mucus. The *pyloric glands* are located in the distal 20%, or antrum, of the stomach. The pyloric glands secret mainly mucus, some pepsinogen, and the hormone gastrin.

The oxyntic gland area of the stomach is composed of glands and pits (Fig. 36-10). The surface area and gastric pits are lined with mucus-producing epithelial cells. The bases of the gastric pits contain the parietal (or oxyntic) cells, which secrete hydrochloric acid and intrinsic factor, and the

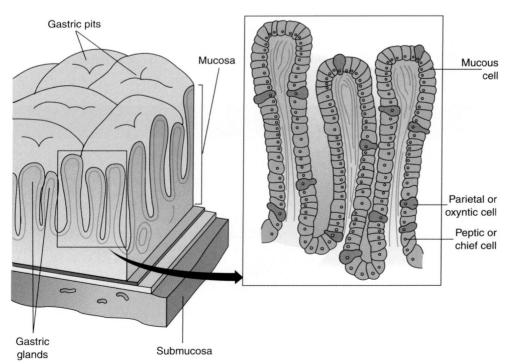

Gastric pits

Mucosa

Mucous cell

Parietal or oxyntic cell

Peptic or chief cell

Gastric glands

Submucosa

FIGURE 36-10 Gastric pit from body of the stomach.

chief (peptic) cells, which secrete large quantities of pepsinogen. There are approximately 1 billion parietal cells in the stomach; together they produce and secrete approximately 20 mEq of hydrochloric acid in several hundred milliliters of gastric juice each hour. The pepsinogen that is secreted by the parietal cells is rapidly converted to pepsin when exposed to the low pH of the gastric juices. Gastric intrinsic factor, which is produced by the parietal cells, is necessary for the absorption of vitamin B_{12}.

One of the important characteristics of the gastric mucosa is resistance to the highly acid secretions that it produces. When the gastric mucosa is damaged by aspirin, nonsteroidal anti-inflammatory drugs (NSAIDs), ethyl alcohol, or bile salts, this impermeability is disrupted, and hydrogen ions move into the tissue. This is called *breaking the mucosal barrier*, and substances that alter gastric mucosal permeability are called *barrier breakers*. As the hydrogen ions accumulate in the mucosal cells, intracellular pH decreases, enzymatic reactions become impaired, and cellular structures are disrupted. The result is local ischemia, vascular stasis, hypoxia, and tissue necrosis. The mucosal surface is further protected by prostaglandins. Aspirin and NSAIDs inhibit prostaglandin synthesis, which also impairs the integrity of the mucosal surface.

Parasympathetic stimulation (through the vagus nerve) and gastrin increase gastric secretions. Histamine increases gastric acid secretions. Research and clinical use of the H_2 receptor antagonists suggest that histamine may be the final common pathway for gastric acid production. Gastric acid secretion and its relation to peptic ulcer are discussed in Chapter 37.

INTESTINAL SECRETIONS

The small intestine secretes digestive juices and receives secretions from the liver and pancreas (see Chapter 38). An extensive array of mucus-producing glands, called *Brunner's glands*, are concentrated at the site where the contents from the stomach and secretions from the liver and pancreas enter the duodenum. These glands secrete large amounts of alkaline mucus that protect the duodenum from the acid content in the gastric chyme and from the action of the digestive enzymes. The activity of Brunner's glands is strongly influenced by ANS activity. For example, sympathetic stimulation causes a marked decrease in mucus production, leaving this area more susceptible to irritation. Between 75% and 80% of peptic ulcers occur at this site.

In addition to mucus, the intestinal mucosa produces two other types of secretions. The first is a serous fluid (pH 6.5 to 7.5) secreted by specialized cells (*i.e.,* crypts of Lieberkühn) in the intestinal mucosal layer. This fluid, which is produced at the rate of 2000 mL/day, acts as a vehicle for absorption. The second type of secretion consists of surface enzymes that aid absorption. These enzymes are the peptidases, or enzymes that separate amino acids, and the disaccharidases, or enzymes that split sugars.

The large intestine usually secretes only mucus. ANS activity strongly influences mucus production in the bowel, as in other parts of the digestive tract. During intense para-

sympathetic stimulation, mucus secretion may increase to the point that the stool contains large amounts of obvious mucus. Although the bowel normally does not secrete water or electrolytes, these substances are lost in large quantities when the bowel becomes irritated or inflamed.

> In summary, the secretions of the gastrointestinal tract include saliva, gastric juices, bile, and pancreatic and intestinal secretions. Each day, more than 7000 mL of fluid is secreted into the digestive tract; all but 50 to 200 mL of this fluid is reabsorbed. Water, derived from the extracellular fluid compartment, is the major component of gastrointestinal tract secretions. Neural, humoral, and local mechanisms contribute to the control of these secretions. The parasympathetic nervous system increases secretion, and sympathetic activity exerts an inhibitory effect. In addition to secreting fluids containing digestive enzymes, the gastrointestinal tract produces and secretes hormones, such as gastrin, secretin, and CCK, that contribute to the control of gastrointestinal function.

Digestion and Absorption

After you have completed this section of the chapter, you should be able to meet the following objectives:

✦ Differentiate digestion from absorption
✦ Relate the characteristics of the small intestine to its absorptive function
✦ Explain the function of intestinal brush border enzymes
✦ Compare the digestion and absorption of carbohydrates, fats, and proteins

Digestion and absorption occur mainly in the small intestine. The stomach is a poor absorptive structure, and only a few lipid-soluble substances, including alcohol, are absorbed from the stomach.

Digestion is the process of dismantling foods into their constituent parts. Digestion requires hydrolysis, enzyme cleavage, and fat emulsification. Hydrolysis is breakdown of a compound that involves a chemical reaction with water. The importance of hydrolysis to digestion is evidenced by the amount of water (7 to 8 L) that is secreted into the gastrointestinal tract daily. The intestinal mucosa is impermeable to most large molecules. Most proteins, fats, and carbohydrates must be broken down into smaller particles before they can be absorbed. Although some digestion of carbohydrates and proteins begins in the stomach, digestion takes place mainly in the small intestine. The breakdown of fats to free fatty acids and monoglycerides takes place entirely in the small intestine. The liver, with its production of bile, and the pancreas, which supplies a number of digestive enzymes, play important roles in digestion.

Absorption is the process of moving nutrients and other materials from the external environment of the gastrointestinal tract into the internal environment. Absorption is accomplished by active transport and diffusion. The ab-

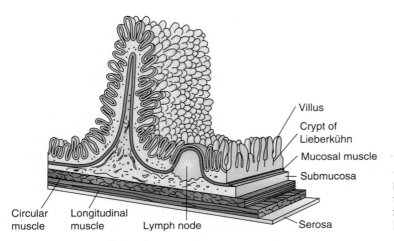

Villus
Crypt of Lieberkühn
Mucosal muscle
Submucosa
Circular muscle
Longitudinal muscle
Lymph node
Serosa

FIGURE 36-11 The mucous membrane of the small intestine. Note the numerous villi on a circular fold. (Chaffee E.E., Lytle I.M. [1980]. *Basic physiology and anatomy* [4th ed.]. Philadelphia: J.B. Lippincott)

sorptive function of the large intestine focuses mainly on water reabsorption. A number of substances require a specific carrier or transport system. For example, vitamin B_{12} is not absorbed in the absence of intrinsic factor, which is secreted by the parietal cells of the stomach. Transport of amino acids and glucose occurs mainly in the presence of sodium. Water is absorbed passively along an osmotic gradient.

The distinguishing characteristic of the small intestine is its large surface area, which in the adult is estimated to be approximately 250 m^2. Anatomic features that contribute to this enlarged surface area are the circular folds that extend into the lumen of the intestine and the villi, which are finger-like projections of mucous membrane, numbering as many as 25,000, that line the entire small intestine (Fig. 36-11). Each villus is equipped with an artery, vein, and lymph vessel (*i.e.*, lacteal), which bring blood to the surface of the intestine and transport the nutrients and other materials that have passed into the blood from the lumen of the intestine (Fig. 36-12). Fats rely largely on the lymphatics for absorption.

Each villus is covered with cells called *enterocytes* that contribute to the absorptive and digestive functions of the small bowel, and goblet cells that provide mucus. The crypts of Lieberkühn are glandular structures that open into the spaces between the villi. The enterocytes have a life span of approximately 4 to 5 days, and it is believed that replacement cells differentiate from progenitor cells located in the area of the crypts. The maturing enterocytes migrate up the villus and eventually are extruded from the tip.

The enterocytes secrete enzymes that aid in the digestion of carbohydrates and proteins. These enzymes are called *brush border enzymes* because they adhere to the border of the villus structures. In this way they have access to the carbohydrates and protein molecules as they come in contact with the absorptive surface of the intestine. This mechanism of secretion places the enzymes where they are needed and eliminates the need to produce enough enzymes to mix with the entire contents that fill the lumen of the small bowel. The digested molecules diffuse through the membrane or are actively transported across the mucosal surface to enter the blood or, in the case of fatty acids, the lacteal.

These molecules are then transported through the portal vein or lymphatics into the systemic circulation.

CARBOHYDRATE ABSORPTION

Carbohydrates must be broken down into monosaccharides, or single sugars, before they can be absorbed from the small intestine. The average daily intake of carbohydrate in the American diet is approximately 350 to 400 g. Starch makes up approximately 50% of this total, sucrose (*i.e.*, table sugar) approximately 30%, lactose (*i.e.*, milk sugar) approximately 6%, and maltose approximately 1.5%.

Digestion of starch begins in the mouth with the action of amylase. Pancreatic secretions also contain an amylase.

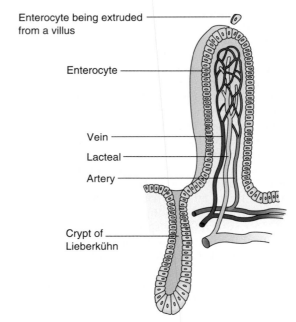

Enterocyte being extruded from a villus
Enterocyte
Vein
Lacteal
Artery
Crypt of Lieberkühn

FIGURE 36-12 A single villus from the small intestine. (Chaffee E.E., Lytle I.M. [1980]. *Basic physiology and anatomy* [4th ed.]. Philadelphia: J.B. Lippincott)

TABLE 36-3 ◆ Enzymes Used in Digestion of Carbohydrates		
Dietary Carbohydrates	**Enzyme**	**Monosaccharides Produced**
Lactose	Lactase	Glucose and galactose
Sucrose	Sucrase	Fructose and glucose
Starch	Amylase	Maltose, maltotriase, and α-dextrins
Maltose and maltotriose	Maltase	Glucose and glucose
α-Dextrins	α-Dextrimase	Glucose and glucose

Amylase breaks down starch into several disaccharides, including maltose, isomaltose, and α-dextrins. The brush border enzymes convert the disaccharides into monosaccharides that can be absorbed (Table 36-3). Sucrose yields glucose and fructose, lactose is converted to glucose and galactose, and maltose is converted to two glucose molecules. When the disaccharides are not broken down to monosaccharides, they cannot be absorbed but remain as osmotically active particles in the contents of the digestive system, causing diarrhea. Persons who are deficient in lactase, the enzyme that breaks down lactose, experience diarrhea when they drink milk or eat dairy products.

Fructose is transported across the intestinal mucosa by facilitated diffusion, which does not require energy expenditure. In this case, fructose moves along a concentration gradient. Glucose and galactose are transported by way of a sodium-dependent carrier system that uses adenosine triphosphate (ATP) as an energy source (Fig. 36-13). Water absorption from the intestine is linked to absorption of osmotically active particles, such as glucose and sodium. It follows that an important consideration in facilitating the transport of water across the intestine (and decreasing diarrhea) after temporary disruption in bowel function is to include sodium and glucose in the fluids that are taken.

FAT ABSORPTION

The average adult eats approximately 60 to 100 g of fat daily, principally as triglycerides containing long-chain fatty acids.

These triglycerides are broken down by pancreatic lipase. Bile salts act as a carrier system for the fatty acids and fat-soluble vitamins A, D, E, and K by forming micelles, which transport these substances to the surface of intestinal villi, where they are absorbed. The major site of fat absorption is the upper jejunum. Medium-chain triglycerides, with 6 to 10 carbon atoms in their structures, are absorbed better than longer-chain of fatty acids because they are more completely broken down by pancreatic lipase and they form micelles more easily. Because they are easily absorbed, medium-chain triglycerides often are used in the treatment of persons with malabsorption syndrome. The absorption of vitamins A, D, E, and K, which are fat-soluble vitamins, requires bile salts.

Fat that is not absorbed in the intestine is excreted in the stool. *Steatorrhea* is the term used to describe fatty stools. It usually indicates that there is 20 g or more of fat in a 24-hour stool sample. Normally, a chemical test is done on a 72-hour stool collection, during which time the diet is restricted to 80 to 100 g of fat per day.

PROTEIN ABSORPTION

Protein digestion begins in the stomach with the action of pepsin. Pepsinogen, the enzyme precursor of pepsin, is secreted by the chief cells in response to a meal and acid pH. Acid in the stomach is required for the conversion of pepsinogen to pepsin. Pepsin is inactivated when it enters the intestine by the alkaline pH.

FIGURE 36-13 The hypothetical sodium-dependent transport system for glucose. Both sodium and glucose must attach to the transport carrier before either can be transported into the cell. The concentration of glucose builds up in the intestinal cell until a diffusion gradient develops, causing glucose to move into the body fluids. Sodium is transported out of the cell by the energy-dependent (ATP) sodium pump. This creates the gradient needed to operate the transport system.

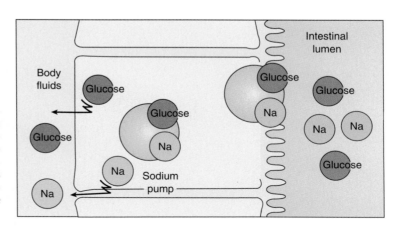

Proteins are broken down further by pancreatic enzymes, such as trypsin, chymotrypsin, carboxypeptidase, and elastase. As with pepsin, the pancreatic enzymes are secreted as precursor molecules. Trypsinogen, which lacks enzymatic activity, is activated by an enzyme located on the brush border cells of the duodenal enterocytes. Activated trypsin activates additional trypsinogen molecules and other pancreatic precursor proteolytic enzymes. The amino acids are liberated intramurally or on the surface of the villi by brush border enzymes that degrade proteins into peptides that are one, two, or three amino acids long. Similar to glucose, many amino acids are transported across the mucosal membrane in a sodium-linked process that uses ATP as an energy source. Some amino acids are absorbed by facilitated diffusion processes that do not require sodium.

In summary, the digestion and absorption of foodstuffs take place in the small intestine. Digestion is the process of dismantling foods into their constituent parts. Digestion requires hydrolysis, enzyme cleavage, and fat emulsification. Proteins, fats, carbohydrates, and other components of the diet are broken down into molecules that can be transported from the intestinal lumen into the body fluids. Absorption is the process of moving nutrients and other materials from the external environment of the gastrointestinal tract into the internal environment. Brush border enzymes break carbohydrates into monosaccharides that can be transported across the intestine into the bloodstream. The digestion of proteins begins in the stomach with the action of pepsin and is further facilitated in the intestine by the pancreatic enzymes, such as trypsin, chymotrypsin, carboxypeptidase, and elastase. Enzymes that break down proteins are released as proenzymes that are activated in the gastrointestinal tract. The absorption of glucose and amino acids is facilitated by a sodium-dependent transport system. Fat in the diet is broken down by pancreatic lipase into triglycerides containing medium- and long-chain fatty acids. Bile salts form micelles that transport these substances to the surface of intestinal villi, where they are absorbed.

Bibliography

Berne R.M., Levy M.N. (1997). *Principles of physiology* (3rd ed., pp. 354–400). St. Louis: C.V. Mosby.

Gershon M.D. (1999). The enteric nervous system: A second brain. *Hospital Practice* 34 (7), 31–52.

Guyton A.C., Hall J.E. (2000). *Textbook of medical physiology* (10th ed., pp. 718–770). Philadelphia: W.B. Saunders.

Johnson L.R. (1997). *Gastrointestinal physiology* (5th ed.). St. Louis: C.V. Mosby.

Rhoades R.A., Tanner G.A. (1996). *Medical physiology* (pp. 487–569). Boston: Little, Brown.

Alterations in Gastrointestinal Function

Gastrointestinal disorders are not cited as the leading cause of death in the United States, nor do they receive the same publicity as heart disease and cancer. However, according to government reports, digestive diseases rank third in the total economic burden of illness, resulting in considerable human suffering, personal expenditures for treatment, lost working hours, and a drain on the nation's economy. It has been estimated that 20 million Americans, or one of every nine persons in the United States, have digestive disease. Even more important is the fact that proper nutrition or a change in health practices could prevent or minimize many of these disorders.

Manifestations of Gastrointestinal Disorders

After you have completed this section of the chapter, you should be able to meet the following objectives:

✦ Describe the physiologic mechanisms involved in anorexia, nausea, and vomiting

✦ Characterize the appearance of blood in vomitus and stool according to the site and extent of bleeding

Several signs and symptoms are common to many types of gastrointestinal disorders. These include anorexia, nausea, vomiting, and gastrointestinal bleeding. Because they occur with so many of the disorders, they are discussed separately as an introduction to the content that follows.

ANOREXIA, NAUSEA, AND VOMITING

Anorexia, nausea, and vomiting are physiologic responses that are common to many gastrointestinal disorders. These responses are protective to the extent that they signal the presence of disease and, in the case of vomiting, remove noxious agents from the gastrointestinal tract. They also can contribute to impaired intake or loss of fluids and nutrients.

Anorexia represents a loss of appetite. Several factors influence appetite. One is hunger, which is stimulated by contractions of the empty stomach. Appetite or the desire for food intake is regulated by the hypothalamus and other associated centers in the brain. Smell plays an important role, as evidenced by the fact that appetite can be stimulated or suppressed by the smell of food. Loss of appetite is associated with emotional factors, such as fear, depression, frustration, and anxiety. Many drugs and disease states cause anorexia. In uremia, for example, the accumulation of nitrogenous wastes in the blood contributes to the development of anorexia. Anorexia often is a forerunner of nausea, and most conditions that cause nausea and vomiting also produce anorexia.

Nausea is an ill-defined and unpleasant subjective sensation. It is the conscious sensation resulting from stimulation of the medullary vomiting center that often precedes or accompanies vomiting. Nausea usually is preceded by anorexia, and stimuli such as foods and drugs that cause anorexia in small doses usually produce nausea when given in larger doses. A common cause of nausea is distention of the duodenum, or upper small intestinal tract. Nausea frequently is accompanied by autonomic nervous system manifestations such as watery salivation and vasoconstriction with pallor, sweating, and tachycardia. Nausea may function as an early warning signal of a pathology.

Vomiting, or emesis, is the sudden and forceful oral expulsion of the contents of the stomach. It usually is preceded by nausea. The contents that are vomited are called *vomitus*. Vomiting, as a basic physiologic protective mechanism, limits the possibility of damage from ingested noxious agents by emptying the contents of the stomach and portions of the small intestine. Nausea and vomiting may represent a total-body response to drug therapy, including overdosage, cumulative effects, toxicity, and side effects.

Vomiting appears to involve two functionally distinct medullary centers: the vomiting center and the chemoreceptor trigger zone. The act of vomiting is integrated by the vomiting center, which is located in the dorsal portion of the reticular formation of the medulla near the sensory nuclei of the vagus. The chemoreceptor trigger zone is located in a small area on the floor of the fourth ventricle, where it is exposed to both blood and cerebrospinal fluid. It is thought to mediate the emetic effects of blood-borne drugs and toxins.

The act of vomiting consists of taking a deep breath, closing the airways, and producing a strong, forceful contraction of the diaphragm and abdominal muscles along with relaxation of the gastroesophageal sphincter. Respiration ceases during the act of vomiting. Vomiting may be accompanied by dizziness, light-headedness, decrease in blood pressure, and bradycardia.

The vomiting center receives input from the gastrointestinal tract and other organs; from the cerebral cortex; from the vestibular apparatus, which is responsible for motion sickness; and from the chemoreceptor trigger zone, which is activated by many drugs and endogenous and exogenous toxins. Hypoxia exerts a direct effect on the vomiting center, producing nausea and vomiting. This direct effect probably accounts for the vomiting that occurs during periods of decreased cardiac output, shock, environmental hypoxia, and brain ischemia caused by increased intracranial pressure. Inflammation of any of the intra-abdominal organs, including the liver, gallbladder, or urinary tract, can cause vomiting because of the stimulation of the visceral afferent pathways that communicate with the vomiting center. Distention or irritation of the gastrointestinal tract also causes vomiting through the stimulation of visceral afferent neurons.

Several neurotransmitters and receptor subtypes are implicated as neuromediators in nausea and vomiting. Dopamine, serotonin (*i.e.*, 5-HT$_3$), and opioid receptors are found in the gastrointestinal tract and in the vomiting and chemoreceptor trigger zone. Dopamine antagonists such as prochlorperazine (Compazine) depress vomiting caused by stimulation of the chemoreceptor trigger zone. Serotonin is believed to be involved in the nausea and emesis associated with cancer chemotherapy and radiation therapy.[1,2] Serotonin receptor antagonists such as granisetron (Kytril) and ondansetron (Zofran) are effective in treating the nausea and vomiting associated with these stimuli. Motion sickness appears to be a central nervous system (CNS) response to vestibular stimuli. Norepinephrine and acetylcholine receptors are located in the vestibular center. The acetylcholine receptors are thought to mediate the impulses responsible for exciting the vomiting center; norepinephrine receptors may have a stabilizing influence that resists motion sickness. Many of the motion sickness drugs (*e.g.*, dimenhydrinate [Dramamine] and meclizine [Antivert and Bonine]) have a strong CNS anticholinergic effect and act on the receptors in the vomiting center and areas related to the vestibular system.

GASTROINTESTINAL TRACT BLEEDING

Bleeding from the gastrointestinal tract can be evidenced by blood that appears in the vomitus or the feces. It can result from disease or trauma to the gastrointestinal structures, from primary diseases of the blood vessels (*e.g.*, esophageal varices, hemorrhoids), or from disorders in blood clotting.

Hematemesis
Blood in the stomach usually is irritating and causes vomiting. Hematemesis refers to blood in the vomitus. It may be bright red or have a "coffee-ground" appearance because of the action of the digestive enzymes.

Melena
Blood that appears in the stool may range in color from bright red to tarry black. Bright red blood usually indicates that the bleeding is from the lower bowel. When it coats the stool, it often is the result of bleeding hemorrhoids.

The word *melena* comes from the Greek word for "black" and refers to the passage of black and tarry stools. These stools have a characteristic odor that is not easily forgotten. Tarry stools usually indicate that the source of the bleeding is above the level of the ileocecal valve, although this is not always the case. Approximately 150 to 200 mL of blood must be present in the stomach to produce a single tarry stool; acute blood loss may produce melena for up to 3 days.[3] With hypermotility of the gastrointestinal tract, bright red blood may be present in the stools even though the bleeding is from the upper gastrointestinal tract.

Occult, or hidden, blood can only be detected by chemical means. It can be caused by gastritis, peptic ulcer, or lesions of the intestine. Occult bleeding can be detected by the use of guaiac-based stool tests that makes use of the pseudoperoxidase activity of hemoglobin. Guaiac turns blue after oxidation by oxidants or peroxidases in the presence of an oxygen donor such as hydrogen peroxide. The likelihood that a guaiac-based test result will be positive is directly proportional to the quantity of fecal heme, which in turn is related to the size and location of the bleeding lesion. Many factors influence guaiac-based tests, including ingestion of vitamin C and dietary factors such as nonhuman heme derived from eating meat or peroxidases from dietary sources.

The blood urea nitrogen (BUN) level frequently is elevated after hematemesis or melena. This results from the breakdown of the blood by the digestive enzymes and the absorption of the nitrogenous end products into the blood. The BUN level usually reaches a peak within 24 hours after the gastrointestinal hemorrhage. It is not elevated when the bleeding is in the colon because digestion does not take place at this level of the digestive system. An elevation in body temperature also may follow gastrointestinal hemorrhage. It usually occurs within 24 hours and may last for a few days to a few weeks.

> In summary, the signs and symptoms of many gastrointestinal tract disorders are manifested by anorexia, nausea, and vomiting. Anorexia, or loss of appetite, may occur alone or may accompany nausea and vomiting. Nausea, which is an ill-defined, unpleasant sensation, signals the stimulation of the medullary vomiting center. It often precedes vomiting and frequently is accompanied by autonomic responses such as salivation and vasoconstriction with pallor, sweating, and tachycardia. The act of vomiting, which is integrated by the vomiting center, involves the forceful oral expulsion of the gastric contents. It is a basic physiologic mechanism that rids the gastrointestinal tract of noxious agents. Disorders that disrupt the integrity of the gastrointestinal tract often cause bleeding, which can be manifested as blood in the vomitus (*i.e.,* hematemesis) or as blood in the stool (*i.e.,* melena).

Disorders of the Esophagus

After you have completed this section of the chapter, you should be able to meet the following objectives:

✦ Define dysphagia, odynophagia, and achalasia
✦ Relate the pathophysiology of gastroesophageal reflux to measures used in diagnosis and treatment of the disorder in adults and children
✦ State the reason for the poor prognosis associated with esophageal cancer

The esophagus is a tube that connects the oropharynx with the stomach. It lies posterior to the trachea and larynx

and extends through the mediastinum, intersecting the diaphragm at the level of the 11th thoracic vertebra.

The esophagus functions primarily as a conduit for passage of food from the pharynx to the stomach, and the structures of its walls are designed for this purpose: the smooth muscle layers provide the peristaltic movements needed to move food along its length, and the epithelial layer secretes mucus, which protects its surface and aids in lubricating food. There are sphincters at either end of the esophagus: an upper esophageal sphincter and a lower esophageal sphincter. The upper esophageal, or pharyngoesophageal, sphincter consists of a circular layer of striated muscle, the cricopharyngeal muscle. The lower esophageal, or gastroesophageal, sphincter is an area approximately 3 cm above the junction with the stomach. The circular muscle in this area normally remains tonically constricted, creating a zone of high pressure that serves to prevent reflux of gastric contents into the esophagus.[4] During swallowing, there is "receptive relaxation" of the lower esophageal sphincter, which allows easy propulsion of the esophageal contents into the stomach. The lower esophageal sphincter passes through an opening, or hiatus, in the diaphragm as it joins with the stomach, which is located in the abdomen. The portion of the diaphragm that surrounds the lower esophageal sphincter helps to maintain the zone of high pressure needed to prevent reflux of stomach contents.[5]

DYSPHAGIA

The act of swallowing depends on the coordinated action of the tongue and pharynx. These structures are innervated by cranial nerves V, IX, X, and XII. *Dysphagia* refers to difficulty in swallowing. If swallowing is painful, it is referred to as *odynophagia.* Dysphagia can result from altered nerve function or from disorders that produce narrowing of the esophagus. Lesions of the CNS, such as a stroke, often involve the cranial nerves that control swallowing. Strictures and cancer of the esophagus and strictures resulting from scarring can reduce the size of the esophageal lumen and make swallowing difficult. Scleroderma, an autoimmune disease that causes fibrous replacement of tissues in the muscularis layer of the gastrointestinal tract, is another important cause of dysphagia.[6] Persons with dysphagia usually complain of choking, coughing, or an abnormal sensation of food sticking in the back of the throat or upper chest when they swallow.

In a condition called *achalasia,* the lower esophageal sphincter fails to relax; food that has been swallowed has difficulty passing into the stomach, and the esophagus above the lower esophageal sphincter becomes enlarged. One or several meals may lodge in the esophagus and pass slowly into the stomach over time. There is danger of aspiration of esophageal contents into the lungs when the person lies down.

Endoscopy, barium esophagoscopy, and videoradiography may be used to determine the site and extent of the swallowing disorder. Esophageal manometry, a procedure in which a small pressure-sensing catheter is inserted into the esophagus, may be done to measure pressures in different parts of the esophagus. Treatment of swallowing disorders depends on the cause and type of altered function that is present. Treatment of dysphagia often involves a multidisciplinary team of health professionals, including a speech therapist. Mechanical dilatation or surgical procedures may be done to enlarge the lower esophageal sphincter in persons with esophageal strictures.

ESOPHAGEAL DIVERTICULUM

A diverticulum of the esophagus is an outpouching of the esophageal wall caused by a weakness of the muscularis layer. An esophageal diverticulum tends to retain food. Complaints that the food stops before it reaches the stomach are common, as are reports of gurgling, belching, coughing, and foul-smelling breath. The trapped food may cause esophagitis and ulceration. Because the condition usually is progressive, correction of the defect often requires surgical intervention.

GASTROESOPHAGEAL REFLUX DISEASE

The term *reflux* refers to backward or return movement. In the context of gastroesophageal reflux, it refers to the backward movement of gastric contents into the esophagus, a condition that causes heartburn. Often referred to as gastroesophageal reflux disease (GERD), it probably is the most common disorder originating in the gastrointestinal tract. Most persons experience heartburn occasionally as a result of reflux. However, for some persons, persistent heartburn can represent reflux disease with esophagitis.

The lower esophageal sphincter regulates the flow of food from the esophagus into the stomach. Both internal and external mechanisms function in maintaining the antireflux function of the lower esophageal sphincter.[5,7] The circular muscles of the distal esophagus constitute the internal mechanisms, and the portion of the diaphragm that surrounds the esophagus constitutes the external mechanism. The oblique muscles of the stomach, located below the lower esophageal sphincter, form a flap that contributes to the antireflux barrier of the internal sphincter. Relaxation of the lower esophageal sphincter is a brain stem reflex that is mediated by the vagus nerve in response to a number of afferent stimuli. Transient relaxation with reflux is common after meals. Gastric distension and meals high in fat increase the frequency of relaxation. Refluxed material is returned to the stomach by secondary peristaltic waves in the esophagus; swallowed saliva neutralizes and washes away the refluxed acid.

Gastroesophageal reflux is thought to be associated with a weak or incompetent lower esophageal sphincter that allows reflux to occur, the irritant effects of the refluxate, and decreased clearance of the refluxed acid from the esophagus after it has occurred.[8,9] In most cases, reflux occurs during transient relaxation of the esophagus. Delayed gastric emptying also may contribute to reflux by increasing gastric volume and pressure with greater chance for reflux. Esophageal mucosal injury is related to the destructive nature of the refluxate and the amount of time it is in contact with mucosa. Acidic gastric fluids (pH < 4.0) are particularly damaging. The gastroesophageal reflux normally is cleared and neutralized by esophageal peristalsis and salivary bicarbonate. Decreased salivation and salivary buffering capacity may contribute to impaired clearing of acid reflux from the esophagus. There is controversy regarding the importance of hiatal hernia (*i.e.,* herniation of the stomach through an enlarged hiatus in the diaphragm) in the pathogenesis of reflux disease. Small hiatal hernias are common and considered to be of no significance in asymptomatic people. However, in cases of severe erosive esophagitis where gastroesophageal reflux and a large hiatal hernia coexist, the hernia may retard esophageal acid clearance and contribute to the disorder.[5,8]

Reflux esophagitis involves mucosal injury to the esophagus, hyperemia, and inflammation. The most frequent symptom of gastroesophageal reflux is heartburn. It frequently is severe, occurring 30 to 60 minutes after eating. It often is made worse by bending at the waist and recumbency and usually is relieved by sitting upright. The severity of heartburn is not indicative of the extent of mucosal injury; only a small percentage of people who complain of heartburn have mucosal injury. Often, the heartburn occurs during the night. Antacids give prompt, although transient relief. Other symptoms include belching and chest pain. The pain usually is located in the epigastric or retrosternal area and often radiates to the throat, shoulder, or back. Because of its location, the pain may be confused with angina. The reflux of gastric contents also may produce respiratory symptoms such as wheezing, chronic cough, and hoarseness. There is considerable evidence linking gastroesophageal reflux with bronchial asthma.[10,11] The proposed mechanisms of reflux-associated asthma and chronic cough include microaspiration and macroaspiration, laryngeal injury, and vagal-mediated bronchospasm.

Complications can result from persistent reflux, which produces a cycle of mucosal damage that causes hyperemia, edema, and erosion of the luminal surface. These complications include strictures and a condition called *Barrett's esophagus.* Strictures are caused by a combination of scar tissue, spasm, and edema. They produce narrowing of the esophagus and cause dysphagia when the lumen becomes sufficiently constricted. Barrett's esophagus is characterized by a reparative process in which the squamous mucosa that normally lines the esophagus gradually is replaced by columnar epithelium resembling that in the stomach or intestines.[8,9] It is associated with increased risk for development of esophageal cancer.

Diagnosis of GERD depends on a history of reflux symptomatology and selective use of diagnostic methods, including radiographic studies using a contrast medium such as barium, esophagoscopy, and ambulatory esophageal pH monitoring.[12] Esophagoscopy involves the passage of a flexible fiberoptic endoscope into the esophagus for the purpose of visualizing the lumen of the upper gastrointestinal tract. It also permits performance of a biopsy, if indicated. For 24-hour pH monitoring, a small tube with a pH electrode is passed through the nose and down into the esophagus. Data from the electrode are recorded in a small, lightweight box worn on a belt around the waist and later are analyzed by computer. The box has a button that the person can press to indicate episodes of heartburn or pain; these can be correlated with episodes of acid reflux.

The treatment of GERD usually focuses on conservative measures. These measures include avoidance of positions and conditions that increase gastric reflux.[12] Avoidance of large meals and foods that reduce lower esophageal sphincter tone (*e.g.*, caffeine, fats, chocolate), alcohol, and smoking is recommended. It is recommended that meals be eaten sitting up and that the recumbent position be avoided for several hours after a meal. Bending for long periods should be avoided, because it tends to increase intra-abdominal pressure and cause gastric reflux. Sleeping with the head elevated helps to prevent reflux during the night. This is best accomplished by placing blocks under the head of the bed or by using a wedge-shaped bolster to elevate the head and shoulders by at least 6 inches. Weight loss usually is recommended in overweight people.

Antacids or a combination of antacids and alginic acid also are recommended for mild disease. Alginic acid produces a foam when it comes in contact with gastric acid; if reflux occurs, the foam rather than acid rises into the esophagus. Histamine type 2 receptor (H_2)–blocking drugs (*e.g.*, cimetidine, ranitidine, nizatidine, famotidine), which inhibit gastric acid production, often are recommended when additional treatment is needed. The proton pump inhibitors (*e.g.*, omeprazole, lansoprazole, rabeprazole, pantoprazole) act by inhibiting the gastric proton pump, which regulates the final pathway for acid secretion. These agents may be used for persons who continue to have daytime symptoms, recurrent strictures, or esophageal ulcerations. Promotility agents (*e.g.*, metoclopramide) may be used to increase lower esophageal pressure and enhance esophageal clearance.[9] Metoclopramide is a dopamine antagonist that may cause neuropsychiatric side effects, limiting its use. Surgical treatment may be indicated in some people.

Gastroesophageal Reflux in Children

Gastroesophageal reflux is a common problem in infants and children. The small reservoir capacity of an infant's esophagus coupled with frequent spontaneous reductions in sphincter pressure contribute to reflux. Regurgitation of at least one episode a day occurs in as many as half of infants aged 0 to 3 months. By 6 months of age it becomes less frequent, and it abates by 2 years of age as the child assumes a more upright posture and eats solid foods.[13,14] Although many infants have minor degrees of reflux, complications occur in 1 of every 300 to 500 children.[13,14] The condition occurs more frequently in children with cerebral palsy, Down syndrome, and other causes of developmental delay.

In most cases, infants with simple reflux are thriving and healthy, and symptoms resolve between 9 and 24 months of age. Pathologic reflux is classified into three categories: (1) regurgitation and malnutrition, (2) esophagitis, and (3) respiratory problems. Symptoms of esophagitis include evidence of pain when swallowing, hematemesis, anemia due to esophageal bleeding, heartburn, irritability, and sudden or inconsolable crying. Parents often report feeding problems in their infants.[13] These infants often are irritable and demonstrate early satiety. Sometimes the prob-

lems progress to actual resistance to feeding. Tilting of the head to one side and arching of the back may be noted in children with severe reflux. The head positioning is thought to represent an attempt to protect the airway or reduce the pain-associated reflux. Sometimes regurgitation is associated with dental caries and recurrent otalgia. The ear pain is thought to occur through referral from the vagus nerve in the esophagus to the ear. A variety of respiratory symptoms are caused by damage to the respiratory mucosa when gastric reflux enters the esophagus. Reflux may cause laryngospasm, apnea, and bradycardia. A relationship between reflux and acute life-threatening events or sudden infant death syndrome has been proposed. However, the association remains controversial and the linkage may be coincidental.[13,14]

Rumination is the repetitive gagging, regurgitation, mouthing, and reswallowing of regurgitated material. Although the cause of the disorder is unknown, it often is associated with mental retardation or altered interaction with the environment (*e.g.*, lack of stimulation in newborn intensive care units or because of altered relationships with caregivers). As with pure reflux, rumination may produce severe esophagitis with signs of iron deficiency anemia, failure to thrive, and head tilting.[14]

Diagnosis of gastroesophageal reflux in infants and children often is based on parental and clinical observations. The diagnosis may be confirmed by esophageal pH probe studies or barium fluoroscopic esophagography. In severe cases, esophagoscopy may be used to demonstrate reflux and obtain a biopsy.

Various treatment methods are available for infants and children with gastroesophageal reflux. Small, frequent feedings are recommended because of the association between gastric volume and transient relaxation of the esophagus. Thickening an infant's feedings with cereal tends to decrease the volume of reflux, decrease crying and energy expenditure, and increase the calorie density of the formula.[13,14] In infants, positioning on the left side seems to decrease reflux. In older infants and children, raising the head of the bed and keeping the child upright may help. Medications usually are not added to the treatment regimen until pathologic reflux has been documented by diagnostic testing.

CANCER OF THE ESOPHAGUS

Carcinoma of the esophagus accounts for approximately 6% of all gastrointestinal cancers. This disease is more common in persons older than 50 years of age, with a male-to-female ratio of approximately 2 : 1.[15]

There are two types of esophageal cancers: squamous cell and adenocarcinomas. Fewer than 50% of esophageal tumors are squamous cell cancers. These cancers are associated more commonly with dietary and environmental influences.[15,16] Most squamous cell cancers in the United States and Europe are attributable to alcohol and tobacco use. Approximately 20% of these squamous cell tumors are located in the upper third, 50% in the middle third, and 25% in the lower third of the esophagus.[15] Adenocarcinomas, which typically arise from Barrett's esophagus, account for more than 50% of esophageal cancers. The incidence of this type of cancer appears to increasing. Adenocarcinomas typically are located in the distal esophagus and may invade the adjacent upper part of the stomach. These tumors usually arise from dysplastic changes that occur in the histologic environment of Barrett's esophagus. Endoscopic surveillance in people with Barrett's esophagus may detect adenocarcinoma at an earlier stage when it is more amenable to curative surgical resection.[16]

Dysphagia is by far the most frequent complaint of persons with esophageal cancer. It is apparent first with ingestion of bulky food, later with soft food, and finally with liquids. Unfortunately, it is a late manifestation of the disease. Weight loss, anorexia, fatigue, and pain on swallowing also may occur.

Treatment includes surgical resection, which provides a means of cure when done in early disease and palliation when done in late disease. Irradiation is used as a palliative treatment. Chemotherapy sometimes is used before surgery to decrease the size of the tumor, and it may be used along with irradiation and surgery in an effort to increase survival.[16]

The prognosis for persons with cancer of the esophagus, although poor, has improved. Even with modern forms of therapy, however, the long-term survival is limited because, in many cases, the disease has already metastasized by the time the diagnosis is made. Better methods of early diagnosis are needed.

In summary, the esophagus is a tube that connects the oropharynx with the stomach; it functions primarily as a conduit for passage of food from the pharynx to the stomach. Dysphagia refers to difficulty in swallowing; it can result from altered nerve function or from disorders that produce narrowing of the esophagus. A diverticulum of the esophagus is an outpouching of the esophageal wall caused by a weakness of the muscularis layer.

Gastrointestinal reflux refers to the backward movement of gastric contents into the esophagus, a condition that causes heartburn. Although most persons experience occasional esophageal reflux and heartburn, persistent reflux can cause esophagitis. Gastroesophageal reflux is a common problem in infants and children. Reflux commonly corrects itself with age, and symptoms abate in most children by 2 years of age. Although many infants have minor degrees of reflux, some infants and small children have significant reflux that interferes with feeding, causes esophagitis, and results in respiratory symptoms and other complications.

Carcinoma of the esophagus, which accounts for 6% of all cancers, is more common in persons older than 50 years of age, and the male-to-female ratio is approximately 2 : 1. There are two types of esophageal cancer: squamous cell and adenocarcinoma. Most squamous cell cancers are attributable to alcohol and tobacco use, whereas adenocarcinomas are more closely linked to esophageal reflux and Barrett's esophagus.

Disorders of the Stomach

After you have completed this section of the chapter, you should be able to meet the following objectives:

✦ Describe the factors that contribute to the gastric mucosal barrier
✦ Characterize the proposed role of *Helicobacter pylori* in the development of chronic gastritis and peptic ulcer and cite methods for diagnosing the infection
✦ Differentiate between the causes and manifestations of acute and chronic gastritis
✦ Describe the predisposing factors in development of peptic ulcer and cite the three complications of peptic ulcer
✦ Describe the goals for pharmacologic treatment of peptic ulcer disease
✦ Cite the etiologic factors in ulcer formation related to Zollinger-Ellison syndrome and stress ulcer
✦ List risk factors associated with gastric cancer

The stomach is a reservoir for contents entering the digestive tract. It lies in the upper abdomen, anterior to the pancreas, splenic vessels, and left kidney. Anteriorly, the stomach is bounded by the anterior abdominal wall and the left inferior lobe of the liver. While in the stomach, food is churned and mixed with hydrochloric acid and pepsin before being released into the small intestine. Normally, the mucosal surface of the stomach provides a barrier that protects it from the hydrochloric acid and pepsin contained in gastric secretions. Disorders of the stomach include gastritis, peptic ulcer, and gastric carcinoma.

GASTRIC MUCOSAL BARRIER

The stomach lining usually is impermeable to the acid it secretes, a property that allows the stomach to contain acid and pepsin without having its wall digested. Several factors contribute to the protection of the gastric mucosa, including an impermeable epithelial cell surface covering, mechanisms for the selective transport of hydrogen and bicarbonate ions, and the characteristics of gastric mucus.[17] These mechanisms are collectively referred to as the *gastric mucosal barrier.*

The gastric epithelial cells are connected by tight junctions that prevent acid penetration, and they are covered with an impermeable hydrophobic lipid layer that prevents diffusion of ionized water-soluble molecules. Aspirin, which is nonionized and lipid soluble in acid solutions, rapidly diffuses across this lipid layer, increasing mucosal permeability and damaging epithelial cells.[18] Gastric irritation and occult bleeding due to gastric irritation occur in a significant number of persons who take aspirin on a regular basis (Fig. 37-1). Alcohol, which also is lipid soluble, disrupts the mucosal barrier; when aspirin and alcohol are taken in combination, as they often are, there is increased risk of gastric irritation. Bile acids also attack the lipid components of the mucosal barrier and afford the potential for gastric irritation when there is reflux of duodenal contents into the stomach.

Gastric Mucosa and Ulcer Development

➤ The stomach is protected by a mucosal barrier that prevents gastric secretions and other destructive agents from injuring the epithelial and deeper layers of the stomach wall.

➤ The integrity of the mucosal layer is maintained by tight cellular junctions and the presence of a protective mucus layer.

➤ Prostaglandins serve as chemical messengers that protect the stomach lining by improving blood flow, increasing bicarbonate secretion, and enhancing mucus production.

➤ Two of the major causes of gastric irritation and ulcer formation are aspirin or nonsteroidal anti-inflammatory drugs (NSAIDs) and infection with *H. pylori*.

➤ Aspirin and NSAIDs exert their destructive effects by irritating the gastric mucosa and inhibiting prostaglandin synthesis.

➤ *H. pylori* is an infectious agent that thrives in the acid environment of the stomach and disrupts the mucosal barrier that protects the stomach from the harmful effects of its digestive enzymes.

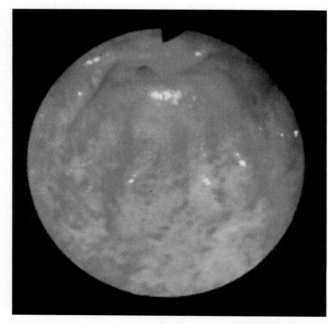

FIGURE 37-1 Erosive gastritis. This endoscopic view of the stomach in a patient who was ingesting aspirin reveals acute hemorrhagic lesions. (From Rubin E., Farber J.L. [1999]. *Pathology* [3rd ed., p. 683]. Philadelphia: Lippincott Williams & Wilkins)

Normally, the secretion of hydrochloric acid by the parietal cells of the stomach is accompanied by secretion of bicarbonate ions (HCO_3^-). For every hydrogen ion (H^+) that is secreted, a HCO_3^- is produced, and as long as HCO_3^- production is equal to H^+ secretion, mucosal injury does not occur. Changes in gastric blood flow, as in shock, tend to decrease HCO_3^- production. This is particularly true in situations in which decreased blood flow is accompanied by acidosis. Aspirin and the nonsteroidal anti-inflammatory drugs (NSAIDs) such as indomethacin and ibuprofen also impair HCO_3^- secretion.

The mucus that protects the gastric mucosa is of two types: water insoluble and water soluble.[17] Water-insoluble mucus forms a thin, stable gel that adheres to the gastric mucosal surface and provides protection from the proteolytic (protein-digesting) actions of pepsin. It also forms an unstirred layer that traps bicarbonate, forming an alkaline interface between the luminal contents of the stomach and its mucosal surface. The water-soluble mucus is washed from the mucosal surface and mixes with the luminal contents; its viscid nature makes it a lubricant that prevents mechanical damage to the mucosal surface. In addition to their effects on mucosal permeability and bicarbonate production, damaging agents such as aspirin and the NSAIDs inhibit and modify the characteristics of gastric mucus.

Prostaglandins, chemical messengers derived from cell membrane lipids, play an important role in protecting the gastric mucosa from injury. The prostaglandins probably exert their effect through improved blood flow, increased bicarbonate ion secretion, and enhanced mucus production. The fact that drugs such as aspirin and the NSAIDs inhibit prostaglandin synthesis may contribute to their ability to produce gastric irritation.[18] Smoking and older age have been associated with reduced gastric and duodenal prostaglandin concentrations; these observations may explain the predisposition to ulcer disease in smokers and older persons.[19]

GASTRITIS

Gastritis refers to inflammation of the gastric mucosa. There are many causes of gastritis, most of which can be grouped under the headings of acute or chronic gastritis.

Acute Gastritis

Acute gastritis refers to a transient inflammation of the gastric mucosa. It is most commonly associated with local irritants such as bacterial endotoxins, caffeine, alcohol, and aspirin. Depending on the severity of the disorder, the mucosal response may vary from moderate edema and hyperemia to hemorrhagic erosion of the gastric mucosa.

The complaints of persons with acute gastritis vary. Persons with aspirin-related gastritis can be totally unaware of the condition or may complain only of heartburn or sour stomach. Gastritis associated with excessive alcohol consumption is a different situation; it often causes transient gastric distress, which may lead to vomiting and, in more severe situations, to bleeding and hematemesis. Gastritis caused by the toxins of infectious organisms, such as the staphylococcal enterotoxins, usually has an abrupt and violent onset, with gastric distress and vomiting ensuing approximately 5 hours after the ingestion of a contaminated food source. Acute gastritis usually is a self-limiting disorder; complete regeneration and healing usually occur within several days.

Chronic Gastritis

Chronic gastritis is a separate entity from acute gastritis. It is characterized by the absence of grossly visible erosions and the presence of chronic inflammatory changes leading eventually to atrophy of the glandular epithelium of the stomach. The changes may become dysplastic and possibly transform into carcinoma. Factors such as chronic alcohol abuse, cigarette smoking, and chronic use of NSAIDs may contribute to the development of the disease.

There are four major types of chronic gastritis: autoimmune gastritis, multifocal atrophic gastritis, *Helicobacter pylori* gastritis, and chemical gastropathy.[20]

Autoimmune Gastritis and Multifocal Atrophic Gastritis. Autoimmune gastritis is the least common form of chronic gastritis. It typically involves the fundus and the body of the stomach and is associated with pernicious anemia. Most persons with the disorder have circulating antibodies to parietal cells and intrinsic factor, and hence this form of chronic gastritis is considered to be of autoimmune origin. Autoimmune destruction of the parietal cells leads to hypochlorhydria or achlorhydria, a high intragastric pH, and hypergastrinemia. Pernicious anemia is a megablastic anemia that is caused by malabsorption of vitamin B_{12} due to a deficiency of intrinsic factor (see Chapter 15). This type of chronic gastritis frequently is associated with other autoimmune disorders such as Hashimoto's thyroiditis and Addison's disease.

Multifocal atrophic gastritis is a disorder of unknown etiology. It is more common than autoimmune gastritis, and is seen more frequently in whites than in other races. It is particularly common in Asia, Scandinavia, and parts of Europe and Latin America. Multifocal atrophic gastritis typically affects the antrum and adjacent areas of the stomach. As with autoimmune gastritis, it is associated with reduced gastric acid secretion, but achlorhydria and pernicious anemia are less common.

Chronic autoimmune gastritis and multifocal atrophic gastritis cause few symptoms related directly to gastric changes. Persons with autoimmune chronic gastritis may develop signs of pernicious anemia. More important is the development of peptic ulcer and increased risk of peptic ulcer and gastric carcinoma. Approximately 2% to 4% of persons with atrophic gastritis eventually develop gastric carcinoma.[15]

Helicobacter Pylori Gastritis. *H. pylori* gastritis is a chronic inflammatory disease of the antrum and body of the stomach. It is the most common type of chronic non-erosive gastritis in the United States. Chronic infection with *H. pylori* can lead to gastric atrophy and intestinal metaplasia. *H. pylori* also can cause peptic ulcer (to be discussed) and has been linked to the development of gastric adenocarcinoma.

H. pylori are small, curved, gram-negative rods (protobacteria) that can colonize the mucus-secreting epithelial

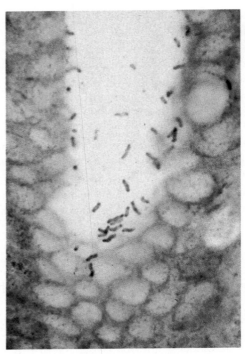

FIGURE 37-2 Infective gastritis. *H. pylori* appears on silver staining as small, curved rods on the surface of the gastric mucosa. (From Rubin E., Farber J.L. [1999]. *Pathology* [3rd ed., p. 687]. Philadelphia: Lippincott Williams & Wilkins)

cells of the stomach[20,21] (Fig. 37-2). *H. pylori* have multiple flagella, which allow them to move through the mucosal layer of the stomach, and they secrete urease, which enables them to produce sufficient ammonia to buffer the acidity of their immediate environment. These properties help to explain why the organism is able to survive in the acidic environment of the stomach. Because the organism adheres only to the mucus-secreting cells of the stomach, it does not usually colonize other parts of the gastrointestinal tract. The exceptions are areas such as Barrett's esophagus and a duodenal ulcer site in which the normal epithelial layer has been replaced with gastric mucosa. *H. pylori* produce an enzyme that degrades mucin and has the capacity to interfere with the local protection of the gastric mucosa against acid. It also may produce toxins that directly damage the mucosa and produce ulceration in other ways.

H. pylori have been isolated from diverse populations throughout the world. The prevalence of infection increases with age, and by 60 years of age, it is estimated that up to one half of the population has serologic evidence of infection.[21] Why some people with *H. pylori* infection develop clinical disease and others do not is unclear. Scientists are studying the different strains of the organism in an attempt to establish whether certain strains are more virulent than others and whether host and environmental factors contribute to the development of clinical disease.[20]

Chemical Gastropathy. Chemical gastropathy is a chronic gastric injury resulting from reflux of alkaline duodenal contents, pancreatic secretions, and bile into the stomach. It is most commonly seen in persons who have had gastro-duodenostomy or gastrojejunostomy surgery. A milder form may occur in persons with gastric ulcer, gallbladder disease, or various motility disorders of the distal stomach.

ULCER DISEASE

Peptic Ulcer Disease

Peptic ulcer is a term used to describe a group of ulcerative disorders that occur in areas of the upper gastrointestinal tract that are exposed to acid-pepsin secretions. The most common forms of peptic ulcer are duodenal and gastric ulcers. Two other forms of gastric ulcers, Zollinger-Ellison syndrome and stress ulcers, have different causes and are discussed separately. Peptic ulcer disease, with its remissions and exacerbations, represents a chronic health problem. Approximately 10% of the population have or will develop peptic ulcer.[9] Duodenal ulcers occur five times more commonly than gastric ulcers. Ulcers in the duodenum occur at any age and frequently are seen in early adulthood. Gastric ulcers tend to affect the older age group, with a peak incidence between 55 and 70 years of age. Both types of ulcers affect men three to four times more frequently than women.

A peptic ulcer can affect one or all layers of the stomach or duodenum (Fig. 37-3). The ulcer may penetrate only the mucosal surface, or it may extend into the smooth muscle layers. Occasionally, an ulcer penetrates the outer wall

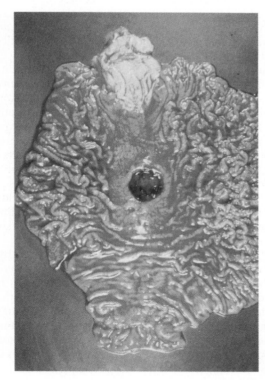

FIGURE 37-3 Gastric ulcer. The stomach has been opened to reveal a sharply demarcated, deep peptic ulcer on the lesser curvature. (From Rubin E., Farber J.L. [1999]. *Pathology* [3rd ed., p. 693]. Philadelphia: Lippincott Williams & Wilkins)

of the stomach or duodenum. Spontaneous remissions and exacerbations are common. Healing of the muscularis layer involves replacement with scar tissue; although the mucosal layers that cover the scarred muscle layer regenerate, the regeneration often is less than perfect, which contributes to repeated episodes of ulceration.

Since the early 1980s, there has been a radical shift in thinking regarding the cause of peptic ulcer. No longer is peptic ulcer thought to result from a genetic predisposition, stress, or dietary indiscretions. Most cases of peptic ulcer are caused by *H. pylori* infection.[22] The second most common cause of peptic ulcer is NSAID and aspirin use.[22] Much of the familial aggregation of peptic ulcer that formerly was credited to genetic factors in the development of peptic ulcer probably is due to intrafamilial infection with *H. pylori* rather than genetic susceptibility.

Since its identification in 1982, *H. pylori* has generated worldwide interest. It has been reported that virtually all persons with duodenal ulcer and 70% of persons with gastric ulcer have *H. pylori* infection.[15] Eradication of the organism can result in resolution of gastritis, with subsequent ulcer healing.

There is a 10% to 20% prevalence of gastric ulcers and a 2% to 5% prevalence of duodenal ulcers among chronic NSAID users. Aspirin appears to be the most ulcerogenic of the NSAIDs. Ulcer development in NSAID users is dose dependent, but some risk occurs even with aspirin doses of 325 mg/day.[9] The pathogenesis of NSAID-induced ulcers is thought to involve mucosal injury and inhibition of prostaglandin synthesis. In contrast to peptic ulcer from other causes, NSAID-induced gastric injury often is without symptoms, and life-threatening complications can occur without warning.

Manifestations. The clinical manifestations of uncomplicated peptic ulcer focus on discomfort and pain. The pain, which is described as burning, gnawing, or cramplike, usually is rhythmic and frequently occurs when the stomach is empty—between meals and at 1 or 2 o'clock in the morning. The pain usually is located over a small area near the midline in the epigastrium near the xiphoid, and may radiate below the costal margins, into the back, or, rarely, to the right shoulder. Superficial and deep epigastric tenderness and voluntary muscle guarding may occur with more extensive lesions. An additional characteristic of ulcer pain is periodicity. The pain tends to recur at intervals of weeks or months. During an exacerbation, it occurs daily for a period of several weeks and then remits until the next recurrence. Characteristically, the pain is relieved by food or antacids.

Complications. The complications of peptic ulcer include hemorrhage, obstruction, and perforation. Hemorrhage is caused by bleeding from granulation tissue or from erosion of an ulcer into an artery or vein. It occurs in up to 10% to 20% of persons with peptic ulcer.[9] Evidence of bleeding may consist of hematemesis or melena. Bleeding may be sudden, severe, and without warning, or it may be insidious, producing only occult blood in the stool. Up to 20% of persons with bleeding ulcers have no antecedent symptoms of pain; this is particularly true in persons receiving NSAIDs. Acute hemorrhage is evidenced by the sudden onset of weakness, dizziness, thirst, cold and moist skin, the desire to defecate, and the passage of loose, tarry, or even red stools and coffee-ground emesis. Signs of circulatory shock develop depending on the amount of blood lost.

Obstruction is caused by edema, spasm, or contraction of scar tissue and interference with the free passage of gastric contents through the pylorus or adjacent areas. There is a feeling of epigastric fullness and heaviness after meals. With severe obstruction, there is vomiting of undigested food.

Perforation occurs when an ulcer erodes through all the layers of the stomach or duodenum wall. Perforation develops in approximately 5% of persons with peptic ulcers, usually from ulcers on the anterior wall of the stomach or duodenum.[9] With perforation, gastrointestinal contents enter the peritoneum and cause peritonitis, or penetrate adjacent structures such as the pancreas. Radiation of the pain into the back, severe night distress, and inadequate pain relief from eating foods or taking antacids in persons with a long history of peptic ulcer may signify perforation. Peritonitis is discussed as a separate topic near the end of this chapter.

Diagnosis. Diagnostic procedures for peptic ulcer include history taking, laboratory tests, radiologic imaging, and endoscopic examination. The history should include careful attention to aspirin and NSAID use. Peptic ulcer should be differentiated from other causes of epigastric pain. Laboratory findings of hypochromic anemia and occult blood in the stools indicate bleeding. X-ray studies with a contrast medium such as barium are used to detect the presence of an ulcer crater and to exclude gastric carcinoma.

Endoscopy (*i.e.*, gastroscopy and duodenoscopy) can be used to visualize the ulcer area and obtain biopsy specimens to test for *H. pylori* and exclude malignant disease. Methods for establishing the presence of *H. pylori* include the C urea breath test using a radioactive carbon isotope (^{13}C or ^{14}C), the stool antigen test, and endoscopic biopsy for urease testing.[9,21] Blood tests to obtain serologic titers of *H. pylori* antibodies also can be done. The serologic test can establish that a person has been infected with *H. pylori,* but it cannot distinguish how recently the infection occurred.

Treatment. The treatment of peptic ulcer has changed dramatically over the past several years, and now aims to eradicate the cause and effect a permanent cure for the disease. Pharmacologic treatment focuses on eradicating *H. pylori*, relieving ulcer symptoms, and healing the ulcer crater. Acid-neutralizing, acid-inhibiting drugs and mucosal protective agents are used to relieve symptoms and promote healing of the ulcer crater. There is no evidence that special diets are beneficial in treating peptic ulcer. Aspirin and NSAID use should be avoided when possible.

Use of medications for eradication of *H. pylori* should be based on an accurate diagnosis of infection. Treatment requires combination therapy that includes two antibiotics and bismuth or a proton pump inhibitor.[9,22] The antibiotics that have shown the greatest efficacy against *H. pylori* are clarithromycin, metronidazole, amoxicillin, and tetracycline. The proton pump inhibitors have direct antimicrobial properties against *H. pylori,* and by raising the intragastric pH they suppress bacterial growth and optimize antibiotic efficacy. Bismuth compounds in a variety of formulations are used to treat dyspepsia, peptic ulcer disease, and diarrhea. The only agent available in the United States is bismuth subsalicylate (*e.g.*, Pepto-Bismol). Bismuth promotes ulcer healing through stimulation of mucosal bicarbonate and prostaglandin production. It also has a direct antibacterial effect against *H. pylori*. Bismuth causes a harmless darkening of the stools.

Among the agents that enhance mucosal defenses are sucralfate and prostaglandin analogs. The drug sucralfate, which is a complex salt of sucrose containing aluminum and sulfate, selectively binds to necrotic ulcer tissue and serves as a barrier to acid, pepsin, and bile. Sucralfate also can directly absorb bile salts. The drug is not absorbed systemically. The drug requires an acid pH for activation and should not be administered with antacids or an H_2 antagonist. Misoprostol, a prostaglandin analog, promotes ulcer healing by stimulating mucus and bicarbonate secretion and by modestly inhibiting acid secretion. It is used as a prophylactic agent to prevent NSAID-induced peptic ulcers. The drug causes dose-dependent diarrhea, and because of its stimulant effect on the uterus, it is contraindicated in women of childbearing age.

There are two pharmacologic methods for reducing gastric acid content. The first involves the neutralization of gastric acid through the use of antacids, and the second a decrease in gastric acid production through the use of H_2 receptor antagonists or proton pump inhibitors. Essentially three types of antacids are used to relieve gastric acidity: calcium carbonate, aluminum hydroxide, and magnesium hydroxide. Many antacids contain a combination of ingredients, such as magnesium aluminum hydroxide. *Calcium preparations* are constipating and may cause hypercalcemia and the milk-alkali syndrome. There also is evidence that oral calcium preparations increase gastric acid secretion after their buffering effect has been depleted. *Magnesium hydroxide* is a potent antacid that also has laxative effects. Approximately 5% to 10% of the magnesium in this preparation is absorbed from the intestine; because magnesium is excreted through the kidneys, this formulation should not be used in persons with renal failure. *Aluminum hydroxide* reacts with hydrochloric acid to form aluminum chloride. It combines with phosphate in the intestine, and prolonged use may lead to phosphate depletion and osteoporosis. Antacids can decrease the absorption, bioavailability, and renal elimination of a number of drugs; this should be considered when antacids are administered with other medications.

Histamine is the major physiologic mediator for hydrochloric acid secretion. The H_2 receptor antagonists (*e.g.*, cimetidine, ranitidine, famotidine, and nizatidine) block gastric acid secretion stimulated by histamine, gastrin, and acetylcholine. The volume of gastric secretion and the concentration of pepsin also are reduced. The proton pump inhibitors (*e.g.*, omeprazole, rabeprazole, pantoprazole, and lansoprazole) inhibit the final stage of hydrogen ion secretion by blocking the action of the gastric parietal cell proton pump (H^+–K^+–ATPase).

The current surgical management of peptic ulcer disease is largely limited to treatment of complications. When surgery is needed, it usually is performed using minimally invasive methods. With bleeding ulcers, hemostasis often can be achieved by endoscopic methods, and endoscopic balloon dilation often is effective in relieving outflow obstruction.

Zollinger-Ellison Syndrome

The Zollinger-Ellison syndrome is a rare condition caused by a gastrin-secreting tumor (gastrinoma). In persons with this disorder, gastric acid secretion reaches such levels that ulceration becomes inevitable.[23] The tumors may be single or multiple; although most tumors are located in the pancreas, a few develop in the submucosa of the stomach or duodenum. Over two thirds of gastrinomas are malignant, and one third have already metastasized at the time of diagnosis.[15] The increased gastric secretions cause symptoms related to peptic ulcer. Diarrhea may result from hypersecretion or from the inactivation of intestinal lipase and impaired fat digestion that occurs with a decrease in intestinal pH.

Hypergastrinemia may also occur in an autosomal dominant disorder called the multiple endocrine neoplasia type 1 (MEN 1) syndrome, which is characterized by multiple endocrine neoplasms. The syndrome is characterized by hyperparathyroidism and multiple endocrine tumors, including gastrinomas. Approximately 20% of gastrinomas are due to MEN 1.

The diagnosis of the Zollinger-Ellison syndrome is based on elevated serum gastrin and basal gastric acid levels and elimination of the MEN 1 syndrome as a cause of the disorder. Proton pump inhibitors are used to control gastric acid secretion. Computed tomography (CT), abdominal ultrasonography, and selective angiography are used to localize the tumor and determine if metastatic disease is present. Surgical removal is indicated when the tumor is malignant and has not metastasized.

Stress Ulcers

A stress ulcer, sometimes called *Curling's ulcer,* refers to gastrointestinal ulcerations that develop in relation to major physiologic stress. Persons at high risk for development of stress ulcers include those with large–surface-area burns, trauma, sepsis, acute respiratory distress syndrome, severe liver failure, and major surgical procedures. These lesions occur most often in the fundus of the stomach and proximal duodenum and are thought to result from ischemia, tissue acidosis, and bile salts entering the stomach in critically ill persons with decreased gastrointestinal tract motility.[24,25] Another form of stress ulcer, called *Cushing ulcer,* consists of gastric, duodenal, and esophageal ulcers arising in persons with intracranial injury, operations, or tumors. They are thought to be caused by hypersecretion of gastric acid resulting from stimulation of vagal nuclei by increased intracranial pressure. These ulcers are associated with a high incidence of perforation.[15]

Stress ulcers develop in approximately 5% to 10% of persons admitted to hospital intensive care units.[15] They usually are manifested by painless upper gastrointestinal tract bleeding. Monitoring and maintaining the gastric pH at 3.5 or higher helps to prevent the development of stress ulcers. H_2 receptor antagonists, proton pump inhibitors, and sucralfate are used in the prevention and treatment of stress ulcers.

CANCER OF THE STOMACH

Although its incidence has decreased during the past 50 years, stomach cancer is the seventh most frequent cause of cancer mortality in the United States. In 2001, it was estimated that approximately 21,700 Americans were diagnosed with stomach cancer and 12,800 died of the disease.[26] The disease is much more common in other countries and regions, principally Japan, Central Europe, the Scandinavian countries, South and Central America, the Soviet Union, China, and Korea. It is the major cause of cancer death worldwide.

Among the factors that increase the risk of gastric cancer are a genetic predisposition, carcinogenic factors in the diet (*e.g.,* N-nitroso compounds and benzopyrene found in smoked and preserved foods), autoimmune gastritis, and gastric adenomas or polyps. The incidence of stomach cancer in the United States has decreased fourfold since 1930, presumably because of improved storage of food with decreased consumption of salted, smoked, and preserved foods.[15,26] Infection with *H. pylori* appears to serve as a cofactor in some types of gastric carcinomas.[15]

Between 50% and 60% of gastric cancers occur in the pyloric region or adjacent to the antrum. Compared with a benign ulcer, which has smooth margins and is concentrically shaped, gastric cancers tend to be larger, are irregularly shaped, and have irregular margins.

Unfortunately, stomach cancers often are asymptomatic until late in their course. Symptoms, when they do occur, usually are vague and include indigestion, anorexia, weight loss, vague epigastric pain, vomiting, and an abdominal mass.

Diagnosis of gastric cancer is accomplished by means of a variety of techniques, including barium x-ray studies, endoscopic studies with biopsy, and cytologic studies (*e.g.,* Papanicolaou smear) of gastric secretions. Cytologic studies can prove particularly useful as routine screening tests for persons with atrophic gastritis or gastric polyps. CT and endoscopic ultrasonography often are used to delineate the spread of a diagnosed stomach cancer.

Surgery in the form of radical subtotal gastrectomy usually is the treatment of choice.[26] Irradiation and chemotherapy have not proved particularly useful as primary treatment modalities in stomach cancer. These methods usually are used for palliative purposes or to control metastatic spread of the disease.

> In summary, disorders of the stomach include gastritis, peptic ulcer, and cancer of the stomach. Gastritis refers to inflammation of the gastric mucosa. Acute gastritis refers to a transient inflammation of the gastric mucosa; it is associated most commonly with local irritants such as bacterial endotoxins, caffeine, alcohol, and aspirin. Chronic gastritis is characterized by the absence of grossly visible erosions and the presence of chronic inflammatory changes leading eventually to atrophy of the glandular epithelium of the stomach. There are four main types of chronic gastritis: autoimmune gastritis, multifocal atrophic gastritis, *H. pylori* gastritis,

and chemical gastropathy. Chronic gastritis increases the risk of stomach cancer.

Peptic ulcer is a term used to describe a group of ulcerative disorders that occur in areas of the upper gastrointestinal tract that are exposed to acid-pepsin secretions, most commonly the duodenum and stomach. There are two main causes of peptic ulcer: *H. pylori* infection and aspirin or NSAID use. *H. pylori* is a "S"-shaped bacterium that colonizes the mucus-secreting epithelial cells of the stomach. The treatment of peptic ulcer focuses on eradication of *H. pylori,* avoidance of gastric irritation from NSAIDs, and conventional pharmacologic treatment directed at symptom relief and ulcer healing.

The Zollinger-Ellison syndrome is a rare condition caused by a gastrin-secreting tumor, in which gastric acid secretion reaches such levels that ulceration becomes inevitable. Stress ulcers, also called *Curling's ulcers,* occur in relation to major physiologic stresses such as burns and trauma and are thought to result from ischemia, tissue acidosis, and bile salts entering the stomach in critically ill persons with decreased gastrointestinal tract motility. Another form of stress ulcer, Cushing ulcers, consists of gastric, duodenal, and esophageal ulcers arising in persons with intracranial injury, operations, or tumors. They are thought to be caused by hypersecretion of gastric acid resulting from stimulation of vagal nuclei by increased intracranial pressure.

Although the incidence of cancer of the stomach has declined over the past 50 years, it remains the seventh leading cause of death in the United States. Because there are few early symptoms with this form of cancer, the disease often is far advanced at the time of diagnosis.

Disorders of the Small and Large Intestines

After you have completed this section of the chapter, you should be able to meet the following objectives:

✦ State the diagnostic criteria for irritable bowel syndrome
✦ Compare the characteristics of Crohn's disease and ulcerative colitis
✦ Relate the use of a high-fiber diet in the treatment of diverticular disease to the etiologic factors for the condition
✦ Describe the rationale for the symptoms associated with appendicitis
✦ Compare the causes and manifestations of small-volume diarrhea and large-volume diarrhea
✦ Explain why a failure to respond to the defecation urge may result in constipation
✦ List five causes of fecal impaction
✦ Differentiate between mechanical and paralytic intestinal obstruction in terms of cause and manifestations

✦ List conditions that cause malabsorption by impaired intraluminal malabsorption, mucosal malabsorption, and lymphatic obstruction
✦ List the risk factors associated with colorectal cancer and cite the screening methods for detection

There are many similarities in conditions that disrupt the integrity and function of the small and large intestines. The walls of the small and large intestines consists of five layers (see Chapter 36, Fig. 36-3): an outer serosal layer; a muscularis layer, which is divided into a layer of circular and a layer of longitudinal muscle fibers; a submucosal layer; and an inner mucosal layer, which lines the lumen of the intestine. Among the conditions that cause altered intestinal function are irritable bowel disease, inflammatory bowel disease, diverticulitis, appendicitis, alterations in bowel motility (*i.e.,* diarrhea, constipation, and bowel obstruction), malabsorption syndrome, and cancer of the colon and rectum.

IRRITABLE BOWEL SYNDROME

The term *irritable bowel syndrome* is used to describe a functional gastrointestinal disorder characterized by a variable combination of chronic and recurrent intestinal symptoms not explained by structural or biochemical abnormalities. There is evidence to suggest that 10% to 20% of people in Western countries have the disorder, although most do not seek medical attention.[27,28]

The condition is characterized by persistent or recurrent symptoms of abdominal pain, altered bowel function, and varying complaints of flatulence, bloatedness, nausea and anorexia, and anxiety or depression. A hallmark of irritable bowel syndrome is abdominal pain that is relieved by defecation and associated with a change in consistency or frequency of stools.

Irritable bowel syndrome is believed to result from dysregulation of intestinal motor and sensory functions modulated by the CNS.[28] Persons with irritable bowel syndrome tend to experience increased motility and abnormal intestinal contractions in response to psychological and physiologic stress. The role that psychological factors play in the disease is uncertain. Although changes in intestinal activity are normal responses to stress, these responses appear to be exaggerated in persons with irritable bowel syndrome. Women tend to be affected more often than men. Menarche often is associated with onset of the disorder. Women frequently notice an exacerbation of symptoms during the premenstrual period, suggesting a hormonal component.

Diagnosis of irritable bowel syndrome is based on continuous or recurrent symptoms of at least 3 months' duration consisting of abdominal pain or discomfort relieved by defecation, a change in the frequency or consistency of stool, and the presence of three or more varying patterns of altered defecation that are present at least 25% of the time.[29] These patterns of defecation include altered stool frequency, altered stool form (*i.e.,* hard or loose, watery stool), altered stool passage (*i.e.,* straining, urgency, or feeling of incomplete evacuation), passage of mucus, and bloating or feeling of abdominal discomfort. A history of lactose intolerance should be considered because intolerance to lactose and other sugars may be a precipitating factor in some persons.

The treatment of irritable bowel syndrome focuses on methods of stress management, particularly those related to symptom production. Reassurance is important. Usually, no special diet is indicated, although adequate fiber intake usually is recommended. Avoidance of offending dietary substances such as fatty and gas-producing foods, alcohol, and caffeine-containing beverages may be beneficial. Various pharmacologic agents, including antispasmodic and anticholinergic drugs, have been used with varying success in treatment of the disorder.

INFLAMMATORY BOWEL DISEASE

The term *inflammatory bowel disease* is used to designate two related inflammatory intestinal disorders: Crohn's disease and ulcerative colitis.[30,31] The prevalence of these diseases ranges from 300,000 to 500,000. Although the two diseases differ sufficiently to be distinguishable, they have many features in common. Both diseases produce inflammation of the bowel, both lack confirming evidence of a proven causative agent, both have a pattern of familial occurrence, and both can be accompanied by systemic manifestations.[20] The distinguishing characteristics of Crohn's disease and ulcerative colitis are summarized in Table 37-1.

The causes of Crohn's disease and ulcerative colitis are largely unknown. The diseases appear to have a familial occurrence, suggesting a hereditary predisposition. There is an increased prevalence of the disease among first-degree relatives. Approximately 15% of persons with inflammatory bowel disease have affected first-degree relatives.[15] One of the common beliefs is that genetic factors predispose to some form of autoimmune reaction, possibly triggered by some relatively innocuous environmental agent such as a dietary antigen or microbial agent. It also is thought that the diseases may have an infectious origin. Research literature implicates many suspect agents, including *Chlamydia*, atypical bacteria, and mycobacteria.[15] Another theory is one of defective immunoregulation in which the mucosal branch of the immune system is stimulated and then fails to down-regulate. Although psychogenic factors may contribute to the severity and onset of both conditions, it seems unlikely that they are the primary cause.

The clinical manifestation of both Crohn's disease and ulcerative colitis are ultimately the result of activation of inflammatory cells with elaboration of inflammatory mediators that cause nonspecific tissue damage. Both diseases are characterized by remissions and exacerbations of diarrhea, fecal urgency, and weight loss. Acute complications such as intestinal obstruction may develop during periods of fulminant disease.

A number of systemic manifestations have been identified in persons with Crohn's disease and ulcerative colitis. These include axial arthritis affecting the spine and sacroiliac joints and oligoarticular arthritis affecting the large joints of the arms and legs; inflammatory conditions of the eye, usually uveitis; skin lesions, especially erythema nodosum; stomatitis; and autoimmune anemia, hypercoagulability of the blood, and sclerosing cholangitis. Occasionally, these systemic manifestations may herald the recurrence of intestinal disease. In children, growth retardation may occur, particularly if the symptoms are prolonged and nutrient intake has been poor.

Crohn's Disease

Crohn's disease is a recurrent, granulomatous type of inflammatory response that can affect any area of the gastrointestinal tract from the mouth to the anus. In nearly 40% of persons with the disease, the lesions are restricted to the small intestine; in 30%, only the large bowel is affected; and in the remaining 30%, the large bowel and small bowel are affected.[15] It is a slowly progressive, relentless, and often disabling disease. Despite the substantial increase in the prevalence of Crohn's disease in the early 1980s, the distribution of affected sites has not changed substantially. The disease usually strikes adolescents and young adults and is most common among persons of European origin, with considerably higher frequency among Ashkenazi Jews.[20]

A characteristic feature of Crohn's disease is the sharply demarcated, granulomatous lesions that are surrounded by

TABLE 37-1 ✦ Differentiating Characteristics of Crohn's Disease and Ulcerative Colitis		
Characteristic	**Crohn's Disease**	**Ulcerative Colitis**
Types of inflammation	Granulomatous	Ulcerative and exudative
Level of involvement	Primarily submucosal	Primarily mucosal
Extent of involvement	Skip lesions	Continuous
Areas of involvement	Primarily ileum, secondarily colon	Primarily rectum and left colon
Diarrhea	Common	Common
Rectal bleeding	Rare	Common
Fistulas	Common	Rare
Strictures	Common	Rare
Perianal abscesses	Common	Rare
Development of cancer	Uncommon	Relatively common

normal-appearing mucosal tissue. When the lesions are multiple, they often are referred to as *skip lesions* because they are interspersed between what appear to be normal segments of the bowel. All the layers of the bowel are involved, with the submucosal layer affected to the greatest extent. The surface of the inflamed bowel usually has a characteristic "cobblestone" appearance resulting from the fissures and crevices that develop and that are surrounded by areas of submucosal edema (Fig. 37-4). There usually is a relative sparing of the smooth muscle layers of the bowel, with marked inflammatory and fibrotic changes of the submucosal layer. The bowel wall, after a time, often becomes thickened and inflexible; its appearance has been likened to a lead pipe or rubber hose. The adjacent mesentery may become inflamed, and the regional lymph nodes and channels may become enlarged.

The clinical course of Crohn's disease is variable; often, there are periods of exacerbations and remissions, with symptoms being related to the location of the lesions. The principal symptoms include intermittent diarrhea, colicky pain (usually in the lower right quadrant), weight loss, fluid and electrolyte disorders, malaise, and low-grade fever. Because Crohn's disease affects the submucosal layer to a greater extent than the mucosal layer, there is less bloody diarrhea than with ulcerative colitis. Ulceration of the perianal skin is common, largely because of the severity of the diarrhea. The absorptive surface of the intestine may be disrupted; nutritional deficiencies may occur, related to the specific segment of the intestine that is involved. When Crohn's disease occurs in childhood, one of its major manifestations may be retardation of growth and physical development.[20]

Complications of Crohn's disease include fistula formation, abdominal abscess formation, and intestinal obstruction. Fistulas are tubelike passages that form connections between different sites in the gastrointestinal tract. They also may develop between other sites, including the bladder, vagina, urethra, and skin. Perineal fistulas that originate in the ileum are relatively common. Fistulas between segments of the gastrointestinal tract may lead to mal-absorption, syndromes of bacterial overgrowth, and diarrhea. They also can become infected and cause abscess formation.

Diagnosis and Treatment. The diagnosis of Crohn's disease requires a thorough history and physical examination. Sigmoidoscopy is used for direct visualization of the affected areas and to obtain biopsies. Measures are taken to exclude infectious agents as the cause of the disorder. This usually is accomplished by the use of stool cultures and examination of fresh stool specimens for ova and parasites. In persons suspected of having Crohn's disease, radiologic contrast studies provide a means for determining the extent of involvement of the small bowel and establishing the presence and nature of fistulas. CT scans may be used to detect an inflammatory mass or abscess.

Treatment methods focus on terminating the inflammatory response and promoting healing, maintaining adequate nutrition, and preventing and treating complications. Several medications have been successful in suppressing the inflammatory reaction, including the corticosteroids, sulfasalazine, metronidazole, 6-mercaptopurine, and cyclosporine. Surgical resection of damaged bowel, drainage of abscesses, or repair of fistula tracts may be necessary.

Sulfasalazine is a topically active agent that has a variety of anti-inflammatory effects. The beneficial effects of the sulfasalazine are attributable to one component of the drug, 5-aminosalicylic acid (5-ASA). Agents containing 5-ASA affect multiple sites in the arachidonic acid pathway critical to the pathogenesis of inflammation. Sulfasalazine contains 5-ASA with sulfapyridine linked to an azo bond. The drug is poorly absorbed from the intestine, and the azo linkage is broken down by the bacterial flora in the ileum and colon to release 5-ASA. Metronidazole is an antibiotic used to treat bacterial overgrowth in the small intestine. Immunosuppressive drugs such as azathioprine and its active derivative, 6-mercaptopurine, also may be used.

In 1999, the U.S. Food and Drug Administration (FDA) approved the drug infliximab for treatment of moderate to severe Crohn's disease that does not respond to standard therapies or for the treatment of open draining fistulas.[32] Infliximab, the first treatment approved specifically for Crohn's disease, is a monoclonal antibody that targets the destruction of tumor necrosis factor-α (TNF-α), a mediator of the inflammatory response. TNF-α is known to be important in granulomatous inflammatory processes such as Crohn's disease.

Nutritional deficiencies are common in Crohn's disease because of diarrhea, steatorrhea, and other malabsorption problems. A nutritious diet that is high in calories, vitamins, and proteins is recommended. Because fats often aggravate the diarrhea, it is recommended that they be avoided. Elemental diets, which are nutritionally balanced but residue free and bulk free, may be given during the acute phase of the illness. These diets are largely absorbed in the jejunum and allow the inflamed bowel to rest. Total parenteral nutrition (*i.e.,* parenteral hyperalimentation) consists of intravenous administration of hypertonic glucose solutions to which amino acids and fats may be added. This form of nutritional therapy may be needed when food cannot be absorbed from the intestine. Because of the hypertonicity of

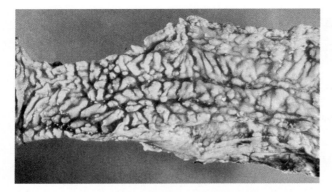

FIGURE 37-4 Crohn's disease. The mucosal surface of the colon displays a "cobblestone" appearance owing to the presence of linear ulcerations and edema and inflammation of the intervening tissue. (From Rubin E., Farber J.L. [1999]. *Pathology* [3rd ed., p. 728]. Philadelphia: Lippincott Williams & Wilkins)

these solutions, they must be administered through a large-diameter central vein.

Fish oil in an enteric-coated preparation has been used to prevent relapses in persons with Crohn's disease.[33] It has been suggested that the oil acts at multiple points in altering the inflammatory process that becomes activated in Crohn's disease, particularly as it relates to the production of messenger molecules of the immune system that attract inflammatory cells.[34]

Ulcerative Colitis

Ulcerative colitis is a nonspecific inflammatory condition of the colon. The disease begins most often between 20 and 25 years of age, but the condition may affect both younger and older persons.[15] Unlike Crohn's disease, which can affect various sites in the gastrointestinal tract, ulcerative colitis is confined to the rectum and colon. The disease usually begins in the rectum and spreads proximally, affecting primarily the mucosal layer, although it can extend into the submucosal layer. The length of proximal extension varies. It may involve the rectum alone (ulcerative proctitis), the rectum and sigmoid colon (proctosigmoiditis), or the entire colon (pancolitis). The inflammatory process tends to be confluent and continuous instead of skipping areas, as it does in Crohn's disease.

Characteristic of the disease are the lesions that form in the crypts of Lieberkühn in the base of the mucosal layer (see Chapter 36, Fig. 36-12). The inflammatory process leads to the formation of pinpoint mucosal hemorrhages, which in time suppurate and develop into *crypt abscesses*. These inflammatory lesions may become necrotic and ulcerate. Although the ulcerations usually are superficial, they often extend, causing large denuded areas (Fig. 37-5). As a result of the inflammatory process, the mucosal layer often develops tonguelike projections that resemble polyps and therefore are called *pseudopolyps*. The bowel wall thickens in response to repeated episodes of colitis.

Diarrhea, which is the characteristic manifestation of ulcerative colitis, varies according to the severity of the disease. There may be up to 30 to 40 bowel movements a day. Because ulcerative colitis affects the mucosal layer of the bowel, the stools typically contain blood and mucus. Nocturnal diarrhea usually occurs when daytime symptoms are severe. There may be mild abdominal cramping and fecal incontinence. Anorexia, weakness, and fatigability are common.

Ulcerative colitis usually follows a course of remissions and exacerbations. The severity of the disease varies from mild to fulminating. Accordingly, the disease has been divided into three types: mild chronic, chronic intermittent, and acute fulminating. The most common form of the disease is the mild chronic, in which bleeding and diarrhea are mild and systemic signs are minimal or absent. This form of the disease usually can be managed conservatively. The chronic intermittent form continues after the initial attack. Compared with the milder form, more of the colon surface usually is involved with the chronic intermittent form, and there are more systemic signs and complications. In approximately 15% of affected persons, the disease assumes a more fulminant course, involves the entire colon, and manifests with severe, bloody diarrhea, fever, and acute abdominal pain. These persons are at risk for development of toxic megacolon, which is characterized by dilatation of the colon and signs of systemic toxicity. It results from extension of the inflammatory response, with involvement of neural and vascular components of the bowel. Contributing factors include use of laxatives, narcotics, and anticholinergic drugs and the presence of hypokalemia.

Cancer of the colon is one of the feared complications of ulcerative colitis. The risk for development of cancer among persons who have had pancolitis for 10 years or more is 20 to 30 times that of the general population.[15]

Diagnosis and Treatment. Diagnosis of ulcerative colitis is based on history and physical examination. The diagnosis usually is confirmed by proctosigmoidoscopy.

Treatment depends on the extent of the disease and severity of symptoms. It includes measures to control the acute manifestations of the disease and prevent recurrence. Some people with mild to moderate symptoms are able to control their symptoms simply by avoiding caffeine, lactose (milk), highly spiced foods, and gas-forming foods. Fiber supplements may be used to decrease diarrhea and rectal symptoms.

The medications used in treatment of ulcerative colitis are similar to those used in the treatment of Crohn's disease. They include the use of nonabsorbable 5-ASA compounds (*e.g.,* mesalamine, olsalaxine). The corticosteroids are used selectively to lessen the acute inflammatory response. Many of these medications can be administered rectally by suppository or enema. Immunosuppressant drugs, such as cyclosporine, may be used to treat persons with severe colitis.

The observation that smokers are less likely to develop ulcerative colitis led to investigation of the use of nicotine patches in the treatment of ulcerative colitis.[35] Although the mechanisms of nicotine's action are unclear, some of the results have been promising.[36]

Surgical treatment (*i.e.,* removal of the rectum and entire colon) with the creation of an ileostomy or ilioanal

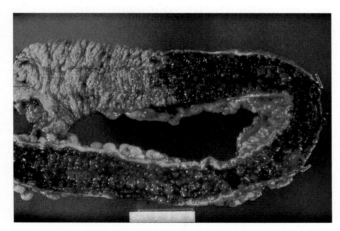

FIGURE 37-5 Ulcerative colitis. Prominent erythema and ulceration of the colon begin in the ascending colon and are most severe in the rectosigmoid area. (From Rubin E., Farber J.L. [1999]. *Pathology* [3rd ed., p. 731]. Philadelphia: Lippincott Williams & Wilkins)

anastomosis may be required for those persons with ulcerative colitis who do not respond to conservative methods of treatment.

INFECTIOUS COLITIS

Two forms of pathogens have emerged as important causes of infectious colitis: *Clostridium difficile* and *Escherichia coli* serotype O157:H7.

Clostridium Difficile Colitis

C. difficile, the agent that causes pseudomembranous colitis associated with antibiotic therapy, has been identified as a common nosocomial pathogen. *C. difficile* is a gram-positive, spore-forming bacillus that is part of normal flora in 2% to 10% of humans.[37] The spores are resistant to the acid environment of the stomach and convert to vegetative forms in the colon. The organism also is resistant to most commonly used antibiotics. Treatment with broad-spectrum antibiotics predisposes to disruption of the normal bacterial flora of the colon, leading to colonization by *C. difficile* along with the release of toxins that cause mucosal damage and inflammation. Almost any antibiotic may cause *C. difficile* colitis, but broad-spectrum antibiotics with activity against gram-negative enteric bacteria are the most frequent agents.[38] After antibiotic therapy has made the bowel susceptible to infection, colonization by *C. difficile* occurs by the oral-fecal route. *C. difficile* infection usually is acquired in the hospital, where the organism is commonly encountered.

C. difficile infection may involve antibiotic-associated colitis without pseudomembrane formation or pseudomembranous colitis. Fortunately, most cases are not severe and do not involve pseudomembrane formation. The infection commonly manifests with diarrhea that is mild to moderate and sometimes is accompanied by lower abdominal cramping. Symptoms usually begin during or shortly after antibiotic therapy has been initiated, although they can be delayed for weeks. In most cases, systemic manifestations are absent, and the symptoms subside after the antibiotic has been discontinued.

The more severe form of the disease, pseudomembranous colitis, is characterized by an adherent inflammatory membrane overlying the areas of mucosal injury. It is a life-threatening form of the disease. Persons with the disease are acutely ill, with lethargy, fever, tachycardia, abdominal pain and distention, and dehydration. The smooth muscle tone of the colon may be lost, resulting in toxic dilatation of the colon. Prompt therapy is needed to prevent perforation of the bowel.

Diagnostic findings include a history of antibiotic use and laboratory tests that confirm the presence of *C. difficile* toxins in the stool. Treatment includes the immediate discontinuation of antibiotic therapy. Specific treatment aimed at eradicating *C. difficile* is used when symptoms are severe or persistent. Metronidazole is the drug of first choice, with vancomycin being reserved for persons who cannot tolerate metronidazole or do not respond to the drug. Both drugs are given orally.[37,38] Metronidazole is absorbed from the upper gastrointestinal tract and may cause side effects. Vancomycin is poorly absorbed, and its actions are limited to the gastrointestinal tract.

Escherichia Coli O157:H7 Infection

E. coli O157:H7 has become recognized as an important cause of epidemic and sporadic colitis. The organism became widely known with a well-publicized outbreak that was associated with undercooked hamburger meat from a national fast-food chain.

E. coli O157:H7 is a strain of *E. coli* found in feces and contaminated milk of healthy dairy and beef cattle, but it also has been found in pork, poultry, and lamb. Infection usually is by food-borne transmission, often by ingesting undercooked hamburger. The organism also can be transferred to nonmeat products such as fruits and vegetables. Person-to-person transmission may occur, particularly in nursing homes, day care settings, and hospitals. The very young and the very old are particularly at risk for the infection and its complications.

The infection may cause no symptoms or cause a variety of manifestations, including acute, nonbloody diarrhea, hemorrhagic colitis, hemolytic-uremic syndrome, and thrombotic thrombocytopenic purpura. The infection often presents with abdominal cramping and watery diarrhea and subsequently may progress to bloody diarrhea. The diarrhea commonly lasts 3 to 7 days or longer, with 10 to 12 diarrheal episodes per day. Fever occurs in up to one third of the cases.

An important aspect of the disease is the production of toxins and the ability to produce toxemia. The two complications of the infection, hemolytic-uremic syndrome and thrombotic thrombocytopenic purpura, reflect the effects of toxins. Hemolytic-uremic syndrome is characterized by hemolytic anemia, thrombocytopenia, and renal failure. It occurs predominantly in infants and young children and is the most common cause of acute renal failure in children.[39] It has a mortality rate of 5% to 10%, and one third of the survivors are left with permanent disability. Thrombotic thrombocytopenic purpura is manifested by thrombocytopenia, renal failure, fever, and neurologic manifestations. It often is regarded as the severe form of the disease that leads to hemolytic-uremic syndrome plus neurologic problems.

No specific therapy is available for *E. coli* O157:H7 infection. Treatment is largely symptomatic and directed toward treating the effects of complications. Antibiotics have not proved useful and may even be harmful, extending the duration of bloody diarrhea.

Because of the seriousness of the infection and its complications, education of the public about techniques for decreasing primary transmission of the infection from animal sources is important. Undercooked meats and unpasteurized milk are sources of transmission. The FDA recommends a minimal internal temperature of 155°F for cooked hamburger. Food handlers and consumers should be aware of the proper methods for handling uncooked meat to prevent cross-contamination of other foods. Particular attention should be paid to hygiene in day care centers and nursing homes, where the spread of infection to the very young and very old may result in severe complications.[39]

DIVERTICULAR DISEASE

Diverticulosis is a condition in which the mucosal layer of the colon herniates through the muscularis layer.[40,41] Often, there are multiple diverticula, and most occur in the sigmoid

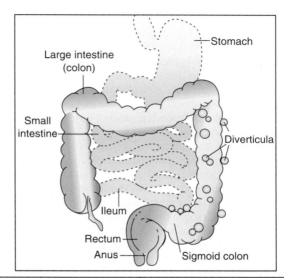

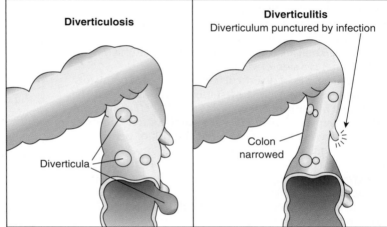

FIGURE 37-6 (**Top**) Location of diverticula in the sigmoid colon. (**Bottom left**) Diverticulosis. (**Bottom right**) Diverticulitis. (National Digestive Diseases Information Clearinghouse. [1989]. *Clearinghouse fact sheet: Diverticulosis and diverticulitis.* NIH publication 90–1163. Washington, DC: US Department of Health and Human Services)

colon (Fig. 37-6). Diverticular disease is common in Western society, affecting approximately 5% to 10% of the population older than 45 years of age and almost 80% of those older than 85 years.[40] Although the disorder is prevalent in the developed countries of the world, it is almost nonexistent in many African nations and underdeveloped countries. This suggests that dietary factors (*e.g.*, lack of fiber content), a decrease in physical activity, and poor bowel habits (*e.g.*, neglecting the urge to defecate), along with the effects of aging, contribute to the development of the disease.

In the colon, the longitudinal muscle does not form a continuous layer, as it does in the small bowel. Instead, there are three separate longitudinal bands of muscle called the *teniae coli*. In a manner similar to the small intestine, bands of circular muscle constrict the large intestine. At each of these constrictive points (approximately every 2.5 cm), the circular muscle contracts, sometimes constricting the lumen of the bowel so that it is almost occluded. The combined contraction of the circular muscle and the lack of a continuous longitudinal muscle layer causes the intestine to bulge outward into pouches called *haustra* (Fig. 37-7). Diverticula develop between the longitudinal muscle bands of the haustra, in the area where the blood vessels pierce the

circular muscle layer to bring blood to the mucosal layer. An increase in intraluminal pressure in the haustra provides the force for creating these herniations. The increase in pressure is thought to be related to the volume of the colonic contents. The scantier the contents, the

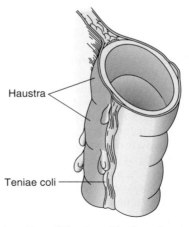

FIGURE 37-7 A portion of the sigmoid colon, showing the haustra and teniae coli.

more vigorous are the contractions and the greater is the pressure in the haustra.

Most persons with diverticular disease remain asymptomatic. The disease often is found when x-ray studies are done for other purposes. When symptoms do occur, they often are attributed to irritable bowel syndrome or other causes. Ill-defined lower abdominal discomfort, a change in bowel habits (*e.g.*, diarrhea, constipation), bloating, and flatulence are common.

Diverticulitis is a complication of diverticulosis in which there is inflammation and gross or microscopic perforation of the diverticulum. One of the most common complaints of diverticulitis is pain in the lower left quadrant, accompanied by nausea and vomiting, tenderness in the lower left quadrant, a slight fever, and an elevated white blood cell count. These symptoms usually last for several days, unless complications occur, and usually are caused by localized inflammation of the diverticula with perforation and development of a small, localized abscess. Complications include perforation with peritonitis, hemorrhage, and bowel obstruction. Fistulas can form, usually involving the bladder (*i.e.*, vesicosigmoid fistula) but sometimes involving the skin, perianal area, or small bowel. Pneumaturia (*i.e.*, air in the urine) is a sign of vesicosigmoid fistula.

The diagnosis of diverticular disease is based on history and presenting clinical manifestations. The disease may be confirmed by barium enema x-ray studies, CT scans, and ultrasonographic studies. CT scans are the safest and most cost-effective method.[40] Because of the risk of peritonitis, barium enema studies should be avoided in persons who are suspected of having acute diverticulitis. Flat abdominal radiographs may be used to detect complications associated with acute diverticulitis.

The usual treatment for diverticular disease is to prevent symptoms and complications. This includes increasing the bulk in the diet and bowel retraining so that the person has at least one bowel movement each day. The increased bulk promotes regular defecation and increases colonic contents and colon diameter, thereby decreasing intraluminal pressure. Acute diverticulitis is treated by withholding solid food and administering a broad-spectrum antibiotic. Surgical treatment is reserved for complications.

APPENDICITIS

Acute appendicitis is extremely common. It is seen most frequently in the 5- to 30-year-old age group, but it can occur at any age. The appendix becomes inflamed, swollen, and gangrenous, and it eventually perforates if not treated. Although the cause of appendicitis is unknown, it is thought to be related to intraluminal obstruction with a fecalith (*i.e.*, hard piece of stool) or to twisting.

Appendicitis usually has an abrupt onset, with pain referred to the epigastric or periumbilical area. This pain is caused by stretching of the appendix during the early inflammatory process. At approximately the same time that the pain appears, there are one or two episodes of nausea. Initially, the pain is vague, but over a period of 2 to 12 hours, it gradually increases and may become colicky. When the inflammatory process has extended to involve the serosal

layer of the appendix and the peritoneum, the pain becomes localized to the lower right quadrant. There usually is an elevation in temperature and a white blood cell count greater than $10,000/mm^3$, with 75% or more polymorphonuclear cells. Palpation of the abdomen usually reveals a deep tenderness in the lower right quadrant, which is confined to a small area approximately the size of the fingertip. It usually is located at approximately the site of the inflamed appendix. The person with appendicitis often is able to place his or her finger directly over the tender area. Rebound tenderness, which is pain that occurs when pressure is applied to the area and then released, and spasm of the overlying abdominal muscles are common.

Treatment consists of surgical removal of the appendix. Complications include peritonitis, localized periappendiceal abscess formation, and septicemia.

ALTERATIONS IN INTESTINAL MOTILITY

The movement of contents through the gastrointestinal tract is controlled by neurons located in the submucosal and myenteric plexuses of the gut (see Chapter 36). The axons from the cell bodies in the myenteric plexus innervate the circular and longitudinal smooth muscle layers of the gut. These neurons receive impulses from local receptors located in the mucosal and muscle layers of the gut and extrinsic input from the parasympathetic and sympathetic nervous systems. As a general rule, the parasympathetic nervous system tends to increase the motility of the bowel, whereas sympathetic stimulation tends to slow its activity.

Disorders of Gastrointestinal Motility

➤ The luminal contents move down the gastrointestinal tract as a result of peristaltic movements regulated by a complex interaction of neural and hormonal control mechanisms.

➤ The enteric nervous system that is incorporated into the wall of the gut controls the basic movement of the gastrointestinal tract, with input from the autonomic nervous system.

➤ Local irritation and the composition and constituents of gastrointestinal contents influence motility through the submucosal afferent neurons of the enteric nervous system. Gastrointestinal wall distention, chemical irritants, osmotic gradients, and bacterial toxins exert many of their effects on gastrointestinal motility through these afferent pathways.

➤ Autonomic influences generated by factors such as medications, trauma, and emotional experiences interact with the enteric nervous system to alter gastrointestinal motility.

The colon has sphincters at both ends: the ileocecal sphincter, which separates it from the small intestine, and the anal sphincter, which prevents the movement of feces to the outside of the body. The colon acts as a reservoir for fecal material. Normally, approximately 400 mL of water, 55 mEq of sodium, 30 mEq of chloride, and 15 mEq of bicarbonate are absorbed each day in the colon. At the same time, approximately 5 mEq of potassium is secreted into the lumen of the colon. The amount of water and electrolytes that remains in the stool reflects the absorption or secretion that occurs in the colon. The average adult ingesting a typical American diet evacuates approximately 200 to 300 g of stool each day.

Diarrhea

The usual definition of *diarrhea* is excessively frequent passage of stools. Diarrhea can be acute or chronic. Diarrhea is considered to be chronic when the symptoms persist for 3 weeks in children or adults and 4 weeks in infants. Acute diarrhea affects 500 million children throughout the world and is the leading cause of death of children younger than 4 years of age.[42] Although diarrheal disease in the United States is less prevalent than it is in other countries, it places a burden on the health care system. Approximately 220,000 children are hospitalized each year for gastroenteritis.[43]

The complaint of diarrhea is a general one and can be related to a number of pathologic and nonpathologic factors. Diarrhea can be acute or chronic. It can be caused by infectious organisms, food intolerance, drugs, or intestinal disease. Acute diarrheas that last less than 4 days are predominantly caused by infectious agents and follow a self-limited course.[44] Chronic diarrheas are those that persist for longer than 3 to 4 weeks. They often are caused by conditions such as inflammatory bowel disease, irritable bowel syndrome, malabsorption syndrome, endocrine disorders (hyperthyroidism, diabetic autonomic neuropathy), or radiation colitis.

Diarrhea commonly is divided into two types, large volume and small volume, based on the characteristics of the diarrheal stool. Large-volume diarrhea results from an increase in the water content of the stool, and small-volume diarrhea results from an increase in the propulsive activity of the bowel. Some of the common causes of small- and large-volume diarrhea are summarized in Chart 37-1. Often, diarrhea is a combination of these two types.

Large-Volume Diarrhea. Large-volume diarrhea can be classified as secretory or osmotic, according to the cause of the increased water content in the feces. Water is pulled into the colon along an osmotic gradient (*i.e.,* osmotic diarrhea) or is secreted into the bowel by the mucosal cells (*i.e.,* secretory diarrhea). The large-volume form of diarrhea usually is a painless, watery type without blood or pus in the stools.

In osmotic diarrhea, water is pulled into the bowel by the hyperosmotic nature of its contents. It occurs when osmotically active particles are not absorbed. In persons with lactase deficiency, the lactose in milk cannot be broken down and absorbed. Magnesium salts, which are contained in milk of magnesia and many antacids, are poorly absorbed

---

> ### CHART 37-1
>
> ### *Causes of Large- and Small-Volume Diarrhea*
>
> #### *Large-Volume Diarrhea*
> Osmotic diarrhea
>   Saline cathartics
>   Lactase deficiency
> Secretory diarrhea
>   Acute infectious diarrhea
>   Failure to absorb bile salts
>   Fat malabsorption
>   Chronic laxative abuse
>   Carcinoid syndrome
>   Zollinger-Ellison syndrome
>   Fecal impaction
>
> #### *Small-Volume Diarrhea*
> Inflammatory bowel disease
>   Crohn's disease
>   Ulcerative colitis
> Infectious disease
>   Shigellosis
>   Salmonellosis
> Irritable colon

---

and cause diarrhea when taken in sufficient quantities. Another cause of osmotic diarrhea is decreased transit time, which interferes with absorption. Osmotic diarrhea usually disappears with fasting.

Secretory diarrhea occurs when the secretory processes of the bowel are increased. Most acute infectious diarrheas are of this type. Enteric organisms cause diarrhea by several ways. Some are noninvasive but secrete toxins that stimulate fluid secretion (*e.g.,* pathogenic *E. coli* or *Vibrio cholerae*). Others (*e.g., Staphylococcus aureus, Bacillus cereus, Clostridium perfringens*) invade and destroy intestinal epithelial cells, thereby altering fluid transport so that secretory activity continues while absorption activity is halted.[45] Diarrhea with vomiting and fever suggests food poisoning, often caused by staphylococcal enterotoxin. Secretory diarrhea also occurs when excess bile acids remain in the intestinal contents as they enter the colon. This often happens with disease processes of the ileum because bile salts are absorbed there. It also may occur with bacterial overgrowth in the small bowel, which interferes with bile absorption. Some tumors, such as those of the Zollinger-Ellison syndrome and carcinoid syndrome, produce hormones that cause increased secretory activity of the bowel.

Small-Volume Diarrhea. Small-volume diarrhea commonly is associated with acute or chronic inflammation or intrinsic disease of the colon, such as ulcerative colitis or Crohn's disease. Small-volume diarrhea usually is evidenced by frequency and urgency and colicky abdominal pain. It commonly is accompanied by tenesmus (*i.e.,* painful straining at stool), fecal soiling of clothing, and awakening during the night with the urge to defecate.

Diagnosis and Treatment. The diagnosis of diarrhea is based on complaints of frequent stools and a history of accompanying factors such as concurrent illnesses, medication use, and exposure to potential intestinal pathogens. Disorders such as inflammatory bowel disease should be considered. If the onset of diarrhea is related to travel outside the United States, the possibility of traveler's diarrhea must be considered.

Although most acute forms of diarrhea are self-limited and require no treatment, diarrhea can be particularly serious in infants and small children, persons with other illnesses, the elderly, and even previously healthy persons if it continues for any length of time. The replacement of fluids and electrolytes therefore is considered to be a primary therapeutic goal in the treatment of diarrhea.

Oral electrolyte replacement solutions can be given in situations of uncomplicated diarrhea that can be treated at home. Complete oral rehydration solutions contain carbohydrate, sodium, potassium, chloride, and base to replace that lost in the diarrheal stool. The effectiveness of oral rehydration therapy is based on the coupled transport of sodium and glucose or other actively transported small organic molecules (see Chapter 36). Oral rehydration therapy can be particularly effective in treating dehydration associated with diarrheal disease in infants and small children. However, cost may be a factor. The bottled oral rehydration products for infants and children that are available in the United States range in price from $3.50 to $5.00 per liter. In severe cases of diarrhea, a child may require several liters per day. The cost can be a sizable burden on socioeconomically disadvantaged families, which are the same families that are at greatest risk for a poor outcome from diarrhea. Less expensive premeasured packets and recipes for preparing replacement solutions are available. The use of oral rehydration therapy also is labor intensive, requiring frequent feeding, sometimes using a spoon.[46] More important, the diarrhea does not promptly cease after oral rehydration has been instituted; this can be discouraging for parents and caregivers who desire early results from their efforts. When oral rehydration is not feasible or adequate, intravenous fluid replacement may be needed.

Evidence suggests that feeding should be continued during diarrheal illness, particularly in children.[43,47] It is recommended that children who require rehydration therapy because of diarrhea be fed an age-appropriate diet. Starch and simple proteins are thought to provide cotransport molecules with little osmotic activity, increasing fluid and electrolyte uptake by intestinal cells. It has been shown that unrestricted diets do not worsen the course or symptoms of mild diarrhea and can decrease stool output. Although there is little agreement on which foods are best, fatty foods and foods high in simple sugars are best avoided. The traditional BRAT diet of bananas, rice, applesauce, and toast usually works well.[43]

Medications used in the treatment of diarrhea include the prescription drugs diphenoxylate and difenoxin (the active metabolite of diphenoxylate) and the over-the-counter drug loperamide. These drugs act by inhibiting gastrointestinal motility via presynaptic opioid receptors in the enteric nervous system. Adsorbents, such as kaolin and pectin, adsorb irritants and toxins from the bowel. These ingredients are included in many over-the-counter antidiarrheal preparations because they adsorb toxins responsible for certain types of diarrhea. Bismuth subsalicylate can be used to reduce the frequency of unformed stools and increase stool consistency, particularly in cases of traveler's diarrhea. The drug is thought to inhibit intestinal secretion caused by enterotoxigenic *E. coli* and cholera toxins. Diarrheal medications should not be used in persons with bloody diarrhea, high fever, or signs of toxicity for fear of worsening the disease. Antibiotics are reserved for persons with identified enteric pathogens.

Constipation

Constipation can be defined as the infrequent passage of stools. The difficulty with this definition arises from the many individual variations of function that are normal. What is considered normal for one person (*e.g.,* two or three bowel movements per week) may be considered evidence of constipation by another. The problem increases with age; there is a sharp rise in health care visits for constipation after 65 years of age.

Constipation can occur as a primary problem or as a problem association with another disease condition. Some common causes of constipation are failure to respond to the urge to defecate, inadequate fiber in the diet, inadequate fluid intake, weakness of the abdominal muscles, inactivity and bed rest, pregnancy, and hemorrhoids. Diseases associated with chronic constipation include neurologic diseases such as spinal cord injury, Parkinson's disease, and multiple sclerosis; endocrine disorders such as hypothyroidism; and obstructive lesions in the gastrointestinal tract. Drugs such as narcotics, anticholinergic agents, calcium channel blockers, diuretics, calcium (antacids and supplements), iron supplements, and aluminum antacids tend to cause constipation. Elderly people with long-standing constipation may develop dilation of the rectum, colon, or both. This condition allows large amounts of stool to accumulate with little or no sensation. Constipation, in the context of a change in bowel habits, may be a sign of colorectal cancer.

Diagnosis of constipation usually is based on a history of infrequent stools, straining with defecation, the passing of hard and lumpy stools, or the sense of incomplete evacuation with defecation.[48] Constipation as a sign of another disease condition should be ruled out. The treatment of constipation usually is directed toward relieving the cause. A conscious effort should be made to respond to the defecation urge. A time should be set aside after a meal, when mass movements in the colon are most likely to occur, for a bowel movement. Adequate fluid intake and bulk in the diet should be encouraged. Moderate exercise is essential, and persons on bed rest benefit from passive and active exercises. Laxatives and enemas should be used judiciously. They should not be used on a regular basis to treat simple constipation because they interfere with the defecation reflex and actually may damage the rectal mucosa.

Fecal Impaction

Fecal impaction is the retention of hardened or putty-like stool in the rectum and colon, which interferes with normal passage of feces. If not removed, it can cause partial or complete bowel obstruction. It may occur in any age group but is more common in incapacitated elderly persons. Fecal impaction may result from painful anorectal disease, tumors, or neurogenic disease; use of constipating antacids or bulk laxatives; a low-residue diet; drug-induced colonic stasis; or prolonged bed rest and debility. In children, a habitual neglect of the urge to defecate because it interferes with play may promote impaction.[49]

The manifestations may be those of severe constipation, but frequently there is a history of watery diarrhea, fecal soiling, and fecal incontinence. This is caused by increased secretory activity of the bowel, representing the body's attempt to break up the mass so that it can be evacuated. The abdomen may be distended, and there may be blood and mucus in the stool. The fecal mass may compress the urethra, giving rise to urinary incontinence. Fecal impaction should be considered in an elderly or immobilized person who develops watery stools with fecal or urinary incontinence.

Digital examination of the rectum is done to assess for the presence of a fecal mass. The mass may need to be broken up and dislodged manually or with the use of a sigmoidoscope. Oil enemas often are used to soften the mass before removal. The best treatment is prevention.

Intestinal Obstruction

Intestinal obstruction designates an impairment of movement of intestinal contents in a cephalocaudal direction. The causes can be categorized as mechanical or paralytic obstruction. Strangulation with necrosis of the bowel may occur and lead to perforation, peritonitis, and sepsis. This is a serious complication and may increase the mortality rate of intestinal obstruction to approximately 25% if surgery is delayed.[9]

Mechanical obstruction can result from a number of conditions, intrinsic or extrinsic, that encroach on the patency of the bowel lumen (Fig. 37-8). Major inciting causes include kinking or compression of bowel due to adhesions

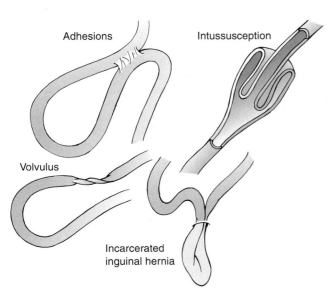

FIGURE 37-8 Causes of mechanical bowel obstruction.

caused by previous surgery or peritonitis or loops of small bowel being incarcerated or trapped in an inguinal or femoral hernia. Less common causes are strictures, tumor, foreign bodies, intussusception, and volvulus. Intussusception involves the telescoping of bowel into the adjacent segment. It is the most common cause of intestinal obstruction in children younger than 2 years of age.[50] The most common form is intussusception of the terminal ileum into the right colon, but other areas of the bowel may be involved. In most cases, the cause of the disorder is unknown. The condition can also occur in adults when an intraluminal mass or tumor acts as a traction force and pulls the segment along as it telescopes into the distal segment. Volvulus refers to a complete twisting of the bowel on an axis formed by its mesentery (see Fig. 37-8). Mechanical bowel obstruction may be a simple obstruction, in which there is no alteration in blood flow, or a strangulated obstruction, in which there is impairment of blood flow and necrosis of bowel tissue.

Paralytic, or adynamic, obstruction results from neurogenic or muscular impairment of peristalsis. Paralytic ileus is seen most commonly after abdominal surgery. It also accompanies inflammatory conditions of the abdomen, intestinal ischemia, pelvic fractures, and back injuries. It occurs early in the course of peritonitis and can result from chemical irritation caused by bile, bacterial toxins, electrolyte imbalances as in hypokalemia, and vascular insufficiency.

The major effects of both types of intestinal obstruction are abdominal distention and loss of fluids and electrolytes. Gases and fluids accumulate in the area; if untreated, the distention resulting from bowel obstruction tends to perpetuate itself by causing atony of the bowel and further distention. Distention is further aggravated by the accumulation of gases. As the process continues, the distention moves proximally (*i.e.,* toward the mouth), involving additional segments of bowel. Either form of obstruction eventually may lead to strangulation (*i.e.,* interruption of blood flow), gangrenous changes, and, ultimately, perforation of the bowel. The increased pressure in the intestine tends to compromise mucosal blood flow, leading to necrosis and movement of blood into the luminal fluids. This promotes rapid growth of bacteria in the obstructed bowel. Anaerobes grow rapidly in this favorable environment and produce lethal endotoxins.

The manifestations of intestinal obstruction depend on the degree of obstruction and its duration. With acute obstruction, the onset usually is sudden and dramatic. With chronic conditions, the onset often is more gradual. The cardinal symptoms of intestinal obstruction are pain, absolute constipation, abdominal distention, and vomiting. With mechanical obstruction, the pain is severe and colicky, in contrast with the continuous pain and silent abdomen of paralytic ileus. There also is borborygmus (*i.e.,* rumbling sounds made by propulsion of gas in the intestine); audible, high-pitched peristalsis; and peristaltic rushes. Visible peristalsis may appear along the course of the distended intestine. Extreme restlessness and conscious awareness of intestinal movements are experienced along with weakness, perspiration, and anxiety. Should strangulation occur, the symptoms change. The character of the pain shifts from the intermittent colicky pain caused by the hyperperistaltic movements of the intestine to a severe and steady type of pain. Vomiting and fluid and electrolyte disorders occur with both types of obstruction.

Diagnosis of intestinal obstruction usually is based on history and physical findings. Abdominal x-ray studies reveal a gas-filled bowel.

Treatment depends on the cause and type of obstruction. Most cases of adynamic obstruction respond to decompression of the bowel through nasogastric suction and correction of fluid and electrolyte imbalances. Strangulation and complete bowel obstruction require surgical intervention.

ALTERATIONS IN INTESTINAL ABSORPTION

Malabsorption is the failure to transport dietary constituents, such as fats, carbohydrates, proteins, vitamins, and minerals, from the lumen of the intestine to the extracellular fluid compartment for transport to the various parts of the body. It can selectively affect a single component, such as vitamin B_{12} or lactose, or its effects can extend to all the substances absorbed in a specific segment of the intestine. When one segment of the intestine is affected, another may compensate. For example, the ileum may compensate for malabsorption in the proximal small intestine by absorbing substantial amounts of fats, carbohydrates, and amino acids. Similarly, the colon, which normally absorbs water, sodium, chloride, and bicarbonate, can compensate for small intestine malabsorption by absorbing additional end products of bacterial carbohydrate metabolism.

The conditions that impair one or more steps involved in digestion and absorption of nutrients can be divided into three broad categories: intraluminal maldigestion, mucosal malabsorption, and lymphatic obstruction. Intraluminal maldigestion involves a defect in processing of nutrients in the intestinal lumen. The most common causes are pancreatic insufficiency, hepatobiliary disease, and intraluminal bacterial growth. Mucosal malabsorption is caused by mucosal lesions that impair uptake and transport of available intraluminal nutrients across the mucosal surface of the intestine. They include disorders such as celiac disease, and Crohn's disease. Lymphatic obstruction interferes with the transport of the products of fat digestion to the systemic circulation after they have been absorbed by the intestinal mucosa. The process can be interrupted by congenital defects, neoplasms, trauma, and selected infectious diseases.

Malabsorption Syndrome
The term *syndrome* implies a common constellation of symptoms arising from multiple causes. Persons with conditions that diffusely affect the small intestine and reduce its absorptive functions share certain common features referred to as *malabsorption syndrome*. Among the causes of malabsorption syndrome are celiac sprue, Crohn's disease, and resection of large segments of the small bowel.

Celiac sprue is a relatively rare chronic disease in which there is a characteristic mucosal lesion of the small intestine and impaired nutrient absorption, which improves when gluten is removed from the diet.[9,15] There is convincing evidence that the disorder is caused by an immunologic re-

sponse to the gliadin fraction of gluten. The condition results in loss of absorptive villi from the small intestine. When the resulting lesions are extensive, they may impair absorption of virtually all nutrients. In approximately one third of the cases, symptoms begin in childhood. The effects of celiac sprue usually are reversed after removal of all wheat, rye, barley, and oat gluten from the diet. Corn and rice products are not toxic and can be used as substitutes.

Persons with intestinal malabsorption usually have symptoms directly referable to the gastrointestinal tract that include diarrhea, steatorrhea, flatulence, bloating, abdominal pain, and cramps. Weakness, muscle wasting, weight loss, and abdominal distention often are present. Weight loss often occurs despite normal or excessive caloric intake. Steatorrheic stools contain excess fat. The fat content causes bulky, yellow-gray, malodorous stools that float in the toilet and are difficult to dispose of by flushing. In a person consuming a diet containing 80 to 100 g of fat each day, excretion of 7 to 9 g of fat indicates steatorrhea.

Along with loss of fat in the stools, there is failure to absorb the fat-soluble vitamins. This can lead to easy bruising and bleeding (*i.e.,* vitamin K deficiency), bone pain, a predisposition to the development of fractures and tetany (*i.e.,* vitamin D and calcium deficiency), macrocytic anemia, and glossitis (*i.e.,* folic acid deficiency). Neuropathy, atrophy of the skin, and peripheral edema may be present. Table 37-2 describes the signs and symptoms of impaired absorption of dietary constituents.

NEOPLASMS

Epithelial cell tumors of the colon and rectum are a major cause of morbidity and mortality worldwide. Although the small intestine accounts for approximately 75% of the length of the gastrointestinal tract, its tumors account for only 3% to 6% of intestinal tumors.[15]

Adenomatous Polyps
An intestinal polyp can be described as a mass that protrudes into the lumen of the gut.[15,20] Polyps can be subdivided according to their attachment to the bowel wall (sessile [raised mucosal nodules] or pedunculated [attached by a stalk]); their histopathologic appearance (hyperplastic or adenomatous); and their neoplastic potential (benign or malignant).[20] The most common types of polyps of the intestine are adenomatous polyps.

Adenomatous polyps (adenomas) are benign neoplasms that arise from the mucosal epithelium of the intestine. They are composed of neoplastic cells that have proliferated in excess of those needed to replace the cells that normally are shed from the mucosal surface (Fig. 37-9). The pathogenesis of adenoma formation involves neoplastic alteration in the replication of the crypt epithelial cells. There may be diminished apoptosis (see Chapter 5), persistence of cell replication, and failure of cell maturation and differentiation of the cells that migrate to the surface of the crypts.[20] Normally, DNA synthesis ceases as the cells reach the upper two thirds of the crypts, after which they mature, migrate to the surface, and become senescent. They then become apoptotic and are shed from the surface.[20] Adenomas arise from a disruption in this sequence, such that the

TABLE 37-2 ✦ Sites of and Requirements for Absorption of Dietary Constituents and Manifestations of Malabsorption

Dietary Constituent	Site of Absorption	Requirements	Manifestations
Water and electrolytes	Mainly small bowel	Osmotic gradient	Diarrhea Dehydration Cramps
Fat	Upper jejunum	Pancreatic lipase Bile salts Functioning lymphatic channels	Weight loss Steatorrhea Fat-soluble vitamin deficiency
Carbohydrates			
Starch	Small intestine	Amylase Maltase Isomaltase α-dextrins	Diarrhea Flatulence Abdominal discomfort
Sucrose	Small intestine	Sucrase	
Lactose	Small intestine	Lactase	
Maltose	Small intestine	Maltase	
Fructose	Small intestine		
Protein	Small intestine	Pancreatic enzymes (*e.g.,* trypsin, chymotrypsin, elastin)	Loss of muscle mass Weakness Edema
Vitamins			
A	Upper jejunum	Bile salts	Night blindness Dry eyes Corneal irritation
Folic acid	Duodenum and jejunum	Absorptive; may be impaired by some drugs (*i.e.,* anticonvulsants)	Cheilosis Glossitis Megaloblastic anemia
B_{12}	Ileum	Intrinsic factor	Glossitis Neuropathy Megaloblastic anemia
D	Upper jejunum	Bile salts	Bone pain Fractures Tetany
E	Upper jejunum	Bile salts	Uncertain
K	Upper jejunum	Bile salts	Easy bruising and bleeding
Calcium	Duodenum	Vitamin D and parathyroid hormone	Bone pain Fractures Tetany
Iron	Duodenum and jejunum	Normal pH (hydrochloric acid secretion)	Iron-deficiency anemia Glossitis

epithelial cells retain their proliferative ability throughout the entire length of the crypt. Alterations in cell differentiation can lead to dysplasia and progression to the development of invasive carcinoma.

More than half of all adenomatous polyps are located in the rectosigmoid colon and can be detected by rectal examination or sigmoidoscopy.[20] The remainder are evenly distributed throughout the rest of the colon. Adenomas can range in size from a barely visible nodule to a large, sessile mass. They can be classified as tubular, villous, or tubulovillous adenomas.

Tubular adenomas, which constitute approximately 65% of benign large bowel adenomas, typically are smooth-surfaced spheres, usually less than 2 cm in diameter, that are attached to the mucosal surface by a stalk.[20] Microscopically, they exhibit closely packed epithelial cells, which may be uniform in appearance or irregular and excessively branched. Although most tubular adenomas display little

epithelial dysplasia, approximately 20% show a range of dysplastic changes, from mild nuclear changes to frank invasive carcinoma. The risk of malignant neoplasia varies with the size of the adenoma. Approximately 1% of tubular adenomas smaller than 1 cm, 10% of those 1 to 2 cm, and 35% of those greater than 2 cm across contain invasive neoplastic carcinoma.

Villous adenomas constitute 10% of adenomas of the colon.[20] They are found predominantly in the rectosigmoid colon. They typically are broad-based, elevated lesions, with shaggy, cauliflower-like surfaces. Microscopically, they are composed of thin, tall, finger-like projections that resemble the villi of the small intestine. In contrast to tubular adenomas, villous adenomas are more likely to contain malignant cells. In polyps less than 1 cm, the risk is 10 times greater than that of a comparable-size tubular adenoma, and one third of all villous adenomas greater than 2 cm contain invasive carcinoma.[20] When invasive carcinoma occurs,

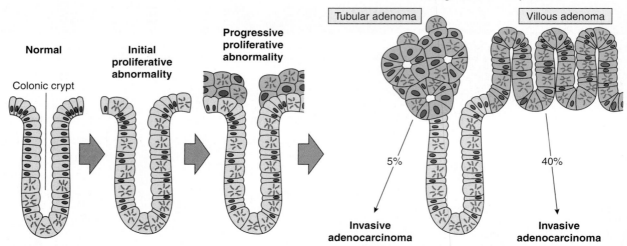

FIGURE 37-9 The histogenesis of adenomatous polyps of the colon. The initial proliferative abnormality of the colonic mucosa, the extension of the mitotic zone in the crypts, leads to accumulation of mucosal cells. The formation of adenomas may reflect epithelial–mesenchymal interactions. (From Rubin E., Farber J.L. [1999]. *Pathology* [3rd ed., p. 739]. Philadelphia: Lippincott Williams & Wilkins.) (Artist: Dimitri Karetnikov)

there is no stalk to isolate the tumor and invasion is directly into the wall of the colon.[15]

Tubulovillous adenomas manifest both tubular and villous architecture. Tubulovillous adenomas are intermediate between tubular and villous adenomas in terms of invasive carcinoma risk.

Most cases of colorectal cancer begin as benign adenomatous colonic polyps. The frequency of polyps increases with age, and the prevalence of adenomatous polyps, which is approximately 20% to 30% before 40 years of age, rises to 40% to 50% after age 60 years.[15] Men and women are equally affected. The peak incidence of adenomatous polyps precedes by some years the peak for colorectal cancer. Programs that provide careful follow-up for persons with adenomatous polyps and removal of all suspect lesions have substantially reduced the incidence of colorectal cancer.[15]

Colorectal Cancer

Colorectal cancer is the second leading cause of cancer death in the United States. In 2001, there was an estimated 98,200 new cases of colorectal cancer and 48,100 deaths from the disease.[51] The death rate for colorectal cancer has been steadily declining since the early 1980s. This may be due to a decreased number of cases because more of the cases are found earlier, and because treatments have improved.

Although the cause of cancer of the colon and rectum is largely unknown, most cases begin as adenomatous polyps. Its incidence increases with age; approximately 80% of persons who develop this form of cancer are older than 50 years of age.[15] Its incidence also is increased among persons with a family history of cancer, persons with Crohn's disease or ulcerative colitis, and those with familial adenomatous polyposis of the colon. Familial adenomatous polyposis is a rare autosomal dominant trait

linked to a mutation in the long arm of chromosome 5. Persons with the disorder develop multiple adenomatous polyps of the colon at an early age. Carcinoma of the colon is inevitable, often by 40 years of age, unless a total colectomy is performed.[20]

Diet also is thought to play a role. Attention has focused on dietary fat intake, refined sugar intake, fiber intake, and the adequacy of such protective micronutrients as vitamins A, C, and E in the diet. It has been hypothesized that a high level of fat in the diet increases the synthesis of bile acids in the liver, which may be converted to potential carcinogens by the bacterial flora in the colon. Bacterial organisms in particular are suspected of converting bile acids to carcinogens; their proliferation is enhanced by a high dietary level of refined sugars. Dietary fiber is thought to increase stool bulk and thereby dilute and remove potential carcinogens. Refined diets often contain reduced amounts of vitamins A, C, and E, which may act as oxygen free radical scavengers.

Reports indicate that aspirin may protect against colorectal cancer.[52] An analysis of the incidence of colorectal cancer in the Nurses Health Study showed a decreased incidence of colorectal cancer among women who took four to six aspirin per week.[53] Although the mechanism of aspirin's action is unknown, it may be related to its effect on the synthesis of prostaglandins, one or more of which may be involved in signal systems that influence cell proliferation or tumor growth. There has been recent interest in what has been termed *chemoprevention* or the use of oral agents such as aspirin or other NSAIDs in the prevention of colorectal cancer.[54, 55] Supplemental folate and calcium, selected vitamins, and postmenopausal hormone replacement therapy (estrogen) also have been proposed as potential chemoprotective agents. All of these agents will require more extensive study before they can be recommended for long-term chemoprevention of colorectal cancer.

Usually, cancer of the colon and rectum is present for a long time before it produces symptoms. Bleeding is a highly significant early symptom, and it usually is the one that causes persons to seek medical care. Other symptoms include a change in bowel habits, diarrhea or constipation, and sometimes a sense of urgency or incomplete emptying of the bowel. Pain usually is a late symptom.

The prognosis for persons with colorectal cancer depends largely on the extent of bowel involvement and on the presence of metastasis at the time of diagnosis. Colorectal cancer commonly is divided into four categories according to the Dukes classification or its variants.[15,20] A stage A tumor is limited to invasion of the mucosal and submucosal layers of the colon and has a 5-year survival rate of almost 100%.[15] A stage B tumor involves the entire wall of the colon, but without lymph node involvement, and has a 5-year survival rate of 43% to 67%.[15] With a stage C tumor, there is invasion of the serosal layer, with involvement of the regional lymph nodes. The 5-year survival rate is approximately 23%.[15] Stage D colorectal cancer involves far-advanced metastasis and has a much poorer prognosis.

Screening, Diagnosis, and Treatment. Among the methods used for the detection of colorectal cancers are stool occult blood tests and digital rectal examination, usually done during routine physical examinations; x-ray studies using barium (*e.g.,* barium enema); and flexible sigmoidoscopy and colonoscopy. Digital rectal examinations are most helpful in detecting neoplasms of the rectum. Rectal examination should be considered a routine part of a good physical examination. The American Cancer Society recommends that all asymptomatic men and women older than 40 years of age should have a digital rectal examination performed annually as a part of their physical examination, and that those older than 50 years should have an annual stool test for occult blood and a flexible sigmoidoscopy examination done every 5 years, as recommended by their physician.[51] Colonoscopy is recommended whenever a screening test is positive.

Almost all cancers of the colon and rectum bleed intermittently, although the amount of blood is small and usually not apparent in the stools. It therefore is feasible to screen for colorectal cancers using commercially prepared tests for occult blood in the stool. This method uses a guaiac-impregnated filter paper. The technique involves preparing two slides per day from different portions of the same stool for 3 to 4 days while the patient follows a high-fiber diet that is free of meat and ascorbic acid. Although the diet is not particularly appealing, this stool test has been shown to be a relatively reliable and inexpensive method of screening for colorectal cancer. Persons with a positive stool occult blood test should be referred to their physicians for further study. Usually, a physical examination, rectal examination, barium enema, and sigmoidoscopy or colonoscopy are done.

Flexible sigmoidoscopy involves examination of the rectum and sigmoid colon with a hollow, lighted tube that is inserted through the rectum. The procedure is performed without sedation and is well tolerated. Approximately 40% of cancers and polyps are out of the reach of the sigmoidoscope, emphasizing the need for fecal occult blood tests. Polyps can be removed or tissue can be obtained for biopsy during the procedure.

Colonoscopy provides a means for direct visualization of the rectum and colon. Compared to the sigmoidoscopy, the flexible tube used in colonoscopy is long enough to reach the full length of the colon. The colonoscope is equipped with a fiber-optic viewing system that provides for direct visualization and photographing of the inside of the entire colon. This method is used for screening persons at high risk for developing cancer of the colon (*e.g.,* those with ulcerative colitis) and for those with symptoms. Colonoscopy also is useful for obtaining a biopsy and for removing polyps. Although this method is one of the most accurate for detecting early colorectal cancers, it is not suitable for mass screening because it is expensive and time consuming and must be done by a person who is highly trained in the use of the instrument.

Carcinoembryonic antigen (CEA) can be used as a marker for colorectal cancer. However, blood levels are of little screening or diagnostic value because they become elevated only after the tumor has reached considerable size. Moreover, CEA is produced by other types of cancers and noncancerous conditions such as alcoholic cirrhosis, pancreatitis, and ulcerative colitis. This marker is of greatest value for monitoring tumor recurrence in persons after resection of the primary tumor.[15,51]

The only recognized treatment for cancer of the colon and rectum is surgical removal. Preoperative radiation therapy may be used and has in some cases demonstrated increased 5-year survival rates. Postoperative adjuvant chemotherapy with 5-fluorouracil (5-FU), 5-FU plus levamisole (an anthelmintic agent that appears to modulate the cellular immune response); or 5-FU with leucovorin (a folic acid derivative) may be used. Radiation therapy and chemotherapy are used as palliative treatment methods.

> In summary, disorders of the small and large intestines include irritable bowel syndrome, inflammatory bowel disease, diverticular disease, disorders of motility (*i.e.,* diarrhea, constipation, fecal impaction, and intestinal obstruction), alterations in intestinal absorption, and colorectal cancer.
>
> Irritable bowel syndrome is a functional disorder characterized by a variable combination of chronic and recurrent intestinal symptoms not explained by structural or biochemical abnormalities. The term *inflammatory bowel disease* is used to designate two inflammatory conditions: Crohn's disease, which affects the small and large bowel, and ulcerative colitis, which affects the colon and rectum. Both are chronic diseases characterized by remissions and exacerbations of diarrhea, weight loss, fluid and electrolyte disorders, and systemic signs of inflammation.
>
> Infectious forms of colitis include those caused by *C. difficile,* which is associated with antibiotic therapy, and *E. coli* O157:H7, which is found in undercooked hamburger and unpasteurized milk. Diverticular disease

includes diverticulosis, which is a condition in which the mucosal layer of the colon herniates through the muscularis layer, and diverticulitis, in which there is inflammation and gross or microscopic perforation of the diverticulum.

Diarrhea and constipation represent disorders of intestinal motility. Diarrhea, characterized by excessively frequent passage of stools, can be divided into large-volume diarrhea, characterized by an increased water content in the feces, and small-volume diarrhea, associated with intrinsic bowel disease and frequent passage of small stools. Constipation can be defined as the infrequent passage of stools; it commonly is caused by failure to respond to the urge to defecate, inadequate fiber or fluid intake, weakness of the abdominal muscles, inactivity and bed rest, pregnancy, hemorrhoids, and gastrointestinal disease. Fecal impaction is the retention of hardened or putty-like stool in the rectum and colon, which interferes with normal passage of feces. Intestinal obstruction designates an impairment of movement of intestinal contents in a cephalocaudal direction as the result of mechanical or paralytic mechanisms.

Malabsorption results from the impaired absorption of nutrients and other dietary constituents from the intestine. It can involve a single dietary constituent, such as vitamin B_{12}, or extend to involve all of the substances absorbed in a particular part of the small intestine. Malabsorption can result from disease of the small bowel and disorders that impair digestion and in some cases obstruct the lymph flow by which fats are transported to the general circulation.

Colorectal cancer, the second most common fatal cancer, is seen most commonly in persons older than 50 years of age. Most, if not all, cancers of the colon and rectum arise in preexisting adenomatous polyps. Programs that provide careful follow-up for persons with adenomatous polyps and removal of all suspect lesions have substantially reduced the incidence of colorectal cancer.

Disorders of the Peritoneum

After you have completed this section of the chapter, you should be able to meet the following objectives:

✦ Describe the characteristics of the peritoneum that increase its vulnerability to and protect it against the effects of peritonitis
✦ Describe the manifestations of peritonitis

PERITONITIS

Peritonitis is an inflammatory response of the serous membrane that lines the abdominal cavity and covers the visceral organs. It can be caused by bacterial invasion or chemical irritation. Most commonly, enteric bacteria enter the peritoneum because of a defect in the wall of one of the abdominal organs. The most common causes of peritonitis are perforated peptic ulcer, ruptured appendix, perforated diverticulum, gangrenous bowel, pelvic inflammatory disease, and gangrenous gallbladder. Other causes are abdominal trauma and wounds. Generalized peritonitis, although no longer the overwhelming problem it once was, is still a leading cause of death after abdominal surgery.

The peritoneum has several characteristics that increase its vulnerability to or protect it from the effects of peritonitis. One weakness of the peritoneal cavity is that it is a large, unbroken space that favors the dissemination of contaminants. For the same reason, it has a large surface that permits rapid absorption of bacterial toxins into the blood. The peritoneum is particularly well adapted for producing an inflammatory response as a means of controlling infection. It tends, for example, to exude a thick, sticky, and fibrinous substance that adheres to other structures, such as the mesentery and omentum, and that seals off the perforated viscus and aids in localizing the process. Localization is enhanced by sympathetic stimulation that limits intestinal motility. Although the diminished or absent peristalsis that occurs tends to give rise to associated problems, it does inhibit the movement of contaminants throughout the peritoneal cavity.

One of the most important manifestations of peritonitis is the translocation of extracellular fluid into the peritoneal cavity (through weeping or serous fluid from the inflamed peritoneum) and into the bowel as a result of bowel obstruction. Nausea and vomiting cause further losses of fluid. The fluid loss may encourage development of hypovolemia and shock. The onset of peritonitis may be acute, as with a ruptured appendix, or it may have a more gradual onset, as occurs in pelvic inflammatory disease. Pain and tenderness are common symptoms. The pain usually is more intense over the inflamed area. The person with peritonitis usually lies still because any movement aggravates the pain. Breathing often is shallow to prevent movement of the abdominal muscles. The abdomen usually is rigid and sometimes described as boardlike because of reflex muscle guarding. Vomiting is common. Fever, an elevated white blood cell count, tachycardia, and hypotension are common. Hiccups may develop because of irritation of the phrenic nerve. Paralytic ileus occurs shortly after the onset of widespread peritonitis and is accompanied by abdominal distention. Peritonitis that progresses and is untreated leads to toxemia and shock.

Treatment

Treatment measures for peritonitis are directed toward preventing the extension of the inflammatory response, correcting the fluid and electrolyte imbalances that develop, and minimizing the effects of paralytic ileus and abdominal distention. Surgical intervention may be needed to remove an acutely inflamed appendix or close the opening in a perforated peptic ulcer. Oral fluids are forbidden. Nasogastric suction, which entails the insertion of a tube placed through the nose into the stomach or intestine, is used to decompress the bowel and relieve the abdominal distention. Fluid and electrolyte replacement is essential. These fluids are prescribed on the basis of frequent blood chemistry determinations. Antibiotics are given to combat infection. Narcotics often are needed for pain relief.

> In summary, peritonitis is an inflammatory response of the serous membrane that lines the abdominal cavity and covers the visceral organs. It can be caused by bacterial invasion or chemical irritation resulting from perforation of the viscera or abdominal organs. It is characterized by severe pain, fluid and electrolyte disorders, paralytic intestinal obstruction, and sepsis. The treatment of peritonitis focuses on preventing the extension of the inflammatory response, correcting the fluid and electrolyte imbalances that develop, and minimizing the effects of bowel obstruction.

Related Web Sites

American College of Gastroenterology   www.acg.gi.org
American Gastroenterological Association   www.gastro.org
CancerNet—Digestive/gastrointestinal cancers   cancernet.nci.
  nih.gov/location.html#digestive
National Digestive Diseases Information Clearinghouse
  www.niddk.nih.gov/health/digest/nddic.htm

References

1. Koda-Kimble M.A, Young L.Y. (1996). Nausea and vomiting. In Young L.Y., Koda-Kimble M.A. (Eds.), *Applied therapeutics: The clinical use of drugs* (6th ed., pp. 105-1–105-11). Vancouver, WA: Applied Therapeutics.
2. Grélot L., Miller A.D. (1994). Vomiting: Its ins and outs. *NIPS* 9, 142–147.
3. Rockey D.C. (1999). Occult gastrointestinal bleeding. *New England Journal of Medicine* 341, 38–46.
4. Guyton A.C., Hall J.E. (2000). *Textbook of medical physiology* (10th ed., pp. 728–737). Philadelphia: W.B. Saunders.
5. Mittal R.K. (1998). The spectrum of diaphragmatic hernia. *Hospital Practice* 33 (11), 65–79.
6. Spieker M.R. (2000). Evaluating dysphagia. *American Family Physician* 61, 3639–3648.
7. Mittal R.K., Balaban D.H. (1997). The esophagogastric junction. *New England Journal of Medicine* 336, 924–931.
8. Katzka D.A., Rustgi A.K. (2000). Gastroesophageal reflux disease and Barrett's esophagus. *Medical Clinics of North America* 84, 1137–1161.
9. McQuaid K.R. (2001). Alimentary tract. In Tierney L.M., McPhee S.J., Papadakis M. (Eds.), *Current medical diagnosis and treatment 2001* (40th ed., pp. 585–569, 604–615, 618–621, 624–665). New York: Lange Medical Books/McGraw-Hill.
10. Alexander J.A., Hunt L.W., Patel A.M. (1999). Prevalence, pathophysiology, and treatment of patients with asthma and gastroesophageal reflux disease. *Mayo Clinic Proceedings* 75, 1055–1063.
11. Patterson P.E., Harding S.M. (1999). Gastroesophageal reflux disorders and asthma. *Current Opinion in Pulmonary Medicine* 5, 63–67.
12. Scott M., Gelhot A.R. (1999). Gastroesophageal reflux disease: Diagnosis and management. *American Family Physician* 59, 1161–1169, 1199.
13. Mason D.B. (2000). Gastroesophageal reflux in children. *Nursing Clinics of North America* 35, 15–36.
14. Herbst J.J. (2000). The esophagus. In Behrman R.E., Kliegman R.M., Jenson H.B. (Eds.). *Nelson textbook of pediatrics* (16th ed., pp. 1125–1126). Philadelphia: W.B. Saunders.
15. Cotran R.S., Kumar V.S., Collins T. (1999). *Pathologic basis of disease* (6th ed., pp. 776–787, 813–814, 826–836, 927). Philadelphia: W.B. Saunders.
16. National Cancer Institute. (2001). Esophageal cancer. [On-line]. Available: http://www.cancernet.nci.nih.gov/cancer_Types/Esophageal_Cancer.shtml.
17. Fromm D. (1987). Mechanisms involved in gastric mucosal resistance to injury. *Annual Review of Medicine* 38, 119–128.
18. Wolfe M.M., Lichtenstein D.R., Singh G. (1999). Gastrointestinal toxicity of nonsteroidal antiinflammatory drugs. *New England Journal of Medicine* 340, 1888–1899.
19. Cryer B., Lee E., Feldman M. (1992). Factors influencing mucosal prostaglandin concentrations: Role of smoking and aging. *Annals of Internal Medicine* 116, 636–640.
20. Hamilton S.R., Farber J.L., Rubin E. (1999). The gastrointestinal tract. In Rubin E., Farber J.L. (Eds.), *Pathology* (3rd ed., pp. 688–695, 727–746). Philadelphia: Lippincott Williams & Wilkins.
21. Shiotani A., Nurgalieva Z.Z., Yamaoka Y., Graham D.Y. (2000). *Helicobacter pylori. Medical Clinics of North America* 84, 1125–1136.
22. Soll A.H. (1996). Medical treatment of peptic ulcer disease: Practice guidelines. *Journal of the American Medical Association* 275, 622–629.
23. Fass R., Rosen H.R., Walsh J.H. (1995). Zollinger-Ellison syndrome: Diagnosis and management. *Hospital Practice* 30 (11), 73–80.
24. Zuckerman G.R., Cort D., Schuman R.B. (1988). Stress ulcer syndrome. *Journal of Intensive Care Medicine* 3, 21–31.
25. Konopad E., Noseworthy T. (1988). Stress ulceration: A serious complication in critically ill patients. *Heart and Lung* 17, 339–347.
26. National Cancer Institute. (2001). Gastric cancer. [On-line]. Available: http://www.cancernet.nci.nih.gov/cancer_Types/Stomach_(Gastric)_Cancer.shtml.
27. Rothenstein R.D. (2000). Irritable bowel syndrome. *Medical Clinics of North America* 85, 1247–1257.
28. Dalton C.B., Drossman D.A. (1997). Diagnosis and treatment of irritable bowel syndrome. *American Family Physician* 55, 875–880, 883–885.
29. Thompson W.G., Doteval G., Drossman D.A., et al. (1989). Irritable bowel syndrome: Guidelines for diagnosis. *Gastrointestinal International* 2, 92–95.
30. Stotland B.R., Stein R.B., Lichtenstein G.R. (2000). Advances in inflammatory bowel disease. *Medical Clinics of North America* 84, 1107–1123.
31. Botoman V.A., Bonner G.F., Botoman D.A. (1998). Management of inflammatory bowel disease. *American Family Physician* 57, 57–68, 71–72.
32. Lewis C. (1999). Crohn's disease: New drug may help when others fail. *FDA Consumer Magazine.* [On-line]. Available: http://www.fda.gov/fdac/features/1999/599_crohn.html.
33. Belluzzi A., Brignola C., Campieri M., Pera A., Baschis S., Miglioli M. (1996). Effect of enteric-coated fish-oil preparation on relapses in Crohn's disease. *New England Journal of Medicine* 334, 1557–1560.
34. Hodgson H.J. (1996). Keeping Crohn's disease quiet. *New England Journal of Medicine* 334, 1599–1600.
35. Bonner G.F. (1996). Current medical therapy for inflammatory bowel disease. *Southern Medical Journal* 89, 556–566.
36. Hanauer S.B. (1994). Nicotine for colitis: The smoke has not yet cleared. *New England Journal of Medicine* 341, 38–46.

37. Kelly C.P., Pothoulakis C., LaMont J.T. (1994). *Clostridium difficile* colitis. *New England Journal of Medicine* 330, 257–261.

38. Mylonakis E., Ryan E.T., Claderswood S.B. (2001). *Clostridium difficile*-associated diarrhea: A review. *Archives of Internal Medicine* 161, 525–533.

39. Greenwald D.A., Brandt L.J. (1997). Recognizing *E. coli* O157:H7 infection. *Hospital Practice* 32, 123–140.

40. Ferzoco L.B., Raptopoulos V., Silen W. (1998). Acute diverticulitis. *New England Journal of Medicine* 338, 1521–1526.

41. Van Ness M., Peller C. (1991). Acute diverticular disease: Diagnosis and management. *Hospital Practice* 26 (3A), 83–91.

42. Gishan F.K. (2000). Chronic diarrhea. In Bierman R.E., Kliegman R.M., Jenson H.B. (Eds.), *Nelson textbook of pediatrics* (16th ed., pp. 1171–1176). Philadelphia: W.B. Saunders.

43. Limbos M.A., Lieberman J.M. (1995). Management of acute diarrhea in children. *Contemporary Pediatrics* 12 (12), 68–88.

44. Schiller L.R. (2000). Diarrhea. *Medical Clinics of North America* 84, 1259–1275.

45. Field M., Rao M.C., Chang E.B. (1989). Intestinal electrolyte transport and diarrheal disease (part 2). *New England Journal of Medicine* 321, 879–883.

46. Avery M.E., Snyder J.D. (1990). Oral therapy for acute diarrhea. *New England Journal of Medicine* 323, 891–894.

47. American Academy of Pediatrics, Subcommittee on Acute Gastroenteritis. (1996). Practice parameter: The management of acute gastroenteritis in young children. *Pediatrics* 97 (3), 424–435.

48. Wald A. (2000). Constipation. *Medical Clinics of North America* 84, 1231–1246.

49. Wrenn K. (1989). Fecal impaction. *New England Journal of Medicine* 321, 658–662.

50. Wyllie R. (2000). Ileus, adhesions, intussusception, and closed-loop obstruction. In Bierman R.E., Kliegman R.M., Jenson H.B. (Eds.), *Nelson textbook of pediatrics* (16th ed., pp. 1142–1143). Philadelphia: W.B. Saunders.

51. American Cancer Society. (2001). Colon and rectal cancer. [On-line]. Available: http://www3.cancer.org/cancerinfo.

52. Giovannucci E., Egan K.M., Hunter D.J., Stamfer M.J., Colditz G.A., Willett W.C., et al. (1995). Aspirin and the risk of colorectal cancer in women. *New England Journal of Medicine* 333, 609–614.

53. Marcus A.J. (1995). Aspirin as prophylaxis against colorectal cancer. *New England Journal of Medicine* 333, 656–657.

54. Pasi J.A., Mayer R.J. (2000). Chemoprevention of colorectal cancer. *New England Journal of Medicine* 342, 1960–1966.

55. Bond J.H. (2000). Colorectal cancer update. *Medical Clinics of North America* 84, 1163–1182.

Chapter 38

Alterations in Function of the Hepatobiliary System and Exocrine Pancreas

The liver, the gallbladder, and the exocrine pancreas are classified as accessory organs of the gastrointestinal tract. In addition to producing digestive secretions, the liver and the pancreas have other important functions. The endocrine pancreas, for example, supplies the insulin and glucagon needed in cell metabolism, whereas the liver synthesizes glucose, plasma proteins, and blood clotting factors and is responsible for the degradation and elimination of drugs and hormones, among other functions. This chapter focuses on functions and disorders of the liver, the biliary tract and gallbladder, and the exocrine pancreas.

The Liver and Hepatobiliary System

After you have completed this section of the chapter, you should be able to meet the following objectives:

✦ Describe the lobular structures of the liver
✦ Trace the movement of blood flow into, through, and out of the liver

✦ Describe the function of the liver in terms of carbohydrate, protein, and fat metabolism
✦ State the origin of ammonia and describe the function of the liver in terms of its detoxification
✦ Characterize the function of the liver in terms of bilirubin elimination and describe the pathogenesis of unconjugated and conjugated hyperbilirubinemia
✦ Relate the mechanism of bile formation and elimination to the development of cholestasis
✦ List four laboratory tests used to assess liver function and relate them to impaired liver function

The liver is the largest visceral organ in the body, weighing approximately 1.3 kg (3 lb) in the adult. It is located below the diaphragm and occupies much of the right hypochondrium (Fig. 38-1). The falciform ligament, which extends from the peritoneal surface of the anterior abdominal wall between the umbilicus and diaphragm, divides the liver into two lobes, a large right lobe and a small left lobe. There are two additional lobes on the visceral surface of the liver: the caudate and quadrate lobes. Except for the portion that is in the epigastric area, the liver is con-

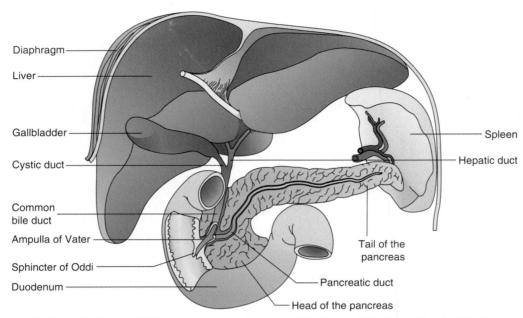

FIGURE 38-1 The liver and biliary system, including the gallbladder and bile ducts. (Chaffee E.E., Lytle I.M. [1980]. *Basic physiology and anatomy* [4th ed.]. Philadelphia: J.B. Lippincott)

tained within the rib cage and in healthy persons cannot normally be palpated. The liver is surrounded by a tough fibroelastic capsule called *Glisson's capsule.*

The liver is unique among the abdominal organs in having a dual blood supply—the hepatic artery and the portal vein. Approximately 300 mL of blood per minute enters the liver through the hepatic artery; another 1050 mL/minute enters by way of the valveless portal vein, which carries blood from the stomach, the small and the large intestines, the pancreas, and the spleen[1] (Fig. 38-2). Although the blood from the portal vein is incompletely saturated with oxygen, it supplies approximately 60% to 70% of the oxygen needs of the liver. The venous outflow from the liver is carried by the valveless hepatic veins, which empty into the inferior vena cava just below the level of the diaphragm. The pressure difference between the hepatic vein and the portal vein normally is such that the liver stores approximately 450 mL of blood.[1] This blood can be shifted back into the general circulation during periods of hypovolemia and shock. In congestive heart failure, in which the pressure in the vena cava increases, blood backs up and accumulates in the liver.

The *lobules* are the functional units of the liver. Each lobule is a cylindrical structure that measures approximately 0.8 to 2 mm in diameter and several millimeters long. There are approximately 50,000 to 100,000 lobules in the liver.[1] Each lobule is organized around a central vein that empties into the hepatic veins and from there into the vena cava. The terminal bile ducts and small branches of the portal vein and hepatic artery are located at the periphery of the lobule. Plates of hepatic cells radiate centrifugally from the central vein like spokes on a wheel (Fig. 38-3). These hepatic plates are separated by wide, thin-walled channels, called *sinusoids*, that extend from the periphery of the lobule to its

central vein. The sinusoids are supplied by blood from the portal vein and hepatic artery. Because the plates of hepatic cells are no more than two layers thick, every cell is exposed to the blood that travels through the sinusoids. Thus, the hepatic cells can remove substances from the blood or can release substances into the blood as it moves through the sinusoids.

The venous sinusoids are lined with two types of cells: the typical endothelial cells and Kupffer's cells. *Kupffer's cells* are reticuloendothelial cells that are capable of removing and phagocytizing old and defective blood cells, bacteria, and other foreign material from the portal blood as it flows through the sinusoid. This phagocytic action removes the enteric bacilli and other harmful substances that filter into the blood from the intestine.

The lobules also are supplied by small tubular channels, called *bile canaliculi*, that lie between the cell membranes of adjacent hepatocytes. The bile produced by the hepatocytes flows into the canaliculi and then to the periphery of the lobules, which drain into progressively larger ducts, until it reaches the right and left hepatic ducts. The intrahepatic and extrahepatic bile ducts often are collectively referred to as the *hepatobiliary tree.* These ducts unite to form the common duct (see Fig. 38-1). The common duct, which is approximately 10 to 15 cm long, descends and passes behind the pancreas and enters the descending duodenum. The pancreatic duct joins the common duct at a short dilated tube called *hepatopancreatic ampulla* (ampulla of Vater) which empties into the duodenum through the duodenal papilla. Muscle tissue at the junction of the papilla, called the *sphincter of Oddi*, regulates the flow of bile into the duodenum. When this sphincter is closed, bile moves back into the common duct and gallbladder.

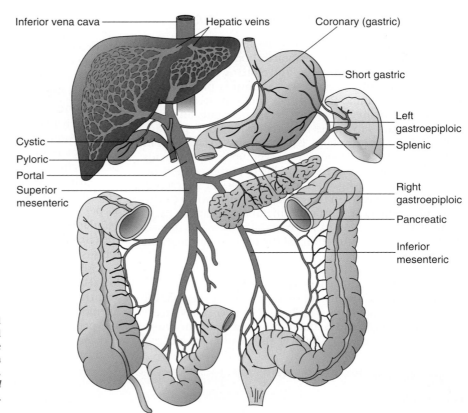

FIGURE 38-2 The portal circulation. Blood from the gastrointestinal tract, spleen, and pancreas travels to the liver by way of the portal vein before moving into the vena cava for return to the heart. (Chaffee E.E., Lytle I.M. [1980]. *Basic physiology and anatomy* [4th ed.]. Philadelphia: J.B. Lippincott)

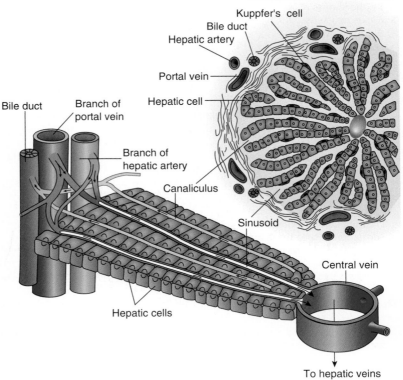

FIGURE 38-3 A section of liver lobule showing the location of the hepatic veins, hepatic cells, liver sinusoids, and branches of the portal vein and hepatic artery. (Chaffee E.E., Lytle I.M. [1980]. *Basic physiology and anatomy* [4th ed.]. Philadelphia: J.B. Lippincott)

METABOLIC FUNCTIONS OF THE LIVER

The liver is one of the most versatile and active organs in the body. It produces bile; metabolizes hormones and drugs; synthesizes proteins, glucose, and clotting factors; stores vitamins and minerals; changes ammonia produced by deamination of amino acids to urea; and converts fatty acids to ketones. The liver degrades excess nutrients and converts them into substances essential to the body. It builds carbohydrates from proteins, converts sugars to fats that can be stored, and interchanges chemical groups on amino acids so that they can be used for a number of purposes. In its capacity for metabolizing drugs and hormones, the liver serves as an excretory organ. In this respect, the bile, which carries the end-products of substances metabolized by the liver, is much like the urine, which carries the body wastes filtered by the kidneys. The functions of the liver are summarized in Table 38-1.

Carbohydrate Metabolism

The liver plays an essential role in carbohydrate metabolism and glucose homeostasis (Fig. 38-4). The liver stores excess glucose as glycogen and releases it into the circulation when blood glucose levels fall. The liver also synthesizes glucose from amino acids, glycerol, and lactic acid as a means of maintaining blood glucose during periods of fasting or increased need. The liver also converts excess carbohydrates to triglycerides for storage in adipose tissue.

Protein Synthesis and Conversion of Ammonia to Urea

The liver is an important site for protein synthesis and degradation. Amino acids used for protein synthesis are derived from dietary proteins, metabolic turnover of endogenous proteins (mainly muscle), and direct hepatic synthesis.

Although the muscle contains the greatest amount of protein, the liver has the greatest rate of protein synthesis per gram of tissue. It produces the proteins for its own cellular needs and secretory proteins that are released into the circulation. The most important of these secretory proteins is albumin.

Albumin contributes significantly to the plasma colloidal osmotic pressure (see Chapter 31) and to the binding and transport of numerous substances, including some hormones, fatty acids, bilirubin, and other anions. The liver also produces other important proteins, such as fibrinogen and the blood clotting factors.

TABLE 38-1 ◆ Functions of the Liver and Manifestations of Altered Function

Function	Manifestations of Altered Function
Production of bile salts	Malabsorption of fat and fat-soluble vitamins
Elimination of bilirubin	Elevation in serum bilirubin and jaundice
Metabolism of steroid hormones	
Sex hormones	Disturbances in gonadal function, including gynecomastia in the male
Glucocorticoids	Signs of increased cortisol levels (*i.e.,* Cushing's syndrome)
Aldosterone	Signs of hyperaldosteronism (*e.g.,* sodium retention and hypokalemia)
Metabolism of drugs	Decreased drug metabolism
	Decreased plasma binding of drugs owing to a decrease in albumin production
Carbohydrate metabolism	Hypoglycemia may develop when glycogenolysis and gluconeogenesis are impaired
Stores glycogen and synthesizes glucose from amino acids, lactic acid, and glycerol	Abnormal glucose tolerance curve may occur because of impaired uptake and release of glucose by the liver
Fat metabolism	
Formation of lipoproteins	Impaired synthesis of lipoproteins
Conversion of carbohydrates and proteins to fat	
Synthesis, recycling, and elimination of cholesterol	Altered cholesterol levels
Formation of ketones from fatty acid	
Protein metabolism	
Deamination of proteins	
Formation of urea from ammonia	Elevated blood ammonia levels
Synthesis of plasma proteins	Decreased levels of plasma proteins, particularly albumin, which contributes to edema formation
Synthesis of clotting factors (fibrinogen, prothrombin, factors V, VII, IX, X)	Bleeding tendency
Storage of mineral and vitamins	Signs of deficiency of fat-soluble and other vitamins that are stored in the liver
Filtration of blood and removal of bacteria and particulate matter by Kupffer's cells	Increased exposure of the body to colonic bacteria and other foreign matter

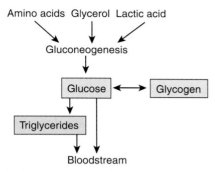

FIGURE 38-4 Hepatic pathways for storage and synthesis of glucose and conversion of glucose to fatty acids.

Through a variety of anabolic and catabolic processes, the liver is the major site of amino acid interconversion (Fig. 38-5). Hepatic catabolism and degradation involves two major reactions: transamination and deamination. In *transamination*, an amino group (NH_2) is transferred to an acceptor substance. As a result of transamination, amino acids can participate in the intermediary metabolism of carbohydrates and lipids. During periods of fasting or starvation, amino acids are used for producing glucose (*i.e.*, gluconeogenesis). Most of the nonessential amino acids are

synthesized in the liver by transamination. The process of transamination is catalyzed by *aminotransferases*, enzymes that are found in high amounts in the liver.

Oxidative *deamination* involves the removal of the amino groups from the amino acids and conversion of amino acids to ketoacids and ammonia. This occurs mainly by transamination, in which the amino groups are transferred to another acceptor substance. The acceptor substance can then transfer the amino group to still another substance or release it as ammonia. Ammonia is very toxic to body tissues, particularly neurons. The ammonia that is released during deamination is removed from the blood almost immediately and converted to urea. Essentially all urea formed in the body is synthesized by the urea cycle in the liver and is then excreted by the kidneys.[2] Although urea is mostly excreted by the kidneys, some diffuses into the intestine, where it is converted to ammonia by enteric bacteria. The intestinal production of ammonia also results from bacterial deamination of unabsorbed amino acids and protein derived from the diet, exfoliated cells, or blood in the gastrointestinal tract. Ammonia produced in the intestine is absorbed into the portal circulation and transported to the liver, where it is converted to urea before being released into the blood. Intestinal production of ammonia is increased after ingestion of high-protein foods and gastrointestinal bleeding. In advanced liver disease, urea synthesis often is impaired, leading to an accumulation of blood ammonia and subsequent reduction in blood urea nitrogen.

Pathways of Lipid Metabolism

Although most cells of body metabolize fat, certain aspects of lipid metabolism occur mainly in the liver, including oxidation of fatty acids to supply energy for other body functions; the synthesis of large quantities of cholesterol, phospholipids, and most lipoproteins; and the formation of triglycerides from carbohydrates and proteins (Fig. 38-6). To derive energy from neutral fats, the fat must first be split into glycerol and fatty acids, and then the fatty acids split by *beta oxidation* into two-carbon acetyl-coenzyme A (acetyl-CoA) units. Although beta oxidation can take place in most body cells, it occurs more rapidly in the hepatic cells. Acetyl- CoA is readily channeled into the citric acid cycle to produce adenosine triphosphate (ATP). The liver itself cannot use all the acetyl-CoA that is formed; instead, two molecules of acetyl-CoA are condensed to form acetoacetic acid, a highly soluble ketoacid that is released into the bloodstream and transported to other tissues, where it is used for energy. During periods of starvation, ketones become a major source of energy as fatty acids released from adipose tissue are converted to ketones by the liver.

Acetyl-CoA units from fat metabolism also are used to synthesize cholesterol and bile acids in the liver. Cholesterol has several fates in the liver. It can be esterified and stored; it can be exported bound to lipoproteins; or it can be converted to bile acids. The rate-limiting step in cholesterol synthesis is that which is catalyzed by 3-hydroxy-

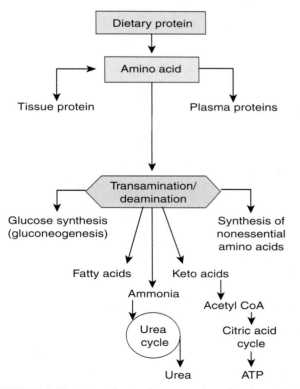

FIGURE 38-5 Hepatic pathways for conversion of amino acids to proteins, nucleic acids, ketone bodies, and glucose. The urea cycle converts ammonia generated by the deamination of amino acids to urea.

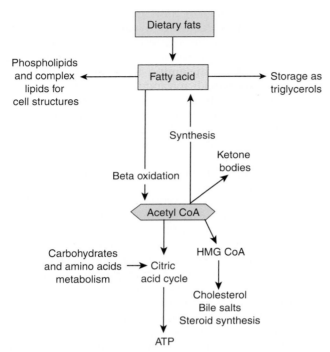

FIGURE 38-6 Hepatic pathways for fat metabolism. Beta oxidation breaks fatty acids into two carbon acetyl-coenzyme A (acetyl-CoA) units that are used in the citric acid cycle to generate adenosine triphosphate (ATP) or are used in the synthesis of ketone bodies and cholesterol.

3-methylglutaryl-coenzyme A reductase (HMG-CoA reductase). The HMG-CoA reductase inhibitors, or statins (fluvastatin, lovastatin, pravastatin, atorvastatin), that are used to to treat high cholesterol levels act by inhibiting this step in cholesterol synthesis (see Chapter 22).

Almost all the fat synthesis in the body from carbohydrates and proteins occurs in the liver. As fat is synthesized in the liver, it is transported as triglycerides in the lipoproteins to adipose tissue to be stored.

BILE PRODUCTION AND CHOLESTASIS

The secretion of bile is essential for digestion of dietary fats and absorption of fats and fat-soluble vitamins from the intestine. The liver produces approximately 600 to 1200 mL of yellow-green bile daily.[1] Bile contains water, bile salts, bilirubin, cholesterol, and certain products of organic metabolism. Of these, only bile salts, which are formed from cholesterol, are important in digestion. The other components of bile depend on the secretion of sodium, chloride, bicarbonate, and potassium by the bile ducts.

The liver forms approximately 0.6 g of bile salts daily.[1] Bile salts serve an important function in digestion; they aid in emulsifying dietary fats, and they are necessary for the formation of the micelles that transport fatty acids and fat-soluble vitamins to the surface of the intestinal mucosa for absorption. Approximately 94% of bile salts that enter the intestine are reabsorbed into the portal circulation by an active transport process that takes place in the distal ileum.

From the portal circulation, the bile salts pass into the liver, where they are recycled. Normally, bile salts travel this entire circuit approximately 18 times before being expelled in the feces.[1] This system for recirculation of bile is called the *enterohepatic circulation*.

Cholestasis

Cholestasis represents a decrease in bile flow through the intrahepatic canaliculi and a reduction in secretion of water, bilirubin, and bile acids by the hepatocytes. As a result, the materials normally transferred to the bile, including bilirubin, cholesterol, and bile acids, accumulate in the blood.[3,4] The condition may be caused by intrinsic liver disease, in which case it is referred to as *intrahepatic cholestasis*, or by obstruction of the large bile ducts, a condition known as *extrahepatic cholestasis*.

A number of mechanisms are implicated in the pathogenesis of cholestasis. Primary biliary cirrhosis and primary sclerosing cholangitis are caused by disorders of the small intrahepatic canaliculi and bile ducts. In the case of extrahepatic obstruction, such as that caused by conditions such cholelithiasis, common duct strictures, or obstructing neoplasms, the effects begin with increased pressure in the large bile ducts. Genetic disorders involving the transport of bile into the canaliculi also can result in cholestasis.

The morphologic features of cholestasis depend on the underlying cause. Common to all types of obstructive and hepatocellular cholestasis is the accumulation of bile pigment in the liver. Elongated green-brown plugs of bile are visible in the dilated bile canaliculi. Rupture of the canaliculi leads to extravasation of bile and subsequent degenerative changes in the surrounding hepatocytes. Prolonged obstructive cholestasis leads not only to fatty changes in the hepatocytes but to destruction of the supporting connective tissue, giving rise to bile lakes filled with cellular debris and pigment.[3] Unrelieved obstruction leads to portal tract fibrosis and ultimately to end-stage biliary cirrhosis.

Pruritus is the most common presenting symptom in persons with cholestasis, probably related to an elevation in plasma bile acids. Skin xanthomas (focal accumulations of cholesterol) may occur, the result of hyperlipidemia and impaired excretion of cholesterol. A characteristic laboratory finding is an elevated serum alkaline phosphatase level, an enzyme present in the bile duct epithelium and canalicular membrane of hepatocytes. Other manifestations of reduced bile flow relate to intestinal absorption, including nutritional deficiencies of fat-soluble vitamins A, D, K.

BILIRUBIN ELIMINATION AND JAUNDICE

Bilirubin is the substance that gives bile its color. It is formed from senescent red blood cells. In the process of degradation, the hemoglobin from the red blood cell is broken down to form biliverdin, which is rapidly converted to free bilirubin (Fig. 38-7). Free bilirubin, which is insoluble in plasma, is transported in the blood attached to plasma albumin. Even when it is bound to albumin, this bilirubin is still called *free bilirubin*. As it passes through the liver, free bilirubin is released from the albumin carrier molecule and moved into

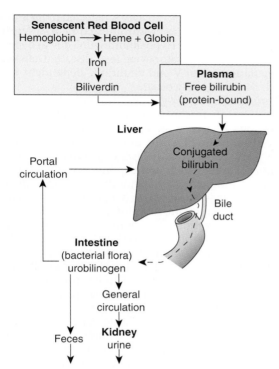

FIGURE 38-7 The process of bilirubin formation, circulation, and elimination.

the hepatocytes. Inside the hepatocytes, free bilirubin is converted to conjugated bilirubin, making it soluble in bile. Conjugated bilirubin is secreted as a constituent of bile, and in this form it passes through the bile ducts into the small intestine. In the intestine, approximately one half of the bilirubin is converted into a highly soluble substance called *urobilinogen* by the intestinal flora. Urobilinogen is either absorbed into the portal circulation or excreted in the feces. Most of the urobilinogen that is absorbed is returned to the liver to be reexcreted into the bile. A small amount of urobilinogen, approximately 5%, is absorbed into the general circulation and then excreted by the kidneys.

Usually, only a small amount of bilirubin is found in the blood; the normal level of total serum bilirubin is 0.1 to 1.2 mg/dL. Laboratory measurements of bilirubin usually measure the free and the conjugated bilirubin as well as the total bilirubin. These are reported as the direct (conjugated) bilirubin and the indirect (unconjugated or free) bilirubin.

Jaundice

Jaundice (*i.e.*, icterus) results from an abnormally high accumulation of bilirubin in the blood, as a result of which there is a yellowish discoloration to the skin and deep tissues. Jaundice becomes evident when the serum bilirubin levels rise above 2.0 to 2.5 mg/dL.[3,4] Because normal skin has a yellow cast, the early signs of jaundice often are difficult to detect, especially in persons with dark skin. Bilirubin has a special affinity for elastic tissue. The sclera of the eye, which contains considerable elastic fibers, usually is one of the first structures in which jaundice can be detected.

The four major causes of jaundice are excessive destruction of red blood cells, impaired uptake of bilirubin by the liver cells, decreased conjugation of bilirubin, and obstruction of bile flow in the canaliculi of the hepatic lobules or in the intrahepatic or extrahepatic bile ducts. From an anatomic standpoint, jaundice can be categorized as prehepatic, intrahepatic, and posthepatic. Chart 38-1 lists the common causes of prehepatic, hepatic, and posthepatic jaundice.

The major cause of prehepatic jaundice is excessive hemolysis of red blood cells. Hemolytic jaundice occurs when red blood cells are destroyed at a rate in excess of the liver's ability to remove the bilirubin from the blood. It may follow a hemolytic blood transfusion reaction or may occur in diseases such as hereditary spherocytosis, in which the red cell membranes are defective, or in hemolytic disease of the newborn (see Chapter 15). Neonatal hyperbilirubinemia results an increased production of bilirubin in newborn infants and their limited ability to excrete it.[5] Premature infants are at particular risk because their red cells have a shorter lifespan and higher turnover rate. In prehepatic jaundice, there is mild jaundice, the unconjugated bilirubin is elevated, the stools are of normal color, and there is no bilirubin in the urine.

Intrahepatic or hepatocellular jaundice is caused by disorders that directly affect the ability of the liver to remove bilirubin from the blood or conjugate it so it can be eliminated in the bile. Gilbert's disease is inherited as a dominant trait and results in a reduced removal of biliru-

---

CHART 38-1

Causes of Jaundice

Prehepatic (Excessive Red Blood Cell Destruction)
Hemolytic blood transfusion reaction
Hereditary disorders of the red blood cell
   Sickle cell anemia
   Thalassemia
   Spherocytosis
Acquired hemolytic disorders
Hemolytic disease of the newborn
Autoimmune hemolytic anemias

Intrahepatic
Decreased bilirubin uptake by the liver
Gilbert's disease
Decreased conjugation of bilirubin
Hepatocellular liver damage
   Hepatitis
   Cirrhosis
   Cancer of the liver
Drug-induced cholestasis

Posthepatic (Obstruction of Bile Flow)
Structural disorders of the bile duct
Cholelithiasis
Congenital atresia of the extrahepatic bile ducts
Bile duct obstruction caused by tumors

bin from the blood; the disorder is benign and fairly common. Affected persons have no symptoms other than a slightly elevated unconjugated bilirubin and mild jaundice. Conjugation of bilirubin is impaired whenever liver cells are damaged, when transport of bilirubin into liver cells becomes deficient, or when the enzymes needed to conjugate the bile are lacking. Liver diseases such as hepatitis and cirrhosis are the most common causes of intrahepatic jaundice. Drugs such as the anesthetic agent halothane, oral contraceptives, estrogen, anabolic steroids, isoniazid, and chlorpromazine may also be implicated in this type of jaundice. Intrahepatic or hepatocellular jaundice usually interferes with all phases of bilirubin metabolism—uptake, conjugation, and excretion. Both the conjugated and unconjugated bilirubin are elevated, the urine often is dark because of bilirubin in the urine, and the alkaline phosphatase is slightly elevated. Alkaline phosphatase is produced by the bile duct epithelium and canalicular membranes of hepatocytes and excreted with the bile; when bile flow is obstructed, the blood alkaline phosphatase level becomes elevated. The aminotransferases are increased in hepatocellular damage and viral hepatitis.

Posthepatic or obstructive jaundice, also called *cholestatic jaundice*, occurs when bile flow is obstructed between the liver and the intestine, with the obstruction located at any point between the junction of the right or left hepatic duct and the point where the bile duct opens into the intestine. Among the causes are strictures of the bile duct, gallstones, and tumors of the bile duct or the pancreas. Conjugated bilirubin levels usually are elevated; the stools are clay colored because of the lack of bilirubin in the bile; the urine is dark; the levels of serum alkaline phosphatase are markedly elevated; and the aminotransferase levels are slightly increased. Blood levels of bile acids often are elevated in obstructive jaundice. As the bile acids accumulate in the blood, pruritus develops. A history of pruritus preceding jaundice is common in obstructive jaundice.

TESTS OF HEPATOBILIARY FUNCTION

The history and physical examination, in most instances, provide clues about liver function. Diagnostic tests help to evaluate liver function and the extent of liver damage. Laboratory tests commonly are used to assess liver function and confirm the diagnosis of liver disease.

Liver function tests, including serum levels of liver enzymes, are used to assess injury to liver cells, the liver's ability to synthesize proteins, and the excretory functions of the liver.[6,7] Elevated serum enzyme tests usually indicate liver injury earlier than other indicators of liver function. The key enzymes are alanine aminotransferase (ALT) and aspartate aminotransferase (AST), which are present in liver cells. ALT is liver specific, whereas AST is derived from organs other than the liver. In most cases of liver damage, there are parallel rises in ALT and AST. The most dramatic rise is seen in cases of acute hepatocellular injury, as occurs with viral hepatitis, hypoxic or ischemic injury, acute toxic injury, or Reye's syndrome.

The liver's synthetic capacity is reflected in measures of serum protein levels and prothrombin time (*i.e.*, synthesis of coagulation factors). Hypoalbuminemia due to depressed synthesis may complicate severe liver disease. Deficiencies of coagulation factor V and vitamin K–dependent factors (II, VII, IX, and X) may occur.

Serum bilirubin, γ-glutamyltransferase (GGT), and alkaline phosphatase measure hepatic excretory function. Alkaline phosphatase is present in the membranes between liver cells and the bile duct and is released by disorders affecting the bile duct.[6] GGT is thought to function in the transport of amino acids and peptides into liver cells; it is a sensitive indicator of hepatobiliary disease. Measurement of GGT may be helpful in diagnosing alcohol abuse.[7]

Ultrasonography provides information about the size, composition, and blood flow of the liver. It has largely replaced cholangiography in detecting stones in the gallbladder or biliary tree. Computed tomography (CT) scanning provides information similar to that obtained by ultrasound. Magnetic resonance imaging (MRI) has proved to be useful in some disorders. Selective angiography of the celiac, superior mesenteric, or hepatic artery may be used to visualize the hepatic or portal circulation. A liver biopsy affords a means of examining liver tissue without surgery. There are several methods for obtaining liver tissue: percutaneous liver biopsy, which uses a suction, cutting, or spring-loaded cutting needle; laparoscopic liver biopsy; and fine-needle biopsy, which is performed under ultrasound or CT guidance.[8] The type of method used is based on number of specimens that is needed and the amount of tissue that is required for evaluation. Laparoscopic liver biopsy provides the means for examining abdominal masses, evaluating ascites of unknown cause, and staging liver cancers.

In summary, the hepatobiliary system consists of the liver, gallbladder, and bile ducts. The liver is the largest and, in functions, one of the most versatile organs in the body. It is located between the gastrointestinal tract and the systemic circulation; venous blood from the intestine flows through the liver before it is returned to the heart. In this way, nutrients can be removed for processing and storage, and bacteria and other foreign matter can be removed by Kupffer's cells before the blood is returned to the systemic circulation.

The liver synthesizes fats, glucose, and plasma proteins. Other important functions of the liver include the deamination of amino acids, conversion of ammonia to urea, and the interconversion of amino acids and other compounds that are important to the metabolic processes of the body. The liver produces approximately 600 to 1200 mL of yellow-green bile daily. Bile serves as an excretory vehicle for bilirubin, cholesterol, and certain products of organic metabolism and it contains bile salts that are essential for digestion of fats and absorption of fat-soluble vitamins. The liver also removes, conjugates, and secretes bilirubin into the bile. Jaundice occurs when bilirubin accumulates in the blood. It can occur because of excessive red blood cell destruction, failure of the liver to remove and conjugate the bilirubin, or obstructed biliary flow.

Liver function tests, including serum aminotransferase levels, are used to assess injury to liver cells. Serum bilirubin, GGT, and alkaline phosphatase measure hepatic excretory function. Ultrasonography, CT scans, and MRI are used to evaluate liver structures. Angiography may be used to visualize the hepatic or portal circulation, and a liver biopsy may be used to obtain tissue specimens for microscopic examination.

Alterations in Hepatic and Biliary Function

After you have completed this section of the chapter, you should be able to meet the following objectives:

✦ State the three ways by which drugs and other substances are metabolized or inactivated in the liver and provide examples of liver disease related to the toxic effects of drugs and chemical agents
✦ Compare hepatitis A, B, C, D, and E in terms of source of infection, incubation period, acute disease manifestations, development of chronic disease, and the carrier state
✦ Define chronic hepatitis and compare the pathogenesis of chronic autoimmune and chronic viral hepatitis
✦ Characterize the metabolism of alcohol by the liver and state metabolic mechanisms that can be used to explain liver injury
✦ Summarize the three patterns of injury that occur with alcohol-induced liver disease.
✦ Describe the pathogenesis of intrahepatic biliary tract disease
✦ Characterize the liver changes that occur with cirrhosis
✦ Describe the physiologic basis for portal hypertension and relate it to the development of ascites, esophageal varices, and splenomegaly
✦ Relate the functions of the liver to the manifestations of liver failure.
✦ Characterize etiologies of hepatocellular cancer and state the reason for the poor prognosis in persons with this type of cancer
✦ Discuss the indications for liver transplantation and the obstacles confronting persons in need of a transplant

The structures of the hepatobiliary system are subject to many of the same pathologic conditions that affect other body systems: injury from drugs and toxins; infection, inflammation, and immune responses; metabolic disorders; and neoplasms. This section focuses on alterations in liver function due to drug-induced injury; viral and autoimmune hepatitis; intrahepatic biliary tract disorders; alcohol-induced liver disease; cirrhosis, portal hypertension, and liver failure; and cancer of the liver.

DRUG-INDUCED LIVER DISEASE

By virtue of its many enzyme systems that are involved in biochemical transformations and modifications, the liver has an important role in the metabolism of many drugs

 Diseases of the Liver

➤ Diseases of the liver can affect the hepatocytes or the biliary drainage system.

➤ Diseases of hepatocytes impair the metabolic and synthetic functions of the liver, causing disorders in carbohydrate, protein, and fat metabolism; metabolism and removal of drugs, hormones, toxins, ammonia, and bilirubin from the blood; and the interconversion of amino acids and synthesis of proteins. Elevations in serum aminotransferase levels signal the presence of hepatocyte damage.

➤ Diseases of the biliary drainage system obstruct the flow of bile and interfere with the elimination of bile salts and bilirubin, producing cholestatic liver damage because of the backup of bile into the lobules of the liver. Elevations in bilirubin and alkaline phosphatase signal the presence of cholestatic liver damage.

➤ Cirrhosis, portal hypertension, and liver failure represent end-stage manifestations of disease conditions that cause injury to the lobular structures of the liver and their replacement with fibrotic tissue.

and chemical substances. The liver is particularly important in terms of metabolizing lipid-soluble substances that cannot be directly excreted by the kidneys. Because the liver is central to metabolic disposition of virtually all drugs and foreign substances, drug-induced liver toxicity is a potential complication of many medications.

Drug and Hormone Metabolism
Two major types of reactions are involved in the hepatic detoxification and metabolism of drugs and other chemicals: phase 1 reactions, which involve chemical modification or inactivation of a substance, and phase 2 reactions, which involve conversion of lipid-soluble substances to water-soluble derivatives.[9,10] Often, the two types of reactions are linked. Many phase 1 reactants are not soluble and must therefore undergo a subsequent phase 2 reaction to be eliminated. These reactions, which are called *biotransformations*, are important considerations in drug therapy.

Phase 1 reactions result in chemical modification of reactive drug groups by oxidation, reduction, hydroxylation, or other chemical reactions. Most drug-metabolizing enzymes are located in the lipophilic membranes of the smooth endoplasmic reticulum of liver cells (see Chapter 4). When these membranes are broken down and separated in the laboratory, they reform into vesicles called *microsomes*. The enzymes in these membranes are often referred to as *microsomal enzymes*. Most oxidative reactions are carried out by the products of a gene superfamily (CYP) that has nearly 300 members.[9] These genes code for a group of microsomal isoenzymes that make up the cytochrome P450 system. The gene products of many of the CYP genes have been identified and traced to the metabolism of specific drugs and to potential interactions among drugs. Each family of genes is responsible for certain drug-metabolizing processes, and each member of the family undertakes specific drug-metabolizing functions. For example, the CYP3 gene family contains an A subfamily and several genes numbered 1, 2, 3, and so forth. The primary enzyme for the metabolism of erythromycin in humans is P450 3A4.[9]

Many gene members of the P450 system can have their activity induced or suppressed as they undergo the task of metabolizing drugs. For example, drugs such as alcohol and barbiturates can induce certain members to increase enzyme production, accelerating drug metabolism and decreasing the pharmacologic action of the drug and of coadministered drugs that use the same member of the P450 system. In the case of drugs metabolically transformed to reactive intermediates, enzyme induction may exacerbate drug-mediated tissue toxicity. Enzymes in the cytochrome system also can be inhibited by drugs. For example, imidazole-containing drugs such as cimetidine (a histamine type 2 receptor–blocking drug that is used to reduce gastric acid secretion) and ketoconazole (an antifungal agent) effectively inhibit the metabolism of testosterone.[9] Environmental pollutants also are capable of inducing P450 gene activity. For example, exposure to benzo[a]pyrene, which is present in tobacco smoke, charcoal-broiled meat, and other organic pyrolysis products, is known to induce members of the cytochrome P450 family and alter the rates of metabolism of some drugs.

Phase 2 reactions, which involve the conversion of lipid-soluble derivatives to water-soluble substances, may follow phase 1 reactions or proceed independently. Conjugation, catalyzed by endoplasmic reticulum enzymes that couple the drug with an activated endogenous compound to render it more water soluble, is one of the most common phase 2 reactions. Although many water-soluble drugs and endogenous substances are excreted unchanged in the urine or bile, lipid-soluble substances tend to accumulate in the body unless they are converted to less active compounds or water-soluble metabolites. In general, the conjugates are more soluble than the parent compound and are pharmacologically inactive. Because the endogenous substrates used in the conjugation process are obtained from the diet, nutrition plays a critical role in phase 2 reactions.

An alternative cytochrome P450–dependent conjugation pathway is important in detoxifying reactive metabolic intermediates. This pathway uses a thiol or sulfur-containing substance called *glutathione*, which is used in conjugating drugs that form potentially harmful electrophilic groups.[10] Glutathione is depleted in the detoxification process and must be constantly replenished by compounds from the diet or by cysteine-containing drugs such as N-acetylcysteine.[9] The glutathione pathway is central to the detoxification of a number of compounds, including the over-the-counter pain medication acetaminophen (*e.g.*, Tylenol). Acetaminophen metabolism involves a phase 2 reaction. Normally, the capacity of the phase 2 reactants is much greater than that required for metabolizing recommended doses of the drug. However, in situations of acetaminophen overdose, the capacity of the phase 2 system is exceeded and the drug is transformed into toxic metabolites that can cause necrosis of the liver if allowed to accumulate. In this situation, the glutathione pathway plays a critical role in the detoxification of these metabolites. Because the glutathione stores are rapidly depleted, the drug N-acetylcysteine, which serves as a glutathione substitute, is used as an antidote for acetaminophen overdose.[10] Chronic alcohol ingestion decreases glutathione stores and increases the risk of acetaminophen toxicity.

In addition to its role in metabolism of drugs and chemicals, the liver also is responsible for hormone inactivation or modification. Insulin and glucagon are inactivated by proteolysis or deamination. Thyroxine and triiodothyronine are metabolized by reactions involving deiodination. Steroid hormones such as the glucocorticoids are first inactivated by a phase 1 reaction and then conjugated by a phase 2 reaction.

Drug-Induced Liver Disease

As the major drug-metabolizing and detoxifying organ in the body, the liver is subject to potential damage from the enormous array of pharmaceutical and environmental chemicals. Many of the widely used therapeutic drugs, including over-the-counter "natural" products, can cause hepatic injury. Of the numerous remedies, medicinal agents, chemicals, and herbal remedies in existence, more than 600 are recognized as being capable of producing hepatic injury.[11] Numerous host factors contribute to the susceptibility to drug-induced liver disease, including genetic predisposition, age differences, underlying chronic liver disease, diet and alcohol consumption, and the use of multiple interacting drugs. Early identification of drug-induced liver disease is important because withdrawal of the drug is curative in most cases.

Drugs and chemicals can exert their effects by causing hepatocyte injury and death or by cholestatic liver damage due to injury of biliary drainage structures. Drug reactions can be predictable based on the drug's chemical structure and metabolites or unpredictable (idiosyncratic) based on individual characteristics of the person receiving the drug.

Direct Hepatotoxic Injury. Some drugs are known to have toxic effects on the liver based on their chemical structure and the way they are metabolized in the liver. Direct hepatic damage often is age and dose dependent. Direct hepatotoxic reactions usually are a recognized characteristic of certain drugs. They usually result from drug metabolism and the generation of toxic metabolites. Because of the greater activity of the drug-metabolizing enzymes in the central zones of the liver, these agents typically cause centrilobular necrosis. Examples of drugs that cause direct hepatotoxicity are acetaminophen, isoniazid, and phenytoin, as well as a number of chemical agents, including carbon tetrachloride. Of the approximately 2000 cases of fulminant hepatic failure that occur each year, approximately one third are due to drugs; acetaminophen is the cause in 20% of cases.[11] The injury is characterized by marked elevations in ALT and AST values with minimally elevated alkaline phosphatase. Bilirubin levels invariably are increased, and the prognosis often is worse when hepatocellular necrosis is accompanied by jaundice.

Idiosyncratic Reactions.   In contrast to direct hepatotoxic drug reactions, idiosyncratic reactions are unpredictable, not related to dose, and sometimes accompanied by features suggesting an allergic reaction. In some cases, the reaction results directly from a metabolite that is produced only in certain persons based on a genetic predisposition. For example, certain people are capable of rapid acetylation of isoniazid, a antituberculosis drug. These people have increased likelihood of toxic reactions resulting from acetylhydrazine, which is transformed to a toxic metabolite.[10] Other drugs that are associated with idiosyncratic reactions are methyldopa, quinidine, ketoconazole, and the anesthetic gas halothane.

Cholestatic Reactions.   Cholestatic drug reactions result in decreased secretion of bile or obstruction of the biliary tree. Acute intrahepatic cholestasis is one of the most frequent types of idiosyncratic drug reactions. Among the drugs credited with causing cholestatic drug reactions are estradiol, chlorpromazine, rifampin, amoxicillin/clavulanic acid, erythromycin, nafcillin, and captopril. Typically, cholestatic drug reactions are characterized by an early onset of jaundice and pruritus, with little alteration in the person's general feeling of well-being. Most instances of acute drug-induced cholestasis subside once the drug is withdrawn.

Chronic Hepatitis.   Some drugs produce a more indolent form of liver damage that closely resembles autoimmune hepatitis. Early identification of drug-related chronic hepatitis often is difficult; cirrhosis may develop before the hepatitis is diagnosed. Identifying the responsible drug that caused the liver damage may be difficult retrospectively if the person has been consuming alcohol or taking several drugs.

HEPATITIS

Hepatitis refers to inflammation of the liver. It can be caused by reactions to drugs and toxins; by infectious disorders such as malaria, infectious mononucleosis, salmonellosis, and amebiasis that cause primary infections of extrahepatic tissues and secondary hepatitis; and by hepatotropic viruses that primarily affect liver cells or hepatocytes.

Viral Hepatitis

The known hepatotropic viruses include hepatitis A virus (HAV), hepatitis B virus (HBV), the hepatitis B–associated delta virus (HDV), hepatitis C virus (HCV), and hepatitis E virus (HEV). Although all of these viruses cause acute hepatitis, they differ in the mode of transmission and incubation period; mechanism, degree, and chronicity of liver damage; and ability to evolve to a carrier state. The presence of viral antigens and antigen antibodies can be determined through laboratory tests. Epidemiologic studies have indicated that some cases of infectious hepatitis are due to other agents. A viral agent similar to HCV has been cloned and

identified as hepatitis G virus (HGV). Evidence of HGV has been found in 1% to 2% of blood donors in the United States. However, HGV does not appear to cause liver disease or exacerbations of liver disease.[3]

There are two mechanisms of liver injury in viral hepatitis: direct cellular injury and induction of immune responses against the viral antigens. The mechanisms of injury have been most closely studied in HBV. It is thought that the extent of inflammation and necrosis depends on the individual's immune response. Accordingly, a prompt immune response during the acute phase of the infection would be expected to cause cell injury but at the same time eliminate the virus. Thus, people who respond with fewer symptoms and a marginal immune response are less likely to eliminate the virus, and hepatocytes expressing the viral antigens persist, leading to the chronic or carrier state. Fulminant hepatitis would be explained in terms of an accelerated immune response with severe liver necrosis.

The clinical course of viral hepatitis involves a number of syndromes, including asymptomatic infection with only serologic evidence of disease; acute hepatitis; the carrier state without clinically apparent disease or with chronic hepatitis; chronic hepatitis with or without progression to cirrhosis; or fulminating disease (>1% to 3%) with rapid onset of liver failure. Not all hepatotoxic viruses provoke each of the clinical syndromes.

The manifestations of acute hepatitis can be divided into three phases: the prodromal or preicterus period, the icterus period, and the convalescent period. The manifestations of the prodromal period vary from abrupt to insidious, with general malaise, myalgia, arthralgia, easy fatigability, and severe anorexia out of proportion to the degree of illness. Gastrointestinal symptoms such as nausea, vomiting, and diarrhea or constipation may occur. Abdominal pain is usually mild and is felt on the right side. Chills and fever may mark an abrupt onset. In persons who smoke, there may be a distaste for smoking that parallels the anorexia. Serum levels of AST and ALT show variable increases during the preicterus phase of acute hepatitis and precede a rise in bilirubin that accompanies the onset of the icterus or jaundice phase of infection. The icterus phase, if it occurs, usually follows the prodromal phase by 5 to 10 days. Jaundice is less likely to occur with HCV infection. The prodromal symptoms may become worse with the onset of jaundice, followed by progressive clinical improvement. Severe pruritus and liver tenderness are common during the icterus period. The convalescent phase is characterized by an increased sense of well-being, return of appetite, and disappearance of jaundice. The acute illness usually subsides gradually over a 2- to 3-week period, with complete clinical recovery by approximately 9 weeks in hepatitis A and 16 weeks in uncomplicated hepatitis B.

Infection with HBV and HCV can produce a *carrier state* in which the person does not have symptoms but harbors the virus and can therefore transmit the disease. Evidence also indicates a carrier state for HDV infection. There is no carrier state for HAV infection. There are two types of carriers: healthy carriers who have few or no ill effects, and those with chronic disease who may or may not have symptoms. Factors that increase the risk of becoming a carrier are age at time of infection and immune status. The carrier state for infections that occur early in life, as in infants of HBV-infected mothers, may be as high as 90% to 95%, compared with 1% to 10% of infected adults.[3] Other persons at high risk for becoming carriers are those with impaired immunity, those who have received multiple transfusions or blood products, those who are on hemodialysis, and drug addicts.

Hepatitis A.   Hepatitis A, formerly called *infectious hepatitis*, is caused by the small, unenveloped, RNA-containing HAV. It usually is a benign, self-limited disease, although it can cause acute fulminant hepatitis and death from liver failure in rare cases. The onset of symptoms usually is abrupt and includes fever, malaise, nausea, anorexia, abdominal discomfort, dark urine, and jaundice. The likelihood of having symptoms is related to age.[12] Children younger than 6 years often are asymptomatic. The illness in older children and adults usually is symptomatic and jaundice occurs in approximately 90% of cases. Symptoms usually last approximately 2 months but can last longer. HAV does not cause chronic hepatitis or induce a carrier state. Although the disease does not cause chronic hepatitis, the costs in terms of medical expenses and lost productivity and wages are substantial. Between 11% and 22% of persons with HAV are hospitalized, and adults with the disease lose an average of 27 days of work.[12]

Hepatitis A has a brief incubation period (15 to 45 days) and usually is transmitted by the fecal-oral route.[3,4,13] The virus replicates in the liver, is excreted in the bile, and shed in the stool. The fecal shedding of HAV occurs up to 2 weeks before the development of symptoms and ends as the immunoglobulin M (IgM) levels rise.[3] The disease often occurs sporadically or in epidemics. Drinking contaminated milk or water and eating shellfish from infected waters are fairly common routes of transmission. At special risk are persons traveling abroad who have not previously been exposed to the virus. Because young children are asymptomatic, they play an important role in the spread of the disease. Institutions housing large numbers of persons (usually children) sometimes are stricken with an epidemic of hepatitis A. Oral behavior and lack of toilet training promote viral infection among children attending preschool day care centers, who then carry the virus home to older siblings and parents. Hepatitis A usually is not transmitted by transfusion of blood or plasma derivatives, presumably because its short period of viremia usually coincides with clinical illness, so that the disease is apparent and blood donations are not accepted.

Serologic Markers.   Antibodies to HAV (anti-HAV) appear early in the disease and tend to persist in the serum (Fig. 38-8). The IgM antibodies (see Chapter 18) usually appear during the first week of symptomatic disease and begin to decline in a few months. Their presence coincides with a decline in fecal shedding of the virus. Peak levels of IgG antibodies occur after 1 month of illness and may persist for years; they provide long-term protective immunity against reinfection. The presence of IgM anti-HAV is indicative of acute hepatitis A, whereas IgG anti-HAV merely documents past exposure.

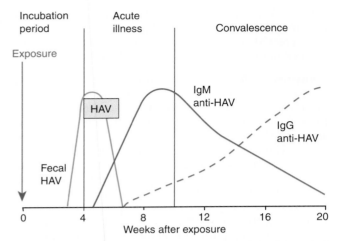

FIGURE 38-8 The sequence of fecal shedding of the hepatitis A virus (HAV), HAV viremia, and HAV antibody (IgM and IgG anti-HAV) changes in hepatitis A.

Two commercially prepared HAV vaccines are available. These vaccines contain formalin-inactivated virus grown in cell culture.[12] Vaccination is intended to replace the use of immune globulin in persons at high risk for HAV exposure. These include international travelers to regions where sanitation is poor and endemic HAV infections are high, children living in communities with high rates of HAV infection, homosexually active men, and users of illicit drugs. Persons with preexisting chronic liver disease also may benefit from immunization. A public health benefit also may be derived from vaccinating persons with increased potential for transmitting the disease (*e.g.,* food handlers). The Centers for Disease Control and Prevention (CDC) has recently recommended vaccination of children in states, counties, and communities with high rates of infection.[12] Because the vaccine is of little benefit in prevention of hepatitis in persons with known HAV exposure, immune globulin (IgG) is recommended for these persons.

Hepatitis B.   Hepatitis B, formerly referred to as *serum hepatitis*, is caused by a double-stranded DNA virus (HBV).[3,4,14,15] The complete virion, also called a *Dane particle,* consists of an outer envelope and an inner nucleocapsid that contains HBV DNA and DNA polymerase (Fig. 38-9). Hepatitis B can produce acute hepatitis, chronic hepatitis, progression of chronic hepatitis to cirrhosis, fulminant hepatitis with massive hepatic necrosis, and the carrier state. It also participates in the development of hepatitis D (delta hepatitis).

The CDC estimates that there are 200,000 to 300,000 new cases of hepatitis B each year and 1 to 1.25 million chronic carriers in the United States.[16] At particular risk of becoming carriers are infants born to hepatitis B–infected mothers. The CDC also estimates that each year in the United States there are 4000 to 5000 deaths from hepatitis B–related cirrhosis and hepatocellular carcinoma. These figures are dwarfed by a much higher frequency of hepatitis B on a global scale. For example, the infection is endemic in regions of Africa and Southeast Asia.

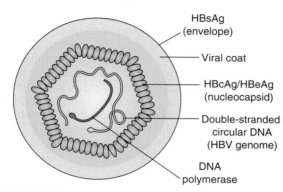

FIGURE 38-9 The hepatitis B virus.

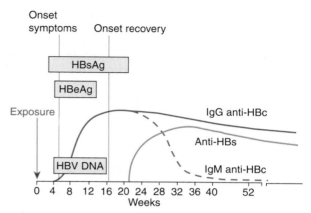

FIGURE 38-10 The sequence of hepatitis B virus (HBV) viral antigens (HBsAg, HbeAg), HBV DNA, and HBV antibody (IgM, IgG, anti-HBc, and anti-HBs) changes in acute resolving hepatitis B.

Hepatitis B has a longer incubation period and represents a more serious health problem than hepatitis A. The HBV usually is transmitted through inoculation with infected blood or serum. However, the viral antigen can be found in most body secretions and can be spread by oral or sexual contact. In the United States, most persons with hepatitis B acquire the infection as adults or adolescents. The disease is highly prevalent among injecting drug users, persons with multiple sex partners, and men who have sex with men.[17] Health care workers are at risk owing to blood exposure and accidental needle injuries. Although the virus can be spread through transfusion or administration of blood products, routine screening methods have appreciably reduced transmission through this route. The risk of hepatitis B in infants born to HBV-infected mothers ranges from 10% to 85%, depending on the mother's HBV core antigen (HBeAg) status. Infants who become infected have a 90% risk of becoming chronic carriers, and up to 25% will die of chronic liver disease as adults.[16]

Serologic Markers. Three well-defined antigens are associated with the virus: two core antigens, HBcAg and HBeAg, which are contained in the nucleocapsid, and a third, surface antigen, HBsAg, which is found in the outer envelope of the virus (see Fig. 38-9). These HBV antigens evoke specific antibodies: anti-HBs, anti-HBc, and anti-HBe. These antigens and their antibodies serve as serologic markers for following the course of the disease (Fig. 38-10).

The *HBsAg* is the viral antigen measured most routinely in blood. It is produced in abundance by infected liver cells and released into the serum. HBsAg is the earliest serologic marker to appear; it appears before the onset of symptoms and is an indicator of acute or chronic infection. The HBsAg level begins to decline after the onset of the illness and usually is undetectable in 3 to 6 months. Persistence beyond 6 months indicates continued viral replication, infectivity, and risk of chronic hepatitis. *Anti-HBs*, a specific antibody to HBsAg, occurs in most individuals after clearance of HBsAg and after successful immunization for hepatitis B. There often is a delay in appearance of anti-HBs after clearance of HBsAg. During this period of serologic gap, called the *window period*, infectivity has been demonstrated. Development of anti-HBs signals recovery from HBV infection, noninfectivity, and protection from future HBV infection. Anti-HBs is the antibody present in persons who have been successfully immunized for HBV.

The HBeAg is thought to be a cleavage product of the viral core antigen; it may be found in the serum as a soluble protein and is an active marker for the disease and shedding of complete virions into the bloodstream. It appears during the incubation period, shortly after the appearance of HBsAg, and is found only in the presence of HBsAg. HBeAg usually disappears before HBsAg. The antibody to HBeAg, *anti-HBe*, begins to appear in the serum at about the time that HBeAg disappears, and its appearance signals the onset of resolution of the acute illness. The clinical usefulness of the antigen and its antibody lies in their predictive value as markers for infectivity.

The *HBcAg* does not circulate in the blood; therefore, it is not a useful marker for the disease. Although the antigen is not found in the blood, its antibodies (anti-HBc) are the first to be detected. They appear toward the end of the incubation period and persist during the acute illness and for several months to years after that. The initial HBcAg antibody is IgM; it serves as a marker for recent infection and is followed in 6 to 18 months by IgG antibodies. These antibodies are not protective and are detectable in the presence of chronic disease.

The presence of viral DNA (HBV DNA) in the serum is the most certain indicator of hepatitis B infection. It is transiently present during the presymptomatic period and for a brief time during the acute illness. The presence of DNA polymerase, the enzyme used in viral replication, usually is transient but may persist for years in persons who are chronic carriers and is an indication of continued infectivity.

Vaccination. Hepatitis B vaccine provides long-term protection against HBV infection.[18] Hepatitis immune globulin may be effective for unvaccinated persons who are exposed to the infection if given within 7 days of exposure. Hepatitis vaccination is recommended for preexposure and postexposure prophylaxis.

The hepatitis B vaccine is produced by recombinant DNA technology. The CDC recommends vaccination of all children ages 0 to 18 years as a means of preventing HBV transmission.[17] The vaccine also is recommended for all persons who are at high risk for exposure to the virus, health care workers exposed to blood (required by Occupational Health and Safety Administration regulations), clients and staff of institutions for the developmentally disabled, patients on hemodialysis, recipients of certain blood products, household contacts and sexual partners of HBV carriers, adoptees from countries where HBV is endemic, international travelers, injecting drug users, sexually active homosexual and bisexual men, heterosexual men and women having sex with multiple partners, and inmates of long-term correctional agencies. It is recommended that persons with end-stage renal disease be vaccinated before they require hemodialysis and that universal hepatitis B vaccination of teenagers be implemented in communities where injecting drug use, pregnancy among teenagers, and sexually transmitted diseases are common. The CDC also recommends that all pregnant women be routinely tested for HBsAg during an early prenatal visit and that infants born to HBsAg-positive mothers receive appropriate doses of hepatitis immune globulin and hepatitis B vaccine.[16]

Hepatitis C. Hepatitis C is the most common cause of chronic hepatitis, cirrhosis, and hepatocellular cancer in the world.[19–21] Before 1990, the main route of transmission was through contaminated blood transfusions or blood products. With implementation of HCV testing in blood banks, the risk of HCV infection from blood transfusion has decreased to 0.03%.[19] There are approximately 3.9 million persons infected with the virus.[20,21] Most of these people are chronically infected and unaware of their infection because they are not clinically ill. Infected persons serve a source of infection to others and are at risk for chronic liver disease during the first two or more decades after initial infection.

Formerly known as *non-A, non-B hepatitis*, hepatitis C is caused by a single-stranded RNA virus (HCV) that is distantly related to the viruses that cause yellow fever and dengue fever. There are at least 6 genotypes and more than 50 subtypes of the virus.[22] Genotype 1 is associated with more severe liver disease. It is likely that the wide diversity of genotypes contributes to the pathogenicity of the virus, allowing it to escape the actions of host immune mechanisms and antiviral medications, and to the difficulties in developing a preventative vaccine.[21,23] Currently, injecting drug use is thought to be the single most important risk factor for HCV infection. There also is concern that transmission of small amounts of blood during tattooing, acupuncture, and body piercing may facilitate the transmission of HCV.[23] The incidence of sexual and vertical transmission is uncertain. Occupational exposure through incidents such as unintentional needle sticks can result in infection. However, the prevalence of HCV among health care, emergency medical, and public safety workers who are exposed to blood in the workplace is reported to be no greater than in the general public.[20,21] Sporadic cases of HCV hepatitis of unknown source account for approximately 40% of cases.

The incubation period for HCV infection ranges from 15 to 150 days (average, 50 days). Clinical symptoms with acute hepatitis C tend to be milder than those seen in persons with other types of viral hepatitis. Children and adults who acquire the infection usually are asymptomatic, or have a nonspecific clinical disease characterized by fatigue, malaise, anorexia, and weight loss. Jaundice is uncommon, and only 25% to 30% of symptomatic adults have jaundice.[23] These symptoms usually last for 2 to 12 weeks. Unlike hepatitis A and B viral infections, fulminant hepatic failure is rare and only a few cases have been reported. The most alarming aspects of HCV infection are its high rate of persistence and ability to induce chronic hepatitis and cirrhosis. HCV also increases the risk for development of hepatocellular cancer.

Serologic Markers. Both antibody and viral tests are available for detecting the presence of hepatitis C infection (Fig 38-11). Antibody testing has the advantage of being readily available and having a relatively lower cost. False-negative results can occur in immunocompromised people and early in the course of the disease before antibodies develop. Direct measurement of HCV in the serum remains the most accurate test for infection. The viral tests are highly sensitive and specific, but more costly than antibody tests. With newer antibody testing methods, infection often can be detected as early as 6 to 8 weeks after exposure, and as early as 1 to 2 weeks with viral tests that use the polymerase chain reaction testing methods (see Chapter 17). Unlike hepatitis A and B, antibodies to HCV are not protective, but they serve as markers for the disease. At present, there is no vaccine that protects against HCV infection.

Hepatitis D. Hepatitis D virus, or the delta hepatitis agent, is a defective RNA virus. It can cause acute or chronic hepatitis. Infection depends on concomitant infection with hepatitis B, specifically the presence of HBsAg. Acute hepatitis D occurs in two forms: coinfection that occurs simultaneously with acute hepatitis B and as a superinfection in which hepatitis D is imposed on chronic

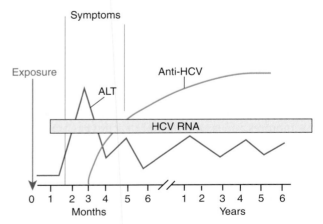

FIGURE 38-11 The sequence of serologic changes in chronic hepatitis C with persistence of hepatitis C virus (HCV) RNA and exacerbations and remissions of clinical symptoms designated by changes in serum alanine amino transferase (ALT) levels.

hepatitis B or hepatitis B carrier state.[24] The delta agent often increases the severity of HBV infection. It can convert mild HBV infection into severe, fulminating hepatitis, cause acute hepatitis in asymptomatic carriers, or increase the tendency for progression to chronic hepatitis and cirrhosis.

The routes of transmission of hepatitis D are similar to those for hepatitis B. In the United States, infection is restricted largely to persons at high risk for HBV infection, particularly injecting drug users and persons receiving clotting factor concentrates. The greatest risk is in HBV carriers; these persons should be informed about the dangers of HDV superinfection.

Hepatitis D is diagnosed by detection of antibody to HDV (anti-HDV) in the serum or HDV RNA in the serum. There is no specific treatment for hepatitis D. Because the infection is linked to hepatitis B, prevention of hepatitis D should begin with prevention of hepatitis B through vaccination.

Hepatitis E. Hepatitis E virus is an unenveloped, single-stranded RNA virus. It is transmitted by the fecal-oral route and causes manifestations of acute hepatitis that are similar to hepatitis A. It does not cause chronic hepatitis or the carrier state. Its distinguishing feature is the high mortality rate (approximately 20%) among pregnant women, owing to the development of fulminant hepatitis. The infection occurs primarily in developing areas such as India, other Southeast Asian countries, parts of Africa, and Mexico. The only reported cases in the United States have been in persons who have recently been in an endemic area.

Chronic Hepatitis

Chronic hepatitis is defined as chronic inflammatory reaction of the liver of more than 3 to 6 months' duration. It is characterized by persistently elevated serum aminotransferase levels and characteristic histologic findings on liver biopsy. The causes of chronic hepatitis include HBV, HCV, HDV, autoimmune hepatitis, and hepatitis associated with certain medications.[25,26]

Chronic Viral Hepatitis. Chronic viral hepatitis is the principal cause of chronic liver disease, cirrhosis, and hepatocellular cancer in the world and now ranks as the chief reason for liver transplantation in adults.[27] Of the hepatotropic viruses, only three are known to cause chronic hepatitis—HBV, HCV, and HDV.

The clinical features of chronic viral hepatitis are highly variable and not predictive of outcome. The most common symptoms are fatigue, malaise, loss of appetite, and occasional bouts of jaundice. Elevation of serum aminotransferase concentrations depends on the level of disease activity.

Chronic hepatitis B accounts for 5% to 10% of chronic liver disease and cirrhosis in the United States.[26,27] Hepatitis B is less likely than hepatitis C to progress to chronic infection. Chronic hepatitis B is characterized by the persistence of HBV DNA and usually by HBeAg in the serum, indicating active viral replication. Many persons are asymptomatic at the time of diagnosis, and elevated serum aminotransferase levels are the first sign of infection. Chronic hepatitis D depends on concurrent infection with HBV.

Chronic hepatitis C accounts for most cases of chronic viral hepatitis. HCV infection becomes chronic in 75% to 80% of cases.[21] Chronic HCV infection often smolders over a period of years, silently destroying liver cells. Most persons with chronic hepatitis C are asymptomatic, and diagnosis usually follows a finding of elevated serum aminotransferase levels, a tender liver, or complaints of fatigue or nonspecific weakness. Because the course of acute hepatitis C often is mild, many persons do not recall the events of the acute infection.

Treatment. There are no simple and effective treatment methods for chronic viral hepatitis.[27,28] Persons with chronic hepatitis B who have evidence of active viral replication may be treated with a course of recombinant interferon alfa-2b. Approximately 40% of persons treated with interferon alfa-2b respond to the treatment and approximately 60% of these eventually clear HBsAg from their serum and liver and develop anti-HBs in their serum, indicating that they are cured of the infection.[25] The nucleoside analog lamivudine may be used as a substitute for interferon alfa.[27] Lamivudine can be given orally and usually is well tolerated, even after being given for prolonged periods.[25] However, 15% to 30% of responders experience a mild relapse during therapy as the virus becomes resistant to the drug. Moreover, hepatitis activity may resume once the drug is discontinued, suggesting that long-term therapy may be required. In persons with concurrent hepatitis D infection, recombinant interferon alfa-2a may lead to normalization of aminotransferase levels, histologic improvement, and elimination of HDV RNA from the serum in approximately 50% of cases, but relapse is common after the therapy is stopped.[25] Lamivudine is not effective in chronic hepatitis D.

Treatment of chronic hepatitis C usually is considered for persons younger than 70 years of age with elevated serum aminotransferase levels and more than minimal inflammation or fibrosis on liver biopsy.[25] Treatment consists of a course of treatment with recombinant human interferon alfa-2b or alfa-2a followed by a course of "consensus" interferon (a synthetic interferon in which the amino acid positions have been reassigned). Ribavirin, a nucleoside analog, may be added to the treatment regimen. Treatment with interferon alfa-2a and ribavirin is costly and the side effects, which include flulike symptoms, are almost universal. More serious side effects, which include psychiatric symptoms (depression), thyroid dysfunction, and bone marrow depression, are less common.

Liver transplantation is a treatment option for end-stage liver disease due to viral hepatitis. Liver transplantation has been more successful in persons with hepatitis C than those with hepatitis B. Although the graft often is reinfected, the disease seems to progress more slowly.

Autoimmune Hepatitis. Chronic autoimmune hepatitis is a chronic inflammatory liver disease of unknown origin, but it is associated with circulating autoantibodies and high serum gamma globulin levels. Autoimmune hepatitis accounts for only approximately 10% of chronic hepatitis in the United States, a decrease from previously reported rates that probably reflects not a true change in incidence but better methods of detecting viral pathogens.

The pathogenesis of the disorder is one of a genetically predisposed person exposed to an environmental agent that triggers an autoimmune response directed at liver cell antigens.[29] The resulting immune response produces a necrotizing inflammatory response that eventually leads to destruction of liver cells and development of cirrhosis. The factors surrounding the genetic predisposition and the triggering events that lead to the autoimmune response are unclear. Autoimmune hepatitis is mainly a disease of young women, although it can occur at any age and in men or women.

Clinical manifestations of the disorder cover a spectrum that extends from no apparent symptoms to the signs accompanying liver failure. In asymptomatic cases, the disorder may be discovered when abnormal serum enzyme levels are discovered during performance of routine screening tests.

The differential diagnosis includes measures to exclude other causes of liver disease, including hepatitis B and C. A characteristic laboratory finding is that of a marked elevation in serum gamma globulins. A biopsy is used to confirm the diagnosis. Corticosteroid drugs and immunosuppressant drugs are the treatment of choice for this type of hepatitis. Liver transplantation may be the only treatment for end-stage disease.

INTRAHEPATIC BILIARY DISORDERS

Intrahepatic biliary diseases disrupt the flow of bile through the liver, causing cholestasis and biliary cirrhosis. Among the causes of intrahepatic biliary disease are primary biliary cirrhosis, primary sclerosing cholangitis, and secondary biliary cirrhosis.

Primary Biliary Cirrhosis

Primary biliary cirrhosis involves inflammation and scarring of small intrahepatic bile ducts, portal inflammation, and progressive scarring of liver tissue.[30] The disease is seen most commonly in women 30 to 65 years of age and accounts for 2% to 5% of cases of cirrhosis. Familial occurrences of the disease are found between parents and children and among siblings. Abnormalities of cell-mediated and humoral immunity suggest an autoimmune mechanism. Antimitochondrial antibodies are found in 98% of persons with the disease, but their role in the pathogenesis of the disease is unclear.[30,31] Up to 84% of persons with primary biliary cirrhosis have at least one other autoimmune disorder, such as scleroderma, Hashimoto's thyroiditis, rheumatoid arthritis, or Sjögren's syndrome.

The disorder is characterized by an insidious onset and progressive scarring and destruction of liver tissue. The liver becomes enlarged and takes on a green hue because of the accumulated bile. The earliest symptoms are unexplained pruritus or itching, weight loss, and fatigue, followed by dark urine and pale stools. Jaundice is a late manifestation of the disorder, as are other signs of liver failure. Serum alkaline phosphatase levels are elevated in persons with primary biliary cirrhosis.

Treatment is largely symptomatic. Bile acid–binding drugs are used as a treatment for itching. Some persons have responded to ultraviolet B light, methyltestosterone, cimetidine, phenobarbital, and prednisone. There is no generally accepted treatment for the underlying disease. Clinical trials using ursodiol, a drug that increases bile flow and decreases the toxicity of bile contents, have shown a decreased rate of clinical deterioration with drug treatment. Colchicine, which acts to prevent leukocyte migration and phagocytosis, and methotrexate, a drug with immunosuppressive properties, have had some reported benefit in improving symptoms. However, liver transplantation remains the only treatment for advanced disease. Primary biliary cirrhosis does not recur after liver transplantation if appropriate immunosuppression is used.[30]

Primary Sclerosing Cholangitis

Cholangitis involves inflammation of hepatic bile ducts. Primary sclerosing cholangitis is a chronic cholestatic disease of unknown origin that causes destruction and fibrosis of intrahepatic and extrahepatic bile ducts.[32] Bile flow is obstructed (*i.e.*, cholestasis), and the bile retention destroys hepatic structures. The disease commonly is associated with inflammatory bowel disease, occurs more often in men than women, and is seen most commonly in the third to fifth decades of life. Primary sclerosing cholangitis, although much less common than alcoholic cirrhosis, is the fourth leading indication for liver transplantation in adults in the United States.[32]

Most persons with the disorder are initially asymptomatic, with the disorder being detected during routine liver function tests that reveal elevated levels of serum alkaline phosphatase or GGT. Alternatively, some persons present with progressive fatigue, jaundice, and pruritus. The later stages of the disease are characterized by cirrhosis, portal hypertension, and liver failure.[32] Ten-year survival rates range from 50% to 75%. Other than measures aimed at symptom relief, the only treatment is liver transplantation.

Secondary Biliary Cirrhosis

Secondary biliary cirrhosis results from prolonged obstruction of the extrabiliary tree. The most common cause is cholelithiasis. Other causes of secondary biliary cirrhosis are malignant neoplasms of the biliary tree or head of the pancreas and strictures of the common duct caused by previous surgical procedures. Extrahepatic biliary cirrhosis may benefit from surgical procedures designed to relieve the obstruction.

ALCOHOL-INDUCED LIVER DISEASE

The spectrum of alcoholic liver disease includes fatty liver disease, alcoholic hepatitis, and cirrhosis. Alcoholic cirrhosis causes 200,000 deaths annually and is the fifth leading cause of death in the United States.[3] Most deaths from alcoholic cirrhosis are attributable to liver failure, bleeding esophageal varices, or kidney failure. It has been estimated that there are 10 million alcoholics in the United States. Only approximately 10% to 15% of alcoholics develop cirrhosis, however, suggesting that other conditions such as genetic and environmental factors contribute to its occurrence.

Metabolism of Alcohol

Alcohol is absorbed readily from the gastrointestinal tract; it is one of the few substances that can be absorbed from the stomach. As a substance, alcohol fits somewhere between a food and a drug. It supplies calories but cannot be broken down or stored as protein, fat, or carbohydrate. As a food, alcohol yields 7.1 kcal/g, compared with the 4 kcal/g produced by metabolism of an equal amount of carbohydrate.[33] Between 80% and 90% of the alcohol a person drinks is metabolized by the liver. The rest is excreted through the lungs, kidneys, and skin.

Alcohol metabolism proceeds simultaneously by three pathways: the alcohol dehydrogenase (ADH) system, located in the cytoplasm of the hepatocytes; the microsomal ethanol-oxidizing system (MEOS), located in the endoplasmic reticulum; and catalase, located in the peroxisomes (see Chapter 4).[34] The ADH and MEOS pathways produce specific metabolic and toxic disturbances, and all three pathways result in the production of acetaldehyde, a very toxic metabolite.[35]

The MEOS pathway, which is located in the smooth endoplasmic reticulum, produces acetaldehyde and free radicals. Prolonged and excessive alcohol ingestion results in enzyme induction and increased activity of the MEOS. One of the most important enzymes of the MEOS, a member of the cytochrome P450 system, also oxidizes a number of other compounds, including various drugs (*e.g.*, acetaminophen, isoniazid), toxins (*e.g.*, carbon tetrachloride, halothane), vitamins A and D, and carcinogenic agents (*e.g.*, aflatoxin, nitrosamines). Increased activity of this system enhances the susceptibility of persons with heavy alcohol consumption to the hepatotoxic effects of industrial toxins, anesthetic agents, chemical carcinogens, vitamins, and acetaminophen.[36]

The metabolic end-products of alcohol metabolism (*e.g.*, acetaldehyde, free radicals) are responsible for a variety of metabolic alterations that can cause liver injury. Acetaldehyde, for example, has multiple toxic effects on liver cells and liver function. Age and sex play a role in metabolism of alcohol and production of harmful metabolites. Women appear to be more predisposed to alcohol-induced liver damage than men. The ADH system is depressed by testosterone; women tend to produce greater amounts of acetaldehyde than men.[35] Endogenous and exogenous (*i.e.*, contraceptive agents) female hormones may also increase the hepatotoxic effects of alcohol through the cytochrome P450 system. Age also appears to affect the alcohol-metabolizing abilities of the liver and the resistance to hepatotoxic effects. Liver injury is related to the average amount of daily consumption and the duration of alcohol abuse. In general, a daily intake of less than 80 g of alcohol in men and 40 g in women seldom results in liver disease.[36]

Alcohol metabolism requires a cofactor, nicotinamide adenine dinucleotide (NAD), that is necessary for many other metabolic processes, including the metabolism of pyruvates, urates, and fatty acids. Because alcohol competes for the use of NAD, it tends to disrupt other metabolic functions of the liver. The preferential use of NAD for alcohol metabolism can result in increased production and accumulation of lactic acid in the blood. By reducing the availability of NAD, alcohol also impairs the liver's ability to form glucose from amino acids and other glucose precursors. Alcohol-induced hypoglycemia can develop when excessive alcohol ingestion occurs during periods of depleted liver glycogen stores. This may become a particular problem for the alcoholic who has been vomiting and has not eaten for several days.

Alcoholic Liver Disease

The metabolism of alcohol leads to chemical attack on certain membranes of the liver, but whether the damage is caused by acetaldehyde or other metabolites is unknown. Acetaldehyde is known to impede the mitochondrial electron transport system, which is responsible for oxidative metabolism and generation of ATP; as a result, the hydrogen ions that are generated in the mitochondria are shunted into lipid synthesis and ketogenesis. Abnormal accumulations of these substances are found in hepatocytes (*i.e.*, fatty liver) and blood. Binding of acetaldehyde to other molecules impairs the detoxification of free radicals and synthesis of proteins. Acetaldehyde also promotes collagen synthesis and fibrogenesis. The lesions of hepatocellular injury tend to be most prevalent in the centrilobular area that surrounds the central vein where the pathways for alcohol metabolism are concentrated. This is the part of the lobule that has the lowest oxygen tension; it is thought that the low oxygen concentration in this area of the liver may contribute to the damage.

Even after alcohol intake has stopped and all alcohol has been metabolized, the processes that damage liver cells may continue for many weeks and months. Clinical and chemical effects often become worse before the disease resolves. Usually, the accumulation of fat disappears within a few weeks, and cholestasis and inflammation also subside. However, fibrosis and scarring remain. The liver lobules become distorted as new liver cells regenerate and form nodules.

Although the mechanism by which alcohol exerts its toxic effects on liver structures is somewhat uncertain, the changes that develop can be divided into three stages: fatty changes, alcoholic hepatitis, and cirrhosis.[3,4] Because these three patterns of hepatocellular injury may occur independently of one another and occur in other types of end-stage liver disease, they are discussed separately.

Fatty Liver. One of the main effects of alcohol is the accumulation of fat in hepatocytes, a condition called *steatosis* (Fig. 38-12). The pathogenesis of fatty liver is not completely understood and can depend on the amount of alcohol consumed, dietary fat content, body stores of fat, hormonal status, and other factors. When alcohol is present, it becomes the preferred fuel for the liver, displacing fuel substrates such as fatty acids. Most of the fat deposited in the liver is derived from the diet. In the fasting state, lipids are derived from endogenous fat stores. Alcohol increases lipolysis and delivery of free fatty acids to the liver. In the liver, alcohol increases fatty acid synthesis, decreases mitochondrial oxidation of fatty acids, increases production of triglycerides, and impairs the release of lipoproteins.

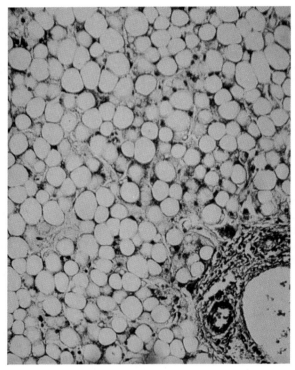

FIGURE 38-12 Alcoholic fatty liver. A photomicrograph shows the cytoplasm of almost all the hepatocytes to be distended by fat, which displaces the nucleus to the periphery. Note the absence of inflammation and fibrosis. (Rubin E., Farber J.L. [1999]. *Pathology* [3rd ed., p. 791]. Philadelphia: Lippincott Williams & Wilkins)

During the fatty liver stage, the liver becomes yellow and enlarges owing to excessive fat accumulation. There is evidence that ingestion of large amounts of alcohol can cause fatty liver changes even with an adequate diet. For example, young, nonalcoholic volunteers had fatty liver changes after 2 days of consuming 18 to 24 oz of alcohol, even though adequate carbohydrates, fats, and proteins were included in the diet.[37] The fatty changes that occur with ingestion of alcohol usually do not produce symptoms and are reversible after the alcohol intake has been discontinued.

Alcoholic Hepatitis. Alcoholic hepatitis is the intermediate stage between fatty changes and cirrhosis. It often is seen after an abrupt increase in alcohol intake and is common in "spree" drinkers. Alcoholic hepatitis is characterized by inflammation and necrosis of liver cells. This stage usually is characterized by hepatic tenderness, pain, anorexia, nausea, fever, jaundice, ascites, and liver failure, but some individuals may be asymptomatic. The condition is always serious and sometimes fatal. The immediate prognosis correlates with severity of liver cell injury. In some cases, the disease progresses rapidly to liver failure and death. The mortality rate in the acute stage ranges from 10% to 30%.[4] In persons who survive and continue to drink, the acute phase often is followed by persistent alcoholic hepatitis with progression to cirrhosis in a matter of 1 to 2 years.[4]

Alcoholic Cirrhosis. With repeated bouts of drinking and hepatitis, liver injury may progress to cirrhosis. The gross appearance of the early cirrhotic liver is one of fine, uniform nodules on its surface. The condition has traditionally been called *micronodular* or *Laennec cirrhosis*. With more advanced cirrhosis, regenerative processes cause the nodules to become larger and more irregular in size and shape. As this happens, the nodules cause the liver to become relobulized through the formation of new portal tracts and venous outflow channels. The nodules may compress the hepatic veins, curtailing blood flow out of the liver and producing portal hypertension, extrahepatic portosystemic shunts, and cholestasis. Cirrhosis designates the onset of end-stage alcoholic liver disease.

CIRRHOSIS, PORTAL HYPERTENSION, AND LIVER FAILURE

The most severe clinical consequence of liver disease is hepatic failure. It may result from sudden and massive hepatic destruction, as in fulminant hepatitis, or it may be the result of progressive damage to the liver, as occurs in cirrhosis. Whatever the sequence, 80% to 90% of hepatic functional capacity must be lost before hepatic failure occurs.[3] In many cases, the progressive decompensating aspects of the disease are hastened by intercurrent conditions such as gastro-intestinal bleeding, systemic infection, electrolyte disturbances, or superimposed diseases such as heart failure.

Cirrhosis

Cirrhosis represents the end stage of chronic liver disease in which much of the functional liver tissue has been replaced by fibrous tissue. It is characterized by diffuse fibrosis and conversion of normal liver architecture into structurally abnormal nodules.[3,4] The fibrous tissue replaces normally functioning liver tissue and forms constrictive bands that disrupt flow in the vascular channels and biliary duct systems of the liver. The disruption of vascular channels predisposes to portal hypertension and its complications; obstruction of biliary channels and exposure to the destructive effects of bile stasis; and loss of liver cells, leading to liver failure.

Although cirrhosis usually is associated with alcoholism, it can develop in the course of other disorders, including viral hepatitis, toxic reactions to drugs and chemicals, biliary obstruction, and cardiac disease. Cirrhosis also accompanies metabolic disorders that cause the deposition of minerals in the liver. Two of these disorders are hemochromatosis (*i.e.*, iron deposition) and Wilson's disease (*i.e.*, copper deposition).

The manifestations of cirrhosis are variable, ranging from asymptomatic hepatomegaly to hepatic failure. Often there are no symptoms until the disease is far advanced. The most common signs and symptoms of cirrhosis are weight loss (sometimes masked by ascites), weakness, and anorexia. Diarrhea frequently is present, although some persons may complain of constipation. Hepatomegaly and jaundice also are common signs of cirrhosis. There may be abdominal pain because of liver enlargement or stretching of Glisson's capsule. This pain is located in the epigastric area or in the upper right quadrant and is described as dull, aching, and causing a sensation of fullness.

The late manifestations of cirrhosis are related to portal hypertension and liver cell failure. Splenomegaly, ascites, and portosystemic shunts (*i.e.,* esophageal varices, anorectal varices, and caput medusae) result from portal hypertension. Other complications include bleeding due to decreased clotting factors, thrombocytopenia due to splenomegaly, gynecomastia and a feminizing pattern of pubic hair distribution in men because of testicular atrophy, spider angiomas, palmar erythema, and encephalopathy with as-terixis and neurologic signs. The manifestations of cirrhosis are discussed in the section that follows and are summarized in Table 38-2.

Portal Hypertension

Portal hypertension is characterized by increased resistance to flow in the portal venous system and sustained portal vein pressure above 12 mm Hg (normal, 5 to 10 mm Hg).[4,38] Normally, venous blood returning to the heart from the abdominal organs collects in the portal vein and travels through the liver before entering the vena cava. Portal hypertension can be caused by a variety of conditions that increase resistance to hepatic blood flow, including pre-hepatic, posthepatic, and intrahepatic obstructions (with *hepatic* referring to the liver lobules rather than the entire liver).[4] Prehepatic causes of portal hypertension include portal vein thrombosis and external compression due to cancer or enlarged lymph nodes that produce obstruction of the portal vein before it enters the liver.

Posthepatic obstruction refers to any obstruction to blood flow through the hepatic veins beyond the liver lobules, either within or distal to the liver. It is caused by conditions such as thrombosis of the hepatic veins, veno-occlusive disease, and severe right-sided heart failure that impede the outflow of venous blood from the liver. *Budd-Chiari syndrome* refers to congestive disease of the liver caused by occlusion of the portal veins and their tributaries. The principal cause of the Budd-Chiari syndrome is thrombosis of the hepatic veins, in association with diverse conditions such as polycythemia vera, hypercoagulability states associated with malignant tumors, pregnancy, bacterial infection, metastatic disease of the liver, and trauma. *Hepatic veno-occlusive disease* is a variant of the Budd-Chiari syndrome seen most commonly in persons treated with certain cancer chemotherapeutic drugs, hepatic irradiation, or bone marrow transplantation, possibly because of graft-versus-host disease.[4]

TABLE 38-2 ✦ Manifestations of Portal Cirrhosis

Primary Alteration in Function	Manifestation
Portal Hypertension	
Development of collateral vessels	Esophageal varices
	Hemorrhoids
	Caput medusae (dilated cutaneous veins around the umbilicus)
Portal vein obstruction and decreased levels of serum albumin	Ascites
	Peripheral edema
Splenomegaly	Anemia
	Leukopenia
	Thrombocytopenia
Hepatorenal syndrome	Elevated serum creatinine
	Azotemia
	Oliguria
Portosystemic shunting of blood	Hepatic–systemic encephalopathy
Hepatocellular Dysfunction	
Impaired metabolism of sex hormones	Female: menstrual disorders
	Male: testicular atrophy, gynecomastia, decrease in secondary sex characteristics
	Skin disorders: vascular spiders and palmar erythema
Impaired synthesis of plasma proteins	Decreased levels of serum albumin with development of edema and ascites
	Decreased carrier proteins for hormones and drugs
Decreased synthesis of blood clotting factors	Bleeding tendencies
Failure to remove and conjugate bilirubin from the blood	Jaundice
Impaired bile synthesis	Malabsorption of fats and fat-soluble vitamins
Impaired metabolism of drugs cleared by the liver	Risk of drug reactions and toxicities
Impaired gluconeogenesis	Abnormal glucose tolerance
Decreased ability to convert ammonia to urea	Elevated blood ammonia levels, encephalopathy

Intrahepatic causes of portal hypertension include conditions that cause obstruction of blood flow within the liver. In alcoholic cirrhosis, which is the major cause of portal hypertension, bands of fibrous tissue and fibrous nodules distort the architecture of the liver and increase the resistance to portal blood flow, which leads to portal hypertension.

Complications of portal hypertension arise from the increased pressure and dilatation of the venous channels behind the obstruction. In addition, collateral channels open that connect the portal circulation with the systemic circulation. The major complications of the increased portal vein pressure and the opening of collateral channels are ascites, splenomegaly, and the formation of portosystemic shunts with bleeding from esophageal varices.

Ascites. Ascites occurs when the amount of fluid in the peritoneal cavity is increased, and is a late-stage manifestation of cirrhosis and portal hypertension.[39] It is not uncommon for persons with advanced cirrhosis to present with an accumulation of 15 L or more of ascitic fluid. Those who gain this much fluid often experience abdominal discomfort, dyspnea, and insomnia. Some persons may have difficulty walking or living independently.[40]

Although the mechanisms responsible for the development of ascites are not completely understood, several factors seem to contribute to fluid accumulation, including an increase in capillary pressure due to portal hypertension and obstruction of venous flow through the liver, salt and water retention by the kidney, and decreased colloidal osmotic pressure due to impaired synthesis of albumin by the liver. Diminished blood volume (*i.e.*, underfill theory) and excessive blood volume (*i.e.*, overfill theory) have been used to explain the increased salt and water retention by the kidney. According to the underfill theory, a contraction in the effective blood volume constitutes an afferent signal that causes the kidney to retain salt and water. The effective blood volume may be reduced because of loss of fluid into the peritoneal cavity or because of vasodilatation caused by the presence of circulating vasodilating substances. The overfill theory proposes that the initial event in the development of ascites is renal retention of salt and water caused by disturbances in the liver itself. These disturbances include failure of the liver to metabolize aldosterone, causing an increase in salt and water retention by the kidney. Another likely contributing factor in the pathogenesis of ascites is a decreased colloidal osmotic pressure, which limits reabsorption of fluid from the peritoneal cavity (see Chapter 31).

Treatment of ascites usually focuses on dietary restriction of sodium and administration of diuretics. Water intake also may need to be restricted. Because of the many limitations in sodium restriction, the use of diuretics has become the mainstay of treatment for ascites. Two classes of diuretics are used: a diuretic that acts in the distal part of nephron to inhibit aldosterone-dependent sodium reabsorption, and a loop diuretic such as furosemide. Combination therapy with a loop-acting and a distal-acting diuretic has been shown to have important synergistic effects in persons with cirrhosis.[41] Oral potassium supplements often are given to prevent hypokalemia. The upright position is associated with the activation of the renin-angiotensin-aldosterone system; therefore, bed rest may be recommended for persons with a large amount of ascites.[41] Large-volume paracentesis (removal of 5 L or more of ascitic fluid) may be done in persons with massive ascites and pulmonary compromise. Because the removal of fluid produces a decrease in vascular volume along with increased plasma renin activity and aldosterone-mediated sodium and water reabsorption by the kidneys, its effects are only temporary. Therefore, a volume expander such as albumin usually is administered at the time of paracentesis to maintain the effective circulating volume. Large-volume paracentesis may be done daily until ascites is largely resolved.[15] A transjugular intrahepatic portosystemic shunt may be inserted in persons with refractory ascites (to be discussed).[25]

Spontaneous bacterial peritonitis is a complication in persons with both cirrhosis and ascites. The infection is serious and carries a high mortality rate even when treated with antibiotics. Presumably, the peritoneal fluid is seeded with bacteria from the blood or lymph or from passage of bacteria through the bowel wall. Symptoms include fever and abdominal pain. Other symptoms include worsening of hepatic encephalopathy, diarrhea, hypothermia, and shock. It is diagnosed by a neutrophil count of 250/mm³ or higher and a protein concentration of 1 g/dL or less in the ascitic fluid.[25]

Splenomegaly. The spleen enlarges progressively in portal hypertension because of shunting of blood into the splenic vein. The enlarged spleen often gives rise to sequestering of significant numbers of blood elements and development of a syndrome known as *hypersplenism*. Hypersplenism is characterized by a decrease in the life span and a subsequent decrease in all the formed elements of the blood, leading to anemia, thrombocytopenia, and leukopenia. The decreased life span of the blood elements is thought to result from an increased rate of removal because of the prolonged transit time through the enlarged spleen.

Portosystemic Shunts. With the gradual obstruction of venous blood flow in the liver, the pressure in the portal vein increases, and large collateral channels develop between the portal and systemic veins that supply the lower rectum and esophagus and the umbilical veins of the falciform ligament that attaches to the anterior wall of the abdomen. The collaterals between the inferior and internal iliac veins may give rise to hemorrhoids. In some persons, the fetal umbilical vein is not totally obliterated; it forms a channel on the anterior abdominal wall (Fig. 38-13). Dilated veins around the umbilicus are called *caput medusae*. Portopulmonary shunts also may develop and cause blood to bypass the pulmonary capillaries, interfering with blood oxygenation and producing cyanosis.

Clinically, the most important collateral channels are those connecting the portal and coronary veins that lead to reversal of flow and formation of thin-walled varicosities in the submucosa of the esophagus (Fig. 38-14). These thin-walled *esophageal varices* are subject to rupture, producing massive and sometimes fatal hemorrhage. Impaired hepatic synthesis of coagulation factors and decreased platelet levels (*i.e.*, thrombocytopenia) due to splenomegaly may further complicate the control of esophageal bleeding. Esophageal

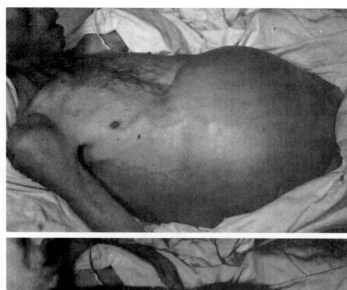

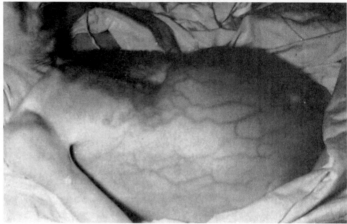

FIGURE 38-13 Collateral abdominal veins on the anterior abdominal wall in a patient with alcoholic liver disease as recorded by black and white photography (**top**) and infrared photography (**bottom**). (Schiff L. [1982]. *Diseases of the liver.* Philadelphia: J.B. Lippincott)

varices develop in approximately 65% of persons with advanced cirrhosis and cause massive hemorrhage and death in approximately half of them.[3]

Treatment of portal hypertension and esophageal varices is directed at prevention of initial hemorrhage, management of acute hemorrhage, and prevention of recurrent variceal hemorrhage. Pharmacologic therapy is used to lower portal venous pressure and prevent initial hemorrhage. β-Adrenergic–blocking drugs (*e.g.*, propranolol) commonly are used for this purpose. These agents reduce portal venous pressure by decreasing splanchnic blood flow and thereby decreasing blood flow in collateral channels. Long-acting nitrates may be used to decrease the risk of variceal rebleeding in people who cannot tolerate β blockers.

Several methods are used to control acute hemorrhage, including administration of octreotide or vasopressin, balloon tamponade, endoscopic injection sclerotherapy, vessel ligation, or esophageal transection. Octreotide, a long-acting synthetic analog of somatostatin, reduces splanchnic and hepatic blood flow and portal pressures in persons with cirrhosis. The drug, which is given intravenously, provides control of variceal bleeding in up to 80% of cases. Vasopressin, a hormone from the posterior pituitary, is a nonselective vasoconstrictor that also can be used to control variceal bleeding. Because octreotide has fewer side effects

and appears to be more effective than vasopressin, it has become the drug of choice for pharmacologic management of acute variceal bleeding.[42] Balloon tamponade provides compression of the varices and is accomplished through the insertion of a tube with inflatable gastric and esophageal balloons. After the tube has been inserted, the balloons are inflated; the esophageal balloon compresses the bleeding esophageal veins, and the gastric balloon helps to maintain the position of the tube. During endoscopic sclerotherapy, the varices are injected with a sclerosing solution that obliterates the vessel lumen.

Prevention of recurrent hemorrhage focuses on lowering portal venous pressure and diverting blood flow away from the easily ruptured collateral channels. Two procedures may be used for this purpose: the surgical creation of a portosystemic shunt or transjugular intrahepatic portosystemic shunt (TIPS). *Surgical portosystemic shunt* procedures involve the creation of an opening between the portal vein and a systemic vein. These shunts have a considerable complication rate, and TIPS has evolved as the preferred treatment for refractory portal hypertension. The technique involves insertion of an expandable metal stent between a branch of the hepatic vein and the portal vein using a catheter inserted through the internal jugular vein. A limitation of the procedure is that stenosis and thrombosis of

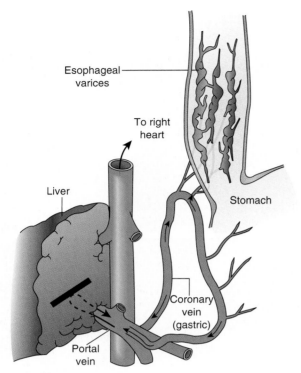

FIGURE 38-14 Obstruction of blood flow in the portal circulation, with portal hypertension and diversion of blood flow to other venous channels, including the gastric and esophageal veins.

the stent occurs in most cases over time, with consequent risk of rebleeding. A complication that is associated with the creation of a portosystemic shunt is hepatic encephalopathy, which is thought to result when ammonia and other neurotoxic substances from the gut pass directly into the systemic circulation without going through the liver.

Liver Failure

Although the liver is among the organs most frequently damaged, only approximately 10% of hepatic tissue is required for the liver to remain functional. The manifestations of liver failure reflect the various functions of the liver, including hematologic disorders, endocrine disorders, skin disorders, hepatorenal syndrome, and hepatic encephalopathy. *Fetor hepaticus* refers to a characteristic musty, sweetish odor of the breath in the patient in advanced liver failure, resulting from the metabolic byproducts of the intestinal bacteria.

Hematologic Disorders. Liver failure can cause anemia, thrombocytopenia, coagulation defects, and leukopenia. Anemia may be caused by blood loss, excessive red blood cell destruction, and impaired formation of red blood cells. A folic acid deficiency may lead to severe megaloblastic anemia. Changes in the lipid composition of the red cell membrane increase hemolysis. Because factors V, VII, IX, X, prothrombin, and fibrinogen are synthesized by the liver, their decline in liver disease contributes to bleeding disorders. Malabsorption of the fat-soluble vitamin K contributes further to the impaired synthesis of these clotting

factors. Thrombocytopenia often occurs as the result of splenomegaly. The person with liver failure is subject to purpura, easy bruising, hematuria, and abnormal menstrual bleeding, and is vulnerable to bleeding from the esophagus and other segments of the gastrointestinal tract.

Endocrine Disorders. The liver metabolizes the sex hormones. Endocrine disorders, particularly disturbances in gonadal function, are common accompaniments of cirrhosis and liver failure. Women may have menstrual irregularities (usually amenorrhea), loss of libido, and sterility. In men, testosterone levels usually fall, the testes atrophy, and loss of libido, impotence, and gynecomastia occur. A decrease in aldosterone metabolism may contribute to salt and water retention by the kidney, along with a lowering of serum potassium resulting from increased elimination of potassium.

Skin Disorders. Liver failure brings on numerous skin disorders. These lesions, called variously *vascular spiders*, *telangiectases*, *spider angiomas*, and *spider nevi*, are seen most often in the upper half of the body. They consist of a central pulsating arteriole from which smaller vessels radiate. Palmar erythema is redness of the palms, probably caused by increased blood flow from higher cardiac output. Clubbing of the fingers may be seen in persons with cirrhosis. Jaundice usually is a late manifestation of liver failure.

Hepatorenal Syndrome. The hepatorenal syndrome refers to a functional state of renal failure sometimes seen during the terminal stages of liver failure with ascites. It is characterized by progressive azotemia, increased serum creatinine levels, and oliguria. Although the basic cause is unknown, a decrease in renal blood flow is believed to play a part. Ultimately, when renal failure is superimposed on liver failure, azotemia and elevated levels of blood ammonia occur; this condition is thought to contribute to hepatic encephalopathy and coma.

Hepatic Encephalopathy. Hepatic encephalopathy refers to the totality of central nervous system manifestations of liver failure. It is characterized by neural disturbances ranging from a lack of mental alertness to confusion, coma, and convulsions. A very early sign of hepatic encephalopathy is a flapping tremor called *asterixis*. Various degrees of memory loss may occur, coupled with personality changes such as euphoria, irritability, anxiety, and lack of concern about personal appearance and self. Speech may be impaired, and the patient may be unable to perform certain purposeful movements. The encephalopathy may progress to decerebrate rigidity and then to a terminal deep coma.

Although the cause of hepatic encephalopathy is unknown, the accumulation of neurotoxins, which appear in the blood because the liver has lost its detoxifying capacity, is believed to be a factor. Hepatic encephalopathy develops in approximately 10% of persons with portosystemic shunts.

One of the suspected neurotoxins is ammonia. A particularly important function of the liver is the conversion of ammonia, a byproduct of protein and amino acid metabolism, to urea. The ammonium ion is produced in abundance in the intestinal tract, particularly in the colon, by the bacterial degradation of luminal proteins and amino acids. Normally, these ammonium ions diffuse into the portal blood and are transported to the liver, where they are converted to urea before entering the general circulation. When the blood from the intestine bypasses the liver or the liver is unable to convert ammonia to urea, ammonia moves directly into the general circulation and from there to the cerebral circulation. Hepatic encephalopathy may become worse after a large protein meal or gastrointestinal tract bleeding. Narcotics and tranquilizers are poorly metabolized by the liver, and administration of these drugs may cause central nervous system depression and precipitate hepatic encephalopathy.

A nonabsorbable antibiotic, such as neomycin, may be given to eradicate bacteria from the bowel and thus prevent this cause of ammonia production. Another drug that may be given is lactulose. It is not absorbed from the small intestine but moves directly to the large intestine, where it is catabolized by colonic bacteria to small organic acids that cause production of large, loose stools with a low pH. The low pH favors the conversion of ammonia to ammonium ions, which are not absorbed by the blood. The acid pH also inhibits the degradation of amino acids, proteins, and blood.

Treatment

The treatment of liver failure is directed toward eliminating alcohol intake when the condition is caused by alcoholic cirrhosis; preventing infections; providing sufficient carbohydrates and calories to prevent protein breakdown; correcting fluid and electrolyte imbalances, particularly hypokalemia; and decreasing ammonia production in the gastrointestinal tract by controlling protein intake. In many cases, liver transplantation remains the only effective treatment.

Liver Transplantation.   Liver transplantation rapidly is becoming a realistic form of treatment for many persons with irreversible chronic liver disease, fulminant liver failure, and certain metabolic disorders that result in end-stage liver disease. The introduction of cyclosporine in 1980 markedly improved the survival rate of persons with liver transplants. Careful selection of potential recipients and improved preoperative management further contributed to the improved transplantation results. In 1983, the National Institutes of Health Consensus Conference concluded that liver transplantation had become an accepted therapeutic modality, prompting many states and private insurance companies to pay for the procedure.[43] Currently, survival rates exceed 85% at 1 year and 70% at 5 years.[44] The shortage of donor organs severely limits the number of transplantations that are done, and many persons die each year while waiting for a transplant.[45]

Criteria for liver transplantation include the presence of a chronic liver disease for which all forms of therapy have failed. Conditions for which liver transplantation has been done are metabolic diseases of the liver such as Wilson's disease, primary biliary cirrhosis, chronic active hepati-

tis, sclerosing cholangitis, and biliary atresia in children. The agents used to prevent liver transplant rejection—cyclosporine, corticosteroid drugs, and azathioprine—are the same ones used to maintain other whole-organ grafts such as heart and kidney transplants.

CANCER OF THE LIVER

Primary liver tumors are relatively rare in the United States, accounting for approximately 0.5% to 2% of all cancers.[3] The American Cancer Society estimates that over 16,000 new cases of primary liver and intrahepatic cancer will be diagnosed during 2001, and over 14,000 people will die of the disease during the same period.[46] In contrast to many other cancers, the number of people who develop liver cancer and die of it is increasing. Liver cancer is approximately 10 times more common in developing countries in Southeast Asia and Africa. In many of these countries, it is the most common type of cancer.

There are two major types of primary liver cancer: hepatocellular carcinoma, which arises from the liver cells, and cholangiocarcinoma, which is a primary cancer of bile duct cells.[3] Hepatocellular cancer is one of the few cancers for which an underlying etiology can be identified in most cases, and is unique because it usually occurs in a background of chronic liver disease.[47] Among the factors identified as etiologic agents in liver cancer are chronic viral hepatitis (HBV, HCV, HDV), cirrhosis, long-term exposure to aflatoxin, and drinking water contaminated with arsenic. The global distribution of hepatocellular carcinoma is strongly linked to HBV infection. In countries where HBV is endemic, there is a high risk of hepatocellular carcinoma, with an age of onset between 20 to 40 years. In the Western world, where HBV is less common, 85% to 90% of cases of hepatocellular carcinoma are associated with cirrhosis. Just how these environmental and chemical agents contribute to the development of liver cancer is still unclear. With HBV and HCV, both of which become integrated into the host DNA, repeated cycles of cell death and regeneration afford the potential for development of cancer-producing mutations. Aflatoxins, produced by food spoilage molds in certain areas endemic for hepatocellular carcinoma, are particularly potent carcinogenic agents.[3] They are activated by hepatocytes and their products incorporated into the host DNA with the potential for producing cancer-producing mutations. A particularly susceptible site for aflatoxin is the p53 tumor suppressor gene (see Chapter 8).

The manifestations of hepatocellular cancer often are insidious in onset and masked by those related to cirrhosis or chronic hepatitis. The initial symptoms include weakness, anorexia, weight loss, fatigue, bloating, a sensation of abdominal fullness, and a dull, aching abdominal pain. Ascites, which often obscures weight loss, is common. Jaundice, if present, usually is mild. There may be a rapid increase in liver size and worsening of ascites in persons with pre-existing cirrhosis. Usually, the liver is enlarged when these symptoms appear, and there is a low fever without apparent cause. Serum α-fetoprotein, a serum protein present during fetal life, normally is barely detectable in the serum after the age of 2 years, but it is present in 60% to 75% of cases of hepatocellular carcinoma.[3]

Cholangiocarcinoma occurs much less frequently than hepatocellular carcinoma. The etiology, clinical features, and prognosis vary considerably with the part of the biliary tree that is the site of origin. Cholangiocarcinoma is not associated with same risk factors as hepatocellular carcinoma. Instead, most of the risk factors revolve around long-standing inflammation and injury of the bile duct epithelium. Cholangiocarcinoma often presents with pain, weight loss, anorexia, and abdominal swelling or awareness of a mass in the right hypochondrium. Tumors affecting the central or distal bile ducts may present with jaundice.

Diagnostic methods include CT scans and MRI. Liver biopsy is used to confirm the diagnosis.

Primary cancers of the liver usually are far advanced at the time of diagnosis; the 5-year survival rate is approximately 1%, and most patients die within 6 months. The treatment of choice is subtotal hepatectomy, if conditions permit. Chemotherapy and radiation therapy are largely palliative. Although liver transplantation may be an option for people with well-compensated cirrhosis and small tumors, it often is impractical because of the shortage of donor organs.

Metastatic tumors of the liver are much more common than primary tumors. Common sources include colorectal cancer and spread from the breast, lung, or urogenital cancers. In addition, tumors of neuroendocrine origin spread to the liver. It often is difficult to distinguish primary from metastatic tumors with the use of CT scans, MRI, or ultrasonography. Usually the diagnosis is confirmed by biopsy.

In summary, the liver is subject to most of the disease processes that affect other body structures, such as vascular disorders, inflammation, metabolic diseases, toxic injury, and neoplasms. As the major drug-metabolizing and detoxifying organ in the body, the liver is subject to potential damage from the enormous array of pharmaceutical and environmental chemicals. Drugs and chemicals can exert their effects by causing hepatocyte injury and death or by cholestatic liver damage due to injury of biliary drainage structures. Drug reactions can be predictable based on the drug's chemical structure and metabolites, or unpredictable (idiosyncratic) based on individual characteristics of the person receiving the drug. Early identification of drug-induced liver disease is important because withdrawal of the drug is curative in most cases.

Hepatitis is characterized by inflammation of the liver. Acute viral hepatitis is caused by hepatitis viruses A, B, C, D, and E. Although all these viruses cause acute hepatitis, they differ in terms of mode of transmission, incubation period, mechanism, degree and chronicity of liver damage, and the ability to evolve to a carrier state. HBV, HCV, and HDV have the potential for progression to the carrier state, chronic hepatitis, and hepatocellular carcinoma.

Intrahepatic biliary diseases disrupt the flow of bile through the liver, causing cholestasis and biliary cirrhosis. Among the causes of intrahepatic biliary diseases are primary biliary cirrhosis, primary sclerosing cholangitis, and secondary biliary cirrhosis. Because alcohol competes for use of intracellular cofactors normally needed by the liver for other metabolic processes, it tends to disrupt the metabolic functions of the liver. The spectrum of alcoholic liver disease includes fatty liver disease, alcoholic hepatitis, and cirrhosis.

Cirrhosis represents the end stage of chronic liver disease in which much of the functional liver tissue has been replaced by fibrous tissue. The fibrous tissue replaces normally functioning liver tissue and forms constrictive bands that disrupt flow in the vascular channels and biliary duct systems of the liver. The disruption of vascular channels predisposes to portal hypertension and its complications, loss of liver cells, and eventual liver failure. Portal hypertension is characterized by increased resistance to flow and increased pressure in the portal venous system; the pathologic consequences of the disorder include ascites, the formation of collateral bypass channels (*e.g.*, esophageal varices) from the portosystemic circulation, and splenomegaly. Liver failure represents the end stage of a number of liver diseases and occurs when less than 10% of liver tissue is functional. The manifestations of liver failure reflect the various functions of the liver, including hematologic disorders, disruption of endocrine function, skin disorders, hepatorenal syndrome, and hepatic encephalopathy. With the introduction of the immunosuppressant agent cyclosporine, liver transplantation is becoming a more realistic form of treatment for end-stage liver disease.

Cancers of the liver include metastatic and primary neoplasms. Primary hepatic neoplasms are rare, accounting for less than 2% of cancers, and those involving the hepatocytes or liver cells are commonly associated with underlying diseases of the liver such as cirrhosis and chronic hepatitis. Liver cancer usually is far advanced at the time of diagnosis; the 5-year survival rate is approximately 1%.

Disorders of the Gallbladder and Exocrine Pancreas

After you have completed this section of the chapter, you should be able to meet the following objectives:

✦ Explain the function of the gallbladder in regulating the flow of bile into the duodenum

✦ Describe the formation of gallstones

✦ Describe the clinical manifestations of acute and chronic cholecystitis

✦ Characterize the effects of choledocholithiasis and cholangitis on bile flow and the potential for hepatic and pancreatic complications

✦ Cite the possible causes and describe the manifestations and treatment of acute pancreatitis

✦ Describe the manifestations of chronic pancreatitis

✦ State the reason for the poor prognosis in pancreatic cancer

DISORDERS OF THE GALLBLADDER

The gallbladder is a distensible, pear-shaped, muscular sac located on the ventral surface of the liver. It has a smooth muscle wall and is lined with a thin layer of absorptive cells. The cystic duct joins the gallbladder to the common duct (see Fig. 38-1). The function of the gallbladder is to store and concentrate bile. When full, it can hold 30 to 60 mL of bile.[1]

Entrance of food into the intestine causes contraction of the gallbladder and relaxation of the *sphincter of Oddi*. The stimulus for gallbladder contraction is primarily hormonal. Products of food digestion, particularly lipids, stimulate the release of a gastrointestinal hormone called *cholecystokinin* from the mucosa of the duodenum. Cholecystokinin provides a strong stimulus for gallbladder contraction. The role of other gastrointestinal hormones in bile release is less clearly understood. Passage of bile into the intestine is regulated largely by the pressure in the common duct. Normally, the gallbladder regulates this pressure. It collects and stores bile as it relaxes and the pressure in the common bile duct decreases, and it empties bile into the intestine as the gallbladder contracts, producing an increase in common duct pressure. After gallbladder surgery, the pressure in the common duct changes, causing the common duct to dilate. The flow of bile then is regulated by the sphincters in the common duct.

Two common disorders of the biliary system are cholelithiasis (*i.e.,* gallstones) and inflammation of the gallbladder (cholecystitis) or common bile duct (cholangitis). At least 10% of adults have gallstones. Approximately twice as many women as men have gallstones, and there is an increased prevalence with age—after 60 years of age, 10% to 15% among men and 20% to 40% among women.[48]

Composition of Bile and Formation of Gallstones

Gallstones are caused by precipitation of substances contained in bile, mainly cholesterol and bilirubin. Bile contains bile salts, cholesterol, bilirubin, lecithin, fatty acids, and water and the electrolytes normally found in the plasma. The cholesterol found in bile has no known function; it is assumed to be a byproduct of bile salt formation, and its presence is linked to the excretory function of bile. Normally insoluble in water, cholesterol is rendered soluble by the action of bile salts and lecithin, which combine with it to form micelles. In the gallbladder, water and electrolytes are absorbed from the liver bile, causing the bile to become more concentrated. Because neither lecithin nor bile salts are absorbed in the gallbladder, their concentration increases along with that of cholesterol; in this way, the solubility of cholesterol is maintained.

The bile of which gallstones are formed usually is supersaturated with cholesterol or bilirubinate. Approximately 75% of gallstones are composed primarily of cholesterol; the other 25% are black or brown pigment stones consisting of calcium salts with bilirubin.[48] Many stones have a mixed composition. Figure 38-15 shows a gallbladder with numerous cholesterol gallstones.

Three factors contribute to the formation of gallstones: abnormalities in the composition of bile, stasis of bile, and inflammation of the gallbladder. The formation of choles-

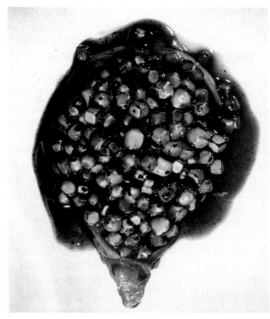

FIGURE 38-15 Cholesterol gallstones. The gallbladder has been opened to reveal numerous yellow cholesterol gallstones (Rubin E., Farber J.L. [1999]. *Pathology* [3rd ed., p. 791]. Philadelphia: Lippincott Williams & Wilkins)

terol stones is associated with obesity and occurs more frequently in women, especially women who have had multiple pregnancies or who are taking oral contraceptives. All of these factors cause the liver to excrete more cholesterol into the bile. Estrogen reduces the synthesis of bile acid in women. Gallbladder sludge (thickened gallbladder mucoprotein with tiny trapped cholesterol crystals) is thought to be a precursor of gallstones. Sludge frequently occurs with pregnancy, starvation, and rapid weight loss.[48] Drugs that lower serum cholesterol levels, such as clofibrate, also cause increased cholesterol excretion into the bile. Malabsorption disorders stemming from ileal disease or intestinal bypass surgery, for example, tend to interfere with the absorption of bile salts, which are needed to maintain the solubility of cholesterol. Inflammation of the gallbladder alters the absorptive characteristics of the mucosal layer, allowing excessive absorption of water and bile salts. Cholesterol gallstones are extremely common among Native Americans, which suggests that a genetic component may have a role in gallstone formation. Pigment stones containing bilirubin are seen in persons with hemolytic disease (*e.g.,* sickle cell disease) and hepatic cirrhosis.

Manifestations. Many persons with gallstones have no symptoms. Gallstones cause symptoms when they obstruct bile flow. Small stones (*e.g.,* <8 mm in diameter) pass into the common duct, producing symptoms of indigestion and biliary colic. Larger stones are more likely to obstruct flow and cause jaundice. The pain of biliary colic usually is abrupt in onset and increases steadily in intensity until it reaches a climax in 30 to 60 minutes. The upper right quadrant, or epigastric area, is the usual location of the pain, often with referred pain to the back, above the waist, the right shoulder, and the right scapula or the midscapular region. A few persons experience pain on the left side. The pain usually persists for 2 to 8 hours and is followed by soreness in the upper right quadrant.

Acute and Chronic Cholecystitis

The term *cholecystitis* refers to inflammation of the gallbladder. Both acute and chronic cholecystitis are associated with cholelithiasis. Acute cholecystitis may be superimposed on chronic cholecystitis.

Acute cholecystitis almost always is associated with complete or partial obstruction. It is believed that the inflammation is caused by chemical irritation from the concentrated bile, along with mucosal swelling and ischemia resulting from venous congestion and lymphatic stasis. The gallbladder usually is markedly distended. Bacterial infections may arise secondary to the ischemia and chemical irritation. The bacteria reach the injured gallbladder through the blood, lymphatics, or bile ducts or from adjacent organs. Among the common pathogens are staphylococci and enterococci. The wall of the gallbladder is most vulnerable to the effects of ischemia, as a result of which mucosal necrosis and sloughing occur. The process may lead to gangrenous changes and perforation of the gallbladder.

Chronic cholecystitis results from repeated episodes of acute cholecystitis or chronic irritation of the gallbladder by stones. It is characterized by varying degrees of chronic inflammation. Gallstones almost always are present. Cholelithiasis with chronic cholecystitis may be associated with acute exacerbations of gallbladder inflammation, common duct stone, pancreatitis, and, rarely, carcinoma of the gallbladder.

Manifestations.   The signs and symptoms of acute cholecystitis vary with the severity of obstruction and inflammation. Pain, initially similar to that of biliary colic, is characteristic of acute cholecystitis. It often is precipitated by a fatty meal and may initiate with complaints of indigestion. It does not, however, subside spontaneously and responds poorly or only temporarily to potent analgesics. When the inflammation progresses to involve the peritoneum, the pain becomes more pronounced in the right upper quadrant. The right subcostal region is tender, and the muscles that surround the area spasm. Approximately 75% of patients have vomiting, and approximately 25% have jaundice.[25] Fever and an abnormally high white blood cell count attest to inflammation. Total serum bilirubin, aminotransferase, and alkaline phosphatase levels usually are elevated.

The manifestations of chronic cholecystitis are more vague than those of acute cholecystitis. There may be intolerance to fatty foods, belching, and other indications of discomfort. Often, there are episodes of colicky pain with obstruction of biliary flow caused by gallstones. The gallbladder, which in chronic cholecystitis usually contains stones, may be enlarged, shrunken, or of normal size.

Diagnosis and Treatment.   The methods used to diagnose gallbladder disease include ultrasonography, nuclear scanning (cholescintigraphy), and oral cholecystography.[48]

Ultrasonography is widely used in diagnosing gallbladder disease and has largely replaced the oral cholecystogram in most medical centers. It can detect stones as small as 1 to 2 cm, and its overall accuracy in detecting gallbladder disease is high. In addition to stones, ultrasonography can detect wall thickening, which indicates inflammation. It also can rule out other causes of right upper quadrant pain such as tumors. Cholescintigraphy, also called a *gallbladder scan*, relies on the ability of the liver to extract a rapidly injected radionuclide, technetium-99m, bound to one of several iminodiacetic acids, that is excreted into the bile ducts. Serial scanning images are obtained within several minutes of the injection of the tracer and every 10 to 15 minutes during the next hour. The gallbladder scan is highly accurate in detecting acute cholecystitis. Oral cholecystography is a radiologic technique that uses oral tablets containing a radiopaque contrast medium that is absorbed from the gut, excreted in the bile, and becomes concentrated in the gallbladder. The person being tested must follow a fat-free diet for 1 to 2 days before the test. The dye is taken 10 to 14 hours before the examination; it may produce nausea and vomiting in 5% to 10% of persons and diarrhea in as many as 25%.

Gallbladder disease usually is treated by removing the gallbladder or by dissolving the stones or fragmenting them. Laparoscopic cholecystectomy has become the treatment of choice for symptomatic gallbladder disease.[49] The procedure involves insertion of a laparoscope through a small incision near the umbilicus, and surgical instruments are inserted through several stab wounds in the upper abdomen. Although the procedure requires more time than the older open surgical procedure, it usually requires only 1 night in the hospital. A major advantage of the procedure is that patients can return to work in 1 to 2 weeks, compared with 4 to 6 weeks after open cholecystectomy.[48] The gallbladder stores and concentrates bile, and its removal usually does not interfere with digestion.

The bile acids—chenodeoxycholic acid and ursodeoxycholic acid—have proved capable of dissolving gallstones and may be used to treat asymptomatic cholelithiasis.[48] They act by desaturating cholesterol in solution in the bile. For the treatment to be effective, the stones must be predominantly cholesterol and not be calcified. The treatment dissolves most stones within 1 or 2 years. Chenodeoxycholic acid is associated with elevation of low-density lipoproteins, dose-related diarrhea, and elevated levels of liver enzymes (*i.e.*, ALT and AST). The drug is not recommended for women of childbearing age because it may adversely affect the fetal liver. Ursodeoxycholic acid appears to have less effect on liver enzymes and produces less diarrhea. This method of treatment is considered only for people who either refuse or are poor risks for surgery.[48]

Extracorporeal shock-wave lithotripsy uses sound waves to pulverize gallstones so that they can be passed through the bile duct.[48] The procedure is suitable only for radiolucent stones because the shock waves must be focused on each stone. Although not a common complication, stone fragments can become trapped in the bile duct. Adjunctive bile acid therapy often is used to speed dissolution of stone fragments.

Choledocholithiasis and Cholangitis

Choledocholithiasis refers to stones in the common duct and cholangitis to inflammation of the common duct. Common duct stones usually originate in the gallbladder, but can form spontaneously in the common duct. The stones frequently are clinically silent unless there is obstruction.

The manifestations of choledocholithiasis are similar to those of gallstones and acute cholecystitis. There is a history of acute biliary colic and right upper abdominal pain, with chills, fever, and jaundice associated with episodes of abdominal pain. Bilirubinuria and an elevated serum bilirubin are present if the common duct is obstructed.

Complications include acute suppurative cholangitis accompanied by pus in the common duct. It is characterized by the presence of an altered sensorium, lethargy, and septic shock.[25] Acute suppurative cholangitis represents an endoscopic or surgical emergency. Common duct stones also can obstruct the outflow of the pancreatic duct, causing a secondary pancreatitis.

Diagnosis and Treatment. Ultrasonography, CT scans, and radionuclide imaging may be used to demonstrate dilatation of bile ducts and impaired blood flow. Endoscopic ultrasonography and magnetic resonance cholangiography are used for detecting common duct stones. Both percutaneous transhepatic cholangiography (PTC) and endoscopic retrograde cholangiopancreatography (ERCP) provide a direct means for determining the cause, location, and extent of obstruction. PTC involves the injection of dye directly into the biliary tree. It requires the insertion of a thin, flexible needle through a small incision in the skin with advancement into the biliary tree. ERCP involves the passage of an endoscope into the duodenum and the passage of a catheter into the ampulla of Vater. ERCP can be used to enlarge the opening of the sphincter of Oddi, which may allow the lodged stone to pass, or an instrument may be inserted into the common duct to remove the stone.

Common duct stones in persons with cholelithiasis usually are treated by stone extraction followed by laparoscopic cholecystectomy. Antibiotic therapy, with an agent that penetrates the bile, is used to treat the infection. Emergency decompression of the common duct, usually by ERCP, may be necessary for persons who are septic or fail to improve with antibiotic treatment.

Cancer of the Gallbladder

Cancer of the gallbladder is found in approximately 2% of persons operated on for biliary tract disease. The onset of symptoms usually is insidious, and they resemble those of cholecystitis; the diagnosis often is made unexpectedly at the time of gallbladder surgery. Because of their ability to produce chronic irritation of the gallbladder mucosa, it is believed that gallstones play a role in the development of gallbladder cancer. The 5-year survival rate is only approximately 3%.[3]

DISORDERS OF THE EXOCRINE PANCREAS

The pancreas lies transversely in the posterior part of the upper abdomen. The head of the pancreas is at the right of the abdomen; it rests against the curve of the duodenum in the area of the ampulla of Vater and its entrance into the duodenum. The body of the pancreas lies beneath the stomach. The tail touches the spleen. The pancreas is virtually hidden because of its posterior position; unlike many other organs, it cannot be palpated. Because of the position of the pancreas and its large functional reserve, symptoms from conditions such as cancer of the pancreas do not usually appear until the disorder is far advanced.

The pancreas is both an endocrine and exocrine organ. Its function as an endocrine organ is discussed in Chapter 41. The exocrine pancreas is made up of lobules that consist of acinar cells, which secrete digestive enzymes into a system of microscopic ducts. These ducts are terminal branches of larger ducts that drain into the main pancreatic duct, which extends from left to right through the substance of the pancreas (see Fig. 38-1). In most persons, the main pancreatic duct empties into the ampulla of Vater, although in some it empties directly into the duodenum. The pancreatic ducts are lined with epithelial cells that secrete water and bicarbonate and thereby modify the fluid and electrolyte composition of the pancreatic secretions.

The pancreatic secretions contain proteolytic enzymes that break down dietary proteins, including trypsin, chymotrypsin, carboxypolypeptidase, ribonuclease, and deoxyribonuclease. The pancreas also secretes pancreatic amylase, which breaks down starch, and lipases, which hydrolyze neutral fats into glycerol and fatty acids. The pancreatic enzymes are secreted in the inactive form and become activated in the intestine. This is important because the enzymes would digest the tissue of the pancreas itself if they were secreted in the active form. The acinar cells secrete a trypsin inhibitor, which prevents trypsin activation. Because trypsin activates other proteolytic enzymes, the trypsin inhibitor prevents subsequent activation of those other enzymes.

Two types of pancreatic disease are discussed in this chapter: acute and chronic pancreatitis and cancer of the pancreas.

Acute Pancreatitis

Acute pancreatitis is a severe, life-threatening disorder associated with the escape of activated pancreatic enzymes into the pancreas and surrounding tissues. These enzymes cause fat necrosis, or autodigestion, of the pancreas and produce fatty deposits in the abdominal cavity with hemorrhage from the necrotic vessels. Although a number of factors are associated with the development of acute pancreatitis, most cases result from gallstones (stones in the common duct) or alcohol abuse.[50-52] In the case of biliary tract obstruction due to gallstones, pancreatic duct obstruction or biliary reflux is believed to activate the enzymes in the pancreatic duct system. The precise mechanisms whereby alcohol exerts its action are largely unknown. Alcohol is known to be a potent stimulator of pancreatic secretions, and it also is known to cause partial obstruction of the sphincter of Oddi. Acute pancreatitis also is associated with hyperlipidemia, hyperparathyroidism, infections (particularly viral), abdominal and surgical trauma, and drugs such as steroids and thiazide diuretics.

Acute pancreatitis may be classified histologically as interstitial edematous or as necrotizing according to inflammatory changes in the pancreatic tissue.[51] Acute necrotizing pancreatitis usually is associated with necrosis of peripancreatic fat. It represents a severe form of acute pancreatitis with a mortality rate of 23%, compared with 6% for acute non-necrotizing pancreatitis.[51] The mortality rate is even higher in patients in whom the necrotic tissue becomes infected. It is thought that infection occurs primarily as a result of bacterial spread from the colon.

The onset of acute pancreatitis usually is abrupt and dramatic, and it may follow a heavy meal or an alcoholic binge. The most common initial symptom is severe epigastric and abdominal pain that radiates to the back. The pain is aggravated when the person is lying supine; it is less severe when the person is sitting and leaning forward. Abdominal distention accompanied by hypoactive bowel sounds is common. An important disturbance related to acute pancreatitis is the loss of a large volume of fluid into the retroperitoneal and peripancreatic spaces and the abdominal cavity. Tachycardia, hypotension, cool and clammy skin, and fever often are evident. Signs of hypocalcemia may develop, probably as a result of the precipitation of serum calcium in the areas of fat necrosis. Mild jaundice may appear after the first 24 hours because of biliary obstruction.

Total serum amylase is the test used most frequently in the diagnosis of acute pancreatitis. Serum amylase levels rise within the first 24 hours after onset of symptoms and remain elevated for 48 to 72 hours. The serum lipase level also is elevated during the first 24 to 48 hours, but remains elevated for 5 to 14 days. Urinary clearance of amylase is increased. Because the serum amylase level may be elevated as a result of other serious illnesses, the urinary level of amylase is often measured. The white blood cell count may be increased, and hyperglycemia and an elevated serum bilirubin level may be present. Plain radiographs of the abdomen may be used for detecting gallstones or abdominal complications. CT scans and dynamic contrast-enhanced CT of the pancreas are used to detect necrosis and fluid accumulation.

Complications include acute respiratory distress syndrome and acute tubular necrosis. Hypocalcemia occurs in approximately 25% of patients. Age older than 55 years, an elevated white blood cell count ($>16,000/\mu L$), and elevated levels of blood glucose (>200 mg/dL), serum lactate dehydrogenase (>350 IU/L), and AST (>250 IU/L) at the time of diagnosis are associated with a poorer prognosis, as are a decrease in hematocrit and serum calcium, increased fluid sequestration (>6 L), an arterial oxygen tension less than 60 mm Hg, and a base deficit greater than 4 mEq/L that develop within the first 48 hours.[51]

The treatment consists of measures directed at pain relief, "putting the pancreas to rest," and restoration of lost plasma volume. Antibiotic prophylaxis is used to prevent infection of necrotic pancreatic tissue. Meperidine (Demerol) rather than morphine usually is given for pain relief because it causes fewer spasms of the sphincter of Oddi. Papaverine,

nitroglycerin, barbiturates, or anticholinergic drugs may be given as supplements to provide smooth muscle relaxation. Oral foods and fluids are withheld, and gastric suction is instituted to treat distention of the bowel and prevent further stimulation of the secretion of pancreatic enzymes. Intravenous fluids and electrolytes are administered to replace those lost from the circulation and to combat hypotension and shock. Intravenous colloid solutions are given to replace the fluid that has become sequestered in the abdomen and retroperitoneal space. Percutaneous peritoneal lavage has been tried as an early treatment of acute pancreatitis with encouraging results. If a pancreatic abscess develops, it must be drained, usually through the flank.

A pseudocyst is a collection of pancreatic fluid in the peritoneal cavity enclosed in a layer of inflammatory tissue. Autodigestion or liquefaction of pancreatic tissue may be the cause. The pseudocyst most often is connected to a pancreatic duct, so that it continues to increase in mass. The symptoms depend on its location; for example, jaundice may occur when a cyst develops near the head of the pancreas, close to the common duct. Pseudocysts may resolve or, if they persist, may require surgical intervention.

Chronic Pancreatitis

Chronic pancreatitis is characterized by progressive destruction of the pancreas. It can be divided into two types: chronic calcifying pancreatitis and chronic obstructive pancreatitis.[53] In chronic calcifying pancreatitis, calcified protein plugs (*i.e.*, calculi) form in the pancreatic ducts. This form is seen most often in alcoholics. Alcohol damages pancreatic cells directly and also increases the concentration of proteins in the pancreatic secretions, which eventually leads to formation of protein plugs.[54] Other causes of chronic pancreatitis are cystic fibrosis and chronic obstructive pancreatitis owing to stenosis of the sphincter of Oddi. In obstructive pancreatitis, lesions are more prominent in the head of the pancreas. The disease usually is caused by cholelithiasis and sometimes is relieved by removal of the sphincter of Oddi.

Chronic pancreatitis is manifested in episodes that are similar, albeit of lesser severity, to those of acute pancreatitis. Patients have persistent, recurring episodes of epigastric and upper left quadrant pain; the attacks often are precipitated by alcohol abuse or overeating. Anorexia, nausea, vomiting, constipation, and flatulence are common. Eventually the disease progresses to the extent that endocrine and exocrine pancreatic functions become deficient. At this point, signs of diabetes mellitus and the malabsorption syndrome (*e.g.*, weight loss, fatty stools [steatorrhea]) become apparent.[53]

Treatment consists of measures to treat coexisting biliary tract disease. A low-fat diet usually is prescribed. The signs of malabsorption may be treated with pancreatic enzymes. When diabetes is present, it is treated with insulin. Alcohol is forbidden because it frequently precipitates attacks. Because of the frequent episodes of pain, narcotic addiction is a potential problem in persons with chronic pancreatitis. Surgical intervention sometimes is needed to relieve the pain and usually focuses on relieving any obstruction that may be present. In advanced cases, a subtotal or total pancreatectomy may be necessary.[25]

Cancer of the Pancreas

Pancreatic cancer is now the fourth leading cause of death in the United States, with more than 28,000 deaths attributed to the neoplasm each year.[55] Considered to be one of the most deadly malignancies, pancreatic cancer is associated with a death : incidence ratio of approximately 0.99. The risk of pancreatic cancer increases after the age of 50 years, with most cases occurring between the ages of 60 and 80 years. The incidence and mortality rates for both male and female African Americans are higher than for whites.

The cause of pancreatic cancer is unknown. Smoking appears to be a major risk factor.[55,56] The incidence of pancreatic cancer is twice as high among smokers than nonsmokers. The second most important factor appears to be diet. There appears to be an association of pancreatic cancer with an increasing total calorie intake and a high intake of fat, meat, salt, dehydrated foods, fried foods, refined sugars, soy beans, and nitrosamines. Data from animal studies indicate that nitrosamines and tobacco smoke are carcinogenic in the pancreas. A protective effect has been ascribed to a diet containing dietary fiber, vitamin C, fresh fruits and vegetables, and no preservatives. Diabetes and chronic pancreatitis also are associated with pancreatic cancer, although neither the nature nor the sequence of the possible cause-and-effect relation has been established.[56,57] Genetic alterations appear to play a role. There appears to be an association between pancreatic cancer and certain genetic disorders, including nonpolyposis colon cancer, familial breast cancer with the BRCA2 gene mutation (see Chapter 8), ataxia-telangiectasia syndrome, familial atypical multiple mole–melanoma syndrome, and hereditary pancreatitis.[55] There has been a recent focus on the molecular genetics of pancreatic cancer, and more insights into the genetic mechanisms involved in pancreatic cancer undoubtedly will be forthcoming.

Cancer of the pancreas usually has an insidious onset. Pain, jaundice, and weight loss constitute the classic presentation of the disease.[48] The most common pain is a dull epigastric pain often accompanied by back pain, often worse in the supine position, and relieved by sitting forward. Duodenal obstruction with nausea and vomiting is a late sign.

Because of the proximity of the pancreas to the common duct and the ampulla of Vater, cancer of the head of the pancreas tends to obstruct bile flow; this causes distention of the gallbladder and jaundice. Jaundice frequently is the presenting symptom of a person with cancer of the head of the pancreas, and it usually is accompanied by complaints of pain and pruritus. Cancer of the body of the pancreas usually impinges on the celiac ganglion, causing pain. The pain usually worsens with ingestion of food or with assumption of the supine position. Cancer of the tail of the pancreas usually has metastasized before symptoms appear.

Ultrasonography and CT scanning are the most frequently used diagnostic methods to confirm the disease. Intravenous and oral contrast–enhanced spiral CT is the preferred method for imaging the pancreas. Percutaneous fine-needle aspiration cytology of the pancreas has been one of the major advances in the diagnosis of pancreatic cancer. Unfortunately, the smaller and more curable tumors are most likely to be missed by this procedure. ERCP may be used for evaluation of persons with suspected pancreatic cancer and obstructive jaundice.

Most cancers of the pancreas have metastasized by the time of diagnosis. Surgical resection of the tumor is done when the tumor is localized, or as a palliative measure. Radiation therapy may be useful when the disease is not resectable but appears to be localized. The use of irradiation and chemotherapy for pancreatic cancer continues to be investigated. Pain control is one of the most important aspects in the management of persons with end-stage pancreatic cancer.

In summary, the biliary tract serves as a passageway for the delivery of bile from the liver to the intestine. This tract consists of the bile ducts and gallbladder. The most common causes of biliary tract disease are cholelithiasis and cholecystitis. Three factors contribute to the development of cholelithiasis: abnormalities in the composition of bile, stasis of bile, and inflammation of the gallbladder. Cholelithiasis predisposes to obstruction of bile flow, causing biliary colic and acute or chronic cholecystitis. Cancer of the gallbladder, which has a poor 5-year survival rate, occurs in 2% of persons with biliary tract disease.

The pancreas is an endocrine and exocrine organ. Diabetes mellitus is the most common disorder of the endocrine pancreas, and it occurs independently of disease of the exocrine pancreas. The exocrine pancreas produces digestive enzymes that are secreted in an inactive form and transported to the small intestine through the main pancreatic duct, which usually empties into the ampulla of Vater and then into the duodenum through the sphincter of Oddi. The most common diseases of the exocrine pancreas are acute and chronic forms of pancreatitis, and cancer. Acute and chronic types of pancreatitis are associated with biliary reflux and chronic alcoholism. Acute pancreatitis is a dramatic and life-threatening disorder in which there is auto-digestion of pancreatic tissue. Chronic pancreatitis causes progressive destruction of the endocrine and exocrine pancreas. It is characterized by episodes of pain and epigastric distress that are similar to but less severe than those that occur with acute pancreatitis. Cancer of the pancreas is the fourth leading cause of death in the United States. It usually is far advanced at the time of diagnosis, and the 5-year survival rate is less than 3%.

References

1. Guyton A., Hall J.E. (2000). *Textbook of medical physiology* (10th ed., pp. 781–802). Philadelphia: W.B. Saunders.
2. Rose S. (1998). *Gastrointestinal and hepatic pathophysiology*. Madison, CT: Fence Creek Publishing.
3. Crawford J.M. (1999). The liver and biliary tract. In Kumar V., Cotran R.S., Collins T. (Eds.), *Robbins pathologic basis of disease* (6th ed., pp. 845–901). Philadelphia: W.B. Saunders.
4. Rubin E., Farber J.L. (1999). The liver and biliary system. In Rubin E., Farber J.L. (Eds.), *Pathophysiology* (3rd ed., pp. 757–838). Philadelphia: Lippincott Williams & Wilkins.

5. Denery P.A., Seidman D.S., Stevenson D.K. (2001). Neonatal hyperbilirubinemia. *New England Journal of Medicine* 344, 581–590.

6. Herlong H.F. (1994). Approach to the patient with abnormal liver enzymes. *Hospital Practice* 29 (11), 32–38.

7. Pratt D.S., Kaplan M.M. (2000). Evaluation of abnormal liver-enzyme results in asymptomatic patients. *New England Journal of Medicine* 342, 1266–1271.

8. Bravo A., Sheth S.G., Chopra S. (2001). Liver biopsy. *New England Journal of Medicine* 344, 495–500.

9. Katzung B.G. (2001). *Basic and clinical pharmacology* (8th ed., pp. 51–63). New York: Lange Medical Books/McGraw-Hill.

10. Lee W.M. (1995). Drug-induced hepatotoxicity. *New England Journal of Medicine* 333, 1118–1127.

11. Lewis J.H. (2000). Drug-induced liver disease. *Medical Clinics of North America* 84, 1275–1311.

12. Advisory Committee on Immunization Practices. (1999). Prevention of hepatitis A through active and passive immunization. *Morbidity and Mortality Weekly Report* 48 (RR-12), 1–25.

13. Kemmer N.M., Miskovsky E.P. (2000). Hepatitis A. *Infectious Disease Clinics of North America* 14, 605–615.

14. Lee W.M. (1997). Hepatitis B virus infection. *New England Journal of Medicine* 337, 1733–1745.

15. Befeler A.S., DiBisceglie A.M. (2000). Hepatitis B. *Infectious Disease Clinics of North America* 14, 617–632.

16. Centers for Disease Control. (1991). Hepatitis B virus: A comprehensive strategy for eliminating transmission in the United States through universal childhood vaccination. *Morbidity and Mortality Weekly Report* 40 (RR-13), 1–25.

17. Advisory Committee on Immunization Practices. (1999). Notice to readers update: Recommendations to prevent hepatitis B transmission—United States. *Morbidity and Mortality Weekly Report* 48 (2), 33–34.

18. Lemon S.M., Thomas D.L. (1997). Vaccines to prevent viral hepatitis. *New England Journal of Medicine* 336, 196–203.

19. Sharara A.I., Hunt C.M., Hamilton J.D. (1996). Hepatitis C. *Annals of Internal Medicine* 125, 658–665.

20. Alter M.J., Kruszon-Moran D., Nainam O.V., McQuillan G.M., Gao F., Moyer L., Kaslow R.A., Margolis H.S. (1999). The prevalence of hepatitis C virus infection in the United States 1988 through 1994. *New England Journal of Medicine* 341, 556–562.

21. Centers for Disease Control and Prevention. (1998). Recommendations for prevention and control of hepatitis C virus (HCV) infection and HCV-related chronic disease. *Morbidity and Mortality Weekly Report* 47 (RR-19), 1–25.

22. Liang T.J., Reheman B., Seeff L.B., Hoofnagle J.H. (2000). Pathogenesis, natural history, treatment, and prevention of hepatitis C. *Annals of Internal Medicine* 132, 296–305.

23. Cheney C.P., Chopra S., Graham C. (2000). Hepatitis C. *Infectious Disease Clinics of North America* 14, 633–659.

24. Hoffnagle J.H. (1989). Type D (delta) hepatitis. *Journal of the American Medical Association* 261, 1321–1325.

25. Friedman S. (2001). Liver, biliary tract and pancreas. In Tierney L.M., McPhee S.J., Papadakis M.A. (Eds.), *Current medical diagnosis and treatment* (40th ed., 662–705). New York: Lange Medical Books/McGraw-Hill.

26. Maddrey W.C. (1994). Chronic viral hepatitis: Diagnosis and management. *Hospital Practice* 29 (2), 117–132.

27. Hoofnagle J.H., DiBisceglie A.M. (1997). The treatment of chronic hepatitis. *New England Journal of Medicine* 336, 347–355.

28. Lin O.S., Keeffe E.B. (2001). Current treatment strategies for chronic hepatitis B and C. *Annual Review of Medicine* 52, 29–49.

29. Krawitt E.L. (1996). Autoimmune hepatitis. *New England Journal of Medicine* 334, 897–902.

30. Kaplan M.M. (1996). Primary biliary cirrhosis. *New England Journal of Medicine* 335, 1570–1580.

31. Gershwin E., Mackay J.R. (1995). New knowledge in primary biliary cirrhosis. *Hospital Practice* 30 (8), 29–36.

32. Lee Y.-M., Kaplan M.M. (1995). Primary sclerosing cholangitis. *New England Journal of Medicine* 332, 924–932.

33. Lieber C.S. (2000). Alcohol: Its metabolism and interaction with nutrients. *Annual Review of Nutrition* 20, 395–430.

34. Alchord J.L. (1995). Alcohol and the liver. *Scientific American Science and Medicine* 2 (2), 16–25.

35. Lieber C.S. (1994). Alcohol and the liver: 1994 update. *Gastroenterology* 106, 1085–1105.

36. Lieber C.S. (1988). Biochemical and molecular basis for alcohol-induced injury to the liver and other tissues. *New England Journal of Medicine* 319, 1639–1650.

37. Rubin E., Lieber C.S. (1968). Alcohol-induced hepatic injury in non-alcoholic volunteers. *New England Journal of Medicine* 278, 869–876.

38. Trevillyan J., Carroll P.J. (1997). Management of portal hypertension and esophageal varices in alcoholic cirrhosis. *American Family Physician* 55, 1851–1858.

39. Roberts L.R., Kamath P.S. (1996). Ascites and hepatorenal syndrome: Pathophysiology and management. *Mayo Clinic Proceedings* 71, 874–881.

40. Epstein M. (1995). Renal sodium retention in liver disease. *Hospital Practice* 30(9), 33–41.

41. Garcia N., Sanyal A.J. (2001). Minimizing ascites: Complications of cirrhosis signals clinical deterioration. *Postgraduate Medicine* 109 (2), 91–103.

42. Hegab A.M., Luketic V.A. (2001). Bleeding esophageal varices. *Postgraduate Medicine* 109 (2), 75–89.

43. National Institutes of Health. (1983). National Institutes of Health Consensus Conference Statement on Liver Transplantation. *Hepatology* 4 (Suppl.), 107S–111S.

44. Rosen H.R., Martin P. (1999). Liver transplantation. In Schiff E.R., Sorrell M.F., Maddrey W.C. (Eds.), *Schiff's diseases of the liver* (8th ed., pp. 1589–1615). Philadelphia: Lippincott Williams & Wilkins.

45. Rosen R.H., Shackleton C.R., Martin P. (1996). Indications and timing of liver transplantation. *Medical Clinics of North America* 80, 1069–1102.

46. American Cancer Society. (2001). Liver cancer (updated January 30, 20001). [On-line]. Available: http://www3.cancer.org.

47. Bisceglie A.M. (1999). Malignant neoplasms of the liver. In Schiff E.R., Sorrell M.F., Maddrey W.C. (Eds.), *Schiff's diseases of the liver* (8th ed., pp. 1281–1300). Philadelphia: Lippincott Williams & Wilkins.

48. Johnston D.E., Kaplan M.M. (1993). Pathogenesis and treatment of gallstones. *New England Journal of Medicine* 328, 412–421.

49. Birkett D.H. (1993). Laparoscopic cholecystectomy with common duct exploration. *Hospital Practice* 28 (5), 37–44.

50. Steinberg W., Jenner S. (1994). Acute pancreatitis. *New England Journal of Medicine* 330, 1198–1210.

51. Baron T.H., Morgan D.E. (1999). Acute necrotizing pancreatitis. *New England Journal of Medicine* 340, 1412–1417.

52. Cartmell M.T., Kingsnorth A.N. (2000). Acute pancreatitis. *Hospital Medicine* 61, 382–385.

53. Steer M.L., Waxman L., Freeman S. (1995). Chronic pancreatitis. *New England Journal of Medicine* 332, 1482–1490.

54. Isla A.M. (2000). Chronic pancreatitis. *Hospital Medicine* 61, 386–389.

55. Lillemoe K.D. (2000). Pancreatic cancer: State-of-the-art care. *CA: A Cancer Journal for Clinicians* 50, 241–268.

56. Warshaw A.I., Castillo C.F. (1992). Pancreatic carcinoma. *New England Journal of Medicine* 326, 455–465.

57. Wanebo H.J., Vezeridis M.P. (1996). Pancreatic cancer in perspective. *Cancer* 76, 580–587.

Endocrine Function

By the end of the Middle Ages, a great storehouse of anatomic knowledge existed; however, this repository had been culled from a combination of incomplete observations, religious beliefs, extrapolation from animal structures, and philosophical guesswork. Scientists slavishly adhered to these teachings, many of which were the products of the early Greeks (such as Aristotle and Galen), even though personal experience provided them with contradictory evidence.

The endocrine system fell victim to the outdated theories postulated long before. Even when some of its parts were discovered, their importance went unrecognized. For example, the pituitary gland, first noted in 1524 by Jacob Berengar of Carpi, was considered to be necessary to the cooling function of the brain. The brain was thought to secrete *pituita*, phlegm (mucous), and discharge it from the nose as part of its cooling process. The gland received its name from Andreas Vesalius, who referred to it in his text *De Fabrica (1543)* as *glandula pituitam cerebri excipiens*, or the gland that receives the phlegm from the brain. It was not until the late 19th and early 20th centuries that the field of endocrinology had its beginnings. It was then that the importance of the pituitary gland was finally realized, and it was called the master endocrine gland.

Chapter 39

Mechanisms of Endocrine Control

Glenn Matfin, Safak Guven, and Julie A. Kuenzi

The endocrine system is involved in all of the integrative aspects of life, including growth, sex differentiation, metabolism, and adaptation to an ever-changing environment. This chapter focuses on general aspects of endocrine function, organization of the endocrine system, hormone receptors and hormone actions, and regulation of hormone levels.

The Endocrine System

After you have completed this section of the chapter, you should be able to meet the following objectives:

✦ Characterize a hormone
✦ State a difference between the synthesis of protein hormones and that of steroid hormones
✦ Describe mechanisms of hormone transport and inactivation
✦ State the function of a hormone receptor and state the difference between cell surface hormone receptors and intracellular hormone receptors
✦ Describe the role of the hypothalamus in regulating pituitary control of endocrine function
✦ State the major difference between positive and negative feedback control mechanisms
✦ Describe methods used in diagnosis of endocrine disorders

The endocrine system uses chemical substances called *hormones* as a means of regulating and integrating body functions. The endocrine system participates in the regulation of digestion, use, and storage of nutrients; growth and development; electrolyte and water metabolism; and reproductive functions. Although the endocrine system once was thought to consist solely of discrete endocrine glands, it is now known that a number of other tissues release chemical messengers that modulate body processes. The functions of the endocrine system are closely linked with those of the nervous system and the immune system. For example, neurotransmitters such as epinephrine can act as neurotransmitters or as hormones. The functions of the immune system also are closely linked with those of the endocrine system. The immune system responds to foreign agents by means of chemical messengers (cytokines, *e.g.*, interleukins, interferons) and complex receptor mechanisms (see Chapter 18). The immune system also is extensively regulated by hormones such as the adrenal corticosteroid hormones.

HORMONES

Hormones generally are thought of as chemical messengers that are transported in body fluids. They are highly specialized organic molecules produced by endocrine organs that exert their action on specific target cells. Hormones do not initiate reactions; they are modulators of systemic and cellular responses. Most hormones are present in body fluids at all times, but in greater or lesser amounts depending on the needs of the body.

A characteristic of hormones is that a single hormone can exert various effects in different tissues or, conversely, a single function can be regulated by several hormones. For example, estradiol, which is produced by the ovary, can act on the ovarian follicles to promote their maturation, on the uterus to stimulate its growth and maintain the cyclic changes in the uterine mucosa, on the mammary gland to stimulate ductal growth, on the hypothalamic-pituitary system to regulate the secretion of gonadotropins and prolactin, and on general metabolic processes to affect adipose tissue distribution. Lipolysis, which is the release of free fatty acids from adipose tissue, is an example of a single function that is regulated by several hormones, including the catecholamines, glucagon, secretin, and prolactin. Table 39-1 lists the major functions and sources of body hormones.

Paracrine and Autocrine Actions

In the past, hormones were described as chemical substances that were released into the bloodstream and transported to distant target sites, where they exerted their action. Although many hormones travel by this mechanism, some hormones and hormone-like substances never enter the bloodstream but instead act locally in the vicinity in which they are released. When they act locally on cells other than those that produced the hormone, the action is called *paracrine*. The action of sex steroids on the ovary is a paracrine action. Hormones also can exert an *autocrine* action on the cells from which they were produced. For example, the release of insulin from pancreatic beta cells can inhibit its release from the same cells. *Juxtacrine* refers to a mechanism whereby a cytokine that is embedded in, bound to, or associated with the plasma membrane of one cell interacts with a specific receptor in a juxtaposed cell.

Eicosanoids and Retinoids

A group of compounds that have a hormone-like action are the eicosanoids, which are derived from polyunsaturated fatty acids in the cell membrane. Among these, *arachidonic acid* is the most important and abundant precursor of the various eicosanoids. The most important of the eicosanoids are the prostaglandins, leukotrienes, and thromboxanes. These fatty acid derivatives are produced by most body cells, are rapidly cleared from the circulation, and are thought to act mainly by paracrine and autocrine mechanisms. Eicosanoid synthesis often is stimulated in response to hormones, and they serve as mediators of hormone action.

Retinoids (*e.g.*, retinoic acid) also are derived from fatty acids and have an important role in regulating nuclear receptor action.

Structural Classification

Hormones have diverse structures ranging from single amino acids to complex proteins and lipids. Hormones usually are divided into four categories according to their structures: (1) amines and amino acids; (2) peptides, polypeptides, glycoproteins, and proteins; (3) steroids; and (4) fatty acid derivatives (Table 39-2). The first category, the amines, includes norepinephrine, epinephrine, and dopamine, which are derived from a single amino acid (*i.e.*, tyrosine), and the thyroid hormones, which are derived from two iodinated tyrosine amino acid residues. The second category, the peptides, polypeptides, glycoproteins, and proteins, can be as small as thyrotropin-releasing hormone (TRH), which contains three amino acids, and as large and complex as growth hormone (GH) and follicle-stimulating hormone (FSH), which have approximately 200 amino acids. Glycoproteins are large peptide hormones associated with a carbohydrate (*e.g.*, FSH). The third category comprises the steroid hormones, which are derivatives of cholesterol. The fourth category, the fatty acid derivatives, includes the eicosanoids and retinoids.

Synthesis and Transport

The mechanisms for hormone synthesis vary with hormone structure. Protein and peptide hormones are synthesized and stored in granules or vesicles in the cytoplasm of the cell until secretion is required. The lipid-soluble steroid hormones are released as they are synthesized.

Protein and peptide hormones are synthesized in the rough endoplasmic reticulum in a manner similar to the synthesis of other proteins (see Chapter 4). The appropriate amino acid sequence is dictated by messenger RNAs from the nucleus. Usually, synthesis involves the production of a precursor hormone, which is modified by the addition of peptides or sugar units. These precursor hormones often contain extra peptide units that ensure proper folding of the molecule and insertion of essential linkages. If extra amino acids are present, as in insulin, the precursor hormone is called a *prohormone*. After synthesis and sequestration in the endoplasmic reticulum, the protein and peptide

Hormones

➤ Hormones function as chemical messengers, moving through the blood to distant target sites of action, or acting more locally as paracrine or autocrine messengers that incite more local effects.

➤ Most hormones are present in body fluids at all times, but in greater or lesser amounts depending on the needs of the body.

➤ Hormones exert their actions by interacting with high-affinity receptors, which in turn are linked to one or more effector systems in the cell. Some hormone receptors are located on the surface of the cell and act through second messenger mechanisms, and others are located in the cell, where they modulate the synthesis of enzymes, transport proteins, or structural proteins.

TABLE 39-1 ✦ **Major Action and Source of Selected Hormones**

Source	Hormone	Major Action

Hypothalamus	Releasing and inhibiting hormones
	  Corticotropin-releasing hormone (CRH)
	  Thyrotropin-releasing hormone (TRH)
	  Growth hormone-releasing hormone (GHRH)
	  Gonadotropin-releasing hormone (GnRH)
		Controls the release of pituitary hormones

Anterior pituitary	Growth hormone (GH)	Stimulates growth of bone and muscle, promotes protein synthesis and fat metabolism, decreases carbohydrate metabolism
	Adrenocorticotropic hormone (ACTH)	Stimulates synthesis and secretion of adrenal cortical hormones
	Thyroid-stimulating hormone (TSH)	Stimulates synthesis and secretion of thyroid hormone
	Follicle-stimulating hormone (FSH)	Female: stimulates growth of ovarian follicle, ovulation Male: stimulates sperm production
	Luteinizing hormone (LH)	Female: stimulates development of corpus luteum, release of oocyte, production of estrogen and progesterone Male: stimulates secretion of testosterone, development of interstitial tissue of testes
Posterior pituitary	Antidiuretic hormone (ADH)	Increases water reabsorption by kidney
	Oxytocin	Stimulates contraction of pregnant uterus, milk ejection from breasts after childbirth
Adrenal cortex	Mineralocorticosteroids, mainly aldosterone	Increases sodium absorption, potassium loss by kidney
	Glucocorticoids, mainly cortisol	Affects metabolism of all nutrients; regulates blood glucose levels, affects growth, has anti-inflammatory action, and decreases effects of stress
	Adrenal androgens, mainly dehydroepiandrosterone (DHEA) and androstenedione	Have minimal intrinsic androgenic activity; they are converted to testosterone and dihydrotestosterone in the periphery
Adrenal medulla	Epinephrine Norepinephrine	Serve as neurotransmitters for the sympathetic nervous system
Thyroid (follicular cells)	Thyroid hormones: triiodothyronine (T_3), thyroxine (T_4)	Increase the metabolic rate; increase protein and bone turnover; increase responsiveness to catecholamines; necessary for fetal and infant growth and development
Thyroid C cells	Calcitonin	Lowers blood calcium and phosphate levels
Parathyroid glands	Parathyroid hormone	Regulates serum calcium
Pancreatic islet cells	Insulin	Lowers blood glucose by facilitating glucose transport across cell membranes of muscle, liver, and adipose tissue
	Glucagon	Increases blood glucose concentration by stimulation of glycogenolysis and glyconeogenesis
	Somatostatin	Delays intestinal absorption of glucose
Gastrointestinal tract	Gastrin	Stimulates release of hydrochloric acid in stomach
	Cholecystokinin	Stimulates release of pancreatic secretions
	Secretin	Stimulates release of pancreatic enzymes, gallbladder contraction
Kidney	1,25-Dihydroxyvitamin D	Stimulates calcium absorption from the intestine
	Renin	Activates renin-angiotensin-aldosterone system
	Erythropoietin	Increases red blood cell production
Heart	Atrial natriuretic peptide (ANP)	Produces natriuresis
Ovaries	Estrogen	Affects development of female sex organs and secondary sex characteristics
	Progesterone	Influences menstrual cycle; stimulates growth of uterine wall; maintains pregnancy
	Inhibin	Inhibits FSH secretion by anterior pituitary

(continued)

TABLE 39-1 ✦ Major Action and Source of Selected Hormones (Continued)

Source	Hormone	Major Action
Testes	Androgens, mainly testosterone	Affect development of male sex organs and secondary sex characteristics; aid in sperm production
	Inhibin	Inhibits FSH secretion by anterior pituitary
Placenta	Human chorionic gonadotropin	Maintains pregnancy
Adipose cells	Leptin	Decreases appetite and food intake, increases sympathetic activity and metabolic rate, decreases insulin secretion to reduce fat storage
	Resistin	Suppresses insulin's ability to stimulate glucose uptake by adipose cells (see Chapter 41)

hormones move into the Golgi complex, where they are packaged in granules or vesicles. It is in the Golgi complex that prohormones are converted into hormones.

Steroid hormones are synthesized in the smooth endoplasmic reticulum, and steroid-secreting cells can be identified by their large amounts of smooth endoplasmic reticulum. Certain steroids serve as precursors for the production of other hormones. In the adrenal cortex, for example, progesterone and other steroid intermediates are enzymatically converted into aldosterone, cortisol, or androgens (see Chapter 40).

Hormones that are released into the bloodstream circulate as either free, unbound molecules or as hormones attached to transport carriers (Fig. 39-1). Peptide hormones and protein hormones usually circulate unbound in the blood. Steroid hormones and thyroid hormone are carried by specific carrier proteins synthesized in the liver. The extent of carrier binding influences the rate at which hormones leave the blood and enter the cells. The half-life of a hormone—the time it takes for the body to reduce the concentration of the hormone by one half—is positively correlated with its percentage of protein binding. Thyroxine, which is more than 99% protein bound, has a half-life of 6 days. Aldosterone, which is only 15% bound, has a half-life of only 25 minutes. Drugs that compete with a hormone for binding with transport carrier molecules increase hormone action by increasing the availability of the active unbound hormone. For example, aspirin competes

TABLE 39-2 ✦ Classes of Hormones Based on Structure

Amines and Amino Acids	Peptides, Polypeptides, and Proteins	Steroids	Fatty Acid Compounds
Dopamine	Corticotropin-releasing hormone (CRH)	Aldosterone	Eicosanoids
Epinephrine	Growth hormone–releasing hormone (GHRH)	Glucocorticoids	Retinoids
Norepinephrine	Thyrotropin-releasing hormone (TRH)	Estrogens	
Thyroid hormone	Adrenocorticotropic hormone (ACTH)	Testosterone	
	Follicle-stimulating hormone (FSH)	Progesterone	
	Luteinizing hormone (LH)	Androstenedione	
	Thyroid-stimulating hormone (TSH)	1,25-Dihydroxyvitamin D	
	Growth hormone (GH)	Dihydrotestosterone (DHT)	
	Antidiuretic hormone (ADH)	Dehydroepiandrosterone	
	Oxytocin	(DHEA)	
	Insulin		
	Glucagon		
	Somatostatin		
	Calcitonin		
	Parathyroid hormone		
	Cholecystokinin		
	Gastrin		
	Secretin		
	Angiotensin II		
	Atrial natriuretic peptide (ANP)		
	Prolactin		
	Erythropoietin		
	Leptin		

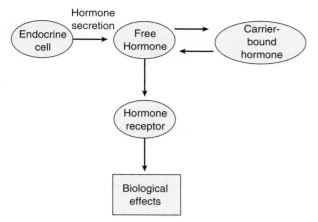

FIGURE 39-1 Relationship of free and carrier-bound hormone.

with thyroid hormone for binding to transport proteins; when the drug is administered to persons with excessive levels of circulating thyroid hormone, such as during thyroid crisis, serious effects may occur.

Metabolism and Elimination

Metabolism of hormones and their precursors can generate more or less active products or it can degrade them to inactive forms. In some cases, hormones are eliminated in the intact form. Hormones secreted by endocrine cells must be inactivated continuously to prevent their accumulation. Intracellular and extracellular mechanisms participate in the termination of hormone function. Some hormones are enzymatically inactivated at receptor sites where they exert their action. The catecholamines, which have a very short half-life, are degraded by catechol-*O*-methyl transferase (COMT) and monoamine oxidase (MAO). Because of their short half-life, their production is measured by some of their metabolites. In general, peptide hormones also have a short life span in the circulation. Their major mechanism of degradation is through binding to cell surface receptors, with subsequent uptake and degradation by enzymes in the cell membrane or inside the cell. Peptide hormones have a short life span and are inactivated by enzymes that split peptide bonds. Steroid hormones are bound to protein carriers for transport and are inactive in the bound state. Their activity depends on the availability of transport hormones. Unbound adrenal and gonadal steroid hormones are conjugated in the liver, which renders them inactive, and then excreted in the bile or urine. Thyroid hormones also are transported by carrier molecules. The free hormone is rendered inactive by the removal of amino acids (*i.e.*, deamination) in the tissues, and the hormone is conjugated in the liver and eliminated in the bile.

Mechanisms of Action

Hormones produce their effects through interaction with high-affinity receptors, which in turn are linked to one or more effector systems within the cell. These mechanisms involve many of the cell's metabolic activities, ranging from ion transport at the cell surface to stimulation of nuclear transcription of complex molecules. The rate at which hormones react depends on their mechanism of action. The neurotransmitters, which control the opening of ion channels, have a reaction time of milliseconds. Thyroid hormone, which functions in the control of cell metabolism and synthesis of intracellular signaling molecules, requires days for its full effect to occur.

Receptors. Hormones exert their action by binding to high-affinity receptors located either on the surface or inside the target cells. The function of these receptors is to recognize a specific hormone and translate the hormonal signal into a cellular response. The structure of these receptors varies in a manner that allows target cells to respond to one hormone and not to others. For example, receptors in the thyroid are specific for thyroid-stimulating hormone, and receptors on the gonads respond to the gonadotropic hormones.

The response of a target cell to a hormone varies with the *number* of receptors present and with the *affinity* of these receptors for hormone binding. A variety of factors influence the number of receptors that are present on target cells and their affinity for hormone binding.

There are approximately 2000 to 100,000 hormone receptor molecules per cell. The number of hormone receptors on a cell may be altered for any of several reasons. Antibodies may destroy or block the receptor proteins. Increased or decreased hormone levels often induce changes in the activity of the genes that regulator receptor synthesis. For example, decreased hormone levels often produce an increase in receptor numbers by means of a process called *up-regulation*; this increases the sensitivity of the body to existing hormone levels. Likewise, sustained levels of excess hormone often bring about a decrease in receptor numbers by *down-regulation*, producing a decrease in hormone sensitivity. In some instances, the reverse effect occurs, and an increase in hormone levels appears to recruit its own receptors, thereby increasing the sensitivity of the cell to the hormone. The process of up-regulation and down-regulation of receptors is regulated largely by inducing or repressing the transcription of receptor genes.

The affinity of receptors for binding hormones also is affected by a number of conditions. For example, the pH of the body fluids plays an important role in the affinity of insulin receptors. In ketoacidosis, a lower pH reduces insulin binding.

Some hormone receptors are located on the surface of the cell and act through second messenger mechanisms, and others are located within the cell, where they modulate the synthesis of enzymes, transport proteins, or structural proteins. The receptors for thyroid hormones, which are found in the nucleus, are thought to be directly associated with controlling the activity of genes located on one or more of the chromosomes. Chart 39-1 lists hormones that act through the two types of receptors.

Surface Receptors. Because of their low solubility in the lipid layer of cell membranes, peptide hormones and catecholamines cannot readily cross the cell membrane. Instead, these hormones interact with surface receptors in a manner that incites the generation of an intracellular

CHART 39-1

Hormone–Receptor Interactions

Second Messenger Interactions

Glucagon
Insulin
Epinephrine
Parathyroid hormone
Thyroid-stimulating hormone (TSH)
Adrenocorticotropic hormone (ACTH)
Follicle-stimulating hormone (FSH)
Luteinizing hormone (LH)
Antidiuretic hormone (ADH)
Secretin

Intracellular Interactions

Estrogens
Testosterone
Progesterone
Adrenal cortical hormones
Thyroid hormones

signal or message. The intracellular signal system is termed the *second messenger*, and the hormone is considered to be the first messenger (Fig. 39-2). For example, the first messenger glucagon binds to surface receptors on liver cells to incite glycogen breakdown by way of the second messenger system.

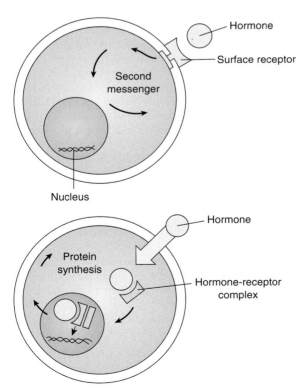

FIGURE 39-2 The two types of hormone–receptor interactions: the surface receptor (**top**) and the intracellular receptor (**bottom**).

The most widely distributed second messenger is cyclic adenosine monophosphate (cAMP). cAMP is formed from cellular adenosine triphosphate (ATP) by the enzyme adenylate cyclase, a membrane-bound enzyme that is located on the inner aspect of the cell membrane. Adenylate cyclase is functionally coupled to various cell surface receptors by the regulatory actions of G proteins (see Chapter 4). A second messenger similar to cAMP is cyclic GMP, derived from guanine triphosphate (GTP). As a result of binding to specific cell receptors, many peptide hormones incite a series of enzymatic reactions that produce an almost immediate increase in cAMP. Some hormones act to decrease cAMP levels and have an opposite effect.

In some cells, binding of hormones or neurotransmitters to surface receptors acts directly rather than through a second messenger to open ion channels in the cell membrane. The influx of ions serves as an intracellular signal to convey the hormonal message to the cell interior. In many instances, activation of hormone receptors results in the opening of calcium channels. The increasing cytoplasmic concentration of calcium may result in direct activation of calcium-dependent enzymes or calcium-calmodulin complexes with their attendant effects.

Intracellular Receptors. A second type of receptor mechanism is involved in mediating the action of hormones such as the steroid and thyroid hormones, which are transported in body fluids attached to carrier proteins (see Fig. 39-2). These hormones are lipid soluble and pass freely through the cell membrane. They then attach to intracellular receptors and form a hormone-receptor complex that travels to the cell nucleus. The hormone-messenger complex then activates or suppresses intracellular mechanisms such as gene activity, with subsequent production or inhibition of messenger RNA and protein synthesis.

CONTROL OF HORMONE LEVELS

Hormone secretion varies widely over a 24-hour period. Some hormones, such as GH and adrenocorticotropic hormone (ACTH), have diurnal fluctuations that vary with the sleep-wake cycle (Fig. 39-3). Others, such as the female sex hormones, are secreted in a complicated cyclic manner. The levels of hormones such as insulin and antidiuretic hormone (ADH) are regulated by feedback mechanisms that monitor substances such as glucose (insulin) and water (ADH) in the body. The levels of many of the hormones are regulated by feedback mechanisms that involve the hypothalamic-pituitary-target cell system.

Hypothalamic-Pituitary Regulation

The hypothalamus and pituitary (*i.e.,* hypophysis) form a unit that exerts control over many functions of several endocrine glands as well as a wide range of other physiologic functions. These two structures are connected by blood flow in the hypophyseal portal system, which begins in the hypothalamus and drains into the anterior pituitary gland, and by the nerve axons that connect the supraoptic and

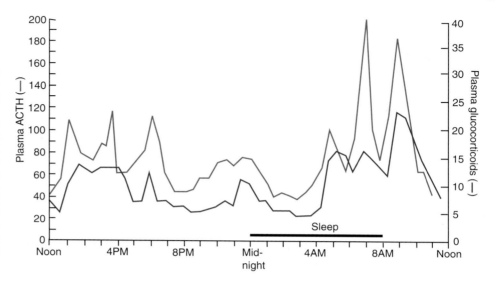

FIGURE 39-3 Pulsatile changes in the concentration of adrenocorticotropic hormone (ACTH) and glucocorticoids over a 24-hour period. The amplitude of the pulses of ACTH and glucocorticoids is lower in the evening hours and then increases greatly during the early morning hours. This is due to the diurnal oscillation of the hypothalamic-pituitary axis. (Modified from Krieger D.T. [1979]. Rhythms of CRF, ACTH and corticosteroids. In Krieger D.T. (Ed.), *Endocrine rhythms* [pp. 123–142]. New York: Raven)

paraventricular nuclei of the hypothalamus with the posterior pituitary gland (Fig. 39-4). The pituitary is enclosed in the sella turcica ("Turkish saddle") and is bridged over by the diaphragma sellae. Embryologically, the anterior pituitary gland developed from glandular tissue and the posterior pituitary developed from neural tissue.

Hypothalamic Hormones. The synthesis and release of anterior pituitary hormones are largely regulated by the action of releasing or inhibiting hormones from the hypothalamus, which is the coordinating center of the brain for endocrine, behavioral, and autonomic nervous system function. It is at the level of the hypothalamus that

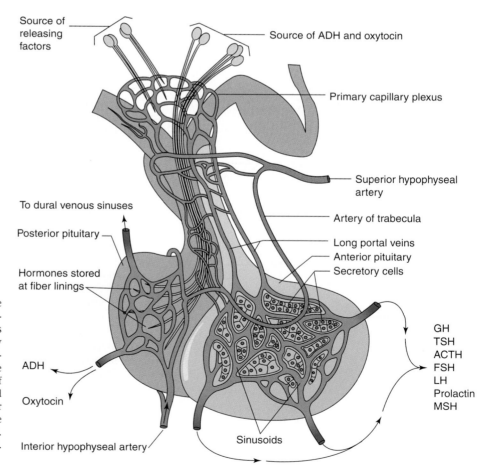

FIGURE 39-4 The hypothalamus and the anterior and posterior pituitary. The hypothalamic releasing or inhibiting hormones are transported to the anterior pituitary by way of the portal vessels. ADH and oxytocin are produced by nerve cells in the supraoptic and paraventricular nuclei of the hypothalamus and then transported through the nerve axon to the posterior pituitary, where they are released into the circulation. (Chaffee E.E., Lytle I.M. [1980]. *Basic physiology and anatomy* [4th ed.]. Philadelphia: J.B. Lippincott)

emotion, pain, body temperature, and other neural input are communicated to the endocrine system (Fig. 39-5). The posterior pituitary hormones, ADH and oxytocin, are synthesized in the cell bodies of neurons in the hypothalamus that have axons that travel to the posterior pituitary. The release and function of ADH are discussed in Chapter 31.

The hypothalamic hormones that regulate the secretion of anterior pituitary hormones include GH-releasing hormone (GHRH), somatostatin, dopamine, TRH, corticotropin-releasing hormone (CRH), and gonadotropin-releasing hormone (GnRH). With the exception of GH and prolactin, most of the pituitary hormones are regulated by hypothalamic stimulatory hormones. GH secretion is stimulated by GHRH; thyroid hormone by thyroid-stimulating hormone (TSH); ACTH by CRH; and luteinizing hormone (LH) and FSH by GnRH. Somatostatin functions as an inhibitory hormone for GH and TSH. Prolactin secretion is inhibited by dopamine; thus, persons receiving antipsychotic drugs that block dopamine often have increased prolactin levels.

The activity of the hypothalamus is regulated by both hormonally mediated signals (*e.g.*, negative feedback signals) and by neuronal input from a number of sources. Neuronal signals are mediated by neurotransmitters such as acetylcholine, dopamine, norepinephrine, serotonin,

γ-aminobutyric acid, and opioids. Cytokines that are involved in immune and inflammatory responses, such as the interleukins, also are involved in the regulation of hypothalamic function. This is particularly true of the hormones involved in the hypothalamic-pituitary-adrenal axis. Thus, the hypothalamus can be viewed as a bridge by which signals from multiple systems are relayed to the pituitary gland.

Pituitary Hormones.   The pituitary gland has been called the *master gland* because its hormones control the functions of many target glands and cells. Hormones produced by the anterior pituitary control body growth and metabolism (GH), function of the thyroid gland (TSH), glucocorticoid hormone levels (ACTH), function of the gonads (FSH and LH), and breast growth and milk production (prolactin). Melanocyte-stimulating hormone, which is involved in the control of pigmentation of the skin, is produced by the pars intermedia of the pituitary gland. The functions of many of these hormones are discussed in other parts of book (*e.g.*, thyroid hormone, GH, and the corticosteroids in Chapter 40, the sex hormones in Chapters 42 and 44, and ADH from the posterior pituitary in Chapter 31).

Feedback Regulation

The level of many of the hormones in the body is regulated by negative feedback mechanisms. The function of this type of system is similar to that of the thermostat in a heating system. In the endocrine system, sensors detect a change in the hormone level and adjust hormone secretion so that body levels are maintained within an appropriate range. When the sensors detect a decrease in hormone levels, they initiate changes that cause an increase in hormone production; when hormone levels rise above the set point of the system, the sensors cause hormone production and release to decrease. For example, an increase in thyroid hormone is detected by sensors in the hypothalamus or anterior pituitary gland, and this causes a reduction in the secretion of TSH, with a subsequent decrease in the output of thyroid hormone from the thyroid gland. The feedback loops for the hypothalamic-pituitary feedback mechanisms are illustrated in Figures 39-5 and 39-6.

Exogenous forms of hormones (given as drug preparations) can influence the normal feedback control of hormone production and release. One of the most common examples of this influence occurs with the administration of the corticosteroid hormones, which causes suppression of the hypothalamic-pituitary-target cell system that regulates the production of these hormones.

Although the levels of most hormones are regulated by negative feedback mechanisms, a small number are under positive feedback control, in which rising levels of a hormone cause another gland to release a hormone that is stimulating to the first. There must, however, be a mechanism for shutting off the release of the first hormone, or its production would continue unabated. An example of such a system is that of the female ovarian hormone estradiol. Increased estradiol production during the follicular stage of

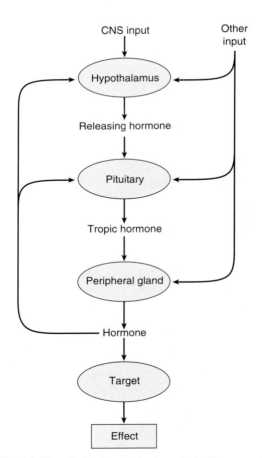

FIGURE 39-5 Hypothalamic–pituitary control of hormone levels.

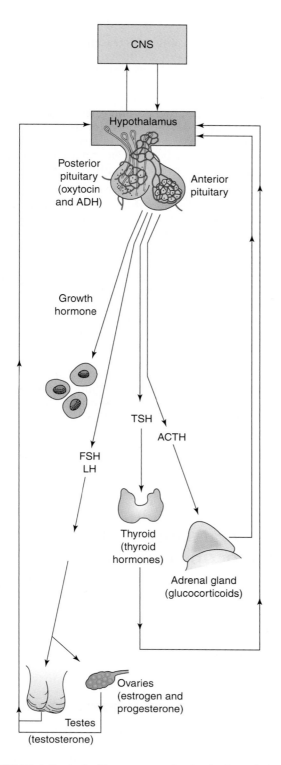

CNS

Hypothalamus

Posterior
pituitary
(oxytocin
and ADH)

Anterior
pituitary

Growth
hormone

TSH

ACTH

FSH
LH

Thyroid
(thyroid
hormones)

Adrenal gland
(glucocorticoids)

Ovaries
(estrogen and
progesterone)

Testes
(testosterone)

FIGURE 39-6 Control of hormone production by hypothalamic–pituitary–target cell feedback mechanism. Hormone levels from the target glands regulate the release of hormones from the anterior pituitary by means of a negative feedback system.

the menstrual cycle causes increased gonadotropin (FSH) production by the anterior pituitary gland. This stimulates further increases in estradiol levels until the demise of the follicle, which is the source of estradiol, results in a fall in gonadotropin levels.

In addition to positive and negative feedback mechanisms that monitor changes in hormone levels, some hormones are regulated by the level of the substance they regulate. For example, insulin levels normally are regulated in response to blood glucose levels, and those of aldosterone in response to body levels of sodium and potassium. Other factors such as stress, environmental temperature, and nutritional status can alter feedback regulation of hormone levels.

DIAGNOSTIC TESTS

Several techniques are available for assessing endocrine function and hormone levels. One technique measures the effect of a hormone on body function. Measurement of blood glucose, for example, reflects insulin levels and is an indirect method of assessing insulin availability. Another method is to measure hormone levels.

Blood Tests

Hormones circulating in the plasma were first detected by bioassays using the intact animal or a portion of tissue from the animal. At one time, female rats or male frogs were used to test women's urine for the presence of human chorionic gonadotropin, which is produced by the placenta during pregnancy. Unfortunately, most bioassays lack the precision, sensitivity, and specificity to measure low concentrations of hormones in plasma, and they are inconvenient to perform.

Blood hormone levels provide information about hormone levels at a specific time. For example, blood insulin levels can be measured along with blood glucose after administration of a challenge dose of glucose to measure the time course of change in blood insulin levels.

Real progress in measuring plasma hormone levels came more than 40 years ago with the use of competitive binding and the development of radioimmunoassay (RIA) methods. This method uses a radiolabeled form of the hormone and a hormone antibody that has been prepared by injecting an appropriate animal with a purified form of the hormone. The unlabeled hormone in the sample being tested competes with the radiolabeled hormone for attachment to the binding sites of the antibody. Measurement of the radiolabeled hormone-antibody complex then provides a means of arriving at a measure of the hormone level in the sample. Because hormone binding is competitive, the amount of radiolabeled hormone-antibody complex that is formed decreases as the amount of unlabeled hormone in the sample is increased. Newer techniques of RIA have been introduced, including the immunoradiometric assay (IRMA). IRMA uses two antibodies instead of one. These two antibodies are directed against two different parts of the molecule, and therefore IRMA assays are more specific. RIA has several disadvantages, including limited shelf-life of the radiolabeled hormone and the cost for the disposal of radioactive waste.

Nonradiolabeled methods have been developed in which the antigen of the hormone being measured is linked to an enzyme-activated label (*e.g.*, fluorescent label, chemiluminescent label) or latex particles that can be agglutinated with an antigen and measured. The enzyme-linked immunosorbent assays (ELISA) use antibody-coated plates and an enzyme-labeled reporter antibody. Binding of the hormone to the enzyme-labeled reporter antibody produces a colored reaction that can be measured using a spectrophotometer.

Urine Tests

Measurements of urinary hormone or hormone metabolite excretion often are done on a 24-hour urine sample and provide a better measure of hormone levels during that period than hormones measured in an isolated blood sample. The advantages of a urine test include the relative ease of obtaining urine samples and the fact that blood sampling is not required. The disadvantage is that reliably timed urine collections often are difficult to obtain. For example, a person may be unable to urinate at specific timed intervals, and urine samples may be accidentally discarded or inaccurately preserved. Because many urine tests involve the measure of a hormone metabolite rather than the hormone itself, drugs or disease states that alter hormone metabolism may interfere with the test result. Some urinary hormone metabolite measurements include hormones from more than one source and are of little value in measuring hormone secretion from a specific source. For example, urinary 17-ketosteroids are a measure of both adrenal and gonadal androgens.

Stimulation and Suppression Tests

Stimulation tests are used when hypofunction of an endocrine organ is suspected. A tropic or stimulating hormone can be administered to test the capacity of an endocrine organ to increase hormone production. The capacity of the target gland to respond is measured by an increase in the appropriate hormone. For example, the function of the hypothalamic-pituitary-thyroid system can be evaluated through stimulation tests using TRH and measuring TSH response. Failure to effect an increase in TSH after a TRH stimulation test suggests inadequate production of TSH by the pituitary.

Suppression tests are used to determine if negative feedback control mechanisms are intact. For example, a glucocorticoid hormone can be administered to persons suspected of having hypercortisolism to assess the capacity to inhibit CRH.

Genetic Tests

Deoxyribonucleic acid (DNA) analysis is being increasingly used for the identification of affected family members in a kindred harboring a known mutation (*e.g.*, looking for the RET protooncogene in certain multiple endocrine neoplasia syndromes).

Imaging

Imaging studies are gaining increasing importance in the diagnosis and follow-up of endocrine diseases. Magnetic resonance imaging (MRI) and computed tomography scans are especially useful for imaging endocrine glands and endocrine tumors. Nuclear scanning also is widely used for assessing thyroid, parathyroid, and adrenal disorders. Ultrasound scanning is recommended for managing thyroid nodules. Positron emission tomography scanning is being used more widely for parathyroid detection after failed parathyroid surgery for hyperparathyroidism.

> In summary, the endocrine system acts as a communication system that uses chemical messengers, or hormones, for the transmission of information from cell to cell and from organ to organ. Hormones act by binding to receptors that are specific for the different types of hormones. Many of the endocrine glands are under the regulatory control of other parts of the endocrine system. The hypothalamus and the pituitary gland form a complex integrative network that joins the nervous system and the endocrine system; this central network controls the output from many of the other glands in the body.
>
> Endocrine function can be assessed directly by measuring hormone levels, or indirectly by assessing the effects that a hormone has on the body (*e.g.*, assessment of insulin function through blood glucose). Imaging techniques are increasingly used to visualize endocrine structures, and genetic techniques are used to determine the presence of genes that contribute to the development of endocrine disorders.

General Aspects of Altered Endocrine Function

After you have completed this section of the chapter, you should be able to meet the following objectives:

✦ Describe the mechanisms of endocrine hypofunction and hyperfunction and differentiate primary, secondary, and tertiary endocrine disorders

✦ Describe the clinical features and causes of hypopituitarism

HYPOFUNCTION AND HYPERFUNCTION

Disturbances of endocrine function usually can be divided into two categories: hypofunction and hyperfunction. Hypofunction of an endocrine gland can occur for a variety of reasons. Congenital defects can result in the absence or impaired development of the gland or the absence of an enzyme needed for hormone synthesis. The gland may be destroyed by a disruption in blood flow, infection, inflammation, autoimmune responses, or neoplastic growth. There may be a decline in function with aging, or the gland may atrophy as the result of drug therapy or for unknown reasons. Some endocrine-deficient states are associated with receptor defects: hormone receptors may be absent, the receptor binding of hormones may be defective, or the cellular responsiveness to the hormone may be impaired. It is suspected that in some cases a gland may produce a biologically inactive hormone or that an active hormone may be destroyed by circulating antibodies before it can exert its action.

Hyperfunction usually is associated with excessive hormone production. This can result from excessive stimulation and hyperplasia of the endocrine gland or from a hormone-producing tumor of the gland. An ectopic tumor can produce hormones; for example, certain bronchogenic tumors produce hormones such as ADH and ACTH.

Primary, Secondary, and Tertiary Disorders

Endocrine disorders in general can be divided into primary, secondary, and tertiary groups. *Primary defects* in endocrine function originate in the target gland responsible for producing the hormone. In *secondary disorders* of endocrine function, the target gland is essentially normal, but its function is altered by defective levels of stimulating hormones or releasing factors from the pituitary system. For example, adrenalectomy produces a primary deficiency of adrenal corticosteroid hormones. Removal or destruction of the pituitary gland eliminates ACTH stimulation of the adrenal cortex and brings about a secondary deficiency. A *tertiary disorder* results from hypothalamic dysfunction (as may occur with craniopharyngiomas or cerebral irradiation); thus, both the pituitary and target organ are understimulated.

Hypopituitarism

Hypopituitarism, which is characterized by a decreased secretion of pituitary hormones, is a condition that affects many of the other endocrine systems. Typically, 70% to 90% of the anterior pituitary must be destroyed before hypopituitarism becomes clinically evident. The cause may be congenital or result from a variety of acquired abnormalities (Chart 39-2). The manifestations of hypopituitarism usually occur gradually, but it can present as an acute and life-threatening condition. Patients usually complain of being chronically unfit, with weakness, fatigue, loss of appetite, impairment of sexual function, and cold intolerance. However, ACTH deficiency (secondary adrenal failure) is the most serious endocrine deficiency, leading to weakness, nausea, anorexia, fever, and postural hypotension (see discussion of addisonian crisis in Chapter 40). Hypopituitarism is associated with increased morbidity and mortality.

Anterior pituitary hormone loss tends to follow a typical sequence, especially with progressive loss of pituitary reserve due to tumors or previous pituitary radiation therapy (which may take 10 to 20 years to produce hypopituitarism). The sequence of loss of pituitary hormones can be remembered by the mnemonic "*Go Look For The Adenoma,*" for *GH* (GH secretion typically is first to be lost), *LH* (results in sex hormone deficiency), *FSH* (causes infer-

---

> **CHART 39-2**
>
> ### *Causes of Hypopituitarism*
>
> - Tumors and mass lesions—pituitary adenomas, cysts, metastatic cancer, and other lesions
> - Pituitary surgery or radiation
> - Infiltrative lesions and infections—hemochromatosis, lymphocytic hypophysitis
> - Pituitary infarction—infarction of the pituitary gland after substantial blood loss during childbirth (Sheehan's syndrome)
> - Pituitary apoplexy—sudden hemorrhage into the pituitary gland
> - Genetic diseases—rare congenital defects of one or more pituitary hormones
> - Empty sella syndrome—an enlarged sella turcica that is not entirely filled with pituitary tissue
> - Hypothalamic disorders—tumors and mass lesions (*e.g.*, craniopharyngiomas and metastatic malignancies), hypothalamic radiation, infiltrative lesions (*e.g.*, sarcoidosis), trauma, infections

---

tility), *TSH* (leads to secondary hypothyroidism), and *ACTH* (usually the last to become deficient, results in secondary adrenal insufficiency).

Treatment of hypopituitarism includes treating any identified underlying cause. Hormone deficiencies should be treated as dictated by baseline, and more sophisticated pituitary testing where appropriate (and safe). Cortisol replacement is started when ACTH deficiency is present (see Chapter 40); thyroid replacement when TSH deficiency is detected; and sex hormone replacement when LH and FSH are deficient. GH replacement is being used increasingly to treat GH deficiency.

Assessment of Hypothalamic-Pituitary Function

The assessment of hypothalamic-pituitary function has been made possible by many newly developed imaging and radioimmunoassay methods. Assessment of the baseline status of the hypothalamic-pituitary-target cell hormones involves measuring the following (ideally performed at 8:00 AM): (1) serum cortisol, (2) serum prolactin, (3) serum thyroxine and TSH, (4) serum testosterone (male)/serum estrogen (female) and serum LH/FSH, (5) serum GH/insulin-like growth factor-1, and (6) plasma osmolality and urine osmolality. Imaging studies (*e.g.*, MRI of the hypothalamus/pituitary) also should be performed as required. When further information regarding pituitary function is required, combined hypothalamic-pituitary function tests are undertaken (although these are performed less often today). These tests consist mainly of hormone stimulation tests (*e.g.*, rapid ACTH stimulation test) or suppression tests (*e.g.*, GH suppression test).

It often is important to test pituitary function, especially if pituitary adenomas are discovered and surgery or radiation treatment is being considered. Investigations include both static and dynamic testing, and radiologic assessment as required. Any of the systems discussed previously may be affected by either deficiency or excess of the usual hormones secreted. Deficiency of hypothalamic-pituitary-target cell hormones can result from various pathologies and results in hypopituitarism (see Chart 39-2).

In summary, endocrine disorders are the result of hypofunction or hyperfunction of an endocrine gland. They can occur as a primary defect in hormone production by a target gland or as a secondary or tertiary disorder resulting from a defect in the hypothalamic-pituitary system that controls a target gland's function. Hypopituitarism, which is characterized by a decreased secretion of pituitary hormones, is a condition that affects many of the other endocrine systems. Depending on the extent of the disorder, it can result in decreased levels of GH, thyroid hormones, adrenal corticosteroid hormones, and testosterone in the male and of estrogens and progesterone in the female.

Bibliography

DeGroot L.J., Jameson J.L. (Eds.). (2001). *Endocrinology*. Philadelphia: W.B. Saunders.

Greenspan F.S., Gardner D.G. (2001). *Basic and clinical endocrinology* (6th ed.). Norwalk, CT: Appleton & Lange.

Griffin J.E., Sergio R.O. (Eds.). (2000). *Textbook of endocrine physiology* (4th ed.). New York: Oxford University Press.

Kacsoh B. (2000). *Endocrine physiology*. New York: McGraw-Hill.

Neal J.M. (2000). *Basic endocrinology*. Malden, MA: Blackwell Science.

Nussey S.S., Whitehead S.A. (2001). *Endocrinology—an integrated approach*. London: Bios.

Chapter 40

Alterations in Endocrine Control of Growth and Metabolism

Glenn Matfin, Safak Guven, and Julie A. Kuenzi

Growth and Growth Hormone Disorders

After you have completed this section of the chapter, you should be able to meet the following objectives:

✦ State the effects of a deficiency in growth hormone
✦ Differentiate genetic short stature from constitutional short stature
✦ State the mechanisms of short stature in hypothyroidism, poorly controlled diabetes mellitus, treatment with adrenal glucocorticosteroid hormones, malnutrition, and psychosocial dwarfism
✦ List three causes of tall stature
✦ Relate the functions of growth hormone to the manifestations of acromegaly and adult-onset growth hormone deficiency
✦ Discuss the classification of pituitary tumors
✦ Explain why children with isosexual precocious puberty are tall-statured children but short-statured adults

Several hormones are essential for normal body growth and maturation, including growth hormone (GH), insulin, thyroid hormone, and androgens. In addition to its actions on carbohydrate and fat metabolism, insulin plays an essential role in growth processes. Children with diabetes, particularly those with poor control, often fail to grow normally even though GH levels are normal. When levels of thyroid hormone are lower than normal, bone growth and epiphyseal closure are delayed. Androgens such as testosterone and dihydrotestosterone exert anabolic growth effects through their actions on protein synthesis. Glucocorticoids at excessive levels inhibit growth, apparently because of their antagonistic effect on GH secretion.

GROWTH HORMONE

Growth hormone, also called *somatotropin*, is a 191–amino-acid polypeptide hormone synthesized and secreted by special cells in the anterior pituitary called *somatotropes*. For many years, it was thought that GH was produced primarily during periods of growth. However, this has proved to be incorrect because the rate of GH production in adults is almost as great as in children. GH is necessary for growth and contributes to the regulation of metabolic functions. All aspects of cartilage growth are stimulated by GH; one of the most striking effects of GH is on linear bone growth, resulting from its action on the epiphyseal growth plates of long bones. The width of bone increases because of enhanced periosteal growth; visceral and endocrine organs, skeletal and cardiac muscle, skin, and connective tissue all undergo increased growth in response to GH. In many instances, the increased growth of visceral and endocrine organs is accompanied by enhanced functional capacity. For example, increased growth of cardiac muscle is accompanied by an increase in cardiac output.

In addition to its effects on growth, GH facilitates the rate of protein synthesis by all of the cells of the body; it enhances fatty acid mobilization and increases the use of fatty acids for fuel; and it maintains or increases blood glucose levels by decreasing the use of glucose for fuel. GH has an initial effect of increasing insulin levels. However, the predominant effect of prolonged GH excess is to increase glucose levels despite an insulin increase. This is because GH induces a resistance to insulin in the peripheral tissues, inhibiting the uptake of glucose by muscle and adipose tissues.

Many of the effects of GH depend on a family of peptides called *insulin-like growth factors* (IGF), also called *somatomedins*, which are produced mainly by the liver. GH cannot directly produce bone growth; instead, it acts indirectly by causing the liver to produce IGF. These peptides act on cartilage and bone to promote their growth. At least four IGFs have been identified; of these, IGF-1 (somatomedin C) appears to be the more important in terms of growth, and it is the one that usually is measured in laboratory tests. The IGFs have been sequenced and have structures that are similar to that of proinsulin. This undoubtedly explains the insulin-like activity of the IGFs and the weak action of insulin on growth. IGF levels are themselves influenced by a family of at least six binding factors called *IGF-binding proteins* (IGFBPs).

GH is carried unbound in the plasma and has a half-life of approximately 20 to 50 minutes. The secretion of GH is regulated by two hypothalamic hormones: GH-releasing hormone (GHRH), which increases GH release, and somatostatin, which inhibits GH release. A third hormone, the recently identified ghrelin, also may be important. These hypothalamic influences (*i.e.*, GHRH and somatostatin) are tightly regulated by neural, metabolic, and hormonal factors. The secretion of GH fluctuates over a 24-hour period, with peak levels occurring 1 to 4 hours after onset of sleep (*i.e.*, during sleep stages 3 and 4). The nocturnal sleep bursts, which account for 70% of daily GH secretion, are greater in children than in adults.

GH secretion is stimulated by hypoglycemia, fasting, starvation, increased blood levels of amino acids (particularly arginine), and stress conditions such as trauma, excitement, emotional stress, and heavy exercise. GH is inhibited by increased glucose levels, free fatty acid release, cortisol, and obesity. Impairment of secretion, leading to growth retardation, is not uncommon in children with severe emotional deprivation.

SHORT STATURE AND GROWTH HORMONE DEFICIENCY

Short stature is a condition in which the attained height is well below the fifth percentile or linear growth is below normal for age and sex. Short stature, or growth retardation, has a variety of causes, including chromosomal abnormalities such as Turner's syndrome (see Chapter 7), GH deficiency, hypothyroidism, and panhypopituitarism (see Chapter 39). Other conditions known to cause short stature include protein-calorie malnutrition, chronic diseases such as renal failure and poorly controlled diabetes mellitus, malabsorption syndromes, and certain therapies such as corticosteroid administration. Emotional disturbances can lead to functional endocrine disorders, causing psychosocial dwarfism. The causes of short stature are summarized in Chart 40-1.

Two forms of short stature, genetic short stature and constitutional short stature, are not disease states but variations from population norms. Genetically short children tend to be well proportioned and to have a height close to the midparental height of their parents. The midparental height for boys can be calculated by adding 13 cm (5 inches)

CHART 40-1

Causes of Short Stature

Variants of Normal
Genetic or "familial" short stature
Constitutional short stature

Low Birth Weight (e.g., intrauterine growth retardation)
Endocrine Disorders
Growth hormone (GH) deficiency
   Primary GH deficiency
      Idiopathic GH deficiency
      Pituitary agenesis
   Secondary GH deficiency (panhypopituitarism)
   Biologically inactive GH production
   Deficient IGF-1 production in response to normal or
      elevated GH (Laron-type dwarfism)
Hypothyroidism
Diabetes mellitus in poor control
Glucocorticoid excess
   Endogenous (Cushing's disease)
   Exogenous (glucocorticoid drug treatment)
Abnormal mineral metabolism (*e.g.*, pseudohypoparathyroidism)

Chronic Illness and Malnutrition
Chronic organic or systemic disease (*e.g.*, asthma, especially when treated with glucocorticoids; heart or renal disease)
Nutritional deprivation
Malabsorption syndrome

Functional Endocrine Disorders (Psychosocial Dwarfism)
Chromosomal Disorders (e.g., Turner's Syndrome)
Skeletal Abnormalities (e.g., achondroplasia)
Unusual Syndromes

to the height of the mother, adding the father's height, and dividing the total by two. For girls, 13 cm (5 inches) is subtracted from the father's height, the result is added to the mother's height, and the total is divided by two. Ninety-five percent of normal children are within 8.5 cm of the midparental height. *Constitutional short stature* is a term used to describe children (particularly boys) who have moderately short stature, thin build, delayed skeletal and sexual maturation, and absence of other causes of decreased growth. *Catch-up growth* is a term used to describe an abnormally high growth rate that occurs as a child approaches normal height for age. It occurs after the initiation of therapy for GH deficiency and hypothyroidism and the correction of chronic diseases.

Psychosocial dwarfism involves a functional hypopituitarism and is seen in some emotionally deprived children. These children usually present with poor growth, potbelly, and poor eating and drinking habits. Typically, there is a history of disturbed family relationships in which the child has been severely neglected or disciplined. Often, the neglect is confined to one child in the family. GH function usually returns to normal after the child is removed from the constraining environment. The prognosis depends on improvement in behavior and catch-up growth. Family therapy usually is indicated, and foster care may be necessary.

Accurate measurement of height is an extremely important part of the physical examination of children. Completion of the developmental history and growth charts is essential. Growth curves and growth velocity studies also are needed. Diagnosis of short stature is not made on a single measurement, but is based on actual height and on velocity of growth and parental height.

The diagnostic procedures for short stature include tests to exclude nonendocrine causes. If the cause is hormonal, extensive hormonal testing procedures are initiated. Usually, GH and IGF-1 levels are determined (IGFBP-3 levels also are useful). Tests can be performed using insulin (to induce hypoglycemia), levodopa, and arginine, all of which stimulate GH secretion so that GH reserve can be evaluated. Because administration of pharmacologic agents can result in false-negative responses, two or more tests usually are performed. If a prompt rise in GH is realized, the child is considered normal. Physiologic tests of GH reserve (*e.g.*, GH response to exercise) also can be performed. Levels of IGF-1 usually reflect those of GH and may be used to indicate GH deficiency. Radiologic films are used to assess bone age, which most often is delayed. Lateral skull x-rays may be used to evaluate the size and shape of the sella turcica (*i.e.*, depression in the sphenoid bone that contains the pituitary gland) and determine if a pituitary tumor exists. However, magnetic resonance imaging (MRI) or computed axial tomography (CT) scans of the hypothalamic-pituitary area are recommended if a lesion is clinically suspected. After the cause of short stature has been determined, treatment can be initiated.

Growth Hormone Deficiency in Children

There are several forms of GH deficiency that present in childhood. Children with idiopathic GH deficiency lack

Growth Hormone

➤ Growth hormone (GH), which is produced by somatotropes in the anterior pituitary, is necessary for linear bone growth in children. It also stimulates cells to increase in size and divide more rapidly; it enhances amino acid transport across cell membranes and increases protein synthesis; and it increases the rate at which cells use fatty acids and decreases the rate at which they use carbohydrates.

➤ The effects of GH on cartilage growth require insulin-like growth factors (IGFs), also called *somatomedins,* which are produced mainly by the liver.

➤ In children, GH deficiency interferes with linear bone growth, resulting in short stature or dwarfism. In a rare condition called *Laron-type dwarfism,* GH levels are normal or elevated, but there is a hereditary defect in IGF production.

➤ GH excess in children results in increased linear bone growth, or gigantism. In adults, GH excess results in overgrowth of the cartilaginous parts of the skeleton, enlargement of the heart and other organs of the body, and metabolic disturbances resulting in altered fat metabolism and impaired glucose tolerance.

the hypothalamic GHRH but have adequate somatotropes, whereas children with pituitary tumors or agenesis of the pituitary lack somatotropes. The term *panhypopituitarism* refers to conditions that cause a deficiency of all of the anterior pituitary hormones (see Chapter 39). In a rare condition called *Laron-type dwarfism,* GH levels are normal or elevated, but there is a hereditary defect in IGF production that can be treated directly with IGF-1 replacement.

Congenital GH deficiency is associated with normal birth length, followed by a decrease in growth rate that can be identified by careful measurement during the first year and that becomes obvious by 1 to 2 years of age. Persons with classic GH deficiency have normal intelligence, short stature, obesity with immature facial features, and some delay in skeletal maturation. Puberty often is delayed, and males with the disorder have microphallus (abnormally small penis), especially if the condition is accompanied by gonadotropin-releasing hormone (GnRH) deficiency. In the neonate, GH deficiency can lead to hypoglycemia and seizures; if adrenocorticotropic hormone (ACTH) deficiency also is present, the hypoglycemia often is more severe. Acquired GH deficiency develops in later childhood; it may be caused by a hypothalamic-pituitary tumor, particularly if it is accompanied by other pituitary hormone deficiencies.

When short stature is caused by a GH deficiency, GH replacement therapy is the treatment of choice. GH is species specific, and only human GH is effective in humans. GH previously was obtained from human cadaver pituitaries, but now is produced by DNA technology and is available in adequate supply. In 1985, the National Hormone and Pituitary Program halted the distribution of human GH derived from cadaver pituitaries in the United States after receiving reports that several recipients died of Creutzfeldt-Jakob disease (see Chapter 50). The disease, which is caused by a prion protein, was thought to be transmitted by cadaver GH preparations. GH is administered subcutaneously in multiple weekly doses during the period of active growth, and can be continued into adulthood.

Children with short stature due to Turner's syndrome and chronic renal insufficiency also are treated with GH. GH therapy may be considered for children with short stature but without GH deficiency. Several studies suggest that short-term treatment with GH increases the rate of growth in these children. Although the effect of GH on adult height is not great, it can result in improved psychological well-being. There are concerns about misuse of the drug to produce additional growth in children with normal GH function who are of near-normal height. Guidelines for use of the hormone continue to be established.

Growth Hormone Deficiency in Adults

There are two categories of GH deficiency in adults: (1) GH deficiency that was present in childhood, and (2) GH deficiency that developed during adulthood, mainly as the result of hypopituitarism resulting from a pituitary tumor or its treatment. GH levels also can decline with aging, and there has been interest in the effects of declining GH levels in the elderly (described as the *somatopause*). GH replacement obviously is important in the growing child; however, the role in adults (especially for the somatopause) is being assessed. Some of the differences between childhood and adult-onset GH deficiency are described in Table 40-1.

TABLE 40-1 ✦ Differences Between Childhood and Adult-Onset Growth Hormone Deficiency

Characteristic	Childhood Onset	Adult Onset
Adult height	↓	NL
Body fat	↑	↑
Lean body mass	↓↓	↓
Bone mineral density	↓	NL, ↓
Insulin-like growth factor (IGF)-1	↓↓	NL, ↓
IGF binding protein-3	↓	NL
Low-density lipoprotein cholesterol	↑	↑
High-density lipoprotein cholesterol	NL, ↓	↓

NL, normal

Several studies have shown that cardiovascular mortality is increased in GH-deficient adults. Increased arterial intima–media thickness and a higher prevalence of atherosclerotic plaques and endothelial dysfunction have been reported in both childhood and adult GH deficiency. The GH deficiency syndrome is associated with a cluster of cardiovascular risk factors, including central adiposity (increased waist–hip ratio), increased visceral fat, insulin resistance, and dyslipidemia. These features also are associated with the *metabolic syndrome* ("syndrome X"; see Chapter 41). In addition to these so-called traditional cardiovascular risk factors, nontraditional cardiovascular risk factors (*e.g.*, C-reactive protein and interleukin-6, which are markers of the inflammatory pathway) also are elevated. GH therapy can improve many of these factors.

The diagnosis of GH deficiency in adults is made by finding subnormal serum GH responses to two provocative stimuli (this is the "official" response; however, in reality, at least one stimulation test is needed). Measurements of the serum IGF-1 or basal GH do not distinguish reliably between normal and subnormal GH secretion in adults. Insulin-induced hypoglycemia is the gold standard test for GH reserve (see discussion of Addison's disease for details). The L-dopa test probably is the next best test. Other stimulation tests involve the use of arginine or arginine plus GHRH, clonidine (an alpha adrenergic agonist), glucagon, or GHRH.

The approval of several recombinant human GH preparations (*e.g.*, Humatrope, Genotropin) for treating adults with GH deficiency allows physicians in the United States and elsewhere to prescribe this treatment. In the United States, persons with GH deficiency acquired as an adult must meet at least two criteria for therapy: a poor GH response to at least two standard stimuli, and hypopituitarism due to pituitary or hypothalamic damage. Difficulties can occur with the diagnosis of adult-onset GH deficiency, determining the GH dosage to be given, and monitoring the GH therapy.

GH replacement therapy may lead to increased lean body mass and decreased fat mass, increased bone mineral density, increased glomerular filtration rate, decreased lipid levels, increased exercise capacity, and improved sense of well-being in GH-deficient adults. The most common side effects of GH treatment in adults with hypopituitarism are peripheral edema, arthralgias and myalgias, carpal tunnel syndrome, paresthesias, and decreased glucose tolerance. Side effects appear to be more common in people who are older and heavier and are overtreated, as judged by a high serum IGF-1 concentration during therapy. Women seem to tolerate higher doses better then men.

TALL STATURE

Just as there are children who are short for their age and sex, there also are children who are tall for their age and sex. Normal variants of tall stature include genetic tall stature and constitutional tall stature. Children with exceptionally tall parents tend to be taller than children with shorter parents. The term *constitutional tall stature* is used to describe a child who is taller than his or her peers and is growing at a velocity that is within the normal range for bone age. Other causes of tall stature are genetic or chromosomal disorders such as Marfan's syndrome or XYY syndrome (see Chapter 7). Endocrine causes of tall stature include sexual precocity because of early onset of estrogen and androgen secretion and excessive GH.

Exceptionally tall children (*i.e.*, genetic tall stature and constitutional tall stature) can be treated with sex hormones—estrogens in girls and testosterone in boys—to effect early epiphyseal closure. Such treatment is undertaken only after full consideration of the risks involved. To be effective, such treatment must be instituted 3 to 4 years before expected epiphyseal fusion.

PITUITARY TUMORS AND GROWTH HORMONE EXCESS

Pituitary tumors can be divided into primary or secondary tumors (*i.e.*, metastatic lesions). Tumors of the pituitary can be further divided into functional tumors that secrete pituitary hormones and nonfunctional tumors that do not secrete hormones. They can range in size from small lesions that do not enlarge the gland (microadenomas, <10 mm) to large, expansive tumors (macroadenomas, >10 mm) that erode the sella turcica and impinge on surrounding cranial structures. Small, nonfunctioning tumors are found in approximately 25% of adult autopsies. Benign adenomas account for most of the functioning anterior pituitary tumors. Carcinomas of the pituitary are less common tumors. Functional adenomas can be subdivided according to cell type and the type of hormone secreted (Table 40-2).

Gigantism

Growth hormone excess occurring before puberty and the fusion of the epiphyses of the long bones results in *gigantism*. Excessive secretion of GH by somatotrope adenomas causes gigantism in the prepubertal child. It occurs when the epiphyses are not fused and high levels of IGF stimulate excessive skeletal growth. Fortunately, the condition is rare because of early recognition and treatment of the adenoma.

Acromegaly

When GH excess occurs in adulthood or after the epiphyses of the long bones have fused, the condition is referred to as *acromegaly*. Acromegaly results from excess levels of GH that stimulate the hepatic secretion of IGF-1, which causes most of the clinical manifestations of acromegaly. The annual incidence of acromegaly is 3 to 4 cases per 1 million people, with a mean age at the time of diagnosis of 40 to 45 years.

The most common cause (95%) of acromegaly is a somatotrope adenoma. Approximately 75% of persons with acromegaly have a somatotrope macroadenoma at the time of diagnosis, and most of the remainder have microadenomas. The other causes of acromegaly (<5%) are excess secretion of GHRH by hypothalamic tumors, ectopic GHRH secretion by nonendocrine tumors such as carcinoid tumors or small cell lung cancers, and ectopic secretion of GH by nonendocrine tumors.

The disorder usually has an insidious onset, and symptoms often are present for a considerable period before a diagnosis is made. When the production of excessive GH occurs after the epiphyses of the long bones have closed, as in the adult, the person cannot grow taller, but the soft tissues continue to grow. Enlargement of the small bones of the hands and feet and of the membranous bones of the face and skull results in a pronounced enlargement of the hands and feet, a broad and bulbous nose, a protruding lower jaw, and a slanting forehead. The teeth become splayed, causing a disturbed bite and difficulty in chewing. The cartilaginous structures in the larynx and respiratory tract also become enlarged, resulting in a deepening of the voice and tendency to develop bronchitis. Vertebral changes often lead to kyphosis, or hunchback. Bone overgrowth often leads to arthralgias and degenerative arthritis of the spine, hips, and knees. Virtually every organ of the body is increased in size. Enlargement of the heart and accelerated atherosclerosis may lead to an early death.

The metabolic effects of excess levels of GH include alterations in fat and carbohydrate metabolism. GH causes increased release of free fatty acids from adipose tissue, leading to increased concentration of free fatty acids in body fluids. In addition, GH enhances the formation of ketones and the utilization of free fatty acids for energy in preference to use of carbohydrates and proteins. GH exerts multiple effects on carbohydrate metabolism, including decreased glucose uptake by tissues such as skeletal muscle and adipose tissue, increased glucose production by the liver, and increased insulin secretion. Each of these changes results in GH-induced insulin resistance (see Chapter 41). This leads to glucose intolerance, which stimulates the beta cells of the pancreas to produce additional insulin. Long-term elevation of GH results in overstimulation of the beta cells, causing them literally to "burn out." Impaired glucose tolerance occurs in as many as 50% to 70% of persons with acromegaly; overt diabetes mellitus subsequently can result.

The pituitary gland is located in the pituitary fossa of the sphenoid bone (*i.e.*, sella turcica), which lies directly

TABLE 40-2 ✦ Frequency of Adenomas of the Anterior Pituitary		
Cell Type	**Hormone**	**Frequency (%)**
Lactotrope	Prolactin (PRL)	32
Somatotrope	Growth hormone (GH)	21
Lactotrope/ somatotrope	Mixed PRL/GH	6
Corticotrope	Adrenocorticotropic hormone (ACTH)	13
Gonadotrope	Follicle-stimulating hormone (FSH) Luteinizing hormone (LH)	<4
Thyrotrope	Thyroid-stimulating hormone (TSH)	
Nonfunctional tumors		25

below the optic nerve. Almost all persons with acromegaly have a recognizable adenohypophysial tumor. Enlargement of the pituitary gland eventually causes erosion of the surrounding bone, and because of its location, this can lead to headaches, visual field defects resulting from compression of the optic nerve, and palsies of cranial nerves III, IV, and VI. Compression of other pituitary structures can cause secondary hypothyroidism, hypogonadism, and adrenal insufficiency (see Chapter 39 for discussion of hypopituitarism). Other manifestations include excessive sweating with an unpleasant odor, oily skin, heat intolerance, moderate weight gain, muscle weakness and fatigue, menstrual irregularities, and decreased libido. Hypertension is relatively common. Paresthesias may develop because of nerve entrapment and compression caused by excess soft tissue and accumulation of subcutaneous fluid (especially carpal tunnel syndrome). Acromegaly also is associated with an increased risk of colonic polyps and colorectal cancer. The mortality rate of patients with acromegaly is two to three times the expected rate, mostly from cardiovascular diseases and cancer. The cardiovascular disease results from the combination of cardiomyopathy, hypertension, insulin resistance and hyperinsulinemia, and hyperlipidemia.

Acromegaly often develops insidiously, and only a small number of persons seek medical care because of changes in appearance. The diagnosis of acromegaly is facilitated by the typical features of the disorder—enlargement of the hands and feet and coarsening of facial features. Laboratory tests to detect elevated levels of GH not suppressed by a glucose load are used to confirm the diagnosis. CT and MRI scans can detect and localize the pituitary lesions. Because most of the effects of GH are mediated by IGF-1, IGF-1 levels may provide information about disease activity.

The treatment goals for acromegaly focus on the correction of metabolic abnormalities, and include normalization of the GH response to an oral glucose load; normalization of IGF-1 levels to age- and sex-matched control levels; removal or reduction of the tumor mass; relieving the central pressure effects; improvement of adverse clinical features; and normalization of the mortality rate. Pituitary tumors can be removed surgically using the transsphenoidal approach or, if that is not possible, a transfrontal craniotomy. Radiation therapy may be used, but remission (reduction in GH levels) may not occur for several years after therapy. Radiation therapy also significantly increases the risk of hypopituitarism, hypothyroidism, hypoadrenalism, and hypogonadism.

Octreotide acetate, an analog of somatostatin that produces feedback inhibition of GH, has been effective in the medical management of acromegaly. However, the medication must be given subcutaneously three times per week for effective dosing. Newer, longer-acting analogs of somatostatin are now available, including Sandostatin LAR, which is a sustained-release formulation of octreotide that effectively inhibits GH secretion for 30 days after a single intramuscular injection of 20 to 30 mg. Lanreotide also is available in a long-acting formulation that has comparable efficacy to octreotide when injected intramuscularly two to three times per month. Bromocrip-

tine, a long-acting dopamine agonist, reduces GH levels and has been used with some success in the medical management of acromegaly. However, high doses often are required, and side effects may be troublesome. Several newly available dopamine agonists (*e.g.,* cabergoline, quinagolide) also can be considered as an alternative or adjunctive therapy.

ISOSEXUAL PRECOCIOUS PUBERTY

Precocious sexual development may be idiopathic or may be caused by gonadal, adrenal, or hypothalamic tumors. Isosexual precocious puberty is defined as early activation of the hypothalamic-pituitary-gonadal axis, resulting in the development of appropriate sexual characteristics and fertility. Sexual development is considered precocious and warrants investigation when it occurs before 8 years of age for girls and before 9 years of age for boys. These criteria were revised recently to age 7 years for breast development in white girls and 6 years in black girls, based on an office pediatric study of more than 17,000 American girls. However, it currently is recommended that the classic age limits be used until this work is confirmed in other populations. Benign and malignant tumors of the central nervous system (CNS) can cause precocious puberty. These tumors are thought to remove the inhibitory influences normally exerted on the hypothalamus during childhood. CNS tumors are found more often in boys with precocious puberty than in girls. In girls, most cases are idiopathic.

Diagnosis of precocious puberty is based on physical findings of early thelarche (*i.e.,* beginning of breast development), adrenarche (*i.e.,* beginning of augmented adrenal androgen production), and menarche (*i.e.,* beginning of menstrual function) in girls. The most common sign in boys is early genital enlargement. Radiologic findings may indicate advanced bone age. Persons with precocious puberty usually are tall for their age as children but short as adults because of the early closure of the epiphyses. CAT or MRI should be used to exclude intracranial lesions.

Depending on the cause of precocious puberty, the treatment may involve surgery, medication, or no treatment. The treatment of choice is administration of a long-acting GnRH agonist. Constant levels of the hormone cause a decrease in pituitary responsiveness to GnRH, leading to decreased secretion of gonadotropic hormones and sex steroids. Parents often need education, support, and anticipatory guidance in dealing with their feelings and the child's physical needs and in relating to a child who appears older than his or her years.

> In summary, a number of hormones are essential for normal body growth and maturation, including GH, insulin, thyroid hormone, and androgens. GH exerts its growth effects through a group of IGFs. GH also exerts an effect on metabolism and is produced in the adult and in the child. Its metabolic effects include a decrease in peripheral use of carbohydrates and an increased mobilization and use of fatty acids.

In children, alterations in growth include short stature, isosexual precocious puberty, and tall stature. Short stature is a condition in which the attained height is well below the fifth percentile or the linear growth velocity is below normal for a child's age or sex. Short stature can occur as a variant of normal growth (*i.e.*, genetic short stature or constitutional short stature) or as the result of endocrine disorders, chronic illness, malnutrition, emotional disturbances, or chromosomal disorders. Short stature resulting from GH deficiency can be treated with human GH preparations. In adults, GH deficiency represents a deficiency carried over from childhood or one that develops during adulthood as the result of a pituitary tumor or its treatment. GH levels also can decline with aging, and there has been interest in the effects of declining GH levels in the elderly (described as the *somatopause*).

Tall stature refers to the condition in which children are tall for their age and sex. It can occur as a variant of normal growth (*i.e.*, genetic tall stature or constitutional tall stature) or as the result of a chromosomal abnormality or GH excess. GH excess in adults results in acromegaly, which involves proliferation of bone, cartilage, and soft tissue along with the metabolic effects of excessive hormone levels. Isosexual precocious puberty defines a condition of early activation of the hypothalamic-pituitary-gonadal axis (*i.e.*, before 8 years of age in girls and 9 years of age in boys), resulting in the development of appropriate sexual characteristics and fertility. It causes tall stature during childhood but results in short stature in adulthood because of the early closure of the epiphyses.

Thyroid Disorders

After you have completed this section of the chapter, you should be able to meet the following objectives:

✦ Characterize the synthesis, transport, and regulation of thyroid hormone
✦ Diagram the hypothalamic-pituitary-thyroid feedback system
✦ Describe tests in the diagnosis and management of thyroid disorders
✦ Relate the functions of thyroid hormone to hypothyroidism and hyperthyroidism
✦ Describe the effects of congenital hypothyroidism
✦ Characterize the manifestations and treatment of myxedematous coma and thyroid storm

CONTROL OF THYROID FUNCTION

The thyroid gland is a shield-shaped structure located immediately below the larynx in the anterior middle portion of the neck. It is composed of a large number of tiny, saclike structures called *follicles* (Fig. 40-1). These are the functional units of the thyroid. Each follicle is formed by a single layer of epithelial (follicular) cells and is filled with a secretory substance called *colloid*, which consists largely of a glycoprotein-iodine complex called *thyroglobulin*.

The thyroglobulin that fills the thyroid follicles is a large glycoprotein molecule that contains 140 tyrosine amino acids. In the process of thyroid synthesis, iodine is attached to these tyrosines. Both thyroglobulin and iodide are secreted into the colloid of the follicle by the follicular cells.

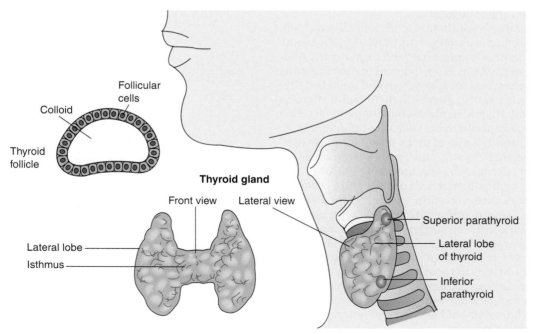

FIGURE 40-1 The thyroid gland and the follicular structure. (Chaffee E.E., Lytle I.M. [1980]. *Basic physiology and anatomy* [4th ed.]. Philadelphia: J.B. Lippincott)

HO—⬡—CH₂CH COOH
         |
         NH₂
Tyrosine

HO—⬡—CH₂CH COOH
  I |
         NH₂
Monoiodotyrosine

HO—⬡—O—⬡—CH₂CH COOH
  I   I |
                   NH₂
Triiodotyrosine (T₃)

HO—⬡—CH₂CH COOH
  I |
  I   NH₂
Diiodotyrosine

HO—⬡—O—⬡—CH₂CH COOH
  I   I |
  I   I   NH₂
Thyroxine (T₄)

FIGURE 40-2 Chemistry of thyroid hormone production.

The thyroid is remarkably efficient in its use of iodide. A daily absorption of 100 to 200 μg of dietary iodide is sufficient to form normal quantities of thyroid hormone. In the process of removing it from the blood and storing it for future use, iodide is pumped into the follicular cells against a concentration gradient. As a result, the concentration of iodide in the normal thyroid gland is approximately 40 times that in the blood.

Once inside the follicle, most of the iodide is oxidized by the enzyme peroxidase in a reaction that facilitates combination with a tyrosine molecule to form monoiodotyrosine and then diiodotyrosine (Fig. 40-2). Two diiodotyrosine residues are coupled to form thyroxine (T_4), or a monoiodotyrosine and a diiodotyrosine are coupled to form triiodothyronine (T_3). Only T_4 (90%) and T_3 (10%) are released into the circulation. There is evidence that T_3 is the active form of the hormone and that T_4 is converted to T_3 before it can act physiologically.

Thyroid hormones are bound to thyroid-binding globulin and other plasma proteins for transport in the blood. Only the free hormone enters cells and regulates the pituitary feedback mechanism. Protein-bound thyroid hormone forms a large reservoir that is slowly drawn on as free thyroid hormone is needed. There are three major thyroid-binding proteins: thyroid hormone–binding globulin (TBG) thyroxine-binding prealbumin (TBPA), and albumin. More than 99% of T_4 and T_3 is carried in the bound form. TBG carries approximately 70% of T_4 and T_3; TBPA binds approximately 10% of circulating T_4 and lesser amounts of T_3; and albumin binds approximately 15% of circulating T_4 and T_3.

A number of disease conditions and pharmacologic agents can decrease the amount of binding protein in the plasma or influence the binding of hormone. Congenital TBG deficiency is an X-linked trait that occurs in 1 of every 2500 live births. Corticosteroid medications and systemic disease conditions such as protein malnutrition, nephrotic syndrome, and cirrhosis decrease TBG concentrations. Medications such as phenytoin, salicylates, and diazepam can affect the binding of thyroid hormone to normal concentrations of binding proteins.

The secretion of thyroid hormone is regulated by the hypothalamic-pituitary-thyroid feedback system (Fig. 40-3).

In this system, thyrotropin-releasing hormone (TRH), which is produced by the hypothalamus, controls the release of thyroid-stimulating hormone (TSH) from the anterior pituitary gland. TSH increases the overall activity of the thyroid gland by increasing thyroglobulin breakdown and the release of thyroid hormone from follicles into the bloodstream, activating the iodide pump, increasing the oxidation of iodide and the coupling of iodide to tyrosine, and increasing the number and the size of the follicle cells. The effect of TSH on the release of thyroid hormones occurs within approximately 30 minutes, but the other effects require days or weeks.

Increased levels of thyroid hormone act in the feedback inhibition of TRH or TSH. High levels of iodide (*e.g.,* from iodide-containing cough syrup or kelp tablets) also cause a temporary decrease in thyroid activity that lasts for several weeks, probably through a direct inhibition of TSH on the thyroid. Cold exposure is one of the strongest stim-

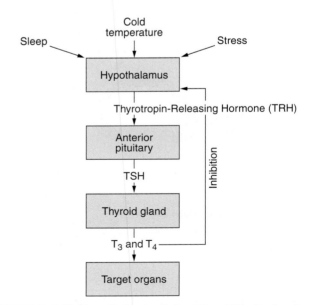

FIGURE 40-3 The hypothalamic-pituitary-thyroid feedback system, which regulates the body levels of thyroid hormone.

uli for increased thyroid hormone production and probably is mediated through TRH from the hypothalamus. Various emotional reactions also can affect the output of TRH and TSH and therefore indirectly affect secretion of thyroid hormones.

Actions of Thyroid Hormone

All the major organs in the body are affected by altered levels of thyroid hormone. Thyroid hormone has two major functions: it increases metabolism and protein synthesis, and it is necessary for growth and development in children, including mental development and attainment of sexual maturity.

Metabolic Rate.   Thyroid hormone increases the metabolism of all body tissues except the retina, spleen, testes, and lungs. The basal metabolic rate can increase by 60% to 100% above normal when large amounts of T_4 are present. As a result of this higher metabolism, the rate of glucose, fat, and protein use increases. Lipids are mobilized from adipose tissue, and the catabolism of cholesterol by the liver is increased. Blood levels of cholesterol are decreased in hyperthyroidism and increased in hypothyroidism. Muscle proteins are broken down and used as fuel, probably accounting for some of the muscle fatigue that occurs with hyperthyroidism. The absorption of glucose from the gastrointestinal tract is increased. Because vitamins are essential parts of metabolic enzymes and coenzymes, an increase in metabolic rate "speeds up" the use of vitamins and tends to cause vitamin deficiency.

Cardiovascular Function.   Cardiovascular and respiratory functions are strongly affected by thyroid function.

Thyroid Hormone

➤ Thyroid hormone increases the metabolism and protein synthesis in nearly all of the tissues of the body.

➤ It also is necessary for brain development and growth in infants and small children. Infants born with decreased or absent thyroid function have impaired mental and physical development.

➤ When hypothyroidism occurs in older children or adults, it produces a decrease in metabolic rate, an accumulation of a hydrophilic mucopolysaccharide substance (myxedema) in the connective tissues throughout the body, and an elevation in serum cholesterol.

➤ Hyperthyroidism has an effect opposite that of hypothyroidism. It produces an increase in metabolic rate and oxygen consumption, increased use of metabolic fuels, and increased sympathetic nervous system responsiveness.

With an increase in metabolism, there is a rise in oxygen consumption and production of metabolic end products, with an accompanying increase in vasodilatation. Blood flow to the skin, in particular, is augmented as a means of dissipating the body heat that results from the higher metabolism. Blood volume, cardiac output, and ventilation all are increased as a means of maintaining blood flow and oxygen delivery to body tissues. Heart rate and cardiac contractility are enhanced as a means of maintaining the needed cardiac output. On the other hand, blood pressure is likely to change little because the increase in vasodilatation tends to offset the increase in cardiac output.

Gastrointestinal Function.   Thyroid hormone enhances gastrointestinal function, causing an increase in motility and production of gastrointestinal secretions that often results in diarrhea. An increase in appetite and food intake accompanies the higher metabolic rate that occurs with increased thyroid hormone levels. At the same time, weight loss occurs because of the increased use of calories.

Neuromuscular Effects.   Thyroid hormone has marked effects on neural control of muscle function and tone. Slight elevations in hormone levels cause skeletal muscles to react more vigorously, and a drop in hormone levels causes muscles to react more sluggishly. In the hyperthyroid state, a fine muscle tremor is present. The cause of this tremor is unknown, but it may represent an increased sensitivity of the neural synapses in the spinal cord that control muscle tone.

In the infant, thyroid hormone is necessary for normal brain development. The hormone enhances cerebration; in the hyperthyroid state, it causes extreme nervousness, anxiety, and difficulty in sleeping.

Evidence suggests a strong interaction between thyroid hormone and the sympathetic nervous system. Many of the signs and symptoms of hyperthyroidism suggest overactivity of the sympathetic division of the autonomic nervous system, such as tachycardia, palpitations, and sweating. Tremor, restlessness, anxiety, and diarrhea also may reflect autonomic nervous system imbalances. Drugs that block sympathetic activity have proved to be valuable adjuncts in the treatment of hyperthyroidism because of their ability to relieve some of these undesirable symptoms.

Tests of Thyroid Function

Various tests aid in the diagnosis of thyroid disorders. Measures of T_3, T_4, and TSH have been made available through immunoassay methods. The free T_4 test measures the unbound portion of T_4 that is free to enter cells to produce its effects. The resin uptake test is an inverse test of TBG. The test involves adding radiolabeled T_3 or T_4 to a serum sample and allowing it to compete with the T_3 or T_4 in the sample for binding sites on TBG. The mixture is then added to a thyroid hormone–binding resin and the resin assayed for uptake of the labeled T_3 or T_4. A high resin test result indicates that the serum sample contains low amounts of TBG or high T_4 levels. TSH levels are used to differentiate between primary and secondary thyroid disorders. T_3, T_4, and free T_4 levels are low in primary hypothyroidism, and the TSH level is elevated.

The radioiodine (^{123}I) uptake test measures the ability of the thyroid gland to remove and concentrate iodine from the blood. Thyroid scans (*i.e.*, ^{123}I, ^{99m}Tc-pertechnetate) can be used to detect thyroid nodules and determine the functional activity of the thyroid gland. Ultrasonography can be used to differentiate cystic from solid thyroid lesions, and CT and MRI scans are used to demonstrate tracheal compression or impingement on other neighboring structures.

Alterations in Thyroid Function

An alteration in thyroid function can represent a hypofunctional or a hyperfunctional state. The manifestations of these two altered states are summarized in Table 40-3. Disorders of the thyroid may be due to a congenital defect in thyroid development, or they may develop later in life, with a gradual or sudden onset.

Goiter is an increase in the size of the thyroid gland. It can occur in hypothyroid, euthyroid, and hyperthyroid states. Goiters may be diffuse, involving the entire gland without evidence of nodularity, or they may contain nodules. Diffuse goiters usually become nodular. Goiters may be toxic, producing signs of extreme hyperthyroidism, or thyrotoxicosis, or they may be nontoxic. Diffuse nontoxic and multinodular goiters are the result of compensatory hypertrophy and hyperplasia of follicular epithelium from some derangement that impairs thyroid hormone output.

The degree of thyroid enlargement usually is proportional to the extent and duration of thyroid deficiency. Multinodular goiters produce the largest thyroid enlargements and often are associated with thyrotoxicosis. When sufficiently enlarged, they may compress the esophagus and trachea, causing difficulty in swallowing, a choking sensation, and inspiratory stridor. Such lesions also may compress the superior vena cava, producing distention of the veins of the neck and upper extremities, edema of the eyelids and conjunctiva, and syncope with coughing.

HYPOTHYROIDISM

Hypothyroidism can occur as a congenital or an acquired defect. Congenital hypothyroidism develops prenatally and is present at birth. Acquired hypothyroidism develops later in life because of primary disease of the thyroid gland or secondary to disorders of hypothalamic or pituitary origin.

Congenital Hypothyroidism

Congenital hypothyroidism is a common cause of preventable mental retardation. It affects approximately 1 of 4000 infants. Hypothyroidism in the infant may result from a congenital lack of the thyroid gland or from abnormal biosynthesis of thyroid hormone or deficient TSH secretion. With congenital lack of the thyroid gland, the infant usually appears normal and functions normally at birth, because hormones have been supplied in utero by the mother. The manifestations of untreated congenital hypothyroidism are referred to as *cretinism*. However, the term does not apply to the normally developing infant in whom replacement thyroid hormone therapy was instituted shortly after birth.

TABLE 40-3 ✦ Manifestations of Hypothyroid and Hyperthyroid States		
Level of Organization	**Hypothyroidism**	**Hyperthyroidism**
Basal metabolic rate	Decreased	Increased
Sensitivity to catecholamines	Decreased	Increased
General features	Myxedematous features Deep voice Impaired growth (child)	Exophthalmos Lid lag Decreased blinking
Blood cholesterol levels	Increased	Decreased
General behavior	Mental retardation (infant) Mental and physical sluggishness Somnolence	Restlessness, irritability, anxiety Hyperkinesis Wakefulness
Cardiovascular function	Decreased cardiac output Bradycardia	Increased cardiac output Tachycardia and palpitations
Gastrointestinal function	Constipation Decreased appetite	Diarrhea Increased appetite
Respiratory function	Hypoventilation	Dyspnea
Muscle tone and reflexes	Decreased	Increased, with tremor and fibrillatory twitching
Temperature tolerance	Cold intolerance	Heat intolerance
Skin and hair	Decreased sweating Coarse and dry skin and hair	Increased sweating Thin and silky skin and hair
Weight	Gain	Loss

Thyroid hormone is essential for normal brain development and growth, almost half of which occurs during the first 6 months of life. If untreated, congenital hypothyroidism causes mental retardation and impairs growth. Long-term studies show that closely monitored T_4 supplementation begun in the first 6 weeks of life results in normal intelligence. Fortunately, neonatal screening tests have been instituted to detect congenital hypothyroidism during early infancy. Screening usually is done in the hospital nursery. In this test, a drop of blood is taken from the infant's heel and analyzed for T_4 and TSH.

Transient congenital hypothyroidism has been recognized more frequently since the introduction of neonatal screening. It is characterized by high TSH levels and low thyroid hormone levels. The fetal and infant thyroids are sensitive to iodine excess. Iodine crosses the placenta and mammary glands and is readily absorbed by infant skin. Transient hypothyroidism may be caused by maternal or infant exposure to substances such as povidone-iodine used as a disinfectant (*i.e.*, vaginal douche or skin disinfectant, in the nursery). Antithyroid drugs such as propylthiouracil, methimazole, and carbimazole also cross the placenta and block fetal thyroid function.

Congenital hypothyroidism is treated by hormone replacement. Evidence indicates that it is important to normalize T_4 levels as rapidly as possible because a delay is accompanied by poorer psychomotor and mental development. Dosage levels are adjusted as the child grows. Infants with transient hypothyroidism usually can have the replacement therapy withdrawn at 6 to 12 months. When early and adequate treatment regimens are followed, the risk of mental retardation in infants detected by screening programs essentially is nonexistent.

Acquired Hypothyroidism and Myxedema

Hypothyroidism in older children and adults causes a general slowing down of metabolic processes and myxedema. Myxedema implies the presence of a nonpitting mucous type of edema caused by an accumulation of a hydrophilic mucopolysaccharide substance in the connective tissues throughout the body. The hypothyroid state may be mild, with only a few signs and symptoms, or it may progress to a life-threatening condition called *myxedematous coma*. It can result from destruction or dysfunction of the thyroid gland (*i.e.*, primary hypothyroidism), or it can be a secondary disorder caused by impaired hypothalamic or pituitary function.

Primary hypothyroidism is much more common than secondary (and tertiary) hypothyroidism. It may result from thyroidectomy (*i.e.*, surgical removal) or ablation of the gland with radiation. Certain goitrogenic agents, such as lithium carbonate (*i.e.*, used in the treatment of manic-depressive states) and the antithyroid drugs propylthiouracil and methimazole in continuous dosage can block hormone synthesis and produce hypothyroidism with goiter. Large amounts of iodine (*i.e.*, ingestion of kelp tablets or iodide-containing cough syrups, or administration of iodide-containing radiographic contrast media or the cardiac drug amiodarone, which contains 75 mg of iodine per 200-mg tablet, and is being increasingly implicated in causing thy-roid problems) also can block thyroid hormone production and cause goiter, particularly in persons with autoimmune thyroid disease. Iodine deficiency, which can cause goiter and hypothyroidism, is rare in the United States because of the widespread use of iodized salt and other iodide sources.

The most common cause of hypothyroidism is Hashimoto's thyroiditis, an autoimmune disorder in which the thyroid gland may be totally destroyed by an immunologic process. It is the major cause of goiter and hypothyroidism in children. Hashimoto's thyroiditis is predominantly a disease of women, with a female-to-male ratio of 5:1. The course of the disease varies. At the onset, only a goiter may be present. In time, hypothyroidism usually becomes evident. Although the disorder usually causes hypothyroidism, a hyperthyroid state may develop midcourse in the disease. The transient hyperthyroid state is caused by leakage of preformed thyroid hormone from damaged cells of the gland. Subacute thyroiditis, which can occur in up to 10% of pregnancies postpartum (postpartum thyroiditis), also can result in hypothyroidism.

Hypothyroidism affects almost all of the organ systems in the body. The manifestations of the disorder are related largely to two factors: the hypometabolic state resulting from thyroid hormone deficiency, and myxedematous involvement of body tissues. Although the myxedema is most obvious in the face and other superficial parts, it also affects many of the body organs and is responsible for many of the manifestations of the hypothyroid state (Fig. 40-4).

The hypometabolic state associated with hypothyroidism is characterized by a gradual onset of weakness and fatigue, a tendency to gain weight despite a loss of appetite,

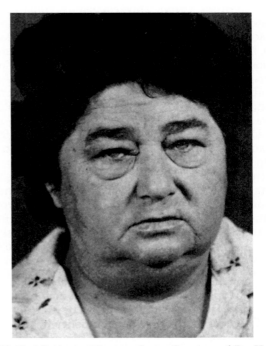

FIGURE 40-4 Patient with myxedema. Courtesy of Dr. Herbert Langford. (From Guyton A. [1981]. *Medical physiology* [6th ed., p. 941]. Philadelphia: W.B. Saunders. Reprinted by permission)

and cold intolerance. As the condition progresses, the skin becomes dry and rough and acquires a pale yellowish cast, which primarily results from carotene deposition, and the hair becomes coarse and brittle. There can be loss of the lateral one third of the eyebrows. Gastrointestinal motility is decreased, producing constipation, flatulence, and abdominal distention. Nervous system involvement is manifested in mental dullness, lethargy, and impaired memory.

As a result of myxedematous fluid accumulation, the face takes on a characteristic puffy look, especially around the eyes. The tongue is enlarged, and the voice is hoarse and husky. Myxedematous fluid can collect in the interstitial spaces of almost any organ system. Pericardial or pleural effusion may develop. Mucopolysaccharide deposits in the heart cause generalized cardiac dilatation, bradycardia, and other signs of altered cardiac function. The signs and symptoms of hypothyroidism are summarized in Table 40-3.

Diagnosis of hypothyroidism is based on history, physical examination, and laboratory tests. A low serum T_4, low resin T_3, and elevated TSH levels are characteristic of primary hypothyroidism. The tests for antithyroid antibodies should be done when Hashimoto's thyroiditis is suspected (antithyroid peroxidase is the preferred test). A TRH stimulation test may be helpful in differentiating pituitary (secondary hypothyroidism) from hypothalamic (tertiary hypothyroidism) disease.

Hypothyroidism is treated by replacement therapy with synthetic preparations of T_3 or T_4. Most people are treated with T_4. Serum TSH levels are used to estimate the adequacy of T_4 replacement therapy. When the TSH level is normalized, the T_4 dosage is considered satisfactory (for primary hypothyroidism only).

Myxedematous Coma. Myxedematous coma is a life-threatening, end-stage expression of hypothyroidism. It is characterized by coma, hypothermia, cardiovascular collapse, hypoventilation, and severe metabolic disorders that include hyponatremia, hypoglycemia, and lactic acidosis. It occurs most often in elderly women who have chronic hypothyroidism from a spectrum of causes. The fact that it occurs more frequently in winter months suggests that cold exposure may be a precipitating factor. The severely hypothyroid person is unable to metabolize sedatives, analgesics, and anesthetic drugs, and buildup of these agents may precipitate coma.

Treatment includes aggressive management of precipitating factors; supportive therapy such as management of cardiorespiratory status, hyponatremia, and hypoglycemia; and thyroid replacement therapy. Prevention is preferable to treatment and entails special attention to high-risk populations, such as women with a history of Hashimoto's thyroiditis. These persons should be informed about the signs and symptoms of severe hypothyroidism and the need for early medical treatment.

HYPERTHYROIDISM

Hyperthyroidism, or thyrotoxicosis, results from excessive delivery of thyroid hormone to the peripheral tissues. The most common cause of hyperthyroidism is Graves' disease, which is accompanied by ophthalmopathy (exophthalmos, *i.e.*, bulging of the eyeballs) and goiter. Other causes of hyperthyroidism are multinodular goiter, adenoma of the thyroid, and, occasionally, ingestion of excessive thyroid hormone. Iodine-containing agents can induce hyperthyroidism as well as hypothyroidism. Thyroid crisis, or storm, is an acutely exaggerated manifestation of the hyperthyroid state.

Many of the manifestations of hyperthyroidism are related to the increase in oxygen consumption and use of metabolic fuels associated with the hypermetabolic state, as well as to the increase in sympathetic nervous system activity that occurs. The fact that many of the signs and symptoms of hyperthyroidism resemble those of excessive sympathetic nervous system activity suggests that thyroid hormone may heighten the sensitivity of the body to the catecholamines or that it may act as a pseudocatecholamine. With the hypermetabolic state, there are frequent complaints of nervousness, irritability, and fatigability. Weight loss is common despite a large appetite. Other manifestations include tachycardia, palpitations, shortness of breath, excessive sweating, muscle cramps, and heat intolerance. The person appears restless and has a fine muscle tremor. Even in persons without exophthalmos, there is an abnormal retraction of the eyelids and infrequent blinking such that they appear to be staring. The hair and skin usually are thin and have a silky appearance. The signs and symptoms of hyperthyroidism are summarized in Table 40-3.

The treatment of hyperthyroidism is directed toward reducing the level of thyroid hormone. This can be accomplished with eradication of the thyroid gland with radioactive iodine, through surgical removal of part or all of the gland, or the use of drugs that decrease thyroid function and thereby the effect of thyroid hormone on the peripheral tissues. Eradication of the thyroid with radioactive iodine is used more frequently than surgery. The β-adrenergic–blocking drug propranolol often is administered to block the effects of the hyperthyroid state on sympathetic nervous system function. It is given in conjunction with other antithyroid drugs such as propylthiouracil and methimazole. These drugs prevent the thyroid gland from converting iodine to its organic (hormonal) form and block the conversion of T_4 to T_3 in the tissues. Iodinated contrast agents (iopanoic acid and ipodate sodium) may be given orally to block thyroid hormone synthesis and release as well as the peripheral conversion of T_4 and T_3. These agents may be used in treatment of thyroid storm or in persons who are intolerant of propylthiouracil or methimazole.

Graves' Disease

Graves' disease is a state of hyperthyroidism, goiter, and ophthalmopathy (or, less commonly, dermopathy). The onset usually is between the ages of 20 and 40 years, and women are five times more likely to develop the disease than men. Graves' disease is an autoimmune disorder characterized by abnormal stimulation of the thyroid gland by thyroid-stimulating antibodies (thyroid-stimulating immunoglobulins [TSI]) that act through the normal TSH receptors. It may be associated with other autoimmune disorders such as myasthenia gravis and pernicious anemia.

The disease is associated with human leukocyte antigen (HLA)-DR3 and HLA-B8, and a familial tendency is evident.

The exophthalmos, which occurs in up to one third of persons with Graves' disease, is thought to result from a cytokine-mediated activation of fibroblasts in orbital tissue behind the eyeball. Humoral autoimmunity also is important; an ophthalmic immunoglobulin may exacerbate lymphocytic infiltration of the extraocular muscles. The ophthalmopathy of Graves' disease can cause severe eye problems, including paralysis of the extraocular muscles; involvement of the optic nerve, with some visual loss; and corneal ulceration because the lids do not close over the protruding eyeball. The exophthalmos usually tends to stabilize after treatment of the hyperthyroidism. However, ophthalmopathy can worsen acutely after radioiodine treatment. Many physicians use glucocorticoid treatment for several weeks surrounding the radioiodine treatment if the patient had signs of ophthalmopathy. Other experts do not to use radioiodine therapy under these circumstances, but prefer antithyroid therapy with drugs (which may decrease the immune activation in the condition). Unfortunately, not all of the ocular changes are reversible with treatment. Ophthalmopathy also can be aggravated by smoking, which should be strongly discouraged. Figure 40-5 depicts a woman with Graves' disease.

Thyroid Storm

Thyroid storm, or crisis, is an extreme and life-threatening form of thyrotoxicosis, rarely seen today because of improved diagnosis and treatment methods. When it does occur, it is seen most often in undiagnosed cases or in persons with hyperthyroidism who have not been adequately treated. It often is precipitated by stress such as an infection (usually respiratory), by diabetic ketoacidosis, by physical or emotional trauma, or by manipulation of a hyperactive thyroid gland during thyroidectomy. Thyroid storm is manifested by a very high fever, extreme cardiovascular effects (*i.e.*, tachycardia, congestive failure, and angina), and severe CNS effects (*i.e.*, agitation, restlessness, and delirium). The mortality rate is high.

Thyroid storm requires rapid diagnosis and implementation of treatment. Peripheral cooling is initiated with cold packs and a cooling mattress. For cooling to be effective, the shivering response must be prevented. General supportive measures to replace fluids, glucose, and electrolytes are essential during the hypermetabolic state. A β-adrenergic–blocking drug, such as propranolol, is given to block the undesirable effects of T_4 on cardiovascular function. Glucocorticoids are used to correct the relative adrenal insufficiency resulting from the stress imposed by the hyperthyroid state and to inhibit the peripheral conversion of T_4 to T_3. Propylthiouracil or methimazole may be given to block thyroid synthesis. Aspirin increases the level of free thyroid hormones by displacing the hormones from their protein carriers, and should not be used during thyroid storm. The iodide-containing radiographic contrast medium sodium ipodate also can be useful for blocking thyroid hormone production.

> In summary, thyroid hormones play a role in the metabolic process of almost all body cells and are necessary for normal physical and mental growth in the infant and young child. Alterations in thyroid function can manifest as a hypothyroid or a hyperthyroid state. Hypothyroidism can occur as a congenital or an acquired defect. Congenital hypothyroidism leads to mental retardation and impaired physical growth unless treatment is initiated during the first months of life. Acquired hypothyroidism leads to a decrease in metabolic rate and an accumulation of a mucopolysaccharide substance in the intercellular spaces; this substance attracts water and causes a mucous type of edema called *myxedema*. Hyperthyroidism causes an increase in metabolic rate and alterations in body function similar to those produced by enhanced sympathetic nervous system activity. Graves' disease is characterized by the triad of hyperthyroidism, goiter, and ophthalmopathy.

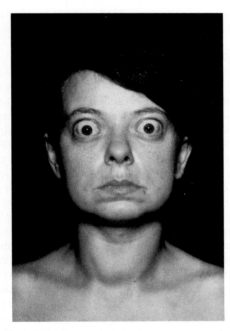

FIGURE 40-5 Graves' disease. A young woman with hyperthyroidism presented with a mass in the neck and exophthalmos. (Rubin E., Farber J.L. [1999]. *Pathology* [3rd ed., p. 1167]. Philadelphia: Lippincott Williams & Wilkins)

Disorders of Adrenal Cortical Function

After you have completed this section of the chapter, you should be able to meet the following objectives:

✦ Describe the function of the adrenal cortical hormones and their feedback regulation
✦ State the underlying cause of the adrenogenital syndrome
✦ Relate the functions of the adrenal cortical hormones to Addison's disease (*i.e.*, adrenal insufficiency) and Cushing's syndrome (*i.e.*, cortisol excess)

CONTROL OF ADRENAL CORTICAL FUNCTION

The adrenal glands are small, bilateral structures that weigh approximately 5 g each and lie retroperitoneally at the apex of each kidney (Fig. 40-6). The medulla or inner portion of the gland secretes epinephrine and norepinephrine and is part of the sympathetic nervous system. The cortex forms the bulk of the adrenal gland and is responsible for secreting three types of hormones: the glucocorticoids, the mineralocorticoids, and the adrenal sex hormones. Because the sympathetic nervous system also secretes epinephrine and norepinephrine, adrenal medullary function is not essential for life, but adrenal cortical function is. The total loss of adrenal cortical function is fatal in 4 to 14 days if untreated. This section of the chapter describes the synthesis and function of the adrenal cortical hormones and the effects of adrenal cortical insufficiency and excess.

Biosynthesis, Transport, and Metabolism

More than 30 hormones are produced by the adrenal cortex. Of these hormones, aldosterone is the principal mineralocorticoid, cortisol (hydrocortisone) is the major glucocorticoid, and androgens are the chief sex hormones. All of the adrenal cortical hormones have a similar structure in that all are steroids and are synthesized from acetate and cholesterol. Each of the steps involved in the synthesis of the various hormones requires a specific enzyme (Fig. 40-7). The secretion of the glucocorticoids and the adrenal androgens is controlled by the ACTH secreted by the anterior pituitary gland.

Cortisol and the adrenal androgens are secreted in an unbound state and bind to plasma proteins for transport in the circulatory system. Cortisol binds largely to corticosteroid-binding globulin and to a lesser extent to albumin. Aldosterone circulates mostly bound to albumin. It has been suggested that the pool of protein-bound hormones may extend the duration of their action by delaying metabolic clearance.

The main site for metabolism of the adrenal cortical hormones is the liver, where they undergo a number of metabolic conversions before being conjugated and made water soluble. They are then eliminated in either the urine or the bile.

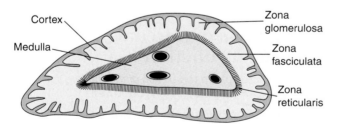

FIGURE 40-6 The adrenal gland, showing the medulla and the three layers of the cortex. The zona glomerulosa is the outer layer of the cortex and is primarily responsible for mineralocorticoid production. The middle layer, the zona fasciculata, and the inner layer, the zona reticularis, produce the glucocorticoids and the adrenal sex hormones.

Adrenal Sex Hormones

The adrenal sex hormones are synthesized primarily by the zona reticularis and the zona fasciculata of the cortex (see Fig. 40-6). These sex hormones probably exert little effect on normal sexual function. There is evidence, however, that the adrenal sex hormones (the most important of which is dehydroepiandrosterone) contribute to the pubertal growth of body hair, particularly pubic and axillary hair in women. They also may play a role in the steroid hormone economy of the pregnant woman and the fetal-placental unit. Dehydroepiandrosterone sulfate (DHEAS) is increasingly being used in the treatment of both Addison's disease (to be discussed) and adults who have decreased levels of DHEAS. Adrenal androgens are physiologically important in women with Addison's disease, and replacement with 25 to 50 mg of DHEAS daily should be considered. Because the testes produce these hormones, there is no rationale for using it in men. The levels of DHEAS decline to approximately one-sixth the levels of a 20-year-old by 60 years of age (the *adrenopause*). The significance if this is unknown, but replacement may improve general well-being and sexuality, and have other important effects in women. The value of routine replacement of DHEAS in the adrenopause is largely unproven.

Mineralocorticoids

The mineralocorticoids play an essential role in regulating potassium and sodium levels and water balance. They are produced in the zona glomerulosa, the outer layer of cells of the adrenal cortex. Aldosterone secretion is regulated by the renin-angiotensin mechanism and by blood levels of potassium. Increased levels of aldosterone promote sodium retention by the distal tubules of the kidney while increasing urinary losses of potassium. The influence of aldosterone on fluid and electrolyte balance is discussed in Chapter 31.

Glucocorticoids

The glucocorticoid hormones, mainly cortisol, are synthesized in the zona fasciculata and the zona reticularis of the adrenal gland. The blood levels of these hormones are regulated by negative feedback mechanisms of the hypothalamic-pituitary-adrenal (HPA) system (Fig. 40-8). Just as other pituitary hormones are controlled by releasing factors from the hypothalamus, corticotropin-releasing hormone (CRH) is important in controlling the release of ACTH. Cortisol levels increase as ACTH levels rise and decrease as ACTH levels fall. There is considerable diurnal variation in ACTH levels, which reach their peak in the early morning (around 6 to 8 AM) and decline as the day progresses (see Fig. 39-3). This appears to be due to rhythmic activity in the CNS, which causes bursts of CRH secretion and, in turn, ACTH secretion. This diurnal pattern is reversed in people who work during the night and sleep during the day. The rhythm also may be changed by physical and psychological stresses, endogenous depression, manic-depressive psychosis, and liver disease or other conditions that affect cortisol metabolism. One of the earliest signs of Cushing's syndrome, a disorder of cortisol excess, is the loss of diurnal variation in CRH and ACTH secretion.

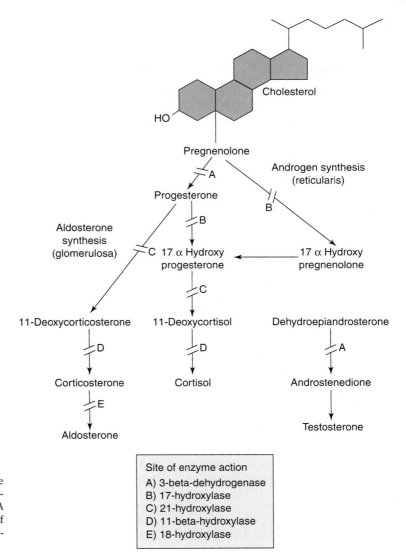

FIGURE 40-7 Predominant biosynthetic pathways of the adrenal cortex. Critical enzymes in the biosynthetic process include 11-beta-hydroxylase and 21-hydroxylase. A deficiency in one of these enzymes blocks the synthesis of hormones dependent on that enzyme and routes the precursors into alternative pathways.

The glucocorticoids perform a necessary function in response to stress and are essential for survival. When produced as part of the stress response, these hormones aid in regulating the metabolic functions of the body and in controlling the inflammatory response. The actions of cortisol are summarized in Table 40-4. Many of the anti-inflammatory actions attributed to cortisol result from the administration of pharmacologic levels of the hormone.

Metabolic Effects. Cortisol stimulates glucose production by the liver, promotes protein breakdown, and causes mobilization of fatty acids. As body proteins are broken down, amino acids are mobilized and transported to the liver, where they are used in the production of glucose (*i.e.,* gluconeogenesis). Mobilization of fatty acids converts cell metabolism from the use of glucose for energy to the use of fatty acids instead. As glucose production by the liver rises and peripheral glucose use falls, a moderate resistance to insulin develops. In persons with diabetes and those who are diabetes prone, this has the effect of raising the blood glucose level.

Psychological Effects. The glucocorticoid hormones appear to be involved directly or indirectly in emotional behavior. Receptors for these hormones have been identified in brain tissue, which suggests that they play a role in the regulation of behavior. Persons treated with adrenal cortical hormones have been known to display behavior ranging from mildly aberrant to psychotic.

Immunologic and Inflammatory Effects. Cortisol influences multiple aspects of immunologic function and inflammatory responsiveness. Large quantities of cortisol are required for an effective anti-inflammatory action. This is achieved by the administration of pharmacologic rather than physiologic doses of synthetic cortisol. The increased cortisol blocks inflammation at an early stage by decreasing capillary permeability and stabilizing the lysosomal membranes so that inflammatory mediators are not released. Cortisol suppresses the immune response by reducing humoral and cell-mediated immunity. With this lessened inflammatory response comes a reduction in fever. During the

Adrenal Cortical Hormones

➤ The adrenal cortex produces three types of steroid hormones: the mineralocorticoids (principally aldosterone), which function in sodium, potassium, and water balance; the glucocorticoids (principally cortisol), which aid in regulating the metabolic functions of the body and in controlling the inflammatory response, and are essential for survival in stress situations; and the adrenal sex hormones (principally androgens), which serve mainly as a source of androgens for women.

➤ The manifestations of primary adrenal cortical insufficiency are related mainly to mineralocorticoid deficiency (impaired ability to regulate salt and water elimination) and glucocorticoid deficiency (impaired ability to regulate blood glucose and control the effects of the immune and inflammatory responses).

➤ Adrenal cortical excess results in derangements in glucose metabolism, disorders of sodium and potassium regulation (increased sodium retention and potassium loss), impaired ability to respond to stress because of inhibition of inflammatory and immune responses, increased gastric acid secretion with gastric ulceration and bleeding, and signs of increased androgen levels such as hirsutism.

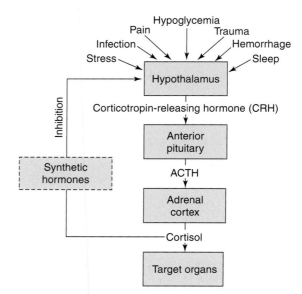

FIGURE 40-8 The hypothalamic-pituitary-adrenal (HPA) feedback system that regulates glucocorticoid (cortisol) levels. Cortisol release is regulated by ACTH. Stress exerts its effects on cortisol release through the HPA system and the corticotropin-releasing hormone (CRH), which controls the release of ACTH from the anterior pituitary gland. Increased cortisol levels incite a negative feedback inhibition of ACTH release. Pharmacologic doses of synthetic steroids inhibit ACTH release by way of the hypothalamic CRH.

healing phase, cortisol suppresses fibroblast activity and thereby lessens scar formation. Cortisol also inhibits prostaglandin synthesis, which may account in large part for its anti-inflammatory actions.

Suppression of Adrenal Function

A highly significant aspect of long-term therapy with pharmacologic preparations of the adrenal cortical hormones is adrenal insufficiency on withdrawal of the drugs. The deficiency results from suppression of the HPA system. Chronic suppression causes atrophy of the adrenal gland, and the abrupt withdrawal of drugs can cause acute adrenal insufficiency. Recovery to a state of normal adrenal function may be prolonged, requiring up to 12 months or more.

Tests of Adrenal Function

Several diagnostic tests can be used to evaluate adrenal cortical function and the HPA system. Blood levels of cortisol, aldosterone, and ACTH can be measured using immunoassay methods. A 24-hour urine specimen measures the excretion of 17-ketosteroids, 17-ketogenic steroids, and 17-hydroxycorticosteroids. These metabolic end-products of the adrenal hormones and the male androgens provide information about alterations in the biosynthesis of the adrenal cortical hormones. The 24-hour urinary free cortisol is an excellent screening test for Cushing's syndrome.

Suppression and stimulation tests afford a means of assessing the state of the HPA feedback system. For example, a test dose of ACTH can be given to assess the response of the adrenal cortex to stimulation. Similarly, administration of dexamethasone, a synthetic glucocorticoid drug, provides a means of measuring negative feedback suppression of ACTH. Adrenal tumors and ectopic ACTH-producing tumors usually are unresponsive to ACTH suppression by dexamethasone. CRH tests can be used to diagnose a pituitary ACTH-secreting tumor (*i.e.*, Cushing's disease), especially when combined with inferior petrosal venous sampling (this allows the blood drainage of the pituitary to be sampled directly). Metyrapone (Metopirone) blocks the final step in cortisol synthesis, resulting in the production of 11-dehydroxycortisol, which does not inhibit ACTH. This test measures the ability of the pituitary to release ACTH. The gold standard test for assessing the HPA axis is the insulin hypoglycemic stress test.

CONGENITAL ADRENAL HYPERPLASIA

Congenital adrenal hyperplasia (CAH), or the adrenogenital syndrome, describes a congenital disorder caused by an autosomal recessive trait in which a deficiency exists in any of the enzymes necessary for the synthesis of cortisol. A common characteristic of all types of CAH is a defect in the synthesis of cortisol that results in increased levels of ACTH and adrenal hyperplasia. The increased levels of ACTH overstimulate the pathways for production of adrenal androgens. Mineralocorticoids may be produced in exces-

TABLE 40-4 ✦ Actions of Cortisol

Major Influence	Effect on Body
Glucose metabolism	Stimulates gluconeogenesis Decreases glucose use by the tissues
Protein metabolism	Increases breakdown of proteins Increases plasma protein levels
Fat metabolism	Increases mobilization of fatty acids Increases use of fatty acids

Anti-inflammatory action (pharmacologic levels)	Stabilizes lysosomal membranes of the inflammatory cells, preventing the release of inflammatory mediators
	Decreases capillary permeability to prevent inflammatory edema
	Depresses phagocytosis by white blood cells to reduce the release of inflammatory mediators
	Suppresses the immune response
	   Causes atrophy of lymphoid tissue
	   Decreases eosinophils
	   Decreases antibody formation
	   Decreases the development of cell-mediated immunity
	Reduces fever
	Inhibits fibroblast activity

Psychic effect	May contribute to emotional instability
Permissive effect	Facilitates the response of the tissues to humoral and neural influences, such as that of the catecholamines, during trauma and extreme stress

sive or insufficient amounts, depending on the precise enzyme deficiency. Infants of both sexes are affected. Males seldom are diagnosed at birth unless they have enlarged genitalia or lose salt and manifest adrenal crisis. In female infants, an increase in androgens is responsible for creating the virilization syndrome of ambiguous genitalia with an enlarged clitoris, fused labia, and urogenital sinus (Fig. 40-9). In male and female children, other secondary sex characteristics are normal, and fertility is unaffected if appropriate therapy is instituted.

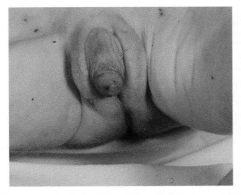

FIGURE 40-9 A female infant with congenital adrenal hyperplasia demonstrating virilization of the genitalia with hypertrophy of the clitoris and partial fusion of labioscrotal folds. (Rubin E., Farber J.L. [1999]. *Pathology* [3rd ed., p. 1186]. Philadelphia: Lippincott Williams & Wilkins)

The two most common enzyme deficiencies are 21-hydroxylase (accounting for >90% of cases) and 11-β-hydroxylase deficiency. The clinical manifestations of both deficiencies are largely determined by the functional properties of the steroid intermediates and the completeness of the block in the cortisol pathway.

A spectrum of 21-hydroxylase deficiency states exists, ranging from simple virilizing CAH to a complete salt-losing enzyme deficiency. Simple virilizing CAH impairs the synthesis of cortisol, and steroid synthesis is shunted to androgen production. Persons with these deficiencies usually produce sufficient aldosterone or aldosterone intermediates to prevent signs and symptoms of mineralocorticoid deficiency. The salt-losing form is accompanied by deficient production of aldosterone and its intermediates. This results in fluid and electrolyte disorders after the fifth day of life, including hyponatremia, hyperkalemia, vomiting, dehydration, and shock.

The 11-β-hydroxylase deficiency is rare and manifests a spectrum of severity. Affected persons have excessive androgen production and impaired conversion of 11-deoxycorticosterone to corticosterone. The overproduction of 11-deoxycorticosterone, which has mineralocorticoid activity, is responsible for the hypertension that accompanies this deficiency. Diagnosis of adrenogenital syndrome depends on the precise biochemical evaluation of metabolites in the cortisol pathway and on clinical signs and symptoms.

Medical treatment of adrenogenital syndrome includes oral or parenteral cortisol replacement. Fludrocortisone acetate, a mineralocorticoid, also may be given to children who are salt losers. Depending on the degree of virilization, reconstructive surgery during the first 2 years of life is indicated to reduce the size of the clitoris, separate the labia, and exteriorize the vagina. Surgery has provided excellent results and does not impair sexual function.

ADRENAL CORTICAL INSUFFICIENCY

There are two forms of adrenal insufficiency: primary and secondary (see Table 40-5 for distinguishing features). Primary adrenal insufficiency, or Addison's disease, is caused by destruction of the adrenal gland. Secondary adrenal insufficiency results from a disorder of the HPA system.

Primary Adrenal Cortical Insufficiency

In 1855, Thomas Addison, an English physician, provided the first detailed clinical description of primary adrenal insufficiency, now called *Addison's disease*. The use of this term is reserved for primary adrenal insufficiency in which adrenal cortical hormones are deficient and ACTH levels are elevated because of lack of feedback inhibition.

Addison's disease is a relatively rare disorder in which all the layers of the adrenal cortex are destroyed. Autoimmune destruction is the most common cause of Addison's disease in the United States. Before 1950, tuberculosis was the major cause of Addison's disease in the United States, and it continues to be a major cause of the disease in countries where it is more prevalent. Rare causes include metastatic carcinoma, fungal infection (particularly histoplasmosis), cytomegalovirus infection, amyloid disease, and hemochromatosis. Bilateral adrenal hemorrhage may occur in persons taking anticoagulants, during open heart surgery, and during birth or major trauma. Adrenal insufficiency can be caused by acquired immunodeficiency syndrome, in which the adrenal gland is destroyed by a variety of opportunistic infectious agents.

Addison's disease, like type 1 diabetes mellitus, is a chronic metabolic disorder that requires lifetime hormone replacement therapy. The adrenal cortex has a large reserve capacity, and the manifestations of adrenal insufficiency usually do not become apparent until approximately 90% of the gland has been destroyed. These manifestations are related primarily to mineralocorticoid deficiency, glucocorticoid deficiency, and hyperpigmentation resulting from elevated ACTH levels. Although lack of the adrenal androgens (*i.e.*, DHEAS) exerts few effects in men because the testes produce these hormones, women have sparse axillary and pubic hair.

Mineralocorticoid deficiency causes increased urinary losses of sodium, chloride, and water, along with decreased excretion of potassium. The result is hyponatremia, loss of extracellular fluid, decreased cardiac output, and hyperkalemia. There may be an abnormal appetite for salt. Orthostatic hypotension is common. Dehydration, weakness, and fatigue are common early symptoms. If loss of sodium and water is extreme, cardiovascular collapse and shock ensue. Because of a lack of glucocorticoids, the person with Addison's disease has poor tolerance to stress. This deficiency causes hypoglycemia, lethargy, weakness, fever, and gastrointestinal symptoms such as anorexia, nausea, vomiting, and weight loss.

Hyperpigmentation results from elevated levels of ACTH. The skin looks bronzed or suntanned in exposed and unexposed areas, and the normal creases and pressure points tend to become especially dark. The gums and oral mucous membranes may become bluish-black. The amino acid sequence of ACTH is strikingly similar to that of melanocyte-stimulating hormone; hyperpigmentation occurs in greater than 90% of persons with Addison's disease and is helpful in distinguishing the primary and secondary forms of adrenal insufficiency.

The daily regulation of the chronic phase of Addison's disease usually is accomplished with oral replacement therapy, with higher doses being given during periods of stress. The pharmacologic agent that is used should have both glucocorticoid and mineralocorticoid activity. Mineralocorticoids are needed only in primary adrenal insufficiency. Hydrocortisone usually is the drug of choice. In mild cases,

---

TABLE 40-5 ◆ Clinical Findings of Adrenal Insufficiency

Finding	Primary	Secondary/Tertiary
Anorexia and weight loss	Yes (100%)	Yes (100%)
Fatigue and weakness	Yes (100%)	Yes (100%)
Gastrointestinal symptoms, nausea, diarrhea	Yes (50%)	Yes (50%)
Myalgia, arthralgia, abdominal pain	Yes (10%)	Yes (10%)
Orthostatic hypotension	Yes	Yes
Hyponatremia	Yes (85%–90%)	Yes (60%)
Hyperkalemia	Yes (60%–65%)	No
Hyperpigmentation	Yes (>90%)	No
Secondary deficiencies of testosterone, growth hormone, thyroxine, antidiuretic hormone	No	Yes
Associated autoimmune conditions	Yes	No

hydrocortisone alone may be adequate. Fludrocortisone (a mineralocorticoid) is used for persons who do not obtain a sufficient salt-retaining effect from hydrocortisone. DHEAS replacement also may be helpful in the female patient.

Because persons with the disorder are likely to have episodes of hyponatremia and hypoglycemia, they need to have a regular schedule for meals and exercise. Persons with Addison's disease also have limited ability to respond to infections, trauma, and other stresses. Such situations require immediate medical attention and treatment. All persons with Addison's disease should be advised to wear a medical alert bracelet or medal.

Secondary Adrenal Cortical Insufficiency

Secondary adrenal insufficiency can occur as the result of hypopituitarism or because the pituitary gland has been surgically removed (see discussion of hypopituitarism in Chapter 39). Tertiary adrenal insufficiency results from a hypothalamic defect. However, a far more common cause than either of these is the rapid withdrawal of glucocorticoids that have been administered therapeutically. These drugs suppress the HPA system, with resulting adrenal cortical atrophy and loss of cortisol production. This suppression continues long after drug therapy has been discontinued and can be critical during periods of stress or when surgery is performed.

Acute Adrenal Crisis

Acute adrenal crisis is a life-threatening situation. If Addison's disease is the underlying problem, exposure to even a minor illness or stress can precipitate nausea, vomiting, muscular weakness, hypotension, dehydration, and vascular collapse. The onset of adrenal crisis may be sudden, or it may progress over a period of several days. The symptoms may occur suddenly in children with salt-losing forms of the adrenogenital syndrome. Massive bilateral adrenal hemorrhage causes an acute fulminating form of adrenal insufficiency. Hemorrhage can be caused by meningococcal septicemia (*i.e.*, Waterhouse-Friderichsen syndrome), adrenal trauma, anticoagulant therapy, adrenal vein thrombosis, or adrenal metastases.

Adrenal insufficiency is treated with hormone replacement therapy that includes a combination of glucocorticoids and mineralocorticoids. For acute adrenal insufficiency, the *five S's* of management should be followed: (1) *S*alt replacement, (2) *S*ugar (dextrose) replacement, (3) *S*teroid replacement, (4) *S*upport of physiologic functioning, and (5) *S*earch for and treat the underlying cause (*e.g.*, infection). Extracellular fluid volume should be restored with several liters of 0.9% saline and 5% dextrose. Corticosteroid replacement is accomplished through the intravenous administration of either dexamethasone or hydrocortisone. Dexamethasone is preferred acutely for two reasons: it is long acting (12 to 24 hours) and it does not interfere with measurement of serum or urinary steroids during subsequent corticotropin (ACTH) stimulation tests. Thereafter, hydrocortisone often is given intramuscularly at 6-hour intervals and then tapered over 1 to 3 days to maintenance levels. Oral hydrocortisone replacement therapy can be resumed once the saline infusion

has been discontinued and the person is taking food and fluids by mouth. Mineralocorticoid therapy is not required when large amounts of hydrocortisone are being given, but as the dose is reduced it usually is necessary to add fludrocortisone. Corticosteroid replacement therapy is monitored using heart rate and blood pressure measurements; serum electrolyte values, and titration of plasma renin activity into the upper-normal range.

GLUCOCORTICOID HORMONE EXCESS (CUSHING'S SYNDROME)

The term *Cushing's syndrome* refers to the manifestations of hypercortisolism from any cause. Three important forms of Cushing's syndrome result from excess glucocorticoid production by the body. One is a pituitary form, which results from excessive production of ACTH by a tumor of the pituitary gland. This form of the disease was the one originally described by Cushing; therefore; it is called *Cushing's disease*. The second form is the adrenal form, caused by a benign or malignant adrenal tumor. The third form is ectopic Cushing's, caused by a nonpituitary ACTH-secreting tumor. Certain extrapituitary malignant tumors such as small cell carcinoma of the lung may secrete ACTH or, rarely, CRH, and produce Cushing's syndrome. Cushing's syndrome also can result from long-term therapy with one of the potent pharmacologic preparations of glucocorticoids; this form is called *iatrogenic Cushing's syndrome*.

The major manifestations of Cushing's syndrome represent an exaggeration of the many actions of cortisol (see Table 40-4). Altered fat metabolism causes a peculiar deposition of fat characterized by a protruding abdomen; subclavicular fat pads or "buffalo hump" on the back; and a round, plethoric "moon face" (Fig. 40-10). There is muscle weakness, and the extremities are thin because of protein breakdown and muscle wasting. In advanced cases,

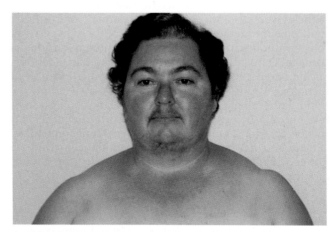

FIGURE 40-10 Cushing's syndrome. A woman who suffered from a pituitary adenoma that produced ACTH exhibits a moon face, buffalo hump, increased facial hair, and thinning of the scalp hair. (Rubin E., Farber J.L. [1999]. *Pathology* [3rd ed., p. 1193]. Philadelphia: Lippincott Williams & Wilkins)

the skin over the forearms and legs becomes thin, having the appearance of parchment. Purple striae, or stretch marks, from stretching of the catabolically weakened skin and subcutaneous tissues are distributed over the breast, thighs, and abdomen. Osteoporosis may develop because of destruction of bone proteins and alterations in calcium metabolism, resulting in back pain, compression fractures of the vertebrae, and rib fractures. As calcium is mobilized from bone, renal calculi may develop.

Derangements in glucose metabolism are found in approximately 75% of patients, with clinically overt diabetes mellitus occurring in approximately 20%. The glucocorticoids possess mineralocorticoid properties; this causes hypokalemia as a result of excessive potassium excretion and hypertension resulting from sodium retention. Inflammatory and immune responses are inhibited, resulting in increased susceptibility to infection. Cortisol increases gastric acid secretion, which may provoke gastric ulceration and bleeding. An accompanying increase in androgen levels causes hirsutism, mild acne, and menstrual irregularities in women. Excess levels of the glucocorticoids may give rise to extreme emotional lability, ranging from mild euphoria and absence of normal fatigue to grossly psychotic behavior.

Diagnosis of Cushing's syndrome depends on the finding of cortisol hypersecretion. The determination of 24-hour excretion of cortisol in urine provides a reliable and practical index of cortisol secretions. One of the prominent features of Cushing's syndrome is loss of the diurnal pattern of cortisol secretion. Cortisol determinations often are made on three blood samples: one taken in the morning, one in late afternoon or early evening, and a third drawn the following morning after a midnight dose of dexamethasone. Measurement of the plasma levels of ACTH, measurement of 24-hour urinary 17-ketosteroids, 17-ketogenic steroids, and 17-hydroxycorticosteroids, and suppression or stimulation tests of the HPA system often are made. MRI or CT scans afford a means for locating adrenal or pituitary tumors.

Untreated, Cushing's syndrome produces serious morbidity and even death. The choice of surgery, irradiation, or pharmacologic treatment is determined largely by the cause of the hypercortisolism. The goal of treatment for Cushing's syndrome is to remove or correct the source of hypercortisolism without causing any permanent pituitary or adrenal damage. Transsphenoidal removal of a pituitary adenoma or a hemihypophysectomy is the preferred method of treatment for Cushing's disease. This allows removal of only the tumor rather than the entire pituitary gland. After successful removal, the person must receive cortisol replacement therapy for 6 to 12 months or until adrenal function returns. Patients also may receive pituitary radiation therapy, but the full effects of treatment may not be realized for 3 to 12 months. Unilateral or bilateral adrenalectomy may be done in the case of adrenal adenoma. When possible, ectopic ACTH-producing tumors are removed. Pharmacologic agents that block steroid synthesis (*i.e.*, etomidate, mitotane, ketoconazole, metyrapone, and aminoglutethimide) may be used to treat persons with ectopic tumors that cannot be resected. Many of these patients also require *Pneumocystis carinii* pneumonia prophylaxis because of the profound immunosuppression caused by the excessive glucocorticoid.

INCIDENTAL ADRENAL MASS

An incidentaloma is a mass lesion found unexpectedly in an adrenal gland by an imaging procedure (done for other reasons), most commonly CAT (but also MRI and ultrasonography). They have been increasingly recognized since the early 1980s. The prevalence of adrenal incidentalomas at autopsy is approximately 10 to 100 per 1000. In CAT series, 0.4% to 0.6% are the usual figures published. Incidentalomas also can occur in other organs (*e.g.*, pituitary, thyroid). The two most important questions are is the mass malignant, and is the mass hormonally active (*i.e.*, is it functioning)?

Primary adrenal carcinoma is quite rare, but other cancers, particularly lung cancers, commonly metastasize to the adrenal gland (other cancers include breast, stomach, pancreas, colon, kidney, melanomas, and lymphomas). The size and imaging characteristics of the mass may help determine whether the tumor is benign or malignant. The risk of cancer is high in adrenal masses larger than 6 cm. Many experts recommend surgical removal of masses larger than 4 cm, particularly in younger patients.

In summary, the adrenal cortex produces three types of hormones: mineralocorticoids, glucocorticoids, and adrenal sex hormones. The mineralocorticoids along with the renin-angiotensin mechanism aid in controlling body levels of sodium and potassium. The glucocorticoids have anti-inflammatory actions and aid in regulating glucose, protein, and fat metabolism during periods of stress. These hormones are under the control of the HPA system. The adrenal sex hormones exert little effect on daily control of body function, but they probably contribute to the development of body hair in women. The adrenogenital syndrome describes a genetic defect in the cortisol pathway resulting from a deficiency of one of the enzymes needed for its synthesis. Depending on the enzyme involved, the disorder causes virilization of female infants and, in some instances, fluid and electrolyte disturbances because of impaired mineralocorticoid synthesis.

Chronic adrenal insufficiency (Addison's disease) can be caused by destruction of the adrenal gland or by dysfunction of the HPA system. Adrenal insufficiency requires replacement therapy with cortical hormones. Acute adrenal insufficiency is a life-threatening situation. Cushing's syndrome refers to the manifestations of excessive cortisol levels. This syndrome may be a result of pharmacologic doses of cortisol, a pituitary or adrenal tumor, or an ectopic tumor that produces ACTH. The clinical manifestations of Cushing's syndrome reflect the very high level of cortisol that is present.

An incidentaloma is a mass lesion found unexpectedly in an adrenal gland by an imaging procedure done for other reasons. They are being recognized with increasing frequency, emphasizing the need for correct diagnosis and treatment.

Bibliography

DeGroot L.J., Jameson J.L. (Eds.). (2001). *Endocrinology*. Philadelphia: W.B. Saunders.

Greenspan F.S., Gardner D.G. (2001). *Basic and clinical endocrinology* (6th ed.). New York: Lange Medical Books/McGraw-Hill.

Griffin J.E., Sergio R.O. (Eds.). (2000). *Textbook of endocrine physiology* (4th ed.). New York: Oxford University Press.

Kacsoh B. (2000) *Endocrine physiology*. New York: McGraw-Hill.

Neal J.M. (2000). *Basic endocrinology*. Malden, MA: Blackwell Science.

Nussen S.S., Whitehead S.A. (2001). *Endocrinology—an integrated approach*. London: Bios.

Growth Disorders

Abs R., Verhelst J., Maitero D., Van Acker K., Nobels F., Coolens J.L., Mahler O., Beckers A. (1998). Cabergoline in the treatment of acromegaly: A study in 64 patients. *Journal of Clinical Endocrinology and Metabolism* 83, 374–378.

Ezzat S. (1997). Acromegaly. *Endocrinology and Metabolism Clinics of North America* 26, 703–723.

Giustina A., Barkan A., Casanaeva F.F., Cavagnini F., Frohman L., Ho K., Veldhius J., Wass J., VonWerdon K., Mehmed C. (2000). Criteria for cure of acromegaly: A consensus statement. *Journal of Clinical Endocrinology and Metabolism* 85, 526–529.

Kaplowitz P.B., Oberfield S.E. (1999). Reexamination of the age limit for defining when puberty is precocious in girls in the United States: Implications for evaluation and treatment. *Pediatrics* 104, 936–941.

Laron Z. (1995). Laron syndrome (primary GH resistance) from patient to laboratory to patient. *Journal of Clinical Endocrinology and Metabolism* 80, 1526–1531.

Lebrethon M.C., Bourguignon J.P. (2001). Central and peripheral isosexual precocious puberty. *Current Opinion in Endocrinology and Diabetes* 8, 17–22.

Orrego J.J., Barkan A.L. (2000). Pituitary disorders: Drug treatment options. *Drugs* 59, 93–106.

Root A. (2001). The tall, rapidly growing infant, child, and adolescent. *Current Opinion in Endocrinology and Diabetes* 8, 6–16.

Sesmilo G., Biller B.M., Levadot J., Hayden D., Hanson G., Rifai N., Klibanski A. (2000). Effects of GH administration on inflammatory and other cardiovascular risk markers in men with GH deficiency. *Annals of Internal Medicine* 133, 111–122.

Shimon I., Melmed S. (1998). Management of pituitary tumors. *Annals of Internal Medicine* 129, 472–483.

Utiger R.D. (2000). Treatment of acromegaly. *New England Journal of Medicine* 342, 1210–1211.

Vance M.L. (1994). Hypopituitarism. *New England Journal of Medicine* 330, 1651–1662.

Vance M.L., Mauras, N. (1999). Growth hormone therapy in adults and children. *New England Journal of Medicine* 341, 1206–1215.

Thyroid Disorders

Arlt W., Callies F., Van Vlymen J.C., Koehler I., Reincke M., Bidlingmaier M., et al. (1999). Dehydroepiandrosterone replacement in women with adrenal insufficiency. *New England Journal of Medicine* 341, 1013–1020.

Dayan C.M. (2001). Interpretation of thyroid function tests. *The Lancet* 357, 619–624.

McKenna T.J. (2001). Grave's disease. *The Lancet* 357, 1793–1796.

Toft A.D. (1994). Thyroxine therapy. *New England Journal of Medicine* 331, 174–180.

Weetman A.P. (2000). Graves' disease. *New England Journal of Medicine* 343, 1236–1248.

Adrenal Disorders

Ackermann J.C., Silverman B.L. (2001). Dehydroepiandrosterone replacement for patients with adrenal insufficiency. *The Lancet* 357, 1381–1382.

Aron D.C. (Ed). (2000). Endocrine incidentalomas. *Endocrinology and Metabolism Clinics of North America* 29, 1–230.

Betterle C., Greggio N.A., Volpato M. (1998). Autoimmune polyglandular syndrome type 1. *Journal of Clinical Endocrinology and Metabolism* 83, 1049–1055.

Boscaro M. (2001). Cushing's syndrome. *Lancet* 357, 783–791.

Mantero F., Terzola M., Arnold G., Osella G., Masina A.M., Ali A., Giovangnett M., Opoder A., Angela A. (2000). A survey on adrenal incidentaloma in Italy: Study Group on Adrenal Tumors of the Italian Society of Endocrinology. *Journal of Clinical Endocrinology and Metabolism* 85, 637–644.

Oelker W. (1996). Adrenal insufficiency. *New England Journal of Medicine* 335, 1206–1212.

Orth D.N. (1995). Cushing's syndrome. *New England Journal of Medicine* 332, 791–803.

Ten S., New M., Maclaren N. (2001). Addison's disease 2001. *Journal of Endocrinology and Metabolism* 86, 2909–2922.

Utiger R.D. (1997). Treatment, and retreatment of Cushing's disease. *New England Journal of Medicine* 336, 215–217.

White P.C., Speiser P.W. (2000). Congenital adrenal hyperplasia due to 21-hydroxylase deficiency. *Endocrine Reviews* 21, 245–291.

Chapter 41

Diabetes Mellitus

Safak Guven, Julie A. Kuenzi, and Glenn Matfin

Diabetes mellitus is a chronic health problem affecting more than 15.7 million people in the United States.[1] The direct and indirect costs of untreated diabetes are $98 billion in health care costs per year, a decline in people's quality of life, and high rates of disabilities. People with diabetes constitute 3.1% of the U.S. population but incur 11.9% of total care expenditures. Direct and indirect costs related to disabilities totaled $77.1 billion in 1997.[1]

The disease affects people in all age groups and from all walks of life. It is more prevalent among African Americans (9.6%) and Hispanic Americans (10.9%) compared with whites (6.2%).[1] The acute complications of diabetes are the most common causes of medical emergencies resulting from metabolic disease. Diabetes is a significant risk factor in coronary heart disease and stroke, and it is the leading cause of blindness and end-stage renal disease, as well as a major contributor to lower extremity amputations.

Hormonal Control of Blood Glucose

After you have completed this section of the chapter, you should be able to meet the following objectives:

✦ Characterize the actions of insulin with reference to glucose, fat, and protein metabolism
✦ Explain what is meant by *counterregulatory hormones* and describe the actions of glucagon, epinephrine, growth hormone, and the adrenal cortical hormones in regulation of blood glucose levels

The body uses glucose, fatty acids, and other substrates as fuel to satisfy its energy needs. Although the respiratory and circulatory systems combine efforts to furnish the body with the oxygen needed for metabolic purposes, it is the liver, in concert with the endocrine pancreas, that controls the body's fuel supply (Fig. 41-1).

The pancreas is made up of two major tissue types: the acini and the islets of Langerhans (Fig. 41-2). The acini secrete digestive juices into the duodenum, and the islets of Langerhans secrete hormones into the blood. Each islet is composed of beta cells that secrete insulin, alpha cells that secrete glucagon, and delta cells that secrete somatostatin. Insulin lowers the blood glucose concentration by facilitating the movement of glucose into body tissues. Glucagon maintains blood glucose by increasing the release of glucose from the liver into the blood. Somatostatin inhibits the release of insulin and glucagon. Somatostatin also decreases

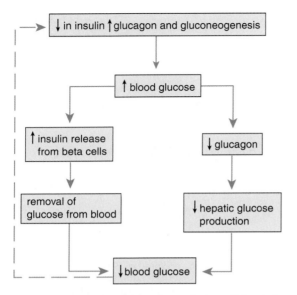

FIGURE 41-1 Hormonal and hepatic regulation of blood glucose.

gastrointestinal activity after ingestion of food. By decreasing gastrointestinal activity, somatostatin is thought to extend the time during which food is absorbed into the blood, and by inhibiting insulin and glucagon, it is thought to extend the use of absorbed nutrients by the tissues.[2]

BLOOD GLUCOSE

Body tissues obtain glucose from the blood. In nondiabetic individuals, fasting blood glucose levels are tightly regulated between 80 and 90 mg/dL. After a meal, blood glucose levels rise, and insulin is secreted in response to this rise in glucose. Approximately two thirds of the glucose that is ingested with a meal is removed from the blood and

stored in the liver as glycogen. Between meals, the liver releases glucose as a means of maintaining blood glucose within its normal range.

Glucose is an optional fuel for tissues such as muscle, adipose tissue, and the liver, which largely use fatty acids and other fuel substrates for energy. Glucose that is not needed for energy is stored as glycogen or converted to fat. When tissues such as those in the liver and skeletal muscle become saturated with glycogen, the additional glucose is converted into fatty acids and then stored as triglycerides in fat cells. When blood glucose levels fall below normal, as they do between meals, glycogen is broken down by a process called *glycogenolysis*, and glucose is released. Glycogen stored in the liver can be released into the bloodstream. Although skeletal muscle has glycogen stores, it lacks the enzyme glucose-6-phosphatase that allows glucose to be broken down sufficiently to pass through the cell membrane and enter the bloodstream, limiting its usefulness to the muscle cell. In addition to mobilizing its glycogen stores, the liver synthesizes glucose from amino acids, glycerol, and lactic acid in a process called *gluconeogenesis*. Glucose metabolism is discussed more fully in Chapter 11.

In contrast to other body tissues such the liver and skeletal muscle, which use fatty acids and other substrates for fuel, the brain and nervous system rely almost exclusively on glucose for their energy needs. Because the brain can neither synthesize nor store more than a few minutes' supply of glucose, normal cerebral function requires a continuous supply from the circulation. Severe and prolonged hypoglycemia can cause brain death, and even moderate hypoglycemia can result in substantial brain dysfunction. The body maintains a system of counterregulatory mechanisms to counteract hypoglycemia-producing situations and ensure brain function and survival. The physiologic mechanisms that prevent or correct hypoglycemia include the actions of the counterregulatory hormones: glucagon, the catecholamines, growth hormone, and the glucocorticoids.

GLUCOSE-REGULATING HORMONES

Insulin

Although several hormones are known to increase blood glucose levels, insulin is the only hormone known to have a direct effect in lowering blood glucose levels. The actions of insulin are threefold: it promotes glucose uptake by target cells and provides for glucose storage as glycogen, it prevents fat and glycogen breakdown, and it inhibits gluconeogenesis and increases protein synthesis (Table 41-1). Fat is the most efficient form of fuel storage. It provides 9 kcal/g of stored energy, compared with the 4 kcal/g provided by carbohydrates and proteins. Insulin acts to promote fat storage by increasing the transport of glucose into fat cells. It also facilitates triglyceride synthesis from glucose in fat cells and inhibits the intracellular breakdown of stored triglycerides. Insulin also inhibits protein breakdown and increases protein synthesis by increasing the active transport of amino acids into body cells. Insulin inhibits gluconeogenesis, or the building of glucose from

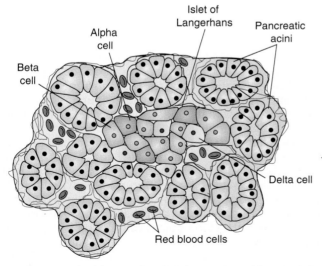

FIGURE 41-2 Islet of Langerhans in the pancreas. (Guyton A.C., Hall J.E. [1996]. *Textbook of medical physiology* [9th ed., p. 972]. Philadelphia: W.B. Saunders)

TABLE 41-1 ✦ Actions of Insulin and Glucagon on Glucose, Fat, and Protein Metabolism

	Insulin	Glucagon
Glucose		
Glucose transport	Increases glucose transport into skeletal muscle and adipose tissue	
Glycogen synthesis	Increases glycogen synthesis	Promotes glycogen breakdown
Gluconeogenesis	Decreases gluconeogenesis	Increases gluconeogenesis
Fats		
Triglyceride synthesis	Increases triglyceride synthesis	
Triglyceride transport into adipose tissue	Increases fatty acid transport into adipose cells	Enhances lipolysis in adipose tissue, liberating fatty acids and glycerol for use in gluconeogenesis
Activation of adipose cell lipase	Inhibits adipose cell lipase	Activates adipose cell lipase
	Activates lipoprotein lipase in capillary walls	
Proteins		
Amino acid transport	Increases active transport of amino acids into cells	Increases transport of amino acids into hepatic cells
Protein synthesis	Increases protein synthesis by increasing transcription of messenger RNA and accelerating protein synthesis by ribosomal RNA	Increases breakdown of proteins into amino acids for use in gluconeogenesis
Protein breakdown	Decreases protein breakdown by enhancing the use of glucose and fatty acids as fuel	Increases conversion of amino acids into glucose precursors

new sources, mainly amino acids. When sufficient glucose and insulin are present, protein breakdown is minimal because the body is able to use glucose and fatty acids as a fuel source. In children and adolescents, insulin is needed for normal growth and development.

Insulin is produced by the pancreatic beta cells in the islets of Langerhans. The active form of the hormone is composed of two polypeptide chains—an A chain and a B chain (Fig. 41-3). Active insulin is formed in the beta cells from a larger molecule called *proinsulin*. In converting proinsulin to insulin, enzymes in the beta cell cleave proinsulin at specific sites to form two separate substances: active insulin and a biologically inactive C-peptide (connecting peptide) chain that joined the A and B chains

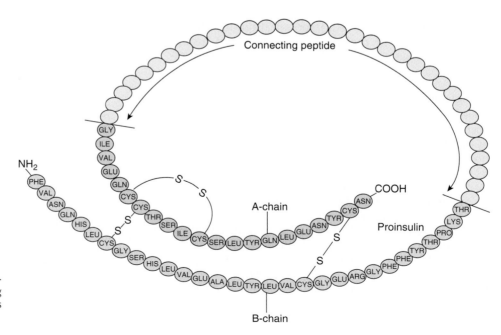

FIGURE 41-3 Structure of proinsulin. With removal of the connecting peptide (C-peptide), proinsulin is converted to insulin.

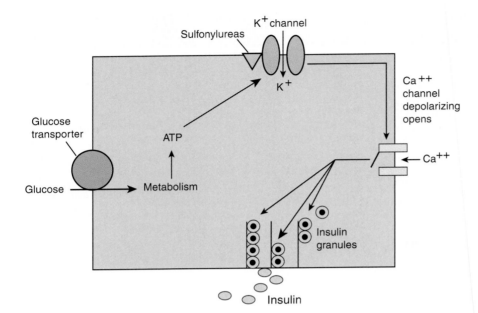

K+ channel

Sulfonylureas

Glucose transporter

ATP

Glucose → Metabolism

K+

Ca++ channel depolarizing opens

Ca++

Insulin granules

Insulin

FIGURE 41-4 One model of control of release of insulin by the pancreatic beta cells and the action of the sulfonylurea agents. In the resting beta cell with low ATP levels, potassium diffuses through the ATP-gated channels maintaining the resting membrane potential. As blood glucose rises and is transported into the beta cell via the glucose transporter, ATP rises causing the potassium channels to close and depolarization to occur. Depolarization results in opening of the voltage-gated calcium channels, which results in insulin secretion. (Modified from Karam J.H. [1992]. Type II diabetes and syndrome X. *Endocrine and Metabolic Clinics of North America* 21, 339)

before they were separated. Active insulin and the inactive C-peptide chain are packaged into secretory granules and released simultaneously from the beta cell. The C-peptide chains can be measured clinically, and this measurement can be used to study beta cell activity. For example, injected (exogenous) insulin in a person with type 2 diabetes would provide few or no C-peptide chains, whereas insulin (endogenous) secreted by the beta cells would be accompanied by the secretion of C-peptide chains.

The release of insulin from the pancreatic beta cells is regulated by blood glucose levels, increasing as blood glucose levels rise and decreasing when blood glucose levels decline. Blood glucose enters the beta cell by means of the glucose transporter, is phosphorylated by an enzyme called *glucokinase* and metabolized to form the adenosine triphosphate (ATP) needed to close the potassium channels and depolarize the cell. Depolarization, in turn, results in opening of the calcium channels and insulin secretion (Fig. 41-4).[3] Secretion of insulin occurs in an oscillatory or pulsatile fashion. After exposure to glucose, which is a nutrient secretagogue, a first-phase release of stored preformed insulin occurs, followed by a second-phase release of newly synthesized insulin (Fig. 41-5). Diabetes may result from dysregulation or deficiency in any of the steps involved in this process (*e.g.*, impaired function of the glucose transporters, intracellular metabolic defects, glucokinase deficiency). Serum insulin levels begin to rise within minutes after a meal, reach a peak in approximately 3 to 5 minutes, and then return to baseline levels within 2 to 3 hours.

Insulin secreted by the beta cells enters the portal circulation and travels directly to the liver, where approximately 50% is used or degraded. Insulin, which is rapidly bound to peripheral tissues or destroyed by the liver or kidneys, has a half-life of approximately 15 minutes once it is released into the general circulation. To initiate its effects

on target tissues, insulin binds to a membrane receptor. The insulin receptor is a combination of four subunits—a larger α subunit that extends outside the cell membrane and is involved in insulin binding, and smaller β subunit that is predominantly inside the cell membrane and contains a kinase enzyme that becomes activated during insulin binding (Fig. 41-6). Activation of the kinase enzyme results in autophosphorylation of the β subunit itself. Phosphorylation of the β subunit in turn activates some enzymes and inactivates others, thereby directing the desired intracellular effect of insulin on glucose, fat, and protein metabolism.

Because cell membranes are impermeable to glucose, they require a special carrier, called a *glucose transporter*, to move glucose from the blood into the cell. These trans-

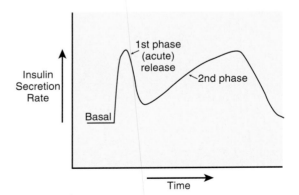

Insulin Secretion Rate

1st phase (acute) release

2nd phase

Basal

Time

FIGURE 41-5 Biphasic insulin response to a constant glucose stimulus. The peak of the first phase in humans is 3 to 5 minutes; the second phase begins at 2 minutes and continues to increase slowly for at least 60 minutes or until the stimulus stops. (From Ward W.K., Beard J.C., Halter J.B., Pfeifer M.A., Porte D. Jr. [1984]. Pathology of insulin secretion in non-insulin-dependent diabetes mellitus. *Diabetes Care* 7, 491–502. Used with permission.)

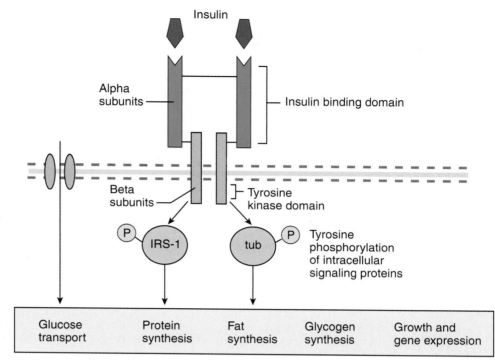

FIGURE 41-6 Insulin receptor. Insulin binds to the alpha subunits of the insulin receptor, which increases glucose transport and causes autophosphorylation of the beta subunit of the receptor, which induces tyrosine kinase activity. Tyrosine phosphorylation, in turn, activates a cascade of intracellular signaling proteins that mediate the effects of glucose on glucose, fat, and protein metabolism.

porters move glucose across the cell membrane at a faster rate than would occur by diffusion alone. Considerable research has revealed a family of glucose transporters termed *GLUT-1*, *GLUT-2*, and so forth.[4] GLUT-4 is the insulin-dependent glucose transporter for skeletal muscle and adipose tissue. It is sequestered inside the membrane of these cells and thus is unable to function as a glucose transporter until a signal from insulin causes it to move from its inactive site into the cell membrane, where it facilitates glucose entry. GLUT-2 is the major transporter of glucose into beta cells and liver cells. It has a low affinity for glucose and acts as a transporter only when plasma glucose levels are relatively high, such as after a meal. GLUT-1 is present in all tissues. It does not require the actions of insulin and is important in transport of glucose into the nervous system.

Glucagon

Glucagon, a polypeptide molecule produced by the alpha cells of the islets of Langerhans, maintains blood glucose between meals and during periods of fasting. Like insulin, glucagon travels through the portal vein to the liver, where it exerts its main action. Unlike insulin, glucagon produces an increase in blood glucose. The most dramatic effect of glucagon is its ability to initiate *glycogenolysis* or the breakdown of liver glycogen as a means of raising blood glucose, usually within a matter of minutes. Glucagon also increases the transport of amino acids into the liver and stimulates their conversion into glucose, a process called *gluconeogenesis*. Because liver glycogen stores are limited, gluconeogenesis is important in maintaining blood glucose levels over time. Other actions of glucagon occur only when the hormone is present in high concentrations, usually well

above those normally present in the blood. At high concentrations, glucagon activates adipose cell lipase, making fatty acids available for use as energy.[2] At very high concentrations, glucagon can increase the strength of the heart, increase blood flow to some tissues, including the kidneys, enhance bile section, and inhibit gastric acid secretion (see Table 41-1).

As with insulin, glucagon secretion is regulated by blood glucose. A decrease in blood glucose concentration to a hypoglycemic level produces an immediate increase in glucagon secretion, and an increase in blood glucose to hyperglycemic levels produces a decrease in glucagon secretion. High concentrations of amino acids, as occur after a protein meal, also can stimulate glucagon secretion. In this way, glucagon increases the conversion of amino acids to glucose as a means of maintaining the body's glucose levels. Glucagon levels also increase during strenuous exercise as a means of preventing a decrease in blood glucose.

Catecholamines

The catecholamines, *epinephrine* and *norepinephrine*, help to maintain blood glucose levels during periods of stress. Epinephrine inhibits insulin release and promotes glycogenolysis by stimulating the conversion of muscle and liver glycogen to glucose. Muscle glycogen cannot be released into the blood; nevertheless, the mobilization of these stores for muscle use conserves blood glucose for use by other tissues such as the brain and the nervous system. During periods of exercise and other types of stress, epinephrine inhibits insulin release from the beta cells and thereby decreases the movement of glucose into muscle cells. The catecholamines also increase lipase activity and thereby increase mobilization of fatty acids; this process conserves glucose. The blood glucose–elevating effect of epinephrine is an important homeostatic mechanism during periods of hypoglycemia.

Growth Hormone

Growth hormone has many metabolic effects. It increases protein synthesis in all cells of the body, mobilizes fatty acids from adipose tissue, and antagonizes the effects of insulin. Growth hormone decreases cellular uptake and use of glucose, thereby increasing the level of blood glucose. The increased blood glucose level stimulates further insulin secretion by the beta cells. The secretion of growth hormone normally is inhibited by insulin and increased levels of blood glucose. During periods of fasting, when both blood glucose levels and insulin secretion fall, growth hormone levels increase. Exercise, such as running and cycling, and various stresses, including anesthesia, fever, and trauma, increase growth hormone levels.

Chronic hypersecretion of growth hormone, as occurs in acromegaly (see Chapter 40), can lead to glucose intolerance and the development of diabetes mellitus. In people who already have diabetes, moderate elevations in growth hormone levels that occur during periods of stress and periods of growth in children can produce the entire spectrum of metabolic abnormalities associated with poor regulation, despite optimized insulin treatment.

Glucocorticoid Hormones

The glucocorticoid hormones, which are synthesized in the adrenal cortex along with other corticosteroid hormones, are critical to survival during periods of fasting and starvation. They stimulate gluconeogenesis by the liver, sometimes producing a 6- to 10-fold increase in hepatic glucose production. These hormones also moderately decrease tissue use of glucose. In predisposed persons, the prolonged elevation of glucocorticoid hormones can lead to hyperglycemia and the development of diabetes mellitus. In people with diabetes, even transient increases in cortisol can complicate control.

There are several steroid hormones with glucocorticoid activity; the most important of these is cortisol, which accounts for approximately 95% of all glucocorticoid activity (see Chapter 40). Cortisol levels increase during periods of stress, such as that produced by infection, pain, trauma, surgery, prolonged and strenuous exercise, and acute anxiety. Hypoglycemia is a potent stimulus for cortisol secretion.

> In summary, energy metabolism is controlled by a number of hormones, including insulin, glucagon, epinephrine, growth hormone, and the glucocorticoids. Of these hormones, only insulin has the effect of lowering the blood glucose level. Insulin's blood glucose–lowering action results from its ability to increase the transport of glucose into body cells and to decrease hepatic production and release of glucose into the bloodstream. Other hormones—glucagon, epinephrine, growth hormone, and the glucocorticoids—maintain or increase blood glucose concentrations and are referred to as *counterregulatory hormones*. Glucagon and epinephrine promote glycogenolysis. Glucagon and the glucocorticoids increase gluconeogenesis. Growth hormone decreases the peripheral use of glucose. Insulin has the effect of decreasing lipolysis and the use of fats as a fuel source; glucagon and epinephrine increase fat use.

Diabetes Mellitus

After you have completed this section of the chapter, you should be able to meet the following objectives:

✦ Compare the distinguishing features of type 1 and type 2 diabetes mellitus, list causes of other specific types of diabetes, and cite the criteria for gestational diabetes

✦ Relate the physiologic functions of insulin to the manifestations of diabetes mellitus

✦ Discuss the role of diet and exercise in the management of diabetes mellitus.

✦ Characterize the actions of oral hypoglycemic agents in terms of the lowering of blood glucose

✦ Describe the clinical manifestations of diabetic ketoacidosis and their physiologic significance

✦ Describe the clinical condition resulting from the nonketotic hyperosmolar state

✦ Name and describe the types (according to duration of action) of insulin

✦ Relate the actions of the oral hypoglycemic agents to alterations in glucose metabolism that occur in persons with type 2 diabetes

✦ Describe the clinical manifestations of insulin-induced hypoglycemia and state how these may differ in elderly people

✦ Describe alterations in physiologic function that accompany diabetic peripheral neuropathy, retinopathy, and nephropathy

✦ Describe the causes of foot ulcers in people with diabetes mellitus

✦ Explain the relation between diabetes mellitus and infection

The term *diabetes* is derived from a Greek word meaning "going through" and *mellitus* from the Latin word for "honey" or "sweet." Reports of the disorder can be traced back to the first century AD, when Aretaeus the Cappadocian described the disorder as a chronic affection characterized by intense thirst and voluminous, honey-sweet urine: "the melting down of flesh into urine." It was the discovery of insulin by Banting and Best in 1922 that transformed the once-fatal disease into a manageable chronic health problem.[5]

Diabetes is a disorder of carbohydrate, protein, and fat metabolism resulting from an imbalance between insulin availability and insulin need. It can represent an absolute insulin deficiency, impaired release of insulin by the pancreatic beta cells, inadequate or defective insulin receptors, or the production of inactive insulin or insulin that is destroyed before it can carry out its action. A person with uncontrolled diabetes is unable to transport glucose into fat and muscle cells; as a result, the body cells are starved, and the breakdown of fat and protein is increased.

CLASSIFICATION AND ETIOLOGY

Although diabetes mellitus clearly is a disorder of insulin availability, it probably is not a single disease. A revised system for the classification of diabetes was developed in 1997 by the Expert Committee on the Diagnosis and Classification of Diabetes Mellitus.[6] The intent of the revised system, which replaces the 1979 classification system, was to move away from a system that focused on the type of pharmacologic treatment used in management of diabetes to one based on disease etiology. The revised system continues to include type 1 and type 2 diabetes, but uses Arabic rather than Roman numerals and eliminates the use of "insulin-dependent" and "non–insulin-dependent" diabetes mellitus (Table 41-2). Type 2 diabetes currently accounts for about 90% of the cases of diabetes. Included in the classification system are the categories of gestational diabetes mellitus (GDM; *i.e.*, diabetes that develops during pregnancy) and other specific types of diabetes, many of which occur secondary to other conditions (*e.g.*, Cushing's syndrome, hematochromatosis, pancreatitis, acromegaly).

The revised classification system also includes a system for diagnosing diabetes according to stages of glucose intolerance[6] (Table 41-3). The revised criteria have retained the former category of *impaired glucose tolerance* (IGT) and have added a new category of *impaired fasting blood glucose* (IFG). The categories of IFG and IGT refer to metabolic stages intermediate between normal glucose homeostasis and diabetes. A fasting blood glucose of 110 mg/dL or less or a 2-hour oral glucose tolerance test result of less than 140 mg/dL is considered normal. IFG is defined as a fasting blood glucose of 110 mg/dL or greater but less than 126 mg/dL. IGT reflects abnormal blood glucose measurements (≥140 mg/dL but <200 mg/dL) 2 hours after an oral glucose load.[6] Approximately 5% of people with IFG and IGT

progress to diabetes each year. IFG and IGT are associated with increased risk of atherosclerotic heart disease. Calorie restriction and weight reduction are important in overweight people in this class.[7]

Type 1 Diabetes Mellitus

Type 1 diabetes mellitus is characterized by destruction of the pancreatic beta cells.[8] Type 1 diabetes is subdivided into two types: type 1A, immune-mediated diabetes, and type 1B, idiopathic diabetes. In the United States and Europe, approximately 10% of people with diabetes mellitus have type 1 diabetes, with 95% of them having type 1A, immune-mediated diabetes.

Type 1A diabetes is characterized by autoimmune destruction of beta cells. This type of diabetes, formerly called *juvenile diabetes*, occurs more commonly in young persons but can occur at any age. Type 1 diabetes is a catabolic disorder characterized by an absolute lack of insulin, an elevation in blood glucose, and a breakdown of body fats and proteins. The absolute lack of insulin in people with type 1 diabetes mellitus means that they are particularly prone to the development of ketoacidosis. One of the actions of insulin is the inhibition of *lipolysis* (*i.e.*, fat breakdown) and release of free fatty acids (FFA) from fat cells. In the absence of insulin, ketosis develops when these fatty acids are released from fat cells and converted to ketones in the liver.

Because of the loss of the first-phase insulin (preformed insulin) response, all people with type 1A diabetes require exogenous insulin replacement to reverse the catabolic state, control blood glucose levels, and prevent ketosis. The rate of beta cell destruction is quite variable, being rapid in some individuals and slow in others. The rapidly progressive form commonly is observed in children, but also may occur in adults. The slowly progressive form usually occurs in adults and is sometimes referred to as *latent autoimmune diabetes in adults*.

It has been suggested that type 1A, immune-mediated diabetes results from a genetic predisposition (*i.e.*, diabetogenic genes), a hypothetical triggering event that involves an environmental agent that incites an immune response, and immunologically mediated beta cell destruction. Much evidence has focused on the inherited major histocompatibility complex (MHC) genes that encode three human leukocyte antigens (HLA-DP, HLA-DQ, and HLA-DR) found on the surface of body cells (see Chapter 18). Susceptibility to type 1 diabetes also has been associated with HLA-DR3 and HLA-DR4.[3] It appears that what is inherited as part of the HLA genotype in people with type 1 diabetes is a susceptibility to an abnormal immune response that affects the beta cells. On the other hand, resistance to the development of type 1 diabetes has been traced to other HLA subtypes: DR11, DR15, and DQB1. In addition to the major susceptibility gene for type 1 diabetes in the MHC region on chromosome 6, an insulin gene regulating beta cell replication and function has been identified on chromosome 11. Type 1 diabetes–associated autoantibodies may exist for years before the onset of hyperglycemia. There are two major types of autoantibodies: insulin autoantibodies (IAAs), and islet

---

 Diabetes Mellitus

➤ Diabetes mellitus is a disorder of carbohydrate, fat, and protein metabolism brought about by impaired beta cell synthesis or release of insulin, or the inability of tissues to use glucose.

➤ Type 1 diabetes results from loss of beta cell function and an absolute insulin deficiency.

➤ Type 2 diabetes results from impaired ability of the tissues to use insulin accompanied by a relative lack of insulin or impaired release of insulin in relation to blood glucose levels.

TABLE 41-2 ✦ Etiologic Classification of Diabetes Mellitus

Type	Subtypes	Etiology of Glucose Intolerance
I. Type 1*	*(Beta cell destruction usually leading to absolute insulin deficiency)*	
	A. Immune-mediated	Autoimmune destruction of beta cells
	B. Idiopathic	Unknown
II. Type 2*	*(May range from predominantly insulin resistance with relative insulin deficiency to a predominantly secretory defect with insulin resistance)*	
III. Other specific types	A. Genetic defects of beta cell function†	
	1. Chromosome 12, HNF-1α (formerly MODY 3)	Regulates HNF-4α expression; reduces insulin response of beta cell to glucose
	2. Chromosome 7, glucokinase (formerly MODY 2).	Defect in signaling insulin secretion due to defect in glucokinase generation
	3. Chromosome 20, HNF-4α (formerly MODY 1)	Transcription factor; reduces insulin response of beta cell to glucose
	B. Genetic defects in insulin action†	Mutation in insulin receptor
	1. Type A insulin resistance	Pediatric syndromes that have mutations in insulin receptor
	2. Leprechaunism	
	3. Rabson-Mendenhall syndrome	Postreceptor defect in signal transduction
	4. Lipoatrophic diabetes	
	C. Diseases of the exocrine pancreas†	
	1. Pancreatitis	Conditions of the exocrine pancreas that result in loss or destruction of insulin-producing beta cells
	2. Trauma/pancreatectomy	
	3. Neoplasms	
	4. Cystic fibrosis	
	D. Endocrinopathies†	
	1. Acromegaly	Diabetogenic effects of excess hormone levels
	2. Cushing's syndrome	
	3. Glucogonoma	
	4. Hyperthyroidism	
	5. Somatostatinoma	
	E. Drug- or chemical-induced†	
	1. Vacor	Toxic destruction of beta cells
	2. Pentamide (intravenous)	Toxic destruction of beta cells
	3. Nicotinic acid	Impaired insulin action
	4. Glucocorticosteroids	Increased glucose synthesis; insulin resistance
	5. Thyroid hormone	Impaired insulin action
	6. Diazoxide	Impaired insulin secretion
	7. β-Adrenergic agonists	Increased hepatic glucose output
	β-Adrenergic blockers	Impaired insulin secretion and sensitivity
	8. Thiazide diuretics	Impaired insulin secretion due to potassium loss
	9. Phenytoin (Dilantin)	Direct inhibition of insulin secretion
	10. α-Interferon	Production of islet cell antibodies
	F. Infections†	
	1. Congenital rubella	Beta cell injury followed by an autoimmune reaction
	2. Cytomegalovirus	
	G. Uncommon forms of immune-mediated diabetes†	
	1. "Stiff-man" syndrome	Autoimmune disorder of central nervous system with immune-mediated beta cell destruction
	2. Anti-insulin receptor antibodies	Destruction of insulin receptors
	H. Other genetic syndromes sometimes associated with diabetes†	
	1. Down syndrome	Disorders of glucose tolerance related to defects associated with chromosomal abnormalities
	2. Klinefelter's syndrome	
	3. Turner's syndrome	
IV. Gestational diabetes mellitus (GDM)	*(Any degree of glucose intolerance with onset or first recognition during pregnancy)*	Combination of insulin resistance and impaired insulin secretion

HNF, hepatocyte nuclear factor; MODY, maturity-onset diabetes of the young.
*Patients with any form of diabetes may require insulin treatment at some stage of their disease. Such use of insulin does not, of itself, classify the patient.
†Not inclusive.
(Adapted from The Expert Committee on the Diagnosis and Classification of Diabetes Mellitus. [1997]. Report of the Expert Committee on the Diagnosis and Classification of Diabetes Mellitus. *Diabetes Care 70*, 1183–1197)

TABLE 41-3 ◆ National Diabetes Data Group for Interpretation of Fasting Plasma Glucose and Oral Glucose Tolerance With Use of Venous Plasma or Serum Using a 75-g Carbohydrate Load

Test	Normoglycemic	IFG	IGT	Diabetes Mellitus
Fasting plasma glucose (mg/dL)	<110	≥110–<126		≥126
Two-hour postload glucose (mg/dL)*	<140		≥140–<200	≥200
Other				Symptoms of diabetes mellitus and random plasma glucose ≥200

IFG, impaired fasting blood glucose; IGT, impaired glucose tolerance.
A diagnosis of diabetes mellitus must be confirmed on a subsequent day by any one of three methods included in the chart. In clinical settings, the fasting plasma glucose test is greatly preferred because of ease of administration, convenience, acceptability to patients, and lower cost. Fasting is defined as no caloric intake for at least 8 hours.
*This test requires the use of a glucose load containing the equivalent of 75 g of anhydrous glucose dissolved in water.

cell autoantibodies and antibodies directed at other islet autoantigens, including glutamic acid decarboxylase (GAD) and the protein tyrosine phosphatase IA-2.[9] Testing for antibodies to GAD or IA-2 and for IAAs using sensitive radiobinding assays can identify more than 85% of cases of new or future type 1 diabetes with 98% specificity.[10] The appearance of IAAs may precede that of antibodies to GAD or IA-2, and IAAs may be the only antibodies detected at diagnosis in young children. Therefore, it is recommended that determination of IAAs be included in primary testing of children younger than 10 years of age to maximize sensitivity. Strategies for full evaluation of the risk of developing future type 1 diabetes should include determination of at least three of the four best-established markers, IAAs, islet cell autoantibodies, and antibodies to GAD and IA-2, as well as a test of the first-phase insulin response. These people also may have other autoimmune disorders such as Graves' disease, rheumatoid arthritis, and Addison's disease.

The fact that type 1 diabetes is thought to result from an interaction between genetic and environmental factors has led to research into methods directed at prevention and early control of the disease. These methods include the identification of genetically susceptible persons and early intervention in newly diagnosed persons with type 1 diabetes. After the diagnosis of type 1 diabetes, there often is a short period of beta cell regeneration, during which symptoms of diabetes disappear and insulin injections are not needed. This is sometimes called the *honeymoon period*. Immune interventions designed to interrupt the destruction of beta cells before development of type 1 diabetes are being investigated in the Diabetes Prevention Trial, which is trying to find a way to prevent complete and irreversible beta cell failure.

The term *idiopathic type 1B diabetes* is used to describe those cases of beta cell destruction in which no evidence of autoimmunity is present. Only a small number of people with type 1 diabetes fall into this category; most are of African or Asian descent. Type 1B diabetes is strongly inherited. People with the disorder have episodic ketoacidosis due to varying degrees of insulin deficiency with periods of absolute insulin deficiency that may come and go.

Type 2 Diabetes Mellitus

Type 2 diabetes mellitus describes a condition of fasting hyperglycemia that occurs despite the availability of insulin. In contrast to type 1 diabetes, type 2 diabetes is not associated with HLA markers or autoantibodies. Most people with type 2 diabetes are older and overweight. The metabolic abnormalities that contribute to hyperglycemia in people with type 2 diabetes include impaired insulin secretion, peripheral insulin resistance, and increased hepatic glucose production. Insulin resistance initially stimulates insulin secretion from the beta cells in the pancreas to overcome the increased demand to maintain a normoglycemic state. In time, the insulin response by the beta cells declines because of exhaustion. This results in elevated postprandial blood glucose levels. During the evolutionary phase, an individual with type 2 diabetes may become insulinopenic because of beta cell failure. Because people with type 2 diabetes do not have an absolute insulin deficiency, they are less prone to develop ketoacidosis as compared to people with type 1 diabetes.

There also is evidence to suggest that insulin resistance not only contributes to the hyperglycemia in persons with type 2 diabetes, but may play a role in other metabolic abnormalities. These include high levels of plasma triglycerides, low levels of high-density lipoproteins, hypertension, abnormal fibrinolysis, and coronary heart disease. This constellation of abnormalities often is referred to as the *insulin resistance syndrome*, *syndrome X*, or *the metabolic syndrome*.[11] Insulin resistance and increased risk of developing type 2 diabetes are also increased in women with polycystic ovary disease (see Chapter 45).[12]

Approximately 80% of persons with type 2 diabetes are overweight. The presence of obesity and the type of obesity are important considerations in the development of type 2 diabetes. It has been found that people with upper body obesity are at greater risk for developing type 2 diabetes than persons with lower body obesity (see Chapter 11). Obese people have increased resistance to the action of insulin and impaired suppression of glucose production by the liver, resulting in both hyperglycemia and hyperinsulinemia. The increased insulin resistance has been attributed to increased visceral (intra-abdominal) fat detected on computed tomography scan.[13] In addition to increased insulin resistance, insulin release from beta cells in response to glucose is impaired. Over time, insulin resistance may improve with weight loss, to the extent that many people with type 2 diabetes can be managed with a weight-reduction program and exercise.

It has been theorized that the insulin resistance and increased glucose production in obese people with type 2 diabetes may stem from an increased concentration of FFA. Accordingly, the slight increase in insulin secretion that occurs in these people leads to adipose cell lipase activation and subsequent FFA release into the circulation. This has several consequences. First, FFAs act at the level of the beta cell to stimulate more insulin secretion. Second, they act at the level of the peripheral tissues to inhibit glucose uptake and glycogen storage through a reduction in muscle glycogen synthetase activity. Third, an FFA-mediated increase in insulin delivery to the liver through the portal vein counteracts the FFA-mediated stimulation of hepatic glucose production.[14] Thus, an increase in FFA that occurs in obese individuals with a genetic predisposition to type 2 diabetes eventually may lead to beta cell exhaustion and an inability to secrete insulin. The resultant decrease in insulin secretion in turn causes hepatic overproduction of glucose and peripheral underutilization of glucose (Fig. 41-7).

Another proposed link to the insulin resistance associated with obesity is an adipose cell messenger (adiocytokine) called *adiponectin*. Adiponectin is secreted by adipose tissue and circulates in the blood. It has been shown that decreased levels of adiponectin coincides with insulin resistance in mouse models of obesity and type 2 diabetes. Moreover, there is evidence that the expression of adiponectin mRNA might be partially regulated by a nuclear receptor (PPAR-γ, to be discussed) that leads to the regulation of genes controlling FFA levels and glucose metabolism. In skeletal muscle, adiponectin has been shown to decrease tissue triglyceride content by increasing the utilization of fatty acids as a fuel source. Since its level is low in obese individuals, the replenishment of adiponectin may be considered as an alternative treatment for the treatment of insulin resistance in the future.[15,16]

The fact that lifestyle plays an important role in the pathogenesis of type 2 diabetes has led to an increased emphasis on prevention. The findings of the Diabetes Prevention Program (DPP), a recently completed research project involving 27 centers in the United States, found that diet and exercise dramatically delay the onset of type 2 diabetes.[17] Participants randomly assigned to an intensive lifestyle modification program (low-fat diet and exercising 150 minutes a week) reduced their risk of getting type 2 diabetes by 58%. The study also found that participants assigned to treatment with the oral diabetic drug, metformin, reduced their risk of getting diabetes by 31%.

Other Specific Types

The category of other specific types of diabetes, formerly known as *secondary diabetes*, describes diabetes that is associated with certain other conditions and syndromes.

Such diabetes can occur with pancreatic disease or the removal of pancreatic tissue and with endocrine diseases, such as acromegaly, Cushing's syndrome, or pheochromocytoma. Endocrine disorders that produce hyperglycemia do so by increasing the hepatic production of glucose or decreasing the cellular use of glucose. Several specific types of diabetes are associated with monogenetic defects in beta cell function. These specific types of diabetes, which resemble type 2 diabetes but occur at an earlier age (usually before 25 years of age), were formerly referred to as *maturity-onset diabetes of the young* (MODY).[18]

Environmental agents that have been associated with altered pancreatic beta cell function include viruses (*e.g.*, mumps, congenital rubella, coxsackievirus) and chemical toxins. Among the suspected chemical toxins are the nitrosamines, which sometimes are found in smoked and cured meats. The nitrosamines are related to streptozocin, which is used to induce diabetes in experimental animals, and to the rat poison Vacor, which can produce diabetes when ingested by humans.

Several diuretics—thiazides and loop diuretics—elevate blood glucose. These diuretics increase potassium loss, which is thought to impair insulin release. Other drugs known to cause hyperglycemia are diazoxide, glucocorticoids, levodopa, oral contraceptives, sympathomimetics, phenothiazines, phenytoin, and total parenteral nutrition (*i.e.*, hyperalimentation). Drug-related increases in blood glucose usually are reversed after the drug has been discontinued.

Gestational Diabetes

Gestational diabetes mellitus refers to glucose intolerance that is detected first during pregnancy. It occurs to various degrees in 2% to 5% of pregnancies. It most frequently affects women with a family history of diabetes; with glycosuria; with a history of stillbirth or spontaneous abortion, fetal anomalies in a previous pregnancy, or a previous large- or heavy-for-date baby; and who are obese, of advanced maternal age, or have had five or more pregnancies. However, because these risk factors fail to identify approximately 50% of people with GDM, all pregnant women are candidates for screening for glucose tolerance. The American Diabetes Association (ADA) Clinical Practice Recommendations suggest that pregnant women who have not been identified as having glucose intolerance before the 24th week have a screening glucose tolerance test between the 24th and 28th week of pregnancy.[19] On the other hand, women who are younger than 25 years of age, were of normal body weight before pregnancy, have no family history of diabetes or poor obstetric outcome, and are not members of a high-risk ethnic/racial group (*e.g.*, Hispanic, Native American, Asian, African American) may not need to be screened. This screening test consists of 50 g of glucose given without regard to the last meal and followed in 1 hour by a venous blood sample for glucose concentration. If the blood glucose level is greater than 140 mg/dL, then a 100-g 3-hour glucose tolerance test is indicated to establish the diagnosis of GDM. This test should be performed after an overnight fast.

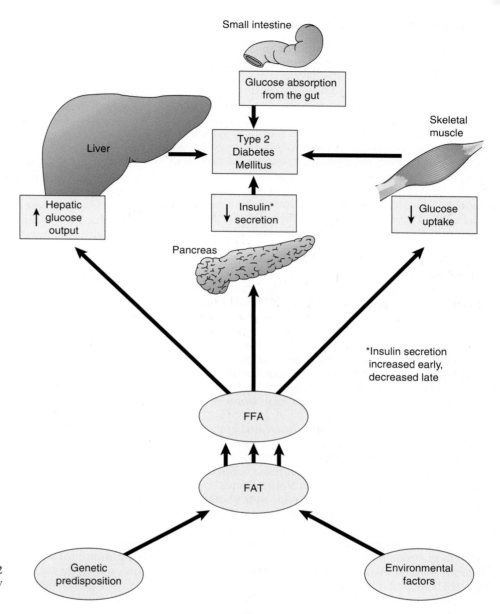

FIGURE 41-7 Pathogenesis of type 2 diabetes mellitus. FFA, free fatty acids.

Diagnosis and careful medical management are essential because women with GDM are at higher risk for complications of pregnancy, mortality, and fetal abnormalities.[20] Fetal abnormalities include macrosomia (*i.e.*, large body size), hypoglycemia, hypocalcemia, polycythemia, and hyperbilirubinemia.

Treatment of GDM includes close observation of mother and fetus because even mild hyperglycemia has been shown to be detrimental to the fetus. Maternal fasting and postprandial blood glucose levels should be measured regularly. Fetal surveillance depends on the degree of risk for the fetus. The frequency of growth measurements and determinations of fetal distress depends on available technology and gestational age. All women with GDM require nutritional guidance because nutrition is the cornerstone of therapy. The nutrition plan should

provide the necessary nutrients for maternal and fetal health, result in normoglycemia and proper weight gain, and prevent ketosis.[20] If dietary management alone does not achieve a fasting blood glucose level no greater than 105 mg/dL or a 2-hour postprandial blood glucose no greater than 120 mg/dL, the Third International Workshop on GDM recommends therapy with human insulin. Oral antidiabetic agents may be teratogenic and are not recommended in pregnancy. Self-monitoring of blood glucose levels is essential.

Women with GDM are at increased risk of developing diabetes 5 to 10 years after delivery. Women in whom GDM is diagnosed should be followed after delivery to detect diabetes early in its course. These women should be evaluated during their first postpartum visit with a 2-hour oral glucose tolerance test with a 75-g glucose load.

MANIFESTATIONS OF DIABETES

Diabetes mellitus may have a rapid or an insidious onset. In type 1 diabetes, signs and symptoms often arise suddenly. Type 2 diabetes usually develops more insidiously; its presence may be detected during a routine medical examination or when a patient seeks medical care for other reasons.

The most commonly identified signs and symptoms of diabetes are referred to as the *three polys*—polyuria (*i.e.,* excessive urination), polydipsia (*i.e.,* excessive thirst), and polyphagia (*i.e.,* excessive hunger). These three symptoms are closely related to the hyperglycemia and glycosuria of diabetes. Glucose is a small, osmotically active molecule. When blood glucose levels are sufficiently elevated, the amount of glucose filtered by the glomeruli of the kidney exceeds the amount that can be reabsorbed by the renal tubules; this results in glycosuria accompanied by large losses of water in the urine. Thirst results from the intracellular dehydration that occurs as blood glucose levels rise and water is pulled out of body cells, including those in the thirst center. Cellular dehydration also causes dryness of the mouth. This early symptom may be easily overlooked in people with type 2 diabetes, particularly in those who have had a gradual increase in blood glucose levels. Polyphagia usually is not present in people with type 2 diabetes. In type 1 diabetes, it probably results from cellular starvation and the depletion of cellular stores of carbohydrates, fats, and proteins.

Weight loss despite normal or increased appetite is a common occurrence in people with uncontrolled type 1 diabetes. The cause of weight loss is twofold. First, loss of body fluids results from osmotic diuresis. Vomiting may exaggerate the fluid loss in ketoacidosis. Second, body tissue is lost because the lack of insulin forces the body to use its fat stores and cellular proteins as sources of energy. In terms of weight loss, there often is a marked difference between type 2 diabetes and type 1 diabetes. Weight loss is a frequent phenomenon in people with uncontrolled type 1 diabetes, whereas many people with uncomplicated type 2 diabetes have problems with obesity.

Other signs and symptoms of hyperglycemia include recurrent blurred vision, fatigue, paresthesias, and skin infections. In type 2 diabetes, these often are the symptoms that prompt a person to seek medical treatment. Blurred vision develops as the lens and retina are exposed to hyperosmolar fluids. Lowered plasma volume produces weakness and fatigue. Paresthesias reflect a temporary dysfunction of the peripheral sensory nerves. Chronic skin infections are common in people with type 2 diabetes. Hyperglycemia and glycosuria favor the growth of yeast organisms. Pruritus and vulvovaginitis resulting from candidal infections are common initial complaints in women with diabetes.

DIAGNOSIS AND MANAGEMENT

The diagnosis of diabetes mellitus in nonpregnant adults is based on fasting blood glucose levels, random blood glucose tests, or the results of a glucose challenge test (see Table 41-3). Testing for diabetes should be considered in all individuals 45 years of age and older. Testing should be considered at a younger age in people who are obese, have a first-degree relative with diabetes, are members of a high-risk group, women who have delivered an infant weighing more than 9 pounds or been diagnosed with GDM, have hypertension or hyperlipidemia, or have met the criteria for IGT or IFG on previous testing.[21]

Blood Tests

Blood glucose measurements are used in both the diagnosis and management of diabetes. Diagnostic tests include the fasting blood glucose, random blood glucose, and the glucose tolerance test. Laboratory and capillary or "finger stick" glucose tests are used for glucose management in people with diagnosed diabetes. Glycosylated hemoglobin (HbA$_{1c}$) provides a measure of glucose control over time. Table 41-4 lists whole-blood and plasma glucose, as well as HbA$_{1c}$ values for glycemic control for people with diabetes.[22]

Fasting Blood Glucose Test. The fasting blood glucose has been suggested as the preferred diagnostic test because of ease of administration, convenience, patient acceptability, and cost.[6] Glucose levels are measured after food has been withheld for 8 to 12 hours. If the fasting plasma glucose level is higher than 126 mg/dL on two occasions, diabetes is diagnosed. A fasting plasma glucose level below 110 mg/dL is normal. A level between 110 mg/dL and 126 mg/dL is significant and is defined as impaired fasting glucose (IFG) (see Table 41-3).

Random Blood Glucose Test. A random blood glucose is one that is done without regard to meals or time of day. A random blood glucose concentration that is unequivocally elevated (>200 mg/dL) in the presence of classic symptoms of diabetes such as polydipsia, polyphagia, polyuria, and blurred vision is diagnostic of diabetes mellitus at any age.

Glucose Tolerance Test. The oral glucose tolerance test is an important screening test for diabetes. The test measures the body's ability to store glucose by removing it from the blood. In men and women, the test measures the plasma glucose response to 75 g of concentrated glucose solution at selected intervals, usually 1 hour and 2 hours. In pregnant women, a glucose load of 100 g is given (see the Gestational Diabetes section) with an additional 3-hour plasma glucose determination. In people with normal glucose tolerance, blood glucose levels return to normal within 2 to 3 hours after ingestion of a glucose load, in which case it can be assumed that sufficient insulin is present to allow glucose to leave the blood and enter body cells. Because a person with diabetes lacks the ability to respond to an increase in blood glucose by releasing adequate insulin to facilitate storage, blood glucose levels rise above those observed in normal people and remain elevated for longer periods (see Table 41-3).

Capillary Blood Tests and Self-Monitoring of Capillary Blood Glucose Levels. Technologic advances have provided the means for monitoring blood glucose levels by using a drop of capillary blood. This procedure has provided health professionals with a rapid and economical

TABLE 41-4 ✦ Glycemic Control for People With Diabetes

	Normal	Goal	Additional Action Suggested
Whole blood values			
Average preprandial glucose (mg/dL)*	<100	80–120	<80/>140
Average bedtime glucose (mg/dL)*	<110	100–140	<100/>160
Plasma values			
Average preprandial glucose (mg/dL)†	<110	90–130	<90/>150
Average bedtime glucose (mg/dL)†	<120	110–150	<110/>180
HbA$_{1c}$ (%)	<6	<7	>8

The values shown in this table are by necessity generalized to the entire population of individuals with diabetes. Patients with comorbid diseases, the very young and older adults, and others with unusual conditions or circumstances may warrant different treatment goals. These values are for nonpregnant adults. "Additional action suggested" depends on the individual patient's circumstances. Such actions may include enhanced diabetes self-management education, comanagement with a diabetes team, referral to an endocrinologist, change in pharmacologic therapy, initiation or increase in self-monitored blood glucose, or more frequent contact with the patient. HbA$_{1c}$ is referenced to a nondiabetic range of 4.0% to 6.0% (mean, 5.0%, standard deviation 0.5%).
*Measurement of capillary blood glucose.
†Values calibrated to plasma glucose.
(From American Diabetes Association. [2000]. Position statement. *Diabetes Care* 23 [Suppl. 1], S33.)

means for monitoring blood glucose and has given people with diabetes a way of maintaining near-normal blood glucose levels through self-monitoring of blood glucose. These methods use a drop of capillary blood obtained by pricking the finger or forearm with a special needle or small lancet. Small trigger devices make use of the lancet virtually painless. The drop of capillary blood is placed on or absorbed by a reagent strip, and glucose levels are determined electronically using a glucose meter.

Laboratory tests that use plasma for measurement of blood glucose give results that are 10% to 15% higher than the finger stick method, which uses whole blood. Many blood glucose monitors approved for home use and some test strips now calibrate blood glucose readings to plasma values. It is important that people with diabetes know whether their monitors or glucose strips provide whole-blood or plasma test results.

Glycosylated Hemoglobin Test. This test measures the amount of HbA$_{1c}$ (*i.e.*, hemoglobin into which glucose has been incorporated) in the blood. Hemoglobin normally does not contain glucose when it is released from the bone marrow. During its 120-day life span in the red blood cell, hemoglobin normally becomes glycosylated to form glycohemoglobins A$_{1a}$ and A$_{1b}$ (2% to 4%) and A$_{1c}$ (4% to 6%). In uncontrolled diabetes or diabetes with hyperglycemia, there is an increase in the level of HbA$_{1c}$. The ADA recommends initiating corrective measures for HbA$_{1c}$ levels greater than 8%. However, after the United Kingdom Prospective Diabetes Study (UKPDS) study, the goal has been redefined as lowering the HbA$_{1c}$ to less than 7.0%, or even achieving normal glycemic levels of less than 6.0%.[23] Because glucose entry into the red blood cell is not insulin dependent, the rate at which glucose becomes attached to the hemoglobin molecule depends on blood glucose. Glycosylation is essentially irreversible, and the level of HbA$_{1c}$ present in the blood provides an index of blood glucose levels over the previous 2 to 3 months.

Urine Tests

The ease, accuracy, and convenience of self-administered blood glucose monitoring techniques have made urine testing for glucose obsolete for most people with diabetes. These tests only reflect urine glucose levels and are influenced by such factors as the renal threshold for glucose, fluid intake and urine concentration, urine testing methodologies, and some drugs. Because of these factors, the ADA recommends that all people who use insulin should self-monitor their blood glucose, not urine glucose.[21] Unlike glucose tests, urine ketone determinations remain an important part of monitoring diabetic control, particularly in people with type 1 diabetes who are at risk for developing ketoacidosis, and in pregnant diabetic women to check the adequacy of nutrition and glucose control.

Dietary Management

The desired outcomes of glycemic control in both type 1 and type 2 diabetes is normalization of blood glucose as a means of preventing short- and long-term complications. Treatment plans usually involve nutrition therapy, exercise, and antidiabetic agents. People with type 1 diabetes require insulin therapy from the time of diagnosis. Weight loss and dietary management may be sufficient to control blood glucose levels in people with type 2 diabetes. However, they require follow-up care because insulin secretion from the beta cells may decrease or insulin resistance may persist, in which case oral antidiabetic agents are prescribed. Among the methods used to achieve these goals are education in self-management and problem solving. Individual treatment goals should take into account the person's age and other disease conditions, the person's capacity to understand and carry out the treatment regime, and socioeconomic factors that might influence compliance with the treatment plan. Optimal control of type 2 diabetes is associated with prevention or delay of chronic diabetes complications.[24]

Nutrition Therapy. Dietary management usually is prescribed to meet the specific needs of each person with diabetes. Goals and principles of diet therapy differ between type 1 and type 2 diabetes, as well as for lean and obese people. Integral to diabetes management is a prescribed plan for nutrition therapy.[25] Therapy goals include maintenance of near-normal blood glucose levels, achievement of optimal lipid levels, adequate calories to maintain and attain reasonable weights, prevention and treatment of chronic diabetes complications, and improvement of overall health through optimal nutrition.

A coordinated team effort, including the person with diabetes, is needed to individualize the nutrition plan. The diabetic diet has undergone marked changes over the years, particularly in the recommendations for distribution of calories among carbohydrates, proteins, and fats. There no longer is a specific diabetic or ADA diet but rather a dietary prescription based on nutrition assessment and treatment goals. Information is assessed regarding metabolic parameters and medical history of factors such as renal impairment and gastrointestinal autonomic neuropathy. Evaluating the effectiveness of the meal plan requires monitoring metabolic parameters such as blood glucose, HbA_{1c}, lipids, blood pressure, body weight, and quality of life. Self-management education is essential for the person with diabetes to facilitate understanding of the associations among food, exercise, medication, and blood glucose. For a person with type 1 diabetes, the usual food intake is assessed and used as a basis for adjusting insulin therapy to fit with the person's lifestyle. Eating consistent amounts and types of food at specific and routine times is encouraged. Home blood glucose monitoring is used to fine-tune the plan. Newer forms of therapy, such as multiple daily insulin injections and the use of an insulin pump, provide many options.

The registered dietitian plays an essential role in the diabetes care team and is able to select from a variety of methods such as carbohydrate counting, food exchanges, healthy food choices, and total available glucose to tailor the meal plan to meet individual needs. Simpler recommendations have been associated with improved client understanding and dietary adherence. Carbohydrate counting uses product label information that is easily available to people with diabetes.[26] Regardless of food source, total grams of carbohydrate are counted, placing an emphasis on the nutrient that most affects blood glucose control.

Most people with type 2 diabetes are overweight. Nutrition therapy goals focus on achieving glucose, lipid, and blood pressure goals, and weight loss if indicated. Mild to moderate weight loss (5 to 10 kg or 10 to 20 pounds) has been shown to improve diabetes control, even if desirable weight is not achieved.[27]

Nutrition therapy also is tailored to control for other dietary components. Because diabetes is a risk factor for cardiovascular disease, it is recommended that less than 10% of daily calories should be obtained from saturated fat and that dietary cholesterol be limited to 300 mg or less. Periodic fasting lipid panels may identify concomitant lipid disorders. If lipid disorders are identified, appropriate modifications according to the Third Report of the National Cholesterol Education Program (NECP III) on detection, evaluation, and treatment of high blood cholesterol should be followed.[28] For example, with a low-density lipoprotein cholesterol elevation, a diet with less than 7% of total calories from saturated fat, with 25% to 35% of daily calories obtained from fat, and a cholesterol intake of less than 200 mg/day is recommended. For people with diabetic nephropathy, some studies suggest lowering the intake of protein to 10% of daily calories. Recommendations for dietary sodium are the same as for the general population: 2400 to 3000 mg/day as a baseline; less than 2400 mg/day if mild to moderate hypertension is present; and less than 2000 if severe hypertension or nephropathy exists. The ADA provides literature with more detailed information on diet therapy and patient education. Included is the method of calculating individual meal plans. Registered dietitians are valuable resources to the nurse, physician, and person with diabetes and should be included in nutritional planning.

Exercise

The benefits of exercise include cardiovascular fitness and psychological well-being. For many people with type 2 diabetes, the benefits of exercise include a decrease in body fat, better weight control, and improvement in insulin sensitivity. The resulting improvement in glucose tolerance may free them from the use of antidiabetic drugs. Exercise is so important in diabetes management that a planned program of regular exercise usually is considered an integral part of the therapeutic regimen for every person with diabetes.

For people without diabetes, the uptake of glucose into the exercising muscle increases 7- to 20-fold during short-term exercise, and blood glucose levels are maintained by an adrenergically induced decrease in insulin release from beta cells and increased breakdown of liver glycogen stores mediated by counterregulatory hormones. When exercise is prolonged for more than 2 hours, the exercising muscles obtain the greater amount of their energy from fatty acids, and glucose release from the liver is derived from gluconeogenesis.

In people with diabetes, the beneficial effects of exercise are accompanied by an increased risk of hypoglycemia. Although muscle uptake of glucose increases significantly, the ability to maintain blood glucose levels is hampered by failure to suppress the absorption of injected insulin and activate the counterregulatory mechanisms that maintain blood glucose. Not only is there an inability to suppress insulin levels, but insulin absorption may increase. This increased absorption is more pronounced when insulin is injected into the subcutaneous tissue of the exercised muscle, but it occurs even when insulin is injected into other body areas. Even after exercise ceases, insulin's lowering effect on blood glucose levels continues. In some people with type 1 diabetes, the symptoms of hypoglycemia occur many hours after cessation of exercise. This may occur because subsequent insulin doses (in people using multiple daily insulin injections) are not adjusted to accommodate the exercise-induced decrease in blood glucose. The cause of hypoglycemia in people who do not administer a subsequent insulin dose is unclear. It may be related to the fact that the liver and skeletal muscles increase their uptake of glucose after exercise as a means of replenishing their glycogen stores, or that the liver and skeletal muscles are more sensitive to insulin during this time. People with diabetes should be aware that delayed hypoglycemia can occur after exercise and that they may need to alter their diabetes medication dose, their carbohydrate intake, or both.

Although of benefit to people with diabetes, exercise must be weighed on the risk-benefit scale. Before beginning an exercise program, persons with diabetes should undergo an appropriate evaluation for macrovascular and microvascular disease.[29] The goal of exercise is safe participation in activities consistent with an individual's lifestyle. As with nutrition guidelines, exercise recommendations need to individualized. Considerations include the potential for hypoglycemia, hyperglycemia, ketosis, cardiovascular ischemia and dysrhythmias (particularly silent ischemic heart disease), exacerbation of proliferative retinopathy, and lower extremity injury. For those with chronic diabetes, the complications of vigorous exercise can be harmful and cause eye hemorrhage and other problems. For people with type 1 diabetes who exercise during periods of poor control (*i.e.*, when blood glucose is elevated, exogenous insulin levels are low, and ketonemia exists), blood glucose and ketone rise to even higher levels because the stress of exercise is superimposed on preexisting insulin deficiency and increased counterregulatory hormone activity.

In general, sporadic exercise has only transient benefits; a regular exercise or training program is the most beneficial. It is better for cardiovascular conditioning and can maintain a muscle–fat ratio that enhances peripheral insulin receptivity.

Antidiabetic Agents

There are two categories of antidiabetic agents: oral medications and insulin. Because people with type 1 diabetes are deficient in insulin, they are in need of exogenous insulin replacement therapy from the start. People with type 2 diabetes have increased hepatic glucose production; decreased peripheral utilization of glucose; decreased utilization of ingested carbohydrates; and over time, impaired insulin secretion from the pancreas (Fig. 41-8). The oral antidiabetic agents used in the treatment of type 2 diabetes attack each one of these areas and sometimes all.[30] If good glycemic control cannot be achieved with a combination of oral agents, insulin can be used with the oral agents or by itself.

Oral Antidiabetic Agents. Oral antidiabetic agents approved by the U.S. Food and Drug Administration (FDA) fall into four categories: beta cell stimulator agents (sulfonylureas, repaglinide, and nateglinide), biguanides, α-glucosidase inhibitors, and thiazolidinediones (TZDs)[31] (Fig. 41-9).[31]

Sulfonylureas. The sulfonylureas were discovered accidentally in 1942, when scientists noticed that one of the sulfonamide drugs being developed at the time caused hypoglycemia. These drugs reduce blood glucose by stimulating the release of insulin from beta cells in the pancreas and increasing the sensitivity of peripheral tissues to insulin. These agents are effective only when some residual beta cell function remains. Sulfonylurea receptors in beta cells of the pancreas are linked to potassium-adenosine triphosphate (ATP) channels; when the drug attaches to the

receptors, these channels close, and a coupled reaction leads to an influx of calcium. The influx of calcium triggers secretion of insulin from the beta cells (see Fig. 41-4).

The sulfonylureas are used in the treatment of type 2 diabetes and cannot be substituted for insulin in people with type 1 diabetes, who have an absolute insulin deficiency. Slight modifications in the basic structure of the members of this drug group produce agents that have similar qualitative actions but markedly different potencies. The sulfonylureas traditionally are grouped into first- and second-generation agents (Table 41-5). These agents differ in dosage and duration of action. The second-generation drugs (glyburide, glipizide, glimepiride) are considerably more potent that the first-generation drugs (tolbutamide, acetohexamide, tolazamide, chlorpropamide). The second-generation agents are used more widely than the first-generation agents.

Because the sulfonylureas increase the rate at which glucose is removed from the blood, it is important to recognize that they can cause hypoglycemic reactions. This problem is more common in elderly people with impaired hepatic and renal function who are taking the longer-acting sulfonylureas.

Repaglinide and Nateglinide. Repaglinide (Prandin) and nateglinide (Starlix) are nonsulfonylurea beta cell stimulators that require the presence of glucose for their main action. These agents exert their action by closing the ATP-dependent potassium channel in the beta cells (see Fig. 41-4). Insulin release is glucose dependent and diminishes at low glucose levels. These agents, which are rapidly absorbed from the gastrointestinal tract, are taken shortly before meals (repaglinide 15 to 30 minutes and nateglinide 15 to 30 minutes). Both repaglinide and nateglinide can produce hypoglycemia; thus, proper timing of meals in relation to drug administration is important.

Biguanides. The biguanides are older oral antidiabetic drugs. Metformin (Glucophage) is the most significant agent in this group. Phenformin, the earlier form of the drug, was used extensively in the 1960s but was removed from the U.S. market in 1977 because of the occurrence of lactic acidosis in people treated with it. After more than a decade of use in Europe as well as Canada and other countries, metformin was approved by the FDA in 1995. Unlike its precursor, phenformin, metformin rarely results in lactic acidosis (0.03 cases per 1000 patients). Metformin inhibits hepatic glucose production and increases the sensitivity of peripheral tissues to the actions of insulin. This medication does not stimulate insulin secretion, which explains the absence of hypoglycemia. Secondary benefits of metformin therapy include weight loss and improved lipid profiles. Whereas the primary action of the sulfonylurea drugs is to increase insulin secretion, metformin exerts its beneficial effects on glycemic control through increased peripheral use of glucose and decreased hepatic glucose production (main effect). To decrease the risk of lactic acidosis, metformin is contraindicated in people with elevated serum creatinine levels (1.5 mg/dL in men, 1.4 mg/dL in women), clinical and laboratory evidence of hepatic disease, and any condition associated with hypoxemia or dehydration. Metformin sometimes is combined with other

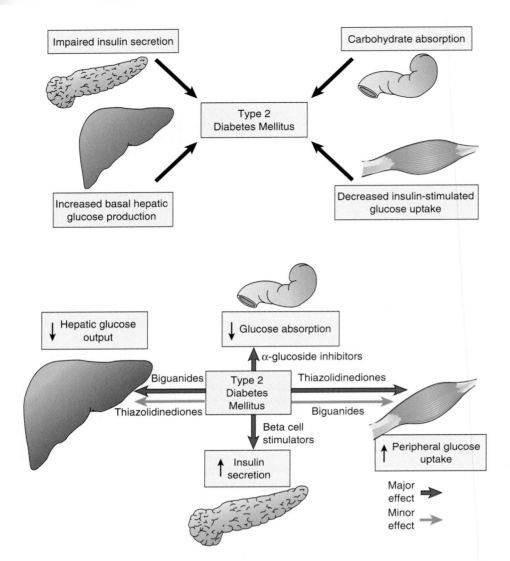

FIGURE 41-8 (**Top**) Mechanisms of elevated blood glucose in type 2 diabetes. (**Bottom**) Action sites of oral hypoglycemic agents and mechanisms of lowering blood glucose in type 2 diabetes mellitus.

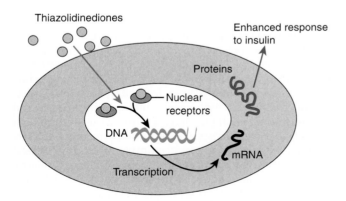

FIGURE 41-9 Action of the thiazolidinediones on activation of the PPARγ receptor that regulates gene transcription of proteins that regulate glucose uptake and reduce fatty acid release.

oral agents such as a sulfonylurea to improve blood glucose control.[32,33]

α-*Glucosidase Inhibitors.* In patients with type 2 diabetes, sulfonylureas, biguanides, or both may have beneficial effects on fasting plasma glucose levels. However, postprandial hyperglycemia persists in more than 60% of patients and probably accounts for sustained increases in HbA_{1c} levels. An alternative approach to the problem of postprandial hyperglycemia is the use of drugs such as acarbose (Precose) and miglitol (Glyset), inhibitors of α-glucosidase, which is a small intestine brush border enzyme that breaks down complex carbohydrates. By delaying the breakdown of complex carbohydrates, the α-glucosidase inhibitors delay the absorption of carbohydrates from the gut and blunt the postprandial increase in plasma glucose and insulin levels. Although not a problem with monotherapy or combination therapy with a biguanide, hypoglycemia may occur with concurrent sulfonylurea treatment. If hypoglycemia does occur, it should be treated with glucose (dextrose) and not

TABLE 41-5 ✦ Oral Beta Cell Stimulator Agents: Dosage Range and Duration of Action

Beta Cell Stimulator Agent	Total Daily Dosage (mg)	Duration (hr)
First-generation sulfonylureas*		
Chlorpropamide (Diabinese)	100–500	60
Second-generation sulfonylureas		
Glipizide (Glucotrol, generic)	2.5–40	12–24
Glipizide extended-release (Glucotrol XL)	5–20	24
Glyburide (DiaBeta, Micronase, generic)	1.25–20	16–24
Glyburide (Glynase Pres Tab)	1.5–12	24
Glimepiride (Amaryl)	0.5–8	18–24
Meglitinides		
Repaglinide (Prandin)	0.5–16	5
D-phenylalanine derivatives		
Nateglinide (Starlix)	90–360	3–4

*List is not inclusive.

sucrose (table sugar), whose breakdown may be blocked by the action of the α-glucosidase inhibitors.

Thiazolidinediones. The TZDs (or glitazones) are the only class of drugs that directly target insulin resistance, a fundamental defect in the pathophysiology of type 2 diabetes. The TZDs improve glycemic control by increasing insulin sensitivity in the insulin-responsive tissues—liver, skeletal muscle, and fat—allowing the tissues to respond to endogenous insulin more efficiently without increased output from already dysfunctional beta cells. A secondary effect is the suppression of hepatic glucose production. Rosiglitazone (Avandia), the most potent TZD insulin sensitizer, and pioglitazone (Actos) were approved by the FDA in 1999. Another TZD, troglitazone, was approved in 1997, but because of hepatic safety concerns, it is no longer available, having been withdrawn worldwide in March 2000. As of March 2001, postmarketing analysis of both rosiglitazone and pioglitazone has shown no indication of similar liver dysfunction. Rosiglitazone and pioglitazone both are approved for use as monotherapy and in combination therapy. Because of the problem with liver toxicity, liver enzymes should be measured according to the guidelines.

The mechanism of action of the TZDs is complex and not fully understood. The action of the TZDs is associated with binding to a nuclear receptor, the *peroxisome proliferator–activated receptor*-γ[34] (PPAR-γ; see Fig. 41-9). Binding of the TZDs to the PPAR-γ receptor begins a cascade of events that lead to regulation of genes involved in lipid and glucose metabolism. These include insulin-responsive genes such as the GLUT-4, lipoprotein lipase, and resistin genes. The result is an increase in the number of GLUT-4 transporters and increased insulin-mediated uptake of glucose in the peripheral tissues. A newly described protein produced by adipocytes, called *resistin*, may be a part of the missing link in explaining insulin resistance in persons with type 2 diabetes. Resistin suppresses insulin's ability to stimulate glucose uptake by adipose cells. The TZDs seem to decrease insulin resistance, in part, by suppressing the production of resistin by adipocytes.[35] Additional effects of TZDs are numerous, and include correction of many of the abnormal metabolic features associated with type 2 diabetes. This includes a decrease in FFA and triglycerides, microalbuminuria, blood pressure, inflammatory mediators (*e.g.*, fibrinogen and C-reactive protein), and procoagulation factors.[36] The TZDs also have the potential for preventing beta cell exhaustion by reducing FFAs and blood glucose levels.

Insulin. Type 1 diabetes mellitus always requires treatment with insulin, and many people with type 2 diabetes eventually require insulin therapy. Insulin is destroyed in the gastrointestinal tract and must be administered by injection. All insulins are measured in units, and the international unit of insulin is defined as the amount of insulin required to lower the blood glucose of a fasting 2-kg rabbit from 145 mg to 120 mg/dL. Most types of insulin are available in U-100 strength (*i.e.*, 100 units of insulin/1 mL). Insulin preparations are categorized according to onset, peak, and duration of action. An inhaled form of insulin is in the clinical trial stage.

During the past several decades, many pharmaceutical companies have entered the insulin-manufacturing market. After much research, human insulin has become available, providing an alternative to previous forms of insulin that were obtained from bovine and porcine sources. The manufacture of human insulin uses recombinant DNA. Beef insulin differs from human insulin by three amino acids, and pork insulin differs by only one amino acid. Many people with diabetes develop antibodies to beef and pork insulin. Improvements in the purification techniques for insulin extracted from animal pancreases have made it possible to reduce or eliminate many of the contaminants that could incite antibody formation. However, synthetic human insulin is widely available and generally used. A change from pork or beef to human insulin should be carefully monitored because hypoglycemia can occur owing to increased receptivity to the human insulin.

There are three principal types of insulin: short-acting, intermediate-acting, and long-acting (Table 41-6). The short-acting insulins fall into two categories: short-acting and ultra–short-acting. Insulin injection (Regular) is a short-acting soluble crystalline insulin whose effects begin within 30 minutes after subcutaneous injection and generally last for 4 to 6 hours. The ultra–short-acting insulins (insulin lispro [Humalog] and insulin aspart [Novolog]) are produced by recombinant technology with an amino acid substitution. These insulins have a more rapid onset, peak, and duration of action than short-acting Regular insulin. The ultra–short-acting insulins, which are used in combination with an intermediate- or long-acting insulin, are usually administered immediately prior to a meal. Intermediate-acting insulins (NPH and Lente) have a slower onset and duration of action. Since the intermediate-acting insulins require several hours to reach therapeutic levels, their use in type 1 diabetes requires supplementation with an ultra–short- or short-acting insulin. The long-acting Ultralente insulin has an even longer onset and duration of action than the intermediate-acting insulins. As with intermediate-acting insulins, it is used in combination with the shorter-acting insulins. Glargine (Lantus) is a new long-acting human insulin analog. It has a slower, more prolonged absorption than NPH insulin and provides a relatively constant concentration over 24 hours. Glargine is usually taken as a single bedtime dose and is used in combination with preprandial injections of a short-acting insulin. All forms of insulin have the potential of producing hypoglycemia or "insulin reaction" as a side effect (to be discussed).

Two intensive treatment regimens—multiple daily injections and continuous subcutaneous infusion of insulin (CSII)—closely simulate the normal pattern of insulin secretion by the body. With each method, a basal insulin level is maintained, and bolus doses of short-acting insulin are delivered before meals. The choice of management is determined by the patient in collaboration with the health care team.

Multiple Daily Injections. With multiple daily injections, the basal insulin requirements are met by long-acting insulin or by intermediate-acting insulin administered once or twice daily. Boluses of short-acting insulin are used before meals. The development of convenient injection devices (*e.g.*, pen injector) has made it easier for people with diabetes to comply with the multiple doses of short-acting insulin that are administered before meals.

Continuous Subcutaneous Insulin Infusion. With the CSII (insulin pump) method, the basal insulin requirements are met by continuous infusion of subcutaneous insulin, the rate of which can be varied to accommodate diurnal variations. The CSII technique involves the insertion of a small needle or plastic catheter into the subcutaneous tissue of the abdomen. Tubing from the catheter is connected to a syringe set into a small infusion pump worn on a belt or in a jacket pocket. The computer-operated pump then delivers one or more set basal amounts of insulin. In addition to the basal amount delivered by the pump, a bolus amount of insulin may be delivered when needed (*e.g.*, before a meal) by pushing a button.

Self-monitoring of blood glucose levels is a necessity when using this method of management. Each basal and bolus dose is determined individually and programmed into the infusion pump computer. Although the pump's safety has been proven, strict attention must be paid to signs of hypoglycemia. However, investigations have found CSII therapy to be associated with a marked and sustained reduction in the rate of severe hypoglycemia. Ketotic episodes caused by pump failure, catheter clogging, and infections at the needle site also are possible complications.

Candidate selection is crucial to the successful use of the insulin pump. Only people who are highly motivated to do frequent blood glucose tests and make daily insulin adjustments are candidates for this method of treatment.[37] Use of an insulin pump requires an intensive therapy program that is best implemented with the support of a diabetes health care team (Chart 41-1). The diabetologist, nurse educator, and dietitian are key team members; a social worker or psychologist and exercise physiologist are helpful additions to the team.

Pancreas or Islet Cell Transplantation

Pancreas or islet cell transplantation is not a lifesaving procedure. It does, however, afford the potential for significantly improving the quality of life. The most serious

TABLE 41-6 ✦ **Activity Profile of Insulin Preparations in the United States**				
Type	**Insulin Preparations**	**Onset (hr)***	**Peak (hr)***	**Duration (hr)***
Short Acting	Lispro Insulin Solution (Humalog)	0.25	0.5–1.5	3
	Insulin Aspart Injection (NovoLog)	0.25–0.5	0.6–1	3–5
	Insulin Injection (Regular)	0.5–1	1–4	4–6
Intermediate Acting	Isophane Insulin Suspension (NPH)	1–4	4–12	12–16
	Insulin Zinc Suspension (Lente)	2.5–4	4–8	16–20
Long Acting	Extended Insulin Zinc Suspension (Ultralente)	4–10	12–16	20–30
	Insulin Glargine (Lantus)	1	Continuous	24

*The times listed are variable, with differences from one injection to another because of multiple factors that influence insulin pharmacokinetics.

problems are the requirement for immunosuppression and the need for diagnosis and treatment of rejection. Investigators are looking for methods of transplanting islet cells and protecting the cells from destruction without the use immunosuppressive drugs.[38,39]

ACUTE COMPLICATIONS

The three major acute complications of diabetes are diabetic ketoacidosis (DKA), hyperglycemic hyperosmolar nonketotic (HHNK) syndrome, and hypoglycemia.

Diabetic Ketoacidosis

Diabetic ketoacidosis occurs when ketone production by the liver exceeds cellular use and renal excretion. DKA most commonly occurs in a person with type 1 diabetes, in whom the lack of insulin leads to mobilization of fatty acids from adipose tissue because of the unsuppressed adipose cell lipase activity that breaks down triglycerides into fatty acids and glycerol. The increase in fatty acid levels leads to ketone production by the liver (Fig. 41-10). It can occur at the onset of the disease, often before the disease has been diagnosed. For example, a mother may bring a child into the clinic or emergency department with reports of lethargy, vomiting, and abdominal pain, unaware that the child has diabetes. Stress increases the release of gluconeogenic hormones and predisposes the person to the development of ketoacidosis. DKA often is preceded by physical or emotional stress, such as infection, pregnancy, or extreme anxiety. In clinical practice, ketoacidosis also occurs with the omission or inadequate use of insulin.

The three major metabolic derangements in DKA are hyperglycemia, ketosis, and metabolic acidosis. The defin-

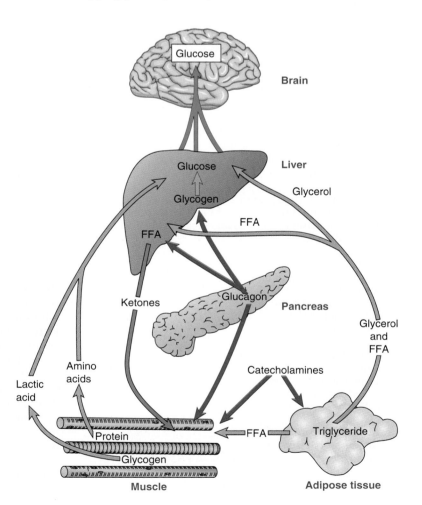

FIGURE 41-10 Mechanisms of diabetic ketoacidosis. Diabetic ketoacidosis is associated with very low insulin levels and extremely high levels of glucagon, catecholamines, and other counter-regulatory hormones. Increased levels of glucagon and the catecholamines (*red arrows*) lead to mobilization of substrates (*blue arrows*) for gluconeogenesis and ketogenesis by the liver (*green arrows*). Gluconeogenesis in excess of that needed to supply glucose for the brain and other glucose-dependent tissues produces a rise in blood glucose levels. Mobilization of free fatty acids (FFA) from triglyceride stores in adipose tissue leads to accelerated ketone production and ketosis.

itive diagnosis of DKA consists of hyperglycemia (blood glucose levels >250 mg/dL), low bicarbonate (<15 mEq/L), and low pH (<7.3), with ketonemia (positive at 1 : 2 dilution) and moderate ketonuria[40,41] (Chart 41-2). Hyperglycemia leads to osmotic diuresis, dehydration, and a critical loss of electrolytes. Hyperosmolality of extracellular fluids from hyperglycemia leads to a shift of water and potassium from the intracellular to the extracellular compartment. Extracellular sodium concentration frequently is low or normal despite enteric water losses because of the intracellular-extracellular fluid shift. This dilutional effect is referred to as *pseudohyponatremia*. Serum potassium levels may be normal or elevated, despite total potassium depletion resulting from protracted polyuria and vomiting. Metabolic acidosis is caused by the excess ketoacids that require buffering by bicarbonate ions; this leads to a marked decrease in serum bicarbonate levels.

Compared with an insulin reaction, DKA usually is slower in onset and recovery is more prolonged. The person typically has a history of 1 or 2 days of polyuria, polydipsia, nausea, vomiting, and marked fatigue, with eventual stupor that can progress to coma. Abdominal pain and tenderness may be experienced without abdominal disease. The breath has a characteristic fruity smell because of the presence of the volatile ketoacids. Hypotension and tachycardia may be present because of a decrease in blood volume. A number of the signs and symptoms that occur in DKA are related to compensatory mechanisms. The heart rate increases as the body compensates for a decrease in blood volume, and the rate and depth of respiration increase (*i.e.*, Kussmaul's respiration) as the body attempts to prevent further decreases in pH. Metabolic acidosis is discussed further in Chapter 32.

The goals in treating DKA are to improve circulatory volume and tissue perfusion, decrease serum glucose, correct the acidosis, and correct electrolyte imbalances. These objectives usually are accomplished through the administration of insulin and intravenous fluid and electrolyte replacement solutions. Because insulin resistance accompanies severe acidosis, low-dose insulin therapy is used. An initial loading dose of regular insulin often is given intravenously, followed by continuous low-dose infusion. Frequent laboratory tests are used to monitor blood glucose and serum electrolyte levels and to guide fluid and electrolyte replacement. It is important to replace fluid and electrolytes and correct pH while bringing the blood glucose concentration to a normal level. Too rapid a drop in blood glucose may cause hypoglycemic symptoms and cerebral edema. A sudden change in the osmolality of extracellular fluid occurs when blood glucose is lowered too rapidly, and this can cause cerebral edema. Serum potassium levels often fall as acidosis is corrected and extracellular potassium moves into the intracellular compartment; at this time, it may be necessary to add potassium to the intravenous infusion. Identification and treatment of the underlying cause, such as infection, also are important. With the better understanding of the pathogenesis of DKA and more uniform agreement on diagnosis and treatment, the mortality rate has been reduced to less than 5%.

Hyperglycemic Hyperosmolar Nonketotic Syndrome

The HHNK syndrome is characterized by hyperglycemia (blood glucose >600 mg/dL), hyperosmolarity (plasma osmolarity >310 mOsm/L) and dehydration, the absence of ketoacidosis, and depression of the sensorium.[41] HHNK syndrome may occur in various conditions, including type 2 diabetes, acute pancreatitis, severe infection, myocardial infarction, and treatment with oral or parenteral nutrition solutions. It is seen most frequently in people with type 2 diabetes. Two factors appear to contribute to the hyperglycemia that precipitates the condition: an increased resistance to the effects of insulin and an excessive carbohydrate intake.

In hyperosmolar states, the increased serum osmolarity has the effect of pulling water out of body cells, including brain cells. The condition may be complicated by thromboembolic events arising because of the high serum osmolality. The most prominent manifestations are dehydration, neurologic signs and symptoms, and excessive thirst (Chart 41-3). The neurologic signs include grand mal seizures, hemiparesis, Babinski's reflexes, aphasia, muscle fasciculations, hyperthermia, hemianopia, nystagmus, and visual hallucinations. The onset of HHNK syndrome often is insidious, and because it occurs most frequently in older people, it may be mistaken for a stroke.

The treatment of HHNK syndrome requires judicious medical observation and care because water moves back into brain cells during treatment, posing a threat of cerebral edema. Extensive potassium losses that also have occurred during the diuretic phase of the disorder require

---

CHART 41-2

Signs and Symptoms of Diabetic Ketoacidosis

Onset 1 to 24 hours
Laboratory findings
    Blood glucose greater than 250 mg/dL
    Ketonemia and presence of ketones in the urine
    Decreased plasma pH (<7.3) and bicarbonate
        (<15 mEq/L)
Dehydration caused by hyperglycemia
    Warm, dry skin
    Dry mucous membranes
    Tachycardia
    Weak, thready pulse
    Acute weight loss
    Hypotension
Ketoacidosis
    Anorexia, nausea, and vomiting
    Odor of ketones on the breath
    Depression of the central nervous system
        Lethargy and fatigue
        Stupor
        Coma
    Abdominal pain
Compensatory responses
    Rapid, deep respirations (Kussmaul's respiration)

CHART 41-3

Signs and Symptoms of Hyperglycemic Hyperosmolar Nonketotic Syndrome

Onset insidious; 24 hours to 2 weeks
Laboratory findings
    Blood glucose greater than 600 mg/dL
    Serum osmolarity 310 mOsm/L or greater
Severe dehydration
    Dry skin and mucous membranes
    Extreme thirst
Neurologic manifestations
    Depressed sensorium lethargy to coma
    Neurologic deficits
        Positive Babinski's sign
        Paresis or paralysis
        Sensory impairment
        Hyperthermia
        Hemianopia
Seizures

CHART 41-4

Signs and Symptoms of Insulin Reaction

Sudden onset
Laboratory findings
    Blood glucose less than 50 mg/dL
Impaired cerebral function (caused by decreased glucose
    availability for brain metabolism)
    Feeling of vagueness
    Headache
    Difficulty in problem solving
    Slurred speech
    Impaired motor function
    Change in emotional behavior
    Seizures
    Coma
Autonomic nervous system responses
    Hunger
    Anxiety
    Hypotension
    Sweating
    Vasoconstriction of skin vessels (skin is pale and cool)
    Tachycardia

correction. Because of the problems encountered in the treatment and the serious nature of the disease conditions that cause HHNK syndrome, the prognosis for this disorder is less favorable than that for ketoacidosis.

Hypoglycemia

Hypoglycemia, or an insulin reaction, occurs from a relative excess of insulin in the blood and is characterized by below-normal blood glucose levels.[42,43] It occurs most commonly in people treated with insulin injections, but prolonged hypoglycemia also can result from some oral hypoglycemic agents.

Hypoglycemia usually has a rapid onset and progression of symptoms (Chart 41-4). The signs and symptoms of hypoglycemia can be divided into two categories: those caused by altered cerebral function and those related to activation of the autonomic nervous system. Because the brain relies on blood glucose as its main energy source, hypoglycemia produces behaviors related to altered cerebral function. Headache, difficulty in problem solving, disturbed or altered behavior, coma, and seizures may occur. At the onset of the hypoglycemic episode, activation of the parasympathetic nervous system often causes hunger. The initial parasympathetic response is followed by activation of the sympathetic nervous system; this causes anxiety, tachycardia, sweating, and constriction of the skin vessels (*i.e.*, the skin is cool and clammy).

There is wide variation in the manifestation of signs and symptoms; not every person with diabetes manifests all or even most of the symptoms. The signs and symptoms of hypoglycemia are more variable in children and in elderly people. Elderly people may not display the typical autonomic responses associated with hypoglycemia but frequently develop signs of impaired function of the central nervous system, including mental confusion. Some people develop hypoglycemic unawareness. Unawareness of hypoglycemia should be suspected in people who do not report symptoms when their blood glucose concentrations are less than 50 to 60 mg/dL. This occurs most commonly in people who have a longer duration of diabetes and HbA$_{1c}$ levels within the normal range.[42,44] Some medications, such as β-adrenergic–blocking drugs, interfere with the sympathetic response normally seen in hypoglycemia.

Many factors precipitate an insulin reaction in a person with type 1 diabetes, including error in insulin dose, failure to eat, increased exercise, decreased insulin need after removal of a stress situation, medication changes, and a change in insulin site. Alcohol decreases liver gluconeogenesis, and people with diabetes need to be cautioned about its potential for causing hypoglycemia, especially if it is consumed in large amounts or on an empty stomach.

The most effective treatment of an insulin reaction is the immediate ingestion of a concentrated carbohydrate source, such as sugar, honey, candy, or orange juice. Alternative methods for increasing blood glucose may be required when the person having the reaction is unconscious or unable to swallow. Glucagon may be given intramuscularly or subcutaneously. Glucagon acts by hepatic glycogenolysis to raise blood sugar. The liver contains only a limited amount of glycogen (approximately 75 g); glucagon is ineffective in people whose glycogen stores have been depleted. Some people report becoming nauseated after glucagon administration, which also could be in response to the severe hypoglycemia. A small amount of glucose gel (available in most pharmacies) may be inserted into the buccal pouch when glucagon is unavailable. Monosaccharides such as glucose, which can be absorbed directly into the bloodstream, work best for this purpose. It is important not to overtreat hypoglycemia and cause hyperglycemia.

Treatment usually consists of an initial administration of 15 to 20 g of glucose, which can be repeated as necessary. Complex carbohydrates can be administered after the acute reaction has been controlled to sustain blood glucose levels. In situations of severe or life-threatening hypoglycemia, it may be necessary to administer glucose (20 to 50 mL of a 50% solution) intravenously.

COUNTERREGULATORY MECHANISMS AND THE SOMOGYI EFFECT AND DAWN PHENOMENON

The Somogyi effect describes a cycle of insulin-induced posthypoglycemic episodes. In 1924, Joslin and associates noticed that hypoglycemia was associated with alternate episodes of hyperglycemia.[45] It was not until 1959 that Somogyi presented the results of his 20 years of studies, which confirmed the observation that "hypoglycemia begets hyperglycemia." In people with diabetes, insulin-induced hypoglycemia produces a compensatory increase in blood levels of catecholamines, glucagon, cortisol, and growth hormone. These counterregulatory hormones cause blood glucose to become elevated and produce some degree of insulin resistance. The cycle begins when the increase in blood glucose and insulin resistance is treated with larger insulin doses. The hypoglycemic episode often occurs during the night or at a time when it is not recognized, rendering the diagnosis of the phenomenon more difficult.

Research suggests that even rather mild insulin-associated hypoglycemia, which may be asymptomatic, can cause hyperglycemia in those with type 1 diabetes through the recruitment of counterregulatory mechanisms, although the insulin action does not wane. A concomitant waning of the effect of insulin (*i.e.*, end of the duration of action), when it occurs, exacerbates posthypoglycemic hyperglycemia and accelerates its development. These findings may explain the labile nature of the disease in some people with diabetes. Measures to prevent hypoglycemia and the subsequent activation of counterregulatory mechanisms include a redistribution of dietary carbohydrates and an alteration in insulin dose or time of administration.[46]

The dawn phenomenon is characterized by increased levels of fasting blood glucose or insulin requirements, or both, between 5 and 9 AM without antecedent hypoglycemia. It occurs in people with type 1 or type 2 diabetes. It has been suggested that a change in the normal circadian rhythm for glucose tolerance, which usually is higher during the later part of the morning, is altered in people with diabetes.[47] Growth hormone has been suggested as a possible factor. When the dawn phenomenon occurs alone, it may produce only mild hyperglycemia, but when it is combined with the Somogyi effect, it may produce profound hyperglycemia.

CHRONIC COMPLICATIONS

The chronic complications of diabetes include neuropathies, disorders of the microcirculation (*i.e.*, neuropathies, nephropathies, and retinopathies), macrovascular complications, and foot ulcers. These disorders occur in the insulin-

independent tissues of the body—tissues that do not require insulin for glucose entry into the cell. This probably means that intracellular glucose concentrations in many of these tissues approach or equal those in the blood. The level of chronic glycemia is the best-established concomitant factor associated with diabetic complications.[24,48–50] The Diabetes Control and Complications Trial (DCCT), which was conducted with 1441 people with type 1 diabetes, has demonstrated that the incidence of retinopathy, nephropathy, and neuropathy can be reduced by intensive diabetic treatment.[51] Similar results have been demonstrated by the UKPDS in people with type 2 diabetes.[23,52]

Theories of Pathogenesis

The interest among researchers in explaining the causes and development of chronic lesions in a person with diabetes has led to a number of theories. Several of these theories have been summarized to prepare the reader for understanding specific chronic complications.

Polyol Pathway. A polyol is an organic compound that contains three or more hydroxyl (OH) groups. The polyol pathway refers to the intracellular mechanisms responsible for changing the number of hydroxyl units on a glucose molecule. In the sorbitol pathway, glucose is transformed first to sorbitol and then to fructose. Although glucose is converted readily to sorbitol, the rate at which sorbitol can be converted to fructose and then

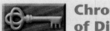

Chronic Complications of Diabetes

➤ The chronic complications of diabetes result from elevated blood glucose levels and associated impairment of lipid and other metabolic pathways.

➤ Diabetic nephropathy, which is a leading cause of end-stage renal disease, is associated with the increased work demands and microalbuminemia imposed by poorly controlled blood glucose levels.

➤ Diabetic retinopathy, which is a leading cause of blindness, is closely linked to elevations in blood glucose and hyperlipidemia seen in persons with uncontrolled diabetes.

➤ Diabetic peripheral neuropathies, which affect both the somatic and autonomic nervous systems result from the demyelinating effect of long-term uncontrolled diabetes.

➤ Macrovascular disorders such as coronary heart disease, stroke, and peripheral vascular disease reflect the combined effects of unregulated blood glucose levels, elevated blood pressure, and hyperlipidemia.

➤ The chronic complications of diabetes are best prevented by measures aimed at tight control of blood glucose levels, maintenance of normal lipid levels, and control of hypertension.

metabolized is limited. Sorbitol is osmotically active, and it has been hypothesized that the presence of excess intracellular amounts may alter cell function in those tissues that use this pathway (*e.g.*, lens, kidneys, nerves, blood vessels). In the lens, for example, the osmotic effects of sorbitol cause swelling and opacity. Increased sorbitol also is associated with a decrease in myoinositol and reduced adenosine triphosphatase activity. The reduction of these compounds may be responsible for the peripheral neuropathies caused by Schwann cell damage.

Formation of Abnormal Glycoproteins. Glycoproteins, or what could be called *glucose proteins*, are normal components of the basement membrane in smaller blood vessels and capillaries. It has been suggested that the increased intracellular concentration of glucose associated with uncontrolled blood glucose levels in diabetes favors the formation of abnormal glycoproteins. These abnormal glycoproteins are thought to produce structural defects in the basement membrane of the microcirculation and to contribute to eye, kidney, and vascular complications.

Problems With Tissue Oxygenation. Proponents of the tissue oxygenation theories suggest that many of the chronic complications of diabetes arise because of a decrease in oxygen delivery in the small vessels of the microcirculation. Among the factors believed to contribute to this inadequate oxygen delivery is a defect in red blood cell function that interferes with the release of oxygen from the hemoglobin molecule. In support of this theory is the finding of a two- to threefold increase in HbA_{1c} in some people with diabetes. In HbA_{1c}, a glycoprotein is substituted for valine in the β chain, causing a high affinity for oxygen. The concentration of the red blood cell glycolytic intermediate, 2,3-diphosphoglycerate (2,3-DPG), declines during the acidotic and recovery phases of DKA; 2,3-DPG reduces hemoglobin's affinity for oxygen. An increase in HbA_{1c} and a decrease in 2,3-DPG increase the hemoglobin's affinity for oxygen, and less oxygen is released for tissue use.

Peripheral Neuropathies

Although the incidence of peripheral neuropathies is high among people with diabetes, it is difficult to document exactly how many people are affected by these disorders because of the diversity in clinical manifestations and because the condition often is far advanced before it is recognized. Results of the DCCT study showed that intensive therapy can reduce the incidence of clinical neuropathy by 60% compared with conventional therapy.[53,54]

Two types of pathologic changes have been observed in connection with diabetic peripheral neuropathies. The first is a thickening of the walls of the nutrient vessels that supply the nerve, leading to the assumption that vessel ischemia plays a major role in the development of these neural changes. The second finding is a segmental demyelinization process that affects the Schwann cell. This demyelinization process is accompanied by a slowing of nerve conduction.

It appears that the diabetic peripheral neuropathies are not a single entity. The clinical manifestations of these disorders vary with the location of the lesion. Although there are several methods for classifying the diabetic peripheral neuropathies, a simplified system divides them into the somatic and autonomic nervous system neuropathies (Chart 41-5).

Somatic Neuropathy. A distal symmetric polyneuropathy, in which loss of function occurs in a stocking-glove pattern, is the most common form of peripheral neuropathy. Somatic sensory involvement usually occurs first and usually is bilateral, symmetric, and associated with diminished perception of vibration, pain, and temperature, particularly to the lower extremities. In addition to the discomforts associated with the loss of sensory or motor function, lesions in the peripheral nervous system predispose a person with diabetes to other complications. The loss of feeling, touch, and position sense increases the risk of falling. Impairment of temperature and pain sensation increases the risk of serious burns and injuries to the feet.

Painful diabetic neuropathy involves the somatosensory neurons that carry pain impulse. This disorder, which causes hypersensitivity to light touch and occasionally severe "burning pain," particularly at night, can become physically and emotionally disabling.[54,55]

Autonomic Neuropathy. With autonomic nervous system neuropathies, there are defects in vasomotor responses, decreased cardiac responses, impaired motility of the gastrointestinal tract, inability to empty the bladder, and sexual dysfunction.[56] Defects in vasomotor reflexes

---

CHART 41-5

Classification of Diabetic Peripheral Neuropathies

Somatic
Polyneuropathies (bilateral sensory)
  Paresthesias, including numbness and tingling
  Impaired pain, temperature, light touch, two-point
    discrimination, and vibratory sensation
  Decreased ankle and knee-jerk reflexes
Mononeuropathies
  Involvement of a mixed nerve trunk that includes
    loss of sensation, pain, and motor weakness
Amyotrophy
  Associated with muscle weakness, wasting, and severe
    pain of muscles in the pelvic girdle and thigh

Autonomic
Impaired vasomotor function
  Postural hypotension
Impaired gastrointestinal function
  Gastric atony
  Diarrhea, often postprandial and nocturnal
Impaired genitourinary function
  Paralytic bladder
  Incomplete voiding
  Impotence
  Retrograde ejaculation
Cranial nerve involvement
  Extraocular nerve paralysis
  Impaired pupillary responses
  Impaired special senses

can lead to dizziness and syncope when the person moves from the supine to the standing position. Gastroparesis (impaired emptying of the stomach) can lead to alternating bouts of diarrhea, particularly at night, and constipation. Incomplete emptying of the bladder predisposes to urinary stasis and bladder infection and increases the risk of renal complications.

In the male, disruption of sensory and autonomic nervous system function may cause sexual dysfunction (see Chapter 43). Diabetes is the leading physiologic cause of erectile dysfunction, and it occurs in both type 1 and type 2 diabetes. Of the 5 million men with diabetes in the United States, 30% to 60% have erectile dysfunction.[57,58]

Nephropathies

Diabetic nephropathy is the leading cause of end-stage renal disease (ESRD), accounting for 40% of new cases.[1] In the United States, 33% of all people who seek renal replacement therapy (see Chapter 34) have diabetes.[59] The complication affects people with both type 1 and type 2 diabetes. According to the reports of the U.S. Renal Data System, the increase in ESRD since the early 1980s has been predominantly among people with type 2 diabetes.[60]

The term *diabetic nephropathy* is used to describe the combination of lesions that often occur concurrently in the diabetic kidney. The most common kidney lesions in people with diabetes are those that affect the glomeruli. Various glomerular changes may occur in people with diabetic nephropathy, including capillary basement membrane thickening, diffuse glomerular sclerosis, and nodular glomerulosclerosis (see Chapter 33). Changes in the capillary basement membrane take the form of thickening of basement membranes along the length of the glomeruli. Diffuse glomerulosclerosis consists of thickening of the basement membrane and the mesangial matrix. Nodular glomerulosclerosis, also called *intercapillary glomerulosclerosis* or *Kimmelstiel-Wilson disease*, is a form of glomerulosclerosis that involves the development of nodular lesions in the glomerular capillaries of the kidneys, causing impaired blood flow with progressive loss of kidney function and, eventually, renal failure. Nodular glomerulosclerosis is thought to occur only in people with diabetes. Changes in the basement membrane in diffuse glomerulosclerosis and Kimmelstiel-Wilson syndrome allow plasma proteins to escape in the urine, causing proteinuria and the development of hypoproteinemia, edema, and others signs of impaired kidney function.

Not all people with diabetes develop clinically significant nephropathy; for this reason, attention is focusing on risk factors for the development of this complication. Among the suggested risk factors are genetic and familial predisposition, elevated blood pressure, poor glycemic control, smoking, hyperlipidemia, and microalbuminemia.[59,61] Diabetic nephropathy occurs in family clusters, suggesting a familial predisposition, although this does not exclude the possibility of environmental factors shared by siblings. The risk for development of ESRD also is greater among Native Americans, Hispanics (especially Mexican Americans), and African Americans.[61] Kidney enlargement, nephron hypertrophy, and hyperfiltration occur early in the disease,

suggesting increased work of the kidneys in reabsorbing excessive amounts of glucose. One of the first manifestations of diabetic nephropathy is an increase in urinary albumin excretion (*i.e.,* microalbuminuria), which is easily assessed by laboratory methods. Microalbuminuria is defined as a urine protein loss between 30 and 300 mg/day. The risk of microalbuminuria increases abruptly with hemoglobin A_{1c} levels above 8.1%[61] (Fig. 41-11). Both systolic and diastolic hypertension accelerates the progression of diabetic nephropathy. Even moderate lowering of blood pressure can decrease the risk of ESRD.[61] Smoking increases the risk of ESRD in both diabetic and nondiabetic people. People with type 2 diabetes who smoke have a greater risk of microalbuminemia, and their rate of progression to ESRD is approximately twice as rapid as in those who do not smoke.[61]

Measures to prevent diabetic nephropathy or its progression in persons with diabetes include achievement of glycemic control, maintenance of blood pressure in the midnormal range (125 to 130/75 to 85 mm Hg), prevention or reduction in the level of proteinuria, and smoking cessation in people who smoke.[59,61]

Retinopathies

Diabetes is the leading cause of acquired blindness in the United States. Although people with diabetes are at increased risk for development of cataracts and glaucoma, retinopathy is the most common pattern of eye disease. Diabetic retinopathy is estimated to be the most frequent cause of newly diagnosed blindness among Americans between the ages of 20 and 74 years.[62] Diabetic retinopathy

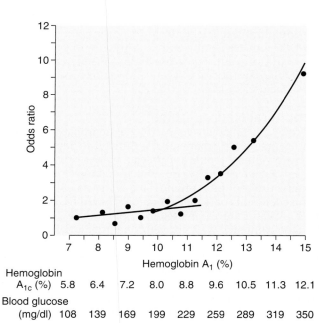

Hemoglobin A_{1c} (%)	5.8	6.4	7.2	8.0	8.8	9.6	10.5	11.3	12.1
Blood glucose (mg/dl)	108	139	169	199	229	259	289	319	350

FIGURE 41-11 Relationship between mean hemoglobin A_1 and the risk of microalbuminuria in patients with type 2 diabetes mellitus. (Krolewski A.S., Laffel L.M.B., Krolewski M., et al. [1995]. Glycosylated hemoglobin and the risk of microalbuminuria in patients with insulin-dependent diabetes mellitus. *New England Journal of Medicine* 332(19), 1251–1255)

is characterized by abnormal retinal vascular permeability, microaneurysm formation, neovascularization and associated hemorrhage, scarring, and retinal detachment (see Chapter 54).[62,63] Twenty years after the onset of diabetes, nearly all people with type 1 diabetes and more than 60% of people with type 2 diabetes have some degree of retinopathy. Pregnancy, puberty, and cataract surgery can accelerate these changes.[62,63,64]

Although there has been no extensive research on risk factors associated with diabetic retinopathy, they appear to be similar to those for other complications. Among the suggested risk factors associated with diabetic retinopathy are poor glycemic control, elevated blood pressure, and hyperlipidemia. The strongest case for control of blood glucose comes from the UKPDS study, which demonstrated a reduction in retinopathy with improved glucose control.[23]

Because of the risk of retinopathy, it is important that people with diabetes have regular dilated eye examinations. They should have an initial examination for retinopathy shortly after the diagnosis of diabetes is made. The recommendation for follow-up examinations is based on the type of examination that was done and the findings of that examination. People with persistently elevated glucose levels or proteinuria should be examined yearly.[62] Women who are planning a pregnancy should be counseled on the risk of development or progression of diabetic retinopathy. Women with diabetes who become pregnant should be followed closely throughout pregnancy. This does not apply to women who develop GDM because such women are not at risk for development of diabetic retinopathy.

People with macular edema, moderate to severe nonproliferative retinopathy, or any proliferative retinopathy should receive the care of an ophthalmologist. Methods used in the treatment of diabetic retinopathy include the destruction and scarring of the proliferative lesions with laser photocoagulation. The Diabetic Retinopathy Study provides evidence that photocoagulation may delay or prevent visual loss in more than 50% of eyes with proliferative retinopathy.[65]

Macrovascular Complications

Diabetes mellitus is a major risk factor for coronary artery disease, cerebrovascular disease, and peripheral vascular disease. The prevalence of these macrovascular complications is increased two- to fourfold in people with diabetes

Multiple risk factors for macrovascular disease, including obesity, hypertension, hyperglycemia, hyperinsulinemia, hyperlipidemia, altered platelet function, and elevated fibrinogen levels, frequently are found in people with diabetes. The prevalence of coronary artery disease, stroke, and peripheral vascular disease is substantially increased in people with diabetes, even in the absence of these risk factors. There appear to be differences between type 1 and type 2 diabetes in terms of duration of disease and the development of macrovascular disease. In people with type 2 diabetes, macrovascular disease may be present at the time of diagnosis. In type 1 diabetes, the attained age and the duration of diabetes appear to correlate with the degree of macrovascular disease. The reason for these discrepancies has been attributed to the IGT that exists before actual diagnosis of type 2 diabetes.[50,66]

Diabetic Foot Ulcers

Foot problems are common among people with diabetes and may become severe enough to cause ulceration, infection, and, eventually, a need for amputation. Foot problems have been reported as the most common complication leading to hospitalization among people with diabetes. In a controlled study of 854 outpatients with diabetes followed in a general medical clinic, foot problems accounted for 16% of hospital admissions over a 2-year period and 23% of total hospital days.[67] In people with diabetes, lesions of the feet represent the effects of neuropathy and vascular insufficiency. Approximately 60% to 70% of people with diabetic foot ulcers have neuropathy without vascular disease, 15% to 20% have vascular disease, and 15% to 20% have neuropathy and vascular disease.[67]

Distal symmetric neuropathy is a major risk factor for foot ulcers. People with sensory neuropathies have impaired pain sensation and often are unaware of the constant trauma to the feet caused by poorly fitting shoes, improper weight bearing, hard objects or pebbles in the shoes, or infections such as athlete's foot. Neuropathy prevents people from detecting pain; they are unable to adjust their gait to avoid walking on an area of the foot where pressure is causing trauma and necrosis. Motor neuropathy with weakness of the intrinsic muscles of the foot may result in foot deformities, which lead to focal areas of high pressure. When the abnormal focus of pressure is coupled with loss of sensation, a foot ulcer can occur. Common sites of trauma are the back of the heel, the plantar metatarsal area, or the great toe, where weight is borne during walking (Fig. 41-12).

All persons with diabetes should receive a full foot examination at least once a year. This examination should include assessment of protective sensation, foot structure and biomechanics, vascular status, and skin integrity.[68] Evaluation of neurologic function should include a somatosensory test using either the Semmes-Weinstein monofilament or vibratory sensation. The Semmes-Weinstein monofilament is a simple, inexpensive device for testing

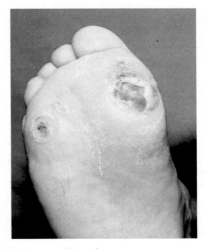

FIGURE 41-12 Neuropathic ulcers occur on pressure points in areas with diminished sensation in diabetic polyneuropathy. Pain is absent (and therefore the ulcer may go unnoticed). (Bates B.B. [1995]. *A guide to physical examination and history taking* [6th ed.]. Philadelphia: J.B. Lippincott)

sensory status (Fig. 41-13). The monofilament is held in the hand or attached to a handle at one end. When the unattached or unsupported end of the monofilament is pressed against the skin until it buckles or bends slightly, it delivers 10 g of pressure at the point of contact.[68] The test consists of having the person being tested report at which of two moments he or she is being touched by the monofilament. For example, the examiner will call out "one" and then "two" and briefly touch the monofilament to the site at one of the two test times. Between 4 and 10 sites per foot are touched. An incorrect response at even one site indicates increased risk of neuropathy and foot complications.

Because of the constant risk of foot problems, it is important that people with diabetes wear shoes that have been fitted correctly and inspect their feet daily, looking for blisters, open sores, and fungal infection (*e.g.*, athlete's foot) between the toes. If their eyesight is poor, a family member should do this for them. In the event a lesion is detected, prompt medical attention is needed to prevent serious complications. Specially designed shoes have been demonstrated to be effective in preventing relapses in people with previous ulcerations.[69] Smoking should be avoided because it causes vasoconstriction and contributes to vascular disease. Because cold produces vasoconstriction, appropriate foot coverings should be used to keep the feet warm and dry. Toenails should be cut straight across to prevent ingrown toenails. The toenails often are thickened and deformed, requiring the services of a podiatrist.

INFECTIONS

Although not specifically an acute or a chronic complication, infections are a common concern of people with diabetes. Certain types of infections occur with increased frequency in people with diabetes: soft tissue infections of the extremities, osteomyelitis, urinary tract infections and pyelonephritis, candidal infections of the skin and mucous surfaces, dental caries and infections, and tuberculosis.[70] Controversy exists about whether infections are more common in people with diabetes or whether infections

seem more prevalent because they often are more serious in people with diabetes.

Suboptimal response to infection in a person with diabetes is caused by the presence of chronic complications, such as vascular disease and neuropathies, and by the presence of hyperglycemia and altered neutrophil function. Sensory deficits may cause a person with diabetes to ignore minor trauma and infection, and vascular disease may impair circulation and delivery of blood cells and other substances needed to produce an adequate inflammatory response and effect healing. Pyelonephritis and urinary tract infections are relatively common in persons with diabetes, and it has been suggested that these infections may bear some relation to the presence of a neurogenic bladder or nephrosclerotic changes in the kidneys. Hyperglycemia and glycosuria may influence the growth of microorganisms and increase the severity of the infection. Diabetes and elevated blood glucose levels also may impair host defenses such as the function of neutrophils and immune cells. Polymorphonuclear leukocyte function, particularly adherence, chemotaxis, and phagocytosis, are depressed in persons with diabetes, particularly those with poor glycemic control.

> In summary, diabetes mellitus is a disorder of carbohydrate, protein, and fat metabolism resulting from an imbalance between insulin availability and insulin need. The disease can be classified as type 1 diabetes, in which there is destruction of beta cells and an absolute insulin deficiency, or type 2 diabetes, in which there is a lack of insulin availability or effectiveness. Type 1 diabetes can be further subdivided into type 1A immune-mediated diabetes, which is thought to be caused by autoimmune mechanisms, and type 1B idiopathic diabetes, for which the cause is unknown. Other specific types of diabetes include secondary forms of carbohydrate intolerance, which occur secondary to some other condition, such as pancreatic disorders, that destroy beta cells, or endocrine diseases such as Cushing's syndrome, which cause increased production of glucose by the liver and decreased use of glucose by the tissues. GDM develops during pregnancy, and although glucose tolerance often returns to normal after childbirth, it indicates an increased risk for development of diabetes.
>
> The diagnosis of diabetes mellitus is based on clinical signs of the disease, fasting blood glucose levels, random plasma glucose measurements, and results of the glucose tolerance test. Self-monitoring provides a means of maintaining near-normal blood glucose levels through frequent testing of blood glucose and adjustment of insulin dosage. Glycosylation involves the irreversible attachment of glucose to the hemoglobin molecule; the measurement of HbA$_{1c}$ provides an index of blood glucose levels over several months.
>
> The treatment of diabetes includes diet, exercise, and, in many cases, the use of an antidiabetic agent. Dietary management focuses on maintaining a well-balanced diet, controlling calories to achieve and

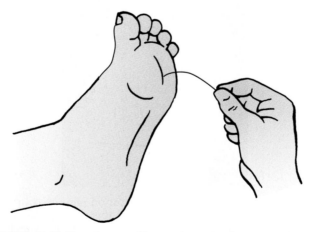

FIGURE 41-13 Use of a monofilament in testing for impaired sensation in the foot of a person with diabetes.

maintain an optimum weight, and regulating the distribution of carbohydrates, proteins, and fats. Two types of antidiabetic agents are used in the management of diabetes: injectable insulin and oral diabetic drugs. Type 1, and sometimes type 2, diabetes requires treatment with injectable insulin. Oral diabetic drugs include the beta cell stimulating agents, biguanides, α-glucosidase inhibitors, and TZDs. These drugs require a functioning pancreas and may be used in the treatment of type 2 diabetes. The benefits of exercise include cardiovascular fitness and psychological well-being. Many people with type 2 diabetes benefit from a decrease in body fat, better weight control, and an improvement in insulin sensitivity. In people with type 1 diabetes, the benefits of exercise are accompanied by a risk of hypoglycemia. The metabolic disturbances associated with diabetes affect almost every body system. The acute complications of diabetes include DKA, HHNK coma, and hypoglycemia. The chronic complications of diabetes affect the non–insulin-dependent tissues, including the retina, blood vessels, kidneys, peripheral nervous system, and feet.

Related Web Sites

American Association of Clinical Endocrinologists—Diabetes management guidelines www.aace.com/clin/guides/diabetes_2000.pdf

American Diabetes Association—Diabetes Information www.diabetes.org/ada/diabetesinfo.asp

Diabetes Care Online Journal care.diabetesjournals.org/

National Institute of Diabetes and Digestive and Kidney Diseases www.niddk.nih.gov/index.htm

References

1. American Diabetes Association. (2000). Diabetes facts and figures. [On-line]. Available: http://www.diabetes.org/
2. Guyton A., Hall J.E. (2000). *Medical physiology* (10th ed., pp. 884–898). Philadelphia: W.B. Saunders.
3. Greenspan F.S., Gardner D.G. (2001). *Basic and clinical endocrinology* (6th ed., pp. 623–633), New York: Lange Medical Books/McGraw-Hill.
4. Shepard P.R., Kahn B. (1999). Glucose transporters and insulin action. *New England Journal of Medicine* 341, 248–256.
5. Goldfine I.R., Youngren J.F. (1998). Contributions of the *American Journal of Physiology* to the discovery of insulin. *American Journal of Physiology* 274, E207–E209.
6. Expert Committee on the Diagnosis and Classification of Diabetes Mellitus. (1997). Report of the Expert Committee on the Diagnosis and Classification of Diabetes Mellitus. *Diabetes Care* 20, 1183–1199.
7. Atkinson M.A., Eisenbarth G.S. (2001). Type 1 diabetes: New perspectives on disease pathogenesis and treatment. *The Lancet* 358, 221–229.
8. Tataranni C., Bogardus C. (2001). Changing habits to delay diabetes. *New England Journal of Medicine* 344, 1390–1391.
9. Atkinson M.A. (2000). The $64,000 question in diabetes continues. *Lancet* 356, 4–5.
10. Bingley P.J., Bonifacio E., Ziegler A.G., Schatz D.A., Atkinson M.A., Eisenbarth G.S. (2001). Proposed guidelines for screening for risk of type 1 diabetes. *Diabetes Care* 24, 398.
11. Davidson M.B. (1995). Clinical implications of insulin resistance syndromes. *American Journal of Medicine* 99, 420–426.
12. Peppard H.R., Marfori J., Iuorno M.J., Nestler J.E. (2001). Prevalence of polycystic ovary syndrome among premenopausal women with type 2 diabetes. *Diabetes Care* 24, 1050–1052.
13. Guven S., El-Bershawi A., Sonnenberg G.E., Wilson C.R., Krakower G.R., Kissebah A.H. (1999). Persistent elevation in plasma leptin level in ex-obese with normal body mass index: Relation to body composition and insulin sensitivity. *Diabetes* 48, 347–352.
14. Boder G. (2001). Free fatty acids—the link between obesity and insulin resistance. *Endocrine Practice* 7, 44–51.
15. Yamauchi T., Kamon J., Waki H., Terauchi Y., Kubota N., Hara K., et. al. (2001). The fat-derived hormone adiponectin reverses insulin resistance associated with both lipoatrophy and obesity. *Nature Medicine* 7(8), 941–946.
16. Kissebah A.H., Sonneberg G.F., Myklebust J., Goldstein M., Broman K., James R.G., et. al. (2000). Quantitative trait loci on chromosomes 3 and 17 influence phenotypes of metabolic syndrome. Proceedings of the National Academy of Science U.S.A. 97(26), 14478–14483.
17. Chamberlain J., DeMouy J. (2001). Diet and exercise dramatically delay type 2 diabetes: Diabetes medication metformin also effective. National Institute Diabetes & Digestive & Kidney Diseases. [On-line.] Available: http://www.niddk.nih.gov/welcome/releases/8_8_01.htm. Accessed 9/22/01.
18. Winter W. E., Kamura M., House D.W. (1999). Monogenic diabetes mellitus in youth: The MODY syndrome. *Metabolic Clinics of North America* 28, 765–785.
19. American Diabetes Association. (2000). Gestational diabetes mellitus. *Diabetes Care* 23 (Suppl. 1), S77–S79.
20. Kjos S.L., Buckanan T.A. (1999). Gestational diabetes mellitus. *New England Journal of Medicine* 341, 1749–1756.
21. American Diabetes Association. (2000). Report of the Expert Committee on the Diagnosis and Classification of Diabetes Mellitus. *Diabetes Care* 23 (Suppl. 1), S14.
22. American Diabetes Association. (2000). Tests of glycemia in diabetes. *Diabetes Care* 23 (Suppl. 1), S80–S82.
23. UKPDS Group. (1998). Intensive blood-glucose control with sulfonylureas or insulin compared with conventional treatment and risk of complications in patients with type 2 diabetes (UKPDS 33). *Lancet* 352, 837–853.
24. Shichiri M., Kishikquq H., Ohkubo Y., Wake N. (2000). Long-term results of Kumamoto Study on optimal diabetes control in type 2 diabetes patients. *Diabetes Care* 23 (Suppl. 2), B21–B29.
25. American Diabetes Association. (2000). Nutrition recommendations and principles for people with diabetes mellitus (Position Statement). *Diabetes Care* 23 (Suppl. 1), S43–S46.
26. Gillespie S., Kulkairni K., Daly A. (1998). Using carbohydrate counting in diabetes clinical practice. *Journal of the American Dietetic Association* 98, 897–905.
27. Markovic T.P., Jenkins A.B., Campbell L.U., Furhler S.M., Kraeger E.W., Chisholm D.J. (1998). The determinants of glycemic responses to diet restriction and weight loss and obesity in NIDDM. *Diabetes Care* 21, 687–694.
28. Grundy S.M., Panel Chair. (2001). Third Report of the National Cholesterol Education Program (NCEP) Expert Panel on Detection, Evaluation, and Treatment of High Blood Cholesterol in Adults (Adult Treatment Panel III). (NIH Publication No. 01-3670.) Bethesda, MD: National Institutes of Health.

29. American Diabetes Association. (2000). Diabetes mellitus and exercise. *Diabetes Care* 23 (Suppl. 1), S50–S54.

30. Lebovitz H.E. (1999). Insulin secretogogues: Old and new. *Diabetes Reviews* 7, 139–153.

31. Vaaler S. (2000). Optimal glycemic control in type 2 diabetes patients. *Diabetes Care* 23 (Suppl. 2), B30.

32. Mudalion S., Heniz R.R. (1999). Combination therapy for type 2 diabetes. *Endocrine Practice* 5, 208–219.

33. Bell D.S.H., Ouolle F. (2000). How long can insulin therapy be avoided in the patient with type 2 diabetes mellitus by use of combination metformin and a sulfonylurea. *Endocrine Practice* 6, 293–295.

34. Schoonjans J., Auwerx J. (2000). Thiazolidinediones: An update. *Lancet* 355, 1008–1010.

35. Flier J.S. (2001). The missing link in diabetes. *Nature* 409, 292–293.

36. Parulkar A.A., Pendergrass M.L., Granda-Ayla R., Lee T.R., Fonseca V.A. (2001). Nonhypoglycemic effects of thiazolidinediones. *Annals of Internal Medicine* 134, 61–71.

37. American Diabetes Association. (2000). Continuous subcutaneous insulin infusion. *Diabetes Care* 23 (Suppl. 1), S90.

38. American Diabetes Association. (2000). Pancreas transplantation for patients with type 1 diabetes. *Diabetes Care* 23 (Suppl. 1), S85.

39. Shapiro J., Lakey J., Ryan E., Korbutt G., Toth E., Warnock G., Knereman N., Rajotte R. (2000). Islet transplantation with type 1 diabetes mellitus using glucocorticoid-free immunosuppressive regimen. *New England Journal of Medicine* 343, 230–238.

40. Kitabachi A.E., Wall B.M. (1995). Diabetic ketoacidosis. *Medical Clinics of North America* 79, 9–35.

41. Kitabachi A.E., Umpierrez G.E., Murphy M.B., Barrett E.J., Kreisberg R.A., Malone J.I., Wall B.M. (2001). Management of hyperglycemic crisis in patients with diabetes. *Diabetes Care* 24, 131–153.

42. Cryer P.E., Fisher J.N., Shamoon H. (1994). Hypoglycemia. *Diabetes Care* 17, 734–755.

43. Birrer R.B. (2000). The many facets of hypoglycemia. *Emergency Medicine* 3, 63–77.

44. Bolli G.B., Fanelli C.G. (1995). Unawareness of hypoglycemia. *New England Journal of Medicine* 333, 1771–1772.

45. Somogyi M. (1957). Exacerbation of diabetes in excess insulin action. *American Journal of Medicine* 26, 169–191.

46. Bolli G.B., Gotterman I.S., Campbell P.J. (1984). Glucose counterregulation and waning of insulin in the Somogyi phenomenon (posthypoglycemic hyperglycemia). *New England Journal of Medicine* 311, 1214–1219.

47. Bolli G.B., Gerich J.E. (1984). The dawn phenomenon: A common occurrence in both non-insulin and insulin dependent diabetes mellitus. *New England Journal of Medicine* 310, 746–750.

48. Strowling S.M., Raskin P. (1995). Glycemic control and complications of diabetes. *Diabetes Reviews* 3, 337–357.

49. Klein R., Klein, B.E.K., Moss S.E. (1996). Relation of glycemic control to diabetic microvascular complications in diabetes mellitus. *Annals of Internal Medicine* 124, 90–96.

50. Estacio R.O., Jeffero B.W., Gifford N., Schrier R.W. (2000). Effect of blood pressure control on diabetic neovascular complications in patients with hypertension and type 2 diabetes. *Diabetes Care* 23 (Suppl. 2), B54–B64.

51. The Diabetes Control and Complications Trial Research Group. (1993). The effect of intensified treatment of diabetes on the development and progression of long-term complications in insulin-dependent diabetes mellitus. *New England Journal of Medicine* 329, 955–977.

52. Stratton I.M., Adler A.I., Neil H.A., Mathews D.R., Manley S.E., Cull C.S., Hadden S., Turner R.C., Holman R.R. (2000). Association of glycaemia with macrovascular and microvascular complications in type 2 diabetes (UKPDS 35) Group: Prospective observational study. *British Medical Journal* 321, 405–412.

53. Said G. (1996). Diabetic neuropathy: An update. *Neurology* 243, 431–440.

54. Vinik A.I., Milicevik Z. (1996). Recent advances in the diagnosis and treatment of diabetic neuropathy. *Endocrinologist* 6, 443–461.

55. Dejaard A. (1998). Pathophysiology and treatment of diabetic neuropathy. *Diabetic Medicine* 15, 97.

56. Vinik A.I. (1999). Diabetic neuropathy: Pathogenesis and therapy. *American Journal of Medicine* 107 (Suppl. 2B), 17S–26S.

57. Spoilett G.R. (1999). Assessment and management of erectile dysfunction in men with diabetes. *Diabetes Educator* 25 (1), 65–73.

58. Lipshultz L.I. (1999). Treatment of erectile dysfunction in men. *Journal of the American Medical Association* 281, 465–466.

59. American Diabetes Association. (2000). Diabetic nephropathy. *Diabetes Care* 23 (Suppl. 1), S69–S72.

60. Renal Data System. (1998, April). *USRDS 1998 annual data report*. NIH publication 98:3176. Bethesda, MD: National Institute of Diabetes and Digestive and Kidney Diseases.

61. Ritz E., Orth S.R. (1999). Nephropathy in patients with type 2 diabetes mellitus. *New England Journal of Medicine* 341, 1127–1133.

62. Krolewski A.S., Laffel L.M.B., Krolewski M., et al. (1995). Glycosylated hemoglobin and the risk of microalbuminemia in patients with insulin-dependent diabetes mellitus. *New England Journal of Medicine* 332, 1251–1255.

63. American Diabetes Association. (2000). Diabetic retinopathy. *Diabetes Care* 23 (Suppl. 1), S73–S76.

64. Ferris F.L., Davis M.D., Aiello L.M. (1999). Treatment of diabetic retinopathy. *New England Journal of Medicine* 341, 667–678.

65. Aiello L.P., Gardner T.W., King G.L., Blankenship G., Cavallerano J.D., Ferris F.L. III, Klein R. (1998). Diabetic retinopathy (Technical Review). *Diabetes Care* 21, 143–156.

66. Chen Y.-D.I., Reaven G.M. (1997). Insulin resistance and atherosclerosis. *Diabetes Reviews* 5, 331–342.

67. American Diabetes Association. (2000). Preventative foot care in people with diabetes. *Diabetes Care* 23 (Suppl. 1), S55–S56.

68. (2000). A simple screen for diabetic foot neuropathy. *Emergency Medicine* 4, 23–25.

69. Levin M.E. (1995). Preventing amputations in patients with diabetes. *Diabetes Care* 18, 1384–1394.

70. Joshi N., Caputo G.M., Weitekamp M.R., Karchmer A.W. (1999). Infections in patients with diabetes mellitus. *New England Journal of Medicine* 341, 1906–1912.

Genitourinary and Reproductive Function

There is a long history of misunderstanding and myths about human reproduction, especially the female reproductive system. Early on, the uterus was deemed the most important structure of the female reproductive anatomy. One of the first representations of the uterus appears in ancient Egyptian hieroglyphs (c. 2900 BC). Its importance was a direct result of the understanding that it was from the uterus that a child was born. That a woman was the carrier of the next generation was enough to establish her importance to society. However, society also imposed harsh restrictions on women that made it difficult, if not impossible, for further understanding. Until the Renaissance, custom and manners dictated that a woman's body could not be represented unless it was fully clothed.

To a regrettable extent, the associations made in ancient times that surmised a destiny for women based on the anatomy peculiar to their sex still affect how women are viewed today. The Greek philosopher Plato (427?–347? BC) postulated that the unused womb became "indignant" and wandered around the body, inhibiting the body's "spirits," or life force, and causing disease. The reasonings of Aristotle (384–322 BC) were equally fanciful. It was he, believing as others of the time did that women were irrational and prone to emotional outbursts, who provided the nomenclature for the womb, naming it *hystera* (ustera). Their concept that emotional excitability or instability was the domain of women is confirmed by another word that was coined by the Greeks: hysteria.

Chapter 42

Structure and Function of the Male Reproductive System

The male genitourinary system is composed of the paired gonads, or testes, genital ducts, accessory organs, and penis. The dual function of the testes is to produce male sex androgens (*i.e.*, male sex hormones), mainly testosterone, and spermatozoa (*i.e.*, male germ cells). The internal accessory organs produce the fluid constituents of semen, and the ductile system aids in the storage and transport of spermatozoa. The penis functions in urine elimination and sexual function. This chapter focuses on the structure of the male reproductive system, spermatogenesis and control of male reproductive function, neural control of sexual function, and changes in function that occur at puberty and as a result of the aging process.

Structure of the Male Reproductive System

After you have completed this section of the chapter, you should be able to meet the following objectives:

✦ Characterize the embryonic development of the male reproductive organs and genitalia
✦ Describe the structure and function of the testes and scrotum, the genital ducts, accessory organs, and penis

EMBRYONIC DEVELOPMENT

The sex of a person is determined at the time of fertilization by the sex chromosomes. In the early stages of embryonic development, the tissues from which the male and female reproductive organs develop are undifferentiated. Until approximately the seventh week of gestation, it is impossible to determine whether the embryo is male or female unless the chromosomes are studied. Until this time, the male and female genital tracts consist of two wolffian ducts, from which the male genitalia develop, and two müllerian ducts, from which the female genital structures develop. During this period of gestation, the gonads (*i.e.*, ovaries and testes) also are undifferentiated.

Between the sixth and eighth weeks of gestation, the testes begin development under the influence of the Y chromosome. During this time, the testicular cells of the male embryo begin producing an antimüllerian hormone and testosterone. The antimüllerian hormone inhibits development of the female genital organ from the müllerian ducts. Testosterone stimulates the wolffian ducts to develop into the epididymis, vas deferens, and seminal vesicles. Testosterone also is the precursor of a third hormone, dihydrotestosterone, which functions in the formation of the male urethra, prostate, and external genitalia. In the absence of testosterone, a male embryo with an XY chromosomal pattern develops female genitalia.

Testicular development and the embryonic production of testosterone require a Y chromosome. Gonadal sex is determined by a testis-determining gene (or genes) located on the short arm of the Y chromosome. In the presence of the testis-determining gene, the embryonic gonads develop into testes, and in its absence, the gonads develop into ovaries.

TESTES AND SCROTUM

The testes, or male gonads, are two egg-shaped structures located outside the abdominal cavity in the scrotum. Embryologically, the testes develop in the abdominal cavity and then descend through the inguinal canal into a pouch of peritoneum (which becomes the tunica vaginalis) in the scrotum during the seventh to ninth months of fetal life. As they descend, the testes pull their arteries, veins, lymphatics, nerves, and conducting excretory ducts with them. These structures are encased by the cremaster muscle and layers of fascia that constitute the spermatic cord. The descent of the testes is thought to be mediated by testosterone, which is active during this stage of development. After descent of the testes, the inguinal canal closes almost completely. Failure of this canal to close predisposes to the development of an inguinal hernia later in life.

The testes are enclosed in a double-layered membrane, the tunica vaginalis, which is derived embryologically from the abdominal peritoneum (Fig. 42-1). An outer covering, the tunica albuginea, is a tough, white, fibrous sheath that resembles the sclera of the eye. The tunica albuginea protects the testes and gives them their ovoid shape. The

cremaster muscles, which are bands of skeletal muscle arising from the internal oblique muscles of the trunk, elevate the testes. The testes receive their arterial blood supply from the long testicular arteries, which branch from the aortic artery. The testicular veins, which drain the testes, arise from a venous network called the *pampiniform plexus* that surrounds the testicular artery. The testes are innervated by fibers from both divisions of the autonomic nervous system. Associated sensory nerves transmit pain impulses, resulting in excruciating pain, especially when the testes are hit forcibly.

The scrotum, which houses the testes, is made up of a thin outer layer of skin that forms rugae, or folds, and is continuous with the perineum and outer skin of the groin. Under the outer skin lies a thin layer of fascia and smooth muscle (*i.e.*, dartos muscle). This layer contains a septum that separates the two testes. The dartos muscle responds to changes in temperature. When it is cold, the muscle contracts, bringing the testes closer to the body, and the scrotum becomes shorter and heavily wrinkled. When it is warmer, the muscle relaxes, allowing the scrotum to fall away from the body.

The location of the testes in the scrotum is important for sperm production, which is optimal at 2°C to 3°C below body temperature. Two systems maintain the temperature of the testes at a level consistent with sperm production. One is the pampiniform plexus of testicular veins that surround the testicular artery. This plexus absorbs heat from the arterial blood, cooling it as it enters the testes. The other is the cremaster muscles, which respond to decreases in testicular temperature by moving the testes closer to the body. Prolonged exposure to elevated temperatures, as a result of

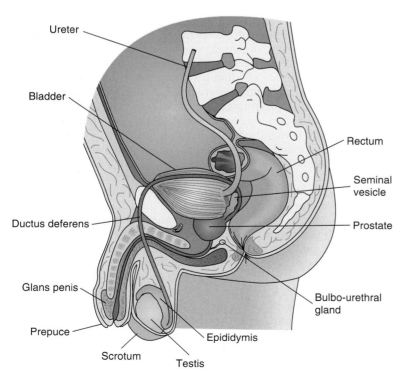

FIGURE 42-1 The structures of the male reproductive system, including the testes, the scrotum, and the excretory ducts. (Chaffee E.E., Lytle I.M. [1990]. *Basic physiology and anatomy* [4th ed.]. Philadelphia: J.B. Lippincott)

Labels on figure: Ureter, Bladder, Ductus deferens, Glans penis, Prepuce, Scrotum, Testis, Epididymis, Bulbo-urethral gland, Prostate, Seminal vesicle, Rectum

prolonged fever or the dysfunction of thermoregulatory mechanisms, can impair spermatogenesis. Some tight-fitting undergarments hold the testes against the body and are thought to contribute to a decrease in sperm counts and infertility by interfering with the thermoregulatory function of the scrotum. Cryptorchidism, the failure of the testes to descend into the scrotum, also exposes the testes to the higher temperature of the body.

GENITAL DUCT SYSTEM

Internally, the testes are composed of several hundred compartments or lobules (Fig. 42-2). Each lobule contains one or more coiled seminiferous tubules. These tubules are the site of sperm production. As the tubules lead into the efferent ducts, the seminiferous tubules become the rete testis. From the rete testis, 10,000 to 20,000 efferent ducts emerge to join the epididymis, which is the final site for sperm maturation. Because the spermatozoa are not motile at this stage of development, peristaltic movements of the ductal walls of the epididymis aid in their movement. The spermatozoa continue their migration through the ductus deferens, also called the *vas deferens*. The ampulla of the vas deferens serves as a storage reservoir for sperm. Sperm are stored in the ampulla until they are released through the penis during ejaculation (Fig. 42-3). Spermatozoa can be stored in the genital ducts for as long as 42 days and still maintain their fertility. Surgical disconnection of the vas deferens in the scrotal area (*e.g.*, vasectomy) serves as an effective method of male contraception. Because sperm are stored in the ampulla, men can remain fertile for 4 to 5 weeks after performance of a vasectomy.

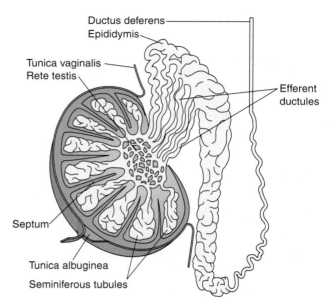

FIGURE 42-2 The parts of the testes and epididymis. (Chaffee E.E., Lytle I.M. [1990]. *Basic physiology and anatomy* [4th ed.]. Philadelphia: J.B. Lippincott)

ACCESSORY ORGANS

The male accessory organs consist of the seminal vesicles, the prostate gland, and the bulbourethral glands. Spermatozoa are transported through the reproductive structures by movement of the seminal fluid, which is combined with secretions from the genital ducts and accessory organs. The spermatozoa plus the secretions from the genital ducts

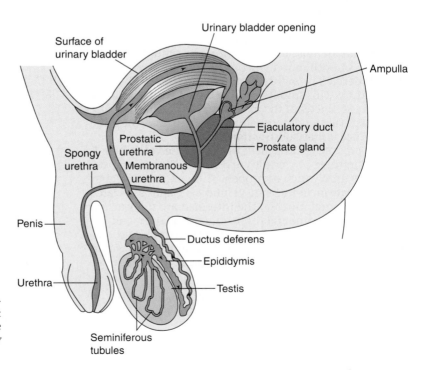

FIGURE 42-3 The excretory ducts of the male reproductive system and the path that sperm follows as it leaves the testis and travels to the urethra. (Chaffee E.E., Lytle I.M. [1990]. *Basic physiology and anatomy* [4th ed.]. Philadelphia: J.B. Lippincott)

and accessory organs make up the semen (from the Latin word meaning *seed*).

The seminal vesicles consist of two highly tortuous tubes that secrete fluid for the semen. Each of the paired seminal vesicles is lined with secretory epithelium containing an abundance of fructose, prostaglandins, and several other proteins. The fructose secreted by the seminal vesicles provides the energy for sperm motility. The prostaglandins are thought to assist in fertilization by making the cervical mucus more receptive to sperm and by causing reverse peristaltic contractions in the uterus and fallopian tubes to move the sperm toward the ovaries.

Each seminal vesicle joins its corresponding vas deferens to form the ejaculatory duct, which enters the posterior part of the prostate and continues through until it ends in the prostatic portion of the urethra. During the emission phase of coitus, each vesicle empties fluid into the ejaculatory duct, adding bulk to the semen. Approximately 70% of the ejaculate originates in the seminal vesicles.

The prostate is a fibromuscular and glandular organ lying just inferior to the bladder. The prostate gland secretes a thin, milky, alkaline fluid containing citric acid, calcium, acid phosphate, a clotting enzyme, and a profibrinolysin. During ejaculation, the capsule of the prostate contracts, and the added fluid increases the bulk of the semen. Both vaginal secretions and the fluid from the vas deferens are strongly acidic. Because sperm mobilization occurs at a pH of 6.0 to 6.5, the alkaline nature of the prostatic secretions is essential for successful fertilization of the ovum. The bulbourethral or Cowper's glands lie on either side of the membranous urethra and secrete an alkaline mucus, which further aids in neutralizing acids from the urine that remain in the urethra.

The prostate gland also functions in the elimination of urine and consists of a thin, fibrous capsule that encloses the circularly oriented smooth muscle fibers and collagenous tissue that surround the urethra where it joins the bladder. The segment of urethra that traverses the prostate gland is called the *prostatic urethra*. It is lined by a thin, longitudinal layer of smooth muscle that is continuous with the bladder wall. The smooth muscle incorporated with the prostate gland is derived primarily from the longitudinal bladder musculature. This smooth muscle represents the true involuntary sphincter of the male posterior urethra. Because the prostate surrounds the urethra, enlargement of the gland can produce urinary obstruction.

The prostate gland is made up of many secretory glands arranged in three concentric areas surrounding the prostatic urethra, into which they open. The component glands of the prostate include the small mucosal glands associated with the urethral mucosa, the intermediate submucosal glands that lie peripheral to the mucosal glands, and the large main prostatic glands that are situated toward the outside of the gland. It is the overgrowth of the mucosal glands that causes benign prostatic hyperplasia in older men (see Chapter 43).

PENIS

The penis is the external genital organ through which the urethra passes. Anatomically, the external penis consists of a shaft that ends in a tip called the *glans* (Fig. 42-4). The

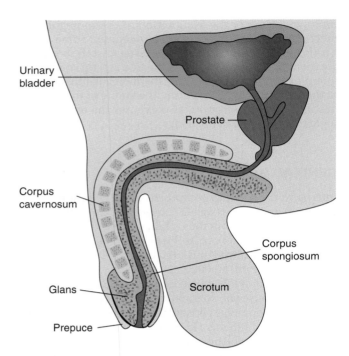

FIGURE 42-4 Sagittal section of the penis, showing the prepuce, glans, corpus cavernosum, and corpus spongiosum.

loose skin of the penis shaft folds to cover the glans, forming the prepuce, or foreskin. The glans of the penis contains many sensory nerves, making this the most sensitive portion of the penile shaft. It is the foreskin that is removed during circumcision.

The cylindrical body or shaft of the penis is composed of three masses of erectile tissue held together by fibrous strands and covered with a thin layer of skin. The two lateral masses of tissue are called the *corpora cavernosa*. The third, ventral mass is called the *corpus spongiosum*. The corpora cavernosa and corpus spongiosum are cavernous sinuses that normally are relatively empty but become engorged with blood during penile erection.

In summary, the male reproductive system consists of a pair of gonads (*i.e.*, testes), a system of excretory ducts (*i.e.*, seminiferous tubules and efferent ducts), the accessory organs (*i.e.*, epididymis, seminal vesicles, prostate, and Cowper's glands), and the penis. The sex of a person is determined by the sex chromosomes at the time of fertilization. During the seventh week of gestation, the XY chromosome pattern in the male embryo is responsible for the development of the testes, with the subsequent production of testosterone and testosterone-stimulated development of the internal and external male genital structures. Before this period of embryonic development, the tissues from which the male and female reproductive structures develop are undifferentiated. In the absence of testosterone production, the male embryo with an XY chromosomal pattern develops female genitalia.

Male Reproductive System

➤ The male genitourinary system functions in both urine elimination and reproduction.

➤ The testes function in both production of male germ cells (spermatogenesis) and secretion of the male sex hormone, testosterone.

➤ The ductile system (epididymides, vas deferens, and ejaculatory ducts) transports and stores sperm, and assists in their maturation; and the accessory glands (seminal vesicles, prostate gland, and bulbourethral glands) prepare the sperm for ejaculation.

➤ The urethra, which is enclosed in the penis, is the terminal portion of the male genitourinary system. Because it conveys both urine and semen, it serves both urinary and reproductive functions.

Spermatogenesis and Hormonal Control of Male Reproductive Function

After you have completed this section of the chapter, you should be able to meet the following objectives:

✦ Describe the process of spermatogenesis
✦ State the functions of testosterone
✦ Draw a diagram illustrating the secretion, site of action, and feedback control of gonadotropin-releasing hormone, luteinizing hormone, and follicle-stimulating hormone
✦ Describe the function of follicle-stimulating hormone in terms of spermatogenesis

During childhood, the gonads remain essentially quiescent. At puberty, the male gonads and testes begin to mature and to carry out spermatogenesis and hormone production. At approximately 10 or 11 years of age, the adenohypophysis, or anterior pituitary, under the control of the hypothalamus begins to secrete the gonadotropins that stimulate testicular function and cause the interstitial cells of Leydig to begin producing testosterone. Approximately the same time, hormonal stimulation induces mitotic activity of the germ cells that develop in sperm. After cell maturation has begun, the testes begin to enlarge rapidly as the individual tubules grow. Full maturity and spermatogenesis usually are attained by 15 or 16 years of age.

SPERMATOGENESIS

Spermatogenesis refers to the generation of spermatozoa or sperm. It begins at an average age of 13 years and continues throughout the reproductive years of a man's life. Spermatogenesis occurs in the seminiferous tubules of the testes. These tubules, if placed end to end, would measure approximately 750 feet. The outer layer of the seminiferous tubules is made up of connective tissue and smooth muscle; the inner lining is composed of Sertoli's cells, which are embedded with sperm in various stages of development. Sertoli's cells secrete a special fluid that contains nutrients to bathe and nourish the immature germ cells; they provide digestive enzymes that play a role in spermiation (*i.e.*, converting the spermatocytes to sperm); and they are thought to play a role in shaping the head and tail of the sperm. Sertoli's cells also secrete several hormones, including müllerian inhibitory factor, which is secreted by the testes during fetal life to inhibit development of fallopian tubes; estradiol, the principal feminizing sex hormone, which seems to be required in the male for spermatogenesis; and inhibin, which controls the function of Sertoli's cells through feedback inhibition of follicle-stimulating hormone (FSH) from the anterior pituitary gland.

In the first stage of spermatogenesis, small and unspecialized diploid germinal cells located immediately adjacent to the tubular wall, called the *spermatogonia*, undergo rapid mitotic division and provide a continuous source of new germinal cells. As these cells multiply, the more mature spermatogonia divide into two daughter cells, which grow and become the primary spermatocytes—the precursors of sperm. Over several weeks, large primary spermatocytes divide by a process called *meiosis* to form two smaller secondary spermatocytes. Each of the secondary spermatocytes divides to form two spermatids, each containing 23 chromosomes. Meiosis is a unique form of cell division that occurs only in the gonads. It consists of two consecutive nuclear divisions with formation of four daughter cells, each containing a single set of 23 chromosomes rather than a pair of 46 chromosomes, as occurs during mitotic cell division in other body cells (see Chapter 6).

The spermatid elongates into a spermatozoon, or mature sperm cell, with a head and tail (Fig. 42-5). The outside of the anterior two thirds of the head, called the *acrosome*, contains enzymes necessary for penetration and fertilization of the ovum. The to-and-fro flagellar motion of the tail imparts movement to the sperm. The energy for this process is supplied by the mitochondria in the tail. Normal sperm move in a straight line at a velocity of 1 to 4 mm/minute. This allows them to move through the female genital tract. When the sperm grow to full size, they move to the epididymis to mature further and gain mobility. A small quantity of sperm can be stored in the epididymis, but most are stored in the vas deferens or the ampulla of the vas deferens. With excessive sexual activity, storage may be no longer than a few days. The sperm can live for many weeks in the male genital tract; however, in the female genital tract, their life expectancy is 1 or 2 days. Frozen sperm have been preserved for years.

The entire process of spermatogenesis takes approximately 60 to 70 days. The sperm count in a normal ejaculate is approximately 100 million to 400 million. Infertility may occur when insufficient numbers of motile, healthy sperm are present.

HORMONAL CONTROL OF MALE REPRODUCTIVE FUNCTION

Testosterone and Other Male Sex Hormones
The male sex hormones are called *androgens*. The testes secrete several male sex hormones, including *testosterone, di-*

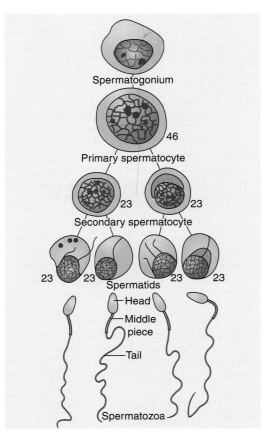

FIGURE 42-5 The various stages of spermatogenesis. (Chaffee E.E., Lytle I.M. [1990]. *Basic physiology and anatomy* [4th ed.]. Philadelphia: J.B. Lippincott)

---

hydrotestosterone, and *androstenedione.* Testosterone, which is the most abundant of these hormones, is considered the main testicular hormone. The adrenal cortex also produces androgens, although in much smaller quantities (<5% of the total male androgens) than those produced in the testes. The testes also secrete small quantities of estradiol and estrone.

Testosterone is produced and secreted by the interstitial Leydig's cells in the testes. It is metabolized in the liver and excreted by the kidneys. In the bloodstream, testosterone exists in a free (unbound) or a bound form. The bound form is attached to plasma proteins, including albumin and the sex hormone–binding protein produced by the liver. Only approximately 2% of circulating testosterone is unbound and therefore able to enter the cell and exert its metabolic effects. Much of the testosterone that becomes fixed to the tissues is converted to dihydrotestosterone, especially in certain target tissues such as the prostate gland. Some of the actions of testosterone depend on this conversion, whereas others do not. Testosterone also can be aromatized or converted to estradiol in the peripheral tissues.

Testosterone exerts a variety of biologic effects in the male (Chart 42-1). In the male embryo, testosterone is essential for the appropriate differentiation of the internal and external genitalia, and it is necessary for descent of the testes in the fetus. Testosterone is essential to the development of primary and secondary male sex characteristics during puberty and for the maintenance of these characteristics during adult life. It causes growth of pubic, chest, and facial hair; it produces changes in the larynx that result in the male bass voice; and it increases the thickness of the skin and increases the activity of the sebaceous glands, predisposing to acne.

All or almost all of the actions of testosterone and other androgens result from increased protein synthesis in target tissues. Androgens function as anabolic agents in males and females to promote metabolism and musculoskeletal growth. Testosterone and the androgens have a great effect on the development of increasing musculature during puberty, with boys averaging approximately a 50% increase in muscle mass compared with girls.

Androgens and Athletic Performance. Because of the great effect that testosterone and other androgens have on body musculature, synthetic androgens sometimes are used by athletes to improve their appearance and muscle performance. Frequently, these agents are taken in doses that far exceed physiologic levels. This practice has been strongly discouraged because of potential harmful effects. Among the undesired or harmful effects of supraphysiologic doses of androgens are acne, decreased testicular size, and azoospermia. These effects may persist for months after use of the agents have ceased. Because testosterone can be aromatized to estradiol in the peripheral tissues, androgens can induce mild gynecomastia. The undesired effects of androgens depend on the type and dose administered. Alkylated androgens at high doses can cause hepatocellular and intrahepatic cholestasis that occasionally results in severe jaundice and liver damage. Alkylated androgens also may lower high-density lipoprotein (HDL) and may increase low-density lipoprotein (LDL) levels. The behavioral effects of anabolic-androgenic steroids also have received attention. Increased and decreased libido, increased aggression, and a variety of psychotic symptoms have been described. In preadolescents who have not yet achieved their full height, increased androgen levels can cause premature close of the epiphyseal growth plates.

Recently, attention has focused on oral androstenedione and dehydroepiandrosterone (DHEA) products that are available over the counter and often are marketed as a safe natural alternative to androgens for building muscle. Androstenedione and DHEA exert only weak androgenic activity, but their main purpose is to act as a key precursor for testosterone after peripheral conversion. For example, androstenedione normally is produced by the adrenal gland and converted to testosterone through the action of 17β-hydroxysteroid dehydrogenase, which is found in most body tissues. However, the interconversion of androstenedione is complex. In addition to being a precursor for testosterone, androstenedione may be converted into estrogens directly. The testosterone that is produced also can be converted to estradiol. A randomized, controlled study measured the short-term effect of androstenedione supplementation on serum hormone levels and muscle development during an 8-week resistance training program in young normotestosterogenic men. The results from this study indicated that androstenedione supplementation did not significantly increase serum testosterone levels or skeletal muscle adaptation. It did, however, elevate serum levels of estrone and estradiol, suggesting that a significant proportion of the ingested androstenedione underwent conversion to these estrogens. Although this study was carefully controlled in terms of drug dose, it is known that many athletes take doses that exceed the clinically recommended amount. Whether large doses of these over-the-counter products can produce some of the serious side effects seen with standard anabolic steroids is largely unknown.

Action of the Hypothalamic and Anterior Pituitary Hormones

The hypothalamus and the anterior pituitary gland play an essential role in promoting spermatogenic activity in the testes and maintaining the endocrine function of the testes by means of the gonadotropic hormones. The synthesis and release of the gonadotropic hormones from the pituitary gland are regulated by gonadotropin-releasing factor, which is synthesized by the hypothalamus and secreted into the hypothalamohypophysial portal circulation (Fig. 42-6).

Two gonadotropic hormones are secreted by the pituitary gland: FSH and luteinizing hormone (LH). In the male, LH also is called *interstitial cell-stimulating hormone*. The production of testosterone by the interstitial cells of Leydig is regulated by LH (see Fig. 42-6). FSH binds selectively to Sertoli's cells surrounding the seminiferous tubules, where it functions in the initiation of spermatogenesis. Under the influence of FSH, Sertoli's cells produce androgen-binding protein, plasminogen activator, and inhibin. Androgen-binding protein binds testosterone and serves as a carrier of testosterone in Sertoli's cells and as a storage site for testosterone. Although FSH is necessary for the initiation of spermatogenesis, full maturation of the spermatozoa requires

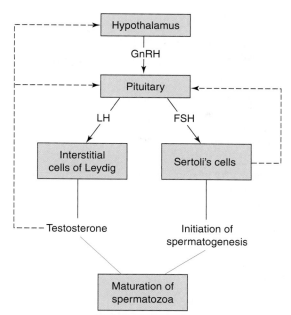

FIGURE 42-6 Hypothalamic-pituitary feedback control of spermatogenesis and testosterone levels in the male.

testosterone. Androgen-binding protein also serves as a carrier of testosterone from the testes to the epididymis. Plasminogen activator, which converts plasminogen to plasmin, functions in the final detachment of mature spermatozoa from Sertoli's cells.

Circulating levels of the gonadotropic hormones are regulated in a negative feedback manner by testosterone. High levels of testosterone suppress LH secretion through a direct action on the pituitary and an inhibitory effect on the hypothalamus. FSH is thought to be inhibited by a substance called *inhibin*, produced by Sertoli's cells. Inhibin suppresses FSH release from the pituitary gland. The pituitary gonadotropic hormones and Sertoli's cells in the testes form a classic negative feedback loop in which FSH stimulates inhibin and inhibin suppresses FSH. Unlike the cyclic hormonal pattern in the female, in the male, FSH, LH, and testosterone secretion and spermatogenesis occur at relatively unchanging rates during adulthood.

In summary, the function of the male reproductive system is under the negative feedback control of the hypothalamus and the anterior pituitary gonadotropic hormones FSH and LH. Spermatogenesis is initiated by FSH, and the production of testosterone is regulated by LH. Testosterone, the major male sex hormone, is produced by the interstitial Leydig's cells in the testes. In addition to its role in the differentiation of the internal and external genitalia in the male embryo, testosterone is essential for the development of secondary male characteristics during puberty, the maintenance of these characteristics during adult life, and spermatozoa maturation.

Neural Control of Sexual Function and Aging Changes

After you have completed this section of the chapter, you should be able to meet the following objectives:

✦ Describe the autonomic nervous system control of erection, emission, and ejaculation
✦ Describe changes in the male reproductive system that occur with aging

In the male, the stages of the sexual act involve erection, emission, ejaculation, and detumescence. The physiology of the sexual act involves a complex interaction between spinal cord reflexes, higher neural centers, the vascular system, and the endocrine system.

NEURAL CONTROL

The most important source of impulse stimulation for initiating the male sexual act is the glans penis, which contains a highly organized sensory system. Afferent impulses from sensory receptors in the glans penis pass through the pudendal nerve to ascending fibers in the spinal cord by way of the sacral plexus. Stimulation of other perineal areas, such as the anal epithelium, the scrotum, and the testes, can transmit signals to higher brain centers, such as the limbic system and cerebral cortex, through the cord, adding to sexual satisfaction.

The psychic element to sexual stimulation, such as thinking sexual thoughts, can cause erection and ejaculation. Although psychic involvement and higher-center functions contribute to the sex act, they are not necessary for sexual performance. Genital stimulation can produce erection and ejaculation in some men with complete transection of the spinal cord (see Chapter 49).

Erection involves the shunting of blood into the corpus cavernosum. It is controlled by the sympathetic, parasympathetic, and nonsympathetic-nonparasympathetic systems. Nitric oxide is the locally released nonsympathetic-nonparasympathetic mediator that produces relaxation of vascular smooth muscle. In the flaccid or detumescent state, sympathetic discharge through α-adrenergic receptors maintains contraction of the arteries that supply the penis and vascular sinuses of the corpora cavernosa and corpus spongiosum (Fig. 42-7). Parasympathetic stimulation produces erection by inhibiting sympathetic neurons that cause detumescence and by stimulating the release of nitric oxide to effect a rapid relaxation of the smooth muscle in the sinusoidal spaces of the corpus cavernosum. During sexual stimulation, parasympathetic impulses also cause the urethral and bulbourethral glands to secrete mucus to aid in lubrication. Parasympathetic innervation is effected through the pelvic nerve and sacral segments of the spinal cord. Sympathetic innervation exits the spinal cord at the L1 and L2 levels. Erectile dysfunction can be caused by disease or dysfunction of the brain, spinal cord, cavernous or pudendal nerves, or terminal nerve endings or receptors (see Chapter 43).

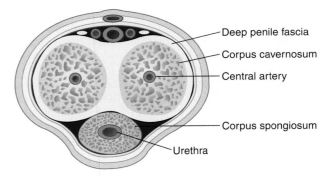

FIGURE 42-7 Erectile tissue of the penis.

Emission and ejaculation, which constitute the culmination of the male sexual act, are a function of the sympathetic nervous system. As with erection, emission and ejaculation are mediated through spinal cord reflexes. With increasing intensity of the sexual stimulus, reflex centers of the spinal cord begin to emit sympathetic impulses that leave the cord at the L1 and L2 level and pass through the hypogastric plexus to the genital organs to initiate emission, which is the forerunner of ejaculation. Emission causes the sperm to move from the epididymis to the urethra. Efferent impulses from the spinal cord produce contraction of smooth muscle in the vas deferens and ampulla that move sperm forward and close the internal urethral sphincter to prevent retrograde ejaculation into the bladder.

Ejaculation represents the expulsion of the sperm from the urethra. It involves contraction of the seminal vesicles and prostate gland, which add fluid to the ejaculate and propel it forward. Ejaculation is accompanied by contraction of the ischiocavernous and bulbocavernous muscles at the base of the penis. The filling of the internal urethra elicits signals that are transmitted through the pudendal nerves from the spinal cord, giving the sudden feeling of fullness of genital organs. Rhythmic increases in pressure in the urethra cause the semen to be propelled to the exterior, resulting in ejaculation. At the same time, rhythmic contractions of the pelvic and trunk muscles produce thrusting movements of the pelvis and penis, which help propel the ejaculate into the vagina.

The period of emission and ejaculation is called *male orgasm*. After ejaculation, erection ceases within 1 to 2 minutes. A man usually ejaculates approximately 2 to 5 mL of semen. The ejaculate may vary with frequency of intercourse. It is less with frequent ejaculation and may increase two to four times its normal amount during periods of abstinence. The semen that is ejaculated is 98% fluid and approximately 2% sperm.

The role of circulating androgens in sexual function remains unclear. It is apparent that sexual desire and performance depend on some threshold level of testosterone; however, this level varies from man to man. Studies of hypogonadal and castrated men show a variety of sexual behavior, ranging from complete loss of libido to normal sexual activity. It may be that the role of testosterone in male sexuality is in the area of sexual interest and motivation, with individual intrapsychic factors playing a significant role.

AGING CHANGES

Like other body systems, the male reproductive system undergoes degenerative changes as a result of the aging process; it becomes less efficient with age. The declining physiologic efficiency of male reproductive function occurs gradually and involves the endocrine, circulatory, and neuromuscular systems. Compared with the marked physiologic change in aging females, the changes in the aging male are more gradual and less drastic. Gonadal and reproductive failure usually are not related directly to age, because a man remains fertile into advanced age; 80- and 90-year-old men have been known to father children.

As the male ages, his reproductive system becomes measurably different in structure and function from that of the younger male. Male sex hormone levels, particularly of testosterone, decrease with age, with the decline starting later on the average than in women. The term *andropause* has been used to describe an ill-defined collection of symptoms in aging men, typically those older than 50 years, who may have a low androgen level. The sex hormones play a part in the structure and function of the reproductive system and other body systems from conception to old age; they affect protein synthesis, salt and water balance, bone growth, and cardiovascular function. Decreasing levels of testosterone affect sexual energy, muscle strength, and the genital tissues. The testes become smaller and lose their firmness. The seminiferous tubules, which produce spermatozoa, thicken and begin a degenerative process that finally inhibits sperm production, resulting in a decrease of viable spermatozoa. The prostate gland enlarges, and its contractions become weaker. The force of ejaculation decreases because of a reduction in the volume and viscosity of the seminal fluid. The seminal vesicle changes little from childhood to puberty. The pubertal increases in the fluid capacity of the gland remain throughout adulthood and decline after 60 years of age. After age 60 years, the walls of the seminal vesicles thin, the epithelium decreases, and the muscle layer is replaced by connective tissue. Age-related changes in the penis consist of fibrotic changes in the trabeculae in the corpus spongiosum, with progressive sclerotic changes in arteries and veins. Sclerotic changes also follow in the corpora cavernosa, with the condition becoming generalized in 55- to 60-year-old men.

As a sexual partner, the aging male exhibits some differences in responsiveness and activity from his younger counterpart. Masters and Johnson studied the significant aging changes in the physiology of the sex act. They observed that frequency of intercourse, intensity of sensation, speed of attaining erection, and force of ejaculation are all reduced.

Erectile dysfunction (see Chapter 43) in the elderly male often is directly related to the general physical condition of the person. Diseases that accompany aging can have direct bearing on male reproductive function. Various cardiovascular, respiratory, hormonal, neurologic, and hematologic disorders can be responsible for secondary impotence. For example, vascular disease affects male potency because it may impair blood flow to the pudendal arteries or their tributaries, resulting in loss of blood volume with subsequent poor distention of the vascular spaces of erectile tissue. Other diseases affecting potency include hypertension, diabetes, cardiac disease, and malignancies of the reproductive organs. In addition, certain medications can have an effect on sexual function.

One of the greatest inhibitors of sexual functioning in older men is the loss of self-esteem and the development of a negative self-image. The emphasis on youth pervades much of our society. The image of success for a man often involves qualities of masculinity and sexual attractiveness. When queried about success, men often mention such things as work, managing money well, participating in sports or other activities, discussing politics or world events, advising younger persons, and being attractive to women. When a man feels good about himself and expresses self-confidence, sexual attractiveness is communicated regardless of age. Many older men live in environments that are not sensitive to the importance of helping them maintain a positive self-image. Premature cessation of the aforementioned esteem-building activities can contribute to loss of libido and zest for life in the elderly man.

Testosterone and other synthetic androgens may be used in older males with low androgen levels to improve muscle strength and vigor. Preliminary studies of androgen replacement in aging males with low androgen levels show an increase in lean body mass and a decrease in bone turnover. Before testosterone replacement therapy is initiated, all men should be screened for prostate cancer. Testosterone is available as an injectable form that is administered every 2 to 3 weeks, or as a transdermal patch or gel. Side effects of replacement therapy may include acne, gynecomastia, and reduced HDL levels. It also may contribute to a worsening of sleep apnea in men who are troubled by this problem.

In summary, the sex act involves erection, emission, ejaculation, and detumescence. The physiology of these functions involves a complex interaction between autonomic-mediated spinal cord reflexes, higher neural centers, and the vascular system. Erection is mediated by the parasympathetic nervous system and emission and ejaculation by the sympathetic nervous system. Like other body systems, the male reproductive system undergoes changes as a result of the aging process. The changes occur gradually and involve parallel changes in endocrine, circulatory, and neuromuscular function. Testosterone levels decrease, the size and firmness of the testes decrease, sperm production declines, and the prostate gland enlarges. There usually is a decrease in frequency of intercourse, intensity of sensation, speed of attaining erection, and force of ejaculation. However, sexual thought, interest, and activity usually continue into old age.

Bibliography

Aboseif S.R., Lue T.F. (1988). Hemodynamics of penile erection. *Urologic Clinics of North America* 15, 1–7.

Braunstein G.D. (2001). Testes. In Greenspan F.S., Gardner D.G. (Eds.), *Basic and clinical endocrinology* (6th ed., pp. 422–452). New York: Lange Medical Books/McGraw-Hill.

Bagatell C.J., Bremner W.J. (1996). Androgens in men: Uses and abuses. *New England Journal of Medicine* 334, 707–714.

Guyton A.C., Hall J. (2000). *Textbook of medical physiology* (10th ed., pp. 916–928). Philadelphia: W.B. Saunders.

Herzog L.W., Alvarez S.R. (1986). The frequency of foreskin problems in uncircumcised children. *American Journal of Diseases of Children* 140, 254.

King D.S., Sharp R.L., Vukovich M.D., Reifenrath R.A., Uhl N.L., Parsons K.A. (1999). Effect of oral androstenedione on serum testosterone and adaptations to resistance training in young men. *Journal of the American Medical Association* 281, 202–228.

Lue T.F. (2000). Male sexual dysfunction. In Tanagho E.A., McAnnich J.W. (Eds.), *Smith's general urology* (15th ed., pp. 788–810). New York: Lange Medical Books/McGraw-Hill.

Masters W.H., Johnson V. (1970). *Human sexual inadequacy* (pp. 337–338). Boston: Little, Brown.

Merry B.J., Holehan A.M. (1994). Aging of the male reproductive system. In Timinas P.S. (Ed.), *Physiological basis of aging and geriatrics* (2nd ed., pp. 171–178). Boca Raton, FL: CRC Press.

Morley J.E., Perry H.M. (1999). Androgen deficiency in aging men. *Medical Clinics of North America* 83, 1279–1289.

Moore K.L., Persaud T.V.N. (1998). *The developing human: Clinically oriented embryology* (6th ed., pp. 323–330). Philadelphia: W.B. Saunders.

Rhoades R.A., Tanner G.A. (1996). *Medical physiology* (pp. 737–756). Boston: Little, Brown.

Tan R.S. (1997). Managing the andropause in aging men. *Clinical Geriatrics* 5 (10), 46–58.

Tanglio E.A. (2000). Embryology of the genitourinary system. In Tanagho E.A., McAnnich J.W. (Eds.), *Smith's general urology* (15th ed., pp. 17–28). New York: Lange Medical Books/McGraw-Hill.

Chapter 43

Alterations in Structure and Function of the Male Genitourinary System

The male genitourinary system is subject to structural defects, inflammation, and neoplasms, all of which can affect urine elimination, sexual function, and fertility. This chapter discusses disorders of the penis, the scrotum and testes, and the prostate.

Disorders of the Penis

After you have completed this section of the chapter, you should be able to meet the following objectives:

✦ State the difference between hypospadias and epispadias
✦ Cite the significance of phimosis
✦ Describe the anatomic changes that occur with Peyronie's disease
✦ Explain the physiology of penile erection and relate it to erectile dysfunction and priapism
✦ Describe the appearance of balanitis xerotica obliterans
✦ List the signs of penile cancer

The penis is the external male genital organ through which the urethra passes to the exterior of the body. It is involved in urinary and sexual function. Disorders of the penis include congenital and acquired defects, inflammatory conditions, and neoplasms.

CONGENITAL AND ACQUIRED DISORDERS

Hypospadias and Epispadias

Hypospadias and epispadias are congenital disorders of the penis resulting from embryologic defects in the development of the urethral groove and penile urethra (Fig. 43-1). In hypospadias, which affects approximately 1 in 300 male infants, the termination of the urethra is on the ventral surface of the penis.[1,2] The testes are undescended in 10% of boys born with hypospadias and chordee (*i.e.,* ventral bowing of the penis), and inguinal hernia also may accompany the disorder. In the newborn with severe hypospadias and cryptorchidism (undescended testes), the differential diagnosis should consider ambiguous genitalia and masculinization that is seen in females with congenital adrenal hyperplasia (see Chapter 40). Because many chromosomal aberrations result in ambiguity of the external genitalia, chromosomal studies often are recommended for male infants with hypospadias and cryptorchidism.[1]

Surgery is the treatment of choice for hypospadias.[1] Circumcision is avoided because the foreskin is used for surgical repair. Factors that influence the timing of surgical repair include anesthetic risk, penile size, and the psychological effects of the surgery on the child. In mild cases, the surgery is done for cosmetic reasons only. In more severe cases, repair becomes essential for normal sexual functioning and to

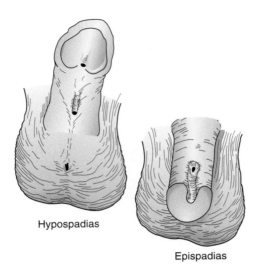

FIGURE 43-1 Hypospadias and epispadias.

prevent the psychological sequelae of having malformed genitalia. In contrast to the practices of several decades ago, when surgical repair often was delayed until the child was 2 to 6 years of age, surgical repair is now done between the ages of 6 to 12 months.

Epispadias, in which the opening of the urethra is on the dorsal surface of the penis, is a less common defect. Although epispadias may occur as a separate entity, it often is associated with exstrophy of the bladder, a condition in which the abdominal wall fails to cover the bladder. The treatment depends on the extent of the developmental defect.

Phimosis and Paraphimosis

Phimosis refers to a tightening of the prepuce or penile foreskin that prevents its retraction over the glans. Embryologically, the foreskin begins to develop during the eighth week of gestation as a fold of skin at the distal edge of the penis that eventually grows forward over the base of the glans.[2] By the 16th week of gestation, the prepuce and the glans are adherent. Only a small percentage of newborns have a fully retractable foreskin. With growth, a space develops between the glans and foreskin, and by 3 years of age, approximately 90% of male children have retractable foreskins.

Because the foreskin of many boys cannot be fully retracted in early childhood, it is important that the area be cleaned thoroughly. There is no need to retract the foreskin forcibly because this could lead to infection, scarring, or paraphimosis. As the child grows, the foreskin becomes retractable, and the glans and foreskin should be cleaned routinely. If symptomatic phimosis occurs after childhood, it can cause difficulty with voiding or sexual activity. Circumcision is then the treatment of choice.[3]

In a related condition called *paraphimosis*, the foreskin is so tight and constricted that it cannot cover the glans. A tight foreskin can constrict the blood supply to the glans and lead to ischemia and necrosis. Many cases of paraphimosis result from the foreskin being retracted for an extended period, as in the case of catheterized uncircumcised males.

Balanitis and Balanoposthitis

Balanitis is an acute or chronic inflammation of the glans penis. *Balanoposthitis* refers to inflammation of the glans and prepuce. It usually is encountered in males with phimosis or a large, redundant prepuce that interferes with cleanliness and predisposes to bacterial growth in the accumulated secretions and smegma (*i.e.*, debris from the desquamated epithelia). If left untreated, the condition may cause ulcerations of the mucosal surface of the glans; these ulcerations may lead to inflammatory scarring of the phimosis and further aggravate the condition.

Acute superficial balanoposthitis is characterized by erythema of the glans and prepuce. An exudate in the form of malodorous discharge may be present. Extension of the erythema and edema may result in phimosis. The condition may result from infection, trauma, or irritation. Infective balanoposthitis may be caused by a wide variety of organisms. Chlamydiae and mycoplasmas have been identified as causative organisms in this disease. The inflammatory reaction is nonspecific, and correct identification of the specific agent requires bacterial smears and cultures.

Balanitis xerotica obliterans is a chronic, sclerosing, atrophic process of the glans penis that occurs in uncircumcised males. It is clinically and histologically similar to the lichen sclerosus that is seen in females. Typically, the lesions consist of whitish plaques on the surface of the glans penis and the prepuce. The foreskin is thickened and fibrous and is not retractable. Treatment measures include circumcision and topical or intralesional injections of corticosteroids.[4]

Peyronie's Disease

Peyronie's disease involves a localized and progressive fibrosis of unknown origin that affects the tunica albuginea (*i.e.*, the tough, fibrous sheath that surrounds the corpora cavernosa) of the penis. It is named after Francois de la Peyronie, who, in 1743, described a patient who had "rosary beads of scar tissue to cause upward curvature of the penis during erection."[5] The disorder is characterized initially by an inflammatory process that results in dense fibrous plaque formation. The plaque usually is on the dorsal midline of the shaft, causing upward bowing of the shaft during erection (Fig. 43-2). Some men may develop scarring on both the dorsal and ventral aspects of the shaft, causing the penis to be straight but shortened or have a lateral bend.[5] The fibrous tissue prevents lengthening of the involved area during erection, making intercourse difficult and painful. The disease usually occurs in middle-aged or elderly men. Although the cause of the disorder is unknown, the dense microscopic plaques are consistent with findings of severe vasculitis.[6] Up to 47% of men with Peyronie's disease have another condition associated with fascial tissue fibrosis, such as Dupuytren's contracture (fibrosis of the palmar fascia).[5]

The manifestations of Peyronie's disease include painful erection, bent erection, and the presence of a hard mass at the site of fibrosis. Approximately two thirds of men complain of pain as a symptom. The pain is thought to be generated by inflammation of the adjacent fascial tissue and usually disappears as the inflammation resolves.

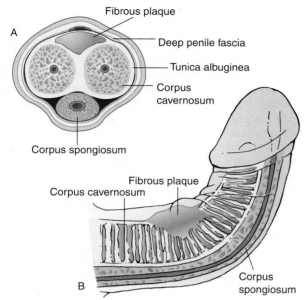

FIGURE 43-2 Peyronie's disease. (**A**) Penile cross-section showing plaque between the corpora. (**B**) Penile curvature.

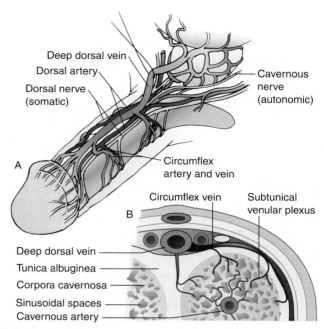

FIGURE 43-3 Anatomy and mechanism of penile erection. (**A**) Innervation and arterial and venous blood supply to penis. (**B**) Cross-section of the sinusoidal system of the corpora cavernosa.

During the first year or so after formation of the plaque, while the scar tissue is undergoing the process of remodeling, penile distortion may increase, remain static, or resolve and disappear completely.[5] The some cases, the scar tissue may progress to calcification and formation of bone-like tissue.

Diagnosis is based on history and physical examination. Doppler ultrasonography may be used to assess causation of the disorder. Although surgical intervention can be used to correct the disorder, it often is delayed, because in many cases the disorder is self-limiting.[6] Less invasive treatments include the administration of oral agents with antioxidant properties. Such agents include vitamin D, potassium aminobenzoate, and colchicine. Experimental intralesional treatments include corticosteroids, collagenase, and the calcium channel blocker, verapamil. Various modes of energy transfer, including ultrasound and short-wave diathermy, also have been used. At present, these methods have been inadequately studied and most have met with variable degrees of success.[5]

DISORDERS OF ERECTILE FUNCTION

Erection is a neurovascular process involving the autonomic nervous system, neurotransmitters and endothelial relaxing factors, the vascular smooth muscle of the arteries and veins supplying the penile tissue, and the trabecular smooth muscle of the sinusoids of the corpora cavernosa (Fig. 43-3). The penis is innervated by both the autonomic and somatic nervous systems. In the pelvis, the sympathetic and parasympathetic components of the autonomic nervous systems merge to form what are called the *cavernous nerves*.[7] Erection is under the control of parasympathetic nervous system, and ejaculation and detumescence (penile relaxation) are under

sympathetic nervous system control. Somatic innervation, which occurs through the pudendal nerve, is responsible for penile sensation and contraction and relaxation of the extracorporeal striated muscles (bulbocavernous and ischiocavernous).[7]

Penile erection is the first effect of male sexual stimulation, whether psychological or physical. It involves increased inflow of blood into the corpora cavernosa due to relaxation of the trabecular smooth muscle that surrounds the sinusoidal spaces and compression of the veins controlling outflow of blood from the venous plexus. Erection is mediated by parasympathetic impulses that pass from the sacral segments of the spinal cord through the pelvic nerves to the penis. Parasympathetic stimulation results in release of nitric oxide, a nonadrenergic-noncholinergic neurotransmitter, which causes relaxation of trabecular smooth muscle of the corpora cavernosa. This relaxation permits inflow of blood into the sinuses of the cavernosa at pressures approaching those of the arterial system. Because the erectile tissues of the cavernosa are surrounded by a nonelastic fibrous covering, high pressure in the sinusoids causes ballooning of the erectile tissue to such an extent that the penis becomes hard and elongated. At the same time, contraction of the somatic-innervated ischiocavernous muscles forcefully compresses the blood-filled corpora cavernosa, producing a further rise in intercavernous pressures. During this phase of erection, inflow and outflow of blood cease.

Parasympathetic innervation must be intact and nitric oxide synthesis must be active for erection to occur. Nitric oxide activates guanyl cyclase, an enzyme that increases the concentration of cyclic guanosine monophosphate (cGMP), which in turn causes smooth muscle relaxation. Other smooth muscle relaxants (*e.g.*, prostaglandin E_1 analogs and α-adrenergic antagonists), if present in high enough concentrations, can independently cause sufficient cavernosal relaxation to result in erection. Many of the drugs that have been developed to treat erectile dysfunction act at the levels of these mediators.

Detumescence or penile relaxation is largely a sympathetic nervous system response. It can result from a cessation of neurotransmitter release, the breakdown of second messengers such as cGMP, or sympathetic discharge during ejaculation. Contraction of the trabecular smooth muscle opens the venous channels so that the trapped blood can be expelled and penile flaccidity return.

Erectile Dysfunction

"Erectile dysfunction is defined as the inability to achieve and maintain an erection sufficient to permit satisfactory sexual intercourse."[8] It has been estimated that the disorder affects 20 to 30 million men in the United States.[9] Erectile dysfunction is commonly classified as psychogenic, organic, or mixed psychogenic or organic.[9,10] The latter is the most common.

Psychogenic Causes. Psychogenic causes of erectile dysfunction include performance anxiety, a strained relationship with a sexual partner, depression, and overt psychotic disorders such as schizophrenia. Depression is a common cause of erectile dysfunction.[9]

Organic Causes. Organic causes span a wide range of pathologies. They include neurogenic, hormonal, vascular, drug-induced, and cavernous impairment etiologies.

Neurogenic disorders such as Parkinson's disease, stroke, and cerebral trauma often contribute to erectile dysfunction by decreasing libido or preventing the initiation of erection. In spinal cord injury, the extent of neural impairment depends on the level, location, and extent of the lesion. Somatosensory involvement of the genitalia is essential to the reflex mechanisms involved in erection; this becomes important with aging and conditions such as diabetes that impair peripheral nerve function.

Hormonal causes of erectile dysfunction include a decrease in androgen levels. Androgen levels may be decreased because of aging. Hypoprolactinemia from any cause interferes with both reproduction and erectile function. This is because prolactin acts centrally to inhibit dopaminergic activity, which is a stimulus for release of the hypothalamic gonadotropin-releasing hormone that controls the release of pituitary gonadotropic hormones.

Common risk factors for generalized penile arterial insufficiency include hypertension, hyperlipidemia, cigarette smoking, diabetes mellitus, and pelvic irradiation.[9] In hypertension, erectile function is impaired not so much by the increased blood pressure as by the associated stenotic arterial lesions. Focal stenosis of the common penile artery most often occurs in men who sustained blunt pelvic or perineal trauma (*e.g.*, from bicycling accidents). Failure of the veins to close completely during an erection (veno-occlusive dysfunction) may occur in men with large venous channels that drain the corpora cavernosa. Other disorders that impair venous occlusion are degenerative changes involving the tunica albuginea, as in Peyronie's disease. Poor relaxation of the trabecular smooth muscle may accompany anxiety with excessive adrenergic tone.

Many drugs are reported to cause erectile dysfunction, including antidepressant, antipsychotic, and antihypertensive medications. Cigarette smoking can induce vasoconstriction and penile venous leakage because of its effects on cavernous smooth muscle.[9] Alcohol in small amounts may increase libido and improve erection; however, in large amounts it can cause central sedation, decreased libido, and transient erectile dysfunction.

Aging is known to increase the risk of erectile dysfunction.[11] After 50 years of age, the overall prevalence of erectile dysfunction is reported to be greater than 50%.[12] Many of the pathologic processes that contribute to erectile dysfunction are more common in older men, including diabetes, hyperlipidemia, vascular disease, and the long-term effects of cigarette smoking. Age-related declines in testosterone also may play a role. Psychosocial problems such as depression, esteem issues, partner relationships, history of substance abuse, and anxiety and fear of performance failure also may contribute to erectile dysfunction in older men.[12]

Diagnosis and Treatment. A diagnosis of erectile dysfunction requires careful history (medical, sexual, and psychosocial), physical examination, and laboratory tests aimed at determining what other tests are needed to rule out organic causes of the disorder. Because many medications, including prescribed, over-the-counter, and illicit drugs, can cause erectile dysfunction, a careful drug history is indicated.

Treatment methods include psychosexual counseling, androgen replacement therapy, oral and intracavernous drug therapy, vacuum constriction devices, surgical treatment (prosthesis and vascular surgery).[9,10,13] Among the commonly prescribed drugs are sildenafil, yohimbine, alprostadil, and phentolamine. Sildenafil (Viagra) is a selective inhibitor of phosphodiesterase type 5, the enzyme that inactivates cGMP. Yohimbine, an α_2-adrenergic receptor antagonist, acts at the adrenergic receptors in brain centers associated with libido and penile erection. Both sildenafil and yohimbine are taken orally. Alprostadil, a prostaglandin E analog, acts by producing relaxation of cavernous smooth muscle. It is either injected directly into the cavernosa or placed in the urethra as a minisuppository. Phentolamine, an α_2-adrenergic receptor antagonist, also is administered by intracavernous injection.

Priapism

Priapism is an involuntary, prolonged, abnormal and painful erection that is not associated with sexual excitement. Priapism is a true urologic emergency because the prolonged erection can result in ischemia and fibrosis of the erectile tissue with significant risk of subsequent impotence. Priapism can occur at any age, in the newborn as well as other age groups. Sickle cell disease or neoplasms are the most common cause in boys between 5 and 10 years of age.

Priapism is caused by impaired blood flow in the corpora cavernosa of the penis. Two mechanisms for priapism have been proposed: low-flow (ischemic) priapism, in which there is stasis of blood flow in the corpora cavernosa with a resultant failure of detumescence, and high-flow (nonischemic) priapism, which involves persistent arterial flow into the corpora cavernosa.[14] In high-flow priapism, there is no hypoxia of local tissue, the penis is less rigid, the pain is less than in stasis priapism, and permanent corporal fibrosis and cellular damage are rare.[14]

Priapism is classified as primary (idiopathic) or secondary to a disease or drug effect. Primary priapism is the result of conditions such as trauma, infection, and neoplasms. Secondary causes include hematologic conditions such as leukemia, sickle cell disease, and thrombocytopenia; neurologic conditions such as stroke, spinal cord injury, and other central nervous system lesions; and renal failure. Between 6% to 12% of males with sickle cell disorders are affected by priapism.[14] The relative deoxygenation and stasis of cavernosal blood during erection is thought to increase sickling. Various medications, such as antihypertensive drugs, anticoagulant drugs, antidepressant drugs, alcohol, and marijuana, can contribute to the development of priapism. Androstenedione, sold as an over-the-counter drug to enhance muscle building and athletic performance, has been implicated in the disorder.[15] Currently, intracavernous injection therapy for erectile dysfunction is one of the more common causes of priapism.

The diagnosis of priapism usually is based on clinical findings. Blood gas studies using intracavernal aspirate may be helpful in differentiating ischemic low-flow priapism from nonischemic high-flow priapism. Corporeal cavernosonography, Doppler studies of penile blood flow, penile ultrasonography, and computed tomography (CT) scans may be used to determine intrapelvic pathology.

Initial treatment measures include analgesics, sedation, and hydration. Urinary retention may necessitate catheterization. Local measures include ice packs and cold saline enemas, aspiration and irrigation of the corpus cavernosum with plain or heparinized saline, or instillation of α-adrenergic drugs. If less aggressive treatment does not produce detumescence, a temporary surgical shunt may be established between the corpus cavernosum and the corpus spongiosum.

The prognosis for whether fibrosis or erectile failure will occur is determined by the severity and duration of blood stasis. In high-flow priapism, the damaging effects of decreased oxygen tension and intracavernal blood pressure are less pronounced than in stasis priapism. Normal erectile potency can be restored even after a long duration of high-flow priapism. Persistent stasis priapism, in contrast, is known to result in impaired erectile function and tissue fibrosis unless resolved within 24 to 48 hours of onset.[14]

CANCER OF THE PENIS

Squamous cell cancer of the penis is most common in men between 45 and 60 years of age. In the United States, it accounts for less than 1% of male genital tumors; however, in other countries, it accounts for 10% to 20% of male cancers.[16,17] When it is diagnosed early, penile cancer is highly curable. The greatest hindrance to early diagnosis is a delay in seeking medical attention.

The cause of penile cancer is unknown. Several risk factors have been suggested, including poor hygiene, human papillomavirus (HPV) infections, ultraviolet radiation exposure, and immunodeficiency states. There is an association between penile cancer and poor genital hygiene and phimosis. This type of cancer is rare in Jewish and Muslim men, who are circumcised routinely. One theory postulates that smegma accumulation under the phimotic foreskin may produce chronic inflammation, leading to carcinoma. The HPVs have been implicated in the genesis of several genital cancers, including cancer of the penis.[16] Ultraviolet radiation also is thought have a carcinogenic effect on the penis.[16] Males who were treated for psoriasis with ultraviolet A or B therapies (*i.e.,* PUVA or PUVB) have had a reported increased incidence of genital squamous cell carcinomas. Because of this observation, it is suggested that men should shield their genital area when using tanning salons. Immunodeficiency states also may play a role in the pathogenesis of penile cancer. Approximately 18% of men with AIDS-related Kaposi's sarcoma have lesions of the penis or genitalia.[16]

Dermatologic lesions with precancerous potential include balanitis xerotica obliterans and giant condylomata acuminata.[17] Balanitis xerotica obliterans is a white, patchy lesion that originates on the glans and usually progresses to involve the meatus. It commonly is observed in middle-aged diabetic men. Giant condylomata acuminata are cauliflower-like lesions arising from the prepuce or glans that result from HPV infection.

Approximately 95% of penile cancers are squamous cell carcinoma.[16] It thought to progress from an in situ lesion to an invasive carcinoma. Bowen's disease and erythroplasia of Queyrat are penile lesions with histologic features of carcinoma in situ.[17] Bowen's disease appears as a solitary, thickened, gray-white, opaque plaque with shallow ulceration and crusting. It commonly involves the skin of the shaft of penis and the scrotum. Erythroplasia of Queyrat involves the mucosal surface of the glans or prepuce. It is characterized by single or multiple, shiny red, sometimes velvety plaques.[17] These lesions require careful follow-up because of their potential to progress to invasive carcinoma.

Invasive carcinoma of the penis begins as a small lump or ulcer. If phimosis is present, there may be painful swelling, purulent drainage, or difficulty urinating. Palpable lymph nodes may be present in the inguinal region. Diagnosis usually is based on physical examination and biopsy results. Cavernosonography, CT scans, and magnetic resonance imaging (MRI) may be used in the diagnostic workup.

Treatment options vary according to stage, size, location, and invasiveness of the tumor. Carcinoma in situ may be treated conservatively with fluorouracil cream application or laser treatment. Conservative treatment requires frequent follow-up examinations.[17] Surgery remains the mainstay of treatment for invasive carcinoma. Superficial primary lesions that are freely movable, do not invade the corpora, and show no evidence of metastatic disease can be treated with sleeve resection. Partial or total penectomy is indicated for invasive lesions. Bilateral lymph node dissection is indicated in stage III tumors with lymph node involvement.

Cumulative data reveal that men with penile cancer have an overall 5-year survival rate of 65% to 90%.[17] The most important prognostic indicator is the lymph node status. For men with tumor-positive inguinal lymph nodes, the 5-year survival rate is 30% to 50%, and with positive iliac nodes, it is 20%.[17]

> In summary, disorders of the penis can be congenital or acquired. Hypospadias and epispadias are congenital defects in which there is malpositioning of the urethral opening: it is located on the ventral surface in hypospadias and on the dorsal surface in epispadias. Phimosis is the condition in which the opening of the foreskin is too tight to permit retraction over the glans. Balanitis is an acute or chronic inflammation of the glans penis, and balanoposthitis is an inflammation of the glans and prepuce. Peyronie's disease is characterized by the growth of a band of fibrous tissue on top of the penile shaft. Erectile dysfunction is defined as the inability to achieve and maintain an erection sufficient to permit satisfactory sexual intercourse. It can be caused by psychogenic factors, organic disorders, or mixed psychogenic and organic conditions. Priapism is prolonged, painful, and nonsexual erection that can lead to thrombosis with ischemia and necrosis of penile tissue. Cancer of the penis accounts for less than 1% of male genital cancers in the United States. Although the tumor is slow growing and highly curable when diagnosed early, the greatest hindrance to successful treatment is a delay in seeking medical attention.

Disorders of the Scrotum and Testes

After you have completed this section of the chapter, you should be able to meet the following objectives:

✦ State the physical manifestations of cryptorchidism
✦ Describe the potential risks associated with cryptorchidism
✦ Compare the cause, appearance, and significance of hydrocele, hematocele, spermatocele, and varicocele
✦ State the difference between extravaginal and intravaginal testicular torsion
✦ Describe the symptoms of epididymitis
✦ State the manifestations and possible complications of mumps orchitis
✦ Relate environmental factors to development of scrotal cancer
✦ State the cell types involved in seminoma, embryonal carcinoma, teratoma, and choriocarcinoma tumors of the testes

The scrotum is a skin-covered pouch that contains the testes and their accessory organs. Defects of the scrotum and testes include cryptorchidism, disorders of the scrotal sac, vascular disorders, inflammation of the scrotum and testes, and neoplasms.

CONGENITAL AND ACQUIRED DISORDERS

Cryptorchidism

Cryptorchidism, or undescended testes, occurs when one or both of the testicles fail to move down into the scrotal sac. The condition is bilateral in 10% to 20% of cases. The testes develop intra-abdominally in the fetus and usually descend into the scrotum through the inguinal canal during the seventh to ninth months of gestation.[2] The undescended testes may remain in the lower abdomen or at a point of descent in the inguinal canal (Fig. 43-4).

The incidence of cryptorchidism is directly related to birth weight and gestational age; infants who are born prematurely or are small for gestational age have the highest incidence of the disorder. Up to one third of premature infants

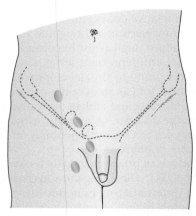

FIGURE 43-4 Possible locations of undescended testicles.

and 3% to 5% of full-term infants are born with undescended testicles.[18,19] The cause of cryptorchidism in full-term infants is poorly understood. Most cases are idiopathic, but some may result from genetic or hormonal factors.[18]

The major manifestation of cryptorchidism is the absence of one or more of the testes from the scrotum. The testis either is not palpable or can be felt external to the inguinal ring. Spontaneous descent often occurs during the first 3 months of life, and by 6 months of age the incidence decreases to 0.8%.[1,19] Spontaneous descent rarely occurs after 6 months of age.[1]

In children with cryptorchidism, histologic abnormalities of the testes reflect intrinsic defects in the testicle or adverse effects of the extrascrotal environment. The undescended testicle is normal at birth, but pathologic changes can be demonstrated at 6 to 12 months.[1] There is a delay in germ cell development, changes in the spermatic tubules, and reduced number of Leydig cells. These changes are progressive over time if the testes remain undescended. When the disorder is unilateral, it also may produce morphologic changes in the contralateral descended testis.

The consequences of cryptorchidism include infertility, malignancy, and the possible psychological effects of an empty scrotum. Indirect inguinal hernias usually accompany the undescended testes but rarely are symptomatic. Recognition of the condition and early treatment are important steps in preventing adverse consequences.

The risk of malignancy in the undescended testis is four to six times higher than in the general population.[1,19] The increased risk of testicular cancer is not significantly affected by orchiopexy, hormonal therapy, or late spontaneous descent after the age of 2 years. Orchiopexy, however, does allow for earlier detection of a testicular malignancy by positioning the testis in a more easily palpable location.

As a group, males with unilateral or bilateral cryptorchidism usually have decreased sperm counts, poorer-quality sperm, and lower fertility rates than men whose testicles descend normally. The likelihood of decreased fertility increases when the condition is bilateral. Unlike the risk of testicular cancer, there seems to be some advantage to early orchiopexy for protection of fertility.[1,19]

Diagnosis and Treatment. Diagnosis is based on careful examination of the genitalia in male infants. Undescended testes due to cryptorchidism should be differentiated from retractable testes that retract into the inguinal canal in response to an exaggerated cremaster muscle reflex. Retractable testes usually are palpable at birth but become nonpalpable later. They can be brought down with careful palpation in a warm room. Retractable testes usually assume a scrotal position during puberty. They have none of the complications associated with undescended testicles due to cryptorchidism.[1]

Improved techniques for testicular localization include ultrasonography (*i.e.*, visualization of the testes by recording the pulses of ultrasonic waves directed into the tissues), gonadal venography and arteriography (*i.e.*, radiography of the veins and arteries of the testes after the injection of a contrast medium), and laparoscopy (*i.e.*, examination of the interior of the abdomen using a visualization instrument). Adrenal hyperplasia in a genetic female should be considered in a phenotypically male infant with bilateral nonpalpable testicles (see Chapter 40).

The treatment goals for the child with cryptorchidism include measures to enhance future fertility potential, placement of the gonad in a favorable place for cancer detection, and improved cosmetic appearance. Regardless of the type of treatment used, it should be carried out between 6 months and 2 years of age.[1,18] Treatment modalities for children with unilateral or bilateral cryptorchidism include initial hormone therapy with human chorionic gonadotropin (hCG) or luteinizing hormone-releasing hormone (LHRH), a hypothalamic hormone that stimulates production of the gonadotropic hormones by the anterior pituitary gland. For children who do not respond to hormonal treatment, surgical placement and fixation of the testes in the scrotum (*i.e.*, orchiopexy) have proved effective. Approximately 95% of infants who have orchiopexy for a unilateral undescended testis will be fertile, compared with a 30% to 50% fertility rate in uncorrected males.[20]

Treatment of males with undescended testis should include lifelong follow-up, considering the sequelae of testicular cancer and infertility. Parents need to be aware of the potential issues of infertility and increased risk of testicular cancer. On reaching puberty, boys should be instructed in the necessity of testicular self-examination.

Hydrocele

The testes and epididymis are completely surrounded by the tunica vaginalis, a serous pouch derived from the peritoneum during fetal descent of the testes into the scrotum. The tunica vaginalis has an outer parietal layer and a deeper visceral layer that adheres to the dense fibrous covering of the testes, the tunica albuginea. A space exists between these two layers that typically contains a few milliliters of clear fluid. A hydrocele forms when excess fluid collects between the layers of the tunica vaginalis (Fig. 43-5). It may be unilateral or bilateral and can develop as a primary congenital defect or as a secondary condition. Acute hydrocele may develop after local injury, epididymitis or orchitis, gonorrhea, lymph obstruction, or germ cell testicular tumor,

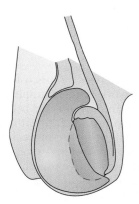

FIGURE 43-5 Hydrocele.

or as a side effect of radiation therapy. Chronic hydrocele is more common. Fluid collects about the testis, and the mass grows gradually. Its cause is unknown, and it usually develops in men older than 40 years of age.

Most cases of hydrocele in male infants and children are caused by a patent processus vaginalis, which is continuous with the peritoneal cavity. In many cases they are associated with an indirect inguinal hernia.[21] Most hydroceles of infancy close spontaneously; therefore, they are not repaired before the age of 1 year. If the hydrocele persists beyond 2 years of age, surgical treatment usually is indicated.

Hydroceles are palpated as cystic masses that may attain massive proportions. If there is enough fluid, the mass may be mistaken for a solid tumor. Transillumination of the scrotum (*i.e.*, shining a light through the scrotum for the purposes of visualizing its internal structures) or ultrasonography can help to determine whether the mass is solid or cystic and whether the testicle is normal.[22] A dense hydrocele that does not illuminate should be differentiated from a testicular tumor. If a hydrocele develops in a young man without apparent cause, careful evaluation is needed to exclude cancer or infection.

In an adult male, a hydrocele is a relatively benign condition. The condition often is asymptomatic, and no treatment is necessary. When symptoms do occur, the feeling may be that of heaviness in the scrotum or pain in the lower back. In cases of secondary hydrocele, the primary condition is treated. If the hydrocele is painful or cosmetically undesirable, surgical correction is indicated. Surgical repair may be done inguinally or transcrotally.

Hematocele

A hematocele is an accumulation of blood in the tunica vaginalis, which causes the scrotal skin to become dark red or purple. It may develop as a result of an abdominal surgical procedure, scrotal trauma, a bleeding disorder, or a testicular tumor.

Spermatocele

A spermatocele is a painless, sperm-containing cyst that forms at the end of the epididymis. It is located above and posterior to the testis, is attached to the epididymis, and is separate from the testes. Spermatoceles may be solitary or multiple and usually are less than 1 cm in diameter. They are freely movable and should transilluminate. Spermatoceles rarely cause problems, but a large one may become painful and require excision.

Varicocele

A varicocele is characterized by varicosities of the pampiniform plexus, a network of veins supplying the testes. The left side is more commonly affected because the left internal spermatic vein inserts into the left renal vein at a right angle, whereas the right spermatic vein usually enters the inferior vena cava. Incompetent valves are more common in the left internal spermatic veins, causing a reflux of blood back into the veins of the pampiniform plexus. The force of gravity resulting from the upright position also contributes to venous dilatation. If the condition persists, there may be

damage to the elastic fibers and hypertrophy of the vein walls, as occurs in formation of varicose veins in the leg. Sperm concentration and motility are decreased in 65% to 75% of men with varicocele.[22]

Varicoceles rarely are found before puberty, and the incidence is highest in men between 15 and 35 years of age. Symptoms of varicocele include an abnormal feeling of heaviness in the left scrotum, although many varicoceles are asymptomatic. Usually, the varicocele is readily diagnosed on physical examination with the patient in the standing and recumbent positions. Typically, the varicocele disappears in the lying position because of venous decompression into the renal vein. Scrotal palpation of a varicocele has been compared to feeling a "bag of worms." Small varicoceles sometimes are difficult to identify. Valsalva's maneuver (*i.e.*, forced expiration against a closed glottis) may be used to accentuate small varicosities.[22] A hand-held Doppler stethoscope is used while the patient performs Valsalva's maneuver. If the varicocele is present, a distinct venous rush is heard because of the sudden occurrence of retrograde blood flow. Other diagnostic aids include real-time ultrasonography, radioisotope scanning, spermatic venography, and scrotopenography.

Treatment options include surgical ligation or sclerosis using a percutaneous transvenous catheter under fluoroscopic guidance. Both can be performed as outpatient procedures. The benefits of the percutaneous technique include a slightly lower recurrence rate and more rapid return to full physical activity. It has been shown that 40% of men with abnormalities in their semen and a varicocele show some degree of improvement in fertility after obliteration of the dilated veins.[22] Aside from improving fertility, other reasons for surgery include the relief of the sensation of "heaviness" and cosmetic improvement.

Testicular Torsion

Testicular torsion is a twisting of the spermatic cord that suspends the testis (Fig. 43-6). It is the most common acute scrotal disorder in the pediatric and young adult popu-

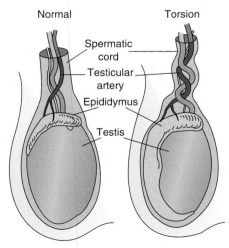

FIGURE 43-6 Testicular torsion.

lation. Testicular torsion can be divided into two distinct clinical entities, depending on the level of spermatic cord involvement: extravaginal and intravaginal torsion.[20,23]

Extravaginal torsion, which occurs almost exclusively in neonates, is the less common form of testicular torsion.[20] It occurs when the testicle and the fascial tunicae that surround it rotate around the spermatic cord at a level well above the tunica vaginalis. The torsion probably occurs during fetal or neonatal descent of the testes before the tunica adheres to the scrotal wall. At birth or shortly thereafter, a firm, smooth, painless scrotal mass is identified. The scrotal skin appears red, and some edema is present. Differential diagnosis is relatively easy because testicular tumors, epididymitis, and orchitis are exceedingly rare in neonates; a hydrocele is softer and can be transilluminated, and physical examination can exclude the presence of hernia. The use of surgical treatment (orchiopexy and orchiectomy) is controversial. There are multiple animal studies indicating that failure to remove the torsed testes may produce an autoimmune response that affects the normal testis.[20,23]

Intravaginal torsion is considerably more common than extravaginal torsion. It occurs when the testis rotates on the long axis in the tunica vaginalis. In most cases, congenital abnormalities of the tunica vaginalis or spermatic cord exist. The tunica vaginalis normally surrounds the testes and epididymis, allowing the testicle to rotate freely in the tunica. Although anomalies of suspension vary, the epididymal attachment may be loose enough to permit torsion between the testis and the epididymis. More commonly, the testis rotates about the distal spermatic cord. Because this abnormality is developmental, bilateral anomalies are common.

Intravaginal torsion occurs most frequently between the ages of 8 and 18 years and rarely is seen after 30 years of age. Patients usually present in severe distress within hours of onset and often have nausea, vomiting, and tachycardia. The affected testis is large and tender, with pain radiating to the inguinal area. Extensive cremaster muscle contraction causes a thickening of the spermatic cord.

Testicular torsion must be differentiated from epididymitis, orchitis, and trauma to the testis. On physical examination, the testicle often is high in the scrotum and in an abnormal orientation. These changes are caused by the twisting and shortening of the spermatic cord. The degree of scrotal swelling and redness depends on the duration of symptoms. The testes are firm and tender. The cremasteric reflex, normally elicited by stroking the medial aspect of the thigh and observing testicular retraction, frequently is absent.[23] Color Doppler ultrasonography is increasingly used in the evaluation of suspected testicular torsion.[22,23]

Intravaginal testicular torsion is a true surgical emergency, and early recognition and treatment are necessary if the testicle is to be saved. Treatment includes surgical detorsion and orchiectomy. Orchiectomy is carried out when the testis is deemed nonviable after surgical detorsion. Testicular salvage rates are directly related to the duration of torsion. Because the opposite testicle usually is affected by the same abnormal attachments, prophylactic fixation of that testis often is performed.

INFECTION AND INFLAMMATION

Epididymitis

Epididymitis is an inflammation of the epididymis, the elongated cordlike structure that lies along the posterior border of the testis, whose function is the storage, transport, and maturation of spermatozoa. There are two major types of epididymitis: sexually transmitted infections associated with urethritis and primary nonsexually transmitted infections associated with urinary tract infections and prostatitis. Most cases of epididymitis are caused by bacterial pathogens.

In primary nonsexual infections, the pressure associated with voiding or physical strain may force pathogen-containing urine from the urethra or prostate up the ejaculatory duct and through the vas deferens and into the epididymis. Infections also may reach the epididymis through the lymphatics of the spermatic cord. In rare cases, organisms from other foci of infection reach the epididymis through the bloodstream. In children, the disorder usually is associated with congenital urinary tract abnormalities and infection with gram-negative rods. Sexually transmitted acute epididymitis occurs mainly in young men without underlying genitourinary disease and is most commonly caused by *Chlamydia trachomatis* and *Neisseria gonorrhoeae* (singly or in combination). In men older than 35 years of age, epididymitis often is associated with pathogens such as *Escherichia coli*, *Pseudomonas*, and gram-positive cocci.

Epididymitis is characterized by unilateral pain and swelling, accompanied by erythema and edema of the overlying scrotal skin that develops over a period of 24 to 48 hours. Initially, the swelling and induration are limited to the epididymis. However, the distinction between the testis and epididymis becomes less evident as the inflammation progresses, and the testis and epididymis become one mass. There may be tenderness over the groin (spermatic cord) or in the lower abdomen. Fever and complaints of dysuria occur in approximately one half of cases. Whether urethral discharge is present depends on the organism causing the infection; it usually accompanies gonorrheal infections, is common in chlamydial infections, and is less common in infections caused by gram-negative organisms.

Laboratory findings usually reveal an elevated white blood cell count. Urinalysis and urine culture are important in the diagnosis of epididymitis, with bacteriuria and pyuria suggestive of the disorder. The cause of epididymitis can be differentiated by Gram's stain examination or culture of a midstream urine specimen or a urethral specimen.

Treatment during the acute phase (which usually lasts for 3 to 4 days) includes bed rest, scrotal elevation and support, and antibiotics.[23] Bed rest with scrotal support improves lymphatic drainage. The choice of antibiotics is determined by age, physical findings, urinalysis, Gram's stain results, cultures, and sexual history. Oral analgesics and antipyretics usually are indicated. Sexual activity or physical strain may exacerbate the infection and worsen the symptoms, and should be avoided.

Orchitis

Orchitis is an infection of the testes. It can be precipitated by a primary infection in the genitourinary tract, or the infection can be spread to testes through the bloodstream or the lymphatics. Epididymitis with subsequent infection of the testis is commonly related to genitourinary tract infections (cystitis, urethritis, genitoprostatitis) that travel to the epididymis and testis through the vas deferens or the lymphatics of the spermatic cord.

Orchitis can develop as a complication of a systemic infection, such as parotitis (*i.e.*, mumps), scarlet fever, or pneumonia. Probably the best known of these complications is orchitis caused by the mumps virus. Mumps orchitis does not occur in prepubertal boys. However, approximately 20% to 35% of adolescent boys and young men with mumps develop this form of orchitis.[24] The onset of mumps orchitis is sudden; it usually occurs approximately 3 to 4 days after the onset of the parotitis and is characterized by fever, painful enlargement of the testes, and small hemorrhages into the tunica albuginea. Unlike epididymitis, the urinary symptoms are absent. The symptoms usually run their course in 7 to 10 days. Microscopically, an acute inflammatory response is seen in the seminiferous tubules, with proliferation of neutrophils, lymphocytes, and histiocytes causing distention of the tubules. The residual effects seen after the acute phase include hyalinization of the seminiferous tubules and atrophy of the testes. Spermatogenesis is irreversibly impaired in approximately 30% of testes damaged by mumps orchitis.[24] If both testes are involved, permanent sterility results, but androgenic hormone function usually is maintained.

NEOPLASMS

Tumors can develop in the scrotum or the testes. Benign scrotal tumors are common and often do not require treatment. Carcinoma of the scrotum is rare and usually is associated with exposure to carcinogenic agents. Almost all solid tumors of the testes are malignant.

Scrotal Cancer

Cancer of the scrotum was the first cancer directly linked to a specific occupation when, in the 1800s, it was associated with chimney sweeps.[25] Studies have linked this cancer to exposure to tar, soot, and oils. Most squamous cell cancers of the scrotum are linked to poor hygiene and chronic inflammation. Exposure to ultraviolet A radiation (*e.g.*, PUVA) or HPV also has been associated with the disease. The mean age of presentation with the disease is 60 years, often preceded by 20 to 30 years of chronic irritation.

In the early stages, cancer of the scrotum may appear as a small tumor or wartlike growth that eventually ulcerates. The thin scrotal wall lacks the tissue reactivity needed to block the malignant process; more than one half of the cases seen involve metastasis to the lymph nodes. Because this tumor does not respond well to chemotherapy or irradiation, the treatment includes wide local excision of the tumor with inguinal and femoral node dissection.[26] The prognosis correlates with lymph node involvement.

Testicular Cancer

Testicular cancer accounts for 1% of all male cancers and 3% of male urogenital cancers. Although relatively rare, it is the most common cause of cancer in the 15- to 34-year-old age group.[20,27,28] In the past, testicular cancer was a leading cause of death among males entering their most productive years. However, since the late 1970s, advances in therapy have transformed an almost invariably fatal disease into one that is highly curable. With the exception of men with advanced metastatic disease at the time of presentation or those who relapse after primary chemotherapy, most men with these tumors are cured with available therapy. The prognosis and extent of treatment required for testicular cancer are related to the stage of the disease at the time of presentation.

Although the cause of testicular cancer is unknown, several predisposing influences may be important: cryptorchidism, genetic factors, and disorders of testicular development.[20] The strongest association has been with cryptorchid testis. Approximately 10% of testicular tumors are associated with cryptorchidism. The higher the location of the undescended testis, the greater the risk.[20] Genetic predisposition also appears to be important. Family clustering of the disorder has been described, although a well-defined pattern of inheritance has not been established. Men with disorders of testicular development, including those with Klinefelter's syndrome and testicular feminization, have a higher risk of germ cell tumors.

Approximately 95% of malignant tumors arising in the testis are germ cell tumors.[20,27,28] Germ cell tumors can be classified as seminomas and nonseminomas based on their origin in primordial germ cells and their ability to differentiate in vivo. Because these tumors derive from germ cells in the testis, they are multipotential (able to differentiate into different tissue types) and often secrete polypeptide hormones or enzymes representing earlier stages of development.

Seminomas are the most common type of testicular tumors. They account for approximately 50% of germ cell tumors and are most frequent in the fourth decade of life.[27] They almost never occur in infants or small children.[20] Seminomas are thought to arise from the seminiferous epithelium of the testes and are the type of germ cell tumor most likely to produce a uniform population of cells.

The nonseminoma tumors include embryonal carcinoma, teratoma, choriocarcinoma, and yolk cell carcinoma derivatives. Nonseminoma tumors usually contain more than one cell type and are less differentiated than seminomas. Embryonal carcinomas are the least differentiated of the tumors, with totipotential capacity to differentiate into other nonseminomatous cell types. They occur most commonly in the 20- to 30-year-old age group. Choriocarcinoma is a rare and highly malignant form of testicular cancer that is identical to tumors that arise in placental tissue. Yolk sac tumors mimic the embryonic yolk sac histologically. They are the most common type of testicular tumors in infants and children up to 3 years of age, and in this age group have a very good prognosis.[20] Teratomas are composed of somatic cell types from two or more germline layers (ectoderm, mesoderm, or endoderm). They constitute less than 2% to 3% of germ cell tumors and can occur at any age from infancy to old age. They usually behave as benign tumors in children; in adults, they often contain minute foci of cancer cells.

Often the first sign of testicular cancer is a slight enlargement of the testicle that may be accompanied by some degree of discomfort. This may be an ache in the abdomen or groin or a sensation of dragging or heaviness in the scrotum. Frank pain may be experienced in the later stages, when the tumor is growing rapidly and hemorrhaging occurs. Testicular cancer can spread when the tumor may be barely palpable. Signs of metastatic spread include swelling of the lower extremities, back pain, cough, hemoptysis, or dizziness. Gynecomastia (breast enlargement) may result from hCG-producing tumors.

Early diagnosis of testicular cancer is important because a delay in seeking medical attention often results in presentation with a later stage of the disease and decreased treatment effectiveness. Recognition of the importance of prompt diagnosis and treatment has resulted in the development of a procedure for testicular self-examination and an emphasis on public education programs about this type of cancer. The American Cancer Society strongly advocates that every young adult male examine his testes at least once each month as a means of early detection of testicular cancer. The examination should be done after a warm bath or shower, when the scrotal skin is relaxed. To do this self-examination, each testicle is examined with the fingers of both hands by rolling the testicle between the thumb and fingers to check for the presence of any lumps. If any lump, nodule, or enlargement is noted, it should be brought immediately to the attention of a physician.

The diagnosis of testicular cancer requires a thorough urologic history and physical examination. A painless testicular mass may be cancer. Conditions that produce an intrascrotal mass similar to testicular cancer include epididymitis, orchitis, hydrocele, or hematocele. The examination for masses should include palpation of the testes and surrounding structures, transillumination of the scrotum, and abdominal palpation. Testicular ultrasonography can be used to differentiate testicular masses. The intravenous pyelogram may be used to evaluate kidney structure. CT scans and MRI are used in assessing metastatic spread.

The clinical staging (TNM classification) for testicular cancer is as follows: stage I, tumor confined to testes, epididymis, or spermatic cord; stage II, tumor spread to retroperitoneal lymph nodes below the diaphragm; and stage III, metastases outside the retroperitoneal nodes or above the diaphragm (see Chapter 8). Staging procedures include CT scans of the chest, abdomen, and pelvis; ultrasonography for detection of bulky inferior nodal metastases; venacavography; and lymphangiography. Radiographic methods are used to detect metastatic spread.

Tumor markers, assayed by immunoassay methods that measure protein antigens produced by malignant cells, provide information about the existence of a tumor and the type of tumor present. These markers may detect tumors that are too small to be found on physical examination or radiographs. Three tumor markers are useful in evaluating the tumor response: α-fetoprotein, a glycoprotein that normally is present in fetal serum in large amounts; hCG, a hormone that normally is produced by the placenta in pregnant women; and lactate dehydrogenase (LDH), a cellular enzyme normally found in muscle, liver, kidney, and brain. During embryonic development, the totipotential germ cells of the testes travel down normal differentiation pathways and produce different protein products. The reappearance of these protein markers in the adult suggests activity of the undifferentiated cells in a testicular germ cell tumor.

The basic treatment of all testicular cancers includes orchiectomy, which is done at the time of diagnostic exploration. The widely used surgical procedure is the unilateral radical orchiectomy through an inguinal incision. Surgical therapy is advantageous because it enables precise staging of the disease. Recommendations for further therapy (*e.g.*, retroperitoneal dissection, chemotherapy, radiation therapy) are based on the pathologic findings from the surgical procedure.

Treatment after orchiectomy depends on the histologic characteristics of the tumor and the clinical stage of the disease. Seminomas are highly radiosensitive; the treatment of stage I or II seminoma is irradiation of the retroperitoneal and homolateral lymph nodes to the level of the diaphragm. Patients with bulky retroperitoneal or distant metastases often are treated with multiagent chemotherapy. Seminoma is probably the most curable of all solid tumors. Men with nonseminomatous tumors usually are managed with observation, chemotherapy, or retroperitoneal lymph node dissection. Rigorous follow-up in all men with testicular cancer is necessary to detect recurrence, most of which occur within the first year.[28] Testicular cancer is a disease in which even recurrence is highly treatable. With appropriate treatment, the prognosis for men with testicular cancer is excellent. The 5-year survival rate for patients with stage I and II disease exceeds 95%.[20] Even patients with more advanced disease have excellent chances for long-term survival.

Therapy for testicular cancer can have potentially adverse effects on sexual functioning. Men who have retroperitoneal lymph node dissection may experience retrograde ejaculation or failure to ejaculate because of severing of the sympathetic plexus. Infertility may result from retrograde ejaculation or as a result of retroperitoneal lymph node dissection or the toxic effects of chemotherapy or radiotherapy on the germ cells in the remaining testis.[27] Sperm banking should be considered for men undergoing these treatments.

In summary, disorders of the scrotum and testes include cryptorchidism (*i.e.*, undescended testicles), hydrocele, hematocele, spermatocele, varicocele, and testicular torsion. Inflammatory conditions can involve the scrotal sac, epididymis, or testes. Tumors can arise in the scrotum or the testes. Scrotal cancers usually are associated with exposure to petroleum products such as tar, pitch, and soot. Testicular cancers account for 1% of all male cancers and 3% of cancers of the male genitourinary system. With current treatment methods, a large percentage of men with these tumors can be cured. Testicular self-examination is recommended as a means of early detection of this form of cancer.

Disorders of the Prostate

After you have completed this section of the chapter, you should be able to meet the following objectives:

◆ Compare the pathology and symptoms of acute bacterial prostatitis, chronic bacterial prostatitis, and chronic prostatitis/pelvic pain syndrome.

◆ Describe the urologic manifestations and treatment of benign prostatic hyperplasia

◆ List the methods used in the diagnosis and treatment of prostatic cancer

The prostate is a firm, glandular structure that surrounds the urethra. It produces a thin, milky, alkaline secretion that aids sperm motility by helping to maintain an optimum pH. The contraction of the smooth muscle in the gland promotes semen expulsion during ejaculation.

PROSTATITIS

Prostatitis refers to a variety of inflammatory disorders of the prostate gland, some bacterial and some not. It may occur spontaneously, as a result of catheterization or instrumentation, or secondary to other diseases of the male genitourinary system. As an outcome of 1995 and 1998 consensus conferences, the National Institutes of Health has established a classification system with four categories of prostatitis syndromes: acute bacterial prostatitis, chronic bacterial prostatitis, chronic prostatitis/pelvic pain syndrome, and asymptomatic inflammatory prostatitis.[29] Men with asymptomatic inflammatory prostatitis have no subjective symptoms, and are detected incidentally on biopsy or examination of prostatic fluid.

Acute Bacterial Prostatitis

Acute bacterial prostatitis often is considered a subtype of urinary tract infection. The most likely etiology of acute bacterial prostatitis is an ascending urethral infection or reflux of infected urine into the prostatic ducts. The most common organism is *E. coli*. Other frequently found species include *Pseudomonas*, *Klebsiella*, and *Proteus*. Less frequently, the infection is caused by *Staphylococcus aureus*, *Streptococcus faecalis*, *Chlamydia*, or anaerobes such as *Bacteroides* species.[30,31]

The manifestations of acute bacterial prostatitis include fever and chills, malaise, myalgia, arthralgia, frequent and urgent urination, dysuria, and urethral discharge. Dull, aching pain often is present in the perineum, rectum, or sacrococcygeal region. The urine may be cloudy and malodorous because of urinary tract infection. Rectal examination reveals a swollen, tender, warm prostate with scattered soft areas. Prostatic massage produces a thick discharge with white blood cells that grows large numbers of pathogens on culture.

Treatment of acute bacterial prostatitis depends on the severity of symptoms. It usually includes antibiotics, bed rest, adequate hydration, antipyretics, analgesics (often narcotics) or spasmolytic drugs to alleviate pain, and stool softeners. Men who are extremely ill, such as those with sepsis, may require hospitalization. A suprapubic catheter may be indicated if voiding is difficult or painful.

Acute prostatitis usually responds to appropriate antimicrobial therapy chosen in accordance with the sensitivity of the causative agents in the urethral discharge. Depending on the urine culture results, antibiotic therapy usually is continued for at least 4 weeks. Because acute prostatitis often is associated with anatomic abnormalities, a thorough urologic examination usually is performed after treatment is completed.

A persistent fever indicates the need for further investigation for an additional site of infection or a prostatic abscess. CT scans and transrectal ultrasonography of the prostate are useful in the diagnosis of prostatic abscesses. Prostatic abscesses, which are relatively uncommon since the advent of effective antibiotic therapy, are found more commonly in males with diabetes mellitus. Because prostatic abscesses usually are associated with bacteremia, prompt drainage by transperitoneal or transurethral incision followed by appropriate antimicrobial therapy usually is indicated.[30]

Chronic Bacterial Prostatitis

In contrast to acute bacterial prostatitis, chronic bacterial prostatitis is a subtle disorder that is difficult to treat. Men with the disorder typically have recurrent urinary tract infections with persistence of the same strain of pathogenic bacteria in prostatic fluid and urine. Organisms responsible for chronic bacterial prostatitis usually are the gram-negative enterobacteria (*E. coli*, *Proteus*, or *Klebsiella*) or *Pseudomonas*. Occasionally, a gram-positive organism such as *S. faecalis* is the causative organism. Infected prostatic calculi may develop and contribute to the chronic infection.

The symptoms of chronic prostatitis are variable and include frequent and urgent urination, dysuria, perineal discomfort, and low back pain. Occasionally, myalgia and arthralgia accompany the other symptoms. Secondary epididymitis sometimes is associated with the disorder. Many men experience relapsing lower or upper urinary tract infections because of recurrent invasion of the bladder by the prostatic bacteria. Bacteria may exist in the prostate gland even when the prostatic fluid is sterile. The most accurate method of establishing a diagnosis is by localizing cultures. This method is based on sequential collections of the first part of the voided urine (urethral specimen), midstream specimen (bladder specimen), the expressed prostatic secretion (obtained by prostatic massage), and the urine voided after prostatic massage. The last two specimens are considered prostatic urine. A positive expressed prostatic specimen establishes the diagnosis of bacterial prostatitis, excluding nonbacterial prostatitis.

Even after an accurate diagnosis has been established, treatment of chronic prostatitis often is difficult and frustrating. Unlike their action in the acutely inflamed prostate, antibacterial drugs penetrate poorly into the chronically inflamed prostate. Long-term therapy (3 to 4 months) with an appropriate low-dose oral antimicrobial agent often is used to treat the infection. Transurethral prostatectomy may be indicated when the infection is not cured or adequately controlled by medical therapy, particularly when prostate stones are present.

Chronic Prostatitis/Chronic Pelvic Pain Syndrome

Chronic prostatitis/pelvic pain syndrome is both the most common and least understood of the prostatitis syndromes.[32] The category is divided into two types, inflammatory and noninflammatory, based on the presence of leukocytes in the prostatic fluid. The inflammatory type was previously referred to as *nonbacterial prostatitis*, and the noninflammatory type as *prostatodynia*.

Inflammatory Prostatitis. A large group of men with prostatitis have pains along the penis, testicles, and scrotum; painful ejaculation; low back pain; rectal pain along the inner thighs; urinary symptoms; decreased libido; and impotence, but they have no bacteria in the urinary system. Men with nonbacterial prostatitis often have inflammation of the prostate with an elevated leukocyte count and abnormal inflammatory cells in their prostatic secretions. The cause of the disorder is unknown, and efforts to prove the presence of unusual pathogens (*e.g.*, mycoplasmas, chlamydiae, trichomonads, viruses) have been largely unsuccessful. It also is thought that nonbacterial prostatitis may be an autoimmune disorder.

Noninflammatory Prostatitis. Men with noninflammatory prostatitis or prostatodynia have symptoms resembling those of nonbacterial prostatitis but have negative urine culture results and no evidence of prostatic inflammation (*i.e.*, normal leukocyte count). The cause of noninflammatory prostatitis is unknown, but because of the absence of inflammation, the search for the cause of symptoms has been directed toward extraprostatic sources. In some cases, there is an apparent functional obstruction of the bladder neck near the external urethral sphincter; during voiding, this results in higher than normal pressures in the prostatic urethra that cause intraprostatic urine reflux and chemical irritation of the prostate by urine. In other cases, there is an apparent myalgia (*i.e.*, muscle pain) associated with prolonged tension of the pelvic floor muscles. Emotional stress also may play a role.

Treatment. Treatment methods for chronic prostatitis/pelvic pain syndrome are highly variable and require further study. Antibiotic therapy is used when an occult infection is suspected. Treatment often is directed toward symptom control. Sitz baths and nonsteroidal anti-inflammatory agents may provide some symptom relief. In men with irritative urination symptoms, anticholinergic agents (*e.g.*, oxybutynin) or α-adrenergic blocking agents (*e.g.*, prazosin, terazosin, doxazosin, or tamsulosin) may be beneficial. Reassurance can be helpful. It is important that these men know that the condition is neither infectious or contagious, nor is it known to cause cancer.[31]

HYPERPLASIA AND NEOPLASMS

Benign Prostatic Hyperplasia

Benign prostatic hyperplasia (BPH) is an age-related, nonmalignant enlargement of the prostate gland. It is characterized by the formation of large, discrete lesions in the periurethral region of the prostate rather than the peripheral zones, which commonly are affected by prostate cancer (Fig. 43-7). BPH is one of the most common diseases of aging men. It has been reported that 25% of men older than 55 years of age and 50% of men older than 75 years of age experience symptoms of BPH.[33]

The exact cause of the BPH is unknown. Potential risk factors include age, family history, race, ethnicity, and hormonal factors. The incidence of BPH increases with advanced age, is highest in African Americans, and lowest in native Japanese. Men with a family history of BPH are reported to have had larger prostates that those of control subjects, and higher rates of BPH were found in monozygotic twins than in dizygotic twins.[33]

Both androgens (testosterone) and estrogens appear to contribute to the development of BPH. The prostate consists of a network of glandular elements embedded in smooth muscle and supporting tissue, with testosterone being the most important factor for prostatic growth. Dihydrotestosterone (DHT), the biologically active metabolite of testosterone, is thought to be the ultimate mediator of prostatic hyperplasia, with estrogen serving to sensitize the prostatic tissue to the growth-producing effects of DHT. Free plasma

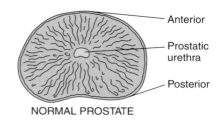

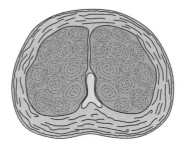

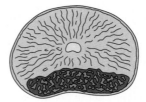

FIGURE 43-7 Normal prostate, nodular benign prostatic hypertrophy, and cancer of the prostate. (Rubin E., Farber J.L. [1999]. *Pathology* [3rd ed., p. 954]. Philadelphia: Lippincott Williams & Wilkins.) (Artist: Dimitri Karetnikov)

testosterone enters prostatic cells, where at least 90% is converted into DHT by the action of 5α-reductase. The discovery that DHT is the active factor in BPH is the rationale for use of 5α-reductase inhibitors in the treatment of the disorder. Although the exact source estrogen is uncertain, small amounts of estrogen are produced in the male. It has been postulated that a relative increase in estrogen levels that occurs with aging may facilitate the action of androgens in the prostate despite a decline in testicular output of testosterone.

The anatomic location of the prostate at the bladder neck contributes to the pathophysiology and symptomatology of BPH. There are two prostatic components to the obstructive properties of BPH and development of lower urinary tract symptoms: dynamic and static.[33–35] The static component of BPH is related to an increase in prostatic size, and gives rise to symptoms such as a weak urinary stream, postvoid dribbling, frequency of urination, and nocturia. The dynamic component of BPH is related to prostatic smooth muscle tone. α_1-Adrenergic receptors are the main receptors for the smooth muscle component of the prostate. The recognition of the role of α_1-adrenergic receptor on neuromuscular function in the prostate is the basis for use of α_1-adrenergic receptor blockers in treating BPH. A third component, detrusor instability and impaired bladder contractility, may contribute to the symptoms of BPH independent of the outlet obstruction created by an enlarged prostate.[34–36] It has been suggested that some of the symptoms of BPH might be related to a decompensating or aging bladder rather than being primarily related to outflow obstruction. An example is the involuntary contraction that results in urgency and an attempt to void that occurs because of small bladder volume.[34]

The clinical significance of BPH resides in its tendency to compress the urethra and cause partial or complete obstruction of urinary outflow. As the obstruction increases, acute retention may occur with overdistention of the bladder. The residual urine in the bladder causes increased frequency of urination and a constant desire to empty the bladder, which becomes worse at night. With marked bladder distention, overflow incontinence may occur with the slightest increase in intra-abdominal pressure. The resulting obstruction to urinary flow can give rise to urinary tract infection, destructive changes of the bladder wall, hydroureter, and hydronephrosis. Hypertrophy and changes in bladder wall structure develop in stages. Initially, the hypertrophied fibers form trabeculations and then herniations, or sacculations; finally, diverticula develop as the herniations extend through the bladder wall (see Chapter 42, Fig. 42-4). Because urine seldom is completely emptied from them, these diverticula are readily infected. Back pressure on the ureters and collecting system of the kidneys promotes hydroureter, hydronephrosis, and danger of eventual renal failure.

Diagnosis. It is now thought that the single most important factor in the evaluation and treatment of BPH is the man's own experiences related to the disorder. The American Urological Society Symptom Index consists of seven questions about symptoms regarding incomplete emptying, frequency, intermittency, urgency, weak stream, straining, and nocturia.[37] Each question is rated with a score of 0 (mild) to 7 (severe). A maximum score of 35 indicates severe symptoms. Total scores below 7 are considered mild; those between 8 and 20, moderate; and scores over 20, severe. A final question relates to quality of life due to urinary problems.

In 1994, the Agency for Health Care Policy and Research published clinical practice guidelines for management of BPH.[38] These guidelines suggest that the initial evaluation of men for a diagnosis of BPH includes history, physical examination, digital rectal examination, urinalysis, blood tests for serum creatinine and prostate-specific antigen (PSA), and urine flow rate. Blood and urine analyses are used as adjuncts to determine BPH complications. Urinalysis is done to detect bacteria, white blood cells, or microscopic hematuria in the presence of infection and inflammation. The serum creatinine test is used as an estimate of the glomerular filtration rate and renal function. The PSA test is used to screen for prostatic cancer. These evaluation measures, along with the symptom index, are used to describe the extent of obstruction, determine if other diagnostic tests are needed, and establish the need for treatment.

The digital rectal examination is used to examine the external surface of the prostate. Enlargement of the prostate due to BPH usually produces a large, palpable prostate with a smooth, rubbery surface. Hardened areas of the prostate gland suggest cancer and should be biopsied. An enlarged prostate found during a rectal examination does not always correlate with the degree of urinary obstruction. Some men can have greatly enlarged prostate glands with no urinary obstruction, but others may have severe symptoms without a palpable enlargement of the prostate.

Residual urine measurement may be made by ultrasonography or postvoiding catheterization for residual urine volume. Residual urines greater than 100 mL are considered high. Uroflowometry provides an objective measure of urine flow rate. The patient is asked to void with a relatively full bladder (at least 150 mL) into a device that electronically measures the force of the stream and urine flow rate. A urinary flow rate of greater than 14 mL/second is

Hyperplasia and Cancer of the Prostate

➤ Benign prostatic hyperplasia is an age-related enlargement of the prostate gland with formation of large, discrete lesions in the periurethral region of the prostate. These lesions compress the urethra and produce symptoms of dysuria or difficulty urinating.

➤ Prostatic cancer begins in the peripheral zones of the prostate gland and usually is asymptomatic until the disease is far advanced and the tumor has eroded the outer prostatic capsule and spread to adjacent pelvic tissues or metastasized.

considered normal, and less than 10 mL/second is indicative of obstruction.

Transabdominal or transrectal diagnostic ultrasonography can be used to evaluate the kidneys, ureters, and bladder. Abdominal radiographs may be used to reveal the size of the gland. Urethrocystoscopy is indicated in men with a history of hematuria, stricture disease, urethral injury, or prior lower urinary tract surgery. It is used to evaluate the length and diameter of the urethra, the size and configuration of the prostate, and bladder capacity. It also detects the presence of trabeculations, bladder stones, and small bladder cancers. CT scans, MRI studies, and radionuclide scans are reserved for rare instances of tumor detection.

Treatment. Treatment of BPH is determined by the degree of symptoms that the condition produces and complications due to obstruction. When a man develops mild symptoms related to BPH, a "watch and wait" stance often is taken. The condition does not always run a predictable course; it may remain stable or even improve.

Until the 1980s, surgery was the mainstay of treatment to alleviate urinary obstruction due to BPH. Currently, there is an emphasis on less invasive methods of treatment, including use of pharmacologic agents. However, when more severe signs of obstruction develop, treatment is indicated to provide comfort and avoid serious renal damage.

Pharmacologic management includes the use of 5α-reductase inhibitors and α$_1$-adrenergic blocking drugs.[33,34,39] The 5α-reductase inhibitors such as finasteride reduce prostate size by blocking the effect of androgens on the prostate. The side effects of finasteride are minimal but include impotence and decreased libido (<5% of patients). The presence of α-adrenergic receptors in prostatic smooth muscle has prompted the use of α$_1$-adrenergic blocking drugs (prozasin, terazosin, doxazosin, and tamsulosin) to relieve prostatic obstruction and increase urine flow.

The surgical removal of an enlarged prostate can be accomplished by the transurethral, suprapubic, or perineal approach. The transurethral prostatectomy (TURP) is the most commonly used technique in the United States. With this approach, an instrument is introduced through the urethra, and prostate tissue removed using a resectoscope and electrocautery. Immediate complications of TURP include the inability to urinate, postoperative hemorrhage or clot retention, and urinary tract infection. Late complications of TURP include impotence, incontinence, and bladder neck contractures. Retrograde ejaculation is another problem that may occur because of resection of bladder neck tissue.

Several alternative procedures for treatment of BPH have been developed. A new surgical approach is the transurethral incision of the prostate (TUIP). This procedure involves making one or two incisions in the bundle of smooth muscle where the prostate gland is attached to the bladder. The gland is split to reduce pressure on the urethra. TUIP is helpful for smaller prostate glands that cause obstruction. Many different techniques of laser surgery are available. Two main energy sources have been used, neodymium-yttrium-aluminum garnet (YAG) and holmium-YAG.[33]

Other new and experimental techniques that can be used to treat BPH include transurethral vaporization, transurethral microwave therapy, transurethral needle ablation, high-intensity focused ultrasound, and transurethral ultrasound-guided laser-induced prostatectomy. Most of these procedure are minimally invasive, and each has advantages and disadvantages when considered as an alternative measure in treatment of BPH.

A balloon dilation approach for removing the obstruction is another new technique. Transrectal ultrasonography is used to monitor balloon dilation of the prostate. Although the procedure may improve symptom score and flow rates, the effects usually are transitory.

For men who have heart or lung disease or a condition that precludes major surgery, a stent may be used to widen and maintain the patency of the urethra. A stent is a device made of tubular mesh that is inserted under local or regional anesthesia. Within several months, the lining of the urethra grows to cover the inside of the stent.

Prostatic Cancer

Prostatic cancer is the most common male cancer in the United States and is second to lung cancer as a cause of cancer-related death in men. The American Cancer Society estimates that during 2001, approximately 198,000 men in the United States were diagnosed with prostate cancer and 31,500 men died of the disorder.[40] The increase in diagnosed cases is thought to reflect earlier diagnosis because of the widespread use of PSA testing since the early 1990s.[40] The incidence of prostate cancer varies markedly from country to country and varies among races in the same country.[40] African-American men have the highest reported incidence for prostate cancer at all ages. Prostate cancer also tends to be diagnosed at a later stage in African-American men.[33] Asians and Native American men have the lowest rate. Prostate cancer also is a disease of aging. The incidence increases rapidly after 50 years of age; more that 80% of all prostate cancers are diagnosed in men older than 65 years of age.[40]

The precise cause of prostatic cancer is unclear. As with other cancers, it appears that the development of prostate cancer is a multistep process involving genes that control cell differentiation and growth. Several risk factors, such as age, race, heredity, and environmental influences, are suspected of playing a role.[18,41] Male hormone levels also may play a role. There is insufficient evidence linking socioeconomic status, infectious agents, smoking, vasectomy, sexual behavior, or BPH to the pathogenesis of prostate cancer.

The incidence of prostate cancer appears to be higher in relatives of men with prostate cancer. It has been estimated that men who have an affected first-degree relative (*e.g.,* father, brother) and an affected second-degree relative (*e.g.,* grandfather, uncle) have an eightfold increase in risk.[42] It has been suggested that dietary patterns, including increased dietary fats, may alter the production of sex hormones and increase the risk of prostate cancer. Supporting the role of dietary fats as a risk factor for prostate cancer has been the observation that the diet of Japanese men, who have a low rate of prostate cancer, is much lower in fat content than that of U.S. men, who have a much higher incidence.

In terms of hormonal influence, androgens are believed to play a role in the pathogenesis of prostate cancer.[18] Evidence favoring a hormonal influence includes the presence of steroid receptors in the prostate, the requirement of sex hormones for normal growth and development of the prostate, and the fact that prostate cancer almost never develops in men who have been castrated. The response of prostatic cancer to estrogen administration or androgen deprivation further supports a correlation between the disease and testosterone levels.

Prostatic adenocarcinomas, which account for 98% of all primary prostatic cancers, are commonly multicentric and located in the peripheral zones of the prostate[41] (see Fig. 43-7). The high frequency of invasion of the prostatic capsule by adenocarcinoma relates to its subcapsular location. Invasion of the urinary bladder is less frequent and occurs later in the clinical course. Metastasis to the lung reflects lymphatic spread through the thoracic duct and dissemination from the prostatic venous plexus to the inferior vena cava. Bony metastases, particularly to the vertebral column, ribs, and pelvis, produce pain that often presents as a first sign of the disease.

Most men with early-stage prostate cancer are asymptomatic. The presence of symptoms often suggests locally advanced or metastatic disease. Depending on the size and location of prostatic cancer at the time of diagnosis, there may be changes associated with the voiding pattern similar to those found in BPH. These include urgency, frequency, nocturia, hesitancy, dysuria, hematuria, or blood in the ejaculate. On physical examination, the prostate is nodular and fixed. Bone metastasis often is characterized by low back pain. Pathologic fractures can occur at the site of metastasis. Men with metastatic disease may experience weight loss, anemia, or shortness of breath.

Screening.   Because early cancers of the prostate usually are asymptomatic, screening tests are important. The screening tests currently available are digital rectal examination, PSA testing, and transrectal ultrasonography. PSA is a glycoprotein secreted into the cytoplasm of benign and malignant prostatic cells that is not found in other normal tissues or tumors. However, a positive PSA test indicates only the possible presence of prostate cancer. It also can be positive in cases of BPH and prostatitis. It has been reported that one third of men with elevated PSA levels have prostate cancer determined by biopsy, and two thirds do not.[43] Measures to increase the specificity of PSA testing in terms of predicting prostate cancer are being developed and evaluated. For example, because PSA levels increase with age, age-specific ranges have been established.[44] PSA velocity (a change of PSA level over time) and PSA density (*i.e.,* PSA level/prostate volume as measured by rectal ultrasonography) are being evaluated as a method of predicting the presence of prostate cancer in men with a positive PSA test result.[44]

The American Cancer Society and the American Urological Association recommend that men 50 years of age or older should undergo annual measurement of PSA and rectal examination for early detection of prostate cancer.[40] Men at high risk for prostate cancer, such as blacks and those with a strong family history, should undergo annual screening beginning at 45 years of age.[40]

A new approach, transrectal ultrasonography, may detect cancers that are too small to be detected by physical examination. This method is not used for first-line detection because of its expense, but it may benefit men who are at high risk for development of prostate cancer.

Diagnosis.   The diagnosis of prostate cancer is based on history and physical examination and confirmed through biopsy methods. Transrectal ultrasonography, a continuously improving method of imaging, is used to guide a biopsy needle and document the exact location of the biopsied tissue. It also is used for providing staging information.[33] Newly developed small probes for transrectal MRI have been shown to be effective in detecting the presence of cancer in the prostate. This method may prevent unnecessary biopsies and is expected to be used increasingly in the early diagnosis of prostatic cancer. Radiologic examination of the bones of the skull, ribs, spine, and pelvis can be used to reveal metastases, although radionuclide bone scans are more sensitive. Excretory urograms are used to delineate changes due to urinary tract obstruction and renal involvement. Lymphangiography often is done to determine pelvic node metastases.

Staging.   Cancer of the prostate, like other forms of cancer, is graded and staged (see Chapter 8). Prostatic adenocarcinoma commonly is classified using the Gleason grading system.[18,41] Well-differentiated tumors are assigned a grade of 1, and poorly differentiated tumors a grade of 5. In 1992, the American Joint Committee on Cancer and the International Union Against Cancer adopted the TNM system for staging prostate cancer. Primary-stage tumors (T1) are asymptomatic and discovered on histologic examination of prostatic tissue specimens; T2 tumors are palpable on digital examination but are confined to the prostate gland; T3 tumors have extended beyond the prostate; and T4 tumors have pushed beyond the prostate to involve adjacent structures. Regional lymph node (N) and distant metastasis (M) are described as Nx or Mx (cannot be assessed), N0 or M0 (not present), and N1 or M1 (present).[33,45,46]

Two tumor markers, PSA and serum acid phosphatase, are important in the staging and management of prostatic cancer. In untreated cases, the level of PSA correlates with the volume and stage of disease. A rising PSA after treatment is consistent with progressive disease, whether it is locally recurring or metastatic. Measurement of PSA is used to detect recurrence after total prostatectomy. Because the prostate is the source of PSA, levels of the antigen should drop to zero after surgery; a rising PSA indicates recurring disease. Serum acid phosphatase is less sensitive than PSA and is used less frequently. However, it is more predictive of metastatic disease and may be used for that purpose.

Treatment.   Cancer of the prostate is treated by surgery, radiation therapy, and hormonal manipulations.[33,45,46] Chemotherapy has shown limited effectiveness in the treatment of prostate cancer. Treatment decisions are based on tumor grade and stage and on the age and health of the man. Expectant therapy (watching and waiting) may be used if the tumor is not producing symptoms, is expected to grow slowly, and is small and contained in one area of the prostate. This approach is particularly suited for men who are elderly or have other health problems. Most men with an anticipated survival greater than 10 years are considered for surgical or radiation therapy.[46] Radical prostatectomy involves complete removal of the seminal vesicles, prostate, and ampullae of the vas deferens. Refinements in surgical techniques have allowed maintenance of continence in most men and erectile function in selected cases. Radiation therapy can be delivered by a variety of techniques, including external beam radiation therapy and transperineal implantation of radioisotopes.

Metastatic disease often is treated with androgen deprivation therapy. Androgen deprivation may be induced at several levels along the pituitary-gonadal axis using a variety of methods or agents. Orchiectomy or estrogen therapy often is effective in reducing symptoms and extending survival. The LHRH analogs (*e.g.*, leuprolide, buserelin, nafarelin) block luteinizing hormone release from the pituitary and reduce testosterone levels without orchiectomy or estrogen therapy. When given continuously and in therapeutic doses, these drugs desensitize LHRH receptors in the pituitary, thereby preventing the release of luteinizing hormone. The antiandrogens (*i.e.*, flutamide and bicalutamide) block the uptake and actions of androgens in the target tissues. Complete androgen blockade can be achieved by combining an antiandrogen with an LHRH agent or orchiectomy. In men with metastatic prostate cancer, treatment with a combination of an LHRH agonist and flutamide seems to increase survival, particularly in those with minimal disease. Although testosterone is the main circulating androgen, the adrenal gland also secrets androgens. Inhibitors of adrenal androgen synthesis (*i.e.*, ketoconazole, aminoglutethimide, and glucocorticosteroids) may be used for treating men with advanced prostatic cancer who present with spinal cord compression, bilateral ureteral obstruction, or disseminated intravascular clotting. Palliative care includes adequate pain control and focal irradiation of symptomatic or unstable bone disease.

In summary, the prostate is a firm, glandular structure that surrounds the urethra. Inflammation of the prostate occurs as an acute or a chronic process. Chronic prostatitis probably is the most common cause of relapsing urinary tract infections in men. BPH is a common disorder in men older than 50 years of age. Because the prostate encircles the urethra, BPH exerts its effect through obstruction of urinary outflow from the bladder. Advances in the treatment of BPH include laser surgery, balloon dilatation, prostatic stents, and pharmacologic treatment using 5α-reductase inhibitors such as finasteride, which reduce prostate size by blocking the effects of androgen on the prostate, and α$_1$-adrenergic receptor blockers, which inhibit contraction of prostatic smooth muscle.

Prostatic cancer is the most common male cancer in the United States and is second to lung cancer as a cause of cancer-related death in men. A recent increase in diagnosed cases is thought to reflect earlier diagnosis because of widespread use of PSA testing. The incidence of prostate cancer increases with age and is greater in African Americans of all ages. Most prostate cancers are asymptomatic and are incidentally discovered on rectal examination. Screening for prostate cancer has become recognized as a method for early identification of prostate cancer. The American Cancer Society suggests that every man 50 years of age or older should have a rectal examination and PSA test done as part of his annual physical examination. Cancer of the prostate, like other forms of cancer, is graded according to the histologic characteristics of the tumor and staged clinically using the TNM system. Treatment, which is based on the extent of the disease, includes surgery, radiation therapy, and hormonal manipulation.

References

1. Behrman R., Kleigman R.M., Nelson W. (2000). *Nelson textbook of pediatrics* (15th ed., pp. 1546–1549, 1650–1651). Philadelphia: W.B. Saunders.
2. Moore K.L., Persaud T.V.N. (1998). *The developing human: Clinically oriented embryology* (6th ed., pp. 338–339). Philadelphia: W.B. Saunders.
3. Duckett J.W., Snow B.W. (1986). Disorders of the urethra and penis. In Walsh P.C., Gittes R.F, Permutter A.D. (Eds.), *Campbell's urology* (5th ed., pp. 200–239). Philadelphia: W.B. Saunders.
4. Vohra S., Badlani G. (1992). Balanitis and balanoposthitis. *Urologic Clinics of North America* 19, 143–147.
5. Fitkin J., Ho G.T. (1999). Peyronie's disease: Current management. *American Family Physician* 60, 549–554.
6. McAninch J.W. (2000). Disorders of the penis and male urethra. In Tanagho E.A., McAninch J.W. (Eds.), *Smith's general urology* (15th ed., pp. 663–675). New York: Lange Medical Books/McGraw-Hill.
7. Anderson K.E., Wagner G. (1995). Physiology of penile erection. *Physiology Review* 75, 191–236.
8. NIH Consensus Development Panel on Impotence. (1993). NIH Consensus Conference: Impotence. *Journal of the American Medical Association* 270, 83–90.
9. Lue T.F. (2000). Erectile dysfunction. *New England Journal of Medicine* 342, 1802–1813.
10. Levine L.A. (2000). Diagnosis and treatment of erectile dysfunction. *American Journal of Medicine* 109 (Suppl. 9A), 3S–12S.
11. Kaiser F.E. (1999). Erectile dysfunction in the aging man. *Medical Clinics of North America* 83, 1267–1278.
12. Feldman H.A., Goldstein J., Hatzichristou D.G., Krane R.J., McKinley J.B. (1994). Impotence and its medical and psychosocial effects. Results of the Massachusetts Male Aging Study. *Journal of Urology* 151, 54–61.
13. Kim E.D., Lipshultz L.I. (1997). Advances in treatment of organic erectile dysfunction. *Hospital Practice* 32(4), 101–120.
14. Harmon W.J., Nehra A. (1997). Priapism: Diagnosis and treatment. *Mayo Clinic Proceedings* 72, 350–355.
15. Kachhi P.N., Henderson S.O. (2000). Priapism after androstenedione intake for athletic performance enhancement. *Annals of Emergency Medicine* 35, 391–393.
16. Krieg R., Hoffman R. (1999). Current management of unusual genitourinary cancers: Part 1. Penile cancer. *Oncology* 13, 1347–1352.

17. Presti J.C., Herr H.W. (2000). Genital tumors. In Tanagho E.A., McAninch J.W. (Eds.), *Smith's general urology* (15th ed., pp. 430–434). New York: Lange Medical Books/McGraw-Hill.

18. Cotran R.S., Kumar V., Collins T. (1999). *Robbins pathologic basis of disease* (6th ed., pp. 1015–1016, 1018–1024, 1029–1033). Philadelphia: W.B. Saunders.

19. Docimo S.G., Silver R.I., Cromie W. (2000). The undescended testicle: Diagnosis and management. *American Family Physician* 62, 2037–2048.

20. Pillai S.B., Besner G.E. (1998). Pediatric testicular problems. *Pediatric Clinics of North America* 45, 813–818.

21. Kapur P., Caty M.G., Glick P.L. (1998). Pediatric hernias and hydroceles. *Pediatric Clinics of North America* 45, 773–789.

22. McAninch J.W. (2000). Disorders of the testis, scrotum, and spermatic cord. In Tanagho E.A., McAninch J.W. (Eds.), *Smith's general urology* (15th ed., pp. 684–693). New York: Lange Medical Books/McGraw-Hill.

23. Galejs L.E., Kass E.J. (1999). Diagnosis and treatment of acute scrotum. *American Family Physician* 59, 817–824.

24. Meares E.M. (1995). Nonspecific infections of the genitourinary tract. In Tanagho E.A., McAninch J.W. (Eds.), *Smith's general urology* (14th ed., pp. 237–238). Norwalk, CT: Appleton & Lange.

25. Mebcow M.M. (1975). Percivall Pott (1713–1788): 200th anniversary of first report of occupation-induced cancer of the scrotum in chimney sweepers (1745). *Urology* 6, 745.

26. Lowe F.C. (1992). Squamous cell carcinoma of the scrotum. *Urologic Clinics of North America* 19, 297–405.

27. Bosl G.J. (1997). Testicular germ-cell cancer. *New England Journal of Medicine* 337, 242–252.

28. Kinade S. (1999). Testicular cancer. *American Family Physician* 59, 2539–2544.

29. Krieger J.N., Nyberg L., Nickel J.C. (1999). NIH consensus definition and classification of prostatitis. *Journal of the American Medical Association* 282, 721–725.

30. McRae S.N., Shortliffe L.M.D. (2000). Bacterial infections of the genitourinary system. In Tanagho E.A., McAninch J.W. (Eds.), *Smith's general urology* (15th ed., pp. 254–259). New York: Lange Medical Books/McGraw-Hill.

31. Stevermer J.J., Easley S.K. (2000). Treatment of prostatitis. *American Family Physician* 61, 3015–3026.

32. Collins M.M., MacDonald R., Wilt T.J. (2000). Diagnosis and treatment of chronic abacterial prostatitis: A systemic review. *Annals of Internal Medicine* 133, 367–381.

33. Presti J.C. (2000). Neoplasms of the prostate gland. In Tanagho E.A., McAninch J.W. (Eds.), *Smith's general urology* (15th ed., pp. 399–406). New York: Lange Medical Books/McGraw-Hill.

34. Zida A., Rosenblum M., Crawford E.D. (1999). Benign prostatic hyperplasia: An overview. *Urology* 53 (Suppl. 3A), 1–6.

35. Roberts R.G., Hartlaub P.P. (1999). Evaluation of dysuria in men. *American Family Physician* 60, 865–872.

36. Elbadawi A. (1998). Voiding dysfunction in benign prostatic hyperplasia: Trends, controversies and recent revelations: Pathology and pathophysiology. *Urology* 51 (Suppl. 5A), 73–82.

37. Agency of Health Care Policy and Research. (1994). *Clinical practice guidelines for benign prostatic hyperplasia.* AHCPR publication no. 94-0582. Rockville, MD: U.S. Department of Health and Human Services.

38. Barry M.J., et al. (1992). The American Urological Association Index of Benign Prostatic Hypertrophy. *Journal of Urology* 148, 1549–1557.

39. Albertson P.C. (1997). Prostate disease in older men: Benign hyperplasia. *Hospital Practice* May 15, 61–81.

40. American Cancer Society. (2001). Prostate cancer resource center. [On-line]. Available: http://www.cancer.org.

41. Peterson R.O. (1999). The urinary tract and male reproductive system. In Rubin E., Farber J.L. (Eds.), *Pathology* (3rd ed., pp. 956–960). Philadelphia: Lippincott Williams & Wilkins.

42. Steinberg G.D., Carter B.S., Beaty T.L., Fowler F.L. Jr., O'Leary M.P., Brus Kewitz R.C., et al. (1990). The familial aggregation of prostate cancer: A case control study [Abstract]. *Journal of Urology* 143, 131A.

43. Woolf S.H. (1995). Screening for prostate cancer with prostate specific antigen: An examination of the evidence. *New England Journal of Medicine* 333, 1401–1405.

44. Brawer M.K. (1999). Prostate-specific antigen: Current status. *CA—A Cancer Journal for Clinicians* 49, 264–265.

45. Garnick M.B., Fair W.R. (1998). Combating prostate cancer. *Scientific American* 279(6), 74–83.

46. Stoller M.L., Presti J.C., Carroll P.R. (2001). Urology. In Tierney L.M., McPhee S.J., Papadakis M.A. (Eds.), *Current medical diagnosis and treatment* (40th ed., pp. 956–961). New York: Lange Medical Books/McGraw-Hill.

Chapter 44

Structure and Function of the Female Reproductive System

Patricia McCowen Mehring

The female genitourinary system consists of internal paired ovaries, uterine tubes, uterus, vagina, external mons pubis, labia majora, labia minora, clitoris, urethra, and perineal body. Although the female urinary structures are anatomically separate from the genital structures, their anatomic proximity provides a means for cross-contamination and shared symptomatology between the two systems (Fig. 44-1). This chapter focuses on the internal and external genitalia. It includes a discussion of hormonal and physical changes that occur throughout the life cycle in response to the gonadotropic hormones. The reader is referred to a specialty text for a discussion of pregnancy.

Reproductive Structures

After you have completed this section of the chapter, you should be able to meet the following objectives:

✦ Describe the anatomic relation of the structures of the external genitalia
✦ Name the three layers of the uterus and describe their function
✦ Cite the location of the ovaries in relation to the uterus, fallopian tubes, broad ligaments, and ovarian ligaments
✦ Explain the function of the fallopian tubes
✦ State the function of endocervical secretions

EXTERNAL GENITALIA

The external genitalia are located at the base of the pelvis in the perineal area and include the mons pubis, labia majora, labia minora, clitoris, and perineal body. The urethra and anus, although not genital structures, usually are considered in a discussion of the external genitalia. The external genitalia, also known collectively as the *vulva,* are diagrammed in Figure 44-2.

The *mons pubis* is a rounded, skin-covered fat pad located anterior to the symphysis pubis. Puberty stimulates an increase in the amount of fat and the development of darker and coarser hair over the mons. Normal pubic hair distribution in the female follows an inverted triangle with the base centered over the mons. Hair color and texture varies from person to person and among racial groups. There is an abundance of sebaceous glands in the skin that can become infected owing to normal variations in glandular secretions or poor hygiene. The mons pubis is the most common site of pubic lice infestation in the female. The *labia majora* (singular, labium majus) are analogous to the male scrotum. These structures are the outermost lips of the vulva, beginning anteriorly at the base of the mons pubis and ending posteriorly at the anus. The labia majora are composed of folds of skin and fat and become covered with hair at the onset of puberty. Before puberty, the labia majora have a skin covering similar to that covering the abdomen. With sufficient hormonal stimulation, the labia of

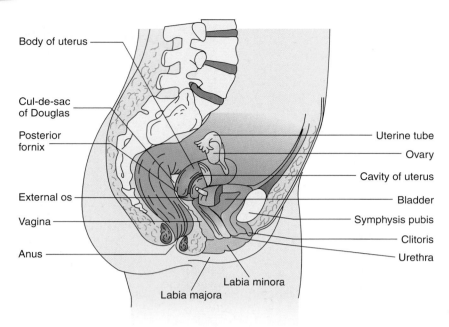

FIGURE 44-1 Female reproductive system as seen in sagittal section. (Chaffee E.E., Lytle I.M. [1980]. *Basic physiology and anatomy* [4th ed.]. Philadelphia: J.B. Lippincott)

a mature woman close over the urethral and vaginal openings; this can change after childbirth or surgery.

The *labia minora* (singular, labium minus) are located between the labia majora. These delicate cutaneous structures are smaller than the labia majora and are composed of skin, fat, and some erectile tissue. Unlike the skin of the labia majora, that of the labia minora is hairless and usually light pink. The labia minora begin anteriorly at the hood of the clitoris and end posteriorly at the base of the vagina. During sexual arousal, the labia minora become distended with blood; with resolution, the labia throb and then return

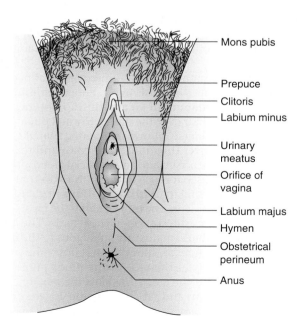

FIGURE 44-2 External genitalia of the female. (Chaffee E.E., Lytle I.M. [1980]. *Basic physiology and anatomy* [4th ed.]. Philadelphia: J.B. Lippincott)

to normal size. The sebaceous glands secrete an odoriferous fluid in the presence or absence of sexual arousal. The clitoris is located below the clitoral hood, or prepuce, which is formed by the joining of the two labia minora. The female clitoris is an erectile organ, rich in vascular and nervous supply. Analogous to the male penis, it is a highly sensitive organ that becomes distended during sexual stimulation.

The area between labia minora is called the *vestibule*. Located in the vestibule are the urethral and vaginal openings and Bartholin's lubricating glands. The *urethra,* or urinary meatus, is the external opening of the internal urinary bladder. The urethra is located posterior to the clitoris and usually is closer to the vaginal opening than to the clitoris. The urethral opening is the site of *Skene's glands,* which have a lubricating function. The vaginal orifice, commonly known as the *introitus,* is the opening between the external and internal genitalia. The size and shape of the opening are determined by a connective tissue membrane called the *hymen* that surrounds the introitus. The opening may be oval, circular, or sievelike and may be partially or completely occluded. Occlusion may occur because of the presence of an intact or partially intact hymen. Contrary to popular notion, an intact hymen does not indicate virginity because this tissue can be stretched without tearing. At puberty, an intact hymen may require surgical intervention to permit discharge of menstrual fluids.

The *perineal body* is that tissue located posterior to the vaginal opening and anterior to the anus. It is composed of fibrous connective tissue and is the site of insertion of several perineal muscles.

INTERNAL GENITALIA

Vagina

Connecting the internal and external genitalia is a fibromuscular tube called the *vagina.* The vagina, which is essentially free of sensory nerve fibers, is located behind the

The Female Genitourinary System

➤ The female reproductive system, which consists of the external and internal genitalia, has both sexual and reproductive functions.

➤ The external genitalia (labia majora, labia minora, clitoris, and vestibular glands) surround the openings of the urethra and vagina. Although the female urinary and genital structures are anatomically separate, their close proximity provides a means for cross-contamination and shared symptomatology.

➤ The internal genitalia of the female reproductive system are specialized to participate in sexual intercourse (the vagina), to produce and maintain the female egg cells (the ovaries), to transport these cells to the site of fertilization (the fallopian tubes), to provide a favorable environment for development of the offspring (the uterus), and to produce the female sex hormones (the ovaries).

ing of the vaginal mucosa and an increased glycogen content of the epithelial cells. The glycogen is fermented to lactic acid by the lactobacilli (*i.e., Döderlein's bacilli*) that are part of the normal vaginal flora, accounting for the mildly acid pH of vaginal fluid. The vaginal ecology can be disrupted at many levels, rendering it susceptible to infection. Pregnancy and the use of oral contraceptive agents increase the amount of estrogen in the system. Diabetes or a prediabetic state may increase the glycogen content of the cells. The use of systemic antibiotics may decrease the number of lactobacilli in the vagina.

Decreased estrogen stimulation after menopause causes the vaginal mucosa to become thin and dry, often resulting in dyspareunia (*i.e., painful intercourse*), atrophic vaginitis, and occasionally in vaginal bleeding. Estrogen levels can be estimated by means of vaginal scrapings obtained during a routine pelvic examination. The scrapings are used for a test, known as the *maturation index,* which examines the cellular structure and configuration of the vaginal epithelial cells. The maturation index determines the ratio of parabasal (least mature), intermediate, and superficial (most mature) cells. Typically, this index is 0-40-60 during the reproductive years. With diminished estrogen levels, there is a shift to the left, producing an index of 30-40-30 during the perimenopausal period and an index of 75-25-0 during the postmenopausal period.

urinary bladder and urethra and anterior to the rectum. The uterine cervix projects into the vagina at its upper end, forming recesses called *fornices.* The vagina functions as a route for discharge of menses and other secretions. It also serves as an organ of sexual fulfillment and reproduction.

The membranous vaginal wall forms two longitudinal folds and several transverse folds, or rugae. The vagina is lined with mucus-secreting stratified squamous epithelial cells. Vaginal tissue usually is moist, with a pH maintained within the bacteriostatic range of 3.8 to 4.2.

The epithelial cells of the vagina, like other tissues of the reproductive system, respond to changing levels of the ovarian sex hormones. Estrogen stimulates the proliferation and maturation of the vaginal mucosa; this results in a thicken-

Uterus and Cervix

The uterus is a thick-walled muscular organ. This pear-shaped, hollow structure is located between the bladder and the rectum. The uterus can be divided into three parts: the portion above the insertion of the fallopian tubes, called the *fundus;* the lower, constricted part, called the *cervix;* and the portion between the fundus and the cervix, called the *body of the uterus* (Fig. 44-3). The uterus is supported on both sides by four sets of ligaments: the *broad ligaments,* which run laterally from the body of the uterus to the pelvic side walls; the *round ligaments,* which run from the fundus laterally into each labium majus; the *uterosacral ligaments,* which run from the uterocervical junction to the sacrum; and the *cardinal* or *transverse cervical* ligaments.

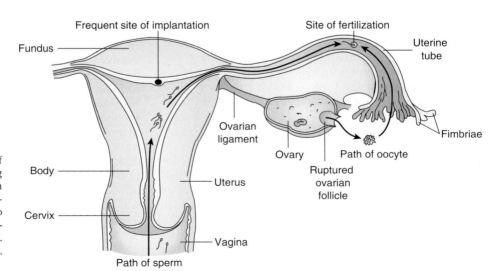

FIGURE 44-3 Schematic drawing of female reproductive organs, showing the path of the oocyte as it moves from the ovary into the fallopian (uterine) tube; the path of sperm is also shown, as is the usual site of fertilization. (Chaffee E.E., Lytle I.M. [1980]. *Basic physiology and anatomy* [4th ed.]. Philadelphia: J.B. Lippincott)

The wall of the uterus is composed of three layers: the perimetrium, the myometrium, and the endometrium. The *perimetrium* is the outer serous covering that is derived from the abdominal peritoneum. This outer layer merges with the peritoneum that covers the broad ligaments. Anteriorly, the perimetrium is reflected over the bladder wall, forming the vesicouterine pouch; posteriorly, it extends to form the *cul-de-sac,* or *pouch of Douglas.* Because of the proximity of the perimetrium to the urinary bladder, infection of this organ often causes uterine symptoms, particularly during pregnancy.

The middle muscle layer, the *myometrium,* forms the major portion of the uterine wall. It is continuous with the myometrium of the fallopian tubes and the vagina and extends into all the supporting ligaments with the exception of the broad ligaments. The inner fibers of the myometrium run in various directions, giving it an interwoven appearance. Contractions of these muscle fibers help to expel menstrual flow and the products of conception during miscarriage or childbirth. When pain accompanies the contractions associated with menses, it is called *dysmenorrhea.* The myometrium has an amazing ability to change length during pregnancy and labor, increasing the uterine capacity more than 4000 times.[1]

The *endometrium,* the inner layer of the uterus, is continuous with the lining of the fallopian tubes and vagina. The endometrium is made up of a basal and a superficial layer. The superficial layer is shed during menstruation and regenerated by cells of the basal layer. Ciliated cells promote the movement of tubal-uterine secretions out of the uterine cavity into the vagina.

The round *cervix* is the neck of the uterus that projects into the vagina. The cervix is a firm structure, composed of a connective tissue matrix of glands and muscular tissue elements, that becomes soft and pliable under the influence of hormones produced during pregnancy. Glandular tissue provides a rich supply of protective mucus that changes in character and quantity during the menstrual cycle and during pregnancy. The cervix is richly supplied with blood from the uterine artery and can be a site of significant blood loss during delivery.

The opening of the cervix, the os, forms a pathway between the uterus and the vagina. The vaginal opening is called the *external os* and the uterine opening, the *internal os.* The space between these two openings is the endocervical canal. Secretions from the columnar epithelium of the endocervix protect the uterus from infection, alter receptivity to sperm, and form a mucoid "plug" during pregnancy. The endocervical canal provides a route for menstrual discharge and sperm entrance.

Fallopian Tubes

The *fallopian,* or uterine, tubes are slender, cylindrical structures attached bilaterally to the uterus and supported by the upper folds of the broad ligament. The end of the fallopian tube nearest the ovary forms a funnel-like opening with fringed, finger-like projections, called *fimbriae,* that pick up the ovum after its release into the peritoneal cavity after ovulation (see Fig. 44-3). The fallopian tubes are formed of smooth muscle and lined with a ciliated, mucus-producing epithelial layer. The beating of the cilia, along with contractile movements of the smooth muscle, propels the nonmobile ovum toward the uterus. If coitus has occurred recently, fertilization normally occurs in the middle to outer portion of the fallopian tube. Besides providing a passageway for ova and sperm, the fallopian tubes provide for drainage of tubal secretions into the uterus.

Ovaries

By the third month of fetal life, the *ovaries* have fully developed and descended to their permanent pelvic position. Remnants of the primitive genital system provide lateral supporting attachments to the uterus; in the mature female, these supporting structures evolve into the round and suspensory ligaments. Remnants that do not evolve may form cysts, which may become symptomatic later in life.

Oogenesis is the process of generation of ova by mitotic division that begins at the sixth week of fetal life. These primitive germ cells ultimately provide the 1 to 2 million oocytes that are present in the ovaries at birth. At puberty, this number is reduced through cell death to approximately 300,000.

The neonate's ovaries are smooth, pale, and elongated. They become shorter, thicker, and heavier before the onset of menarche, which is initiated by pituitary influence. The initial hormonal stimulus for this development is believed to come from ovarian rather than systemic estrogen.

In the adult, the ovaries are flat, almond-shaped structures that are 3 to 5 cm long and weigh 2 to 3 g. They are located on either side of the uterus below the fimbriated ends of the two oviducts, or fallopian tubes. The ovaries are attached to the posterior surface of the broad ligament and to the uterus by the ovarian ligament. They are covered with a thin layer of surface epithelium that is continuous with the lining of the peritoneum. The integrity of this covering is periodically broken at the time of ovulation.

The ovaries, like the male testes, have a dual function: they store the female germ cells, or ova, and produce the female sex hormones, estrogen and progesterone. Unlike the male gonads, which produce sperm throughout a man's reproductive life, the female gonads contain a fixed number of ova at birth that diminishes throughout a woman's life.

Structurally, the mature ovary is divided into a highly vascular inner medulla, which contains supporting connective tissue, and an outer cortex of stroma and epithelial follicles (*i.e.,* vesicles), which contain the primary oocytes, or germ cells. After puberty, the pituitary gonadotropic hormones—follicle-stimulating hormone (FSH) and the luteinizing hormone (LH)—stimulate the primordial follicles to develop into *mature graafian follicles.* The graafian follicle produces estrogen, which begins to stimulate the development of the endometrium in the uterus. Although several follicles begin to develop during each ovulatory cycle, only one or two complete the entire developmental process and rupture to release a mature ovum. After ovulation, the follicle becomes luteinized; as the corpus luteum, it produces estrogen and progesterone to support the endometrium until conception occurs or the cycle begins again.

In summary, the female reproductive system consists of internal paired ovaries, uterine tubes, uterus, vagina, external mons pubis, labia majora, labia minora, clitoris, urethra, and perineal body. The genitourinary system as a whole serves sexual and reproductive functions throughout the life cycle. The uterus is a thick-walled, muscular organ. The wall of the uterus is composed of three layers: the outer perimetrium; the myometrium or muscle layer, which is continuous with the myometrium of the fallopian tubes and the vagina; and the inner lining or endometrium, which is continuous with the lining of the fallopian tubes and vagina. The gonads, or ovaries, which are internal in the female (unlike the testes in the male), have the dual function of storing the female germ cells, or ova, and producing the female sex hormones. Through the regulation and release of sex hormones, the ovaries influence the development of secondary sexual characteristics, regulation of menstrual cycles, maintenance of pregnancy, and advent of menopause.

Menstrual Cycle

After you have completed this section of the chapter, you should be able to meet the following objectives:

- ✦ Describe the feedback control of estrogen and progesterone levels by means of gonadotropin-releasing hormone, LH, FSH, and ovarian follicle function
- ✦ List the actions of estrogen and progesterone
- ✦ Describe the four functional compartments of the ovary
- ✦ Relate FSH and LH levels to the stages of follicle development and to estrogen and progesterone production
- ✦ Describe the endometrial changes that occur during the menstrual cycle
- ✦ Describe the composition of normal cervical mucus and the changes that occur during the menstrual cycle
- ✦ Describe the physiology of normal menopause

Between menarche (*i.e.,* first menstrual bleeding) and menopause (*i.e.,* last menstrual bleeding), the female reproductive system undergoes cyclic changes called the *menstrual cycle.* This includes the maturation and release of oocytes from the ovary during ovulation and periodic vaginal bleeding resulting from the shedding of the endometrial lining. It is not necessary for a woman to ovulate to menstruate; anovulatory cycles do occur. The menstrual cycle produces changes in the breasts, uterus, skin, ovaries, and perhaps other, unidentified tissues. The maintenance of the cycle affects biologic and sociologic aspects of a woman's life, including fertility, reproduction, sexuality, and femaleness.

HORMONAL CONTROL

Normal menstrual function results from interactions among the central nervous system, hypothalamus, anterior pituitary, ovaries, and associated target tissues. Although each part of the system is essential to normal function, the ovaries are primarily responsible for controlling the cyclic changes and the length of the menstrual cycle. In most women in the middle reproductive years, menstrual bleeding occurs every 25 to 35 days, with a median length of 28 days.

The hormonal control of the menstrual cycle is complex. For example, the biosynthesis of estrogens that occurs in adipose tissue may be a significant source of the hormone. There is evidence that a certain minimum body weight (48 kg) and fat content (16% to 24%) are necessary for menarche to occur and for the menstrual cycle to be maintained. This is supported by the observation of amenorrhea in women with anorexia nervosa, chronic disease, and malnutrition and in those who are long-distance runners. In women with anorexia nervosa, gonadotropin and estradiol secretion, including LH release and responsiveness to the hypothalamic gonadotropin-releasing hormone (GnRH), can revert to prepubertal levels. With resumption of weight gain and attainment of sufficient body mass, the normal hormonal pattern usually is reinstated. Obesity or significant weight gain also is associated with oligomenorrhea or amenorrhea and infertility, although the mechanism is not well understood.

Hypothalamic and Pituitary Hormones

Growth, prepubertal maturation, the reproductive cycle, and sex hormone secretion in males and females are regulated by FSH and LH from the anterior pituitary gland (Fig. 44-4). Because these hormones promote the growth of cells in the ovaries and testes as a means of stimulating the production of sex hormones, they are called the *gonadotropic hormones.* The secretion of LH and FSH is stimulated by GnRH from the hypothalamus. In addition to LH and FSH, the anterior pituitary secretes a third hormone called *prolactin.* The primary function of prolactin is the stimulation of lactation in the postpartum period. During pregnancy, prolactin, along with other hormones such as estrogen, progesterone, insulin, and cortisol, contributes to breast development in preparation for lactation. Although prolactin does not appear to play a physiologic role in ovarian

 Menstrual Cycle

➤ The menstrual cycle begins at menarche and continues until menopause. It includes the maturation and release of oocytes from the ovary during ovulation and periodic vaginal bleeding resulting from the shedding of the endometrial lining.

➤ The menstrual cycle is controlled by rhythmic synthesis and release of ovarian hormones (the estrogens and progesterone) under feedback control from the hypothalamic gonadotropin-releasing hormone and the anterior pituitary gonadotropic follicle-stimulating and luteinizing hormones.

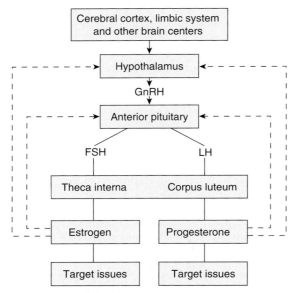

FIGURE 44-4 Hypothalamic-pituitary feedback control of estrogen and progesterone levels in the female.

function, hyperprolactinemia leads to hypogonadism. This may include an initial shortening of the luteal phase with subsequent anovulation, oligomenorrhea or amenorrhea, and infertility. The hypothalamic control of prolactin secretion is primarily inhibitory, and dopamine is the most important inhibitory factor. Hyperprolactinemia may occur as an adverse effect of drug treatment using phenothiazine derivatives (*i.e.,* antipsychotic drugs that block dopamine receptors).

Ovarian Hormones

The ovaries produce estrogens, progesterone, and androgens. Ovarian hormones are secreted in a cyclic pattern as a result of the interaction between the hypothalamic GnRH and the pituitary gonadotropic hormones, FSH and LH. The steroid sex hormones enter cells by passive diffusion, bind to specific receptor proteins in the cytoplasm, and then move to the nucleus, where they bind to specific sites on the chromosomes. These hormones exert their effects through gene-hormone interactions, which stimulate the synthesis of specific messenger ribonucleic acid (mRNA). In addition, estrogen appears to have the ability to influence cell activity through other nongenomic mechanisms. These nongenomic effects take place in cells that have no steroid receptors, possibly mediated by other membrane receptors. This may explain in part some of the nonreproductive effects of estrogen. An example of a nongenomic cardioprotective effect would be the antioxidant activity of estrogen in preventing endothelial injury that can lead to platelet adherence.[2] The number of hormonal receptor sites on a cell is not fixed; evidence suggests that they are constantly being removed and replaced. An increase or a decrease in the number of receptors can serve as a mechanism for regulating hormonal activity. For example, estrogen may induce the development of an increased number of estrogen receptors in some tissues and may stimulate the synthesis of progesterone receptors in others. In contrast, progesterone may cause a reduction in the number of estrogen and progesterone receptors.

The recent discovery of a second type of estrogen receptor (ER_2) that is different in structure, tissue distribution, and expression from ER_1 helps to expand our understanding of the mechanism of action of estrogen in the body. The ER_2 appears to be an activator of estrogen response, whereas the ER_1 appears to modulate or inhibit the action of estrogen.[3] Likewise, the progesterone receptor has two major forms (A and B), expressed by a single gene, but promoted differently in a complex system of transcription regulation.

Estrogens.   Estrogens are a family of structurally related female sex hormones synthesized and secreted by cells in the ovaries and, in small amounts, by cells in the adrenal cortex. Androgens can be converted to estrogens peripherally, especially in fat tissue. Three estrogens occur naturally in humans: estrone (E1), estradiol (E2), and estriol (E3). Of these, estradiol is the most biologically potent and the most abundantly secreted product of the ovary. Estrogens are secreted throughout the menstrual cycle. Two peaks occur: one before ovulation and one in the middle of the luteal phase. Estrogens are transported in the blood bound to specific plasma globulins (which can also bind testosterone), inactivated and conjugated in the liver, and then excreted in the bile.

Estrogens are necessary for the normal female physical maturation. In concert with other hormones, estrogens provide for the reproductive processes of ovulation, implantation of the products of conception, pregnancy, parturition, and lactation by stimulating the development and maintaining the growth of the accessory organs. In the absence of androgens, estrogens stimulate the intrauterine development of the vagina, uterus, and uterine tubes from the embryonic müllerian system. They also stimulate the stromal development and ductal growth of the breasts at puberty, are responsible for the accelerated pubertal skeletal growth phase and for closure of the epiphyses of the long bones, contribute to the growth of axillary and pubic hair, and alter the distribution of body fat to produce the typical female body contours, including the accumulation of body fat around the hips and breasts. Larger quantities of estrogen stimulate pigmentation of the skin in the nipple, areolar, and genital regions.

In addition to their effects on the growth of uterine muscle, estrogens play an important role in the development of the endometrial lining. During anovulatory cycles, continued exposure to estrogens for prolonged periods leads to abnormal hyperplasia of the endometrium and abnormal bleeding patterns. When estrogen production is poorly coordinated during the normal menstrual period, inappropriate bleeding and shedding of the endometrium also can occur (see Chapter 45).

Estrogens have a number of important extragenital metabolic effects. They are responsible for maintaining the normal structure of skin and blood vessels in women. Estrogens decrease the rate of bone resorption by antagonizing the effects of parathyroid hormone on bone; for this reason, osteoporosis is a common problem in estrogen-deficient postmenopausal women. In the liver, estrogens increase the synthesis of transport proteins for thyroxine, estrogen, testosterone, and other hormones. Estrogens also affect the composition of the plasma lipoproteins. They produce an increase in high-density lipoproteins (HDLs), a slight reduction in low-density lipoproteins (LDLs), and a reduction in cholesterol levels (see Chapter 22). Estrogens have additional cardioprotective actions, including direct antiatherosclerotic effects on the arterial wall (augmentation of vasodilating and antiplatelet aggregation factors such as nitric oxide and prostacyclin), vasodilation through endothelium-independent mechanisms, antioxidant activity, reduced levels of angiotensin-converting enzyme and renin, reduction of homocysteine levels, improved peripheral glucose metabolism with subsequent decreased circulating insulin levels, and direct effects on cardiac function (*i.e.,* increased left ventricular diastolic filling and stroke volume output). Estrogens increase plasma triglyceride levels and they enhance the coagulability of blood by effecting increased circulating levels of plasminogen and factors II, VII, IX, and X.

Estrogens appear to have both neurotropic and neuroprotective effects on cognitive function and memory. Studies indicate possible prevention of Alzheimer's disease through anti-inflammatory mechanisms to prevent vascular injury, increased cerebral blood flow, and altered brain activation. Estrogens promote dendritic branching and enhance presynaptic and postsynaptic signal transmission through increased production of neurotransmitters and receptors.[4]

The estrogens cause moderate retention of sodium and water. Most women retain sodium and water and gain weight just before menstruation. This occurs because the estrogens facilitate the movement of intravascular fluids into the extracellular spaces, producing edema and increased sodium and water retention by the kidneys because of the decreased plasma volume. The actions of estrogens are summarized in Table 44-1.

Progesterone. Although the word *progesterone* refers to a substance that maintains pregnancy, progesterone is secreted as part of the normal menstrual cycle. The corpus luteum of the ovary secretes large amounts of progesterone after ovulation, and the adrenal cortex secretes small amounts. The hormone circulates in the blood attached to a specific plasma protein. It is metabolized in the liver and conjugated for excretion in the bile.

The local effects of progesterone on reproductive organs include the glandular development of the lobular and alveolar tissue of the breasts and the cyclic glandular development of the endometrium. Progesterone also can compete with aldosterone at the level of the renal tubule, causing a decrease in sodium reabsorption, with a resultant increase in secretion of aldosterone by the adrenal cortex, as occurs in pregnancy. Although the mechanism is uncertain, progesterone increases basal body temperature and is responsible for the increase in body temperature that occurs with ovulation. Smooth muscle relaxation under the influence of progesterone plays an important role in maintaining pregnancy by decreasing uterine contractions and is responsible for many of the common discomforts of pregnancy, such as edema, nausea, constipation, flatulence, and headaches. The increased progesterone present during pregnancy and the luteal phase of the menstrual cycle enhances the ventilatory response to carbon dioxide, leading to a measurable change in arterial and alveolar carbon dioxide (PCO_2) levels.

Androgens. The normal female produces androgens, estrogens, and progesterone. Approximately 25% of these androgens are secreted from the ovaries, 25% from the adrenal cortex, and 50% from ovarian or adrenal precursors. In the female, androgens contribute to normal hair growth at puberty and may have other important metabolic effects.

TABLE 44-1 ✦ Actions of Estrogens

General Function	Specific Actions
Growth and development	
Reproductive organs	Stimulate development of vagina, uterus, and fallopian tubes in utero and of secondary sex characteristics during puberty
Skeleton	Accelerate growth of long bones and closure of epiphyses at puberty
Reproductive processes	
Ovulation	Promote growth of ovarian follicles
Fertilization	Alter the cervical secretions to favor survival and transport of sperm
	Promote motility of sperm within the fallopian tubes by decreasing mucus viscosity
Implantation	Promote development of endometrial lining in the event of pregnancy
Vagina	Proliferate and cornify vaginal mucosa
Cervix	Increase mucus consistency
Breasts	Stimulate stromal development and ductal growth
General metabolic effects	
Bone resorption	Decrease rate of bone resorption
Plasma proteins	Increase production of thyroid and other binding globulins
Lipoproteins	Increase high-density and slightly decrease low-density lipoproteins

OVARIAN FOLLICLE DEVELOPMENT AND OVULATION

The tissues of the adult ovary can be conveniently divided into four compartments, or units: the stroma, or supporting tissue; the interstitial cells; the follicles; and the corpus luteum. The *stroma* is the connective tissue substance of the ovary in which the follicles are distributed. The *interstitial cells* are estrogen-secreting cells that resemble the Leydig's cells, or interstitial cells, of the testes.

Beginning at puberty, a cyclic rise in the anterior pituitary hormones FSH and LH stimulates the development of several graafian, or mature, follicles. Follicles at all stages of development can be found in both ovaries, except in menopausal women (Fig. 44-5). Most follicles exist as primary follicles, each of which consists of a round oocyte surrounded by a single layer of flattened, epithelium-derived granulosa cells and a basement membrane. The primary follicles constitute an inactive pool of follicles from which all the ovulating follicles develop. Under the influence of endocrine stimulation, 6 to 12 primary follicles develop into secondary follicles once every ovulatory cycle. During the development of the secondary follicle, the primary oocyte increases in size, and the granulosa cells proliferate to form a multi-layered wall around it. During this time, a membrane called the *zona pellucida* develops and surrounds the oocyte and small pockets of fluid begin to appear between the granulosa cells. Blood vessels, however, do not penetrate the basement membrane; the granulosa cell layer remains avascular until after ovulation has occurred.

As the follicles mature, FSH stimulates the development of the cell layers. Cells from the surrounding stromal tissue align themselves to form a cellular wall called the *theca*. The cells of the theca become differentiated into two layers: an inner theca interna, which lies adjacent to the follicular cells, and an outer theca externa. As the follicle enlarges, a single large cavity, or *antrum,* is formed, and a portion of the granulosa cells and the oocytes are displaced to one side of the follicle by the fluid that accumulates. The secondary oocyte remains surrounded by a crown of granulosa cells, the corona radiata. As the follicle ripens, ovarian estrogen is produced by the granulosa cells. Selection of a dominant follicle occurs with the conversion to an estrogen micro-environment. The lesser follicles, although continuing to produce some estrogen, atrophy or become atretic. The dominant follicle accumulates a greater mass of granulosa cells, and the theca becomes richly vascular, giving the follicle a hyperemic appearance. High levels of estrogen exert a negative feedback effect on FSH, inhibiting multiple follicular development and causing an increase in LH levels. This represents the follicular stage of the menstrual cycle. As estrogen suppresses FSH, the actions of LH predominate, and the mature follicle (measuring approximately 20 mm) bursts; the oocyte, along with the corona radiata, is ejected from the follicle. The ovum normally is then picked up and transported through the fallopian tube toward the uterus.

After ovulation, the follicle collapses, and the luteal stage of the menstrual cycle begins. The granulosa cells are invaded by blood vessels and yellow lipochrome-bearing cells from the theca layer. A rapid accumulation of blood and fluid forms a mass called the *corpus luteum*. Leakage of this blood onto the peritoneal surface that surrounds the ovary is thought to contribute to the *mittelschmerz* ("middle [or intermenstrual] pain") of ovulation. During the luteal

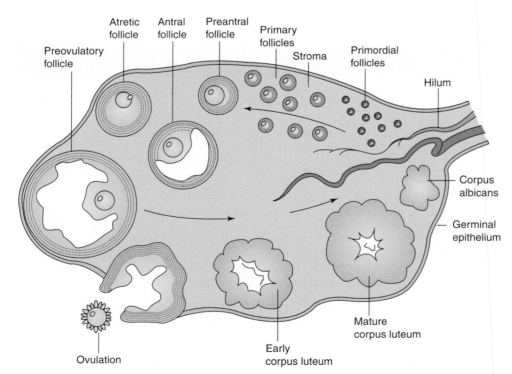

FIGURE 44-5 Schematic diagram of an ovary, showing the sequence of events in the origin, growth, and rupture of an ovarian follicle and the formation and retrogression of a corpus luteum. The atretic follicles are those that show signs of degeneration and death.

stage, progesterone is secreted from the corpus luteum. If fertilization does not take place, the corpus luteum atrophies and is replaced by white scar tissue called the *corpus albicans;* the hormonal support of the endometrium is withdrawn and menstruation occurs. In the event of fertilization, a hormone called *human chorionic gonadotropin* is produced by the trophoblastic cells in the blastocyst. This hormone prevents luteal regression. The corpus luteum remains functional for 3 months and provides hormonal support for pregnancy until the placenta is fully functional. Figure 44-6 shows the hormonal changes that occur during the development of the ovarian follicle and ovulation.

ENDOMETRIAL CHANGES

The endometrium consists of two distinct layers, or zones, that are responsive to hormonal stimulation: a basal layer and a functional layer. The *basal layer* lies adjacent to the myometrium and is not sloughed during menstruation. The *functional layer* arises from the basal layer and undergoes proliferative changes and menstrual sloughing. It can be subdivided into two components: a thin, superficial, compact layer and a deeper spongiosa layer that makes up most of the secretory and fully developed endometrium. The endometrial cycle can be divided into three phases: the proliferative, or preovulatory, phase, during which the glands and

stroma of the superficial layer grow rapidly under the influence of estrogen; the secretory, or postovulatory, phase, during which progesterone produces glandular dilation and active mucus secretion and the endometrium becomes highly vascular and edematous; and the menstrual phase, during which the superficial layer degenerates and sloughs off.

CERVICAL MUCUS

Cervical mucus is a complex, heterogeneous secretion produced by the glands of the endocervix. It is composed of 92% to 98% water and 1% inorganic salts, mainly sodium chloride. The mucus also contains simple sugars, polysaccharides, proteins, and glycoproteins. Its pH usually is alkaline, ranging from 6.5 to 9.0. Its characteristics are strongly influenced by serum levels of estrogen and progesterone. Estrogen stimulates the production of large amounts of clear, watery mucus through which sperm can penetrate most easily. Progesterone, even in the presence of estrogen, reduces the secretion of mucus. During the luteal phase of the menstrual cycle, mucus is scant, viscous, and cellular (see Fig. 44-6).

Two methods are used to examine the properties of cervical mucus and correlate them with hormonal activity. *Spinnbarkeit* is the property that allows cervical mucus to be stretched or drawn into a thread. Spinnbarkeit can be estimated by stretching a sample of cervical mucus between two glass slides and measuring the maximum length of the thread before it breaks. At midcycle, spinnbarkeit usually exceeds 10 cm. A second method of estimating hormonal levels is *ferning,* or arborization. Ferning refers to the characteristic microscopic pattern that results from the crystallization of the inorganic salts in the cervical mucus when it is dried. As the estrogen levels increase, the composition of the cervical mucus changes, so that dried mucus begins to demonstrate ferning in the later part of the follicular phase. The absence of ferning can indicate inadequate estrogen stimulation of the endocervical glands or inhibition of the endocervical glands by increased secretion of progesterone. Persistent ferning throughout the menstrual cycle suggests anovulatory cycles or insufficient progesterone secretion.

MENOPAUSE

Menopause is the cessation of menstrual cycles. Like menarche, it is more of a process than a single event. Most women stop menstruating between 48 and 55 years of age. *Perimenopause* (the years immediately surrounding menopause) precedes menopause by approximately 4 years and is characterized by menstrual irregularity and other menopausal symptoms. *Climacteric* is a more encompassing term that refers to the entire transition to the nonreproductive period of life. Premature ovarian failure describes the approximately 1% of women who experience menopause before the age of 40. A woman who has not menstruated for a full year or has an FSH level greater than 30 mIU/mL is considered menopausal.

Menopause results from the gradual cessation of ovarian function and the resultant diminished levels of estrogen.

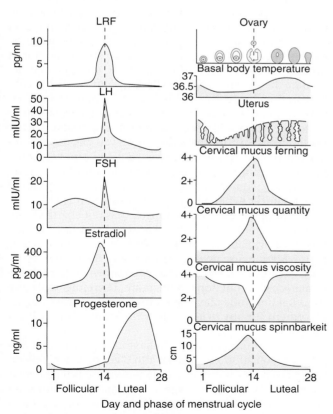

FIGURE 44-6 Hormonal and morphologic changes during the normal menstrual cycle. (Hershman J.M. [1982]. *Endocrine pathophysiology* [2nd ed.]. Philadelphia: Lea & Febiger)

Although estrogens derived from the adrenal cortex continue to circulate in a woman's body, they are insufficient to maintain the secondary sexual characteristics in the same manner as ovarian estrogens. As a result, breast tissue, body hair, skin elasticity, and subcutaneous fat decrease; the ovaries and uterus diminish in size; and the cervix and vagina become pale and friable. Problems that can arise as a result of this urogenital atrophy include vaginal dryness, urinary stress incontinence, urgency, nocturia, vaginitis, and urinary tract infection. The woman may find intercourse painful and traumatic, although some type of vaginal lubrication may be helpful.

Systemically, a woman may experience significant vasomotor instability secondary to the decrease in estrogens and the relative increase in other hormones, including FSH, LH, GnRH, dehydroepiandrosterone, and androstenedione, epinephrine, corticotropin, β-endorphin, growth hormone, and calcitonin gene-related peptide. This instability may give rise to "hot flashes," palpitations, dizziness, and headaches as the blood vessels dilate. Despite the association with these biochemical changes, the underlying cause of hot flashes is unknown.[5] Tremendous variation exists in the onset, frequency, severity, and length of time that women experience hot flashes. When they occur at night and are accompanied by significant perspiration, they are referred to as *night sweats*. Insomnia as well as frequent awakening because of vasomotor symptoms can lead to sleep deprivation. A woman may experience irritability, anxiety, and depression as a result of these uncontrollable and unpredictable events.

Consequences of long-term estrogen deprivation include osteoporosis due to an imbalance in bone remodeling (*i.e.,* bone resorption occurs at a faster rate than bone formation), and an increased risk for cardiovascular disease (atherosclerosis is accelerated), which is the leading cause of death for women after menopause. Hormone replacement therapy (HRT) to slow the rate of bone loss is the gold standard for prevention and treatment of osteoporosis in women. Other therapies include bisphosphonates, calcitonin, raloxifene (a selective estrogen receptor modulator that works only on certain estrogen receptors, but not others), calcium, and fluoride (see Chapter 58).

HRT has been associated with a 50% reduction in coronary heart disease mortality rates. Secondary prevention in women with established heart disease is less clear. Estrogen replacement is associated with protection in long-term users but may increase risk of a second cardiovascular event within the first year of HRT use through an increased incidence of deep vein thrombosis and pulmonary emboli.[6] Research also points to other potential advantages to long-term HRT, including reduced risk of Alzheimer's disease (leading cause of lost independence and institutionalization),[7] decreased risk of colon cancer (third leading cause of cancer death among women),[8] less tooth loss,[9] and lower incidence of macular degeneration (leading cause of legal blindness in the U.S.).[10]

HRT continues to be controversial with women. An association between the use of estrogen replacement therapy (continuous estrogen only [ERT]) and the development of endometrial cancer was noted in the 1970s. It is now known that unopposed estrogen can lead to the development of endometrial hyperplasia, which in some cases can increase a woman's risk for endometrial cancer. HRT that involves the use of both estrogen and progesterone is not associated with endometrial cancer. When used cyclically, progesterone is added for 10 to 14 days to mature any endometrium that has developed in response to the estrogen. Progesterone withdrawal results in endometrial shedding (*i.e.,* a cyclic bleeding episode). When used continuously, a small amount of progesterone is added to the daily estrogen regimen. This continuous exposure to progesterone inhibits endometrial development. Eventually, the continuous regimen results in no bleeding; however, it can be associated with irregular bleeding and spotting until the lining becomes atrophic. Prevention of endometrial hyperplasia either by shedding the endometrial buildup or by preventing its development minimizes the risk of endometrial cancer. Despite reassurance, some women still worry that estrogen causes cancer.

The association with breast cancer is the other area of concern, and the data are not as clear here despite over 50 years of study. When evaluating the many studies reporting estimated risks of breast cancer associated with ERT/HRT, most of the confidence intervals cross the relative risk of 1 and therefore are not statistically significant.[11] However, new studies linking estrogen and breast cancer continue to make front-page news, and consequently the worry persists. Current theory postulates that these studies are in fact detection studies rather than incidence studies, which would explain why some show a positive correlation between estrogen and breast cancer, whereas other studies do not. If unknown cancer cells exist in the breast, estrogen may accelerate the growth of those cells to a point where the cancer can then be detected. This is not necessarily bad news. Once cancer is detected, it can be treated. All mortality studies to date show a lower death rate among women using hormones at the time the breast cancer was diagnosed compared with those women who were not on hormones at the time of diagnosis. The risk–benefit ratio must be carefully weighed by women, taking into account their individual circumstances, when making decisions about HRT.

Although the age of menopause has not changed substantially from the early 1900s, life expectancy has. Women today will live almost one third of their lives after menopause. Menopause now represents only the end of reproductive capability. Estrogen has been shown to participate in many other functions in the body. Therefore, replacing this vital hormone may be no different than providing replacement for any other endocrine organ failure within the body.

Societal mores influence behaviors. A society that emphasizes youthfulness, fitness, and vigor may not look on aging as a positive process, and menopause is regarded as a hallmark of advancing age. A woman who focuses her energy on beauty and youth may feel frustrated or depressed by the natural aging process. A woman who values her other, nonphysical attributes may welcome advancing age as a time when she may more fully develop as a person.

In summary, between the menarche and menopause, the female reproductive system undergoes cyclic changes called the *menstrual cycle*. The normal menstrual function results from complex interactions among the hypothalamus, which produces GnRH; the anterior pituitary gland, which synthesizes and releases FSH, LH, and prolactin; the ovaries, which synthesize and release estrogens, progesterone, and androgens; and associated target tissues, such as the endometrium and the vaginal mucosa. Although each component of the system is essential for normal functioning, the ovarian hormones are largely responsible for controlling the cyclic changes and length of the menstrual cycle. Estrogens are necessary for normal female physical maturation, for growth of ovarian follicles, for generation of a climate that is favorable to fertilization and implantation of the ovum, and for promoting the development of the endometrium in the event of pregnancy. Estrogens also have a number of extragenital effects, including prevention of bone resorption and regulation of the composition of cholesterol-carrying lipoproteins (HDL and LDL) in the blood. The functions of progesterone include the glandular development of the lobular and alveolar tissue of the breasts and the cyclic glandular development of the endometrium, and maintenance of pregnancy. Androgens contribute to hair distribution in the female and may have important metabolic effects.

Breasts

After you have completed this section of the chapter, you should be able to meet the following objectives:

- ✦ Describe the anatomy of the female breast
- ✦ Describe the influence of hormones on breast development
- ✦ Characterize the changes in breast structure that occur with pregnancy, lactation, and menopause

Although anatomically separate, the breasts are functionally related to the female genitourinary system in that they respond to the cyclic changes in sex hormones and produce milk for infant nourishment. The breasts also are important for their sexual function and for cosmetic appearance. Breast cancer represents the most common malignancy among women in the United States. The high rate of breast cancer has drawn even greater attention to the importance of the breasts throughout the life span.

STRUCTURE

The breasts, or mammary tissues, are located between the third and seventh ribs of the anterior chest wall and are supported by the pectoral muscles and superficial fascia. They are specialized glandular structures that have an abundant shared nervous, vascular, and lymphatic supply (Fig. 44-7). What are commonly called breasts are two parts of a single anatomic breast. This contiguous nature of breast tissue is important in health and illness. Men and women alike are born with rudimentary breast tissue, with the ducts lined with epithelium. In women, the pituitary release of FSH, LH, and prolactin at puberty stimulates the ovary to produce and release estrogen. This estrogen stimulates the growth and proliferation of the ductile system. With the onset of ovulatory cycles, progesterone release stimulates the growth and development of ductile and alveolar secretory epithelium. By adolescence, the breasts have developed characteristic fat deposition patterns and contours.

Structurally, the breast consists of fat, fibrous connective tissue, and glandular tissue. The superficial fibrous connective tissue is attached to the skin, a fact that is important in the visual observation of skin movement over the breast during breast self-examination. The breast mass is supported by the fascia of the pectoralis major and minor muscles and by the fibrous connective tissue of the breast. Fibrous tissue ligaments, called *Cooper's ligaments*, extend from the outer boundaries of the breast to the nipple area in a radial manner, like the spokes on a wheel (see Fig. 44-7).

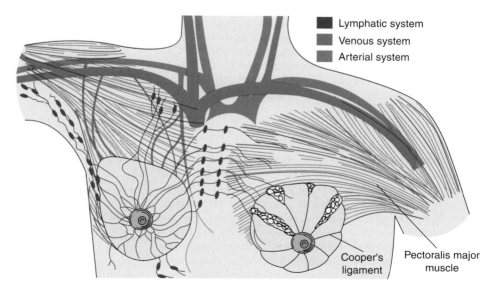

Lymphatic system
Venous system
Arterial system

Cooper's ligament

Pectoralis major muscle

FIGURE 44-7 The breasts, showing the shared vascular and lymphatic supply as well as the pectoral muscles.

These ligaments further support the breast and form septa that divide the breast into 15 to 25 lobes. Each lobe consists of grapelike clusters, alveoli or glands, which are interconnected by ducts. The alveoli are lined with secretory cells capable of producing milk or fluid under the proper hormonal conditions (Fig. 44-8). The route of descent of milk and other breast secretions is from alveoli to duct, to intralobar duct, to lactiferous duct and reservoir, to nipple. Breast milk is produced secondary to complex hormonal changes associated with pregnancy. Fluid is produced and reabsorbed during the menstrual cycle. The breasts respond to the cyclic changes in the menstrual cycle with fullness and discomfort.

The nipple is made up of epithelial, glandular, erectile, and nervous tissue. Areolar tissue surrounds the nipple and is recognized as the darker, smooth skin between the nipple and the breast. The small bumps or projections on the areolar surface known as *Montgomery's tubercles* are sebaceous glands that keep the nipple area soft and elastic. At puberty and during pregnancy, increased levels of estrogen and progesterone cause the areola and nipple to become darker and more prominent and Montgomery's glands to become more active. The erectile tissue of the nipple is responsive to psychological and tactile stimuli, which contributes to the sexual function of the breasts.

There are many individual variations in breast size and shape. The shape and texture vary with hormonal, genetic, nutritional, and endocrine factors and with muscle tone, age, and pregnancy. A well-developed set of pectoralis muscles supports the breast mass higher on the chest wall. Poor posture, significant weight loss, and lack of support may cause the breasts to droop.

PREGNANCY

During pregnancy, the breasts are significantly altered by increased levels of estrogen and progesterone. Estrogen stimulates increased vascularity of the breasts and the growth and extension of the ductile structures, causing "heaviness" of the breasts. Progesterone causes marked budding and growth of the alveolar structures. The alveolar epithelium assumes a secretory state in preparation for lactation. The progesterone-induced changes that occur during pregnancy may confer some protection against cancer. Cellular changes that occur in the alveolar lining are thought to change the susceptibility of these cells to estrogen-mediated changes later in life.

LACTATION

During lactation, milk is secreted by alveolar cells, which are under the influence of the anterior pituitary hormone prolactin. Milk ejection from the ductile system occurs in response to the release of oxytocin from the posterior pituitary. The suckling of the infant provides the stimulus for milk ejection. Suckling produces feedback to the hypothalamus, stimulating the release of oxytocin from the posterior pituitary. Oxytocin causes contraction of the myoepithelial cells lining the alveoli and ejection of milk into

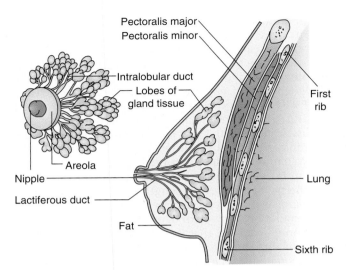

FIGURE 44-8 The breast, showing the glandular tissue and ducts of the mammary glands. (Chaffee E.E., Lytle I.M. [1980]. *Basic physiology and anatomy* [4th ed.]. Philadelphia: J.B. Lippincott)

the ductal system. A woman may have breast leakage for 3 months to 1 year after the termination of breast-feeding as breast tissue and hormones regress to the nonlactating state. Overzealous breast stimulation with or without pregnancy can likewise cause breast leakage.

CHANGES WITH MENOPAUSE

At the onset of menopause, the levels of estrogen and progesterone are gradually reduced, and the breasts regress because of loss of glandular tissue. The lobular-alveolar structures atrophy, leaving fat, connective tissue, and ducts. The breasts become pendulous with the decrease in tissue mass.

In summary, the breast is a complex structure of variable size, consistency, and composition. Although anatomically distinct, the breasts are functionally related to the female genitourinary system in that they respond to cyclic changes in sex hormones and produce milk for infant nourishment. Breast tissue is not static but changes throughout the life cycle with development of the alveolar structures in preparation for lactation during pregnancy, milk production during pregnancy, and replacement of glandular tissue with adipose tissue during menopause.

Related Web Sites

American College of Obstetricians and Gynecologists
    www.acog.org
National Osteoporosis Foundation   www.nof.org
North American Menopause Society   www.menopause.org

References

1. Benson R.C., Pernoll M.L. (1994). *Handbook of obstetrics and gynecology* (9th ed.). New York: McGraw-Hill.
2. Revelli A., Massobrio M., Tesarik J. (1998). Nongenomic actions of steroid hormones in reproductive tissue. *Endocrine Review* 19, 3–17.
3. Hall J.M., McDonnell D.P. (1999). The estrogen receptor β-isoform (ER beta) of the human estrogen receptor modulates ER alpha transcriptional activity and is the key regulator of the cellular response to estrogens and anti-estrogens. *Endocrinology* 140, 5566–5578.
4. Speroff L., Glass R.H., Kase N.G. (1999). *Clinical gynecologic endocrinology and infertility* (6th ed., pp. 64–66, 664, 667, 684). Philadelphia: Lippincott Williams & Wilkins.
5. Rebar R., Gass M. (2000). Hormonal changes and symptomatic management. *Clinical Bulletins in Menopause* 1, 2.
6. Speroff L. (2000). Postmenopausal HRT and CHD: Clinical implications of recent randomized trial results. *Contemporary Obstetrics/Gynecology* 8, 89–104.
7. Seifer D.B., Kennard E.A. (1999). *Menopause: Endocrinology and management* (p. 100). Totowa, NJ: Humana Press.
8. Nanda K., Bostoc L.A., Hasselblad V., Simmel D.L. (1999). Hormone replacement therapy and the risk of colorectal cancer: A meta-analysis. *Obstetrics and Gynecology* 93, 880–888.
9. Grodstein F., Colditz G.A., Stampfer M.J. (1996). Postmenopausal hormone use and tooth loss: A prospective study. *Journal of the American Dental Association* 127, 370–377.
10. The Eye-Disease Case-Control Study Group. (1992). Risk factors for neurovascular age-related macular degeneration. *Archives of Ophthalmology* 110, 1701–1708.
11. Speroff L. (2000). Postmenopausal estrogen-progestin therapy and breast cancer: A clinical response to an epidemiologic report. *Contemporary Obstetrics/Gynecology* 3, 103–121.

Chapter 45

Alterations in Structure and Function of the Female Reproductive System

Patricia McCowen Mehring

Disorders of the female genitourinary system have widespread effects on physical and psychological function, affecting sexuality and reproductive function. The reproductive structures are located close to other pelvic structures, particularly those of the urinary system, and disorders of the reproductive system may affect urinary function. This chapter focuses on infection and inflammation, benign conditions, and neoplasms of the female reproductive structures; disorders of pelvic support and uterine position; and alterations in menstruation. An overview of infertility also is included.

Disorders of the External Genitalia and Vagina

After you have completed this section of the chapter, you should be able to meet the following objectives:

✦ Compare the extragenital abnormalities associated with vulvitis, Bartholin's cyst, epidermal cysts, nevi, vulvar dystrophy, vulvodynia, and cancer of the vulva

✦ State the role of Döderlein's bacilli in maintaining the normal ecology of the vagina

◆ Describe the conditions that predispose to vaginal infections and the methods used to prevent and treat these infections
◆ Cite the association between diethylstilbestrol and adenocarcinoma of the vagina

DISORDERS OF THE EXTERNAL GENITALIA

Vulvitis and Folliculitis

Vulvitis is characterized by inflammation and pruritus (itching) of the vulva. It is not considered a specific disease but typically accompanies other local and systemic disorders. The cause often is an irritating vaginal discharge. *Candida albicans*, a yeast, is the most common cause of chronic vulvar pruritus, particularly in women with diabetes mellitus. Vulvitis also may be a component of sexually transmitted diseases (STDs) such as herpes genitalis and human papillomavirus (HPV) infection (*i.e.*, condyloma). Local dermatologic reactions to chemical irritants, such as laundry products, perfumed soaps or sprays, and spermicides, or to allergens such as poison ivy, also can cause inflammation. Vulvar itching may be caused by atrophy that is part of the normal aging process.

Management of vulvitis focuses on appropriate treatment of underlying causes and comfort measures to relieve the irritation. These include keeping the area clean and dry; using warm sitz baths with baking soda, wet dressings, or Burow's solution soaks (a mild astringent); or applying a mild hydrocortisone cream for the immediate relief of symptoms.

Folliculitis is an infection that involves the hair follicles of the mons or labia majora. The infection, characterized by small red papules or pustules surrounding the hair shaft, is relatively common because of the density of bacteria in this area and the occlusive nature of clothing covering the genitalia. Treatment includes thorough cleaning of the area with germicidal soap, followed by the application of a mild bacterial ointment (*e.g.*, Neosporin or Polysporin).

Bartholin's Gland Cyst and Abscess

Bartholin's cyst is a fluid-filled sac that results from the occlusion of the duct system in Bartholin's gland. When the cyst becomes infected, the contents become purulent; if the infection goes untreated, an abscess can result. The obstruction that causes cyst and abscess formation most commonly follows a bacterial, chlamydial, or gonococcal infection. Cysts can attain the size of an orange and frequently recur (Fig. 45-1). Abscesses can be extremely tender and painful. Asymptomatic cysts require no treatment. The treatment of symptomatic cysts consists of the administration of appropriate antibiotics, local application of moist heat, and incision and drainage. Cysts that frequently are abscessed or are large enough to cause blockage of the introitus may require surgical intervention (*i.e.*, marsupialization, a procedure that involves removal of a wedge of vulvar skin and the cyst wall).[1]

Epidermal Cysts

Epidermal cysts (*i.e.*, sebaceous or inclusion cysts) are common semisolid tumors of the vulva. These small nodules are

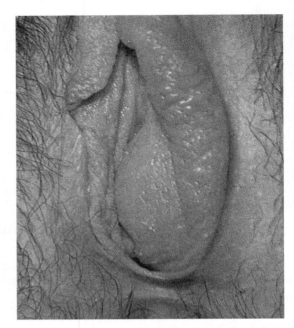

FIGURE 45-1 Bartholin's gland cyst. The 4-cm lesion is located to the right of and posterior to the vaginal introitus. (Rubin E., Farber J.L. [1999]. *Pathology* [3rd ed., p. 970]. Philadelphia: Lippincott Williams & Wilkins)

lined with keratinizing squamous epithelium and contain cellular debris with a sebaceous appearance and odor. Epidermal cysts may be solitary or multiple and have a yellow appearance when stretched or compressed. They usually resolve spontaneously, and treatment is unnecessary unless they become infected or significantly enlarged.

Nevi

Nevi (moles) occur on the vulva as elsewhere on the body. They can be singular or multiple, flat or raised, and may vary in degree of pigmentation from flesh colored to dark brown or black. Nevi are asymptomatic but should be observed for changes that could indicate cancer. Nevi may resemble melanomas or basal cell carcinomas, and excisional biopsy is recommended when doubt exists (see Chapter 61).

Vulvar Dystrophy

Vulvar dystrophy, characterized by white lesions of the vulva, is a common condition that once was considered to be precancerous. The lesions may be categorized as lichen sclerosus, squamous cell hyperplasia, or other dermatoses, depending on clinical and histologic characteristics. Lichen sclerosus patches are hypopigmented, parchment-thin, and atrophic. Hyperplastic lesions are thick, gray-white plaques. Both types of lesions can be pruritic. Treatment for lichen sclerosus includes topical testosterone propionate or topical corticosteroid in combination with a vulvar drying regimen. Hyperplastic areas respond well to a combination corticosteroid (*e.g.*, betamethasone valerate) and antipruritic cream (*e.g.*, crotamiton [Eurax]) and to the removal of any irritants (*e.g.*, detergents, perfumes). Lichen sclerosus frequently recurs, and lifetime maintenance therapy may be required. Hyperplastic areas that occur in the field of lichen sclerosus may be sites of malignant change and warrant close follow-up and possible biopsy.[2]

Vulvodynia

Vulvodynia is a syndrome of unexplained vulvar pain, also referred to as *vulvar pain syndrome* or *burning vulva syndrome*. It is a chronic disorder characterized by burning, stinging, irritation, and rawness. Several forms or subsets of vulvodynia have been identified. Because vulvodynia is a multi-faceted condition, certain subsets may coexist with others. Pain at onset of intercourse (*i.e.*, insertional dyspareunia), localized point tenderness near the vaginal opening, and sensitivity to tampon placement, tight-fitting pants, bicycling, or prolonged sitting are characteristic of *vulvar vestibulitis*. When the condition demonstrates episodic flares that occur only before menses or after coitus, it is referred to as *cyclic vulvovaginitis*. Symptoms that are in general non-cyclic and pruritic and develop progressively during the perimenopausal or postmenopausal years are characteristic of *vulvar dermatoses*.

Vulvar dysesthesia, also known as *idiopathic* or *essential vulvodynia*, involves severe, constant, widespread burning that interferes with daily activities. Although the cause is unknown, the quality of pain with vulvar dysesthesia resembles reflex sympathetic dystrophy (see Chapter 48) or pudendal neuralgia and possibly is the result of myofascial restrictions affecting sacral and pelvic floor enervation. Surface electromyography-assisted pelvic floor muscle rehabilitation has been shown to be an effective and long-term cure for dysesthetic vulvodynia.[3]

Possible causes for other forms of vulvodynia include candidal hypersensitivity related to chronic recurrent yeast infections; chemical irritation or drug effects, especially prolonged use of topical steroid creams; the irritating effects of elevated urinary levels of calcium oxalate; immunoglobulin A deficiency; and dermatoses such as lichen sclerosus, lichen planus, or squamous cell hyperplasia. Herpes simplex virus may be related to episodic vulvodynia, and long-term viral suppressive therapy may be of benefit to women with known herpes simplex virus infection who experience multiple outbreaks each year. Previous links to HPV infection have not been supported by studies, and the finding of subclinical HPV infection in women with vulvodynia now is thought to be a secondary or unrelated phenomenon.

Treatment for this chronic, often debilitating problem is aimed at symptom relief and elimination of suspected underlying problems. Careful history taking and physical assessment are essential for differential diagnosis and treatment. Regimens can include long-term vaginal or oral anti-fungal therapy, avoidance of potential irritants, cleaning with water only or a gentle soap, sitz baths with baking soda, emollients such as vitamin E or vegetable oil for lubrication, low-oxalate diet plus calcium citrate supplements (calcium binds oxalate in the bowel and citrate inhibits the formation of oxalate crystals), topical anesthetic or steroid ointments, antidepressants, physical therapy, and surgery. Psychosocial support often is needed because this condition can cause strain in sexual, family, and work relationships. Vulvo-dynia often needs to be managed from a multidimensional, chronic pain perspective.[4]

Cancer of the Vulva

Carcinoma of the vulva accounts for approximately 4% of all cancers of the female genitourinary system.[5] Invasive carcinoma occurs most frequently in women who are 60 years of age or older, and its incidence has remained relatively stable since the early 1980s. The mean age for carcinoma in situ is 20 years younger than for invasive carcinoma (45 to 50 years), and the incidence of occurrence for this type of cancer almost doubled between 1973 and 1987.[6]

Approximately 90% of vulvar malignancies are squamous cell carcinomas. Less common types of cancer found on the vulva include adenocarcinoma in the form of extramammary Paget's disease (intraepithelial or invasive) or carcinoma of Bartholin's gland, basal cell carcinoma, and malignant melanoma.[5]

Vulvar intraepithelial neoplasia (VIN), which is a precursor lesion of squamous cell carcinoma, represents a spectrum of neoplastic changes that range from minimal cellular atypia to invasive cancer.

A significant rise in the incidence of VIN among women in their third and fourth decades appears to be caused by the oncogenic (cancer-promoting) potential of certain strains of HPV that are sexually transmitted. VIN lesions may take many forms. The lesions may be singular or multicentric, macular, papular, or plaquelike. VIN frequently is multicentric, and 10% to 30% are associated with squamous neoplasms in the vagina and cervix.[7] Microscopically, VIN presents as a proliferative process characterized by cells with abnormal epithelial maturation, nuclear enlargement, and nuclear atypia. The same system that is used for grading cervical cancer is used for vulvar cancer. The extent of replacement of epithelial cells by abnormal cells determines the grade of involvement (VIN I, II, or III). The grading of vulvar cancers uses the same scale as cervical cancers[2,8] (Table 45-1). Full-thickness replacement, VIN III, is synonymous with carcinoma in situ. Spontaneous resolution of VIN lesions has occurred. The risk of progression to invasive cancer increases in older women and in immunosuppressed women.

A second form of VIN, which is seen more often in older women, often is preceded by chronic vulvar irritation or lichen sclerosus.[6] If left untreated, many of these women develop invasive cell carcinoma after 6 to 7 years.[8] The etiology of this form of VIN is largely unknown, but it infrequently is associated with HPV.

The initial lesion of squamous cell vulvar carcinoma may appear as an inconspicuous thickening of the skin, a small raised area or lump, or an ulceration that fails to heal. It may be single or multiple and vary in color from white to velvety red or black. The lesions may resemble eczema or dermatitis and may produce few symptoms, other than pruritus, local discomfort, and exudation. A recurrent, persistent, pruritic vulvitis may be the only complaint. The symptoms frequently are treated with various home remedies before medical treatment is sought. The lesion often becomes secondarily infected, and this causes pain and discomfort. The malignant lesion gradually spreads super-

TABLE 45-1 ✦ Cervical Intraepithelial Neoplasia Grading System

Grade	Extent of Involvement	Differentiation of Lesion
CIN I (mild dysplasia)	Initial one third of epithelial layer	Well differentiated
CIN II (moderate dysplasia)	Initial two thirds of epithelial layer	Less well differentiated
CIN III (severe dysplasia or carcinoma in situ [CIS])	Full-thickness involvement	Undifferentiated

(Data from Rubin E., Farber J.L. [1999]. *Pathology* [3rd ed., pp. 982–983]. Philadelphia: Lippincott Williams & Wilkins)

ficially or as a deep furrow involving all of one labial side. Because there are many lymph channels around the vulva, the cancer metastasizes freely to the regional lymph nodes. The most common extension is to the superficial inguinal, deep femoral, and external iliac lymph nodes.

Early diagnosis is important in the treatment of vulvar carcinoma. Because malignant lesions can vary in appearance and commonly are mistaken for other conditions, biopsy and treatment often are delayed. Treatment is primarily wide surgical excision of the lesion for noninvasive cancer and vulvectomy with node resection for invasive cancer. Local chemotherapeutic agents (*e.g.*, fluorouracil) and colposcopically guided laser therapy are used to treat focal areas of cancer in cases where surgery is contraindicated. The 5-year survival rate for women with lesions less than 3 cm in diameter and minimal node involvement is approximately 90% after surgical treatment. Follow-up visits every 3 months for the first 2 years after surgery and every 6 months thereafter are important to detect recurrent disease or a second primary cancer. The 5-year survival rate for patients who have larger lesions in conjunction with pelvic lymphadenopathy drops to 30% to 55% after surgical treatment. Outlook for survival diminishes with increasing nodal involvement.[5]

DISORDERS OF THE VAGINA

The normal vaginal ecology depends on the delicate balance of hormones and bacterial flora. Normal estrogen levels maintain a thick, protective squamous epithelium that contains glycogen. Döderlein's bacilli, part of the normal vaginal flora, metabolize glycogen, and in the process produce the lactic acid that normally maintains the vaginal pH below 4.5. Disruptions in these normal environmental conditions predispose to infection.

Vaginitis

Vaginitis is inflammation of the vagina; it is characterized by vaginal discharge and burning, itching, redness, and swelling of vaginal tissues. Pain often occurs with urination and sexual intercourse. Vaginitis may be caused by chemical irritants, foreign bodies, and infectious agents. The causes of vaginitis differ in various age groups. In premenarchal girls, most vaginal infections have nonspecific causes, such as poor hygiene, intestinal parasites, or the presence of foreign bodies. *C. albicans*, *Trichomonas vaginalis*, and bacterial vaginosis are the most common causes of vaginitis in the childbearing years, and some of these organisms can be transmitted sexually (see Chapter 46).[9,10] In postmenopausal women, atrophic vaginitis is the most common form.

Atrophic vaginitis is an inflammation of the vagina that occurs after menopause or removal of the ovaries and their estrogen supply. Estrogen deficiency results in a lack of regenerative growth of the vaginal epithelium, rendering these tissues more susceptible to infection and irritation.[9] Döderlein's bacilli disappear, and the vaginal secretions become less acidic. The symptoms of atrophic vaginitis include itching, burning, and painful intercourse. These symptoms usually can be reversed by local application of estrogen.

Every woman has a normal vaginal discharge during the menstrual cycle, but it should not cause burning or itching or have an unpleasant odor. These symptoms suggest inflammation or infection. Because these symptoms are common to the different types of vaginitis, precise identification of the organism is essential for proper treatment. A careful history should include information about systemic disease conditions, the use of drugs such as antibiotics that foster the growth of yeast, dietary habits, stress, and other factors that alter the resistance of vaginal tissue to infections. A physical examination usually is done to evaluate the nature of the discharge and its effects on the genital structures.

Microscopic examination of a saline wet-mount smear (prepared by placing a sample of vaginal mucus in one to two drops of normal saline) is the primary means of identifying the organism responsible for the infection. A small amount of 10% potassium hydroxide (KOH) is added to a second specimen on the slide to aid in the identification of *C. albicans*.[9,10] KOH destroys the cellular material, making the epithelial cells become increasingly transparent so that the hyphae and buds that are characteristic of *Candida* become much easier to see. Culture methods may be needed when the organism is not apparent on the wet-mount preparation.

The prevention and treatment of vaginal infections depend on proper health habits and accurate diagnosis and treatment of ongoing infections. Measures to prevent infection include development of daily hygiene habits that keep the genital area clean and dry, maintenance of normal vaginal flora and healthy vaginal mucosa, and avoidance of contact with organisms known to cause vaginal infections. Perfumed products, such as feminine deodorant sprays, douches, bath powders, soaps, and even toilet paper, can be irritating and may alter the normal vaginal flora. Tight clothing prevents the dissipation of body heat and evaporation of skin moisture and promotes favorable conditions for irritation and the growth of pathogens. Nylon and other synthetic undergarments, pantyhose, and swimsuits hold body moisture next to the skin and harbor infectious organisms, even after they have been washed. Cotton undergarments that withstand hot water and bleach (*i.e.*, a fungicide) may be preferable for women to prevent such infections. Swimsuits and other garments that cannot withstand hot water or bleaching should be hung in the sunlight to dry. Women should be taught to wipe the perineal area from front to back to avoid bringing rectal contamination into the vagina. Avoiding sexual contact whenever an infection is known to exist or suspected should limit that route of transmission.

Cancer of the Vagina

Primary cancers of the vagina are extremely rare. They account for approximately 3% of all cancers of the female reproductive system. Like vulvar carcinoma, carcinoma of the vagina is largely a disease of older women. Approximately half of women are 60 years of age or older at the time of diagnosis. The exception to that is the clear cell adenocarcinoma associated with diethylstilbestrol (DES) exposure in utero, which is associated with an average age at diagnosis of 19 years.[11] Vaginal cancers may result from local extension of cervical cancer, from local irritation such as occurs with prolonged use of a pessary, or from exposure to sexually transmitted herpesvirus or HPV.

Approximately 85% to 90% of vaginal cancers are squamous cell carcinomas, with other common types being adenocarcinomas, sarcomas, and melanomas.[12] Maternal ingestion of DES in early pregnancy has been associated with the development of clear cell adenocarcinoma in female offspring who were exposed in utero. Between 1940 and 1971, DES, a nonsteroidal synthetic estrogen, commonly was prescribed to prevent miscarriage.[11] The incidence of clear cell adenocarcinoma of the vagina is low, approximately 0.1%, in young women who were exposed to DES in utero. Although only a small percentage of girls exposed to estrogen actually develop clear cell adenocarcinoma, 75% to 90% of them develop benign adenosis (*i.e.*, ectopic extension of cervical columnar epithelium into the vagina, which normally is stratified squamous epithelium), which may predispose to cancer. Most DES-exposed daughters are now between 30 and 60 years of age, so the number of new cases should be decreasing. Because the upper age limit for this type of cancer is unknown, there is no age at which a DES-exposed daughter can be considered risk free.[11]

The most common symptom of vaginal carcinoma is abnormal bleeding. Twenty percent of women are asymptomatic, with the cancer being discovered during a routine pelvic examination. The anatomic proximity of the vagina to other pelvic structures (*e.g.*, urethra, bladder, rectum) permits early spread to these areas. Pelvic pain, dysuria, constipation, and vaginal discharge can be associated symptoms. Vaginal squamous cell carcinoma most often is detected in the upper posterior one third of the vagina, with adenocarcinoma more often found on the lower anterior and lateral vaginal vault. Cancer can develop anywhere in

the vagina, and visualization during physical examination always should cover the entire vault. Women should continue to have vaginal cytology studies (Papanicolaou's test [Pap smear]) every 3 to 5 years after hysterectomy to exclude development of vaginal cancer. Diagnosis requires biopsy of suspect lesions or areas.

Treatment of vaginal cancer must take into consideration the type of cancer, the size, location, and spread of the lesion, and the woman's age. Local excision, laser vaporization, or a loop electrode excision procedure (LEEP) can be considered with stage 0 squamous cell cancer. Radical surgery and radiation therapy are both curative with more advanced cancers. When there is upper vaginal involvement, radical surgery may be required. This includes a total hysterectomy, pelvic lymph node dissection, partial vaginectomy, and placement of a graft from the buttock to the area from which the vagina was excised. Vaginal reconstruction often is possible to allow for sexual intercourse. The ovaries usually are preserved unless they are diseased. Extensive lesions and those located in the middle or lower vaginal area usually are treated by radiation therapy, which can be intracavitary, interstitial, or external beam. The prognosis depends on the stage of the disease, the involvement of lymph nodes, and the degree of mitotic activity of the tumor. With appropriate treatment and follow-up, the 5-year survival rate for tumors confined to vagina (stage I) is 80%, whereas it is only 20% for those with extensive spread (stages III and IV).[7]

> In summary, the surface of the vulva is affected by disorders that affect skin on other parts of the body. These disorders include inflammation (*i.e.*, vulvitis and folliculitis), epidermal cysts, and nevi. Although these disorders are not serious, they can be distressing because they produce severe discomfort and itching. Bartholin's cysts are the result of occluded ducts in Bartholin's glands. They often are painful and can become infected. Vulvar dystrophies are characterized by thinning and hyperplastic thickening of vulvar tissues. Vulvodynia is a chronic vulvar pain syndrome with several classifications and variable treatment results. Cancer of the vulva, which accounts for 4% of all female genitourinary cancers, is associated with HPV infections.
>
> The normal vaginal ecology depends on the delicate balance of hormones and bacterial flora. Normal estrogen levels maintain a thick protective squamous epithelium that contains glycogen. Döderlein's bacilli, which are part of the normal vaginal flora, metabolize glycogen and, in the process, produce the lactic acid that normally maintains the vaginal pH below 4.5. Disruptions in these normal environmental conditions predispose to vaginal infections. Vaginitis or inflammation of the vagina is characterized by vaginal discharge and burning, itching, redness, and swelling of vaginal tissues. It may be caused by chemical irritants, foreign bodies, and infectious agents. Primary cancers of the vagina are less common, accounting for 3% of all cancers of the female reproductive system. Daughters of women treated with DES to prevent miscarriage are at increased risk for development of adenocarcinoma of the vagina.

Disorders of the Cervix and Uterus

After you have completed this section of the chapter, you should be able to meet the following objectives:

✦ Describe the importance of the cervical transformation zone in the development of cervical cancer
✦ Compare the lesions associated with nabothian cysts and cervical polyps
✦ List the complications of untreated cervicitis
✦ Compare the age distribution and risk factors for cervical and endometrial cancer
✦ Characterize the development of cervical cancer, from the appearance of atypical cells to the development of invasive cervical cancer
✦ Relate the importance of Papanicolaou's test in early detection and decreased incidence of deaths from cervical cancer
✦ Describe the methods used in the treatment of cervical cancer
✦ Compare the pathology and manifestations of endometriosis and adenomyosis
✦ Cite the major early symptom of endometrial cancer
✦ Compare intramural and subserosal leiomyomas

DISORDERS OF THE UTERINE CERVIX

The cervix is composed of two distinct types of tissue. The exocervix, or visible portion, is covered with stratified squamous epithelium, which also lines the vagina. The endocervical canal is lined with columnar epithelium. The junction of these two tissue types (*i.e.*, squamocolumnar junction) appears at various locations on the cervix at different points in a woman's life (Fig. 45-2). During periods of high estrogen production, particularly fetal existence, menarche, and the first pregnancy, the cervix everts or turns outward, exposing the columnar epithelium to the vaginal environment. The combination of estrogen and low vaginal pH leads to a gradual transformation from columnar to squamous epithelium—a process called *metaplasia* (see Chapter 5). The dynamic area of change where metaplasia takes place is called the *transformation zone*. The process of

transformation is increased by trauma and infections occurring during the reproductive years.[7] As the squamous epithelium expands and obliterates the surface columnar papillae, it covers and obstructs crypt openings, with trapping of mucus in the deeper crypts (glands) to form retention cysts, called *nabothian cysts*. These are benign cysts that require no treatment unless they become so numerous that they cause cervical enlargement. The nabothian cyst farthest away from the external cervical os indicates the outer aspect of the transformation zone.

The transformation zone is a critical area for the development of cervical cancer. During metaplasia, the newly developed squamous epithelial cells are vulnerable to development of dysplasia and genetic change if exposed to carcinogenic agents (*i.e.*, cancer-producing substances). *Dysplasia* means disordered growth or development. Although initially a reversible cell change, untreated dysplasia can develop into carcinoma. The transformation zone is the area of the cervix that must be sampled to have an adequate Pap smear and the area most carefully examined during colposcopy.

Cervicitis and Cervical Polyps

Cervicitis is an acute or chronic inflammation of the cervix. Acute cervicitis may result from the direct infection of the cervix or may be secondary to a vaginal or uterine infection. It may be caused by a variety of infective agents, including *C. albicans*, *T. vaginalis*, *Neisseria gonorrhoeae*, *Gardnerella vaginalis*, *Chlamydia trachomatis*, *Ureaplasma urealyticum*, and herpes simplex virus. *C. trachomatis* is the organism most commonly associated with mucopurulent cervicitis. Chronic cervicitis represents a low-grade inflammatory process. It is common in parous women and may be a sequela to minute lacerations that occur during childbirth, instrumentation, or other trauma. The organisms usually are of a nonspecific type, often staphylococcal, streptococcal, or coliform bacteria.

With acute cervicitis, the cervix becomes reddened and edematous. Irritation from the infection results in copious mucopurulent drainage and leukorrhea. The symptoms of chronic cervicitis are less well defined: the cervix may be ulcerated or normal in appearance; it may contain nabothian cysts; the cervical os may be distorted by old lac-

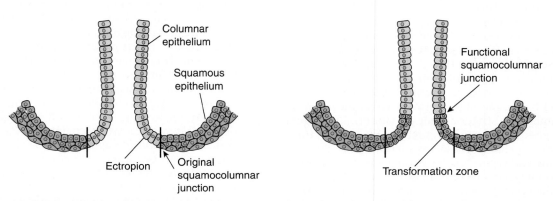

FIGURE 45-2 The transformation zone of the cervix. (Rubin E., Farber J.L. [1999]. *Pathology* [3rd. ed., p. 978]. Philadelphia: Lippincott Williams & Wilkins)

erations or everted to expose areas of columnar epithelium; and a mucopurulent drainage may be present.

Untreated cervicitis may extend to include the development of pelvic cellulitis, low back pain, painful intercourse, cervical stenosis, dysmenorrhea, and further infection of the uterus or fallopian tubes. Depending on the causative agent, acute cervicitis is treated with appropriate antibiotic therapy. Diagnosis of chronic cervicitis is based on vaginal examination, colposcopy, cytologic (Pap) smears, and occasionally on biopsy to exclude malignant changes. The treatment usually involves cryosurgery or cauterization, which causes the tissues to slough and leads to eradication of the infection. Colposcopically guided laser vaporization of abnormal epithelium is the newest but most expensive treatment for cervicitis.

Polyps are the most common lesions of the cervix. They can be found in women of all ages, but their incidence is higher during the reproductive years. Polyps are soft, velvety red lesions; they usually are pedunculated and often are found protruding through the cervical os. They usually develop as a result of inflammatory hyperplasia of the endocervical mucosa. Polyps typically are asymptomatic but may have associated postcoital bleeding. Most are benign, but they should be removed and examined by a pathologist to exclude malignant change.

Cancer of the Cervix

Cervical cancer is readily detected and, if detected early, is the most easily cured of all the cancers of the female reproductive system. According to the American Cancer Society, an estimated 12,800 cases of invasive cervical cancer were diagnosed in 2000, with approximately 4600 deaths from cervical cancer during the same period.[13] By comparison, there were four times as many new cases of cervical carcinoma in situ (*i.e.*, precancerous lesion) diagnosed, indicating that a large number of potentially invasive cancers are cured by early detection and effective treatment. The death rate has steadily declined over the past 50 years with the introduction of more sensitive and readily available screening methods (*e.g.*, Pap smear, colposcopy, cervicography), consistent use of a standardized grading system that guides treatment, and more effective treatment methods. However, the mortality rate is more than twice as high for black women than for white women. The 5-year survival rate for all patients with cervical cancer is 70%. For women with localized disease, the 5-year survival rate is 92%, but only 53% of cancers are discovered that early.[13]

Carcinoma of the cervix is considered a STD. It is rare among celibate women. Risk factors include early age at first intercourse, multiple sexual partners, a promiscuous male partner, smoking, and a history of STDs.[14–16] A preponderance of evidence suggests a causal link between HPV infection and uterine cancer. Certain strains of HPV have been identified in invasive carcinoma of the cervix, whereas others are associated more often with dysplasia or carcinoma in situ. The strongest link is with HPV types 16, 18, 31, and 33.[7] Because these viruses are spread by sexual contact, their association with cervical cancer provides a tempting hypothesis to explain the relation between sexual practices and cervical cancer. HPV is discussed further

in Chapter 46. Other factors such as smoking, nutrition, and coexisting sexual partners may play a contributing role in determining whether a woman with HPV infection develops cervical cancer.

One of the most important advances in the early diagnosis and treatment of cancer of the cervix was made possible by the observation that this cancer arises from precursor lesions, which begin with the development of atypical cervical cells. These atypical cells gradually progress to carcinoma in situ and to invasive cancer of the cervix. Atypical cells differ from normal cervical squamous epithelium. There are changes in the nuclear and cytoplasmic parts of the cell and more variation in cell size and shape (*i.e.*, dysplasia). Carcinoma in situ is localized to the epithelial layer, whereas invasive cancer of the cervix spreads to deeper layers.

A system of grading devised to describe the dysplastic changes of cancer precursors uses the term *cervical intraepithelial neoplasia* (CIN). The CIN system grades according to extent of involvement of the epithelial thickness of the cervix (see Table 45-1). After cancer has been diagnosed, the general preference is to use the International Federation of Gynecology and Obstetrics (FIGO) classification system to describe the histologic and clinical stage of the disease[8] (Table 45-2). The development of an internationally accepted grading system has significantly increased the database for cervical cancer and the consistency of that database.

The atypical cellular changes that precede frank neoplastic changes consistent with cancer of the cervix can be recognized by a number of direct and microscopic techniques, including the Pap smear, colposcopy, and cervicography. The precursor lesions can exist in a reversible form, which may regress spontaneously (approximately

---

 Gynecologic Cancers

➤ Cancers of the vulva, cervix, endometrium, and ovaries represent a spectrum of malignancies.

➤ Cancers of the vulva and cervix are mainly squamous cell carcinomas. Certain types of sexually transmitted human papillomaviruses are risk factors for cervical intraepithelial neoplasia, which can be a precursor lesion of invasive carcinoma.

➤ Endometrial cancers, which are seen most frequently in women 55 to 65 years of age, are strongly associated with conditions that produce excessive estrogen stimulation and endometrial hyperplasia.

➤ Ovarian cancer is the second most common female cancer and the most lethal. The most significant risk factors for ovarian cancers are the length of time that a woman's ovarian cycles are not suppressed by pregnancy, lactation, or oral contraceptive use, and family history.

TABLE 45-2 ✦ Stages of Gynecologic Cancer	
Stage	**Description***
0	Rarely used; refers to preinvasive lesions
I	Cancer is confined to organ in which it originated
II	Cancer involves some of the structures surrounding the organ of origin
III	Regional spread of cancer with lymph node involvement
IV	Distant spread of cancer with metastasis

*This table represents a generic staging system used for most gynecologic cancers. The International Federation of Gynecology and Obstetrics (FIGO) system is a defined staging system used for each specific site and can be found in most cancer textbooks.

TABLE 45-3 ✦ Epithelial Cell Abnormalities

Squamous Cell

ASCUS: atypical squamous cells of undetermined significance
   Favor reactive (probably benign)
   Favor dysplasia (consider same as SIL)
LSIL: low-grade squamous intraepithelial lesion
   Includes human papillomavirus effect and mild dysplasia (CIN I)
HSIL: high-grade squamous intraepithelial lesion
   Includes moderate and severe dysplasia of carcinoma in situ (CIN II and III)
SCC: squamous cell carcinoma

Glandular Cell

Presence of endometrial cells
   Out of phase in a menstruating woman
   In a postmenopausal woman
   No menstrual history available
AGCUS: atypical glandular cells of undetermined significance
   Endometrial
   Endocervical
   Not otherwise specified
Adenocarcinoma
   Specify site: endometrial, endocervical, extrauterine, not specified

CIN, cervical intraepithelial neoplasia.

60%), persist (30%), or progress and undergo malignant change (10%). Only approximately 1% of lesions progress to invasive carcinoma. Cancers of the cervix have a long latent period; untreated dysplasia gradually progresses to carcinoma in situ, which may remain static for 7 to 10 years before it becomes invasive. After the preinvasive period, growth may be rapid, and survival rates decline significantly depending on the extent of disease at the time of diagnosis.[17]

The purpose of the Pap smear (see Chapter 8) is to detect the presence of abnormal cells on the surface of the cervix or in the endocervix. This test detects precancerous and cancerous lesions. Although the American Cancer Society has suggested that the Pap smear need not be done annually if there have been three negative tests in succession, many clinicians maintain that performing an annual test is the safest course to follow. If the woman has risk factors, such as previous HPV infection, DES exposure in utero, or a strong family history of cervical cancer, more frequent Pap smears may be recommended.

It has been estimated that approximately 15% to 25% of women with intraepithelial lesions have normal Pap smear results.[16] Care must be taken to obtain an adequate smear from the transformation zone that includes endocervical cells and to ensure that the cytologic examination is done by a competent laboratory. New techniques of specimen collection, slide preparation and processing, and computer-assisted evaluation of Pap smears are being evaluated and offer hope of improved accuracy in diagnosis of precancerous cervical changes.

The accepted format for reporting cervical and vaginal cytologic diagnoses, called *The Bethesda System* (TBS), was developed during a National Cancer Institute Workshop in 1989 and updated in 1991.[18] TBS includes three components: a statement of specimen adequacy (*i.e.*, satisfactory, satisfactory but limited by . . . , unsatisfactory); general categorization (*i.e.*, within normal limits or other); and a descriptive diagnosis of findings (infection, reactive and reparative changes, hormonal balance, and epithelial cell abnormalities). Table 45-3 presents terms used to describe epithelial cell abnormalities.

In June 1992, the National Cancer Institute convened a workshop of experts to develop guidelines for management of abnormal cervical cytologic results based on the classifications in TBS. The minimally abnormal Pap smear (*i.e.*, atypical squamous cells of undetermined significance [ASCUS], low-grade squamous intraepithelial lesion [LSIL]) presents the greatest challenge to clinicians. The uncertain significance of ASCUS often is related to inflammation, atrophy, or other temporary or reversible processes. Even squamous intraepithelial lesions (SIL) regress spontaneously in approximately 60% of patients, and costly evaluation or aggressive treatment may not be warranted. Follow-up with repeat Pap smears at 3- to 6-month intervals usually is appropriate. If compliance with follow-up observation is uncertain, colposcopy, endocervical curettage, or directed biopsy may be used to confirm the presence of a lesion so treatment can be selected.[19]

The presence of normal endometrial cells in a cervical cytologic sample during the luteal phase of the menstrual cycle or during the postmenopausal period has been associated with endometrial disease and warrants further evaluation with endometrial biopsy. This demonstrates that shedding of even normal cells at an inappropriate time may indicate disease. Because adenocarcinoma of the cervix is being detected more frequently, especially in women younger than 35 years of age, a Pap smear result of atypical glandular cells of undetermined significance (AGCUS) warrants further evaluation by endocervical or endometrial curettage, hysteroscopy, or, ultimately, a cone biopsy if the abnormality cannot be located or identified through other means.

Diagnosis of cervical cancer requires pathologic confirmation. Pap smear results demonstrating SIL often require further evaluation by colposcopy. This is a vaginal examination that is done using a colposcope, an instrument that affords a well-lit and magnified stereoscopic view of the cervix. During colposcopy, the cervical tissue may be stained with an iodine solution (*i.e.*, Schiller's test) or acetic acid solution to accentuate topographic or vascular changes that can differentiate normal from abnormal tissue. A biopsy sample may be obtained from suspect areas and examined microscopically.

A final diagnostic tool in areas where colposcopy is not readily available is cervicography, a noninvasive photographic technique that provides permanent objective documentation of normal and abnormal cervical patterns. Acetic acid (5%) is applied to the cervix, a cervicography camera is used to take photographs, and the projected cervicogram (*i.e.*, slide after film developing) can be sent for expert evaluation. In one study, the cervicogram was found to give a greater yield of CIN than Pap smear alone in patients with previous abnormal pap smears.[20]

Before the availability of colposcopy, many women with abnormal Pap smears required surgical cone biopsy for further evaluation. Cone biopsy involves the removal of a cone-shaped wedge of cervix, including the entire transformation zone and at least 50% of the endocervical canal. Postoperative hemorrhage, infection, cervical stenosis, infertility, and incompetent cervix are possible sequelae that warrant avoidance of this procedure unless it is truly necessary. Diagnostic conization still is indicated when a lesion is partly or completely beyond colposcopic view or colposcopically directed biopsy fails to explain the cytologic findings.

The LEEP, a refinement of loop diathermy techniques dating back to the 1940s, is quickly becoming the first-line management for SIL. This outpatient procedure allows for the simultaneous diagnosis and treatment of dysplastic lesions found on colposcopy. It uses a thin, rigid, wire loop electrode attached to a generator that blends high-frequency, low-voltage current for cutting and a modulated higher voltage for coagulation. In skilled hands, this wire can remove the entire transformation zone, providing adequate treatment for the lesion while obtaining a specimen for further histologic evaluation. The width and depth of the tissue excised are controlled by the size and shape of the loop and the speed and pressure that is applied during the procedure. This can help avoid the problems that can occur after surgical cone biopsy (*e.g.*, stenosis, incompetent cervix). Bleeding can be minimized by fulguration of the base with electrocoagulation or by applying a thin layer of Monsel's gel (*i.e.*, chemical cautery). Although long-term results are not available, this procedure, which requires only local anesthesia, appears to provide a lower-cost, office-based alternative to cone biopsy.

Early treatment of cervical cancer involves removal of the lesion by one of various techniques. Biopsy or local cautery may be therapeutic in and of itself. Electrocautery, cryosurgery, or carbon dioxide laser therapy may be used to treat moderate to severe dysplasia that is limited to the exocervix (*i.e.*, squamocolumnar junction clearly visible). Therapeutic conization becomes necessary if the lesion extends into the endocervical canal and can be done surgically or with LEEP in the physician's office.[18]

Depending on the stage of involvement of the cervix, invasive cancer is treated with radiation therapy, surgery, or both. External beam irradiation and intracavitary cesium irradiation (*i.e.*, insertion of a closed metal cylinder containing cesium) can be used in the treatment of cervical cancer. Intracavitary radiation provides direct access to the central lesion and increases the tolerance of the cervix and surrounding tissues, permitting curative levels of radiation to be used. External beam radiation eliminates metastatic disease in pelvic lymph nodes and other structures, as well as shrinking the cervical lesion to optimize the effects of intracavitary radiation. Surgery can include extended hysterectomy (*i.e.*, removal of the uterus, fallopian tubes, ovaries, and upper portion of the vagina) without pelvic lymph node dissection, radical hysterectomy with pelvic lymph node dissection, or pelvic exenteration (*i.e.*, removal of all pelvic organs, including the bladder, rectum, vulva, and vagina). The choice of treatment is influenced by the stage of the disease as well as the woman's age and health.[17]

DISORDERS OF THE UTERUS

Endometritis

Inflammation or infection of the endometrium is an ill-defined entity that produces variable symptoms. The presence of plasma cells is required for diagnosis. Endometritis can occur as a postpartum or postabortal infection, with gonococcal or chlamydial salpingitis, or after instrumentation or surgery, or can be associated with an intrauterine device or tuberculosis.[10] Causative organisms, in addition to *N. gonorrhoeae*, *Chlamydia*, and *Mycobacterium tuberculosis*, include *Escherichia coli*, *Proteus*, *Pseudomonas*, *Klebsiella*, *Bacteroides*, and *Mycoplasma* species. Abnormal vaginal bleeding, mild to severe uterine tenderness, fever, malaise, and foul-smelling discharge have been associated with endometritis, but the clinical picture is variable. Treatment involves oral or intravenous antibiotic therapy, depending on the severity of the condition.

Endometriosis

Endometriosis is the condition in which functional endometrial tissue is found in ectopic sites outside the uterus. The site may be the ovaries, broad ligaments, pouch of Douglas (cul-de-sac), pelvis, vagina, vulva, perineum, or intestines. Rarely, endometrial implants have been found in the nostrils, umbilicus, lungs, and limbs.

The cause of endometriosis is unknown. There appears to have been an increase in its incidence in the developed Western countries during the past four to five decades. Approximately 10% to 15% of premenopausal women have some degree of endometriosis. The incidence may be higher in women with infertility (25% to 40%)[21] or women younger than 20 years of age with chronic pelvic pain (45% to 70%).[22] It is more common in women who have postponed childbearing. Risk factors for endometriosis may include early menarche; regular periods with shorter cycles (<27 days), longer duration (>7 days), or heavier flow; increased menstrual pain; and other first-degree relatives with the condition.

Several theories attempt to account for endometriosis. One theory suggests that menstrual blood containing fragments of endometrium is forced upward through the fallopian tubes into the peritoneal cavity. Retrograde menstruation is not an uncommon phenomenon, and it is unknown why endometrial cells implant and grow in some women but not in others. Another proposal is that dormant, immature cellular elements spread over a wide area during embryonic development persist into adult life and that the ensuing metaplasia accounts for the development of ectopic endometrial tissue. Another theory suggests that the endometrial tissue may metastasize through the lymphatics or vascular system. Altered cellular immunity and genetic components also have been studied as contributing factors to the development of endometriosis.[21]

The gross pathologic changes that occur in endometriosis differ with location and duration. In the ovary, the endometrial tissue may form cysts (*i.e.*, endometriomas filled with old blood that resembles chocolate syrup [chocolate cysts]). Rupture of these cysts can cause peritonitis and adhesions. Elsewhere in the pelvis, the tissue may take the form of small hemorrhagic lesions that may be black, bluish, or red and clear or opaque. Some may be surrounded by scar tissue. These ectopic implants respond to hormonal stimulation in the same way normal endometrium does, becoming proliferative, then secretory, and finally undergoing menstrual breakdown. Bleeding into the surrounding structures can cause pain and the development of significant pelvic adhesions. Extensive fibrotic tissue can develop and cause bowel obstruction.

Endometriosis may be difficult to diagnose because its symptoms mimic those of other pelvic disorders. The severity of the symptoms does not always reflect the extent of the disease. The classic triad of dysmenorrhea, dyspareunia, and infertility strongly suggests endometriosis. Accurate diagnosis can be accomplished only through laparoscopy. This minimally invasive surgery allows direct visualization of pelvic organs to determine the presence and extent of endometrial lesions.

Treatment goals for endometriosis are pain management or restoration of fertility. Treatment modalities fall into three categories: pain relief, endometrial suppression, and surgery. In young, unmarried women, simple observation and antiprostaglandin analgesics (*i.e.*, nonsteroidal antiinflammatory drugs) may be sufficient treatment. The use of hormones to induce physiologic amenorrhea is based on the observation that pregnancy affords temporary relief by inducing atrophy of the endometrial tissue. This can be accomplished through administration of progesterone, oral contraceptive pills, danazol (a synthetic androgen), or long-acting gonadotropin-releasing hormone analogues that inhibit the pituitary gonadotropins and suppress ovulation.[23,24]

Surgery is the most definitive therapy for many women with endometriosis. In the past, laparoscopic cautery was limited to mild endometriosis without significant adhesions. More extensive treatment required laparotomy. With the advent of carbon dioxide, potassium-titanyl-phosphate (KTP), neodynium–yttrium-aluminum garnet (Nd-YAG), argon, and holmium-YAG lasers, in-depth treatment of endometriosis or pelvic adhesions can be accomplished by means of laparoscopy. Advantages of laser surgery include better hemostasis, more precision in vaporizing lesions with less damage to surrounding tissue, and better access to areas that are not well visualized or would be difficult to reach with cautery. Each type of laser has distinct properties that allow it to be useful for tissue vaporization under different conditions. The KTP laser is particularly useful for endometriosis because of its flexible fiberoptic delivery system, which allows tissue incision and vaporization in addition to photocoagulation, and its green beam, which makes visualization and fine focusing easier. Carbon dioxide permits the operator to excise easily with extreme accuracy and control and causes less peripheral tissue damage than other wavelengths. The Nd-YAG laser allows for a contact mode that avoids direct application of laser energy to tissues. Lasers are expensive instruments and require skill to use effectively. Some hospitals and surgeons have turned to other therapies in an effort to conserve financial resources. Electrosurgical, thermal, and ultrasonic ablation techniques are under investigation.[23] Radical treatment involves total hysterectomy and bilateral salpingo-oophorectomy (*i.e.*, removal of the fallopian tubes and ovaries) when the symptoms are unbearable or the woman's childbearing is completed.

Treatment offers relief but not cure. Recurrence of endometriosis is not uncommon, regardless of the treatment (except for radical surgery). Recurrence rates appear to correlate with severity of disease. With medical treatment, recurrence rates after 7 years ranged from 34% in women with mild disease to 74% in those with severe disease. Recurrence rates of 20% to 40% have been reported within 5 years after surgery.[24] Pregnancy may delay but does not preclude recurrence.

Adenomyosis

Adenomyosis is the condition in which endometrial glands and stroma are found within the myometrium, interspersed between the smooth muscle fibers. In contrast to endometriosis, which usually is a problem of young, infertile women, adenomyosis typically is found in multiparous women in their late fourth or fifth decade. It is thought that events associated with repeated pregnancies, deliveries, and uterine involution may cause the endometrium to be displaced throughout the myometrium. Adenomyosis frequently coexists with uterine myomas or endometrial hyperplasia. The diagnosis of adenomyosis often occurs as an incidental finding in a uterus removed for symptoms suggestive of myoma or hyperplasia. Up to 70% of these women have a retrospective history of painful, heavy periods.[25] Although in the past the diagnosis was made primarily through careful history and the pelvic examination findings of an enlarged, boggy uterus, magnetic resonance imaging is now considered an excellent diagnostic tool for confirming this condition. Adenomyosis resolves with menopause. Conservative therapy using oral contraceptives or gonadotropin-releasing hormone (GnRH) agonists is the first choice for treatment. Hysterectomy (with preservation of the ovaries in premenopausal women) is considered when this approach fails.[25]

Endometrial Cancer

Endometrial cancer is the most common cancer found in the female pelvis; it occurs more than twice as often as cervical cancer. In 2000, the American Cancer Society estimated that approximately 36,000 women were diagnosed with endometrial cancer and 6500 died of the disorder.[13] Endometrial cancer occurs more frequently in older women (peak ages of 55 to 65 years), with only a 2% to 5% incidence among women younger than 40 years of age.

Prolonged estrogen stimulation with excessive growth (*i.e.*, hyperplasia) of endometrium has been identified as a major risk factor for endometrial cancer. Obesity, anovulatory cycles, conditions that alter estrogen metabolism, estrogen-secreting neoplasms, and unopposed estrogen therapy all increase the risk of endometrial cancer.[26,27]

Estrogens are synthesized in body fats from adrenal and ovarian androgen precursors. Endometrial hyperplasia and endometrial cancer appear to be related to obesity. The degree of risk correlates with body weight, with the risk increasing 10-fold for women who are more than 50 pounds overweight.[8] Ovulatory dysfunction that causes infertility at any age or occurs with declining ovarian function in perimenopausal women also can result in unopposed estrogen and increase the risk of endometrial cancer. Diabetes mellitus, hypertension, and polycystic ovary syndrome are conditions that alter estrogen metabolism and elevate estrogen levels.

Endometrial cancer risk also is increased in women with estrogen-secreting granulosa cell tumors and in those receiving unopposed estrogen therapy. A sharp rise in endometrial cancer was seen in the 1970s among middle-aged women who had received unopposed estrogen therapy (*i.e.*, estrogen therapy without progesterone) for menopausal symptoms. It was later determined that it was not the estrogen exposure that increased the risk of cancer, but that the hormone was administered without progesterone. It is the presence of progesterone in the second half of the menstrual cycle that matures the endometrium and the withdrawal of progesterone that ultimately results in endometrial sloughing. Long-term unopposed estrogen exposure without periodic addition of progesterone allows for continued endometrial growth. Hyperplasia may develop, with or without the presence of atypical cells, and can progress to carcinoma if left untreated. Hyperplasia usually regresses after treatment with cyclic progesterone. Sequential oral contraceptives (estrogen alone for 15 days followed by 7 days of combined estrogen and progestin) were withdrawn from the market in the 1970s because of potential risk of endometrial hyperplasia. In contrast, combination oral contraceptives (estrogen and progestin in each pill) effectively prevent hyperplasia and decrease the risk of cancer by 50%.[26] Tamoxifen, a drug that blocks estrogen receptor sites and is used in treatment of breast cancer, exerts a weak estrogenic effect on the endometrium and represents another exogenous risk factor for endometrial cancer.

A small subset of women in whom endometrial cancer develops do not exhibit increased estrogen levels or pre-existing hyperplasia. These women usually acquire the disease at an older age. These tumors arise from clones of cancer-initiated mutant cells and are more poorly differentiated. This type of endometrial cancer usually has a poorer prognosis than that associated with prolonged estrogen stimulation and endometrial hyperplasia.[26]

The major symptom of endometrial hyperplasia or overt endometrial cancer is abnormal, painless bleeding. In menstruating women, this takes the form of bleeding between periods or excessive, prolonged menstrual flow. In postmenopausal women, any bleeding is abnormal and warrants investigation. Abnormal bleeding is an early warning sign of the disease, and because endometrial cancer tends to be slow growing in its early stages, the chances of cure are good if prompt medical care is sought. Later signs of uterine cancer may include cramping, pelvic discomfort, postcoital bleeding, lower abdominal pressure, and enlarged lymph nodes. Although the Pap smear can identify a small percentage of endometrial cancers, it is not a good screening test for this gynecologic cancer. Endometrial biopsy (*i.e.*, tissue sampling obtained in an office procedure by direct aspiration of the endometrial cavity) is far more accurate; 80% to 90% of endometrial cancers are identified if adequate tissue is obtained. Dilatation and curettage (D & C), which consists of dilating the cervix and scraping the uterine cavity, is the definitive procedure for diagnosis because it provides a more thorough evaluation. Transvaginal ultrasonography used to measure the endometrial thickness is being evaluated as an initial test for postmenopausal bleeding because it is less invasive than endometrial biopsy and less costly than D & C when biopsy is not possible.

The prognosis for endometrial cancer depends on the clinical stage of the disease when it is discovered and its histologic grade and type. Surgery and radiation therapy are the most successful methods of treatment for endometrial cancer. When used alone, radiation therapy has a 20% lower cure rate than surgery for stage I disease. It may be the best option, however, in women who are not good surgical candidates. Total abdominal hysterectomy with bilateral salpingo-oophorectomy plus sampling of regional lymph nodes and peritoneal washings for cytologic evaluation of occult disease is the treatment of choice whenever possible. Postoperative radiation therapy may be added in cases of advanced disease for more complete treatment and to prevent recurrence or metastasis, although the benefits of this as adjuvant therapy are still controversial. With early diagnosis and treatment, the 5-year survival rate is approximately 90%. This decreases to 20% for more advanced stages of the disease.[7]

Leiomyomas

Leiomyomas are benign neoplasms of smooth muscle origin. They also are known as *myomas* and sometimes are called *fibroids*. These are the most common form of pelvic tumor and are believed to occur in one of every four or five women older than 35 years of age. They are seen more often and their rate of growth is more rapid in black women than in white women. Leiomyomas usually develop in the corpus of the uterus; they may be submucosal, subserosal, or intramural (Fig. 45-3). Intramural fibroids are embedded in the myometrium. They are the most common type of fibroid, and present as a symmetric enlargement of the nonpregnant uterus. Subserosal tumors are located beneath the perimetrium of the uterus. These tumors are recognized as irregular projections on the uterine surface; they may become pedunculated, displacing or impinging on other

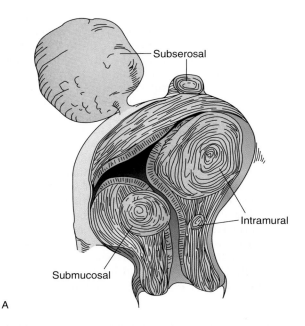

A

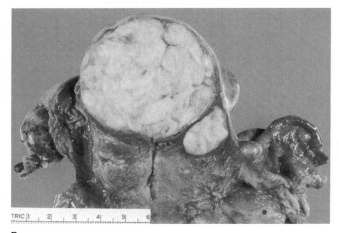

B

FIGURE 45-3 (**A**) Submucosal, intramural, and subserosal leiomyomas. (**A** redrawn from Green T.H. [1977]. *Gynecology: Essentials of clinical practice* [3rd ed.]. Boston: Little, Brown.) (**B**) A bisected uterus displays a prominent, sharply circumscribed, fleshy tumor. (Rubin E., Farber J.L. [1999]. *Pathology* [3rd ed., p. 999]. Philadelphia: Lippincott Williams & Wilkins)

genitourinary structures and causing hydroureter or bladder problems. Submucosal fibroids displace endometrial tissue and are more likely to cause bleeding, necrosis, and infection than either of the other types.

Leiomyomas are asymptomatic approximately half of the time and may be discovered during a routine pelvic examination, or they may cause menorrhagia (excessive menstrual bleeding), anemia, urinary frequency, rectal pressure/constipation, abdominal distention, and infrequently pain. Their rate of growth is variable, but they may increase in size during pregnancy or with exogenous estrogen stimulation (*i.e.*, oral contraceptives or menopausal estrogen replacement therapy). Interference with pregnancy is rare unless the tumor is submucosal and interferes with implantation

or obstructs the cervical outlet. These tumors may outgrow their blood supply, become infarcted, and undergo degenerative changes. Most leiomyomas regress with menopause, but if bleeding, pressure on the bladder, pain, or other problems persist, hysterectomy may be required. Myomectomy (removal of just the tumors) can be done to preserve the uterus for future childbearing. Cesarean section may be recommended if the uterine cavity is entered during myomectomy. GnRH (*e.g.*, leuprolide [Lupron]) may be used to suppress leiomyoma growth before surgery. Uterine artery embolization done by an interventional radiologist is a nonsurgical therapy for management of heavy bleeding.[28]

> In summary, disorders of the cervix and uterus include inflammatory conditions (*i.e.*, cervicitis and endometritis), cancer (*i.e.*, cervical and endometrial cancer), endometriosis, and leiomyomas. Cervicitis is an acute or chronic inflammation of the cervix. Acute cervicitis may result from the direct infection of the cervix or may be secondary to a vaginal or uterine infection. It may be caused by a variety of infective agents. Chronic cervicitis represents a low-grade inflammatory process resulting from trauma or nonspecific infectious agents. Cervical cancer is readily detected, and if detected early, it is the most easily cured of all the cancers of the female reproductive system. It arises from precursor lesions that can be detected on a Pap smear; the condition can be cured if detected and treated early.
>
> Endometritis represents an ill-defined inflammation or infection of the endometrium that produces variable symptoms. Endometriosis is the condition in which functional endometrial tissue is found in ectopic sites outside the uterus such as the ovaries, broad ligaments, pouch of Douglas (cul-de-sac), pelvis, vagina, vulva, perineum, or intestines. It causes dysmenorrhea, dyspareunia, and infertility. Adenomyosis is the condition in which endometrial glands and stroma are found in the myometrium, interspersed between the smooth muscle fibers. Endometrial cancer is the most common cancer found in the female pelvis; it occurs more than twice as often as cervical cancer. Prolonged estrogen stimulation with hyperplasia of the endometrium has been identified as a major risk factor for endometrial cancer.
>
> Leiomyomas are benign uterine wall neoplasms of smooth muscle origin. They can develop in the corpus of the uterus and can be submucosal, subserosal, or intramural. Submucosal fibroids displace endometrial tissue and are more likely to cause bleeding, necrosis, and infection than either of the other types.

Disorders of the Fallopian Tubes and Ovaries

After you have completed this section of the chapter, you should be able to meet the following objectives:

✦ List the common causes and symptoms of pelvic inflammatory disease

✦ State the causative factors associated with tubal pregnancy

- ✦ Describe the symptoms of a tubal pregnancy
- ✦ State the underlying cause of ovarian cysts
- ✦ Differentiate benign ovarian cyst from polycystic ovary syndrome (previously called *Stein-Leventhal syndrome*)
- ✦ List the hormones produced by the three types of functioning ovarian tumors
- ✦ State the reason that ovarian cancer may be difficult to detect in an early stage

PELVIC INFLAMMATORY DISEASE

Pelvic inflammatory disease (PID) is an inflammation of the upper reproductive tract that involves the uterus (endometritis), fallopian tubes (salpingitis), or ovaries (oophoritis). Most women with acute salpingitis have *N. gonorrhoeae* or *C. trachomatis* identified in the reproductive tract. PID is a polymicrobial infection and the cause varies by geographic location and population. In addition to the primary causative agents already mentioned, *Mycoplasma hominis*, *Ureaplasma urealyticum*, *Bacteroides*, *Peptostreptococcus*, *E. coli*, *Haemophilus influenzae*, and *Streptococcus agalactiae* may be involved.[29] The organisms ascend through the endocervical canal to the endometrial cavity, and then to the tubes and ovaries. The endocervical canal is slightly dilated during menstruation, allowing bacteria to gain entrance to the uterus and other pelvic structures. After entering the upper reproductive tract, the organisms multiply rapidly in the favorable environment of the sloughing endometrium and ascend to the fallopian tube.

Factors that predispose women to the development of PID include an age of 16 to 24 years, unmarried status, nulliparity, history of multiple sexual partners, and previous history of PID. Although the use of an intrauterine contraceptive device (IUD) has been associated with a three- to fivefold increased risk for development of PID, studies have shown that women with only one sexual partner who are at low risk of acquiring STDs have no significant risk for development of PID from using an IUD.

The symptoms of PID include lower abdominal pain, which may start just after a menstrual period; purulent cervical discharge; adnexal tenderness; and an exquisitely painful cervix. New-onset breakthrough bleeding on oral contraceptives, Depo-Provera, or Norplant has recently been associated with PID. Fever (>101°F), increased erythrocyte sedimentation rate, and an elevated white blood cell count (>10,000 cells/mL) commonly are seen, even though the woman may not appear acutely ill. A newer test involves measurement of C-reactive protein in the blood. Elevated C-reactive protein levels equate with inflammation. Laparoscopy is the gold standard for diagnosis of PID, but clinical criteria have a positive predictive value of 65% to 90% compared with laparoscopy.[29] Minimal criteria for a presumptive diagnosis of PID require only the presence of lower abdominal, adnexal, and cervical motion tenderness.

Treatment may involve hospitalization with intravenous administration of antibiotics. If the condition is diagnosed early, outpatient antibiotic therapy may be sufficient. Antibiotic regimens should be selected according to STD treatment guidelines, which are published every 4 years by the Centers for Disease Control and Prevention (CDC).[30] Treatment is aimed at preventing complications, which can include pelvic adhesions, infertility, ectopic pregnancy, chronic abdominal pain, and tubo-ovarian abscesses. Accurate diagnosis and appropriate antibiotic therapy may decrease the severity and frequency of PID sequelae. The CDC recommends empiric treatment with a presumptive diagnosis of PID, while waiting for confirmation by culture or other definitive test results.

ECTOPIC PREGNANCY

Although pregnancy is not discussed in detail in this text, it is reasonable to mention ectopic pregnancy because it represents a true gynecologic emergency and should be considered when a woman of reproductive age presents with the complaint of pelvic pain. Ectopic pregnancy occurs when a fertilized ovum implants outside the uterine cavity. The most common site for ectopic pregnancy is the fallopian tube (Fig. 45-4). According to the CDC, between 1970 and 1992, the number of ectopic pregnancies increased from 17,800 to 108,800, and the rate of occurrence among women aged 15 to 44 years rose from 4.5 to 19.7 per 1000 reported pregnancies (*i.e.*, live births, abortions, and ectopic pregnancies). Although ectopic pregnancy is the leading cause of maternal mortality in the first trimester and accounts for 10% to 15% of all maternal deaths in the United States, the death rate has steadily declined to a rate of 3.8 per 10,000 ectopic pregnancies in 1992.[31]

The cause of ectopic pregnancy is delayed ovum transport, which may result from decreased tubal motility or distorted tubal anatomy (*i.e.*, narrowed lumen, convolutions, or diverticula). Factors that may predispose to the development of an ectopic pregnancy include PID, therapeutic abortion, tubal ligation or tubal reversal, previous ectopic

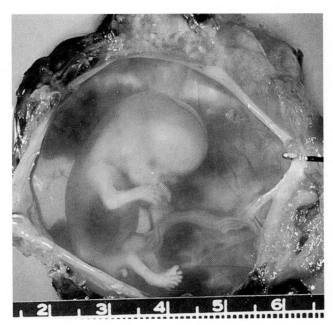

FIGURE 45-4 Ectopic pregnancy. An enlarged fallopian tube has been opened to disclose a minute fetus. (Rubin E., Farber J.L. [1999]. *Pathology* [3rd ed., p. 1001]. Philadelphia: Lippincott Williams & Wilkins)

pregnancy, intrauterine exposure to DES, infertility, and the use of fertility drugs to induce ovulation. Contraceptive failure with progestin-only birth control pills or the "morning-after pill" also has been associated with ectopic pregnancy.

The site of implantation in the tube (*e.g.*, isthmus, ampulla) may determine the onset of symptoms and the timing of diagnosis. As the tubal pregnancy progresses, the surrounding tissue is stretched. The pregnancy eventually outgrows its blood supply, at which point the pregnancy terminates or the tube itself ruptures because it can no longer contain the growing pregnancy. Symptoms can include lower abdominal discomfort—diffuse or localized to one side—which progresses to severe pain caused by rupture, spotting, syncope, referred shoulder pain from bleeding into the abdominal cavity, and amenorrhea. Physical examination usually reveals adnexal tenderness; an adnexal mass is found in only 50% of cases. Although rarely used today, culdocentesis (*i.e.*, needle aspiration from the culde-sac) may reveal blood if rupture has occurred. Quantitative β-human chorionic gonadotropin (hCG) pregnancy tests may detect lower-than-normal hCG production. Pelvic ultrasound studies after 5 weeks' gestation may demonstrate an empty uterine cavity or presence of the gestational sac outside the uterus. Definitive diagnosis may require laparoscopy. Differential diagnosis for this type of pelvic pain includes ruptured ovarian cyst, threatened or incomplete abortion, PID, acute appendicitis, and degenerating fibroid.

Treatment usually is surgical: a laparoscopic salpingostomy to remove the ectopic pregnancy if the fallopian tube has not ruptured or salpingectomy to remove the tube if it has. In salpingostomy, a linear incision is made in the tube and allowed to heal closed without suturing to decrease scar tissue formation; this procedure preserves fertility but requires careful surgical technique to minimize the risk of recurrent ectopic pregnancies. Laparoscopic treatment of ectopic pregnancy is well tolerated and more cost effective than laparotomy because of shorter convalescence and the reduced need for postoperative analgesia. When possible, it is the preferred method of treatment. In laparotomy, an open incision is made into the abdominopelvic cavity; this procedure becomes necessary when there is uncontrolled internal bleeding, when the ectopic site cannot be visualized through the laparoscope, or when the surgeon is not trained in operative laparoscopy.

Methotrexate, a chemotherapeutic agent, has been successfully used to eliminate residual ectopic pregnancy tissue after laparoscopy, in cases where the pregnancy is diagnosed early and is unruptured, or when surgery is contraindicated. There are several methotrexate regimens and no standardized protocol as yet. The drug is given for 1 to 8 days and is better tolerated when given orally. Adverse effects can include oral lesions, transient elevation of liver enzyme levels, and anemia. Close follow-up with weekly monitoring of hCG levels is necessary until the pregnancy is completely resolved.[32]

CANCER OF THE FALLOPIAN TUBE

Although a common site of metastases, primary cancer of the fallopian tube is rare, accounting for less than 1% of all female genital tract cancers. Fewer than 3000 cases have been reported worldwide. Most primary tubal cancers are papillary adenocarcinomas, and these tumors develop bilaterally in 40% to 50% of patients.

Symptoms are uncommon, but intermittent serosanguineous vaginal discharge, abnormal vaginal bleeding, and colicky low abdominal pain have been reported. An adnexal mass may be present; however, the preoperative diagnosis in most cases is leiomyoma or ovarian tumor. Management is similar to that for ovarian cancer and usually includes total hysterectomy, bilateral salpingo-oophorectomy, and pelvic lymph node dissection. More extensive procedures may be warranted, depending on the stage of the disease. Two thirds of patients are diagnosed at stage I or II. The 5-year survival rate in these cases is approximately 60%, but drops to 10% if metastasis has occurred.[33]

BENIGN OVARIAN CYSTS AND TUMORS

The ovaries have a dual function: they produce germ cells, or ova, and they synthesize the female sex hormones. Disorders of the ovaries frequently cause menstrual and fertility problems. Benign conditions of the ovaries can present as primary lesions of the ovarian structures or as secondary disorders related to hypothalamic, pituitary, or adrenal dysfunction.

Ovarian Cysts

Cysts are the most common form of ovarian tumor. Many are benign. A follicular cyst is one that results from occlusion of the duct of the follicle. Each month, several follicles begin to develop and are blighted at various stages of development. These follicles form cavities that fill with fluid, producing a cyst. The dominant follicle normally ruptures to release the egg (*i.e.*, ovulation) but occasionally persists and continues growing. Likewise, a luteal cyst is a persistent cystic enlargement of the corpus luteum that is formed after ovulation and does not regress in the absence of pregnancy. Functional cysts are asymptomatic unless there is substantial enlargement or bleeding into the cyst. This can cause considerable discomfort or a dull, aching sensation on the affected side. The cyst may become twisted or may rupture into the intra-abdominal cavity. These cysts usually regress spontaneously.

Ovarian dysfunction associated with infrequent or absent menses in obese, infertile women was first reported in the 1930s by Stein and Leventhal, for whom the syndrome was originally named. Polycystic ovary syndrome (PCOS) is characterized by numerous cystic follicles or follicular cysts. Once thought to be relatively rare, it appears that this clinical entity is one of the most common endocrinologic disorders among women in the reproductive years. PCOS is characterized by varying degrees of hirsutism, obesity, and infertility, and often is associated with hyperinsulinemia or insulin resistance. This syndrome has been the subject of considerable research. Chronic anovulation, causing amenorrhea or irregular menses, is now thought to be the underlying cause of the bilaterally enlarged "polycystic" ovaries. Hence, the appearance of the ovary is a sign, not the disease itself.[34] The precise etiology of this condition is still being debated. A possible genetic basis has been suggested with an autosomal dominant mode of inheritance and premature balding as the phenotype in males.[34]

Most women with PCOS have elevated luteinizing hormone (LH) levels with normal estrogen and follicle-stimulating hormone (FSH) production. Elevated levels of testosterone, dehydroepiandrosterone sulfate (DHAS), or androstenedione are not uncommon, and these women occasionally have hyperprolactinemia or hypothyroidism. Persistent anovulation results in an estrogen environment that alters the hypothalamic release of GnRH. Increased sensitivity of the pituitary to GnRH results in increased LH secretion and suppression of FSH. This altered LH:FSH ratio often is used as a diagnostic criterion for this condition, but it is not universally present. The presence of some FSH allows for new follicular development; however, full maturation is not attained, and ovulation does not occur. The elevated LH level also results in increased androgen production, which in turn prevents normal follicular development and contributes to the vicious cycle of anovulation.[34] The association between hyperandrogenism and insulin resistance is now well recognized. Evidence suggests that the hyperinsulinemia may lead to the excess androgen production, and several reports have shown that normal ovulation and sometimes pregnancy have occurred when women with hyperandrogenism were treated with insulin-sensitizing drugs.[36–38] The diagnosis can be suspected from the clinical picture. Confirmation with ultrasonography or laparoscopic visualization of the ovaries is not required. When fertility is desired, the condition usually is treated by the administration of the hypothalamic-pituitary–stimulating drug clomiphene citrate or injectable gonadotropins to induce ovulation. These drugs must be used carefully because they can induce extreme enlargement of the ovaries. An insulin-sensitizing drug may be used before or concurrent with ovulation-inducing medications.[36] Weight loss also may be beneficial in restoring normal ovulation when obesity is present. When medication is ineffective, laser surgery to puncture the multiple follicles may restore normal ovulatory function, although adhesion formation is a potential problem. If fertility is not desired, oral contraceptives or cyclic progesterone can induce regular menses and prevent the development of endometrial hyperplasia caused by unopposed estrogen. Chronic anovulation can increase a woman's risk of endometrial cancer, cardiovascular disease, and hyperinsulinemia leading to diabetes mellitus. Treatment is essential for anyone with this condition.

Benign and Functioning Ovarian Tumors

Serous cystadenoma and mucinous cystadenoma are the most common benign ovarian neoplasms. Some of these adenomas, however, are considered to have low malignant potential. They are asymptomatic unless their size is sufficient to cause abdominal enlargement. Endometriomas are the "chocolate cysts" that develop secondary to ovarian endometriosis (see the endometriosis section earlier in this chapter). Ovarian fibromas are connective tissue tumors composed of fibrocytes and collagen. They range in size from 6 to 20 cm. Cystic teratomas, or dermoid cysts, are derived from primordial germ cells and are composed of various combinations of well-differentiated ectodermal,

mesodermal, and endodermal elements. Not uncommonly, they contain sebaceous material, hair, or teeth. Treatment for all ovarian tumors is surgical excision. Ovarian tissue that is not affected by the tumor can be left intact if frozen-section analysis does not reveal malignancy. When ovarian tumors are very large, as is frequently the case with serous or mucinous cystadenomas, the entire ovary must be removed.

The three types of functioning ovarian tumors are estrogen secreting, androgen secreting, and mixed estrogen-androgen secreting. These tumors may be benign or cancerous. One such tumor, the granulosa cell tumor, is associated with excess estrogen production. When it develops during the reproductive period, the persistent and uncontrolled production of estrogen interferes with the normal menstrual cycle, causing irregular and excessive bleeding, endometrial hyperplasia, or amenorrhea and fertility problems. When it develops after menopause, it causes postmenopausal bleeding, stimulation of the glandular tissues of the breast, and other signs of renewed estrogen production. Androgen-secreting tumors (*i.e.*, Sertoli-Leydig cell tumor or androblastoma) inhibit ovulation and estrogen production. They tend to cause hirsutism and development of masculine characteristics, such as baldness, acne, oily skin, breast atrophy, and deepening of the voice. The treatment is surgical removal of the tumor.

OVARIAN CANCER

Ovarian cancer is the second most common female genitourinary cancer and the most lethal. In 2000, 23,100 new cases of ovarian cancer were reported in the United States, two thirds of which were in advanced stages of the disease. Most of these women die of the disease (14,000 women in 2000).[13] The incidence of ovarian cancer increases with age, being greatest between 65 and 84 years of age. Ovarian cancer is difficult to diagnose, and up to 75% of women have metastatic disease before the time of discovery.

The most significant risk factor for ovarian cancer appears to be ovulatory age—the length of time during a woman's life when her ovarian cycle is not suppressed by pregnancy, lactation, or oral contraceptive use. The incidence of ovarian cancer is much lower in countries where women bear numerous children than in the United States. Family history also is a significant risk factor for ovarian cancer. Women with two or more first- or second-degree relatives who have had *site-specific ovarian cancer* have up to a 50% risk for development of the disease. There are two other types of inherited risk for ovarian cancer: *breast-ovarian cancer syndrome*, where both breast and ovarian cancer occur among first- and second-degree relatives, and *family cancer syndrome* or *Lynch syndrome II*, in which male or female relatives have a history of colorectal, endometrial, ovarian, pancreatic, or other types of cancer.[39,40] The breast cancer (BRCA) susceptibility genes, BRAC1 and BRCA2, which are tumor suppressors, are incriminated in 5% to 10% of hereditary ovarian cancers despite being identified as "breast cancer genes." Susceptibility to ovarian cancer is transmitted as an autosomal dominant characteristic; therefore, a mutated gene from either parent is sufficient to cause the problem. Most men who pass on the BRCA mutations do not themselves manifest male breast cancer.[41] A high-fat Western diet and use of powders containing talc in the genital area are other factors that have been linked to the development of ovarian cancer.

Cancer of the ovary is complex because of the diversity of tissue types that originate in the ovary. As a result of this diversity, there are several types of ovarian cancers. Malignant neoplasms of the ovary can be divided into three categories: epithelial tumors, germ cell tumors, and gonadal stromal tumors. Epithelial tumors account for approximately 90% of cases. These different cancers display various degrees of virulence, depending on the type of tumor and degree of differentiation involved. A well-differentiated cancer of the ovary may have produced symptoms for many months and still be found operable at the time of surgery. A poorly differentiated tumor may have been clinically evident for only a few days but found to be widespread and inoperable. Often no correlation exists between the duration of symptoms and the extent of the disease.

Most cancers of the ovary produce no symptoms, or the symptoms are so vague that the woman seldom seeks medical care until the disease is far advanced. These vague discomforts include abdominal distress, flatulence, and bloating, especially after ingesting food. These gastrointestinal manifestations may precede other symptoms by months. Many women take antacids or bicarbonate of soda for a time before consulting a physician. The physician also may dismiss the woman's complaints as being caused by other conditions, further delaying diagnosis and treatment. It is not fully understood why the initial symptoms of ovarian cancer are manifested as gastrointestinal disturbances. It is thought that biochemical changes in the peritoneal fluids may irritate the bowel or that pain originating in the ovary may be referred to the abdomen and be interpreted as a gastrointestinal disturbance. Clinically evident ascites (*i.e.*, fluid in the peritoneal cavity) is seen in approximately one fourth of women with malignant ovarian tumors and is associated with a worse prognosis.

No good screening tests or other early methods of detection exist for ovarian cancer. The serum tumor marker CA-125 is a cell surface antigen; its level is elevated in 80% to 90% of women with stage II to IV nonmucinous ovarian epithelial cancers. The result is negative, however, for as many as 50% of women with stage I disease. In a postmenopausal woman with a pelvic mass, an elevated CA-125 has a positive predictive value of greater than 70% for cancer. It also can be used in monitoring therapy and recurrences when preoperative levels have been elevated. Despite its role in diagnostic evaluation and follow-up, CA-125 is not cancer or tissue specific for ovarian cancer. Levels also are elevated in the presence of endometriosis, uterine fibroids, pregnancy, liver disease, and other benign conditions and with cancer of the endometrium, cervix, fallopian tube, and pancreas. Because it lacks sensitivity and specificity, CA-125 has limited value as a single screening test, but combining CA-125 with other serum tumor markers (*e.g.*, CA-15-3, TAG 72.3) may improve specificity.[42]

Transvaginal ultrasonography (TVS) has been used to evaluate ovarian masses for malignant potential. As a screening test, it has demonstrated 80% to 90% sensitivity and 83% to 95% specificity. Because the lifetime risk for development of ovarian cancer is 1 in 70 women with family history of the disease, the cost of universal screening for ovarian cancer using the available technology has been estimated at $1 million to save one woman.[43] The National Institutes of Health Consensus Panel convened in 1995 recommended no widespread screening of women for ovarian cancer. CA-125 with TVS is suggested only for women who are part of a family with hereditary ovarian cancer syndrome (*i.e.*, two or more affected first-degree relatives), or less than 1% of all women.[44] Other authors recommend that screening of the normal population be conducted in research settings to add to our knowledge in this area.[42] Molecular biologic studies have identified tumor suppressor genes that may play a role in the cause of ovarian cancer. Further evaluation in this area is ongoing and may eventually lead to identification of appropriate screening techniques for ovarian cancer.

When ovarian cancer is suspected, surgical evaluation is required for diagnosis, complete and accurate staging, and cytoreduction and debulking procedures to reduce the size of the tumor. At the time of surgery, the uterus, fallopian tubes, ovaries, and omentum are removed; the liver, diaphragm, retroperitoneal and aortic lymph nodes, and peritoneal surface are examined and biopsies are taken as needed. Cytologic washings are done to test for cancerous cells in the peritoneal fluid. Recommendations regarding treatment beyond surgery and prognosis depend on the stage of the disease. Women with limited disease (*i.e.*, well-differentiated stage Ia or Ib) usually do not require adjuvant treatment; women with intermediate disease (*i.e.*, stage Ib or II) or advanced disease (*i.e.*, stage III or IV) can benefit from chemotherapy with cisplatin and cyclophosphamide. When this combination therapy fails, salvage chemotherapy with newer drugs such as paclitaxel (Taxol) may prolong survival. Irradiation no longer plays a major role in treatment of ovarian cancer because of the difficulty in irradiating the entire abdomen without causing life-threatening damage to vital organs.

The lack of accurate screening tools and the resistant nature of ovarian cancers significantly affects success of treatment and survival. The 5-year survival rate is 94.6% for women whose ovarian cancer is detected and treated early; however, only 25% of all cases are detected at the localized stage. Overall, the 5-year survival rate is 50.4%.[45]

In summary, PID is an inflammation of the upper reproductive tract that involves the uterus (endometritis), fallopian tubes (salpingitis), or ovaries (oophoritis). It is most commonly caused by *N. gonorrhoeae* or *C. trachomatis*. Accurate diagnosis and appropriate antibiotic therapy are aimed at preventing complications such as pelvic adhesions, infertility, ectopic pregnancy, chronic abdominal pain, and tubo-ovarian abscesses.

Ectopic pregnancy occurs when a fertilized ovum implants outside the uterine cavity; the common site is the fallopian tube. Causes of ectopic pregnancy are delayed ovum transport resulting from complications of PID, therapeutic abortion, tubal ligation or tubal reversal, previous ectopic pregnancy, or other conditions such as use of fertility drugs to induce ovulation. It represents a true gynecologic emergency, often necessitating surgical intervention. Cancer of the fallopian tube is rare; the diagnosis is difficult, and the condition usually is well advanced when diagnosed.

Disorders of the ovaries include benign cysts, functioning ovarian tumors, and cancer of the ovary; they usually are asymptomatic unless there is substantial enlargement or bleeding into the cyst, or the cyst becomes twisted or ruptures. Polycystic ovarian disease is characterized by numerous cystic follicles or follicular cysts; it causes various degrees of hirsutism, obesity, and infertility. Benign ovarian tumors consist of endometriomas, which are chocolate cysts that develop secondary to ovarian endometriosis; ovarian fibromas, which are connective tissue tumors composed of fibrocytes and collagen; and cystic teratomas or dermoid cysts, which are derived from primordial germ cells and are composed of various combinations of well-differentiated ectodermal, mesodermal, and endodermal elements. Functioning ovarian tumors are of three types: estrogen secreting, androgen secreting, and mixed estrogen–androgen secreting, and may be benign or cancerous. Cancer of the ovary is the second most common female genitourinary cancer and the most lethal. It can be divided into three categories: epithelial tumors, germ cell tumors, and gonadal stromal tumors. There are no effective screening methods for ovarian cancer, and often the disease is well advanced at the time of diagnosis.

Disorders of Pelvic Support and Uterine Position

After you have completed this section of the chapter, you should be able to meet the following objectives:

✦ Characterize the function of the supporting ligaments and pelvic floor muscles in maintaining the position of the pelvic organs, including the uterus, bladder, and rectum

✦ Describe the manifestations of cystocele, rectocele, and enterocele

✦ Explain how uterine anteflexion, retroflexion, and retroversion differ from normal uterine position

✦ Describe the cause and manifestations of uterine prolapse

The uterus and the pelvic structures are maintained in proper position by the uterosacral ligaments, round ligaments, broad ligament, and cardinal ligaments. The two cardinal ligaments maintain the cervix in its normal position. The uterosacral ligaments normally hold the uterus in a forward position (Fig. 45-5). The broad ligament suspends the uterus, fallopian tubes, and ovaries in the pelvis. The vagina is encased in the semirigid structure of the strong supporting fascia. The muscular floor of the pelvis is a strong, slinglike structure that supports the uterus, vagina, urinary bladder, and rectum (Fig. 45-6). In the female anat-

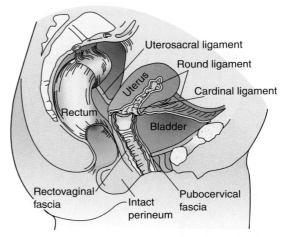

FIGURE 45-5 Normal support of the uterus and vagina. (Rock J.A., Thompson J.D. [1992]. *Te Linde's operative gynecology* [7th ed.]. Philadelphia: J.B. Lippincott)

omy, nature is faced with the problems of supporting the pelvic viscera against the force of gravity and increases in intra-abdominal pressure associated with coughing, sneezing, defecation, and laughing while at the same time allowing for urination, defecation, and normal reproductive tract function, especially the delivery of an infant. Three supporting structures are provided for the abdominal pelvic diaphragm. The bony pelvis provides support and protection for parts of the digestive tract and genitourinary structures, and the peritoneum holds the pelvic viscera in place. The main support for the viscera, however, is the pelvic diaphragm, made up of muscles and connective tissue that stretch across the bones of the pelvic outlet. The openings that must exist for the urethra, rectum, and vagina cause an inherent weakness in the pelvic diaphragm. Congenital or acquired weakness of the pelvic diaphragm results in widening of these openings, particularly the vagina, with the possible herniation of pelvic viscera through the pelvic floor (*i.e.*, prolapse).

Relaxation of the pelvic outlet usually comes about because of overstretching of the perineal supporting tissues during pregnancy and childbirth. Although the tissues are stretched only during these times, there may be no difficulty until later in life, such as the fifth or sixth decade, when further loss of elasticity and muscle tone occurs. Even in a woman who has not borne children, the combination of aging and postmenopausal changes may give rise to problems related to relaxation of the pelvic support structures. The three most common conditions associated with this relaxation are cystocele, rectocele, and uterine prolapse. These may occur separately or together.

CYSTOCELE

Cystocele is a herniation of the bladder into the vagina. It occurs when the normal muscle support for the bladder is weakened, and the bladder sags below the uterus. The vaginal wall stretches and bulges downward because of the force

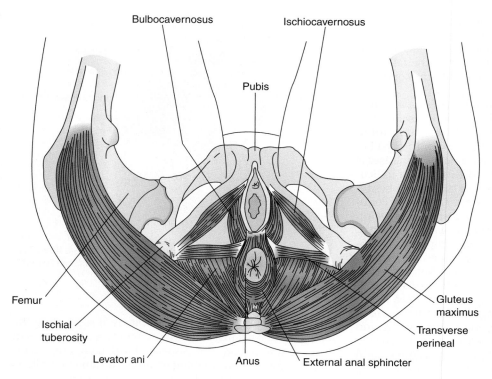

Bulbocavernosus

Ischiocavernosus

Pubis

Femur

Ischial
tuberosity

Levator ani

Anus

External anal sphincter

Gluteus
maximus

Transverse
perineal

FIGURE 45-6 Muscles of the pelvic floor (female perineum). (Chaffee E.E., Lytle I.M. [1980]. *Basic physiology and anatomy* [4th ed.]. Philadelphia: J.B. Lippincott)

of gravity and the pressure from coughing, lifting, or straining at stool. The bladder herniates through the anterior vaginal wall, and a cystocele forms (Fig. 45-7).

The symptoms include an annoying bearing-down sensation, difficulty in emptying the bladder, frequency and urgency of urination, and cystitis. Stress incontinence may occur at times of increased abdominal pressure, such as

Intra-abdominal
pressure on fundus

Uterus

Round ligament

Uterosacral
ligament

Cardinal ligament

Rectum

Bladder

Urethra

Rectocele

Fascia

Relaxed
perineum

Cystocele

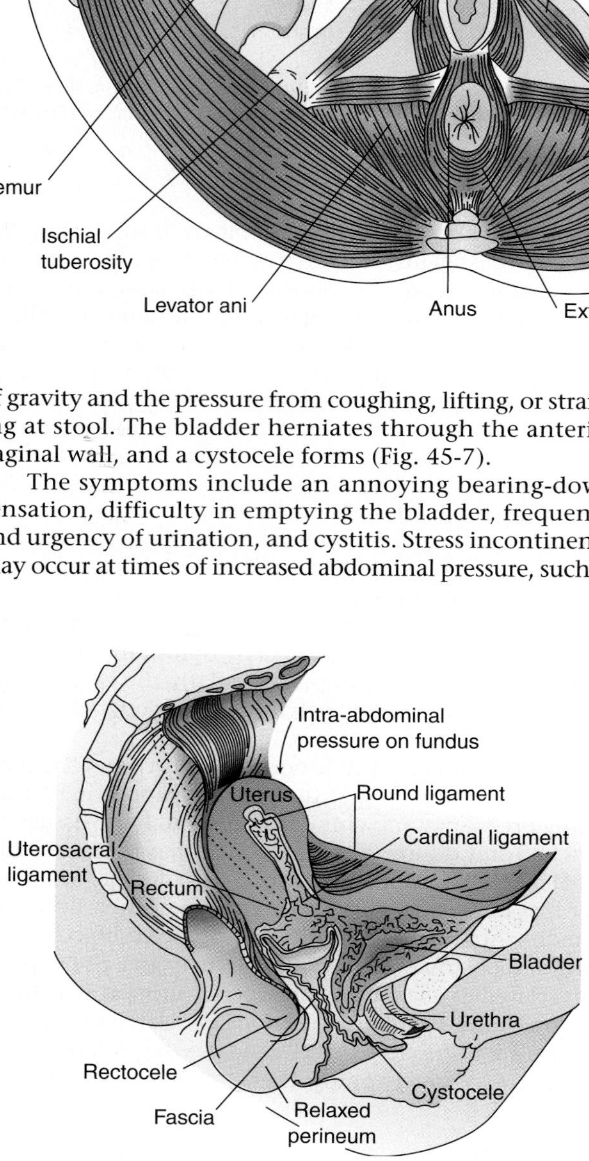

FIGURE 45-7 Relaxation of pelvic support structures with descent of the uterus as well as formation of cystocele and rectocele. (Rock J.A., Thompson J.D. [1992]. *Te Linde's operative gynecology* [7th ed.]. Philadelphia: J.B. Lippincott)

during squatting, straining, coughing, sneezing, laughing, or lifting.

RECTOCELE AND ENTEROCELE

Rectocele is the herniation of the rectum into the vagina. It occurs when the posterior vaginal wall and underlying rectum bulge forward, ultimately protruding through the introitus as the pelvic floor and perineal muscles are weakened. The symptoms include discomfort because of the protrusion of the rectum and difficulty in defecation (see Fig. 45-7). Digital pressure (*i.e.*, splinting) on the bulging posterior wall of the vagina may become necessary for defecation.

The area between the uterosacral ligaments just posterior to the cervix may weaken and form a hernial sac into which the small bowel protrudes when the woman is standing. This defect, called an *enterocele*, may extend into the rectovaginal septum. It may be congenital or acquired through birth trauma. Enterocele can be asymptomatic or cause a dull, dragging sensation and occasionally cause low backache.

UTERINE PROLAPSE

Uterine prolapse is the bulging of the uterus into the vagina that occurs when the primary supportive ligaments (*i.e.*, cardinal ligaments) are stretched. Prolapse is ranked as first, second, or third degree, depending on how far the uterus protrudes through the introitus. First-degree prolapse shows some descent, but the cervix has not reached the introitus. In second-degree prolapse, the cervix or part of the uterus has passed through the introitus. The entire uterus protrudes through the vaginal opening in third-degree prolapse (*i.e.,* procidentia).

The symptoms associated with uterine prolapse result from irritation of the exposed mucous membranes of the cervix and vagina and the discomfort of the protruding mass. Prolapse often is accompanied by perineal relaxation, cystocele, or rectocele. Like cystocele, rectocele, and enterocele, it occurs most commonly in multiparous women because childbearing is accompanied by injuries to pelvic structures and uterine ligaments. It also may result from pelvic tumors and neurologic conditions, such as spina bifida and diabetic neuropathy, that interrupt the innervation of pelvic muscles. A pessary may be inserted to hold the uterus in place and may stave off surgical intervention in women who want to have children or in older women for whom the surgery may pose a significant health risk.

TREATMENT OF PELVIC SUPPORT DISORDERS

Most of the disorders of pelvic relaxation require surgical correction. These are elective surgeries and usually are deferred until after the childbearing years. The symptoms associated with the disorders often are not severe enough to warrant surgical correction. In other cases, the stress of surgery is contraindicated because of other physical disorders; this is particularly true of older women, in whom many of these disorders occur.

There are a number of surgical procedures for the conditions that result from relaxation of pelvic support structures. Removal of the uterus through the vagina (vaginal hysterectomy) with appropriate repair of the vaginal wall (colporrhaphy) often is done when uterine prolapse is accompanied by cystocele or rectocele. A vesicourethral suspension may be done to alleviate the symptoms of stress incontinence. Repair may involve abdominal hysterectomy along with anteroposterior repair. Kegel exercises, which strengthen the pubococcygeus muscle, may be helpful in cases of mild cystocele or rectocele or after surgical repair to help maintain the improved function.

VARIATIONS IN UTERINE POSITION

Variations in the position of the uterus are common. Some variations are innocuous; others, which may be the result of weakness and relaxation of the perineum, give rise to various problems that compromise the structural integrity of the pelvic floor, particularly after childbirth.

The uterus usually is flexed approximately 45 degrees anteriorly, with the cervix positioned posteriorly and downward in the anteverted position. When the woman is standing, the angle of the uterus is such that it lies practically horizontal, resting lightly on the bladder. Asymptomatic, normal variations in the axis of the uterus in relation to the cervix (*i.e.,* flexion) and physiologic dis-

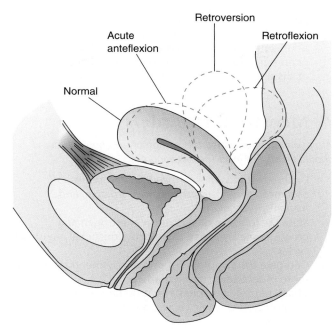

FIGURE 45-8 Variations in uterine position.

placements that arise after pregnancy or with pathology of the cul-de-sac include anteflexion, retroflexion, and retroversion (Fig. 45-8). An anteflexed uterus is flexed forward on itself. Retroflexion is flexion backward at the isthmus. Retroversion describes the condition in which the uterus inclines posteriorly while the cervix remains tilted forward. Simple retroversion of the uterus is the most common displacement, found in 30% of normal women. It usually is a congenital condition caused by a short anterior vaginal wall and relaxed uterosacral ligaments; together, these force the uterus to fall back into the cul-de-sac. Retroversion also can follow certain diseases, such as endometriosis and PID, which produce fibrous tissue adherence with retraction of the fundus posteriorly. Large leiomyomas also may cause the uterus to move into a posterior position. Dyspareunia with deep penetration or low back pain with menses can be associated with retroversion. Most symptoms in these women are caused by the associated condition (*e.g.,* adhesions, fibroids) rather than congenital retroversion.

In summary, alterations in pelvic support frequently occur because of weaknesses and relaxation of the pelvic floor and perineum. Cystocele and rectocele involve herniation of the bladder or rectum into the vagina. Uterine prolapse occurs when the uterus bulges into the vagina. Pelvic relaxation disorders typically result from overstretching of the perineal supporting muscles during pregnancy and childbirth. The loss of elasticity in these structures that is a normal accompaniment of aging contributes to these problems. Variations in uterine position are common; they include anteflexion, retroflexion, and retroversion. These disorders, which often are innocuous, can be the result of a congenital shortness of the vaginal wall, development of fibrous adhesions secondary to endometriosis or PID, or displacement caused by large uterine leiomyomas.

Menstrual Disorders

After you have completed this section of the chapter, you should be able to meet the following objectives:

✦ Define the terms *amenorrhea, hypomenorrhea, oligomenorrhea, menorrhagia, metrorrhagia,* and *menometrorrhagia*

✦ State the function of alterations in estrogen and progesterone levels as a cause of dysfunctional menstrual cycles

✦ Compare the symptoms of primary dysmenorrhea with those of secondary dysmenorrhea

✦ Characterize the manifestations of the premenstrual syndrome, its possible causes, and the methods of treatment

DYSFUNCTIONAL MENSTRUAL CYCLES

Although unexplained uterine bleeding can occur for many reasons, such as pregnancy, abortion, bleeding dyscrasias, and neoplasms, the most frequent cause in the nonpregnant female is what is commonly called *dysfunctional menstrual cycles* or *bleeding.* Dysfunctional cycles may take the form of amenorrhea (absence of menstruation), hypomenorrhea (scanty menstruation), oligomenorrhea (infrequent menstruation, periods more than 35 days apart), menorrhagia (excessive menstruation), or metrorrhagia (bleeding between periods). Menometrorrhagia is heavy bleeding during and between menstrual periods.

Dysfunctional menstrual cycles are related to alterations in the hormones that support normal cyclic endometrial changes. Estrogen deprivation causes retrogression of a previously built-up endometrium and bleeding. Such bleeding often is irregular in amount and duration, with the flow varying with the time and degree of estrogen stimulation and with the degree of estrogen withdrawal. A lack of progesterone can cause abnormal menstrual bleeding; in its absence, estrogen induces development of a much thicker endometrial layer with a richer blood supply. The absence of progesterone results from the failure of any of the developing ovarian follicles to mature to the point of ovulation, with the subsequent formation of the corpus luteum and production and secretion of progesterone.

Periodic bleeding episodes alternating with amenorrhea are caused by variations in the number of functioning ovarian follicles present. If sufficient follicles are present and active and if new follicles assume functional capacity, high levels of estrogen develop, causing the endometrium to proliferate for weeks or even months. In time, estrogen withdrawal and bleeding develop. This can occur for two reasons: an absolute estrogen deficiency may develop when several follicles simultaneously degenerate, or a relative de-

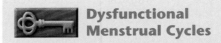

Dysfunctional Menstrual Cycles

➤ The pattern of menstrual bleeding tends to be fairly consistent in most healthy women with regard to frequency, duration, and amount of flow.

➤ Dysfunctional bleeding in postpubertal women can take the form of absent or scanty periods, infrequent periods, excessive and irregular periods, excessive bleeding during periods, and bleeding between periods.

➤ When the basic pattern of bleeding is changed it is most often due to a lack of ovulation and disturbances in the pattern of hormone secretion.

➤ When the basic pattern is undisturbed and there are superimposed episodes of bleeding or spotting, the etiology is more likely to be related to organic lesions or hematologic disorders.

ficiency may develop as the needs of the enlarged endometrial tissue mass exceed the capabilities of the existing follicles, even though estrogen levels remain constant. Estrogen and progesterone deficiency are associated with the absence of ovulation, hence the term *anovulatory bleeding.* Because the vasoconstriction and myometrial contractions that normally accompany menstruation are caused by progesterone, anovulatory bleeding seldom is accompanied by cramps, and the flow frequently is heavy. Anovulatory cycles are common among adolescents during the first several years after menarche, when ovarian function is becoming established, and among perimenopausal women, whose ovarian function is beginning to decline.

Dysfunctional menstrual cycles can originate as a primary disorder of the ovaries or as a secondary defect in ovarian function related to hypothalamic–pituitary stimulation. The latter can be initiated by emotional stress, marked variation in weight (*i.e.,* sudden gain or loss), or nonspecific endocrine or metabolic disturbances. Organic causes of irregular menstrual bleeding include endometrial polyps, submucosal myoma (*i.e.,* fibroid), blood dyscrasia, infection, endometrial cancer, polycystic ovarian disease, and pregnancy.

The treatment of dysfunctional bleeding depends on what is identified as the probable cause. The minimum evaluation should include a detailed history with emphasis on bleeding pattern and a physical examination. Endocrine studies (FSH : LH ratio, prolactin, testosterone, DHAS), β-hCG pregnancy test, endometrial biopsy, D & C with or without hysteroscopy, and progesterone withdrawal tests may be needed for diagnosis. If organic problems are excluded and alterations in hormone levels are the primary cause, treatment may include the use of oral contraceptives, cyclic progesterone therapy, or long-acting progesterone injections.

AMENORRHEA

There are two types of amenorrhea: primary and secondary. Primary amenorrhea is the failure to menstruate by 16 years of age, or by 14 years of age if failure to menstruate is accompanied by absence of secondary sex characteristics. Secondary amenorrhea is the cessation of menses for at least 6 months in a woman who has established normal menstrual cycles. Primary amenorrhea usually is caused by gonadal dysgenesis, congenital müllerian agenesis, testicular feminization, or a hypothalamic-pituitary-ovarian axis disorder. Causes of secondary amenorrhea include ovarian, pituitary, or hypothalamic dysfunction; intrauterine adhesions (*i.e.*, Asherman's syndrome); infections (*e.g.*, tuberculosis, schistosomiasis); pituitary tumor; anorexia nervosa; or strenuous physical exercise, which can alter the critical body fat–muscle ratio needed for menses to occur.[46]

Diagnostic evaluation resembles that for dysfunctional uterine bleeding, with the possible addition of a computed tomographic scan to exclude a pituitary tumor. Treatment is based on correcting the underlying cause and inducing menstruation with cyclic progesterone or combined estrogen-progesterone regimens.

DYSMENORRHEA

Dysmenorrhea is pain or discomfort with menstruation. Although not usually a serious medical problem, it causes some degree of monthly disability for a significant number of women. There are two forms of dysmenorrhea: primary and secondary. Primary dysmenorrhea is menstrual pain that is not associated with a physical abnormality or pathology.[47] It usually occurs with ovulatory menstruation beginning 6 months to 2 years after menarche. Symptoms may begin 1 to 2 days before menses, peak on the first day of flow, and subside within several hours to several days. Severe dysmenorrhea may be associated with systemic symptoms such as headache, nausea, vomiting, diarrhea, fatigue, irritability, dizziness, and syncope. The pain typically is described as dull, lower abdominal aching or cramping, spasmodic or colicky in nature, often radiating to the lower back, labia majora, or upper thighs.

Secondary dysmenorrhea is menstrual pain caused by specific organic conditions, such as endometriosis, uterine fibroids, adenomyosis, pelvic adhesions, IUDs, or PID. Laparoscopy often is required for diagnosis of secondary dysmenorrhea if medication for primary dysmenorrhea is ineffective.

Treatment for primary dysmenorrhea is directed at symptom control. Although analgesic agents such as aspirin and acetaminophen may relieve minor uterine cramping or low back pain, prostaglandin synthetase inhibitors, such as ibuprofen, naproxen, mefenamic acid, and indomethacin, are more specific for dysmenorrhea and the treatment of choice if contraception is not desired. Ovulation suppression and symptomatic relief of dysmenorrhea can be instituted simultaneously with the use of oral contraceptives. Relief of secondary dysmenorrhea depends on identifying the cause of the problem. Medical or surgical intervention may be needed to eliminate the problem.

PREMENSTRUAL SYNDROME

The *premenstrual syndrome* (PMS) is a distinct clinical entity characterized by a cluster of physical and psychological symptoms limited to 3 to 14 days preceding menstruation and relieved by onset of the menses. According to surveys, 25% to 40% of the adult female population in the United States experience mild to moderate monthly symptoms that they attribute to PMS; 2% to 8% report extreme or severe symptoms.[48] How many of these women have symptoms that are severe enough to warrant treatment is unknown. The incidence of PMS seems to increase with age. It is less common in women in their teens and twenties, and most of the women seeking help for the problem are in their mid-thirties. There is some dispute about whether PMS occurs more frequently in women who have not had children or in those who have had children. The disorder is not culturally distinct; it affects non-Westerners and Westerners.

The physical symptoms of PMS include painful and swollen breasts, bloating, abdominal pain, headache, and backache. Psychologically, there may be depression, anxiety, irritability, and behavioral changes. In some cases, there are puzzling alterations in motor function, such as clumsiness and altered handwriting. Women with PMS may report one or several symptoms, with symptoms varying from woman to woman and from month to month in the same patient. Signs and symptoms associated with this disorder are summarized in Table 45-4. PMS can significantly affect a woman's ability to perform at normal levels. She may lose time from or function ineffectively at work. Family responsibilities and relationships may suffer. Students have had lower grades during the premenstrual period. More crimes are committed by females during the premenstrual phase of the cycle, and more lives are lost to suicide during this period. The term *premenstrual dysphoric disorder* is a psychiatric diagnosis that has been developed to distinguish those women whose symptoms are severe enough to interfere significantly with activities of daily living or where the symptoms are not relieved with the onset of menstruation, as is usually the case with PMS.[49]

Although the causes of PMS are poorly documented, they probably are multifactorial. Like dysmenorrhea, it is only recently that PMS has been recognized as a bona fide disorder rather than merely a psychosomatic illness. There has been a tendency to link the disorder with endocrine imbalances such as hyperprolactinemia, estrogen excess, and alteration in the estrogen-progesterone ratio. Prolactin concentration affects sodium and water retention, is higher in the luteal phase than in the follicular phase, and can be increased by estrogens, stress, hypoglycemia, pregnancy, and oral contraceptives.[50] Estrogens stimulate anxiety and nervous tension, and increased progesterone levels may produce depression. The role of hormonal factors in the cause of PMS is supported by two well-established phenomena. First, women who have undergone a hysterectomy but not an oophorectomy may have cyclic symptoms that resemble PMS. Second, PMS symptoms are rare in postmenopausal women. Research has failed to confirm these theories.

Other hypotheses suggest that increased aldosterone may contribute to symptoms associated with fluid retention

TABLE 45-4 ♦ Symptoms of Premenstrual Syndrome (PMS) by System

Body System	Symptoms
Cerebral	Irritability, anxiety, nervousness, fatigue, and exhaustion; increased physical and mental activity; lability; crying spells; depressions; inability to concentrate
Gastrointestinal	Craving for sweets or salts, lower abdominal pain, bloating, nausea, vomiting, diarrhea, constipation
Vascular	Headache, edema, weakness, or fainting
Reproductive	Swelling and tenderness of the breasts, pelvic congestion, ovarian pain, altered libido
Neuromuscular	Trembling of the extremities, changes in coordination, clumsiness, backache, leg aches
General	Weight gain, insomnia, dizziness, acne

(*e.g.*, headache, bloating, breast tenderness, weight gain); that pyridoxine (vitamin B_6) deficiency may lead to estrogen excess or decreased production of the neurotransmitters dopamine and serotonin, which may contribute to PMS symptoms; or that decreased prostaglandin E_1 concentrations can lead to abnormal sensitivity to prolactin, with associated fluid retention, irritability, and depression. In addition, increased appetite, binge eating, fatigue, and depression have been associated with altered endorphin activity and subclinical hypoglycemia.[50] There also is evidence that learned beliefs about menstruation can contribute to the production of PMS or at least affect the woman's response to the symptoms.

Diagnosis focuses on identification of the symptom clusters by means of prospective charting for at least 3 months. A complete history and physical examination are necessary to exclude other physical causes of the symptoms. Depending on the symptom pattern, blood studies, including thyroid hormones, glucose, and prolactin assays, may be done. Psychosocial evaluation is helpful to exclude emotional illness that is merely exacerbated premenstrually.

In the past, the treatment of PMS has been largely symptomatic. Attempts have been made to effect weight loss and reduce fluid retention through the use of diuretics. Tranquilizer drugs were used to treat mood changes, and pain was treated with mild analgesics. Treatment still is directed to some extent toward somatic complaints. Relief of somatic pain does not, however, totally resolve PMS suffering. The latest approach is to recommend an integrated program of personal assessment by diary, regular exercise, avoidance of caffeine, and a diet low in simple sugars and high in lean proteins. Additional therapeutic regimens include vitamin or mineral supplements (particularly pyridoxine, vitamin E, and magnesium), natural progesterone supplements, low-dose monophasic oral contraceptives, GnRH agonists, bromocriptine for prolactin suppression, danazol (a synthetic androgen), spironolactone (an aldosterone antagonist and steroidogenesis inhibitor), evening primrose oil (which contains linoleic acid, a precursor of prostaglandin E_1), and lithium for marked functional impairment

from affective symptoms.[50] Few other treatments have been adequately evaluated in randomized, controlled trials. The use of selective serotonin reuptake inhibitors, however, has demonstrated significant improvement in overall symptoms compared with placebo.[51]

The daily use of prescribed relaxation techniques during the premenstrual period can improve physical and emotional symptoms.[50] Management includes education and support directed toward lifestyle changes. Drug therapy should be used cautiously until well-controlled studies establish criteria for use and effective treatment results. The placebo effect may account for symptom relief in a significant number of women. It is unlikely that a single cause or treatment for PMS will be found. Evaluation and management should focus on identifying and controlling the individual symptom clusters when possible.

In summary, menstrual disorders include dysfunctional menstrual cycles, dysmenorrhea, and PMS. Dysfunctional menstrual cycles occur when the hormonal support of the endometrium is altered. Estrogen deprivation causes retrogression of a previously built-up endometrium and bleeding. A lack of progesterone can cause abnormal menstrual bleeding; in its absence, estrogen induces development of a much thicker endometrial layer with a richer blood supply. The absence of progesterone results from the failure of any of the developing ovarian follicles to mature to the point of ovulation, with the subsequent formation of the corpus luteum and production and secretion of progesterone. Dysfunctional menstrual cycles produce amenorrhea, oligomenorrhea, metrorrhagia, or menorrhagia. Dysmenorrhea is characterized by pain or discomfort during menses. It can occur as a primary or secondary disorder. Primary dysmenorrhea is not associated with other disorders and begins soon after menarche. Secondary dysmenorrhea is caused by a specific organic condition, such as endometriosis or pelvic adhesions. It occurs in women with previously painless menses. PMS represents a cluster of physical and psychological symptoms that precede menstruation by 1 to 2 weeks. The true incidence and nature of PMS has been recognized only recently, and its cause and methods for treatment are still under study.

Disorders of the Breast

After you have completed this section of the chapter, you should be able to meet the following objectives:

✦ Describe changes in breast function that occur with galactorrhea, mastitis, and ductal ectasia
✦ Describe the manifestations of fibrocystic disease and state why it is often referred to as a "catchall" for breast irregularities
✦ Cite the risk factors for breast cancer, the importance of breast self-examination, and recommendations for mammography
✦ Describe the methods used in the diagnosis and treatment of breast cancer

Most breast disease may be described as benign or cancerous. Breast tissue is never static; the breast is constantly responding to changes in hormonal, nutritional, psychological, and environmental stimuli that cause continual cellular changes. Benign breast conditions are nonprogressive; some forms of benign disease, however, increase the risk of malignant disease. In light of this, strict adherence to a dichotomy of benign versus malignant disease may not always be appropriate. This dichotomy, however, is useful for the sake of simplicity and clarity.

GALACTORRHEA

Galactorrhea is the secretion of breast milk in a nonlactating breast. Galactorrhea may result from vigorous nipple stimulation during lovemaking, exogenous hormones, internal hormonal imbalance, or local chest infection or trauma. A pituitary tumor may produce large amounts of prolactin and cause galactorrhea. Galactorrhea occurs in men and women and usually is benign. Observation may be continued for several months before diagnostic hormonal screening.

MASTITIS

Mastitis is inflammation of the breast. It most frequently occurs during lactation but may also result from other conditions.

In the lactating woman, inflammation results from an ascending infection that travels from the nipple to the ductile structures. The most common organisms isolated are *Staphylococcus* and *Streptococcus*.[8] The offending organisms originate from the suckling infant's nasopharynx or the mother's hands. During the early weeks of nursing, the breast is particularly vulnerable to bacterial invasion because of minor cracks and fissures that occur with vigorous suckling. Infection and inflammation cause obstruction of the ductile system. The breast area becomes hard, inflamed, and

tender if not treated early. Without treatment, the area becomes walled off and may abscess, requiring incision and drainage. It is advisable for the mother to continue breast-feeding during antibiotic therapy to prevent this.

Mastitis is not confined to the postpartum period; it can occur as a result of hormonal fluctuations, tumors, trauma, or skin infection. Cyclic inflammation of the breast occurs most frequently in adolescents, who commonly have fluctuating hormone levels. Tumors may cause mastitis secondary to skin involvement or lymphatic obstruction. Local trauma or infection may develop into mastitis because of ductal blockage of trapped blood, cellular debris, or the extension of superficial inflammation.

The treatment for mastitis symptoms may include application of heat or cold, excision, aspiration, mild analgesics, antibiotics, and a supportive brassiere or breast binder.

DUCTAL DISORDERS

Ductal ectasia manifests in older women as a spontaneous, intermittent, usually unilateral, grayish-green nipple discharge. Palpation of the breast increases the discharge. Ectasia occurs during or after menopause and is symptomatically associated with burning, itching, pain, and a pulling sensation of the nipple and areola. The disease results in inflammation of the ducts and subsequent thickening. The treatment requires removal of the involved ductal mass.

Intraductal papillomas are benign epithelial tissue tumors that range in size from 2 mm to 5 cm. Papillomas usually manifest with a bloody nipple discharge. The tumor may be palpated in the areolar area. The papilloma is probed through the nipple, and the involved duct is removed.

FIBROADENOMA AND FIBROCYSTIC DISEASE

Fibroadenoma is seen in premenopausal women, most commonly in the third and fourth decade. The clinical findings include a firm, rubbery, sharply defined round mass. On palpation, the mass "slides" between the fingers and is easily movable. These masses usually are singular; only 15% are multiple or bilateral. Fibroadenoma is asymptomatic and usually found by accident. It is not thought to be precancerous. Treatment involves simple excision.

The term *fibrocystic breast disease* is the most frequent lesion of the breast. It is most common in women 30 to 50 years of age and is rare in postmenopausal women not receiving hormone replacement.[52] Fibrocystic disease usually presents as nodular (*i.e.*, "shotty"), granular breast masses that are more prominent and painful during the luteal or progesterone-dominant portion of the menstrual cycle. Discomfort ranges from heaviness to exquisite tenderness, depending on the degree of vascular engorgement and cystic distention.

Fibrocystic disease encompasses a wide variety of lesions and breast changes. Microscopically, fibrocystic disease refers to a constellation of morphologic changes manifested by (1) cystic dilation of terminal ducts, (2) relative increase in fibrous tissue, and (3) variable proliferation of terminal duct epithelial elements.[8] Autopsy studies have demonstrated some degree of fibrocystic change in 60% to 80% of adult women in the United States.[8] Symptomatic fibrocystic disease, in which large, clinically detectable cysts are present, is much less common, occurring in approximately 10% of the adult women between 35 and 50 years of age.[8] Although fibrocystic disease often has been thought to increase the risk of breast cancer, only certain variants in which proliferation of the epithelial components is demonstrated represent a true risk. Fibrocystic disease with giant cysts and proliferative epithelial lesions with atypia are more common in women who are at increased risk for developing breast cancer. The nonproliferative form of fibrocystic disease that does not carry an increased risk for development of cancer is more common.

Diagnosis of fibrocystic disease is made by physical examination, biopsy (*i.e.*, aspiration or tissue sample), and mammography. The presence of diffuse radiographic densities, lumpy breasts, or premenstrual breast pain correlate poorly with the presence or degree of fibrocystic change. Instead, a diagnosis of fibrocystic disease should be based on the results of a microscopic examination of a biopsy specimen. Fine-needle aspiration may be used, but if a suspect mass that was nonmalignant on cytologic examination does not resolve over several months, it should be removed surgically. Any discrete mass or lump on the breast should be viewed as possible carcinoma, and cancer should be excluded before instituting the conservative measures used to treat fibrocystic disease. The use of mammography for diagnosis in high-risk groups younger than 35 years of age on a routine basis is still controversial. Mammography may be helpful in establishing the diagnosis, but increased breast tissue density in women with fibrocystic disease may make an abnormal or cancerous mass difficult to discern among the other structures. Hand-held ultrasonography can be useful in clarifying inconclusive mammographic densities.

Treatment for fibrocystic breast disease usually is symptomatic. Aspirin, mild analgesics, and local application of heat or cold may be recommended. Some physicians attempt to aspirate prominent or persistent cysts and send any fluid obtained to the laboratory for cytologic analysis. Women are advised to avoid foods that contain xanthines (*e.g.*, coffee, cola, chocolate, and tea) in their daily diets, particularly premenstrually. Vitamin E may be helpful in reducing mastalgia (breast pain), and women should be encouraged to wear a good supporting brassiere. Danazol can be used for women with severe pain, although the potential for adverse effects warrants trying other methods first.

BREAST CANCER

Cancer of the breast is the most common female cancer. One in eight women in the United States will have breast cancer in her lifetime. In 2000, breast cancer affected 182,800 American women and killed almost 40,800 women.[13] Although the breast cancer mortality rate has shown a slight decline, it is second only to lung cancer as a cause of cancer-related deaths in women. An additional 400 deaths occurred from breast cancer in males.[13] Incidence rates for carcinoma

in situ have increased dramatically since the mid-1970s because of recommendations regarding mammography screening. The decline in the breast cancer mortality rate since 1989 is due to this earlier diagnosis as well as improvements in cancer treatments.[53]

Risk factors for breast cancer include sex, increasing age, personal or family history of breast cancer (*i.e.*, at highest risk are those with multiple affected first-order relatives), history of benign breast disease (*i.e.*, primary "atypical" hyperplasia), and hormonal influences that promote breast maturation and may increase the chance of cell mutation (*i.e.*, early menarche, late menopause, and no term pregnancies or first child after 30 years of age).[54] Most women with breast cancer have no identifiable risk factors.

Approximately 8% of all breast cancers are hereditary.[54] Two breast cancer susceptibility genes—BRCA1 on chromosome 17 and BRCA2 on chromosome 13—may account for most inherited forms of breast cancer (see Chapter 8). BRAC1 is known to be involved in tumor suppression. A woman with known mutations in BRCA1 has a lifetime risk of 56% to 85% for breast cancer and an increased risk of ovarian cancer. BRCA2 is another susceptibility gene that carries an elevated cancer risk similar to that with BRCA1.[55] A task force organized by the National Institutes of Health and the National Genome Research Institute has proposed a set of provisional consensus recommendations for monitoring known carriers of BRCA1 and BRCA2 mutations.[56] The task force recommended that known carriers should begin monthly breast self-examination (BSE) at 18 years of age and begin having annual mammograms at 25 years of age.

Detection

Cancer of the breast may manifest clinically as a mass, a puckering, nipple retraction, or unusual discharge. Many cancers are found by women themselves through BSE—sometimes when only a thickening or subtle change in breast contour is noticed. The variety of symptoms and potential for self-discovery underscore the need for regular, systematic self-examination. BSE should be done routinely by women older than 20 years of age. Premenopausal women should conduct the examination right after menses. This time is most appropriate in relation to cyclic breast changes that occur in response to fluctuations in hormone levels. Postmenopausal women and women who have had a hysterectomy should perform the examination on the same day of every month. Examination should be done in the shower or bath or at bedtime. The most important aspect of BSE is to devise a regular, systematic, convenient, and consistent method of examination. As an adjunct to BSE, women should have a clinical examination by a trained health professional at least every 3 years between 20 and 40 years of age, and annually after 40 years of age.

Mammography is the only effective screening technique for the early detection of clinically inapparent lesions. A generally slow-growing form of cancer, breast cancer may have been present for 2 to 9 years before it reaches 1 cm, the smallest mass normally detected by palpation. Mammography can disclose lesions as small as 1 mm and the clustering of calcifications that may warrant biopsy to exclude cancer. The American Cancer Society recommends annual evaluation for women after 40 years of age. Approximately 40% of breast cancers can be detected only by palpation and another 40% only by mammography.[13] The most comprehensive approach to screening is a combination of BSE, clinical evaluation by a health professional, and mammography.

Diagnosis and Classification

Procedures used in the diagnosis of breast cancer include physical examination, mammography, ultrasonography, percutaneous needle aspiration, stereotactic needle biopsy (*i.e.*, core biopsy), and excisional biopsy. Figure 45-9 illustrates the appearance of breast cancer on mammography. Breast cancer often manifests as a solitary, painless, firm, fixed lesion with poorly defined borders. It can be found anywhere in the breast but is most common in the upper outer quadrant. Because of the variability in presentation, any suspect change in breast tissue warrants further investigation. The diagnostic use of mammography enables additional definition of the clinically suspect area (*e.g.*, appearance, character, calcification). Placement of a wire marker under radiographic guidance can ensure accurate surgical biopsy of nonpalpable suspect areas. Ultrasonography is useful as a diagnostic adjunct to differentiate cystic from solid tissue in women with nonspecific thickening.

Fine-needle aspiration is a simple in-office procedure that can be performed repeatedly in multiple sites and with minimal discomfort. It can be accomplished by stabilizing a palpable mass between two fingers or in conjunction with hand-held sonography to define cystic masses or fibrocystic changes and to provide specimens for cytologic examination. Fine-needle aspiration can identify the presence of malignant cells, but it cannot differentiate in situ from infiltrating cancers. Stereotactic needle biopsy is an outpatient procedure done with the guidance of a mammography machine. After the lesion is localized radiologically, a large-bore needle is mechanically thrust quickly into the area, removing a core of tissue. Discomfort is similar to that with ear piercing, and even when multiple cores are obtained, healing occurs quite rapidly. Cells are available for histologic evaluation with a 96% accuracy in detecting cancer. This procedure is less costly than excisional biopsy. Excisional biopsy to remove the entire lump provides the only definitive diagnosis of breast cancer, and often is therapeutic without additional surgery. Magnetic resonance imaging techniques, positron emission tomography, and computer-based or digital mammography are being evaluated as additional diagnostic modalities for breast cancer.

Tumors are classified histologically according to tissue characteristics and staged clinically according to tumor size, nodal involvement, and presence of metastasis. It is recommended that estrogen and progesterone receptor analysis be performed on surgical specimens. Information about the

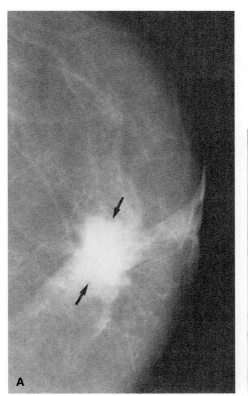
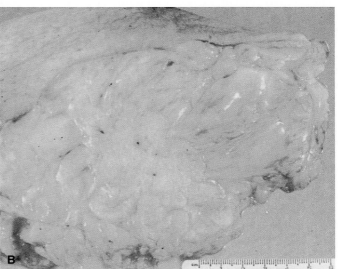

FIGURE 45-9 Carcinoma of the breast. (**A**) Mammogram. An irregularly shaped, dense mass (*arrows*) is seen in this otherwise fatty breast. (**B**) Mastectomy specimen. The irregular white, firm mass in the center is surrounded by fatty tissue. (Rubin E., Farber J.L. [1999]. *Pathology* [3rd ed., p. 1042]. Philadelphia: Lippincott Williams & Wilkins)

presence or absence of estrogen and progesterone receptors can be used in predicting tumor responsiveness to hormonal manipulation. High levels of both receptors improve the prognosis and increase the likelihood of remission.

Treatment

The treatment methods for breast cancer are controversial. They may include surgery, chemotherapy, radiation therapy, and hormonal manipulation. Radical mastectomy (*i.e.*, removal of the entire breast, underlying muscles, and all axillary nodes) rarely is used today as a primary surgical therapy unless breast cancer is advanced at the time of diagnosis. Modified surgical techniques (*i.e.*, mastectomy plus axillary dissection or lumpectomy for breast conservation) accompanied by chemotherapy or radiation therapy have achieved outcomes comparable with those obtained with radical surgical methods and constitute the preferred treatment methods.

The prognosis is related more to the extent of nodal involvement than to the extent of breast involvement. Greater nodal involvement requires more aggressive postsurgical treatment, and many cancer specialists believe that a diagnosis of breast cancer is not complete until dissection and testing of the axillary lymph nodes has been accomplished. A newer technique for evaluating lymph node involvement is a sentinel lymph node biopsy. A radioactive substance or dye is injected into the region of the tumor. In theory, the dye is carried to the first (sentinel) node to receive lymph from the tumor.[57,58] This would therefore be the node most likely to contain cancer cells if the cancer has spread. If the sentinel node biopsy is positive, more nodes are removed. If it is negative, further lymph node evaluation may not be needed. It is not always possible to identify the sentinel node.

Adjuvant systemic therapy refers to the administration of chemotherapy or hormonal therapy to women without detectable metastatic disease. The goal of this therapy depends on nodal involvement, menopausal status, and hormone receptor status. Adjuvant systemic therapy has been widely studied and has demonstrated benefits in reducing rates of recurrence and death from breast cancer.[53] Tamoxifen is a nonsteroidal antiestrogen that binds to estrogen receptors and blocks the effects of estrogens on the growth of malignant cells in the breast. Studies have shown decreased cancer recurrence, decreased mortality rates, and increased 5-year survival rates in women with estrogen receptor–positive tissue samples who have been treated with the drug. Autologous bone marrow transplantation and peripheral stem cell transplantation are experimental therapies that may be used for treatment of advanced disease or in women at increased risk for recurrence. Immunotherapy, using a drug called trastuzumab (Herceptin), is used to stop the growth of breast tumors that express the HER2/neu receptor on their cell surface. The HER2/neu receptor binds an epidermal growth factor that contributes to cancer cell growth. Trastuzumab is a recombinant DNA-derived monoclonal antibody that binds to the HER2/neu receptor, thereby inhibiting proliferation of tumor cells that overexpress the receptor gene.[53,57]

The 5-year survival rate for localized cancer is 96%; with nodal involvement, it is approximately 75%; and it is

approximately 21% with distant metastasis. Five-year survival rates by age at diagnosis range from 81% for women younger than 45 years to 87% for women older than 65 years of age.[45]

Paget's Disease

Paget's disease accounts for 1% of all breast cancers. The disease presents as an eczemoid lesion of the nipple and areola (Fig. 45-10). Paget's disease usually is associated with an infiltrating, intraductal carcinoma. When the lesion is limited to the nipple only, the rate of axillary metastasis is approximately 5%. Complete examination is required and includes a mammogram and biopsy. Treatment depends on the extent of spread.

> In summary, the breasts are subject to benign and malignant disease. Mastitis is inflammation of the breast, occurring most frequently during lactation. Galactorrhea is an abnormal secretion of milk that may occur as a symptom of increased prolactin secretion. Ductal ectasia and intraductal papilloma cause abnormal drainage from the nipple. Fibroadenoma and fibrocystic disease are characterized by abnormal masses in the breast that are benign. By far the most important disease of the breast is breast cancer, which is a significant cause of death of women. BSE and mammography afford a woman the best protection against breast cancer. They provide the means for early detection of breast cancer and, in many cases, allow early treatment and cure.

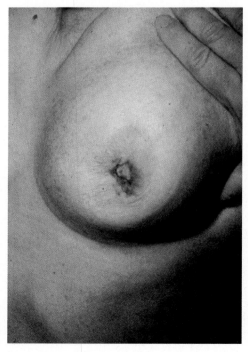

FIGURE 45-10 Paget's disease of the nipple. An erythematous, scaly, and weeping "eczema" involves the nipple. (Rubin E., Farber J.L. [1999]. *Pathology* [3rd ed., p. 1043]. Philadelphia: Lippincott Williams & Wilkins)

Infertility

After you have completed this section of the chapter, you should be able to meet the following objectives:

✦ Provide a definition of infertility
✦ List male and female factors that contribute to infertility
✦ Briefly describe methods used in the treatment of infertility

Infertility is the inability to conceive a child after 1 year of unprotected intercourse. It affects approximately 15% of couples in the United States. Primary infertility refers to situations in which there has been no prior conception. Secondary infertility is infertility that occurs after one or more previous pregnancies. Sterility is the inability to father a child or to become pregnant because of congenital anomalies, disease, or surgical intervention. Approximately 1% to 2% of U.S. couples are affected by sterility.

The complexity of the process that must occur to achieve a pregnancy is taken for granted by most couples. For some couples, pregnancy occurs far too easily, whereas for others, no amount of money, hard work, love, patience, or medical resources seems to be able to bring about this amazing, desired event. Although a full discussion of the diagnosis and treatment of infertility is beyond the scope of this book, an overview of the areas in which problems can occur is presented.

The causes of infertility are almost equally divided between male factors (30% to 40%), female factors (30% to 40%), and combined factors (30% to 40%). In approximately 10% to 15% of infertile couples, the cause remains unknown even after a full workup.

MALE FACTORS

For pregnancy to occur, the male must be able to provide sperm in sufficient quantity, delivered to the upper end of the vagina, with adequate motility to traverse the female reproductive tract. The male contribution to this process is assessed by means of a semen analysis, which evaluates volume of semen (normally 2 to 5 mL), sperm density (20 million/mL), motility (50% good progressive), viability (50%), morphology (60% normal), and viscosity (full liquefaction within 20 minutes). The specimen is best collected by masturbation into a sterile container after 3 days of abstinence. Because of variability in specimens, abnormal results should lead to a repeat test before the need for treatment is presumed.

Azoospermia is the absence of sperm; oligospermia refers to decreased numbers of sperm; and asthenospermia refers to poor motility of sperm. Tests of sperm function include cervical mucus penetration tests (*e.g.*, postcoital test, Penetrak), sperm penetration assay (*i.e.*, Hamster Zona Free Ovum test), and sperm antibody testing.

The causes of male infertility include varicocele, ejaculatory dysfunction, hyperprolactinemia, hypogonadotropic hypogonadism, infection, immunologic problems (*i.e.*, antisperm antibodies), obstruction, and congenital anomalies. Risk factors for sperm problems include a history of mumps orchitis, cryptorchidism (*i.e.*, undescended testes), testicular torsion, hypospadias, previous urologic surgery, infection, and exposure to known gonadotoxins.[59] Treatment depends on the cause and may include surgery, medication, or the use of artificial insemination to deliver a more concentrated specimen directly to the cervical canal or uterine fundus. Artificial insemination with donor sperm can be offered if the male is sterile and this is an alternative acceptable to the husband and wife.

FEMALE FACTORS

The female contribution to pregnancy is more complex, requiring production and release of a mature ovum capable of being fertilized; production of cervical mucus that assists in sperm transport and maintains sperm viability in the female reproductive tract; patent fallopian tubes with the motility potential to pick up and transfer the ovum to the uterine cavity; development of an endometrium that is suitable for the implantation and nourishment of a fertilized ovum; and a uterine cavity that allows for growth and development of a fetus. Each of these factors is discussed briefly, along with an overview of diagnostic tests and treatment.

Ovulatory Dysfunction

In a normally menstruating female, ovulatory cycles begin several months to a year after menarche. Release of FSH from the pituitary causes the development of several primordial follicles in the ovary. At some point, a dominant follicle is selected and the remaining follicles undergo atresia. When the dominant follicle has become large enough to contain a mature ovum (16 to 20 mm in diameter) and is producing sufficient estradiol to ensure adequate proliferation of the endometrium, production of LH increases (*i.e.*, the LH surge), and the increased LH level induces release of the ovum from within the follicle (*i.e.*, ovulation).

After ovulation, under the influence of LH, the former follicle luteinizes and begins producing progesterone in addition to estradiol. The progesterone stimulates the development of secretory endometrium, which has the capability to nourish a fertilized ovum if one should implant.

The presence of progesterone after ovulation causes a rise in the woman's basal body temperature (BBT). This thermogenic property of progesterone provides the basis for the simplest, most inexpensive beginning test of ovulatory function—the measurement of BBT. Women should be able to detect at least a 0.4°F rise in their BBT (at rest) after ovulation that should be maintained throughout the luteal phase. This biphasic temperature pattern demonstrates that ovulation has taken place, where in the cycle it occurred, and the length of the luteal phase. BBT can be influenced by many other factors, including restless sleep, alcohol intake, drug use, fever due to illness, and change in usual rising time. However, as an initial step in the infertility investigation, it can provide useful information to direct other forms of testing.

Endometrial biopsy, the removal of a sample of the endometrium during an office procedure, provides histologic evidence of secretory endometrium and the level of maturation of the lining. In a normal cycle, the luteal phase should be 14 days long. Without pregnancy and the subsequent secretion of hCG, the corpus luteum begins to degenerate 7 to 10 days after the LH surge. The luteal phase of the cycle is so consistent that a pathologist can tell by evaluating a section of endometrium that it is representative of a particular day of the luteal phase. The pathologist's assessment of maturation is compared with the arrival of the next menses. If a discrepancy of more than 2 days exists, the woman is said to have a luteal phase defect (LPD). This diagnosis indicates that, although ovulation is occurring, endometrial development is insufficient and implantation may not be possible. Pregnancy requires fertilization and implantation. LPD also can be suggested by an abnormal serum progesterone level 7 days after ovulation. It can be treated directly with supplemental progesterone after ovulation or with the use of clomiphene citrate to stimulate increased pituitary production of FSH and LH.

Anovulation (no ovulation) and oligo-ovulation (irregular ovulation) are other forms of ovulatory dysfunction. These problems can be identified by the tests for LPD previously described. Ovulatory problems can be primary problems of the ovary or secondary problems related to endocrine dysfunction. When disturbances in ovulation are confirmed, it is reasonable to evaluate other endocrine functions before initiating treatment. If the results of tests for pituitary hormones (*e.g.*, FSH, LH, prolactin), thyroid studies, and tests of adrenal function (*e.g.*, DHAS, androstenedione) are normal, ovulatory dysfunction is primary and should respond to treatment. Abnormalities in any of the other endocrine areas should be further evaluated as needed and treated appropriately. Hyperprolactinemia responds well to bromocriptine, but pituitary microadenoma may need to be excluded first. Hypothyroidism requires thyroid replacement, and hyperthyroidism requires suppressive therapy and, sometimes, surgical intervention with thyroid replacement later. Adrenal suppression can be instituted with dexamethasone, a glucocorticoid analogue. Normal ovulatory function may resume without further intervention; if not, treatment can be concurrent with management of other endocrine problems.

Cervical Mucus Problems

High preovulatory levels of estradiol stimulate the production of large amounts of clear, stretchy cervical mucus that aids the transport of sperm into the uterine cavity and helps to maintain an environment that keeps the sperm viable for up to 72 hours. Insufficient estrogen production (*i.e.*, inherent or secondary to treatment with clomiphene citrate, an antiestrogen), cervical abnormalities from disease or invasive procedures (*e.g.*, DES exposure, stenosis, conization), and cervical infection (*e.g.*, chlamydial infection, mycoplasmal infection, gonorrhea) can adversely affect the production of healthy cervical mucus.

A postcoital test (Sims-Huhner) involves evaluation of the cervical mucus 1 to 8 hours after intercourse within the 48 hours before ovulation. A sample of cervical mucus is obtained using a special syringe and evaluated grossly for amount, clarity, and stretch (*i.e.*, spinnbarkeit) and microscopically for cellularity, number and quality of motile sperm, and the presence of ferning after the sample has air

dried on the slide. To obtain good-quality mucus, it is essential to obtain the sample within the 48 hours before ovulation. Tests may have to be repeated in the same cycle or in subsequent cycles to ensure appropriate timing.

If inadequate estrogen effect is seen (poor-quality mucus), supplemental oral estrogen can be given in the first 9 days of the next cycle, and the test can be repeated. Administration of mucolytic expectorants (1 teaspoon four times daily, starting on day 10 and continuing until ovulation is confirmed) also may improve the quality of the mucus. If mucus is good but sperm are inadequate in number or motility, further evaluation of the male may be needed. The man and woman should be tested for antisperm antibodies when repeated postcoital tests reveal that the sperm are all dead or agglutinated. Artificial insemination with the husband's sperm can bypass the cervical mucus.

Cervical cultures for gonorrhea, chlamydial infection, and mycoplasmal infection should be obtained with the postcoital test if they have not already been acquired. If the cultures give positive results, treatment should be instituted as needed.

Uterine Cavity Abnormalities

Alterations in the uterine cavity can occur because of DES exposure, submucosal fibroids, cervical polyps, bands of scar tissue, or congenital anomalies (*e.g.*, bicornuate septum, single horn). These defects may be suspected from the patient's history or pelvic examination but require hysterosalpingography (*i.e.*, x-ray study in which dye is placed through the cervix to outline the uterine cavity and demonstrate tubal patency) or hysteroscopy (*i.e.*, study in which a lighted fiberoptic endoscope placed through the cervix under general anesthesia allows direct visualization of the uterine cavity) for confirmation. Treatment is surgical when possible.

Tubal Factors

Tubal patency is required for fertilization and can be disrupted secondary to PID, ectopic pregnancy (*i.e.*, after salpingectomy or salpingostomy), large myomas, endometriosis, pelvic adhesions, and previous tubal ligation. Hysterosalpingography can reveal the location and type of any blockage, such as fimbrial, cornual, or hydrosalpinx. Microsurgical repair sometimes is possible.

Even when tubal patency is demonstrated, tubal disease may make ovum pickup impossible. Contrary to popular belief, the ovum is not extruded directly into the fallopian tube. The tube must be free to move to engulf the ovum after release. Pelvic adhesions from previous infection, surgery, or endometriosis can interfere with the tube's mobility. Laparoscopic evaluation of the pelvis is needed for diagnosis. Laser ablation or cautery can be used to lyse adhesions and remove endometriosis through the laparoscope or, if severe, by means of laparotomy.

NEW TECHNOLOGIES

In vitro fertilization (IVF) was developed in 1978 for women with significantly damaged or absent tubes to provide them with an opportunity for pregnancy where none normally exists. The ovaries are superstimulated to produce multiple follicles using clomiphene citrate, human menopausal menotropins (*e.g.*, Pergonal, Humegon), pure FSH (*e.g.*, Gonal F, Follistim, Fertinex), or a combination of these drugs. Follicular maturation is monitored by means of ultrasonography and assay of serum estradiol levels. When preovulatory criteria are met, an injection of hCG is given to simulate an LH surge; 35 hours later, the follicles are aspirated laparoscopically or, more often, by the ultrasound-guided transvaginal route. The follicular fluid is evaluated microscopically for the presence of ova. When found, they are removed and placed into culture media in an incubator.

The eggs are inseminated with sperm from the husband that have been prepared by a washing technique that removes the semen, begins the capacitation process, and allows the strongest sperm to be used for fertilization. When very low numbers of normal motile sperm are available, microsurgical techniques can be used to assist with fertilization. A procedure called *partial zona dissection* involves the creation of a small opening in the layer (*i.e.*, zona pellucida) that surrounds the egg. With subzonal insertion, several sperm are inserted into the space just beneath the protective layer. The most definitive form of micromanipulation is a procedure called *intracytoplamsic sperm injection*, where a single spermatozoa is injected directly into the cytoplasm of the egg.

Between 12 and 24 hours after insemination, the ova are evaluated for signs of fertilization. If signs are present, the ova are returned to the incubator, and 48 to 72 hours after egg retrieval, the fertilized eggs are placed back into the woman's uterus by means of a transcervical catheter. A procedure similar to partial zona dissection can be performed just before embryo transfer to help the fertilized egg escape from the zona pellucida. This "assisted hatching" improves the chances of implantation. In an effort to reduce the number of multiple births resulting from this type of technology, the embryos may be grown to the blastocyst stage and transferred back to the uterus on the fifth day after fertilization. Because many embryos will not advance to the blastocyst stage in vitro, this therapy usually is limited to those women who have produced a significant number of embryos.

Hormonal supplementation of the luteal phase often is used to increase the possibility of implantation. The overall live delivery rate for 1997, as reported by the Society for Assisted Reproductive Technology and American Society for Reproductive Medicine, was 27.9% per egg retrieval.[59] Indications for IVF have been expanded to include male factors (*i.e.*, severe oligospermia or asthenospermia), immunologic infertility, severe endometriosis, and idiopathic infertility (*i.e.*, infertility of unknown cause). The substantial risk of multiple births with IVF procedures has been reduced with the availability of cryopreservation, which allows freezing of excess embryos and limits the number of fresh embryos transferred. The live delivery rate in 1997 after frozen embryo transfer was 18.8%.[59]

An outgrowth of IVF technology is gamete intrafallopian transfer (GIFT), which uses similar ovarian stimulation protocols and egg retrieval procedures but uses laparoscopy to place ovum and sperm directly into the fallopian tube. This procedure requires at least one patent fallopian tube and was developed primarily to increase the pregnancy rate in women with idiopathic infertility. The basic premises are that if a transportation problem is interfering with ovum pickup, GIFT could solve that problem, and that implantation may result more often if fertilization occurs in the body. The live delivery rate for 1997 was 30.0%.[59] The multiple birth rate with GIFT is similar to that with IVF.

Newer reproductive technologies include zygote intrafallopian transfer (ZIFT) and tubal embryo transplant (TET). With ZIFT, the zygote is placed laparosopically into the fallopian tube after the traditional IVF procedure. With TET, the embryos are transferred into the fallopian tubes transcervically using ultrasound guidance or by means of hysteroscopy. The theoretic advantages of these procedures involve tubal factors that may facilitate implantation. The live delivery rate for ZIFT-related procedures in 1997 was 28.0%.[59]

By 2000, more than 400,000 infants had been born worldwide using some type of assisted reproductive technology, with almost 100,000 births being made possible with the use of intracytoplamsic sperm injection. Future research will focus on understanding and improving the implantation process.

In summary, infertility is the inability to conceive a child after 1 year of unprotected intercourse. Male factors are related to number and motility of sperm and their ability to penetrate the cervical mucus and the ovum. Causes of male infertility include varicocele, ejaculatory dysfunction, hyperprolactinemia, hypogonadotropic hypogonadism, infection, immunologic problems (*i.e.*, anti-sperm antibodies), obstruction, and congenital anomalies. Risk factors for sperm disorders include a history of mumps orchitis, cryptorchidism (undescended testes), testicular torsion, hypospadias, previous urologic surgery, infection, and exposure to known gonadotoxins.

The female contribution to pregnancy is more complex, requiring production and release of a mature ovum capable of being fertilized; production of cervical mucus that assists in sperm transport and maintains sperm viability in the female reproductive tract; patent fallopian tubes with the mobility potential to pick up and transfer the ovum to the uterine cavity; development of an endometrium that is suitable for the implantation and nourishment of a fertilized ovum; and a uterine cavity that allows for growth and development of a fetus.

Evaluation and treatment of infertility can be lengthy and highly stressful for the couple. Options for therapy continue to expand, but newer treatment modalities, such as IVF, GIFT, ZIFT, and TET are expensive, and financial resources can be strained while couples seek to fulfill their sometimes elusive dream of having a child.

Related Web Sites

American Cancer Society   www.cancer.org
Centers for Disease Control and Prevention   www.cdc.org
DES (diethylstilbestrol) Action   www.desaction.org

Medscape Women's Health   womenshealth.medscape.com/
  Home/Topics/WomensHealth/womenshealth.html
National Cancer Institutes CancerNet   cancernet.nci.nih.gov
National Cancer Institutes Publications Locator   www.cancer.
  gov/publications
National Women's Health Resource Center   www.
  healthywomen.org

References

1. Hill A.D., Lense J.J. (1998). Office management of Bartholin gland cysts and abscesses. *American Family Physician* 57, 1611–1620.
2. Wilkinson E.J., Stone I.K. (1995). *Atlas of vulvar disease.* (pp. 16, 33–35, 101). Baltimore: Williams & Wilkins.
3. Glazer H.I. (2000). Dysesthetic vulvodynia: Long term follow-up after treatment with surface electromyography-assisted pelvic floor muscle rehabilitation. *Journal of Reproductive Medicine* 45, 798–802.
4. Masheb R.M., Nash J.M., Brondolo E., Kerns R.D. (2000). Vulvodynia: An introduction and critical review of a chronic pain condition. *Pain* 86, 3–10.
5. Cancer Resource Center. (2001). *Vulvar cancer.* The American Cancer Society. [On-line]. Available: http://www.cancer.org/cancerinfo. Accessed March 2, 2001.
6. Chi D.S. (1998). *The diagnosis and management of vulvar cancer.* Medscape Oncology Web site. [On-line]. Available: http://www.medscape.com/medscape/oncology/journal/1990/v01.n4585.chi. Accessed February 21, 2001.
7. Cotran R.S., Kumar V., Collins T. (1999). *Robbins pathologic basis of disease* (6th ed., pp. 1034–1035, 1042–1044, 1061–1062, 1067–1069). Philadelphia: W.B. Saunders.
8. Rubin E., Farber J.L. (1999). *Pathology* (3rd ed., pp. 971–973, 994, 1033–1035). Philadelphia: Lippincott Williams & Wilkins.
9. Sobel J.D. (1997). Vaginitis. *New England Journal of Medicine* 337, 1896–1903.
10. Egan M.E., Lipsky M. (2000). Diagnosis of vaginitis. *American Family Physician* 62, 1095–1104.
11. Cancer Resource Center. (2001). *Vaginal cancer.* The American Cancer Society. [On-line]. Available: http://www.cancer.org/cancerinfo. Accessed March 2, 2001.
12. National Cancer Institute, National Institute of Child Health and Human Development, National Institutes of Health. (1995). *Clear cell carcinoma: Resource guide for DES-exposed daughters and their families* (pp. 3, 5, 24). Rockville, MD: National Institutes of Health.
13. American Cancer Society. (2000). *Cancer facts and figures 2000.* New York: Author.
14. Richards L.A., Klemm P. (2000). An inpatient cervical cancer screening program to reach underserved women. *Journal of Obstetric, Gynecologic, and Neonatal Nursing* 29, 465–473.
15. Canavan T.P., Doshi N.R. (2000). Cervical cancer. *American Family Practitioner* 61, 169–176.
16. Cannistra S.A., Niloff J.M. (1996). Cancer of the uterine cervix. *New England Journal of Medicine* 334, 1030–1038.
17. Scott J.R., DiSaia P.J., Hammond C.B., Spellacy W.N. (1999). *Danforth's obstetrics and gynecology* (8th ed., pp. 589, 815, 818). Philadelphia: Lippincott Williams & Wilkins.
18. Herbst A.L. (1992). The Bethesda system for cervical/vaginal cytologic diagnoses. *Clinical Obstetrics and Gynecology* 35, 22–27.
19. Kurman R.J., et al. (1994). Interim guidelines for management of abnormal cytology. *JAMA* 271, 1866–1869.
20. Eskridge C., Begneaud W.P., Landwehr C. (1998). Cervicography combined with repeat Papanicolaou test as triage for low grade cytologic abnormalities. *Obstetrics and Gynecology* 92, 351–355.
21. Lessey B.A. (2000). Medical management of endometriosis and infertility. *Fertility and Sterility* 73, 1089–1096.
22. Propst A.M., Laufer M.R. (2000). Diagnosing and treating adolescent endometriosis. *Contemporary Nurse Practitioner* Spring, 11–18.
23. Feste J.R., Schattman G.L. (2000). Laparoscopy and endometriosis: Preventing complications and improving outcomes. In *Changing perspectives: A new outlook on gynecologic disorders. Symposia proceedings 2000* (p. 40–42). Medical Education Collaborative.
24. American College of Obstetricians and Gynecologists. (1999). Medical management of endometriosis. ACOG Practice Bulletin no. 11. In *2001 Compendium of selected publications* (pp. 982, 986). Washington, DC: Author.
25. Seltzer V.L., Pearse W.H. (1999). *Women's primary health care: Office practice and procedures* (2nd ed., pp. 230–231, 320, 325). New York: McGraw-Hill.
26. Finan M.A., Kline R.C. (1998). Current management of endometrial cancer. *Contemporary Obstetrics and Gynecology,* 12, 86–97.
27. Canavan T.P., Doshi N.R. (1999). Endometrial cancer. *American Family Practitioner* 59, 3069–3077.
28. Hutchins F.J. (1998). Fibroids in primary care. *The Clinical Advisor* 9, 29.
29. Mott A.M. (2000). Prevention and management of pelvic inflammatory disease by primary care providers. *American Journal of Nurse Practitioners* 8, 7–13.
30. Centers for Disease Control and Prevention. (1998). 1998 Guidelines for treatment of sexually transmitted diseases. *Morbidity and Mortality Weekly Report* 47 (RR-1), 79–86.
31. Centers for Disease Control and Prevention. (1995). Current trends for ectopic pregnancy—United States, 1990–1992. *Morbidity and Mortality Weekly Report* 44 (RR-3), 46–48.
32. Tenore J.L. (2000). Ectopic pregnancy. *American Family Physician* 61, 1080–1088.
33. Ng P., Lawton F. (1998). Fallopian tube carcinoma: A review. *Annals of the Academy of Medicine, Singapore* 27, 693–697.
34. Speroff L., Glass R.H., Kase N.G. (1999). *Clinical gynecologic endocrinology and infertility* (6th ed., pp. 497–503), Philadelphia: Lippincott Williams & Wilkins.
35. Velzquez E., Acosta A., Mendoza S.G. (1997). Menstrual cyclicity after metformin in polycystic ovary syndrome. *Obstetrics and Gynecology* 90, 392–395.
36. Nestler J.E., Jakubowicz D.J., Evans W.S., Pasquali R. (1998). Effects of metformin on spontaneous and clomiphene-induced ovulation in the polycystic ovary syndrome. *New England Journal of Medicine* 338, 1876–1880.
37. Ehrmann D.A., et al. (1997). Troglitazone improves defects in insulin action, insulin secretion, ovarian steroidogenesis and fibrinolysis in women with polycystic ovary syndrome. *Journal of Clinical Endocrinology and Metabolism* 82, 2108–2116.
38. American Society for Reproductive Medicine. (2000). *Use of insulin sensitizing agents in the treatment of polycystic ovary syndrome.* Practice Committee Report. Birmingham, AL: Author.
39. Piver M.S., Eltabbakh G. (1998). *Myths and fact about ovarian cancer: What you need to know* (pp. 17–18). Huntington, NY: PRR.
40. Partridge E.E., Barnes M.N. (1999). Epithelial ovarian cancer: Prevention, diagnosis, and treatment. *CA—A Cancer Journal for Clinicians* 49, 297–320.

41. Frank T.S. (1998). Identifying women with inherited risk for ovarian cancer: Who and why? *Contemporary OB/Gyn* 12, 27–50.

42. Gershenson D.M., McGuire W.P. (1998). *Ovarian cancer: Controversies in management* (pp. 9, 14). New York: Churchill Livingstone.

43. Igoe B.A. (1997). Symptoms attributed to ovarian cancer by women with the disease. *Nurse Practitioner* 22(7), 122, 127–128, 130.

44. National Institutes of Health Consensus Development Panel on Ovarian Cancer. (1995). Ovarian cancer: Screening and follow-up. *Journal of the American Medical Association* 273, 491–497.

45. National Cancer Institute. (2000). *SEER Cancer statistics review 1973–1997* (pp. 370, 122). [On-line]. Available: http://www.seer.cancer.gov.

46. American College of Obstetricians and Gynecologists. (2000). Management of anovulatory bleeding. ACOG Practice Bulletin no. 14. In *2001 Compendium of selected publications* (pp. 961–968). Washington, DC: Author.

47. Coco A.S. (1999). Primary dysmenorrhea. *American Family Practitioner* 60, 489–496.

48. Stair W.L., Lrmmel L.L., Shannon M.T. (1995). *Women's primary health care: Protocols for practice* (pp. 12–153). Washington, DC: American Nurses Publishing.

49. Frye G.M., Silverman S.D. (2000). Is it premenstrual syndrome? Keys to focused diagnosis, therapies for multiple symptoms. *Postgraduate Medicine* 107(5), 151–159.

50. Moline M.L., Zendell S.M. (2000). Evaluating and managing premenstrual syndrome. *Medscape Women's Health* 5(2). [On-line]. Available: http://www.medscape.com/MedscapeWomensHealth/journal/2000/v05,n02.

51. Dimmock P.W., Wyatt K.M., Jones P.W., O'Brien P.M.S. (2000). Efficacy of selective serotonin-reuptake inhibitors in pre-menstrual syndrome: A systemic review. *Lancet* 356, 1131–1136.

52. Giuliano A.E. (2001). Benign breast disorders. In Tierney L.M., McPhee S.J., Papadakis M.A. (Eds.), *Current medical diagnosis and treatment* (40th ed., pp. 706–707). New York: Lange Medical Books/McGraw-Hill.

53. McCance K.L., Jorde L.B. (1998). Evaluating the genetic risk of breast cancer. *Nurse Practitioner* 23(8), 14–16, 19–20, 23–27.

54. Apantaku L.M. (2000). Breast cancer diagnosis and screening. *American Family Physician* 62, 596–606.

55. Rosenthal T.C., Puck S.M. (1999). Screening for genetic risk of breast cancer. *American Family Physician* 59, 99–104.

56. Burke W., Daly M., Garber J., Bokin J., Kahn M.J., Lynch P., et al. (1997). Recommendations for follow-up care of individuals with an inherited predisposition to cancer: II. BRCA1 and BRCA2. Cancer Genetics Studies Consortium. *Journal of the American Medical Association* 227, 997–1003.

57. Hortobagyi G.N. (1998). Treatment of breast cancer. *New England Journal of Medicine* 339, 974–984.

58. McMasters K.M., Guilliano A.E., Ross M.I., Reintgen D.S., Hunt K.K., Byrd D.R., Klimberg V.S., Whitworth P.W., Tafra L.C., Edwards M.J. (1998). Sentinel-lymph-node biopsy for breast cancer: Not yet the standard of care. *New England Journal of Medicine* 339, 990–996.

59. Society of Assisted Reproductive Technology. (2000). Assisted reproductive technology of the United States: 1997 results generated from the American Society of Reproductive Medicine/Society for Assisted Reproductive Technology Registry. *Fertility and Sterility* 74, 641–654.

Chapter 46

Sexually Transmitted Diseases

Patricia McCowen Mehring

Infections of the External Genitalia

Human Papillomavirus
(Condylomata Acuminata)
Genital Herpes
Molluscum Contagiosum
Chancroid

Granuloma Inguinale
Lymphogranuloma Venereum

Vaginal Infections

Candidiasis
Trichomoniasis
Bacterial Vaginosis
(Nonspecific Vaginitis)

Vaginal-Urogenital-Systemic Infections

Chlamydial Infections
Gonorrhea
Syphilis

The incidence and types of sexually transmitted diseases (STDs), as reported in the professional literature and public health statistics, are increasing. The incidence of disease is based on clinical reports, however, and many STDs are not reportable or not reported. The agents of transmission include bacteria, chlamydiae, viruses, fungi, protozoa, parasites, and unidentified microorganisms (see Chapter 17). Portals of entry include the mouth, genitalia, urinary meatus, rectum, and skin. All STDs are more common in persons who have more than one sexual partner, and it is not uncommon for a person to be concurrently infected with more than one type of STD. This chapter discusses the manifestations of STDs in men and women in terms of infections of the external genitalia, vaginal infections, and infections that have systemic effects and genitourinary manifestations. Human immunodeficiency virus (HIV) infection is presented in Chapter 20.

Infections of the External Genitalia

After you have completed this section of the chapter, you should be able to meet the following objectives:

✦ Define what is meant by a sexually transmitted disease (STD)
✦ Give a reason why the reported incidence of STDs may not accurately reflect the true incidence
✦ List common portals of entry for STDs

✦ Name the organisms responsible for condylomata acuminata, genital herpes, molluscum contagiosum, chancroid, granuloma inguinale, and lymphogranuloma venereum
✦ State the significance of condyloma acuminata
✦ Explain the recurrent infections in genital herpes

Some STDs primarily affect the mucocutaneous tissues of the external genitalia. These include human papillomavirus (HPV) infection, genital herpes, molluscum contagiosum, chancroid, granuloma inguinale, and lymphogranuloma venereum (LGV).

HUMAN PAPILLOMAVIRUS (CONDYLOMATA ACUMINATA)

Condylomata acuminata, or *genital warts*, are caused by HPV. Although recognized for centuries, HPV-induced genital warts have become one of the fastest-growing STDs of the past decade. The Centers for Disease Control and Prevention (CDC) estimates that 20 million Americans carry the virus and that up to 5.5 million new cases are diagnosed each year.[1] The current prevalence of HPV is difficult to determine because it is not a reportable disease in all states.

A 1998 American Medical Association consensus conference on external genital warts identified four specific types of warts: *condyloma acuminata* (cauliflower-shaped lesions that tend to appear on moist skin surfaces such as the vaginal introitus or anus); *keratotic warts* (display a thick, horny layer; develop on dry, fully keratinized skin such as

Sexually Transmitted Disease

➤ Sexually transmitted diseases (STDs) are spread by sexual contact and involve both male and female partners. Portals of entry include the mouth, genitalia, urinary meatus, rectum, and skin. All STDs are more common in persons who have more than one sexual partner, and it is not uncommon for a person to be concurrently infected with more than one type of STD.

➤ In general, STDs due to bacterial pathogens can be successfully treated and the pathogen eliminated by antimicrobial therapy. However, many of these pathogens are developing antibiotic resistance.

➤ STDs due to viral pathogens such as the human papillomavirus (HPV) and genital herpes simplex virus infections (HSV-1 and HSV-2) are not eliminated by current treatment modalities and persist with risk of recurrence (HSV infections) or increased cancer risk (HPV).

➤ Untreated, STDs such as chlamydial infection and gonorrhea can spread to involve the internal genital organs with risk of complications and infertility.

➤ Intrauterine or perinatally transmitted STDs can have potentially fatal or severely debilitating effects on a fetus or an infant.

the penis, scrotum, or labia majora); *papular warts* (smooth surface, typically develop on fully keratinized skin); and *flat warts* (macular, sometimes faintly raised, usually invisible to the naked eye, occur on either fully or partially keratinized skin). Flat warts sometimes can be visualized by applying a 5% acetic acid solution to opacify the lesions ("aceto-whitening"). However, this procedure is no longer routinely used because of the high number of both false-positive and false-negative results with this technique. Biopsy may be required to differentiate warts from other hyperkeratotic or precancerous lesions.[2]

A relation between HPV and genital (*i.e.*, cervix, vulva, and penis) neoplasms has become increasingly apparent since the early 1980s. With newer technologies, HPV DNA has been identified in 99.7% of cervical cancers worldwide.[3] One hundred types of HPV have been identified, 33 of which affect the anogenital area. Of the high-risk types, type 16 and type 18 appear to be the most virulent and are associated with most invasive squamous cell cancers. Types 31, 33, 35, 39, 45, 51, 52, 56, and 58 are less common but also have demonstrated some malignant potential in squamous intraepithelial lesions. In contrast, types 6 and 11 are found in most external genital warts but usually are benign, with only a low potential for dysplasia. Only a subset of women

infected with HPV go on to develop cancer. There may be variants of even the most virulent HPV, type 16, with differing oncogenic potential. Cofactors that may increase the risk for cancer include smoking, immunosuppression, and exposure to hormonal alteration (*e.g.*, pregnancy, oral contraceptives).[4] The association with premalignant and malignant changes has increased the concern about diagnosis and treatment of this viral infection.

HPV infection begins with viral inoculation into a stratified squamous epithelium, where infection stimulates the replication of the squamous epithelium, producing the various HPV-proliferative lesions. The incubation period for HPV-induced genital warts ranges from 6 weeks to 8 months. Subclinical infection occurs more frequently than visible genital warts among men and women. Infection often is indirectly diagnosed on the cervix by Papanicolaou testing (Pap smear), colposcopy, or biopsy. Both spontaneous resolution and infection with new HPV types are common. Although reinfection from sexual partners has been considered as a reason for the high prevalence of this disease, it is now thought that reinfection with the same HPV type is infrequent. Instead, it is thought that HPV may be a lifelong infection.

Genital condylomas should be considered in any woman who presents with the primary complaint of vulvar pruritus or who has had an abnormal Pap smear. Microscopic examination of a wet-mount slide preparation and cultures are used to exclude associated vaginitis. Acetic acid soaks may be used before inspecting the vulva under magnification, and specimens for biopsy can be taken from questionable areas. Colposcopic examination of the cervix and vagina may be advised as a follow-up measure when there is an abnormal Pap smear or when HPV lesions are identified on the vulva. Evaluation and treatment of sexual partners may be suggested, although this may be difficult considering that warts often do not become clinically apparent for several years after exposure.

No treatment to date has been shown to eradicate the virus from the body.[5] Treatment goals therefore are aimed at elimination of symptomatic warts, surveillance for malignancy and premalignant changes, and education and counseling to decrease psychosocial distress.[6] Prevention of HPV transmission through condom use has not been adequately demonstrated. Prophylactic vaccines for genital HPV infection are under development and may eventually offer the best opportunity for prevention or eradication of this sexually transmitted precursor to neoplasia.

The CDC identifies several pharmacologic treatments for symptomatic removal of visible genital warts, including patient-applied therapies (podofilox and imiquimod) and provider-administered therapies (podophyllin and trichloroacetic acid).[5] Podophyllin, a topical cytotoxic agent, has long been used for treatment of visible external growths. Multiple applications may be required for resolution of lesions. The amount of drug used and the surface area treated should be limited with each treatment session to avoid systematic absorption and toxicity. This treatment is contraindicated in pregnancy for the same reason. An alternative therapy is the topical application of a solution of trichloroacetic acid. This weak destructive agent produces an initial burning in the affected area, followed in several days by a sloughing of the superficial tissue. Several applications 1 to 2 weeks apart may be necessary to eradicate the lesion. Podofilox is a topical patient-applied antimitotic agent that results in visible necrosis of wart tissue. It is applied twice a day for 3 days, followed by 4 days of nontreatment for a total of four cycles. The safety of podofilox during pregnancy has not been established. Imiquimod cream is a new type of therapeutic agent that stimulates the body's immune system (*i.e.*, production of interferon-α and other cytokines). This cream is applied at home three times a week for up to 16 weeks. It must be washed off 6 to 10 hours after application to avoid excessive skin reaction. It is a category B drug and therefore potentially safe for use in pregnancy. Interferon, in the form of a topical application or as an intralesional injection, has not shown any advantage over other available forms of treatment. Sexual abstinence is suggested during any type of treatment to enhance healing.

Genital warts also may removed using cryotherapy, laser surgery, or electrocautery. Because it can penetrate deeper than other forms of therapy, cryotherapy (*i.e.*, freezing therapy) often is the treatment of choice for cervical HPV lesions. Laser surgery can be used to remove large or widespread lesions of the cervix, vagina, or vulva, or lesions that have failed to respond to other first-line methods of treatment. Electrosurgical treatment has become more widespread for these types of lesions because it is more readily available in outpatient settings and is much less expensive than laser.

GENITAL HERPES

Herpesviruses are large, encapsulated viruses that have a double-stranded genome. There are nine types of herpesviruses, belonging to three groups, that cause infections in humans: neurotropic α-group viruses, including herpes simplex virus type 1 (HSV-1; usually associated with cold sores) and HSV-2 (usually associated with genital herpes); varicella-zoster virus (causes chickenpox and shingles); and lymphotropic β-group viruses, including cytomegalovirus (causes cytomegalic inclusion disease), Epstein-Barr virus (causes infectious mononucleosis and Burkitt's lymphoma), and human herpesvirus type 8 (the apparent cause of Kaposi's sarcoma).[7]

Genital herpes is caused by the herpes simplex virus. Because herpesvirus infection is not reportable in all states, reliable data on its true incidence (estimated number of new cases every year) and prevalence (estimated number of people currently infected) are lacking. From the late 1970s to early 1990s, genital herpes prevalence increased 30%. Incidence rates have been relatively stable since 1990, with an estimated 1 million new cases occurring each year. Recent estimates in the United States indicate 45 million people (one in five adolescents or adults) are infected with genital herpes.[1] Genital infections affect 17% of men and 26% of women in the United States.[8] Women have a greater mucosal surface area exposed in the genital area and therefore are at greater risk of acquiring the infection.

Both HSV-1 and HSV-2 are genetically similar, both cause a similar set of primary and recurrent infections, and both can cause genital lesions. Both viruses replicate in the skin and mucous membranes at the site of infection (oropharynx or genitalia), where they cause vesicular lesions of the epidermis and infect the neurons that innervate the area. HSV-1 and HSV-2 are *neurotropic* viruses, meaning that they grow in neurons and share the biologic property of latency. Latency refers to the ability to maintain disease potential in the absence of clinical signs and symptoms. In genital herpes, the virus ascends through the peripheral nerves to the sacral dorsal root ganglia (Fig. 46-1). The virus can remain dormant in the dorsal root ganglia, or it can reactivate, in which case the viral particles are transported back down the nerve root to the skin, where they multiply and cause a lesion to develop. During the dormant or latent period, the virus replicates in a different manner so that the immune system or available treatments have no effect on it. It is not known what reactivates the virus. It may be that the body's defense mechanisms are altered. Numerous studies have shown that host responses to infection influence initial development of the disease, severity of infection, development and maintenance of latency, and frequency of HSV recurrences.

HSV is transmitted by contact with infectious lesions or secretions. HSV-1 is transmitted by oral secretions, and infections frequently occur in childhood, with most persons (50% to 90%) being infected by adulthood.[9] HSV-1 may be spread to the genital area by autoinoculation after poor hand washing or through oral intercourse. HSV-2 usually is transmitted by sexual contact but can be passed to an infant during childbirth if the virus is actively being shed from the genital tract. Most cases of HSV-2 infection are subclinical, manifesting as truly asymptomatic or symptomatic but unrecognized infections. These subclinical infections can occur in people who have never had a symptomatic outbreak or

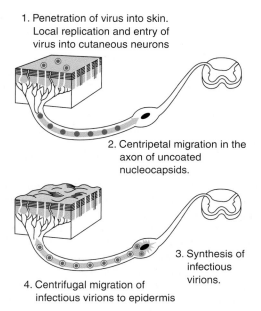

1. Penetration of virus into skin. Local replication and entry of virus into cutaneous neurons

2. Centripetal migration in the axon of uncoated nucleocapsids.

3. Synthesis of infectious virions.

4. Centrifugal migration of infectious virions to epidermis

FIGURE 46-1 Pathogenesis of primary mucocutaneous herpes simplex virus infection. (Corey L., Spear P.G. [1986]. Infections with herpes simplex viruses. Pt. 1. *New England Journal of Medicine* 314, 686)

between recognized clinical recurrences. Up to 70% of genital herpes is spread through asymptomatic shedding by people who do not realize they have the infection.[8] This "unknown" transmission of the virus to sex partners explains why this infection has reached epidemic proportions throughout the world. Because HSV is readily inactivated at room temperature and by drying, aerosol and fomite spread are unusual means of transmission.[4]

The incubation period for HSV is 2 to 10 days. Genital HSV infection may manifest as a primary, nonprimary, or recurrent infection. *Primary infections* are infections that occur in a person who is seronegative for antibody to HSV-1 or HSV-2. *Initial nonprimary infections* refer to the first clinical episode in a person who is seropositive for antibodies to the opposite HSV type (usually genital herpes in someone seropositive to HSV-1). *Recurrent infections* refer to the second or subsequent outbreak due to the same virus type. HSV-2 is responsible for greater than 90% of recurrent genital herpes infections.[6] Approximately 40% of apparent initial cases are actually first-recognized recurrences in persons with long-standing infection.[6]

The initial symptoms of primary genital herpes infections include tingling, itching, and pain in the genital area, followed by eruption of small pustules and vesicles. These lesions rupture on approximately the fifth day to form wet ulcers that are excruciatingly painful to touch and can be associated with dysuria, dyspareunia, and urine retention. Involvement of the cervix and urethra is seen in more than 80% of women with primary infections.[10] In men, the infection can cause urethritis and lesions of the penis and scrotum. Rectal and perianal infections are possible with anal contact. Systemic symptoms associated with primary infections include fever, headache, malaise, muscle ache, and lymphadenopathy. Primary infections may be debilitating enough to require hospitalization, particularly in women.

Untreated primary infections typically are self-limited and last for approximately 2 to 4 weeks. The symptoms usually worsen for the first 10 to 12 days. This period is followed by a 10- to 12-day interval during which the lesions crust over and gradually heal. Nonprimary episodes of genital herpes manifest with less severe symptoms that usually are of shorter duration and have fewer systemic manifestations. Except for the greater tendency of HSV-2 to recur, the clinical manifestations of HSV-2 and genital HSV-1 are similar. Recurrent HSV infection results from reactivation of the virus stored in the dorsal root ganglia of the infected dermatomes. An outbreak may be preceded by a prodrome of itching, burning, or tingling at the site of future lesions. Because the person has already developed immune lymphocytes from the primary infection, recurrent episodes have fewer lesions, fewer systemic symptoms, less pain, and a shorter duration (7 to 10 days). Frequency and severity of recurrences vary from person to person. Numerous factors, including emotional stress, lack of sleep, overexertion, other infections, vigorous or prolonged coitus, and premenstrual or menstrual distress have been identified as triggering mechanisms.

Diagnosis of genital herpes is based on the symptoms, appearance of the lesions, and identification of the virus from cultures taken from the lesions. Depending on the laboratory, a preliminary culture report takes from 2 to 5 days, and a final negative report takes from 10 to 12 days to establish. The stability of the virus in transport media is good for 48 to 72 hours, making mail transport possible. The likelihood of obtaining a positive culture decreases with each day that has elapsed after a lesion develops. The chance of obtaining a positive culture from a crusted lesion is slight, and patients suspected of having genital herpes should be instructed to have a culture within 48 hours of development of new lesions.

Serology tests are used as a means of determining past infection through the presence of specific HSV-2 antibodies in the blood. Noncommercial Western blot assay remains the serologic gold standard for research settings. New, commercially available serology tests provide accurate type-specific HSV-2 antibody results and allow for widespread screening to identify subclinical disease or asymptomatic HSV carriers. Nearly all persons with HSV-2 antibodies reactivate virus periodically and potentially can transmit the infection.[4] Seropositivity for HSV-2 is associated with viral shedding in the genital tract, even in individuals with no reported history of genital herpes.[11]

There is no known cure for genital herpes, and the methods of treatment are largely symptomatic. The antiviral drugs acyclovir, valacyclovir, and famciclovir have become the cornerstone for management of genital herpes. By interfering with viral DNA replication, these drugs decrease the frequency of recurrences, shorten the duration of active lesions, reduce the number of new lesions formed, and decrease viral shedding with primary infections. Valacyclovir, the active component of acyclovir, and famciclovir have greater bioavailability, which enables improved dosing schedules and increased compliance. Episodic intervention reduces the duration of viral shedding and the healing time for recurrent lesions. Continuous antiviral suppressive therapy may be advised when more than six outbreaks occur within 1 year. These drugs are well tolerated, with few adverse effects. This long-term suppressive therapy does not limit latency, and reactivation of the disease frequently occurs after the drug is discontinued. The use of long-term suppressive therapy to reduce asymptomatic shedding and therefore interrupt transmission is under study. Topical treatment with antibacterial soaps, lotions, dyes, ultrasonography, and ultraviolet light has been tried with little success. Sometimes symptomatic relief can be obtained with cool compresses (*i.e.*, Burow's soaks), sitz baths, topical anesthetic agents, and oral analgesic drugs.

Good hygiene is essential to prevent secondary HSV infection. Fastidious hand washing is recommended to avoid hand-to-eye spread of the infection. HSV infection of the eye is the most frequent cause of corneal blindness in the United States. To prevent spread of the disease, intimate contact should be avoided until lesions are completely healed.

Half of infants born vaginally to mothers experiencing a primary HSV infection at the time of delivery will be infected, compared with only 4% of those born to women with recurrent infection. Approximately 60% of infected neonates die in the neonatal period and 50% of the survivors have significant sequelae. Active infection during labor may necessitate cesarean delivery. Recommendations from the American College of Obstetricians and Gynecologists direct care providers to obtain cultures when a woman has active lesions during pregnancy. Vaginal delivery is acceptable if visible lesions are not present at the onset of labor.

MOLLUSCUM CONTAGIOSUM

Molluscum contagiosum is a common viral disease of the skin that gives rise to multiple umbilicated papules. The disease is mildly contagious; it is transmitted by skin-to-skin contact, fomites, and autoinoculation. Lesions are domelike and have a dimpled appearance. A curdlike material can be expressed from the center of the lesion. Necrosis and secondary infection are possible. Diagnosis is based on the appearance of the lesion and microscopic identification of intracytoplasmic molluscum bodies. Molluscum is a benign and self-limited disease.

Spontaneous regression of mature lesions followed by continued emergence of new lesions is common with molluscum, and in the absence of therapy this cycle may persist for 6 months to 3 years. Recurrence is frequent after treatment; therefore, the goal of therapy is to hasten the resolution of individual lesions and reduce the likelihood of further spread.[12] When indicated, treatment consists of removing the top of the papule with a sterile needle or scalpel, expressing the contents of each lesion, and applying alcohol or silver nitrate to the base. Electrodesiccation, cryosurgery, laser ablation, and surgical biopsy are alternative treatments but seldom are needed unless lesions are large or extend over a wide area. A new approach to therapy is the application of imiquimod 1% cream to lesions. This self-applied therapy is the first to show efficacy in patients with immunosuppressive diseases such as AIDS.[12]

CHANCROID

Chancroid (*i.e.*, soft chancre) is a disease of the external genitalia and lymph nodes. The causative organism is the gram-negative bacterium *Haemophilus ducreyi*, which causes acute ulcerative lesions with profuse discharge. This disease has become uncommon in the United States, with only 143 reported cases in 1999.[1] It typically occurs in discrete outbreaks rather than as an endemic disease in this country. It is more prevalent in Southeast Asia, the West Indies, and North Africa. A highly infectious disease, chancroid usually is transmitted by sexual intercourse or through skin and mucous membrane abrasions. Autoinoculation may lead to multiple chancres.

Lesions begin as macules, progress to pustules, and then rupture. This painful ulcer has a necrotic base and jagged edges. In contrast, the syphilitic chancre is nontender and indurated. Subsequent discharge can lead to further infection of self or others. On physical examination, lesions and regional lymphadenopathy (*i.e.*, buboes) may be found. Secondary infection may cause significant tissue destruction. Diagnosis usually is made clinically, but may be confirmed through culture. Gram stain rarely is used today because it is insensitive and nonspecific. Polymerase chain reactions

(PCR) methods may soon be available commercially for definitive identification of *H. ducreyi* (see Chapter 17 for an explanation of PCR methods). The organism has shown resistance to treatment with sulfamethoxazole alone and to tetracycline. The CDC recommends treatment with azithromycin, erythromycin, or ceftriaxone.[5]

GRANULOMA INGUINALE

Granuloma inguinale (*i.e.*, granuloma venereum) is caused by a gram-negative bacillus, *Calymmatobacterium donovani*, which is a tiny, encapsulated intracellular parasite. This disease is almost nonexistent in the United States. It is found most frequently in India, Brazil, the West Indies, and parts of China, Australia, and Africa.

Granuloma inguinale causes ulceration of the genitalia, beginning with an innocuous papule. The papule progresses through nodular or vesicular stages until it begins to break down as pink, granulomatous tissue. At this final stage, the tissue becomes thin and friable and bleeds easily. There are complaints of swelling, pain, and itching. Extensive inflammatory scarring may cause late sequelae, such as lymphatic obstruction with the development of enlarged and elephantoid external genitalia. The liver, bladder, bone, joint, lung, and bowel tissue may become involved. Genital complications include tubo-ovarian abscess, fistula, vaginal stenosis, and occlusion of vaginal or anal orifices. Lesions may become neoplastic.

Diagnosis is made through the identification of Donovan bodies (*i.e.*, large mononuclear cells filled with intracytoplasmic gram-negative rods) in tissue smears, biopsy samples, or culture. A 3-week period of treatment with doxycycline, tetracycline, erythromycin, or gentamicin is used in treating the disorder.[5]

LYMPHOGRANULOMA VENEREUM

Lymphogranuloma venereum is an acute and chronic venereal disease caused by *Chlamydia trachomatis* types L1, L2, and P3. The disease, although found worldwide, has a low incidence outside the tropics. Most cases reported in the United States are in men.

The lesions of LGV can incubate for a few days to several weeks and thereafter cause small, painless papules or vesicles that may go undetected. An important characteristic of the disease is the early (1 to 4 weeks later) development of large, tender, and sometimes fluctuant inguinal lymph nodes called *buboes*. There may be flulike symptoms with joint pain, rash, weight loss, pneumonitis, tachycardia, splenomegaly, and proctitis. In later stages of the disease, a small percentage of affected persons develop elephantiasis of the external genitalia, caused by lymphatic obstruction or fibrous strictures of the rectum or urethra from inflammation and scarring. Urethral involvement may cause pyuria and dysuria. Cervicitis is a common manifestation of primary LGV, and could extend to perimetritis or salpingitis, which are known to occur in other chlamydial infections.[4] Anorectal structures may be compromised to the point of incontinence. Complications of LGV may be minor or extensive, involving compromise of whole systems or progression to a cancerous state.

Diagnosis usually is accomplished by means of a complement fixation test for LGV-specific *Chlamydia* antibodies. High titers for this antibody differentiate this group from other chlamydial subgroups. Treatment involves 3 weeks of doxycycline, tetracycline, or erythromycin.[5] Surgery may be required to correct sequelae such as strictures or fistulas or to drain fluctuant lymph nodes.

In summary, STDs that primarily affect the external genitalia include HPV (condyloma acuminata), genital herpes (HSV-2), molluscum contagiosum, chancroid, granuloma inguinale, and LGV. The lesions of these infections occur on the external genitalia of male and female sexual partners. Of concern is the relation between HPV and genital neoplasms. Genital herpes is caused by a neurotropic virus (HSV-2) that ascends through the peripheral nerves to reside in the sacral dorsal root ganglia. The herpesvirus can be reactivated, producing recurrent lesions in genital structures that are supplied by the peripheral nerves of the affected ganglia. There is no permanent cure for herpes infections. Molluscum contagiosum is a benign and self-limited infection that is only mildly contagious. Chancroid, granuloma inguinale, and LGV produce external genital lesions with various degrees of inguinal lymph node involvement. These diseases are uncommon in the United States.

Vaginal Infections

After you have completed this section of the chapter, you should be able to meet the following objectives:

✦ State the difference between wet-mount slide and culture methods of diagnosis of STDs
✦ Compare the signs and symptoms of infections caused by *Candida albicans*, *Trichomonas vaginalis*, and bacterial vaginosis

Candidiasis, trichomoniasis, and bacterial vaginosis are vaginal infections that can be sexually transmitted. Although these infections can be transmitted sexually, the male partner usually is asymptomatic.

CANDIDIASIS

Also called *yeast infection*, *thrush*, and *moniliasis*, *candidiasis* is the second leading cause of vulvovaginitis in the United States. Approximately 75% of reproductive-age women in the United States experience one episode in their lifetime; 40% to 45% experience two or more infections.[4]

The causative organism is *Candida*, a genus of yeastlike fungi. The species most commonly identified is *Candida albicans*, but other candidal species, such as *Candida glabrata* and *Candida tropicalis*, have caused symptoms. Another 18 separate strains of *C. albicans* with various levels of virulence have been identified.[13] These organisms are present in 20%

to 55% of healthy women without causing symptoms, and alteration of the host vaginal environment usually is necessary before the organism can cause pathologic effects.[4] Although vulvovaginal candidiasis usually is not transmitted sexually, it is included in the CDC STD treatment guidelines because it often is diagnosed in women being evaluated for STDs.[5] The possibility of sexual transmission has been recognized for many years; however, candidiasis requires a favorable environment for growth. The gastrointestinal tract also serves as a reservoir for this organism, and candidiasis can develop through autoinoculation in women who are not sexually active. Although studies have documented the presence of *Candida* on the penis of male partners of women with vulvovaginal candidiasis, few men develop balanoposthitis that requires treatment.

Causes for the overgrowth of *C. albicans* include antibiotic therapy, which suppresses the normal protective bacterial flora; high hormone levels owing to pregnancy or the use of oral contraceptives, which cause an increase in vaginal glycogen stores; and diabetes mellitus or HIV infection, because they compromise the immune system. Food allergies, hypothyroidism, endocrine disorders, dietary influences, tight-fitting clothing, and douching also have been suggested as possible contributors to the development of vulvovaginal candidiasis. However, there is little evidence to support these etiologies.

In obese persons, *Candida* may grow in skin folds underneath the breast tissue, the abdominal flap, and the inguinal folds. Vulvar pruritus accompanied by irritation, dysuria, dyspareunia, erythema, and an odorless, thick, cheesy vaginal discharge are the predominant symptoms of the infection. Accurate diagnosis is made by identification of budding yeast filaments (*i.e.*, hyphae) or spores on a wet-mount slide using 20% potassium hydroxide (Fig. 46-2). The pH of the discharge, which is checked with litmus paper, typically is less than 4.5. When the wet-mount technique is negative but the clinical manifestations are suggestive of candidiasis, a culture may be necessary.

Antifungal agents such as clotrimazole, miconazole, butaconazole, and terconazole, in various forms, are effec-

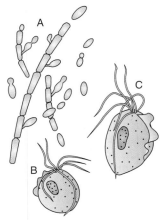

FIGURE 46-2 Organisms that cause vaginal infections. (**A**) *Candida albicans* (blastospores and pseudohyphae). (**B,C**) *Trichomonas vaginalis*.

tive in treating candidiasis. These drugs, with the exception of terconazole, are available without prescription for use by women who have had a previously confirmed diagnosis of candidiasis. Oral fluconazole has been shown to be as safe and effective as the standard intravaginal regimens.[5] Gentian violet solution (1%) applied to the vagina by swabs or tampon (not recommended in pregnant women), boric acid vaginal suppositories, or boric acid soaks to the vulva are treatment adjuncts. Tepid sodium bicarbonate baths, clothing that allows adequate ventilation, and the application of cornstarch to dry the area may increase comfort during treatment. Chronic vulvovaginal candidiasis, defined as four or more mycologically confirmed episodes within 1 year, affects approximately 5% of women and is difficult to manage. Subsequent prophylaxis (maintenance therapy) often is required for long-term management of this problem.[14]

Candidiasis can be confused with Döderlein cytolysis—an excess of lactobacilli—which can present with a similar clinical picture. In the case of Döderlein cytolysis, wet-mount and culture techniques show only excessive lactobacilli, but no yeast. Treatment for Döderlein cytolysis involves use of a sodium bicarbonate douche two to three times each week to raise the vaginal pH and decrease the symptoms.

TRICHOMONIASIS

An anaerobic protozoan that can be transmitted sexually, *Trichomonas vaginalis* is shaped like a turnip and has three or four anterior flagella (see Fig. 46-2). Trichomonads can reside in the paraurethral glands of both sexes. Males harbor the organism in the urethra and prostate and are asymptomatic. Although 10% to 25% of women are asymptomatic, trichomoniasis is a common cause of vaginitis when some imbalance allows the protozoan to proliferate. Five million cases of trichomoniasis were diagnosed in 1999.[1] This extracellular parasite feeds on the vaginal mucosa and ingests bacteria and leukocytes. The infection causes a copious, frothy, malodorous, green or yellow discharge. There commonly is erythema and edema of the affected mucosa, with occasional itching and irritation. Sometimes, small hemorrhagic areas, called *strawberry spots*, appear on the cervix.

Diagnosis is made microscopically by identification of the protozoan on a wet-mount slide preparation. The pH of the discharge usually is greater than 6.0. Special culture media are available for diagnosis, but are costly and not needed for diagnosis.

Because the organism resides in other urogenital structures besides the vagina, systemic treatment is recommended. The treatment of choice is oral metronidazole (Flagyl), a medication that is effective against anaerobic protozoans.[5] Metronidazole is chemically similar to disulfiram (Antabuse), a drug used in the treatment of alcohol addiction that causes nausea, vomiting, flushing of the skin, headache, palpitations, and lowering of the blood pressure when alcohol is ingested. Alcohol should be avoided during and for 24 to 48 hours after treatment. Gastrointestinal disturbances and a metallic taste in the mouth are potential adverse effects of the drug. Metronidazole has not been proven safe for use during pregnancy and is used only after the first trimester for fear of potential teratogenic effects. Sexual partners should be treated to avoid reinfection, and abstinence is recommended until the full course of therapy is completed.

BACTERIAL VAGINOSIS (NONSPECIFIC VAGINITIS)

Considerable controversy exists regarding the organisms responsible for a vaginal infection that produces a characteristic fishy- or ammonia-smelling discharge yet fails to produce an inflammatory response that is characteristic of most infections. A number of terms have been used to describe the nonspecific vaginitis that cannot be attributed to one of the accepted pathogenic organisms, such as *T. vaginalis* or *C. albicans*.

In 1955, Gardner and Dukes isolated an organism from women with this type of vaginitis and proposed the name *Haemophilus vaginalis*, apparently because the gram-negative organism required blood for growth.[15] In 1963, gram-positive isolates were found, and the organism was renamed *Corynebacterium vaginale*. Because the organism did not meet all the criteria of corynebacteria, it was renamed *Gardnerella vaginalis* in 1980, after its original discoverer, and admitted to a taxonomic genus of its own. The development of a special agar on which *G. vaginalis* could be cultured led to the discovery that 40% to 70% of women harbor this organism as part of their normal vaginal flora. Further study revealed that abnormal discharge frequently contained highly motile, crescent-shaped rods called *Mobiluncus* and many more anaerobic than aerobic bacteria. It has been suggested that the presence of anaerobes, which produce ammonia or amines from amino acids, favors the growth of *G. vaginalis* by raising vaginal pH. Because of the presence of anaerobic bacteria and the lack of an inflammatory response, a new term, *bacterial vaginosis*, was proposed.[4] Bacterial vaginosis is characterized by absence of the normal lactobacillus species in the vagina and an overgrowth of other organisms, including *G. vaginalis*, *Mobiluncus* species, *Mycoplasma hominis*, and numerous anaerobes.[6]

Bacterial vaginosis is the most prevalent form of vaginal infection seen by health care professionals. Its relation to sexual activity is not clear. Sexual activity is believed to be a catalyst rather than a primary mode of transmission, and endogenous factors play a role in the development of symptoms. The predominant symptom of bacterial vaginosis is a thin, grayish-white discharge that has a foul, fishy odor. Burning, itching, and erythema usually are absent because the bacteria has only minimal inflammatory potential. Bacterial vaginosis may be carried asymptomatically by men and women.

The diagnosis is made when at least three of the following characteristics are present: homogeneous discharge, production of a fishy, amine odor when a 10% potassium hydroxide solution is dropped onto the secretions, vaginal pH above 4.5 (usually 5.0 to 6.0), and appearance of characteristic "clue cells" on wet-mount microscopic studies. *Clue cells* are squamous epithelial cells covered with masses of coccobacilli, often with large clumps of organisms floating free from the cell. Because *G. vaginalis* can be a normal vaginal flora, cultures should not be done routinely. They are of limited clinical value because it is believed that the condition is caused by a combination of *G. vaginalis* and anaerobic bacteria.

The mere presence of *G. vaginalis* in an asymptomatic woman is not an indication for treatment. When indicated, treatment is aimed at eradicating the anaerobic component of bacterial vaginosis to reestablish the normal balance of the vaginal flora. The CDC recommends oral metronidazole, although failure rates may range from 30% to 70%. Alternative therapies include metronidazole vaginal gel, clindamycin vaginal cream, or oral clindamycin. Treatment of sexual partners is not recommended.[5]

Pelvic inflammatory disease (PID), preterm labor, premature rupture of membranes, chorioamnionitis, and postpartum endometritis have been linked to the organisms associated with bacterial vaginosis. Oral or cream clindamycin formulations can be used for treatment during the first trimester of pregnancy; oral or vaginal metronidazole can be used after the first trimester for treatment failures. Routine screening for bacterial vaginosis is not advocated, but symptomatic women should be treated.

> In summary, candidiasis, trichomoniasis, and bacterial vaginosis are common vaginal infections that become symptomatic because of changes in the vaginal ecosystem. Only trichomoniasis is spread through sexual contact. Trichomoniasis is caused by an anaerobic protozoan. The infection incites the production of a copious, frothy, yellow or green, malodorous discharge. Candidiasis, also called a *yeast infection*, is the form of vulvovaginitis with which women are most familiar. *Candida* can be present without producing symptoms; usually some host factor, such as altered immune status, contributes to the development of vulvovaginitis. It can be treated with over-the-counter medications. Bacterial vaginosis is the most common cause of vaginal discharge. It is a nonspecific type of infection that produces a characteristic fishy-smelling discharge. The infection is thought to be caused by the combined presence of *G. vaginalis* and anaerobic bacteria. The anaerobe raises the vaginal pH, thereby favoring the growth of *G. vaginalis*.

Vaginal-Urogenital-Systemic Infections

After you have completed this section of the chapter, you should be able to meet the following objectives:

- ✦ Compare the signs and symptoms of gonorrhea in the male and female
- ✦ Describe the three stages of syphilis
- ✦ State the genital and nongenital complications that can occur with chlamydial infections, gonorrhea, and syphilis
- ✦ State the treatment for chlamydial urogenital infections, gonorrhea, nonspecific urogenital infections, and syphilis

Some STDs infect male and female genital and extragenital structures. Among the infections of this type are chlamydial infections, gonorrhea, and syphilis. Many of these infections also pose a risk to infants born to infected mothers. Some infections, such as syphilis, may be spread to the infant while in utero; others, such as chlamydial and gonorrheal infections, can be spread to the infant during the birth process.

CHLAMYDIAL INFECTIONS

Chlamydia trachomatis is an obligate intracellular bacterial pathogen that is closely related to gram-negative bacteria. It resembles a virus in that it requires tissue culture for isolation, but like a bacteria, it has RNA and DNA and is susceptible to some antibiotics. *C. trachomatis* causes a wide variety of genitourinary infections, including nongonococcal urethritis in men and PID in women. The closely related organisms *Chlamydia pneumoniae* and *Chlamydia psittaci* cause mild and severe pneumonia, respectively. *C. trachomatis* can be serologically subdivided into types A, B, and C, which are associated with trachoma and chronic keratoconjunctivitis; types D through K, which are associated with genital infections and their complications; and types L1, L2, and L3, which are associated with LGV. *C. trachomatis* can cause significant ocular disease in neonates; it is a leading cause of blindness in underdeveloped countries. In these countries, the organism is spread primarily by flies, fomites, and nonsexual personal contact. In industrial countries, the organism is spread almost exclusively by sexual contact and therefore affects primarily the genitourinary structures.

Chlamydial infection is the most prevalent STD in the U.S. Although chlamydial infections are not reportable in all states, their incidence is estimated to be more than twice that of gonorrhea. According to CDC estimates, chlamydial infections occur at a rate of 3 million new cases each year, predominantly among individuals younger than 25 years of age.[1] Reported rates for chlamydial infections are higher in women largely because of these screening efforts, although actual occurrence rates are thought to be the same for men and women.[16] In the United States, costs associated with managing chlamydial infections and their complications exceed 2 billion dollars annually.[16] Rates are believed to be declining owing to increased efforts to screen and treat this infection.

Chlamydiae exist in two forms: elementary bodies, which are the infectious particles capable of entering uninfected cells, and the initiator or reticulate bodies, which multiply by binary fission to produce the inclusions identified in stained cells. The 48-hour growth cycle starts with attachment of the elementary body to the susceptible host cell, after which it is ingested by a process that resembles phagocytosis (Fig. 46-3). Once inside the cell, the elementary body is organized into the reticulate body, the metabolically active form of the organism that is capable of reproduction. The reticulate body is not infectious and cannot survive outside the body. The reticulate bodies divide in the cell for up to 36 hours and then condense to form new elementary bodies, which are released when the infected cell bursts.

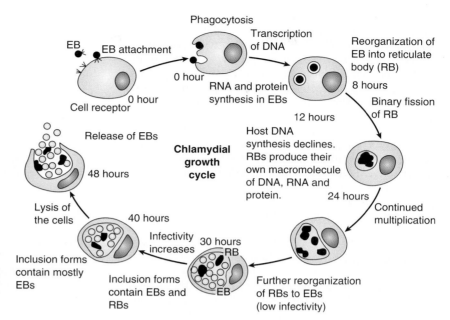

FIGURE 46-3 Chlamydial growth cycle. EB, elementary body; RB, reticulate body. (Thompson S.E., Washington A.E. [1983]. Epidemiology of sexually transmitted *Chlamydia trachomatis* infections. *Epidemiologic Reviews* 5, 96–123)

The signs and symptoms of chlamydial infection resemble those produced by gonorrhea. The most significant difference between chlamydial and gonococcal salpingitis is that chlamydial infections may be asymptomatic or subclinically nonspecific. In women, chlamydial infections may cause urinary frequency, dysuria, and vaginal discharge. The most common symptom is a mucopurulent cervical discharge. The cervix itself frequently hypertrophies and becomes erythematous, edematous, and extremely friable. Seventy-five percent of women and 50% of men with chlamydial infection have no symptoms; therefore, most cases are undiagnosed, unreported, and untreated.[16] This can lead to greater fallopian tube damage and increase the reservoir for further chlamydial infections. Approximately 40% of women with an untreated chlamydial infection develop PID, and 1 in 5 of these women becomes infertile. Research has identified a possible link between three specific serotypes of chlamydiae and an increased risk for cervical cancer. The mechanism by which this occurs is unclear.[17]

In men, chlamydial infections cause urethritis, including meatal erythema and tenderness, urethral discharge, dysuria, and urethral itching. Prostatitis and epididymitis with subsequent infertility may develop. The most serious complication that can develop with nongonococcal urethritis is Reiter's syndrome, a systemic condition characterized by urethritis, conjunctivitis, arthritis, and mucocutaneous lesions (see Chapter 59).

Routine screening for sexually active adolescents and young adults has been suggested by the CDC in an effort to minimize these serious sequelae of asymptomatic infection. Between 25% and 50% of infants born to mothers with cervical chlamydial infections develop ocular disease (*i.e.*, inclusion conjunctivitis), and 10% to 20% develop chlamydial pneumonitis.

Diagnosis of chlamydial infections takes several forms. The identification of polymorphonuclear leukocytes on Gram stain of male discharge or cervical discharge is presumptive evidence. The two available serologic tests, the complement fixation and microimmunofluorescent tests, can be misleading. Complement fixation tests are the most useful in diagnosing LGV. The microimmunofluorescent test is more sensitive for *C. trachomatis* types D through K, but it does not distinguish among acute, chronic, or carrier states. The high rates of anti-chlamydial antibodies in sexually active populations render serodiagnosis inconclusive. Tissue culture tests are definitive but slow (requiring at least 3 days), costly, and not always available. Once thought to be the testing standard, tissue culture has been shown to be less sensitive than other, newer methods. Nonculture methods, such as direct fluorescent antibody test and an enzyme-linked immunosorbent assay, which use antibodies against an antigen in the *Chlamydia* cell wall, are available. These are less expensive, rapid tests that require less sophisticated laboratory techniques, with sensitivity ranging from 70% to 100% and specificity from 94% to 100% for either type of test. The positive predictive value of these tests is excellent among high-risk groups, but false-positive results occur more often in populations with lower risks.

Amplified DNA probe assays, such as the PCR, ligase chain reaction (LCR), or transcription-mediated amplification (TMA), have demonstrated specificities of near 100% (same as culture) and sensitivities of 90% to 95%. Sensitivity of cell culture has been estimated at 70% to 85% for endocervical specimens and 50% to 75% for male urethral specimens. Because amplified DNA testing can be performed on urine and swab specimens from the distal vagina as well as the traditional endocervical and urethral specimens, this easy, convenient means of accurate detection has become the diagnostic method of choice.[6,18,19] DNA hybridization assay using RNA as the target tests for *C. trachomatis* and *N. gonorrhoeae* in a single test. RNA is a "naturally amplified" target with up to 10,000 copies per cell, compared with DNA with only 1 copy per cell. The test extracts target RNA from the specimen (endocervical or male urethral swab) and mixes it with a labeled DNA probe that will combine with RNA of *Chlamydia* or *Neisseria* to produce a chemiluminescent signal that is measured objectively by an optical scanner. Specimens are stable at room temperature for up to 7 days, making the assay cost effective when conducted at a moderate- to high-volume laboratory.[19] Cost often is a factor in determining which type of testing to use.

The CDC recommends the use of azithromycin or doxycycline in the treatment of chlamydial infection; penicillin is ineffective. Erythromycin or amoxicillin is the preferred choice in pregnancy.[5] Antibiotic treatment of both sexual partners simultaneously is recommended. Abstinence from sexual activity is encouraged to facilitate cure.

GONORRHEA

Gonorrhea is a reportable disease caused by the bacterium *N. gonorrhoeae*. In 1999, there were 360,076 reported cases of gonorrhea in the United States. Of these reported cases, more than 90% involved persons between 15 and 44 years of age, with the heaviest concentration among young adults (15 to 24 years of age).[16] There are an estimated 650,000 new cases every year.[1] Although the incidence of gonorrhea has declined steadily from its peak in 1975, there was an increase in occurrence between 1997 and 1998. Improved screening efforts as well as greater use of more sensitive nonculture methods of testing may have contributed to this increase. Higher rates of occurrence among homosexual men were documented in several states, leading to a concern that a rise in unsafe sexual behavior may be occurring because of the availability of highly active antiretroviral agents for treatment of HIV infection.[20]

The gonococcus is a pyogenic (*i.e.*, pus-forming), gram-negative diplococcus that evokes inflammatory reactions characterized by purulent exudates. Humans are the only natural host for *N. gonorrhoeae*. The organism grows best in warm, mucus-secreting epithelia. The portal of entry can be the genitourinary tract, eyes, oropharynx, anorectum, or skin.

Transmission usually is by heterosexual or homosexual intercourse. Autoinoculation of the organism to the conjunctiva is possible. Neonates born to infected mothers can acquire the infection during passage through the birth canal and are in danger of developing gonorrheal conjunctivitis, with resultant blindness, unless treated promptly. An amniotic infection syndrome characterized by premature rupture of the membranes, premature delivery, and increased risk of infant morbidity and mortality has been identified as an additional complication of gonococcal infections in pregnancy. Genital gonorrhea in young children should raise the possibility of sexual abuse.

The infection commonly manifests 2 to 7 days after exposure. It typically begins in the anterior urethra, accessory urethral glands, Bartholin's or Skene's glands, and the cervix. If untreated, gonorrhea spreads from its initial sites upward into the genital tract. In males, it spreads to the prostate and epididymis; in females, it commonly moves to the fallopian tubes. Pharyngitis may follow oral-genital contact. The organism also can invade the bloodstream (*i.e.*, disseminated gonococcal infection), causing serious sequelae such as bacteremic involvement of joint spaces, heart valves, meninges, and other body organs and tissues.

Persons with gonorrhea may be asymptomatic and may unwittingly spread the disease to their sexual partners. Men are more likely to be symptomatic than women. In men, the initial symptoms include urethral pain and a creamy, yellow, sometimes bloody discharge. The disorder may become chronic and affect the prostate, epididymis, and periurethral glands. Rectal infections are common in homosexual men. In women, recognizable symptoms include unusual genital or urinary discharge, dysuria, dyspareunia, pelvic pain or tenderness, unusual vaginal bleeding (including bleeding after intercourse), fever, and proctitis. Symptoms may occur or increase during or immediately after menses because the bacterium is an intracellular diplococcus that thrives in menstrual blood but cannot survive long outside the human body. There may be infections of the uterus and development of acute or chronic infection of the fallopian tubes (*i.e.*, salpingitis), with ultimate scarring and sterility.

Diagnosis is based on the history of sexual exposure and symptoms. It is confirmed by identification of the organism on Gram stain or culture. A Gram stain usually is an effective means of diagnosis in symptomatic men (*i.e.*, those with discharge). In women and asymptomatic men, a culture usually is preferred because the Gram stains often are unreliable. A specimen should be collected from the appropriate site (*i.e.*, endocervix, urethra, anal canal, or oropharynx), plated onto selective Thayer-Martin media, and placed in a carbon dioxide environment. *N. gonorrhoeae* is a fastidious organism with specific nutrient and environmental needs. Optimal growth requires a pH of 7.4, temperature of 35.5°C, and an atmosphere that contains 2% to 10% carbon dioxide.[21] The accuracy of culture results is affected if transport is delayed or growth requirements are not available. Culture detects more than 95% of male urethral gonorrhea and 80% to 90% of cervical, rectal, and pharyngeal infections.[6] An enzyme immunoassay for detecting gonococcal antigens (Gonozyme) is available but has several requirements that limit its usefulness. Detection by means of amplified DNA probes (PCR, LCR, TMA) is possible using urine and urethral swab specimens. The sensitivity of these probes is similar to that of culture, and they may be cost effective in high-risk populations. A nucleic acid probe–based assay for detecting *N. gonorrhoeae* in cervical specimens has demonstrated 93% sensitivity (similar to culture) and 98.5% specificity.[22]

Testing for other STDs, particularly syphilis and chlamydial infections, is suggested at the time of examination. Pregnant women are routinely screened at the time of their first prenatal visit; high-risk populations should have repeat cultures during the third trimester. Neonates are routinely treated with various antibacterial agents applied to the conjunctiva within 1 hour of birth to protect against undiagnosed gonorrhea and other diseases.

Penicillin-resistant strains of *N. gonorrhoeae* are prevalent worldwide and strains with other kinds of antibiotic resistance continue to evolve and spread. The current treatment recommendation to combat tetracycline- and penicillin-resistant strains of *N. gonorrhoeae* is ceftriaxone in a single injection or cefixime, ciprofloxacin, or ofloxacin in a single oral dose. All are equally effective and should be followed with azithromycin or doxycycline for chlamydiae. All sex partners within 60 days before discovery of the infection should be contacted, tested, and treated. Test of cure is not required with observed single-dose therapy. Patients are instructed to refrain from intercourse until therapy is completed and symptoms are no longer present.[5]

SYPHILIS

Syphilis is a reportable disease caused by a spirochete, *Treponema pallidum*. During 1999, 6657 new cases of primary and secondary syphilis were reported in the United States (2.5 per 100,000 population). This is the lowest rate ever reported, and it now appears that syphilis transmission is primarily concentrated in a few geographic areas.[23] This represents a steady decline from the 50,000 cases reached in 1990 after an epidemic resurgence of this problem between 1985 and 1990. Syphilis continues to disproportionately affect minority populations. Although the 1999 rate for blacks declined by 10% over the previous year, it was still 30 times the rate reported in whites. The rate for Hispanics increased 20%, primarily among men. The National Plan to Eliminate Syphilis was launched in 1999 with a goal of reducing primary and secondary syphilis to fewer than 1000 cases and increasing the number of syphilis-free counties to 90% by 2005. Federal funding is available to support this effort.[23]

T. pallidum is spread by direct contact with an infectious, moist lesion, usually through sexual intercourse. Bacteria-laden secretions may transfer the organism during kissing or intimate contact. Skin abrasions provide another possible portal of entry. There is rapid transplacental transmission of the organism from the mother to the fetus after 16 weeks' gestation, so that active disease in the mother during pregnancy can produce congenital syphilis in the fetus. Untreated syphilis can cause prematurity, stillbirth, and congenital defects and active infection in the infant. Once treated for syphilis, a pregnant woman usually is followed throughout pregnancy by repeat testing of serum titers.

The clinical disease is divided into three stages: primary, secondary, and tertiary. Primary syphilis is characterized by the appearance of a chancre at the site of exposure. Chancres typically appear within 3 weeks of exposure but may incubate for 1 week to 3 months. The primary chancre begins as a single, indurated, button-like papule up to several centimeters in diameter that erodes to create a clean-based ulcerated lesion on an elevated base. These lesions usually are painless and located at the site of sexual contact. Primary syphilis is readily apparent in the male, where the lesion is on the penis or scrotum. Although chancres can develop on the external genitalia in females, they are more common on the vagina or cervix, and primary syphilis therefore may go untreated. There usually is an accompanying regional lymphadenopathy. The disease is highly contagious at this stage, but because the symptoms are mild, it frequently goes unnoticed. The chancre usually heals within 3 to 12 weeks, with or without treatment.

The timing of the second stage of syphilis varies even more than that of the first, lasting from 1 week to 6 months. The symptoms of a rash (especially on the palms and soles), fever, sore throat, stomatitis, nausea, loss of appetite, and inflamed eyes may come and go for a year but usually last for 3 to 6 months. Secondary manifestations may include alopecia and genital condylomata lata. Condylomata lata are elevated, red-brown lesions that may ulcerate and produce a foul discharge. They are 2 to 3 cm in diameter, contain many spirochetes, and are highly infectious.

After the second stage, syphilis frequently enters a latent phase that may last the lifetime of the person or progress to tertiary syphilis at some point. Persons can be infective during the first 1 to 2 years of latency.

Tertiary syphilis is a delayed response of the untreated disease. It can occur as long as 20 years after the initial infection. Only approximately one third of those with untreated syphilis progress to the tertiary stage of the disease, and symptoms develop in approximately one half of these. Approximately one third undergo spontaneous cure, and the remaining one third continue to have positive serologic tests but do not develop structural lesions.[19] When syphilis does progress to the symptomatic tertiary stage, it commonly takes one of three forms: development of localized destructive lesions called *gummas*, development of cardiovascular lesions, or development of central nervous system lesions. The syphilitic gumma is a peculiar, rubbery, necrotic lesion that is caused by noninflammatory tissue necrosis. Gummas can occur singly or multiply and vary in size from microscopic lesions to large, tumorous masses. They most commonly are found in the liver, testes, and bone. Central nervous system lesions can produce dementia, blindness, or injury to the spinal cord, with ataxia and sensory loss (*i.e.*, tabes dorsalis). Cardiovascular manifestations usually result from scarring of the medial layer of the thoracic aorta with aneurysm formation. These aneurysms produce enlargement of the aortic valve ring with aortic valve insufficiency.

T. pallidum does not produce endotoxins or exotoxins but evokes a humoral immune response that provides the basis for serologic tests. Two types of antibodies—nonspecific and specific—are produced. The nonspecific antibodies can be detected by flocculation tests such as the Venereal Disease Research Laboratory (VDRL) test or the rapid plasma reagin (RPR) test. Because these tests are nonspecific, positive results can occur with diseases other than syphilis. The tests are easy to perform, rapid, and inexpensive and frequently are used as screening tests for syphilis. Results become positive 4 to 6 weeks after infection or 1 to 3 weeks after the appearance of the primary lesion. Because these tests are quantitative, they can be used to measure the degree of disease activity or treatment effectiveness. The VDRL titer usually is high during the secondary stage of the disease and becomes less so during the tertiary stage. A falling titer during treatment suggests a favorable response. The fluorescent treponemal antibody absorption test or microhemagglutinin test is used to detect specific antibodies to *T. pallidum*. These qualitative tests are used to determine whether a positive result on a nonspecific test such as the VDRL is attributable to syphilis. The test results remain positive for life.

T. pallidum cannot be cultured. The diagnosis of syphilis is based on serologic tests or dark-field microscopic examination with identification of the spirochete in specimens collected from lesions. Because the disease's incubation period may delay test sensitivity, serologic tests usually are repeated after 6 weeks if the initial test results were negative.

The treatment of choice for syphilis is penicillin. Because of the spirochetes' long generation time, effective tissue levels of penicillin must be maintained for several weeks. Long-acting injectable forms of penicillin are used. Tetracycline or doxycycline is used for treatment in persons who are sensitive to penicillin. Pregnant patients should be desensitized and treated with penicillin because erythromycin does not treat fetal infection. Sexual partners should be evaluated and treated prophylactically even though they may show no sign of infection. All treated individuals should be reexamined clinically and serologically at 6 and 12 months after completing therapy; more frequent monitoring (3-month intervals) is suggested for individuals with HIV infection.[5]

> In summary, the vaginal-urogenital-systemic STDs—chlamydial infections, gonorrhea, and syphilis—can severely involve the genital structures and manifest as systemic infections. Gonorrheal and chlamydial infections can cause a wide variety of genitourinary complications in men and women, and both can cause ocular disease and blindness in neonates born to infected mothers. Syphilis is caused by a spirochete, *T. pallidum*. It can produce widespread systemic effects and is transferred to the fetus of infected mothers through the placenta.

Related Web Sites

American Social Health Association   www.ashastd.org
Centers for Disease Control and Prevention National Center for HIV, STD and TB Prevention   www.cdc.gov/nchstp/od/nchstp.html
JAMA Women's Health STD Information Center   www.ama-assn.org/special/std/std.htm
STI Online—Web site of the *Journal of Sexually Transmitted Infections*   sti.bmjjournals.com

References

1. Cates W. Jr. (1999). Estimates of the incidence and prevalence of STDs in the US. *Sexually Transmitted Diseases* 4 (Suppl.), S2–S7.
2. Beutner K.R, Reitano M.V., Richwald G.A, Wiley D.J. (1998). External genital warts: Report of the American Medical Association Consensus Conference. *Clinical Infectious Diseases* 27, 796–806.
3. Richart R.M. (2000). Genital warts: The clinical challenge. *Medical Economics* (CME Suppl. Fall), 4–14.
4. Holmes K.K, Per-Anders M., Sparling P.F., Lemon S.M., Stamm W.E., Piott P., et al. (1999). *Sexually transmitted disease* (3rd ed., pp. 347, 287, 290, 424, 563–564, 629, 820–821) New York: McGraw-Hill.
5. Centers for Disease Control and Prevention. (1998). 1998 Guidelines for treatment of sexually transmitted diseases. *Morbidity and Mortality Weekly Report* 47 (RR-1), 1–118.
6. Handsfield H.H. (2001). *Color atlas and synopsis of sexually transmitted diseases* (pp. 13, 23, 71, 87, 163). New York: McGraw-Hill.
7. Cotran R.S., Kumar V., Collins T. (1999). *Robbins pathologic basis of disease* (6th ed., pp. 359–361). Philadelphia: W.B. Saunders.
8. Flemming D.T., McQuillan G.M., Johnson R.E., Nahmias A.J., Aral S.O., Lee F.K., St Louis M.E. (1997). Herpes simplex virus type 2 in the United States, 1976 to 1994. *New England Journal of Medicine* 337, 1105–1111.
9. Rubin E., Farber J.L. (1999). *Pathology* (3rd ed.). Philadelphia: Lippincott Williams & Wilkins.
10. Scott J.R., DiSaia P.J., Hammond C.B., Spellacy W.N. (1999). *Danforth's obstetrics and gynecology* (8th ed., pp. 402–403). Philadelphia: Lippincott Williams & Wilkins.
11. Wald A., Zeh J., Selke S., Warren T., Ryncarz A.J., Ashley R., Krieger J.N., Corey L. (2000). Reactivation of genital herpes simplex virus type 2 infection in asymptomatic seropositive persons. *New England Journal of Medicine* 342, 844–850.
12. Soper D.E. (2000). Skin diseases: Molluscum contagiosum. *Contemporary Obstetrics/Gynecology* 9, 95–96.
13. Robertson W.H. (1988). Mycology of vulvovaginitis. *American Journal of Obstetrics and Gynecology* 158, 989–991.
14. Ringdahl E.N. (2000). Treatment of recurrent vulvovaginal candidiasis. *American Family Physician* 61, 3306–3317.
15. Gardner H.L., Dukes C.D. (1955). *Haemophilus vaginalis* vaginitis. *American Journal of Obstetrics and Gynecology* 69, 962.
16. Centers for Disease Control and Prevention. (2000). *Tracking the hidden epidemics: Trends in STDs in the United States.* [On-line]. Available: http://www.cdc.gov/nchstp/dstd/dstdp.html. Accessed March 28, 2001.
17. Antilla T., Saiku P., Koskela P., Bloigu A., et al. (2001). Serotypes of *Chlamydia trachomatis* and risk for development of cervical squamous cell carcinoma. *Journal of the American Medical Association* 285, 47–51.
18. Hooten T.M. (2000). STDs: Testing, testing. In Program and Abstracts of the 38th Annual Meeting of the Infectious Diseases Society of America, September 7–10, 2000, New Orleans, Louisiana.
19. Chapin K. (1999). Probing the STDs. *American Journal of Nursing* 99 (7), 24AAA–24DDD.
20. Centers for Disease Control and Prevention. (2000). Gonorrhea–United States, 1998. *Morbidity and Mortality Weekly Report* 49, 538.
21. Sweet R.L., Gibbs R.S. (1995). *Infectious diseases of the female genital tract* (3rd ed., pp. 103–122). Baltimore: Williams & Wilkins.
22. Schacter J., Hook R.W. III, McCormack W.M., Quinn T.C., et al. (1999). Ability of hybrid capture II test to identify *Chlamydia trachomatis* and *Neisseria gonorrhoeae* in cervical specimens. *Journal of Clinical Microbiology* 37, 3668–3671.
23. Centers for Disease Control and Prevention. (2001). Primary and secondary syphilis—United States, 1999. *Morbidity and Mortality Weekly Report* 50, 113–117.

Neural Function

For centuries, the nervous system was ignored or even deemed unimportant. Aristotle (384–322 BC), the great Greek philosopher, decreed that the heart was the seat of the soul, whereas the brain—which he assumed was composed largely of water—simply cooled it. Although Galen (AD 130–200) was able to show that the spinal cord was essential to many sensations and movements, his experiments were conducted only on animals. Not until the 1500s, when the Flemish anatomist Andreas Vesalius (1514–1564) dissected "the heads of executed criminals . . . still warm," was the overarching importance of the human brain and spinal cord established.

Investigations continued with scientists debating whether the brain should be considered as a whole or as consisting of separate areas, each responsible for specific functions. Progress in brain research took an impressive, if accidental, leap in 1841, when an explosion at a railroad work site in Vermont shot an iron rod into the left cheek of Phineas Gage, through his brain, and out the top of his head. Gage survived the accident, but it became clear to all who knew him that he had changed greatly. Formerly a conscientious, hardworking man, he became fitful, obstinate, foul-mouthed, and capricious. Gage died in 1860, and an autopsy showed destruction of the left lobe of his brain and damage to his right lobe. Scientists concluded that his personality change was the result of the grievous damage to the frontal lobes, an observation that supported the then-emerging concept that different parts of the brain serve different functions.

Chapter 47

Organization and Control of Neural Function

Edward W. Carroll and Robin L. Curtis

The nervous system, in coordination with the endocrine system, provides the means by which cell and tissue functions are integrated into a solitary, surviving organism. It controls skeletal muscle movement and helps to regulate cardiac and visceral smooth muscle activity. The nervous system enables the reception, integration, and perception of sensory information; it provides the substratum necessary for intelligence, anticipation, and judgment; and it facilitates adjustment to an ever-changing external environment. No part of the nervous system functions independently from other parts. In the human, who is a thinking and feeling creature, the effects of emotion can exert a strong influence on neural and hormonal control of body function. However, alterations in neural and endocrine function, particularly at the biochemical level, also can exert a strong influence on psychological behavior. This chapter is divided into five parts: nervous tissue cells, the development and organization of the nervous system, neuronal communication, the spinal cord, the brain, and the autonomic nervous system.

Nervous Tissue Cells

After you have completed this section of the chapter, you should be able to meet the following objectives:

✦ Differentiate between the central and peripheral nervous systems

✦ List the three parts of a neuron and describe their structure and function

◆ Name the supporting cells in the central nervous system and peripheral nervous system and state their functions

◆ Describe the energy requirements of nervous tissue

The nervous system can be divided into two parts: the central nervous system (CNS) and the peripheral nervous system (PNS). The CNS consists of the brain and spinal cord, which are protected by the skull and vertebral column. The PNS is found outside these structures. Inherent in the basic design of the nervous system is the provision for the concentration of computational and control functions in the CNS. In this design, the PNS functions as an input-output system for relaying input to the CNS and for transmitting output messages that control effector organs, such as muscles and glands.

Nervous tissue contains two types of cells: neurons and supporting cells. The neurons are the functional cells of the nervous system. They exhibit membrane excitability and conductivity and secrete neurotransmitters and hormones, such as epinephrine and antidiuretic hormone. The supporting cells, such as Schwann cells in the PNS and the glial cells in the CNS, protect the nervous system and provide metabolic support for the neurons.

NEURONS

The functioning cells of the nervous system are called *neurons*. Neurons have three distinct parts: the cell body, and its cytoplasm-filled processes, the dendrites and axons (Fig. 47-1). These processes form the functional connections, or synapses, with other nerve cells, with receptor cells, or with effector cells. Axonal processes are particularly designed for rapid communication with other neurons and the many body structures innervated by the nervous system. Afferent, or sensory, neurons transmit information from the PNS to the CNS. Efferent neurons, or motoneurons, carry information away from the CNS. Interspersed between the afferent and efferent neurons is a network of interconnecting neurons (interneurons or internuncial neurons) that modulate and control the body's response to changes in the internal and external environments.

The cell body, or soma, of a neuron contains a large, vesicular nucleus with one or more distinct nucleoli and a well-developed rough endoplasmic reticulum. A neuron's nucleus has the same DNA and genetic code content that is present in other cells of the body, and its nucleolus, which is composed of portions of several chromosomes, produces RNA associated with protein synthesis. The cytoplasm contains large masses of ribosomes that are prominent in most neurons. These acidic RNA masses, which are involved in protein synthesis, stain as dark Nissl bodies with basic histologic stains (see Fig. 47-1).

The dendrites (*i.e.*, "treelike") are multiple, branched extensions of the nerve cell body; they conduct information toward the cell body and are the main source of information for the neuron. The dendrites and cell body are studded with synaptic terminals that communicate with axons and dendrites of other neurons (Fig. 47-2).

Axons are long efferent processes that project from the cell body and carry impulses away from the cell. Most neurons have only one axon; however, axons may exhibit multiple branching that results in many axonal terminals. The cytoplasm of the cell body extends to fill the dendrites and the axon (see Fig. 47-1). The proteins and other materials used by the axon are synthesized in the cell body and then flow down the axon through its cytoplasm.

The cell body of the neuron is equipped for a high level of metabolic activity. This is necessary because the cell body must synthesize the cytoplasmic and membrane constituents required to maintain the function of the axon and its terminals. Some of these axons extend for a distance of 1 to 1.5 m and have a volume that is 200 to 500 times greater than the cell body itself. Two axonal transport systems, one slow and one rapid, move molecules from the cell body through the cytoplasm of the axon to its terminals. Replacement proteins and nutrients slowly diffuse from the cell body, where they are synthesized, down the axon, moving at the rate of approximately 1 mm/day. Other molecules, such as some neurosecretory granules or their precursors, are conveyed by a rapid, energy-dependent active transport system, moving at the rate of approximately 400 mm/day. Often, membrane-bound vesicles containing neurosecretory granules (*e.g.*, neurotransmitters, neuromodulators, and neurohormones) are moved to the axon synaptic terminals by the active transport process. For example, rapid axonal transport carries antidiuretic hormones and oxytocin from hypothalamic neurons through their axons to the posterior pituitary, where the hormones are released into the blood. A reverse rapid (*i.e.*, retrograde) axonal transport system moves materials, including target cell messenger molecules, from axonal terminals back to the cell body.

SUPPORTING CELLS

Supporting cells of the nervous system, the Schwann and satellite cells of the PNS and the several types of glial cells of the CNS, give the neurons protection and metabolic support. The supporting cells segregate the neurons into isolated metabolic compartments, which are required for normal neural function. Astrocytes, together with the tightly joined endothelial cells of the capillaries in the CNS, contribute to what is called the *blood-brain barrier*. This term is used to emphasize the impermeability of the nervous system to large or potentially harmful molecules.

Recent information suggests that many glial cells have functions other than protection and support. Evidence suggests that Schwann cells release developmental signals in embryonic nervous tissue that are crucial for the survival of neonatal neurons. Postnatally, Schwann cells synthesize and release self-regulating autocrine substances that bind to receptors on their cell surface, enabling them to survive without axons. The survival of Schwann cells is essential for the successful regeneration of damaged peripheral nerves. Schwann cells and astrocytes respond to neuronal activity

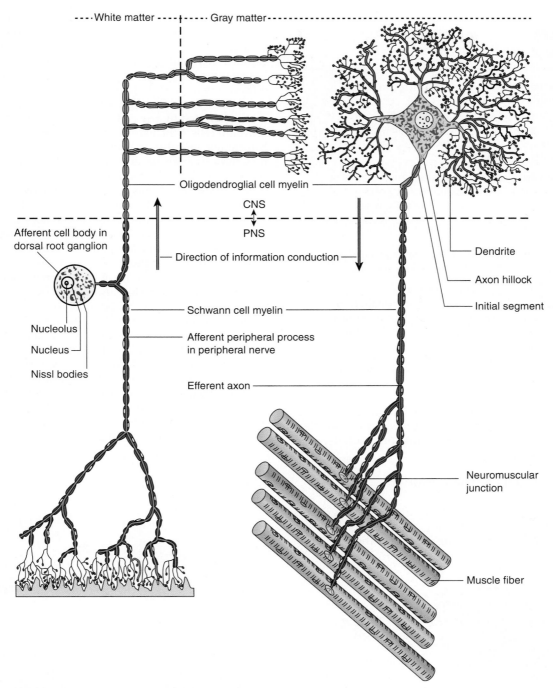

FIGURE 47-1 Afferent and efferent neurons.

by elevating their internal calcium (Ca^{2+}) ion concentrations, triggering the release of glial neurotransmitters, thus influencing feedback regulation of neuronal activity and synaptic strength.

The many-layered myelin wrappings of Schwann cells of the PNS and the oligodendroglia of the CNS produce the myelin sheaths that serve to increase the velocity of nerve impulse conduction in axons. Myelin has a high lipid con-

tent, which gives it a whitish color, and the name *white matter* is given to the masses of myelinated fibers of the spinal cord and brain. Besides its role in increasing conduction velocity, the myelin sheath is essential for the survival of larger neuronal processes, perhaps by the secretion of neurotrophic compounds. In some pathologic conditions, such as multiple sclerosis in the CNS and Guillain-Barré syndrome in the PNS, the myelin may degenerate or be de-

The Structural Organization of the Nervous System

➤ The nervous system is divided into two parts: the central nervous system (CNS), consisting of the brain and spinal cord, which are located in the skull and spinal column, and the peripheral nervous system, which is located outside these structures.

➤ The nervous system contains two major types of cells: neurons, which are functioning cells of the nervous system, and supporting cells, which protect the nervous system and supply metabolic support.

➤ The neurons consist of a cell body with cytoplasm-filled processes, the dendrites, and the axons.

➤ There are two types of neurons: afferent neurons or sensory neurons, which carry information to the CNS, and efferent neurons or motoneurons, which carry information from the CNS to the effector organs.

stroyed, leaving a section of the axonal process without myelin while leaving the nearby Schwann or oligodendroglial cells intact. Unless remyelination takes place, the axon eventually dies.

Supporting Cells of the Peripheral Nervous System
Schwann cells and satellite cells are the two types of supporting cells in the PNS. Normally, the nerve cell bodies in the PNS are collected into ganglia, such as the dorsal root

and autonomic ganglia. Each of the cell bodies and processes of the peripheral nerves is separated from the connective tissue framework of the ganglion by a single layer of flattened capsular cells called *satellite cells*. Satellite cells secrete a basement membrane that protects the cell body from the diffusion of large molecules.

The processes of larger afferent and efferent neurons are surrounded by the cell membrane and cytoplasm of Schwann cells, which are close relatives of the satellite cells. During myelination, the Schwann cell wraps around the nerve process many times in a "jelly roll" fashion (Fig. 47-3). Schwann cells line up along the neuronal process, and each of these cells forms its own discrete myelin segment. The end of each myelin segment attaches to the cell membrane of the axon by means of intercellular junctions. Successive Schwann cells are separated by short extracellular fluid gaps called the *nodes of Ranvier*, where the myelin is missing and voltage-gated sodium channels are concentrated (Fig. 47-4). The nodes of Ranvier increase nerve conduction by allowing the impulse to jump from node to node through the extracellular fluid in a process called *saltatory conduction* (from the Latin *saltare*, "to jump"). In this way, the impulse can travel more rapidly than it could if it were required to move systematically along the entire nerve process. This increased conduction velocity greatly reduces reaction time, or time between the application of a stimulus and the subsequent motor response. The short reaction time is of particular importance in peripheral nerves with long distances (sometimes 1 to 1.5 m) for conduction between the CNS and distal effector organs.

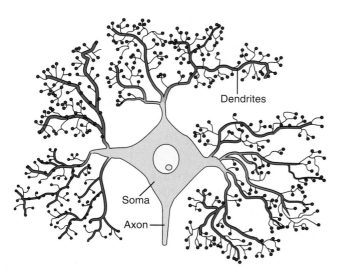

FIGURE 47-2　A typical motoneuron, showing presynaptic terminals on the neuronal soma and dendrites. Notice the single axon.

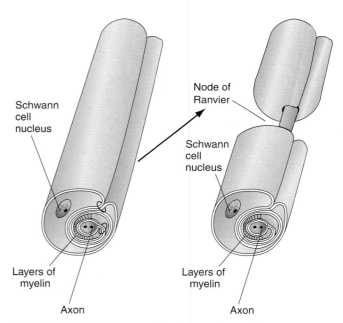

FIGURE 47-3　The Schwann cell migrates down a larger axon to a bare region, settles down, and encloses the axon in a fold of its plasma membrane. It then rotates around and around, wrapping the axon in many layers of plasma membrane, with most of the Schwann cell cytoplasm squeezed out. The resultant thick, multiple-layered coating around the axon is called myelin.

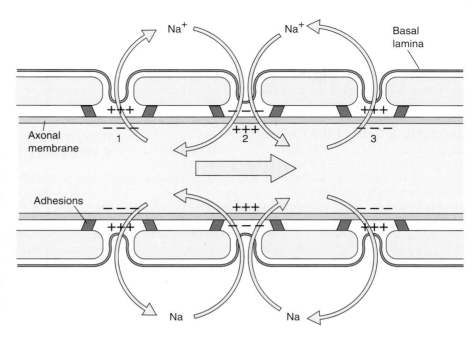

FIGURE 47-4 Schematic drawing of a longitudinal section of a myelinated axon in the peripheral nervous system. Schwann cells insulate the axon, decreasing flow through the membrane. Action potentials occur at the nodes of Ranvier, which are unmyelinated areas of the basal lamina between the Schwann cells. The impulses jump from node to node in a process called saltatory conduction, which greatly increases the velocity of conduction. (1) represents the trailing hyperpolarized region behind the action potential, (2) the hypopolarized region at the action potential, and (3) the leading hyperpolarized area ahead of the action potential. The Schwann cell adhesions (*red*) to the plasma membrane of the axon block the leakage of current under the myelin.

Each of the Schwann cells along a peripheral nerve is encased in a continuous tube of basement membrane, which in turn is surrounded by a multilayered sheath of loose connective tissue known as the *endoneurium* (Fig. 47-5). The endoneurial sheath, which is essential to the regeneration of peripheral nerves, provides a collagenous tube through which a regenerating axon can again reach its former target. The endoneurial sheath does not penetrate the CNS. The absence of the endoneurial sheaths is thought to be a major factor in the limited axonal regeneration of CNS nerves compared with those of the PNS.

The endoneurial sheaths are bundled with blood vessels into small bundles or clusters of nerves called *fascicles*. In the nerve, the fascicles consisting of bundles of nerve fibers are surrounded by another protective covering called the *perineurium*. Usually, several fascicles are further surrounded by the heavy, protective *epineurial sheath* of the peripheral nerve. The protective layers that surround the

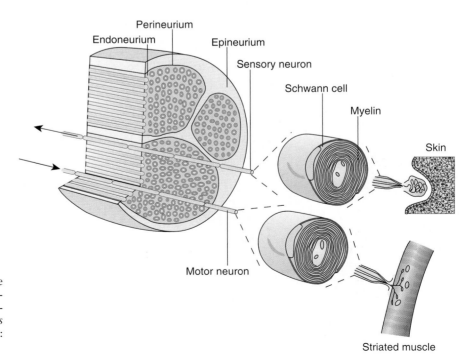

FIGURE 47-5 Section of a peripheral nerve containing axons of both afferent (sensory) and efferent (motor) neurons. (Modified from Cormack D.H. [1987]. *Ham's histology* [9th ed., p. 374]. Philadelphia: J.B. Lippincott)

peripheral nerve processes are continuous with the connective tissue capsule of the sensory nerve endings and the connective tissue that surrounds the effector structures, such as the skeletal muscle cell. Centrally, the connective tissue layers continue along the dorsal and ventral roots of the nerve and fuse with the meninges that surround the spinal cord and brain.

Supporting Cells of the Central Nervous System

Supporting cells of the CNS consist of the oligodendroglia, astroglia, microglia, and ependymal cells. The *oligodendroglial* cells form the myelin in the CNS. Instead of forming a myelin covering for a single axon, these cells reach out with several processes, each wrapping around and forming a multilayered myelin segment around several different axons (Fig. 47-6). The coverings of axons in the CNS function in increasing the velocity of nerve conduction, similar to the peripheral myelinated fibers.

A second type of glial cell, the *astroglia*, is particularly prominent in the gray matter of the CNS. These large cells have many processes, some reaching to the surface of the capillaries, others reaching to the surface of the nerve cells, and still others filling most of the intercellular space of the CNS. The astrocytic linkage between the blood vessels and the neurons may provide a transport mechanism for the exchange of oxygen, carbon dioxide, and metabolites. The astrocytes also have an important role in sequestering cations such as calcium and potassium from the intercellular fluid. Astrocytes can fill their cytoplasm with microfibrils (*i.e.*, fibrous astrocytes), and masses of these cells form the special type of scar tissue called *gliosis* that develops in the CNS when tissue is destroyed.

A third type of glial cell, the *microglia*, is a small phagocytic cell that is available for cleaning up debris after cellular damage, infection, or cell death. The fourth type of cell, the *ependymal* cell, forms the lining of the neural tube cavity, the ventricular system. In some areas, these cells combine with a rich vascular network to form the *choroid plexus*, where production of the cerebrospinal fluid (CSF) takes place.

METABOLIC REQUIREMENTS OF NERVOUS TISSUE

Nervous tissue has a high rate of metabolism. Although the brain comprises only 2% of the body's weight, it receives approximately 15% of the resting cardiac output and consumes 20% of its oxygen. Despite its substantial energy requirements, the brain can neither store oxygen nor engage in anaerobic metabolism. An interruption in the blood or oxygen supply to the brain rapidly leads to clinically observable signs and symptoms. Without oxygen, brain cells continue to function for approximately 10 seconds. Unconsciousness occurs almost simultaneously with cardiac arrest, and the death of brain cells begins within 4 to 6 minutes. Interruption of blood flow also leads to the accumulation of metabolic byproducts that are toxic to neural tissue.

Glucose is the major fuel source for the nervous system, but neurons have no provision for storing glucose. Ketones can provide for limited temporary energy requirements; however, these sources are rapidly depleted. Unlike muscle cells, neurons have no glycogen stores and must rely on glucose from the blood or the glycogen stores of supporting glial cells. Persons receiving insulin for diabetes may

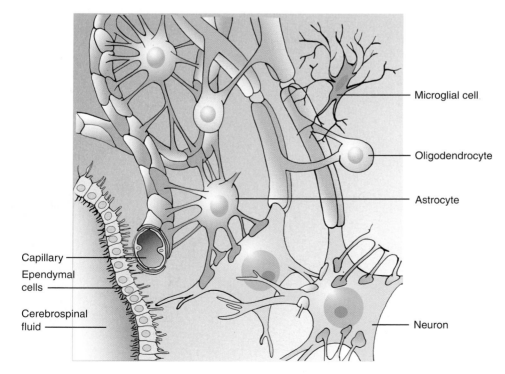

Capillary

Ependymal cells

Cerebrospinal fluid

Microglial cell

Oligodendrocyte

Astrocyte

Neuron

FIGURE 47-6 The cells of the central nervous system (CNS). Diagrammatic view of relationships between the glial elements (astrocyte, oligodendrocyte, microglial cell, and the ependymal cells), the capillaries, the cerebral spinal fluid, and the cell bodies of CNS neurons.

experience signs of neural dysfunction and unconsciousness (*i.e.*, insulin reaction or shock) when blood glucose drops because of insulin excess (see Chapter 41).

In summary, nervous tissue is composed of two types of cells: neurons and supporting cells. Neurons are composed of three parts: a cell body, which controls cell activity; the dendrites, which conduct information toward the cell body; and the axon, which carries impulses from the cell body. The supporting cells consist of Schwann and satellite cells of the PNS and the glial cells of the CNS. Supporting cells protect and provide metabolic support for the neurons and aid in segregating them into isolated compartments, which is necessary for normal neuronal function. The function of the nervous system demands a high amount of metabolic energy. Glucose is the major fuel for the nervous system. The brain comprises only 2% of body weight but receives 15% of the resting cardiac output.

Nerve Cell Communication

After you have completed this section of the chapter, you should be able to meet the following objectives:

✦ Describe the functional importance of ion channels and relate this to the different phases of an action potential
✦ Differentiate electrical from chemical synapses
✦ Describe the interaction of the presynaptic and post-synaptic terminals
✦ Relate excitatory and inhibitory postsynaptic potentials to the process of spatial and temporal summation of membrane potentials
✦ Briefly describe how neurotransmitters are synthesized, stored, released, and inactivated

Neurons are characterized by the ability to communicate with other neurons and body cells through pulsed electrical signals called *impulses*. An impulse, or action potential, represents the movement of electrical charge along the axon membrane. This phenomenon, sometimes called *conductance*, is based on the rapid flow of charged ions through the plasma membrane. In excitable tissue, ions such as sodium, potassium, and calcium move through the membrane channels and carry the electrical charges involved in the initiation and transmission of such impulses.

ACTION POTENTIALS

The cell membranes of excitable tissue, including neurons, contain ion channels that are responsible for generating action potentials. These membrane channels are guarded by voltage-dependent gates that open and close with changes in the membrane potential. Separate voltage-gated channels exist for the sodium, potassium, and calcium ions. Each type of ion channel has a characteristic membrane potential that opens and closes its channels. There also are ligand-gated channels that respond to chemical messengers such as neurotransmitters, mechanically gated channels respond

to physical changes in the cell membrane, and light-gated channels that respond to fluctuations in light levels.

Nerve signals are transmitted by action potentials, which are abrupt, pulsatile changes in the membrane potential that last a few ten thousandths to a few thousandths of a second. Action potentials can be divided into three phases: the resting or polarized state, depolarization, and repolarization (Fig. 47-7).

The resting phase is the undisturbed period of the action potential during which the nerve is not transmitting impulses. During this period, the membrane is said to be *polarized* because of the large separation of charge (*i.e.*, positive on the outside and negative on the inside). The resting membrane potential for large nerve fibers is approximately –90 mV. However, in small neurons and in many neurons in the CNS, the resting membrane potential often is as little as –40 to –60 mV. The resting phase of the membrane potential continues until some event causes the membrane to increase its permeability to sodium.

The threshold potential represents the membrane potential at which neurons or other excitable tissues are stimulated to fire. In large nerve fibers, the sodium channels open approximately at –60 mV, which is the threshold for initiation of an action potential. When the threshold

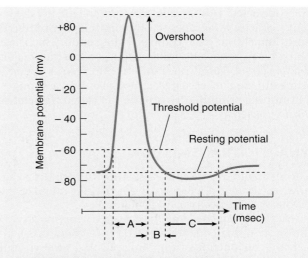

A = Absolute refractory period (active potential and partial recovery)
B = Relative refractory period
C = Positive relative refractory period

FIGURE 47-7 Time course of the action potential recorded at one point of an axon with one electrode inside and one on the outside of the plasma membrane. The rising part of the action potential is called the spike. The rising phase plus approximately the first half of the repolarization phase is equal to the absolute refractory period (*A*). The portion of the repolarization phase that extends from the threshold to the resting membrane potential represents the relative refractory period (*B*). The remaining portion of the repolarization phase to the resting membrane potential is equal to the negative after potential (*C*). Hyperpolarization is equal to the positive relative refractory period.

potential is reached, the gatelike structures in the ion channels open. Below the threshold potential, these gates remain tightly closed. The gates are either fully open or fully closed (all-or-none). Under ordinary circumstances, the threshold stimulus is sufficient to open large numbers of ion channels, triggering massive depolarization of the membrane (the action potential).

Depolarization is characterized by the flow of electrically charged ions. During the depolarization phase, the membrane suddenly becomes permeable to sodium ions; the rapid inflow of sodium ions produces local currents that travel through the adjacent cell membrane, causing the sodium channels in this part of the membrane to open. In neurons, the sodium ion gate remains open only for approximately a quarter of a millisecond, and closes quickly. During this phase of the action potential, the inner face of the membrane becomes positive (approximately +30 to +45 mV).

Repolarization is the phase during which the polarity of the resting membrane potential is reestablished. This is accomplished with closure of the sodium channels and opening of the potassium channels. The outflow of positively charged potassium ions across the cell membrane returns the membrane potential to negativity. The sodium–potassium pump gradually reestablishes the resting ionic concentrations on each side of the membrane. Membranes of excitable cells must be sufficiently repolarized before they can be reexcited. During repolarization, the membrane remains refractory (*i.e.*, does not fire) until repolarization is approximately one-third complete. This period, which lasts approximately one half a millisecond, is called the *absolute refractory period*. During one portion of the recovery period, the membrane can be excited, although only by a stronger-than-normal stimulus. This period is called *the relative refractory period*.

SYNAPTIC TRANSMISSION

Neurons communicate with each other through structures known as *synapses*. Two types of synapses are found in the nervous system: electrical and chemical.

Electrical synapses permit the passage of current-carrying ions through small openings called *gap junctions* that penetrate the cell junction of adjoining cells and allow current to travel in either direction. The gap junctions allow an action potential to pass directly and quickly from one neuron to another. They may link neurons having close functional relationships into circuits.

The most common type of synapse is the *chemical synapse*. Chemical synapses involve special presynaptic and postsynaptic membrane structures, separated by a synaptic cleft (Fig. 47-8). The presynaptic terminal secretes one and often several chemical messenger molecules (*i.e.*, neurotransmitters or neuromodulators) into the synaptic cleft. The neurotransmitters diffuse into the synaptic cleft and unite with receptors on the postsynaptic membrane; this causes excitation or inhibition of the postsynaptic neuron by producing either hypopolarization or hyperpolarization of the postsynaptic membrane. Hypopolarization in-

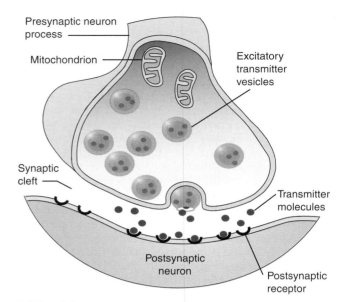

FIGURE 47-8 A synapse showing the synaptic vesicles in the presynaptic neuron, release of the transmitter, and binding of the transmitter to the receptors on the membrane surface of the postsynaptic neuron.

creases the excitability of the postsynaptic neuron by bringing the membrane potential closer to the threshold potential so that a smaller subsequent stimulus is needed to cause the neuron to fire. Hyperpolarization, on the other hand, brings the membrane potential further from threshold and has the opposite effect. It has an inhibitory effect and decreases the likelihood that an action potential will be generated.

In contrast to an electrical synapse, a chemical synapse serves as a rectifier, permitting only one-way communication. One-way conduction is a particularly important characteristic of chemical synapses. It is this specific transmission of signals to discrete and highly localized areas of the nervous system that allows it to perform the myriad functions of sensation, motor control, and memory.

Chemical synapses are the slowest component in progressive communication through a sequence of neurons, such as in a spinal reflex. In contrast to the conduction of electrical action potentials, each successive event at the chemical synapse—transmitter secretion, diffusion across the synaptic cleft, interaction with postsynaptic receptors, and generation of a subsequent action potential in the postsynaptic neuron—consumes time. On the average, conduction across a chemical synapse requires approximately 0.3 milliseconds.

A neuron's cell body and dendrites are covered by thousands of synapses, any or many of which can be active at any moment. Because of the interaction of this rich synaptic input, each neuron resembles a little integrator, in which circuits of many neurons interact with one another. It is the complexity of these interactions and the subtle integrations involved in producing behavioral responses that gives the system its intelligence. This complexity also is what makes the prediction of stimulus-response associations difficult without a millisecond-to-millisecond knowledge of the excitatory and inhibitory activity that takes place on the surfaces of each neuron in a functional circuit. It is amazing that predictions are possible at all considering the number of these tiny integrators. It is even more astounding that the basic microcircuitry present in the nervous system is reproduced reliably during the development of each new organism.

Chemical synapses exhibit several relationships. Axons can synapse with dendrites (axodendritic), with the cell body (axosomatic), or to the axon (axoaxonic). Dendrites can synapse with axons (dendroaxonic), other dendrites (dendrodendritic), or the soma of other neurons (dendrosomatic). Synapses between the nerve cell body and axons (somatoaxonic synapses) also have been observed. Synapses occurring between the soma of neighboring neurons (somasomatic) are uncommon, with the exception of some between efferent nuclei. The mechanism of communication between the presynaptic and the postsynaptic neuron is similar in all types of synapses; the action potential sweeps into the axonal terminals of the afferent neuron and triggers the rapid release of neurotransmitter molecules from the axonal, or presynaptic, surface. Conversion of action potentials into neurotransmitter release is called *coupling*, and although it is not completely understood, it is believed that the release of calcium ions is involved.

Excitatory and Inhibitory Postsynaptic Potentials

Many CNS neurons possess thousands of synapses on their dendritic or somatic surfaces, each of which can produce partial excitation or inhibition of the postsynaptic neuron. When the combination of a neurotransmitter with a receptor site causes partial depolarization of the postsynaptic membrane, it is called an *excitatory postsynaptic potential* (EPSP). In other synapses, the combination of a transmitter with a receptor site is inhibitory in the sense that it causes the local nerve membrane to become hyperpolarized and less excitable. This is called an *inhibitory postsynaptic potential* (IPSP).

Action potentials do not begin in the membrane adjacent to the synapse. They begin in the initial segment of the axon, near the *axon hillock*, that lies just before the first myelin segment. The initial segment of the axon is more excitable than the rest of the neuron. The local currents resulting from an EPSP (sometimes called a *generator potential*) usually are insufficient to reach threshold and cause depolarization of the axon's initial segment. However, if several EPSPs occur simultaneously, the area of depolarization can become large enough and the currents at the initial segment can become strong enough to exceed the threshold potential and initiate an action potential. This summation of depolarized areas is called *spatial summation*. EPSPs also can summate and cause an action potential if they occur in rapid succession. This temporal aspect of the occurrence of two or more EPSPs is called *temporal summation*.

IPSPs also can undergo spatial and temporal summation with each other and with EPSPs, reducing the effectiveness of the latter by a roughly algebraic summation. If the sum of EPSPs and IPSPs keeps the depolarization at the initial segment below threshold levels, the generation of an action potential does not occur.

The spatial and temporal summation involved during synaptic activity serves as a sensitive and complicated switch that requires the right combination of incoming activity before the cell can elicit an action potential. The occurrence and frequency of action potentials in axons is in an all-or-none language (*i.e.,* digital language), which varies only as to the presence or absence of such impulses and their frequency. Action potentials permit rapid communication over long distances. However, it is the capacity for integration of excitatory and inhibitory synaptic bombardment of the soma and dendrites that gives the neuron and the nervous system the capability for complexity, memory, and intelligence.

MESSENGER MOLECULES

Neurotransmitters are the chemical messenger molecules of the nervous system. The process of neurotransmission involves the synthesis, storage, and release of a neurotransmitter; the reaction of the neurotransmitter with a receptor; and termination of the receptor action (Fig. 47-9). Newer research methods, including staining techniques and the use of radiolabeled antibodies, have allowed scientists to study and gain answers in each of these areas.

Both the nervous system and the endocrine system use chemical molecules as messengers. As more information is

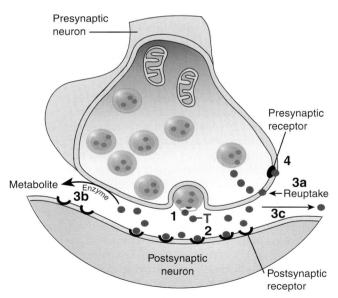

FIGURE 47-9 Schematic illustration of (1) neurotransmitter (T) release; (2) binding of transmitter to postsynaptic receptor; termination of transmitter action by (3a) reuptake of transmitter into the presynaptic terminal, (3b) enzymatic degradation, or (3c) diffusion away from the synapse; and (4) binding of transmitter to presynaptic receptors for feedback regulation of transmitter release.

obtained about the chemical messengers of these systems, the distinction between them becomes less evident. Many neurons, such as those in the adrenal medulla, secrete transmitters into the bloodstream, and it has been found that other neurons possess receptor sites for hormones. Many hormones have turned out to be neurotransmitters. Vasopressin (also known as *antidiuretic hormone*), a peptide hormone released from the posterior pituitary gland, acts as a hormone in the kidney and as a neurotransmitter for nerve cells in the hypothalamus. More than a dozen of these cell-to-cell and blood-borne messengers can relay signals in the nervous system or the endocrine system.

Neurotransmitters are synthesized in the cytoplasm of the axon terminal. The synthesis of transmitters may require one or more enzyme-catalyzed steps (*e.g.*, one for acetylcholine and three for norepinephrine). Neurons are limited as to the type of transmitter they can synthesize by their enzyme systems.

After synthesis, the neurotransmitter molecules are stored in the axon terminal in tiny, membrane-bound sacs called *synaptic vesicles*. There may be thousands of vesicles in a single terminal, each containing 10,000 to 100,000 transmitter molecules. The vesicle protects the neurotransmitters from enzyme destruction in the nerve terminal. The arrival of an impulse at a nerve terminal causes the vesicles to move to the cell membrane and release their transmitter molecules into the synaptic space.

Neurotransmitters exert their actions through specific proteins, called *receptors*, embedded in the postsynaptic membrane. These receptors are tailored precisely to match the size and shape of the transmitter. In each case, the interaction between a transmitter and receptor results in a specific physiologic response. The action of a transmitter is determined by the type of receptor to which it binds. For example, acetylcholine is excitatory when it is released at a myoneural junction, and it is inhibitory when it is released at the sinoatrial node in the heart. Receptors are named according to the type of neurotransmitter with which they interact. For example, a *cholinergic receptor* is a receptor that binds acetylcholine.

Rapid removal of a transmitter, once it has exerted its effects on the postsynaptic membrane, is necessary to maintain precise control of neural transmission. A released transmitter can undergo one of three fates: it can be broken down into inactive substances by enzymes; it can be taken back up into the presynaptic neuron in a process called *reuptake*; or it can diffuse away into the intercellular fluid until its concentration is too low to influence postsynaptic excitability. Acetylcholine, for example, is rapidly broken down by acetylcholinesterase into acetic acid and choline, with the choline being taken back into the presynaptic neuron for reuse in acetylcholine synthesis. The catecholamines are largely taken back into the neuron in an unchanged form for reuse. Catecholamines also can be degraded by enzymes in the synaptic space or in the nerve terminals.

Neurotransmitters are small molecules that incorporate a positively charged nitrogen atom; they include several amino acids, peptides, and monoamines. Amino acids are the building blocks of proteins and are present in body fluids. Peptides are low–molecular-weight molecules that are made up of two or more amino acids. They include substance P and the endorphins and enkephalins, which are involved in pain sensation and perception (see Chapter 48). A monoamine is an amine molecule containing one amino group (NH_2). Serotonin, dopamine, norepinephrine, and epinephrine are monoamines synthesized from amino acids. Fortunately, the blood-brain barrier protects the nervous system from circulating amino acids and other molecules with potential neurotransmitter activity.

Much needs to be learned about the role of amino acids and peptides as neurotransmitters. For example, several amino acids (especially glutamic acid and aspartic acid) appear to exert powerful excitatory effects on synaptic transmission; they often are called *excitatory amino acids*. Glycine, another amino acid, is known to have strong inhibitory effects. One of the most common inhibitory transmitters is γ-aminobutyric acid (GABA). This amino acid is unique in that it is synthesized almost exclusively in the brain and spinal cord. It has been established that almost a third of the synapses use GABA. Adding to the already complicated nature of neurotransmitters, it is puzzling that the same amino acid can function as both a neurotransmitter and as a building block for protein synthesis.

The actions of most neurotransmitters are localized in specific clusters of neurons with axons that project to highly specific brain regions. As more has been learned about the location and mechanism of action of the various neurotransmitters, it is becoming increasingly clear that many disease conditions have their origin in altered neurotransmitter physiology. In some cases, there is evidence of degeneration or dysfunction of the neurons producing the neurotransmitters; in other cases, there is an apparent alteration in the postsynaptic response to the neurotransmitter. For example, the neurons containing dopamine are concentrated in regions of the midbrain known as the *substantia nigra* and *ventral tegmentum*. Many of these dopamine-containing neurons project their axons to areas of the forebrain thought to be involved in regulation of emotional behavior. Other dopamine fibers terminate in regions near the middle of the brain called the *corpus striatum*. The latter fibers are thought to play an essential role in the performance of complex motor movements. Degeneration of the dopamine fibers in this area of the brain leads to the tremor and rigidity that are characteristic of Parkinson's disease. Some forms of mental illness, such as schizophrenia, are thought to involve abnormal release of or response to neurotransmitters in the brain. Pharmacologic methods of supplying neurotransmitters (*e.g.*, in Parkinson's disease) or modifying their actions (*e.g.*, with psychoactive drugs) are used to treat some of these disorders. Undoubtedly, more specific treatment methods will become available as more is learned about the transmission of neural information.

Other classes of messenger molecules, known *neuromodulators*, also may be released from axon terminals. Neuromodulator molecules react with presynaptic or postsynaptic receptors to alter the release of or response to neurotransmitters. Neuromodulators may act on postsynaptic receptors to produce slower and longer-lasting changes in membrane excitability. This alters the action of the faster-acting neurotransmitter molecules by enhancing or decreasing their effectiveness. By combining with autoreceptors on its own presynaptic membrane, a transmitter can act as a neuromodulator to augment or inhibit further nerve activity. In some nerves, such as the peripheral sympathetic nerves, a messenger molecule can have both transmitter and modulator functions. For example, norepinephrine can activate an α_1-adrenergic postsynaptic receptor to produce vasoconstriction, or stimulate an α_2-adrenergic presynaptic receptor to inhibit further norepinephrine release.

Neurohumoral mediators reach their target cells through the bloodstream and produce an even slower action than the neuromodulators. Neurotrophic or nerve growth factors are required to maintain the long-term survival of the postsynaptic cell and are secreted by axon terminals independent of action potentials. Examples include lower motoneurons (LMNs) to muscle cell trophic factors and neuron-to-neuron trophic factors in the sequential synapses of CNS sensory neurons. Trophic factors from target cells that enter the axon and are necessary for the long-term survival of presynaptic neurons also have been demonstrated. Target cell-to-neuron trophic factors probably have great significance in establishing specific neural connections during normal embryonic development.

> In summary, neurons are characterized by the ability to communicate with other neurons and body cells through pulsed electrical signals called *action potentials*. The cell membranes of neurons contain ion channels that are responsible for generating action potentials. These channels are guarded by voltage-dependent gates that open and close with changes in the membrane potential. Action potentials are divided into three parts: the resting membrane potential, during which the membrane is polarized but no electrical activity occurs; the depolarization phase, during which sodium channels open, allowing rapid inflow of the sodium ions that generate the electrical impulse; and the repolarization phase, during which the membrane is permeable to the potassium ion, allowing for the efflux of potassium ions and return to the resting membrane potential. The membrane threshold represents the membrane potential at which the sodium channels open, heralding the onset of an action potential. Once initiated, an action potential travels rapidly along the cell's axonal membrane to trigger transmitter release from the next neuron in the sequence.
>
> Synapses are structures that permit communication between neurons. Two types of synapses have been identified: electrical and chemical. Electrical synapses consist of gap junctions between adjacent cells that allow action potentials to move rapidly from one cell to another. Chemical synapses involve special presynaptic and postsynaptic structures, separated by a synaptic cleft. They rely on chemical messengers, released from the presynaptic neuron, that cross the synaptic cleft and then interact with receptors on the postsynaptic neuron.
>
> Neurotransmitters are chemical messengers that control neural function; they selectively cause excitation or inhibition of action potentials. Three major types of neurotransmitters are known: amino acids such as glutamic acid and GABA, peptides such as the endorphins and enkephalins, and monoamines such as epinephrine and norepinephrine. Neurotransmitters interact with cell membrane receptors to produce either excitatory or inhibitory actions. Neuromodulators are chemical messengers that react with membrane receptors to produce slower and longer-acting changes in membrane permeability. Neurotrophic or growth factors, also released from presynaptic terminals, are required to maintain the long-term survival of postsynaptic neurons.

Developmental Organization of the Nervous System

After you have completed this section of the chapter, you should be able to meet the following objectives:

- ✦ Cite the significance of the hierarchy of control levels of the CNS
- ✦ Use the segmental approach to explain the development of the nervous system and the organization of the postembryonic nervous system
- ✦ Define the terms *afferent, efferent, ganglia, association neuron, cell column,* and *tract*
- ✦ State the origin and destination of nerve fibers contained in the dorsal and ventral roots
- ✦ State the structures innervated by general somatic afferent, special visceral afferent, general visceral afferent, special somatic afferent, general visceral efferent, pharyngeal efferent, and general somatic efferent neurons

The development of the nervous system can be traced far back into evolutionary history. During its development, newer functional features and greater complexity resulted from the modification and enlargement of more primitive structures. Survival of the species depended on the rapid reaction to environmental danger, to potential food sources, or to a sexual partner.

The front, or rostral, end of the CNS became specialized for sensing the external environment and controlling reactions to it. In time, the ancient organization, which is largely retained in the spinal cord segments, was expanded in the forward segments of the nervous system. Of these, the most forward segments have undergone the most radical modification and have developed into the forebrain: the diencephalon and the cerebral hemispheres. The dominance of the front end of the CNS is reflected in a hierarchy of control levels: brain stem over spinal cord, and forebrain over brain stem. Throughout evolution, newer functions were added to the surface of functionally more ancient systems. As newer functions became concentrated at the rostral end of the nervous system, they also became more vulnerable to injury.

Three basic principles underlie the functioning of the nervous system: no portion of the nervous system functions independently of the other parts; newer systems control older systems; and the newer systems are more vulnerable to injury. These principles provide a basis for understanding the many manifestations of injuries and diseases of the nervous system.

EMBRYONIC DEVELOPMENT

The nervous system appears very early in embryonic development (week 3). This early development is essential because it influences the development and organization of many other body systems, including the axial skeleton, skeletal muscles, and sensory organs such as the eyes and ears. During later fetal life and thereafter, the nervous system provides communication, signal processing, integrative, and memory functions. The early induction and later, lifelong communication functions of the nervous system are at the center of the integrity, survival, and individuality of each person.

During the second week of development, embryonic tissue consists of two layers, the endoderm and the ectoderm. At the beginning of third week, the ectoderm begins to invaginate and migrates between the two layers, forming a third layer called the *mesoderm* (Fig. 47-10). The mesoderm along the entire midline of the embryo forms a specialized rod of embryonic tissue called the *notochord*. The notochord and adjacent mesoderm provide

the necessary induction signal for the overlying ectoderm to differentiate and form a thickened structure called the *neural plate*, the primordium of the nervous system. The neural plate develops an axial groove (*i.e.*, neural groove) that sinks into the underlying mesoderm; its walls fuse across the top, forming an ectodermal tube called the *neural tube*. This process, called *closure*, occurs during the later third and fourth weeks of gestation and is vital to the survival of the embryo. During development, the neural tube develops into the CNS, the notochord becomes the foundation around which the vertebral column ultimately develops, and the surface ectoderm separates from the neural tube and fuses over the top to become the outer layer of skin. Closure of the neural tube begins at the cervical and high thoracic levels and zippers rostrally toward the cephalic end of the embryo and caudally toward the sacrum. The last locations for completion of closure are at the rostral-most end of brain (*i.e.*, anterior neuropore, 25 days) and the lumbosacral region (*i.e.*, posterior neuropore, 27 days).

As the neural tube closes, ectodermal cells called *neural crest cells* migrate away from the dorsal surface of the neural tube to become the progenitors of the neurons and supporting cells of the PNS (see Fig. 47-10). Some of these cells gather into clusters to form the *dorsal root ganglia* at the sides of each spinal cord segment and the *cranial ganglia* in most brain segments. Neurons of these ganglia be-

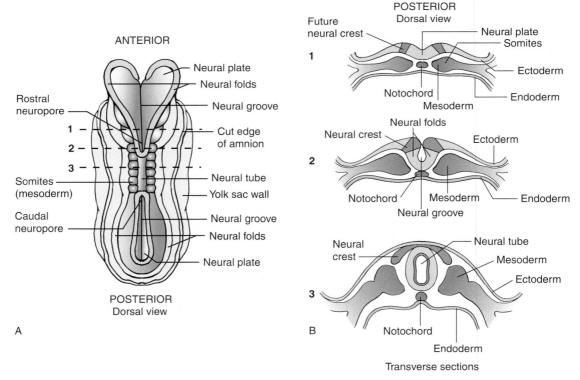

FIGURE 47-10 Folding of the neural tube. (**A**) Dorsal view of a six somite embryo (22–23 days) showing the neural folds, groove and the fused neural tube. The anterior neuropore closes at about day 26 and the posterior neuropore at about day 28. (**B**) Three cross-sections taken at the levels indicated in (**A**). The sections indicate where the neural tube is just beginning to form.

come the afferent or sensory neurons of the PNS. Other neural crest cells become the pigment cells of the skin or contribute to the formation of the meninges, many structures of the face, and the peripheral ganglion cells of the autonomic nervous system. The latter include cells of the adrenal cortex.

During development, the more rostral part of the embryonic neural tube—approximately 10 segments—undergoes extensive modification and enlargement to form the brain (Fig. 47-11). In the early embryo, 3 swellings, or primary vesicles, develop, subdividing these 10 segments into the prosencephalon, or forebrain, containing the first 2 segments; the mesencephalon, or midbrain, which develops from segment 3; and the rhombencephalon, or hindbrain, which develops from segments 4 to 10.

The 10 rostral brain segments represent modifications of the spinal cord neural tube and often are called, collectively, the *brain stem*. The brain stem does not include later-developed outgrowths—the cerebral hemispheres, the optic nerve and retina, and the cerebellum. The central canal of the prosencephalon develops two pairs of lateral outpouchings that carry the neural tube with them: the optic cup, which becomes the optic nerve and retina, and the telencephalic vesicles, which become the olfactory bulbs and the cerebral hemispheres. In the neural tube, the central canal extends into the cerebral hemispheres as enlarged CSF-filled cavities, the first and second (lateral) ventricles. The remaining neural tube of these three segments is called the *diencephalon*; it develops into the thalamus and hypothalamus. The neurohypophysis (posterior pituitary) grows as a midline ventral outgrowth at the junctions of segments 1 and 2. A dorsal outgrowth, the pineal body, develops between segments 2 and 3.

All brain segments, except segment 2, retain some portion of the basic segmental organization of the nervous system. The evolutionary development of the brain is reflected in the cranial and upper cervical paired segmental nerves. This reflects the original pattern of a segmented neural tube, each segment of which has multiple paired branches containing a grouping of component axons. One segment would have paired branches to body muscles and another set to visceral structures, and so on. The classic pattern of spinal nerve organization, which consists of a pair of dorsal and a pair of ventral roots, is a later evolutionary development that has not occurred in the cranial nerves. Consequently, the cranial nerves, which are arbitrarily numbered 1 through 12, retain the ancient pattern, with more than one cranial nerve branching from a single segment. The truly segmental nerve pattern of the cranial nerves is altered because all branches from segment 2 and most of the branches from segment 1 are missing. The second cranial nerve, also called the *optic nerve*, is not a segmental nerve. It is a brain tract connecting the retina (modified brain) with the first forebrain segment from which it developed.

Soma and Viscera. All body tissues and organs have developed from the three embryonic layers (*i.e.*, endoderm, ectoderm, and mesoderm) that were present during the third week of embryonic life. The body is organized into the soma and viscera (Fig. 47-12). The *soma,* or body wall, includes all of the structures derived from the embryonic ectoderm, such as the epidermis of the skin and the CNS. The mesodermal connective tissues of the soma include the dermis of the skin, skeletal muscle, bone, and the outer lining of the body cavity (*i.e.*, parietal pleura and peritoneum). The nervous system innervates all somatic structures as well as the internal structures making up the viscera. The *viscera* includes the great vessels derived from the intermediate mesoderm, the urinary system, and the gonadal structures; it also includes the inner lining of the body cavities, such as the visceral pleura and peritoneum, and the mesodermal tissues that surround the endoderm-lined gut and its derivative organs (*e.g.*, lungs, liver, pancreas).

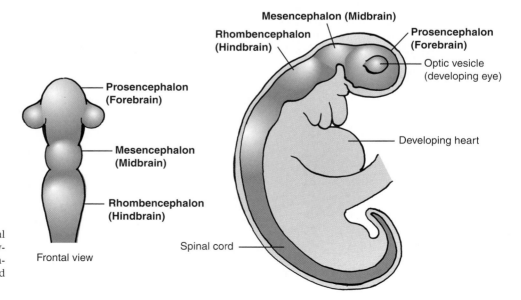

FIGURE 47-11 A lateral and frontal view of 5-week-old embryo showing the brain vesicles and three embryonic divisions of the brain and brainstem.

Prosencephalon (Forebrain)

Mesencephalon (Midbrain)

Rhombencephalon (Hindbrain)

Frontal view

Mesencephalon (Midbrain)

Rhombencephalon (Hindbrain)

Prosencephalon (Forebrain)

Optic vesicle (developing eye)

Developing heart

Spinal cord

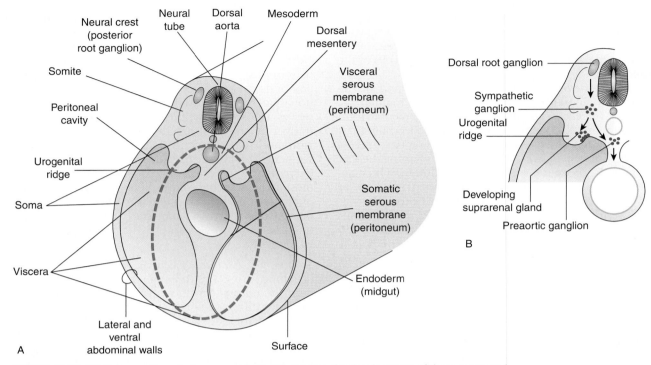

FIGURE 47-12 (**A**) Cross-section of a human embryo, illustrating the development of the somatic and visceral structures. (**B**) The derivatives of the neural crest: the dorsal root ganglia, sympathetic trunk ganglia, preaortic and paravertebral trunk ganglia, as well as the adrenal medulla and the enteric or organ plexus.

SEGMENTAL ORGANIZATION

The early pattern of segmental development is presented as a framework for understanding the nervous system. Developmentally, the basic organizational pattern of the body is that of a longitudinal series of segments, each repeating the same fundamental pattern (Fig. 47-13). Although the early muscular, skeletal, vascular, and excretory systems and the nerves that supply the somatic and visceral structures have the same segmental pattern, it is the nervous system that most clearly retains this organization in postnatal life. The CNS and its associated peripheral nerves consist of approximately 43 segments, 33 of which form the spinal cord and spinal nerves, and 10 of which form the brain and its cranial nerves.

Each segment of the CNS is accompanied by bilateral pairs of bundled nerve fibers, or roots, a ventral pair and a dorsal pair. The paired dorsal roots connect a pair of dorsal root ganglia and their corresponding CNS segment. The dorsal root ganglia contain many afferent nerve cell bodies, each having two axon-like processes—one that ends in a peripheral receptor and the other that enters the central neural segment. The axon-like process that enters the central neural segment communicates with a neuron called an

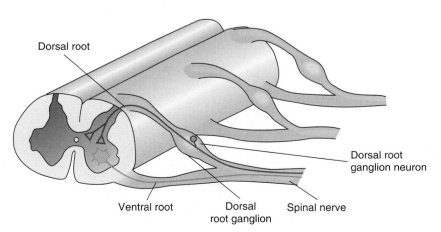

FIGURE 47-13 In this diagram of three segments of the spinal cord, three dorsal roots enter the dorsal lateral surface of the cord, and three ventral roots exit. The dorsal root ganglion contains dorsal root ganglion cells, whose axons bifurcate: one process enters the spinal cord in the dorsal root, and the other extends peripherally to supply the skin and muscle of the body. The ventral root is formed by axons from motoneurons in the spinal cord. (Conn P.M. [1995]. *Neuroscience in medicine* (p. 199). Philadelphia: J.B. Lippincott)

input association (IA) *neuron*. Somatic afferent (SA) neurons transmit information from the soma to somatic IA (SIA) neurons, and visceral afferent (VA) neurons transmit information from the viscera to visceral IA (VIA) neurons. The paired ventral roots of each segment are bundles of axons that provide efferent output to effector sites such as the muscles and glandular cells of the body segment.

On cross-section, the hollow embryonic neural tube can be divided into a central canal, or ventricle, containing CSF, and the wall of the tube. The latter develops into an inner gray cellular portion, which is functionally divided into longitudinal columns of neurons called the *cell columns*. These cell columns contain nerve cell bodies that are surrounded by a superficial white matter region containing the longitudinal tract systems of the CNS. These tract systems are composed of many nerve cell processes. The dorsal half of the gray matter is called the *dorsal horn*. It contains sensory IA neurons that receive afferent information from the dorsal roots. The ventral portion, or ventral horn, contains efferent neurons that communicate by way of the ventral roots with effector cells of the body segment. Many

CNS neurons develop axons that grow longitudinally as tract systems that communicate between neighboring and distal segments of the neural tube.

Cell Columns

The organizational structure of the nervous system can be best explained and simplified as a pattern in which functionally specific PNS and CNS neurons are repeated as parallel cell columns running lengthwise along the nervous system. In this organizational pattern, afferent neurons, dorsal horn cells, and ventral horn cells are organized as a bilateral series of 11 cell columns. A box of 22 colored beverage straws can be used as a model to represent the cell columns. In this model, the right and left sides are each represented in mirror fashion by a set of 11 colored straws. If these straws were cut crosswise (equivalent to a transverse section through the nervous system) at several places along their length, the spatial relations among the different colored straws would be repeated in each section.

The cell columns on each side can be further grouped according to their location in the PNS: four in the dorsal ganglia that contain sensory neurons; four in the dorsal horn containing sensory IA neurons; and three in the ventral horn that contain motoneurons (Fig. 47-14). Each column of dorsal root ganglia projects to its particular column of IA neurons in the dorsal horn. IA neurons distribute afferent information to local reflex circuitry and to more rostral and elaborate segments of the CNS. The ventral horns contain output association (OA) neurons and LMNs. The LMNs provide the final circuitry for organizing efferent nerve activity.

Between the IA neurons and the OA neurons are networks of small internuncial neurons (interneurons) arranged in complex circuits. Internuncial neurons provide the discreteness, appropriateness, and intelligence of responses to stimuli. Most of the billions of CNS cells in the spinal cord and brain gray matter are internuncial neurons.

Dorsal Horn Cell Columns. Four columns of afferent (sensory) neurons in the dorsal root ganglia directly innervate four corresponding columns of IA neurons in the dorsal horn. These columns are categorized as special and general afferents: special somatic afferent, general somatic afferent, special visceral afferent, and general visceral afferent.

Special somatic afferent fibers are concerned with internal sensory information such as joint and tendon sensation (*i.e.*, proprioception). Neurons in the special SIA column cells relay their information to local reflexes concerned with posture and movement. These neurons also relay information to the cerebellum, contributing to coordination of movement, and to the forebrain, contributing to experience. Afferents innervating the labyrinth and derived auditory end organs of the inner ear also belong to the special somatic afferent category.

General somatic afferents innervate the skin and other somatic structures, responding to stimuli such as those that produce pressure or pain. General SIA column cells relay the sensory information to protective and other reflex circuits and project the information to the forebrain, where it is perceived as painful, warm, cold, and the like.

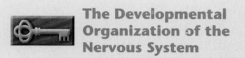

The Developmental Organization of the Nervous System

➤ Embryologically, the nervous system begins its development as a hollow tube, the cephalic portion of which becomes the brain and the more caudal part the spinal cord.

➤ In the process of development, the basic organizational pattern of the body is that of a longitudinal series of segments, each repeating the same basic fundamental organizational pattern: a body wall or soma containing the axial skeleton and a neural tube, which develops into the nervous system.

➤ On cross section, the embryonic neural tube develops into a central canal surrounded by gray matter or cellular portion (cell columns) and the white matter, or tract system of the central nervous system (CNS).

➤ As the nervous system develops, it becomes segmented, with a repeating pattern of afferent neuron axons forming the dorsal roots of each succeeding segmental nerve, and the exiting efferent neurons forming the ventral roots of each succeeding segmental nerve.

➤ The nerve cells in the gray matter are arranged longitudinally in cell columns, with afferent sensory neurons located in the dorsal columns and efferent motor neurons located in the ventral columns.

➤ The axons of the cell column neurons project out into the white matter of the CNS, forming the longitudinal tract systems.

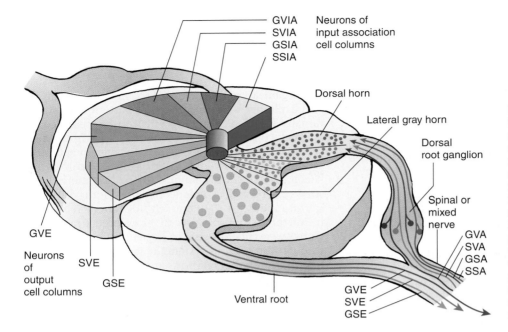

FIGURE 47-14 Cell columns of the central nervous system. The cell columns in the dorsal horn contain input association (IA) neurons for the general visceral afferent (GVA), special visceral afferent (SVA), special sensory afferent (SSA), and general somatic afferent (GSA) neurons with cell bodies in the dorsal root ganglion. The cell columns in the ventral horn contain the general visceral efferent (GVE), pharyngeal efferent (PE), and general somite efferent (GSE) neurons and their output association (OA) neurons.

Special visceral afferent cells innervate specialized gut-related receptors, such as the taste buds and receptors of the olfactory mucosa. Their central processes communicate with special VIA column neurons that project to reflex circuits producing salivation, chewing, swallowing, and other responses. Forebrain projection fibers from these association cells provide sensations of taste (*i.e.*, gustation) and smell (*i.e.*, olfaction).

General visceral afferent neurons innervate visceral structures such as the gastrointestinal tract, urinary bladder, and heart and great vessels; they project to the general VIA column, which relays information to vital reflex circuits and sends information to the forebrain regarding visceral sensations such as stomach fullness, bladder pressure, and sexual experience.

Ventral Horn Cell Columns.

The ventral horn contains three longitudinal cell columns: general visceral efferent, pharyngeal efferent, and general somatic efferent. Each of these cell columns contains OA and efferent neurons. The OA neurons coordinate and integrate the function of the efferent motoneuron cells of its column.

General visceral efferent neurons transmit the efferent output of the autonomic nervous system and are called *preganglionic neurons*. These neurons are structurally and functionally divided into either the sympathetic or the parasympathetic nervous systems. Their axons project through the segmental ventral roots to innervate smooth and cardiac muscle and glandular cells of the body, most of which are in the viscera. In the viscera, three additional neural crest–derived cell columns are present on each side of the body. These become the postganglionic neurons of the autonomic nervous system. In the sympathetic nervous system, the columns are represented by the paravertebral or sympathetic chain ganglia and the prevertebral series of ganglia

(*e.g.*, celiac ganglia) associated with the dorsal aorta. For the parasympathetic system, these become the enteric plexus in the wall of the gut-derived organs and a series of ganglia in the head.

Pharyngeal efferent neurons innervate the branchial arch skeletal muscles: the muscles of mastication, facial expression, and muscles of the pharynx and larynx. Pharyngeal efferent neurons also innervate muscles responsible for moving the head.

The *general somatic efferent* neurons supply somite-derived muscles of the body and head, which include the skeletal muscles of the body, limbs, tongue, and extrinsic eye muscles (see Fig. 47-14). These efferent neurons transmit the commands of the CNS to peripheral effectors, the skeletal muscles. They are the "final common pathway neurons" in the sequence leading to motor activity. They often are called *LMNs* because they are under the control of higher levels of the CNS, including precise control by upper motoneurons (UMNs).

Longitudinal Tracts

The gray matter of the cell columns in the CNS is surrounded by bundles of myelinated axons (*i.e.*, white matter) and unmyelinated axons that travel longitudinally along the length of the neural axis. This white matter can be divided into three layers: an inner, a middle, and an outer layer (Fig. 47-15). The inner layer, or *archilayer*, contains short fibers that project for a maximum of approximately five segments before reentering the gray matter. The middle layer, or *paleolayer*, projects to six or more segments. Archilayer and paleolayer fibers have many branches, or collaterals, that enter the gray matter of intervening segments. The outer layer, or *neolayer*, contains large-diameter axons that can travel the entire length of the nervous system (Table 47-1). *Suprasegmental* is a term that refers to higher

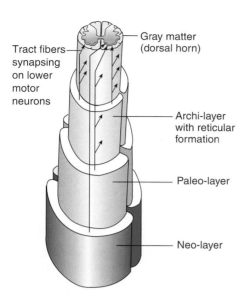

Tract fibers synapsing on lower motor neurons

Gray matter (dorsal horn)

Archi-layer with reticular formation

Paleo-layer

Neo-layer

FIGURE 47-15 The three concentric subdivisions of the tract systems of the white matter. Migration of neurons into the archilayer converts it into the reticular formation of the white matter.

levels of the CNS, such as the brain stem and cerebrum and structures above a given CNS segment. Paleolayer and neolayer fibers have suprasegmental projections.

The longitudinal layers are arranged in bundles, or fiber tracts, that contain axons that have the same destination, origin, and function (Fig. 47-16). These longitudinal tracts are named systematically to reflect their origin and destination; the origin is named first, and the destination is named second. For example, the spinothalamic tract originates in the spinal cord and terminates in the thalamus. The corticospinal tract originates in the cerebral cortex and ends in the spinal cord.

The Inner Layer. The inner layer of white matter contains the axons of neurons that connect neighboring segments of the nervous system. Axons of this layer permit the pool of motoneurons of several segments to work together as a functional unit. They also allow the afferent neurons of one segment to trigger reflexes that activate motor units in neighboring and in the same segments. In terms of evolution, this is the oldest of the three layers, and it is sometimes called the *archilayer*. It is the first of the longitudinal layers to become functional, and its circuitry may be limited to reflex types of movements, including reflex movements of the fetus (*i.e.*, quickening) that begin during the fifth month of intrauterine life.

The inner layer of the white matter differs from the other two layers in one important aspect. Many neurons in the embryonic gray matter migrate out into this layer, resulting in a rich mixture of neurons and local fibers called the *reticular formation*. The circuitry of most reflexes is contained in the reticular formation. In the brain stem, the reticular formation becomes quite large and contains major portions of vital reflexes, such as those controlling respiration, cardiovascular function, swallowing, and vomiting. A functional system called the *reticular activating system* operates in the lateral portions of the reticular formation of the medulla, pons, and especially the midbrain. Information converging from all sensory modalities, including those of the somesthetic, auditory, visual, and visceral afferent nerves, bombards the neurons of this system.

The reticular activating system has descending and ascending portions. The descending portion communicates with all spinal segmental levels through paleolevel reticulospinal tracts and serves to facilitate many cord-level reflexes. For example, it speeds reaction time and stabilizes postural reflexes. The ascending portion accelerates brain activity, particularly thalamic and cortical activity. This is reflected by the appearance of awake brain-wave patterns. Sudden stimuli result in protective and attentive postures and cause increased awareness.

The Middle Layer. The middle layer of the white matter contains most of the major fiber tract systems required for sensation and movement. It contains the ascending spinoreticular and spinothalamic tracts. This layer consists of larger-diameter and longer suprasegmental fibers, which ascend to the brain stem and are largely functional at birth. In terms of evolutionary development, these tracts are quite old, and this layer is sometimes called the *paleolayer*. It facilitates many primitive functions, such as the auditory

TABLE 47-1 ✦ Characteristics of the Concentric Subdivisions of the Longitudinal Tracts in the White Matter of the Central Nervous System

Characteristics	Archilayer Tracts	Paleolayer Tracts	Neolayer Tracts
Segmental span	Intersegmental (<5 segments)	Suprasegmental (≥5 segments)	Suprasegmental
Number of synapses	Multisynaptic	Multisynaptic but fewer than archilayer tracts	Monosynaptic with target structures
Conduction velocity	Very slow	Fast	Fastest
Examples of functional systems	Flexor withdrawal reflex circuitry	Spinothalamic tracts	Corticospinal tracts

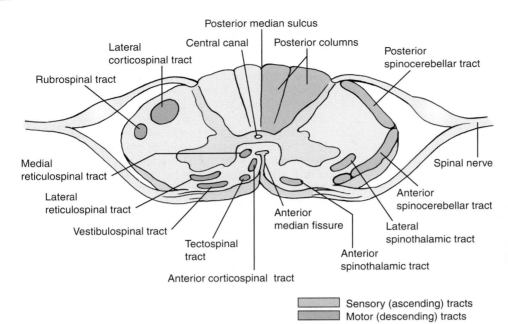

Posterior median sulcus

Central canal Posterior columns

Lateral
corticospinal tract

Posterior
spinocerebellar tract

Rubrospinal tract

Medial
reticulospinal tract

Spinal nerve

Lateral
reticulospinal tract

Anterior
spinocerebellar tract

Vestibulospinal tract

Anterior
median fissure

Lateral
spinothalamic tract

Tectospinal
tract

Anterior
spinothalamic tract

Anterior corticospinal tract

Sensory (ascending) tracts
Motor (descending) tracts

FIGURE 47-16 Transverse section of the spinal cord showing selected sensory and motor tracts. The tracts are bilateral but are only indicated on one half of the cord.

startle reflex, which occurs in response to loud noises. This reflex consists of turning the head and body toward the sound, dilating the pupils of the eyes, catching of the breath, and quickening of the pulse.

The Outer Layer. The outer layer of the tract systems is the newest of the three layers with respect to evolutionary development, and it is sometimes called the *neolayer*. It becomes functional approximately the second year of life, and it includes the pathways needed for bladder training. Myelination of these suprasegmental tracts, which include many pathways required for delicate and highly coordinated skills, is not complete until approximately the fifth year of life. This includes the development of tracts needed for fine manipulative skills, such as the finger–thumb coordination required for using tools and the toe movements needed for acrobatics. Neolayer tracts are the most recently evolved systems and, being more superficial on the brain and spinal cord, are the most vulnerable to injury. When neolayer tracts are damaged, the paleolayer and archilayer tracts often remain functional, and rehabilitation methods can result in effective use of the older systems. Delicacy and refinement may be lost, but basic function remains. For example, when the corticospinal system, an important neolayer system that permits the fine manipulative control required for writing, is damaged, the remaining paleolayer systems, if intact, permit the grasping and holding of objects. The hand can still be used to perform its basic function, but the individual manipulation of the fingers is permanently lost.

Collateral Communication Pathways. Axons in the archilayer and paleolayer characteristically possess many collateral branches that move into the gray cell columns or synapse with fibers of the reticular formation as the axon passes each succeeding CNS segment. Should a major axon be destroyed at some point along its course, these collater-

als provide multisynaptic alternative pathways that bypass the local damage. Neolayer tracts do not possess these collaterals but instead project mainly to the target neurons with which they communicate. Because of this, damage to the neolayer tracts causes permanent loss of function. Damage to the archilayer or paleolayer systems usually is followed by slow return of function, presumably through the collateral connections.

In summary, development of the nervous system can be traced far back into evolutionary history. The CNS develops from the ectoderm of the early embryo by formation of a hollow tube that closes along its longitudinal axis and sinks below the surface. This hollow tube forms the ventricles of the brain and spinal canal, and the side wall develops to form the brain stem and spinal cord. The brain stem and spinal cord are subdivided into the dorsal horn, which contains neurons that receive and process incoming or afferent information, and the ventral horn, which contains efferent motoneurons that handle the final stages of output processing. The PNS develops from ectodermal cells called *neural crest cells* that migrate away from the dorsal surface of the forming neural tube.

Throughout life, the organization of the nervous system retains many patterns established during early embryonic life. This segmental pattern of early embryonic development is retained in the fully developed nervous system. Each of the 43 or more body segments is connected to corresponding CNS or neural tube segments by segmental afferent and efferent neurons. Afferent neuronal processes enter the CNS through the dorsal root ganglia and the dorsal roots. Afferent neurons of the dorsal root ganglia are of four types: general somatic afferent, special somatic afferent, general visceral afferent, and special visceral afferent. Each of these afferent neurons synapses with its appropriate IA neurons in the cell columns of the dorsal horn (*e.g.*, general somatic afferents synapse with neurons in the general somatic afferent IA cell column). Efferent fibers from motoneurons in the ventral horn exit the CNS in the ventral roots. General somatic efferent neurons are LMNs that innervate somite-derived skeletal muscles, and general visceral efferent neurons are preganglionic fibers that synapse with postganglionic fibers that innervate visceral structures. This pattern of afferent and efferent neurons, which in general is repeated in each segment of the body, forms parallel cell columns running lengthwise through the CNS and PNS.

Longitudinal communication between CNS segments is provided by neurons that send the axons into nearby segments by means of the innermost layer of the white matter, the ancient archilayer system of fibers. These cells provide coordination between neighboring segments. Neurons have invaded this layer, and the mix of these cells and axons is called the *reticular formation*. The reticular formation is the location of many important reflex circuits of the spinal cord brain stem. Paleolayer tracts, located outside this layer, provide the longitudinal communication between more distant segments of the nervous system; this layer includes most of the important ascending and descending tracts. The recently evolved neolayer systems, which become functional during infancy and childhood, travel outside the white matter and provide the means for very delicate and discriminative function. The outer position of the neolayer tracts and their lack of collateral and redundant pathways make them the most vulnerable to injury.

The Spinal Cord

After you have completed this section of the chapter, you should be able to meet the following objectives:

✦ Describe the longitudinal and transverse structures of the spinal cord

✦ Trace an afferent and efferent neuron from its site in the periphery through its entrance into or exit from the spinal cord

✦ Explain muscle tone and posture using the myotatic or stretch reflex

In the adult, the spinal cord is found in the upper two thirds of the spinal canal of the vertebral column (Fig. 47-17). It extends from the foramen magnum at the base of the skull to a cone-shaped termination, the conus medullaris, usually at the level of the first or second lumbar vertebra (L1 or L2) in the adult. The dorsal and ventral roots of the more caudal portions of the cord elongate during development and angle downward from the cord, forming what is called the *cauda equina* (from the Latin for "horse's tail"). The filum terminale, which is composed of non-neural tissues and the pia mater, continues caudally and attaches to the second sacral vertebra (S2).

The spinal cord is somewhat oval on transverse section. Internally, the gray matter has the appearance of a butterfly or the letter "H" on cross section (Fig. 47-18). Some neurons that make up the gray matter of the cord have processes or axons that leave the cord, enter the peripheral nerves, and supply tissues such as autonomic ganglia or skeletal muscles. The white matter of the cord that surrounds the gray matter contains nerve fiber tracts or descending axons that transmit information between segments of the cord or from higher levels of the CNS, such as the brain stem or cerebrum.

The extensions of the gray matter that form the letter "H" are called the *horns*. Those that extend posteriorly are called the *dorsal horns*, and those that extend anteriorly are called the *ventral horns*. The dorsal horns contain IA neurons that receive afferent impulses through the dorsal roots and other connecting neurons. Ventral horns contain OA neurons and the efferent LMNs that leave the cord through the ventral roots.

The spinal cord contains many small internuncial neurons that surround the efferent motoneurons and synapse with the cell body or dendrites of the efferent cells. Action potentials of these internuncial neurons exert excitatory or inhibitory effects on the LMNs. Although some CNS systems communicate directly with the LMNs, most LMN activity is controlled by systems communicating through excitatory or inhibitory internuncial neurons. These internuncial neurons rep-resent the final stage of communication between elaborate CNS neuronal circuits and the skeletal muscle cells of the motor unit.

The central portion of the cord, which connects the dorsal and ventral horns, is called the *intermediate gray matter*. The intermediate gray matter surrounds the central canal. In the thoracic area, the small, slender projections that emerge from the intermediate gray matter are called the *intermediolateral columns* of the horns. These columns contain the visceral OA neurons and the efferent neurons of the sympathetic nervous system.

The gray matter is proportional to the amount of tissue innervated by a given segment of the cord (see Fig. 47-18). Larger amounts of gray matter are present in the lower lumbar and upper sacral segments, which supply the lower extremities, and in the fifth cervical segment to the first thoracic segment, which supply the upper limbs. The white matter in the spinal cord also increases progressively toward the brain because ever more ascending fibers are added and the number of descending axons is greater.

The spinal cord and the dorsal and ventral roots are covered by a connective tissue sheath, the pia mater, which also contains the blood vessels that supply the white and gray matter of the cord (Fig. 47-19). On the lateral sides of the spinal cord, extensions of the pia mater, the denticulate ligaments, attach the sides of the spinal cord to the bony walls of the spinal canal. Thus, the cord is suspended by both the denticulate ligaments and the segmental nerves. A fat- and vessel-filled epidural space intervenes between the spinal dura mater and the inner wall of the spinal canal. Each vertebral body has two pedicles that extend posteriorly and support the laterally oriented transverse processes of the

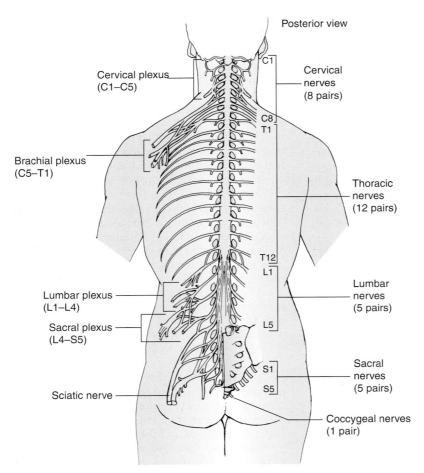

Posterior view

Cervical plexus (C1–C5)

Brachial plexus (C5–T1)

Lumbar plexus (L1–L4)

Sacral plexus (L4–S5)

Sciatic nerve

C1

C8
T1

T12
L1

L5

S1

S5

Cervical nerves (8 pairs)

Thoracic nerves (12 pairs)

Lumbar nerves (5 pairs)

Sacral nerves (5 pairs)

Coccygeal nerves (1 pair)

FIGURE 47-17 Dorsal view of the spinal cord including portions of the major spinal nerves and some of the components of the major nerve plexuses.

neural laminae, which arch medially and fuse to continue as the spinal processes.

The spaces between the vertebral bodies are filled with fibrocartilaginous discs and stabilized with tough ligaments. A gap, the intervertebral foramen, occurs between each two succeeding pedicles, allowing for the exit of the segmental nerves and passage of blood vessels. The spinal cord lives in the protective confines of this series of concentric flexible tissue and body sheaths. Supporting structures of the spinal cord are discussed further in Chapter 49.

Early in fetal life, the spinal cord extends the entire length of the vertebral column and the spinal nerves exit through the intervertebral foramina (openings) near their level of origin. Because the vertebral column and spinal dura grow faster than the spinal cord, a disparity develops between each succeeding cord segment and the exit of its dorsal and ventral nerve roots through the corresponding intervertebral foramina. In the newborn, the cord terminates at the level of L2 or L3. In the adult, the cord usually terminates in the inferior border of L1, and the arachnoid and its enclosed subarachnoid space, which is filled with CSF, do not close down on the filum terminale until they reach the level of S2 (Fig. 47-20). This results in the formation of a pocket of CSF, the *dural cisterna spinalis*, which extends from approximately L2 to S2. Because this area

contains an abundant supply of CSF and the spinal cord does not extend this far, the area often is used for sampling the CSF. A procedure called a *spinal tap*, or puncture, can be done by inserting a special needle into the dural sac at L3 or L4. The spinal roots, which are covered with pia mater, are in little danger of trauma from the needle used for this purpose.

SPINAL NERVES

The peripheral nerves that carry information to and from the spinal cord are called *spinal nerves*. There are 32 or more pairs of spinal nerves (*i.e.*, 8 cervical, 12 thoracic, 5 lumbar, 5 sacral, and 2 or more coccygeal); each pair is named for the segment of the spinal cord from which it exits. Because the first cervical spinal nerve exits the spinal cord just above the first cervical vertebra (C1), the nerve is given the number of the bony vertebra just below it. The numbering is changed for all lower levels, however. An extra cervical nerve, the C8 nerve, exits above the T1 vertebra, and each subsequent nerve is numbered for the vertebra just above its point of exit (see Fig. 47-20).

Each spinal cord segment communicates with its corresponding body segment through the paired segmental spinal nerves (see Fig. 47-13). Each spinal nerve, accompanied by the blood vessels supplying the spinal cord, enters

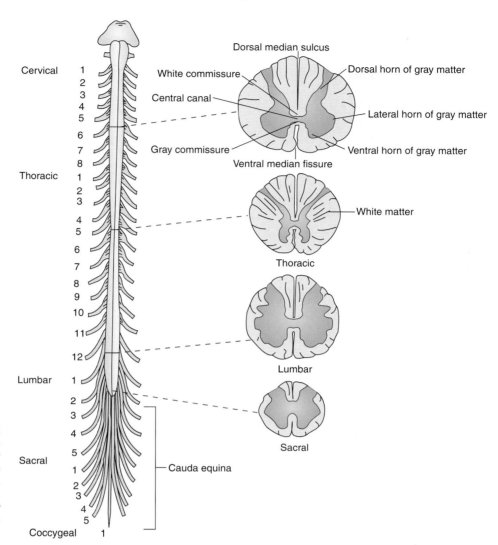

FIGURE 47-18 Cross-sectional views of the spinal cord, showing regional variations in gray matter and increasing white matter as the cord ascends. (Chaffee E.E., Lytle I.M. [1980]. *Basic physiology and anatomy* [4th ed., p. 233]. Philadelphia: J.B. Lippincott)

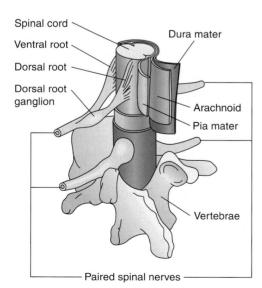

FIGURE 47-19 Spinal cord and meninges. (Chaffee E.E., Lytle I.M. [1980]. *Basic physiology and anatomy* [4th ed., p. 234]. Philadelphia: J.B. Lippincott)

the spinal canal through an intervertebral foramen, where it divides into two branches, or roots. One branch enters the dorsolateral surface of the cord (*i.e.*, dorsal root), carrying the axons of afferent neurons into the CNS. The other branch leaves the ventrolateral surface of the cord (*i.e.*, ventral root), carrying the axons of efferent neurons into the periphery. These two branches or roots fuse at the intervertebral foramen, forming the mixed spinal nerve—"mixed" because it has both afferent and efferent axons.

After emerging from the vertebral column, the spinal nerve divides into two branches or *rami* (singular, *ramus*): a small dorsal primary ramus and a larger ventral primary ramus (Fig. 47-21). The thoracic and upper lumbar spinal nerves also lead to a third branch, the ramus communicans, which contains sympathetic axons supplying the blood vessels, the genitourinary system, and the gastrointestinal system. The dorsal ramus contains sensory fibers from the skin and motor fibers to muscles of the back. The anterior primary ramus contains motor fibers that innervate the skeletal muscles of the anterior body wall and the legs and arms.

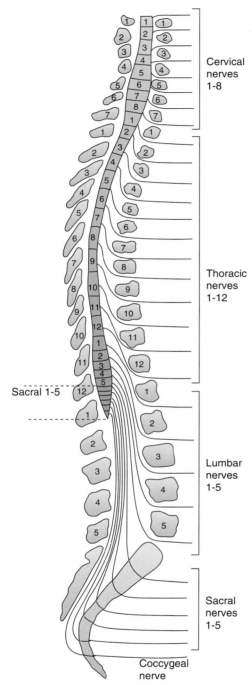

FIGURE 47-20 Relation of segments of the spinal cord and spinal nerves to the vertebral column. (Barr M.L., Kiernan J.A. [1998]. *The human nervous system: An anatomic viewpoint* [5th ed., p. 65]. Philadelphia: J.B. Lippincott)

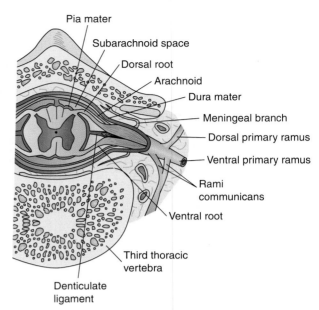

FIGURE 47-21 Cross-section of vertebral column at the level of the third thoracic vertebra, showing the meninges, the spinal cord, and the origin of a spinal nerve and its branches or rami. (Chaffee E.E., Lytle I.M. [1980]. *Basic physiology and anatomy* [4th ed., p. 235]. Philadelphia: J.B. Lippincott)

supply the skin and muscles of the various parts of the body. The PNS contains four major plexuses: the cervical plexus, the brachial plexus, the lumbar plexus, and the sacral plexus.

SPINAL REFLEXES

A *reflex* is a highly predictable relationship between a stimulus and an elicited motor response. Its anatomic basis consists of an afferent neuron, the connection or synapse with CNS interneurons that communicate with the effector neuron, and the effector neuron that innervates a muscle or organ. Reflexes are essentially "wired in" to the CNS in that normally they are always ready to function; with training, most reflexes can be modulated to become parts of more complicated movements. A reflex may involve neurons in a single cord segment (*i.e.*, segmental reflexes), several or many segments (*i.e.*, intersegmental reflexes), or structures in the brain (*i.e.*, suprasegmental reflexes). Two important types of spinal motor reflexes are discussed in this chapter: the myotatic reflex and the withdrawal reflex.

Myotatic or Stretch Reflex

The myotatic or stretch reflex controls muscle tone and helps maintain posture. Specialized sensory nerve terminals in skeletal muscles and tendons relay information on muscle stretch and joint tension to the CNS. This information, which drives postural reflex mechanisms, also is relayed to the thalamus and the sensory cortex and is experienced as *proprioception*, the sense of body movement and position. To provide this information, the muscles and their tendons

Spinal nerves do not go directly to skin and muscle fibers; instead, they form complicated nerve networks called *plexuses*. A plexus is a site of intermixing nerve branches. Many spinal nerves enter a plexus and connect with other spinal nerves before exiting from the plexus. Nerves emerging from a plexus form progressively smaller branches that are supplied with two types of sensory receptors: muscle spindle receptors and Golgi tendon organs. The muscle spindles, which are distributed throughout the belly of a muscle, provide information about muscle length and rate of stretch. The *Golgi tendon organs* are found in muscle tendons and transmit information about muscle tension.

Essentially all skeletal muscles contain many specialized stretch receptor apparatuses called *muscle spindles* (Fig. 47-22). The muscle spindles consist of a group of specialized miniature skeletal muscle fibers called *intrafusal fibers* that are encased in a connective tissue capsule and attached to muscle fibers (*i.e.*, extrafusal fibers) of a skeletal muscle. Two types of intrafusal fibers exist: nuclear bag fibers, named for the large amount of nuclei in their middle, and nuclear chain fibers, in which the nuclei are arranged in a single row. These fibers are supplied by two types of afferent endings: large-diameter primary, or *type Ia*, and smaller secondary, or *type II* fibers. The type Ia fibers, which are stimulated by the rate and amount of stretch, have endings that wind helically around the middle of the spindle intrafusal fibers, where no contractile elements are present. The endings of the type II fibers, which are stimulated only by the degree of stretch, are wound around the contractile elements of the intrafusal fibers, near the end of the spindle.

The extrafusal fibers and the intrafusal fibers are innervated by motoneurons that reside in the ventral horns of the spinal cord. Extrafusal fibers are innervated by large alpha motoneurons that produce contraction of the muscle. The intrafusal fibers are innervated by two types of gamma motoneurons: dynamic gamma axons with endings on the nuclear bag fibers and static gamma axons that innervate the nuclear chain fibers. The intrafusal fibers are equipped to monitor dynamic and static changes in muscle function.

The intrafusal muscle fibers in a spindle function as "skinniness" receptors. When a skeletal muscle is stretched, the spindle and its intrafusal fibers are stretched and therefore become more slender. Increased slenderness of the intrafusal fibers results in an increased firing rate of its afferent fibers. The rate of firing is proportional to the degree of spindle stretch and therefore of extrafusal muscle length. Axons of the spindle afferent neurons enter the spinal cord through the several branches of the dorsal root. Some branches end in the segment of entry and others ascend in the dorsal column of the cord to the medulla of the brain stem. Segmental branches make connections, along with other branches, that pass directly to the anterior gray matter of the spinal cord and establish monosynaptic contact with each of the LMNs that have motor units in the muscle containing the spindle receptor. This produces an opposing muscle contraction. This single-synapse, or monosynaptic, connection is the only known instance of a direct afferent-to-efferent reflex in the nervous system. Another segmental branch of the same afferent neuron innervates an internuncial neuron that is inhibitory to motor units of antagonistic muscle groups. Inhibition of these muscle units helps in opposing muscle stretch.

Branches of the afferent axon also ascend the spinal cord, sending collateral branches into the dorsal horn of the adjacent segments influencing reflex function at each level. The intersegmental reflexes are particularly important

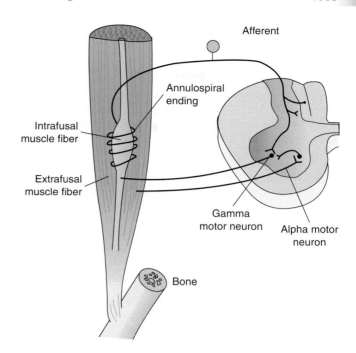

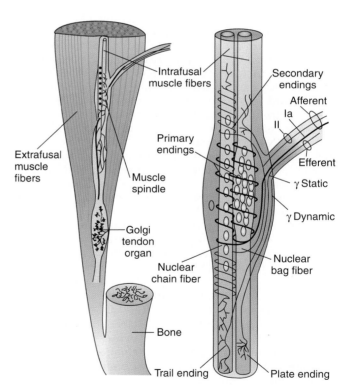

FIGURE 47-22 (Top) Spinal cord innervation of muscle spindle and Golgi tendon organ. Cell bodies from both the alpha motoneurons that innervate the extrafusal muscle fibers and the gamma (γ) fibers that innervate the intrafusal fibers reside in the ventral horns of the spinal cord and are activated by the same afferent systems. (**Bottom**) Golgi tendon organ and extrafusal muscle fibers (*left*) and the nuclear bag fiber and nuclear chain fiber of the interfusal fibers of the muscle spindle (*right*). (Modified from Rhoades R.A., Tanner G.A. [1996]. *Medical physiology.* [p. 94]. Boston: Little, Brown)

in coordinating hand, leg, neck, and limb movements. Ascending fibers from the stretch reflex ultimately provide information about muscle length to the cerebellum and cerebral cortex.

The role of afferent spindle fibers is to inform the CNS of the status of muscle length. When a skeletal muscle lengthens or shortens against tension, a feedback mechanism needs to be available for readjustment such that the spindle apparatus remains sensitive to moment-to-moment changes in muscle stretch, even while changes in muscle length are occurring. This is accomplished by the gamma motoneurons that adjust spindle fiber length to match the length of the extrafusal muscle fiber. Descending fibers of motor pathways synapse with and simultaneously activate both alpha and gamma motoneurons so that the sensitivity of the spindle fibers is coordinated with muscle movement.

In the muscles that are supporting body weight, the stretch reflex operates continuously, producing a continuous resistance to passive stretch called *muscle tone*. An abnormal increase or decrease in muscle tone suggests that the stretch reflex is not functioning normally or that the excitability of the alpha LMNs innervating the muscle is abnormal. Reduced excitability of the stretch reflex results in decreased muscle tone, or hypotonia, ranging from postural weakness to total flaccid paralysis. It can result from decreased function of the descending facilatory systems controlling the gamma LMNs that innervate the muscle or damage to the stretch reflex or peripheral nerves innervating the muscle. Hypertonia, or spasticity, is an abnormal increase in muscle tone. It can result from increased excitation or loss of inhibition of the spindle's gamma LMNs or changes in the segmental spinal cord circuitry controlling the stretch reflex. The result is strong facilitation of transmission in the monosynaptic reflex pathway from Ia sensory fibers to the alpha LMNs. It is characterized by hyperactive tendon reflexes and an increase in resistance to rapid muscle stretch. An active muscle contraction occurs only during rapid stretch; when the muscle is held in a lengthen position, the reflex contraction subsides. Spasticity commonly occurs with UMN lesions such as those that exist after spinal shock in persons with spinal cord injury (see Chapter 49). Rigidity is a greatly increased resistance to movements in all directions. It is caused by increased activation of the alpha LMNs innervating the extrafusal muscle fibers and does not depend on the dorsal root innervation of the intrafusal spindle fibers.

The muscle tone in the agonist and antagonist muscles around a joint provides for a fixed, stable situation. Central control over the gamma LMN mechanism permits increases or decreases in muscle tone in anticipation of changes in the muscle force required to oppose ongoing conditions, such as when weight is about to be lifted. The CNS, through its coordinated control of the muscle's alpha LMNs and the spindle's gamma LMNs, can suppress the stretch reflex. This occurs during centrally programmed movements such as pitching a baseball, permitting the muscle to produce its greatest range of motion. Without this programmed adjustability of the stretch reflex, any movement is immediately opposed and prevented. All reflex and learned movement patterns involve programmed control of gamma

Assessment of Deep Tendon Reflexes

The status of the stretch reflex can be determined by assessing muscle tone and deep tendon reflexes. Clinically, muscle tone is evaluated by asking a person to relax while supporting the limb except at the joint that is being examined. The distal part of the extremity is then moved passively around the joint. Normally, there is a mild resistance to movement. A method for assessing muscle stretch excitability is to tap the tendon of a muscle briskly with a reflex hammer, which is normally immediately followed by a sudden contraction or *muscle jerk*, as illustrated. The stretch reflex has been "tricked" by the sudden tug on the tendon. A synchronous burst of afferent Ia nerve activity from the many spindles in the muscle results in essentially simultaneous firing of a large number of lower motoneuron units. The stretch reflex was tricked into responding, as though the muscle had been suddenly stretched. These muscle jerk reflexes are called *deep tendon reflexes* (DTRs). They usually are checked at the wrists, elbows, knees, and Achilles tendons.

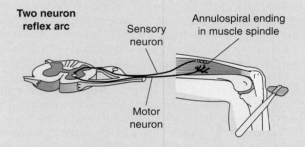

Two neuron reflex arc
Sensory neuron
Annulospiral ending in muscle spindle
Motor neuron

Testing the stretch reflex with a reflex hammer.

The DTRs can provide much information in a brief period. A normal-range DTR indicates that the afferent peripheral process in the peripheral muscle and nerves is normal; the dorsal root ganglion function is normal; the dorsal root function is normal; and the dorsal, intermediate, and ventral horns are functioning appropriately, as are the ventral root and lower motoneuron cell body and axon. It also means that the neuromuscular synapse is functioning normally; the muscle fibers are capable of normal contraction; and suprasegmental input is normal. Using this method of assessment, it is possible to test the function of many spinal nerves and spinal cord segments and some of the cranial nerves and brain stem segments in a short time. If abnormality of excitability is detected, further tests are required to determine the nature and location of the pathologic process.

efferents, resulting in continuous readjustments of stretch reflex sensitivity in agonists, antagonists, and synergists as the movement progresses. The status of the stretch reflex can be determined by assessing muscle tone and deep tendon reflexes.

Inverse Myotatic Reflex

The *inverse myotatic reflex*, most prominent in antigravity extensor muscles, reduces the strength of alpha LMN–driven muscle contraction when the force generated by the muscle threatens the integrity of the muscle or tendon. This protective reflex, which consists of two or more synapses in its path, has a very high threshold and activates inhibitory interneurons in the ventral horn that decrease the firing rate of alpha LMNs. Type II muscle spindle afferents in the Golgi tendon apparatus and nociceptive afferents from the connective tissue of muscle and tendon units drive this high-threshold protective reflex. The inverse myotatic reflex also has a contralateral component. If, for example, the inverse myotatic reflex produced relaxation of the quadriceps in one leg, the contralateral component would produce contraction in the quadriceps of the other leg. The inverse myotatic reflex provides postural stability to ambulatory movements. For example, when the inverse myotatic reflex produces relaxation of antigravity muscles (with flexion) of one leg as we walk, the contralateral component produces contraction and extension of the opposite leg.

In persons with spastic paralysis, the inverse myotatic reflex becomes hyperactive and produces what is called the *clasp-knife reaction*. If an examiner were passively to flex the lower limb of such a person at the knee, increasing resistance would be encountered. This resistance would continue to increase until, at some point, it would abruptly cease and the leg could then be passively flexed. Similar signs are seen in spastic upper limbs.

Withdrawal Reflex

The withdrawal reflex is stimulated by a damaging (nociceptive) stimulus and quickly moves the body part away from the offending stimulus, usually by flexing a limb part (Fig. 47-23). The withdrawal reflex is a powerful reflex, taking precedence over other reflexes associated with locomotion. Any of the major joints may be involved, depending on the site of afferent stimulation. All the joints of an extremity (*e.g.*, finger, wrist, elbow, shoulder) typically are involved. This complex, polysynaptic reflex also shifts postural support to the opposite side of the body with a crossed extensor reflex and simultaneously alerts the forebrain to the offending stimulus event. The withdrawal reflex also can produce contraction of muscles other than the extremities. For example, irritation of the abdominal viscera may cause contraction of the abdominal muscles.

In summary, in the adult, the spinal cord is in the upper two thirds of the spinal canal of the vertebral column. On transverse section, the spinal cord has an oval shape and the internal gray matter has the appearance of a

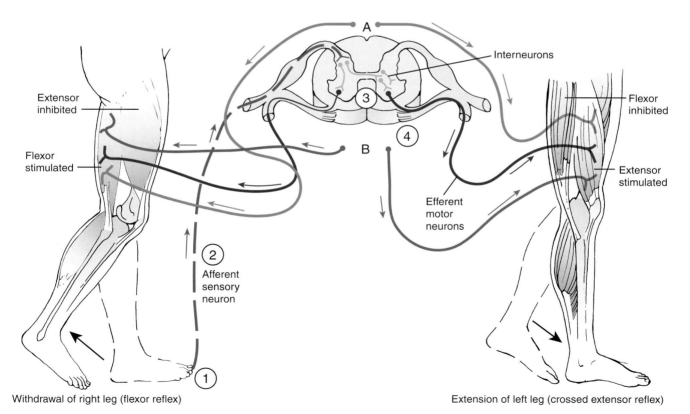

Withdrawal of right leg (flexor reflex)

Extension of left leg (crossed extensor reflex)

FIGURE 47-23 Crossed extensor reflex. Ipsilateral and contralateral circuitry, including interneurons, are shown for one spinal segment: (1) stepping on a painful object, (2) excitation of afferent sensory neurons, (3) integration of spinal cord circuitry, and (4) excitation of efferent motor neurons. Lower motoneuron outputs from more rostral (**A**) and more caudal (**B**) segments are also indicated. These outputs are via ascending and descending interneurons. Inhibitory circuits are not shown.

butterfly or letter "H." The dorsal horns contain the IA neurons and receive afferent information from dorsal root and other connecting neurons. The ventral horns contain the OA neurons and efferent LMNs that leave the cord by the ventral roots.

Thirty-two pairs of spinal nerves (*i.e.*, 8 cervical, 12 thoracic, 5 lumbar, 5 sacral, and 2 or more coccygeal) are present. Each pair communicates with its corresponding body segments. The spinal nerves and the blood vessels that supply the spinal cord enter the spinal canal through an intervertebral foramen. After entering the foramen, they divide into two branches, or roots, one of which enters the dorsolateral surface of the cord (*i.e.*, dorsal root), carrying the axons of afferent neurons into the CNS. The other root leaves the ventrolateral surface of the cord (*i.e.*, ventral root), carrying the axons of efferent neurons into the periphery. These two roots fuse at the intervertebral foramen, forming the mixed spinal nerve.

A reflex provides a highly reliable relation between a stimulus and a motor response. Its anatomic basis consists of an afferent neuron, the connection or synapse with CNS neurons that communicate with the effector neuron, and the effector neuron that innervates a muscle or organ. Reflexes are essentially "wired in" to the CNS in that normally they always are ready to function; with training, most reflexes can be modulated to become parts of more complicated movements.

Two important types of spinal motor reflexes are the myotatic or stretch reflex and the withdrawal reflex. The myotatic reflex controls muscle tone and is important in maintaining posture. The withdrawal reflex is stimulated by any tissue-threatening or damaging stimulus and quickly moves the body part away from the offending stimulus. Hundreds of reflexes exist, including those involved in stepping, gagging, swallowing, and inspiration. These are polysynaptic and complex, except for the disynaptic inverse myotatic reflex and monosynaptic stretch reflex.

The Brain

After you have completed this section of the chapter, you should be able to meet the following objectives:

✦ List the structures of the hindbrain, midbrain, and forebrain and describe their functions
✦ Name the cranial nerves and cite their location and function
✦ State the characteristics of the dominant and non-dominant hemispheres of the brain
✦ Describe the characteristics of the CSF and trace its passage through the ventricular system
✦ Contrast and compare the blood-brain and CSF-brain barriers

The brain is divided into three regions, the hindbrain, the midbrain, and the forebrain. The hindbrain includes the medulla oblongata, the pons, and its dorsal outgrowth, the

cerebellum. Midbrain structures include two pairs of dorsal enlargements, the superior and inferior colliculi. The forebrain, which consists of two hemispheres and is covered by the cerebral cortex, contains central masses of gray matter, the basal ganglia, and the rostral end of the neural tube, the diencephalon with its adult derivatives—the thalamus and hypothalamus.

An important concept is that the more rostral, recently developed parts of neural tube gain dominance or control over regions and functions at lower levels. They do not replace the more ancient circuitry but merely dominate it. After damage to the more vulnerable parts of the forebrain, as occurs with brain death, a brain stem–controlled organism remains that is capable of breathing and may survive if the environmental temperature is regulated and nutrition and other aspects of care are provided. However, all aspects of intellectual function, experience, perception, and memory usually are permanently lost. The organization of content in this section moves from the more ancient circuitry of the hindbrain to the more dominant and recently developed structures of the forebrain.

HINDBRAIN

The term *brain stem* often is used to include the hindbrain, pons, and midbrain. These regions of the neural tube have the organization of spinal cord segments, except that more of the longitudinal cell columns are present, reflecting the increased complexity of the cranial segmental nerves. In the brain stem, the structure and function of the reticular formation have been greatly expanded. In the pons and medulla, the reticular formation contains networks controlling basic breathing, eating, and locomotion functions. Higher-level integration of these functions occurs in the midbrain. The reticular formation is surrounded on the outside by the long tract systems that connect the forebrain with lower parts of the CNS (Fig. 47-24).

Medulla

The *medulla oblongata* represents the caudal five segments of the brain part of the neural tube; the cranial nerve branches entering and leaving it have functions similar to the spinal segmental nerves. Although the ventral horn areas in the medulla are quite small, the dorsal horn areas are enlarged, processing a large amount of the information pouring through the cranial nerves. The segmental peripheral nerve components of the medulla can be divided into those leaving the neural tube ventromedially (*i.e.*, hypoglossal and abducens cranial nerves) or dorsolaterally (*i.e.*, vagus, spinal accessory, glossopharyngeal, and vestibulocochlear cranial nerves). Because pathologic signs and symptoms reflect the spatial segregation of brain stem components, neurologic syndromes resulting from trauma, tumors, aneurysms, and cerebrovascular accidents often are classified as ventral or dorsolateral syndromes.

The general somatic efferent LMNs of the lower segments of the medulla supply the extrinsic and intrinsic muscles of the tongue by means of the *hypoglossal nerve*, or *cranial nerve XII* (Table 47-2). Damage to the hypoglossal nerve results in weakness or paralysis of tongue muscles.

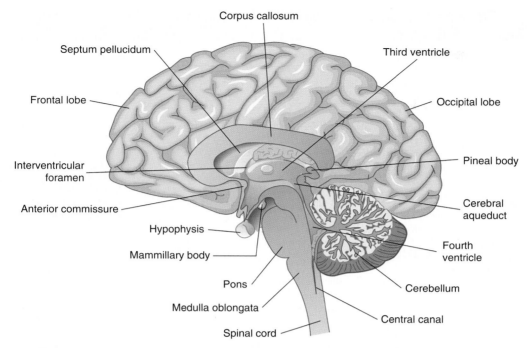

FIGURE 47-24 Midsagittal section of the brain. (Chaffee E.E., Lytle I.M. [1980]. *Basic physiology and anatomy* [4th ed., p. 214]. Philadelphia: J.B. Lippincott)

When the tongue is protruded, it deviates toward the damaged and therefore weaker side because of the greater protrusion strength on the normal side. Axons of the hypoglossal nerve exit the medulla adjacent to two long, longitudinal ridges along the medial undersurface of the medulla. These ridges, called the *pyramids*, contain the corticospinal fibers, most of which cross to descend in the lateral column to the opposite side of the spinal cord. Lesions of the ventral surface of the caudal medulla result in the syndrome of alternating hypoglossal hemiplegia. These lesions are characterized by signs of ipsilateral (*i.e.*, same side) denervation of the tongue and contralateral (*i.e.*, opposite side) weakness or paralysis of both the upper and lower extremities.

The *vagus nerve*, or *cranial nerve X*, has several afferent (sensory) and efferent (motor) components. General somatic afferent neurons innervate the external ear, whereas special visceral afferent neurons innervate the pharyngeal taste buds. Sensory and motor components of the nerve innervate the pharynx, the gastrointestinal tract (from the laryngeal pharynx to the mid-transverse colon), the heart, the spleen, and the lungs. Initiation of many essential reflexes and normal functions depends on intact vagal innervation. For example, 80% of the fibers of the vagus are afferents, some of which are involved in vomiting and hiccup reflexes and in ongoing feedback during swallowing and speech. The unilateral loss of vagal function can result in slowed gastrointestinal motility, a permanently husky voice, and deviation of the uvula away from the damaged side. Bilateral loss of vagal function can seriously damage reflex maintenance of cardiovascular and respiratory reflexes. Swallowing may become difficult and, occasionally, paralysis of laryngeal structures causes life-threatening airway obstruction.

The sternocleidomastoid, a powerful head-turning muscle, and the trapezius muscle, which elevates the shoulders, are innervated by the *spinal accessory nerve*, or *cranial nerve XI*, with LMNs in the upper four cervical spinal segments. Intermediate rootlets from these segmental levels combine and enter the cranial cavity through the foramen magnum and exit the jugular foramen with cranial nerves IX and X. Loss of spinal accessory nerve function results in drooping of the shoulder on the damaged side and weakness when turning the head to the opposite side.

The dorsolateral *glossopharyngeal nerve*, or *cranial nerve IX*, contains the same components as the vagus nerve but for a more rostral segment of the gastrointestinal tract and the pharynx. This nerve provides the special visceral sensory innervation of the taste buds of the oral pharynx and the back of the tongue; the afferent innervation of the oral pharynx and the baroreceptors of the carotid sinus; the efferent innervation of the otic ganglion, which controls the salivary function of the parotid gland; and the efferent innervation of the stylopharyngeus muscles of the pharynx. This cranial nerve seldom is damaged, but when it is, anesthesia of the ipsilateral oral pharynx develops along with dry mouth resulting from reduced salivation.

The special sensory afferent *vestibulocochlear nerve*, or *cranial nerve VIII*, formerly called the *auditory nerve*, is attached laterally at the junction of the medulla oblongata and the pons, often called the *caudal pons*. It consists of two distinct fiber divisions, the cochlear and vestibular divisions, both of which are sensory. The cochlear division arises from cell bodies in the cochlea in the inner ear and transmits impulses related to the sense of hearing. The vestibular divi-

TABLE 47-2 ✦ The Segmental Nerves and Their Components

Segment and Nerve	Component	Innervation	Function
1. Forebrain			
I. Olfactory	SVA	Receptors in olfactory mucosa	Reflexes, olfaction (smell)
2. II. Optic nerve		Optic nerve and retina (part of brain system, not a peripheral nerve)	
3. Midbrain			
V. Trigeminal (V₁) ophthalmic division	SSA	Muscles: upper face: forehead, upper lid	Facial expression, proprioception
	GSA	Skin, subcutaneous tissue; conjunctiva; frontal/ethmoid sinuses	Somesthesia Reflexes (blink)
III. Oculomotor	GVE	Iris sphincter Ciliary muscle	Pupillary constriction Accommodation
	GSE	Extrinsic eye muscles	Eye movement, lid movement
4. Pons			
V. Trigeminal (V₂) maxillary division	SSA	Muscles: facial expression	Proprioception Reflexes (sneeze), somesthesia
	GSA	Skin, oral mucosa, upper teeth, hard palate, maxillary sinus	
V. Trigeminal (V₃) mandibular division	SSA	Lower jaw, muscles: mastication	Proprioception, jaw jerk
	GSA	Skin, mucosa, teeth, anterior ⅔ of tongue	Reflexes, somesthesia
	PE	Muscles: mastication tensor tympani tensor veli palantini	Mastication: speech Protects ear from loud sound Tenses soft palate
IV. Trochlear	GSE	Extrinsic eye muscle	Moves eye down and in
5. Caudal Pons			
VIII. Vestibular, cochlear (vestibulocochlear)	SSA	Vestibular end organs Organ of Corti	Reflexes, sense of head position Reflexes, hearing
VII. Facial nerve, intermedius portion	GSA	External auditory meatus	Somesthesia
	GVA	Nasopharynx	Gag reflex: sensation
	SVA	Taste buds of anterior ⅔ of tongue	Reflexes: gustation (taste)
	GVE	Nasopharynx	Mucous secretion, reflexes
		Lacrimal, sublingual, submandibular glands	Lacrimation, salivation
Facial nerve	PE	Muscles: facial expression, stapedius	Facial expression Protects ear from loud sounds
VI. Abducens	GSE	Extrinsic eye muscle	Lateral eye deviation
6. Middle Medulla			
IX. Glossopharyngeal	SSA	Stylopharyngeus muscle	Proprioception
	GSA	Posterior external ear	Somesthesia
	SVA	Taste buds of posterior ⅓ of tongue	Gustation (taste)
	GVA	Oral pharynx	Gag reflex: sensation
	GVE	Parotid gland; pharyngeal mucosa	Salivary reflex: mucous secretion
	PE	Stylopharyngeus muscle	Assists swallowing
7,8,9,10. Caudal Medulla			
X. Vagus	SSA	Muscles: pharynx, larynx	Proprioception
	GSA	Posterior external ear	Somesthesia
	SVA	Taste buds, pharynx, larynx	Reflexes, gustation
	GVA	Visceral organs (esophagus to mid-transverse colon, liver, pancreas, heart, lungs)	Reflexes, sensation
	GVE	Visceral organs as above	Parasympathetic efferent
	PE	Muscles: pharynx, larynx	Swallowing, phonation, emesis
XIII. Hypoglossal	GSE	Muscles of tongue	Tongue movement, reflexes

(continued)

TABLE 47-2 ✦ The Segmental Nerves and Their Components (Continued)

Segment and Nerve	Component	Innervation	Function
Spinal Segments			
C1–C4 Upper Cervical	PE	Muscles: sternocleidomastoid, trapezius	Head, shoulder movement
XI. Spinal accessory nerve			
Spinal nerves	SSA	Muscles of neck	Proprioception, DTRs
	GSA	Neck, back of head	Somesthesia
	GSE	Neck muscles	Head, shoulder movement
C5–C8 Lower Cervical	SSA	Upper limb muscles	Proprioception, DTRs
	GSA	Upper limbs	Reflexes, somesthesia
	GSE	Upper limb muscles	Movement, posture
T1–L2 Thoracic,	SSA	Muscles: trunk, abdominal wall	Proprioception
Upper Lumbar	GSA	Trunk, abdominal wall	Reflexes, somesthesia
	GVA	All of viscera	Reflexes and sensation
	GVE	All of viscera	Sympathetic reflexes, vasomotor control, sweating, piloerection
	GSE	Muscles: trunk, abdominal wall, back	Movement, posture, respiration
L2–S1 Lower Lumbar,	SSA	Lower limb muscles	Proprioception, DTRs
Upper Sacral	GSA	Lower trunk, limbs, back	Reflexes, somesthesia
	GSE	Muscles: trunk, lower limbs, back	Movement, posture
S2–S4 Lower Sacral	SSA	Muscles: pelvis, perineum	Proprioception
	GSA	Pelvis, genitalia	Reflexes, somesthesia
	GVA	Hindgut, bladder, uterus	Reflexes, sensation
	GVE	Hindgut, visceral organs	Visceral reflexes, defecation, urination, erection
S5–Co2 Lower Sacral,	SSA	Perineal muscles	Proprioception
Coccygeal	GSA	Lower sacrum, anus	Reflexes, somesthesia
	GSE	Perineal muscles	Reflexes, posture

Afferent (sensory) components: SSA, special somatic afferent; GSA, general somatic afferent; SVA, special visceral afferent; GVA, general visceral afferent.
Efferent (motor) components: GVE, general visceral efferent (autonomic nervous system); PE, pharyngeal efferent; GSE, general somatic efferent; DTRs, deep tendon reflexes.

sion arises from two ganglia that innervate cell bodies in the utricle, saccule, and semicircular canals and transmits impulses related to head position and movement of the body through space. Irritation of the cochlear division results in tinnitus (*i.e.*, ringing of the ears); destruction of the nerve results in nerve deafness. Injury to the vestibular division leads to vertigo, nystagmus, and some postural instability (see Chapter 55).

Another segmental branch of the caudal pons, the *facial nerve*, or *cranial nerve VII*, and its intermediate component (the intermedius) contain both afferent and efferent functional components. The nervus intermedius, containing the general somatic afferent, special visceral afferent, general visceral afferent, and general visceral efferent neurons, innervates the nasopharynx and taste buds of the palate. It also innervates the anterior two thirds of the tongue, the submandibular and sublingual salivary glands, the lacrimal glands, and mucous membranes of the nose and roof of the mouth. Loss of this branch of the facial nerve can lead to eye dryness with risk of corneal scarring and blindness. The pharyngeal effer-

ent LMNs of the facial nerve proper innervate muscles that control facial expression, such as wrinkling of the brow and smiling. Unilateral loss of facial nerve function results in flaccid paralysis of the muscles of half the face, a condition called *Bell's palsy*. The facial nerve passes through a bony tunnel behind the middle ear cavity. Sometimes, Bell's palsy has been attributed to inflammatory reactions involving the facial nerve in or near this bony tunnel. Because such injuries result from pressure caused by edematous tissue, the integrity of the endoneurial sheath is retained, and regeneration with full recovery of all muscles usually occurs within several months.

Another segmental nerve branch of the caudal pons, the *abducens nerve*, or *cranial nerve VI*, sends LMNs out ventrally on either side of the pyramids and then forward into the orbit to innervate the lateral rectus muscle of the eye. As the name suggests, the abducens nerve abducts the eye (lateral or outward rotation); peripheral damage to this nerve results in medial strabismus, which is a weakness or loss of eye abduction (see Chapter 54).

Pons

The pons (from the Latin for "bridge") develops from the fifth neural tube segment. The central canal of the spinal cord, which is enlarged in the pons and rostral medulla, forms the fourth ventricle (see Fig. 47-24). An enlarged area on the ventral surface of the pons contains the pontine nuclei, which receive information from all parts of the cerebral cortex. The axons of these neurons form a massive bundle that swings around the lateral side of the fourth ventricle to enter the cerebellum. In the pons, the reticular formation is large and contains the circuitry for masticating food and manipulating the jaws during speech.

The *trigeminal nerve*, or *cranial nerve V*, which has sensory and motor subdivisions, exits the brain stem laterally on the forward surface of the pons. The trigeminal is the main sensory nerve conveying the modalities of pain, temperature, touch, and proprioception to the superficial and deep regions of the face. Regions innervated include the skin of the anterior scalp and face, the conjunctiva and orbit, the meninges, the paranasal sinuses, and the mouth, including the teeth and the anterior two thirds of the tongue. The LMNs of the trigeminal nerve innervate skeletal muscles involved with mastication and contribute to swallowing and speech, movements of the soft palate, and tension of the tympanic membrane through the tensor tympani muscle. The tensor tympani has a protective reflex function, dampening movement of the middle ear ossicles during high-intensity sound.

CEREBELLUM

The cerebellum is located in the posterior fossa of the cranium superior to the pons (see Fig. 47-24). It is separated from the cerebral hemispheres by a fold of dura mater, the tentorium cerebelli. The cerebellum consists of a small unpaired median portion, called the *vermis*, and two large lateral masses, the *cerebellar hemispheres*. In contrast to the brain stem with its external white matter and internal gray nuclei, the cerebellum, like the cerebrum, has an outer cortex of gray matter overlying the white matter. Next to the fourth ventricle, several masses of gray matter, called the *deep cerebellar nuclei*, border the roof of the fourth ventricle. Cells of the cerebellar cortex and deep nuclei interact, and axons from the latter send information to many regions, particularly to the motor cortex by means of a thalamic relay. Synergistic (*i.e.*, temporal and spatial smoothing) functions of the cerebellum participate in all movements of limbs, trunk, head, larynx, and eyes, whether the movement is part of a voluntary movement or of a highly learned semiautomatic or automatic movement. During highly skilled movements, the motor cortex sends signals to the cerebellum, informing it about the movement that is to be performed. The cerebellum makes continuous adjustments, resulting in smoothness of movement, particularly during the delicate maneuvers. Highly skillful movement requires extensive motor training, and considerable evidence suggests many of these learned movement patterns involve cerebellar circuits.

The cerebellum receives proprioceptor input from the vestibular system; feedback from the muscles, tendons, and joints; and indirect signals from the somesthetic, visual, and auditory systems that provide background information for ongoing movement. Sensory and motor information from a given area of the body is sent to the same area in the cerebellum. In this way, the cerebellum can assess continuously the status of each body part—position, rate of movement, and forces such as gravity that are opposing movement. The cerebellum compares what is actually happening with what is intended to happen. It then transmits the appropriate corrective signals back to the motor system, instructing it to increase or decrease the activity of the participating muscle groups so that smooth and accurate movements can be performed.

Another function of the cerebellum is the dampening of muscle movement. All body movements are basically pendular (*i.e.*, swinging back and forth). As movement begins, momentum develops and must be overcome before the movement can be stopped. This momentum would cause movements to overshoot if they were not dampened. In the intact cerebellum, automatic signals stop movement precisely at the intended point. The cerebellum analyzes proprioceptive information to predict the future position of moving parts, their rapidity of movement, and the projected time course of the movement. This allows the cerebellum to inhibit agonist muscles and excite antagonist muscles when movement approaches the intended target.

MIDBRAIN

The midbrain develops from the fourth segment of the neural tube, and its organization is similar to that of a spinal segment. The central canal is reestablished as the cerebral aqueduct, connecting the fourth ventricle with the third ventricle (see Fig. 47-24). Two general somatic efferent cranial nerves, the oculomotor nerve, or cranial nerve III, and the trochlear nerve, or cranial nerve IV, exit the midbrain.

Two prominent bundles of nerve fibers, the *cerebral peduncles*, pass along the ventral surface of the midbrain. These fibers include the corticospinal tracts and are the main motor pathways between the forebrain and the pons. On the dorsal surface, four "little hills," the *superior* and *inferior colliculi*, are areas of cortical formation. The inferior colliculus is involved in directional turning and, to some extent, in experiencing the direction of sound sources. The superior colliculi are essential to the reflex mechanisms that control conjugate eye movements when the visual environment is surveyed.

The ventral central gray matter (*i.e.*, ventral horn) of the midbrain contains the LMNs that innervate most of the skeletal muscles that move the optic globe and raise the eyelids. These axons leave the midbrain through the *oculomotor nerve*, or *cranial nerve III*. This nerve also contains the parasympathetic LMNs that control pupillary constriction and ciliary muscle focusing of the lens. Damage to the ventrally exiting cranial nerve III and to the adjacent cerebral peduncle, which contains the corticospinal axon system on one side, results in paralysis of eye movement combined with contralateral hemiplegia.

A small group of cells in the ventral part of the caudal central gray matter contains the *trochlear nerve*, or *cranial nerve IV*, which innervates the superior oblique eye muscle. This muscle moves the upper part of the eye downward and toward the nose when the eye is adducted, or turned inward. The trochlear nerve exits the dorsal surface of the midbrain and decussates (crosses over) before exiting the brain stem. Lesions of the trochlear nerve affect downward gaze on the side opposite the denervated muscle, producing diplopia, or double vision. Walking downstairs becomes particularly difficult. Because the superior oblique muscle has inward rotation of the optic globe as its major function, persons with trochlear nerve damage usually carry their heads tilted to the side of damage.

FOREBRAIN

The most rostral part of the brain, the forebrain consists of the telencephalon, or "end brain," and the diencephalon, or "between brain." The diencephalon forms the core of the forebrain, and the telencephalon forms the cerebral hemispheres.

Diencephalon

Three of the most forward brain segments form an enlarged dorsal horn and ventral horn with a narrow, deep, enlarged central canal—the third ventricle—separating the two sides. This region is called the *diencephalon*. The dorsal horn part of the diencephalon is the thalamus and subthalamus, and the ventral horn part is the hypothalamus (Fig. 47-25). The optic nerve, or cranial nerve II, and retina are outgrowths of the diencephalon. The structure and function of the optic nerve are presented in Chapter 53.

The thalamus consists of two large, egg-shaped masses, one on either side of the third ventricle. The thalamus is divided into several major parts, and each part is divided into distinct nuclei, which are the major relay stations for information going to and from the cerebral cortex. All sensory pathways have direct projections to thalamic nuclei, which convey the information to restricted areas of the sensory cortex. Coordination and integration of peripheral sensory stimuli occur in the thalamus, along with some crude interpretation of highly emotion-laden auditory experiences that not only occur but can be remembered. For example, a person can recover from a deep coma in which cerebral cortex activity is minimal and remember some of what was said at the bedside.

The thalamus also plays a role in relaying critical information regarding motor activities to and from selected areas of the motor cortex. Two neuronal circuits are significant in this regard. One is the pathway from the cerebral cortex to the pons and cerebellum and then, by way of the thalamus, back to the motor cortex. The second is the feedback circuit that travels from the cortex to the basal ganglia, then to the thalamus, and from the thalamus back to the cortex. The subthalamus also contains movement control systems related to the basal ganglia.

Through its connections with the ascending reticular activating system, the thalamus processes neural influences that are basic to cortical excitatory rhythms (*i.e.*, those recorded on the electroencephalogram), to essential sleep-wakefulness cycles, and to the process of attending to stimuli. Besides their cortical connections, the thalamic nuclei have connections with each other and with neighboring nonthalamic brain structures such as the limbic system. Through their connections with the limbic system, some thalamic nuclei are involved in the relation between stimuli and the emotional responses they evoke.

The ventral horn portion of the diencephalon is the hypothalamus, which borders the third ventricle and includes a ventral extension, the neurohypophysis (*i.e.*, posterior pituitary). The hypothalamus is the area of master-level integration of homeostatic control of the body's internal environment. Maintenance of blood gas concentration,

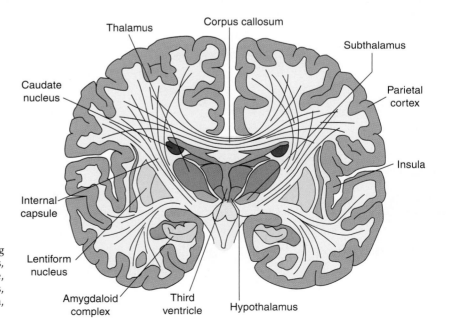

FIGURE 47-25 Frontal section of the brain passing through the third ventricle, showing the thalamus, subthalamus, hypothalamus, internal capsule, corpus callosum, basal ganglia (caudate nucleus, lenticular nucleus), amygdaloid complex, insula, and parietal cortex.

Thalamus
Corpus callosum
Subthalamus
Caudate nucleus
Parietal cortex
Insula
Internal capsule
Lentiform nucleus
Amygdaloid complex
Third ventricle
Hypothalamus

water balance, food consumption, and major aspects of endocrine and autonomic nervous system control require hypothalamic function.

The internal capsule is a broad band of projection fibers that lies between the thalamus medially and the basal ganglia laterally (see Fig. 47-25). It contains all of the fibers that connect the cerebral cortex with deeper structures, including the basal ganglia, thalamus, midbrain, pons, medulla, and spinal cord.

Cerebral Hemispheres

The two cerebral hemispheres are lateral outgrowths of the diencephalon. The cerebral hemispheres contain the lateral ventricles (*i.e.*, ventricles I and II), which are connected with the third ventricle of the diencephalon by a small opening called the *interventricular foramen* (*i.e.*, foramen of Monro). Axons of the olfactory nerve, or cranial nerve I, terminate in the most ancient portion of the cerebrum—the olfactory bulb, where initial processing of olfactory information occurs. Projection axons from the olfactory bulb relay information through the olfactory tracts to the thalamus and to other parts of the cerebral cortex (*i.e.*, orbital cortex), where olfactory-related reflexes and olfactory experience occur.

The *corpus callosum* is a massive commissure, or bridge, of myelinated axons that connects the cerebral cortex of the two sides of the brain. Two smaller commissures, the anterior and posterior commissures, connect the two sides of the more specialized regions of the cerebrum and diencephalon.

The surfaces of the hemispheres are lateral (side), medial (area between the two sides of the brain), and basal (ventral). The cerebral cortex observed laterally is the recently evolved six-layered neocortex. The surface of the hemispheres contains many ridges and grooves. A *gyrus* is the ridge between two grooves, and the groove is called a *sulcus* or *fissure*. The cerebral cortex is arbitrarily divided into lobes named after the bones that cover them: the frontal, parietal, temporal, and occipital lobes (Fig. 47-26).

Basal Ganglia

A section through the cerebral hemispheres reveals the surface of the cerebral cortex, a subcortical layer of white matter made up of masses of myelinated axons and deep masses of gray matter: the basal ganglia that border the lateral ventricle. The basal ganglia lie on either side of the internal capsule, just lateral to the thalamus. The basal ganglia comprise the comma-shaped *caudate* (tailed) nucleus, the shield-shaped *putamen*, and the *globus pallidus* (*i.e.*, "pale globe"). The term *striatum* (*i.e.*, "striped body") refers to the caudate plus the putamen. Together, the globus pallidus and putamen make up the *lentiform* (lens-shaped) *nucleus*.

The basal ganglia supply axial and proximal unlearned and learned postures and movements, which enhance and add gracefulness to UMN-controlled manipulative movements. These background movement functions are called *associated movements*. Intact and functional basal ganglia provide arm swinging during walking and running. Basal ganglia also are involved in follow-through movements that accompany throwing a ball or swinging a club. As with the motor cortex, the nuclei on the left side control movement on the right side of the body, and vice versa. Circuits connecting the premotor cortex and supplementary motor cortex, the basal ganglia, and parts of the thalamus provide associated movements that accompany highly skilled behaviors. Parkinson's disease, Huntington's chorea, and some forms of cerebral palsy, among other dysfunctions involving the basal ganglia, result in a frequent or continuous release of abnormal postural or axial and proximal movement patterns. If damage to the basal ganglia is localized to one side, the movements occur on the opposite side of the body. These automatic movement patterns stop only in sleep, but in some conditions, the movements are so violent that getting to sleep becomes difficult.

Frontal Lobe

The frontal lobe extends from the frontal pole to the central sulcus (*i.e.*, fissure) and is separated from the temporal

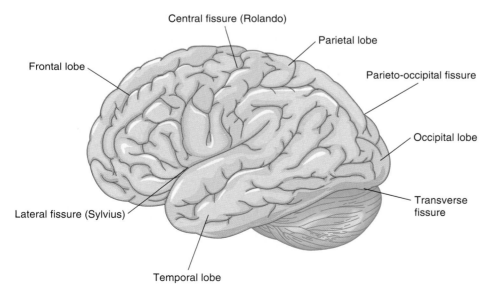

FIGURE 47-26 Lateral aspect of the left cerebral and cerebellar hemispheres. (Chaffee E.E., Lytle I.M. [1980]. *Basic physiology and anatomy* [4th ed., p. 204]. Philadelphia: J.B. Lippincott)

Central fissure (Rolando)

Parietal lobe

Frontal lobe

Parieto-occipital fissure

Occipital lobe

Lateral fissure (Sylvius)

Transverse fissure

Temporal lobe

lobe by the lateral sulcus. The frontal lobe can be subdivided rostrally into the frontal pole and laterally into the superior, middle, and inferior gyri, which continue on the undersurface over the eyes as the orbital cortex. These areas are associated with the medial thalamic nuclei, which also are related to the limbic system. In terms of function, the prefrontal cortex is thought to be involved in anticipation and prediction of consequences of behavior. This "future-oriented" region is particularly depressed by many drugs, including alcohol.

The precentral gyrus (area 4), next to the central sulcus, is the *primary motor cortex* (Fig. 47-27). This area of the cortex provides precise movement control for distal flexor muscles of the hands and feet and of the phonation apparatus required for speech. Just rostral to the precentral gyrus is a region of the frontal cortex called the *premotor* or *motor association cortex*. This region (area 8 and rostral area 6) is involved in the planning of complex learned movement patterns, and damage to these areas results in dyspraxia or apraxia. Such people can manipulate a screwdriver, for instance, but cannot use it to loosen a screw. The primary motor cortex and the association motor cortex are connected with lateral thalamic nuclei, through which they receive feedback information from the basal ganglia and cerebellum. On the medial surface of the hemisphere, the premotor area includes a *supplementary motor cortex* involved in the control of bilateral movement patterns requiring great dexterity.

Parietal Lobe

The parietal lobe of the cerebrum lies behind the central sulcus (*i.e.*, postcentral gyrus) and above the lateral sulcus. The strip of cortex bordering the central sulcus is called the *primary somatosensory cortex* (areas 3, 1, and 2) because it receives very discrete sensory information from the lateral nuclei of the thalamus. Just behind the primary sensory cortex is the *somesthetic association cortex* (areas 5 and 7), which is connected with the thalamic nuclei and with the primary

sensory cortex. This region is necessary for somesthetic perception (*i.e.*, appreciation of the meaningfulness [gnosis] of integrated sensory information from various sensory systems), especially concerning perception of "where" the stimulus is in space and in relation to body parts. Localized lesions of this region can result in the inability to recognize the meaningfulness of an object (*i.e.*, agnosia). With the person's eyes closed, a screwdriver can be felt and described as to shape and texture. Nevertheless, the person cannot integrate the sensory information required to identify it as a screwdriver (*i.e.*, astereognosis). Somesthetic functions of the sensory cortex are discussed further in Chapter 48.

Temporal Lobe

The temporal lobe lies below the lateral sulcus and merges with the parietal and occipital lobes. It includes the temporal pole and three primary gyri, the superior, middle, and inferior gyri. It is separated from the limbic areas on the ventral surface by the collateral or rhinal sulcus. The primary auditory cortex (area 41) involves the part of the superior temporal gyrus that extends into the lateral sulcus (see Fig. 47-27). This area is particularly important in discrimination of sounds entering opposite ears. It receives auditory input projections by way of the inferior colliculus of the midbrain and a ventrolateral thalamic nucleus. The more exposed part of the superior temporal gyrus involves the auditory association or perception area (area 22). The gnostic aspects of hearing (*e.g.*, the meaning of a certain sound pattern) require the function of this area. The remaining portion of the temporal cortex is less defined functionally, but apparently is important in long-term memory recall. This is particularly true with respect to perception and memory of complex sensory patterns such as geometric figures and faces (*i.e.*, recognition of "what" or "who" the stimulus is). Irritation or stimulation can result in vivid hallucinations of long-past events. These higher-order temporal and parietal cortical regions are connected with a large, recently evolved dorsal lateral thalamic nuclear complex.

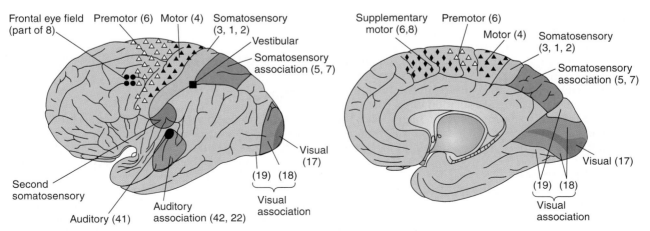

FIGURE 47-27 Motor and sensory areas of the cerebral cortex. (**Left**) The lateral view of the left (dominant) side is drawn as though the lateral sulcus had been pried open, exposing the insula. (**Right**) The diagram represents the areas in a brain that has been sectioned in the median plane. (Reproduced by permission from Nolte J. [1981]. *The human brain*. St. Louis: C.V. Mosby)

The cortices of the frontal, parietal, and temporal lobes, surrounding the older cortex of the insula, located deep in the lateral fissure, represent the most recently evolved parts of the cerebral cortex. These areas contain primary and association functions for motor control and somesthesias for the lips and tongue and for audition; they are particularly involved in speech mechanisms.

Occipital Lobe

The occipital lobe lies posterior to the temporal and parietal lobes and is only arbitrarily separated from them. The medial surface of the occipital lobe contains a deep sulcus extending from the limbic lobe to the occipital pole, the *calcarine sulcus*, which is surrounded by the primary visual cortex (area 17). Stimulation of this cortex causes the experience of bright lights (phosphenes) in the visual field. Just superior and inferior and extending onto the lateral side of the occipital pole is the *visual association cortex* (areas 18 and 19). This area is closely connected with the primary visual cortex and with complex nuclei of the thalamus. Integrity of the association cortex is required for gnostic visual function, by which the meaningfulness of visual experience, including experiences of color, motion, depth perception, pattern, form, and location in space, takes place.

The neocortical areas of the parietal lobe, between the somesthetic and the visual cortices, have a function in relating the texture, or "feel," and location of an object with its visual image. Between the auditory and visual association areas, the *parieto-occipital region* is necessary for relating the meaningfulness of a sound and image to an object or person.

Limbic System

The medial aspect of the cerebrum is organized into concentric bands of cortex, the *limbic system* (*limbic* = borders), which surrounds the connection between the lateral and third ventricles. The innermost band just above and below the cut surface of the corpus callosum is folded out of sight but is an ancient, three-layered cortex ending as the hippocampus in the temporal lobe. Just outside the folded area is a band of transitional cortex, which includes the cingulate and the parahippocampal gyri (Fig. 47-28). This limbic lobe has reciprocal connections with the medial and the intralaminar nuclei of the thalamus, with the deep nuclei of the cerebrum (*e.g.*, amygdaloid nuclei, septal nuclei), and with the hypothalamus. Overall, this region of the brain is involved in emotional experience and in the control of emotion-related behavior. Stimulation of specific areas in this system can lead to feelings of dread, high anxiety, or exquisite pleasure. It also can result in violent behaviors, including attack, defense, or explosive and emotional speech.

Cerebral Dominance

Cerebral dominance refers to the fact that control of certain learned forms of behavior is exerted primarily by one of the two cerebral hemispheres. Handedness, perception of language, performance of speech, and appreciation of spatial relations are primarily expressions of one or the other hemisphere. By convention, speech is used to designate the dominant hemisphere. The dominant hemisphere has a

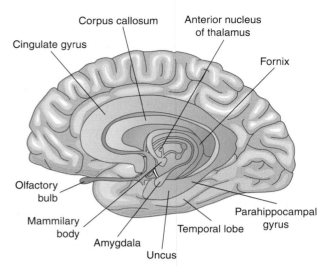

FIGURE 47-28 The limbic system includes the limbic cortex (cingulate gyrus, parahippocampal gyrus, uncus) and associated subcortical structures (thalamus, hypothalamus, amygdala). (Chaffee E.E., Lytle I.M. [1980]. *Basic physiology and anatomy* [4th ed., p. 211]. Philadelphia: J.B. Lippincott)

major role in verbal and analytic abilities; the nondominant hemisphere has a lesser role in these functions and a major role in nonverbal and spatial abilities. Although it is assumed that the dominance of speech and handedness are assigned to the same hemisphere, this is not always the case. In clinical practice, communication dominance is the determinant of cerebral dominance. In most persons, even left-handed persons, the left hemisphere is the dominant hemisphere for speech. Because of substantial overlap, the concept of strict lateralization may not be appropriate other than in primary sensory areas.

The interhemispheric communication pathways are largely undeveloped at birth. The communication between the two hemispheres increases with age and is well developed by the second or third year of life. Cerebral dominance probably develops gradually throughout childhood. This explains why a child with an injury to the normally dominant hemisphere often can be trained to become left-handed and proficient in speech, but an older person with similar deficits finds such learning difficult or impossible.

MENINGES

Inside the skull and vertebral column, the brain and spinal cord are loosely suspended and protected by several connective tissue sheaths called the *meninges* (Fig. 47-29). The surfaces of the spinal cord, brain, and segmental nerves are covered with a delicate connective tissue layer called the *pia mater* (Latin for "delicate mother"). The surface blood vessels and those that penetrate the brain and spinal cord are encased in this protective tissue layer. A second, very delicate, nonvascular, and waterproof layer, called the *arachnoid*, encloses the entire CNS (Fig. 47-30). The arachnoid layer is named for its spider web appearance. The CSF is contained in the subarachnoid space. Immediately out-

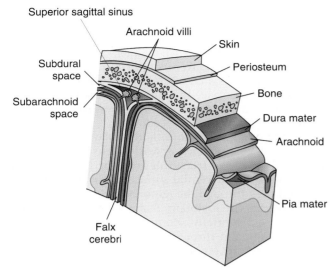

FIGURE 47-29 The cranial meninges. Arachnoid villi, shown with-in the superior sagittal sinus, are one site of cerebrospinal fluid absorption into the blood. (Chaffee E.E., Lytle I.M. [1980]. *Basic physiology and anatomy* [4th ed., p. 218]. Philadelphia: J.B. Lippincott)

side the arachnoid is a continuous sheath of strong connective tissue, the *dura mater* (*i.e.,* "tough mother"), which provides the major protection for the brain and spinal cord. The cranial dura often splits into two layers, with the outer layer serving as the periosteum of the inner surface of the skull.

The inner layer of the dura forms two major folds. The first, a longitudinal fold called the *falx cerebri*, separates the cerebral hemispheres and fuses with a second transverse fold, called the *tentorium cerebelli* (Fig. 47-31). The tentorium cerebelli acts as a hammock, supporting the occipital lobes above the cerebellum. The tentorium forms a tough septum, separating the anterior and middle cranial fossae, which

contain the cerebral hemispheres, from the posterior fossa, found interiorly and containing the brain stem and cerebellum. The tentorium attaches to the petrous portion of the temporal bone and the dorsum sellae of the cranial floor, with a semicircular gap, or incisura, formed at the midline to permit the midbrain to pass forward from the posterior fossa. This compartmentalization is the basis for the commonly used terms *supratentorial* (*i.e.,* above the tentorium) and *infratentorial* (*i.e.,* below the tentorium). The cerebral hemispheres and the diencephalon are supratentorial structures, and the pons, cerebellum, and medulla are infratentorial structures.

The tentorium and falx cerebri normally support and protect the brain, which floats in the CSF within the enclosed space. During extreme trauma, however, the sharp edges of these folds can damage the brain. Space-occupying lesions such as enlarging tumors or hematomas can squeeze the brain against these edges or through the incisura of the tentorium (*i.e.,* herniation). As a result, brain tissue can be compressed, contused, or destroyed, often causing permanent deficits (see Chapter 50).

VENTRICULAR SYSTEM AND CEREBROSPINAL FLUID

The ventricular system is a series of CSF-filled cavities in the brain (Fig. 47-32). The CSF provides a supporting and protective fluid in which the brain and spinal cord float. CSF helps maintain a constant ionic environment that serves as a medium for diffusion of nutrients, electrolytes, and metabolic end-products into the extracellular fluid surrounding CNS neurons and glia. Filling the ventricles, the CSF supports the mass of the brain. Because it fills the subarachnoid space surrounding the CNS, a physical force delivered to either the skull or spine is to some extent diffused and cushioned.

The lining of the ventricles and central canal of the spinal cord is called the *ependyma*. There is a tremendous

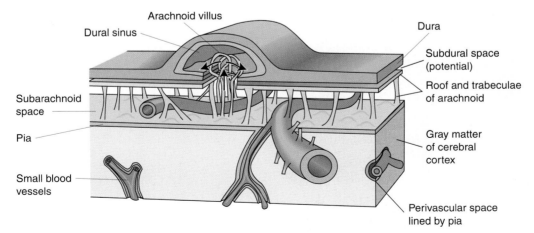

FIGURE 47-30 Schematic diagram of the three connective tissue membranes (pia, arachnoid, and dura) constituting the meninges of the central nervous system. Cerebrospinal fluid is resorbed (*arrows*) by way of the arachnoid villi projecting into the dural sinuses. (From Cormack D.H. [1987]. *Ham's histology* [9th ed., p. 367]. Philadelphia: J.B. Lippincott)

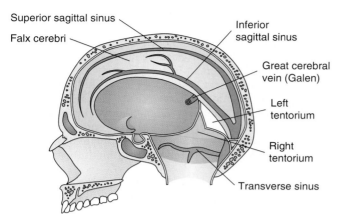

FIGURE 47-31 Cranial dura mater. The skull is open to show the falx cerebri and the right and left portions of the tentorium cerebelli, as well as some of the cranial venous sinuses. (Chaffee E.E., Lytle I.M. [1980]. *Basic physiology and anatomy* [4th ed., p. 219]. J.B. Lippincott)

expansion of the ependyma in the roof of the lateral, third and fourth ventricles. The CSF is produced by tiny reddish masses of specialized capillaries from the pia mater, called the *choroid plexus*, that project into the ventricles. CSF is an ultrafiltrate of blood plasma, composed of 99% water with other constituents, making it close to the composition of the brain extracellular fluid (Table 47-3). Humans secrete approximately 500 mL of CSF each day. However, only approximately 150 mL is in the ventricular system at any one time, meaning that the CSF is continuously being absorbed.

The CSF produced in the ventricles must flow through the interventricular foramen, the third ventricle, the cerebral aqueduct, and the fourth ventricle to exit from the neural tube. Three openings, or foramina, allow the CSF to pass into the subarachnoid space. Two of these, the foramina of Luschka, are located at the lateral corners of the fourth ventricle. The third, the medial foramen of Magendie, is in the midline at the caudal end of the fourth ventricle (see Fig. 47-32). Approximately 30% of the CSF passes down into the subarachnoid space that surrounds the spinal cord, mainly on its dorsal surface, and moves back up to the cranial cavity along its ventral surface.

Reabsorption of CSF into the vascular system occurs along the sides of the superior sagittal sinus in the anterior and middle fossa. To reach this area, the CSF must pass along the sides and ventral surface of the medulla and pons and then through the tentorial incisura or opening that surrounds the midbrain. Some of the CSF exits the posterior fossa ventrally, along the sides of the basilar artery rostrally and through a CSF cistern between the midbrain peduncles (*i.e.*, basilar cistern). The major part of the flow continues along the sides of the hypothalamus to the region of the optic chiasm and then laterally and superiorly along the lateral fissure and over the parietal cortex to the superior sagittal sinus region. Here, the waterproof arachnoid has protuberances, the arachnoid villi, that penetrate the inner dura and venous walls of the superior sagittal sinus.

The reabsorption of CSF into the vascular system occurs through a pressure gradient. The normal CSF pressure is approximately 130 H_2O (10 mm Hg) in the lateral recumbent position, although it may be as low as 65 mm H_2O to as high as 195 mm H_2O, even in healthy persons. The microstructures of the arachnoid villi are such that if the CSF pressure falls below approximately 50 mm H_2O, the passageways collapse, and reverse flow is blocked. The arachnoid villi function as one-way valves, permitting CSF outflow into the blood but not allowing blood to pass into the arachnoid spaces.

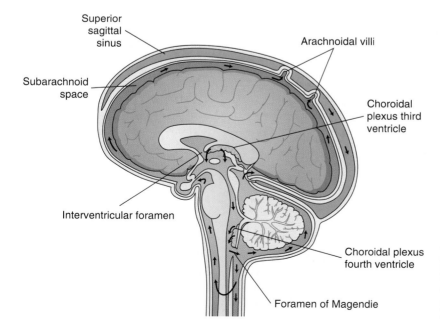

FIGURE 47-32 The flow of cerebrospinal fluid from the time of its formation from blood in the choroid plexuses until its return to the blood in the superior sagittal sinus. Plexuses in the lateral ventricles are not illustrated. (Chaffee E.E., Lytle I.M. [1980]. *Basic physiology and anatomy* [4th ed., p. 221]. Philadelphia: J.B. Lippincott)

TABLE 47-3 ✦ Composition of Cerebrospinal Fluid Compared With Plasma

Substance	Plasma	Cerebrospinal Fluid
Protein mg/dL	6000.00	20.00
Na^+ mEq/L	145.00	141.00
CL^- mEq/L	101.00	124.00
K^+ mEq/L	4.50	2.90
HCO_3^- mEq/L	25.00	24.00
pH	7.4	7.32
Glucose mg/dL	92.00	61.00

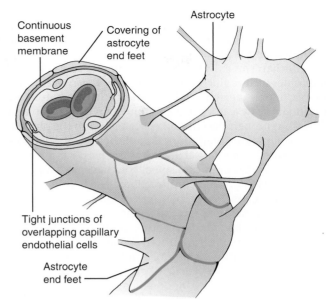

FIGURE 47-33 The three components of the blood–brain barrier: the astrocyte and astrocytic feet that encircle the capillary, the capillary basement membrane, and the tight junctions that join the overlapping capillary endothelial cells.

BLOOD-BRAIN AND CEREBROSPINAL FLUID–BRAIN BARRIERS

Maintenance of a chemically stable environment is essential to the function of the brain. In most regions of the body, extracellular fluid undergoes small fluctuations in pH and concentrations of hormones, amino acids, and potassium ions during routine daily activities such as eating and exercising. If the brain were to undergo such fluctuations, the result would be uncontrolled neural activity, because some substances such as amino acids act as neurotransmitters, and ions such as potassium influence the threshold for neural firing. Two barriers, the blood-brain barrier and the CSF-brain barrier, provide the means for maintaining the stable chemical environment of the brain. Only water, carbon dioxide, and oxygen enter the brain with relative ease; the transport of other substances between the brain and the blood is slow.

Blood-Brain Barrier

The blood-brain barrier depends on the unique characteristics of the brain capillaries. The endothelial cells of brain capillaries are joined by continuous tight junctions. In addition, most brain capillaries are completely surrounded by a basement membrane and by the processes of supporting cells of the brain, called *astrocytes* (Fig. 47-33). The blood-brain barrier permits passage of essential substances while excluding unwanted materials. Reverse transport systems remove materials from the brain. Large molecules such as proteins and peptides are largely excluded from crossing the blood-brain barrier. Acute cerebral lesions, such as trauma and infection, increase the permeability of the blood-brain barrier and alter brain concentrations of proteins, water, and electrolytes.

The blood-brain barrier prevents many drugs from entering the brain. Most highly water-soluble compounds are excluded from the brain, especially molecules with high ionic charge such as many of the catecholamines. In contrast, many lipid-soluble molecules cross the lipid layers of the blood-brain barrier with ease. Some drugs, such as the antibiotic chloramphenicol, are highly lipid soluble and therefore enter the brain readily. Other medications have a low solubility in lipids and enter the brain slowly or not at all. Alcohol, nicotine, and heroin are very lipid soluble and

rapidly enter the brain. Some substances that enter the capillary endothelium are converted by metabolic processes to a chemical form incapable of moving into the brain.

The cerebral capillaries are much more permeable at birth than in adulthood, and the blood-brain barrier develops during the early years of life. In severely jaundiced infants, bilirubin can cross the immature blood-brain barrier, producing kernicterus and brain damage (see Chapter 15). In adults, the mature blood-brain barrier prevents bilirubin from entering the brain, and the nervous system is not affected.

Cerebrospinal Fluid–Brain Barrier

The ependymal cells covering the choroid plexus are linked together by tight junctions, forming a blood-CSF barrier to diffusion of many molecules from the blood plasma of choroid plexus capillaries to the CSF. Water is transported through the choroid epithelial cells by osmosis. Oxygen and carbon dioxide move into the CSF by diffusion, resulting in partial pressures roughly equal to those of plasma. The high sodium and low potassium contents of the CSF are actively regulated and kept relatively constant. Lipids and nonpeptide hormones diffuse through the barrier rather easily, but most large molecules, such as proteins, peptides, many antibiotics, and other medications, do not normally get through. The choroid epithelium uses energy in the form of adenosine triphosphate to secrete actively many components into the CSF, including proteins; sodium ions; a number of micronutrients such as vitamins C, B_6 (pyridoxine), and folate; and ribonucleosides and deoxyribonucleosides. Because the resultant CSF has a relatively high sodium content, the negatively charged chloride and bicarbonate diffuse into the CSF along an ionic gradient. The choroid cells also generate bicarbonate from carbon dioxide in the blood. The generation of bicarbonate is important to the regulation of the pH of the CSF.

Mechanisms exist that facilitate the transport of other molecules such as glucose without energy expenditure. Ammonia, a toxic metabolite of neuronal activity, is converted to glutamine by astrocytes. Glutamine moves by facilitated diffusion through the choroid epithelium into the plasma. This exemplifies a major function of the CSF, that of providing a means of removal of toxic waste products from the CNS. Because the brain and spinal cord have no lymphatic channels, the CSF serves this function.

There are several specific areas of the brain where the blood-CSF barrier does not exist. One area is at the caudal end of the fourth ventricle (*i.e.*, area postrema), where specialized receptors for the carbon dioxide level of the CSF influence respiratory function. Another area consists of the walls of the third ventricle, which permit hypothalamic neurons to monitor blood glucose levels. This mechanism permits hypothalamic centers to respond to these blood glucose levels, contributing to hunger and eating behaviors.

In summary, in the process of development, the most rostral part of the embryonic neural tube develops to form the brain. The brain can be divided into three parts, hindbrain, midbrain, and forebrain. The hindbrain, consisting of the medulla oblongata, pons, and cerebellum, contains the neuronal circuits for the eating, breathing, and locomotive functions required for survival. Cranial nerves XII, XI, X, IX, VIII, VII, VI, and V are located in the hindbrain. The midbrain contains cranial nerves III and IV. The forebrain is the most rostral part of the brain; it consists of the diencephalon and the telencephalon. The dorsal horn part of the diencephalon comprises the thalamus and subthalamus, and the ventral horn part is the hypothalamus. The cerebral hemispheres are the lateral outgrowths of the diencephalon. Although there may be considerable overlap, one of the hemispheres is the more dominant hemisphere; it has a major role in verbal and analytic abilities. The less dominant hemisphere has a major role in nonverbal and spatial abilities.

The cerebral hemispheres are arbitrarily divided into lobes—the frontal, parietal, temporal, and occipital lobes—named after the bones of the skull that cover them. The prefrontal premotor area and primary motor cortex are located in the frontal lobe; the primary sensory cortex and somesthetic association area are in the parietal cortex; the primary auditory cortex and the auditory association area are in the temporal lobe; and the primary visual cortex and association visual cortex are in the occipital lobe. The limbic system, which is involved in emotional experience and release of emotional behaviors, is located in the medial aspect of the cerebrum. These cortical areas are reciprocally connected with underlying thalamic nuclei through the internal capsule. Thalamic involvement is essential for normal forebrain function.

The brain is enclosed and protected by the pia mater, arachnoid, and dura mater. The protective CSF in which the brain and spinal cord float isolates them from minor and moderate trauma. The CSF is secreted into the ventricles, circulates through the ventricular system, passes outside to surround the brain, and is reabsorbed into the venous system through the arachnoid villi. The CSF-brain barrier and the blood-brain barrier protect the brain from substances in the blood that would disrupt brain function.

The Autonomic Nervous System

After you have completed this section of the chapter, you should be able to meet the following objectives:

- ◆ State the function of the autonomic nervous system
- ◆ Compare the sensory and motor components of the autonomic nervous system with those of the CNS
- ◆ Compare the anatomic location and functions of the sympathetic and parasympathetic nervous systems
- ◆ Describe neurotransmitter synthesis, release, and degradation, and receptor function in the sympathetic and parasympathetic nervous systems

The ability to maintain homeostasis and perform the activities of daily living in an ever-changing physical environment is largely vested in the autonomic nervous system (ANS). The ANS functions at the subconscious level and is involved in regulating, adjusting, and coordinating vital visceral functions such as blood pressure and blood flow, body temperature, respiration, digestion, metabolism, and elimination. The ANS is strongly affected by emotional influences and is involved in many of the expressive aspects of behavior. Blushing, pallor, palpitations of the heart, clammy hands, and dry mouth are several emotional expressions that are mediated through the ANS. Biofeedback and relaxation exercises have been used for modifying the subconscious functions of the ANS.

As with the somatic nervous system, the ANS is represented in both the CNS and the PNS. Traditionally, the ANS has been defined as a general efferent system innervating visceral organs. The efferent outflow from the ANS has two divisions: the sympathetic nervous system and the parasympathetic nervous system. The afferent input to the ANS is provided by visceral afferent neurons, usually not considered to be part of the ANS.

The functions of the sympathetic nervous system include maintaining body temperature and adjusting blood flow and blood pressure to meet the changing needs of the body that occur with activities of daily living, such as moving from the supine to the standing position. The sympathoadrenal system also can discharge as a unit when there is a critical threat to the integrity of the individual—the so-called fight-or-flight response. During a stress situation, the heart rate accelerates; the blood pressure rises; blood flow shifts from the skin and gastrointestinal tract to the skeletal

The Autonomic Nervous System (ANS)

➤ The ANS functions at the subconscious level and is responsible for maintaining homeostatic functions of the body.

➤ The ANS has two divisions: the sympathetic and parasympathetic systems. Although the two divisions function in concert, they are generally viewed as having opposite and antagonistic actions.

➤ The sympathetic division functions in maintaining vital functions and responding when there is a critical threat to the integrity of the individual—the "fight-or-flight" response.

➤ The parasympathetic nervous system is concerned with conservation of energy, resource replenishment, and maintenance of organ function during periods of minimal activity.

➤ The outflow of the both divisions of the ANS consists of a two-neuron pathway: a preganglionic and a postganglionic neuron. Acetylcholine is the neurotransmitter for the preganglionic neurons for both ANS divisions, as well as the postganglionic neurons of the parasympathetic nervous system. Norepinephrine and epinephrine are the neurotransmitters for the sympathetic postganglionic neurons.

muscles and brain; blood sugar increases; the bronchioles and pupils dilate; the sphincters of the stomach and intestine and the internal sphincter of the urethra constrict; and the rate of secretion of exocrine glands that are involved in digestion diminishes. Emergency situations often require vasoconstriction and shunting of blood away from the skin and into the muscles and brain, a mechanism that, should a wound occur, provides for a reduction in blood flow and preservation of vital functions needed for survival. Sympathetic function often is summarized as catabolic in that its actions predominate during periods of pronounced energy expenditure, such as when survival is threatened.

In contrast to the sympathetic nervous system, the functions of the parasympathetic nervous system are concerned with conservation of energy, resource replenishment and storage (*i.e.*, anabolism), and maintenance of organ function during periods of minimal activity. The parasympathetic nervous system slows heart rate, stimulates gastrointestinal function and related glandular secretion, promotes bowel and bladder elimination, and contracts the pupil, protecting the retina from excessive light during periods when visual function is not vital to survival. The two divisions of the ANS usually are viewed as having opposite and antagonistic actions (*i.e.*, if one activates, the other inhibits a function). Exceptions are functions, such as sweating and

regulation of arteriolar blood vessel diameter, that are controlled by a single division of the ANS, in this case the sympathetic nervous system.

The sympathetic and parasympathetic nervous systems are continually active. The effect of this continual or basal (baseline) activity is referred to as *tone*. The tone of an effector organ or system can be increased or decreased and usually is regulated by a single division of the ANS. For example, vascular smooth muscle tone is controlled by the sympathetic nervous system. Increased sympathetic activity produces local vasoconstriction from increased vascular smooth muscle tone, and decreased activity results in vasodilatation due to decreased tone. In structures such as the sinoatrial node and atrioventricular node of the heart, which are innervated by both divisions of the ANS, one division predominates in controlling tone. In this case, the tonically active parasympathetic nervous system exerts a constraining or braking effect on heart rate, and when parasympathetic outflow is withdrawn, similar to releasing a brake, the heart rate increases. The increase in heart rate that occurs with vagal withdrawal can be further augmented by sympathetic stimulation. Table 47-4 describes the responses of effector organs to sympathetic and parasympathetic impulses.

AUTONOMIC EFFERENT PATHWAYS

The outflow of both divisions of the ANS follows a two-neuron pathway. The first motoneuron, called the *preganglionic neuron*, lies in the intermediolateral cell column in the ventral horn of the spinal cord or its equivalent location in the brain stem. The second motoneuron, called the *postganglionic neuron*, synapses with a preganglionic neuron in an autonomic ganglion located in the PNS. The two divisions of the ANS differ in terms of location of preganglionic cell bodies, relative length of preganglionic fibers, general function, nature of peripheral responses, and preganglionic and postganglionic neuromediators (see Table 47-4). This two-neuron outflow pathway and the interneurons in the autonomic ganglia that add further modulation to ANS function are features distinctly different from the arrangement in somatic motor innervation (Fig. 47-34).

Most visceral organs are innervated by both sympathetic and parasympathetic fibers. Exceptions include structures such as blood vessels and sweat glands that have input from only one division of the ANS. The fibers of the sympathetic nervous system are distributed to effectors throughout the body, and as a result, sympathetic actions tend to be more diffuse than those of the parasympathetic nervous system, in which there is a more localized distribution of fibers. The preganglionic fibers of the sympathetic nervous system may traverse a considerable distance and pass through several ganglia before synapsing with postganglionic neurons, and their terminals make contact with a large number of postganglionic fibers. In some ganglia, the ratio of preganglionic to postganglionic cells may be 1:20; because of this, the effects of sympathetic stimulation are diffuse. There is considerable overlap, and one ganglion cell may be supplied by several preganglionic fibers. In contrast to the sympathetic nervous system, the parasympathetic

TABLE 47-4 ✦ Characteristics of the Sympathetic and Parasympathetic Nervous Systems

Characteristic	Sympathetic Outflow	Parasympathetic Outflow
Location of preganglionic cell bodies	T1–T12, L1 and L2	Cranial nerves: III, VII (intermedius), IX, X; sacral segments 2, 3, and 4
Relative length of preganglionic fibers	Short—to paravertebral chain of ganglia or to aortic prevertebral of ganglia	Long—to ganglion cells near or in the innervated organ
General function	Catabolic—mobilizes resources in anticipation of challenge for survival (preparation for "fight-or-flight" response)	Anabolic—concerned with conservation, renewal, and storage of resources
Nature of peripheral response	Generalized	Localized
Transmitter between preganglionic terminals and postganglionic neurons	ACh	ACh
Transmitter of post-ganglionic neuron	ACh (sweat glands and skeletal muscle vasodilator fibers); norepinephrine (most synapses); norepinephrine and epinephrine (secreted by adrenal gland)	ACh

ACh, acetylcholine.

nervous system has its postganglionic neurons located very near or in the organ of innervation. Because the ratio of preganglionic to postganglionic communication often is 1:1, the effects of the parasympathetic nervous system are much more circumscribed.

Sympathetic Nervous System

The neurons of the sympathetic nervous system are located primarily in the thoracic and upper lumbar segments (T1 to L2) of the spinal cord; hence, the sympathetic nervous system often is referred to as the *thoracolumbar division* of

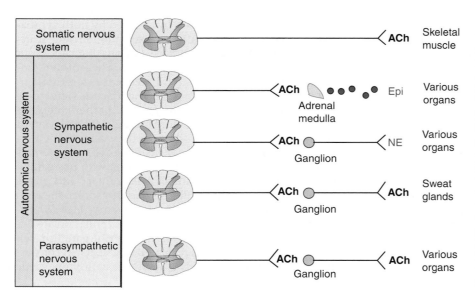

FIGURE 47-34 Comparison of the neurotransmission in the somatic and autonomic nervous systems. In the somatic nervous system, all motor neurons release acetylcholine (ACh) as their neurotransmitter. In the autonomic nervous system, both sympathetic and parasympathetic preganglionic neurons release ACh as their neurotransmitter. Parasympathetic postganglionic neurons release ACh at the site of organ innervation. Most postganglionic neurons of the sympathetic nervous system release norepinephrine (NE) at the site of organ innervation. The principal neurotransmitter released by the adrenal gland is epinephrine (Epi) which travels to the site of organ innervation by way of the bloodstream. The postganglionic neurons innervating the sweat gland are sympathetic fibers that use ACh as their neurotransmitter.

the ANS. These preganglionic neurons, which are located primarily in the ventral horn intermediolateral cell column, have axons that are largely myelinated and relatively short. The postganglionic neurons of the sympathetic nervous system are located in the paravertebral ganglia of the sympathetic chain of ganglia that lie on either side of the vertebral column, or in prevertebral sympathetic ganglia such as the celiac ganglia (Fig. 47-35). In addition to postganglionic efferent neurons, the sympathetic ganglia contain neurons of the internuncial, short-axon type, similar to those associated with complex circuitry in the brain and spinal cord. Many of these inhibit and others modulate preganglionic-to-postganglionic transmission. The full significance of these modulating circuits awaits further investigation.

The axons of the preganglionic neurons leave the spinal cord through the ventral root of the spinal nerves (T1 to L2), enter the ventral primary rami, and leave the spinal nerve through white rami of the rami communicantes to reach the paravertebral ganglionic chain (Fig. 47-36). In the sympathetic chain of ganglia, preganglionic fibers may synapse with neurons of the ganglion it enters, pass up or down the chain and synapse with one or more ganglia, or pass through the chain and move outward through a splanchnic nerve to terminate in one of the prevertebral ganglia (*i.e.*, celiac, superior mesenteric, or inferior mesenteric) that are scattered along the dorsal aorta and its branches.

Preganglionic fibers from the thoracic segments of the cord pass upward to form the cervical chain connecting the inferior, middle, and superior cervical sympathetic ganglia with the rest of the sympathetic chain at lower levels. Postganglionic sympathetic axons of the cervical and lower lumbosacral chain ganglia spread further through nerve plexuses along continuations of the great arteries. Cranial structures, particularly blood vessels, are innervated by the spread of postganglionic axons along the external and internal carotid arteries into the face and the cranial cavity. The sympathetic fibers from T1 pass in general up the sympathetic chain into the head; those from T2 pass into the neck; those from T1 to T5 pass to the heart: those from T3, T4, T5, and T6 pass to the thoracic viscera; those from T7, T8, T9, T10, and T11 pass to the abdominal viscera; and those from T12, L1, L2, and L3 pass to the kidneys and pelvic organs. Many of the preganglionic fibers from the fifth to the last thoracolumbar segment pass through the paravertebral ganglia to continue as the splanchnic nerves. Most of these fibers do not synapse until they reach the celiac or superior mesenteric ganglion; others pass to the adrenal medulla.

The adrenal medulla, which is part of the sympathetic nervous system, contains postganglionic sympathetic neurons that secrete sympathetic neurotransmitters directly into the bloodstream. Some of the postganglionic fibers, all of which are unmyelinated, from the paravertebral ganglionic chain reenter the segmental nerve through unmyelinated branches, called *gray rami*, of all segmental nerves and are then distributed to all parts of the body wall in the spinal nerve branches. These fibers innervate the sweat glands, piloerector muscles of the hair follicles, all of the blood vessels of the skin and skeletal muscles, and the CNS itself.

Parasympathetic Nervous System

The preganglionic fibers of the parasympathetic nervous system, also referred to as the *craniosacral division* of the ANS, originate in some segments of the brain stem and sacral segments of the spinal cord (see Fig. 47-35). The central regions of origin are the midbrain, pons, medulla oblongata, and the sacral part of the spinal cord. The midbrain outflow passes through the oculomotor nerve (cranial nerve III) to the ciliary ganglion that lies in the orbit behind the eye; it supplies the pupillary sphincter muscle of each eye and the ciliary muscles that control lens thickness for accommodation. Caudal pontine outflow comes from preganglionic fibers of the intermedius component of the facial nerve (cranial nerve VII) complex, which synapse in the submandibular ganglia, supplying the submandibular and sublingual glands, and the pterygopalatine ganglia, supplying the lacrimal and nasal glands. The medullary outflow develops from cranial nerves VII, IX, and X. Fibers in the glossopharyngeal nerve (cranial nerve IX) synapse in the otic ganglia, which supply the parotid salivary glands. Approximately 75% of parasympathetic efferent fibers are carried in the vagus nerve (cranial nerve X). The vagus nerve provides parasympathetic innervation for the heart, trachea, lungs, esophagus, stomach, small intestine, proximal half of the colon, liver, gallbladder, pancreas, kidneys, and upper portions of the ureters.

Sacral preganglionic axons leave the S2 to S4 segmental nerves by gathering into the pelvic nerves, also called the *nervi erigentes*. The pelvic nerves leave the sacral plexus on each side of the cord and distribute their peripheral fibers to the bladder, uterus, urethra, prostate, distal portion of the transverse colon, descending colon, and rectum. The sacral parasympathetic fibers also supply the venous outflow from the external genitalia to facilitate erectile function.

With the exception of cranial nerves III, VII, and IX, which synapse in discrete ganglia, the long parasympathetic preganglionic fibers pass uninterrupted to short postganglionic fibers located in the organ wall. In the walls of these organs, postganglionic neurons send axons to smooth muscle and glandular cells that modulate their functions.

The gastrointestinal tract has its own intrinsic network of ganglionic cells located between the smooth muscle layers, called *enteric* (or *intramural*) *plexus*, which controls local peristaltic movements and secretory functions. This network of parasympathetic postganglionic neurons and interneurons runs from the upper portion of the esophagus to the internal anal sphincter. Local afferent sensory neurons respond to mechanical and chemical stimuli and communicate these influences to motor fibers in the enteric plexus. The number of neurons in the enteric neural network (10^8) is so large that it approximates that of the spinal cord. It is thought that this enteric nervous system is capable of independent function without control from CNS fibers. The CNS has a modulating role, by way of preganglionic innervation of the plexus, converting local peristalsis to longer-distance movements, thereby speeding the transit of intestinal contents.

CENTRAL INTEGRATIVE PATHWAYS

General visceral afferent fibers accompany the sympathetic and parasympathetic outflow into the spinal and cranial nerves, bringing chemoreceptor, pressure, organ capsule

Sympathetic   **Parasympathetic**

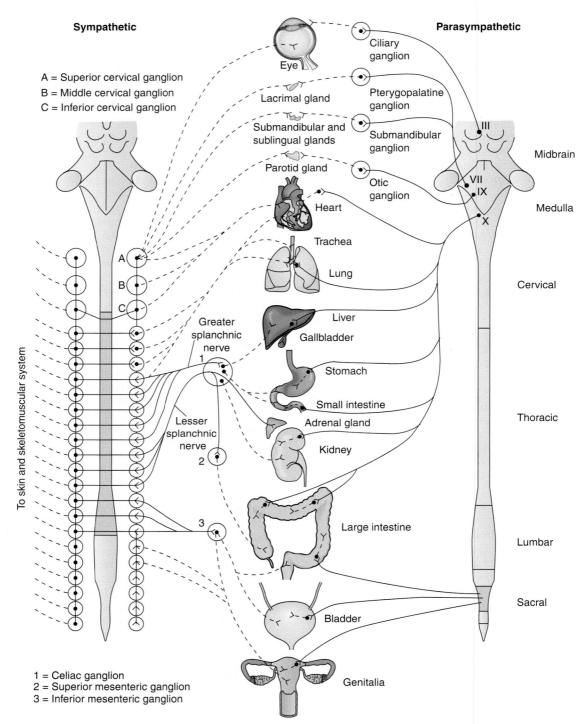

A = Superior cervical ganglion
B = Middle cervical ganglion
C = Inferior cervical ganglion

Eye

Ciliary ganglion

Lacrimal gland

Pterygopalatine ganglion

Submandibular and sublingual glands

Submandibular ganglion

Parotid gland

Otic ganglion

Heart

Trachea

Lung

Liver

Gallbladder

Stomach

Small intestine

Adrenal gland

Kidney

Large intestine

Bladder

Genitalia

III

VII
IX

X

Midbrain

Medulla

Cervical

Thoracic

Lumbar

Sacral

A

B

C

Greater splanchnic nerve

1

Lesser splanchnic nerve

2

3

To skin and skeletomuscular system

1 = Celiac ganglion
2 = Superior mesenteric ganglion
3 = Inferior mesenteric ganglion

FIGURE 47-35 The autonomic nervous system. The involuntary organs are depicted with their parasympathetic innervation (craniosacral) indicated on the right and sympathetic innervation (thoracolumbar) on the left. Preganglionic fibers are *solid lines;* postganglionic fibers are *dashed lines.* For purposes of illustration, the sympathetic outflow to the skin and skeletomuscular system is shown separately (to the far left); effectors include sweat glands, pilomotor muscles and blood vessels of the skin, and blood vessels of the skeletal muscles and bones. (Modified from Hemer L. [1983]. *The human brain and spinal cord*: Functional neuroanatomy and dissection guide. New York: Springer-Verlag)

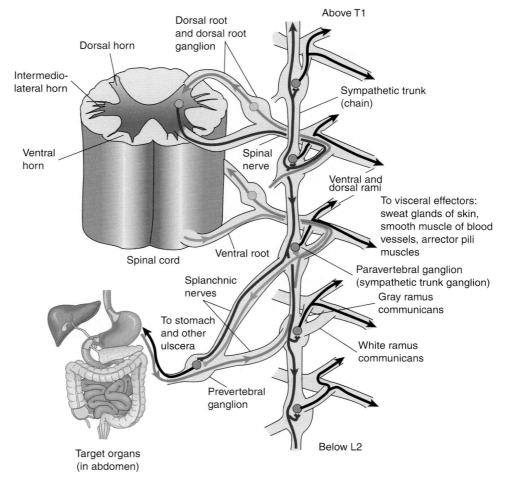

FIGURE 47-36 Sympathetic pathways. Sympathetic fibers leave the spinal cord by way of the ventral root of the spinal nerves, enter the ventral primary rami, and pass through the white rami to the prevertebral or paravertebral ganglia of the sympathetic chain, where they synapse with postganglionic neurons. Some postganglionic fibers from the paravertebral ganglia reenter the segmental nerves through the gray rami and are then distributed in the spinal nerve branches. Other postganglionic neurons travel directly to their destination in the various effector organs. General visceral afferents carry information from the effector organs through the white rami to the dorsal root ganglia and into the dorsal horn of the spinal cord.

stretch, and nociceptive information from organs of the viscera to the brain stem, thoracolumbar cord, and sacral cord. Local reflex circuits relating visceral afferent and autonomic efferent activity are integrated into a hierarchic control system in the spinal cord and brain stem. Progressively greater complexity in the responses and greater precision in their control occur at each higher level of the nervous system. Most visceral reflexes contain contributions from the LMNs that innervate skeletal muscles as part of their response patterns. The distinction between purely visceral and somatic reflex hierarchies becomes less and less meaningful at the higher levels of hierarchic control and behavioral integration.

For most autonomic-mediated functions, the hypothalamus serves as the major control center. The hypothalamus, which has connections with the cerebral cortex, the limbic system, and the pituitary gland, is in a prime position to receive, integrate, and transmit information to other areas of the nervous system. The neurons concerned with thermoregulation, thirst, and feeding behaviors are found in the hypothalamus. The hypothalamus also is the site for integrating neuroendocrine function. Hypothalamic releasing and inhibiting hormones control the secretion of anterior pituitary hormones (*i.e.*, thyroid- stimulating

hormone, corticotropin, growth hormone, luteinizing hormone, follicle-stimulating hormone, and prolactin). The supraoptic nuclei of the hypothalamus are involved in water metabolism through synthesis of antidiuretic hormone and its release from the posterior pituitary gland (see Chapter 31). Oxytocin, which causes contraction of the pregnant uterus and milk letdown during breast-feeding, is synthesized in the hypothalamus and released from the posterior pituitary gland in a manner similar to that of antidiuretic hormone.

The organization of many life-support reflexes occurs in the reticular formation of the medulla and pons. These areas of reflex circuitry, often called *centers*, produce complex combinations of autonomic and somatic efferent functions required for the respiration, gag, cough, sneeze, swallow, and vomit reflexes, as well as for the more purely autonomic control of the cardiovascular system. At the hypothalamic level, these reflexes are integrated into more general response patterns such as rage, defensive behavior, eating, drinking, voiding, and sexual function. Forebrain and especially limbic system control of these behaviors involves inhibiting or facilitating release of the response patterns according to social pressures during learned emotion-provoking situations.

Reflex adjustments of cardiovascular and respiratory function occur at the level of the brain stem. A prominent example is the carotid sinus baroreflex. Increased blood pressure in the carotid sinus increases the discharge from afferent fibers that travel by way of the ninth cranial nerve to cardiovascular centers in the brain stem. These centers increase the activity of descending efferent vagal fibers that slow heart rate, while inhibiting sympathetic fibers that increase heart rate and blood vessel tone. One of the striking features of ANS function is the rapidity and intensity with which it can change visceral function. Within 3 to 5 seconds, it can increase heart rate to approximately twice its resting level. Bronchial smooth muscle tone is largely controlled by parasympathetic fibers carried in the vagus nerve. These nerves produce mild to moderate constriction of the bronchioles.

Other important ANS reflexes are located at the level of the spinal cord. As with other spinal reflexes, these reflexes are modulated by input from higher centers. When there is loss of communication between the higher centers and the spinal reflexes, as occurs in spinal cord injury, these reflexes function in an unregulated manner (see Chapter 49). There is uncontrolled sweating, vasomotor instability, and reflex bowel and bladder function.

AUTONOMIC NEUROTRANSMISSION

The generation and transmission of impulses in the ANS occur in the same manner as in other neurons. There are self-propagating action potentials with transmission of impulses across synapses and other tissue junctions by way of neurohumoral transmitters. However, the somatic motoneurons that innervate skeletal muscles divide into many branches, with each branch innervating a single muscle fiber; in contrast, the distribution of postganglionic fibers of the ANS forms a diffuse neural plexus at the site of innervation. The membranes of the cells of many smooth muscle fibers are connected by conductive protoplasmic bridges, called *gap junctions*, that permit rapid conduction of impulses through whole sheets of smooth muscle, often in repeating waves of contraction. Autonomic neurotransmitters released near a limited portion of these fibers provide a modulating function extending to a large number of effector cells. The muscle layers of the gut and of the bladder wall are examples. In some instances, isolated smooth muscle cells are individually innervated by the ANS, such as the piloerector cells that elevate the hair on the skin during cold exposure.

The main neurotransmitters of the autonomic nervous system are acetylcholine and the catecholamines, epinephrine and norepinephrine. Acetylcholine is released at all of the sites of preganglionic transmission in the autonomic ganglia of sympathetic and parasympathetic nerve fibers and at the sites of postganglionic transmission in parasympathetic nerve endings. It also is released at sympathetic nerve endings that innervate the sweat glands and cholinergic vasodilator fibers found in skeletal muscle. Norepinephrine is released at most sympathetic nerve endings. The adrenal medulla, which is a modified prevertebral sym-

pathetic ganglion, produces epinephrine along with small amounts of norepinephrine. Dopamine, which is an intermediate compound in the synthesis of norepinephrine, also acts as a neurotransmitter. It is the principal inhibitory transmitter of internuncial neurons in the sympathetic ganglia. It also has vasodilator effects on renal, splanchnic, and coronary blood vessels when given intravenously and is sometimes used in the treatment of shock (see Chapter 26).

A considerable number of neurons secreting peptide molecules have been identified in ANS ganglia, especially in the enteric plexus and in postganglionic ANS terminals of the sympathetic and parasympathetic systems. Many of these are secreted by internuncial neurons or as additional transmitters or "cotransmitters" by preganglionic and postganglionic neurons. Binding at postsynaptic neuropeptide receptors usually does not result in action potentials; instead, it alters the membrane potential or receptor numbers, producing long-term (minutes to hours) changes in responsiveness to the neurotransmitter. For example, dual secretion of norepinephrine and neuropeptide Y in some sympathetic vasoconstrictor terminals results in longer vasomotor constriction. Similarly, some parasympathetic postganglionic acetylcholine-secreting neurons can secrete vasoactive intestinal peptide as a cotransmitter that potentiates postsynaptic actions. Many neuropeptides involved in peripheral ANS function are under active investigation, including substance P, cholecystokinin, somatostatin, and neurotensin.

Acetylcholine and Cholinergic Receptors

Acetylcholine is synthesized in the cholinergic neurons from choline and acetyl coenzyme A (acetyl CoA; Fig. 47-37). After acetylcholine is secreted by the cholinergic nerve endings, it is rapidly broken down by the enzyme acetylcholinesterase. The choline molecule is transported back into the nerve ending, where it is used again in the synthesis of acetylcholine.

Receptors that respond to acetylcholine are called *cholinergic receptors*. There are two types of cholinergic receptors: muscarinic and nicotinic. Muscarinic receptors are present on the innervational targets of postganglionic fibers of the parasympathetic nervous system and the sweat glands, which are innervated by the sympathetic nervous system. Nicotinic receptors are found in autonomic ganglia and the end plates of skeletal muscle. Acetylcholine has an excitatory effect on muscarinic and nicotinic receptors, except for those in the heart and lower esophagus, where it has an inhibitory effect. The drug atropine is an antimuscarinic or muscarinic cholinergic-blocking drug that prevents the action of acetylcholine at excitatory and inhibitory muscarinic receptor sites. Because it is a muscarinic-blocking drug, it exerts little effect at nicotinic receptor sites.

Catecholamines and Adrenergic Receptors

The catecholamines, which include norepinephrine, epinephrine, and dopamine, are synthesized in the axoplasm of sympathetic nerve terminal endings from the amino acid tyrosine (see Fig. 47-37). In the process of catecholamine synthesis, tyrosine is hydroxylated (*i.e.*, has a hydroxyl group added) to form DOPA, DOPA is decarboxylated

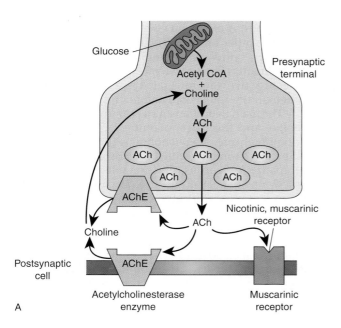

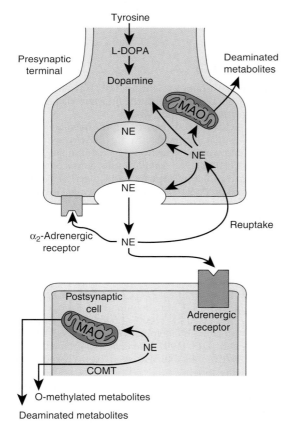

FIGURE 47-37 Schematic illustration of cholinergic parasympathetic (**A**) and noradrenergic sympathetic (**B**) neurotransmitter synthesis, release, receptor binding, neurotransmitter degradation, and metabolite transport back into the presynaptic neuron (acetylcholine) and reuptake (norepinephrine). (Adapted from Rhoades R.A., Tanner G.A. [1996]. *Medical physiology*. Boston: Little, Brown)

(*i.e.*, has a carboxyl group removed) to form dopamine, and dopamine is hydroxylated to form norepinephrine. In the adrenal gland, an additional step occurs during which norepinephrine is methylated (*i.e.*, a methyl group is added) to form epinephrine.

Each of the steps in sympathetic neurotransmitter synthesis requires a different enzyme, and the type of neurotransmitter that is produced depends on the types of enzymes that are available in a nerve terminal. For example, the postganglionic sympathetic neurons that supply blood vessels synthesize norepinephrine, but postganglionic neurons in the adrenal medulla produce epinephrine or norepinephrine. Epinephrine accounts for approximately 80% of the catecholamines released from the adrenal gland. The synthesis of epinephrine by the adrenal medulla is influenced by the glucocorticoid secretion from the adrenal cortex. These hormones are transported through an intraadrenal vascular network from the adrenal cortex to the adrenal medulla, where they cause the sympathetic neurons to increase their production of epinephrine through increased enzyme activity. Thus, any stress situation sufficient to evoke increased levels of glucocorticoids also increases epinephrine levels. As the catecholamines are synthesized, they are stored in vesicles. The final step of norepinephrine synthesis occurs in these vesicles. When an action potential reaches an axon terminal, the neurotransmitter molecules are released from the storage vesicles. The storage vesicles provide a means for concentrated storage of the catecholamines and protect them from the cytoplasmic enzymes that degrade the neurotransmitters.

In addition to neuronal synthesis, there is a second major mechanism for replenishment of norepinephrine in sympathetic nerve terminals. This mechanism consists of the active recapture or reuptake of the released neurotransmitter into the nerve terminal. Between 50% and 80% of the norepinephrine that is released during an action potential is removed from the synaptic area by an active reuptake process. This process terminates the action of the neurotransmitter and allows it to be reused by the neuron. The remainder of the released catecholamines diffuses into the surrounding tissue fluids or is degraded by two special enzymes: catechol-*O*-methyltransferase, which is diffusely present in all tissues, and monoamine oxidase (MAO), which is found in the nerve endings themselves. Some drugs, such as the tricyclic antidepressants, are thought to increase the level of catecholamines at the site of nerve endings in the brain by blocking the reuptake process. Others, such as the MAO inhibitors, decrease the enzymatic degradation of the neurotransmitters and increase their levels.

Catecholamines can cause excitation or inhibition of smooth muscle contraction, depending on the site, dose, and type of receptor present. Norepinephrine has potent excitatory activity and low inhibitory activity. Epinephrine is potent as both an excitatory and an inhibitory agent.

The excitatory or inhibitory responses of organs to sympathetic neurotransmitters are mediated by interaction with special structures in the cell membrane called *receptors*. In 1948, Ahlquist proposed the designations α and β for the receptor sites where catecholamines produce their excitatory (α) and inhibitory (β) effects.

In vascular smooth muscle, excitation of α receptors causes vasoconstriction, and excitation of β receptors causes vasodilatation. Endogenously and exogenously administered norepinephrine produces marked vasoconstriction of the blood vessels in the skin, kidneys, and splanchnic circulation that are supplied with α receptors. The β receptors are most prevalent in the heart, the blood vessels of skeletal muscle, and the bronchioles. Blood vessels in skeletal muscle have α and β receptors. In these vessels, high levels of norepinephrine produce vasoconstriction; low levels produce vasodilatation. The low levels are thought to have a diluting effect on norepinephrine levels in the arteries of these blood vessels so that the β effect predominates. In vessels with few receptors, such as those that supply the brain, norepinephrine has little effect.

α-Adrenergic receptors have been further subdivided into α_1 and α_2 receptors, and β-adrenergic receptors into β_1 and β_2 receptors. β_1-Adrenergic receptors are found primarily in the heart and can be selectively blocked by β_1 receptor–blocking drugs. β_2-Adrenergic receptors are found in the bronchioles and in other sites that have β-mediated functions. The α_1 receptors are found primarily in postsynaptic effector sites; they mediate responses in vascular smooth muscle. The α_2 receptors are mainly located presynaptically and can inhibit the release of norepinephrine from sympathetic nerve terminals. The α_2 receptors are abundant in the CNS and are thought to influence the central control of blood pressure.

The various classes of adrenergic receptors provide a mechanism by which the same adrenergic neurotransmitter can have many selective effects on different effector cells. This mechanism also permits neurotransmitters carried in the bloodstream, whether from neuroendocrine secretion by the adrenal gland or from subcutaneously or intravenously administered drugs, to produce the same effects.

The catecholamines that are produced and released from sympathetic nerve endings are referred to as *endogenous neuromediators*. Sympathetic nerve endings also can be activated by exogenous forms of these neuromediators, which reach the nerve endings by way of the bloodstream after being injected into the body or administered orally. These drugs mimic the action of the neuromediators and are said to have a *sympathomimetic action*. Other drugs can selectively block the receptor sites on the neurons and temporarily prevent the neurotransmitter from exerting its action.

In summary, the ANS regulates, adjusts, and coordinates the visceral functions of the body. The ANS, which is divided into the sympathetic and parasympathetic systems, is an efferent system. It receives its afferent input from visceral afferent neurons. The ANS has CNS and PNS components. The outflow of the sympathetic and parasympathetic nervous system follows a two-neuron pathway, which consists of a preganglionic neuron located in the CNS and a postganglionic neuron located outside the CNS. Sympathetic fibers leave the CNS at the thoracolumbar level, and the parasympathetic fibers leave at the craniosacral level. In general, the sympathetic and parasympathetic nervous systems have opposing effects on visceral function—if one excites, the other inhibits. The hypothalamus serves as the major control center for most ANS functions; local reflex circuits relating visceral afferent and autonomic efferent activity are integrated in a hierarchic control system in the spinal cord and brain stem.

The main neurotransmitters for the ANS are acetylcholine and the catecholamines, epinephrine and norepinephrine. Acetylcholine is the transmitter for all preganglionic neurons, for postganglionic parasympathetic neurons, and for selected postganglionic sympathetic neurons. The catecholamines are the neurotransmitters for most postganglionic sympathetic neurons. The neurotransmitters exert their target action through specialized cell surface receptors—cholinergic receptors that bind acetylcholine and adrenergic receptors that bind the catecholamines. The cholinergic receptors are divided into nicotinic and muscarinic receptors, and adrenergic receptors are divided into α and β receptors. Different receptors for the same transmitter at various sites in the same tissue or in other tissues result in differences in tissue responses to the same transmitter. This arrangement also permits the use of pharmacologic agents that act at specific receptor types.

Bibliography

Araque A., Parpura V., Sanzgiri, R.P., Haydon P.G. (1999). Tripartite synapses: Glia, the unacknowledged partner. *Trends in Neuroscience* 22, 208–215.

Atkins D.L. (1998). *Synapses. Step 4: Exploration of the neuron.* [On-line]. Available: http://gwis2.circ.gwu.edu/~atkins/Neuroweb/synapse.html. Accessed August 10, 2001.

Brodal P. (1998). *The central nervous system: Structure and function* (2nd ed.). New York: Oxford University Press.

Carlson B.M. (1994). *Human embryology and developmental biology* (pp. 204–240). St. Louis: C.V. Mosby.

Dambska M., Wisniewski K.E. (1999). *Normal and pathologic development of the human brain and spinal cord.* London: John Libbey & Company.

Farnabee M.J. (2001). The nervous system. [On-line]. Available: http://gened. emc.maricopa.edu/bio/bio181/BIOBK/BioBookNERV.html. Accessed August 10, 2001.

Gartner L.P., Hiatt J.L. (1997). *Color textbook of histology* (pp. 155–185). Philadelphia: W.B. Saunders.

Guyton A.C., Hall J.E. (2000). *Textbook of medical physiology* (10th ed.). Philadelphia: W.B. Saunders.

Haines D.E. (Ed.). (1997). *Fundamental neuroscience* (pp. 115–121, 126–127, 146–148, 443–454). New York: Churchill Livingstone.

Jessen K.R., Mirsky R. (1999). Schwann cells and their precursors emerge as major regulators of nerve development. *Trends in Neuroscience* 22, 402–410.

Matthews G.G. (1998). *Neurobiology: Molecules, cells, and systems.* Malden, MA: Blackwell Science.

Moore K.L, Persaud T.V.N. (1998). *The developing human: Clinically oriented embryology* (6th ed., pp. 63–82, 451–490). Philadelphia: W.B. Saunders.

Parent A. (1996). *Carpenter's human neuroanatomy* (9th ed., pp. 186–192, 268–292, 748–756). Baltimore: Williams & Wilkins.

Sadler T.W. (2000). *Langman's medical embryology* (8th ed,. pp. 83–111, 345–381, 411–458). Philadelphia: Lippincott Williams & Wilkins.

Sanes D.H., Reh T.A., Harris W.A. (2000). *Development of the nervous system*. San Diego: Academic Press.

Virtual Vermont Internet Magazine. (2001). Vermont history: Phineas Gage's tamping iron. [On-line]. Available: http://www.virtualvermont.com/history/pgage.html. Accessed August 10, 2001.

WGBH. (1998). Probing the brain—you try it. Mapping the motor cortex: a history. [On-line]. Available: http://www.pbs.org/wgbh/aso/tryit/brain/cortexhistory.html. Accessed August 10, 2001.

Wong-Riley M.T.T. (2000). *Neuroscience secrets*. Philadelphia: Hanley & Belfus.

Zigmond M.J., Bloom E.F., Landis S.C., Roberts J.L., Squire L.R. (1999). *Fundamental neuroscience*. San Diego: Academic Press.

Chapter 48

Somatosensory Function and Pain

Elizabeth C. Devine

Sensory mechanisms provide individuals with a continuous stream of information about their bodies, the outside world, and the interactions between the two. The somatosensory component of the nervous system provides an awareness of body sensations such as touch, temperature, limb position, and pain. Other sensory components of the nervous system include the special senses of vision, hearing, smell, and taste, which are discussed in other chapters. The sensory receptors for somatosensory function consist of discrete nerve endings in the skin and other body tissues. Between 2 and 3 million sensory neurons deliver a steady stream of encoded information. Only a small proportion of this information reaches awareness; most provides input essential for a myriad of reflex and automatic mechanisms that keep us alive and manage our functioning.

This chapter is organized into two distinct parts. The first part describes the organization and control of somatosensory function, and the second focuses on pain as a somatosensory modality.

Organization and Control of Somatosensory Function

After you have completed this section of the chapter, you should be able to meet the following objectives:

✦ Describe the four major classes of somatosensory modalities

◆ Describe the organization of the somatosensory system in terms of first-, second-, and third-order neurons
◆ Characterize the structure and function of the dorsal root ganglion neurons in terms of sensory receptors, conduction velocities, and spinal cord projections
◆ Compare the discriminative pathway with the antero-lateral pathway, and explain the clinical usefulness of this distinction
◆ Describe the sensory homunculus in the cerebral cortex
◆ Compare the tactile, thermal, and position sense modalities in terms of receptors, adequate stimuli, ascending pathways, and central integrative mechanisms
◆ Describe the role of clinical examination in assessing somatosensory function

The somatosensory system is designed to provide the central nervous system (CNS) with information about the body. Sensory neurons can be divided into three types that vary in distribution and the type of sensation detected: general somatic, special somatic, and general visceral afferent neurons. *General somatic afferent neurons* have branches with widespread distribution throughout the body and with many distinct types of receptors that result in sensations such as pain, touch, and temperature. *Special somatic afferent neurons* have receptors located primarily in muscles, tendons, and joints. These receptors sense position and movement of the body. *General visceral afferent neurons* have receptors on various visceral structures and sense fullness and discomfort.

SENSORY SYSTEMS

Sensory systems can be conceptualized as a serial succession of neurons consisting of first-order, second-order, and third-order neurons. *First-order neurons* transmit sensory information from the periphery to the CNS. *Second-order neurons* communicate with various reflex networks and sensory pathways in the spinal cord and travel directly to the thalamus. *Third-order neurons* relay information from the thalamus to the cerebral cortex (Fig. 48-1).

This organizing framework corresponds with the three primary levels of neural integration in the somatosensory system: the sensory units, which contain the sensory receptors; the ascending pathways; and the central processing centers in the thalamus and cerebral cortex. Sensory information usually is relayed in a cephalad direction by the three orders of neurons; along the way, it also is processed. Many interneurons process and modify the sensory information at the level of the second- and third-order neurons, and many more participate before coordinated and appropriate learned-movement responses occur. The number of participating neurons increases exponentially from the primary through the secondary and the secondary through the tertiary levels.

The Sensory Unit

The somatosensory experience arises from information provided by a variety of receptors distributed throughout the body. There are four major modalities of sensory experience: discriminative touch, which is required to identify the size

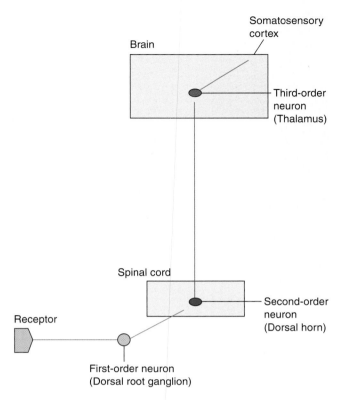

FIGURE 48-1 Arrangement of first-order, second-order, and third-order neurons of the somatosensory system.

  The Somatosensory System

➤ The somatosensory system relays information about four major modalities: touch, temperature, pain, and body position.

➤ The system is organized segmentally into dermatomes, with each segment supplied by a single dorsal root ganglion that contains the neuronal cell bodies for the sensory units of the segment.

➤ Somatosensory information is sequentially transmitted over three types of neurons: first-order neurons, which transmit information from sensory receptors to dorsal horn neurons; second-order CNS association neurons, which communicate with various reflex circuits and transmit information to the thalamus; and third-order neurons, which forward the information from the thalamus to the sensory cortex.

➤ The integrity of the somatosensory system can be evaluated on a segment-by-segment basis by using a pinprick to elicit a person's report of pain sensation and observing for the withdrawal reflex.

and shape of objects and their movement across the skin; temperature sensation; sense of movement of the limbs and joints of the body; and nociception, or pain sense.

Each of the somatosensory modalities is mediated by a distinct system of receptors and pathways to the brain; however, all somatosensory information from the limbs and trunk shares a common class of sensory neurons called *dorsal root ganglion neurons*. Somatosensory information from the face and cranial structures is transmitted by the trigeminal sensory neurons, which function in the same manner as the dorsal root ganglion neurons. The cell body of the dorsal root ganglion neuron, its peripheral branch (which innervates a small area of periphery), and its central axon (which projects to the CNS) form a *sensory unit*. Individual dorsal root ganglion neurons respond selectively to specific types of stimuli because of their specialized peripheral terminals, or receptors.

The fibers of different dorsal root ganglion neurons conduct impulses at varying rates, ranging from 0.5 to 120 m/second. This rate depends on the diameter of the nerve fiber. There are three types of nerve fibers that transmit somatosensory information: types A, B, and C (Table 48-1). Type A fibers, which are myelinated, have the fastest rate of conduction. They are further divided into type Aα, type Aβ, and type Aδ fibers. Type A fibers convey cutaneous pressure and touch sensation, cold sensation, mechanical pain, and heat pain. Type B fibers, which also are myelinated, transmit information from cutaneous and subcutaneous mechanoreceptors. The unmyelinated type C fibers have the smallest diameter and the slowest rate of conduction. They convey warm-hot sensation and mechanical and chemical as well as heat- and cold-induced pain sensation. Type Aα and Aδ fibers transmit information about muscle length and tendon stretch (discussed in Chapter 47).

Dermatomal Pattern of Dorsal Root Innervation

The somatosensory innervation of the body, including the head, retains a basic segmental organizational pattern that was established during embryonic development. Thirty-three paired spinal (*i.e.,* segmental) nerves provide sensory and motor innervation of the body wall, the limbs, and the viscera (see Chapter 47). Sensory input to each spinal cord segment is provided by sensory neurons with cell bodies in the dorsal root ganglia.

The region of the body wall that is supplied by a single pair of dorsal root ganglia is called a *dermatome*. These dorsal root ganglion–innervated strips occur in a regular sequence moving upward from the second coccygeal segment through the cervical segments, reflecting the basic segmental organization of the body and the nervous system (Fig. 48-2). The cranial nerves that innervate the head send their axons to equivalent nuclei in the brain stem. Neighboring dermatomes overlap one another sufficiently so that a loss of one dorsal root or root ganglion results in reduced but not total loss of sensory innervation of a dermatome (Fig. 48-3). Dermatome maps are helpful in interpreting the level and extent of sensory deficits that are the result of segmental nerve and spinal cord damage.

Spinal Circuitry and Ascending Neural Pathways

On entry into the spinal cord, the central axons of the somatosensory neurons branch extensively and project to nuclei in the spinal gray matter. Some branches become involved in local spinal cord reflexes and directly initiate motor reflexes (*e.g.,* flexor-withdrawal reflex). Two parallel pathways, the *discriminative pathway* and the *anterolateral*

TABLE 48-1 ◆ Somatosensory Modalities, Receptor Types, and Fiber Group

Sensory Modality	Receptor Type	Fiber Group
Touch	Cutaneous and subcutaneous mechanoreceptors	
Stroking, fluttering	Meissner's corpuscle	Aα, β
Pressure, texture	Merkel disk receptor	Aα, β
Vibration	Pacinian corpuscle	Aα, β
Skin stretch	Ruffini's ending	Aα, β
Hair movement	Hair follicle end-organ	Aα, β
Temperature	Thermal receptors	
Skin cooling (33° to 6°C)	Cool receptors	Aδ
Skin warming (34° to 44°C)	Warm receptors	C
Hot temperature (>45°C)	Heat nociceptors	Aδ
Cold temperature (<5°C)	Cold nociceptors	C
Pain	Nociceptors	
Sharp, pricking pain	Mechanical	Aδ
Burning pain	Thermal-mechanical	Aδ
Freezing pain	Thermal-mechanical	C
Slow, burning pain	Polymodal (mechanical, chemical, and thermal)	C

(Developed from Kandel E.R., Schwartz J.H., Jessell T.M. [2000]. *Principles of neural science* [4th ed., p. 432]. New York: McGraw-Hill)

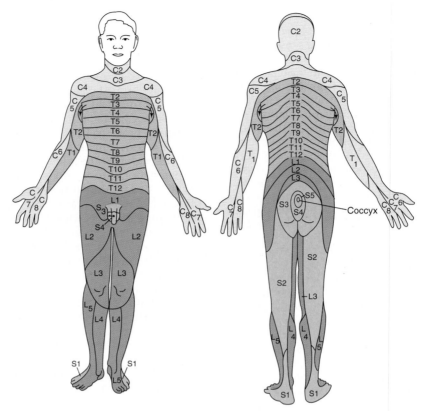

FIGURE 48-2 Cutaneous distribution of spinal nerves (dermatomes). (Barr, M. [1993]. *The human nervous system*. New York: Harper & Row)

---

pathway, carry the information from the spinal cord to the thalamic level of sensation, each taking a different route through the CNS. The discriminative pathway crosses at the base of the medulla and the anterolateral pathway crosses within the first few segments of entering the spinal cord. These pathways relay information to the brain for three purposes: perception, arousal, and motor control. Having a two-pathway system has several advantages. It adds rich-

ness to the sensory input by allowing the sensory information to be handled in two different ways, and it ensures that if one pathway is damaged, the other still can provide input.

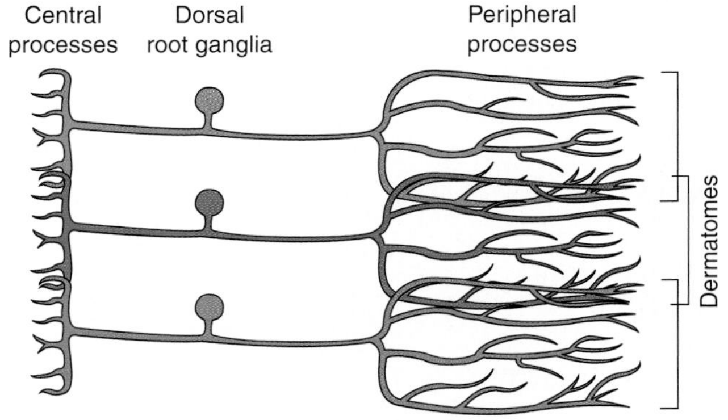

The Discriminative Pathway.   The discriminative pathway is used for the rapid transmission of sensory information such as discriminative touch. It contains branches of primary afferent axons that travel up the ipsilateral (*i.e.,* same side) dorsal columns of the spinal cord white matter and synapse with highly evolved somatosensory input association neurons in the medulla. The discriminative pathway uses only three neurons to transmit information from a sensory receptor to the somatosensory strip of parietal cerebral cortex of the opposite side of the brain: (1) the primary dorsal root ganglion neuron, which projects its central axon to the dorsal column nuclei; (2) the dorsal column neuron, which sends its axon through a rapid conducting tract, called the *medial lemniscus,* that crosses at the base of the medulla and travels to the thalamus on the opposite side of the brain, where basic sensation begins; and (3) the thalamic neuron, which projects its axons through the somatosensory radiation to the primary sensory cortex (Fig. 48-4). The medial lemniscus is joined by fibers from the sensory nucleus of the trigeminal nerve (cranial nerve V) that supplies the face. Sensory information arriving at the sensory cortex by this route can be discretely localized and discriminated in terms of intensity.

Central processes   Dorsal root ganglia   Peripheral processes

Dermatomes

FIGURE 48-3 The dermatomes formed by the peripheral processes of adjacent spinal nerves overlap on the body surface. The central processes of these fibers also overlap in their spinal distribution.

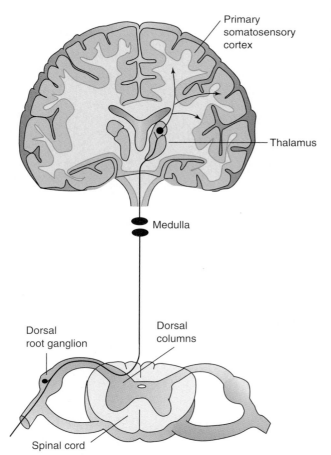

FIGURE 48-4 Discriminative pathway. This pathway is an ascending system for rapid transmission of sensations that relate joint movement (kinesthesis), body position (proprioception), vibration, and delicate touch. Primary afferents travel up the dorsal columns of the spinal cord white matter and synapse with somatosensory input association neurons in the medulla. Secondary neurons project through the brain stem to the thalamus and synapse with tertiary neurons, which relay the information to the primary somatosensory cortex on the opposite side of the brain.

One of the distinct features of the discriminative pathway is that it relays precise information regarding spatial orientation. This is the only pathway taken by the sensations of muscle and joint movement, vibration, and delicate discriminative touch, as is required to differentiate correctly the location of touch on the skin at two neighboring points (*i.e.,* two-point discrimination). One of the important functions of the discriminative pathway is to integrate the input from multiple receptors. The sense of shape and size of an object in the absence of visualization, called *stereognosis,* is based on precise afferent information from muscle, tendon, and joint receptors. For example, a screwdriver is perceived as being different from a knife in terms of its texture (tactile sensibility) and shape based on the relative position of the fingers as they move over the object. This complex interpretive perception requires that the discriminative system must be functioning optimally and that higher-order parietal association cortex processing and prior learning must

have occurred. If the discriminative somatosensory pathway is functional but the parietal association cortex has become discretely damaged, the person can correctly describe the object but does not recognize that it is a screwdriver. This deficit is called *astereognosis.*

The Anterolateral Pathway. The anterolateral pathways (anterior and lateral spinothalamic pathways) consist of bilateral multisynaptic slow-conducting tracts. These pathways provide for transmission of sensory information such as pain, thermal sensations, crude touch, and pressure that does not require discrete localization of signal source or fine discrimination of intensity. The fibers of the anterolateral pathway originate in the dorsal horns at the level of the segmental nerve, where the dorsal root neurons enter the spinal cord. They cross in the anterior commissure, within a few segments of origin, to the opposite anterolateral pathway, where they ascend upward toward the brain. The spinothalamic tract fibers synapse with several nuclei in the thalamus, but en route they give off numerous branches that travel to the reticular activating system of the brain stem. These projections provide the basis for increased wakefulness or awareness after strong somatosensory stimulation and for the generalized startle reaction that occurs with sudden and intense stimuli. They also stimulate autonomic nervous system responses, such as a rise in blood pressure and heart rate, dilation of the pupils, and the pale, moist skin that results from constriction of the cutaneous blood vessels and activation of the sweat glands.

There are two subdivisions in the anterolateral pathway: the *neospinothalamic tract* and the *paleospinothalamic tract* (Fig. 48-5). The neospinothalamic tract, which carries bright pain, consists of a sequence of at least three neurons with long axons. It provides for relatively rapid transmission of sensory information to the thalamus. The paleospinothalamic tract, which is phylogenetically older than the neospinothalamic system, consists of bilateral, multisynaptic slow-conducting tracts that transmit sensory signals that do not require discrete localization of signal source or discrimination of fine gradations in intensity. This slower-conducting pathway also projects into the intralaminar nuclei of the thalamus, which have close connections with the limbic cortical systems. This circuitry gives touch its affective or emotional aspects, such as the particular unpleasantness of heavy pressure and the peculiar pleasantness of the tickling and gentle rubbing of the skin.

Central Processing of Somatosensory Information

Perception, or the final processing of somatosensory information, involves awareness of the stimuli, localization and discrimination of their characteristics, and interpretation of their meaning. As sensory information reaches the thalamus, it begins to enter the level of consciousness. In the thalamus, the sensory information is roughly localized and perceived as a crude sense. The full localization, discrimination of the intensity, and interpretation of the meaning of the stimuli require processing by the somatosensory cortex.

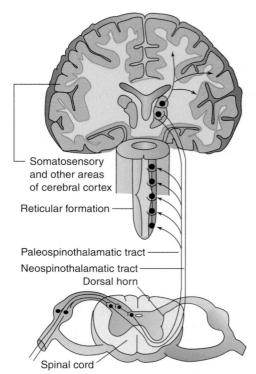

FIGURE 48-5 Neospinothalamic and paleospinothalamic subdivisions of the anterolateral sensory pathway. The neospinothalamic tract runs to the thalamic nuclei and has fibers that project to the somatosensory cortex. The paleospinothalamic tract sends collaterals to the reticular formation and other structures, from which further fibers project to the thalamus. These fibers influence the hypothalamus and the limbic system as well as the cerebral cortex. (From Rodman M.J., Smith D.W. [1979]. *Pharmacology and drug therapy in nursing.* [2nd ed.]. Philadelphia: J.B. Lippincott)

The somatosensory cortex is located in the parietal lobe, which lies behind the central sulcus and above the lateral sulcus (Fig. 48-6). The strip of parietal cortex that borders the central sulcus is called the *primary somatosensory cortex* because it receives primary sensory information by way of direct projections from the thalamus. A distorted map of the body and head surface, called the *sensory homunculus,* reflects the density of cortical neurons devoted to sensory input from afferents in corresponding peripheral areas. As depicted in Figure 48-7, most of the cortical surface is devoted to areas of the body such as the thumb, forefinger, lips, and tongue, where fine touch and pressure discrimination are essential for normal function.

Parallel to and just behind the primary somatosensory cortex (*i.e.,* toward the occipital cortex) lie the somatosensory association areas, which are required to transform the raw material of sensation into meaningful learned perception. Most of the perceptive aspects of body sensation, or somesthesia, require the function of this parietal association cortex. The perceptive aspect, or meaningfulness, of a stimulus pattern involves the integration of present sensation with past learning. For instance, a person's past learning plus present tactile sensation provides the perception of sitting on a soft chair rather than on a hard bicycle seat.

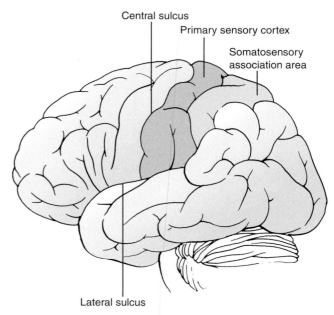

FIGURE 48-6 Primary somatosensory and association somatosensory cortex.

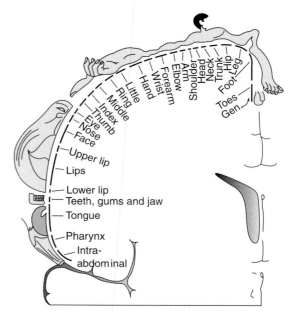

FIGURE 48-7 Homunculus, as determined by stimulation studies on the human cortex during surgery. (Penfield E., Rasmussen T. [1955]. *The cerebral cortex of man.* New York: Macmillan. Copyright © by Macmillan Publishing Co., Inc., renewed 1978 by Theodore Rasmussen)

SENSORY MODALITIES

Somatosensory experience can be divided into *modalities,* a term used for qualitative, subjective distinctions between sensations such as touch, heat, and pain. Such experiences require the function of sensory receptors and forebrain structures in the thalamus and cerebral cortex. Sensory experience also involves quantitative sensory discrimination or the ability to distinguish between different levels of sensory stimulation.

The receptive endings of different afferent neurons are particularly sensitive to specific forms of physical and chemical energy. They can initiate action potentials to many forms of energy at high energy levels, but they usually are highly tuned to be differentially sensitive to low levels of a particular energy type. For instance, a receptive ending may be particularly sensitive to a small increase in local skin temperature. Stimulating the ending with electric current or strong pressure also can result in action potentials. The amount of energy required, however, is much greater than it is for a change in temperature. Other afferent sensory terminals are most sensitive to slight indentations of the skin, and their signals are subjectively interpreted as touch. Cool versus warm, sharp versus dull pain, and delicate touch versus deep pressure are all based on different populations of afferent neurons or on central integration of simultaneous input from several differently tuned afferents. For example, the sensation of itch results from a combination of high activity in pain- and touch-sensitive afferents, and the sensation of tickle requires a gently moving tactile stimulus over cool skin.

When information from different primary afferents reaches the forebrain, where subjective experience occurs, the qualitative differences between warmth and touch are called *sensory modalities*. Although the receptor-detected information is relayed to the thalamus and cortex over separate pathways, the experience of a modality, such as cold versus warm, is uniquely subjective.

Stimulus Discrimination

The ability to discriminate the location of a somesthetic stimulus is called *acuity* and is based on the sensory field in a dermatome innervated by an afferent neuron. High acuity (*i.e.,* the ability to make fine discriminations of location) requires a high density of innervation by afferent neurons. For example, acuity is high on the thumb but lower on the back of the hand. High acuity also requires a projection system through the CNS to the forebrain that preserves distinctions between levels of activity in neighboring sensory fields. Receptors or receptive endings of primary afferent neurons differ as to the intensity at which they begin to fire. This threshold usually is lower than the stimulus threshold required for first brain-level perception of subjective sensation (*i.e.,* subjective threshold). For instance, when a single hair on the back of the hand is bent progressively, some bending occurs before action potentials appear in the primary afferent neuron (*i.e.,* afferent threshold). The hair must be bent further and the action potentials must increase in frequency before a person is able reliably to detect the bending of the hair (*i.e.,* subjective sensation threshold). For highly developed discriminative systems, under ideal conditions, these thresholds may correspond closely.

Many factors, such as attention and emotion, can greatly elevate the subjective threshold. After the subjective threshold is reached, the intensity of the experienced sensation is based on the rate of impulse generation in the afferent neuron, such that gradations in stimulus intensity are discriminated proportional to the logarithm of stimulus strength. This means that, after the subjective threshold has been reached, greater changes in stimulus strength are needed for further discrimination. This is known as the *Weber-Fechner principle*. For example, after the subjective threshold has been reached, a person could have difficulty detecting a less than 1-g increase in weight when holding a 30-g weight or a less than 10-g increase when holding a 300-g weight. In each case, the ratio of change (*i.e.,* logarithm) remains approximately 1 to 30.[1] This relation holds true for all sensory systems, including the somesthetic system, and is based on characteristics of the receptor endings.

Some afferent neurons maintain a more or less steady rate of firing to a continuous stimulus. This is true for afferents from muscles, tendons, and joints, where continuous feedback information is necessary for maintaining posture. These slow-adapting afferent neurons contrast with rapid-adapting afferent neurons, which signal only the onset, sudden change, and conclusion of a stimulus. Rapid-adapting afferent neurons are required to signal moving, brief, or vibrating stimuli.

Tactile Sensation

The tactile system, which relays sensory information regarding touch, pressure, and vibration, is considered the basic somatosensory system. Loss of temperature or pain sensitivity leaves the person with no awareness of deficiency. However, if the tactile system is lost, total anesthesia (*i.e.,* numbness) of the involved body part results.

Touch sensation results from stimulation of tactile receptors in the skin and in tissues immediately beneath the skin, pressure from deformation of deeper tissues, and vibration from rapidly repetitive sensory signals. There are at least six types of specialized tactile receptors in the skin and deeper structures: free nerve endings,[2] Meissner's corpuscles, Merkel's disks, pacinian corpuscles, hair follicle end-organs, and Ruffini's end-organs[1,2] (Fig. 48-8).

Free nerve endings are found in skin and many other tissues, including the cornea. They detect touch and pressure. *Meissner's corpuscle* is an elongated encapsulated nerve ending that is present in nonhairy parts of the skin. It is particularly abundant in the fingertips, lips, and other areas where the sense of touch is highly developed. *Merkel's disks* are dome-shaped receptors found in nonhairy areas and in hairy parts of the skin. In contrast to Meissner's corpuscles, which adapt within a fraction of a second, Merkel's disks transmit an initial strong signal that diminishes in strength but is slow in adapting. For this reason, Meissner's corpuscles are particularly sensitive to the movement of very light objects over the surface of the skin and to low-frequency vibration. Merkel's disks are responsible for giving steady-state signals that allow for continuous determination of touch against the skin.

The *pacinian corpuscle* is located immediately beneath the skin and deep in the fascial tissues of the body. This type of receptor, which is stimulated by rapid movements of the tissues and adapts within a few hundredths of a second, is important in detecting tissue vibration. The *hair follicle end-organ* consists of afferent unmyelinated fibers entwined around most of the length of the hair follicle. These

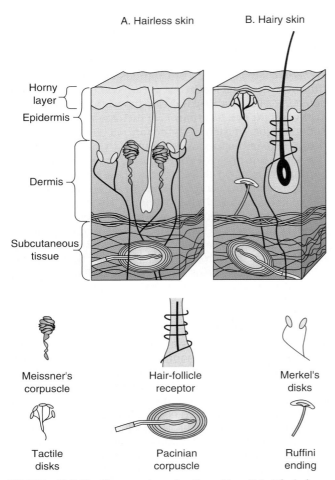

A. Hairless skin   B. Hairy skin

Horny layer
Epidermis
Dermis
Subcutaneous tissue

Meissner's corpuscle
Hair-follicle receptor
Merkel's disks

Tactile disks
Pacinian corpuscle
Ruffini ending

FIGURE 48-8 Tactile receptors in the skin. (Modified from Schmidt R.F. [1981]. *Fundamentals of sensory physiology* [2nd ed.]. New York: Springer-Verlag)

receptors, which are rapidly adapting, detect movement on the surface of the body. *Ruffini's end-organs* are found in the skin and deeper structures, including the joint capsules. These receptors, which have multibranched encapsulated endings, have very little adaptive capacity and are important for signaling continuous states of deformation, such as heavy and continuous touch and pressure.

Almost all the specialized touch receptors, such as Merkel's disks, Meissner's corpuscles, hair follicle end-organs, pacinian corpuscles, and Ruffini's end-organs, transmit their signals in large myelinated nerve fibers (*i.e.*, type Aα, β) that have transmission velocities ranging from 25 to 70 m/second. Most free nerve endings transmit signals by way of small myelinated fibers (*i.e.*, type Aδ) with conduction velocities of 10 to 30 m/second.

The sensory information for tactile sensation enters the spinal cord through the dorsal roots of the spinal nerves. All tactile sensation that requires rapid transmission is transmitted through the discriminative pathway to the thalamus by way of the medial lemniscus. This includes touch sensation requiring a high degree of localization or fine gradations of intensity, vibratory sensation, and sensation that signals movement against the skin. In addition to the ascending discriminative pathway, tactile sensation uses the more primitive and crude anterolateral pathway. The afferent axons that carry tactile information up the dorsal columns have many branches or collaterals, and some of these synapse in the dorsal horn near the level of dorsal root entry. After several synapses, axons are projected up both sides of the anterolateral aspect of the spinal cord to the thalamus. Few fibers travel all the way to the thalamus. Most synapse on reticular formation neurons that then send their axons on toward the thalamus. The lateral nuclei of the thalamus are capable of contributing a crude, poorly localized sensation from the opposite side of the body. From the thalamus, some projections travel to the somatosensory cortex, especially to the side opposite the stimulus.

Because of these multiple routes, total destruction of the pathway seldom occurs. The only time this crude alternative system becomes essential is when the discriminative pathway is damaged. Then, despite projection of the anterolateral system information to the somatosensory cortex, only a poorly localized, high-threshold sense of touch remains. Such persons lose all sense of joint and muscle movement, body position, and two-point discrimination.

Thermal Sensation

Thermal sensation is discriminated by three types of receptors: cold receptors, warmth receptors, and pain receptors. The cold and warmth receptors are located immediately under the skin at discrete but separate points, each serving an area of approximately 1 mm². In some areas, there are more cold receptors than warmth receptors. For example, the lips have 15 to 25 cold receptors per square centimeter, compared with 3 to 5 in the same-sized area of the finger.[1] There are correspondingly fewer warmth receptors in these areas. The different gradations of heat and cold result from the relative degrees of stimulation of the different types of nerve endings. The thermal receptors are very sensitive to differences between the temperature of skin and temperature of objects that are touched. Warmth receptors respond proportionately to increases in skin temperature above resting values of 34°C and cool receptors to temperatures below 34°C.[3] The thermal pain receptors are stimulated only by extremes of temperature such as "freezing cold" (temperatures below 5°C) and "burning hot" (temperatures above 45°C) sensations.[3] With the exception of pain receptors, thermal receptors tend to adapt rapidly during the first few minutes and then more slowly during the next 30 minutes or so. However, these receptors do not appear to adapt completely, as evidenced by the experience of an intense sense of heat on entering a tub of hot water or the extreme degree of cold initially sensed when going outside on a cold day.

Dorsal root ganglion afferents, with receptive thermal endings in the skin, send their central axons into the segmental dorsal horn of the spinal cord. Cranial nerves that innervate the face and inside of the mouth send their axons to homologous, or equivalent, nuclei of the brain stem. On entering the dorsal horn, thermal signals are processed by second-order input association neurons. These association neurons activate projection neurons whose axons then cross to the opposite side of the cord and ascend in the multisynaptic, slow-conducting anterolateral system to the opposite side of the brain. Thalamic and cortical somatosensory regions for temperature are mixed with those for tactile sensibility.

Conduction of thermal information through peripheral nerves is quite slow compared with the rapid tactile afferents that travel through the discriminative system. If a person places a foot in a tub of hot water, the tactile sensation occurs well in advance of the burning sensation. The foot has been removed from the hot water by the local withdrawal reflex well before the excessive heat is perceived by the forebrain. Local anesthetic agents block the small-diameter afferents that carry thermal sensory information before they block the large-diameter axons that carry discriminative touch information.

Position Sensation

Position sense refers to the sense of limb and body movement and position without using vision. It is mediated by input from proprioceptive receptors (muscle spindle receptors and Golgi tendon organs) found primarily in muscles, tendons, and joint capsules (see Chapter 47). There are two submodalities of proprioception: the stationary or static component (limb position sense) and the dynamic aspects of position sense (kinesthesia). Both of these depend on constant transmission of information to the CNS regarding the degree of angulation of all joints and the rate of change in angulation. In addition, stretch-sensitive receptors in the skin (Ruffini's end-organs, pacinian corpuscles, and Merkel's cells) also signal postural information. Signals from these receptors are processed through the dorsal column–medial lemniscus pathway. In addition to the transmission of signals from the periphery to the cerebral cortex, the signals are processed in the thalamus before reaching the cerebral cortex. Lesions affecting the posterior column impair position sense. The vestibular system also plays an essential role in position sense. The vestibular system's role and the diseases affecting it and thus impairing position sense are discussed in Chapter 55.

CLINICAL ASSESSMENT OF SOMATOSENSORY FUNCTION

Clinically, neurologic assessment of somatosensory function can be done by testing the integrity of spinal segmental nerves. A pinpoint pressed against the skin of the sole of the foot that results in a withdrawal reflex and a complaint of skin pain confirms the functional integrity of the afferent terminals in the skin, the entire pathway through the peripheral nerves of the foot, leg, and thigh to the sacral (S1) dorsal root ganglion, and through the dorsal root into the spinal cord segment. It confirms that the somatosensory input association cells receiving this information are functioning and that the reflex circuitry of the cord segments (L5 to S2) is functioning. In addition, the lower motor neurons of the L4 to S1 ventral horn can be considered operational, and their axons through the ventral roots, the mixed peripheral nerve, and the motor neuron to the muscles producing the withdrawal response can be considered intact and functional. The communication between the lower motor neuron and the muscle cells is functional, and these muscles have normal responsiveness and strength.

Testing is done at each segmental level, or dermatome, moving upward along the body and neck from coccygeal segments through the high cervical levels to test the functional integrity of all the spinal nerves. Similar dermatomes cover the face and scalp, and these, although innervated by cranial segmental nerves, are tested in the same manner.

The observation of a normal withdrawal reflex rules out peripheral nerve disease, disorders of the dorsal root and ganglion, diseases of the myoneural junction, and severe muscle diseases. Normal reflex function also indicates that many major descending CNS tract systems are functioning within normal limits. If the person is able to report the pinprick sensation and accurately identify its location, many ascending systems through much of the spinal cord and brain also are functioning normally, as are basic intellect and speech mechanisms.

The integrity of the discriminative dorsal column–medial lemniscus pathway compared with the anterolateral tactile pathways is tested with the person's eyes closed by gently brushing the skin with a wisp of cotton, touching an area with one or two sharp points, touching corresponding parts of the body on each side simultaneously or in random sequence, and passively bending the person's finger one way and then another in random order. If only the anterolateral pathway is functional, the tactile threshold is markedly elevated, two-point discrimination and proprioception are missing, and the patient has difficulty discriminating which side of the body received stimulation.

In summary, the somatosensory component of the nervous system provides an awareness of body sensations such as touch, temperature, position sense, and pain. There are three primary levels of neural integration in the somatosensory system: the sensory units containing the sensory receptors, the ascending pathways, and the central processing centers in the thalamus and cerebral cortex. A sensory unit consists of a single dorsal root ganglion neuron, its receptors, and its central axon that terminates in the dorsal horn of the spinal cord or medulla. The part of the body innervated by the somatosensory afferent neurons of one set of dorsal root ganglia is called a *dermatome*. Ascending pathways include the discriminative pathway, which crosses at the base of the medulla, and the anterolateral pathway, which crosses within the first few segments of entering the spinal cord. Perception, or the final processing of somatosensory information, involves centers in the thalamus and somatosensory cortex. In the thalamus, the sensory information is crudely localized and perceived. The full localization, discrimination of the intensity, and interpretation of the meaning of the stimuli require processing by the somatosensory cortex. A distorted map of the body and head surface, called the *sensory homunculus,* reflects the density of cortical neurons devoted to sensory input from afferents in corresponding peripheral areas.

The tactile system relays the sensations of touch, pressure, and vibration. It uses two anatomically separate pathways to relay touch information to the opposite side of the forebrain: the dorsal column discriminative pathway and the anterolateral pathway. Delicate touch, vibration, position, and movement sensations use the discriminative pathway to reach the thalamus, where third-order relay occurs to the primary somatosensory strip of parietal cortex. Crude tactile sensation is carried by the bilateral slow-conducting anterolateral pathway. Temperature sensations of warm-hot and cool-cold are the result of stimulation to thermal receptors of sensory units projecting to the thalamus and cortex through the anterolateral system on the opposite side of the body. Proprioception is the sense of limb and body movement and position without using vision. Proprioceptive information is processed through the rapid-transmitting dorsal column–medial lemniscus pathway. Testing of the ipsilateral dorsal column (discriminative touch) system or the contralateral temperature projection systems permits diagnostic analysis of the level and extent of damage in spinal cord lesions.

Pain

After you have completed this section of the chapter, you should be able to meet the following objectives:

+ Differentiate among the specificity, pattern, gate control, and neuromatrix theories of pain
+ Characterize the response of nociceptors to stimuli that produce pain
+ State the difference between the Aδ- and C-fiber neurons in the transmission of pain information
+ Trace the transmission of pain signals with reference to the neospinothalamic, paleospinothalamic, and reticulospinal pathways, including the role of chemical mediators and factors that modulate pain transmission
+ Describe the function of endogenous analgesic mechanisms as they relate to transmission of pain information
+ Compare pain threshold and pain tolerance
+ Differentiate acute pain from chronic pain in terms of mechanisms, manifestations, and treatment
+ Describe the mechanisms of referred pain, and list the common sites of referral for cardiac and other types of visceral pain
+ Describe three methods for assessing pain
+ Describe the proposed mechanisms of pain relief associated with the use of heat, cold, transcutaneous electrical nerve stimulation, and acupuncture and acupressure
+ State the mechanisms whereby non-narcotic and narcotic analgesics, tricyclic antidepressants, and antiseizure drugs relieve pain

Pain is an "unpleasant sensory and emotional experience associated with actual and potential tissue damage, or described in terms of such damage."[4] The early work by Sir Charles Sherrington[5] introduced the important concept that pain perception and reaction to pain can be separated. This is particularly important for clinical pain because suffering is more heavily influenced by the reaction to pain than by actual pain intensity. Attention, motivation, past experience, and the meaning of the situation can influence the individual's reaction to pain. Thus, pain involves anatomic structures, physiologic behaviors, as well as psychological, social, cultural, and cognitive factors.

Pain is a common symptom that varies widely in intensity and spares no age group. When pain is extremely severe, it disrupts a person's customary behavior and can consume all of a person's attention. It can be equally devastating for infants and children, young and middle-aged adults, as well as the young-old and the old-old. Both acute pain and chronic pain can be major health problems. Acute pain often results from injury, surgery, or invasive medical procedures. It also can be a presenting symptom for some infections (*e.g.,* pharyngitis, appendicitis, and otitis media). Chronic pain can be symptomatic of a wide range of health problems (*e.g.,* arthritis, back injury, or cancer). In recent epidemiologic surveys, approximately 46% of adults reported having chronic pain.[6] Results from the National Health Interview Survey revealed that 13.7% of the population limits daily activities because of chronic pain conditions.[7]

The experience of pain depends on both sensory stimulation and perception. The perception of pain can be heavily influenced by the endogenous analgesia system that modulates the sensation of pain. This is perhaps most dramatically illustrated by the phenomenon of soldiers injured in battle or athletes injured during a game who do not perceive major injuries as painful until they leave the battlefield or the game.

Pain can be either nociceptive or neuropathic in origin. When nociceptors (pain receptors) are activated in response to actual or impending tissue injury, *nociceptive pain* is the consequence. *Neuropathic pain,* on the other hand, arises from direct injury to nerves. Tissue and nerve injury can result in a wide range of symptoms. These include pain from noninjurious stimuli to the skin (*allodynia*), extreme sensitivity to pain (*hyperalgesia*), and the absence of pain from stimuli that normally would be painful (*analgesia*). The latter, although not painful, can be extremely serious (*e.g.,* in diabetic persons with peripheral neuropathy) because the normally protective early warning system for the presence of tissue injury is absent.

PAIN THEORIES

Traditionally, two theories have been offered to explain the physiologic basis for the pain experience. The first, *specificity theory,* regards pain as a separate sensory modality evoked by the activity of specific receptors that transmit information to pain centers or regions in the forebrain where pain is experienced.[8] The second theory includes a group of theories collectively referred to as *pattern theory.* It proposes that pain receptors share endings or pathways with other sensory modalities, but that different patterns of activity (*i.e.,* spatial or temporal) of the same neurons can be used to signal painful and nonpainful stimuli.[8] For example, light touch applied to the skin would produce the sensation of touch through low-frequency firing of the receptor; intense pressure would produce pain through high-frequency firing of the same receptor. Both theories focus on the neurophysiologic basis of pain, and both probably apply. Specific nociceptive afferents have been identified; however, almost all afferent stimuli, if driven at a very high frequency, can be experienced as painful.

Gate control theory, a modification of specificity theory, was proposed by Melzack and Wall in 1965 to meet the challenges presented by the pattern theories. This theory postulated the presence of neural gating mechanisms at the segmental spinal cord level to account for interactions between pain and other sensory modalities.[9] The original gate control theory proposed a spinal-cord–level network of transmission or projection cells and internuncial neurons that inhibits the transmission cells, forming a segmental level gating mechanism that could block projection of pain information to the brain.

According to the gate control theory, the internuncial neurons involved in the gating mechanism are activated by large-diameter, faster-propagating fibers that carry tactile information. The simultaneous firing of the large-diameter touch fibers has the potential for blocking the transmission of impulses from the small-diameter myelinated and unmyelinated pain fibers. Pain therapists have long known that pain intensity can be temporarily reduced during active tactile stimulation. For example, repeated sweeping of a soft-bristled brush on the skin (*i.e.,* brushing) over or near a painful area may result in pain reduction for several minutes to several hours.

Pain modulation is now known to be a much more complex phenomenon than that proposed by the original gate control theory. Tactile information is transmitted by small- and large-diameter fibers. Major interactions between sensory modalities, including the so-called gating phenomenon, occur at several levels of the CNS rostral to the input segment. Perhaps the most puzzling aspect of locally applied stimuli, such as brushing, that can block the experience of pain is the relatively long-lasting effect (minutes to hours) of such treatments. This prolonged effect has been difficult to explain on the basis of specificity theories, including the gate control theory. Other important factors include the effect of endogenous opioids and their receptors at the segmental and brain stem level, descending feedback modulation, altered sensitivity, learning, and culture. Despite this complexity, the Melzack and Wall theory has served a useful purpose. It excited interest in pain and stimulated research and clinical activity related to the pain-modulating systems.

More recently, Melzack has developed the *neuromatrix theory* to address further the brain's role in pain as well as the multiple dimensions and determinants of pain.[10] This theory is particularly useful in understanding chronic pain and phantom limb pain, in which there is not a simple one-to-one relationship between tissue injury and pain experience. The neuromatrix theory proposes that the brain contains a widely distributed neural network, called the *body-self neuromatrix,* that contains somatosensory, limbic, and thalamocortical components. Genetic and sensory influences determine the synaptic architecture of an individual's neuromatrix that integrates multiple sources of input and yields the neuro-signature pattern that evokes the sensory, affective, and cognitive dimensions of pain experience and behavior. These multiple sources include somatosensory inputs; other sensory inputs affecting interpretation of the situation; phasic and tonic inputs from the brain addressing such things as attention, expectation, culture, and personality; intrinsic neural inhibitory modulation; and various components of stress-regulation systems. This theory may open entire new areas of research such as an understanding of the role that cortisol plays in chronic pain, the effect estrogen has on pain mediated through the release of peripheral cytokines, and the reported increase in chronic pain that occurs with age.

PAIN MECHANISMS AND PATHWAYS

Pain usually is viewed in the context of tissue injury. The term *nociception,* which means "pain sense," comes from the Latin word *nocere* ("to injure"). Nociceptive stimuli are objectively defined as stimuli of such intensity that they cause or are close to causing tissue damage. Researchers often use the withdrawal reflex (*e.g.,* the reflexive withdrawal of a body part from a tissue-damaging stimulus) to determine when a stimulus is nociceptive. Stimuli used include pressure from a sharp object, strong electric current to the skin, or application of heat or cold of approximately 10°C above or below normal skin temperature. At low levels of intensity these noxious stimuli do activate nociceptors (pain receptors), but typically are perceived as painful only when the intensity reaches a level where tissue damage occurs or is imminent.

The mechanisms of pain are many and complex. As with other forms of somatosensation, the pathways are composed of first-, second-, and third-order neurons. The first-order neurons and their receptive endings detect stimuli that threaten the integrity of innervated tissues. Second-order neurons are located in the spinal cord and process nociceptive information. Third-order neurons project pain information to the brain. The thalamus and cortex integrate and modulate pain as well as the person's subjective reaction to the pain experience.

Pain Receptors and Mediators

Nociceptors, or pain receptors, are sensory receptors that are activated by noxious insults to peripheral tissues. Structurally, the receptive endings of the peripheral pain fibers are free nerve endings. These receptive endings, which are widely distributed in the skin, dental pulp, periosteum, meninges, and some internal organs, translate the noxious stimuli into action potentials that are transmitted by a dorsal root ganglion to the dorsal horn of the spinal cord. Nociceptive action potentials are transmitted through two types of afferent nerve fibers: myelinated Aδ fibers and unmyelinated C fibers. The larger Aδ fibers have considerably greater conduction velocities, transmitting impulses at a rate of 10 to 30 m/second. The C fibers are the smallest of all peripheral nerve fibers; they transmit impulses at the rate of 0.5 to 2.5 m/second. Pain conducted by Aδ fibers traditionally is called *fast pain* and typically is elicited by mechanical or thermal stimuli. C-fiber pain often is described as *slow-wave pain* because

Pain Sensation

➤ Pain is both a protective and an unpleasant physical and emotionally disturbing sensation originating in pain receptors that respond to a number of stimuli that threaten tissue integrity.

➤ There are two pathways for pain transmission:

  ➤ The pathway for fast, sharply discriminated pain that moves directly from the receptor to the spinal cord using myelinated Aδ fibers and from the spinal cord to the thalamus using the neospinothalamic tract

  ➤ The pathway for slow, continuously conducted pain that is transmitted to the spinal cord using unmyelinated C fibers and from the spinal cord to the thalamus using the more circuitous and slower-conducting paleospinothalamic tract

➤ The central processing of pain information includes transmission to the somatosensory cortex, where pain information is perceived and interpreted, the limbic system, where the emotional components of pain are experienced, and to brain stem centers, where autonomic nervous system responses are recruited.

➤ Modulation of the pain experience occurs by way of the endogenous analgesic center in the midbrain, the pontine noradrenergic neurons, and the nucleus raphe magnus in the medulla, which sends inhibitory signals to dorsal horn neurons in the spinal cord.

it is slower in onset and longer in duration. It typically is incited by chemical stimuli or by persistent mechanical or thermal stimuli. The slow postexcitatory potentials generated in C fibers are now believed to be responsible for central sensitization to chronic pain.

Stimulation of Nociceptors.   Unlike other sensory receptors, nociceptors respond to several forms of stimulation, including mechanical, thermal, and chemical. Some receptors respond to a single type of stimuli (mechanical or thermal) and others, called *polymodal receptors,* respond to all three types of stimuli (mechanical, thermal, and chemical). Mechanical stimuli can arise from intense pressure applied to skin or from the violent contraction or extreme stretch of a muscle. Both extremes of heat and cold can stimulate nociceptors. Chemical stimuli arise from a number of sources, including tissue trauma, ischemia, and inflammation. A wide range of chemical mediators are released from injured and inflamed tissues, including hydrogen and potassium ions, prostaglandins, leukotrienes, histamine, bradykinin, acetylcholine, and serotonin. These chemical mediators produce their effects by directly stimulating nociceptors or

sensitizing them to the effects of nociceptive stimuli; perpetuating the inflammatory responses that lead to the release of chemical agents that act as nociceptive stimuli; or inciting neurogenic reflexes that increase the response to nociceptive stimuli. For example, bradykinin, histamine, serotonin, and potassium activate and also sensitize nociceptors. Adenosine triphosphate, acetylcholine, and platelets act alone or in concert to sensitize nociceptors through other chemical agents such as prostaglandins. Aspirin and other nonsteroidal analgesic drugs are effective in controlling pain because they block the enzyme needed for prostaglandin synthesis.

Nociceptive stimulation that activates C fibers can cause a response known as *neurogenic inflammation* that produces vasodilation and an increased release of chemical mediators to which nociceptors respond. This mechanism is thought to be mediated by a dorsal root neuron reflex that produces retrograde transport and release of chemical mediators, which in turn causes increasing inflammation of peripheral tissues. This reflex can set up a vicious cycle, which has implications for persistent pain and hyperalgesia.[11] Local anesthetics (*e.g.,* procaine [Novocain]) can prevent the spread of sensitization and secondary hyperalgesia due to stimulation of cutaneous nociceptors by blocking the dorsal root neuron reflex.[12]

Mediators in the Spinal Cord.   In the spinal cord, the transmission of impulses between the nociceptive neurons and the dorsal horn neurons is mediated by chemical neurotransmitters released from central nerve endings of the nociceptive neurons. Some of these neurotransmitters are amino acids (*e.g.,* glutamate), others are amino acid derivatives (*e.g.,* norepinephrine), and still others are low–molecular-weight peptides composed of two or more amino acids. The amino acid glutamate is a major excitatory neurotransmitter released from the central nerve endings of the nociceptive neurons. Substance P, a neuropeptide, also is released in the dorsal horn by C fibers in response to nociceptive stimulation. Substance P elicits slow excitatory potentials in dorsal horn neurons. Unlike glutamate, which confines its action to the immediate area of the synaptic terminal, some neuropeptides released in the dorsal horn can diffuse some distance because they are not inactivated by reuptake mechanisms. In persistent pain, this may help to explain the excitability and unlocalized nature of many painful conditions. Neuropeptides such as substance P also appear to prolong and enhance the action of glutamate. If these neurotransmitters are released in large quantities or over extended periods, they can lead to secondary hyperalgesia, a condition in which the second-order neurons are overly sensitive to low levels of noxious stimulation. Understanding how chemical mediators function in nociception is an active area of research that has implications for the development of new treatments for pain.

Spinal Cord Circuitry and Pathways

On entering the spinal cord through the dorsal roots, the pain fibers bifurcate and ascend or descend one or two segments before synapsing with association neurons in the dorsal horn. From the dorsal horn, the axons of association projection neurons cross through the anterior commissure to the opposite side and then ascend upward in the previously described neospinothalamic and paleospinothalamic pathways.

The faster-conducting fibers in the neospinothalamic tract (*i.e.*, discriminative pain pathway) are associated mainly with the transmission of sharp-fast pain information to the thalamus. In the thalamus, synapses are made and the pathway continues to the contralateral parietal somatosensory area to provide the precise location of the pain. Typically, the pain is experienced as bright, sharp, or stabbing in nature. There is also a local cord-level withdrawal reflex that is designed to remove endangered tissue from a damaging stimulus.

The paleospinothalamic tract is a slower-conducting, multisynaptic tract concerned with the diffuse, dull, aching, and unpleasant sensations that commonly are associated with chronic and visceral pain. This information travels through the small, unmyelinated C fibers. Fibers of this system also project up the contralateral (*i.e.*, opposite) anterolateral pathway to terminate in several thalamic regions, including the intralateral nuclei, which project to the limbic system. It is associated with the emotional or affective-motivational aspects of pain. Spinoreticular fibers from this pathway project bilaterally to the reticular formation of the brain stem. This component of the paleospinothalamic system facilitates avoidance reflexes at all levels. It also contributes to an increase in the electroencephalographic activity associated with alertness and indirectly influences hypothalamic functions associated with sudden alertness, such as increased heart rate and blood pressure. This may explain the tremendous arousal effects of certain pain stimuli.

Dorsal horn (second-order) neurons are divided primarily into two types: wide–dynamic-range (WDR) neurons that respond to low intensity stimuli and nociceptive-specific neurons that respond only to noxious or nociceptive stimuli. When stimuli are increased to a noxious level, the WDR neurons respond more intensely. After more severe damage to peripheral sensory afferents, Aδ and C fibers respond more intensely as they are increasingly stimulated. When C fibers are repetitively stimulated at a rate of once per second, each stimulus produces a progressively increasing response from WDR neurons. This phenomenon of amplification of transmitted signals has been called *windup* and may explain why pain sensation appears to increase with repeated stimulation. Windup and sensitization of dorsal horn neurons have implications for appropriate and early, or even preemptive, pain therapy to avoid the possibility of spinal cord neurons becoming hypersensitive or subject to firing spontaneously.[11,13]

Brain Centers and Pain Perception

The basic sensation of hurtfulness, or pain, occurs at the level of the thalamus. In the neospinothalamic system, interconnections between the lateral thalamus and the somatosensory cortex are necessary to add precision and discrimination to the pain sensation. Association areas of the parietal cortex are essential to the learned meaningfulness of the pain experience. For example, if a person is stung on the index finger by a bee and only the thalamus is functional, the person complains of pain somewhere on the hand. With

the primary sensory cortex functional, the person can localize the pain to the precise area on the index finger. With the association cortex functional, the person can interpret the buzzing and sight of the bee that preceded the pain as being related to the bee sting. The paleospinothalamic system projects diffusely from the intralaminar nuclei of the thalamus to large areas of the limbic cortex. These connections probably are associated with the hurtfulness and the mood-altering and attention-narrowing effect of pain.

Central Pathways for Pain Modulation

A major advance in understanding pain was the discovery of neuroanatomic pathways that arise in the midbrain and brain stem, descend to the spinal cord, and modulate ascending pain impulses. One such pathway begins in an area of the midbrain called the *periaqueductal gray* (PAG) region. Through research it was found that focal stimulation of the midbrain PAG regions produced a state of analgesia. The resultant analgesia lasted for many hours and was sufficient to permit abdominal surgery, although levels of consciousness and reactions to auditory and visual stimuli remained unaffected. A few years later, opioid receptors were found to be highly concentrated in this and other regions of the CNS where electrical stimulation produced analgesia. Because of these findings, the PAG area of the midbrain often is referred to as the *endogenous analgesia center.*

The PAG area receives input from widespread areas of the CNS, including the cerebral cortex, hypothalamus, brain stem reticular formation, and spinal cord by way of the paleospinothalamic and neospinothalamic tracts. This region is intimately connected to the limbic system, which is associated with emotional experience. The neurons of the PAG area in the midbrain have axons that descend into an area called the *nucleus raphe magnus* (NRM) in the rostral medulla. The axons of these NRM neurons project to the dorsal horn of the spinal cord, where they terminate in the same layers as the entering primary pain fibers (Fig. 48-9). Stimulation of the NRM is thought to inhibit pain transmission by dorsal horn projection neurons.[14] There also is evidence of nor-adrenergic neurons that can inhibit transmission of pain impulses at the level of the spinal cord. Studies indicate that the rostral pons also has noradrenergic neurons with axons that project to the NRM and to the dorsal horn cells of the spinal cord.[15] The discovery that norepinephrine can block pain transmission led to studies directed at the combined administration of opioids and clonidine, a central-acting α-adrenergic agonist for pain relief.

Serotonin also has been identified as a neuromodulator in the NRM medullary nuclei that project to the spinal cord. It has been shown that tricyclic antidepressant compounds, such as amitriptyline, have analgesic properties independent of their antidepressant effects. These drugs, which enhance the effects of serotonin by blocking its presynaptic uptake, have been found to be effective in the management of certain types of chronic pain.[16]

Endogenous Analgesic Mechanisms

There is evidence that the endogenous opioid peptides, morphine-like substances synthesized in many regions of the CNS, modulate pain in the CNS. Three families of

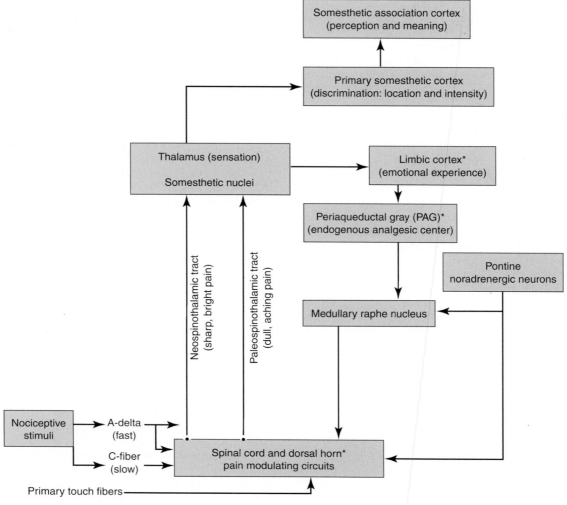

FIGURE 48-9 Primary pain pathways. The transmission of incoming nociceptive impulses is modulated by dorsal horn circuitry that receives input from peripheral touch receptors and from descending pathways that involve the limbic cortical systems (orbital frontal cortex, amygdala, and hypothalamus), periaqueductal endogenous analgesic center in the midbrain, pontine noradrenergic neurons, and the raphe nucleus in the medulla.

opioid peptides have been identified—the enkephalins, endorphins, and dynorphins. Each family is derived from a distinct precursor polypeptide and has a characteristic anatomic distribution. Although each family usually is located in different groups of neurons, occasionally more than one family is present in the same neuron. For example, proenkephalin peptides are present in areas of the spinal cord and PAG that are related to perception of pain, in the hippocampus and other areas of the brain that modulate emotional behavior, in structures in the basal ganglia that modulate motor control, and in brain stem neurons that regulate autonomic nervous system responses. Although the endogenous opioid peptides appear to function as neurotransmitters, their full significance in pain control and other physiologic functions is not completely understood. Probably of greater importance in understanding mechanisms of pain control has been the characterization of receptors that bind the endogenous opioid peptides. The

identification of these receptors has facilitated a more thorough understanding of the actions of available opioid drugs, such as morphine, and it also has facilitated ongoing research into the development of newer preparations that are more effective in relieving pain and have fewer side effects.

PAIN THRESHOLD AND TOLERANCE

Pain threshold and tolerance affect an individual's response to a painful stimulus. Although the terms often are used interchangeably, pain threshold and pain tolerance have distinct meanings. *Pain threshold* is closely associated with the point at which a stimulus is perceived as painful. *Pain tolerance* relates more to the total pain experience; it is defined as the maximum intensity or duration of pain that a person is willing to endure before the person wants something done about the pain. Psychological, familial, cultural, and environmental factors significantly influence the amount of pain a person is willing to tolerate. The threshold to pain is fairly uniform from one person to another, whereas pain tolerance is extremely variable.[11] Separation and identification of the role of each of these two aspects of pain continue to pose fundamental problems for the pain management team and for pain researchers.

TYPES OF PAIN

The most widely accepted classifications of pain are according to source or location, referral, and duration (acute or chronic). Classification based on associated medical diagnosis (*e.g.,* surgery, trauma, cancer, sickle cell disease, fibromyalgia) is useful in planning appropriate interventions.

Cutaneous and Deep Somatic Pain

Cutaneous pain arises from superficial structures, such as the skin and subcutaneous tissues. A paper cut on the finger is an example of easily localized superficial, or cutaneous, pain. It is a sharp, bright pain with a burning quality and may be abrupt or slow in onset. It can be localized accurately and may be distributed along the dermatomes. Because there is an overlap of nerve fiber distribution between the dermatomes, the boundaries of pain frequently are not as clear-cut as the dermatomal diagrams indicate.

 Types of Pain

➤ Pain can be classified according to location (cutaneous or deep and visceral), site of referral, and duration.

➤ Cutaneous pain is a sharp, burning pain that has its origin in the skin or subcutaneous tissues.

➤ Deep pain is a more diffuse and throbbing pain that originates in structures such as the muscles, bones, and tendons and radiates to the surrounding tissues.

➤ Visceral pain is a diffuse and poorly defined pain that results from stretching, distention, or ischemia of tissues in a body organ.

➤ Referred pain is pain that originates at a visceral site but is perceived as originating in part of the body wall that is innervated by neurons entering the same segment of the nervous system.

➤ Acute pain is a self-limiting pain that lasts less than 6 months.

➤ Chronic pain is persistent pain that lasts longer than 6 months, lacks the autonomic and somatic responses associated with acute pain, and is accompanied by loss of appetite, sleep disturbances, depression, and other debilitating responses.

Deep somatic pain originates in deep body structures, such as the periosteum, muscles, tendons, joints, and blood vessels. This pain is more diffuse than cutaneous pain. Various stimuli, such as strong pressure exerted on bone, ischemia to a muscle, and tissue damage, can produce deep somatic pain. This is the type of pain a person experiences from a sprained ankle. Radiation of pain from the original site of injury can occur. For example, damage to a nerve root can cause a person to experience pain radiating along its fiber distribution.

Visceral Pain

Visceral, or splanchnic, pain has its origin in the visceral organs. Common examples of visceral pain are renal colic, pain caused by cholecystitis, pain associated with acute appendicitis, and peptic ulcer pain. Although the viscera are diffusely and richly innervated, cutting or burning of viscera, as opposed to similar noxious stimuli applied to cutaneous or superficial structures, is unlikely to cause pain. Instead, strong abnormal contractions of the gastrointestinal system, distention, or ischemia affecting the walls of the viscera can induce severe visceral pain. Anyone who has had severe gastrointestinal distress or ureteral colic can readily attest to the misery involved.

Visceral pain is transmitted by small unmyelinated pain fibers that travel with the axons of the autonomic nervous system and project to visceral input association neurons of the cord or brain stem. In addition to sending projections to the forebrain, these input association neurons also project through the paleospinal and spinoreticular pathways into visceral reflex circuits. Visceral pain typically is accompanied by autonomic nervous system responses such as nausea, vomiting, sweating, and pallor and, less commonly, is followed by shock.

Ascending pathways resulting in the experience of visceral pain have three different overlapping general visceral afferent sources: pharynx through lower esophagus that travel along cranial nerves IX and X; stomach through mid-transverse colon that travel along T1 to L2; and below the mid-transverse colon that travel along S2 to S4. The peripheral general visceral afferent pathways involved travel with the parasympathetic distribution for the upper and lower viscera and with the sympathetic distribution for the intervening viscera. Pain from the viscera may be localized only with difficulty. There are several explanations for this. First, innervation of visceral organs is poorly represented at the forebrain levels (*i.e.,* perception). A second possible explanation is that the brain does not easily learn to localize sensations that originate in organs that are only imprecisely visualized. For example, a cut on the third finger of the right hand can be readily seen, identified, and localized, whereas an inflamed internal organ can be localized only vaguely. A third explanation is that sensory information from thoracic and abdominal viscera can travel by two pathways to the CNS.

Referred Pain

Referred pain is pain that is perceived at a site different from its point of origin but innervated by the same spinal segment. It is hypothesized that visceral and somatic afferent neurons converge on the same dorsal horn projection neurons (Fig. 48-10). For this reason, it can be difficult for the brain to correctly identify the original source of pain. Pain that originates in the abdominal or thoracic viscera is diffuse and poorly localized and often perceived at a site far removed from the affected area. For example, the pain associated with myocardial infarction commonly is referred to the left arm, neck, and chest.

Referred pain may arise alone or concurrent with pain located at the origin of the noxious stimuli. This lack of correspondence between the location of the pain and the location of the painful stimuli can make diagnosis difficult. Although the term *referred* usually is applied to pain that originates in the viscera and is experienced as if originating from the body wall, it also may be applied to pain that arises from somatic structures. For example, pain referred to the chest wall could be caused by nociceptive stimulation of the peripheral portion of the diaphragm, which receives somatosensory innervation from the intercostal nerves. An understanding of pain referral is of great value in diagnosing illness. The typical pattern of pain referral can be derived from our understanding that the afferent neurons from visceral or deep somatic tissue enter the spinal cord at the same level as the afferent neurons from the cutaneous areas to which the pain is referred (Fig. 48-11).

The sites of referred pain are determined embryologically with the development of visceral and somatic structures that share the same site for entry of sensory information into the CNS and then move to more distant locations. For example, a person with peritonitis may complain of pain in the shoulder. Internally, there is inflammation of the peritoneum that lines the central part of the diaphragm. In the embryo, the diaphragm originates in the neck, and its central portion is innervated by the phrenic nerve, which enters the cord at the level of the third to fifth segments (C3 to C5). As the fetus develops, the diaphragm descends to its adult position between the thoracic and abdominal cavities, while maintaining its embryonic pattern

of innervation. Thus, fibers that enter the spinal cord at the C3 to C5 level carry information from both the neck area and the diaphragm, and the diaphragmatic pain is interpreted by the forebrain as originating in the shoulder or neck area.

Although the visceral pleura, pericardium, and peritoneum are said to be relatively free of pain fibers, the parietal pleura, pericardium, and peritoneum do react to nociceptive stimuli. Visceral inflammation can involve parietal and somatic structures, and this may give rise to diffuse local or referred pain. For example, irritation of the parietal peritoneum resulting from appendicitis typically gives rise to pain directly over the inflamed area in the lower right quadrant. Such stimuli can evoke pain referred to the umbilical area.

Muscle spasm, or *guarding,* occurs when somatic structures are involved. Guarding is a protective reflex rigidity; its purpose is to protect the affected body parts (*e.g.,* an abscessed appendix or a sprained muscle). This protective guarding may cause blood vessel compression and give rise to the pain of muscle ischemia, causing local and referred pain.

Acute and Chronic Pain

It is common to classify pain according to its duration. Pain research of the past three decades has emphasized the importance of differentiating acute pain from chronic pain. The diagnosis and therapy for each is distinctive because they differ in cause, function, mechanisms, and psychological sequelae (Table 48-2).

Acute Pain. The classic definition of acute pain is pain that lasts less than 6 months. This somewhat arbitrary cutoff point reflects the notion that acute pain is the result of a tissue-damaging event, such as trauma or surgery, and usually is self-limited, ending when the injured tissues heal. The purpose of acute pain is to serve as a warning system.

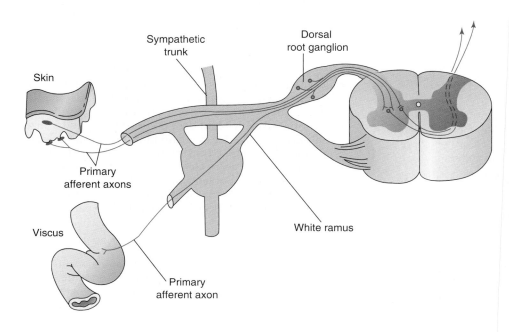

FIGURE 48-10 Convergence of cutaneous and visceral inputs onto the same second-order projection neuron in the dorsal horn of the spinal cord. Although virtually all visceral inputs converge with cutaneous inputs, most cutaneous inputs do not converge with other sensory inputs. (From Conn P.M. [1995]. *Neuroscience in medicine.* Philadelphia: J.B. Lippincott)

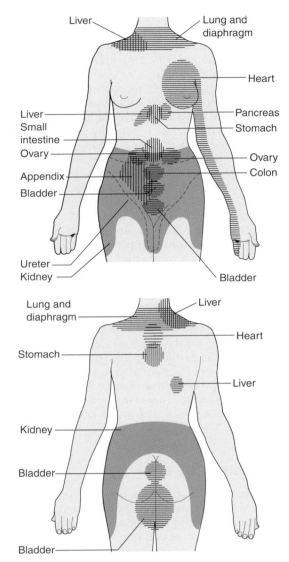

FIGURE 48-11 Areas of referred pain. (**Top**) Anterior view. (**Bottom**) Posterior view. (From Chaffee E.E., Lytle I.M. [1980]. *Basic physiology and anatomy* [4th ed.]. Philadelphia: J.B. Lippincott)

TABLE 48-2 ◆ Characteristics of Acute and Chronic Pain		
Characteristic	**Acute Pain**	**Chronic Pain**
Onset	Recent	Continuous or intermittent
Duration	Short duration (<6 months)	6 months or more
Autonomic responses	Consistent with sympathetic fight-or-flight response* Increased heart rate Increased stroke volume Increased blood pressure Increased pupillary dilation Increased muscle tension Decreased gut motility Decreased salivary flow (dry mouth)	Absence of autonomic responses
Psychological component	Associated anxiety	Increased irritability Associated depression Somatic preoccupation Withdrawal from outside interests Decreased strength of relationships
Other types of response		Decreased sleep Decreased libido Appetite changes

*Responses are approximately proportional to intensity of the stimulus.

Besides alerting the person to the existence of actual or impending tissue damage, it prompts a search for professional help. The pain's location, radiation, intensity, and duration as well as those factors that aggravate or relieve it provide essential diagnostic clues.

Acute pain can lead to anxiety and secondary reflex musculoskeletal spasms, which in turn tend to worsen the pain.[17] Interventions that alleviate the pain usually alleviate the anxiety and musculoskeletal spasms as well. Inadequately treated pain can provoke physiologic responses that alter circulation and tissue metabolism and produce physical manifestations, such as tachycardia, reflective of increased sympathetic activity. Inadequately treated acute pain tends to decrease mobility and respiratory movements such as deep breathing and coughing to the extent that it may complicate or delay recovery.

Chronic Pain. Chronic pain classically has been defined as pain lasting 6 months or longer. In practice, however, one does not wait an arbitrary 6 months before deciding that the pain is chronic; rather, one considers the normal expected healing time for the underlying cause of the pain. The International Association for the Study of Pain defines chronic pain as that which persists beyond the expected normal time of healing.[17] Chronic pain can be quite variable. It may be unrelenting and extremely severe, as in metastatic bone pain. It can be relatively continuous with or without periods of escalation, as with some forms of back pain. Some conditions with recurring episodes of acute pain are particularly problematic because they have characteristics of both acute and chronic pain. These include the pain associated with sickle cell crisis or migraine headaches.

Chronic pain is a leading cause of disability in the United States. Unlike acute pain, persistent chronic pain usually serves no useful function. To the contrary, it imposes physiologic, psychological, familial, and economic stresses and may exhaust a person's resources. In contrast to acute pain, psychological and environmental influences may play an important role in the development of behaviors associated with chronic pain. Chronic pain often is associated with loss of appetite, sleep disturbances, and depression.[18] The physiology of chronic pain is poorly understood.

Persons with chronic pain may not exhibit the somatic, autonomic, or affective behaviors often associated with acute pain. With chronic pain, it is particularly important to heed the person's own description of the pain because the expected psychophysiologic responses may or may not be present. As painful conditions become prolonged and continuous, autonomic nervous system responses decrease. Decreased pain tolerance, which may result from the depletion of serotonin and endorphins, and depression are common in individuals with chronic pain. The link between depression and decreased pain tolerance may be explained by the similar manner in which both respond to changes in the biologic pathways of serotonergic and noradrenergic systems.[18] Tricyclic antidepressants and other medications with serotonergic and noradrenergic effects have been shown to relieve a variety of chronic pain syndromes (*e.g.,* peripheral neuropathic pain, facial pain, and fibrositis), lending credence to the theory that chronic pain and depression share a common biologic pathway.[18]

ASSESSMENT OF PAIN

Careful assessment of pain assists clinicians in diagnosing, managing, and relieving the patient's pain. Assessment includes such things as the nature, severity, location, and radiation of the pain. As with other disease states, it is preferable to eliminate the cause of the pain rather than simply to treat the symptom. A careful history often provides information about the triggering factors (*i.e.,* injury, infection, or disease) and the site of nociceptive stimuli (*i.e.,* peripheral receptor or visceral organ). Although the observation of facial expression and posture may provide additional information, the *Clinical Practice Guideline No. 1. Acute Pain Management: Operative and Medical Procedures and Trauma* (released in 1992 by the Agency for Health Care Policy and Research [AHCPR], currently the Agency for Healthcare Research and Quality, Public Health Service, U.S. Department of Health and Human Services) emphasizes that "the single most reliable indicator of the existence and intensity of acute pain—and any resultant affective discomfort or distress—is the patient's self report."[19] A comprehensive pain history should include pain onset; description, localization, radiation, intensity, quality, and pattern of the pain; anything that relieves or exacerbates it; and the individual's personal reaction to the pain.

Unlike many other bodily responses, such as temperature and blood pressure, the nature, severity, and distress of pain cannot be measured objectively. To overcome this problem, various methods have been developed for quantifying a person's pain. Most of these are based on the patient's report. They include numeric pain intensity, visual analog, and verbal descriptor scales. Most pain questionnaires assess a single aspect of pain such as pain intensity. For example, a *numeric pain intensity* scale would have patients select which number best represents the intensity of their pain, where 0 represents no pain and 10 represents the most intense pain imaginable. A *visual analog* scale also can

be used; it is a straight line, often 10 cm in length, with a word description (*e.g.,* "no pain" or "the most intense pain imaginable") at each of the ends of the line representing the continuum of pain intensity. Patients are asked to choose a point on the continuum that represents the intensity of their pain. The response can be quantified by measuring the line to determine the distance of the mark, measured in millimeters, from the "no pain" end of the line. *Verbal descriptor* scales consist of several numerically ranked choices of words such as none = 0, slight = 1, mild = 2, moderate = 3, and severe = 4. The word chosen is used to determine the numeric representation of pain severity on an ordinal scale.

Some pain questionnaires are multidimensional (*e.g.,* the McGill Pain Questionnaire) in that they include several sections or sets of questions that are scored into subscales that quantify various aspects of pain. The McGill Pain Questionnaire[20] is divided into four parts. The first part uses a drawing of the body on which the person indicates the location of pain. The second part uses a list of 20 words to describe the sensory, affective, evaluative, and other qualities of pain, with the selected words being given a numeric score (*e.g.,* words implying the least pain are assigned a value of 1, moderate pain a value of 2, and so on). The third part asks the person to select words such as *brief, momentary,* and *constant* to describe the pattern of pain. The fourth part of the instrument evaluates the present pain intensity on a scale with scores from 0 to 5. The Memorial Pain Assessment Card, another multidimensional instrument, can be used to determine the intensity of pain, mood, and effectiveness of analgesia.[21]

MANAGEMENT OF PAIN

The therapeutic approaches to acute and chronic pain differ markedly. In acute pain, therapy is directed at providing pain relief by interrupting the nociceptive stimulus. Because the pain is self-limited, in that it resolves as the injured tissues heal, long-term therapy usually is not needed. Chronic pain management is much more complex and is based on multiple considerations, including life expectancy.

Acute Pain

Acute pain should be aggressively managed and pain medication provided before the pain becomes severe. This allows the person to be more comfortable and active and to assume a greater role in directing his or her own care. Part of the reluctance of health care workers to provide adequate relief for acute pain has been fear of addiction. However, addiction to opioid medications is thought to be virtually nonexistent when these drugs are prescribed for acute pain. Usually, less medication is needed when the drug is given before the pain becomes severe and the pain pathways become sensitized.

The AHCPR guidelines, which addresses pain from surgery, medical procedures, and trauma, emphasizes the need for (1) a collaborative, interdisciplinary approach to pain control, which includes members of the health care team and input from the patient and the patient's family when appropriate; (2) an individualized, proactive pain control plan developed before surgery (if possible) by patients and providers; (3) the assessment and frequent reassessment of the patient's pain, facilitated by a pain management log or flow sheet; (4) the use of drug and nondrug therapies to control or prevent pain; and (5) a formal, institutional approach to management of acute pain with clear lines of responsibility.

Chronic Pain

Management of chronic pain requires early attempts to prevent pain and adequate therapy for acute bouts of pain. Specific treatment depends on the cause of the pain, the natural history of the underlying health problem, as well as the life expectancy of the individual. If the organic illness causing the pain cannot be cured, then noncurative methods of pain control become the cornerstone of treatment. Treatment methods for chronic pain can include neural blockade, electrical modalities (*e.g.*, transcutaneous electrical nerve stimulation), physical therapy, cognitive behavioral interventions, and non-narcotic and narcotic medications. Non-narcotic medications such as tricyclic antidepressants, antiseizure medications, and nonsteroidal anti-inflammatory drugs (NSAIDs) serve as useful adjuncts to opioids for the treatment of different types of chronic pain. Chronic pain is best handled by a multidisciplinary team that includes specialists in areas such as anesthesiology, nursing, physical therapy, social services, and surgery.

Cancer is a common cause of chronic pain. The goal of chronic cancer pain management should be pain alleviation and prevention. Preemptive therapy tends to reduce sensitization of pain pathways and provides for more effective pain control. In 1994, the AHCPR published Clinical Practice Guideline No. 9, *Management of Cancer Pain.*[21] This guideline highlights the fact that pain control remains a significant problem despite the advances in understanding and management of pain. The report emphasizes that pain control merits high priority because pain diminishes activity, appetite, and sleep and can further weaken a person already debilitated with cancer. It also emphasizes that pain interferes with productive employment, enjoying recreation, and taking an active part in family life. As with the AHCPR acute pain guideline, the cancer pain guideline also emphasizes the need for a collaborative multidisciplinary approach to cancer pain management. Clinically useful interventions are described in the guideline. Some of these (*e.g.*, analgesics, adjuvant drugs, cognitive or behavioral strategies, physical modalities, and nerve blocks) are used for many forms of chronic pain. Depending on the form and stage of the cancer, other treatments such as palliative radiation, antineoplastic therapies, and palliative surgery may help to control the pain. The AHCPR guideline also stresses that written patient education materials at an appropriate reading level should be provided. The World Health Organization has created an analgesic ladder for cancer pain that assists clinicians in choosing the appropriate analgesic.[22]

Nonpharmacologic Treatment

A number of nonpharmacologic methods of pain control often are used in pain management. These include cognitive-behavioral interventions, physical agents such as heat and cold, and electroanalgesia. Often these methods are used in addition to analgesics rather than as the only form of pain management.

Cognitive-Behavioral Interventions.   Cognitive-behavioral interventions, which often are helpful for individuals experiencing acute as well as chronic pain, include relaxation, distraction, cognitive reappraisal, imagery, meditation, and biofeedback. If the person is having surgery or a painful procedure, it is ideal to teach these techniques before the pain begins (*e.g.*, before surgery). If the person is already in severe pain, the use of cognitive-behavioral interventions should be based on the person's ability to master the technique as well as his or her response to the intervention. For example, it would be a more appropriate adjunct to analgesics for a terminally ill person in severe pain to use self-selected relaxing music rather than trying to teach that person an intervention requiring more attention (*e.g.*, meditation or cognitive reappraisal).

Relaxation is one of the best-evaluated cognitive-behavioral approaches to pain relief. The relaxation method need not be complex. Relatively simple strategies, such as slow rhythmic breathing and brief jaw relaxation procedures, have been successful in decreasing self-reported pain and analgesic use.

Distraction (*i.e.*, focusing a person's attention on stimuli other than painful stimuli or negative emotions) does not eliminate pain, but it can make pain more tolerable. It may serve as a type of sensory shielding whereby attention to pain is sacrificed to pay attention to other stimuli that are easily perceived. Examples of distraction include counting, repeating phrases or poems, and engaging in activities that require concentration, such as projects, activities, work, conversation, or describing pictures. Television, adventure movies, music, and humor also can provide distraction. *Cognitive reappraisal* is a form of self-distraction or cognitive control in which individuals focus their attention on the positive aspects of the experience and away from their pain. Individuals using distraction may not appear to be in severe pain. Nonetheless, it is inappropriate to assume that a person who copes with pain by using distraction does not have pain. Prescribed analgesics should not be denied to patients simply because they appear to be coping with their pain without medication. Appropriate assessment is needed to determine the patient's level of pain and what other interventions for pain may be needed.

Imagery consists of using one's imagination to develop a mental picture. In pain management, therapeutic guided imagery (*i.e.*, goal-directed imaging) is used. It can be used alone or in conjunction with other cognitive behavioral interventions (*e.g.*, relaxation or biofeedback) to develop sensory images that may decrease the perceived intensity of pain. It also can be used to lessen anxiety and reduce muscle tension. *Meditation* also can be used, but it requires practice and the ability to concentrate to be effective.

Biofeedback is used to provide feedback to a person concerning the current status of some body function (*e.g.*, finger temperature, temporal artery pulsation, blood pressure, or muscle tension). It involves a process of learning designed to make the person aware of certain of his or her own body functions for the purpose of modifying these functions at a conscious level. Interest in biofeedback increased with the possibility of using this treatment modality in the management of migraine and tension headaches or for other pain that has a muscle tension component.

Physical Agents. Heat and cold are physical agents that are used to provide pain relief. The choice of physical agent depends on the type of pain being treated and, in many cases, personal preference.

Heat has long been used to relieve pain. Heat dilates blood vessels and increases local blood flow; it also can influence the transmission of pain impulses and increase collagen extensibility. An increase in local circulation can reduce the level of nociceptive stimulation by reducing local ischemia caused by muscle spasm or tension, increase the removal of metabolites and inflammatory mediators that act as nociceptive stimuli, and help to reduce swelling and relieve pressure on local nociceptive endings. The heat sensation is carried to the posterior horn of the spinal cord and may exert its effect by modulating projection of pain transmission. It also may trigger the release of endogenous opioids. Heat also alters the viscosity of collagen fibers in ligaments, tendons, and joint structures so that they are more easily extended and can be stretched further before the nociceptive endings are stimulated. Thus, heat often is applied before therapy aimed at stretching joint structures and increasing range of motion. Care must be taken not to use excessive heat. When excessive heat is used, the heat itself becomes a noxious stimulus, which results in actual or impending tissue damage and pain. In certain conditions, the use of heat is controversial, and in some conditions (*e.g.,* peripheral vascular disease) where increased blood flow or metabolism would be detrimental, the use of heat is contraindicated.

Like heat, the application of *cold* may produce a dramatic reduction in pain. Cold exerts its effect on pain through circulatory and neural mechanisms. The initial response to local application of cold is sudden local vasoconstriction. This initial vasoconstriction is followed by alternating periods of vasodilatation and vasoconstriction during which the body "hunts" for its normal level of blood flow to prevent local tissue damage. This gives rise to the so-called *hunting reflex* whereby the circulation to the cooled area undergoes alternating periods of pallor caused by ischemia and flushing caused by hyperemia.[23] The vasoconstriction is caused by local stimulation of sympathetic fibers and direct cooling of blood vessels, and the hyperemia by local autoregulatory mechanisms. In situations of acute injury, cold is used to produce vasoconstriction and prevent extravasation of blood into the tissues; pain relief results from decreased swelling and decreased stimulation of nociceptive endings. The vasodilatation that follows can be useful in removing substances that stimulate nociceptive endings.

Cold also can have a marked and dramatic effect on pain that results from the spasm–induced accumulation of metabolites in muscle. In terms of pain modulation, cold may reduce afferent activity reaching the posterior horn of the spinal cord by modulating sensory input. The application of cold is a noxious stimulus and may influence the release of endogenous opioids from the PAG area. Cold packs should be flexible to conform to body parts easily, adequately wrapped to protect the skin, and applied no more than 15 minutes at a time. Cold should be used only with great caution in anyone whose circulation is compromised.

Stimulus-Induced Analgesia. Stimulus-induced analgesia is one of the oldest known methods of pain relief. Historical references to the use of electricity to decrease or control pain date back to AD 46, when a Roman physician, Scribonius Largus, described how the stimulus from an electric eel was able to provide pain relief for headache and gout.[24] Electrical stimulation methods of pain relief include transcutaneous electrical nerve stimulation (TENS) and electrical acupuncture. TENS refers to the transmission of electrical energy across the surface of the skin to the peripheral nerve fibers. TENS units have been developed that are convenient, easily transported, and relatively economical to use. Most are approximately the size of a transistor radio or cigarette package. These battery-operated units deliver an electrical current to a target site.

The system usually consists of three parts: a pair of electrodes, lead wires, and a stimulator. The electrical stimulation is delivered in a pulsed waveform that can be varied in terms of pulse amplitude, width, and rate. The type of stimulation used varies with the type of pain being treated. Electrode placement is determined by the physiologic pathways and an understanding of the pain mechanisms involved. They may be placed on either side of a painful area, over an affected dermatome, over an affected peripheral nerve where it is most superficial, or over a nerve trunk. For example, the electrodes commonly are placed medial and lateral to the incision when treating postoperative pain.

There probably is no single explanation for the physiologic effects of TENS. Each specific type of stimulator may have different sites of action and may be explained by more than one theory. The gate control theory was proposed as one possible mechanism. According to this theory, pain information is transmitted by small-diameter Aδ and C fibers. Large-diameter afferent A fibers and small-diameter fibers carry tactile information mediating touch, pressure, and kinesthesia. TENS may function on the basis of differential firing of impulses in the large fibers that carry nonpainful information. Accordingly, increased activity in these larger fibers purportedly modulates transmission of painful information to the forebrain. A second possible explanation is that the high-frequency stimulation (50 to 60 Hz) produced by some units simply acts as a counterirritant.[25] A third possible explanation is that stimulators that produce strong rhythmic contractions may act through the release of endogenous analgesics such as the endorphins and enkephalins that suppress or modulate pain transmission. A fourth, and probably the best, explanation for quick analgesia with brief, intense stimulation is that it acts as a conduction block.[26] TENS has the advantage that it is noninvasive, easily regulated by the person or health professional, and effective in some forms of acute and chronic pain. Its use can be taught before surgery, affording a reduction in postoperative analgesic medication and, possibly, preventing the development of persistent pain.

Acupuncture and Acupressure.   The practice of acupuncture involves introducing needles into specific points on the surface of the body. Charts are available that describe the points of needle placement that are used to relieve pain at certain anatomic sites. In addition to needles, sometimes palpation is used. The practice of acupuncture dates back thousands of years to ancient China, when the stimulation was achieved by using needles made of bone, stone, or bamboo. Annually, approximately 1 million individuals in the United States receive acupuncture, and pain is the major complaint for which they receive it. Acupuncture is widely available in pain clinics even though large, high-quality, randomized studies on the effects of acupuncture for chronic pain are not plentiful.[27] Various theories of how acupuncture achieves analgesia have been proposed, including the gate control theory and the neurohumoral theory, involving the cascade of endorphins and monoamines. This possible physiologic basis for pain relief from acupuncture alone or acupuncture with electrical stimulation has been demonstrated by reversing pain control through the use of the morphine antagonist naloxone.

Acupressure is the means of stimulating acupressure points without using needles. It is particularly popular in Japan, where it is called *shiatsu* (*shi*, meaning "finger," and *atsu*, meaning "pressure").[28] Pressure may be applied with a finger, thumb, or any blunt instrument. Many techniques are used, including massaging in a circular motion for 3 to 5 minutes, pressing inward toward the center of the body and releasing three times, or vibrating the point with fingertip pressure.

Pharmacologic Treatment

Analgesics have been used for many years to relieve pain of short duration, enabling the person to achieve mobility after surgery, for example, when exercises such as coughing and deep breathing may be required. With acute pain, and even more so with chronic pain, the use of analgesics is only one aspect of a comprehensive pain management program. An analgesic drug is a medication that acts on the nervous system to decrease or eliminate pain without inducing loss of consciousness. Analgesic drugs do not cure the underlying cause of the pain, but their appropriate use may prevent acute pain from progressing to chronic pain. The AHCPR cancer pain guideline classifies pain medications into three categories: aspirin, other NSAIDs, and acetaminophen; opioid analgesics; and adjuvant analgesics.[21]

The ideal analgesic would be effective, nonaddictive, and inexpensive. In addition, it would produce minimal adverse effects and not affect the person's level of consciousness. Although long-term treatment with opioids can result in opioid tolerance (*i.e.*, more drug being needed to achieve the same effect) and physical dependence, this should not be confused with addiction. Long-term drug-seeking behavior is rare in persons who are treated with opioids only during the time that they require pain relief. The unique needs and circumstances presented by each person in pain must be addressed to achieve satisfactory pain management. For example, an established history of substance abuse poses a special challenge to pain management, but not an insoluble one.

Non-Narcotic Analgesics.   Common non-narcotic oral analgesic medications include aspirin, other NSAIDs, and acetaminophen. Aspirin, or acetylsalicylic acid, acts centrally and peripherally to block the transmission of pain impulses. It also has antipyretic and anti-inflammatory properties. Aspirin and the other NSAIDs inhibit several forms of prostaglandins through the inhibition of cyclooxygenase, an enzyme in the prostanoid pathway. Prostaglandins affect the sensation of pain by sensitizing nociceptors to chemical mediators such as bradykinin and histamine. Independent of prostaglandins, NSAIDs also decrease the sensitivity of blood vessels to bradykinin and histamine, affect lymphokine production by T lymphocytes, reverse vasodilation, and decrease the release of inflammatory mediators from granulocytes, mast cells, and basophils. Acetaminophen is an alternative to the NSAIDs. Although usually considered equivalent to aspirin as an analgesic and antipyretic agent, it lacks anti-inflammatory properties.

Opioid Analgesics.   The term *opioid* or *narcotic* is used to refer to a group of medications, natural or synthetic, with morphine-like actions. The older term *opiate* was used to designate drugs derived from opium—morphine, codeine, and many other semisynthetic congeners of morphine. The analgesic and psychopharmacologic properties of morphine have been known for centuries. More recently, it was discovered that the brain contains its own (*i.e.*, endogenous) analgesic, morphine-like chemicals that comprise a group of peptides known as *endorphins*. Three distinct families of endogenous opioid peptides have since been identified: *enkephalins*, *endorphins*, and *dynorphins*. Each family of opioid peptides is derived from a distinct precursor molecule (*e.g.*, proenkephalin, proendorphin, prodynorphin). Each of these precursors contains a number of biologically active peptides, opioid and nonopioid. The precursor molecules are found in the CNS and in blood and various other tissues.

The opioids exert their action through opioid receptors. There are three major categories of opioid receptors in the CNS, designated mu (μ, for "morphine"), delta (δ), and kappa (κ).[29] Each of the receptors has been cloned. Receptor subtypes have been proposed: mu_1 and mu_2; $delta_1$ and $delta_2$; and $kappa_1$, $kappa_2$, $kappa_3$. However, genes encoding only one subgroup for each of the families have been isolated and characterized thus far.[29] Analgesia, as well as respiratory depression, miosis, reduced gastrointestinal motility (causing constipation), feelings of well-being or euphoria, and physical dependence result principally from morphine and morphine-like opioid analgesics that act at mu receptors. Delta and kappa receptors also can contribute to pain relief. Although morphine binds to delta and kappa receptors, it is uncertain if this contributes to its analgesic effects. Part of the pain-relieving properties of exogenous opioids such as morphine involves the release of endogenous opioids.[29]

Opioid receptors have been localized using radiolabeled antibodies that bind to unique peptide sequences in each receptor subtype.[29] These studies have found that all three types of the major receptors are present in high concentrations on the primary pain afferents that enter the dorsal horn and on the secondary neurons that transmit the pain information to the brain. This spinal location has been exploited clinically by direct application of opioid analgesics to the spinal cord, which provides regional anesthesia while minimizing the unwanted respiratory depression, nausea and vomiting, and sedation that occur with systemically administered drugs that act at the brain level. Mu receptors also have been found in peripheral terminals of sensory neurons.[29] Thus, opioid drugs also can produce analgesia in sites outside the CNS. Pain associated with inflammation seems to be especially sensitive to these peripheral opioid actions.

As more information becomes available regarding the opioids and their receptors, it seems likely that pain medications can be developed that act selectively at certain receptor sites, providing more effective pain control while producing fewer adverse effects and affording less danger of addiction. For example, it might be possible to develop opioid drugs that produce effective analgesia but not undesirable adverse effects, such as respiratory depression and the most common complication, constipation.

When given for temporary relief of severe pain, such as that occurring after surgery, there is much evidence that opioids given routinely before the pain starts or becomes extreme are far more effective than those administered in a sporadic manner. Persons who are treated in this manner seem to require fewer doses and are able to resume regular activities sooner. Opioids also are used for persons with limited life expectancy. Too often, because of undue concern about the possibility of addiction, many chronic pain sufferers with a short life expectancy receive inadequate pain relief. Most pain experts agree that it is appropriate to provide the level of opioid necessary to relieve the severe, intractable pain of persons whose life expectancy is limited.

Addiction is not considered a problem in patients with cancer.[30] In persons with chronic cancer pain, morphine remains the most useful strong opioid. The World Health Organization has recommended that oral morphine be part of the essential medication list and made available throughout the world as the medication of choice for cancer pain.[31] Oral forms of morphine are well absorbed from the gastrointestinal tract and have a half-life of approximately 2.5 hours and a duration of action of 4 to 6 hours. Liquid forms of the medication usually are given at 4-hour intervals to maintain an adequate blood level for analgesia, while minimizing the potential for toxic side effects. Controlled-release forms of the drug also are available.

Adjuvant Analgesics. Adjuvant analgesics include medications such as tricyclic antidepressants, antiseizure medications, and neuroleptic anxiolytic agents. The fact that the pain suppression system has nonendorphin synapses raises the possibility that potent, centrally acting, nonopiate medications may be useful in relieving pain. Serotonin has been shown to play an important role in producing analgesia. The tricyclic antidepressant medications (*i.e.,* imipramine, amitriptyline, and doxepin) that block the removal of serotonin from the synaptic cleft have been shown to produce pain relief in some persons. These medications are particularly useful in some chronic painful conditions, such as postherpetic neuralgia.

Certain antiseizure medications, such as carbamazepine (Tegretol) and phenytoin (Dilantin), have analgesic effects in some pain conditions. These medications, which suppress spontaneous neuronal firing, are particularly useful in the management of pain that occurs after nerve injury. Other agents, such as the corticosteroids, may be used to decrease inflammation and nociceptive stimuli responsible for pain.

Placebo Response. Sometimes when people receive treatments with no therapeutic benefit (*e.g.,* a sugar pill or an injection of normal saline), they get well or their symptoms are alleviated. This phenomenon is often called the *placebo effect.* The term *placebo* is the Latin word for "I please." The improvement in health status is thought to derive from the person's belief that the treatment will be effective rather than from the specific or therapeutic properties of the placebo itself. For example, a *positive placebo reactor* might report pain relief after the administration of a medication believed to be an analgesic, when in fact it was composed of an inert substance. It is believed that the placebo-derived analgesia may be mediated through endogenous opioid pathways. However, because we cannot predict who will have pain relief from a placebo or if they will have pain relief every time they receive a placebo, the use of placebos in clinical practice without the patient's informed consent raises serious ethical concerns. The Oncology Nursing Society has a position statement asserting that placebos should not be used in the management or assessment of cancer pain.[32] The American Pain Society also proposes that placebos should not be used to assess pain and that the deceptive use of placebos is unethical.[33]

Surgical Intervention

If surgery removes the problem causing the pain, such as a tumor pressing on a nerve or an inflamed appendix, it can be curative. In other instances, surgery is used for symptom management rather than for cure. However, with rare exceptions, noninvasive analgesic approaches should precede invasive palliative approaches.[21] Surgery for severe, intractable pain of peripheral or central origin has met with some success. It can be used to remove the cause or block the transmission of intractable pain from phantom limb pain, severe neuralgia, inoperable cancer of certain types, and causalgia.

> In summary, pain is an elusive and complex phenomenon; it is a symptom common to many illnesses. It is a highly individualized experience that is shaped by a person's culture and previous life experiences, and it is difficult to measure. Traditionally, there have been two principal theories of pain, specificity and pattern theories. Scientifically, pain is viewed within the context of nociception. Nociceptors are receptive nerve endings that respond to noxious stimuli. Pain receptors respond to mechanical, thermal, and chemical stimuli. Nociceptive neurons transmit impulses to the dorsal horn

neurons using chemical neurotransmitters. The neospinothalamic and the paleospinothalamic paths are used to transmit pain information to the brain. Several neuroanatomic pathways as well as endogenous opioid peptides modulate pain in the CNS.

Pain can be classified according to location, referral, and duration as well as associated medical diagnoses. Pain can arise from cutaneous, deep somatic, or visceral locations. Referred pain is pain perceived at a site different from its origin. Acute pain is self-limiting pain that ends when the injured tissue heals, whereas chronic pain is pain that lasts much longer than the anticipated healing time for the underlying cause of the pain. Pain threshold, pain tolerance, age, sex, and other factors affect an individual's reaction to pain.

Treatment modalities for pain include the use of physiologic, cognitive, and behavioral measures; heat and cold; stimulation-induced analgesic methods; and pharmacologic agents singly or in combination. It is becoming apparent that even with chronic pain, the most effective approach is early treatment or even prevention. After pain is present, the greatest success in pain assessment and management is achieved with the use of an interdisciplinary approach.

Alterations in Pain Sensitivity and Special Types of Pain

After you have completed this section of the chapter, you should be able to meet the following objectives:

✦ Define allodynia, hypoesthesia, hyperesthesia, paresthesias, hyperpathia, analgesia, and hypoalgesia
✦ Describe the cause and characteristics and treatment of neuropathic pain, trigeminal neuralgia, postherpetic neuralgia, and complex regional pain syndrome.
✦ Cite possible mechanisms of phantom limb pain

ALTERATIONS IN PAIN SENSITIVITY

Sensitivity and perception of pain varies among persons and in the same person under different conditions and in different parts of the body. Irritation, mild hypoxia, and mild compression of a peripheral nerve often result in hyperexcitability of the sensory nerve fibers or cell bodies. This is experienced as unpleasant hypersensitivity (*i.e., hyperesthesia*) or increased painfulness (*i.e., hyperalgesia*). Possible causes of increased sensitivity to noxious stimuli include a decrease in the threshold of nociceptors, an increase in pain produced by suprathreshold stimuli, and the windup phenomenon. Primary hyperalgesia occurs at the site of injury. Secondary hyperalgesia occurs in nearby uninjured tissue.

Hyperpathia is a syndrome in which the sensory threshold is raised, but when it is reached, continued stimulation, especially if repetitive, results in a prolonged and unpleasant experience. This pain can be explosive and radiates through a peripheral nerve distribution. It is associated with pathologic changes in peripheral nerves, such as localized

ischemia. Spontaneous, unpleasant sensations called *paresthesias* occur with more severe irritation (*e.g.,* the pins-and-needles sensation that follows temporary compression of a peripheral nerve). The general term *dysesthesia* is given to distortions (usually unpleasant) of somesthetic sensation that typically accompany partial loss of sensory innervation.

More severe pathologic processes can result in reduced or lost tactile (*e.g., hypoesthesia, anesthesia*), temperature (*e.g., hypothermia, athermia*), and pain sensation (*i.e., hypalgesia*). *Analgesia* is the absence of pain on noxious stimulation or the relief of pain without loss of consciousness. The inability to sense pain may result in trauma, infection, and even loss of a body part or parts. Inherited insensitivity to pain may take the form of congenital indifference or congenital insensitivity to pain. In the former, transmission of nerve impulses appears normal but appreciation of painful stimuli at higher levels appears to be absent. In the latter, a peripheral nerve defect apparently exists such that transmission of painful nerve impulses does not result in perception of pain. Whatever the cause, persons who lack the ability to perceive pain are at constant risk of tissue damage because pain is not serving its protective function.

Allodynia (Greek *allo,* "other," and *odynia,* "painful") is the term used for the puzzling phenomenon of pain that follows a non-noxious stimulus to apparently normal skin. This term is intended to refer to instances in which otherwise normal tissues may be abnormally innervated or may be referral sites for other loci that give rise to pain with non-noxious stimuli. It may be that an area is hypersensitive because of inflammation, injury, or another cause, and a normally subthreshold stimulus is sufficient to trigger the sensation of pain. This response is thought to be chemically mediated, possibly the result of tissue damage in the surrounding area. *Trigger points* are highly localized points on the skin or mucous membrane that can produce immediate intense pain at that site or elsewhere when stimulated by light tactile stimulation. Myofascial trigger points are foci of exquisite tenderness found in many muscles and can be responsible for pain projected to sites remote from the points of tenderness. Trigger points are widely distributed in the back of the head and neck and in the lumbar and thoracic regions. These trigger points cause reproducible myofascial pain syndromes in specific muscles. These pain syndromes are the major source of pain in clients at chronic pain treatment centers.

SPECIAL TYPES OF PAIN

Neuropathic Pain

When peripheral nerves are affected by injury or disease, it can lead to unusual and sometimes intractable sensory disturbances. These include numbness, paresthesias, and pain. Depending on the cause, few or many axons could be damaged and the condition could be unilateral or bilateral. Causes of neuropathic pain can be categorized according to the extent of peripheral nerve involvement. Conditions that can lead to pain by causing damage to peripheral nerves in a single area include nerve entrapment, nerve compression from a tumor mass, and various neuralgias (*e.g.,* trigeminal, postherpetic, and post-traumatic). Conditions that can lead to pain by causing damage to peripheral nerves in a wide area include diabetes mellitus, long-term alcohol use, hypothyroidism, renal insufficiency, and drug treatment with neurotoxic agents.[34] Injury to a nerve also can lead to a multisymptom, multisystem syndrome called *complex regional pain syndrome* (previously known as *causalgia* or *reflex sympathetic dystrophy*). Nerve damage associated with amputation is believed to be a cause of phantom limb pain.

Neuropathic pain can vary with the extent and location of disease or injury. There may be allodynia or pain that is stabbing, jabbing, burning, or shooting. The pain may be persistent or intermittent. The diagnosis depends on the mode of onset, the distribution of abnormal sensations, the quality of the pain, and other relevant medical conditions (*e.g.,* diabetes, hypothyroidism, alcohol use, rash, or trauma). Injury to peripheral nerves sometimes results in pain that persists beyond the time required for the tissues to heal. Peripheral pathologic processes (*e.g.,* neural degeneration, neuroma formation, and generation of abnormal spontaneous neural discharges from the injured sensory neuron) and neural plasticity (*i.e.,* changes in CNS function) are the primary working hypotheses to explain persistent neuropathic pain.

Treatment methods include measures aimed at restoring or preventing further nerve damage (*e.g.,* surgery to resect a tumor causing nerve compression, improving glycemic control for diabetic patients with painful neuropathies), and interventions for the palliation of pain. Although many adjuvant analgesics are used for neuropathic pain, pain control often is difficult. The initial approach in seeking adequate pain control is to try these drugs in sequence and then in combination. The adjuvant analgesics can be divided into three general classes according to the pain they are used to treat: burning, tingling, or aching pain; stabbing or shooting pain; and neurogenic pain. For pain that is burning, tingling or aching, tricyclic antidepressants, antiarrhythmics (*e.g.,* mexiletine), and the α_2-adrenergic agonist clonidine frequently are used. For the stabbing or shooting pain of neuralgias, antiseizure medications or baclofen, a drug used in treatment of spasticity, may be used. For neurogenic pain that is thought to be exacerbated by sympathetic nervous activity (*e.g.,* post-traumatic nerve pain), medications such as corticosteroids, sympathetic receptor–blocking drugs such as propranolol or phenoxybenzamine, or calcium channel–blocking drugs such as nifedipine may be used. However, successful pain relief has not been demonstrated with any of these drugs.[34]

Poor pain control or unacceptable side effects may lead to a trial with other medications. If there has been a poor response to the adjuvant analgesics, opioids also can be used. However, concerns about side effects and the remote possibility of addiction must be considered. When opioids are used, the use of long-acting opioids with a plan for breakthrough pain is desirable because it addresses the typically continuous nature of neuropathic pain. Using long-acting opioids also avoids the hepatotoxic effect of high doses of acetaminophen that could result from frequent and long-term treatment of severe pain with the oral combination opioid preparations. Nonpharmacologic therapies also are used for neurogenic pain. Electrical stimulation of the peripheral nerve or spinal cord can be used for radiculopathies and neuralgias. As a last resort, neurolysis or neurosurgical blockade sometimes is used.

Neuralgia

Neuralgia is characterized by severe, brief, often repetitive attacks of lightning-like or throbbing pain. It occurs along the distribution of a spinal or cranial nerve and usually is precipitated by stimulation of the cutaneous region supplied by that nerve.

Trigeminal Neuralgia. Trigeminal neuralgia, *or tic douloureux,* is one of the most common and severe neuralgias. It is manifested by facial tics or grimaces and characterized by stabbing, paroxysmal attacks of pain that usually are limited to the unilateral sensory distribution of one or more branches of the trigeminal nerve, most often the maxillary or mandibular divisions. Although intermittent, the pain often is excruciating and may be triggered by light touch.

Carbamazepine, an antiseizure drug, may be used to control the pain of trigeminal neuralgia and may delay or eliminate the need for surgery. Surgical release of vessels, dural structures, or scar tissue surrounding the semilunar ganglion or root in the middle cranial fossa often eliminates the symptoms. If not, destruction or blocking of peripheral branches or the central root of cranial nerve V produces loss of all sensation, including pain. A more satisfactory treatment is sectioning of the descending spinal tract of nerve V in the brain stem. This may be effective because it removes background inflow of impulses on which spontaneous attacks depend. Dissociation of facial sensation occurs, in that the ability to detect pain and temperature disappears, but there is only a slight decrease in ability to detect touch. This neurosurgical procedure provides evidence that the nucleus caudalis of the trigeminal complex is necessary for the transmission of facial pain. Considerable controversy remains regarding the pathophysiology of trigeminal neuralgia. Other interventions include avoidance of precipitating factors (*e.g.,* stimulation of trigger spots) and eye injury due to irritation; provision for adequate nutrition; and avoidance of social isolation.

Postherpetic Neuralgia. Herpes zoster (also called *shingles*) is caused by the same herpesvirus that causes varicella (*i.e.,* chickenpox) and is thought to represent a localized recurrent infection by the varicella virus that has remained latent in the dorsal root ganglia since the initial attack of chickenpox. Reactivation of viral replication is associated with a decline in immunity, such as that which occurs with aging or certain diseases. Postherpetic neuralgia develops in from 10% to 70% of patients with shingles[35]; the risk increases with age. The pain associated with postherpetic neuralgia occurs in the areas of innervation of the infected ganglia.

During the acute attack of herpes zoster, the reactivated virus travels from the ganglia to the skin of the corresponding dermatomes, causing localized vesicular eruption and hyperpathia (*i.e.,* abnormally exaggerated subjective response to pain). In the acute infection, proportionately more of the large nerve fibers are destroyed. Regenerated fibers appear to have smaller diameters. Older patients have pain, dysesthesia, and hyperesthesia after the acute phase; these are increased by minor stimuli. Because there is a relative loss of large fibers with age, elderly persons are particularly prone to suffering because of the shift in the proportion of large- to small-diameter nerve fibers. Normally, the pain of acute herpes zoster tends to resolve spontaneously. Postherpetic neuralgia describes the presence of pain more than 1 month after the onset of herpes zoster.

Early treatment of shingles with high doses of systemic corticosteroids and an oral antiviral drug such as acyclovir or valacyclovir, a medication that inhibits herpesvirus DNA replication, may reduce the incidence of postherpetic neuralgia. Initially, postherpetic neuralgia can be treated with a topical anesthetic agent, lidocaine-prilocaine cream or 5% lidocaine gel. A tricyclic antidepressant medication, such as amitriptyline or desipramine, may be used for pain relief. Regional nerve blockade (*i.e.*, stellate ganglion, epidural, local infiltration, or peripheral nerve block) has been used with limited success. Topical capsaicin preparations have been used with mixed results because many persons are intolerant of the burning sensation that precedes anesthesia after application.[35]

Complex Regional Pain Syndrome

Recently, the International Association for the Study of Pain created the terms *complex regional pain syndrome I* and *complex regional pain syndrome II*. These terms refer, respectively, to reflex sympathetic dystrophy and causalgia. Trauma, frequently minor, to a nerve is the major cause. However, injury to soft tissue or a broken bone also can cause these pain syndromes. The hallmark is pain and mobility problems more severe than the injury warrants. Characteristically, the pain is severe and burning with or without deep aching. Usually, the pain can be elicited with the slightest movement or touch to the affected area, it increases with repetitive stimulation, and it lasts even after the stimulation has stopped. The pain can be exacerbated by emotional upsets or any increased peripheral sympathetic nerve stimulation. All the variations of complex regional pain syndromes include sympathetic components. These are characterized by vascular and trophic (*e.g.*, dystrophic or atrophic) changes to the skin, soft tissue, and bone, and can include rubor or pallor, sweating or dryness, edema (often sharply demarcated), skin atrophy, and, with time, patchy osteoporosis.

According to the clinical practice guideline proposed by the Reflex Sympathetic Dystrophy Syndrome Association of America, the cornerstone of treatment is promoting normal use of the affected part to the extent possible.[36] Initially, oral analgesics (including the adjuvant analgesics), TENS, and physical activity are used. If this does not lead to improvement, treatment by sympathetic blockade may provide relief from pain; it also determines the extent to which the pain is sympathetically maintained. If the block successfully treats the pain, then sympathectomy may be an effective treatment. If not, electrical stimulation of the spinal cord or narcotics may be considered.

Phantom Limb Pain

Phantom limb pain, a type of neurologic pain, follows amputation of a limb or part of a limb. As many as 70% of amputees experience phantom pain.[37] The pain often begins as sensations of tingling, heat and cold, or heaviness, followed by burning, cramping, or shooting pain. It may disappear spontaneously or persist for many years. One of the more troublesome aspects of phantom pain is that the person may experience painful sensations that were present before the amputation, such as that of a painful ulcer or bunion.

Several theories have been proposed as to the causes of phantom pain.[37] One theory is that the end of a regenerating nerve becomes trapped in the scar tissue of the amputation site. It is known that when a peripheral nerve is cut, the scar tissue that forms becomes a barrier to regenerating outgrowth of the axon. The growing axon often becomes trapped in the scar tissue, forming a tangled growth (*i.e.*, neuroma) of small-diameter axons, including primary nociceptive afferents and sympathetic efferents. It has been proposed that these afferents show increased sensitivity to innocuous mechanical stimuli and to sympathetic activity and circulating catecholamines. A related theory moves the source of phantom limb pain to the spinal cord, suggesting that the pain is due to the spontaneous firing of spinal cord neurons that have lost their normal sensory input from the body. In this case, a closed self-exciting neuronal loop in the posterior horn of the spinal cord is postulated to send impulses to the brain, resulting in pain. Even the slightest irritation to the amputated limb area can initiate this cycle. Other theories propose that the phantom limb pain may arise in the brain itself. In one hypothesis, the pain is caused by changes in the flow of signals through somatosensory areas of the brain. In other words, there appears to be plasticity even in the adult CNS. Treatment of phantom limb pain has been accomplished by the use of sympathetic blocks, TENS of the large myelinated afferents innervating the area, hypnosis, and relaxation training.

In summary, pain may occur with or without an adequate stimulus, or it may be absent in the presence of an adequate stimulus—either of which describes a pain disorder. There may be analgesia (absence of pain), hyperalgesia (increased sensitivity to pain), hypoalgesia (a decreased sensitivity to painful stimuli), hyperpathia (an unpleasant and prolonged response to pain), hyperesthesia (an abnormal increase in sensitivity to sensation), hypoesthesia (an abnormal decrease in sensitivity to sensations), paresthesia (abnormal touch sensation such as tingling or "pins and needles" in the absence of external stimuli), or allodynia (pain produced by stimuli that do not normally cause pain).

Neuropathic pain may be due to trauma or disease of neurons in a focal area or in a more global distribution (*e.g.*, from endocrine disease or neurotoxic medications). Neuralgia is characterized by severe, brief, often repetitiously occurring attacks of lightning-like or throbbing pain that occurs along the distribution of a spinal or cranial nerve and usually is precipitated by stimulation of the cutaneous region supplied by that nerve. Trigeminal neuralgia, or tic douloureux, is one of the most common and severe neuralgias. It is manifested by facial tics or grimaces. Postherpetic neuralgia is a chronic pain that can occur after shingles, an infection of the dorsal root ganglia and corresponding areas of innervation by the herpes zoster virus. Complex regional pain syndrome is an extremely painful condition that may follow sudden and traumatic deformation of peripheral nerves. Phantom limb pain, a neurologic pain, can occur after amputation of a limb or part of a limb.

Headache and Associated Pain

After you have completed this section of the chapter, you should be able to meet the following objectives:

◆ State the importance of distinguishing between primary and secondary types of headache

◆ Differentiate between the periodicity of occurrence and manifestations of migraine headache, cluster headache, tension-type headache, and headache due to temporomandibular joint syndrome

◆ Characterize the nonpharmacologic and pharmacologic methods used in treatment of headache

◆ Cite the most common cause of temporomandibular joint pain

HEADACHE

Headache is a common health problem. Seventy-six percent of women and 57% of men report at least one headache a month.[38] Although head and facial pain have characteristics that distinguish them from other pain disorders, they also share many of the same features.

Headache is caused by a number of conditions. Some headaches represent primary disorders and others occur secondary to other disease conditions in which head pain is a symptom. The most common types of primary or chronic headaches are migraine headache, tension-type headache, cluster headache, and chronic daily headache. Although most causes of secondary headache are benign, some are indications of serious disorders such as meningitis, brain tumor, or cerebral aneurysm. The sudden onset of a severe, intractable headache in an otherwise healthy person is more likely related to a serious intracranial disorder, such as subarachnoid hemorrhage or meningitis, than to a chronic headache disorder. Headaches that disturb sleep, exertional headaches, and headaches accompanied by neurologic symptoms such as drowsiness, visual or limb disturbances, or altered mental status also are suggestive of underlying intracranial lesions or other pathology.

The diagnosis and classification of headaches often is difficult. It requires a comprehensive history and physical examination to exclude secondary causes. The history should include factors that precipitate headache, such as foods and food additives, missed meals, and association with the menstrual period. A careful medication history is essential because many medications can provoke or aggravate headaches. Alcohol also can cause or aggravate headache. A headache diary in which the person records his or her headaches and concurrent or antecedent events may be helpful in identifying factors that contribute to headache

onset. Appropriate laboratory and imaging studies of the brain may be done to rule out secondary headaches.

In 1988, the International Headache Society published a proposed classification of headaches that lists diagnostic criteria for both primary headache syndromes and headaches that occur secondary to other medical conditions (see Chart 48-1 for a summary of the components of the system).[39] Migraine, tension-type, and cluster headaches usually present with typical characteristics. Mixed headache syndrome, however, involves an overlapping of symptoms.

Migraine Headache

Migraine headaches affect more than 10 million persons in the United States. They occur more frequently in women than men and result in considerable time lost from work and other activities.[40] Migraine headaches tend to run in families and are thought to be inherited as an autosomal dominant trait with incomplete penetrance.[38]

CHART 48-1

Classification and Diagnostic Criteria for Headache Disorders, Cranial Neuralgias, and Facial Pain

1. Migraine
   1.1 Migraine without aura
   1.2 Migraine with aura
   1.3 Ophthalmoplegic migraine
   1.4 Retinal migraine
   1.5 Childhood periodic syndromes that may be precursors to or associated with migraine
   1.6 Complications with migraine
   1.7 Migrainous disorder not fulfilling above criteria
2. Tension-type headache
   2.1 Episodic tension-type headache
   2.2 Chronic tension-type headache
   2.3 Headache of the tension type not fulfilling the above criteria
3. Cluster headache and chronic paroxysmal hemicrania
4. Miscellaneous headaches unassociated with structural lesion
5. Headache associated with head trauma
6. Headache associated with vascular disorders
7. Headache associated with nonvascular intracranial disorders
8. Headache associated with substances or their withdrawal
9. Headache associated with noncephalic infection
10. Headache associated with metabolic disorder
11. Headache or facial pain associated with disorder of cranium, neck, eyes, ears, nose, sinuses, teeth, mouth, or other facial or cranial structures
12. Cranial neuralgias, nerve trunk pain, and deafferentation pain
13. Headache not classifiable

(Adapted from Oleson J. [1988]. Classification and diagnostic criteria for headache disorders, cranial neuralgias, and facial pain. *Cephalgia* 8 [Suppl 7], 13–19)

There are two categories of migraine headache—migraine without aura, which accounts for approximately 85% of migraines, and migraine with aura, which accounts for most of the remaining migraines. Migraine without aura is a pulsatile, throbbing, unilateral headache that typically lasts 1 to 2 days and is aggravated by routine physical activity. The headache is accompanied by nausea and vomiting, which often is disabling, and a sensitivity to light and sound. Visual disturbances occur quite commonly and consist of visual hallucinations such as stars, sparks, and flashes of light. Migraine with aura has similar symptoms, but with the addition of visual or neurologic symptoms that precede the headache. The aura usually develops over a period of 5 to 20 minutes and lasts less than an hour. Although only a small percentage of persons with migraine experience an aura before an attack, many persons without aura have prodromal symptoms, such as fatigue and irritability, that precede the attack by hours or even days.

Subtypes of migraine include ophthalmoplegic migraine, hemiplegic migraine, aphasic migraine, and retinal migraine, in which transient visual and motor deficits occur. Ophthalmoplegic migraine is characterized by diplopia, due to a transient paralysis of the muscles that control eye movement (usually the third cranial nerve), and localized pain around the eye. Migraine headache also can present as a mixed headache, including symptoms typically associated with tension-type headache or CDH. These are called *transformed migraine* and are difficult to classify.

Migraine headaches occur in children as well as adults. [41,42] Before puberty, migraine headaches are equally distributed between sexes. The essential diagnostic criterion for migraine in children is the presence of recurrent headaches separated by pain-free periods. Diagnosis is based on at least three of the following symptoms or associated findings: abdominal pain, nausea or vomiting, throbbing headache, unilateral location, associated aura (visual, sensory, motor), relief during sleep, and a positive family history. [42] Symptoms vary widely among children, from those that interrupt activities and cause the child to seek relief in a dark environment, to those detectable only by direct questioning. A common feature of migraine in children is intense nausea and vomiting. The vomiting may be associated with abdominal pain and fever; thus, migraine may be confused with other conditions such as appendicitis. More than half of children with migraine undergo spontaneous prolonged remission after their 10th birthday. Because headaches in children can be a symptom of other, more serious disorders, including intracranial lesions, it is important that other causes of headache that require immediate treatment be ruled out.

The mechanisms of migraine attacks are poorly understood. There is increasing evidence in support of a neurogenic basis for migraine. Supporting this neurogenic concept is the frequent presence of premonitory symptoms before the headache begins; the presence of focal neurologic disturbances, which cannot be explained in terms of cerebral blood flow; and the numerous accompanying symptoms, including autonomic and constitutional dysfunction. [38] The pathophysiologic process of migraine probably involves alterations in serotonin function and occurrence of inflam-

matory disturbances in the trigeminal vascular system. [38] Hormonal variations, particularly in estrogen levels, play a role in the pattern of migraine attacks. For many women, migraine headaches coincide with their menstrual periods. The greater predominance of migraine headaches in women is thought to be related to the aggravating effect of estrogen on the migraine mechanism. [38] Dietary substances, such as monosodium glutamate, aged cheese, and chocolate, also may precipitate migraine headaches. The actual triggers for migraine are the chemicals in the food, not allergens. [43]

Treatment. The treatment of migraine headaches includes preventative and abortive nonpharmacologic and pharmacologic treatment. In 1998, the U.S. Headache Consortium, a multidisciplinary panel, produced a set of evidence-based guidelines for the nonpharmacologic and pharmacologic management and prevention of migraine headaches in primary care settings. [44]

Nonpharmacologic treatment includes the avoidance of migraine triggers, such as foods, that precipitate an attack. Many persons with migraines benefit from maintaining regular eating and sleeping habits. Measures to control stress, which also can precipitate an attack, also are important. During an attack, many persons find it helpful to retire to a quiet, darkened room until symptoms subside.

Pharmacologic treatment involves both abortive therapy for acute attacks and preventive therapy. A wide range of medications is used to treat the acute symptoms of migraine headache. [45] These include serotonin receptor agonists (*e.g.,* sumatriptan, naratriptan, rizatriptan, zolmitriptan), ergotamine derivatives (*e.g.,* dihydroergotamine), analgesics (*e.g.,* acetylsalicylic acid, acetaminophen, and NSAIDs such as naproxen sodium), sedatives (*e.g.,* butalbital), and antiemetic medications (*e.g.,* prochlorperazine, metoclopramide). Oral medications may be ineffective for severe migraine headaches because of decreased gastric motility. Both sumatriptan and dihydroergotamine have been approved for intranasal administration. For intractable migraine headache, dihydroergotamine may be administered parenterally with an antiemetic (metoclopramide or prochlorperazine) or opioid analgesic (meperidine or transnasal butorphanol). [45] Frequent use of abortive headache medications may cause rebound headache or perpetuate chronic daily headaches.

Preventative pharmacologic treatment may be necessary if migrainous headaches are disabling or occur more than two or three times a month. In most cases, preventative treatment must be taken daily for months to years. The β-adrenergic blocking medications (*e.g.,* propranolol, metoprolol, timolol, nadolol, atenolol) are usually the first choice for prophylactic treatment because of empiric support for their effectiveness, safety, efficacy, and favorable side effect profile. Several other medications that may be effective prophylactically for migraine headache are antidepressants (amitriptyline, doxepin, imipramine, nortriptyline), selective serotonin reuptake inhibitors (fluoxetine), calcium channel blockers (diltiazem, verapamil), antiseizure medications (divalproex sodium, valproic acid), ergot derivatives (methysergide), and NSAIDs (naproxen sodium). [46] When a decision to discontinue preventive therapy is made, the medications should be gradually withdrawn.

There may be serious side effects with some of the anti-migraine medications. Because of the risk of coronary vasospasm, the 5-HT$_1$ receptor agonists should not be given to persons with coronary artery disease. Ergotamine preparations can cause uterine contractions and should not be given to pregnant women. They also can cause vasospasm, and should be used with caution in persons with peripheral vascular disease.

Cluster Headache

Cluster headaches are relatively infrequent headaches that affect men more often than women. These headaches tend to occur in clusters over weeks or months, followed by a long, headache-free remission period. Typically the symptoms in cluster headaches include severe, unrelenting, unilateral pain located, in order of decreasing frequency, in the orbital, retro-orbital, temporal, supraorbital, and infraorbital region. The pain is of rapid onset and builds to a peak in approximately 10 to 15 minutes, lasting for 15 to 180 minutes. The pain behind the eye radiates to the ipsilateral trigeminal nerve (*e.g.*, temple, cheek, gum). The headache frequently is associated with one or more symptoms such as conjunctival redness, lacrimation, nasal congestion, rhinorrhea, forehead and facial sweating, miosis, ptosis, and eyelid edema. Because of their location and associated symptoms, cluster headaches are often mistaken for sinus infections or dental problems.[43]

The underlying pathophysiologic mechanisms of cluster headaches are unknown. Hypotheses include the interplay of vascular, neurogenic, metabolic, and humoral factors. Although the trigeminovascular system appears to be involved in the pathogenesis of cluster headache, a theory to explain the symptoms, periodicity, and circadian regularity of cluster headaches does not exist. The regularity in the timing of cluster headache may be caused by dysfunction of the hypothalamic biologic clock mechanisms. Ipsilateral lacrimation, nasal stuffiness, and rhinorrhea are thought to result from parasympathetic overactivity. Pain and vasodilation are thought to result from activation of the trigeminovascular system.

Treatment. Because of the relatively short duration and self-limited nature of cluster headache, oral preparations typically take too long to reach therapeutic levels. The most effective treatments are those that act quickly (*e.g.*, oxygen inhalation and subcutaneous sumatriptan). Intranasal lidocaine also may be effective.[38] Oxygen inhalation may be indicated for home use. Prophylactic medications for cluster headaches include ergotamine, verapamil, methysergide, lithium carbonate, corticosteroids, sodium valproate, and indomethacin.

Tension-Type Headache

The most common type of headache is tension-type headache. Unlike migraine and cluster headaches, tension-type headache usually is not sufficiently severe that it interferes with daily activities. Tension-type headaches frequently are described as dull, aching, diffuse, nondescript headaches, occurring in a hatband distribution around the head, and not associated with nausea or vomiting or worsened by activity. They can be infrequent, episodic, or chronic.

The exact mechanisms of tension-type headache are not known and the hypotheses of causation are contradictory. One popular theory is that tension-type headache results from sustained tension of the muscles of the scalp and neck; however, some research has found no correlation between muscle contraction and tension-type headache. Many authorities now believe that tension-type headaches are forms of migraine headache.[38] It is thought that migraine headache may be transformed gradually into chronic tension-type headache. Tension-type headaches also may be caused by oromandibular dysfunction, psychogenic stress, anxiety, depression, and muscular stress. They also may result from overuse of analgesics or caffeine. Daily use of caffeine, whether in beverages or medications, can produce addiction, and a headache can develop in such persons who go without caffeine for several hours.[43]

Treatment. Tension-type headaches often are more responsive to nonpharmacologic techniques, such as biofeedback, massage, acupuncture, relaxation, imagery, and physical therapy, than other types of headache. For persons with poor posture, a combination of range-of-motion exercises, relaxation, and posture improvement may be helpful.[43]

The medications of choice for acute treatment of tension-type headaches are analgesics, including acetylsalicylic acid, acetaminophen, and NSAIDs. Persons with infrequent tension-type headache usually self-medicate using over-the-counter analgesics to treat the acute pain, and do not require prophylactic medication. These agents should be used cautiously because rebound headaches can develop when the medications are taken regularly.

Because the "dividing lines" between tension-type headache, migraine, and chronic daily headache often are vague, addition of medications as well as the entire range of migraine medications may be tried in refractory cases. Other medications used concomitantly with analgesics include sedatives (*e.g.*, butalbital), anxiolytics (*e.g.*, diazepam), and skeletal muscle relaxants (*e.g.*, orphenadrine). Prophylactic treatment can include antidepressants (*e.g.*, amitriptyline, doxepin).

Chronic Daily Headache

The term *chronic daily headache* (CDH) is used to refer to headaches that occur 15 days or more a month, including those due to medication overuse.[47] Little is known about the prevalence and incidence of CDH. Diagnostic criteria for CDH are not provided in the International Headache Society Classification System. The cause of CDH is unknown, although there are several hypotheses. They include transformed migraine headache, evolved tension-type headache, new daily persistent headache, and post-traumatic headache. In many persons, CDH retains certain characteristics of migraine, whereas in others it resembles chronic tension-type headache. CDH may be associated with chronic and episodic tension-type headache. New daily persistent headache may have a fairly rapidly onset, with no history of migraine, tension-type headache, trauma, or psychological stress. Although overuse of symptomatic medications (*e.g.*, analgesics, ergotamine) has been related to CDH, there is a group of patients in whom CDH is unrelated to excessive use of medications.

Treatment. For patients with CDH, a combination of pharmacologic and behavioral interventions may be necessary. As with tension-type headaches, nonpharmacologic techniques, such as biofeedback, massage, acupuncture, relaxation, imagery, and physical therapy, may be helpful. Measures to reduce or eliminate medication overuse may be helpful. Most of the medications used for prevention of CDH have not been examined in well-designed, double-blind studies.

Temporomandibular Joint Pain

A common cause of head pain is temporomandibular joint (TMJ) syndrome. It usually is caused by an imbalance in joint movement because of poor bite, bruxism (*i.e.,* teeth grinding), or joint problems such as inflammation, trauma, and degenerative changes.[48] The pain almost always is referred and commonly presents as facial muscle pain, headache, neck ache, or earache. Referred pain is aggravated by jaw function. Headache associated with this syndrome is common in adults and children and can cause chronic pain problems.

Treatment of TMJ pain is aimed at correcting the problem, and in some cases this may be difficult. The initial therapy for TMJ should be directed toward relief of pain and improvement in function. Pain relief often can be achieved with use of the NSAIDs. Muscle relaxants may be used when muscle spasm is a problem. In some cases, the selected application of heat or cold, or both, may provide relief. Referral to dentist who is associated with a team of therapists, such as a psychologist, physical therapist, or pain specialist, may be indicated.[48]

> In summary, head pain is a common disorder that is caused by a number of conditions. Some headaches represent primary disorders and others occur secondary to another disease state in which head pain is a symptom. Primary headache disorders include migraine headache, tension-type headache, cluster headache, and CDH. Although most causes of secondary headache are benign, some are indications of serious disorders such as meningitis, brain tumor, or cerebral aneurysm. TMJ syndrome is one of the major causes of headaches. It usually is caused by an imbalance in joint movement because of poor bite, teeth grinding, or joint problems such as inflammation, trauma, and degenerative changes.

Pain in Children and Older Adults

After you have completed this section of the chapter, you should be able to meet the following objectives:

✦ State how the pain response may differ in children and older adults
✦ Explain how pain assessment may differ in children and older adults
✦ Explain how pain treatment may differ in children and older adults

Pain frequently is underrecognized and undertreated in both children[49] and the elderly.[50] In addition to the common obstacles to adequate pain management, such as concern about the effects of analgesia on respiratory status and the potential for addiction to opioids, there are additional deterrents to adequate pain management in children and the elderly. With regard to both children and the elderly, there are stereotypic beliefs that they feel less pain than other patients.[51-53] These beliefs may affect a clinician's opinion about the need for pain control. In very young children and confused elderly, there are several additional factors. These include the extreme difficulty of assessing the location and intensity of pain in individuals who are cognitively immature or cognitively impaired, and the argument that even if they feel pain, they do not remember it. Research during the past few decades has added a great deal to the body of knowledge about pain in children and the elderly. It also has provided valuable data to refute previously held misconceptions and has changed markedly the practices of health professionals.[51-53]

Human responsiveness to painful stimuli begins in the neonatal period and continues through the life span. Although the specific and localized behavioral reactions are less marked in the younger neonate or the more cognitively impaired individual, protective or withdrawal reflexes in response to nociceptive stimuli are clearly demonstrated. Pain pathways, cortical and subcortical centers, and neurochemical responses associated with pain transmission are developed and functional by the last trimester of pregnancy. As infants mature and children grow, their responses to pain become more complex and reflective of their maturing cognitive and developmental processes. Children do feel pain and have been shown reliably and accurately to report pain at as young as 3 years of age. They also remember pain, as evidenced in studies of children with cancer, whose distress during painful procedures increases over time without intervention, and in neonates in intensive care units, who demonstrate protective withdrawal responses to a heel stick after repeated episodes.

Among adults, the prevalence of pain in the general population increases with age.[54] It is estimated that from 25% to 50% of community-dwelling elders[55,56] and 80% of individuals in long-term care facilities report experiencing pain.[57] Research is inconsistent about whether there are age-related changes in pain perception. Some apparent age-related differences in pain may be due to differences in willingness to report the pain rather than actual differences in pain. The elderly may be reluctant to report pain so as not to be a burden or out of fear of the diagnoses, tests, medications, or costs that may result from an attempt to diagnose or treat their pain.

PAIN IN CHILDREN

Pain Assessment

The assessment of pain in children is somewhat complicated, but research has led to the development of a variety of developmentally appropriate measurement tools. These include scales with faces of actual children or cartoon faces that can be used to elicit a pain report from young children.

In older children and adolescents, numeric scales (*i.e.,* 1 to 10) and word graphic scales (*i.e.,* "none," "a little," "most I have ever experienced") can be used. Another strategy for assessing a child's pain is to use a body outline and ask the child to indicate where the hurt is located. Particular care must be taken is assessing children's reports of pain because their report may be influenced by a variety of factors, including age, anxiety and fear levels, and parental presence.

Nurses and physicians have reported that they rely most often on physiologic parameters such as heart rate, respiratory rate, and behavior expressions rather than the child's self-report of pain.[58] Relying on indicators of sympathetic nervous system activity and behaviors can be problematic because they can be caused by things other than pain (*e.g.,* anxiety and activity) and they do not always accompany pain, particularly chronic pain. It is unfortunate that there are no objective physiologic parameters that are specific for pain. Given this, pain experts recommend that health professionals consider the child's report of pain as the gold standard and a primary component of their assessment, in addition to their assessment of the child's behavior and physiologic parameters. When individuals are too cognitively immature or cognitively impaired to report pain, behavior and physiologic parameters must be used.

Pain Management

The management of children's pain basically falls into two categories: pharmacologic and nonpharmacologic. In terms of pharmacologic interventions, many of the analgesics used in adults can be used safely and effectively in children and adolescents. However, it is critical when using specific medications to determine that the medication has been approved for use with children and that it is dosed appropriately according to the child's weight. As with any person in pain, the type of analgesic used should be matched to the type and intensity of pain; and whether the patient is a child or adult, the management of chronic pain may require a multidisciplinary team. The overriding principle in all pediatric pain management is to treat each child's pain on an individual basis and to match the analgesic agent with the cause and the level of pain. A second principle involves maintaining the balance between the level of side effects and pain relief such that pain relief is obtained with as little opioid and sedation as possible. One strategy toward this end is to time the administration of analgesia so that a steady blood level is achieved and, as much as possible, pain is prevented. This requires that the child receive analgesia on a regular dosing schedule, not "as needed."

Nonpharmacologic strategies can be very effective in reducing the overall amount of pain and amount of analgesia used. In addition, some nonpharmacologic strategies can reduce anxiety and increase the child's level of self-control during pain. In full-term infants, ingesting 2 mL of a sucrose solution has been found to relieve the pain from a heel stick.[59] Children as young as 4 years of age can use TENS,[60] and they can be taught to use simple distraction and relaxation and other techniques such as application of heat and cold.[61] Other nonpharmacologic techniques can be taught to the child to provide psychological preparation for a painful procedure or surgery. These include positive

self-talk, imagery, play therapy, modeling, and rehearsal. The nonpharmacologic interventions must be developmentally appropriate and, if possible, the child and parent should be taught these techniques when the child is not in pain (*e.g.,* before surgery or a painful procedure) so that it is easier to practice the technique. Research has provided health professionals with a wide variety of pharmacologic and nonpharmacologic options to treat a child's pain. The application of this research is critical if effective and safe pain care is to be provided.

PAIN IN OLDER ADULTS

Pain Assessment

The assessment of pain in the elderly can range from relatively simple in a well-informed, alert, cognitively intact individual with pain from a single source and no comorbidities to extraordinarily difficult in a frail individual with severe dementia and many concurrent health problems. When possible, patient report of pain is the gold standard, but outward signs of pain should be considered as well. Accurately diagnosing pain when the individual has many health problems or some decline in cognitive function can be particularly challenging. In recent years, there has been increased awareness of the need to address issues of pain in individuals with dementia. The Assessment for Discomfort in Dementia Protocol is one example of the efforts to improve assessment and pain management in these individuals. It includes behavioral criteria for assessing pain and recommended interventions for pain. Its use has been shown to improve pain management.[53]

Pain Management

Treatment of pain in the elderly can be complicated. The elderly may have physiologic changes that affect the pharmacokinetics of medications prescribed for pain management. These changes include decreased blood flow to organs, delayed gastric motility, reduced kidney function, and decreased albumin related to poor nutrition. These changes may affect the choice of medications or dosing (*e.g.,* using a lower initial dose of tricyclic antidepressants).[62] Also, the elderly often have many coexisting health problems, leading to polypharmacy. Whenever multiple medications are being taken, there is an increased risk of drug interactions and of noncompliance because of the complexity of the treatment regimen. When prescribing pharmacologic and nonpharmacologic methods of pain management, care must be taken to consider the cause of the pain, the patient's health status, concurrent therapies, and the patient's mental status. Careful monitoring and treatment of side effects is critical.

In summary, children experience and remember pain, and even fairly young children are able accurately and reliably to report their pain. Recognition of this has changed the clinical practice of health professionals involved in the assessment of children's pain. Pain management in children is improving as exaggerated fears and misconceptions concerning the risks of addiction and respiratory depression in children treated with opioids also are dispelled. Pharmacologic (including opioids) and nonpharmacologic pain management interventions have been shown to be effective in children. Nonpharmacologic techniques must be based on the developmental level of the child and should be taught to both children and parents.

Pain is a common symptom in the elderly. Assessment, diagnosis, and treatment of pain in the elderly can be complicated. The elderly may be reluctant or cognitively unable to report their pain. Diagnosis and treatment can be complicated by comorbidities and age-related changes in cognitive and physiologic function.

Related Web Sites

American Academy of Pain Medicine—position and consensus statements (*e.g.,* use of opioids for chronic pain; ethics for pain medicine; quality end of life care) www.painmed.org/productpub/statements

American Pain Society resources for professionals www.ampainsoc.org/links

City of Hope Pain Resource Center—a clearinghouse for information and resources prc.coh.org

Reflex Sympathetic Dystrophy Syndrome Association of America: clinical practice guidelines www.rsds.org/english.htm

Wisconsin Cancer Pain Initiative—links to Agency for Healthcare Research and Quality (formerly AHCPR) acute and chronic pain guidelines and more www.wisc.edu/wcpi

World Health Organization booklet: Cancer Pain Relief and Palliative Care in Children (1998) coninfo.nursing.uiowa.edu/sites/PedsPain/World/WHO_Acrobat.htm

References

1. Guyton A., Hall J.E. (2000). *Textbook of medical physiology* (10th ed., pp. 552–563). Philadelphia: W.B. Saunders.
2. Rhoades R.A., Tanner G.A. (1996). *Medical physiology* (pp. 60–70). Boston: Little, Brown.
3. Kandel E.R., Schwartz J.H., Jessell T.M. (2000). *Principles of neural science* (4th ed., pp. 430–450). New York: McGraw-Hill.
4. Ready L.B. (Chair) (1992). *International Association for the Study of Pain Task Force on Chronic Pain*. Seattle: IASP Publications.
5. Sherrington C. (1947). *The integrative action of the nervous system*. New Haven: Yale University Press.
6. Elliott A.M., Smith B.H., Penny K.I., Smith W.C., Chambers W.A. (1999). The epidemiology of chronic pain in the community. *Lancet* 354, 1248–1252.
7. Lister B.J. (1996). Dilemmas in the treatment of chronic pain. *American Journal of Medicine* 101 (Suppl. 1A), 2S–4S.
8. Bonica J.J. (1991). History of pain concepts and pain theory. *Mount Sinai Journal of Medicine* 58, 191–202.
9. Melzack R., Wall P.D. (1965). Pain mechanisms: A new theory. *Science* 150, 971–979.
10. Melzack R. (1999). From the gate to the neuromatrix. *Pain* 6 (Suppl.), S121–S126.
11. Cross S.A. (1994). Pathophysiology of pain. *Mayo Clinic Proceedings* 69, 375–383.
12. Beeson J., Chaouch A. (1987). Peripheral and spinal mechanisms of nociception. *Physiological Reviews* 67, 67–186.
13. Markenson J.A. (1996). Mechanisms of chronic pain. *American Journal of Medicine* 101 (Suppl. 1A), 6S–18S.
14. Cooper J.R., Bloom F.E., Roth R.H. (1991). *The biochemical basis of neuropharmacology* (6th ed., p. 263). New York: Oxford University Press.
15. Basabaum A.I. (1987). Cytochemical studies of the neural circuitry underlying pain and pain control. *Acta Neurochirurgica (Wien)* 38 (Suppl.), 5–15.
16. Fields H.L., Heinricher M.M., Mason P. (1991). Neurotransmitters in nociceptive modulatory circuits. *Review of Neuroscience* 14, 219–245.
17. Grichnick K., Ferrante F.M. (1991). The difference between acute and chronic pain. *Mount Sinai Journal of Medicine* 58, 217–220.
18. Ruoff G.E. (1996). Depression in the patient with chronic pain. *Journal of Family Practice* 43 (6 Suppl.), S25–S33.
19. Acute Pain Management Guideline Panel. (1992). *Clinical practice guideline no. 1. Acute pain management: Operative or medical procedures and trauma*. AHCPR Publication No. 92-0032. Rockville, MD: Agency for Health Care Policy and Research, Public Health Service, U.S. Department of Health and Human Services.
20. Melzack R. (1975). The McGill Pain Questionnaire: Major properties and scoring methods. *Pain* 1, 277–299.
21. Jacox A., Carr D.B., Payne R., et al. (1994). *Clinical practice guideline no. 9. Management of cancer pain*. AHCPR Publication No. 94-0592. Rockville, MD: Agency for Health Care Policy and Research, Public Health Service, U.S. Department of Health and Human Services.
22. World Health Organization. (1990). *Cancer pain relief and palliative care: Report of the WHO Expert Committee* (Technical Report Series. 804). Geneva, Switzerland: Author.
23. Shepard J.T., Rusch N.J., Vanhoutte P.M. (1983). Effect of cold on the blood vessel walls. *General Pharmacology* 14 (1), 61–64.
24. Hymes A. (1984). A review of the historical area of electricity. In Mannheimer J.S., Lampe G.N. (Eds.), *Clinical transcutaneous electrical stimulation* (pp. 1–5). Philadelphia: F.A. Davis.
25. Anderson S.A. (1979). Pain control by sensory stimulation. In Bonica J.J., Liebeskind J.C., Albe-Fessard D.G. (Eds.), *Advances in pain research and therapy* (pp. 569–585). New York: Raven Press.
26. Ignelzi R.J., Nyquist J.K. (1979). Excitability changes in peripheral nerve fibers after repetitive electrical stimulation: Implications for pain modulation. *Journal of Neurosurgery* 51, 824–833.
27. Ezzo J., Berman B., Hadhazy A., Jadad A.R., Lao L., Singh B.B. (2000). Is acupuncture effective for the treatment of chronic pain: A systematic review. *Pain* 86, 217–225.
28. Wolf S.L. (1984). Neurophysiologic mechanisms of pain modulation: Relevance to TENS. In Mannheimer J.S., Lampe G.N. (Eds.), *Clinical transcutaneous electrical stimulation* (pp. 41–55). Philadelphia: F.A. Davis.
29. Way W.L., Field H.L., Schumacher M.A. (2001). Opioid analgesics and antagonists. In Katzung H. (Ed.), *Basic and clinical pharmacology* (8th ed., pp. 512–531). New York: Lange Medical Books/McGraw-Hill.
30. Melzack R. (1990). The tragedy of needless pain. *Scientific American* 262 (2), 2–8.
31. Swerdlow M., Stjerward J. (1982). Cancer pain relief: An urgent problem. *World Health Forum* 3, 325–330.
32. McCaffery M., Ferrell B.R., Turner M. (1996). Ethical issues in the use of placebos in cancer pain management. *Oncology Nursing Forum* 23, 1587–1593.
33. American Pain Society. (1992). *Principles of analgesic use in the treatment of acute and cancer pain* (3rd ed.). Glenview, IL: Author.

34. Vaillancourt P.D., Langevin H.M. (1999). Painful peripheral neuropathies. *Medical Clinics of North America* 83, 627–643.

35. Kost R.G., Straus S.E. (1996). Postherpetic neuralgia: Pathogenesis, treatment and prevention. *New England Journal of Medicine* 335, 32–42.

36. Reflex Sympathetic Dystrophy Syndrome Association of America. (2000). Clinical practice guideline for treatment of reflex sympathetic dystrophy syndrome. [On-line]. Available: http://www.rsds.org/cpgeng.htm.

37. Melzack R. (1992). Phantom limb. *Scientific American* 226, 120–126.

38. Saper J.R. (1999). Headache disorders. *Medical Clinics of North America* 83, 663–670.

39. Olesen J. (Chair). (1988). Headache Classification Committee of the International Headache Society: The classification and diagnostic criteria for headache disorders, cranial neuralgias, and facial pain. *Cephalalgia* 8 (Suppl. 7), 1–96.

40. Stewart W.F., Lipton R.B., Celentano D.D., Reed M.L. (1992). Prevalence of migraine headache in the United States: Relation to age, income, race, and other other sociodemographic factors. *Journal of the American Medical Association* 267, 64–69.

41. Annequin D., Tourniare B., Massoui H. (2000). Migraine and headache in childhood and adolescence. *Pediatric Clinics of North America* 47, 617–631.

42. Behrman R.E., Kliegman R.M., Jensen H.B. (2000). *Nelson textbook of pediatrics* (16th ed., pp. 1832–1834). Philadelphia: W.B. Saunders.

43. Kunkel R.S. (2000). Managing primary headache syndromes. *Patient Care* January 30. [On-line]. Available: www.patientcareonline.com.

44. The U.S. Headache Consortium Participants. (1998). Evidence-based guidelines for migraine headaches in primary care setting: Pharmacological management of acute attacks. American Academy of Neurology. [On-line]. Available: http://www.aan.com/public/practiceguidelines/05.pdf.

45. Moore K.L., Noble S.L. (1997). Drug treatment for migraine: Part I. Acute therapy and drug-rebound headache. *American Family Physician* 56 (8), 2039–2048.

46. Noble S., Moore K.L. (1997). Drug treatment of migraine: Part II. Preventative therapy. *American Family Physician* 56 (9), 2279–2286.

47. Silberstein S.D., Lipton R.B. (2000). Chronic daily headache. *Current Opinion in Neurology* 13, 277–283.

48. Okeson J.P. (1996). Temporomandibular disorders in the medical practice. *Journal of Family Practice* 43, 347–356.

49. Eland J., Anderson J. (1977). The experience of pain in children. In Jacox A. (Ed.), *Pain: A sourcebook for nurses and other professionals* (pp. 453–473). Boston: Little, Brown.

50. Morrison R.S., Siu A.L. (2000). A comparison of pain and its treatment in advanced dementia and cognitively intact patients with hip fracture. *Journal of Pain and Symptom Management* 19, 240–248.

51. Broome M., Richtsmeier A., Maikler V., Alexander M. (1996). Pediatric pain practices: A survey of health professionals. *Journal of Pain and Symptom Management* 4, 315–319.

52. McCaffery M., Bebee A. (1994). *Pain: Clinical manual for nursing practice.* St Louis: Mosby.

53. Kovach C.R., Weissman, D.E., Griffie J., Matson S., Muchka S. (1999). Assessment and treatment of discomfort for people with late-stage dementia. *Journal of Pain and Symptom Management* 18, 412–419.

54. Bassols A., Bosch F., Campillo M., Banos J.E. (1999). An epidemiological comparison of pain complaints in the general population of Catalonia (Spain). *Pain* 83, 9–16.

55. Brattberg G., Parker M.G., Thorslund M. (1996). A longitudinal study of pain: Reported from middle age to old age. *Clinical Journal of Pain* 13, 144–149.

56. Crook J., Ridofut E., Browne G. (1984). The prevalence of pain complaints in a general population. *Pain* 18, 299–314.

57. Ferrell B.A., Ferrell B.R., Osterweil D. (1990). Pain in the nursing home. *Journal of the American Geriatric Society* 38, 409–414.

58. Watt-Watson J., Donovan M. (1992). *Nursing management of the patient in pain.* Philadelphia: J.B. Lippincott.

59. Haouari N., Wood C., Griffiths G., Levene, M. (1995). The analgesic effect of sucrose in full term infants: A randomized controlled trial. *British Medical Journal* 310, 1498–1500.

60. Merkel S.I., Gutstein H.B., Malviya S. (1999). Use of transcutaneous electrical nerve stimulation in a young child with pain from open perineal lesions. *Journal of Pain and Symptom Management* 18, 376–381.

61. Vessey J., Carlson K., McGill J. (1995). Use of distraction with children during an acute pain experience. *Nursing Research* 43, 369–372.

62. Irving G.A., Wallace M.S. (1997). *Pain management for the practicing physician.* Philadelphia: Churchill Livingstone.

Chapter 49

Alterations in Motor Function

Carol M. Porth and Robin L. Curtis

*E*ffective motor function requires that muscles move and that the mechanics of their movement be programmed in a manner that provides for smooth and coordinated movement. In some cases, purposeless and disruptive movements can be almost as disabling as relative or complete absence of movement. This chapter addresses control of motor function, alterations in function of the neuromuscular unit, alterations in pyramidal or extrapyramidal function, and spinal cord injury. Although motor function relies on continuous input from sensory neurons, the focus of this chapter is on the efferent output that controls movement. Spinal cord injury is presented as an example of a condition that affects multiple motor systems.

Control of Motor Function

After you have completed this section of the chapter, you should be able to meet the following objectives:

✦ Define a motor unit and characterize its mechanism of controlling muscle movement

✦ Define the function of the following muscle types: extensors, flexors, adductors, abductors, rotators, agonists, antagonists, and synergists
✦ Contrast the functions of the pyramidal and extrapyramidal systems
✦ Construct a movement model for voluntary muscle movement that begins in the motor cortex and terminates in the muscle fibers of a motor unit

Movement begins in utero at approximately 21 weeks of gestation with the quickening of the fetus, and the capability for some coordinated movement is present at birth. Maturation of the spinal cord and brain circuitry during the first year or two of life allows the child to defy the force of gravity and learn to sit, then stand, and, in rapid sequence, master the skills of walking, running, jumping, and climbing.

MOTOR FUNCTION

Motor function, whether it involves walking, running, or precise finger movements, requires movement and maintenance of posture. Posture can be described as the relative position of various parts of the body with respect to one another (limb extension, flexion) or to the environment (standing, supine).[1] Posture also can be described as the active muscular resistance to the displacement of the body by gravity or acceleration. The structures that control posture and movement are located throughout the neuromuscular system. The system consists of the neuromuscular unit, which includes the motoneurons, the myoneural junction, and the muscle fibers; the spinal cord, which contains the basic reflex circuitry for posture and movement; and the descending pathways from the brain stem circuits, the cerebellum, basal ganglia, and the motor cortex.

Muscle Groups

Skeletal muscle is composed of muscle cells, or fibers, which contain the interacting actin and myosin filaments that generate the contractile force required for movement (see Chapter 4). In terms of function, muscles can be classified as extensors, muscles that increase the angle of a joint, or flexors, muscles that decrease the angle of a joint. In the legs, groups of extensor muscles work together to resist gravity and function to maintain the upright posture and provide locomotion power. In general, flexor muscle groups assist gravity, participate in withdrawal reflexes, and provide the more delicate aspects of manipulation. Other muscle groups work roughly in pairs: adductors versus abductors, which move a part toward or away from the midline of the body, and rotators, which work in pairs to rotate a part of the limb, the trunk, or the head around each part's longitudinal axis. Many muscles participate in more than one of these functions.

Coordinated movement requires the action of two or more muscle groups: agonists, which promote a movement; antagonists, which oppose it; and synergists, which assist the agonist muscles by stabilizing a joint or contributing additional force to the movement. Some simple types of movement require only a burst of energy from an agonist muscle group. Other types of movements, such as self-terminated actions, require a smooth sequence of movements: agonist, antagonist, and cocontraction of agonist and antagonist to stop and stabilize the end of the movement. Agonist and antagonist contractions are programmed by higher brain centers to fit the situation. Simple movements are programmed before they start so that the movement proceeds from start to finish without modification. Self-terminated movements are more complex; they are programmed to start and then modified as they proceed.

The Motor Unit

The neurons that control motor function are referred to as *motoneurons* or sometimes as *alpha motoneurons*. A motor unit consists of one motoneuron and the group of muscle fibers it innervates in a muscle. The motoneurons supplying a motor unit are located in the ventral horn of the spinal cord and are called *lower motoneurons* (LMNs). The synapse between an LMN and the muscle fibers of a motor unit is called the *neuromuscular junction*. Upper motoneurons (UMNs), which exert control over LMNs, project from the motor strip in the cerebral cortex to the ventral horn and are fully contained within the central nervous system (CNS) (Fig. 49-1).

Axons of the LMNs exit the spinal cord at each segment to innervate skeletal muscle cells, including those of the limbs, back, abdomen, and chest. Each LMN undergoes multiple branching, making it possible for a single LMN to innervate 10 to 2000 muscle cells. In general, large muscles—those containing hundreds or thousands of muscle cells and providing gross motor movement—have large motor units. This sharply contrasts with those that control the hand, tongue, and eye movements, for which the motor units are small and permit very discrete control.

Basic to the understanding of motor control is the concept of the *motor unit*—the LMN and the muscle fibers it innervates—functioning as a unit. All muscles contain thousands of muscle fibers and are innervated by fewer LMNs. When the LMN develops an action potential, all of the muscle fibers in the motor unit it innervates develop action potentials, causing them to contract simultaneously. Thus, an LMN and the muscle fibers it innervates function as a single unit—the basic unit of motor control. All neurally controlled motor functions involve the differential use of combinations of motor units in agonist and antagonist muscles around a joint, manipulating the resultant joint angle. Movement involves some joints being held stable and the joint angle of other joints being changed.

Most skeletal muscle groups fall into two categories based on differences in the chemistry of their contractile proteins and their source of energy.[2] The first type, the *slow-twitch fibers*, have many mitochondria, depend on blood-

Motor Systems

➤ Motor systems require upper motoneurons (UMNs) that project from the motor cortex to the brain stem or spinal cord, where they directly or indirectly innervate the lower motoneurons (LMNs) of the contracting muscles; sensory feedback from the involved muscles that is continuously relayed to the cerebellum, basal ganglia, and sensory cortex; and a functioning neuromuscular junction that links nervous system activity with muscle contraction.

➤ The pyramidal motor system originating in the motor cortex provides control of delicate muscle movement, and the extrapyramidal system originating in the basal ganglia provides the background for the more crude, supportive movement patterns.

➤ The efficiency of the movement by the motor system depends on a background of muscle tone provided by the stretch reflex and vestibular system input to maintain stable postural support.

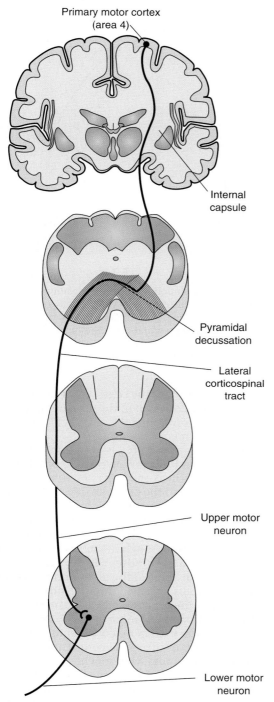

Primary motor cortex
(area 4)

Internal
capsule

Pyramidal
decussation

Lateral
corticospinal
tract

Upper motor
neuron

Lower motor
neuron

FIGURE 49-1 The corticospinal tract. The long axons of motoneurons originating in the primary motor cortex descend through the telencephalon through the internal capsule and traverse the brain stem in a ventral path through the cerebral peduncles and the pyramids. The axons cross in the lower medulla (pyramidal decussation) to the opposite side and continue as the corticospinal tract in the spinal cord, where they synapse on motoneurons and interneurons in the ventral horns. (Modified from Kandel E.R., Schwartz J.H. [1985]. *Principles of neural science* [2nd ed.]. New York: Elsevier)

borne oxygen for energy, and are slow to fatigue. The second type, the *fast-twitch fibers*, depend on muscle glycogen stores that can be rapidly depleted. The fast-twitch fibers are further divided into fast-twitch fatigable and fast-twitch fatigue-resistant fibers. The antigravity postural muscles that use slow-twitch fibers are slow to fatigue. Muscles used for more rapid movements such as jumping and throwing are rich in large, powerful, but rapidly fatiguing fast-twitch motor units.

Most muscles contain motor units with most or all of these muscle fiber types, but the proportions may vary with muscle function. For example, postural muscles and delicate distal flexor muscles are predominantly slow-twitch fibers, whereas the large, proximal limb muscles such as the gastrocnemius are mixed, with many fast-twitch fatigable and fast-twitch fatigue-resistant fiber motor units that can provide brief, high power.

The muscle fibers for each motor unit are uniform as to muscle fiber type (*e.g.*, slow-twitch and fast-twitch). The group of LMNs in the spinal cord ventral horn that have muscle fibers in a particular muscle is called a *motoneuron pool*. When reflex or descending systems activate such a pool, the first motor units to fire are the slow-twitch units. With stronger activation, the fast-twitch fatigue-resistant units begin firing, and then the fast-twitch fatigable units.

The motor system is designed to minimize participation of the forebrain in details of movements, permitting the forebrain to specialize in the planning and motor learning required for precise control of motor function. The recruitment order of slow-twitch, then fast-twitch fatigue-resistant, and finally fast-twitch fatigable motor units provides the automatic sequence for increasing muscle contraction power and for the initial, delicate control of movement.

The Motor Cortex

Delicate, skillful, intentional movement of distal and especially flexor muscles of the limbs and the speech apparatus is initiated and controlled from the motor cortex located in the posterior part of the frontal lobe. It consists of the primary, premotor, and supplementary motor cortex[2,3] (Fig. 49-2). These areas receive information from the thalamus and the somesthetic cortex and, indirectly, from the cerebellum and basal ganglia. The primary motor cortex (area 4), also called the *motor strip*, is located on the rostral surface and adjacent portions of the central sulcus. The primary motor cortex controls discrete muscle movement sequences and is the first level of descending control for precise movements. Discrete lesions in the most posterior part of the primary motor cortex can result in profound weakness in specific distal flexor muscle groups and permanent inability to perform delicate manipulative motor patterns on the opposite side of the body or face. Lesions restricted to the more anterior part of the motor strip result in weakness of larger limb, girdle, and axial muscles.

The premotor cortex (areas 6 and 8), which is located just anterior to the primary motor cortex, sends some fibers into the corticospinal tract but mainly innervates the primary motor strip. A movement pattern to accomplish a particular objective, such as throwing a ball or picking up a fork, is programmed by the prefrontal association cortex and

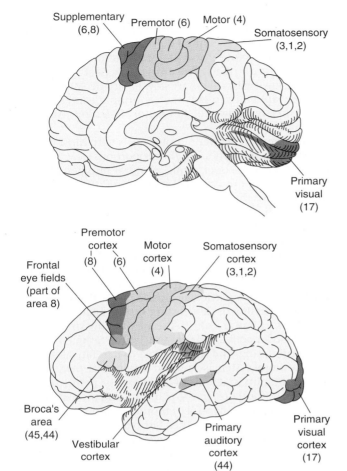

FIGURE 49-2 Primary motor cortex. (**Top**) The location of the primary, premotor, and supplementary cortex on the medial surface of the brain. (**Bottom**) The location of the primary and premotor cortex on the lateral surface of the brain. (Courtesy of Carole Russell Hilmer, C.M.I.)

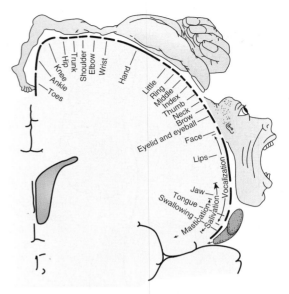

FIGURE 49-3 Representation of the relative extent of motor cortical area 4 devoted to muscles of the various body regions. Medial surface is at the left, lateral fissure is at the right, with pharyngeal and laryngeal muscle representation extending toward the insula. (Penfield E., Rasmussen T. [1968]. *The cerebral cortex in man: A clinical study of localization of function.* New York: Macmillan)

associated thalamic nuclei. The "program" for the movement pattern includes the muscle contraction sequences for complex distal manipulation and for the larger preparative and supportive actions of whole-limb and limb girdle muscles.

The supplementary motor cortex, which contains representations of all parts of the body, is located on the medial surface of the hemisphere (areas 6 and 8) in the premotor region. It is intimately involved in the performance of complex, skillful movements that involve both sides of the body. Bilateral lesions cause long-lasting loss of movements involving both hands or both feet.

The neurons in the primary motor cortex are arranged in a somatotopic array or distorted map of the body called the *motor homunculus* (Fig. 49-3). This map, which shows the degree of representation of the neurons that control voluntary movement of a particular body part, was published by Penfield and Rasmussen in 1950.[4] The mapping was done by electrically stimulating the brain of persons who were undergoing brain surgery. The body parts that require

the greatest dexterity have the largest cortical areas devoted to them. More than one half of the primary motor cortex is concerned with controlling the muscles of the hands, of facial expression, and of speech.[2]

The primary motor cortex is very thick. It contains many layers of pyramid-shaped output neurons that project to the same side of the cortex (*i.e.*, premotor and somesthetic areas), project to the opposite side of the cortex, or descend to subcortical structures such as the basal ganglia and thalamus. The large pyramidal cells located in the fifth layer project to the brain stem and spinal cord. The axons of these UMNs project through the subcortical white matter and internal capsule to the deep surface of the brain stem, through the ventral bulge of the pons, and to the ventral surface of the medulla, where they form a ridge or pyramid (see Fig. 49-1). At the junction between the medulla and cervical spinal cord, 80% or more of the UMN axons cross the midline to form the lateral corticospinal tract in the lateral white matter of the spinal cord. This tract extends throughout the spinal cord, with roughly 50% of the fibers terminating in the cervical segments, 20% in the thoracic segments, and 30% in the lumbosacral segments. Most of the remaining uncrossed fibers travel down the ventral column of the cord, mainly to cervical levels, where they cross and innervate contralateral LMNs.

Monosynaptic innervation of LMNs by UMNs of the primary motor cortex only occurs for the most distal muscles involved with delicate manipulative skills, such as those of the hands and fingers, tongue, mouth, and pharynx. For LMNs of other muscles, the connection is multisynaptic and less discrete. As the UMN axons pass along their long pathways, collateral branches move out and innervate regions of the basal ganglia, the thalamus, the brain stem, and nuclei that project into the cerebellum. The cerebellum matches the temporal smoothness aspect of the ongoing movement against very rapid proprioceptive feedback from the actual movement and sends error signals back to the thalamus and motor cortex for corrective modifications of the ongoing movement. Similarly, sensory feedback to the basal ganglia results in error-correcting feedback for supportive and background aspects of the movement. Slower sensory feedback from the somesthetic cortex permits error correction on the next trial. Ongoing error correction becomes less and less important for well-learned movements that can proceed without sensory feedback.

Movement Model

The performance of skilled motor movements can be represented by the movement model depicted in Figure 49-4. This model involves the use of a repertoire of inherited and learned neural interactions that contribute skill, grace, and temporal smoothness to the movement.

A movement sequence, such as moving a body part to a precise point in three-dimensional space, involves the higher-order functions of the primary motor, premotor, and supplementary motor cortex. The plan is programmed into a sequence of component actions, a learned function performed by the premotor cortex. Complex bilateral movements require the function of the supplementary motor cortex, with the precise control of distal muscle movements being provided by the primary motor cortex. Descending axons from the motor cortex project to the brain stem or spinal cord, where they directly or indirectly innervate

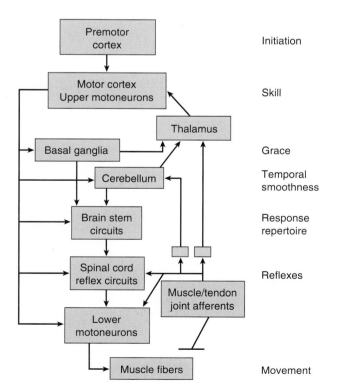

FIGURE 49-4 Diagram of neural pathways for control of motor function. (Courtesy Robin L. Curtis)

LMNs that supply the muscle fibers. The basal ganglia provide the axial and proximal support required for the movement. Continuous sensory feedback from the involved muscles and from all sensory systems are matched against the model, and adjustments for errors in timing or in sequence are continuously relayed from the cerebellum, the basal ganglia, and the primary sensory cortex back to the motor cortex. The programmed movement, which is continuously corrected and adjusted, progresses until the precise goal is accomplished.

The efficiency of the entire motor system depends on optimally functioning motor units on a background of muscle tone provided by the stretch reflex and vestibular system input to maintain stable postural support. The program for motor function involves parallel processing and ongoing interactive communication between these functions. A highly skilled movement is beautiful to behold, but it can be easily damaged or distorted because of the necessary complexity of its control.

Pyramidal and Extrapyramidal Systems

By convention, motor tracts are often classified as belonging to one of two motor systems: the pyramidal and extrapyramidal systems. The pyramidal system consists of the motor pathways originating in the motor cortex and terminating in the corticobulbar fibers in the brain stem and the corticospinal fibers in the spinal cord. The corticospinal fibers traverse the ventral surface of the medulla in a bundle called the *pyramid* before decussating or crossing to the opposite side of the brain at the medulla–spinal cord junction, hence the name *pyramidal system*. Other fibers from the cortex and basal ganglia also project to the brain stem reticular formation and reticulospinal systems, following a more ancient pathway to LMNs of proximal and extensor muscles. These fibers do not decussate in the pyramids, hence the name *extrapyramidal system*.

The pyramidal and extrapyramidal systems have different effects on muscle tone. The pyramidal system is largely excitatory; it provides control of delicate muscle movement. The extrapyramidal system provides the more crude, background supportive movement patterns. In terms of actual function, the pyramidal and extrapyramidal systems do not function independently, but the concept of two separate systems is helpful in understanding motor function. After severe damage to the pyramidal system, the crude movements and slurred speech that remain result from extrapyramidal system function.

DISORDERS OF MOTOR FUNCTION

Disorders of motor function include skeletal muscle weakness and paralysis, which result from lesions in the voluntary motor pathways, including the UMNs of the corticospinal and corticobulbar tracts or the LMNs that leave the CNS and travel by way of the peripheral nerve to the muscle. Muscle tone, which is a necessary component of muscle movement, is a function of the muscle spindle (myotatic) system (see Chapter 47) and the extrapyramidal system, which monitors and buffers input to the LMNs by way of the multisynaptic pathways.

DISORDERS OF MUSCLE TONE

Muscle tone is the normal tension in a muscle as evidenced by the resistance to passive movement around a joint. Disorders of skeletal muscle tone are characteristic of many nervous system pathologies. Any interruption of the myotatic reflex circuit by peripheral nerve injury, pathology of the neuromuscular junction and of skeletal muscle fibers, damage to the corticospinal system, or injury to the spinal cord or spinal nerve root results in disturbance of muscle tone. Muscle tone may be described as less than normal (hypotonia), absent (flaccidity), or excessive (hypertonia, rigidity, spasticity, or tetany). Hypertonicity, rigidity, and spasticity are extremes of hypertonia that include other distinguishing features.

PARESIS AND PARALYSIS

The suffix *plegia* comes from the Greek word for a blow, a stroke, or paralysis. Terms used to describe the extent and anatomic location of motor damage are *paralysis*, meaning loss of movement, and *paresis*, implying weakness or incomplete loss of muscle function. *Monoparesis* or *monoplegia* results from the destruction of pyramidal UMN innervation of one limb; *hemiparesis* or *hemiplegia*, both limbs on one side; *diparesis* or *diplegia* or *paraparesis* or *paraplegia*, both upper or lower limbs; and *tetraparesis* or *tetraplegia,* also called *quadriparesis* or *quadriplegia*, all four limbs (Fig. 49-5). Paresis or paralysis can be further designated as of UMN or LMN origin.

Upper Motoneuron Lesions

A UMN lesion can involve the motor cortex, the internal capsule, or other brain structures through which the corticospinal or corticobulbar tracts descend, or the spinal cord. When the lesion is at or above the level of the pyramids, paralysis affects structures on the opposite side of the body. In UMN disorders involving injury to the L1 level or above, there is an immediate, profound weakness and loss of fine, skilled voluntary lower limb movement, reduced bowel and bladder control, and diminished sexual functioning, followed by an exaggeration of muscle tone. With UMN damage above C5, upper limb movement also is affected.

With UMN lesions, the LMN spinal reflexes remain intact, but communication and control from higher brain centers are lost. Descending excitatory influences from the pyramidal system and some descending inhibitory influences from other cortical regions are lost after injury, resulting in immediate weakness accompanied by the loss of control of delicate, skilled movements. After several weeks, this weakness becomes converted to hypertonicity or spasticity, which is manifested by an initial increased resistance (stiffness) to the passive movement of a joint at the extremes of range of motion followed by a sudden or gradual release of resistance. The spasticity often is greatest in the flexor muscles of the upper limbs and extensor muscles of the lower limbs. Sometimes, a lesion of the pyramidal tract is less severe and results in a relatively minor degree of weakness. In this case, the finer and more skilled movements are most severely impaired.

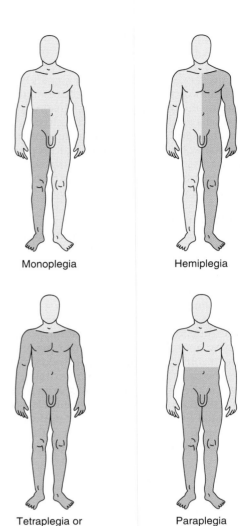

Monoplegia   Hemiplegia

Tetraplegia or   Paraplegia
quadriplegia

FIGURE 49-5 Areas of the body affected by monoplegia, hemiplegia, tetraplegia or quadriplegia, and paraplegia. The *shaded area* shows the extent of motor and sensory loss. (Hickey J.V. [1997]. *The clinical practice of neurological and neurosurgical nursing* [3rd ed.]. Philadelphia: J.B. Lippincott)

Clonus is the rhythmic contraction and alternate relaxation of a limb that is caused by suddenly stretching a muscle and gently maintaining it in the stretched position. It is seen in the hypertonia of spasticity associated with UMN lesions. It is caused by an oscillating stimulation of the muscle spindles that occurs when the spindle fibers are activated by an initial muscle stretch. This results in reflex contraction of the muscle and unloading of the spindle fibers with decreased afferent activity. The reduced spindle fiber activity causes the muscle to relax, which causes the spindle fiber to stretch again, and the cycle starts over.

Lower Motoneuron Lesions

In contrast to UMN lesions, in which the spinal reflexes remain intact, LMN disorders disrupt communication between the muscle and all neural input from spinal cord reflexes, including the stretch reflex, which maintains muscle tone.

Infection or irritation of the cell body of the LMN or its axon can lead to hyperexcitability, which causes spontaneous contractions of the muscle units. These can be observed as twitching and squirming movements on the muscle surface, a condition called *fasciculations*. Toxic agents, such as the tetanus toxin, produce extreme hyperexcitability of the LMN, which results in continuous firing at maximum rate. The resultant sustained contraction of the muscles is called *tetany*. Tetany of muscles on both sides of a joint produces immobility or tetanic paralysis. When a virus, such as the poliomyelitis virus, attacks an LMN, it first irritates the LMN, causing fasciculations to occur. These fasciculations often are followed by death of LMNs. Weakness and severe muscle wasting or denervation atrophy result. If muscles are totally denervated, total weakness and total loss of reflexes, called *flaccid paralysis*, occurs.

With complete LMN lesions, the muscles of the affected limbs, bowel, bladder, and genital areas become atonic, and it is impossible to elicit contraction by stretching the tendons. One of the outstanding features of LMN lesions is the profound development of muscle atrophy. Damage to an LMN with or without spinal cord damage, often called *peripheral nerve injury*, may occur at any level of the spinal cord. For example, a C7 peripheral nerve injury leads to LMN hand weakness only. All segments below the level of injury that have intact LMNs manifest UMN signs. Usually, injury to the spinal cord at the T12 level or below results in LMN injury and flaccid paralysis to all areas below the level of injury. This occurs because the spinal cord ends at the T12 to L1 level, and from this level, the spinal roots of the LMNs continue caudally in the vertebral canal as part of the cauda equina.

In summary, motor function involves the neuromuscular unit, spinal cord circuitry, brain stem neurons, the cerebellum, the basal ganglia, and the motor cortex. A motor unit consists of one LMN and the group of muscle fibers it innervates in the muscle. Delicate, skillful, intentional movement of distal and especially flexor muscles of the limbs and the speech apparatus is initiated and controlled from the motor cortex located in the posterior frontal lobe. It consists of the primary, premotor, and supplementary motor cortex. These areas receive information from the thalamus and somesthetic cortex and, indirectly, from the cerebellum and basal ganglia. The UMNs in the motor cortex send their axons through the subcortical white matter and internal capsule and the deep surface of the brain stem to the ventral surface to the opposite side of the medulla, where they form a pyramid before crossing the midline to form the lateral corticospinal tract in the spinal cord. Skillful movement patterns are planned in the prefrontal cortex, a sequential model is organized in the premotor cortex, and the model is carried out by the primary motor cortex. If the UMN system is severely damaged, delicate and skillful movement is lost, but crude movements still can be made using extrapyramidal systems.

Alterations in musculoskeletal function include weakness resulting from lesions of voluntary UMN pathways of the corticobulbar and corticospinal tracts and the LMNs of the peripheral nerves. Muscle tone is maintained through the combined function of the muscle spindle system and the extrapyramidal system that monitors and buffers UMN innervation of the LMNs. Hypotonia is a condition of less-than-normal muscle tone, and hypertonia or spasticity is a condition of excessive tone. Paresis refers to weakness in muscle function, and paralysis refers to a loss of muscle movement. UMN lesions produce spastic paralysis, and LMN lesions produce flaccid paralysis. Damage to the UMNs of the corticospinal and corticobulbar tracts is a common component of stroke.

Skeletal Muscle and Peripheral Nerve Disorders

After you have completed this section of the chapter, you should be able to meet the following objectives:

+ Describe muscle atrophy and differentiate between disuse and degenerative atrophy
+ Explain the causes of muscle atrophy
+ Describe the pathology associated with Duchenne's muscular dystrophy
+ Relate the clinical manifestations of myasthenia gravis to its cause
+ Trace the steps in regeneration of an injured peripheral nerve
+ Describe the manifestation of peripheral nerve root injury due to a ruptured intervertebral disk
+ Compare the cause and manifestations of peripheral mononeuropathies with peripheral polyneuropathies

SKELETAL MUSCLE DISORDERS

Disorders of skeletal muscle groups involve atrophy and dystrophy. Atrophy describes a decrease in muscle mass. Muscular dystrophy is a primary disorder of muscle tissue and is characterized by defect in the muscle fibers.

Muscle Atrophy

Maintenance of muscle strength requires relatively frequent movements against resistance. Reduced use results in muscle atrophy, which is characterized by a reduction in the diameter of the muscle fibers because of a loss of protein filaments. When a normally innervated muscle is not used for long periods, the muscle cells shrink in diameter, and although the muscle cells do not die, they lose much of their contractile protein and become weakened. This is called *disuse atrophy*, and it occurs with conditions such as immobilization and chronic illness.

The most extreme examples of muscle atrophy are found in persons with disorders that deprive muscles of their innervation. This form is called *denervation atrophy*. During early embryonic development, outgrowing skeletal nerves innervate partially mature muscle cells. If the developing muscle cells are not innervated, they do not mature and eventually die. In the process of innervation, randomly contracting muscle cells become enslaved by the innervating neurons, and from then on, the muscle cell contracts only when stimulated by that particular neuron. If the LMN dies or its axon is destroyed, the skeletal muscle cell is again free of neural domination. When this happens, it begins to have temporary spontaneous contractions, called *fibrillations*, of its own. It also begins to lose its contractile proteins and, after several months, if not reinnervated, it degenerates.

If a peripheral motoneuron is crushed and its endoneurial tube remains intact, regenerating axons can grow down the connective tissue tube to reinnervate the muscle cell. If the nerve is cut, however, scar tissue between the cut ends of the endoneurial tube reduces the likelihood of reinnervation by the original axon, and muscle cell loss is likely to occur. If some intact LMN axons remain in the muscle, nearby denervated muscle cells apparently emit what is called a *trophic signal*, probably a chemical messenger, that signals intact axons to sprout and send outgrowing collaterals into the denervated area and recapture control of some of the denervated muscle fibers. The degree of axonal regeneration that occurs after injury to an LMN depends on the amount of scar tissue that develops at the site of injury and how quickly reinnervation occurs. If reinnervation occurs after the muscle cell has degenerated, no recovery is possible. Peripheral nerve section usually results in some loss of muscle cell function, which is experienced as weakness. Collateral sprout reinnervation results in enlarged motor units and therefore in a reduction in the precision of muscle control after recovery.

Muscular Dystrophy

Muscular dystrophy is a term applied to a number of genetic disorders that produce progressive deterioration of skeletal muscles because of mixed muscle cell hypertrophy, atrophy, and necrosis. They are primary diseases of muscle tissue and probably do not involve the nervous system. As the muscle undergoes necrosis, fat and connective tissue replace the muscle fibers, which increases muscle size and results in muscle weakness. The increase in muscle size resulting from connective tissue infiltration is called *pseudohypertrophy*. The muscle weakness is insidious in onset but continually progressive, varying with the type of disorder.

The most common form of the disease is *Duchenne's muscular dystrophy*, which has an incidence of approximately 3 cases per 100,000 male children. Duchenne's muscular dystrophy is inherited as a recessive single-gene defect on the X chromosome and is transmitted from the mother to her male offspring (see Chapter 7).[5] A spontaneous (mutation) form may occur in females. Another form of dystrophy, *Becker's muscular dystrophy*, is similarly X-linked but manifests later in childhood or adolescence and has a slower course. The Duchenne's muscular dystrophy mutation results in a defective form of a very large protein associated with the muscle cell membrane, called *dystrophin*, which fails to provide the normal attachment site for the contractile proteins. The regeneration of new muscle cells produces more defective cells.

In Duchenne's muscular dystrophy, the postural muscles of the hip and shoulder are affected first, and the child usually has no problems until approximately 3 years of age, when frequent falling begins to occur. Imbalances between agonist and antagonist muscles lead to abnormal postures and the development of contractures and joint immobility. Scoliosis is common. Wheelchairs usually are needed at approximately 7 to 12 years of age.[6] The function of the distal muscles usually is preserved well enough that the child can continue to use eating utensils and a computer keyboard. The function of the extraocular nerves also is well preserved, as is the function of the muscles controlling urination and defecation. Incontinence is an uncommon and late event. Respiratory muscle involvement results in weak and ineffective cough, frequent respiratory infections, and decreasing respiratory reserve. Cardiomyopathy is a common feature of the disease. The severity of cardiac involvement, however, does not necessarily correlate with skeletal muscle weakness. Some patients die early of severe cardiomyopathy, whereas others maintain adequate cardiac function until the terminal stages of the disease. Death from respiratory and cardiac muscle involvement usually occurs in young adulthood.

Observation of the child's voluntary movement and a complete family history provide important diagnostic data for the disease. Serum levels of the enzyme creatine kinase, which leaks out of damaged muscle fibers, can be used to confirm the diagnosis. Muscle biopsy, which shows a mixture of muscle cell degeneration and regeneration and reveals fat and scar tissue replacement, is diagnostic of the disorder. Echocardiography, electrocardiography, and chest radiography are used to assess cardiac function. A specific molecular genetic diagnosis is possible by demonstrating defective dystrophin through the use of immunohistochemical staining of sections of muscle biopsy tissue or by DNA analysis from the peripheral blood. The same methods of DNA analysis may be used on blood samples to establish carrier status in female relatives at risk, such as sisters and cousins. Prenatal diagnosis is possible as early as 12 weeks' gestation by sampling chorionic villi for DNA analysis (see Chapter 7).[6]

Management of the disease is directed toward maintaining ambulation and preventing deformities. Passive stretching, correct or counter posturing, and splints help to prevent deformities. Precautions should be taken to avoid respiratory infections. Although there have been exciting advances in identifying the gene and gene product involved in Duchenne's muscular dystrophy, there is no known cure.

DISORDERS OF THE NEUROMUSCULAR JUNCTION

The transmission of impulses at the neuromuscular junction is mediated by the release of the neurotransmitter acetylcholine from the axon terminals. Acetylcholine binds to specific receptors in the end-plate region of the muscle fiber surface to cause muscle contraction. Studies suggest that there are more than 1 million binding sites per motor end-plate.[7]

Acetylcholine is active in the neuromuscular junction only for a brief period, during which an action potential is generated in the innervated muscle cell. Some of the transmitter diffuses out of the synapse, and the remaining transmitter is rapidly inactivated by an enzyme called *acetylcholinesterase*. This enzyme splits the acetylcholine molecule into choline and acetic acid. The choline is then transported back into the nerve terminal and reused in the synthesis of acetylcholine. The rapid inactivation of acetylcholine allows repeated muscle contractions and gradations of contractile force.

A number of drugs and agents can alter neuromuscular function by changing the release, inactivation, or receptor binding of acetylcholine. Curare acts on the postjunctional membrane of the motor end-plate to prevent the depolarizing effect of the neurotransmitter. Blocking of neuromuscular transmission by curare-type drugs is used during many types of surgical procedures to facilitate relaxation of involved musculature. Drugs such as physostigmine and neostigmine inhibit the action of acetylcholinesterase and allow acetylcholine released from the motoneuron to accumulate. These drugs are used in the treatment of myasthenia gravis.

Toxins from the botulism organism (*Clostridium botulinum*) produce paralysis by blocking acetylcholine release. Spores from the botulism organism may be found in soil-grown foods that are not cooked at temperatures of at least 100°C in home canning procedures. A pharmacologic preparation of the botulism toxin (botulism toxin type A [Botox]) has become available for use in treating eyelid and eye movement disorders such as blepharospasm and strabismus. It also is used for treatment of spasmodic torticollis, spasmodic dysphonias (laryngeal dystonia), and other dystonias. The drug is injected into the target muscle using the electrical activity recorded from the tip of a special electromyographic injection needle to guide the injection. The treatment is not permanent and usually needs to be repeated approximately every 3 months.

The organophosphates (*e.g.*, malathion, parathion) that are used in some insecticides bind acetylcholinesterase to prevent the breakdown of acetylcholine. They produce excessive and prolonged acetylcholine action with a depolarization block of cholinergic receptors, including those of the neuromuscular junction.[8] The organophosphates are well absorbed from the skin, lungs, gut, and conjunctiva of the eye, making them particularly effective as insecticides but also potentially dangerous to humans. Malathion and certain other organophosphates are rapidly metabolized to inactive products in humans and are considered safe for sale to the general public. The sale of other insecticides, such as parathion, which is not effectively metabolized to inactive products, has been banned. Other organophosphate compounds (*e.g.*, soman) were developed as "nerve gases"; if absorbed in high enough concentrations, they have lethal effects from depolarization block and loss of respiratory muscle function.

Myasthenia Gravis

Myasthenia gravis is a disorder of transmission at the neuromuscular junction that affects communication between the motoneuron and the innervated muscle cell. Now recognized as an autoimmune disease, the disorder is caused by antibody-mediated loss of acetylcholine receptors in the neuromuscular junction.[5] The incidence of myasthenia gravis in the United States is 50 to 125 cases per million persons.[9] The disease may occur at any age, but the peak incidence occurs between 20 and 30 years of age, and the disease is approximately three times more common in women than men. A smaller second peak occurs in later life and affects men more often than women. The disorder appears transiently and lasts for days to weeks in approximately 10% of infants born to mothers with myasthenia gravis.

The exact mechanism that triggers the autoimmune response is unknown but is thought to be related to abnormal T-lymphocyte characteristics. Approximately 75% of persons with myasthenia gravis also have thymic abnormalities, such as a thymoma (*i.e.*, thymus tumor) or thymic hyperplasia (*i.e.*, increased thymus weight from an increased number of thymus cells).[9]

In persons with myasthenia gravis who have fewer acetylcholine receptors in the postsynaptic membrane, each release of acetylcholine from the presynaptic membrane results in a lower-amplitude end-plate potential. This results in both muscle weakness and fatigability with sustained effort. Most commonly affected are the eye and preorbital muscles. Either ptosis due to eyelid weakness or diplopia due to weakness of the extraocular muscles is an initial symptom in approximately 50% of persons with the disease.[10] The disease may progress from ocular muscle weakness to generalized weakness, including respiratory muscle weakness. Chewing and swallowing may be difficult, and persons with the disease often choose to eat soft puddings and cereals rather than meats and hard fruit. Weakness in limb movement usually is more pronounced in proximal than in distal parts of the extremity, so that climbing stairs and lifting objects are difficult. As the disease progresses, the muscles of the lower face are affected, causing speech impairment. When this happens, the person often supports the chin with one hand to assist in speaking. In most persons, symptoms are least evident when arising in the morning, but they grow worse with effort and as the day proceeds. Persons with purely ocular manifestations during the initial month of diagnosis usually develop generalized disease within the first 3 years of onset.[10]

Diagnosis. The diagnosis of myasthenia gravis is based on history and physical examination, the anticholinesterase test, nerve stimulation studies, and an assay for acetylcholine receptor antibodies. The anticholinesterase test uses a drug that inhibits acetylcholinesterase, the enzyme that breaks down acetylcholine. Edrophonium (Tensilon), a short-acting acetylcholinesterase inhibitor, commonly is used for the test. The drug, which is administered intravenously, decreases the breakdown of acetylcholine in the neuromuscular junction. When weakness is caused by myasthenia gravis, a dramatic transitory improvement in muscle function occurs. Electrophysiologic studies can be done to demonstrate a decremental muscle response to repetitive 2- or 3-Hz stimulation of motor nerves. An advance in diagnostic methods for myasthenia gravis is single-fiber electromyography, which is available in many medical centers. Single-fiber electromyography detects delayed or failed neuromuscular transmission in muscle fibers supplied by a single nerve fiber.[10] An immunoassay test can be used to detect the presence of acetylcholine receptor antibodies circulating in the blood.

Treatment.   Treatment methods include the use of pharmacologic agents; immunosuppressive therapy, including corticosteroid drugs; management of myasthenic crisis; thymectomy; and plasmapheresis or intravenous immunoglobulin.[9,10] Medications that may exacerbate myasthenia gravis, such as the aminoglycoside antibiotics, should be avoided.[11] Pharmacologic treatment with reversible anticholinesterase drugs inhibits the breakdown of acetylcholine at the neuromuscular junction by acetylcholinesterase. Pyridostigmine and neostigmine are the drugs of choice. Corticosteroid drugs, which suppress the immune response, are used in cases of a poor response to anticholinesterase drugs and thymectomy. Immunosuppressant drugs (*e.g.*, azathioprine, cyosporine) also may be used, often in combination with plasmapheresis.

Plasmapheresis removes antibodies from the circulation and provides short-term clinical improvement. It is used primarily to stabilize the condition of persons in myasthenic crisis or for short-term treatment in persons undergoing thymectomy. Intravenous immunoglobulin also produces improvement in persons with myasthenia gravis. Although the effect is temporary, it may last for weeks to months. The indications for its use are similar to those for plasmapheresis. The mechanism of action of intravenous immunoglobulin is unknown. Intravenous immunoglobulin therapy is very expensive, which limits its use.

Thymectomy, or surgical removal of the thymus, may be used as a treatment for myasthenia gravis. Because the mechanism whereby surgery exerts its effect is unknown, the treatment is controversial. Thymectomy is performed in persons with thymoma, regardless of age, and in persons 50 to 60 years of age or older with recent onset of moderate disease.

Myasthenia Crisis.   Persons with myasthenia gravis may experience a sudden exacerbation of symptoms and weakness known as *myasthenia crisis*.[12] Myasthenia crisis occurs when muscle weakness becomes severe enough to compromise ventilation to the extent that ventilatory support and airway protection are needed. This usually occurs during a period of stress, such as infection, emotional upset, pregnancy, alcohol ingestion, cold, or after surgery. Medications that exacerbate muscle weakness and trigger myasthenia crisis include quinidine, the aminoglycoside antibiotics, β-adrenergic receptor blockers, calcium channel blockers, and magnesium sulfate or citrate. It also can result from inadequate or excessive doses of the anticholinesterase drugs used in treatment of the disorder. However, myasthenic crisis resulting from the need for more medication is virtually indistinguishable from cholinergic crisis resulting from too much medication. In the case of too much medication, cholinergic crisis often is accompanied by nausea, vomiting, pallor, sweating, salivation, colic, diarrhea, miosis, or bradycardia from the muscarinic effects of the anticholinesterase drugs.

Whatever the cause, prompt medical treatment is needed. Options for treatment during crisis include plasmapheresis, intravenous immunoglobulins, immunosuppressant drugs, and corticosteroids. In addition to supportive care, treatment requires removal of underlying triggers such as infection or pharmacologic agents. To determine whether the crisis was precipitated by the disease process or by cholinergic drugs, the Tensilon test is used. If the crisis is myasthenic, the symptoms improve. Provision for respiratory support should be available in either case.

PERIPHERAL NERVE DISORDERS

The peripheral nervous system consists of the motor and sensory branches of the cranial and spinal nerves, the peripheral parts of the autonomic nervous system, and peripheral ganglia. A peripheral neuropathy is any primary disorder of the peripheral nerves. The result usually is muscle weakness, with or without atrophy and sensory changes. The disorder can involve a single nerve (mononeuropathy) or multiple nerves (polyneuropathy).

Unlike the nerves of the CNS, peripheral nerves are fairly strong and resilient. They contain a series of connective tissue sheaths that enclose their nerve fibers. An outer fibrous sheath called the *epineurium* surrounds the medium-sized to large nerves; inside, a sheath called the *perineurium* invests each bundle of nerve fibers, and within each bundle, a delicate sheath of connective tissue known as the *endoneurium* surrounds each nerve fiber (see Chapter 47, Fig. 47-5). Small peripheral nerves lack the epineurial covering. In its endoneurial sheath, each nerve fiber is invested by a segmented sheath of Schwann cells. The Schwann cells produce the myelin sheath that surrounds the peripheral nerves. Each Schwann cell, however, can myelinate only one segment of a single axon—the one that it covers—so that myelination of an entire axon requires the participation of a long line of these cells.

Peripheral Nerve Injury and Repair

Neurons exemplify the general principle that the more specialized the function of a cell type, the less able it is to regenerate. In neurons, cell division ceases by the time of birth, and from then on, the cell body of a neuron is unable to divide and replace itself. Although the entire neuron cannot be replaced, it often is possible for the dendritic and axonal cell processes to regenerate as long as the cell body remains viable.

When a peripheral nerve is destroyed by a crushing force or by a cut that penetrates the nerve, the portion of the nerve fiber that is separated from the cell body rapidly undergoes degenerative changes, whereas the central stump and cell body of the nerve often are able to survive (Fig. 49-6). Because the cell body synthesizes the material required for nourishing and maintaining the axon, it is likely that the loss of these materials results in the degeneration of the separated portion of the nerve fibers.

After injury, the Schwann cells that are distal to the site of damage also are able to survive, but their myelin degenerates in a process called *wallerian degeneration*. The Schwann cells assist other phagocytic cells in the area in the cleanup

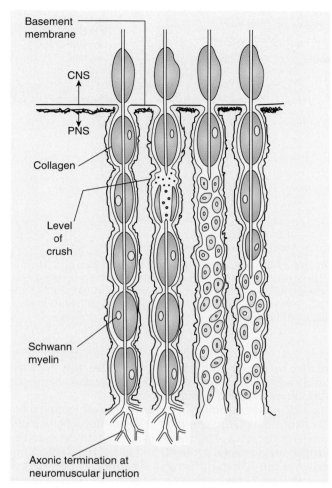

FIGURE 49-6 Sequential stages in efferent axon degeneration and regeneration within its endoneurial tube, following peripheral nerve crush injury.

Basement membrane

CNS

PNS

Collagen

Level of crush

Schwann myelin

Axonic termination at neuromuscular junction

of the debris caused by the degenerating axon and myelin. As they remove the debris, the Schwann cells multiply and fill the empty endoneurial tube. At this point, nothing further happens, unless a regenerating nerve fiber penetrates into the endoneurial tube, in which case the Schwann cells reform the myelin segments around the fiber.

Meanwhile, the cell body of the neuron responds to the loss of part of its nerve fiber by shifting into a phase of greatly increased protein and lipid synthesis. It does this by dispersing the masses of ribosomes, which stain as Nissl granules. They cease to be stainable and disappear in a process called *chromatolysis*. In the process, the nucleus moves away from the axonal side of the cell body, as though displaced by the active synthetic apparatus of the cells. These changes reach their height within approximately 10 days of injury and continue until regrowth of the nerve fiber ceases.

In the process of regeneration, the injured nerve fiber develops one or more new branches from the proximal nerve stump that grow into the developing scar tissue. If a crushing injury has occurred and the endoneurial tube is

intact through the trauma area, the outgrowing fiber will grow back down this tube to the structure that was originally innervated by the neuron. If, however, the injury involves the severing of a nerve, the outgrowing branch must come in contact with its original endoneurial tube if it is to be reunited with its original target structure. The rate of outgrowth of regenerating nerve fibers is approximately 1 to 2 mm/day; the recovery of conduction to a target structure depends on regrowth into the appropriate endoneurial tube and on the distance involved. It can take weeks or months for the regrowing fiber to reach the end-organ and communicative function to be reestablished. More time is required for the Schwann cells to form new myelin segments and for the axon to recover its original diameter and conduction velocity.

The successful regeneration of a nerve fiber in the peripheral nervous system depends on many factors. If a nerve fiber is destroyed relatively close to the neuronal cell body, the chances are that the nerve cell will die, and if it does, it will not be replaced. If a crushing type of injury has occurred, partial or often full recovery of function occurs. Cutting-type trauma to a nerve is an entirely different matter. Connective scar tissue forms rapidly at the wound site, and when it does, only the most rapidly regenerating axonal branches are able to get through to the intact distal endoneurial tubes. A number of scar-inhibiting agents have been used in an effort to reduce this hazard, but have met with only moderate success. In another attempt to improve nerve regeneration, various types of tubular implants have been placed to fill longer gaps in the endoneurial tube.

Perhaps the most difficult problem is the alignment of the proximal and distal endoneurial tubes so that a regenerating fiber can return down its former tube and innervate its former organ. This problem is similar to realigning a large telephone cable that has been cut so that all the wires are reconnected exactly as before the separation. Microscopic alignment of the cut edges during microsurgical repair results in improved success. If an efferent nerve fiber that formerly innervated a skeletal muscle regrows down an endoneurial tube formerly occupied by an afferent fiber and reaches the former sensory area, then its cell body eventually dies. A sensory fiber that grows down an endoneurial tube that connects with a skeletal muscle fiber undergoes the same fate. If, however, these fibers grow down endoneurial tubes that innervate the appropriate type of target organ, reinnervation and function may return, even though the fibers have changed places. Under the best of conditions, a 50% regeneration to the appropriate organ is considered a success after a peripheral nerve has been severed. Even so, considerable function can return with that amount of innervation.

Peripheral Nerve Root Injury

Herniated Intervertebral Disk.   Although back problems commonly are attributed to a herniated disk, most acute back problems are caused by other, less serious conditions. It has been reported that 90% of persons with acute lower back problems of less than 3 months' duration recover spontaneously.[13,14] Thus, the current trend in treatment of acute back problems is to focus on improvement in activity tolerance rather than exclusively on the pain associated with the problem.[14] Persons with signs of a herniated disk are evaluated for the problem.

The intervertebral disk is considered the most critical component of the load-bearing structures of the spinal column (Fig. 49-7). The intervertebral disk consists of a soft, gelatinous center called the *nucleus pulposus*, which is encircled by a strong, ringlike collar of fibrocartilage called the *annulus fibrosus*. The structural components of the disk make it capable of absorbing shock and changing shape while allowing movement. With dysfunction, the nucleus pulposus can be squeezed out of place and herniate through the annulus fibrosus, a condition referred to as a *herniated* or *slipped disk* (Fig. 49-8).

The cervical and lumbar regions are the most flexible area of the spine and most easily injured. Usually, herniation occurs at the lower levels of the lumbar spine, where the mass being supported and the bending of the vertebral column are greatest. Approximately 90% to 95% of lumbar herniations occur in the L4 or L5 to S1 regions. With her-

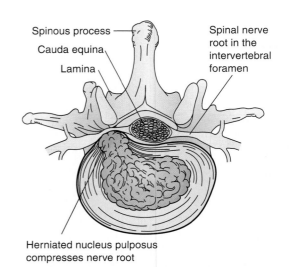

FIGURE 49-8 A prolapsed (herniated) intervertebral disk. The soft central portion of the disk is protruding into the vertebral canal, where it exerts pressure on a spinal nerve root. (Chaffee E.E., Lytle I.M. [1980]. *Basic physiology and anatomy*. [4th ed.]. Philadelphia: J.B. Lippincott)

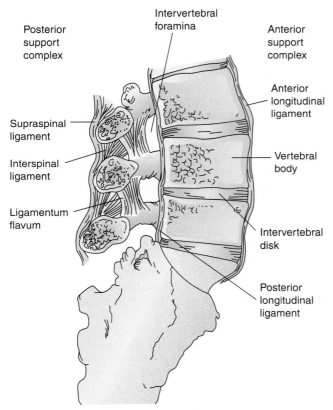

FIGURE 49-7 Soft tissue supporting structures of the spine. Two basic soft tissue units constitute each spinal segment: the anterior support complex, formed by the anterior and posterior longitudinal ligaments, the disk, and the annulus; and the posterior support complex, formed by the supraspinal ligament and interspinal ligament, the ligamentum flavum, and the facet capsules. The intravertebral foramen forms the passageway through which a spinal nerve root travels as it passes from the spinal canal to the periphery.

niations of the cervical spine, the most frequently involved levels are C6 to C7 and C5 to C6.[13] Men have herniated disks more frequently than women.

The intervertebral disk can become dysfunctional because of trauma, the effects of aging, or degenerative disorders of the spine. This results in movement between the articulating vertebral segments and loss of the elastic properties of the disk itself. Trauma accounts for 50% of disk herniations. Trauma results from activities such as lifting while in the flexed position, slipping, falling on the buttocks or back, or suppressing a sneeze. With aging, the gelatinous center of the disk dries out and loses much of its elasticity, causing it to fray and tear. Degenerative processes such as osteoarthritis or ankylosing spondylitis predispose to malalignment of the vertebral column. The anterior longitudinal ligament, which extends along the anterior (ventral) surface of the spinal column, is so strong that nucleus pulposus protrusion anteriorly is rare (see Fig. 49-7). The corresponding posterior longitudinal ligament is less strong and weakest laterally. The most common herniation is directed posteriorly and obliquely toward the intervertebral foramen and its contained spinal nerve root and dorsal root ganglion (see Fig. 49-8). The consequent compression and irritation causes spontaneous firing of sensory afferents and severe pain locally because of injured tissue and pain referred to the area of dermatomal distribution of the spinal nerve root.

The level at which a herniated disk occurs is important. When the injury occurs in the lumbar area, only the cauda equina is irritated or crushed. Because these elongated dorsal and ventral roots contain endoneurial tubes of connective tissue, regeneration of the nerve fibers is likely. However, several weeks or months are required for full recovery to occur because of the distance to the innervated muscle or skin of the lower limbs.

The posterior longitudinal ligament is strongest along the midline so that nucleus pulposus displacement into the spinal canal, possibly compressing or damaging the spinal cord itself, is uncommon. When it does occur, the axons of the ventral white column, including those of the spinothalamic system, are irritated, causing referred pain that can be experienced for many lower segments on the opposite side of the body. Sometimes the entire spinal segment can be damaged, resulting in functional transection of the spinal cord at that skeletal level.

The signs and symptoms of a herniated disk are localized to the area of the body innervated by the nerve roots. Pain is the first and most common symptom of a herniated disk. The nerve roots of L4, L5, S1, S2, and S3 give rise to a syndrome of back pain that spreads down the back of the leg and over the sole of the foot. The pain is intensified by coughing, sneezing, straining, stooping, standing, and the jarring motions that occur during walking or riding. Motor and sensory symptoms also may occur because of nerve root compression. Slight motor weakness may occur, although major weakness is rare. The most common sensory deficits from spinal nerve root compression are paresthesias and numbness, particularly of the leg and foot. Knee and ankle reflexes also may be diminished or absent.

A herniated disk must be differentiated from other causes such as traumatic injury or fracture of the vertebral column, tumor, infection, cauda equina syndrome, or other conditions that cause back pain.[14] Diagnostic measures include history and physical examination. Neurologic assessment includes testing of muscle strength and reflexes. The straight leg test is done in the supine position and is performed by passively raising the person's leg. Normally, it is possible to raise the leg approximately 90 degrees without causing discomfort of the hamstring muscles. The test result is positive if pain is produced when the leg is raised to 60 degrees or less. Other diagnostic methods include radiographs of the back, magnetic resonance imaging (MRI), computed tomography (CT), myelography, and CT-myelography. Myelography, MRI, and CT usually are reserved for persons suspected of having more complex causes of back pain.

Treatment usually is conservative and consists of analgesic medications and education on how to protect the back. Pain relief usually can be provided using nonsteroidal anti-inflammatory drugs, although short-term use of opioid pain medications may be required for severe pain. Muscle relaxants such as diazepam, cyclobenzaprine, carisoprodol, or methocarbamol may be used on a short-term basis. Bed rest, once the mainstay of conservative therapy, is now understood to be ineffective for acute pain. Instruction in the correct mechanics for lifting and methods of protecting the back is important. Conditioning exercises of the trunk muscles, particularly the back extensors, may be recommended for persons with acute low back problems, particularly if the problem persists. Surgical treatment may be indicated when there is documentation of herniation by some imaging procedure, consistent pain, or consistent neurologic deficit that has failed to respond to conservative therapy.

Mononeuropathies

Mononeuropathies usually are caused by localized conditions such as trauma, compression, or infections that affect a single spinal nerve, plexus, or peripheral nerve trunk. Fractured bones may lacerate or compress nerves; excessively tight tourniquets may injure nerves directly or produce ischemic injury; and infections such as herpes zoster may affect a single segmental afferent nerve distribution. Recovery of nerve function usually is complete after compression lesions and incomplete or faulty after nerve transection.

Carpal Tunnel Syndrome.   Carpal tunnel syndrome is an example of a compression-type mononeuropathy that is relatively common. It is caused by compression of the median nerve as it travels with the flexor tendons through a canal made by the carpal bones and transverse carpal ligament (Fig. 49-9). The condition can be caused by a variety of conditions that produce a reduction in the capacity of the carpal tunnel (*i.e.*, bony or ligament changes) or an increase in the volume of the tunnel contents (*i.e.*, inflammation of the tendons, synovial swelling, or tumors).[13] Carpal

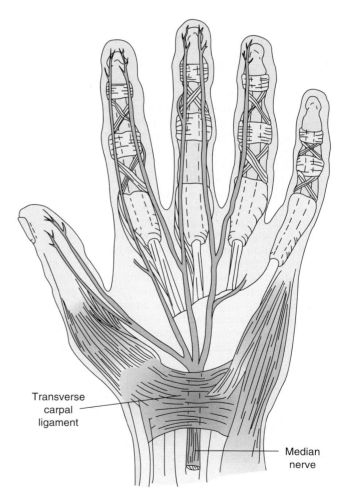

FIGURE 49-9 Carpal tunnel syndrome: compression of the median nerve by the transverse carpal ligament. (Courtesy Carole Russell Hilmer, C.M.I.)

Transverse carpal ligament

Median nerve

tunnel syndrome can be a feature of many systemic diseases such as rheumatoid arthritis, hyperthyroidism, acromegaly, and diabetes mellitus.[15,16] The condition can result from wrist injury; it can occur during pregnancy and use of birth control drugs; and it is seen in persons with repetitive use of the wrist (*i.e.*, flexion-extension movements and stress associated with pinching and gripping motions).

Carpal tunnel syndrome is characterized by pain, paresthesia, and numbness of the thumb and first two and one-half digits of the hand; pain in the wrist and hand, which worsens at night; atrophy of abductor pollicis muscle; and weakness in precision grip. All of these abnormalities may contribute to clumsiness of fine motor activity.

Diagnosis usually is based on sensory disturbances confined to median nerve distribution, a positive Tinel's sign, and a positive Phalen's sign. *Tinel's sign* describes the development of a tingling sensation radiating into the palm of the hand that is elicited by light percussion over the median nerve at the wrist. The *Phalen test* is performed by having the person hold the wrist in complete flexion for approximately a minute; if numbness and paresthesia along the median nerve are reproduced or exaggerated, the test result is considered to be positive. Electromyography and nerve conduction studies often are done to confirm the diagnosis and exclude other causes of the disorder.

Treatment includes avoidance of use, splinting, and anti-inflammatory medications. Measures to decrease the causative repetitive movements should be initiated. Splints may be confined to nighttime use. When splinting is ineffective, corticosteroids may be injected into the carpal tunnel to reduce inflammation and swelling. Surgical intervention consists of operative division of the volar carpal ligaments as a means of relieving pressure on the medial nerve.

Polyneuropathies

Polyneuropathies involve demyelination or axonal degeneration of multiple peripheral nerves that leads to symmetric sensory, motor, or mixed sensorimotor deficits. Typically, the longest axons are involved first, with symptoms beginning in the distal part of the extremities. If the autonomic nervous system is involved, there may be postural hypotension, constipation, and impotence. Polyneuropathies can result from immune mechanisms (*e.g.*, Guillain-Barré syndrome), toxic agents (*e.g.*, arsenic polyneuropathy, lead polyneuropathy, alcoholic polyneuropathy), and metabolic diseases (*e.g.*, diabetes mellitus, uremia). Different causes tend to affect axons of different diameters and to affect sensory, motor, or autonomic neurons to different degrees.

Guillain-Barré Syndrome. Guillain-Barré syndrome is a subacute polyneuropathy. The manifestations of the disease involve an infiltration of mononuclear cells around the capillaries of the peripheral neurons, edema of the endoneurial compartment, and demyelination of ventral spinal roots. The annual incidence of Guillain-Barré syndrome is approximately 1 case per 50,000 persons, and it is more common with increasing age.[17] Approximately 80% to 90% of persons with the disease achieve a spontaneous recovery.

The cause of Guillain-Barré syndrome is unknown. Approximately two thirds of cases follow an infection that is seemingly mundane and often of viral origin.[5] There is an association with preceding gastrointestinal tract infection with *Campylobacter jejuni*.[18] A widely studied outbreak of the disorder followed the swine flu vaccination program of 1976 and 1977.[19] It has been suggested that an altered immune response to peripheral nerve antigens contributes to the development of the disorder.

The disorder is characterized by progressive ascending muscle weakness of the limbs, producing a symmetric flaccid paralysis. Symptoms of paresthesia and numbness often accompany the loss of motor function. The rate of disease progression varies, and there may be disproportionate involvement of the upper or lower extremities. Paralysis may progress to involve the respiratory muscles; approximately 20% of persons with the disorder require ventilatory assistance.[17] Autonomic nervous system involvement that causes postural hypotension, arrhythmias, facial flushing, abnormalities of sweating, and urinary retention is common.

Guillain-Barré syndrome usually is a medical emergency. There may be a rapid development of ventilatory failure and autonomic disturbances that threaten circulatory function. Treatment includes support of vital functions and prevention of complications such as skin breakdown and thrombophlebitis. Clinical trials have shown the effectiveness of plasmapheresis in decreasing morbidity and shortening the course of the disease. Treatment is most effective if initiated early in the course of the disease. High-dose intravenous immunoglobulin therapy also has proved effective.[20]

> In summary, the motor unit consists of the LMN, the neuromuscular junction, and the skeletal muscle that the nerve innervates. Disorders of the neuromuscular unit include muscular dystrophy, myasthenia gravis, and peripheral nerve disorders. *Muscular dystrophy* is a term used to describe a number of disorders that produce progressive deterioration of skeletal muscle. Muscle necrosis is followed by fat and connective tissue replacement. One form, Duchenne's muscular dystrophy, is inherited as a X-linked trait and transmitted by the mother to her male offspring. Myasthenia gravis is a disorder of the neuromuscular junction resulting from a deficiency of functional acetylcholine receptors, which causes weakness of the skeletal muscles. Because the disease affects the neuromuscular junction, there is no loss of sensory function. The most common manifestations are weakness of the eye muscles, with ptosis and diplopia. Weakness of the jaw muscles can make chewing and swallowing difficult. Usually, the proximal muscles and extremities are involved, making it difficult to climb stairs and lift objects. Myasthenia crisis, which involves a sudden and transient weakness, may occur and necessitate mechanical ventilatory assistance.
>
> Disorders of peripheral nerves include mononeuropathies and polyneuropathies. Mononeuropathies involve a single spinal nerve, plexus, or peripheral nerve trunk. Carpal tunnel syndrome, a mononeuropathy, is caused by compression of the medial nerve that passes through the carpal tunnel in the wrist. Poly-

neuropathies involve multiple peripheral nerves and produce symmetric sensory, motor, and mixed sensorimotor deficits. A number of conditions, including immune mechanisms, toxic agents, and metabolic disorders, are implicated as causative agents in polyneuropathies. Guillain-Barré syndrome is a subacute polyneuropathy of uncertain origin. It causes progressive ascending motor, sensory, and autonomic nervous system manifestations. Respiratory involvement may occur and necessitate mechanical ventilation.

Disorders of the Basal Ganglia and Cerebellum

After you have completed this section of the chapter, you should be able to meet the following objectives:

✦ Describe the functional organization of the basal ganglia and communication pathways with the thalamus and cerebral cortex
✦ State the possible mechanisms responsible for the development of Parkinson's disease and characterize the manifestations and treatment of the disorder
✦ Relate the functions of the cerebellum to production of vestibulocerebellar ataxia, decomposition of movement, and cerebellar tremor

DISORDERS OF THE BASAL GANGLIA

The basal ganglia are a group of deep, interrelated subcortical nuclei that play an essential role in control of movement. The basal ganglia receive indirect input from the cerebellum and from all sensory systems, including vision, and direct input from the motor cortex. They function in the organization of inherited and highly learned and rather automatic movement programs, especially those affecting the trunk and proximal limbs. The movements are released when commanded by the motor cortex, contributing gracefulness to cortically initiated and controlled skilled movements. The function of the basal ganglia is not limited to motor functions. They also are involved in cognitive and perception functions.

Disorders of the basal ganglia comprise a complex group of motor disturbances characterized by involuntary movements, alterations in muscle tone, and disturbances in body posture. Unlike disorders of the motor cortex and corticospinal (pyramidal) tract, lesions of the basal ganglia disrupt movement but do not cause paralysis. Because of these and other differences, the basal ganglia and associated structures are often referred to as the *extrapyramidal system*.

Functional Organization of the Basal Ganglia

The structural components of the basal ganglia include the caudate nucleus, putamen, and the globus pallidus in the forebrain. The caudate and putamen are collectively referred to as the *neostriatum*, and the putamen and the globus pallidus form a wedge-shaped region called the *lentiform nucleus*. Two other structures, the *subthalamic nucleus* of the

diencephalon and the *substantia nigra* of the midbrain, are considered part of the basal ganglia (Fig. 49-10). The dorsal part of the substantia nigra contains cells that use dopamine as a neurotransmitter and are rich in a black pigment called *melanin*. The high concentration of melanin gives the structure a black color, hence the name *substantia nigra*. The axons of the substantia nigra form the *nigrostriatal pathway*, which supplies dopamine to the striatum. The dopamine released from the substantia nigra regulates the overall excitability of the striatum and release of other neurotransmitters.

The basal ganglia have input structures that receive afferent information from outside structures, internal circuits that connect the various structures of the basal ganglia, and output structures that deliver information to other brain centers. The neostriatum represents the major input structure for the basal ganglia. Virtually all areas of the cortex and afferents from the thalamus project to the neostriatum. The output areas of the basal ganglia, including the lateral globus pallidus, have ascending and descending components. The major ascending input is transmitted to thalamic nuclei, which process all incoming information that are transmitted to the cerebral cortex. Descending output is directed to the midbrain, brain stem, and spinal cord. The output functions of the basal ganglia are mainly inhibitory. Looping circuits from specific cortical areas pass through the basal ganglia to modulate the excitability of specific thalamic nuclei and control the cortical activity involved in highly learned, automatic, and stereotyped motor functions.

Each region of the cerebral cortex is interconnected with a corresponding region of the ventral row of thalamic nuclei. For the motor and premotor cortex, these nuclei are the ventral lateral (VL) and the ventral anterior (VA) nuclei. The cortex-to-thalamus (corticothalamic) and thalamus-to-cortex (thalamocortical) feedback circuitries are excitatory and, if unmodulated, would produce hyperactivity of the cortical area, causing stiffness and rigidity of the face, body, and limbs, and, if alternating, a continuous tremor (*i.e.,* tremor at rest). The excitability of the thalamic nuclei in this

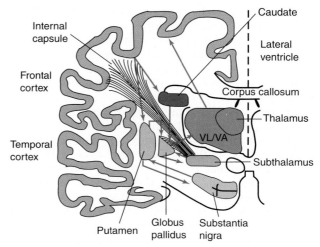

FIGURE 49-10 Basal ganglia.

reciprocal circuit is regulated by other thalamic afferents, many of which depress thalamic excitability.

For many semiautomatic stereotyped movements, thalamic excitability is modulated through inhibition by the basal ganglia. The basal ganglia form a major component of an inhibitory loop from each specific cortical region. Discrete inhibitory cortex-to-basal ganglia and thalamus-to-cortex loops modulate the function of all cerebral cortex regions. These modulatory loops exist for the prefrontal, limbic, premotor, motor, sensory, and parietal higher-order areas of the cerebral cortex. Abnormalities of the modulatory loop that influence motor function have such dramatic results that the role of the basal ganglia often has been relegated to that of the modulation of movement patterns.

The most is known about the inhibitory basal ganglia loop involved in modulating cortical motor control. This loop regulates release of stereotyped movement patterns that add efficiency and gracefulness to precise and delicate cortically controlled movements. These movements include inherited patterns that add efficiency, balance, and gracefulness to motion, such as the swinging of the arms during walking and running, and the highly learned automatic postural and follow-through movements of throwing a ball or swinging a bat. The basic repertoire of many of these complex movement patterns is built into brain stem circuitry under gene control. Individual differences limit the extent to which learning and practice can enhance their perfection. Thus, not everyone can become an accomplished ballerina or gymnast.

There are four functional pathways involving the basal ganglia: (1) a dopamine pathway from the substantia nigra to the striatum; (2) a γ-aminobutyric acid (GABA) pathway from the striatum to the globus pallidus and substantia nigra; (3) acetylcholine-secreting neurons, which are important in networks within the neostriatum; and (4) multiple general pathways from the brain stem that secrete norepinephrine, serotonin, enkephalin, and several other neurotransmitters in the basal ganglia and the cerebral cortex. These pathways provide a balance of inhibitory and excitatory activity. GABA functions as an inhibitory neurotransmitter, and GABAergic neurons participate in the negative feedback loop from the cortex through the basal ganglia and back to the cortex. Dopamine also functions as an inhibitory neurotransmitter. There are multiple glutamine pathways that provide excitatory signals that balance the large number of inhibitory signals transmitted by GABAergic and dopaminergic neurons.

In the cortex-to-basal ganglia and thalamus-to-cortex loop are two pathways that normally balance each other.[21] One permits cortical disinhibition of the thalamus, and the other permits increased inhibition of the thalamus. *Cortical disinhibition* or release of a stereotyped movement pattern requires withdrawal of the inhibitory influence of the globus pallidus on the thalamus. The circuit involves cortical facilitation (glutaminergic action) of the neostriatum, which is inhibitory (GABAergic) to the internal segment of the globus pallidus, which is inhibitory (GABAergic) to the thalamus. Activation of a motor cortex movement pattern involves disinhibition of the thalamus, thereby potentiating cortical activity. The second *thalamic inhibition* circuit involves globus pallidus inhibition (GABAergic) and cortical facilitation of the subthalamic nucleus, which is excitatory (glutaminergic) to the internal segment of the globus pallidus. Increased activity in this circuit increases the inhibitory function of the globus pallidus. Pathologic movement regulation results from damaged function of one or both of these circuits. For example, destruction of the subthalamic nucleus by a stroke results in loss of thalamic inhibition, with a consequent release of violent, flailing (ballistic) limb movements on the contralateral side of the body.

An additional modulating circuit involves a *neostriatal inhibitory projection* (GABAergic) on the substantia nigra. The substantia nigra projects dopaminergic axons back on the neostriatum. A deficiency in the dopaminergic projection of this modulating circuit is implicated in Parkinson's syndrome. The function of the neostriatum also involves local cholinergic interneurons, and their destruction is thought to be related to the choreiform movements of Huntington's chorea, another basal ganglia-related syndrome (see Chapter 50). Precisely how these transmitter-related abnormalities affect the functional microcircuitry of the basal ganglia circuit remains to be elucidated. However, some progress has been made in supplying decreased or missing transmitters, reducing at least temporarily the severity of several extrapyramidal diseases.

Movement Disorders

Reduced function of the basal ganglia loop results in *hyperkinesis*, or release of movement patterns at inappropriate times or sometimes continuously. Pathologically released patterns that often are disabling include rigidity and movement disorders. These movement patterns are not under cortical control and often are referred to as *involuntary movements*. Destruction of the corticospinal system does not eliminate the extrapyramidal movements. These movements are lost during sleep, although they may make getting to sleep difficult.

Descending pathways to the LMNs involved in basal ganglia-related movements involve the corticospinal systems and other descending systems. Although these signs are always on the side of the body opposite to basal ganglia damage, in metabolic or toxic abnormalities the signs usually are bilateral.

Rigidity and Bradykinesia.   Basal ganglia-derived rigidity involves a strong resistance to movement that decreases to stiffness after the movement gets underway. In some instances, forcing a rigid joint to turn is met with a series of sudden releases followed by renewed resistance, a phenomenon called *cog-wheel rigidity*.

Hyperfunction of the basal ganglia inhibitory loop results in excessive inhibition of cortical function, producing *bradykinesia* or *hypokinesis*. The results are slowness in beginning movement, a reduced range and force of the movement ("poverty of movement"), reduced or absent emotional responses, including emotion-related facial expressions, and a loss of the balance and grace-producing movements and postures associated with skilled motion. An example of hypokinesis is seen in severely affected persons with the parkinsonian syndrome.

Involuntary Movements.   Involuntary movements include tremor, tics, choreiform movements, athetoid movements, and ballismus. These disorders are summarized in Table 49-1. *Tremor* is caused by involuntary, oscillating contractions of opposing muscle groups around a joint. It usually is fairly uniform in frequency and amplitude. Certain tremors are considered physiologic in that they are transitory and normally occur under conditions of increased muscle tone, as in highly emotional situations, or they may be related to muscle fatigue or reduced body temperature (*i.e.*, shivering). Toxic tremors are produced by hyperexcitability related to conditions such as thyrotoxicosis. The tremor of Parkinson's disease is caused by degenerative changes in the basal ganglia. *Tics* involve sudden and irregularly occurring contractions of whole muscles or major portions of a muscle. These are particularly evident in the muscles of the face, but can occur elsewhere.

Choreiform movements are sudden, jerky, and irregular but are coordinated and graceful. They can involve the distal limb, face, tongue, or swallowing muscles. Choreiform movements are accentuated by movement and by environmental stimulation; they often interfere with normal movement patterns. The word *chorea* originated from the Greek word meaning "to dance." There may be grimacing movements of the face, raising of the eyebrows, rolling of the eyes, and curling, protrusion and withdrawal of the tongue. In the limbs, the movements largely are distal; there may be piano-playing–type movements with alternating extension and flexion of the fingers. The shoulders may be elevated and depressed or rotated. Movements of the face or limbs may occur alone or, more commonly, in combination.

Athetoid movements are relatively continuous, worm-like twisting and turning motions of the joints of a limb or body. These result from continuous and prolonged contraction of agonist and antagonistic muscle groups. These are normal, smooth, and useful movements, except in extrapyramidal diseases, when they occur continuously in a nonrhythmic, often irregular sequence.

The term *ballismus* originated from a Greek word meaning "to jump around." Ballistic movements are violent, sweeping, flinging motions, especially of the limbs on one side of the body (hemiballismus). They may occur as the result of a small vascular accident involving the subthalamic nucleus on the opposite side of the brain.

Dystonia refers to the abnormal maintenance of a posture resulting from a twisting, turning movement of the limbs, neck, or trunk. These postures often result from simultaneous contraction of agonist and antagonist muscles. Long-sustained simultaneous hypertonia across a joint can result in degenerative changes and permanent fixation in unusual postures. These effects can occur as a side effect of some antipsychotic medications. *Spasmodic torticollis*, the most common type of dystonia, affects the muscles of the neck and shoulder. The condition, which is caused by bilateral and simultaneous contraction of the neck and shoulder muscles, results in unilateral head turning or head extension, sometimes limiting rotation. Elevations of the shoulder commonly accompany the spasmodic movements of the head and neck. Immobility of the cervical vertebrae eventually can lead to degenerative fixation in the twisted posture. Torsional spasm involving the trunk also can occur.

Dyskinesias are rhythmic, repetitive, bizarre movements. They frequently involve the face, mouth, jaw, and tongue, causing grimacing, pursing of the lips, or protrusion

---

TABLE 49-1 ✦ Involuntary Movements Disorders Associated With Extrapyramidal Disorders

Movement Disorder	Characteristics
Tremor	Rhythmic oscillating contractions or movements of whole muscles or major portions of a muscle. They can occur as resting tremors, which are prominent at rest and decrease or disappear with movement; intention tremors, which increase with activity and become worse when the target is reached; and postural tremors, which appear when the affected part is maintained in a stabilized position.
Tics	Irregularly occurring brief, repetitive, stereotyped, coordinated movements such as winking, grimacing, or shoulder shrugging
Chorea	Brief, rapid, jerky, and irregular movements that are coordinated and graceful. The face, head, and distal limbs are most commonly involved. They often interfere with normal movement patterns.
Athetosis	Continuous, slow, wormlike, twisting and turning motions of a limb or body that most commonly involve the face and distal extremities and are often associated with spasticity
Ballismus	Involve violent sweeping, flinging-type limb movements, especially on one side of the body (hemiballismus)
Dystonia	Abnormal maintenance of posture results from a twisting, turning motion of the limbs, neck, or trunk. Motions are similar to athetosis but involve larger portions of the body. They can result in grotesque and twisted postures.
Dyskinesias	Rhythmic, repetitive, bizarre movements that chiefly involve the face, mouth, jaw, or tongue, causing grimacing, pursing of the lips, protrusion of the tongue, opening and closing of the mouth, and deviations of the jaw. The limbs are affected less often.

(From Bates B. [1991]. *A guide to physical examination and history taking* [5th ed., pp. 554–556]. Philadelphia: J.B. Lippincott)

of the tongue. The limbs are affected less often. Tardive dyskinesia is an untoward reaction that can develop with long-term use of some of the antipsychotic medications.

Parkinson's Disease

Parkinson's disease is a degenerative disorder of basal ganglia function that results in variable combinations of tremor, rigidity, and bradykinesia. Up to 1.5 million people in the United States are affected by the disease.[22] It usually begins after 50 years of age; most cases are diagnosed in the sixth and seventh decade of life. Up to 1% of the population older than 65 years of age may be affected with the disorder.[22]

Parkinson's disease is characterized by progressive destruction of the nigrostriatal pathway, with subsequent reduction in striatal concentrations of dopamine. Usually, there has been an 80% loss of dopamine in the striatum by the time symptoms become clinically apparent.[23] Secondary degenerative changes occur in the striatum, particularly in the putamen.

The clinical syndrome arising from the degenerative changes in basal ganglia function often is referred to as *parkinsonism*. Parkinson's disease, the most common form of parkinsonism, is named after James Parkinson, a British physician who first described the disease in a paper he published in 1817 on the "shaking palsy."[24] In the idiopathic form of the disease, dopamine depletion results from degeneration of the dopamine nigrostriatal system. Parkinsonism can also develop as a postencephalitic syndrome, as a side effect of therapy with antipsychotic drugs that block dopamine receptors, as a toxic reaction to a chemical agent, or as an outcome of severe carbon monoxide poisoning. Symptoms of parkinsonism also may accompany conditions such as cerebral vascular disease, brain tumors, or degenerative neurologic diseases that structurally damage the nigrostriatal pathway. The national attention given Muhammad Ali, former world heavyweight boxing champion and 1960 Olympic gold medal winner, as he lighted the Olympic torch for the 1996 Summer Games in Atlanta, not only served as a recognition of one person's remarkable courage in coping with the disease, but as a reminder that Parkinson's disease may have multiple causes, including repeated head trauma.[25]

Postencephalitic parkinsonism was a particular problem in the 1930s and 1940s as a result of an outbreak of lethargic encephalitis (sleeping sickness) that occurred in 1914 to 1918. Drug-induced parkinsonism can follow the administration of antipsychotic drugs in high doses (*e.g.*, phenothiazines, butyrophenones). These drugs block dopamine receptors and dopamine output by the cells of the substantia nigra. Of interest in terms of research was the development of Parkinson's disease in several persons who had attempted to make a narcotic drug and instead synthesized a compound called MPTP (1-methyl-phenyl-2,3,6-tetrahydropyridine).[25] This compound selectively destroys the dopaminergic neurons of the substantia nigra. This incident prompted investigations into the role of toxins that are produced by the body as a part of metabolic processes and those that enter the body from outside sources in the pathogenesis of Parkinson's disease. One theory is that the auto-oxidation of catecholamines such as dopa-

mine during melanin synthesis injures neurons in the substantia nigra. There is increasing evidence that the development of Parkinson's disease may be related to oxidative metabolites of this process and the inability of neurons to render these products harmless. MPTP is an inhibitor of the mitochondrial electron transport system that functions in the inactivation of these metabolites, suggesting that it may produce Parkinson's disease in a manner similar to the naturally occurring disease.[26]

A recent discovery suggests that genetic susceptibility may play a role in the pathogenesis of early-onset (before 45 years of age) Parkinson's disease. A mutation in a gene called the *Parkin gene* has been identified in a high percentage of family members and persons with early-onset Parkinson's disease.[27]

Manifestations. The cardinal manifestations of Parkinson's disease are tremor, rigidity, and bradykinesia or slowness of movement.[28,29] Tremor is the most visible manifestation of the disorder. It is present in 75% of persons at some point in their disease. The tremor affects the distal segments of the limbs, mainly the hands and feet; head, neck, face, lips, and tongue; or jaw. It is characterized by rhythmic, alternating flexion and contraction movements (four to six beats per minute) that resemble the motion of rolling a pill between the thumb and forefinger. The tremor usually is unilateral, occurs when the limb is supported and at rest, and disappears with movement and sleep. The tremor eventually progresses to involve both sides of the body. Although the most noticeable sign of Parkinson's disease, tremor usually is the least disabling because of the dampening effect of purposeful movement.[27]

Rigidity is defined as resistance to movement of both flexors and extensors throughout the full range of motion. It is most evident during passive joint movement, and involves jerky, cog-wheel–type or ratchet-like movements that require considerable energy to perform. Flexion contractions may develop as a result of the rigidity. As with tremor, rigidity usually begins unilaterally but progresses to involve both sides of the body.

Bradykinesia is characterized by slowness in initiating and performing movements and difficulty in sudden, unexpected stopping of voluntary movements. Unconscious associative movements occur in a series of disconnected steps rather than in a smooth, coordinated manner. This is the most disabling of the symptoms of Parkinson's disease. Persons with Parkinson's disease have difficulty initiating walking and difficulty turning. While walking, they may freeze in place and feel as if their feet are glued to the floor, especially when moving through a doorway or preparing to turn. When they walk, they lean forward to maintain their center of gravity and take small, shuffling steps without swinging their arms, and they have difficulty in changing their stride. Loss of postural reflexes predispose them to falling, often backward. Emotional and voluntary facial movements become limited and slow as the disease progresses, and facial expression becomes stiff and masklike. There is loss of the blinking reflex and a failure to express emotion. The tongue, palate, and throat muscles become rigid; the person may drool because of difficulty in moving the saliva to the back of the mouth and swallowing it. The speech becomes slow and monotonous, without modulation and poorly articulated.

Because the basal ganglia also influence the autonomic nervous system, persons with Parkinson's disease often have excessive and uncontrolled sweating, sebaceous gland secretion, and salivation. Autonomic symptoms such as lacrimation, dysphagia, orthostatic hypotension, thermal regulation, constipation, impotence, and urinary incontinence may be present, especially late in the disease. Other advanced-stage parkinsonian manifestations are falls, fluctuations in motor function, neuropsychiatric disorders, and sleep disorders.

Dementia is an important feature associated with Parkinson's disease. It occurs in approximately 20% of persons with the disease and develops late in the course of the disease.[27] The mental state of some persons with Parkinson's disease may be indistinguishable from that seen in Alzheimer's disease. It has been suggested that many of the brain changes in both diseases may result from degeneration of acetylcholine-containing neurons in a region of the brain called the *nucleus basalis of Meynert*, which is the main source of cholinergic innervation of the cerebral cortex. Persons with Parkinson's disease also have other neurochemical disturbances that can account for some of the features of dementia.

Treatment. The approach to treatment of parkinsonism must be highly individualized. It includes nonpharmacologic, pharmacologic, and, when indicated, surgical methods. Nonpharmacologic interventions offer group support, education, daily exercise, and adequate nutrition. Botulism toxin injections may be used in the treatment of dystonias such as eyelid spasm and limb dystonias that frequently are associated with Parkinson's disease.[29]

Pharmacologic treatment usually is determined by the severity of symptoms. Antiparkinson drugs act by increasing the functional ability of the underactive dopaminergic system, or they reduce the excessive influence of excitatory cholinergic neurons. Drugs that increase dopamine levels include levodopa and levodopa with the decarboxylase inhibitor (carbidopa), amantadine, bromocriptine, pergolide, and selegiline. Because dopamine transmission is disrupted in Parkinson's disease, there is a preponderance of cholinergic activity, which may be treated with anticholinergic drugs.

Dopamine does not cross the blood-brain barrier. Administration of levodopa, a precursor of dopamine that does cross the blood-brain barrier, has yielded significant improvement in clinical symptoms of Parkinson's disease and remains the most effective drug for treatment. The evidence of decreased dopamine levels in the striatum in Parkinson's disease led to the administration of large doses of the synthetic compound levodopa, which is absorbed from the intestinal tract, crosses the blood-brain barrier, and is converted to dopamine by centrally acting dopa decarboxylase. Unfortunately, only 1% to 3% of administered levodopa enters the brain unaltered; the remainder is metabolized outside the brain, predominantly by decarboxylation to dopamine, which cannot cross the blood-brain barrier. This means that large doses of levodopa are needed when the drug is used alone, and this leads to many

side effects. However, when levodopa is given in combination with carbidopa, a decarboxylase inhibitor, the peripheral metabolism of levodopa is reduced, plasma levels of levodopa are higher, the plasma half-life is longer, more dopa is available for entry into the brain, and a smaller dose is needed.

A later adverse effect of levodopa treatment is the "on-off phenomenon," in which frequent, abrupt, and unpredictable fluctuations in motor performance occur during the day. These fluctuations include periods of dyskinesia (the "on" response) and periods of bradykinesia (the "off" response). Some fluctuations reflect the timing of drug administration, in which case the on response coincides with peak drug levels and the off response with low drug levels.

Amantadine was introduced as an antiviral agent for prophylaxis of A_2 influenza and was unexpectedly found to cause symptomatic improvement of persons with parkinsonism. Although the exact mechanism of action remains to be elucidated, it may augment release of dopamine from the remaining intact dopaminergic terminals in the nigrostriatal pathway of persons with Parkinson's disease. It is used to treat persons with mild symptoms, but no disability. Bromocriptine, pergolide, pramipexole, and ropinirole are dopamine agonists that act directly to stimulate dopamine receptors. These drugs are used as adjunctive therapy in Parkinson's disease. They often are used for persons who have become refractory to levodopa or have developed an on-off phenomenon.

Selegiline is a monoamine oxidase type B inhibitor that inhibits the metabolic breakdown of dopamine. Selegiline may be used as adjunctive treatment to reduce mild on-off fluctuations in the responsiveness of persons who are receiving levodopa. It has been proposed that in inhibiting dopamine metabolism and the generation of destructive metabolites, selegiline also may delay the progression of the disease.

Anticholinergic drugs (*e.g.*, trihexyphenidyl, benztropine) are thought to restore a "balance" between reduced dopamine and uninhibited cholinergic neurons in the striatum. They are more useful in alleviating tremor and rigidity than bradykinesia. The anticholinergic drugs lessen the tremors and rigidity and afford some improvement of function. However, their potency seems to decrease over time, and increasing the dosage merely increases side effects such as blurred vision, dry mouth, bowel and bladder problems, and some mental changes.

When medical therapy is ineffective in controlling symptoms, pallidectomy performed by stereotactic surgery may be explored. With this surgical procedure, part of the globus pallidum in the basal ganglia is destroyed using an electrical stimulator. Brain mapping is done during the surgery to identify and prevent injury to sensory and motor tracts.

Autotransplantation of adrenal medullary tissue into the caudate has been used with limited success. Results of this procedure have been contradictory, and this approach is highly controversial. More recently, transplantation of embryonic dopamine neurons has met with some success in treatment of severe Parkinson's disease.[30]

DISORDERS OF THE CEREBELLUM

The functions of the cerebellum, or "little brain," are essential for smooth, coordinated, skillful movement. The cerebellum influences voluntary and automatic aspects of movement. It does not initiate activity, but it is responsible for smoothing the temporal and spatial aspects of rapid movement anywhere in the body.

The signs of cerebellar dysfunction can be grouped into three classes: vestibulocerebellar disorders, cerebellar ataxia or decomposition of movement, and cerebellar tremor. These disorders occur on the side of cerebellar damage, whether because of congenital defect, vascular accident, or growing tumor. The abnormality of movement occurs whether the eyes are open or closed. Visual monitoring of movement cannot compensate for cerebellar defects.

Damage to the part of the cerebellum associated with the vestibular system leads to difficulty or inability to maintain a steady posture of the trunk, which normally requires constant readjusting movements. This is seen as an unsteadiness of the trunk, called *truncal ataxia*, and it can be so severe that standing is not possible. The ability to fix the eyes on a target also can be affected. Constant conjugate readjustment of eye position, called *nystagmus*, results and makes reading extremely difficult, especially when the eyes are deviated toward the side of cerebellar damage.

Cerebellar ataxia and tremor are different aspects of defects in the smooth, continuously correcting functions. Cerebellar dystaxia or, if severe, ataxia includes a decomposition of movement; each succeeding component of a complex movement occurs separately instead of being blended into a smoothly proceeding action. Because ethanol specifically affects cerebellar function, persons who are inebriated often walk with a staggering and unsteady gait. Rapid alternating movements such as supination-pronation-supination of the hands are jerky and performed slowly (dysdiadochokinesia). Reaching to touch a target breaks down into small sequential components, each going too far, followed by overcorrection. The finger moves jerkily toward the target, misses, corrects in the other direction, and misses again, until the target is finally reached. This is called *over-and-under reaching*, and the general term is *dysmetria*.

Cerebellar tremor is a rhythmic back-and-forth movement of a finger or toe that worsens as the target is approached. The tremor results from the inability of the damaged cerebellar system to maintain ongoing fixation of a body part and to make smooth, continuous corrections in the trajectory of the movement; overcorrection occurs, first in one direction and then the other. Often, the tremor of an arm or leg can be detected during the beginning of an intended movement. The common term for cerebellar tremor is *intention tremor*. Cerebellar function as it relates to tremor can be assessed by asking a person to touch one heel to the opposite knee, to gently move the toes along the back of the opposite shin, or to move the hand so as to touch the nose with a finger.

Cerebellar function also can affect the motor skills of chewing and swallowing (dysphagia) and of speech (dysarthria). Normal speech requires smooth control of respiratory muscles and highly coordinated control of the laryngeal, lip, and tongue muscles. Cerebellar dysarthria is characterized by slow, slurred speech of continuously varying loudness. Rehabilitative efforts directed by speech therapists include learning to slow the rate of speech and to compensate as much as possible through the use of less-affected muscles.

> In summary, alterations in coordination of muscle movements and abnormal muscle movements result from disorders of the cerebellum and basal ganglia. The basal ganglia organize basic movement patterns into more complex patterns and release them when commanded by the motor cortex, contributing gracefulness to cortically initiated and controlled skilled movements. Disorders of the basal ganglia are characterized by involuntary movements, alterations in muscle tone, and disturbances in posture. These disorders include tremor, tics, hemiballismus, chorea, athetosis, dystonias, and dyskinesias.
>
> Parkinsonism, a disorder of the basal ganglia, is characterized by destruction of the nigrostriatal pathway, with a subsequent reduction in striatal concentrations of dopamine. This results in an imbalance between the inhibitory effects of dopaminergic basal ganglia functions and an increase in the excitatory cholinergic functions. The disorder is manifested by combinations of slowness of movement (*i.e.*, bradykinesia), increased muscle tonus and rigidity, rest tremor, gait disturbances, and impaired autonomic postural responses. The disease usually is slowly progressive over several decades, but the rate of progression varies from 2 to 30 years. The tremor often begins in one or both hands and then becomes generalized. Postural changes and gait disturbances continue to become more pronounced, resulting in significant disability.
>
> The function of the cerebellum is essential for smooth, coordinated movements. Cerebellar disorders include vestibulocerebellar dysfunction, cerebellar ataxia, and cerebellar tremor.

◼ Upper Motoneuron Disorders

After you have completed this section of the chapter, you should be able to meet the following objectives:

♦ Relate the pathologic UMN and LMN changes that occur in amyotrophic lateral sclerosis to the manifestations of the disease

♦ Explain the significance of demyelination and plaque formation in multiple sclerosis

♦ Describe the manifestations of multiple sclerosis

♦ Relate the structures of the vertebral column to mechanisms of spinal cord injury

♦ Explain how loss of UMN function contributes to the muscle spasms that occur after recovery from spinal cord injury

♦ State the effects of spinal cord injury on ventilation and communication, the autonomic nervous system, cardiovascular function, sensorimotor function, and bowel and bladder function

AMYOTROPHIC LATERAL SCLEROSIS

Amyotrophic lateral sclerosis (ALS), also known as *Lou Gehrig's disease* after the famous New York Yankees baseball player, is a devastating neurologic disorder that selectively affects motor function. There are approximately 5000 new cases of ALS in the United States each year.[31] ALS is primarily a disorder of middle to late adulthood, affecting persons between 55 and 60 years of age, with men developing the disease nearly twice as often as women. The disease typically follows a progressive course, with a mean survival period of 2 to 5 years from the onset of symptoms.

ALS affects motoneurons in three locations: the anterior horn cells of the spinal cord; the motor nuclei of the brain stem, particularly the hypoglossal nuclei; and the UMNs of the cerebral cortex.[27] The fact that the disease is more extensive in the distal parts of the affected tracts in the lower spinal cord rather than the proximal parts suggests that affected neurons first undergo degeneration at their distal terminals and that the disease proceeds in a centripetal direction until ultimately the parent nerve cell dies. A remarkable feature of the disease is that the entire sensory system, the regulatory mechanisms of control and coordination of movement, and the intellect remain intact. The neurons for ocular motility and the parasympathetic neurons in the sacral spinal cord also are spared.

The death of LMNs leads to denervation, with subsequent shrinkage of musculature and muscle fiber atrophy. It is this fiber atrophy, called *amyotrophy*, which appears in the name of the disease. The loss of nerve fibers in lateral columns of the white matter of the spinal cord along with fibrillary gliosis imparts a firmness or sclerosis to this CNS tissue; the term *lateral sclerosis* designates these changes.

The cause of LMN and UMN destruction in ALS is uncertain. Five to 10% of cases are familial; the others are believed to be sporadic, with no family history of the disease. Recently, mutations to a gene encoding superoxide dismutase 1 (SOD1) was mapped to chromosome 21. This enzyme functions in the prevention of free radical formation (see Chapter 5). The mutation accounts for 20% of familial ALS, with the remaining 80% being caused by mutations in other genes.[32] Five percent of persons with sporadic ALS also have SOD1 mutations. Possible targets of SOD1-induced toxicity include the neurofilament proteins, which function in the axonal transport of molecules necessary for the maintenance of axons.[32] Another suggested mechanism of pathogenesis in ALS is exotoxic injury through activation of glutamate-gated ion channels, which are distinguished by their sensitivity to *N*-methyl-D-aspartic acid (see Chapter 50). The possibility of glutamate excitotoxicity in the pathogenesis of ALS was suggested by the finding of increased glutamine levels in the cerebrospinal fluid of patients with sporadic ALS.[32] Although autoimmunity has been suggested as a cause of ALS, the disease does not respond to the immunosuppressant agents that normally are used in treatment of autoimmune disorders.

The symptoms of ALS may be referable to UMN or LMN involvement. Manifestations of UMN lesions include weakness, spasticity or stiffness, and impaired fine motor control.[31,33] Dysphagia (difficulty swallowing), dysarthria (impaired articulation of speech), and dysphonia (difficulty making the sounds of speech) may result from brain stem LMN involvement or from dysfunction of UMNs descending to the brain stem. Manifestations of LMN destruction include fasciculations, weakness, muscle atrophy, and hyporeflexia. Muscle cramps involving the distal legs often is an early symptom. The most common clinical presentation is slowly progressive weakness and atrophy in distal muscles of one upper extremity. This is followed by regional spread of clinical weakness, reflecting involvement of neighboring areas of the spinal cord. Eventually, UMNs and LMNs involving multiple limbs and the head are affected. In the more advanced stages, muscles of the palate, pharynx, tongue, neck, and shoulders become involved, causing impairment of chewing, swallowing, and speech. Dysphagia with recurrent aspiration and weakness of the respiratory muscles produces the most significant acute complications of the disease. Death usually results from involvement of cranial and respiratory musculature.

Currently, there is no cure for ALS. Rehabilitation measures assist persons with the disorder to manage their disability, and respiratory and nutritional support allows persons with the disorder to survive longer than would otherwise have been the case. An antiglutamate drug, riluzole, is the only drug approved by the U.S. Food and Drug Administration (FDA) for treatment of ALS. The drug is designed to decrease glutamate accumulation and slow the progression of the disease. In two therapeutic trials, the drug prolonged survival by 3 to 6 months.[32]

DEMYELINATING DISORDERS

Multiple Sclerosis

Multiple sclerosis (MS), a demyelinating disease of the CNS, is a major cause of neurologic disability among young and middle-aged adults. Approximately two thirds of persons with MS experience their first symptoms between 20 and 40 years of age. Sometimes, a diagnosis may be delayed until the fourth or fifth decade because symptoms were short lasting or were not bothersome enough to warrant medical attention. In these cases, a detailed medical history usually reveals that symptoms did appear previously. In approximately 80% of the cases, the disease is characterized by exacerbations and remissions over many years in several different sites in the CNS.[34] Initially, there is normal or near-normal neurologic function between exacerbations. As the disease progresses, there is less improvement between exacerbations and increasing neurologic dysfunction.

Epidemiologic Features. The prevalence of MS varies considerably around the world. The disease is more prevalent in the colder northern latitudes; it is more common in the northern Atlantic states, the Great Lakes region, and the Pacific Northwest than in the southern parts of the United States. Other high-incidence areas include northern Europe, Great Britain, southern Australia, and New Zealand.[34] Estimates of the total number of cases of MS in the United States range from 250,000 to 350,000.[35] The incidence among women is almost double that among men. Migration studies have shown that persons who move from a high-risk area tend to retain the risk of their birthplace if they move after 15 years of age, or adopt the risk of their new home if they migrate as children.[5]

Genetic Factors. Although MS is not directly inherited, there is a familial predisposition in some cases, suggesting a genetic influence on susceptibility. The risk of developing MS is 15 times greater when the disease is present in a first-degree relative.[5] The concordance rate for monozygotic twins is approximately 30%, compared with 5% for dizygotic twins.[34] There also is a strong association between MS and certain human leukocyte antigens[5] (HLA; see Chapter 18). The presence of the HLA-DR2 allele substantially increases the risk for development of MS.[34] Also, the severity and course of the disease may be influenced by genetic factors.

Pathophysiology. The pathophysiology of MS involves the demyelination of nerve fibers in the white matter of the brain, spinal cord, and optic nerve. In the CNS, myelin is formed by the oligodendrocytes, chiefly those lying among the nerve fibers in the white matter. This function is equivalent to that of the Schwann cells in the peripheral nervous system (see Chapter 47). The properties of the myelin sheath—high electrical resistance and low capacitance—permit it to function as an electrical insulator. Demyelinated nerve fibers display a variety of conduction abnormalities, ranging from decreased conduction velocity to conduction blocks, resulting in a variety of symptoms that depend on the location and duration of the lesion.

The lesions of MS consist of hard, sharp-edged demyelinated or sclerotic patches that are macroscopically visible throughout the white matter of the CNS.[27] These lesions, which represent the end result of acute myelin breakdown, are called *plaques.* The lesions have a predilection for the optic nerves, periventricular white matter, brain stem, cerebellum, and spinal cord white matter.[34] In an active plaque, there is evidence of ongoing myelin breakdown. The sequence of myelin breakdown is not well understood, although it is known that the lesions contain small amounts of myelin basic proteins and increased amounts of proteolytic enzymes, macrophages, lymphocytes, and plasma cells. Oligodendrocytes are decreased in number and may be absent, especially in older lesions. Acute, subacute, and chronic lesions often are seen at multiple sites throughout the CNS.

Magnetic resonance imaging has shown that the lesions of MS may occur in two stages: a first stage that involves the sequential development of small inflammatory lesions, and a second stage during which the lesions extend and consolidate and when demyelination and gliosis (scar formation) occur. It is not known whether the inflammatory process, present during the first stage, is directed against the myelin or against the oligodendrocytes that produce myelin. Remyelination of the nervous system was considered to be impossible until the late 1990s. Evidence now suggests that remyelination can occur in the CNS if the process that initiated the demyelination is halted before the oligodendrocyte dies.[35]

Multiple sclerosis generally is believed to be an immune-mediated disorder that occurs in genetically susceptible individuals. However, the sequence of events that initiates the process is largely unknown. The demyelination process in MS is marked by prominent lymphocytic invasion in the lesion. The infiltrate in plaques contains both CD8[+] and CD4[+] T cells as well as macrophages. Both macrophages and cytotoxic CD8[+] T cells are thought to induce oligodendrocyte injury. There also is evidence of antibody-mediated damage involving myelin oligodendroglial protein.[5]

Manifestations and Clinical Course. The interruption of neural conduction in the demyelinated nerves is manifested by a variety of symptoms, depending on the location and extent of the lesion. Areas commonly affected by MS are the optic nerve (visual field), corticobulbar tracts (speech and swallowing), corticospinal tracts (muscle strength), cerebellar tracts (gait and coordination), spinocerebellar tracts (balance), medial longitudinal fasciculus (conjugate gaze function of the extraocular eye muscles), and posterior cell columns of the spinal cord (position and vibratory sensation). Typically, an otherwise healthy person presents with an acute or subacute episode of paresthesias, optic neuritis (*i.e.,* visual clouding or loss of vision in part of the visual field with pain on movement of the globe), diplopia, or specific types of gaze paralysis.

Paresthesias are evidenced as numbness, tingling, a burning sensation, or pressure on the face or involved extremities; symptoms can range from annoying to severe. *Lhermitte's symptom* is an electric shock–like tingling down the back and onto the legs that is produced by flexion of the neck. Pain from spasticity also may be a factor that can be aided by appropriate stretching exercises. Although pain may not be a prominent symptom, approximately 80% of persons with MS experience some pain in the course of the disease. Other common symptoms are abnormal gait, bladder and sexual dysfunction, vertigo, nystagmus, fatigue, and speech disturbance. These symptoms usually last for several days to weeks, and then completely or partially resolve. After a period of normal or relatively normal function, new symptoms appear. Psychological manifestations, such as mood swings, may represent an emotional reaction to the nature of the disease or, more likely, involvement of the white matter of the cerebral cortex. Depression, euphoria, inattentiveness, apathy, forgetfulness, and loss of memory may occur.

Fatigue is one of the most common problems for persons with MS. Fatigue often is described as a generalized low-energy feeling not related to depression and different from weakness. Fatigue has a harmful impact on activities of daily living and sustained physical activity. Interventions such as spacing activities and setting priorities often are helpful.

The course of the disease may fall into one of four categories: relapsing-remitting, secondary progressive, primary progressive, or progressive relapsing.[36,37] The *relapsing-remitting* form of the disease is characterized by episodes of acute worsening with recovery and a stable course between relapses. *Secondary progressive disease* involves a gradual neurologic deterioration with or without superimposed acute relapses in a person with previous relapsing-remitting disease. *Primary progressive disease* is characterized by nearly continuous neurologic deterioration from onset of symptoms. The *progressive relapsing* category of disease involves gradual neurologic deterioration from the onset of symptoms but with subsequent superimposed relapses.

Diagnosis. The diagnosis of MS is based on established clinical and, when necessary, laboratory criteria. Advances in cerebrospinal fluid analysis and MRI have greatly simplified the procedure. A definite diagnosis of MS requires evidence of one of the following patterns: two or more episodes of exacerbation separated by 1 month or more and lasting more than 24 hours, with subsequent recovery; a clinical history of clearly defined exacerbations and remissions, with or without complete recovery, followed by progression of symptoms over a period of at least 6 months; or slow and stepwise progression of signs and symptoms over a period of at least 6 months.[38] Primary progressive MS may be suggested by a progressive course that lasts longer than 6 months. A person who has not had a relapse or progression of symptoms is described as having stable MS.

Magnetic resonance imaging can be used as an adjunct to clinical diagnosis. MRI studies can detect the multiplicity of lesions even when CT scans appear normal. A computer-assisted method of MRI can measure lesion size. Many new areas of myelin abnormality are asymptomatic. Serial MRI studies can be done to detect asymptomatic lesions, monitor the progress of existing lesions, and evaluate the effectiveness of treatment. Although MRI can be used to provide evidence of disseminated lesions in persons with the disease, normal findings do not exclude the diagnosis.[38] Electrophysiologic evaluations (*e.g.,* evoked potential studies) and CT scans may assist in the identification and documentation of lesions.

Although no laboratory test can be used to diagnose MS, examination of the cerebrospinal fluid is helpful. A large percentage of patients with MS have elevated immunoglobulin G (IgG) levels, and some have oligoclonal patterns (*i.e.,* discrete electrophoretic bands) even with normal IgG levels. Total protein or lymphocyte levels may be mildly elevated in the cerebrospinal fluid. These test results can be altered in a variety of inflammatory neurologic disorders and are not specific for MS.

Treatment. Most treatment measures for MS are directed at modifying the course and managing the primary symptoms of the disease. The variety of symptoms, unpredictable course, and lack of specific diagnostic methods have made the evaluation and treatment of MS difficult. Persons who are minimally affected by the disorder require no specific treatment. The person should be encouraged to maintain as healthy a lifestyle as possible, including good nutrition and adequate rest and relaxation. Physical therapy may help maintain muscle tone. Every effort should be made to avoid excessive fatigue, physical deterioration, emotional stress, viral infections, and extremes of environmental temperature, which may precipitate an exacerbation of the disease.

The pharmacologic agents used in the treatment of MS fall into four categories: (1) those used to treat acute symptoms of the disease, (2) those used to modify the course of the disease, (3) those used to interrupt progressive disease, and (4) those used to treat the symptoms of the disorder.[37] Corticosteroids are the mainstay of treatment for acute relapses of MS. These agents are thought to reduce the inflammation, improve nerve conduction, and have important immunologic effects. Long-term administration does not, however, appear to alter the course of the disease and can have harmful side effects. Adrenocorticotropic hormone (ACTH) also may be used in treatment of MS. Plasmapheresis has proved beneficial in some cases.

The agents used to modify the course of the disease include interferon beta and glatiramer acetate.[37] Both agents have shown some benefit in reducing exacerbations in persons with relapsing-remitting MS. Interferon beta is a cytokine that acts as an immune enhancer. Two forms of recombinant interferon beta—1a and 1b—have been approved by the FDA for treatment of MS. Interferon beta-1a is a recombinant form of interferon beta that has an amino acid sequence similar to the natural form of interferon beta. Interferon beta-1b is a nonglycosylated recombinant bacterial product in which serine is substituted for cysteine. Both types of interferon beta are administered by injection (1a, once a week, and 1b, every other day). Both types of interferon beta usually are well tolerated. The most common side effects are flulike symptoms for 24 to 48 hours after each injection, and these usually subside after 2 to 3 months of treatment. Glatiramer acetate is a synthetic polypeptide that simulates parts of the myelin basic protein. Although the exact mechanism of action is unknown, the drug seems to block myelin-damaging T cells by acting as a myelin decoy. The drug is given daily by subcutaneous injection.

Progressive MS may be treated with immunosuppressive drugs such as methotrexate, cyclophosphamide, mitoxantrone, and cyclosporine. Among the medications used to relieve symptoms associated with MS are dantrolene (Dantrium), baclofen (Lioresal), or diazepam (Valium) for spasticity; cholinergic drugs for bladder problems; and antidepressant drugs for depression.

SPINAL CORD INJURY

Despite the protective mechanisms built in during the development of the CNS, spinal cord injury (SCI) continues to occur. It is estimated that the annual incidence of SCI, not including those victims who die at the site of injury, is approximately 11,000 new cases per year.[39] Nationally, the number of people who are alive today and have SCI is estimated to be 183,000 to 230,000. SCI is a disease of young adults. Fifty-five percent of injuries occur in persons in the 16- to 30-year age group.[39] The most frequent cause of SCI is motor vehicle accidents, followed by falls, violence, sports injuries, and other types of injuries, which include attempted suicide and occupational injuries. Of sports-related injuries, 66% are from diving. As age increases, the cause of injury changes, with falls becoming the most frequent cause. Males sustain spinal cord injuries at a rate four times higher than that of females. Alcohol and drugs have been cited as contributing factors in an increasing number of cases.

Injury to the Vertebral Column

The spinal column, which is located in the posterior midline of the body, begins at the base of the skull and ends at the coccyx, or "tailbone." There are 32 to 33 individual and fused vertebral bodies, or vertebrae, that make up the spinal column: 7 cervical, 12 thoracic, 5 lumbar, 5 fused sacral, and 3 or 4 fused coccygeal vertebrae. Each vertebra in the vertebral column, with the exception of the first cervical vertebra, shares common characteristics; each consists of an anterior portion, or body, and a posterior portion, called the *vertebral* or *neural arch* (Fig. 49-11). The vertebral arch or posterior elements are composed of two pedicles, two laminae, a spinous process, two transverse processes, and four articular processes known as *facets*. The transverse foramina in the transverse processes of the cervical vertebrae form passageways for the vertebral artery, vertebral vein, and sympathetic nerves.

The design of the vertebra provides bony support and protection for the cord by forming a vertebral foramen or spinal canal. The size and function of the vertebrae are directly related to their specific location in the spinal column. In general, vertebral bodies increase in size to bear additional weight as they descend along the spinal column. The width of the spinal canal also varies at different levels. The atlas (C1) and the axis (C2) are smaller than the rest of the vertebrae and are formed in a manner that allows flexion, extension, and rotation of the head. The intermediate-sized thoracic vertebrae are heart shaped and limited in movement, making the thoracic spine, especially the lower levels, more rigid. They also possess tubercles for rib attachment. Each vertebra articulates with the next above and below by means of articular processes called *facets*, which function as sliding synovial joints. The facets provide some support and major limitation of movement. They also can be a frequent source of back pain. The design of the lumbar spine allows for powerful flexion and some extension; these lumbar vertebrae are large and heavy to accommodate the attachment of lower limb muscles and the weight of the thorax, neck, and head.

The intervertebral disks and supporting ligaments assist the vertebral column in supporting and protecting the spinal cord (see previous discussion). The intervertebral disks, along with the facet joints, carry all of the compressive loading to which the trunk of the body is subjected. The vertebrae and intervertebral disks are held in place by the ligaments. There are two major longitudinal ligaments that extend from the axis (C2) to the sacrum on the anterior and posterior surfaces of the vertebral bodies and disks (see Fig. 49-7). These ligaments allow adequate motion and maintenance of alignment between vertebrae; protect the spinal cord by limiting motions within well-defined limits; assist the muscles in providing stability to the spine; and protect the spinal cord in traumatic situations associated with high loads and fast speeds. Other fibrous ligaments that attach at various sites between the parts of neighboring vertebrae also support and limit movement of the spinal column, thereby protecting the spinal cord. Additional stabilizing forces are the rib cage, superficial and deep trunk muscles, and the normal curvature of the spine, which is anteriorly convex at the cervical and lumbar regions and posteriorly convex in the thoracic and sacral levels.

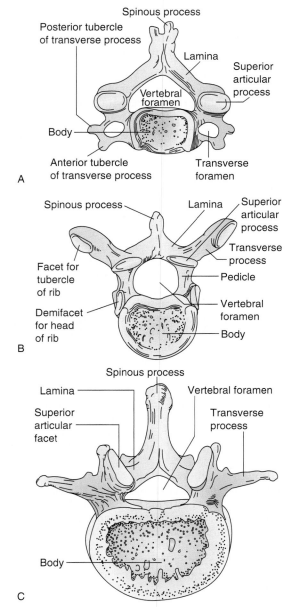

FIGURE 49-11 Views of three types of vertebrae. (**A**) Fourth cervical vertebra, superior aspect; (**B**) sixth thoracic vertebra, superior aspect; (**C**) third lumbar vertebra, superior aspect. (Chaffee E.E., Lytle I.M. [1980]. *Basic physiology and anatomy.* [4th ed.]. Philadelphia: J.B. Lippincott)

Injuries to the vertebral column include fractures, dislocations, and subluxations. A fracture can occur at any part of the bony vertebrae, causing fragmentation of the bone. It most often involves the pedicle, lamina, or processes (*e.g.*, facets). Dislocation or subluxation (partial dislocation) injury causes the vertebral bodies to become displaced, with one overriding another and preventing correct alignment of the vertebral column. The extent of injury to the vertebral column caused by motion or trauma is related to the amount and direction of motion and the rate of application of force causing the motion. Damage to the ligaments or bony vertebrae may make the spine unstable. In an unstable spine, further unguarded movement of the spinal column can impinge on the spinal canal, causing compression or overstretching of neural tissue.

Most injuries result from some combination of compressive force or bending movement (Fig. 49-12). Flexion injuries occur when forward bending of the spinal column exceeds the limits of normal movement. Typical flexion injuries result, for example, when the head is struck from behind, as in a fall with the back of the head as the point of impact. Extension injuries occur with excessive forced bending (*i.e.*, hyperextension) of the spine backward. A typical extension injury involves a fall in which the chin or face is the point of impact, causing hyperextension of the neck. Injuries of flexion and extension occur more commonly in the cervical spine (C4 to C6) than in any other area. Limitations imposed by the ribs, spinous processes, and joint capsules in the thoracic and lumbar spine make this area less flexible and less susceptible to flexion and extension injuries than the cervical spine.

A compression injury, causing the vertebral bones to shatter, squash, or even burst, occurs when there is spinal loading from a high-velocity blow to the top of the head or when landing forcefully on the feet. This typically occurs at the cervical level (*e.g.*, diving injuries) or in the thoracolumbar area (*e.g.*, falling from a distance and landing on the feet). Compression injuries may occur when the vertebrae are weakened by conditions such as osteoporosis and cancer with bone metastasis. Axial rotation injuries can produce highly unstable injuries. Maximal axial rotation occurs in the cervical region, especially between C1 and C2 and at the lumbosacral joint. Coupling of vertebral motions is common in injury when two or more individual motions occur (*e.g.*, lateral bending and axial rotation). The motion produced by the external force is called the *main motion*, and all the accompanying motions are considered *coupled motions*.

Classification and Types of Spinal Cord Injury

Alterations in body function that result from SCI depend on the level of injury and the amount of cord involvement. The American Spinal Injury Association (ASIA) has published *Standards for Neurological and Functional Classification of Spinal Cord Injury*.[40] According to ASIA, *tetraplegia* (a term preferred to *quadriplegia*), refers to impairment or loss of motor or sensory function (or both) in the cervical segments of the cord after damage of neural elements in the spinal canal. Tetraplegia results in impairment of function in the arms, trunk, legs, and pelvic organs (see Fig. 49-4). It does not include peripheral nerve injuries. *Paraplegia* refers to impairment or loss of motor or sensory function (or both) in the thoracic, lumbar, or sacral segments of the spinal cord from damage of neural elements in the spinal canal. With paraplegia, arm functioning is spared, but depending on the level of injury, functioning of the trunk, legs, and pelvic organs may be involved. Paraplegia also refers to conus medullaris and cauda equina injuries, but not injury to peripheral nerves outside the spinal canal.

Further definitions describe the extent of neurologic damage as *complete* or *incomplete* injuries. In an incomplete SCI, partial preservation of sensory and motor function is found below the neurologic level of injury and includes the lowest sacral segment (*e.g.*, sparing of S2 to S4 innervation of myocutaneous and deep anal sensation and rectal sphincter control). The necessary test of motor function is the voluntary contraction of the anal sphincter on digital examination. A complete injury refers to the absence of sensory and motor function, which includes the lowest sacral segment. The myotome and dermatome charts (see Chapter 48, Fig. 48-2) show skeletal muscle and sensory areas

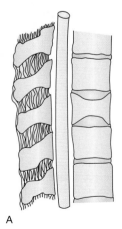
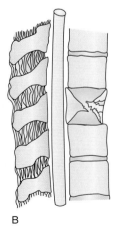
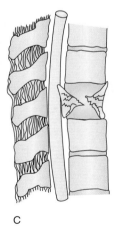

A   B   C

FIGURE 49-12 Progressive degrees of compression fracture. (**A**) Severe compression fracture showing the biconcave profile produced by the adjacent disks. (**B**) A more severe degree of fracture. A vertical fracture has joined the deformed, concave endplates. The anterior body fragment is comminuted and displaced anteriorly. (**C**) A more severe degree of compression fracture. The posterior body fragment is now comminuted and displaced posteriorly into the spinal canal. Neural damage may occur. (Rockwood C.A., Green D.P. [1977]. *Fractures*. Philadelphia: J.B. Lippincott)

of skin innervated by specific spinal cord segments. The prognosis for return of function is better in an incomplete injury because of preservation of axonal function. However, the longer the period since the injury, the less likely it is that improvement will occur.

Incomplete Spinal Cord Injuries

Incomplete SCI implies there is residual motor or sensory function more than three segments below the level of injury.[41] Incomplete injuries may manifest in a variety of patterns but can be organized into certain patterns or "syndromes" that occur more frequently and reflect the predominant area of the cord that is involved. Types of incomplete lesions include the central cord syndrome, anterior cord syndrome, Brown-Séquard syndrome, and the conus medullaris syndrome.

Central Cord Syndrome. A condition called *central cord syndrome* occurs when injury is predominantly in the central gray or white matter of the cord[13] (Fig. 49-13). Because the corticospinal tract fibers are organized with those controlling the arms located more centrally and those controlling the legs located more laterally, some external axonal transmission may remain intact. Motor function of the upper extremities is affected, but the lower extremities may not be affected or may be affected to a lesser degree, with some sparing of sacral sensation. Bowel, bladder, and sexual functions usually are affected to various degrees and may parallel the degree of lower extremity involvement. This syndrome occurs almost exclusively in the cervical cord,

rendering the lesion a UMN lesion with spastic paralysis. Central cord damage is more frequent in elderly persons with narrowing or stenotic changes in the spinal canal that are related to arthritis. Damage also may occur in persons with congenital stenosis. As in any incomplete injury, the prognosis for return of function is better than in complete injury, and improvement seems to affect the lower extremities to a greater degree than the upper extremities because of the nature of the primary injury.

Anterior Cord Syndrome. Anterior artery or anterior cord syndrome usually is caused by damage from infarction of the anterior spinal artery, resulting in damage to the anterior two thirds of the cord[13] (Fig. 49-14). The deficits result in loss of motor function provided by the corticospinal tracts and loss of pain and temperature sensation from damage to the lateral spinothalamic tracts. The spinal gray matter largely depends on blood flow from the anterior spinal artery. Loss of the local gray matter can result in reduction in or loss of local reflexes and localized LMNs of the anterior horn. The posterior one third of the cord is relatively unaffected, preserving the dorsal column axons that convey position, vibration, and touch sensation.

Brown-Séquard Syndrome. A condition called *Brown-Séquard syndrome* results from damage to a hemisection of the anterior and posterior cord[13] (Fig. 49-15). The effect is a loss of voluntary motor function from the corticospinal tract, proprioception loss from the ipsilateral side of the body, and contralateral loss of pain and temperature sen-

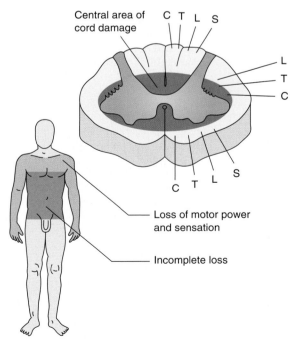

FIGURE 49-13 Central cord syndrome. A cross-section of the cord shows central damage and the associated motor and sensory loss. (C, cervical; T, thoracic; L, lumbar; S, sacral). (Hickey J.V. [1997]. *The clinical practice of neurological and neurosurgical nursing.* [3rd ed.]. Philadelphia: J.B. Lippincott)

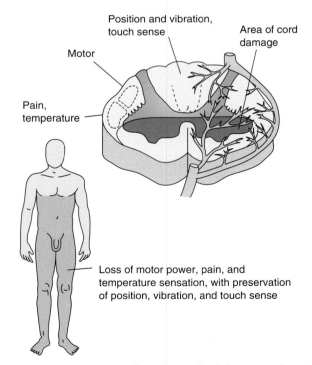

FIGURE 49-14 Anterior cord syndrome. Cord damage and associated motor and sensory loss are illustrated. (Hickey J.V. [1997]. *The clinical practice of neurological and neurosurgical nursing.* [3rd ed.]. Philadelphia: J.B. Lippincott)

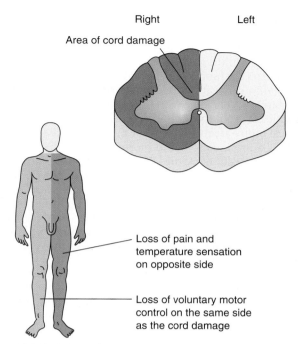

Right   Left

Area of cord damage

Loss of pain and
temperature sensation
on opposite side

Loss of voluntary motor
control on the same side
as the cord damage

FIGURE 49-15 Brown-Séquard syndrome. Cord damage and associated motor and sensory loss are illustrated. (Hickey J.V. [1997]. *The clinical practice of neurological and neurosurgical nursing.* [3rd ed.]. Philadelphia: J.B. Lippincott)

sation from the lateral spinothalamic tracts for all levels below the lesion.

Conus Medullaris Syndrome. Conus medullaris syndrome involves damage to the conus medullaris or the sacral cord (*i.e.*, conus) and lumbar nerve roots in the neural canal. Functional deficits resulting from this type of injury usually result in flaccid bowel, bladder, and sexual function. Sacral segments occasionally show preserved reflexes if only the conus is affected. Motor function in the legs and feet may be impaired without significant sensory impairment. Damage to the lumbosacral nerve roots in the spinal canal usually results in LMN and sensory neuron damage known as *cauda equina syndrome.* Functional deficits present as various patterns of asymmetric flaccid paralysis, sensory impairment, and pain.

Complete Spinal Cord Injuries

Complete SCI implies there is no motor or sensory function more than three levels below the level of injury. Complete cord injuries can result from severance of the cord, disruption of nerve fibers although they remain intact, or interruption of blood supply to that segment, resulting in complete destruction of neural tissue and UMN or LMN paralysis. However, complete severance of the cord is rare. Approximately 3% of persons with complete injuries on initial examination experience some recovery within 24 hours.[41]

Acute Spinal Cord Injury. The pathophysiology of acute SCI can be divided into two types: primary and second-ary.[13,42] The *primary neurologic injury* occurs at the time of mechanical injury and is irreversible. It is characterized by small hemorrhages in the gray matter of the cord, followed by edematous changes in the white matter that lead to necrosis of neural tissue. This type of pathology results from the forces of compression, stretch, and shear associated with fracture or compression of the spinal vertebrae, dislocation of vertebrae (*e.g.*, flexion, extension, subluxation), and contusions due to jarring of the cord in the spinal canal. Penetrating injuries produce lacerations and direct trauma to the cord and may occur with or without spinal column damage. The most frequent penetrating injuries are caused by gunshot and knife wounds. Lacerations occur when there is cutting or tearing of the spinal cord, which injures nerve tissue and causes bleeding and edema. Even in the presence of complete damage to all neural tissue at the site of injury, the spinal cord frequently remains intact, lending support to the concept that mechanisms secondary to the initial injury play a significant role.

Secondary injuries follow the primary injury and promote the spread of injury. Although there is considerable debate about the pathogenesis of secondary injuries, the tissue destruction that occurs ends in progressive neurologic damage. After SCI, several pathologic mechanisms come into play, including vascular damage, neuronal injury that leads to loss of reflexes below the level of injury, and release of vasoactive agents and cellular enzymes. Vascular pathology (*i.e.*, vessel trauma and hemorrhage) can lead to ischemia, increased vascular permeability, and edema. Blood flow to the spinal cord may be further compromised by spinal shock that results from a loss of vasomotor tone and neural reflexes below the level of injury. The release of vasoactive substances (*i.e.*, norepinephrine, serotonin, dopamine, and histamine) from the wound tissue causes vasospasm and impedes blood flow in the microcirculation, producing further necrosis of blood vessels and neurons. The release of proteolytic and lipolytic enzymes from injured cells causes delayed swelling, demyelination, and necrosis in the spinal cord.

As in spine trauma, the greater the magnitude of force applied to the spinal cord, the greater is the associated damage. Some areas of hemorrhage and injury may occur rostral and caudal to the site of impact, and the severity of bony injury or radiographic findings may not always correspond to the extent of neurologic damage. Also, the location of bony injury may not coincide with the clinical findings of motor and sensory deficits, such as a C6 compression fracture with motor and sensory level functioning at C7, C4, or C5.

The goal of management of acute SCI is to reduce the neurologic deficit and prevent any additional loss of neurologic function. The specific steps in resuscitation and initial evaluation can be carried out at the trauma site or in the emergency room, depending on the urgency of the situation.[42,43] Most traumatic injuries to the spinal column render it unstable, mandating measures such as immobilization with collars and backboards and limiting the movement of persons at risk for or with known SCI. Every person with multiple trauma or head injury, including victims of traffic and sporting accidents, should be suspected of having sustained an acute SCI.[42,43] In-line immobilization without traction is recommended. This includes immobilizing the neck in a neutral position in a rigid cervical collar. The person should be "log rolled" onto a rigid backboard, with the head secured by straps or tape.

The nature of the injury determines further methods of stabilization and treatment. In unstable injuries of the cervical spine, cervical traction improves or restores spinal alignment, decompresses neural structures, and facilitates recovery. Fractures and dislocations of the thoracic and lumbar vertebrae may be initially stabilized by restricting the person to bed rest and turning him or her in a log-rolling manner to keep the spine rigid. Gunshot or stab wounds of the spinal column may not produce structural instability and require immobilization. The goal of early surgical intervention for an unstable spine is to provide internal skeletal stabilization so that early mobilization and rehabilitation can occur.

The concept of neuroprotection is aimed at preserving neural function after SCI. One of the more important aspects of early SCI care is the prevention and treatment of spinal or systemic shock and the hypoxia associated with compromised respiration. Correcting hypotension or hypoxia is essential to maintaining circulation to the injured cord.[44] The use of high-dose methylprednisolone has been shown to improve the outcome from SCI when given shortly after injury. Methylprednisolone is a short-acting corticosteroid that has been used extensively in the treatment of inflammatory and allergic disorders. In acute SCI, it is thought to stabilize cell membranes, enhance impulse generation, improve blood flow, and inhibit free radical formation. In a prospective, randomized, double-blind, controlled study, high-dose methylprednisolone treatment, when given within 8 hours of injury, resulted in a significant long-term improvement in motor function.[45] Because methylprednisolone has been identified as an effective initial treatment for SCI in the U.S., it now is considered standard medical treatment to be given within the first 8 hours of injury. Patients who receive methylprednisolone within 3 hours of injury are maintained on the treatment regimen for 24 hours, and those who receive it from 3 to 8 hours after injury continue to receive it for 48 hours.[46]

The success of methylprednisolone in improving neurologic functioning after SCI is expected to lead to the evaluation of other, new agents. One of the agents that has been more extensively studied is GM-1. GM-1, a ganglioside normally found in the CNS, is believed to enhance neuronal sprouting and regeneration and counteract some of the secondary injury processes.[44] Other research involves use of the calcium channel–blocking agents (nimodipine), functional electrical stimulation, and tissue-bridge implants to reactivate damaged motor systems and promote nerve regeneration. Until a cure is found, prevention of injury through health promotion education, early diagnosis, and prompt intervention, as well as rehabilitation to prevent complications and restore optimal functioning, are essential.

Alterations in Functional Abilities

Functional abilities after SCI are subject to various degrees of sensorimotor loss and altered reflex activity based on the level of cord injury and extent of cord damage. Table 49-2 summarizes the functional abilities by level of injury. Motor function in cervical injuries ranges from complete dependence to independence with or without assistive devices in activities of mobility and self-care. The functional levels of cervical injury are related to C5, C6, C7, or C8 innervation. At the C5 level, deltoid and biceps function is spared, allowing full head, neck, and diaphragm control with good shoulder strength and full elbow flexion. At the C6 level, wrist dorsiflexion by the way of wrist extensors is functional, allowing tenodesis, which is the natural bending inward and flexion of the fingers when the wrist is extended and bent backward. Tenodesis is a key movement, because it can be used to pick up objects when finger movement is absent. A functional C7 injury allows full elbow flexion and extension, wrist plantar flexion, and some finger control. At the C8 level, finger flexion is added.

Thoracic cord injuries (T1 to T12) allow full upper extremity control with limited to full control of intercostal and trunk muscles and balance. Injury at the T1 level allows full fine motor control of the fingers. Because of the lack of specific functional indicators at the thoracic levels, the level of injury usually is determined by sensory level testing.

Functional capacity in the L1 through L5 nerve innervations allows hip flexors, hip abductors (L1 to L3), movement of the knees (L2 to L5), and ankle dorsiflexion (L4 to L5). Sacral (S1 to S5) innervation allows for full leg, foot, and ankle control and innervation of perineal musculature for bowel, bladder, and sexual function.

Spinal Reflexes. A reflex is a stereotypic motor response to a particular sensory input. Spinal cord reflexes are integrated within the spinal cord and can function independent of input from higher centers. They include the flexor withdrawal reflex, the reflex control of muscle tone, and bladder emptying. Altered spinal reflex activity in SCI is essentially determined by UMN and LMN lesions. UMNs that are fully contained in the CNS usually are affected by any injury at the T12 level or above. This results in spastic paralysis of the affected skeletal muscle groups and the smooth and skeletal muscles that control bowel, bladder, and sexual functions. LMN injuries interrupt the peripheral sensory neurons or motoneurons that communicate with the reflex center in the spinal cord. They result in a decrease or absence of reflex function. They usually occur with injuries below T12 and result from damage to the peripheral nerves that enter or exit the spinal cord. The LMN injuries cause flaccid paralysis of involved skeletal muscle groups and the smooth and skeletal muscles that control bowel, bladder, and sexual function. However, injuries near the T12 level may result in mixed UMN and LMN deficits (*e.g.,* spastic paralysis of the bowel and bladder with flaccid muscle tone).

Spinal shock or *neurogenic shock* is the term used to describe the state of areflexia that occurs after cord injury.

TABLE 49-2 ✦ Functional Abilities by Level of Cord Injury

Injury Level	Segmental Sensorimotor Function	Dressing, Eating	Elimination	Mobility*
C1	Little or no sensation or control of head and neck; no diaphragm control; requires continuous ventilation	Dependent	Dependent	Limited. Voice or sip-n-puff controlled electric wheelchair
C2 to C3	Head and neck sensation; some neck control. Independent of mechanical ventilation for short periods	Dependent	Dependent	Same as for C1
C4	Good head and neck sensation and motor control; some shoulder elevation; diaphragm movement	Dependent; may be able to eat with adaptive sling	Dependent	Limited to voice, mouth, head, chin, or shoulder-controlled electric wheelchair
C5	Full head and neck control; shoulder strength; elbow flexion	Independent with assistance	Maximal assistance	Electric or modified manual wheel chair, needs transfer assistance
C6	Fully innervated shoulder; wrist extension or dorsiflexion	Independent or with minimal assistance	Independent or with minimal assistance	Independent in transfers and wheelchair
C7 to C8	Full elbow extension; wrist plantar flexion; some finger control	Independent	Independent	Independent; manual wheelchair
T1 to T5	Full hand and finger control; use of intercostal and thoracic muscles	Independent	Independent	Independent; manual wheelchair
T6 to T10	Abdominal muscle control, partial to good balance with trunk muscles	Independent	Independent	Independent; manual wheelchair
T11 to L5	Hip flexors, hip abductors (L1–3); knee extension (L2–4); knee flexion and ankle dorsiflexion (L4–5)	Independent	Independent	Short distance to full ambulation with assistance
S1 to S5	Full leg, foot, and ankle control; innervation of perineal muscles for bowel, bladder, and sexual function (S2–4)	Independent	Normal to impaired bowel and bladder function	Ambulate independently with or without assistance

*Assistance refers to adaptive equipment, setup, or physical assistance.

Spinal shock involves the loss of all or most of the spinal cord reflexes below the level of injury.[47] It involves the motor pathways that control skeletal muscle function, blood vessel tone, and bowel and bladder function. It is characterized by hypotension, bradycardia, hypothermia, and flaccid paralysis with loss of tendon reflexes. These manifestations occur regardless of whether the level of the lesion eventually will produce spastic (UWM) or flaccid (LMN) paralysis. The basic mechanisms accounting for transient spinal shock are unknown. Spinal shock may last for hours, days, or weeks. Usually, if reflex function returns by the time the person reaches the hospital, the neuromuscular changes are reversible. This type of reversible spinal shock may occur in football-type injuries, in which jarring of the spinal cord produces a concussion-like syndrome with loss of movement and reflexes, followed by full recovery within days. In persons in whom the loss of reflexes persists, hypotension and bradycardia may become critical but manageable problems. In general, the higher the level of injury, the greater is the effect.

Ventilation and Communication. Ventilation requires movement of the expiratory and inspiratory muscles, all of which receive innervation from the spinal cord. The main muscle of ventilation, the diaphragm, is innervated by segments C3 to C5 through the phrenic nerves. The intercostal muscles, located between the ribs, are innervated by spinal segments T1 through T7. These muscles function in elevating the rib cage and are needed for coughing and deep breathing. The major muscles of expiration are the

Spastic Versus Flaccid Paralysis

➤ Afferent input from stretch receptors located in muscles and joints is incorporated into spinal cord reflexes that control muscle tone. The activity of the spinal cord reflexes that control muscle tone is constantly monitored and regulated by input from higher brain centers.

➤ Upper motor neuron lesions that interrupt communication between the spinal cord reflexes and higher brain centers result in unregulated reflex activity, increased muscle tone, and spastic paralysis.

➤ Lower motor neuron lesions that interrupt communication between the muscle and the spinal cord reflex result in a loss of reflex activity, decreased or absent muscle tone, and flaccid paralysis.

abdominal muscles, which receive their innervation from levels T6 to T12. By forcing the abdominal viscera against the diaphragm, the muscles exert pressure on the diaphragm and return the thoracic cage to its resting position. Coughing and deep breathing, which are vital to the removal of mucus and foreign particles from the respiratory tract, are facilitated by the elevation of the rib cage and expansion of the anteroposterior and lateral dimensions of the chest wall, followed by strong respiratory and abdominal muscle contraction forcing air out of the lungs.

Although the ability to inhale and exhale may be preserved at various levels of SCI, functional deficits in ventilation are most apparent in the quality of the breathing cycle and the ability to oxygenate tissues, eliminate carbon dioxide, and mobilize secretions. Cord injuries involving C1 to C3 result in a lack of respiratory effort, and affected patients require assisted ventilation. Although a C3 to C5 injury allows partial or full diaphragmatic function, ventilation is diminished because of the loss of intercostal muscle function, resulting in shallow breaths and a weak cough. Below the C5 level, as less intercostal and abdominal musculature is affected, the ability to take a deep breath and cough is less impaired. Maintenance therapy consists of muscle training to strengthen existing muscles for endurance and mobilization of secretions.

With assisted ventilation, whether continuous or intermittent, ensuring adequate communication of needs also is essential. There are several ways of ensuring communication of needs with the use of verbal or nonverbal communication systems. Verbal approaches may consist of fenestrated tracheal tubes to provide air flow and vibration of the vocal cords, talking tracheostomy tubes, diaphragmatic pacing, electrolarynx-type devices, and mechanical ventilation with an air leak. Nonverbal communication techniques include boards or cards displaying the person's most frequently used words, computerized scanning programs, and mouth-stick–controlled devices.

Autonomic Nervous System. Spinal cord injury not only interrupts the function of the somatic nerves that control skeletal muscle function, it interrupts visceral afferent input and autonomic outflow from below the site of injury. This affects parasympathetic outflow from the sacral segments of the spinal cord and the sympathetic outflow from the thoracic and lumbar segments. After SCI, the spinal reflex circuits are largely isolated from the rest of the CNS. Afferent somatic and visceral sensory input that enters the spinal cord through intact segmental nerves is unaffected. Likewise, the efferent outflow from intact reflex centers below the site of injury is largely unaffected. However, the transmission of ascending sensory input to higher centers and descending motor control output from higher centers is blocked at the site of injury. Lacking is the regulation and integration of reflex function from higher autonomic and motor control centers in the brain and brain stem. Interruption of autonomic outflow results in continued function above the level of injury, but the spinal and autonomic reflexes below the level of injury are uncontrolled.

In persons in whom high-level paraplegia or tetraplegia persists beyond the first few hours or days after injury, hypotension and bradycardia may be critical but manageable problems. Circulatory function is impaired by the loss of sympathetic control of heart rate, peripheral vascular resistance, and lack of muscle tone in paralyzed limbs, resulting in sluggish circulating blood flow and venous return. The resulting bradycardia and hypotension usually can be managed with slow fluid resuscitation and body positioning that facilitates venous return. Spinal shock and true hemorrhagic shock (*i.e.*, hypotension and tachycardia) must be differentiated and treated accordingly. Spinal shock usually is self-limited, and the return of reflexes usually occurs in a caudal to rostral direction, with the first returning reflexes being those in the sacral area (*i.e.*, rectal sphincter contraction) followed by those of the lumbar area (*i.e.*, the lower extremities). However, bradycardia and hypotension may persist and become asymptomatic normal parameters. The length of time that it takes to adjust to the altered circulatory status is variable and may be as long as 1 year.

The autonomic regulation of circulatory function and thermoregulation present the most severe problems in SCI. The higher level of injury and the greater the surface area affected, the more profound are the effects on circulation and thermoregulation. Persons with injury at the T6 level or above experience problems in regulating vasomotor tone; those with injuries below the T6 level usually have sufficient sympathetic function to maintain adequate vasomotor function. The level of injury and its corresponding problems may vary among persons and situations, and some dysfunctional effects may be seen at levels below T6. With lower lumbar and sacral injuries, sympathetic function remains essentially unaltered.

The Vasovagal Response. The vagus nerve (cranial nerve X) normally exerts a continuous inhibitory effect on heart rate. Vagal stimulation that causes a marked bradycardia by way of the vagus nerve is called the *vasovagal response.* Visceral afferent input to the vagal centers in the brain stem of persons with tetraplegia or high-level paraplegia can produce marked bradycardia when unchecked by a dysfunctional sympathetic nervous system. Severe bradycardia and even asystole can result when the vasovagal response is elicited by deep endotracheal suctioning or rapid position change. Preventive measures, such as hyperoxygenation before, during, and after suctioning, are advised. Rapid position changes should be avoided or anticipated, and anticholinergic drugs should be immediately available to counteract severe episodes of bradycardia.

Autonomic Dysreflexia. The terms *autonomic dysreflexia* and *autonomic hyperreflexia* refer to an acute episode of exaggerated sympathetic reflex responses that occur in persons with SCI because of a lack of control from higher brain centers. This exaggerated response usually is caused by visceral stimuli that normally cause pain or discomfort in the abdominopelvic region. Autonomic dysreflexia does not occur until spinal shock has resolved and autonomic reflexes return, most often within the first 6 months after injury. It is most unpredictable during the first year after injury but can occur throughout the person's lifetime.

Autonomic dysreflexia usually is characterized by hypertension ranging from mild (20 mm Hg above baseline) to severe (as high as 240/120 mm Hg or higher), bradycardia, and headache ranging from dull to severe and pounding.[13] The condition is associated with injuries at T6 and above. Usually, persons with injuries at the T6 level or below have sufficient sympathetic outflow to control visceral reflexes. In persons with injuries at T6 or above, sympathetic responses that occur at and below that level of the spinal cord are lost, whereas baroreceptor function and parasympathetic control of heart rate remain intact. Unregulated sympathetic activity below the level of injury causes vasospasm, hypertension, skin pallor, and gooseflesh associated with the piloerector response. Continued hypertension produces a baroreflex-mediated vagal slowing of the heart rate to bradycardic levels. There is an accompanying baroreflex-mediated vasodilatation, flushed skin, and profuse sweating above the level of injury, along with headache, nasal stuffiness, and feelings of anxiety. A person may experience one, several, or all of the symptoms with each episode.

The stimuli initiating the dysreflexic response include visceral distention, such as a full bladder or rectum; stimulation of pain receptors, as occurs with pressure ulcers, ingrown toenails, dressing changes, and diagnostic or operative procedures; and visceral contractions, such as ejaculation, bladder spasms, or uterine contractions. In many cases, the dysreflexic response results from a full bladder.

Autonomic dysreflexia is a clinical emergency, and without prompt and adequate treatment, convulsions, loss of consciousness, and even death can occur. The major components of treatment include monitoring blood pressure while removing or correcting the initiating cause or stimulus. The person should be placed in an upright position, and all support hose or binders should be removed to promote venous pooling of blood and reduce venous re-turn, thereby decreasing blood pressure. If the stimuli have been removed or the stimuli cannot be identified and the upright position is established, but the blood pressure remains elevated, drugs that block autonomic function are administered. Persons should be monitored for several hours after the dysreflexic event. Prevention of the type of stimuli that trigger the dysreflexic event is advocated.

Postural Hypotension. Postural, or orthostatic, hypotension usually occurs in persons with injuries at T4 to T6 and above and is related to the interruption of descending control of sympathetic outflow to blood vessels in the extremities and abdomen. Pooling of blood, along with gravitational forces, impairs venous return to the heart, and there is a subsequent decrease in cardiac output when the person is placed in an upright position. This usually occurs when the person is placed in the seated position in bed or transferred from the bed to the wheelchair. The signs of orthostatic hypotension include dizziness, pallor, excessive sweating above the level of the lesion, complaints of blurred vision, and possibly fainting. Because of the disruption in autonomic function at the time of injury, the blood pressure and heart rate already may be low but not produce symptoms. Postural hypotension usually is prevented by slow changes in position and measures to promote venous return.

Temperature Regulation. The central mechanisms for thermoregulation are located in the hypothalamus. In response to cold, the hypothalamus stimulates vasoconstrictor responses in peripheral blood vessels, particularly those of the skin. This results in decreased loss of body heat. Heat production results from increased metabolism, voluntary activity, or shivering. Shivering can almost double the heat production of the body. To reduce heat, hypothalamus-stimulated mechanisms produce vasodilatation of skin blood vessels to dissipate heat and sweating to increase evaporative heat losses.

After SCI, the communication between the thermoregulatory centers in the hypothalamus and the sympathetic effector responses below the level of injury is disrupted; the ability to control blood vessel responses that conserve or dissipate heat is lost, as are the abilities to sweat and shiver. Higher levels of injury tend to produce greater disturbances in thermoregulation. In tetraplegia and high paraplegia, there are few defenses against changes in the environmental temperature, and body temperature tends to assume the temperature of the external environment, a condition known as *poikilothermy.* Persons with lower-level injuries have various degrees of thermoregulation. Disturbances in thermoregulation are chronic and may cause continual loss of body heat. Treatment consists of education in the adjustment of clothing and awareness of how environmental temperatures affect the person's ability to accommodate these changes.

Edema and Deep Vein Thrombosis. Edema and deep vein thrombosis are common problems in persons with SCI. The development of edema is related to decreased peripheral vascular resistance, areflexia or decreased tone in the paralyzed limbs, and immobility that causes increased venous pressure and abnormal pooling of blood in the abdomen, lower limbs, and upper extremities. Orthostatic or dependent edema in the dependent body parts usually is relieved by positioning to minimize gravitational forces or by using compression devices (*e.g.*, support stockings, binders) that encourage venous return.

Deep vein thrombosis also is of concern because of the venous pooling and loss of movement below the level of injury. Although it is seen more frequently in the postacute phase of SCI, it often has its origin during the events surrounding the initial injury. Prevention includes low-dose heparin, measures to prevent venous pooling of blood, especially in the paralyzed limbs (*e.g.*, range of motion and vascular compression devices), and assessment of risk and presence of deep vein thrombosis beginning immediately after injury.

Sensorimotor Function. After the period of spinal shock in a UMN injury, isolated spinal reflex activity and muscle tone that is not under the control of higher centers returns. This may result in hypertonia and spasticity of skeletal muscles below the level of injury, where the normal communication pathways to higher centers for voluntary motor control have been interrupted by the spinal cord lesion. These spastic movements are involuntary instead of voluntary, a distinction that needs to be explained to the spinal cord–injured person and his or her family members. Spastic movements in flexor and extensor patterns, which occur below the level of injury, can be tonic (sustained tone) or clonic (intermittent) and usually are heightened initially after injury, reaching a peak and then becoming stable in approximately 2 years, with further exacerbations caused by other medical conditions.

These movements occur in most spinal injuries above the T12 level in which the stretch reflex arc is preserved. In injuries at T12 or below, the reflex response itself is damaged at the cord or spinal nerve level, preventing spasticity. Spasticity in and of itself is not detrimental to the spinal cord–injured person and may even facilitate maintenance of muscle tone to prevent muscle wasting, improve venous return, and aid in mobility. Spasms become detrimental when they impair safety; reduce the ability to make functional gains in mobility and activities of daily living, such as feeding, dressing, and toileting; and affect vocational and avocational interests. Spasms also may cause trauma to bones and tissues, leading to joint contractures and skin breakdown.

The stimuli for reflex muscle spasm arise from somatic and visceral afferent pathways that enter the cord below the level of injury. The most common of these stimuli are muscle stretching, bladder infections or stones, fistulas, bowel distention or impaction, pressure areas or irritation of the skin, and infections. Because the stimuli that precipitate spasms vary from person to person, careful assessment needs to be done to identify the factors that precipitate spasm in each person. Passive range-of-motion exercises to stretch spastic muscles should be done twice a day, avoiding stimuli that elicit spasm. Antispasmodic medications (*e.g.*, baclofen, dantrium) may be warranted and need to be carefully monitored for effectiveness.[13]

Skin Integrity. The entire surface of the skin is innervated by cranial or spinal nerves organized into dermatomes that show cutaneous distribution. The central and autonomic nervous systems also play a vital role in skin function. Impulses from the peripheral nervous system carry sensory information to the brain and receive information for motor control and reflex activity at each dermatome.

The sympathetic nervous system, through control of vasomotor and sweat gland activity, influences the health of the skin by providing adequate circulation, excretion of body fluids, and temperature regulation. The lack of sensory warning mechanisms and voluntary motor ability below the level of injury, coupled with circulatory changes, place the spinal cord–injured person at major risk for disruption of skin integrity. Significant factors associated with disruption of skin integrity are pressure, shearing forces, and localized trauma and irritation. Relieving pressure, allowing adequate circulation to the skin, and skin inspection are primary ways of maintaining skin integrity. Of all the complications after SCI, skin breakdown is the most preventable.

Pain. Pain after SCI is a diverse and unpredictable experience that, for some persons, can be severe.[48] Initially, pain arises from soft tissues such as the skin, muscles, and joint structures and from fractures and dislocations of bony elements. With healing or decompression of neurologic tissue, much of the pain associated with the injury resolves. For many persons, however, chronic pain syndromes develop. Chronic pain is more common among persons with paraplegia than those with tetraplegia.[48] The mechanisms of drug action and specifics of chronic pain management are discussed in Chapter 48.

Four types of pain syndromes occur after SCI: mechanical, radicular, visceral, and central.[48] Mechanical or fracture pain usually occurs at the level of injury, is related to soft tissue damage, and most commonly is due to damaged facet joints or spinal fracture. It is dull, aching, and often aggravated by movement. Radicular (spinal nerve root) pain presents as an aching or shooting pain that radiates into a more-or-less well-defined nerve root distribution affecting the arm, leg, or trunk. Although the pain occurs in its severest form with incomplete spinal cord lesions, it also occurs with transected cauda equina lesions. The cause of radicular pain is obscure, but it may result from compression or injury of nerve roots by a herniated nucleus pulposus, a fracture fragment, or a dislocated vertebra, or from neuronal hyperexcitability due to local ischemia. Visceral pain involves a poorly localized, burning discomfort of the abdomen and pelvis. It often is related to some intra-abdominal event such as bladder distention or urinary tract infection. It is thought that the cause of visceral pain may be similar to that of central pain. Central pain is a diffuse burning sensation that is experienced in body parts below the level of injury and is aggravated by touch, movement, and visceral distention. The mechanism of central pain is possibly an abnormal firing of deafferented input association or projection neurons. Because this type of pain has resulted from loss of normal sensory input, it often is called *deafferentation* pain.

Bladder Function. Among the most devastating consequences of SCI is the loss of bowel and bladder function. Loss of these functions is apparent immediately after injury and requires much time, expense, material, and human energy for management.

Micturition, or the act of voiding, can be described as the sequence of events involving sensory input that occurs with bladder filling, activation of the spinal reflex voiding center, stimulation and provision of cerebral control, and progression and termination of actual voiding. Although the anatomy and function of the kidneys or production of urine is not greatly altered after SCI, most affected persons experience some loss of bladder function. The physiology of micturition and neurogenic disorders of bladder function are further discussed in Chapter 35.

After resolution of spinal shock, which renders the bladder areflexic, bladder dysfunction is manifested by the disruption of neural pathways between the bladder and the reflex voiding center (*i.e.*, an LMN lesion) or between the reflex voiding center and higher brain centers for communication and coordinated sphincter control (*i.e.*, a UMN lesion). Persons with UMN lesions or spastic bladders lack awareness of bladder filling (*i.e.*, storage) and voluntary control of voiding (*i.e.*, evacuation). In LMN lesions or flaccid bladder dysfunction, lack of awareness of bladder filling and lack of bladder tone render the person unable to void voluntarily or involuntarily. Of specific importance to optimal bladder function is the storage and evacuation of urine under low pressure to prevent damage to the bladder, urethra, and kidneys.

The principal goals of bladder management are to provide low-pressure drainage to the urinary bladder and prevent complications, with consideration of the person's lifestyle, the potential for his or her cooperation, and the degree of support from family and community. Management of neurogenic bladder dysfunction consists of methods of continuous or intermittent drainage, external collection, and manual techniques (*e.g.*, Crede's maneuver, Valsalva's maneuver, bladder tapping).

Bowel Elimination. Bowel elimination is a coordinated function involving the enteric nervous system, the autonomic nervous system, and the CNS. The enteric nervous system consists of a network of nerve fibers in the bowel wall that respond to fecal distention with increased peristalsis. As with micturition, parasympathetic fibers from the S2 to S4 segments of the spinal cord travel by way of the pelvic nerve to innervate the colon, rectum, and internal anal sphincter. Somatic innervation from the same cord segments travels by way of the pudendal nerve to provide for voluntary control of the striated muscles of the external anal sphincter. Parasympathetic stimulation produces an increase in intestinal motility and a decrease in internal sphincter tone. Sympathetic outflow from the thoracic and lumbar segments (T6 to L3) of the spinal cord has the opposite effect, producing a decrease in intestinal motility and an increase in internal sphincter tone. Persons with SCI above S2 to S4 develop spastic functioning of the defecation reflex and loss of voluntary control of the external anal sphincter. Damage to the cord at the S2 to S4

level causes flaccid functioning of the defecation reflex and loss of anal sphincter tone. Even though intrinsic contractile responses are intact, without the defecation reflex, peristaltic movements are ineffective in evacuating stool.

The goal of bowel management after SCI is to establish complete evacuations, which minimize incontinence and complications and afford dignity and independence to the person. The principal methods of bowel management include measures such as a high-fluid and high-fiber diet, mobility at the highest level that is possible, consistent timing of evacuation, privacy, positioning, and chemical (laxatives), mechanical (digital stimulation), and other stimulants (Valsalva's maneuver, peristaltic stimulators).

Sexual Function. Although the physical act of sex itself may change with SCI, the ability to enjoy a sexual and caring relationship with another person remains and can take on greater importance than before injury.

Spinal cord injury at any level abolishes communication pathways between the genital and higher centers. Erotic and emotional feelings and thoughts, however, may still be experienced in areas above the level of injury, especially when the mouth and neck are stimulated. Extragenital circulatory, musculoskeletal, and respiratory responses, such as increased heart rate, breathing, and muscle tone, that are mediated by centers above the level of injury may occur.

Sexual function, as in bladder and bowel control, is mediated by the S2 to S4 segments of the spinal cord. The genital sexual response in SCI, which is manifested by an erection in men and vaginal lubrication in women, may be initiated by mental or touch stimuli, depending on the level of injury. The T11 to L2 cord segments have been identified as the mental-stimuli, or psychogenic, sexual response area, where autonomic nerve pathways in communication with the forebrain leave the cord and innervate the genitalia. The S2 to S4 cord segments have been identified as the sexual-touch, or reflexogenic, reflex center. In T10 or higher injuries (UMN lesion), reflex sexual response to genital touch may occur freely. However, a sexual response to mental stimuli (T11 to L2) does not occur because of the spinal lesion blocking the communication pathway. In an injury at T12 or below (LMN lesion), the sexual reflex center may be damaged, and there may be no response to touch.

In men, the lack of erectile ability or inability to experience penile sensations or orgasm is not a reliable indicator of fertility, which should be evaluated by an expert. In women, fertility is parallel to menses; usually, it is delayed 3 months to 5 months after injury. There are hazards to pregnancy, labor, and birth control devices relative to SCI that require knowledgeable health care providers but need not be prohibitive.

In summary, upper motoneuron lesions are those involving neurons that are fully contained in the CNS. MS is an example of a demyelinating disease in which there is a slowly progressive breakdown of myelin and formation of plaques but sparing of the axis cylinder of the neuron. The cause of MS remains unknown. Geographic distributions and migration studies suggest an environmental influence. Interruption of neural conduction in MS is manifested by a variety of disabling signs and symptoms that depend on the neurons that are affected. The most common symptoms are paresthesias, optic neuritis, and motor weakness. The disease usually is characterized by exacerbations and remissions. Initially, near-normal function returns between exacerbations. The variety of symptoms, course of the disease, and lack of specific diagnostic tests make diagnosis and treatment of the disease difficult. Treatment is largely symptomatic.

Spinal cord injury is a disabling neurologic condition most commonly caused by motor vehicle accidents, falls, and sports injuries. It occurs most frequently in males and in persons younger than 30 years of age. SCI is caused by abnormal motion or trauma to the spinal column, including injuries caused by excessive forward flexion and lateral bending, rotation, and extension of the spinal column. Dysfunctions of the nervous system after SCI comprise various degrees of sensorimotor loss and altered reflex activity based on the level of injury and extent of cord damage. Depending on the level of injury, the physical problems of SCI include spinal shock; ventilation and communication problems; autonomic nervous system dysfunction that predisposes to the vasovagal response, autonomic hyperreflexia, impaired body temperature regulation, and postural hypotension; impaired muscle pump and venous innervation leading to edema of dependent areas of the body and risk of deep vein thrombosis; altered sensorimotor integrity that contributes to uncontrolled muscle spasms, altered pain responses, and threat to skin integrity; alterations in bowel and bladder elimination; and impaired sexual function. The treatment of SCI involves a continuum of care that begins at the moment of injury and continues throughout the person's life.

Related Web Sites

American Parkinson Disease Association
    www.apdaparkinson.com
National Institute of Neurological Disorders and Stroke
    www.ninds.nih.gov
National Multiple Sclerosis Society   www.nmss.org
Spinal Cord Injury Information Center—link to National Spinal
    Cord Injury Statistical Center   www.spinalcord.uab.edu

References

1. Kandel E.R., Schwartz J.H., Jessell T.M. (2000). *Principles of neural science* (4th ed., pp. 816–831). New York: McGraw-Hill.
2. Guyton A., Hall J.E. (2000). *Medical physiology* (10th ed., pp. 634–637, 973). Philadelphia: W.B. Saunders.
3. Conn M.P. (1995). *Neuroscience in medicine* (pp. 312–317). Philadelphia: J.B. Lippincott.
4. Penfield W., Rasmussen T. (1950). *The cerebral cortex of man.* New York: Macmillan.
5. Cotran R.S., Kumar V., Collins T. (1999). *Robbins pathologic basis of disease* (6th ed., pp. 1275–1276, 1281–1282, 1289, 1326–1328). Philadelphia: W.B. Saunders.
6. Sarnat H.B. (2000). Muscular dystrophies. In Behrman R.E., Kliegman R.M., Jenson H.B. (Eds.), *Nelson textbook of pediatrics* (16th ed., pp. 1873–1877). Philadelphia: W.B. Saunders.
7. Berne R.M., Levy M.N. (2000). *Principles of physiology* (p. 43). St. Louis: Mosby.
8. Katzung B.G. (2001). *Basic and clinical pharmacology* (8th ed., pp. 92–102). New York: Lange Medical Books/McGraw-Hill.
9. Drachman D.B. (1994). Myasthenia gravis. *New England Journal of Medicine* 330, 1797–1810.
10. LaPate G., Pestronk A. (1993). Autoimmune myasthenia gravis. *Hospital Practice* 28 (1A), 109–131.
11. Wittbrodt E.T. (1997). Drugs and myasthenia gravis. *Archives of Internal Medicine* 157, 399–408.
12. Bedlack R.S., Sanders D.B. (2000). How to handle myasthenic crisis. *Postgraduate Medicine* 10, 211–222.
13. Hickey J.V. (1997). *Neurological and neurosurgical nursing* (4th ed., pp. 419–465, 469–480). Philadelphia: Lippincott-Raven.
14. Acute Low Back Problems Guideline Panel. (1994). *Acute low back problems in adults: Assessment and treatment.* AHCPR publication no. 95-0642. Rockville, MD: Agency for Health Care Policy and Research, Public Health Service, U.S. Department of Health and Human Services.
15. Dawson D.M. (1993). Entrapment neuropathies of the upper extremities. *New England Journal of Medicine* 329, 2013–2018.
16. Dawson D.M. (1995). Entrapment neuropathies: Clinical overview. *Hospital Practice* 30 (8), 37–44.
17. Hughes R.A.C. (1992). The management of Guillain-Barré syndrome. *Hospital Practice* 27 (3A), 107–125.
18. Langmuir A.D., Bregman D.J., Nathanson N., Victor M. (1984). An epidemic and clinical evaluation of Guillain-Barré syndrome reported in association of swine influenza vaccines. *American Journal of Epidemiology* 119, 841–879.
19. Rees J.H., Saudain S.E., Gregson N.A., Hughes R.A.C. (1995). *Campylobacter jejuni* infection and Guillain-Barré syndrome. *New England Journal of Medicine* 333, 1374–1379.
20. Ropper A.H. (1992). The Guillain-Barré syndrome. *New England Journal of Medicine* 326, 10–16.
21. Haines D. (Ed.). (1997). *Fundamental neuroscience* (p. 372). New York: Churchill Livingstone.
22. Ng D.C. (1996). Parkinson's disease: Diagnosis and treatment. *Western Journal of Medicine* 165, 234–240.
23. Silverstein P.M. (1996). Moderate Parkinson's disease. *Postgraduate Medicine* 99 (1), 53–68.
24. Parkinson J. (1817). *An essay on the shaking palsy.* London: Sherwood, Nelley & Jones.
25. Youdim M.B.H., Riederer P. (1997). Understanding Parkinson's disease. *Scientific American* 276, 52–59.
26. Rubin E., Farber J.L. (1999). *Pathology* (3rd ed., pp. 1496–1498, 1502–1505). Philadelphia: Lippincott Williams & Wilkins.
27. Lücking C.B., Dürr A., Bonifati V., Vaughn J., DeMichele G., Gasser T., et al. (European Consortium on Genetic Susceptibility in Parkinson's Disease Genetic Study Group). (2000). Association between early-onset Parkinson's disease and mutations in the Parkin gene. *New England Journal of Medicine* 342, 1560–1567.
28. Colcher A., Simuni T. (1999). Clinical manifestations of Parkinson's disease. *Medical Clinics of North America* 83, 327–347.

29. Young R. (1999). Update on Parkinson's disease. *American Family Physician* 59 (8), 2155–2167.

30. Freed C.R., Greene P.E., Breeze R.E., Tsai W., DuMouchel W., Dillon S., Winfield H., Culver S., Trojanowski J.O., Eidelberg D., Fahn S. (2001). Transplantation of embryonic dopamine neurons for severe Parkinson's disease. *New England Journal of Medicine* 344, 710–719.

31. Mackin G.A. (1999). Optimizing care of patients with ALS. *Postgraduate Medicine* 105 (4), 143–146.

32. Rowland L.P., Shneider N.A. (2001). Amyotropic lateral sclerosis. *New England Journal of Medicine* 344, 1688–1700.

33. Walling A.D. (1999). Amyotropic lateral sclerosis: Lou Gehrig's disease. *American Family Practitioner* 59 (6), 1489–1496.

34. Noseworthy J.H., Lucchinett C., Rodrequez M., Weinshenker B.G. (2000). Multiple sclerosis. *New England Journal of Medicine* 343, 938–952.

35. Anderson D.W., Ellenberg J.H., Leventhal C.M., Reingold S.C., Rodreguez M., Silberberg D.H. (1992). Revised estimate of multiple sclerosis in the United States. *Annals of Neurology* 31, 333–336.

36. Lublin F.D., Reingold S.C. (1996). Defining the clinical course of multiple sclerosis: Results of an international survey. *Neurology* 46, 907–911.

37. Rudick R.A., Cohen J.A., Weinstock-Guttman B., Kinkel R.P., Ransohoff R.M. (1997). Management of multiple sclerosis. *New England Journal of Medicine* 337, 1604–1611.

38. Brod S.A., Lindsey W., Wolinsky J.S. (1996). Multiple sclerosis: Clinical presentation, diagnosis and treatment. *American Family Physician* 54, 1301–1311.

39. National Spinal Cord Injury Statistical Center. (2001). Spinal cord injury: Facts and figures at a glance. Birmingham: University of Alabama. [On-line]. Available: http://www.spinalcord.uab.edu.

40. American Spinal Injury Association. (1992). *Standards of neurological and functional classification of spinal cord injury.* Chicago: American Spinal Cord Injury Association.

41. Buckley D.A., Guanci M.K. (1999). Spinal cord trauma. *Nursing Clinics of North America* 34, 661–687.

42. Chiles B.W., Cooper P.R. (1996). Acute spinal cord injury. *New England Journal of Medicine* 334, 514–520.

43. Fehling M.G., Louw D. (1996). Initial stabilization and medical management of acute spinal cord injury. *American Family Physician* 42, 155–162.

44. Tator C.H., Fehlings M.G. (1999). Review of clinical trials in neuroprotection in acute spinal cord injury. *Neurosurgical Focus* 6 (1), 1–14.

45. Bracken M.B., Shepard M.J., Collins W.F., Holford T.R., Young W., Haskin D.S., Eisenberg H.M., Flamm E., Leo-Summers L., Maroon J., et al. (1990). A randomized, controlled trial of methylprednisolone or naloxone in the treatment of acute spinal-cord injury: Results of the Second National Acute Spinal Cord Injury Study. *New England Journal of Medicine* 322, 1405–1411.

46. Bracken M.B., Shepard M.J., Collins W.F., Holford T.R., Leo-Summers L., Aldrich E.F., Fazl M., Fehlings M., Herr D.L., et al. (1997). Administration of methylprednisolone for 24 or 48 hours or tirilazad mesylate for 48 hours in the treatment of acute spinal cord injury: Results of the Third National Acute Spinal Cord Injury Study. *Journal of the American Medical Association* 277, 1597–1604.

47. Atkinson P.P., Atkinson J.L.D. (1996). Spinal shock. *Mayo Clinic Proceedings* 71, 384–389.

48. Woolsey R.M. (1986). Chronic pain following spinal cord injury. *Paraplegia* 9 (3–4), 39–41.

Disorders of Brain Function

Diane Book

The brain is protected from external forces by the rigid confines of the skull and the cushioning afforded by the cerebrospinal fluid (CSF). The metabolic stability required by its electrically active cells is maintained by a number of regulatory mechanisms, including the blood-brain barrier and autoregulatory mechanisms that ensure its blood supply. Nonetheless, the brain remains remarkably vulnerable to injury by ischemia, trauma, tumors, degenerative processes, and metabolic derangements.

Mechanisms and Manifestations of Brain Injury

After you have completed this section of the chapter, you should be able to meet the following objectives:

✦ Differentiate cerebral hypoxia from cerebral ischemia and focal from global ischemia

✦ Compare cytotoxic, vasogenic, and interstitial cerebral edema

+ Characterize the role of excitatory amino acids as a common pathway for neurologic disorders
+ State the determinants of intracranial pressure and describe compensatory mechanisms used to prevent large changes in intracranial pressure when there are changes in brain, blood, and cerebrospinal fluid volumes
+ Draw a pressure-volume curve and explain the relation between a change in intracranial volume and intracranial pressure
+ Explain the causes of tentorial herniation of the brain and its consequences
+ Compare the causes of communicating and non-communicating hydrocephalus
+ Define consciousness and trace the rostral-to-caudal progression of consciousness in terms of pupillary changes, respiration, and motor function as the effects of brain dysfunction progress to involve structures in the diencephalon, midbrain, pons, and medulla
+ State two criteria for the diagnosis of brain death

MECHANISMS OF INJURY

Injury to brain tissue can result from a number of conditions, including trauma, tumors, stroke, metabolic derangements, and degenerative disorders. Brain damage resulting from these disorders involves several common pathways, including the effects of ischemia, excitatory amino acid injury, cerebral edema, and injury due to increased intracranial pressure (ICP). In many cases, the mechanisms of injury are interrelated.

Hypoxic and Ischemic Injury

The energy requirements of the brain are provided mainly by adenosine triphosphate (ATP); the ability of the cerebral circulation to deliver oxygen in sufficiently high concentrations to facilitate metabolism of glucose and generate ATP is essential to brain function. Although the brain makes up only 2% of the body weight, it receives one sixth of the resting cardiac output and accounts for 20% of the oxygen consumption.[1] It follows that deprivation of oxygen or blood flow can have a deleterious effect on brain structures.

By definition, *hypoxia* denotes a deprivation of oxygen with maintained blood flow; *ischemia* is a situation of greatly reduced or interrupted blood flow. Hypoxia usually is seen in conditions such as exposure to reduced atmospheric pressure, carbon monoxide poisoning, severe anemia, and failure to oxygenate the blood. Because hypoxia indicates decreased oxygen levels in the tissue, it produces a generalized depressant effect on the brain. The cellular pathophysiologies of hypoxia and ischemia are quite different, and the brain tends to have different sensitivities to the two conditions. Contrary to popular belief, hypoxia is fairly well tolerated, particularly in situations of chronic hypoxia. Neurons are capable of substantial anaerobic metabolism and fairly tolerant of pure hypoxia; it commonly produces euphoria, listlessness, drowsiness, and impaired problem solving. Unconsciousness and convulsions may occur when hypoxia is sudden and severe. However, the effects of severe hypoxia (*i.e.*, anoxia) on brain function

seldom are seen because the condition rapidly leads to cardiac arrest and ischemia.

Ischemia can be focal, as in stroke, or global, as in cardiac arrest. Persons with global ischemia have no collateral circulation during the ischemic event. In contrast, collateral circulation may provide low levels of blood flow during focal ischemia. The residual perfusion may provide sufficient substrates to maintain a low level of metabolic activity, thereby preserving membrane integrity. At the same time, the delivery of glucose under these anaerobic conditions may result in additional lactic acid production and worsening of lactic acidosis.[2]

Global Ischemia. Global ischemia occurs when blood flow is inadequate to meet the metabolic needs of the entire brain, as in cardiac arrest or circulatory shock. The result is a spectrum of neurologic disorders. Unconsciousness occurs within seconds of severe global ischemia, such as that resulting from complete cessation of blood flow, as in cardiac arrest, or with marked decrease in blood flow, as in serious cardiac dysrhythmias. If circulation is restored immediately, consciousness is regained quickly. However, if blood flow is not promptly restored, severe pathologic changes take place. Energy sources, glucose and glycogen, are exhausted in 2 to 4 minutes, and cellular ATP stores are depleted in 4 to 5 minutes. Approximately 50% to 75% of the total energy requirement of neuronal tissue is spent on mechanisms for maintenance of ionic gradients across the cell membrane (*e.g.*, sodium-potassium pump), resulting in fluxes of sodium, potassium, and calcium ions[3] (Table 50-1). Excessive influx of sodium results in neuronal and interstitial edema. The influx of calcium initiates a cascade of events, including release of intracellular and nuclear enzymes that cause cell destruction. When ischemia is sufficiently severe or prolonged, infarction or death of all the cellular elements of the brain occurs.

The pattern of global ischemia reflects the anatomic arrangement of the cerebral vessels and the sensitivity of various brain tissues to oxygen deprivation[4] (Fig. 50-1). Selective neuronal sensitivity to a lack of oxygen is most apparent in the Purkinje cells of the cerebellum and neurons in Sommer's sector of the hippocampus.

TABLE 50-1 ✦ Pathophysiologic Consequences of Impaired Cerebral Perfusion	
Consequences	**Timing**
Depletion of oxygen	10 sec
Depletion of glucose	2–4 min
Conversion to anaerobic metabolism	2–4 min
Exhaustion of cellular ATP	4–5 min
Consequences	
Efflux of potassium	
Influx of sodium	
Influx of calcium	

(Adapted from Richmond T.S. [1997]. Cerebral resuscitation after global brain ischemia: Linking research to practice. *AACN Clinical Issues* 8 [2], 173)

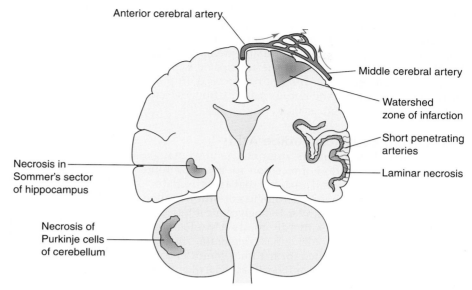

FIGURE 50-1 Consequences of global ischemia. A global insult induces lesions that reflect the vascular architecture (watershed infarcts, laminar necrosis) and the sensitivity of individual neuronal systems (pyramidal cells of Sommer's section, Purkinje cells). (Courtesy of Dmitri Karetnikov, artist). (Rubin E., Farber J.L. [1999]. *Pathology* [3rd ed., p. 1470]. Philadelphia: Lippincott Williams & Wilkins)

The anatomic arrangement of blood vessels predisposes to two types of injury: watershed infarcts and laminar necrosis. Watershed infarcts are concentrated in anatomically vulnerable border zones between the overlapping territories supplied by the major cerebral arteries, notably the middle, anterior, and posterior cerebral arteries. The overlapping territory at the distal ends of these vessels forms extremely vulnerable areas in terms of ischemia, called *watershed zones*. During events such as severe hypotension, these distal territories undergo a profound lowering of blood flow, predisposing to ischemia and infarction of brain tissues. As a consequence, areas of the cortex that are supplied by the major cerebral arteries usually regain function on recovery of adequate blood flow; however, infarctions may occur in the watershed boundary strips, resulting in focal neurologic deficits.[4]

Laminar necrosis occurs in areas supplied by the penetrating arteries. The gray matter of the cerebral cortex receives its major blood supply through short penetrating arteries that emerge at right angles from larger vessels in pia mater and then form a cascade as they repeatedly branch, forming a rich capillary network. An abrupt loss of arterial blood pressure markedly diminishes flow through these capillary channels. Because of the branching arrangement of these vessels, the necrosis that develops is laminar and is most severe in the deeper layers of the cortex.

Although the threshold for ischemic neuronal injury is unknown, there is a period during which neurons can survive if blood flow is reestablished. Unfortunately, brain injury may not be reversible if the duration of ischemia is such that the threshold of injury has been reached. Even after circulation has been reestablished, damage to blood vessels and changes in blood flow can prevent return of adequate tissue perfusion. This period of postischemic hypoperfusion is thought to be associated with mechanisms such as desaturation of venous blood, capillary and venular clotting, or sludging of blood.[2] Because of sludging, blood viscosity increases and there is increased resistance to blood flow. There is evidence of immediate vasomotor paralysis of the surface conducting blood vessels due to extracellular acidosis, followed by ischemic vasoconstriction.

Hypermetabolism due to increased circulating catecholamines also has been implicated as a contributing factor in postischemic hypoperfusion. Catecholamine release results in an increased cerebral metabolic rate and increased need for all energy-producing substrates, which the damaged brain is unable to sustain.

The neurologic deficits that result from global ischemic injury vary widely. If the period of nonflow or low flow is minimal, the neurologic damage usually is minimal to nonexistent. When the period is extensive or resuscitation is lengthy, the early neurologic clinical picture is that of fixed and dilated pupils, abnormal motor posturing, and coma. If the brain recovers, there is gradual improvement in neurologic status, although cognitive and focal deficits usually persist and can prevent a return to the preischemic level of function.

An exception to this time frame is the circumstance of cold-water drowning in which the person, especially a child, is submerged in cold water for longer than 10 minutes.[5] Hypothermia develops and reduces the cerebral metabolic requirements for oxygen; it subsequently serves as a protective mechanism for the neurons. In this case, recovery can be rapid and remarkable, and resuscitation efforts should not be discontinued precipitously.

Treatment of global ischemia is aimed at providing oxygen to the troubled brain and decreasing the metabolic needs of brain tissue during the nonflow state. Methods that decrease brain temperature as a means of decreasing brain metabolism have shown promise.[3] Normovolemic hemodilution may be used to overcome sludging of cerebral blood flow during reperfusion. Because both hypoglycemia and hyperglycemia adversely affect outcome in persons with global ischemia, control of blood glucose within a range of 100 to 200 mg/dL has been advocated.[3,6] Although several pharmacologic agents have been advocated as a means of preventing brain damage in global ischemia, none has proven to be highly effective. In the past, barbiturates were used as a means of decreasing brain metabolism. However, the beneficial effects of barbiturates are minimal unless they are administered before the anticipated ischemia (*e.g.*, before neurosurgery).[2] Interest has focused on pharmacologic agents that could minimize injury from free radicals and excitatory amino acids.

Injury From Excitatory Amino Acids

In many neurologic disorders, injury to neurons may be caused by overstimulation of receptors for specific amino acids such as glutamate and aspartate that act as excitatory neurotransmitters.[7] These neurologic conditions range from acute insults such as stroke, hypoglycemic injury, and trauma to chronic degenerative disorders such as Huntington's disease and possibly Alzheimer's dementia. The term *excitotoxicity* has been coined for the final common pathway for neuronal cell injury and death associated with excessive activity of the excitatory neurotransmitters and their receptor-mediated functions.

Glutamate is the principal excitatory neurotransmitter in the brain, and its interaction with specific receptors is responsible for many higher-order functions, including memory, cognition, movement, and sensation.[7] Many of the actions of glutamate are coupled with receptor-operated ion channels. Glutamate channels are large, complex proteins that bridge the plasma membrane and contain a central pore or channel that, when open, permits ions to diffuse across the cell membrane. One subtype in particular, called the *glutamate* N-*methyl-D-aspartate* (NMDA) receptor, has been implicated in causing central nervous system (CNS) injury. This subtype of glutamate receptor opens a large-diameter calcium channel that permits calcium and sodium ions to enter the cell and allows potassium ions to exit, resulting in prolonged (seconds) action potentials. The uncontrolled opening of NMDA receptor–operated channels produces an increase in intracellular calcium and leads to a series of calcium-mediated processes called the *calcium cascade*. Activation of the calcium cascade leads to the release of intracellular enzymes that cause protein breakdown, free radical formation, lipid peroxidation, fragmentation of DNA, and nuclear breakdown.

The intracellular concentration of glutamate is approximately 16 times that of the extracellular concentration.[7] Normally, extracellular concentrations of glutamate are tightly regulated, with excess amounts removed and actively transported into astrocytes and neurons. During prolonged ischemia, these transport mechanisms become immobilized, causing extracellular glutamate to accumulate. In the case of cell injury and death, intracellular glutamate is released from the damaged cells, causing injury to surrounding cells.

The first sign of glutamate toxicity, which develops within minutes of exposure to excessive amounts of glutamate, is neuronal swelling from the increased amounts of sodium and water entering the cell. The effects of acute toxicity do not necessarily lead to cell death; they are reversible if excess glutamate can be removed or if its effects can be blocked. Later signs of glutamate toxicity result from the effects of excessive levels of intracellular calcium. Neurons die within several hours after exposure to glutamate, at least partly depending on extracellular calcium levels and the inability of the nervous system to remove glutamate from the extracellular spaces.

Central nervous system neurons can be divided into two major categories: macroneurons and microneurons. *Macroneurons* are large cells with long axons that leave the local network of intercommunicating neurons to send action potentials to other regions of the nervous system at distances of centimeters to meters (*e.g.*, upper motoneurons that communicate with lower motoneurons that control leg movement). *Microneurons* are very small cells that are intimately involved in local circuitry. Their axons transmit action potentials to other members of the same local network. In contrast to macroneurons, which number in the thousands, microneurons account for most of the many billions of CNS neurons.

Many macroneurons use glutamate as a neurotransmitter in their excitatory communication with microneurons. Macroneurons synapse on the postsynaptic excitatory amino acid receptors of the microneurons. It is the microneuron network that provides the analytic, integrative, and learning circuitry that is the basis for the higher-order function of the CNS. The microneurons of the cerebral cortex and hippocampus are particularly vulnerable to excessive stimulation of the glutamate NMDA receptors and the neurotoxic effects of increased intracellular calcium levels. Because of their increased vulnerability, many of the small interneurons that make up essential parts of the complex control and memory functions of the brain are selectively damaged, even if the remainder of the brain survives the insult. This pattern may account for the long-term effects of brain insult, which frequently include subtle and noticeable reductions in cognitive and memory functions.

Research is being directed toward attenuating or preventing the accumulation and injurious effects of excitatory amino acids. These pharmacologic strategies, called *neuroprotectants*, may protect viable brain cells from irreversible damage in the setting of excitotoxicity. Some pharmacologic methods being explored block the synthesis or release of excitatory amino acid transmitters; block the NMDA receptors; stabilize the membrane potential to prevent initiation of the calcium cascade using lidocaine and certain barbiturates; and specifically block certain intracellular proteases, endonucleases, and lipases that are known to be cytotoxic.[8,9] Animal studies and human clinical trials are underway looking for methods of preventing brain damage from excitatory amino acids. The drug riluzole, which acts presynaptically to inhibit glutamate release, is used in the treatment of amyotrophic lateral sclerosis (see Chapter 49). Nimodipine, a calcium channel blocker that acts at the level of the NMDA receptor–operated channels, is being investigated for use in subarachnoid hemorrhage and acquired immunodeficiency syndrome dementia.[7] In the setting of ischemic stroke, multiple mechanisms of pharmacologic action, including NMDA receptor blockade, nitric oxide potentiation, and potassium channel opening, are being studied.[10]

Increased Intracranial Volume and Pressure

The brain is enclosed in the rigid confines of the skull, or cranium, making it particularly susceptible to increases in ICP. Increased ICP is a common pathway for brain injury from different types of insults and agents. Excessive ICP can obstruct cerebral blood flow, destroy brain cells, displace brain tissue as in herniation, and otherwise damage delicate brain structures.

The cranial cavity contains blood (approximately 10%), brain tissue (approximately 80%), and CSF (approximately 10%) in the rigid confines of a nonexpandable skull.[11] Each of these three volumes contributes to the ICP, which normally is maintained within a range of 0 to 15 mm Hg when measured in the lateral ventricles. The volumes of each of these components can vary slightly without causing marked changes in ICP. This is because small increases in the volume of one component can be compensated for by a decrease in the volume of one or both of the other two components.[12] This association is called the *Monro-Kellie hypothesis*. Normal fluctuations in ICP occur with respiratory movements and activities of daily living such as straining, coughing, and sneezing.

Abnormal variation in intracranial volume with subsequent changes in ICP can be caused by a volume change in any of the three intracranial components. For example, an increase in tissue volume can result from a brain tumor, brain edema, or bleeding into brain tissue. An increase in blood volume develops when there is vasodilatation of cerebral vessels or obstruction of venous outflow. Excess production, decreased absorption, or obstructed circulation of CSF affords the potential for an increase in the CSF component. When the change in volume is caused by a brain tumor, it tends to occur slowly and usually is localized to the immediate area, whereas the increase resulting from head injury usually develops rapidly.

According to the modified Monro-Kellie hypothesis, reciprocal compensation occurs among the three intracranial compartments.[11] Of the three intracranial volumes, tissue volume is relatively restricted in its ability to undergo change; CSF and blood volume are best able to compensate for changes in ICP. Initial increases in ICP are buffered by a translocation of CSF to the spinal subarachnoid space and increased reabsorption of CSF. The compensatory ability of the blood compartment is limited by the small amount of blood that is in the cerebral circulation. The cerebral blood vessels contain less than 10% of the intracranial volume, most of which is contained in the low-pressure venous system. As the volume-buffering capacity of this compartment becomes exhausted, venous pressure increases and cerebral blood volume and ICP rise. Also, cerebral blood flow is highly controlled by autoregulatory mechanisms, which affect its compensatory capacity. Conditions such as ischemia and elevated partial pressure of carbon dioxide (PCO_2) produce vasodilation of the cerebral blood vessels in an attempt to increase cerebral blood flow. A decrease in PCO_2 has the opposite effect; for this reason, hyperventilation sometimes is used in the treatment of ICP.

Cerebral Compliance and the Impact of Intracranial Pressure. The impact of increases in blood, brain tissue,

or CSF volumes on ICP varies among individuals and depends on the amount of increase that occurs, the effectiveness of compensatory mechanisms, and the compliance of brain tissue. Compliance represents the ratio of change in volume to the resulting change in pressure (compliance = change in volume/change in pressure).[11] The effect of intracranial volume changes (horizontal axis) on ICP changes (vertical axis) are depicted in Figure 50-2.[11] The shape of the curve demonstrates effects of intracranial volume changes on ICP. The ICP remains constant from point A to point B when volume is added to the intracranial space. Because the compensatory mechanisms are adequate, compliance is high in this area of the curve, and there is little change in ICP. From points B to C, the compensatory mechanisms become less efficient; compliance decreases, and ICP begins to rise. At points C to D, the compensatory mechanisms have been exceeded such that even small changes in volume produce large changes in ICP.

Impact of Intracranial Pressure on Cerebral Perfusion Pressure. The cerebral perfusion pressure (CPP), which represents the difference between the mean arterial blood pressure (MABP) and the ICP (CPP = MABP – ICP), is the pressure perfusing the brain.[13] CPP is determined by the pressure gradient between the internal carotid artery and the subarachnoid veins. The MABP and ICP are monitored frequently in persons with brain conditions that increase ICP and impair brain perfusion. Normal CPP ranges from 70 to 100 mm Hg. Brain ischemia develops at levels

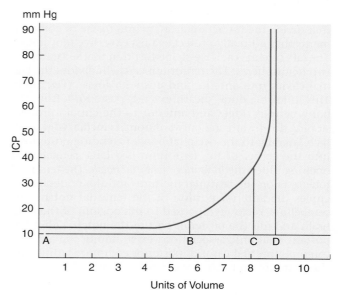

FIGURE 50-2 Pressure–volume curve. From point A to just before B, the ICP remains constant although there is an addition of volume (compliance is high). At point B, even though the ICP is within normal limits, compliance begins to change, as evidenced by the slight rise in ICP. From points B to C, the ICP rises with an increase in volume (low compliance). From points C to D, ICP rises significantly with each minute increase in volume (compliance is lost). (Hickey J.V. [1996]. *Neurological and neurosurgical nursing* [4th ed., p. 296]. Philadelphia: Lippincott-Raven)

below 50 to 70 mm Hg.[11] When the pressure in the cranial cavity approaches or exceeds the MABP, tissue perfusion becomes inadequate, cellular hypoxia results, and, if the pressure is maintained, neuronal death may occur. The highly specialized cortical neurons are the most sensitive to oxygen deficit; a decrease in the level of consciousness is one of the earliest and most reliable signs of increased ICP. The continued cellular hypoxia leads to general neurologic deterioration; the level of consciousness may deteriorate from alertness through confusion, lethargy, obtundation, stupor, and coma.

One of the late reflexes seen with a marked increase in ICP is the CNS ischemic response, which is triggered by ischemia of the vasomotor center in the brain stem. Neurons in the vasomotor center respond directly to ischemia by producing a marked increase in MABP, sometimes to levels as high as 270 mm Hg, accompanied by a widening of the pulse pressure and reflex slowing of the heart rate. These three signs, sometimes called the *Cushing reflex*, are important but late indicators of increased ICP.[14] They result from a severely increased ICP that compresses the blood flow to the brain stem. If the increase in blood pressure initiated by the CNS ischemic reflex is greater than the pressure surrounding the compressed vessels, blood flow is reestablished. The ischemic reflex is a last-ditch effort by the nervous system to maintain the cerebral circulation. The Cushing reflex seldom is seen in modern clinical settings since the advent of ICP monitoring.

Brain Herniation

The brain is protected by the nonexpandable skull and supporting septa, the falx cerebri and the tentorium cerebelli, that divide the intracranial cavity into fossae or compartments that normally protect against excessive movement. The falx cerebri is a sickle-shaped septum that separates the two hemispheres. The tentorium cerebelli divides the cranial cavity into anterior and posterior fossae (Fig. 50-3). This inflexible dural sheath extends posteriorly from the bony petrous ridges and anterior to the clinoid process, sloping downward and outward from its medial edge to attach laterally to the occipital bone. Extending posteriorly into the center of the tentorium is a large semicircular opening called the *incisura* or *tentorial notch*. The temporal lobe rests on the tentorial incisura, and the midbrain occupies the anterior portion of the tentorial notch. The cerebellum is closely opposed to the dorsum of the midbrain and fills the posterior part of the notch. Other important anatomic associations exist among the anterior cerebral, internal carotid, posterior communicating, and the posterior and superior cerebellar arteries, and the in-

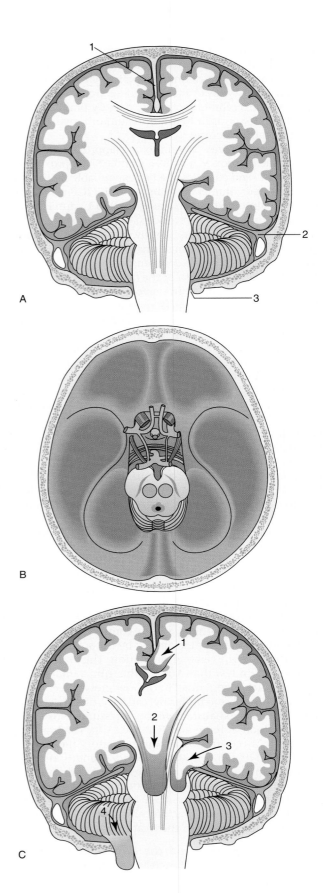

FIGURE 50-3 Supporting septa of the brain and patterns of herniation. (**A**) The falx cerebri [1], tentorium cerebelli [2], foramen magnum [3]. (**B**) The location of the insicura or tentorial notch in relation to the cerebral arteries and oculomotor nerve. (**C**) Herniation of the cingulate gyrus under the falx cerebri [1], central or transtentorial herniation [2], herniation of the temporal lobe into the tentorial notch [3], and infratentorial herniation of the cerebellar tonsils [4]. (Courtesy of Carole Hilmer, C.M.I.)

cisura (see Fig. 50-3B). The oculomotor nerve (cranial nerve III) emerges from the mediolateral surface of each peduncle just caudal to the tentorium.

Brain herniation is displacement of brain tissue under the falx cerebri or through the tentorial notch or incisura of the tentorium cerebelli. A rising ICP created by the increased volume causes displacement of the cerebral tissue toward a less-dense area. The different types of herniation syndromes are based on the area of the brain that has herniated and the structure under which it has been pushed (see Fig. 50-3C). They commonly are divided into two broad categories, supratentorial and infratentorial, based on whether they are located above or below the tentorium.

Supratentorial Herniations. Three major patterns of supratentorial herniation were described by Plum and Posner in their classic work: cingulate or across the falx cerebri, uncal or lateral, and transtentorial or central.[15] Each herniation syndrome has distinguishing features in the early phases, but as the forced downward displacement on the pons and medulla continues, clinical signs become similar. Table 50-2 describes the key structures and clinical signs of these three types of herniations. Any of the supratentorial herniation syndromes can compress vascular and CSF flow, which can further complicate the neurologic manifestations of brain lesions. Downward displacement of the brain in any of the supratentorial herniation syndromes can cause brain stem herniation, in which the medulla herniates into the foramen magnum, which is the opening between the cranial cavity and the vertebral canal. Death is immediate and caused by medullary compression.

Cingulate herniation involves displacement of the cingulate gyrus and hemisphere beneath the sharp edges of the falx cerebri to the opposite side of the brain. Displacement of the falx can compress the local brain tissue and blood supply from the anterior cerebral artery, causing ischemia and edema, which further increase ICP levels. Unilateral or bilateral leg weakness is an early sign of impending cingulate herniation.

Uncal herniation occurs when a lateral mass pushes the brain tissue centrally and forces the medial aspect of the temporal lobe, which contains the uncus and hippocampal gyrus, under the edge of the tentorial incisura, into the posterior fossa. The diencephalon and midbrain are compressed and displaced to the opposite side in uncal herniations. Cranial nerve III (oculomotor nerve) and the posterior cerebral artery frequently are caught between the uncus and the tentorium. The oculomotor nerve controls pupillary constriction. The entrapment of this nerve results in ipsilateral pupillary dilatation, which usually is an early sign of uncal herniation. Consciousness may be unimpaired because the reticular activating system (RAS) has not yet been affected. Deterioration, however, may proceed rather rapidly—making it important to recognize the distinguishing early features of lateral herniations.

As central and lateral herniations progress, there are changes in motor strength and coordination of voluntary movements because of compression of the descending motor pathways. It is not unusual for initial changes in motor function to occur on the side of the damage because of compression of the contralateral cerebral peduncles. This may result in a false localizing sign of hemiparesis on the same side as cranial nerve III, rather than on the opposite side, where the motor nerves have crossed over, as would be expected. As the condition progresses, bilateral positive Babinski responses and respiratory changes (*e.g.,* Cheyne-Stokes respirations, ataxic patterns) occur. Decorticate and decerebrate posturing may develop, followed by dilated, fixed pupils, flaccidity, and respiratory arrest.

Transtentorial or central herniation involves the downward displacement of the cerebral hemispheres, basal ganglia, diencephalon, and midbrain through the tentorial incisura. The diencephalon may be compressed tightly against the midbrain with such force that edema and hemorrhage result. It may or may not be associated with uncal herniation. In the early diencephalic stage, central herniation is manifested by a clouding of consciousness, with bilaterally small pupils (approximately 2 mm in diameter) with a full range of constriction and with motor responses to pain that are purposeful or semipurposeful (localizing) and often asymmetric. The clouding of consciousness is caused by pressure on the RAS in the upper midbrain, which is responsible for wakefulness. The pressure interferes with RAS function, and central herniations are evidenced first by changes in the level of consciousness.

TABLE 50-2 ✦ Key Structures and Clinical Signs of Cingulate, Transtentorial, and Uncal Herniation

Herniation Syndrome	Key Structures Involved	Key Clinical Signs
Cingulate	Anterior cerebral artery	Leg weakness
Transtentorial	Reticular activating system	Altered level of consciousness
	Corticospinal tract	Decorticate posturing
		Rostral–caudal deterioration
Uncal	Cerebral peduncle	Hemiparesis
	Oculomotor nerve	Pupil dilatation
	Posterior cerebral artery	Visual field loss
	Cerebellar tonsil	
	Respiratory center	Respiratory arrest

As the herniation progresses to the late diencephalic stage, painful stimulation results in decorticate posturing, which may be asymmetric (Fig. 50-4), and there is a waxing and waning of respirations with periods of apnea (*i.e.*, Cheyne-Stokes respirations). With midbrain involvement, the pupils are fixed and midsize (approximately 5 mm in diameter), reflex adduction of the eyes is impaired, and pain elicits cerebrate posturing. Respirations change from Cheyne-Stokes breathing to neurogenic hyperventilation, in which the frequency of ventilation may exceed 40 breaths per minute because of uninhibited stimulation of the inspiratory and expiratory centers. Progression to involve the pons and medulla produces fixed, midsized pupils, although with loss of reflex abduction and adduction of the eyes and with no motor response or only leg flexion on painful stimulation.

Infratentorial Herniation.   Infratentorial herniation results from increased pressure in the infratentorial compartment. It often progress rapidly and can cause death because it is likely to involve the lower brain stem centers that control vital cardiopulmonary functions. Herniation may occur superiorly (upward) through the tentorial incisura or inferiorly (downward) through the foramen magnum.

Upward displacement of brain tissue can cause blockage of the aqueduct of Sylvius and lead to hydrocephalus and coma. Downward displacement of the midbrain through the tentorial notch or the cerebellar tonsils through the foramen magnum can interfere with medullary functioning and cause cardiac or respiratory arrest. In cases of preexisting ICP, herniation may occur when the pressure is released from below, such as in a lumbar puncture. If the CSF pathway is blocked and fluid cannot leave the ventricles, the volume expands, and fluid is displaced downward through the tentorial notch. The expanding volume causes all function at a given level to cease as destruction progresses in a rostral-to-caudal direction. The result of this displacement is brain stem ischemia and hemorrhage extending from the diencephalon to the pons. If the lesion expands rapidly, displacement and obstruction occur quickly, leading to irreversible infarction and hemorrhage.

Cerebral Edema

Cerebral edema, or brain swelling, is an increase in tissue volume secondary to abnormal fluid accumulation. There are three types of brain edema: interstitial, vasogenic, and cytotoxic.[11] Interstitial edema is associated with an increase in sodium and water content of the periventricular white matter. Vasogenic edema results from an increase in the extracellular fluid that surrounds brain cells. Cytotoxic edema involves the actual swelling of brain cells themselves. Brain edema may or may not increase ICP. The impact of brain edema depends on the brain's compensatory mechanisms and the extent of the swelling.

Interstitial Edema.   Interstitial edema involves movement of the CSF across the ventricular wall so there is water and sodium in the periventricular white matter. It is seen most commonly in conditions of impaired CSF flow through the ventricles, such as obstructive hydrocephalus or purulent meningitis.

Vasogenic Edema.   Vasogenic edema occurs with conditions that impair function of the blood-brain barrier and allow transfer of water and protein into the interstitial space, such as tumors, prolonged ischemia, hemorrhage, brain injury, and infectious processes (*e.g.*, meningitis). When brain injury occurs, the blood-brain barrier is disrupted and increased permeability occurs. There is almost free diffusion across the capillary membranes. Vasogenic edema occurs primarily in the white matter of the brain, possibly because the white matter is more compliant than the gray matter and offers less resistance to fluid accumulation. Vasogenic edema can displace a cerebral hemisphere and can be responsible for various types of herniation. The functional manifestations of vasogenic edema include focal neurologic deficits, disturbances in consciousness, and severe intracranial hypertension.

Cytotoxic Edema.   Cytotoxic edema involves an increase in fluid in the intracellular space, chiefly the gray matter, although the white matter may be involved. Cytotoxic edema can result from hypo-osmotic states such as water intoxication or severe ischemia that impair the function of

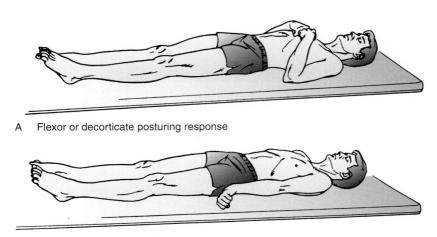

A   Flexor or decorticate posturing response

B   Extensor or decerebrate posturing

FIGURE 50-4 Abnormal posturing. (**A**) Decorticate rigidity. In decorticate rigidity, the upper arms are held at the sides, with elbows, wrists, and fingers flexed. The legs are extended and internally rotated. The feet are plantar flexed. (**B**) Decerebrate rigidity. In decerebrate rigidity, the jaws are clenched and neck extended. The arms are adducted and stiffly extended at the elbows with the forearms pronated, wrists and fingers flexed. (From Fuller J., Schaller-Ayers J. [1994]. *Health assessment: A nursing approach.* [2nd ed.]. Philadelphia: J.B. Lippincott)

the sodium-potassium membrane pump. This causes rapid accumulation of sodium in the cell, followed by movement of water along the osmotic gradient. Major changes in cerebral function, such as stupor and coma, occur with cytotoxic edema. The edema associated with ischemia may be severe enough to produce cerebral infarction with necrosis of brain tissue.

Abnormal conditions such as hypoxia, acidosis, and brain trauma also may result in cytotoxic edema, causing neuronal cell damage and possible death. If blood flow in the brain falls to abnormally low levels, cellular hypoxia results in reduced energy (ATP) production and depletion of energy stores. A low-energy state reduces the function of the membrane ion pumps. Low blood flow also results in the inadequate removal of anaerobic metabolic end-products such as lactic acid, producing extracellular acidosis. The altered osmotic conditions result in water entry and cell swelling. Depending on the nature of the insult, cellular edema can occur in the vascular endothelium or smooth muscle cells, astrocytes, the myelin-forming processes of oligodendrocytes, or neurons. If blood flow is reduced to low levels for extended periods or to extremely low levels for a few minutes, cellular edema can cause the cell membrane to rupture, allowing the escape of intracellular contents into the surrounding extracellular fluid. This leads to damage of neighboring cells.

Cytotoxic edema is a slowly progressive process. When neurons are involved in this cytopathic process, presynaptic and postsynaptic elements become hypopolarized. Presynaptic hypolarization opens voltage-gated calcium channels, producing increased levels of free intracellular calcium and the release of neurotransmitters. The gradual change in membrane potentials brings the presynaptic and postsynaptic neurons into the threshold range, resulting in electrical hyperactivity; this process continues until there is insufficient energy for recovery to the threshold potential, at which time the cells fall into electrical silence. This progression suggests possible mechanisms of seizure generation, loss of neuronal function, and eventual cell death.

Treatment.   Although cerebral edema is viewed as a pathologic process, it does not necessarily disrupt brain function unless it increases the ICP. The localized edema surrounding a brain tumor often responds to corticosteroid therapy (*e.g.*, dexamethasone), but use of these drugs on generalized edema is controversial. The mechanism of action of the corticosteroid drugs in the treatment of cerebral edema is unknown, but in therapeutic doses, they seem to stabilize cell membranes and scavenge free radicals. Osmotic diuretics (*e.g.*, mannitol) may be useful in the acute phase of vasogenic and cytotoxic edema when hypo-osmolarity is present.

Hydrocephalus

Enlargement of the CSF compartment occurs with hydrocephalus, which is defined as an abnormal increase in CSF volume in any part or all of the ventricular system. The two causes of hydrocephalus are decreased absorption or overproduction of CSF. There are two types of hydrocephalus: noncommunicating and communicating.

Noncommunicating or obstructive hydrocephalus occurs when obstruction in the ventricular system prevents the CSF from reaching the arachnoid villi. CSF flow can be obstructed by congenital malformations, from tumors encroaching on the ventricular system, and by inflammation or hemorrhage. The ependyma (*i.e.*, lining of ventricles and CSF-filled spaces) is particularly sensitive to viral infections, particularly during embryonic development; ependymitis is believed to be the cause of congenital aqueductal stenosis.[4]

Communicating hydrocephalus results from impaired reabsorption of CSF from the arachnoid villi into the venous system. Decreased absorption can result from a block in the CSF pathway to the arachnoid villi or a failure of the villi to transfer the CSF to the venous system. It can occur if too few villi are formed, if postinfective (meningitis) scarring occludes them, or if the villi become obstructed with fragments of blood or infectious debris. Adenomas of the choroid plexus can cause an overproduction of CSF. This form of hydrocephalus is much less common than that resulting from decreased absorption of CSF.

Similar pathologic patterns occur with noncommunicating and communicating types of hydrocephalus. The cerebral hemispheres become enlarged, and the ventricular system is dilated beyond the point of obstruction. The gyri on the surface of the brain become less prominent and the white matter is reduced in volume. The presence and extent of the ICP is determined by fluid accumulation and the type of hydrocephalus, the age at onset, and the rapidity and extent of pressure rise. Acute hydrocephalus usually is manifested by increased ICP. Slowly developing hydrocephalus is less likely to produce an increase in ICP, but it may produce deficits such as progressive dementia and gait changes. Computed tomographic (CT) scans are used to diagnose all types of hydrocephalus. The usual treatment is a shunting procedure, which provides an alternative route for return of CSF to the circulation.

When hydrocephalus develops in utero or before the cranial sutures have fused in infancy, the ventricles expand beyond the point of obstruction, the cranial sutures separate, the head expands, and there is bulging of the fontanels (Fig. 50-5). Because the skull is able to expand, signs of increased ICP usually are absent and intelligence usually is spared. Seizures are common, and in severe cases, optic nerve atrophy leads to blindness. Weakness and uncoordinated movement are common. Surgical placement of a shunt allows for diversion of excess CSF fluid, preventing extreme enlargement of the head. Before surgical shunting procedures were available, the weight and size of the enlarged head made ambulation difficult.

In contrast to hydrocephalus that develops in utero or during infancy, head enlargement does not occur in adults, and increases in ICP depend on whether the condition developed rapidly or slowly. Acute-onset hydrocephalus in adults usually is marked by symptoms of increased ICP, including headache and vomiting, followed by papilledema. If the obstruction is not relieved, mental deterioration eventually occurs. The pressure of CSF is not always elevated, and the syndrome of low-pressure hydrocephalus may go undetected. Treatment includes surgical shunting for noncommunicating hydrocephalus. In communicating

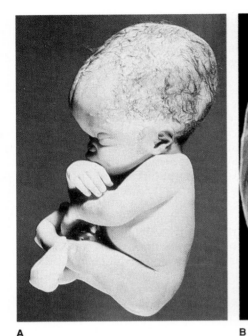
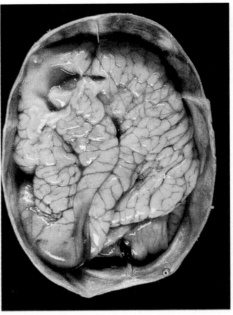

A   **B**

FIGURE 50-5 Congenital hydrocephalus. (**A**) Hydrocephalus occurring before the fusion of the cranial sutures causes pronounced enlargement of the head. (**B**) Removal of the calvarium demonstrates an atrophic and collapsed cerebral cortex. (Rubin E., Farber J.L. [1999]. *Pathology* [3rd ed., p. 1454]. Philadelphia: Lippincott Williams & Wilkins)

hydrocephalus, attempts to clear the arachnoid villi of exudate may be made, and if this is unsuccessful, surgical shunting may be required.

MANIFESTATIONS OF GLOBAL BRAIN INJURY

Brain injury is manifested by alterations in sensory and motor function and by changes in the level of consciousness. Focal injury commonly causes alterations in sensory function (Chapter 48) or motor function (Chapter 49); more global injury tends to result in altered levels of consciousness. Severe injury that seriously compromises brain function may result in brain death.

Consciousness

Consciousness is the state of awareness of self and the environment and of being able to become oriented to new stimuli.[11] The state of consciousness involves arousal and wakefulness and content or cognition, which includes the sum of cognitive functions. Arousal and wakefulness rely on an intact ascending RAS (ARAS) in the brain stem to act as the alerting or awakening element of consciousness. The content and cognitive aspects of consciousness are determined by a functioning cerebral cortex.

Reticular Formation. The reticular formation is a diffuse, primitive system of interlacing nerve cells and fibers that receive input from multiple sensory pathways (Fig. 50-6). Anatomically, the reticular formation constitutes the central core of the brain stem, extending from the medulla through the pons to the midbrain, which is continuous caudally with the spinal cord and rostrally with the subthalamus, the hypothalamus, and the thalamus.[16,17] A unique characteristic of neurons in the reticular formation is their widespread system of collaterals, which make ex-

tensive synaptic contacts and travel long distances in the CNS. Along with this widespread distribution of converging contacts, there is a loss of specificity because many afferent signals contribute to the efferent output of reticular formation neurons.[17]

Ascending fibers of the reticular formation, known as the ARAS, relay activating information to all parts of the cerebral cortex. The flow of information in the ARAS activates the hypothalamic and limbic structures that regulate emotional and behavioral responses such as those that occur in response to pain, and they exert facilitory effects on cortical neurons. Other examples of ARAS activity include the alerting responses to loud noises or a splash of water on the face. Without cortical activation, a person is less able to detect specific stimuli, and the level of consciousness is reduced. Because cortical activation is diffuse,

> **Brain Injury and Levels of Consciousness**

> ➤ Consciousness is a global function that depends on a diffuse neural network that includes activity of the reticular activating system (RAS) and both cerebral hemispheres.

> ➤ Impaired consciousness implies diffuse brain injury to the RAS at any level (medulla through thalamus) or both cerebral hemispheres simultaneously.

> ➤ In contrast, local brain injury causes focal neurologic deficit but does not disrupt consciousness.

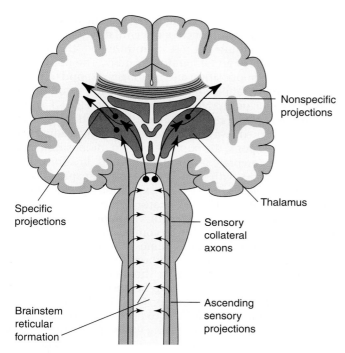

FIGURE 50-6 The brain stem reticular formation and reticular activating system. Ascending sensory tracts send axon collateral fibers to the reticular formation. These give rise to fibers synapsing in the nonspecific nuclei of the thalamus. From there the nonspecific thalamic projections influence widespread areas of the cerebral cortex and limbic system. (Rhoades R.A., Tanner G.A. [1996]. *Medical physiology.* Boston: Little, Brown)

unilateral injury usually does not impair consciousness. The pathways for the ARAS travel through the midbrain, and lesions of the midbrain can interrupt ARAS activity, leading to altered levels of consciousness and coma.

Any deficit in level of consciousness, from mild confusion to stupor or coma, implicates injury to either the RAS

or to both cerebral hemispheres concurrently. For example, consciousness may decline owing to severe systemic metabolic derangements that affect both hemispheres, or from head trauma causing shear injuries to white matter of both the RAS and the cerebral hemispheres. Brain injuries that affect a hemisphere unilaterally and also spare the RAS, such as cerebral infarction, usually do not cause impaired consciousness. Focal injuries disrupt local brain functions and manifest as focal deficits.

Fibers from the RAS also project to the hypothalamus, to the autonomic nervous system, and to motor systems. The hypothalamus plays a predominant role in maintaining homeostasis through integration of somatic, visceral, and endocrine functions. Inputs from the reticular formation, vestibulospinal projections, and other motor systems are integrated to provide a continuously adapting background of muscle tone and posture to facilitate voluntary motor actions. Reticular formation neurons that function in regulation of cardiovascular, respiratory, and other visceral functions are intermingled with those that maintain other reticular formation functions. Cardiovascular neurons are located primarily in the medulla, and those that influence respiratory rhythms are located in the medulla and pons.

Levels of Consciousness.   Level of consciousness reflects an orientation to person, place, and time. A fully conscious person is totally aware of her or his surroundings.[18] Levels of consciousness exist on a continuum that includes consciousness, confusion, delirium, obtundation, stupor, and coma[19] (Table 50-3). Stupor and coma are signs of advanced brain failure. As with failure of other body systems, a wide spectrum of conditions can injure the brain and cause progressive deterioration of consciousness and coma.

Deterioration of brain function from supratentorial lesions tends to follow a rostral-to-caudal progression, which is observed as the brain initially compensates for the injury and subsequently decompensates with the loss of autoregulation and cerebral perfusion. Infratentorial (brain stem)

TABLE 50-3 *Descending Levels of Consciousness and Their Characteristics*	
Level of Consciousness	**Characteristics**
Confusion	Disturbance of consciousness characterized by impaired ability to think clearly, and to perceive, respond to, and remember current stimuli; also disorientation
Delirium	State of disturbed consciousness with motor restlessness, transient hallucinations, disorientation, and sometimes delusions
Obtundation	Disorder of decreased alertness with associated psychomotor retardation
Stupor	A state in which the person is not unconscious but exhibits little or no spontaneous activity
Coma	A state of being unarousable and unresponsive to external stimuli or internal needs; often determined by the Glasgow Coma Scale

(Data from Bates D. [1993]. The management of medical coma. *Journal of Neurology, Neurosurgery, and Psychiatry* 56, 590)

lesions may lead to an early, sometimes abrupt disturbance in consciousness without any orderly rostrocaudal progression of neurologic signs. Table 50-4 describes the key signs in the rostral-to-caudal progression of brain lesions.

The cerebral hemispheres are most susceptible to damage, and the most frequent sign of brain dysfunction is altered level of consciousness and change in behavior. As brain structures in the diencephalon, midbrain, pons, and medulla are affected, additional motor and pupillary signs become evident. Hemodynamic and respiratory instability are the last signs to occur because their regulatory centers are located low in the medulla.

Progressive injury affecting the diencephalon, midbrain, pons, and medulla usually causes a predictable pattern of change in the level of consciousness. The highest level of consciousness is seen in an alert person who is oriented to person, place, and time and is totally aware of the surroundings. The earliest signs of diminution in level of consciousness are inattention, mild confusion, disorientation, and blunted responsiveness. With further deterioration, the delirious or encephalopathic person becomes markedly inattentive and variably lethargic or agitated. The person may progress to become obtunded, and may respond only to vigorous or noxious stimuli, such as shaking. Early respiratory changes include yawning and sighing, with progression to Cheyne-Stokes breathing. These signs are indicative of bilateral hemisphere damage with a danger of tentorial herniation. Although the pupils may respond briskly to light, the full range of eye movements is seen only reflexively when the head is passively rotated from side to side (*i.e.*, oculocephalic reflex or "doll's-head" eye maneuver) or when the caloric test (*i.e.*, instillation of hot or cold water into the ear canal) is done to elicit nystagmus. In the oculocephalic reflex maneuver, intact eye movements are manifested by the eyes rolling in the opposite direction of passive head rotation (see Chapter 53). There is some combative movement and purposeful movement in response to pain. As coma progresses, the bulboreticular facility area becomes more active as fewer inhibitory signals descend from the basal ganglia and cerebral cortex. This results in *flexor* or *decorticate posturing* (see Fig. 50-4).

With progression continuing in a rostrocaudal direction, the midbrain becomes involved. Respirations change from Cheyne-Stokes breathing to neurogenic hyperventilation, in which the frequency of ventilation may exceed 40 breaths per minute because of uninhibited stimulation of the inspiratory and expiratory centers. The pupils become fixed in midposition and no longer respond to stimuli. Muscle excitability increases, producing a condition called *extensor* or *decerebrate posturing* (see Fig. 50-4), in which the arms are rigid and extended with the palms of the hands turned away from the body. As coma advances to involve the pons, the pupils remain in midposition and fixed, and decerebrate posturing continues. Breathing becomes apneustic, with sighs evident in midinspiration or with prolonged inspiration and expiration because of excessive stimulation of the respiratory center.

With medullary involvement, the pupils remain fixed in midposition. Respiration becomes ataxic (*i.e.*, totally uncoordinated and irregular). Apnea may occur because of the loss of responsiveness to carbon dioxide stimulation. Complete ventilatory assistance should be considered for any person with ataxic breathing. Because the medulla has bulboreticular neurons but not facility neurons, the hyperexcitability that gave rise to decorticate and decerebrate posturing disappears, giving way to flaccidity.

In progressive brain deterioration, the person's neurologic capabilities appear to deteriorate in stepwise fashion. Similarly, as neurologic function returns, there appears to be stepwise progress to higher levels of consciousness. An assessment tool called the *Glasgow Coma Scale* often is used to describe levels of coma. This scale uses three aspects of neurologic function—eye opening, verbal response, and motor response—to arrive at a numeric score that represents the level of coma[19,20] (Table 50-5). Studies of interrater reliability have shown that the distinction between degrees of dysfunction in these three components can be made consistently by a range of medical, nursing, and paramedical personnel.[21] One possible exception is assessment of the distinction between "abnormal" and "normal" flexion movements in the motor component of the scale.[21]

Brain Death

Brain death is defined as the irreversible loss of function of the brain, including the brain stem.[22,23] With advances in scientific knowledge and technology that have provided

---

TABLE 50-4 ◆ Key Signs in Rostral-to-Caudal Progression of Brain Lesions

Level of Brain Injury	Key Clinical Signs
Diencephalon	Impaired consciousness (see Table 50-3); small, reactive pupils; intact oculocephalic reflex; decorticate posturing; Cheyne-Stokes respirations
Midbrain	Coma, fixed, midsize pupils; impaired oculocephalic reflex; neurogenic hyperventilation; decerebrate posturing
Pons	Coma, fixed, irregular pupils; dysconjugate gaze; impaired cold caloric stimulation; loss of corneal reflex; hemiparesis/quadriparesis; decerebrate posturing; apneustic respirations
Medulla	Coma, fixed pupils, flaccidity, loss of gag and cough reflexes, ataxic/apneic respirations

TABLE 50-5 ✦ The Glasgow Coma Scale

Test	Score*
Eye Opening (E)	
Spontaneous	4
To call	3
To pain	2
None	1
Motor Response (M)	
Obeys commands	6
Localizes pain	5
Normal flexion (withdrawal)	4
Abnormal flexion (decorticate)	3
Extension (decerebrate)	2
None (flaccid)	1
Verbal Response (V)	
Oriented	5
Confused conversation	4
Inappropriate words	3
Incomprehensible sounds	2
None	1

*GCS Score = E + M + V. Best possible score = 15; worst possible score = 3.

the means for artificially maintaining ventilatory and circulatory function, the definition of death has had to be continually reexamined. In 1968, criteria for irreversible coma were published by a Harvard Medical School Ad Hoc Committee.[24] Advances in treatment, including the development of effective artificial cardiopulmonary support for brain-injured persons, created a need to reevaluate the determination of death. The definitive criteria for brain death that followed in the United States were proposed in 1981 by the President's Commission for the Study of Ethical Problems in Medicine and Biomedical and Behavioral Research.[25] According to these criteria, a diagnosis of death requires cessation of all brain functions, including those of the brain stem, and irreversibility.[25]

In 1995, the Quality of Standards Subcommittee of the American Academy of Neurology published the clinical parameters for determining brain death and procedures for testing persons older than 18 years of age.[26] According to these parameters, "brain death is the absence of clinical brain function when the proximate cause is known and demonstrably irreversible."[26]

Clinical examination must disclose at least the absence of responsiveness, brain stem reflexes, and respiratory effort. Brain death is a clinical diagnosis, and a repeat evaluation at least 6 hours later is recommended.[27] Longer periods of observation of absent brain activity are required in cases of drug overdose (*e.g.*, barbiturates, other CNS depressants), drug toxicity (*e.g.*, neuromuscular blocking drugs, aminoglycoside antibiotics), neuromuscular diseases such as myasthenia gravis, hypothermia, and shock. Medical circumstances may require use of confirmatory tests. In the United States, electroencephalographic (EEG) testing is used to establish brain death. EEG testing should reveal no electrical activity during at least 30 minutes of recording that adheres to the minimal technical criteria for EEG recording in suspected brain death as adopted by the American Electroencephalographic Society, including 16-channel EEG instruments. Other confirmatory tests include conventional angiography (*i.e.*, no intracerebral filling at the level of the carotid bifurcation or circle of Willis), transcranial Doppler ultrasonography, technetium-99m hexamethylpropyleneamineoxime brain scan (*i.e.*, no uptake of isotope in brain parenchyma), and somatosensory evoked potentials.

Medical documentation should include cause and irreversibility of the condition, absence of brain stem reflexes and motor responses to pain, absence of respiration with a PCO_2 of 60 mm Hg or more, and the justification for use of confirmatory tests and their results.[23] Brain stem reflexes that are assessed include the pupillary reaction to light, corneal reflexes, the gag or swallowing reflex, and the oculovestibular reflex. Adequate testing for apnea is important. An acceptable method is ventilation with pure oxygen or an oxygen and carbon dioxide mixture for 10 minutes before withdrawal from the ventilator, followed by passive flow of oxygen. This method allows blood levels of carbon dioxide to rise without hazardously lowering the oxygen content of the blood. If respiratory reflexes are intact, the hypercarbia that develops should stimulate ventilatory effort within 30 seconds when the PCO_2 is greater than 60 mm Hg. A 10-minute period of apnea usually is sufficient to attain this level of PCO_2. Spontaneous breathing efforts indicate that the brain stem is functioning.

Irreversibility implies that brain death cannot be reversed. Some conditions such as drug and metabolic intoxication can cause cessation of brain functions that is completely reversible, even when they produce clinical cessation of brain functions and EEG silence. This needs to be excluded before declaring that a person is brain dead. The clinical examination to determine brain death in children is the same as for adults. However, the brains of infants and small children have increased resistance to damage and may recover substantial function after exhibiting unresponsiveness. Because of limitations on the clinical examination of infants, an observation period of 48 hours is recommended, as well as a confirmatory test, such as EEG or a study of cerebral blood flow.[23]

Persistent Vegetative State

Advances in the care of brain-injured persons during the past several decades have resulted in survival of many persons who previously would have died. Unfortunately, some of these persons remain in what often is called the *persistent vegetative state*. The vegetative state is characterized by loss of all cognitive functions and the unawareness of self and surroundings. Reflex and vegetative functions remain.[27] Persons in the vegetative state must be fed and require full nursing care.

The criteria for diagnosis of vegetative state include the absence of awareness of self and environment and an inability to interact with others; the absence of sustained or reproducible voluntary behavioral responses; lack of language comprehension; sufficiently preserved hypothalamic and brain stem function to maintain life; bowel and bladder incontinence; and variably preserved cranial nerve (*e.g.*, pupillary, oculocephalic, gag) and spinal cord reflexes.[28] The diagnosis of persistent vegetative state requires that the condition has continued for at least 1 month.

In summary, many of the agents that cause brain damage do so through common pathways, including hypoxia or ischemia, accumulation of excitatory neurotransmitters, increased ICP, and cerebral edema. Deprivation of oxygen (*i.e.*, hypoxia) or blood flow (*i.e.*, ischemia) can have deleterious effects on the brain structures. Ischemia can be focal, as in stroke, or global. Global ischemia occurs when blood flow is inadequate to meet the metabolic needs of the brain, as in cardiac arrest. In many neurologic disorders, neuron injury may be caused at least in part by overstimulation of receptors for specific amino acids, such as glutamate and aspartate, that act as excitatory neurotransmitters. Many of the actions of the excitatory neurotransmitters are coupled with glutamate NMDA receptor–operated ion channels that control calcium entry into neurons. Increased intracellular calcium leads to activation of intracellular enzymes that cause protein breakdown, free radical formation, lipid peroxidation, fragmentation of DNA, and nuclear breakdown. Neurons of the cerebral cortex and hippocampus have large numbers of special glutamate NMDA receptors and are particularly vulnerable to injury through this mechanism.

The contents of the cranial cavity, which are enclosed in the rigid confines of the skull, consist of brain tissue, blood, and CSF. The collective volumes of these three intracranial components determine ICP. A variation in volume of any of these components can cause the ICP to rise, affecting cerebral function. Compensatory mechanisms protect the brain from small variations in the volume. Large variations, however, exceed the compensatory mechanisms and may lead to hypoxia, brain herniation, and death. Disorders of cerebral volumes and pressure include increases in brain tissue (*i.e.*, neoplasms), increased extracellular fluid and edema, and increased CSF (*i.e.*, hydrocephalus). Brain herniation is the displacement of brain tissue under the tough dural folds of the falx cerebri or past the incisura or notch of the tentorium cerebelli. Brain herniation commonly is divided into two broad categories, supratentorial and infratentorial, based on location of the herniation.

Brain edema represents an increase in tissue volume from abnormal fluid accumulation. There are three types of brain edema: vasogenic, which results from an increase in extracellular fluid; cytotoxic, which involves the actual swelling of brain cells; and interstitial, which involves an increase in fluid in the periventricular white matter.

Consciousness is a state of awareness of self and environment. It exists on a normal continuum of wakefulness and sleep and a pathologic continuum of wakefulness and coma. Consciousness depends on the normal functioning of the RAS. In progressive brain injury, coma may follow a rostral-to-caudal progression with characteristic changes in levels of consciousness, pupillary response, muscle tone, and respiratory activity occurring as the diencephalon through the medulla are affected.

Brain death is defined as the irreversible loss of function of the brain, including that of the brain stem. Clinical examination must disclose at least the absence of responsiveness, brain stem reflexes, and respiratory effort. Brain death is a clinical diagnosis, and a repeat evaluation and serial examinations at least 6 hours later is recommended. Confirmatory tests include EEG testing, conventional angiography, transcranial Doppler ultrasonography, technetium-99m hexamethylpropyleneamineoxime brain scan, and somatosensory evoked potentials. The vegetative state is characterized by loss of all cognitive functions and the unawareness of self and surroundings. Reflex and vegetative functions remain.

Cerebrovascular Disease

After you have completed this section of the chapter, you should be able to meet the following objectives:

◆ List the major vessels in the cerebral circulation and state the contribution of the internal carotid arteries, the vertebral arteries, and the circle of Willis to the cerebral circulation
◆ Explain autoregulation of cerebral blood flow
◆ Explain the substitution of "brain attack" for stroke in terms of making a case for early diagnosis and treatment
◆ Compare the pathologies of ischemic and hemorrhagic stroke
◆ Explain the significance of transient ischemic attacks, the ischemic penumbra, and watershed zones of infarction and how these conditions relate to ischemic stroke
◆ List the manifestations of stroke and the major vessel involved
◆ Cite the most common cause of subarachnoid hemorrhage and state the complications associated with subarachnoid hemorrhage
◆ Describe the alterations in cerebral vasculature that occur with arteriovenous malformations
◆ Describe the progression of motor deficits that occurs as a result of stroke
◆ Characterize problems of speech and language that can result from stroke
◆ Cite the characteristics of the denial, neglect, or hemiattention syndrome

Cerebrovascular disease encompasses a number of disorders involving vessels in the cerebral circulation. These disorders include stroke and transient ischemic attacks (TIAs), aneurysmal subarachnoid hemorrhage, and arteriovenous malformations.

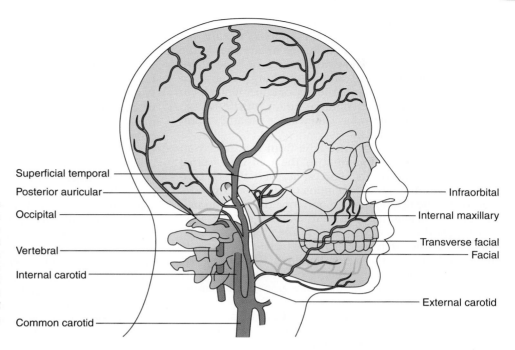

FIGURE 50-7 Branches of the right external carotid artery. The internal carotid artery ascends to the base of the brain. The right vertebral artery is also shown as it ascends through the transverse foramina of the cervical vertebrae. (Chaffee E.E., Lytle I.M. [1980]. *Basic physiology and anatomy* [4th ed.]. Philadelphia: J.B. Lippincott)

Labels in figure:
Superficial temporal
Posterior auricular
Occipital
Vertebral
Internal carotid
Common carotid
Infraorbital
Internal maxillary
Transverse facial
Facial
External carotid

CEREBRAL CIRCULATION

Anatomy and Physiology

The blood flow to the brain is supplied by the two internal carotid arteries anteriorly and the vertebral arteries posteriorly (Fig. 50-7). The internal carotid artery, a terminal branch of the common carotid artery, branches into several arteries: ophthalmic, posterior communicating, anterior choroidal, anterior cerebral, and middle cerebral (Fig. 50-8). Most of the arterial blood in the internal carotid arteries is distributed through the anterior and middle cerebral arteries. The anterior cerebral arteries supply the medial surface of the frontal and parietal lobes cerebrum and the anterior half of the thalamus, the corpus striatum, part of the corpus callosum, and the anterior limb of the internal capsule. The genu and posterior limb of the internal capsule and medial globus pallidus are fed by the anterior choroidal branch of the internal carotid artery. The middle cerebral artery passes laterally, supplying the lateral basal ganglia and the insula, and then emerges on the lateral cortical surface, supplying the inferior frontal gyrus, the motor and premotor frontal cortex concerned with delicate face and hand control. It is the major vascular source for the primary and association somesthetic cortex for the face and hand and the superior temporal gyrus, with the primary and association auditory cortex. It also is a major source of supply for much of the

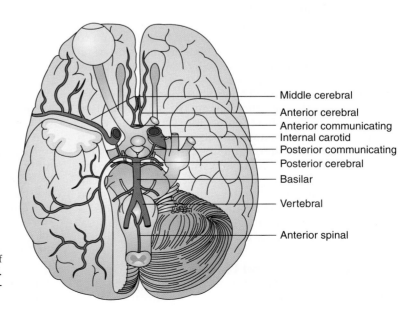

FIGURE 50-8 The circle of Willis as seen at the base of a brain removed from the skull. (Chaffee E.E., Lytle I.M. [1980]. *Basic physiology and anatomy* [4th ed.]. Philadelphia: J.B. Lippincott)

Labels in figure:
Middle cerebral
Anterior cerebral
Anterior communicating
Internal carotid
Posterior communicating
Posterior cerebral
Basilar
Vertebral
Anterior spinal

basal ganglia. The middle cerebral artery is functionally a continuation of the internal carotid; emboli of the internal carotid most frequently become lodged in branches of the middle cerebral artery. The consequences of ischemia of these areas may be most devastating, resulting in damage to the fine manipulative skills of the face or upper limb and to receptive and expressive communication functions (*e.g.,* aphasia). Occlusion of the local branches of the artery result in more restricted deficits.

The two vertebral arteries arise from the subclavian artery and enter the foramina in the transverse spinal processes at the level of the sixth cervical vertebra and continue upward through the foramina of the upper six vertebrae; they wind behind the atlas and enter the skull through the foramen magnum and unite to form the basilar artery, which then diverges to terminate in the posterior cerebral arteries. Branches of the basilar and vertebral arteries supply the medulla, pons, cerebellum, midbrain, and caudal part of the diencephalon. The posterior cerebral arteries supply the remaining occipital and inferior regions of the temporal lobes, and the thalamus.

The distal branches of the internal carotid and vertebral arteries communicate at the base of the brain through the circle of Willis; this anastomosis of arteries can provide continued circulation if blood flow through one of the main vessels is disrupted. Without collateral input, cessation of blood flow in cerebral arteries may result in neural damage as metabolic needs of electrically active cells exceed nutrient supply. Because the vertebral arteries supply the structures in the brain stem that maintain basic life support reflexes, interruption of blood flow in the carotid arteries with preserved vertebral supply may result in severe coma, although not necessarily death.

The cerebral blood is drained by two sets of veins that empty into the dural venous sinuses: the deep (great) cerebral venous system and the superficial venous system. The deep system is well protected, in contrast to the superficial cerebral veins that travel through the pia mater on the surface of the cerebral cortex. These vessels connect directly to the sagittal sinuses in the falx cerebri by way of bridging veins. They travel through the CSF-filled subarachnoid space and penetrate the arachnoid and then the dura to reach the dural venous sinuses. This system of sinuses returns blood to the heart primarily by way of the internal jugular veins. Alternate routes for venous flow also exist; for example, venous blood may exit through the emissary veins that pass through the skull and through veins that traverse various foramina to empty into extracranial veins.

The intracranial venous system has no valves. The direction of flow depends on gravity or the relative pressure in the venous sinuses compared with that of the extracranial veins. Increases in intrathoracic pressure, as can occur with coughing or performance of a Valsalva's maneuver, produce a rise in central venous pressure that is reflected back into the internal jugular veins and to the dural sinuses. This briefly raises the ICP.

Regulation of Cerebral Blood Flow

The blood flow to the brain is maintained at approximately 750 mL/minute or one sixth of the resting cardiac output.[14]

The regulation of blood flow to the brain is controlled largely by autoregulatory or local mechanisms that respond to the metabolic needs of the brain. Cerebral autoregulation has been classically defined as the ability of the brain to maintain constant cerebral blood flow despite changes in systemic arterial pressure. The autoregulation of cerebral blood flow is efficient within an MABP range of approximately 60 to 140 mm Hg.[14] If blood pressure falls below 60 mm Hg, cerebral blood flow becomes severely compromised, and if it rises above the upper limit of autoregulation, blood flow increases rapidly and overstretches the cerebral vessels. In persons with hypertension, this autoregulatory range shifts to a higher level. Autoregulation has been further defined as the ability of the cerebral cortex to adjust cerebral blood flow to satisfy its metabolic needs. Although total cerebral blood flow remains relatively stable throughout marked changes in cardiac output and arterial blood pressure, regional blood flow may change markedly in response to local changes in metabolism.

At least three metabolic factors affect cerebral blood flow: carbon dioxide concentration, hydrogen ion concentration, and oxygen concentration. Increased carbon dioxide or increased hydrogen ion concentrations increase cerebral blood flow; decreased oxygen concentration also increases blood flow. Carbon dioxide, by way of the hydrogen ion concentration, provides a potent stimulus for control of cerebral blood flow—a doubling of the PCO_2 in the blood results in a doubling of cerebral blood flow. Other substances that alter the pH of the brain produce similar changes in cerebral blood flow. Because increased hydrogen ion concentration greatly depresses neural activity, the increase in blood flow is protective in that it washes the hydrogen ions and other acidic materials away from the brain tissue.[12] Profound extracellular acidosis also induces vasomotor paralysis, in which case cerebral blood flow may depend entirely on the systemic arterial blood pressure.

The deep cerebral blood vessels appear to be completely controlled by autoregulation. However, the superficial and major cerebral blood vessels are innervated by the sympathetic nervous system. Under normal physiologic conditions, the sympathetic nervous system exerts little effect on superficial cerebral blood flow because local regulatory mechanisms are so powerful that they compensate almost entirely for the effects of sympathetic stimulation. However, when local mechanisms fail, sympathetic control of cerebral blood pressure becomes important.[14] For example, when the arterial pressure rises to very high levels during strenuous exercise or in other conditions, the sympathetic nervous system constricts the large and intermediate-sized superficial blood vessels as a means of protecting the smaller, more easily damaged vessels. Sympathetic reflexes are believed to cause vasospasm in the intermediate and large arteries in some types of brain damage, such as that caused by rupture of a cerebral aneurysm.

STROKE (BRAIN ATTACK)

Stroke is an acute focal neurologic deficit from a vascular disorder that injures brain tissue. Stroke remains one of the leading causes of mortality and morbidity in the United

States. Each year, 600,000 Americans are afflicted with stroke, and approximately 160,000 of these persons die, while many survivors are left with at least some degree of neurologic impairment.[29] The term *brain attack* has been promoted to highlight that time-dependent tissue damage occurs and to raise awareness of the need for rapid emergency treatment, similar to that with heart attack.

There are two main types of strokes: ischemic stroke and hemorrhagic stroke. Ischemic strokes are caused by an interruption of blood flow in a cerebral vessel and are the most common type of stroke, accounting for 70% to 80% of all strokes. The less common hemorrhagic strokes are caused by bleeding into brain tissue. This type of stroke usually is from a blood vessel rupture caused by hypertension, aneurysms, arteriovenous malformations, head injury, or blood dyscrasias and has a much higher fatality rate than ischemic strokes.

Risk Factors

Among the major risk factors for stroke are age, sex, race, heart disease, hypertension, high cholesterol levels, cigarette smoking, prior stroke, and diabetes mellitus.[29,30] Other risk factors include sickle cell disease, polycythemia, blood dyscrasias, excess alcohol use, cocaine and illicit drug use, obesity, and sedentary lifestyle. The incidence of stroke increases with age, with a 1% per year increased risk for persons 65 to 74 years of age; the incidence of stroke is approximately 19% greater in men than women; and African Americans have a 60% greater risk of death and disability from stroke than whites.[29] Heart disease, particularly atrial fibrillation and other conditions that predispose to clot formation on the wall of the heart or valve leaflets or to paradoxical embolism through right-to-left shunting, predisposes to cardioembolic stroke. Polycythemia, sickle cell disease (during sickle cell crisis), and blood disorders predispose to clot formation in the cerebral vessels. Alcohol can contribute to stroke in several ways: induction of cardiac arrhythmias and defects in ventricular wall motion that lead to cerebral embolism, induction of hypertension, enhancement of blood coagulation disorders, and reduction of cerebral blood flow.[31] Another cause of stroke is cocaine. Cocaine use causes both ischemic and hemorrhagic strokes by inducing vasospasm, enhanced platelet activity, and increased blood pressure, heart rate, body temperature, and metabolic rate. Cocaine stroke victims range in age from newborn (*i.e.*, from maternal cocaine use) to old age.[32]

Elimination or control of risk factors for cerebrovascular disease (*e.g.*, use of tobacco, control of blood lipids and blood sugar, reduction of hypertension) offers the best opportunity to prevent cerebral ischemia from cerebral atherosclerosis. Early detection and treatment offer significant advantages over waiting until a serious event has occurred.

Ischemic Stroke

Ischemic strokes are caused by cerebrovascular obstruction by thrombosis or emboli (Fig. 50-9). Various methods have been used to classify ischemic cerebrovascular disease. A common classification system identifies five stroke subtypes and their frequency; 20% large artery atherosclerotic disease (both thrombosis and arterial emboli); 25% small vessel or penetrating artery disease (so-called *lacunar stroke*); 20% cardiogenic embolism; 30% cryptogenic stroke (undetermined cause); and 5% other, unusual causes[33] (*i.e.*, migraine, dissection, coagulopathy).

Ischemic Penumbra in Evolving Stroke.   During the evolution of a stroke, there usually is a central core of dead or dying cells, surrounded by an ischemic band or area of minimally perfused cells called the *penumbra* (*i.e.*, halo). Brain cells of the penumbra receive marginal blood flow and their metabolic activities are impaired; although the area undergoes an "electrical failure," the structural integrity of the brain cells is maintained.[34] Whether the cells of the penumbra continue to survive depends on the successful timely return of adequate circulation, the volume of toxic products released by the neighboring dying cells, the degree of cerebral edema, and alterations in local blood flow. If the toxic products result in additional death of cells in the penumbra, the core of dead or dying tissue enlarges, and the volume of surrounding ischemic tissue increases.

Transient Ischemic Attacks.   Transient ischemic attacks are characterized by focal ischemic cerebral neurologic deficits that last for less than 24 hours (usually less than 1 to 2 hours). TIA or "ministroke" is equivalent to "brain angina" and reflects a temporary disturbance in focal cerebral blood flow, which reverses before infarction occurs, analogous to angina in relation to heart attack. The term *TIA* and the qualification of a deficit resolving within 24 hours were defined before the mechanisms of ischemic cell damage and the penumbra were known. A more accu-

Stroke/Brain Attack

➤ Stroke is an acute focal neurologic deficit from an interruption of blood flow in a cerebral vessel (ischemic stroke, the most common type) due to thrombi or emboli or to bleeding into the brain tissue (hemorrhagic stroke).

➤ The term *brain attack* as a description for stroke is intended to alert people to the need for immediate treatment at the first sign of a stroke.

➤ During the evolution of an ischemic stroke, there usually is a central core of dead or dying cells surrounded by an ischemic band of minimally perfused cells called a *penumbra*. Whether the cells of the penumbra continue to survive depends on the successful timely return of adequate circulation.

➤ The realization that there is a window of opportunity during which ischemic but viable brain tissue can be salvaged has led to the use of thrombolytic agents in the early treatment of ischemic stroke.

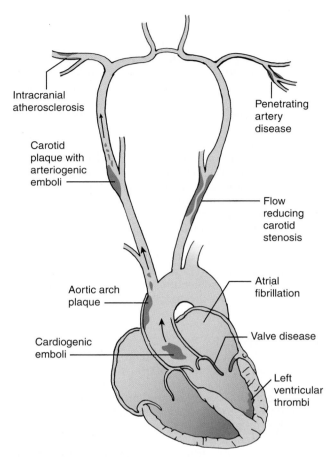

FIGURE 50-9 The most frequent sites of arterial and cardiac abnormalities causing ischemic stroke. (From Albers G.W., Easton D., Sacco R.L., Teal P. [1999]. Antithrombotic and thrombotic therapy for ischemic stroke. *Chest* 114 (5), 684S)

chronic atherosclerosis, with or without embolization of the plaque material distally, or from critical perfusion failure distal to a stenosis (watershed). These infarcts often affect the cortex, causing aphasia or neglect, visual field defects, or the retina (amaurosis fugax). In most cases of stroke, a single cerebral artery and its territories are affected. Usually, thrombotic strokes are seen in older persons and frequently are accompanied by evidence of arteriosclerotic heart or peripheral arterial disease. The thrombotic stroke is not associated with activity and may occur in a person at rest.

Small Vessel Stroke (Lacunar Infarct).   Lacunar infarcts are small (1.5 to 2.0 cm) to very small (3 to 4 mm) infarcts located in the deeper, noncortical parts of the brain or in the brain stem. They are found in the territory of single deep penetrating arteries supplying the internal capsule, basal ganglia, or brain stem. They result from occlusion of the smaller branches of large cerebral arteries, commonly the middle cerebral and posterior cerebral arteries and less commonly the anterior cerebral, vertebral, or basilar arteries. In the process of healing, lacunar infarcts leave behind small cavities, or lacunae (lakes). They are thought to result from arteriolar lipohyalinosis or microatheroma, commonly in the settings of chronic hypertension or diabetes. Six basic causes of lacunar infarcts have been proposed: embolism, hypertension, small vessel occlusive disease, hematologic abnormalities, small intracerebral hemorrhages, and vasospasm. Because of their size and location, lacunar infarcts usually do not cause cortical deficits like aphasia or apraxia. Instead, they produce classic recognizable "lacunar syndromes" such as pure motor hemiplegia, pure sensory hemiplegia, and dysarthria with the clumsy hand syndrome. Because CT scans are not sensitive enough to detect these tiny infarcts, diagnosis used to depend on clinical features alone. The use of magnetic resonance imaging (MRI) has allowed frequent visualization of small vessel infarcts and is obligatory to confirm such a lesion.

Cardiogenic Embolic Stroke.   An embolic stroke is caused by a moving blood clot that travels from its origin to the brain. It usually affects the larger proximal cerebral vessels, often lodging at bifurcations. The most frequent site of embolic strokes is the middle cerebral artery, probably because it offers the path of least resistance, reflecting the large territory of this vessel and its position as the terminus of the carotid artery. Although most cerebral emboli originate from a thrombus in the left heart, they also may originate in an atherosclerotic plaque in the carotid arteries. The embolus travels quickly to the brain and becomes lodged in a smaller artery through which it cannot pass. Embolic stroke usually has a sudden onset with immediate maximum deficit.

Various cardiac conditions predispose to formation of emboli that produce embolic stroke, including rheumatic heart disease, atrial fibrillation, recent myocardial infarction, ventricular aneurysm, mobile aortic arch atheroma and bacterial endocarditis. More recently, the use of transesophageal echocardiography, which better images the interatrial septum, has implicated a patent foramen ovale

rate definition now is a deficit lasting less than 24 minutes, and it may best be described as a zone of penumbra without central infarction. The causes of TIAs are the same as those of ischemic stroke, and include atherosclerotic disease of cerebral vessels and emboli. TIAs are important because they may provide warning of impending stroke. In fact, the risk of stroke after a TIA is similar to the risk after a first stroke, and is maximal immediately after the event: 4% to 8% risk of stroke within 1 month, 12% to 13% risk during the first year, and 24% to 29% risk over 5 years.[35] Diagnosis of TIA before a stroke may permit surgical or medical intervention that prevents an eventual stroke and the associated neurologic deficits.[35]

Large Vessel (Thrombotic) Stroke.   Thrombi are the most common cause of ischemic strokes, usually occurring in atherosclerotic blood vessels. In the cerebral circulation, atherosclerotic plaques are found most commonly at arterial bifurcations. Common sites of plaque formation include larger vessels of the brain, notably the origins of the internal carotid and vertebral arteries, and junctions of the basilar and vertebral arteries. Cerebral infarction can result from an acute local thrombosis and occlusion at the site of

as a source for paradoxical venous emboli to the arterial system. Advances in the diagnosis and treatment of heart disease can be expected to alter favorably the incidence of embolic stroke.

Hemorrhagic Stroke

The most frequently fatal stroke is a spontaneous hemorrhage into the brain substance.[36,37] With rupture of a blood vessel, hemorrhage into the brain tissue occurs, resulting in edema, compression of the brain contents, or spasm of the adjacent blood vessels. The most common predisposing factors are advancing age and hypertension. Other causes of hemorrhage are aneurysm, trauma, erosion of the vessels by tumors, arteriovenous malformations, coagulopathies, vasculitis, and drugs. A cerebral hemorrhage occurs suddenly, usually when the person is active. Vomiting commonly occurs at the onset, and headache sometimes occurs. Focal symptoms depend on which vessel is involved. In the most common situation, hemorrhage into the basal ganglia results in contralateral hemiplegia, with initial flaccidity progressing to spasticity. The hemorrhage and resultant edema exert great pressure on the brain substance, and the clinical course progresses rapidly to coma and frequently to death.

Acute Manifestations of Stroke

The specific manifestations of stroke or TIA are determined by the cerebral artery that is affected, by the area of brain tissue that is supplied by that vessel, and by the adequacy of the collateral circulation. Symptoms of stroke/TIA always are sudden in onset and focal, and usually one-sided. The most common symptom is weakness of the face and arm, sometimes also of the leg. Other frequent stroke symptoms are unilateral numbness, vision loss in one eye (amaurosis fugax) or to one side (hemianopia), language disturbance (aphasia), slurred speech (dysarthria), and sudden, unexplained imbalance or ataxia. In the event of TIA, symptoms rapidly resolve spontaneously, although the underlying mechanisms are the same as for stroke. The specific stroke signs depend on the specific vascular territory compromised (Table 50-6). As a generalization, carotid ischemia causes monocular visual loss or aphasia (dominant hemisphere) or hemineglect (nondominant hemisphere), contralateral sensory or motor loss, or other discrete cortical signs such as apraxia and agnosia. Vertebrobasilar ischemia induces ataxia, diplopia, hemianopia, vertigo, cranial nerve deficits, contralateral hemiplegia, sensory deficits (either contralateral or crossed, *i.e.*, contralateral body and ipsilateral face), and arousal defects. Discrete

---

TABLE 50-6 ✦ Signs and Symptoms of Stroke by Involved Cerebral Artery

Cerebral Artery	Brain Area Involved	Signs and Symptoms*
Anterior cerebral	Infarction of the medial aspect of one frontal lobe if lesion is distal to communicating artery; bilateral frontal infarction if flow in other anterior cerebral artery is inadequate	Paralysis of contralateral foot or leg; impaired gait; paresis of contralateral arm; contralateral sensory loss over toes, foot, and leg; problems making decisions or performing acts voluntarily; lack of spontaneity, easily distracted; slowness of thought; aphasia depends on the hemisphere involved; urinary incontinence; cognitive and affective disorders
Middle cerebral	Massive infarction of most of lateral hemisphere and deeper structures of the frontal, parietal, and temporal lobes; internal capsule; basal ganglia	Contralateral hemiplegia (face and arm); contralateral sensory impairment; aphasia; homonymous hemianopia; altered consciousness (confusion to coma); inability to turn eyes toward paralyzed side; denial of paralyzed side or limb (hemiattention); possible acalculia, alexia, finger agnosia, and left–right confusion; vasomotor paresis and instability
Posterior cerebral	Occipital lobe; anterior and medial portion of temporal lobe	Homonymous hemianopia and other visual defects such as color blindness, loss of central vision, and visual hallucinations; memory deficits, perseveration (repeated performance of same verbal or motor response)
	Thalamus involvement	Loss of all sensory modalities; spontaneous pain; intentional tremor; mild hemiparesis; aphasia
	Cerebral peduncle involvement	Oculomotor nerve palsy with contralateral hemiplegia
Basilar and vertebral	Cerebellum and brain stem	Visual disturbance such as diplopia, dystaxia, vertigo, dysphagia, dysphonia

*Depend on hemisphere involved and adequacy of collaterals.

subsets of these vascular syndromes usually occur, depending on which branches of the involved artery are blocked.

Diagnosis

Accurate diagnosis of stroke is based on a complete history and thorough physical and neurologic examination. A careful history, including documentation of previous TIAs, the time of onset and pattern and rapidity of system progression, the specific focal symptoms (to determine the likely vascular territory), and the existence of any coexisting diseases, can help to determine the type of stroke that is involved. The diagnostic evaluation should aim to determine the presence of hemorrhage or ischemia, identify the stroke or TIA mechanism (large vessel or small vessel atherothrombotic, cardioembolic, other or cryptogenic, hemorrhagic), characterize the severity of clinical deficits, and unmask the presence of risk factors.

Imaging studies document the brain infarction and the anatomy and pathology of the related blood vessels. CT scans and MRI have become essential tools in diagnosing stroke, differentiating cerebral hemorrhage from ischemia and excluding intracranial lesions that mimic stroke clinically. CT scans are a necessary screening tool in the acute setting for rapid identification of hemorrhage, but are insensitive to ischemia within 24 hours, and to any brain stem or small infarcts. MRI is superior for imaging ischemic lesions in all territories. Newer MRI techniques such as perfusion- and diffusion-weighted imaging can reveal cerebral ischemia immediately after onset and identify areas of potentially reversible damage (*i.e.*, penumbra). Arteriography can demonstrate the site of the vascular abnormality and afford visualization of most intracranial vascular areas. Although angiography still is required for invasive treatments and for maximal sensitivity, magnetic resonance angiography (MRA) has largely replaced angiography as a screening tool for vascular lesions.

Two other types of imaging, positron emission tomography and single-photon emission computed tomography, are nuclear studies used to assess the distribution of blood flow and metabolic activity of the brain. These tests rarely are used in routine stroke management because of limited availability, and are applied more often in clinical research of cerebral ischemia.

The introduction of several Doppler ultrasonographic techniques has facilitated the noninvasive evaluation of the cerebral circulation, especially for detection of carotid stenosis. Emitted signals may be uninterrupted (*i.e.*, continuous-wave Doppler) or intermittent (*i.e.*, pulsed-wave Doppler). The flow characteristics of all vessels in the depth of field are demonstrated on the continuous-wave Doppler; the pulsed-wave Doppler samples flow at any depth. Use of these methods has increased because of low cost, ease of application, safety features, continuous technical advances, improved imaging quality, and increased reliability.[34]

Treatment of Stroke

The treatment of acute ischemic stroke changed markedly since the early 1990s, with an emphasis on salvaging brain tissue and minimizing long-term disability. The realization that there is a window of opportunity during which ischemic but viable brain tissue can be salvaged has led to the use of thrombolytic agents in the early treatment of ischemic stroke. Although the results of emergent treatment of hemorrhagic stroke have been less dramatic, continued efforts to reduce disability have been promising.

The use of thrombolytic therapy for stroke was first investigated in the late 1960s and early 1970s, but it was quickly abandoned because of hemorrhagic complications. Because these studies were done before CT scanning was available, exclusion of persons with hemorrhagic stroke was difficult. Patients also were treated many hours after stroke, which now is understood to be beyond the time window of penumbral cell viability. The interest in thrombolytic therapy has increased because of the development of new thrombolytic agents and the availability of diagnostic scanning methods that are able to differentiate between ischemic and hemorrhagic stroke.

Thrombolytic agents include streptokinase, urokinase, recombinant tissue-type plasminogen activator (tPA), p-anisoylated lys-plasminogen-streptokinase activator complex (see Chapter 14). The first agent approved by the U.S. Food and Drug Administration, in 1996, was tPA. A subcommittee of the Stroke Council of the American Heart Association has developed guidelines for the use of tPA for acute stroke.[38-40] These guidelines recommend that in persons with suspected stroke, the diagnosis of hemorrhagic stroke be excluded through the use of CT scanning before administration of thrombolytic therapy, which must be administered within 3 hours of onset of symptoms. The major risk of treatment with thrombolytic agents is intracranial hemorrhage of the infarcted brain. A number of conditions, including use of oral anticoagulant medications, a history of gastrointestinal bleeding, recent myocardial infarction, previous stroke or head injury within 3 months, surgery within the past 14 days, and a blood pressure greater than 200/120 mm Hg, are considered contraindications to thrombolytic therapy.[39]

The successful treatment of stroke depends on education of the public, paramedics, and health care professionals in emergency care facilities about the need for early diagnosis and treatment. As with heart attack, the message should be "do not wait to decide if the symptoms subside but seek immediate treatment." Effective medical and surgical procedures may preserve brain function and prevent disability.

Longer-term treatment is aimed at preventing complications and recurrent stroke and promoting the fullest possible recovery of function. During the acute phase, proper positioning and range-of-motion exercises are essential. Early rehabilitation efforts include all members of the rehabilitation team—physician, nurse, speech therapist, physical therapist, and occupational therapist—and the family.

ANEURYSMAL SUBARACHNOID HEMORRHAGE

Aneurysmal subarachnoid hemorrhage represents bleeding into the subarachnoid space caused by a ruptured cerebral aneurysm. Bleeding into the subarachnoid space can extend well beyond the site of origin, flooding the basal cistern, ventricles, and spinal subarachnoid space.[41–43] Aneurysmal subarachnoid hemorrhages occur most frequently between 30 and 60 years of age and seldom are seen in children. The mortality and morbidity rates with aneurysmal subarachnoid hemorrhage are high. Only approximately one third of persons who experience aneurysmal subarachnoid hemorrhage recover without major disability.[11]

An aneurysm is a bulge at the site of a localized weakness in the muscular wall of an arterial vessel. Most aneurysms are small saccular aneurysms called *berry aneurysms* (Fig. 50-10). They usually occur in the anterior circulation and are found at bifurcations and other junctions of vessels such as those in the circle of Willis. There is angiographic evidence that these aneurysms enlarge with time and produce weakening of the vessel wall, often to the extent that only a thin fibrous vessel wall remains. The probability of rupture increases with the size of the aneurysm; aneurysms larger than 10 mm in diameter have a 50% chance of bleeding per year.[1] Rupture often occurs with acute increases in ICP. Large aneurysms also may cause chronic headache, neurologic deficits, or both. For example, giant aneurysms of the internal carotid artery may cause persistent headache and ptosis because of pressure on the third cranial nerve. Small aneurysms may go unnoticed; intact aneurysms frequently are found at autopsy as an incidental finding.[1]

The cause of aneurysms is unknown. Intracranial aneurysms are thought to arise from a congenital defect in the media of the involved vessels, particularly at bifurcations. Considerable evidence supports the role of genetic factors in the pathogenesis of intracranial aneurysms. Family history seems to be a significant risk factor. Persons with heritable connective tissue disorders such as autosomal dominant polycystic kidney disease, Ehlers-Danlos syndrome, neurofibromatosis type I, and Marfan's syndrome are at particular risk.[1] There also is evidence linking age and environmental factors with the development of aneurysms. For example, intracranial aneurysms are rare in children, and although the mean age for subarachnoid hemorrhage is approximately 50 years, the incidence of hemorrhage increases with age. Of the various environmental factors that may predispose to aneurysmal subarachnoid hemorrhage, cigarette smoking and hypertension appear to constitute the greatest risks.

Subarachnoid hemorrhage is a dreaded complication of cerebral aneurysm. When it occurs, the onset of subarachnoid aneurysmal rupture often is heralded by a sudden and severe headache, described as "the worst headache of my life." Other manifestations of subarachnoid hemorrhage include signs of meningeal irritation such as nuchal rigidity (neck stiffness) and photophobia (light intolerance); cranial nerve deficits, especially cranial nerve II, and sometimes III and IV (diplopia and blurred vision); stroke syndrome; loss of consciousness; increased ICP; and pituitary dysfunction. Bleeding into the subarachnoid space causes meningeal irritation with the resulting signs of headache and nuchal rigidity. The optic nerves are ensheathed in meninges, and meningeal irritation causes photophobia. Occasionally, nausea and vomiting accompany the presenting symptoms. In other cases, there may be no focal neurologic findings. If bleeding is severe, headache may be accompanied by collapse and loss of consciousness. Depending on the course of the bleeding, the headache subsides slowly over a matter of days. Hypertension is a frequent finding and may be the result of the hemorrhage. Cardiac dysrhythmias and noncardiac edema result from massive release of catecholamines triggered by the subarachnoid hemorrhage.

Approximately 50% of persons with subarachnoid hemorrhage have a history of atypical headaches occurring days to weeks before the onset of hemorrhage, suggesting the presence of a small leak.[42,43] These headaches are characterized by sudden onset and often are accompanied by nausea, vomiting, and dizziness. Persons with these symptoms may be mistakenly diagnosed as having tension or migraine headaches.

The complications of aneurysmal rupture include rebleeding, vasospasm with cerebral ischemia, hydrocephalus, hypothalamic dysfunction, and seizure activity. Rebleeding and vasospasm are the most severe and most difficult to treat. Rebleeding, which has its highest incidence on the first day after the initial rupture, results in further and usually catastrophic neurologic deficits.

Vasospasm is a dreaded complication of aneurysmal rupture. The condition is difficult to treat and is associated with a high incidence of morbidity and mortality. Although the description of aneurysm-associated vasospasm is relatively uniform, its proposed mechanisms are controversial. Usually, the condition develops within 3 to 10 days (peak, 7 days) after aneurysm rupture and involves a focal narrowing of the cerebral artery or arteries that can be visualized on arteriography. The neurologic status gradually deteriorates as blood supply to the brain in the region of the spasm is decreased; this usually can be differentiated from the rapid deterioration seen in rebleeding. Vasospasm is

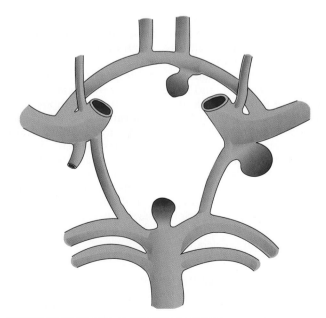

FIGURE 50-10 Locations of berry aneurysms.

treated by attempting to maintain adequate CPP through the use of vasoactive drugs or administration of large amounts of intravenous fluids to increase intravascular volume and produce hemodilution to maintain vessel patency and prevent sludging of blood flow. There is risk of rebleeding from this therapy. Early surgery may provide some protection from vasospasm. Endovascular techniques, including balloon dilatation, have been developed to treat narrowed arterial segments mechanically. Nimodipine, a drug that blocks calcium channels and selectively acts on cerebral blood vessels, may be used to prevent or treat vasospasm.

Another complication of aneurysm rupture is the development of hydrocephalus. It is thought to result from obstruction of the arachnoid villi of the CSF system, which are responsible for reabsorption of CSF. The lysis of blood in the subarachnoid space causes the protein content of the CSF to increase, thereby preventing diffusion of CSF across the arachnoid villi, plugging the system and resulting in hydrocephalus. Occasionally, hydrocephalus can be managed medically by the use of osmotic diuretics, but if neurologic deterioration is significant, surgical placement of a shunt is indicated. Hydrocephalus is diagnosed by serial CT scans, by the increasing size of the ventricles, and by the clinical signs of increased ICP.

The diagnosis of subarachnoid hemorrhage and intracranial aneurysms is made by clinical presentation, CT scan, lumbar puncture, and angiography. The CT scan is the most commonly used diagnostic method for subarachnoid hemorrhage. Lumbar puncture may be used to detect blood in the CSF, but the procedure has a risk of rebleeding and brain herniation. Among the methods used for diagnosis of intracranial aneurysms are conventional angiography, MRA, and helical (spiral) CT angiography. Conventional angiography is the definitive diagnostic tool for detecting the aneurysm. This procedure involves the injection of contrast into an artery so the vessel can be visualized using fluoroscopic or x-ray methods; defects such as vasospasm can be detected. MRA does not require the intravascular administration of contrast. Helical CT angiography has the advantage of screening for new aneurysms in persons with ferromagnetic clips in whom the use of MRI is contraindicated.

The course of treatment after aneurysm rupture depends on the extent of neurologic deficit. Persons with less severe deficits, with or without headache and no neurologic deficits, may undergo cerebral arteriography and early surgery, usually within 24 to 72 hours. A procedure involving craniotomy and clipping often is used. In this procedure, a specially designed silver clip is inserted and tightened around the neck of the aneurysm. This procedure offers protection from rebleeding and may permit removal of the hematoma. Some persons with subarachnoid hemorrhage are managed medically for 10 days or more in an attempt to improve their clinical status before surgery. The use of endovascular techniques such as balloon embolization and platinum coil electrothrombosis is evolving.

Arteriovenous Malformations

Arteriovenous malformations are a complex tangle of abnormal arteries and veins linked by one or more fistulas.[44] These vascular networks lack a capillary bed and the small arteries have a deficient muscularis layer. Arteriovenous malformations have long been thought to arise from failure in development of the capillary network in the embryonic brain. As the child's brain grows, the malformation acquires additional arterial contributions that enlarge to form a tangled collection of thin-walled vessels that shunt blood directly from the arterial to the venous circulation. Learning disorders have been documented in 66% of adults with arteriovenous malformations.[44] Approximately 90% of arteriovenous malformations are in the cerebral hemispheres; one half are superficial, and the others are buried more deeply.

The hemodynamic effects of arteriovenous malformations are twofold. First, blood is shunted from the high-pressure arterial system to the low-pressure venous system without the buffering advantage of the capillary network. The draining venous channels are exposed to high levels of pressure, predisposing them to rupture and hemorrhage. Second, impaired perfusion affects the cerebral tissue adjacent to the arteriovenous malformation. The elevated arterial and venous pressures and lack of a capillary circulation impair cerebral perfusion by producing a high-flow situation that diverts blood away from the surrounding tissue. Clinically, this is evidenced by slowly progressive neurologic deficits. The diversion of blood to the arteriovenous malformation has been referred to as *vascular steal phenomenon.*

Arteriovenous malformations typically present before 40 years of age and affect men and women equally. Rupture of vessels in the malformation accounts for approximately 2% of all strokes.[44] The major clinical manifestations of arteriovenous malformations are hemorrhage, seizures, headache, and progressive neurologic deficits. Approximately 50% of arteriovenous malformations present with intracerebral hemorrhage. Subarachnoid hemorrhage and intraventricular hemorrhage also may occur, but are less frequent than intracerebral hemorrhage. Headaches often are severe, and persons with the disorder may describe them as being throbbing and synchronous with their heart beat. Other, less common symptoms include visual symptoms (*i.e.*, diplopia and hemianopia), hemiparesis, mental deterioration, and speech deficits. Definitive diagnosis often is obtained through cerebral angiography.

Treatment methods include surgical excision, endovascular occlusion, and radiation therapy. Because of the nature of the malformation, each of these methods is accompanied by some risk of complications. If the arteriovenous malformation is accessible, surgical excision usually is the treatment of choice. Endovascular treatment involves the insertion of flow-directed and flow-assisted microcatheters into the cerebral circulation for delivery of embolic materials (*e.g.*, microballoons, sclerosing agents, microcoils, or quick-drying glue) to the arteriovenous malformation site.[44,45] Radiation therapy (also known as *radiosurgery*) may involve the use of a gamma knife, proton beam, or linear accelerator.[44]

LONG-TERM DISABILITIES

Stroke and cerebrovascular disorders often cause long-term disabilities, including motor and sensory deficits, language and speech problems, and a condition called the *hemineglect syndrome.* Although there are many other disorders of motor, sensory, and perceptual function, they are beyond the scope of this text.

Motor Deficits

After a stroke affecting an area of the corticospinal tract such as the motor cortex, posterior limb of the internal capsule, or medullary pyramids, there is profound weakness on the contralateral side. A slight corticospinal lesion may be indicated by clumsiness in carrying out fine movements of the fingers (*e.g.*, buttoning, sewing) rather than obvious weakness. There is a tendency toward foot drop, outward rotation of the leg, and dependent edema in the affected extremities. Putting the extremities through passive range-of-motion exercises helps to maintain the joint function and to prevent edema, shoulder subluxation (*i.e.*, incomplete dislocation), and muscle atrophy. The smooth sequential movement of the exercises also may help to reestablish motor patterns.

When the corticospinal tract has been affected, muscle tone gradually returns after a few weeks, and then spasticity begins to replace the initial flaccidity within 6 to 8 weeks. Spasticity involves an increase in the tone of affected muscles and usually an element of weakness. Because of the distribution of muscle hypertonia with spasticity, the flexor muscles usually are more strongly affected in the upper extremities and the extensor muscles more strongly affected in the lower extremities. Various mechanisms, including disinhibition of segmental and suprasegmental reflexes and reorganization of segmental circuitry, appear to contribute to spasticity. Altered limb posture may be manifested by shoulder adduction, forearm pronation, finger flexion, and knee and hip extension. If no voluntary movement or movement on command appears within a few months, function probably will not return to that extremity. Passive range-of-motion exercises should be continued, and positioning should be directed toward keeping all the joints in functional positions.

Language and Speech Problems

Communication is a complex process by which ideas and feelings are exchanged; it is accomplished by means of various behavioral patterns, gestures, expressions, and symbols. Communication involves memory, reasoning, and emotions, as well as speech and language. Two key aspects of communication are language and speech. Language involves higher-order integrative functions of the forebrain. It is used to communicate thoughts and feeling through the use of symbolic formulations, such as words or numbers, and information is transmitted vocally or graphically. Speech involves the mechanical act of articulating language, the "motor act" of verbal expression.[46] Speech depends on the functional integrity of the peripheral musculature involved and its control by upper and lower motoneurons.

Disorders of language and speech fall into three general categories: disturbances of the central processing mechanisms of language, which result in aphasia; dysfunction of the larynx, pharynx, palate, tongue, lips, or mouth, which results in dysarthria; and apraxia of speech, in which the person is unable to program a sequence of the volitional movements needed for speech despite the absence of motor deficits.[47] Some persons exhibit elements of all three components of speech and language disorders. Aphasia may be localized above the tentorium to the cerebral cortex; dysarthria localizes to any level affecting motor control to the face, oropharynx, or larynx.

Dysarthria. Dysarthria is imperfect articulation of speech sounds or changes in voice pitch or quality, and does not relate to the content of speech. It is caused by disturbed motor control resulting from damage to the nervous system. A person with dysarthria may demonstrate an inability to articulate while still retaining language ability, or may have a concurrent language problem as well.

Aphasia. *Aphasia* is a general term that encompasses varying degrees of inability to comprehend, integrate, and express language. The most common cause is a vascular lesion of the middle cerebral artery of the dominant hemisphere (*i.e.*, the hemisphere responsible for mediation of language). The left hemisphere is dominant in approximately 95% of right-handed and 70% of left-handed persons. The cerebral hemispheres usually function similarly in controlling opposite sides of the body. Language dominance by one hemisphere does not occur before 1 to 2 years of age. Because the other hemisphere appears to take over, unilateral lesions occurring during childhood usually result in only transient language disorders.

Aphasia can be categorized as receptive or expressive, or as fluent or nonfluent. Most aphasias are partial, and a thorough speech evaluation is needed to determine the type and extent of language disorder and appropriate therapy. *Fluency* relates to the ease and spontaneity of conversational speech, and is more strictly defined by the rate of speech. This has been classified as (fluent = many words, nonfluent = few words). Fluent speech requires little or no effort, is articulate, and is of increased quantity. The term *fluent* refers only to the ease and rate of verbal output, and does not relate to the content of speech or the ability of the person to comprehend what is being said. There are three categories of fluent aphasia: Wernicke's, anomic, and conductive aphasia. Wernicke's aphasia is characterized by an inability to comprehend the speech of others and of oneself. Wernicke's aphasia includes deficits of reading. Lesions of the posterior temporal or lower parietal lobe (areas 22 and 39) are associated with receptive, fluent aphasia. Anomic aphasia is speech that is nearly normal except for a difficulty with finding singular words. Conduction aphasia is inappropriate word use manifest as impaired repetition and speech riddled with word substitutions, despite good comprehension and fluency. Conduction aphasia (*i.e.*, disconnection syndrome) results from destruction of the fiber system under the insula that connects Wernicke's and Broca's areas.

Expressive or nonfluent aphasia is characterized by an inability to spontaneously communicate or translate thoughts or ideas into meaningful speech or writing. Speech production is limited, effortful, and halting and often may be poorly articulated because of a concurrent dysarthria. The person may be able, with difficulty, to utter two or three words, especially those with an emotional overlay. Comprehension is normal, and the person seems to be aware of his or her deficits but is unable to correct them. This often leads to frustration, anger, and depression. Expressive aphasia is associated with lesions of Broca's area of the dominant frontal lobe (areas 44 and 45).

Denial or Hemiattention

Because of an inability to analyze and interpret incoming sensory information caused by some the disruptive lesions of the brain and the internal production of abnormal signals, some persons with stroke have a form of denial of illness and a denial of one half of the body and environment on that side of the body (*i.e.*, hemiattention or hemineglect). Such persons are unaware of the deficit. For example, a person with left hemineglect may raise the right arm when asked, but when asked to raise the left arm, he or she may say, "I just did." Spatial orientation often is impaired, and patients have difficulty localizing stimuli, their own limbs, and objects in space. Affected persons may totally disregard stimuli coming from the involved side of the body, even though they can see and hear. The affected side of the body may go unattended and ungroomed (*i.e.*, hemineglect). The person may wash or shave only the unaffected side of the body. When asked to draw a picture of themselves, these persons often draw a person with only one arm and leg. The condition is more common in persons with strokes that affect the nondominant hemisphere side of the brain, usually the right hemisphere, which is more involved with spatial orientation, body image, and inductive modes of reasoning.

> In summary, a stroke, or "brain attack," is an acute focal neurologic deficit caused by a vascular disorder that injures brain tissue. It is the third leading cause of death in the United States and a major cause of disability. There are two main types of stroke: ischemic and hemorrhagic. Ischemic stroke, which is the most common type, is caused by cerebrovascular obstruction by a thrombus or emboli. Hemorrhagic stroke, which is associated with greater morbidity and mortality, is caused by the rupture of a blood vessel and bleeding into the brain. The acute manifestations of stroke depend on the location of the blood vessel that is involved and can include motor, sensory, language, speech, and cognitive disorders. Early diagnosis and treatment with thrombolytic agents has improved the outlook for many persons with ischemic stroke. Treatment of long-term neurologic deficits from stroke is primarily symptomatic, involving the combined efforts of the health care team, the patient, and the family.
>
> A subarachnoid hemorrhage involves bleeding into the subarachnoid space. Most subarachnoid hemorrhages are the result of a ruptured cerebral aneurysm. Presenting symptoms include headache, nuchal rigidity, photophobia, and nausea. Complications include rebleeding, vasospasm, and hydrocephalus. Arteriovenous malformations are congenital abnormal communications between arterial and venous channels that result from failure in development of the capillary network in the embryonic brain. The vessels in the arteriovenous malformations may enlarge to form a space-occupying lesion, become weak and predispose to bleeding, and divert blood away from other parts of the brain; they can cause brain hemorrhage, seizures, headache, and other neurologic deficits.

Trauma, Infections, and Neoplasms

After you have completed this section of the chapter, you should be able to meet the following objectives:

♦ Differentiate primary and secondary brain injuries due to head trauma
♦ Describe the mechanism of brain damage in coup-contrecoup injuries
♦ List the constellation of symptoms involved in the postconcussion syndrome
♦ Compare the manifestations of mild, moderate, and severe head injury
♦ Differentiate among the location, manifestations, and morbidity of epidural, subdural, and intracerebral hematoma
♦ List the sequence of events that occur with meningitis
♦ Describe the symptoms of encephalitis
♦ List the major categories of brain tumors and interpret the meaning of *benign* and *malignant* as related to brain tumors
♦ Describe the general manifestations of brain tumors
♦ List the methods used in diagnosis and treatment of brain tumors

HEAD INJURY

The brain is enclosed in the protective confines of the rigid bony skull. Although the skull affords protection for the tissues of the CNS, it also provides the potential for development of ischemic and traumatic brain injuries. This is because it cannot expand to accommodate the increase in volume that occurs when there is swelling or bleeding in its confines. The bony structures themselves can cause injury to the nervous system. Fractures of the skull can compress sections of the nervous system, or they can splinter and cause penetrating wounds.

The term *head injury* is used to describe all structural damage to the head, and has become synonymous with *brain injury*.[48] In the United States, head injury is the leading cause of death among persons younger than 24 years of age. The main causes of head injury are road accidents, falls, and assaults, and the most common cause of fatal head injuries is road accidents involving vehicles and pedestrians.[49]

Head injuries can involve both closed injuries and open wounds. Skull fractures can be divided into three groups: simple, depressed, and basilar. A *simple* or *linear* skull fracture is a break in the continuity of bone. A *comminuted* skull fracture refers to a splintered or multiple fracture line. When bone fragments are embedded into the brain tissue, the fracture is said to be *depressed*. A fracture of the bones that form the base of the skull is called a *basilar* skull fracture.

Radiologic examination usually is needed to confirm the presence and extent of a skull fracture. This evaluation is important because of the possible damage to the underlying tissues. The ethmoid cribriform plate, through which the olfactory fibers enter the skull, represents the most fragile portion of the neurocranium and is shattered in basal skull fractures. A frequent complication of basilar skull fractures is leakage of CSF from the nose (rhinorrhea) or ear (otorrhea); this occurs because of the proximity of the base of the skull to the nose and ear. This break in protection of the brain becomes a probable source of infection of the meninges or of brain substance. There may be lacerations to the vessels of the dura, with resultant intracranial bleeding. Damage to the cranial nerves (I, II, III, VII, VIII) also may result from basilar skull fractures if the fracture is in the vicinity of the foramen magnum, from which the cranial nerves exit the skull.

Types of Brain Injuries

The effects of traumatic head injuries can be divided into two categories: primary or direct injuries, in which damage is caused by impact, and secondary injuries, in which damage results from the subsequent brain swelling, intracranial hematomas, infection, cerebral hypoxia, and ischemia.

Primary head injuries include concussion, contusion, and laceration. Even if there is no break in the skull, a blow to the head can cause severe and diffuse brain damage. Such closed injuries vary in severity and can be classified as focal or diffuse. Focal injuries include contusion, laceration, and hemorrhage. Diffuse injuries include concussion, contusion, diffuse axonal injury (formerly known as *shearing lesion*), and hypoxic brain injury.

Ischemia is considered to be the most common cause of secondary brain injury. It can cause the hypoxia and hypotension that occur during the resuscitation process or the impairment of regulatory mechanisms by which cerebrovascular responses maintain an adequate blood flow and oxygen supply.[50,51] Insults that occur immediately after injury or in the course of resuscitation efforts are important determinants of the outcome from severe brain injury. More than 25% of patients with severe head injury sustain one or more secondary insults in the time between injury and resuscitation, indicating the need for improved airway management and circulatory status.[50] The significance of secondary injuries depends on the extent of damage caused by the primary injury. Certain secondary injuries have been discussed, such as increased ICP, cerebral edema, and brain herniation.

In mild head injury, there may be momentary loss of consciousness without demonstrable neurologic symptoms or residual damage, except for possible residual amnesia. Microscopic changes usually can be detected in the neurons and glia within hours of injury. *Concussion* is defined as a momentary interruption of brain function with or without loss of consciousness. Although recovery usually takes place within 24 hours, mild symptoms, such as headache, irritability, insomnia, and poor concentration and memory, may persist for months. This is known as the *postconcussion syndrome*. Because these complaints are vague and subjective, they sometimes are regarded as being of psychological origin. An organic basis for the postconcussion syndrome is strongly suspected. Postconcussion syndrome can have a significant effect on activities of daily living and return to employment. Persons with postconcussion syndrome may need cognitive retraining or psychological support.

Moderate head injury is characterized by a longer period of unconsciousness and may be associated with focal manifestations such as hemiparesis, aphasia, and cranial nerve palsy. In this type of injury, many small hemorrhages and some swelling of brain tissue occur. A contusion or bruising of brain tissue often can be visualized on CT scan, whereas a concussion cannot be visualized except microscopically. Contusions often are distributed along the rough, irregular inner surface of the brain and are more likely to occur in the frontal or temporal lobes, resulting in cognitive and motor deficits.

Severe head injury involves more extensive damage to brain structures and a deeper level of coma than moderate head injury. In severe head injury, primary damage to the brain often is instantaneous and irreversible, resulting from shearing and pressure forces that cause diffuse axonal injury, disruption of blood vessels, and tissue damage. It often is accompanied by neurologic deficits such as hemiplegia. Severe head injuries often occur with injury to other parts of the body such as the extremities, chest, and abdomen. Blood may extravasate into the brain; if the contusion is severe, the blood may accumulate, as in intracranial hemorrhage. Similarly, when laceration of the brain directly under the area of injury occurs, especially if the skull is fractured, hemorrhage may be sufficiently extensive to form a hematoma.

Although the skull and CSF provide protection for the brain, they also can contribute to trauma. A form of brain injury that can cause concussion or contusion from bouncing of the brain in the closed confines of the rigid skull is called a *coup-contrecoup injury*. Because the brain floats freely in the CSF, blunt force to the head can cause the brain to accelerate in the skull, then abruptly decelerate on hitting the inner confines of the skull. The direct contusion of the brain at the site of external force is referred to as a *coup* injury, whereas the opposite side of the brain receives the *contrecoup* injury. The brain is thrown against one side of the skull (coup) in one continuous motion, which causes damage immediately below the site of impact (Fig. 50-11). The brain then rebounds and strikes the opposite side of the skull (contrecoup), which causes injury in regions of the brain opposite the side of impact. As the brain strikes the rough surface of the cranial vault, brain tissue, blood vessels, nerve tracts, and other structures are bruised and torn.

Hematomas

Hematomas result from vascular injury and bleeding. Depending on the anatomic position of the ruptured vessel, bleeding can occur in any of several compartments, including the epidural, subdural, and subarachnoid spaces or into the brain itself (intracerebral hematoma).

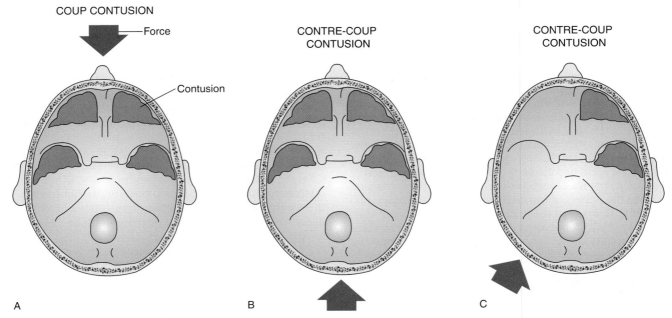

COUP CONTUSION
Force
Contusion

CONTRE-COUP CONTUSION

CONTRE-COUP CONTUSION

A   B   C

FIGURE 50-11 Mechanisms of cerebral contusion in coup-contrecoup injuries. (**A**) A focal area of cerebral injury (coup contusion) at the point of impact. The cerebral hemispheres float in the cerebrospinal fluid. (**B**) Rapid deceleration or, less commonly, acceleration, causes the cortex to forcefully impact into the anterior and middle fossa causing injury to the side of the brain opposite the site of injury (contrecoup contusion). (**C**) The position of a contrecoup contusion is determined by the direction of force and the intracranial anatomy. (Courtesy of Dmitri Karetnikov, artist). (Rubin E., Farber J.L. [1999]. *Pathology* [3rd ed., p. 1461]. Philadelphia: Lippincott Williams & Wilkins)

Epidural Hematoma. Epidural hematomas usually are caused by head injury in which the skull is fractured. An epidural (extradural) hematoma is one that develops between the inner table of the bones of the skull and the dura (Fig. 50-12). It usually results from a tear in an artery, most often the middle meningeal, which is located under the thin temporal bone. Because bleeding is arterial in origin, rapid compression of the brain occurs from the expanding hematoma. Epidural hematoma is more common in a young person because the dura is not so firmly attached to the skull surface as it is in an older person; as a consequence, the dura can be easily stripped away from the inner surface of the skull, allowing the hematoma to form.

Typically, a person with an epidural hematoma presents with a history of head injury and a brief period of unconsciousness followed by a lucid period in which consciousness is regained, followed by rapid progression to unconsciousness. The lucid interval does not always occur, but when it does, it is of great diagnostic value. With rapidly developing unconsciousness, there are focal symptoms related to the area of the brain involved. These symptoms can include ipsilateral (same side) pupil dilatation and contralateral (opposite side) hemiparesis. If the hematoma is not removed, the condition progresses, with increased ICP, tentorial herniation, and death. Prognosis is excellent, however, if the hematoma is removed before loss of consciousness occurs.

Subdural Hematoma. A subdural hematoma develops in the area between the dura and the arachnoid (subdural

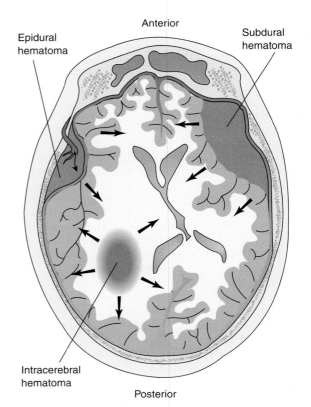

Anterior

Epidural hematoma

Subdural hematoma

Intracerebral hematoma

Posterior

FIGURE 50-12 Location of epidural, subdural, and intracerebral hematomas.

space) and usually is the result of a tear in the small bridging veins that connect veins on the surface of the cortex to dural sinuses. The bridging veins pass from the pial vessels through the CSF-filled subarachnoid space, penetrate the arachnoid and the dura, and empty into the intradural sinuses. These veins are readily snapped in head injury when the brain moves suddenly in relation to the cranium (Fig. 50-13). Bleeding can occur between the dura and arachnoid (*i.e.*, subdural hematoma) or into the CSF-filled subarachnoid space (*i.e.*, subarachnoid hematoma). Subdural hematoma develops more slowly than an epidural hematoma because the tear is in the venous system, whereas epidural hematomas are arterial.

Subdural hematomas are classified as acute, subacute, or chronic. This classification system is based on the approximate time intervals before the appearance of symptoms. Symptoms of acute hematoma are seen within 24 hours of the injury, whereas subacute hematoma does not produce symptoms until 2 to 10 days after injury. Symptoms of chronic subdural hematoma may not arise until several weeks after the injury. These classifications are based partially on pathologic considerations.

Acute subdural hematomas progress rapidly and have a high mortality rate because of the severe secondary injuries related to edema and increased ICP. The high mortality rate has been associated with uncontrolled ICP increase, loss of consciousness, decerebrate posturing, and delay in surgical removal of the hematoma. The clinical picture is similar to that of epidural hematoma, except that there usually is no lucid interval. In subacute hematoma, there may be a period of improvement in the level of consciousness and neurologic symptoms, only to be followed by deterioration if the hematoma is not removed.

Symptoms of chronic subdural hematoma develop weeks after a head injury, so much later that the person may not remember having had a head injury. This is especially true of the older person with fragile vessels whose brain has shrunk away from the dura. Seepage of blood into the subdural space may occur slowly. Because the blood in the subdural space is not absorbed, fibroblastic activity begins, and the hematoma becomes encapsulated. Within this encap-

sulated area, the blood cells are slowly lysed, and a fluid with a high osmotic pressure is formed. This creates an osmotic gradient, with fluid from the surrounding subarachnoid space being pulled into the area; the mass increases in size, exerting pressure on the cranial contents. In some instances, the clinical picture is less defined, with the most prominent symptom being a decreasing level of consciousness indicated by drowsiness, confusion, and apathy. The person also may have headache. Morbidity and mortality rates are higher with acute subdural hematoma than with epidural and intracerebral hematoma.

Intracerebral Hematoma.   Intracerebral hematoma can result from head injury. This type of bleeding occurs in the brain tissue itself. Blood often leaks into the CSF, causing the same problems as a bridging vein bleed, but the phenomenon is more rapid because of the arterial origin. The severe motion that the brain undergoes can cause bleeding in brain tissue, or a contusion can coalesce into a hematoma (see Fig. 50-12). Intracerebral hematoma occurs more frequently in older persons and alcoholics whose brain vessels are more friable. Intracerebral hematomas can occur in any lobe of the brain but are most common in the frontal or temporal lobes. There can be one hematoma or many.

The signs and symptoms produced by an intracerebral hematoma depend on its size and location within the brain. Signs of increased ICP can be manifested if the hematoma is large and encroaching on vital structures. A hematoma in the temporal lobe can be dangerous because of the potential for lateral herniation.

Treatment of an intracerebral hematoma can be medical or surgical. For a large hematoma with a rapidly deteriorating neurologic condition, surgery to evacuate the clot usually is indicated. Surgery may not be needed in someone who is neurologically stable despite neurologic deficits; in this case, the hematoma may resolve much like a contusion.

INFECTIONS

Infections of the CNS may be classified according to the structure involved: the meninges, meningitis; the brain parenchyma, encephalitis; the spinal cord, myelitis; and the brain and spinal cord, encephalomyelitis. They also may be classified by the type of invading organism: bacterial, viral, or other. In general, the pathogens enter the CNS through the bloodstream by crossing the blood-brain barrier or by direct invasion through skull fracture or a bullet hole, or, rarely, by contamination during surgery or lumbar puncture.

Meningitis

Meningitis is an inflammation of the pia mater, the arachnoid, and the CSF-filled subarachnoid space. Inflammation spreads rapidly because of CSF circulation around the brain and spinal cord. The inflammation usually is caused by an infection, but chemical meningitis can occur. There are two types of acute infectious meningitis: acute pyogenic meningitis (usually bacterial) and acute lym-

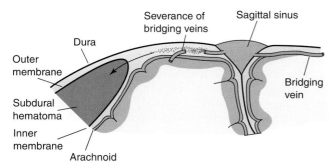

FIGURE 50-13 Mechanism of bleeding in subdural hematoma. (Courtesy of Dmitri Karetnikov, artist). (Rubin E., Farber J.L. [1999]. *Pathology* [3rd ed., p. 1460]. Philadelphia: Lippincott Williams & Wilkins)

phocytic (usually viral) meningitis.[1] Factors responsible for the severity of meningitis include virulence factors of the pathogen, host factors, brain edema, and the presence of permanent neurologic sequelae.

Bacterial Meningitis. In the United States, the incidence of bacterial meningitis is approximately 3 to 10 cases per 100,000 persons, and two thirds of cases are in children younger than 5 years of age. The most common pyogenic infectious agents are *Streptococcus pneumoniae, Haemophilus influenzae, Neisseria meningitidis* (the meningococcus), and *Escherichia coli.* In children younger than 5 years of age, the most common agent of infection is *H. influenzae;* after that age, infection with *S. pneumoniae* is most common.[52] Recently, the frequency of meningitis due to *H. influenzae* in children has declined dramatically because of vaccination against *H. influenza.* The meningococcus can reside asymptomatically in the throat and nasopharynx, and this infection has the highest incidence among children and young adults. Epidemics occur in settings such as the military, where the recruits must reside in close contact. The very young and the very old are at highest risk for pneumococcal meningitis. Meningitis due to *E. coli* occurs most often in the neonate, especially if there is a neural tube defect. Risk factors associated with contracting meningitis include head trauma with basilar skull fractures, otitis media, sinusitis or mastoiditis, neurosurgery, dermal sinus tracts, systemic sepsis, or immunocompromise.

Although antibiotic therapy was introduced approximately 50 years ago, morbidity and mortality rates remain high for bacterial meningitis. Reports indicate that the mortality rate for bacterial meningitis in adults remains at approximately 25%. Similarly, 61% of infants who survive gram-negative bacillary meningitis have developmental and neurologic sequelae.[52]

In the pathophysiology of bacterial meningitis, the bacterial organisms replicate and undergo lysis in the CSF, releasing endotoxins or cell wall fragments. These substances initiate the release of inflammatory mediators (*i.e.,* cytokines), which set the stage for a complex but coordinated sequence of events by which neutrophils bind to cerebral endothelial cells of the blood-brain barrier and damage these cells by the release of toxic oxygen products (free radicals), permitting fluid to move across the capillary wall. Experimental evidence strongly suggests that inflammatory mediators released into the CSF impair the blood-brain barrier to the extent that pathogens, neutrophils, and albumin cross the endothelial wall into the CSF.

The most common symptoms of acute bacterial meningitis are fever and chills; headache; stiff neck; back, abdominal, and extremity pains; and nausea and vomiting. Other signs include seizures, cranial nerve palsies, and focal cerebral signs.[53] A petechial rash is found in most persons with meningococcal meningitis. These petechiae vary from pinhead size to large ecchymoses or even areas of skin gangrene that slough if the person survives. Other types of meningitis also may produce a petechial rash. Persons infected with *H. influenzae* or *S. pneumoniae* may present with difficulty in arousal and seizures, whereas those with *N. meningitidis* infection may present with delirium

or coma.[53] The development of brain edema, hydrocephalus, or increased cerebral blood flow can increase ICP.

Meningeal signs (*e.g.,* photophobia and nuchal rigidity), such as those seen in subarachnoid hemorrhage, also may be present. Two assessment techniques can help determine whether meningeal irritation is present. *Kernig's sign* is resistance to extension of the leg while the person is lying with the hip flexed at a right angle. *Brudzinski's sign* is elicited when flexion of the neck results in flexion of the hip and knee. These postures are caused by stretching of the inflamed meninges from the lumbar level to the head. Stretching of the inflamed meninges is extremely painful, producing resistance to stretching.

Lumbar puncture (*i.e.,* spinal tap) yields a cloudy and purulent CSF under increased pressure. The CSF typically contains large numbers of polymorphonuclear neutrophils (up to 90,000/mm³), increased protein content, and reduced sugar content. Bacteria can be seen on smears and can easily be cultured with appropriate media.

Arthritis, cranial nerve damage (especially the eighth nerve, with resulting deafness), and hydrocephalus may occur as complications of pyogenic meningitis. As the pathogens enter the subarachnoid space, they cause inflammation, characterized by a cloudy, purulent exudate. Thrombophlebitis of the bridging veins and dural sinuses may develop, followed by congestion and infarction in the surrounding tissues. Ultimately, the meninges thicken, and adhesions form. These adhesions may impinge on the cranial nerves, giving rise to cranial nerve palsies, or may impair the outflow of CSF, causing hydrocephalus.

Diagnosis of bacterial meningitis is based on the history and physical examination, along with laboratory data. Data from lumbar punctures are necessary for accurate diagnosis. Treatment includes antibiotics and glucocorticoids. Optimal antibiotic treatment requires that the drug have a bactericidal effect in the CSF. Because bactericidal therapy often results in rapid bacteriolysis of the pathogen, treatment can promote the release of biologically active cell wall products into the CSF (*e.g., H. influenzae* lipopolysaccharide, *S. pneumoniae* cell wall fragments). The release of these cell wall products can increase the products of inflammatory mediators (interleukin-1, interleukin-6, and tumor necrosis factor) that have the potential for exacerbating the abnormalities of the blood-brain barrier and the inflammatory process in the CSF. Because of evidence linking the inflammatory mediators to the pathogenesis of bacterial meningitis, adjunctive glucocorticoid therapy usually is administered with or just before the first dose of antibiotics in infants and children. The adjunctive use of glucocorticoid therapy in adults is controversial.

Persons who have been exposed to someone with meningococcal meningitis should be treated prophylactically with antibiotics.[54] Effective polysaccharide vaccines are available to protect against meningococcal groups A, C, Y, and W-135. These vaccines are recommended for military recruits and college students, who are at increased risk of invasive meningococcal disease.

Viral Meningitis. Viral meningitis manifests in much the same way as bacterial meningitis, but the course is less severe, and the CSF findings are markedly different. There are lymphocytes in the fluid rather than polymorphonuclear cells, the protein content is only moderately elevated, and the sugar content usually is normal. The acute viral meningitides are self-limited and usually require only symptomatic treatment. Viral meningitis can be caused by many different viruses, including mumps, coxsackievirus, Epstein-Barr virus, and herpes simplex type 2. In many cases, the virus cannot be identified.

Encephalitis

Generalized infection of the parenchyma of the brain or spinal cord usually is caused by a virus, but it also may be caused by bacteria, fungi, and other organisms. Less frequent causes of encephalitis are toxic substances such as ingested lead and vaccines for measles, mumps, and rabies, which cause postvaccination encephalitis. Encephalitis caused by human immunodeficiency virus infection is discussed in Chapter 20.

The pathologic picture of encephalitis includes local necrotizing hemorrhage, which ultimately becomes generalized, with prominent edema. There is progressive degeneration of nerve cell bodies. The histologic picture, although rather general, demonstrates some specific characteristics. For example, the poliovirus selectively destroys the cells of the anterior horn of the spinal cord.

Encephalitis, like meningitis, is characterized by fever, headache, and nuchal rigidity. Patients experience a wide range of neurologic disturbances, such as lethargy, disorientation, seizures, dysphagias, focal paralysis, delirium, and coma. The nervous system is subjected to invasion by many viruses, such as arbovirus, poliovirus, and rabies virus. The mode of transmission may be the bite of a mosquito (arbovirus), a rabid animal (rabies virus), or ingestion (poliovirus). A common cause of encephalitis in the United States is herpes simplex virus. Diagnosis of encephalitis is made by clinical history and presenting symptoms, in addition to traditional CSF studies.

BRAIN TUMORS

Brain tumors account for 2% of all cancer deaths. The American Cancer Society estimates that there were 17,200 new cases and more than 13,100 deaths from brain and CNS cancers in 2001.[55] Metastasis to the brain from other sites is even more common. One estimate suggests that more than 100,000 people per year die with symptomatic intracranial metastasis.[56] More adults die each year of brain tumors than of Hodgkin's disease or multiple sclerosis.[57] In children, brain tumors are second only to leukemia as a cause of death from cancer, and they kill approximately 1600 children and young adults annually.

Types of Tumors

For most neoplasms, the term *malignant* is used to describe the tumor's lack of cell differentiation, its invasive nature, and its ability to metastasize. In the brain, however, even a well-differentiated and histologically benign tumor may grow and cause death because of its location.

Brain tumors can be divided into three types: primary intracranial tumors of CNS tissue (*e.g.*, neurons, neuroglia), primary intracranial tumors that originate in the skull cavity but are not derived from the brain tissue itself (*e.g.*, meninges, pituitary gland, pineal gland), and metastatic tumors. Primary intracranial neoplasms of CNS origin can be classified according to the site of origin and histologic type.

Collectively, the neoplasms of astrocyte origin are the most common type of primary brain tumor in the adult. Astrocytomas fall into four clinicopathologic groups: fibrillary astrocytomas, glioblastoma multiforme, pilocytic astrocytomas, and pleomorphic xanthoastrocytomas.[1]

Fibrillary or diffuse astrocytomas account for 80% of adult primary brain tumors. They are most common in middle age, with the anaplastic astrocytomas having a peak incidence in the sixth decade.

Although they usually are found in the cerebral hemispheres, they also can occur in the cerebellum, brain stem, or spinal cord. Astrocytomas of the cerebral hemispheres commonly are divided into three grades of increasing pathologic anaplasia and rapidity of progression: astrocytoma, anaplastic astrocytoma, and glioblastoma multiforme (see Chapter 8 for a discussion of cell differentiation and anaplasia).

Glioblastoma multiforme commonly is used as a synonym for highly malignant forms of astrocytoma (grades III and IV). Astrocytomas have a marked tendency to become more anaplastic with time, so that a tumor beginning as a fibrillary astrocytoma may develop into a glioblastoma. Brain stem gliomas occur in the first two decades of life and account for approximately 20% of brain tumors in this age group.[1]

Pilocytic astrocytomas are distinguished from other astrocytomas by their cellular appearance and their benign behavior. Typically, they occur in children and young adults and usually are located in the cerebellum, but they also can be found in the floor and walls of the third ventricle, the optic chiasm and nerves, and occasionally in the cerebral hemispheres. Pleomorphic xanthoastrocytoma most often occurs as a superficial tumor in the temporal lobe of children and young adults. Seizures are common presenting signs for this type of tumor.

Oligodendrogliomas comprise approximately 5% to 15% of glial tumors. They are most common in middle life and are found in the cerebral hemispheres.[1] In general, persons with oligodendrogliomas have a better prognosis than persons with astrocytomas.

Ependymomas are derived from the single layer of epithelium that lines the ventricles and spinal canal. Although they can occur at any age, they are most likely to occur in the first two decades of life and most frequently affect the fourth ventricle; they constitute 5% to 10% of brain tumors in this age group.[1] The spinal cord is the most common site for ependymomas occurring in middle age.

Meningiomas develop from the meningothelial cells of the arachnoid and are outside the brain. They comprise approximately 20% of primary brain tumors and usually have their onset in the middle or later years of life.[1] Meningiomas are slow-growing, well-circumscribed, and often highly vascular tumors. They usually are benign, and complete removal is possible if the tumor does not involve vital structures. Pituitary adenomas comprise 12% to 14% of brain tumors; they usually are nonmalignant.[1]

Etiology

Although a number of chemical and viral agents can cause brain tumors in laboratory animals, there is no evidence that these agents directly cause brain cancer in humans. Cranial irradiation and exposure to some chemicals may lead to an increased incidence of astrocytomas and meningiomas. There may also be a hereditary factor. Childhood tumors are considered to be developmental in origin.

Manifestations

Intracranial tumors give rise to focal disturbances in brain function and increased ICP. Focal disturbances occur because of brain compression, tumor infiltration, disturbances in blood flow, and brain edema.

Tumors may be located intra-axially (*i.e.*, within brain tissue) or extra-axially (*i.e.*, outside brain tissue). Disturbances in brain function usually are greatest with fast-growing, infiltrative, intra-axial tumors because of compression, infiltration, and necrosis of brain tissue. Extra-axial tumors, such as meningiomas, may reach a large size without producing signs and symptoms. Cysts may form in tumors and contribute to brain compression. Cerebral edema usually is of the vasogenic type, which develops around brain tumors and is characterized by increased brain water and expanded extracellular fluid. The edema is thought to result from increased permeability of tumor capillary endothelial cells.

Because the volume of the intracranial cavity is fixed, brain tumors cause a generalized increase in ICP when they reach sufficient size. Tumors can obstruct the flow of CSF in the ventricular cavities and produce hydrocephalic dilatation of the proximal ventricles and atrophy of the cerebral hemispheres. Complete compensation of ventricular volumes can occur with very slow-growing tumors, but with rapidly growing tumors, increased ICP is an early sign. Depending on the location of the tumor, brain displacement and herniation of the uncus or cerebellum may occur. The clinical manifestations of brain tumors depend on the size and location of the tumor. General signs and symptoms include headache, nausea, vomiting, mental changes, papilledema, visual disturbances (*e.g.*, diplopia), alterations in sensory and motor function, and seizures.

The brain itself is insensitive to pain. The headache that accompanies brain tumors results from compression or distortion of pain-sensitive dural or vascular structures. It may be felt on the same side of the head as the tumor but more commonly is diffuse. In the early stages, the headache, which is caused by irritation, compression, and traction on the dural sinuses or blood vessels, is mild and occurs in the morning when the person awakens. It usually disappears after the person has been up for a short time. The headache becomes more constant as the tumor enlarges and often is worsened by coughing, bending, or sudden movements of the head.

Vomiting occurs with or without preceding nausea and is a common symptom of increased ICP and brain stem compression. Direct stimulation of the vomiting center, which is located in the medulla, may contribute to the vomiting that occurs with brain tumors. The vomiting may be projectile. Vomiting caused by brain tumor usually is unrelated to meals and often is associated with headache. Papilledema (edema of the optic disk) results from increased ICP and obstruction of the CSF pathways. It is associated with decreased visual acuity, diplopia, and deficits in the visual fields. Visual defects associated with papilledema often are the reason that persons with brain tumor seek medical care.

Personality and mental changes are common with brain tumors. Persons with brain tumors often are irritable initially and later become quiet and apathetic. They may become forgetful, seem preoccupied, and appear to be psychologically depressed. Because of the mental changes, a psychiatric consultation may be sought before a diagnosis of brain tumor is made.

Focal signs and symptoms are determined by the location of the tumor. Tumors arising in the frontal lobe may grow to large size, increase the ICP, and cause signs of generalized brain dysfunction before focal signs are recognized. Tumors that impinge on the visual system cause visual loss or visual field defects long before generalized signs develop. Certain areas of the brain have a relatively low threshold for seizure activity; tumors arising in relatively silent areas of the brain may produce focal epileptogenic discharges. Temporal lobe tumors often produce seizures as their first symptom. Hallucinations of smell or hearing and déjà vu phenomena are common focal manifestations of temporal lobe tumors. Brain stem tumors commonly produce upper and lower motoneuron signs, such as weakness of facial muscles and ocular palsies that occur with or without involvement of sensory or long motor tracts. Cerebellar tumors often cause ataxia of gait.

Diagnosis and Treatment

Diagnostic procedures for brain tumor include physical and neurologic examinations, visual field and funduscopic examination, CT scans and MRI, skull x-ray films, technetium pertechnetate brain scans, electroencephalography, and cerebral angiography. Physical examination is used to assess motor and sensory function. Because the visual pathways travel through many areas of the cerebral lobes, detection of visual field defects can provide information about the location of tumors. A funduscopic examination is done to detect papilledema. Although CT scanning is used as a screening test, MRI scans are more sensitive than CT for mass lesions and can be diagnostic when a clinically suspected tumor is not detected by CT scanning. Skull x-ray films are used to detect calcified areas in a neoplasm or erosion of skull structures due to tumors. Approximately 75% of persons with a brain tumor have an abnormal electroencephalogram; in some cases, the results of the test can be used to localize the tumor. Cerebral angiography can be used to locate a tumor and visualize its vascular supply, information that is important when planning surgery. MRA can be used to distinguish vascular masses from tumors.

The three general methods for treatment of brain tumors are surgery, irradiation, and chemotherapy. Surgery is part of the initial management of virtually all brain tumors; it establishes the diagnosis and achieves tumor removal in many cases. The development of microsurgical neuroanatomy, the operating microscope, and advanced stereotactic and ultrasonographic technology; the fusion of imaging systems with resection techniques; and the intraoperative monitoring of evoked potentials have improved the effectiveness of surgical resection.[58] However, removal may be limited by the location of the tumor and its invasiveness. Stereotactic surgery uses three-dimensional coordinates and CT and MRI to localize a brain lesion precisely. Ultrasonographic technology has been used for localizing and removing tumors. The ultrasonic aspirator, which combines a vibrating head with suction, permits atraumatic removal of tumors from cranial nerves and important cortical areas. Intraoperative monitoring of evoked potentials is an important adjunct to some types of surgery. For example, evoked potentials can be used to monitor auditory, visual, speech, or motor responses during surgery done under local anesthesia.

Most malignant brain tumors respond to external irradiation. Irradiation can increase longevity and sometimes can allay symptoms when tumors recur. The treatment dose depends on the tumor's histologic type, radioresponsiveness, and anatomic site and on the level of tolerance of the surrounding tissue. A newer technique called *gamma knife* combines stereotactic localization of tumor with radiosurgery, allowing delivery of high-dose radiation to deep tumors, sparing surrounding brain. Radiation therapy is avoided in treating children younger than 2 years of age because of the long-term effects, which include developmental delay, panhypopituitarism, and secondary tumors.[58]

The use of chemotherapy for brain tumors is somewhat limited by the blood-brain barrier. Chemotherapeutic agents can be administered intravenously, intra-arterially, intrathecally (*i.e.*, into the spinal canal), or intraventricularly. A promising area of improved delivery of chemotherapeutic agents is the use of biodegradable anhydrous wafers impregnated with a drug and implanted into the tumor at the time of surgery. These wafers are constructed so they release the drug over a period of many months.

> In summary, although the skull and the CSF provide protection for the brain, they also can contribute to brain injury through compression and bone splinters that occur with skull fracture and coup-contrecoup injuries. Head injuries may result from penetration or impact, with each type affecting the brain and supporting structures in different ways. Head injuries can be classified as direct, resulting from the immediate effects of injury, skull fracture, concussion, or contusion; or as secondary, resulting from edema, hemorrhage, or infection. Secondary injury may result from epidural, subdural, or intracerebral hematoma formation.
>
> Infections of the CNS may be classified according to the structures involved (*e.g.*, meningitis, encephalitis) or the type of organism causing the infection. The damage caused by infection may predispose to hydrocephalus, seizures, or other neurologic defects.

Brain tumors account for 2% of all cancer deaths and are the second most common type of cancer in children. Brain tumors can arise primarily from intracranial structures, and tumors from other parts of the body often metastasize to the brain. Primary brain tumors can arise from any structure in the cranial cavity. Most begin in brain tissue, but the pituitary, the pineal region, and the meninges also are sites of tumor development. Brain tumors cause focal disturbances in brain function and increase the ICP. Focal disturbances result from brain compression, tumor infiltration, disturbances in blood flow, and cerebral edema. The clinical manifestations of brain tumor depend on the size and location of the tumor. General signs and symptoms include headache, nausea, vomiting, mental changes, papilledema, visual disturbances, alterations in motor and sensory function, and seizures. Diagnostic tests include physical examination, visual field testing and funduscopic examination, CT scans, MRI studies, skull x-ray films, brain scans, electroencephalography, and cerebral angiography. Treatment includes surgery, irradiation, and chemotherapy.

▌ Seizure Disorders

After you have completed this section of the chapter, you should be able to meet the following objectives:

- ✦ Explain the difference between seizure activity and epileptic seizure
- ✦ State four or more causes of seizures other than epilepsy
- ✦ Differentiate between the origin of seizure activity in partial and generalized forms of epilepsy and compare the manifestations of simple partial seizures with those of complex partial seizures and major and minor motor seizures
- ✦ Characterize status epilepticus

Seizures, sometimes called *convulsions*, are paroxysmal motor, sensory, or cognitive manifestations of spontaneous, abnormally synchronous discharges of collections of neurons in the cerebral cortex. This uncontrolled neuronal activity causes signs and symptoms that vary according to the location of the originating focus of seizure activity, involvement of surrounding neurons, and spread to other parts of the brain. These signs and symptoms can include strange sensations and perceptions (*e.g.*, hallucinations), unusual or repetitive muscle movements, autonomic visceral activity, and the onset of a confusional state or loss of consciousness. The neuronal hyperexcitability that results in a seizure occurs regardless of the discrete functions of individual neurons. However, its manifestations depend on the particular population of nerve cells involved.

Approximately 2 million persons in the United States are subject to recurrent seizures.[59] Seizure activity is the most common disorder encountered in pediatric neurology, and among adults, its incidence is exceeded only by cerebrovascular disorders. Age of onset can be a clue to the type or cause of seizure. When there is no other known cause, seizures may be caused by vulnerability of the developing nervous system to seizure activity. In most persons, the first seizure episode occurs before 20 years of age. After 20 years of age, a seizure is caused most often by a structural change, trauma, tumor, or stroke.

ETIOLOGY

A seizure is not a disease but a symptom of an underlying CNS dysfunction. Seizures may occur during almost all serious illnesses or injuries affecting the brain, including infections, tumors, drug abuse, vascular lesions, congenital deformities, and brain injury. A seizure represents the clinical manifestations of an abnormal, uncontrolled electrical discharge from a group of neurons.

Many theories have been proposed to explain the initiation of the abnormal brain electrical activity that occurs with seizures. Seizures may be caused by alterations in cell membrane permeability or distribution of ions across the neuronal cell membranes. Another cause may be decreased

Seizures

➤ Seizures are paroxysmal motor, sensory, or cognitive manifestations of spontaneous, abnormally synchronous electrical discharges from collections of neurons in the cerebral cortex.

➤ Seizures are thought to result directly or indirectly from changes in excitability of single neurons or groups of neurons.

➤ The site of seizure generation and the extent to which the abnormal neural activity is conducted to other areas of the brain determine the type and manifestations of the seizure activity.

➤ Partial seizures originate a small group of neurons in one hemisphere with secondary spread of seizure activity to other parts of the brain. Simple partial seizures usually are confined to one hemisphere and do not involve loss of consciousness. Complex partial seizures begin in a localized area, spread to both hemispheres, and involve impairment of consciousness.

➤ Generalized seizures show simultaneous disruption of normal brain activity in both hemispheres from the onset. They include unconsciousness and varying bilateral degrees of symmetric motor responses with evidence of localization to one hemisphere. Absence seizures are generalized nonconvulsive seizure events that are expressed mainly by brief periods of unconsciousness. Tonic-clonic seizures involve unconsciousness along with both tonic and clonic muscle contractions.

inhibition of cortical or thalamic neuronal activity or structural changes that alter the excitability of neurons. Neurotransmitter imbalances such as an acetylcholine excess or γ-aminobutyric acid (GABA, an inhibitory neurotransmitter) deficiency have been proposed as a cause.

Everyone has a seizure threshold that, when exceeded, can result in seizure activity. Whether seizure activity occurs depends on the individual's seizure threshold and the extent to which it has been altered by pathologic processes. Some individuals have a low seizure threshold and are more likely to experience them, even in response to benign stimuli. The roles of genetic or familial predisposition to seizures and interictal (between seizures) alterations in EEG tracings remain under active investigation. The incidence of certain types of seizure activity is statistically higher in families with a genetic predisposition toward cerebral dysrhythmia, but evidence of cerebral dysrhythmia is not invariably associated with clinical manifestations of a primary seizure disorder.

The terms *seizure disorder* and *epileptic syndrome* often are used interchangeably, although most clinicians prefer *seizure disorder* because of the negative connotations still associated with the term *epilepsy*. A seizure disorder can be defined as a syndrome in which there is a tendency to have recurrent, paroxysmal seizure activity without evidence of a reversible metabolic cause. It is a chronic condition for which long-term medication may be appropriate.

PROVOKED AND UNPROVOKED SEIZURES

Clinically, seizures may be categorized as unprovoked (primary or idiopathic) or provoked (secondary or acute symptomatic).[60] Provoked or symptomatic seizures include febrile seizures, seizures precipitated by systemic metabolic conditions, and those that follow a primary insult to the CNS. Unprovoked or idiopathic seizures are those for which no identifiable cause can be determined.

The most common subgroup of seizures under the category of provoked seizures is that of febrile seizures in children.[61] They are associated with a high fever, usually with a temperature higher than 104°F. In the United States, 3% to 4% of children experience a febrile seizure before the age of 5 years. Of these, approximately 50% have one recurrent febrile seizure, and only small number have numerous recurrent seizures. Treatment includes a careful search for the cause of the fever. Because the risks of treatment (*e.g.*, side effects of medications used to control seizures) often exceed the benefits, anticonvulsant medications may be avoided in these cases.[61]

Seizures precipitated by systemic or metabolic disturbances and by primary CNS insults also fall into the category of provoked seizures. Transient systemic metabolic disturbances may precipitate seizures. Examples include electrolyte imbalances, hypoglycemia, hypoxia, hypocalcemia, and alkalosis. Toxemia of pregnancy, water intoxication, uremia, and CNS infections such as meningitis also may precipitate a seizure. The rapid withdrawal of sedative-hypnotic drugs, such as alcohol or barbiturates, is another cause of seizures. Approximately 5% to 10% of those who sustain a CNS insult, such as occurs with cerebral bleeding, edema, or neuronal damage, experience a seizure at the time. Treatment of the immediate cause of these seizures often results in their disappearance. Long-term prophylactic treatment with anticonvulsant medications remains controversial in these situations.

Multiple episodes or frequent recurrences of apparently unprovoked seizures are considered a seizure disorder, or epilepsy—the less preferred term. These persons are evaluated to determine and possibly treat the underlying dysfunction. In these cases, anticonvulsant therapy may be prescribed to minimize the likelihood of seizures.

CLASSIFICATION

Although a knowledge of the cause is important, seizure management usually is directed toward identifying the seizure type and controlling seizure occurrence. Two classification systems are in use. The first is based on seizure type and the second on the concept of epilepsy and epileptic syndromes.[62] Both systems were developed by the International League Against Epilepsy, and both are based on clinical manifestations and EEG activity. The first, the International Classification of Epileptic Seizures, is based on symptoms during the seizure. It divides seizures into two broad categories: partial seizures, in which the seizure begins in a specific or focal area of one cerebral hemisphere, and generalized seizures, which involve virtually simultaneous onset in both cerebral hemispheres[63] (Chart 50-1).

The second classification system is the International Classification of Epilepsies and Epileptic Syndromes.[63] This system maintains the dichotomy of partial and generalized seizures but substitutes the term *localized-related* for partial seizures. The system further divides epilepsies into idiopathic, symptomatic, and cryptogenic (*i.e.*, suspected to be symptomatic despite absence of definitive proof of an underlying cause). The system also has categories for seizures of undetermined origin such as neonatal seizures and a category of special syndromes such as febrile seizures.

Partial Seizures

Partial or focal seizures are the most common type of seizure among newly diagnosed cases in all groups older than 10 years of age. Partial seizures can be subdivided into three major groups: simple partial (consciousness is not impaired), complex partial (impairment of consciousness), and secondarily generalized partial seizures. These categories are based primarily on current neurophysiologic theories related to seizure propagation and the extent of involvement of the brain's hemispheres.

Simple Partial Seizures. Simple partial seizures usually involve only one hemisphere and are not accompanied by loss of consciousness or responsiveness. These seizures also have been referred to as *elementary partial seizures*, *partial seizures with elementary symptoms*, or *focal seizures*. The 1981 Commission on Classification and Terminology of the International League Against Epilepsy classified simple partial seizures according to motor signs, sensory symptoms, autonomic manifestations, and psychic symptoms.

> ## CHART 50-1
>
> ### *Classification of Epileptic Seizures*
>
> **Partial Seizures**
> Simple partial seizures (no impairment of consciousness)
>   With motor symptoms
>   With sensory symptoms
>   With autonomic signs
>   With psychic symptoms
> Complex partial seizures (impairment of consciousness)
>   Simple partial onset followed by impaired
>   consciousness
>   Impairment of consciousness at onset
> Partial seizures evolving to secondarily generalized
>   seizures
>   Simple partial leading to generalized seizures
>   Complex partial leading to generalized seizures
>
> **Unclassified Seizures**
> Classification not possible because of inadequate or
>   incomplete data
>
> **Generalized Seizures**
> Absence seizures (typical or atypical)
> Atonic seizures
> Myoclonic seizures
> Clonic seizures
> Tonic
> Tonic-clonic seizures
>
> (Adapted from Commission on Classification and Terminology of the International League Against Epilepsy [1981]. Proposal for revised clinical and electroencephalographic classification of epileptic seizures. *Epilepsia* 22, 489)

The observed clinical signs and symptoms depend on the area of the brain where the abnormal neuronal discharge is taking place. If the motor area of the brain is involved, the earliest symptom is motor movement corresponding to the location of onset on the contralateral side of the body. The motor movement may remain localized or may spread to other cortical areas, with sequential involvement of body parts in an epileptic-type "march," known as a *Jacksonian seizure*. If the sensory portion of the brain is involved, there may be no observable clinical manifestations. Sensory symptoms correlating with the location of seizure activity on the contralateral side of the brain may involve somatic sensory disturbance (*e.g.*, tingling and crawling sensations) or special sensory disturbance (*i.e.*, visual, auditory, gustatory, or olfactory phenomena). When abnormal cortical discharge stimulates the autonomic nervous system, flushing, tachycardia, diaphoresis, hypotension or hypertension, or pupillary changes may be evident.

The term *prodrome* or *aura* traditionally has meant a sensory warning sign of impending seizure activity or the onset of seizure that affected persons could describe because they were conscious. The aura itself now is considered part of the seizure. Because consciousness is maintained and only a small portion of the brain is involved, an aura is a simple partial seizure. Simple partial seizures may progress to complex partial seizures or generalized tonic-clonic seizures that result in unconsciousness. Therefore, the aura in simple partial seizure may be considered a warning sign of impending complex partial seizures.

Complex Partial Seizures. Complex partial seizures involve impairment of consciousness and often arise from the temporal lobe. The seizure begins in a localized area of the brain but may progress rapidly to involve both hemispheres. These seizures also may be referred to as *temporal lobe seizures* or *psychomotor seizures*.

Complex partial seizures often are accompanied by automatisms. Automatisms are repetitive, nonpurposeful activity such as lip smacking, grimacing, patting, or rubbing clothing. Confusion during the postictal state (after a seizure) is common. Hallucinations and illusional experiences such as *déjà vu* (familiarity with unfamiliar events or environments) or *jamais vu* (unfamiliarity with a known environment) have been reported. There may be overwhelming fear, uncontrolled forced thinking or a flood of ideas, and feelings of detachment and depersonalization. A person with a complex partial seizure disorder sometimes is misunderstood and believed to require hospitalization for a psychiatric disorder.

Secondarily Generalized Partial Seizures. These seizures are focal at onset but then become generalized as the ictal neuronal discharge spreads, involving deeper structures of the brain, such as the thalamus or the reticular formation. Discharges spread to both hemispheres, resulting in progression to tonic-clonic seizure activity. These seizures may start as simple or complex partial seizures, and may be preceded by an aura. The aura, often a stereotyped peculiar sensation that precedes the seizure, is the result of partial seizure activity. A history of an aura is clinically useful to identify the seizure as partial and not generalized in onset. However, absence of an aura does not reliably exclude a focal onset because many partial seizures generalize too rapidly to generate an aura.

Generalized-Onset Seizures

Generalized-onset seizures are the most common type in young children. These seizures are classified as primary or generalized when clinical signs, symptoms, and supporting EEG changes indicate involvement of both hemispheres at onset. The clinical symptoms include unconsciousness and involve varying bilateral degrees of symmetric motor responses without evidence of localization to one hemisphere.

These seizures are divided into four broad categories: absence seizures (typical and atypical), atonic (akinetic) seizures, myoclonic seizures, and major motor (formerly grand mal) seizures, characterized by tonic, clonic, or tonic-clonic activity.[63]

Absence Seizures. Absence seizures are generalized, nonconvulsive epileptic events and are expressed mainly as disturbances in consciousness. These were referred to as *petit mal seizures*. Absence seizures typically occur only in children and cease in adulthood or evolve to generalized motor seizures. Children may present with a history of school failure that predates the first evidence of seizure episodes. Although typical absence seizures have been characterized as a blank stare, motionlessness, and unresponsiveness,

motion occurs in many cases of absence seizures. This motion takes the form of automatisms such as lip smacking, mild clonic motion (usually in the eyelids), increased or decreased postural tone, and autonomic phenomena. There often is a brief loss of contact with the environment. The seizure usually lasts only a few seconds, and then the person is able to resume normal activity immediately. The manifestations often are so subtle that they may pass unnoticed. Because automatisms and unresponsiveness are common to complex partial seizures, the latter often are mistakenly labeled as "petit mal" seizures.

Atypical absence seizures are similar to typical absence seizures except for greater alterations in muscle tone and less abrupt onset and cessation. In practice, it is difficult to distinguish typical from atypical absence seizures without benefit of supporting EEG findings. However, it is important for the clinician to distinguish between complex partial and absence seizures because the drugs of choice are different. Medications that are effective for partial seizures may increase the frequency of absence seizures.

Atonic Seizures. In akinetic or atonic seizures, there is a sudden, split-second loss of muscle tone leading to slackening of the jaw, drooping of the limbs, or falling to the ground. These seizures also are known as *drop attacks*.

Myoclonic Seizures. Myoclonic seizures involve brief involuntary muscle contractions induced by stimuli of cerebral origin. A myoclonic seizure involves bilateral jerking of muscles, generalized or confined to the face, trunk, or one or more extremities. Tonic seizures are characterized by a rigid, violent contraction of the muscles, fixing the limbs in a strained position. Clonic seizures consist of repeated contractions and relaxations of the major muscle groups.

Tonic-Clonic Seizures. Tonic-clonic seizures, formerly called *grand mal seizures*, are the most common major motor seizure. Frequently, a person has a vague warning (probably a simple partial seizure) and experiences a sharp tonic contraction of the muscles with extension of the extremities and immediate loss of consciousness. Incontinence of bladder and bowel is common. Cyanosis may occur from contraction of airway and respiratory muscles. The tonic phase is followed by the clonic phase, which involves rhythmic bilateral contraction and relaxation of the extremities. At the end of the clonic phase, the person remains unconscious until the RAS begins to function again. This is called the *postictal phase*. The tonic-clonic phases last approximately 60 to 90 seconds.

Unclassified Seizures

Unclassified seizures are those that cannot be placed in one of the previous categories. These seizures are observed in the neonatal and infancy periods. Determination of whether the seizure is focal or generalized is not possible. Unclassified seizures are difficult to control with medication.

DIAGNOSIS AND TREATMENT

The diagnosis of seizure disorders is based on a thorough history and neurologic examination, including a full description of the seizure. The physical examination and laboratory studies help exclude any metabolic disease (*e.g.,* hyponatremia) that could precipitate seizures. Skull radiographs and CT or MRI scans are used to identify structural defects. One of the most useful diagnostic tests is the EEG, which is used to record changes in the brain's electrical activity. It is used to support the clinical diagnosis of epilepsy, to provide a guide for prognosis, and to assist in classifying the seizure disorder.

The first rule of treatment is to protect the person from injury during a seizure, preserve brain function by aborting or preventing seizure activity, and treat any underlying disease. Persons with epilepsy should be advised to avoid situations that could be dangerous or life threatening if seizures occur. Treatment of the underlying disorder may reduce the frequency of seizures.

After the underlying disease is treated, the aim of treatment is to bring the seizures under control with the least possible disruption in lifestyle and minimum side effects from medication. Since the late 1970s, the therapy for epilepsy has changed drastically because of an improved classification system, the ability to measure serum anticonvulsant levels, and the availability of potent new anticonvulsant drugs. With proper drug management, 60% to 80% of persons with epilepsy can obtain good seizure control.

Anticonvulsant Medications

More than 20 drugs are available in the United States for the treatment of epilepsy. This group includes six antiepileptic drugs that were approved for use in the United States since 1996.

Drugs used as first-line therapy for seizure disorders are carbamazepine, phenytoin, ethosuximide, valproate, phenobarbital, primidone, and clonazepam.[64-66] Carbamazepine and phenytoin are the drugs of choice in treating partial seizures. They also are used for tonic-clonic seizures resulting from partial seizures. Ethosuximide is the drug of choice for absence seizures, but it is not effective for tonic-clonic seizures that progress from partial seizures. Valproate is helpful for persons with many of the minor motor seizures and tonic-clonic seizures. Valproate and ethosuximide can be used together. Phenobarbital is used for tonic-clonic seizures, as is primidone. Primidone also is prescribed for simple and complex partial seizures. Absence and myoclonic seizures can be treated with clonazepam. Atonic seizures are highly resistant to therapy. Each of the new drugs—gabapentin, lamotrigine, felbamate, topiramate, levetiracetam, tiagabine, and oxcarbazepine—is approved for use in adults who have partial seizures alone or with secondarily generalized (grand mal) seizures.

Women of childbearing age require special consideration concerning fertility, contraception, and pregnancy. Many of the drugs interact with oral contraceptives; some affect hormone function or decrease fertility. All such women should be advised to take folic acid supplementation. For women with epilepsy who become pregnant, antiseizure drugs increase the risk of congenital abnormalities and other perinatal complications.

Whenever possible, a single drug should be used in epilepsy therapy. Monotherapy eliminates drug interactions

and additive side effects. Determining the proper dose of the anticonvulsant drug is often a long and tedious process, which can be very frustrating for the person with epilepsy. Consistency in taking the medication is essential. Anticonvulsant drugs never should be discontinued abruptly; the dose should be decreased slowly to prevent seizure recurrence. The most frequent cause of recurrent seizures is patient noncompliance with drug regimens. Ongoing education and support are extremely important in the management of seizures. The psychosocial implications of a diagnosis of epilepsy continue to have a large impact on those affected with the disorder.

The neurologist and primary care physician must work together when a person on anticonvulsant medication becomes ill and must take additional medications. Some drugs act synergistically, and others interfere with the actions of anticonvulsant medications. This situation needs to be carefully monitored to avoid overmedication or interference with successful seizure control.

Surgical Therapy

Surgical treatment may be an option for persons with epilepsy that is refractory to drug treatment.[67] With the use of modern neuroimaging and surgical techniques, a single epileptogenic lesion can be identified and removed without leaving a neurologic deficit. The most common surgery consists of removal of the amygdala and anterior part of the hippocampus and entorhinal cortex, as well as a small part of the temporal pole, leaving the lateral temporal neocortex intact. Another surgical procedure involves partial removal of the corpus callosum to prevent spread of a unilateral seizure to a generalized seizure. Modern epilepsy surgery requires a multidisciplinary team of highly skilled surgeons and specialists working together in an epilepsy center. Most procedures require only a few hours in the operating room and a few days' stay in the hospital after surgery. However, surgery for epilepsy is still in its early stages and is considered a treatment modality for only a limited number of persons with epilepsy.

GENERALIZED CONVULSIVE STATUS EPILEPTICUS

Seizures that do not stop spontaneously or occur in succession without recovery are called *status epilepticus*. There are as many types of status epilepticus as there are types of seizures. Tonic-clonic status epilepticus is a medical emergency and, if not promptly treated, may lead to respiratory failure and death.

The disorder occurs most frequently in the young and old. Morbidity and mortality rates are highest in elderly persons and persons with acute symptomatic seizures, such as those related to anoxia or cerebral infarction.[68] Approximately one third of patients have no history of a seizure disorder, and in another one third, status epilepticus occurs as an initial manifestation of epilepsy.[68] If status epilepticus is caused by neurologic or systemic disease, the cause needs to be identified and treated immediately because the seizures probably will not respond until the underlying cause has been corrected.

Treatment consists of appropriate life-support measures. Medications are given to control seizure activity. Intravenously administered diazepam or lorazepam is considered first-line therapy for the condition. The prognosis is related to the underlying cause more than to the seizures themselves.

> In summary, seizures are caused by spontaneous, uncontrolled, paroxysmal, transitory discharges from cortical centers in the brain. Seizures may occur as a reversible symptom of another disease condition or as a recurrent condition called *epilepsy*. Epileptic seizures are classified as partial or generalized seizures. Partial seizures have evidence of local onset, beginning in one hemisphere. They include simple partial seizures, in which consciousness is not lost, and complex partial seizures, which begin in one hemisphere but progress to involve both. Generalized seizures involve both hemispheres and include unconsciousness and rapidly occurring, widespread, bilateral symmetric motor responses. They include minor motor seizures such as absence and akinetic seizures, and major motor or grand mal seizures. Control of seizures is the primary goal of treatment and is accomplished with anticonvulsant medications. Anticonvulsant medications interact with each other and need to be monitored closely when more than one drug is used.

Dementias

After you have completed this section of the chapter, you should be able to meet the following objectives:

+ State the criteria for a diagnosis of dementia
+ Compare the causes associated with Alzheimer's disease, vascular dementia, Pick's disease, Creutzfeldt-Jakob disease, the Wernicke-Korsakoff syndrome, and Huntington's disease
+ Describe the changes in brain tissue that occur with Alzheimer's disease
+ Use the three stages of Alzheimer's disease to describe its progress
+ Cite the difference between Wernicke's disease and the Korsakoff component of the Wernicke-Korsakoff syndrome
+ State the pros and cons for the presymptomatic use of genetic testing for Huntington's disease

Dementia is a syndrome of intellectual deterioration severe enough to interfere with occupational or social performance. It may involve disturbances in memory, language use, perception, and motor skills and may interrupt the ability to learn necessary skills, solve problems, think abstractly, and make judgments. Depression is the most common treatable illness that may masquerade as dementia, and it must be excluded when a diagnosis of dementia is considered (see Chapter 3). This is important because cognitive functioning usually returns to baseline levels after depression is treated. Dementia can be caused by any disorder that per-

manently damages large association areas of the cerebral hemispheres or subcortical areas subserving memory and learning. The dementias include Alzheimer's disease, multi-infarct dementia, Pick's disease, Creutzfeldt-Jakob disease, Wernicke-Korsakoff syndrome, and Huntington's chorea.

ALZHEIMER'S DISEASE

Dementia of the Alzheimer's type occurs in middle or late life and accounts for 50% to 70% of all cases of dementia. The disorder affects approximately 4 million Americans and may be the fourth leading cause of death in the United States.[69] The risk of developing Alzheimer's disease increases with age, and it occurs in nearly half of persons 85 years of age and older. As the elderly population in the United States continues to increase, the number of persons with Alzheimer's-type dementia also is expected to increase.

Pathophysiology

Alzheimer's disease is characterized by cortical atrophy and loss of neurons, particularly in the parietal and temporal lobes (Fig. 50-14). With significant atrophy, there is ventricular enlargement (*i.e.*, hydrocephalus) from the loss of brain tissue.

The major microscopic features of Alzheimer's disease are the presence of amyloid-containing neuritic plaques and neurofibrillary tangles.[4] The neurofibrillary tangles, found in the cytoplasm of abnormal neurons, consist of fibrous proteins that are wound around each other in a helical fashion. These tangles are resistant to chemical or enzymatic breakdown, and they persist in brain tissue long after the neuron in which they arose has died and disappeared. The senile plaques are patches or flat areas composed of clusters of degenerating nerve terminals arranged around a central core of amyloid β-peptide (BAP).[4] These plaques are found in areas of the cerebral cortex that are linked to intellectual function. BAP is a fragment of a much larger membrane-spanning amyloid precursor protein (APP). The function of APP is unclear, but it appears to be associated with the cytoskeleton of nerve fibers. Normally, the degradation of APP involves cleavage in the middle of the BAP portion of the molecule, with both fragments being lost in the extracellular fluid. In Alzheimer's disease, the APP molecule is cut at both ends of the BAP segment, thereby releasing an intact BAP molecule that accumulates in neuritic plaques as amyloid fibrils.[4]

Some plaques and tangles can be found in the brains of older persons who do not show cognitive impairment. The number and distribution of the plaques and tangles appear to contribute to the intellectual deterioration that occurs with Alzheimer's disease. In persons with the disease, the plaques and tangles are found throughout the neocortex and in the hippocampus and amygdala, with relative sparing of the primary sensory cortex.[1] Hippocampal function in particular may be compromised by the pathologic changes that occur in Alzheimer's disease. The hippocampus is crucial to information processing, acquisition of new memories, and retrieval of old memories. The development of neurofibrillary tangles in the entorhinal cortex and su-

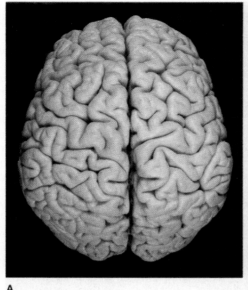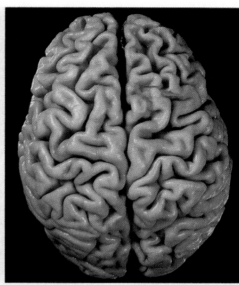

FIGURE 50-14 Alzheimer's disease. (**A**) Normal brain. (**B**) The brain of a patient with Alzheimer's disease shows cortical atrophy, characterized by slender gyri and prominent sulci. (Rubin E., Farber J.L. [1999]. *Pathology* [3rd ed., p. 1511]. Philadelphia: Lippincott Williams & Wilkins)

A   B

perior portion of the hippocampal gyrus interferes with cortical input and output, thereby isolating the hippocampus from the remainder of the cortex and rendering it functionless.

Neurochemically, Alzheimer's disease has been associated with a decrease in the level of choline acetyltransferase activity in the cortex and hippocampus. This enzyme is required for the synthesis of acetylcholine, a neurotransmitter that is associated with memory. The reduction in choline acetyltransferase is quantitatively related to the numbers of neuritic plaques and severity of dementia.

Several drugs have been shown to be effective in slowing the progression of the disease by potentiating the available acetylcholine. The drugs—tacrine, donepezil, rivastigmine, and galantamine—inhibit acetylcholinesterase, preventing the metabolism of endogenous acetylcholine. Thus far, such therapy has not halted disease progression, but it can establish a meaningful plateau in decline.

It is likely that Alzheimer's disease is caused by several factors that interact differently in different persons. Progress on the genetics of inherited early-onset Alzheimer's disease shows that mutations in at least three genes—the APP gene on chromosome 21; presenilin-1 (PS1), a gene on chromosome 14; and presenilin-2 (PS2), a gene on chromosome 1—can cause Alzheimer's disease in certain families.[4,70,71] The APP gene is associated with an autosomal dominant form of early-onset Alzheimer's disease, and can be tested clinically. Persons with Down syndrome (trisomy 21) develop the pathologic changes of Alzheimer's disease and a comparable decline in cognitive functioning at a relatively young age. Virtually all persons with Down syndrome who survive past 50 years of age develop the full-blown pathologic features of dementia. Because the APP gene is located on chromosome 21, it is thought that the additional dosage of the gene product in trisomy 21 predisposes to accumulation of BAP.[4] There is some indication that PS1 and PS2 mutant proteins alter the processing of APP.[4] A fourth gene, an

allele of the apolipoprotein E gene, APOE e4, has been identified as a risk factor for late-onset Alzheimer's disease.

Manifestations

Alzheimer's-type dementia follows an insidious and progressive course. The hallmark symptoms are loss of short-term memory and a denial of such memory loss, with eventual disorientation, impaired abstract thinking, apraxias, and changes in personality and affect. Three stages of Alzheimer's dementia have been identified, each characterized by progressive degenerative changes (Chart 50-2). The *first stage*, which may last for 2 to 4 years, is characterized by short-term memory loss that often is difficult to differentiate from the normal forgetfulness that occurs in the elderly, and usually is reported by caregivers and denied by the patient. Although most elderly have trouble retrieving from memory incidental information and proper names, persons with Alzheimer's disease randomly forget important and unimportant details. They forget where things are placed, get lost easily, and have trouble remembering appointments and performing novel tasks. Mild changes in personality, such as lack of spontaneity, social withdrawal, and loss of a previous sense of humor, occur during this stage.

As the disease progresses, the person with Alzheimer's disease enters the *second* or *confusional stage* of dementia. This stage may last several years and is marked by a more global impairment of cognitive functioning. During this stage, there are changes in higher cortical functioning needed for language, spatial relationships, and problem solving. Depression may occur in persons who are aware of their deficits. There is extreme confusion, disorientation, lack of insight, and inability to carry out the activities of daily living. Personal hygiene is neglected, and language becomes impaired because of difficulty in remembering and retrieving words. Wandering, especially in the late afternoon or early evening, becomes a problem. The *sundown syndrome*, which is characterized by confusion, restlessness, agitation, and wandering, may become a daily occurrence late in the afternoon. Some persons may become hostile and abusive toward family members. Persons who enter this stage become unable to live alone and should be assisted in making decisions about supervised placement with family members or friends or in a community-based facility.

Stage 3 is the terminal stage. It usually is relatively short (1 to 2 years) compared with the other stages, but it has been known to last for as long as 10 years.[72] The person becomes incontinent, apathetic, and unable to recognize family or friends. It usually is during this stage that the person is institutionalized.

Diagnosis and Treatment

Alzheimer's disease is essentially a diagnosis of exclusion. There are no peripheral biochemical markers or tests for the disease. The diagnosis can be confirmed only by microscopic examination of tissue obtained from a cerebral biopsy or at autopsy. The diagnosis is based on clinical findings. Guidelines for the early recognition and assessment of Alzheimer's disease have been published by the Agency for Health Care Policy and Research (AHCPR).[72] A diagnosis of Alzheimer's disease requires the presence of dementia established by clinical examination and documented by results of a Mini-Mental State Examination, Blessed Dementia Test, or similar mental status test; no disturbance in consciousness; onset between ages 40 and 90 years, most often after age 65 years; and absence of systemic or brain disorders that could account for the memory or cognitive deficits.[73] Brain imaging, CT scan, or MRI is done to exclude other brain disease. Metabolic screening should be done for known reversible causes of dementia such as vitamin B_{12} deficiency, thyroid dysfunction, and electrolyte imbalance.

There is no curative treatment for Alzheimer's dementia. Drugs are used primarily to slow the progression and to control depression, agitation, or sleep disorders. Two major goals of care are maintaining the person's socialization and providing support for the family. Self-help groups that provide support for family and friends have become available, with support from the Alzheimer's Disease and Related Disorders Association. Day care and respite centers are available in many areas to provide relief for caregivers and appropriate stimulation for the patient.

Although there is no current drug therapy that is curative for Alzheimer's disease, some show promise in terms of slowing the progress of the disease. The use of pharmacologic agents such as tacrine, donepezil, rivastigmine, and galantamine has been approved for symptomatic therapy in Alzheimer's disease.[74] There also is interest in the use of agents such as antioxidants (*e.g.*, vitamin E, ginkgo), anti-inflammatory agents, and estrogen replacement therapy in women to prevent or delay the onset of the disease.

OTHER TYPES OF DEMENTIA

Vascular Dementia

Dementia associated with cerebrovascular disease does not result directly from atherosclerosis, but rather is caused by multiple infarctions throughout the brain—hence the name vascular or *multi-infarct dementia*. Approximately 20% to 25% of dementias are vascular in origin, and the incidence is closely associated with hypertension. Other contributing factors are arrhythmias, myocardial infarction, peripheral vascular disease, diabetes mellitus, and smoking. The usual onset is between the ages of 55 and 70 years. The disease differs from Alzheimer's dementia in its presentation and tissue abnormalities. The onset may be gradual or abrupt, the course usually is stepwise progression, and there should be focal neurologic symptoms related to local areas of infarction.

Pick's Disease

Pick's disease is a rare form of dementia characterized by atrophy of the frontal and temporal areas of the brain. The neurons in the affected areas contain cytoplasmic inclusions called *Pick bodies*. The average age at onset of Pick's disease is 38 years. The disease is more common in women than men. Behavioral manifestations may be noticed earlier than memory deficits, taking the form of a striking absence of concern and care, a loss of initiative, echolalia (*i.e.*, automatic repetition of anything said to the person), hypotonia, and incontinence. The course of the disease is relentless, with death ensuing within 2 to 10 years. The immediate cause of death usually is infection.

Creutzfeldt-Jakob Disease

Creutzfeldt-Jakob disease is a rare transmissible form of dementia thought to be caused by an infective protein agent called a *prion*[75] (see Chapter 17). Similar diseases occur in animals, including scarpie in sheep and goats, and bovine spongiform encephalitis (BSE; mad cow disease) in cows.

The pathogen is resistant to chemical and physical methods commonly used for sterilizing medical and surgical equipment. The disease reportedly has been transmitted through corneal transplants and human growth hormone obtained from cadavers. The National Hormone and Pituitary Program halted the distribution of human pituitary hormone in 1985 after reports that three young persons who had received the hormone had died of Creutzfeldt-Jakob disease.[76]

Creutzfeldt-Jakob disease causes degeneration of the pyramidal and extrapyramidal systems and is distinguished most readily by its rapid course. Affected persons usually are demented within 6 months of onset. The disease is uniformly fatal, with death often occurring within months, although a few persons may survive for several years.[1] The early symptoms consist of abnormalities in personality and visual-spatial coordination. Extreme dementia, insomnia, and ataxia follow as the disease progresses.[75]

Wernicke-Korsakoff Syndrome

Wernicke-Korsakoff syndrome results from chronic alcoholism. Wernicke's disease is characterized by acute weakness and paralysis of the extraocular muscles, nystagmus, ataxia, and confusion. The affected person also may have signs of peripheral neuropathy. The person has an unsteady gait and complains of diplopia. There may be signs attributable to alcohol withdrawal such as delirium, confusion, and hallucinations. This disorder is caused by a deficiency of thiamine (vitamin B_1), and many of the symptoms are reversed when nutrition is improved with supplemental thiamine.

The Korsakoff component of the syndrome involves the chronic phase with severe impairment of recent memory. There often is difficulty in dealing with abstractions, and the person's capacity to learn is defective. Confabulation (*i.e.*, recitation of imaginary experiences to fill in gaps in memory) probably is the most distinctive feature of the disease. Polyneuritis also is common. Unlike Wernicke's disease, Korsakoff's psychosis does not improve significantly with treatment.

Huntington's Disease

Huntington's disease is a rare hereditary disorder characterized by chronic progressive chorea, psychological changes, and dementia. Although the disease is inherited as an autosomal dominant disorder, the age of onset most commonly is in the fourth and fifth decades.[1] By the time the disease has been diagnosed, the person often has passed the gene on to his or her children.

Huntington's disease produces localized death of brain cells. The first and most severely affected neurons are the caudate nucleus and putamen of the basal ganglia. The neurochemical changes that occur with the disease are complex. The neurotransmitter GABA is an inhibitory neurotransmitter in the basal ganglia. Postmortem studies have shown a decrease of GABA and GABA receptors in the basal ganglia of persons dying of Huntington's disease. Likewise, the levels of acetylcholine, an excitatory neurotransmitter in the basal ganglia, are reduced in persons with Huntington's disease. The dopaminergic pathway of the nigrostriatal system, which is affected in parkinsonism, is preserved in Huntington's disease, suggesting that an imbalance in dopamine and acetylcholine may contribute to manifestations of the disease.

Depression and personality changes are the most common early psychological manifestations; memory loss often is accompanied by impulsive behavior, moodiness, antisocial behavior, and a tendency toward emotional outbursts.[77] Other early signs of the disease are lack of initiative, loss of spontaneity, and inability to concentrate. Fidgeting or restlessness may represent early signs of dyskinesia, followed by choreiform and some dystonic posturing. Eventually, progressive rigidity and akinesia (rather than chorea) develop in association with dementia.

There is no cure for Huntington's disease. The treatment is largely symptomatic. Drugs may be used to treat the dyskinesias and behavioral disturbances.

Study of the genetics of Huntington's disease led to the discovery that the gene for the disease is located on chromosome 4.[4] The discovery of a marker probe for the gene locus has enabled testing that can predict whether a person will develop the disease. The testing procedure requires obtaining DNA samples from the person at risk and from several relatives to determine which member of the gene pair travels with the marker probe for the Huntington's gene in a particular family. DNA for determining the genotype can be obtained from the blood of a consenting person, from amniotic fluid, or from frozen brain tissue from a deceased person.[13] Presymptomatic testing raises many ethical questions, including that of providing a person with knowledge that he or she is carrying a gene that eventually will lead to prolonged physical and mental deterioration.

In summary, cognitive disorders can be caused by any disorder that permanently damages large cortical or subcortical areas of the hemispheres, including Alzheimer's disease, vascular dementia, Pick's disease, Creutzfeldt-Jakob disease, Wernicke-Korsakoff syndrome, and Huntington's disease. Multi-infarct dementia is associated with vascular disease and Pick's disease with atrophy of the frontal and temporal lobes. Creutzfeldt-Jakob disease is a rare transmissible form of dementia. Wernicke-Korsakoff syndrome results from chronic alcoholism. Huntington's disease is a rare hereditary disorder characterized by chronic and progressive chorea, psychological change, and dementia.

By far the most common cause of dementia (50% to 70%) is Alzheimer's disease. The condition is a major health problem among the elderly. It is characterized by cortical atrophy and loss of neurons, the presence of neuritic plaques, granulovacuolar degeneration, and cerebrovascular deposits of amyloid. The disease follows an insidious and progressive course that begins with memory impairment and terminates in an inability to recognize family or friends and the loss of control over bodily functions. The particular tragedy of Alzheimer's disease and other related dementias is that they dissolve the mind and rob the victim of humanity. Simultaneously, these disorders devastate the lives of spouses and other family members, who must endure an insidious loss of the person and a valued relationship.

Related Web Sites

Alzheimer's Association   www.alz.org
American Heart Association   www.americanheart.org
Brain Injury Association   www.biausa.org
Epilepsy Foundation   www.efa.org
National Rehabilitation Information Center   www.naric.com
National Resource Center for Traumatic Brain Injury
      www.neuro.pmr.vcu.edu

References

1. Cotran R.S., Kumar V., Collins T. (1999). *Robbins pathologic basis of disease* (6th ed., pp. 1307, 1312–1313, 1329–1333, 1343–1349). Philadelphia: W.B. Saunders.
2. Meyer F.B. (1992). Brain metabolism, blood flow, and ischemic thresholds. In Awad I.A. (Ed.), *Neurosurgical topics: Cerebrovascular occlusive disease and brain ischemia* (pp. 1–24). Cleveland: American Association of Neurological Surgeons.
3. Richmond T.S. (1997). Cerebral resuscitation after global brain ischemia: Linking research to practice. *AACN Clinical Issues* 8, 171–181.
4. Rubin E., Farber J.L. (1999). *Pathology* (3rd ed., pp. 1470–1473, 1509–1512). Philadelphia: Lippincott Williams & Wilkins.
5. Martin T.G. (1986). Drowning and near-drowning. *Hospital Medicine* 22 (7), 53.
6. Sieber F.E., Traystman R.J. (1992). Special issues: Glucose and the brain. *Critical Care Medicine* 20, 104–116.
7. Lipton S.A., Rosenberg P.A. (1994). Excitatory amino acids as a final common pathway in neurologic disorders. *New England Journal of Medicine* 330, 613–622.
8. Feuerstein G., Hunter J., Barone F.C. (1992). Calcium blockers and neuroprotection. In Marangos P.J., Lal H. (Eds.), *Advances in neuroprotection: Emerging strategies in neuroprotection* (p. 129). Boston: Birkhauser.
9. Sauer D., Massiu L., Allegrini P.R., Amacker H., Schmutz M., Fagg G.E. (1992). Excitotoxicity, cerebral ischemia, and neuroprotection by competitive NMDA receptor antagonists. In Marangos P.J., Lal H. (Eds.), *Advances in neuroprotection: Emerging strategies in neuroprotection* (pp. 93–105). Boston: Birkhauser.
10. Albers G.W., Clark W.M., DeGraba T.J. (1998). *The evolving paradigm of neuronal protection following stroke.* Monograph. Englewood, CO: Postgraduate Institute for Medicine.
11. Hickey J.V. (1996). *The clinical practice of neurological and neurosurgical nursing* (4th ed., pp. 295–327, 569–584). Philadelphia: Lippincott-Raven.
12. Lang E.W., Chestnut R.M. (1995). Intracranial pressure and cerebral perfusion pressure in severe head injury. *New Horizons* 3, 400–409.
13. Ghajar J. (2000). Traumatic brain injury. *Lancet* 356, 923–929.
14. Guyton A.C., Hall J.E. (2000). *Textbook of medical physiology* (10th ed., pp. 192, 671–722). Philadelphia: W.B. Saunders.
15. Plum F., Posner J.B. (1980). *The diagnosis of stupor and coma* (3rd ed.). Philadelphia: F.A. Davis.
16. Conn P.M. (1995). *Neuroscience in medicine* (pp. 232–235). Philadelphia: J.B. Lippincott.
17. Rhoades R.A., Tanner G.A. (1996). *Medical physiology* (pp. 132–133), Boston: Little, Brown.
18. Samuels M.A. (1993). The evaluation of comatose patients. *Hospital Practice* 28, 165–181.
19. Bates D. (1993). The management of medical coma. *Journal of Neurology, Neurosurgery, and Psychiatry* 56, 589–598.
20. Ingersoll G.L., Leyden D.B. (1987). The Glasgow Coma Scale for patients with head injuries. *Critical Care Nursing* 7 (5), 26–32.
21. Teasdale G.M. (2000). Revisiting the Glasgow Coma Scale and Coma Score. *Intensive Care Medicine* 26, 153–154.
22. Wijdicks E.F.M. (1995). Determining brain death in adults. *Neurology* 45, 1003–1011.
23. Wijdicks E.F.M. (2001). The diagnosis of brain death. *New England Journal of Medicine* 344, 1215–1221.
24. Beecher H.K. (1968). A definition of irreversible coma: Report of the Ad Hoc Committee of the Harvard Medical School to Examine the Definition of Brain Death. *Journal of the American Medical Association* 237, 337–340.
25. President's Committee for the Study of Ethical Problems in Medicine and Biomedical and Behavioral Research. (1981). *Defining death: A report on the medical, legal and ethical issues in the determination of death.* Washington, DC: Government Printing Office.
26. Quality Standards Subcommittee of American Academy of Neurology. (1995). Practice parameters for determining brain death in adults. *Neurology* 45, 1012–1014.
27. Celesia G.G. (1993). Persistent vegetative state. *Neurology* 43, 1457–1458.
28. Quality Standards Subcommittee of American Academy of Neurology. (1995). Practice parameters: Assessment and management of patients with persistent vegetative state. *Neurology* 45, 1015–1018.
29. American Stroke Association. (1999). *The latest news about stroke.* Dallas, TX: American Heart Association.
30. Bronner L.L., Kaner D.S., Manson J.E. (1995). Primary prevention of stroke. *New England Journal of Medicine* 333, 1392–1400.
31. Gorelick P.B. (1987). Alcohol and stroke. *Current Concepts in Cerebrovascular Disease* 21 (5), 21.
32. Blank-Reid C. (1996). How to have a stroke at an early age: The effects of crack, cocaine and other illicit drugs. *Journal of Neuroscience Nursing* 28 (1), 19–27.
33. Albers W.A. (Chair). (1998). Antithrombotic and thrombolytic therapy for ischemic stroke. *Chest* 114, 683S–698S.
34. Zambramski J.M., Anson J.A. (1992). Diagnostic evaluation of ischemic cerebrovascular disease. In Awad I.A. (Ed.), *Neurosurgical topics: Cerebrovascular occlusive disease and brain ischemia* (pp. 73–101). Cleveland: American Association of Neurological Surgeons.
35. Gregory W. (Chair AD Hoc Committee on Guidelines for Management of Transient Ischemic Attacks, Stroke Council, American Heart Association). (1999). Supplement to the guidelines for transient ischemic attacks. *Stroke* 30, 2502–2511.
36. Qureshi A.I., Tuhrim S., Broderick J.P., Batjer H.H., Hondo H., Hanley D.F. (2001). Spontaneous intracerebral hemorrhage. *New England Journal of Medicine* 344, 1450–1460.
37. Broderick J.P., Adams H.P., Barson W., Feinberg W., Feldmann E., Grotta J., Kase C., Krieger D., Mayberg M., Tilley B., Zabramski J.M., Zuccarelli M. (1999). American Heart Association Scientific Statement: Guidelines to the management of spontaneous intracerebral hemorrhage. *Stroke* 30, 905–915.
38. Adams H.P. (Chair). (1994). Guidelines for the management of patients with acute ischemic stroke: A statement for healthcare professionals from a Special Writing Group of the Stroke Council, American Heart Association. *Stroke* 25, 1901–1914.
39. Adams H.P. (Chair). (1996). Guidelines for thrombolytic therapy of acute stroke: A supplement to the guidelines for the management of patients with acute ischemic stroke: A statement for healthcare professionals from the Special Writing Group of the Stroke Council, American Heart Association. *Circulation* 94, 1167–1174.
40. Albers G.W. (1997). Management of acute ischemic stroke: An update for primary care physicians. *Western Journal of Medicine* 166, 253–262.

41. Schievink W.I. (1997). Intracranial aneurysms. *New England Journal of Medicine* 336, 28–39.

42. Mayberg M.R. (Chair). (1994). Guidelines for the management of aneurysmal subarachnoid hemorrhage: A statement for healthcare professionals from a Special Writing Group of the Stroke Council, American Heart Association. *Stroke* 25, 2315–2327.

43. Sawin P.D., Loftus C.M. (1997). Diagnosis of spontaneous subarachnoid hemorrhage. *American Family Physician* 55, 145–155.

44. Arteriovenous Malformations Study Group. (1999). Arteriovenous malformations of the brain in adults. *New England Journal of Medicine* 340, 1812–1818.

45. Ogilvy C.S. (Chair, Special Writing Group of the Stroke Council, American Heart Association). (2001). Recommendations for management of intracranial arteriovenous malformations. *Stroke* 32, 1458–1471.

46. Bronstein K.S., Popovich J.M., Stewart-Amidei C. (1991). *Promoting stroke recovery: A research based approach for nurses* (p. 200). St. Louis: C.V. Mosby.

47. Gresham G.E., Duncan P.W., Stason W.B., .dams H.P., Adelman A.M., Alexander D., et al. (1995). *Post-stroke rehabilitation: Clinical practice guidelines no. 16.* AHCPR publication no. 95-0662. Rockville, MD: U.S. Department of Health and Human Services, Public Health Services, Agency for Health Care Policy and Research.

48. White R.J., Likavec M.J. (1992). The diagnosis and initial management of head injury. *New England Journal of Medicine* 327, 1507–1511.

49. Jennett B. (1996). Epidemiology of head injury. *Journal of Neurology, Neurosurgery, and Psychiatry* 60, 362–369.

50. Chestnut R.M. (1995). Secondary brain insults after head injury: Clinical perspectives. *New Horizons* 3, 366–375.

51. Teasdale G.M. (1995). Head injury. *Journal of Neurology, Neurosurgery, and Psychiatry* 58, 526–539.

52. Tunkel A.R., Scheld W.M. (1997). Issues in management of bacterial meningitis. *American Family Physician* 56, 1355–1365.

53. Quagliarello V.J., Scheld W.M. (1997). Treatment of bacterial meningitis. *New England Journal of Medicine* 336, 708–716.

54. Mehta N., Levin M. (2000). Management and prevention of meningococcal disease. *Hospital Practice* 35 (8), 75–86.

55. American Cancer Society. (2001). Brain and spinal cord cancers in adults. [On-line]. Available: http://www3.cancer.org.

56. DeAngelo L.M. (2001). Brain tumors. *New England Journal of Medicine* 344, 114–123.

57. Black P.M. (1991). Brain tumors (second of two parts). *New England Journal of Medicine* 324, 1555–1564.

58. Black P.M. (1991). Brain tumors (first of two parts). *New England Journal of Medicine* 324, 1471–1476.

59. Browne T.R., Holmes G.L. (2001). Epilepsy. *New England Journal of Medicine* 344, 1145–1151.

60. Mosewich R.K., So E.L. (1996). The clinical approach to classification of seizures and epileptic syndromes. *Mayo Clinic Proceedings* 71, 405–441.

61. Haslam R.H. (2000). The nervous system. In Behrman R.E., Kliegman R.M., Jenson H.B. (Eds.). *Nelson textbook of medicine* (16th ed., pp. 1813–1829). Philadelphia: W.B. Saunders.

62. Commission on Classification and Terminology of the International League Against Epilepsy. (1981). Proposal for revised clinical and electroencephalographic classification of epileptic seizures. *Epilepsia* 22, 489–501.

63. Commission on Classification and Terminology of the International League Against Epilepsy. (1989). Proposal for revised classification of epilepsies and epileptic syndromes. *Epilepsia* 30, 389–399.

64. Schachter S.C., Yerby M.S. (1997). Management of epilepsy. *Postgraduate Medicine* 101, 133–153.

65. Brodie M.J., Dichter M.A. (1996). Antiepileptic drugs. *New England Journal of Medicine* 334, 168–175.

66. Dichter M.A., Brodie M.J. (1996). New antiepileptic drugs. *New England Journal of Medicine* 334, 1583–1589.

67. Engel J. (1996). Surgery for seizures. *New England Journal of Medicine* 334, 647–652.

68. Cascino G.D. (1996). Generalized convulsive status epilepticus. *New England Journal of Medicine* 71, 787–792.

69. Morrison-Borgorad M., Phelps C., Buckholtz N. (1996). Alzheimer disease research comes of age. *Journal of the American Medical Association* 277, 837–840.

70. van Duijn C.M. (1996). Epidemiology of the dementias: Recent developments and new approaches. *Journal of Neurology, Neurosurgery, and Psychiatry* 60, 478–488.

71. Lendon C.L., Ashall F., Goate A.M. (1996). Exploring the etiology of Alzheimer's disease using molecular genetics. *Journal of the American Medical Association* 277, 825–831.

72. U.S. Department of Health and Human Services. (1996). *Recognition and initial assessment of Alzheimer's disease and related disorders.* AHCPR publication no. 97-0702. Washington, DC: Public Health Service, Agency for Health Care Policy and Research.

73. Morris J.C. (1997). Alzheimer's disease: A review of clinical assessment and management issues. *Geriatrics* 52 (Suppl. 2), S22–S25.

74. Mayeux R., Sano M. (1999). Treatment of Alzheimer's disease. *New England Journal of Medicine* 341, 1670–1679.

75. Prusiner S.B. (2001). Shattuck lecture: Neurodegenerative diseases and prions. *New England Journal of Medicine* 344, 1516–1526.

76. Rappaport E.B. (1987). Iatrogenic Creutzfeldt-Jakob disease. *Neurology* 37, 1520–1522.

77. Martin J., Gusella J. (1987). Huntington's disease: Pathogenesis and management. *New England Journal of Medicine* 315, 1267–1276.

Chapter 51

Sleep and Sleep Disorders

Neurobiology of Sleep

Neural Structures and Pathways
The Sleep-Wake Cycle
  Brain Waves
  Sleep Stages
  Breathing During Sleep
  Dreaming
Circadian Rhythms
Melatonin

Sleep Disorders

Diagnostic Methods
  Sleep History
  Sleep Log/Diary
  Polysomnography
Dyssomnias
  Circadian Rhythm Disorders
  Insomnia
  Narcolepsy
  Motor Disorders of Sleep
  Obstructive Sleep Apnea

Parasomnias
  Nightmares
  Sleepwalking and Sleep Terrors

**Sleep and Sleep Disorders
in Children and the Elderly**

Sleep Disorders in Children
  Sleep Terrors in Children
  Sleepwalking in Children
Sleep Disorders in the Elderly

As humans, we spend approximately a third of our lives asleep. We all know what sleep feels like. Yet defining sleep, describing what happens when we sleep, and why we sleep is more difficult. Of equal concern is an understanding of factors that interfere with sleep. For many people, the inability to engage in appropriate periods of normal, restful sleep seriously impairs their functioning. The content in this chapter is divided into three parts: (1) the neurobiology of sleep, (2) sleep disorders, and (3) sleep and sleep disorders in children and the elderly.

Neurobiology of Sleep

After you have completed this section of the chapter, you should be able to meet the following objectives:

✦ Cite the major brain structures that are involved in sleep
✦ Describe the different stages of sleep in terms of the electroencephalogram tracing, eye movements, motor movements, heart rate, blood pressure, and cerebral activity
✦ Characterize the circadian rhythm as it relates to sleep and wakefulness
✦ Describe the possible role of melatonin in regulation of sleep

Sleep is part of what is called the *sleep-wake cycle*. In contrast to wakefulness, which is a time of mental activity and energy expenditure, sleep is a period of inactivity and restoration of mental and physical function. It has been suggested that sleep provides time for entering information that has been acquired during periods of wakefulness into memory and for reestablishing communication between various parts of the brain. Sleep also is a time when other body systems restore their energy and repair their tissues. Muscle activity and digestion decrease and sympathetic nervous system activity is diminished. Many hormones, such as growth hormone, are produced in a cyclic manner correlating with the sleep-wake cycle, suggesting that growth and tissue repair may occur during sleep.

NEURAL STRUCTURES AND PATHWAYS

Anatomically, the sleep-wake cycle involves structures in the thalamus, associated areas of the cerebral cortex, and interneurons in the reticular formation of the midbrain, the pons, and the brain stem (Fig. 51-1). The reticular formation of the midbrain, pons, and brain stem monitors and modulates the activity of various circuits controlling wakefulness. The thalamus and the cerebral cortex function in tandem, with all sensory information being relayed to the thalamus and from there to the cerebral cortex. For example, visual

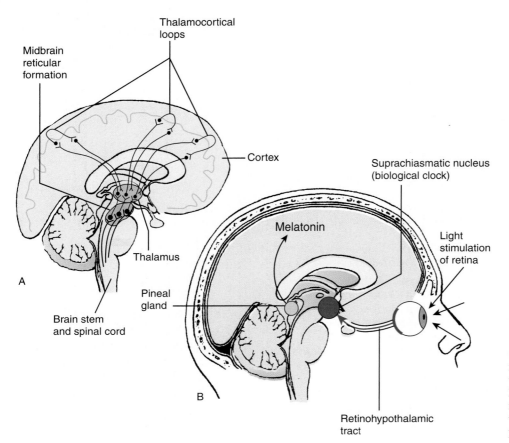

FIGURE 51-1 (A) Brain structures involved in sleep. **(B)** Location of the suprachiasmatic nucleus (biological clod) with input from the retina and its association with the pineal gland and melatonin production.

impulses from the retina go to the thalamus and are then relayed to the visual cortex. The pathways between each sensory area of the thalamus and the cortex form a two-way communication loop called the *thalamocortical loop*.[1] Communication between each sensory area of the thalamus and its companion area in the cortex is kept orderly by several neuronal control systems, including the midbrain reticular formation that controls the level of background activity so that external stimuli can be processed.

THE SLEEP-WAKE CYCLE

The sleep-wake cycle normally consists of a synchronous pattern of wakefulness and sleep. Wakefulness is a state of being aware of the environment—of receiving and responding to information arriving from all the senses, placing that information into memory, and recalling and integrating present experiences with previously stored memories. During wakefulness, both the thalamocortical loop and brain stem centers are active. A full repertoire of motor movements is made possible by corticospinal circuits that travel through the brain stem. Sleep represents a period of diminished consciousness from which a person can be aroused by sensory or other stimuli. It occurs in stages during which the brain remains active, but does not effectively process sensory information.

> ### 🔑 Sleep–Wake Cycle
>
> ➤ The sleep–wake cycle normally consists of a synchronous pattern of wakefulness and sleep.
>
> ➤ Wakefulness and sleep differ in terms of awareness of the environment, motor and eye movements, and brain waves.
>
> ➤ Wakefulness is a state of being aware of the environment, receiving and responding to sensory input, recalling and integrating experiences into memory, and purposeful body movements.
>
> ➤ Sleep, which is a period of inactivity and restoration of mental and physical function, is characterized by alterations between non-REM and REM sleep.
>
> ➤ Non-REM sleep is a quiet type of sleep characterized by a relatively inactive, yet fully regulating brain, and fully movable body, whereas REM sleep is associated with rapid eye movements, loss of muscle movements, and vivid dreaming.

Brain Waves

Many of the advances in understanding the sleep-wake cycle have come about because of the ability to record brain waves through the use of the electroencephalogram (EEG). It was in 1928 that the German psychiatrist Hans Berger successfully recorded continuous electrical activity from the scalp of human subjects.[1] The source of the brain waves is the alternating excitatory and inhibitory nerve activity in postsynaptic neurons.[2] During the recording of an EEG, the postsynaptic potentials are averaged and filtered to improve the quality of the signal. As such, the EEG does not measure the activity of a single neuron, but rather the combined activity and "cross-talk" among many hundreds of neurons responding to a given stimulus.

The normal EEG consists of brain waves of various frequencies (measured in cycles per second, or hertz [Hz]) and amplitude (measured in microvolts [μV]; Fig. 51-2). Four types of EEG rhythms are used to describe brain activity during the sleep-wake cycle: alpha, beta, delta, and theta rhythms.[2,3] The *alpha* rhythm, which has a frequency of 7 to 13 Hz, occurs when a person is awake with eyes closed. When the eyes are open, the EEG becomes desynchronized and the dominant frequency changes to the low-amplitude *beta* rhythm with a frequency of 14 to 32 Hz. The increased frequency of the beta waves is thought to reflect a higher level of brain activity produced by firing of a large number of neurons and the low amplitude a lack of synchronization resulting from nerve activity occurring in many different brain sites at the same time. The *delta* (0.5 to 4 Hz) and *theta* (4 to 7 Hz) rhythms are observed during sleep. The low-frequency, higher-amplitude waves that occur during sleep indicate that fewer neurons are firing and that those that are active are more highly synchronized and less affected by sensory stimulation.

Sleep Stages

There are two types of sleep: rapid eye movement (REM) and non-REM sleep.[2,4] These two types of sleep alternate with each other and are characterized by differences in eye movements, muscle tone and body movements, heart rate and

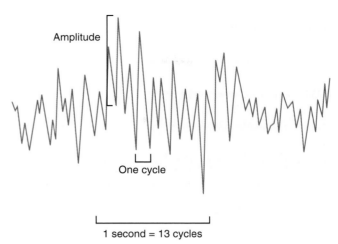

FIGURE 51-2 The amplitude and frequency characteristics of an EEG tracing.

blood pressure, breathing patterns, brain wave activity, and dreaming (Table 51-1).

Non–Rapid Eye Movement Sleep. Non-REM sleep is a quiet type of sleep characterized by a relatively inactive, yet fully regulating brain, and fully movable body. The brain stem coordinates activity between the spinal cord and various reflexes such as swallowing and chewing. Non-REM sleep normally is encountered when the person first becomes drowsy. It is divided into four stages that reflect an increasing depth of sleep (Fig. 51-3). *Stage 1* consists of low-voltage, mixed-frequency EEG activity. It occurs at sleep onset and is a brief (1 to 7 minutes) transitional stage between wakefulness and true sleep. During this stage, persons can be easily aroused simply by touching them, calling their name, or quietly closing a door. In addition to its role at sleep onset, stage 1 serves as a transitional stage for repeated sleep cycles throughout the night. A common sign of severely disrupted sleep is an increase or decrease in stage 1 sleep. *Stage 2*, which lasts approximately 10 to 25 minutes, is a deeper sleep during which EEG activity is interrupted by

TABLE 51-1 ✦ **Electroencephalogram, Eye and Motor Movements, Vital Functions, and Cerebral Activity During Sleep**

Sleep Stage	Electroencephalogram	Eye Movements	Motor Movements	Heart Rate, Blood Pressure, Respirations	Cerebral Activity
Stage 1	Low voltage, mixed frequency	Slow, rolling movements	Moderate activity	Slows	Decreases
Stage 2	Low voltage, 12- to 14-Hz spindles	Slow, rolling movements	Moderate activity	Slows	Decreases
Stages 3 and 4 (deep sleep)	Delta (0.5–2 Hz) waves (slow-wave sleep)	Slow, rolling movements	Moderate activity	Slows	Decreases
REM sleep	Low voltage, mixed frequency	Clusters of rapid eye movements	Suppressed with loss of muscle tone	Increases, variable	Increases

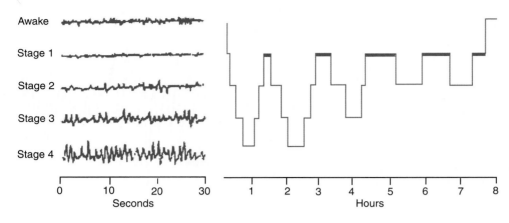

FIGURE 51-3 Brain waves during wakefulness and stages 1, 2, 3, and 4 sleep on the **left** and duration of wakefulness, REM, and non-REM sleep on the **right**. (Adapted from Kryger M.H., Roth T., Dement W.C. [Eds]. [1989]. *Principles and practices of sleep medicine.* Philadelphia: W.B. Saunders)

sleep spindles consisting of bursts of high-frequency (12 to 14 Hz) waves. *Stages 3 and 4* represent deep sleep and are dominated by high-voltage, low-frequency (1 to 3 Hz) waves. Stage 3 usually lasts only a few minutes and is transitional to stage 4, which lasts for approximately 20 to 40 minutes. During deep sleep, the muscles of the body relax and posture is adjusted intermittently. The heart rate and blood pressure decrease and gastrointestinal activity is slowed. An incrementally larger stimulus is required for arousal from slow-wave sleep.

Rapid Eye Movement Sleep. Rapid eye movement sleep is associated with rapid eye movements, loss of muscle movements, and vivid dreaming. External sensory input is inhibited, whereas internal sensory circuits such as those of the auditory and visual systems are aroused. During this time, the brain can replay previous memories but cannot acquire new sensory information (Fig. 51-4). At the same time, motor systems that control body movements are inhibited. There is a loss of muscle movement and muscle tone. The result is an extraordinary set of paradoxes, in

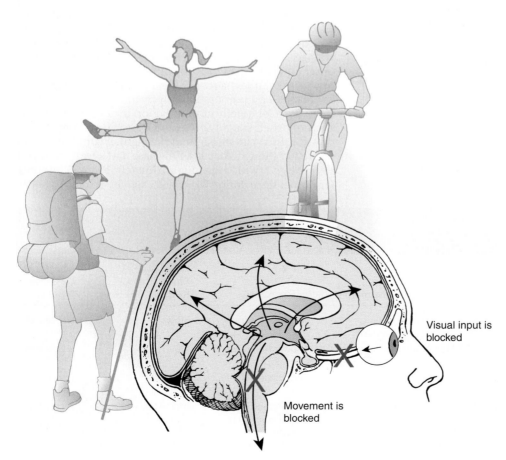

Visual input is blocked

Movement is blocked

FIGURE 51-4 Dreaming during REM sleep when sensory and motor activity are blocked.

which people see things in their dreams, but cannot move. They imagine being engaged in activities such as running, flying, or dancing but are paralyzed.

There also are changes in autonomic nervous system–controlled functions during REM sleep—blood pressure, heart rate, and respirations increase and fluctuate and temperature regulation is lost. Cerebral blood flow and metabolic rate decrease. Sleep-related penile erection occurs during this stage of sleep.

It has been shown that adequate amounts of REM sleep are necessary for normal daytime functioning. Deprivation of REM sleep is associated with anxiety, irritability, inability to concentrate, and, if deprivation is severe enough, disturbed behavior.

Moving Between Sleep Stages. There is a rather predictable pattern of shifting between one non-REM stage and another during a typical night's sleep.[4] At sleep onset, there is a stepwise descent from lighter stage 1 sleep to deeper stage 4 sleep, followed by an abrupt ascent back toward stage 1. However, in place of stage 1, the first REM episode usually occurs. REM sleep is comparatively short (1 to 5 minutes) during the first sleep cycle, but gradually becomes longer across the night. Stages 3 and 4 occupy less time in the second and subsequent sleep cycles and disappear altogether in later cycles.

Breathing During Sleep

Breathing normally changes during sleep. Stages 1 and 2 of non-REM sleep are characterized by a cyclic waning and waxing of tidal volume and respiratory rate, which may include brief periods (5 to 15 seconds) of apnea. This pattern is called *periodic breathing*. Although the amount of periodic breathing that occurs during the first two stages of non-REM sleep differs among healthy persons, it is more common in persons older than 40 years of age.[5] After sleep has stabilized during stages 3 and 4 of non-REM sleep, breathing becomes more regular. Ventilation usually is 1 to 2 L/minute less than during quiet wakefulness; the PCO_2 levels are 2 to 8 mm Hg greater; the PO_2 levels are 5 to 10 mm Hg less; and the pH is 0.03 to 0.05 units less.[6] Involuntary respiratory control mechanisms, such as responses to hypercapnia, hypoxia, and lung inflation, are intact during non-REM sleep and critically important to maintaining ventilation.

During REM sleep, respirations become irregular, but not periodic, and may include short periods of apnea. Breathing during REM sleep has many features of the voluntary control that integrates breathing with acts such as walking, talking, and swallowing. However, their influence on breathing is diminished.

Dreaming

Dreams are recollections of mental activity that occurred during sleep. They occur during all stages of sleep, but are more frequent during REM sleep. Approximately 80% of dreams occur during REM and sleep onset (stages 1 and 2) sleep.[7] Dreams that occur during REM sleep tend to be bizarre with colorful, storybook-like detail.[1] Most nightmares occur during REM sleep. Dreams that occur during stages 1 and 2 of sleep tend to be shorter, have fewer associations, and lack the color and emotion of those that occur during REM sleep.

The purpose of dreaming is unclear. Evidence suggests that dreaming, like other physiologic functions, is important to learning and memory processing.[7] It has been suggested that dreaming may be the result of reprogramming of the central nervous system (*i.e.*, rearranging previous experiences) in preparation for the next day's conscious experiences.

CIRCADIAN RHYTHMS

Normally, sleep and wakefulness occur in a cyclic manner, integrated into the 24-hour light-dark solar day. The term *circadian*, from the Latin *circa* ("about") and *dies* ("day"), is used to describe these 24-hour diurnal rhythms. The function of the circadian time system is to provide a temporal organization for physiologic processes and behaviors as a means of promoting effective adaptation to the environment. At the behavioral level, this is expressed in regular cycles of sleep and waking and body functions such as temperature regulation and hormone secretion based on changes in the 24-hour light-dark solar day.

The daily rhythm of the sleep-wake cycle is part of a time-keeping system created by an internal pacemaker or clock.[8,9] Time isolation experiments, in which people were placed in an environment without time cues, showed that the cycle length of the human internal clock is in general from 23.5 to 26.5 hours.[8] Because the intrinsic cycle tends to be longer than 24 hours, a daily resetting of the circadian clock is necessary to synchronize with the environmental day. This process is called *entrainment* and normally is accomplished by exposure to the light-dark changes of the solar day.

The circadian clock appears to be controlled by a small group of hypothalamic cells, called the *suprachiasmatic nucleus* (SCN), located just above the optic chiasm and lateral to the third ventricle[8–10] (see Fig. 51-1). The SCN, which receives light-dark input from the retina, exhibits a rhythm of neuronal firing that is high during the day and low during the night. Although light serves as the primary stimulus for resetting the circadian clock, other stimuli such as locomotion and activity contribute to its regulation. The major projections from the SCN are to the anterior pituitary, with lesser ones to the basal forebrain and midline thalamus. Projections to the anterior pituitary provide for diurnal regulation of growth hormone and cortisol secretion; those to hypothalamic centers, for changes in metabolism and body temperature; and those to the brain stem reticular formation, for changes in autonomic nervous system regulated functions such as heart rate and blood pressure (Fig. 51-5).

MELATONIN

Melatonin, a hormone produced by the pineal gland, is thought to help regulate the sleep-wake cycle and, possibly, circadian rhythm.[11–13] The pineal gland synthesizes and releases melatonin at night, a rhythm that is under the direct

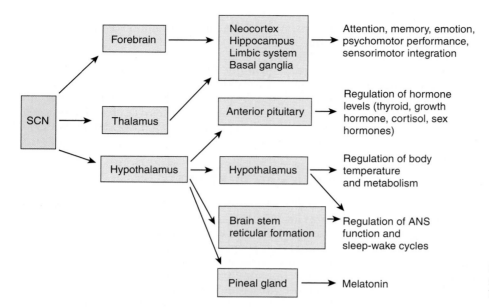

FIGURE 51-5 Projections from the suprachiasmic nucleus (SCN) to the forebrain, thalamus, and hypothalamus.

control of the SCN (see Fig. 51-1). Large numbers of melatonin receptors are present in the SCN, suggesting a feedback loop between the SCN and the pineal gland. Administration of melatonin produces phase-shifting changes in the circadian rhythm, similar to those caused by light. There has been recent interest in the use of melatonin in treatment of various sleep disorders, particularly those related to a shift in the circadian rhythm. Although synthetic preparations are available without prescription in health food stores and pharmacies, their potency, purity, safety, and effectiveness cannot be assured. There also is a lack of clinical trial evidence about appropriate dosage, adverse effects, drug interactions, and the effects of melatonin on various disease states.[12]

Sleep is part of what is called the *sleep-wake cycle*. In contrast to wakefulness, which is a time of mental activity and energy expenditure, sleep is a period of inactivity and restoration of mental and physical function. There are two types of sleep: rapid eye movement (REM) and non-REM sleep. REM sleep is associated with rapid eye movements, loss of muscle movements, and vivid dreaming. External sensory input is inhibited, whereas internal sensory circuits such as those of the auditory and visual systems are aroused. Non-REM sleep is a quiet type of sleep characterized by a relatively inactive, yet fully regulating brain, and a fully movable body. It is divided into four stages that reflect an increasing depth of sleep. Stage 1 is a brief transitional stage that occurs at the onset of sleep, during which a person is easily aroused. Stage 2 is a deeper sleep, lasting approximately 10 to 25 seconds, during which EEG activity is interrupted by sleep spindles consisting of bursts of high-frequency waves. Stages 3 and 4 represent deep sleep, during which the muscles of the body relax, the heart rate and blood pressure decrease, and gastrointestinal activity is slowed.

Normally, sleep and wakefulness occur in a cyclic manner, called the *circadian rhythm*, that is integrated into the 24-hour light-dark solar day. The circadian clock is thought to be controlled by the SCN in the hypothalamus. The SCN, which receives light-dark input from the retina, exhibits a rhythm of neuronal firing that is high during the day and low during the night. Melatonin, a hormone produced by the pineal gland, is thought to help regulate the sleep-wake cycle.

Sleep Disorders

After you have completed this section of the chapter, you should be able to meet the following objectives:

♦ List the four categories of sleep disorders included in the International Classification of Sleep Disorders

♦ Describe the methods used in diagnosis of sleep disorders, including the sleep history, sleep diary, polysomnography, and wrist actigraphy

♦ Characterize the non–24-hour sleep-wake syndrome experienced by visually impaired individuals, sleep disorders associated with acute shifts in the sleep-wake cycle due to intercontinental travel and shift work, and advanced sleep phase and delayed sleep phase circadian rhythm sleep disorders

♦ Describe the causes, manifestations, diagnosis, and treatment of acute and chronic insomnia

♦ Differentiate periodic limb movement disorder and restless legs syndrome in terms of manifestations and treatment

♦ Explain the physiologic mechanisms, contributing factors, and manifestations of obstructive sleep apnea and describe the methods used in diagnosis and treatment of the disorder

♦ Define the term *parasomnias* and relate it to the manifestations of nightmare, sleep terrors, and sleep walking

In 1997, the American Sleep Disorders Association (ASDA) published a revision of the *International Classification of Sleep Disorders* (ICSD), which originally was developed in 1990.[14] The ICSD classifies sleep disorders into four categories: (1) dyssomnias, which are disorders of initiating and maintaining sleep and disorders of excessive sleepiness; (2) parasomnias, which are not responsible for disturbing the sleep-wake cycle but are undesirable phenomena that occur primarily during sleep; (3) sleep disorders associated with other medical or psychiatric disorders; and (4) proposed sleep disorders, such as pregnancy-induced sleep disruptions (Chart 51-1).

DIAGNOSTIC METHODS

The diagnosis of sleep disorders usually is based on adequate sleep history and physical examination. A sleep diary or sleep log often is helpful in describing sleep problems and arriving at a diagnosis.[14,15] In some cases, sleep laboratory studies may be needed to arrive at an accurate diagnosis.

Sleep History

A sleep history is fundamental to the process of identifying the nature of a sleep disorder.[16] The history should include the person's perception of the sleep problem, sleep schedule (*e.g.*, time of retiring and arising); problems with falling asleep and maintaining sleep, quality of sleep, daytime sleepiness and impact of the sleep disorder on daytime functioning, general emotional and physical problems, sleep hygiene (*e.g.*, eating and drinking before retiring), and sleep environment (*e.g.*, bed comfort, room temperature, noise, light). Because drugs such as over-the-counter medications, herbal preparations, and prescription medications can influence sleep, a careful drug history is important. It

---

CHART 51-1

International Classification of Sleep Disorders

Dyssomnias
Intrinsic sleep disorders
Extrinsic sleep disorders
Circadian rhythm sleep disorders

Parasomnias
Arousal disorders
Sleep-wake transition disorders
Parasomnias usually associated with REM sleep
Other parasomnias

Sleep disorders associated with mental, neurologic, or other medical disorders
Associated with mental disorders
Associated with neurologic disorders
Associated with other medical disorders

Proposed sleep disorders

(From American Sleep Disorder Association. [1997]. *The international classification of sleep disorders: Revised*. Rochester, MN: Author.)

---

also is important to obtain information about the use of alcohol, caffeine, tobacco, and illegal substances.

Sleep Log/Diary

A sleep log/diary is a person's written account of his or her sleep experience. It usually is recommended that the diary be kept for at least 2 weeks. The diary should record the person's account of their bedtime, wakeup time, total sleep time, time of sleep onset, time needed to prepare for bed and to fall asleep, use of sleep medications, number of awakenings, subjective assessment of sleep quality, time out of bed in the morning, and daytime naps and symptoms. A number of sample forms are available to health care professionals for distribution to their clients.

Polysomnography

A typical sleep study, or *polysomnography*, involves use of the EEG, electro-oculogram (EOG), electromyogram (EMG), electrocardiogram (ECG), breathing movements, and pulse oximetry.[4] The EOG records eye movements. Because the eye is like a small battery with the retina negative to the cornea, an electrode placed on the skin near the eye records changes in voltage as the eye rotates in its socket. The EMG records the electrical activity from muscle movement. It is recorded from the surface of the skin. It typically is recorded from under the chin because muscles in this area of the body show very dramatic changes associated with the sleep cycle. The ECG is used to measure the heart rate and detect cardiac dysrhythmias. The pulse oximeter (ear or finger) measures arterial oxygen saturation.

The multiple sleep latency test (MSLT) is used to evaluate daytime sleepiness. This test usually is completed the

---

 Sleep Disorders

➤ Sleep disorders, which represent a disruption in the sleep-wake cycle, can be divided into four categories: dyssomnias; parasomnias; sleep disorders associated with mental, neurologic, or other medical conditions; and proposed sleep disorders.

➤ The dyssomnias, which are disorders that produce either excessive sleepiness or difficulty initiating or maintaining sleep, include circadian rhythm disorders, the various types of insomnia, narcolepsy, motor disorders that disrupt sleep, and sleep apnea.

➤ The parasomnias, which are undesirable physical phenomena that occur almost exclusively during sleep or are exaggerated by sleep, include nightmares, sleepwalking, and sleep terrors.

morning after a diagnostic sleep study. An average adult requires 10 or more minutes to fall asleep. An MSLT result of less than 5 minutes is considered abnormal. Polysomnographic recordings are made during three to five naps spaced 2 hours apart during the day. Special attention is paid to how much time elapses from when the lights go out to the first evidence of sleep. This interval is called *sleep latency*.[17]

Wrist actigraphy measures muscle motion and is used to obtain objective measurements of sleep duration and efficiency outside the sleep laboratory. The actigraph is a compact device that is worn on the wrist and is used most often in conjunction with a sleep diary. Depending on the unit that is used, it can collect up to 4 weeks' worth of information.

DYSSOMNIAS

The dyssomnias are disorders that produce either excessive sleepiness or difficulty initiating or maintaining sleep. They represent the major cause of disturbed sleep or impaired wakefulness. They include the circadian rhythm disorders, the various types of insomnia, narcolepsy, motor disorders that disrupt sleep, and sleep apnea.

Circadian Rhythm Disorders

Sleep problems due to alterations in circadian rhythm tend to fall into three categories: non–24-hour sleep-wake syndrome (disorders of visual input and SCN function); acute shifts in the sleep-wake cycle (jet lag and shift work); and changes in sleep phase disorders (advanced and delayed sleep phase disorders).[9,18]

Non–24-Hour Sleep-Wake Syndrome. The non–24-hour sleep-wake syndrome consists of a lack of synchronization between the internal sleep-wake rhythm and the external 24-hour day. Most persons with the disorder are blind or have brain lesions that affect the SCN. Studies have shown that 70% or more of blind persons have chronic sleep-wake complaints.[18]

The non–24-hour syndrome often goes unrecognized. In sighted persons, a neurologic examination, including magnetic resonance imaging to detect possible SNC lesions, often is indicated. The disorder usually is unresponsive to sedative and stimulant medications. Some blind people seem to respond to a schedule of strict 24-hour cues.

Acute Shifts in the Sleep-Wake Cycle. The normal diurnal clock is set for a 24-hour day and resists changes in its pattern by as little as 1 to 2 hours per day. This means that there is a limited range of day lengths to which humans can synchronize. Imposed sleep-wake schedules of less than 23 hours or more than approximately 26 hours, such as those that occur with intercontinental jet travel and switches in the work shift, produce increasing sleep difficulties.

Time Zone Change (Jet Lag) Syndrome. *Jet lag*, a popular term for symptoms of sleep disturbances that occur with air travel that crosses several time zones, is caused by the sudden loss of synchrony between a traveler's intrinsic circadian clock and the local time of the flight's destination. The severity and duration of symptoms vary depending on the

number of times zones crossed, direction of travel (eastward vs. westward), takeoff and arrival times, and age. Most people who cross three or four time zones experience some sleep disturbance, usually lasting two to four nights.

Circadian rhythms take longer to resynchronize to local time after eastward flights than westward flights, presumably because of the longer-than-24-hour intrinsic circadian period in most people.[18] Because the human time system seems to be less flexible in adjusting to sudden time changes after 35 years of age, age also affects adjustment to time zone changes.

Manifestations of jet lag syndrome include insomnia, daytime sleepiness, and decreased alertness and performance. Other symptoms, such as eye and nasal irritation, headache, abdominal distention, dependent edema, and intermittent dizziness, result from cabin conditions and usually remit sooner than symptoms of jet lag. Frequent travelers, such as airline personnel and business travelers, may develop chronic sleep disturbances accompanied by malaise, irritability, and performance impairment. Jet lag usually is milder in infrequent travelers, but may reduce the enjoyment of a vacation or effectiveness of business transactions. Persons with preexisting sleep disorders such as sleep apnea often experience a worsening of symptoms with jet travel.

Management of jet lag focuses on efforts either to maintain the home time schedule or adapt to the new time zone schedule. For persons crossing four or fewer time zones for only a few days, trying to maintain a schedule that is nearer to the home time schedule may be helpful, especially with westward travel. For longer stays, adapting to the new time schedule as quickly as possible is probably a better strategy. Use of artificial light may enhance the adjustment to the time shift. Getting outdoors and engaging in local social events enhances resynchronization by providing social cues and increasing exposure to the new light-dark environment.

Shift Work Sleep Disorder. The sleep disruption of night-shift work can be attributed to a clash between shift demands for wakefulness as part of the work environment and the sleep setting of the worker's intrinsic circadian clock. Shift work usually creates an environment in which some circadian clock-setting cues (*e.g.*, artificial light and rest-activity) are shifted, whereas others (*e.g.*, natural light-dark schedule, family and social routines) are not. This situation almost never allows for a complete shift of the circadian system. To complicate the situation, most night-shift workers revert to a nighttime sleeping schedule on days off. The effect of abruptly attempting to sleep at normal hours after working nights and sleeping days is biologically equivalent to a 6- to 10-hour eastbound jet flight.

Manifestations of sleep disorders of night-shift workers include shortened and interrupted daytime sleep after the night shift, somnolence and napping at work, sleepiness while commuting home, and insomnia on the nights off from work. Shift workers usually sleep less per scheduled sleep period than daytime workers and therefore are in a condition of chronic sleep deprivation.[18,19] Permanent night workers report averaging 6 hours of sleep on work days, approximately an hour less than evening and day workers.[18]

Arriving at a sleep schedule that is most supportive of the worker's intrinsic circadian rhythm often is difficult for night-shift workers. Beginning sleep at noon rather than earlier in the morning may produce a more normal sleep period in relation to shift onset, but exacerbate insomnia on nights off. Sleeping in absolute darkness during daytime by using blackout shades or eye masks may benefit the night worker's sleep.

Change in Sleep Phase Disorders. Change in sleep phase disorders include delayed sleep phase syndrome (DSPS) and advanced sleep phase syndrome (ASPS). The disorders may arise because of developmental changes in the sleep-wake cycle or because of poor sleep habits.

Delayed Sleep Phase Syndrome. The main symptoms of DSPS are extreme difficulty falling sleep at a conventional hour of the night and awakening on time in the morning for school, work, or other responsibilities. Although most chronically sleep-deprived persons are sleepy in the late afternoon or evening, persons with DSPS report greatest alertness at these times of the day.[18]

The disorder is more common in adolescents and in persons older than 50 years of age.[18] In adults, there is evidence of association between some psychopathologic disorders and DSPS. Most cases are adolescents whose frustrated parents cannot wake them up in time for school and have trouble getting them to go to bed at night. Staying up late is fairly common among today's teenagers, who are strongly influenced by peer pressure, defiance of parental rules, and other pressures. It has been suggested that social pressure may contribute to, but may not be the only reason for, changes in a teenager's sleep pattern. Rather, puberty may be accompanied by a lengthening of the intrinsic circadian rhythm, with a corresponding increase in evening wakefulness, which in turn leads to later sleep onset and arising.

Diagnosis of DSPS usually can be made from information in a sleep history and confirmed with a 2-week sleep log or diary. The presence of concurrent psychopathologic disorders or chronic sedative or alcohol use should be considered.

There are no quick remedies for DSPS. In adolescents, common-sense remedies such as setting earlier bedtimes and using multiple alarm clocks for waking up have been used, but with minimal success. The use of bright light may be helpful in maintaining morning wakefulness. For some people, engagement in a regular morning exercise program, such as taking a daily 20- to 30-minute walk outdoors as soon as possible after arising each morning, may prove beneficial. In persons with psychopathologic disorders or sedative abuse, treatment of the underlying disorder is indicated.[18]

Advanced Sleep Phase Syndrome. Advanced sleep phase syndrome (ASPS) basically is the mirror image of DSPS—early sleep onset and early arising. People with ASPS have trouble staying awake in the evening and have to curtail evening activities to avoid falling asleep. Unlike persons with depression, who awaken early with feelings of hopelessness and sadness, the person with ASPS obtains a normal amount of consolidated sleep, and wakes up feeling refreshed.[18]

The pathophysiology of ASPS is presumed to be a partial defect in phase delay capability, with the possibility that persons with the disorder have an inherently fast circadian timing system. This disorder often is found in the elderly. Time isolation studies in middle-aged and older subjects suggest that the circadian timing system shortens with aging, usually beginning sometime in the sixth decade of life.[18]

Diagnosis of ASPS is based on history and information from a sleep log. Other pathologic causes, such as sleep apnea and depression, should be ruled out. The need for treatment depends on how disruptive a person perceives the problem to be. Current treatment methods, which focus largely on sleep schedule changes, are somewhat limited.

Insomnia

Insomnia probably is the most common of all sleep disorders. Every year, approximately 35% of the adult population has difficulty sleeping, and approximately half of these adults consider the problem serious.[15,20-22] Insomnia is more common in women and increases with age, psychological discomfort, and multiple health problems.

Insomnia represents a subjective problem of insufficient or nonrestorative sleep despite an adequate opportunity to sleep, thus differentiating insomnia from sleep deprivation. It includes difficulty falling asleep or maintaining sleep, waking up too early, or nonrefreshing sleep. Insomnia also involves daytime consequences such as tiredness, lack of energy, difficulty concentrating, and irritability.[15] Primary insomnia is sleep difficulty in which other causes of sleep disruption have been ruled out or treated.

Acute or Transient Insomnia. Acute or transient insomnia is characterized by periods of sleep difficulty lasting between one night and a few weeks. The primary consequences of acute insomnia are sleepiness, negative mood, and impairment of performance. The degree of impairment is related to the amount of sleep lost.

Acute insomnia often is caused by emotional and physical discomfort. Some common examples include an unfamiliar or nonconducive sleep environment, stress-related events, and sleep schedule problems. Probably one of the most common causes of acute insomnia is an unfamiliar sleep environment, such as that encountered when traveling. Factors that contribute to a nonconducive sleep environment include excessive noise, extremes of temperature, an uncomfortable sleep surface, or being forced to sleep in an uncomfortable position. Hospital intensive care units with their noise, intensive lighting, and frequent interruptions for monitoring vital signs and providing treatments are excellent examples of nonconducive sleep environments. Common stress-related causes of insomnia are expected occurrences such as being on call or stressful life events. Sleep schedule changes include jet lag and sleep disruption due to shift work.

Chronic Insomnia. Chronic insomnia refers to the subjective experience of inadequate quality or quantity of sleep that has persisted for at least 1 month.[20] Persons with chronic insomnia frequently complain of fatigue; mood changes, such as irritability and depression; difficulty concentrating; and impaired performance.

Chronic insomnia often is related to medical or psychiatric disorders. Factors such as pain, immobility, and hormonal changes associated with pregnancy or menopause also can cause insomnia. Interrupted sleep can accompany other sleep disorders such as restless legs syndrome and sleep apnea. Many health problems worsen during the night. Heart failure, respiratory disease, and gastroesophageal reflux can cause frequent awakening during the night. Mood and anxiety disorders are the most frequent cause of insomnia in persons with psychiatric diagnoses.

A number of drugs can lead to poor-quality sleep. Drugs commonly related to insomnia are caffeine, nicotine, stimulating antidepressants, alcohol, and recreational drugs.[15,20,21] Approximately 10% to 15% of persons with insomnia have problems with chronic substance abuse, including alcohol.[21] Although alcohol initially may induce sleep, it often causes disrupted and fragmented sleep. Sleep also is disrupted in persons undergoing alcohol or sleep medication withdrawal.

Diagnosis and Treatment. The diagnosis of insomnia is aided by a sleep history. Questions should address both sleep and daytime functioning. If the person has a bed partner, it is important to ask if the person snores, has unusual movement during sleep, or is excessively drowsy during the day.[23] Because sleep needs vary from person to person, a 1- to 2-week sleep diary can be useful in diagnosing the sleep problem and in serving as a baseline for treatment effects.[15,20,23] Other factors that need to be explored are the use of drugs such as caffeine, tobacco, and alcohol, as well as prescription and over-the-counter drugs that affect the sleep-wake cycle. Identification of physical and psychological factors that interfere with sleep also is important.

Treatment of insomnia includes education and counseling regarding better sleep habits (sleep hygiene), behavioral therapy aimed at changing maladaptive sleep habits, and the judicious use of pharmacologic interventions. The cause and duration of insomnia are particularly important in deciding on a treatment strategy. With transient insomnia, treatment stresses the development of good sleep hygiene and judicious short-term use of sedatives or hypnotics. Long-term and chronic insomnia require careful assessment to determine the cause of the disorder. Depending on the findings, treatment options include behavioral strategies such as relaxation therapy, sleep restriction therapy, stimulus control therapy, and cognitive therapy. Sedatives and hypnotics, which tend to become less effective with time and may cause dependence, are used with caution.

Sleep hygiene refers to a set of rules and information about personal and environmental activities that affect sleep.[15,20,21] These rules include establishing a regular wakeup time to help set the circadian clock and regularity of sleep onset; maintaining a practice of sleeping only as long as needed to feel refreshed; providing a quiet sleep environment that is neither too hot nor too cold; and avoiding the use of alcohol and caffeine (coffee, colas, tea, chocolate) before retiring for sleep. It is important that the bed and bedroom be identified with sleep and not with reading, watching television, or working. Persons who cannot fall asleep should be instructed to turn on the light and do something else outside the bed, preferably in another room.

Behavioral therapies include relaxation therapy, sleep restriction therapy, stimulus control therapy, and cognitive therapy. Relaxation therapy is based on the premise that persons with insomnia tend to display high levels of physiologic, cognitive, and emotional arousal during both the day and the night.[15] Sleep restriction therapy consists of curtailing the amount of time spent in bed in an effort to increase the sleep efficiency (time asleep/time in bed). People with insomnia often increase their time in bed in the misguided belief that it will provide more opportunity to sleep. Stimulus control therapy focuses on reassociating the bed and bedroom with sleep rather than sleeplessness. Cognitive therapy involves the identification of dysfunctional beliefs and attitudes about sleep and replacing them with more adaptive substitutes.

Pharmacologic treatment usually is reserved for short-term management of insomnia—either as the sole treatment or as adjunctive therapy until the underlying problem can be addressed. The most common type of agents used to promote sleep are the benzodiazepines.[15,20,21,23] There are small differences between the different benzodiazepines in terms of their ability to induce and maintain sleep, depending on their rate of absorption, generation of active metabolites, and rate of elimination. The most common adverse effect of these drugs is anterograde amnesia and, for long-acting agents, residual daytime drowsiness. Sedating antidepressants also may be prescribed, particularly when insomnia is due to depression. Antihistamines have sedative effects and may be used to induce sleep. The most commonly used agents are diphenhydramine and hydroxyzine. Most over-the-counter sleep medications include an antihistamine. Adverse effects of antihistamines include daytime sleepiness, cognitive impairments, and anticholinergic effects. Falls and fractures are more frequent in persons using hypnotic or other psychotherapeutic agents. The usefulness of melatonin in treating insomnia remains to be established.

Narcolepsy

Narcolepsy is a disorder of daytime sleep attacks, cataplexy (brief periods of muscle weakness), hallucinations occurring at the onset of sleep, and sleep paralysis.[17,24–26] Although the disorder is not progressive, it can be disabling and difficult to treat. Sixty to 80% of persons with narcolepsy have fallen asleep while driving, at work, or both.[17,24]

Daytime sleepiness is the most common initial symptom of narcolepsy. Sleepiness is most apparent in boring, sedentary situations and often is relieved by movement. Although the sleepiness that occurs with narcolepsy is similar to that experienced after sleep deprivation, it is different in that no amount of nighttime sleep produces full alertness. The periods of daytime sleep usually are brief, lasting 30 minutes or less, and often are accompanied by brief interruption of speech or irrelevant words, lapses in memory, and nonsensical activities. Cataplexy is characterized by brief periods of muscle weakness brought about by about emotional reactions such as laughter, anger, or fear. Some persons with narcolepsy have brief, intense, often frightening, dreamlike hallucinations (hypnagogic hallucinations) while dozing or falling asleep, and brief periods of sleep paralysis.

The occurrence of REM sleep at sleep onset or within 10 to 15 minutes of sleep onset is the most characteristic and striking manifestation of the disorder. Periods of REM onset sleep are thought to indicate impaired sleep-wake regulation rather than increased need for REM sleep. The sleep paralysis, dreamlike hallucinations, and the loss of muscle tone that occur during cataplexy are similar to behaviors that occur during REM sleep.

Narcolepsy affects men and women equally.[24] Symptoms usually begin in the second or third decade of life. Onset is rare before 5 or after 50 years of age. The onset appears to peak at approximately 15 years of age, with a secondary peak at approximately 36 years.[25] The onset of symptoms often is insidious, with excessive daytime sleepiness preceding the onset of cataplexy. Sometimes it may have an abrupt onset attributed to head trauma, an infection, drug abuse, or pregnancy. Whether these events are causal or coincidental is unknown.

Although the cause of narcolepsy is unknown, there are indications that the disorder may have a genetic component. Persons with narcolepsy have been shown to have an unusually high rate of a specific human leukocyte antigen (HLA) subtype (HLA DQB1-0602). Of persons with severe cataplexy, 85% to 95% have this HLA subtype. Most diseases associated with a specific HLA subtype have an autoimmune component. However, no autoimmune markers have been found to date. Recent research has suggested a link between a newly identified group of neurotransmitters called *hypocretins* and narcolepsy. The hypocretins (hypocretin 1 and hypocretin 2) are secreted by cells in the area of the hypothalamus that is related to wakefulness.[26] A mutation in the hypocretin 2 receptor was shown to cause canine narcolepsy.[27] Although the role of the hypocretin transmitter system in human narcolepsy is unclear, a small preliminary study has shown a lack of hypocretin 1 in the cerebral spinal fluid of 7 out of 9 patients with the disorder.[28] Although these findings are preliminary, they suggest new avenues for research into the cause of narcolepsy.

Usually, sleep laboratory studies are required for accurate diagnosis of narcolepsy. Both daytime and nighttime studies usually are done. Nighttime studies usually are performed after the person has been on a regular sleep schedule for 10 days or more to determine the presence and severity of sleep apnea, limb movement disorders, and nocturnal sleep disturbance. A daytime MSLT usually is done the next day. People with narcolepsy are observed to have a short period of sleep latency (2 to 4 minutes) during daytime studies, along with a rapid onset of REM sleep (usually within 10 minutes). A mean sleep latency of less than 5 minutes and two or more periods of sleep-onset REM during the repeated nap opportunities is considered diagnostic of narcolepsy.[25]

The treatment of narcolepsy focuses on use of stimulant medications such as mazindol, methylphenidate, methamphetamine, and modafinil to counteract daytime sleepiness. Only modafinil, a nonamphetamine stimulant, has been studied and approved for use in treatment of narcolepsy. The mechanism of action of modafinil is unknown, al-though animal studies indicate that drug acts in areas of the brain involved in the sleep-wake cycle. Tricyclic antidepressants may be used to treat the cataleptic attacks. Non-pharmacologic treatment includes prevention of sleep deprivation, regular sleep and wake times, work in a stimulating environment, and avoidance of shift work. Scheduled short naps may be effective in reducing daytime sleepiness.

Motor Disorders of Sleep

A variety of spontaneous movements can occur during sleep. Some occur during normal sleep in all persons at some time. Others are not part of normal sleep patterns and can be disruptive of sleep. Among the abnormal motor disorders are periodic limb movement disorder (PLMD) and restless legs syndrome (RLS).

Limb movements can demonstrate characteristic rates and patterns during certain stages of sleep. Motoneuron depression is minimal during non-REM sleep and maximal during REM sleep. Many movement disorders occur during stage 2 non-REM sleep.

Periodic Limb Movement Disorder. Periodic limb movement disorder is characterized by episodes of repetitive movement of the large toe with flexion of the ankle, knee, and hip during sleep.[29,30] Both lower extremities are usually affected in an asymmetric manner. The condition occurs most frequently during light (stages 1 and 2 non-REM) sleep compared with deep (stages 3 and 4 non-REM) sleep and REM sleep. The disorder frequently accompanies RLS.

Periodic limb movement disorder, which occurs equally in men and women, is found in up to 11% of the population.[29] It rarely is diagnosed before 30 years of age and the prevalence increases with age. It may occur in as many as 44% of persons older than 65 years of age. The cause of PLMD is largely unknown. It has been observed that the movements mimic the Babinski reflex, suggesting removal of an excitatory influence over a subcortical inhibitory system allowing for facilitation of abnormal movements during sleep.[29] Diagnosis of PLMD is facilitated with use of EMG recordings from both tibialis anterior muscles. Four or more consecutive muscle contractions, each lasting 5 to 90 seconds (typically 20 to 40 seconds) and recurring at intervals of 5 to 90 seconds, is indicative of PLMD.

Restless Legs Syndrome. Restless legs syndrome is a neurologic disorder characterized by an irresistible urge to move the legs, usually because of a "creeping," "crawling," or uncomfortable sensation.[29–32] It usually is worse during periods of inactivity and often interferes with sleep. Occasionally the condition occurs during the day after long periods of sitting. The prevalence of the condition peaks in middle age and reportedly occurs in 2% to 15% of the elderly population.[31] Although the prevalence increases with age, it has a variable age of onset and can occur in children.

The disorder, which is thought to have its origin in the central nervous system, can occur as a primary or secondary disorder. There is a high familial incidence of primary RLS, suggesting a genetic disorder. Secondary causes of RLS include iron deficiency, neurologic disorders such as spinal cord and peripheral nerve lesions, pregnancy, uremia, and medications. Although the neurologic basis of RLS has not been determined, it has been suggested that the disorder may involve disruption of descending inhibitory input to brain stem and spinal cord circuits. Based on classes of medications proved to be effective in treating the disorder, there is evidence for involvement of the dopaminergic, adrenergic, and opioid systems in the pathogenesis of the disorder.

Diagnosis of RLS is based on a history of (1) a compelling urge to move the legs, usually associated with paresthesias; (2) motor restlessness, as seen by activities such as pacing, tossing and turning in bed, or rubbing the legs; (3) symptoms that become worse at rest and are relieved by activity; and (4) symptoms that are worse in the evening or at night.[31] Laboratory tests to determine secondary causes of RLS usually are done. Sleep studies usually are not required because the condition can be diagnosed on the basis of history and clinical findings.

Treatment of RLS varies depending on the severity of symptoms. Dopaminergic agents are the first-line drugs for most persons with RLS. These include precursors of dopamine (carbidopa-levodopa), dopamine agonists (pergolide, pramipexole, ropinirole), and facilitating agents (selegiline). Benzodiazepines (*e.g.*, clonazepam, temazepam), opioids (*e.g.*, codeine, hydrocodone), and antiseizure agents (carbamazepine, gabapentin) are alternative agents. Although pharmacologic treatment is helpful for many persons with RLS, those with mild symptoms may not require medications. For many persons, deliberate manipulation of the muscles through ambulation, kicking movements, stretching, or massage may provide relief.[33] Good sleep habits are important.

Obstructive Sleep Apnea

Sleep apnea is a serious, potentially life-threatening disorder characterized by brief periods of apnea or breathing cessation during sleep. There are two types of sleep apnea: obstructive and central. Obstructive apnea, which is caused by upper airway obstruction and characterized by snoring, disrupted sleep, and excessive daytime sleepiness, is the much more common type.[33] Central sleep apnea, which is caused by disorders affecting the respiratory center in the brain, is rare.

Apnea is defined as cessation of airflow through the nose and mouth for 10 seconds or longer. The apneic periods typically last for 15 to 120 seconds, and some persons may have as many as 500 apneic periods per night. An accompanying decrease in the depth and rate of respiration (called *hypopnea*) is associated with a decrease in arterial oxygen saturation. The average number of apnea-hypopnea periods per hour is called the *apnea-hypopnea index* (AHI).[34] An adult may experience up to five events an hour without symptoms. As the AHI increases, so does the severity of symptoms. An AHI of five or greater in combination with reports of excessive daytime sleepiness is indicative of sleep apnea.

All skeletal muscles except the diaphragm undergo a decrease in tone during sleep. This loss of muscle tone is most pronounced during REM sleep. The loss of muscle tone in the upper airways predisposes to airway obstruction as the negative airway pressure produced by contraction of the diaphragm brings the vocal cords together, collapses the

pharyngeal wall, and sucks the tongue back into the throat[35] (Fig. 51-6). Airway collapse is accentuated in persons with conditions that cause narrowing of the upper airway or weakness of the throat muscles.

Conditions that predispose to sleep apnea include male sex, increasing age, and obesity. Alcohol and other drugs that depress the central nervous system tend to increase the severity of obstructive episodes. It has been estimated that sleep apnea affects up to 4% of middle-aged men and 2% of middle-aged women.[5] Most persons who develop sleep apnea are obese. Large neck girth in both male and female snorers is highly predictive of sleep apnea. Men with a neck circumference greater than 17 inches and women with a neck circumference greater than 16 inches are at higher risk for sleep apnea.[34] The pickwickian syndrome, named after the fat boy in Charles Dickens' *The Posthumous Papers of the Pickwick Club*, published in 1837, is characterized by obesity, hypersomnolence, periodic breathing, hypoxemia, and right-sided heart failure.[36]

Obstructive sleep apnea is characterized by loud snoring interrupted by periods of silence. Abnormal gross motor movements during sleep are common. In many cases, the snoring precedes by many years the onset of other signs of

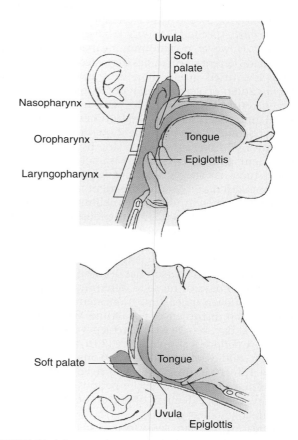

FIGURE 51-6 Principal mechanism of obstructive sleep apnea. When the person is awake (**top**), the airway is kept open by the activity of the pharyngeal musculature. During sleep (**bottom**), this activity is decreased causing airway obstruction, most commonly in the area behind the uvula, soft palate, and posterior tongue.

sleep apnea. Persons with sleep apnea often complain of persistent daytime sleepiness, morning headache, memory and judgment problems, irritability, difficulty concentrating, and depression. They also are more likely to fall asleep at inappropriate times, and have higher rates of automobile and work-related accidents. Men may complain of impotence. In children, a decline in school performance may be the only indication of the problem.

Sleep apnea also is associated with sleep-related cardiac dysrhythmias and hypertension. Usually bradycardia is observed, but ventricular tachycardia may occur in situations of severe hypoxemia. Frequent apneic periods may result in increased systemic and pulmonary blood pressures. The morning blood pressure has been shown to increase almost linearly with increasing apnea episodes. In severe cases, pulmonary hypertension, polycythemia, and cor pulmonale may develop. The signs and symptoms of sleep apnea are summarized in Chart 51-2.

Diagnosis and Treatment. Sleep apnea usually is suspected from a history of snoring, disturbed sleep, and daytime sleepiness. A definitive diagnosis is accomplished with sleep studies done in a sleep laboratory using polysomnography.[5,6,37] Currently, this procedure requires an overnight stay in a sleep laboratory. This procedure consists of EEG and EOG to determine the sleep stages; monitoring of the airflow; an ECG to detect arrhythmias; methods to measure ventilatory effort; and pulse oximetry to detect changes in oxygen saturation. An MSLT may be done to rule out narcolepsy in persons who exhibit excessive daytime sleepiness.

Home evaluation using pulse oximetry and portable monitors may be used to screen for sleep apnea. This method is less expensive than laboratory sleep tests but often is less accurate.[34] It is most useful in persons with severe sleep apnea, in whom the results clearly are positive.

The treatment of sleep apnea is determined by the severity of the condition. Behavioral measures may be the only treatment needed for persons with mild sleep apnea. These include weight loss, eliminating evening alcohol and sedatives, and proper bed positioning. Weight loss often is beneficial for persons with obstructive apnea. In many instances, the disordered breathing events are confined to the supine sleeping position, so that training the person to sleep in the lateral position may help to alleviate the problem.

Oral or dental appliances that displace the tongue forward and move the mandible to a more anterior and forward position may be an option for persons with mild to moderate sleep apnea. Persons who snore but do not have sleep apnea also may use these devices. They should be fitted by a dentist or orthodontist experienced in their use. Side effects of the devices include excessive salivation and temporomandibular joint discomfort.

The application of nasal continuous positive airway pressure (NCPAP) at night has proven helpful in treating obstructive sleep apnea. This method uses an occlusive nasal mask or a device that fits into the nares, an expiratory valve and tubing, and a blower system to generate positive pressure. The main difficulty with NCPAP is that many persons find it unacceptable. Common complaints include dryness of the mouth, claustrophobia, and noise.

Several surgical procedures have been used to correct airway obstruction, including nasal septoplasty (*i.e.*, repair of the nasal septum) and uvulopalatopharyngoplasty (*i.e.*, excision of excess soft tissue on the palate, uvula, and posterior pharyngeal wall). Both of these procedures have met with limited success. Severe cases of sleep apnea may require a tracheostomy (*i.e.*, surgical placement of a tube into the trachea for the purpose of maintaining an open airway). The tracheostomy tube remains occluded during the day and is opened during the night.

PARASOMNIAS

The parasomnias are undesirable physical phenomena that occur almost exclusively during sleep or are exaggerated by sleep.[38] They include nightmares, sleepwalking (somnambulism) and sleep terrors, teeth grinding, and bed-wetting (enuresis). Sleepwalking, sleep terrors, and bed-wetting often are seen in children and may be considered normal to some degree at a certain age. They are less common in adults and may be indicative of other pathologies. For example, sleepwalking and sleep terrors may occur in persons with poorly controlled cardiac insufficiency after myocardial infarction. In rare cases, sleepwalking and sleep terrors may be the first sign of a slowly evolving brain tumor. Finally, sleepwalking and sleep terrors may be triggered by disorders interacting with the sleep-wake cycle. Particularly in the elderly, health problems such as a febrile illness may enhance non-REM sleep nightmares, sleep terrors, and sleepwalking.

Nightmares

Nightmares are vivid and terrifying nocturnal episodes in which the dreamer is abruptly awakened from sleep. Usually there is difficulty returning to sleep. Nightmares affect 20% to 39% of children between 5 and 12 years of age and 5% to 8% of adults.[39] Most nightmares occur during REM sleep. Most REM-altering disorders and medications that affect REM sleep affect dreaming.

Nightmares are a defining symptom of post-traumatic stress disorder (PTSD).[7] These nightmares occur after intensely frightening or highly emotional experiences and are associated with disturbed sleep and daytime hyperarousability. Persons with PTSD report awakening from dreams that involve reliving the trauma. The frequency of

---

> ### CHART 51-2
>
> ### *Signs and Symptoms of Sleep Apnea*
>
> - Noisy snoring
> - Insomnia
> - Abnormal movements during sleep
> - Morning headaches
> - Excessive daytime sleepiness
> - Cognitive and personality changes
> - Sexual impotence
> - Systemic hypertension
> - Pulmonary hypertension, cor pulmonale
> - Polycythemia

PTSD nightmares increases with severity of trauma, and they can persist for long periods after the traumatic experience. It has been reported that 30% of veterans of the Vietnam War are affected by PSTD.[7] Among the civilian population, PTSD affects approximately 25% of persons who have experienced severe emotional and physical trauma or have had a severe medical illness.

Sleepwalking and Sleep Terrors

Sleepwalking and sleep terrors usually occur during stages 3 and 4 of non-REM sleep. Because stages 3 and 4 are more prolonged during the first third of the night, sleepwalking and sleep terrors usually occur during this time. Sleep terrors are characterized by sudden, loud, terrified screaming and prominent autonomic nervous system activation (tachycardia, tachypnea, diaphoresis, and mydriasis). Sleepwalking is characterized by complex automatic behaviors, such as aimless wandering, furniture rearranging, urinating in closets, and going outdoors. During a typical episode, the sleepwalker appears dazed and relatively unresponsive to the communication efforts of others. On awakening, there may be a brief period of confusion or disorientation. The sleepwalker usually has no memory or only a vague awareness of what has happened.

Sleep terrors are more common in children and are discussed later in the chapter. In children, sleepwalking usually is a benign and self-limited disorder. In adults, sleepwalking occurs almost three times more often per year and persists for a longer period than in children. It often is associated with stress or major life events.[40] New-onset sleepwalking in older adults is uncommon and usually is a manifestation of another disorder such as delirium, drug toxicity, or seizure disorders.[40] Although rare, sleepwalking can occur during complex partial seizures.

Diagnosis and treatment of sleepwalking and sleep terrors depend on age. Because most children eventually outgrow the disorders, parents may need simply to be reassured and instructed in safety measures. Insufficient sleep may precipitate episodes of sleepwalking, so parents should make certain that the child goes to bed on time and gets enough sleep. In adults, a through medical, psychiatric, and sleep history should be done to eliminate other causes of the disorder. Because sleepwalking can be dangerous, it is important that the environment be safe. Dangerous objects should be removed and bolts should be placed on doors and windows. No attempt should be made to interrupt the sleepwalking event because such efforts may be frightening.

Pharmacologic treatment includes the selective use of the benzodiazepines (particularly diazepam and clonazepam) or the tricyclic antidepressant imipramine.[40] In elderly persons, treatment focuses on reversing the underlying causes of delirium. Because medications are a frequent cause of delirium in the elderly, a complete drug history should be done with the intent of eliminating medications that might be causing the disorder.

> In summary, the ICSD classifies sleep disorders into four categories: (1) dyssomnias, which are disorders of initiating and maintaining sleep and disorders of excessive sleepiness; (2) parasomnias, which are not responsible for disturbing the sleep-wake cycle but are undesirable phenomena that occur primarily during sleep; (3) sleep disorders associated with other medical/psychiatric disorders; and (4) proposed sleep disorders such as pregnancy-induced sleep disruptions.
>
> The dyssomnias include circadian rhythm sleep disorders, insomnia, narcolepsy, disorders of leg movement, and sleep apnea. Sleep problems due to alterations in circadian rhythm tend to fall into three categories: non–24-hour sleep-wake syndrome (disorders of visual input and SCN function); acute shifts in the sleep-wake cycle (jet lag and shift work); and changes in sleep phase disorders (advanced and delayed sleep phase disorders). Insomnia represents a subjective problem of insufficient or nonrestorative sleep despite an adequate opportunity to sleep. It includes transient and chronic problems in falling asleep and maintaining sleep, waking up too early, or nonrefreshing sleep. Narcolepsy is a disorder of daytime sleep attacks, cataplexy, hallucinations occurring at the onset of sleep, and sleep paralysis. Among the abnormal motor disorders that occur during sleep are PLMD and RLS. PLMD is characterized by episodes of repetitive movement of the large toe with flexion of the ankle, knee, and hip during sleep, usually involving both legs. RLS is a neurologic disorder characterized by an irresistible urge to move the legs, usually owing to a "creeping," "crawling," or uncomfortable sensation. It usually is worse during periods of inactivity and often interferes with sleep. Obstructive sleep apnea is a serious, potentially life-threatening disorder characterized by brief periods of apnea or breathing cessation during sleep, loud snoring interrupted by periods of silence, and abnormal gross motor movements. It is accompanied by complaints of persistent daytime sleepiness, morning headache, memory and judgment problems, irritability, difficulty concentrating, and depression. Sleep apnea also is associated with sleep-related cardiac dysrhythmias and hypertension.
>
> The parasomnias are undesirable physical phenomena that occur almost exclusively during sleep or are exaggerated by sleep. They include nightmares, sleepwalking and sleep terrors, teeth grinding, and bedwetting (enuresis).

Sleep and Sleep Disorders in Children and the Elderly

After you have completed this section of the chapter, you should be able to meet the following objectives:

+ Characterize normal sleep patterns of the infant and small child and relate to the development of sleep disorders
+ Describe the normal changes in sleep stages that occur with aging and relate to sleep problems in the elderly.

It has been said that "sleep is of the brain, by the brain, and for the brain."[1] Thus, sleep changes as the brain develops in the fetus and neonate, matures during adolescence and early adulthood, and begins to decline with aging.

SLEEP DISORDERS IN CHILDREN

A child's circadian rhythms and sleep patterns are established early in life. There is evidence that many of the sleep patterns in the newborn are present at birth.[1] The first behavioral manifestations of sleep patterns occur between 28 to 30 weeks of gestation, when movement of the fetus is interrupted by periods of quiet. At 32 weeks, periods of quiescence begin to occur at regular intervals, suggesting the beginnings of a sleep-wake cycle.

An infant born at full term sleeps approximately 16 to 17 hours a day, half of which is spent in REM sleep. The other half of the infant's sleep resembles adult non-REM sleep.[1,40] Not only does the infant spend more time in REM sleep than adults, but the behavioral manifestations of REM sleep are more exaggerated. This probably is because inhibitory systems in the infant's brain are relatively immature. Thus, an infant's sleep behavior includes a wide range of physical behaviors such as changes in facial expression, cooing sounds, and movement and stretching of the extremities.

Although infants have some capacity to concentrate sleep in one part of the day, this capacity must be developed in the weeks after birth. As development progresses, the infant is able to concentrate sleep during the night and remain awake for longer periods during the day. By 5 to 6 months, the infant may sleep through the night and may nap at predictable times during the day. As the cyclic structure of the sleep-wake cycle progresses, the amount of time spent in REM sleep decreases. By the time the child is 8 months of age, the duration of sleep has decreased to approximately 13 hours and REM sleep occupies only approximately one third of that time. At 12 to 15 years of age, sleep has decreased to approximately 8 hours, with one fourth being spent in REM sleep.

Although complaints of sleep are common among adults, children usually do not complain about sleep problems, although their parents might. The usual concerns of parents include irregular sleep habits, insufficient or too much sleep, nightmares, sleep terrors, sleepwalking, and bed-wetting. Complaints of excessive daytime sleepiness or sleep attacks not accounted for by an inadequate amount of sleep may be due to a more serious health or sleep problem (*e.g.*, narcolepsy), in which case a careful sleep history, physical examination, and other diagnostic tests may be needed. Two of the more common sleep problems of children are discussed in this section of the chapter: sleep terrors and sleepwalking.

Sleep Terrors in Children

Sleep terrors are marked by repeated episodes of awakening from sleep. They usually occur during the first half of sleep in the first interval of non-REM sleep.[41,42] The age of onset usually is between 4 and 12 years. The course is variable, usually occurring at intervals of days or weeks. The disorder gradually resolves in children and usually disappears during adolescence.

In a typical episode, the child sits up abruptly in bed, appears frightened, and demonstrates signs of extreme anxiety, including dilated pupils, excessive perspiration, rapid breathing, and tachycardia. Until the agitation and confusion subside, efforts to comfort or help the child are futile. There usually is no memory of the episode. Occasionally, the child recounts a sense of terror on being aroused during a night terror, but there is only fragmentary recall of dreamlike images. Treatment consists primarily of educating and reassuring the family. The child should be assisted in settling down without awakening. The child must be protected if he or she gets up and walks about during the episodes.

Sleepwalking in Children

Sleepwalking involves repeated episodes of complex motor movements that lead to leaving the bed and walking without the child being conscious of the episode or remembering that it occurred. As with sleep terrors, it normally occurs in non-REM sleep stages 3 and 4 during the first third of the sleep period.

A sleepwalking episode typically lasts for a few minutes to half an hour, during which time the child sits up; makes purposeful movements such as picking at the bed coverings; then proceeds to semipurposeful movements such as getting out of bed, walking around, opening doors, dressing, or going to the bathroom. Often they end up in the parent's bedroom. Commonly, they are unresponsive to the efforts of others to communicate with them. Confusion and disorientation are typical of the events, and on awakening there is no memory of the event. There may be manifestations of extreme autonomic nervous system activity such as tachycardia, rapid breathing, perspiration, and urination.

Approximately 10% to 15% of children have had isolated sleepwalking events.[40] It occurs more commonly in boys than in girls and is more frequent in children in whom there is a family history of sleepwalking. The onset usually is between 4 and 8 years of age, and it lasts several years. Usually symptoms resolve by the end of the teens or in the early twenties. The primary concern is injury during an episode. Children may bump into things, fall down stairs, or even leave their home during an episode.

SLEEP DISORDERS IN THE ELDERLY

Complaints of difficulty sleeping increase with aging. In a National Institute of Aging Study of over 9000 persons aged 65 years and older, over one half of the men and women reported at least one chronic sleep complaint.[42] The consequences of chronic sleep problems in the elderly can be considerable. Left uncorrected, a sleep disorder affects the quality of life. Loss of sleep and use of sedating medications may lead to falls and accidents. Sleep-related disorders of breathing may have serious cardiovascular, pulmonary, and central nervous system effects.

There are a number of changes that occur in the sleep-wake cycle as a person ages. Elderly persons have more fragmented sleep and shorter duration of stage 3 and 4 sleep.

Although REM sleep tends to be preserved, the deepest stages of non-REM sleep frequently are reduced or nonexistent.[43–45] Compared with younger persons, the elderly tend to achieve less total nighttime sleep. They often take longer to fall asleep, they awaken earlier, they have more nighttime arousals. Environmental influences, particularly auditory stimuli, often are more disruptive in the elderly. With an increase in nighttime wakefulness, there is an increase in daytime fatigue and daytime napping.

The causes of sleep disorders in the elderly include age-related sleep changes, secondary sleep disturbances, primary sleep disorders, lack of exercise, and poor sleep habits. Factors that predispose to secondary sleep disturbances include physical and mental illness, medication effects, and emotional stress. A variety of medical illnesses contribute to sleep disorders in the elderly, including arthritic pain, respiratory problems and cardiac disease, and neurologic disorders. Nightmares and nighttime fears are common in elderly persons with Parkinson's disease, particularly those who are receiving levodopa. Psychiatric illness, such as depression, is a common cause of disturbed sleep in this age group. Primary sleep disorders such as sleep apnea, RLS, and PLMD also increase in old age. Many medications have stimulating effects and interfere with sleep. These include some of the antidepressants, decongestants, bronchodilators, corticosteroids, and some antihypertensives. Alcohol use also may serve as a deterrent to sleep in the elderly. Sleep-wake problems may be compounded further by inappropriate interventions initiated by the older person, his or her family, or health care providers.

Sleep also is disturbed in disorders characterized by dementia. Episodes of nocturnal wandering, confusion, and delirium can occur despite normal daytime functioning. Persons with Alzheimer's disease often have increased periods of nighttime awakening and daytime napping.

Diagnosis of sleep disorders in the elderly requires a comprehensive sleep history, inquiries about pain and anxiety or depression, review of current sleep hygiene practices, drug use history, spousal or bed partner reports, a comprehensive physical examination, and appropriate laboratory tests.[45,46] Treatment of a medical disorder and changes in medication regimes and timing of medication doses can improve sleep. Avoidance of alcohol and stimulants before bedtime and improving sleep hygiene are other measures that can be used to improve sleep. Although hypnotics can be used to treat transient insomnia, they often fail to provide long-term relief of chronic sleep disturbances.

In summary, circadian rhythms and sleep patterns are established early in life. In the newborn, REM sleep occurs at sleep onset, and periods of sleep and awakening are distributed throughout the day. As the cyclic structure of the sleep-wake cycle progresses, the amount of time spent in REM sleep decreases. By the time the child is 8 months of age, the duration of sleep has decreased to approximately 13 hours and REM sleep occupies only approximately one third of that time. At 12 to 15 years of age, sleep has decreased to approximately 8 hours, with one fourth being spent in REM

sleep. Although complaints of sleep are common among adults, children usually do not complain about sleep problems, although their parents might. The usual concerns of parents include irregular sleep habits, insufficient or too much sleep, nightmares, sleep terrors, sleepwalking, and bed-wetting.

Complaints of sleep disorders are common in the elderly. The sleep-wake cycle changes with aging, resulting in more fragmented sleep, shorter duration of stage 3 and 4 sleep, and reduced REM sleep. The circadian rhythm of a typical sleep period also changes; elderly persons tend to go to bed earlier in the evening and awaken earlier in the morning. Elderly persons also have more health problems that interrupt sleep, they are apt to be on medications that interfere with sleep, and they are more likely to have sleep disorders such as insomnia, RLS, and sleep apnea. Left uncorrected, sleep disorders in the elderly affect the quality of life. Loss of sleep and use of sedating medications may lead to falls and accidents.

Related Web Sites

American Academy of Sleep Medicine   www.aasmnet.org
American Sleep Apnea Foundation   www.sleepapnea.org
Basics of Sleep Behavior—an entire syllabus with text on sleep
   www.sleephomepages.org/sleepsyllabus
Methodists Hospitals Center for Sleep Disorders
   www.methodisthospitals.org/services/diagnostics/sleep/
   sleep1.html
National Sleep Foundation   www.sleepfoundation.org
Restless Legs Syndrome Foundation   www.rls.org
Sleep Information for Patients and the General Public—
   presented by the research center for division of National
   Institutes of Health that oversees sleep disorders. Rich
   source of government publications on sleep and sleep disorders.   www.nhlbi.nih.gov/health/public/sleep/index.htm
Sleep Research Society   www.srssleep.org
Stanford School of Medicine Center for Narcolepsy
   www.med.stanford.edu/school/psychiatry/narcolepsy

References

1. Hobson J.A. (1989). *Sleep* (pp. 1–21, 74–78, 117–134, 121, 159–169). New York: Scientific American Library.
2. McCarley R.W. (1995). Sleep, dreams, and states of consciousness. In Conn P.M. (Ed.), *Neuroscience in medicine* (pp. 537–583). Philadelphia: J.B. Lippincott.
3. Carskadon M.A., Dement W.C. (1994). Normal human sleep. In Kryger M.H., Roth T., Dement W.C. (Eds.), *Principles and practices of sleep medicine* (2nd ed., pp. 16–25). Philadelphia: W.B. Saunders.
4. Carskadon M.A., Rechtschaffen A. (1994). Monitoring and staging human sleep. In Kryger M.H., Roth T., Dement W.C. (Eds.), *Principles and practices of sleep medicine* (2nd ed., pp. 944–999). Philadelphia: W.B. Saunders.
5. Strollo P.J., Rogers R.M. (1996). Obstructive sleep apnea. *New England Journal of Medicine* 334, 99–104.
6. Berry R.A. (1995). Sleep-related breathing disorders. In George R.B., Light R.W., Matthay M.A., Matthay R.A. (Eds.), *Chest medicine* (3rd ed., pp. 247–268). Baltimore: Williams & Wilkins.

7. Pagel J.F. (2000). Nightmares and disorders of dreaming. *American Family Physician* 61, 2037–2042, 2044.

8. Moore M.C., Czeisler C.A., Richardson G.S. (1983). Circadian timekeeping in health and disease. *New England Journal of Medicine* 309, 469–473.

9. Moore R.Y. (1997). Circadian rhythms: Basic neurobiology and clinical applications. *Annual Review of Medicine* 48, 253–266.

10. Richardson G., Tate B. (2000). Hormonal and pharmacological manipulation of the circadian clock: Recent developments and future strategies. *Sleep* 23 (Suppl. 3), S77–S85.

11. Brzezinski A. (1997). Melatonin in humans. *New England Journal of Medicine* 336, 186–195.

12. Cupp M.J. (1997). Melatonin. *American Family Physician* 56 (5), 1421–1488.

13. Ahrendt J. (2000). Melatonin, circadian rhythms, and sleep. *New England Journal of Medicine* 343, 1114–1115.

14. American Sleep Disorders Association. (1997). *The international classification of sleep disorders*. Rochester, MN: Author.

15. Members of National Heart, Lung, and Blood Institute Working Group on Insomnia. (1998). *Insomnia: Assessment and management in primary care*. NIH publication no. 98-4088. Bethesda, MD: National Institutes of Health.

16. Bootzin R.R., Lehmeyer H., Lillie J.K., Hanawait A.K., Shaver J.L. (1994). *Integrated approach to sleep management* (pp. 16–19). Belle Meade, NJ: Cahners Healthcare Communications.

17. Aldrich M.S. (1992). Narcolepsy. *Neurology* 42 (Suppl. 6), 34–43.

18. Wagner D.R. (1996). Disorders of the circadian sleep-wake cycle. *Neurologic Clinics* 14, 651–669.

19. Pilcher J.J., Lambert B.J., Huffcutt A.I. (2000). Differential effects of permanent and rotating shifts on self-report sleep length: A meta-analytic view. *Sleep* 23, 155–163.

20. Rajput V., Bromley S.M. (1999). Chronic insomnia: A practical review. *American Family Physician* 60, 1431–1442.

21. Meyer T.J. (1998). Evaluation and management of insomnia. *Hospital Practice* 33 (12), 75–86.

22. Vgontzas A.N., Kales A. (1999). Sleep and its disorders. *Annual Review of Medicine* 50, 387–400.

23. Kupfer D.J., Reynold C.F. (1997). Management of insomnia. *New England Journal of Medicine* 336, 341–345.

24. Aldrich M.S. (1990). Narcolepsy. *New England Journal of Medicine* 323, 389–394.

25. Mahowald M.W. (2000). What is causing excessive daytime sleepiness? *Postgraduate Medicine* 107 (3), 108–123.

26. Krahn L.E., Black J.L., Silber M.H. (2001). Narcolepsy: A new understanding of irresistible sleep. *Mayo Clinic Proceedings* 76, 185–194.

27. Lin L., Faraco J., Li R. (1999). The sleep disorder canine narcolepsy is caused by a mutation in hypocretin (oxexin) receptor 2 gene. *Cell* 98, 365–376.

28. Nishino S., Ripley B., Overseem S., Lammers G.J., Mignot E. (2000). Hypocretin (orexin) deficiency in human narcolepsy [Letter]. *Lancet* 355, 39–40.

29. Dyken M.E., Rodnitzky R.L. (1992). Periodic, aperiodic, and rhythmic motor disorders of sleep. *Neurology* 42 (Suppl. 6), 68–74.

30. Trenkwalder C., Walters A.S., Henning W. (1996). Periodic limb movements and restless legs syndrome. *Neurologic Clinics* 14, 629–649.

31. National Center on Sleep Disorders Research. (2000). *Restless legs syndrome: Detection and management in primary care*. NIH publication no. 00-3788. Bethesda, MD: National Institutes of Health.

32. Paulson G.W. (2000). Restless legs syndrome: How to provide symptom relief with drug and nondrug therapies. *Geriatrics* 55 (6), 35–48.

33. Guilleminault C., Stoohs R., Quera-Salva M. (1992). Sleep-related obstructive and nonobstructive apneas and neurologic disorders. *Neurology* 42 (Suppl. 6), 53–60.

34. Members of the National Heart, Lung, and Blood Institute Working Group on Sleep Apnea. (1995). *Sleep apnea: Is your patient at risk?* NIH publication no. 95-3803. Bethesda, MD: National Institutes of Health.

35. Victor L.D. (1999). Obstructive sleep apnea. *American Family Physician* 60, 2279–2286.

36. Burwell C.S., Robin E.D., Whaley R.D., et al. (1956). Extreme obesity associated with alveolar hypoventilation: A pickwickian syndrome. *American Journal of Medicine* 21, 811–818.

37. Ross S.D., Sheinhait I.A., Harrison K.J., Kvasz M., Connelly B.S., Shea S.A., Allen E. (2000). Systematic review and meta-analysis of the literature regarding the diagnosis of sleep apnea. *Sleep* 23, 519–533.

38. Schenck C.H., Mahowald M.W. (2000). Parasomnias. *Postgraduate Medicine* 107 (3), 145–156.

39. Masand R., Popli A.P. (1995). Sleepwalking. *American Family Physician* 51, 649–653.

40. Ferber R. (1996). Childhood sleep disorders. *Neurologic Clinics* 14, 493–451.

41. Garcia J., Wills L. (2000). Sleep disorders in children and teens. *Postgraduate Medicine* 107 (3), 161–178.

42. Foley D.J., Monjan A.A., Brown S.L., Simonsick E.M., Wallace R.B., Blazer D.G. (1995). Sleep complaints among elderly persons: An epidemiologic study of three communities. *Sleep* 18, 425–432.

43. Neubauer D.N. (1999). Sleep problems in the elderly. *American Family Physician* 59, 2551–2559.

44. Ancoli-Israel S. (2000). Insomnia in the elderly: A review for the primary care practitioner. *Sleep* 23 (Suppl. 1), S23–S29.

45. Foreman M.D., Wykle M. (1995). Nursing standard-of-practice protocol: Sleep disturbances in elderly patients. *Geriatric Nursing* 16, 238–243.

46. Vitello M.V. (1999). Effective treatments for age-related sleep disturbances. *Geriatrics* 54 (11), 47–52.

Chapter 52

Neurobiology of Thought, Mood, and Anxiety Disorders

Mary Pat Kunert and Jane Dresser

Psychiatric disorders are characterized by changes in a person's thoughts, mood, or behaviors that preclude ordinary functioning in one or more spheres of life. Throughout the course of history, persons in the healing professions have tried to uncover the causes and find effective treatments for diseases that alter the way in which people experience the world and behave in it. Over the centuries, the pendulum has swung between those practitioners who espouse the view that mental disease arises from inadequate interpersonal relationships and those who espouse the view that mental disease arises from alterations in brain structure or activity. In the late 20th century, and now in the early years of the 21st, the conversation between these two apparently divergent philosophies continues, perhaps to conclude with a new synthesis of nurture versus nature and therefore new and effective therapies for those with mental illness. The purpose of this chapter is to review the evolution in understanding of the pathogenesis and treatment of mental illness, the anatomy of the brain and its integrated regional functions, and the causes, manifestations, and treatment of selected thought and mood disorders.

Evolution in Understanding of Mental Illness

After you have completed this section of the chapter, you should be able to meet the following objectives:

✦ Define the terms *biologic psychiatry* and *psychosocial psychiatry* and compare them in terms of their definitions of the origins of mental disease
✦ Describe the changes in treatment of mental illness over the past three centuries
✦ Describe neuroimaging techniques
✦ Explain the role that heredity plays in the epidemiology and development of mental illness
✦ State categories of antipsychotic drugs and antidepressants

HISTORICAL PERSPECTIVES

Pathogenesis of Mental Illness

Psychiatry was not an organized specialty before the end of the 18th century, but mental disorders are as old as the human race. Artifacts and cave drawings from a half million years ago indicate that what we have come to call psychotic disorders were known then. Over the ages, the explanations of mental disorders have ranged from possession by gods and demons, to the breaking of taboos, to the idea that a harmful substance had entered the body. Persons with psychiatric disorders were treated with prayers, magic, and exorcisms. In some communities, the mentally ill were viewed with fear and often turned out of their homes, villages, and towns. In other communities, families took care of the mentally ill, but often these people were neglected or locked up in barns or cellars.[1]

The history of our understanding of psychiatric illnesses reveals a tension between two schools of thought as to the origin of mental disease. The pendulum has swung between these two apparently opposite viewpoints across the centuries. One view of psychiatric illness is that mental disorders are due to anatomic, developmental, and functional disorders of the brain, and is called *biologic psychiatry*. Another view is that mental disorders are due to impaired psychological development, a consequence of poor child rearing or environmental stress, and is called *psychosocial psychiatry*.[1] These differences of emphasis in terms of the pathogenesis of mental illness are important because the prevailing theory about the origins of mental disease influences what therapies for psychiatric illness predominate.

Early biologic psychiatry in the late 1800s to early 1900s emphasized the correlation of neurologic symptoms with postmortem microscopic study of anatomic changes in the brain. Although this research was of immense importance in terms of regional localization of brain functions (*e.g.*, Wernicke's aphasia), it provided little help to the clinical psychiatrist of the time.

Emil Kraepelin, a German psychiatrist, was the first to begin to classify psychiatric disorders by systematically studying the natural history of the disease. The intent was to be able to predict outcomes. In the sixth edition of his textbook, *Psychiatrie* (1899), Kraepelin laid the groundwork for the *Diagnostic and Statistical Manual of Mental Disorders* (DSM; the current 4th edition [revised] is abbreviated DSM-IV) of the American Psychiatric Association. He divided all mental disorders into 13 groups, including psychoses, which he divided into two distinct groups: those with an affective component, which he called *manic-depressive psychosis*, and those without, which he called *dementia praecox*.[1]

In the mid-20th century, the psychoanalytic view of mental disorders took hold, reaching its zenith in the 1950s and 1960s. Psychiatric illness was explained as the result of unconscious conflicts over events in an individual's past. Alterations in nurture, not nature, were the underlying cause of psychiatric illness.

In the last half of the 20th century, biologic psychiatry became important once again. During the 1970s, techniques of neuroimaging became available that allowed the neuroscientist to visualize brain structures and function.[1] The results of genetic studies examining the correlation between family relationships and incidence of psychiatric illness, in particular the studies of monozygotic and dizygotic twins, suggested that depression and schizophrenia had a strong genetic component. The introduction of chlorpromazine as a treatment for schizophrenia revolutionized psychiatry because although it did not cure psychosis, it did control the symptoms of the disease, increasing the potential for more traditional therapies to work and allowing previously institutionalized individuals to lead much more normal lives. It also suggested strongly that mental illness had a biologic foundation. Chlorpromazine soon was followed by other drugs for psychosis and depression.

This move to biologic psychiatry, however, has not excluded the healing value of the therapist-client relationship. It appears that pharmacotherapy in conjunction with psychotherapy is of greater healing power than either alone. Perhaps the distinction drawn between biologic and psychosocial disease is arbitrary. Indeed, experiments indicate that learning and sensory stimulation or deprivation can in fact weaken or strengthen synaptic connections, which in turn could change brain function and thus behavior, but not necessarily gross anatomy.[2]

Treatment of Mental Illness

Asylums have existed since the Middle Ages, but until the end of the 18th century their only function was custodial. One of the oldest asylums was the Priory of St. Mary of Bethlehem, founded in London in the 13th century. Its name was eventually shortened to *Bedlam*, a term that has become synonymous with madness. The asylum as a therapeutic establishment did not become an important concept until the end of the 18th century.[1]

At this time, madness was viewed as an excessive irritation of the nerves, so establishing a calming environment was crucial. These asylums often had a very rigid schedule of daily activities meant to focus the patient and afford mental rest. It was also during this time that practitioners attempted to systematize the techniques known to establish a therapeutic relationship between the doctor and the patient.

In 1800, patients in asylums numbered in the hundreds at the most. By the mid-1900s, the numbers were in the thousands. Unfortunately, by the early 1900s, asylums had become little more than warehouses for the chronically mentally ill. Whether this was due to the failure of asylums as a therapeutic environment or to the increased number of persons housed in them, overwhelming the available resources, remains a matter of debate. The reason for the increased numbers of persons in the asylum in the 19th century also is debated. Was there an increased incidence of mental illness, or did society become increasingly intolerant of deviant behavior?

This debate exploded in the 1960s, during which several writers suggested that there was no such thing as mental illness but rather a medicalizing of deviance, and that psychiatric institutions were evil. Schizophrenia in this view was a gifted and creative state of consciousness, not an illness. This antipsychiatry attitude, coupled with the advent of psychopharmacology, laid the foundations for the deinstitutionalization of the mentally ill and the move to community psychiatry. Unfortunately, deinstitutionalization was neither carefully planned nor adequately funded, leaving many mentally ill homeless and without proper care.[1]

RESEARCH AND THE ROLE OF NEUROIMAGING

Abnormalities in brain structure and function can contribute to the manifestations of mental illness. Since the early 1970s, imaging techniques have been developed that allow practitioners and researchers to map brain anatomy in exquisite detail and to estimate brain activity by measuring brain blood flow and metabolic rate. These imaging studies have suggested intriguing correlations between brain pathologies and psychiatric manifestations that provide clues to the pathogenesis of mental disorders. Brain imaging techniques, however, remain research tools and have not yet been applied clinically, which means that imaging cannot be used to make a diagnosis of mental illness. The techniques include computed tomography (CT) scans, magnetic resonance imaging (MRI), positron emission tomography (PET), and single-photon emission computed tomography (SPECT).

A CT scan of the brain provides a three-dimensional view of brain structures that can differentiate fine densities. Abnormalities in a CT scan are not diagnostic of any particular mental illness; however, they suggest a brain-based problem. Structural abnormalities of the brain have been measured in people with schizophrenia, mood disorders, and dementias. MRI is used primarily for diagnosis of structural changes in the brain, although newer techniques are able to measure brain function as well. Unlike CT, MRI is able to distinguish between gray and white matter. The basis of PET is the variable brain tissue uptake of an infused radioactive substance. The tissue uptake of the substance depends on tissue type and metabolic activity. Labeled drugs can be infused in PET to study neurotransmitter receptor activity or concentration in the brain. SPECT is similar to PET but is less expensive and uses more stable substances and different detectors to visualize blood flow patterns. This is useful for diagnosis of cerebrovascular accidents and brain tumors.[3,4]

THE ROLE OF HEREDITY IN MENTAL ILLNESS

Who we are and how we express ourselves through behavior depend on the complex influences of genetic and environmental factors on neural development and function. Since the early 1990s, the scientific knowledge base in genetics has grown exponentially and has created new tools to study the role of genetic inheritance in the development of mental illness. Research into the complexities of the regulation of gene expression can only deepen our understanding of the etiology of mental disorders, increase our ability to treat the disorders with more precisely targeted psychotherapeutic drugs, and ultimately lead to the discovery of ways to prevent the development of psychiatric illness.

Epidemiologic studies of twins, of adopted children, and of family histories or pedigrees have shed light on the debate over the relative influence of nurture versus nature in the development of mental illness. Twin studies compared the incidence of mental illness among monozygotic (identical) twins, dizygotic (fraternal) twins, and their siblings. If a disease is at all genetically determined, higher rates of coexistence of the disorder (concordance) would be expected among monozygotic twins as compared to dizygotic twins, nontwin siblings, or the general population. Adoption studies questioned whether children with a genetic history of mental illness, adopted by parents with no history of psychiatric illness, had a greater risk of developing mental illness than children with no genetic history of mental illness who were adopted by parents with a psychiatric illness. Also, if a mental illness has a genetic component, it would be expected that higher numbers of persons in a family would have the disorder than would be found in the general population.[5,6,7] The overwhelming conclusions of these studies have been that both genetic vulnerability and environmental influences play significant roles in the development of mental illness.

For example, studies of twins have shown a 45% concordance for schizophrenia among monozygotic twins, compared with 15% for dizygotic twins or other siblings.[8] In bipolar depression, there is an 80% concordance in monozygotic twins, compared with 10% for siblings. In monozygotic twins living apart, the concordance rate for affective disorders is 40% to 60%.[9] Even the concordance rates among siblings for these two disorders is suggestive of a genetic influence because schizophrenia has approximately a 1% incidence and depression a 5% incidence among the general population.[8,9] The rate of occurrence of either disorder also is higher in the biologic families of adopted children than in the adoptive families. The incidence of suicide is six times higher among biologic relatives of adoptees with depressive illness than among the biologic relatives of normal adoptees.

Although the evidence for a genetic basis for mental illness is compelling, the fact that the concordance among monozygotic twins is not 100% indicates that other factors may be involved in the development of a mental illness. It certainly is highly likely that mental illnesses are polygenic and multifactorial rather than simply inherited through transmission of a classic disordered dominant or recessive mendelian trait (see Chapter 6). In addition, mental disorders exhibit variable expressivity. It is possible that a person with the disease genotype needs to have the right environmental stressors (*i.e.*, viral illness, physical or emotional abuse, substance abuse) to express the disease phenotype, or that there are gene–gene interactions that influence the extent to which a mental illness is manifested.[5]

EMERGENCE OF PSYCHOTROPIC MEDICATIONS

In the 1950s, a French neurosurgeon, Henri Laborit, was searching for a drug that would reduce the affects of preoperative anxiety-induced histamine release in his patients.

Basic Concepts in Mental Illness

➤ Psychiatric disease is characterized by alterations in thought, mood, or behavior that interfere with a person's ability to engage in ordinary social interactions.

➤ There are differences of emphasis concerning the fundamental causes of mental illness. One school of thought views mental illness as arising from impaired psychosocial relationships in early development, and another school of thought conceptualizes mental illness as a disease of the brain.

➤ Neuroimaging techniques are able to detect changes in brain activity through measures of regional blood flow and metabolic rate. Although not diagnostic tools at this time, the results of these examinations may help correlate changes in brain anatomy and function with the symptoms of mental illness.

➤ Heredity plays a role in the development of mental illness. The incidence of depression and schizophrenia is greater among siblings than in the general population.

Through trial and error, he found chlorpromazine to be the most effective calming agent and recommended the drug to his psychiatric colleagues, who subsequently found that high doses of chlorpromazine were efficacious in calming agitated persons with schizophrenia and bipolar disorders. It eventually became clear that chlorpromazine was not simply a tranquilizer but also had some specific antipsychotic effects. Chlorpromazine and related drugs in the phenothiazine class attenuated or abolished delusions, hallucinations, and disordered thinking.

There are now four major groups of antipsychotic agents used to treat schizophrenia, divided into two major categories: the typical and the atypical antipsychotics. The typical antipsychotics include the phenothiazines (chlorpromazine), butyrophenones (haloperidol), and thioxanthenes (chlorprothixene). The atypical antipsychotics, exemplified by clozapine, are more effective in treating the negative symptoms of schizophrenia (to be discussed) and produce fewer extrapyramidal effects. Both categories of drugs exert their effect by blocking dopamine receptors. The atypical antipsychotics also may exert some of their effects through blockade of serotonin (5-HT) receptors.

Psychopharmacology has been particularly productive in developing highly effective treatments for affective disorders. Antidepressants alleviate depressive symptoms by increasing the activity of norepinephrine and serotonin at postsynaptic membrane receptors. The most widely used antidepressants can be divided into three major categories: the monoamine oxidase inhibitors (MAOIs), the tricyclic

compounds, and selective serotonin reuptake inhibitors (SSRIs). MAOIs increase the concentration of serotonin and norepinephrine by reducing the degradation of these neurotransmitters by monoamine oxidase. Tricyclics block the reuptake of serotonin and norepinephrine by the presynaptic membrane, whereas the SSRIs selectively inhibit the reuptake of serotonin.

However, the therapeutic effect of the antipsychotic and antidepressant drugs probably is not entirely due to increasing or decreasing the neural levels of one or more neurotransmitters. For example, the clinical effect of the antidepressants typically is slow (weeks), even though the drugs rapidly block receptors. This suggests that the real mechanism of these drugs may be due to their effects on expression of receptors at the cellular membrane or on other intracellular pathways that regulate protein synthesis.[3]

In summary, psychiatric disorders are characterized by alterations in thought, mood, or behavior that may interfere with a person's ability to engage in ordinary social interactions and may in some instances require temporary or long-term institutionalization. Our understanding of the pathogeneses of mental disease is still in its infancy, and the historical debate over the relative importance of nurture and nature in the development of mental illness continues. It is likely that the cause of mental illness is multifactorial and includes a dynamic interplay among genetic predisposition, alterations in early neurodevelopment, and dysfunctional social interactions in a family.

New diagnostic tools, such as increasingly sophisticated neuroimaging techniques, may help to develop more precise correlations between behavior, thought and mood disorders, and microscopic alterations in brain structure and neuron function. In addition, an increased understanding of the complex interactions among the different parts of the brain will assist in the development of more effective psychotherapies and more efficacious psychotropic drugs.

Anatomic and Neurochemical Basis of Behavior

After you have completed this section of the chapter, you should be able to meet the following objectives:

✦ Name the cerebral cortical structures and structures from the primitive brain involved in thought and emotion
✦ Describe the major functions of each brain structure in terms of thought processes, learning, and emotion
✦ Describe the cortical pathways by which learning and the development of memory occur
✦ Define the terms *synapse*, *synaptic transmission*, and *neuromediator*
✦ Name the major neuromediators in the brain, their major location and source in the brain, and the possible involvement of each in the manifestations of mental illness

BEHAVIORAL ANATOMY OF THE BRAIN

There is increasing scientific evidence that anatomic and biochemical alterations in the brain play a critical role in the behaviors observed in mental illness. The brain is extraordinarily complex, divided into several distinct groups of functional neurons that also are highly interconnected and thus able to influence each other's activity. The information processing happens within nanoseconds. However, for persons with brain injury or illness, information processing may be impaired.

Cerebral Cortical Structures

Frontal Lobe. The frontal lobe is the largest lobe and often is referred to as the chief administrator of the brain. It is responsible for planning, problem solving, intellectual insight, judgment, and expression of emotion. The frontal lobe is highly involved in memory and is central to our sense of being a self and having a unique history. An area of the frontal lobe called the *association cortex* is the main area of the brain responsible for the expression of our personality. Capacity for abstraction and volition depends on frontal lobe function. Table 52-1 summarizes frontal lobe functions.

Persons with frontal lobe damage show distractibility and poor attention. Memory often is impaired and thinking tends to be concrete. Other signs of frontal lobe impairment include apathy, an emotional blunting, and an inability to plan ahead.

Temporal Lobe. The temporal lobe integrates and interprets auditory and spatial information that is critical for recognition of the familiar or the novel, as well as appropriate interpretation of and response to social contexts. Part of appropriate social response is the accurate interpretation of emotions and the ability to respond with a level of emotionality deemed socially congruent. Impulse control, the management of aggression and sexual expression, including the culturally determined stereotypy of what it means to be male or female in a given society, also are temporal lobe

Neurophysiologic Foundations of Mental Illness

➤ The brain is organized into discrete anatomic regions, each with specific, discrete functions related to motor activity, sensual experience, behavior, thought, and emotion. However, the activity of each region of the brain is regulated or modulated by other brain areas through numerous neural connections.

➤ The manifestations of mental illness arise from alterations in brain neuron functioning, destruction of those neurons, or alterations in the neural connections among the brain regions.

functions. Emotion originates in the amygdala of the limbic system (see later), but the modulation and "fine tuning" of that emotion into an appropriate level of intensity occurs in the temporal lobe. Imaging studies indicate that this process occurs almost exclusively in the left temporal lobe in men and in both temporal lobes in women. Table 52-1 summarizes temporal lobe functions.

Parietal Lobe. The parietal lobe is essential in the integration and processing of sensory (visual, tactile, and auditory) input. It is in the parietal lobe that sensory experiences first begin to coalesce into the cognitions we experience as thinking in the frontal lobes. The coordination of spatial awareness occurs in the parietal lobe and involves not only visual content, but the ability to experience, claim, and care for all of one's body. Another important parietal lobe function is to filter out extraneous information. The ability to filter out background and extraneous noise and sensations is critical to normal daily functioning. Table 52-1 summarizes parietal lobe functions.

TABLE 52-1 ✦ Selected Functions of Several Brain Regions

Frontal Lobe	Temporal Lobe	Parietal Lobe	Occipital Lobe
Abstract vs. concrete reasoning	Visual-spatial recognition	Sensory integration and spatial relations	Vision
Motivation–volition	Attention	Bodily awareness	Possible information holding area
Concentration	Motivation	Filtration of background stimuli	
Decision making	Emotional modulation and interpretation	Personality factors and symptom denial	
Purposeful behavior	Impulse and aggression control	Memory and nonverbal memory	
Memory and historical sense of self	Interpretation and meaning of social context	Concept formation	
Sequencing	Aspects of sexual action and meaning		
Making meaning of language			
Speech organization			
Speech production (Broca's area)			
Aspects of emotional response—blunting			

Occipital Lobe.   The occipital lobe is the most posterior of the lobes and is responsible for receiving visual information from the eyes. The association cortex of the occipital lobe is important for the interpretation of visual experiences, including depth perception and location in space. Table 52-1 summarizes occipital lobe functions.

The Limbic System

The limbic system of the brain includes several discrete structures in the deep part of the brain, including the hippocampus, the parahippocampal gyrus, cingulate gyrus, the amygdala, and a bridgelike structure called the *fornix*, which is a bundle of nerve fibers connecting the hippocampus with the hypothalamus. The hippocampus plays a major role in the encoding, consolidation, and retrieval of memories. The amygdala, located deep in the medial temporal lobe, is important in emotional function and regulation and modulation of affective responses. Sexual arousal and aggression also are functions of the amygdala. The hypothalamus, although not strictly an anatomic part of the limbic system, plays a critical role in it because of the extensive connections it has with the limbic system. The hypothalamus has a multitude of regulatory functions related to basic survival needs of the body, such as regulation of body temperature, sleep-rest patterns, hunger, sexual drive, and hormonal secretion.

INTEGRATION OF THOUGHT, MOOD, LEARNING, AND COGNITION

Behavior is altered through environmental cues that are processed through learning and memory. Learning is the process of acquiring knowledge, whereas the process of memory allows storage and retrieval of what has been learned. There are two forms of memory: implicit memory, which is involved in learning reflexive motor and perceptual skills, and explicit memory, which is involved with the processing of factual knowledge of persons, places, and things and the meaning of these facts. Psychiatric patients and brain-injured persons not only experience specific cortical dysfunctions but may experience difficulty in the proposed pathways for learning and memory. These difficulties are likely to influence their behavior and may have an impact on the design of effective interventions.

Information Processing

Information from the senses, end-organs, and endocrine system enters the information processing system through the thalamus. The thalamus initially determines whether the sensory input is familiar or unfamiliar, safe or unsafe. If the input is deemed safe, it simply is forwarded through the information processing pathways. If the input is deemed unsafe, the sympathetic cascade is stimulated through the hypothalamic-pituitary-adrenal (HPA) axis, as discussed elsewhere in this text. Almost immediately after the HPA axis is triggered, an endorphin cascade is stimulated as well, and the input is forwarded through the information pathway.

The amygdala receives the input and generates a primitive and unmodulated emotional response. The amygdala forwards the input to the hippocampus, the seat of short-term memory, without which no new memories would go into long-term storage. In addition, the hippocampus groups and schematizes input in preparation for memory encoding. This grouping and schematizing is extremely important. For example, the hippocampus must keep the input from reading these words separate from the sound of your stereo or the sensations produced by your shirt against your skin. If it did not do that effectively, the music from your stereo would be mixed up with your shirt. Hippocampal atrophy has been noted in diseases in which memory problems play an important role, such as Alzheimer's disease (see Chapter 50) and post-traumatic stress disorder (see Chapter 9).

The prefrontal associative cortex is the next to act on the sensory input. The prefrontal associative area is important for keeping track of where information has been put in long-term memory and is responsible for integrating memories with sensory input for decision making. Think about an apple. How is it shaped? What color is it? Is it on a tree, in the produce department, on a table, in your lunch? How does it smell? How does it taste? What is its texture? Do you have any favorite apple memories? Each of these pieces of "appleness" is stored in different areas of the brain, and it is the job of the prefrontal associative area to ensure that the correct parts come back together so your apple is crunchy, juicy, and delicious, not square, gray, and foul-smelling.

The parietal lobe is the next stop on the information processing pathway. Here, as discussed earlier, background information is filtered out and only that which is essential is forwarded to the frontal lobe, where we first become consciously aware of thinking about the input.

ROLE OF NEUROMEDIATORS

Many of the new advances in the understanding and treatment of mental illness are derived from an increased understanding of how nerve cells in the brain communicate with one another. Nerve cells of discrete brain regions communicate with each other rapidly and over long distances by electrochemical signals that are propagated along the length of each neuron from the dendrites of the cell body down to the axonal terminal. The axon terminal of each neuron has on the average 1000 physical connections with the dendrites of other neurons, and on the average receives signals from 10,000 dendritic connections with other neuronal axons. The point at which two neurons meet is called a *synapse*, and the process by which the signal from one neuron to another is communicated is called *synaptic transmission* or *neurotransmission* (See Fig 47-8). Chemical substances called *neurotransmitters* or *neuromediators* are released from the axonal terminal of one neuron (presynaptic cell), cross the synapse (a space <20 nm), bind to receptors on the postsynaptic cells (cell receiving message from the axonal terminal of another neuron), and cause excitatory or inhibitory actions.[10]

Neurotransmission involves several discrete steps: (1) the synthesis of a transmitter substance, (2) the storage and release of the transmitter, (3) binding of the transmitter to receptors on the postsynaptic membrane, and (4) removal of the transmitter from the synaptic cleft. The classic neurotransmitters include small-molecule transmitters and neuroactive peptides. These molecules typically are stored in vesicles in the presynaptic axonal terminal and released by the process of exocytosis.[11]

The substances generally agreed to be neurotransmitters and that are implicated in mental illness include acetylcholine, the biogenic amines (dopamine, epinephrine, norepinephrine, and serotonin), and amino acids (γ-aminobutyric acid [GABA], glutamate, glycine, and aspartate). Table 52-2 summarizes the major source and effect of each neurotransmitter.

In summary, the symptoms of mental illness arise from alterations in neural functioning or from destruction of neurons in the brain. Because the brain integrates the processes of learning, memory, and emotions, the manifestations of mental disease may be primarily cognitive impairment, emotional impairment, or a combination of both. Psychiatric patients and brain-injured persons not only experience specific cortical dysfunctions but may experience difficulty in the proposed pathways for learning and memory. These difficulties are likely to influence behavior and may have an impact on the design of effective interventions.

Many of the new advances in the understanding and treatment of mental illness are derived from an increased understanding of how nerve cells in the brain communicate with one another. Neurotransmission involves several discrete steps: (1) the synthesis of a transmitter substance, (2) the storage and release of the transmitter, (3) the binding of the transmitter to receptors on the postsynaptic membrane, and (4) the removal of the transmitter from the synaptic cleft. The substances generally agreed to be neurotransmitters and that are implicated in mental illness include acetylcholine, the biogenic amines, and amino acids.

Disorders of Thought and Volition

After you have completed this section of the chapter, you should be able to meet the following objectives:

◆ Define the term *schizophrenia*
◆ Describe the epidemiology of schizophrenia
◆ Describe the manifestations of schizophrenia, both positive and negative symptoms, and their underlying neuropathophysiology
◆ Cite the diagnostic criteria for schizophrenia according to the DSM-IV classification
◆ Describe the treatment for the positive and negative manifestations of schizophrenia

TABLE 52-2 ◆ The Source and Effect of Brain Neuromediators

Neuromediator	Major Source in the Brain	Effect and Implications for Mental Illness
Acetylcholine (Ach)	Formed in many synapses of the brain; in high concentration in basal ganglia and motor cortex Derived from choline	Can be excitatory or inhibitory, depending on the area of the brain Underactivity implicated in Alzheimer's disease
Dopamine (DA)	Substantia nigra and ventral segmental area in the midbrain Derived from tyrosine	Usually excitatory Involved in motivation, thought, and emotional regulation Overactivity thought to be involved in schizophrenia and other psychotic disorders
Norepinephrine (NE) and epinephrine (E)	Locus ceruleus in brain stem Derived from dopamine	Can be excitatory or inhibitory, depending on the area of the brain Noradrenergic pathways to cerebral cortex, limbic system, and brain stem Underactivity thought to be involved in some depressions
Serotonin (5-HT)	Raphe nucleus in the brain stem Derived from tryptophan	Involved in the regulation of attention and complex cognitive functions Pathways to cerebral cortex, limbic system, and brain stem Underactivity thought to be involved in some depressions and obsessive-compulsive disorder
γ-Aminobutyric acid (GABA), glutamate, aspartate, and glycine	No single major source	GABA and glycine usually are inhibitory; glutamate is excitatory Implicated in anxiety disorders

SCHIZOPHRENIA

Epidemiology

Schizophrenia is fairly common, found in approximately 1% of the general population. An additional 2% to 3% has a milder form of the disease, called *schizotypal personality disorder*. Schizophrenia is not "split personality." Although the word *schizophrenia* means "splitting of the mind," it refers to the disconnect between thought and language that occurs in this disease. Schizophrenia accounts for 30% of all hospital admissions, and it is estimated that 30% of the homeless have schizophrenia. The onset of the disorder typically occurs between 20 and 35 years of age, although late-onset schizophrenia occurring between the ages of 66 and 77 years is not uncommon. Men and women seem to be affected equally, but the age of onset for the paranoid subtype is 3 to 4 years later in women than in men. In contrast, the disorganized type appears earlier in women. Risk factors for schizophrenia include having a close relative with schizotypal personality disorder or schizophrenia (first-degree relatives of a person with schizophrenia have a 10-fold greater prevalence of the illness than the population at large), winter/spring birth date, second trimester prenatal influenza infection, and early history of attentional deficits.[12,13]

Manifestations

Schizophrenia is a psychotic disorder with many subtypes characterized by positive or negative symptoms. Positive symptoms are those that reflect the presence of abnormal behaviors and include disorganized, incomprehensible speech; delusions (*e.g.*, that one is being controlled by an outside force); hallucinations (hearing voices is the most common); and grossly disorganized or catatonic behavior. Alterations in speech patterns can include using invented words (neologisms), derailment (moving off the subject), tangentiality (inability to stick to the original point), incoherence (loss of logical connections), or word salad (groups of disconnected words). Frequently, persons with schizophrenia lose the ability to appropriately sort and interpret incoming stimuli, which impairs the ability to appropriately respond to the environment. An enhancement or a blunting of the senses is very common in the early stages of schizophrenia. Sounds may be experienced as louder and more intrusive; colors may be brighter and sharper. In addition, the person with schizophrenia often experiences sensory overload owing to a loss of the ability to screen external sensory stimuli.[12–15]

Delusions and hallucinations may be a natural outgrowth of the inability of the person with schizophrenia to interpret and respond appropriately to stimuli. Delusions are false ideas believed by the affected person that cannot be corrected by reason. They range from simply believing that people are watching them to beliefs that they are being controlled and manipulated by others. Delusions of being a historical figure (*e.g.*, Jesus Christ or the President) also are common. Sometimes the delusions include a belief that the affected person is able to control others with his or her thoughts.[14]

Hallucinations are very common in schizophrenia, especially the auditory type. In these cases, the individual sees and hears things that are not in the external world but nevertheless are very real phenomena to the person experiencing them. Hallucinations may represent the end of the spectrum of increasing intensity of sensual stimuli. Auditory hallucinations range from simple repetitive sounds to many voices speaking at once. Sometimes the voices are pleasant, but often they accuse and curse. When visual hallucinations occur, they usually are in conjunction with auditory hallucinations.[12–14,16]

Negative symptoms reflect the absence of normal social and interpersonal behaviors and include alogia (tendency to speak very little), avolition (lack of motivation for goal-oriented activity), apathy, affective flattening (lack of emotional expression), and anhedonia (an inability to experience pleasure in things that ordinarily are pleasurable). Some persons with schizophrenia have a blunted response to pain. Negative symptoms often are severe and persistent between acute episodes of illness.[12,15]

Paranoid schizophrenia manifests with persecutory or grandiose delusions. Auditory hallucinations are common. Interactions with others are rigid, intense, and controlled. It often has a sudden onset and negative symptoms are not prominent. The prognosis of this form of schizophrenia seems to be better, with less evidence of disturbance in the anatomy of the brain than in those types in which negative symptoms predominate.[17]

Disorganized schizophrenia is characterized by a disintegration of the personality and a predominance of negative symptoms. Socially, the person is withdrawn and inept. Speech often is disorganized and incoherent. Personal grooming is neglected and because behavior is aimless, the person with this disorder often is not able to complete activities of daily living. The person also may have cognitive and psychomotor deficits. In general, the prognosis is not as good as that for the paranoid schizophrenic type.[17]

Catatonic schizophrenia is characterized by intense psychomotor disturbance (retardation or excitement), extreme negativism, and peculiar voluntary movements such as grimacing, posturing, and echolalia (repeating what is said by another) or echopraxia (imitating the movements of others).[17]

Diagnostic Criteria

For a diagnosis of schizophrenia to be made, according to the DSM-IV classification, two or more of the following symptoms must be present for a significant portion of 1 month: delusions, hallucinations, disorganized speech, grossly disorganized or catatonic behavior, or negative symptoms. In addition, one or more areas of functioning must be significantly impaired compared with premorbid abilities, and continuous signs of the disturbance must persist for at least 6 months.[17]

Neurophysiology of Symptoms

The pathogenesis of schizophrenia is unknown. However, abnormalities in brain structure that are characteristic of this disorder are present at the first episode and in unmedicated persons. This suggests that the anatomic alterations are not the result of progressive brain deterioration due to repeated psychotic episodes or to effects of psychotropic drugs, but rather are caused by abnormalities in neurodevelopment in intrauterine and early postnatal life. The lateral and third ventricles are enlarged, the thalamus and hippocampus are somewhat smaller, and the left hemisphere is both smaller and smoother than that of persons without the illness. These changes are accompanied by a change in brain volume averaging 3%. Schizophrenia also is characterized by hypofrontality (reduced metabolic activity in the frontal cortex), although marked decreases in activity can be seen in almost every area of the brain depending on the individual and the particular symptoms being experienced at the time of the scan.

It is not known at what age these differences might be visible with imaging because children usually are not subjected to imaging techniques without a specific event indicating a clinical need for the procedure. Nevertheless, adolescents and young adults who are at high risk for development of schizophrenia because of a strong family history have enlarged ventricles and smaller medial temporal lobes.[18]

An additional anatomic finding is an increased density of dopamine (D_2) receptor sites, particularly in the basal ganglia. With the additional information that effective antipsychotic drugs are dopamine antagonists and that dopamine-releasing agents such as amphetamine can cause psychosis, the "dopamine hypothesis" was developed, which proposes that the symptoms of schizophrenia are due to dopaminergic overactivity. However, this hypothesis cannot explain types of schizophrenia in which negative symptoms predominate or explain the residual symptoms of an acute psychotic episode. In addition, it is possible that the increased density of dopamine receptors found in some studies is related to the effects of antipsychotic drugs. In contrast, there is emerging evidence of a presynaptic dopaminergic autoreceptor abnormality such that there is a dysregulation or hyperresponsiveness of the neurons.[18]

Other transmitters implicated in the development of schizophrenia include a decreased activity of serotonin through the $5-HT_{2A}$ receptor and a decreased activity of glutamate through dysfunction of its *N*-methyl-D-aspartate receptor.

Treatment

The goals of treatment for schizophrenia are to induce a remission, prevent a recurrence, and restore behavioral, cognitive, and psychosocial function to premorbid levels. Initially, in some cases the goal may be primarily to reduce agitation and the risk of physical harm. Both pharmacotherapy and psychotherapy are essential components in the treatment of persons with schizophrenia. The positive symptoms of schizophrenia (delusion, hallucinations, agitation, thought broadcasting, loose associations, suspiciousness, and poor hygiene and dress) are most likely to respond to drug therapy, particularly with the typical antipsychotic drugs. The negative symptoms of schizophrenia respond more favorably to the atypical antipsychotic drugs (*i.e.*, clozapine). Often antipsychotics are combined

with benzodiazepines during the acute phase of treatment to reduce the risk of extrapyramidal effects from large doses of antipsychotic agents. Psychotherapy (individual and group) is particularly important after the acute phase of therapy to help the client gain insight into the illness, to enhance socialization skills, and to support and educate the client in the maintenance of pharmacotherapy.

Thought, Mood, and Anxiety Disorders

➤ Schizophrenia is a psychotic disorder of thought and language. Manifestations include disorganized speech, delusions, visual and auditory hallucinations, and possible catatonic behavior.

➤ Brain changes in schizophrenia include enlarged ventricles, reduced thalamic and hippocampal size, and reduced metabolic activity. Alterations in the neurotransmitters dopamine, serotonin, and glutamate are implicated in the pathogenesis of schizophrenia. Treatment for schizophrenia includes antipsychotic agents and psychotherapy.

➤ Disorders of emotion include unipolar and bipolar depression. Unipolar depression is characterized by a persistent unpleasant mood. Bipolar depression is characterized by alternating periods of depression and mania.

➤ Depression is a mood disorder characterized by feelings of worthlessness and guilt, decreased concentration, alterations in sleep and appetite, and possible suicidal ideation. Mania is characterized by decreased need for food and sleep, labile mood, irritability, and high distractibility.

➤ Brain changes in depression include a reduction in activity in the frontal and temporal lobes and an increased blood flow in the amygdala, a part of the limbic system. Possible alterations in the neurotransmitters serotonin and norepinephrine are implicated in depression. Disturbances in the regulation of cortisol also may play a role. Treatments for depression include psychotherapy, antidepressant drugs, lithium, anticonvulsants, and electroconvulsive therapy.

➤ Anxiety disorders include generalized anxiety disorder, obsessive-compulsive disorder, panic disorder, and social phobia. Panic disorder is characterized by an experience of intense fear with neurologic, cardiac, respiratory, and psychological symptoms. Generalized anxiety disorder is characterized by excessive, uncontrollable worry. Obsessive-compulsive disorder is characterized by repetitive thoughts and compulsions. Social phobia is an intense fear reaction to social interaction.

In summary, schizophrenia is a mental illness classified as a disorder of thought and volition. Schizophrenia and its various subtypes are psychotic mental alterations in which thought and language become disconnected. It is characterized by both positive symptoms and negative symptoms. Positive symptoms are abnormal behaviors (*e.g.*, incomprehensible speech), delusions, and auditory or visual hallucinations. Negative symptoms are abnormal social and interpersonal behaviors (*e.g.*, lack of emotional expression) and an inability to experience pleasure. The onset of the disorder typically occurs between the ages of 20 and 35 years, with an equal incidence in men and women. Risk factors for schizophrenia include having a close relative with schizotypal personality disorder or schizophrenia. The pathogenesis of schizophrenia is unknown, although neuroimaging reveals several anatomic and functional changes in regions of the brain. Abnormalities in neurotransmission have been implicated, including changes in concentration and activity of the neurotransmitters dopamine, serotonin, and glutamate. Treatment includes both psychotherapy and atypical antipsychotic drugs.

Disorders of Mood

After you have completed this section of the chapter, you should be able to meet the following objectives:

+ Define the terms *unipolar depression* and *bipolar depression*
+ Describe the epidemiology of unipolar and bipolar depression
+ Describe the manifestations of unipolar depression, bipolar depression, and mania, and the underlying neuropathophysiology of each
+ Cite the diagnostic criteria for depression according to the DSM-IV classification
+ Describe the treatment modalities for depression

DEPRESSION

Epidemiology

Depression is a disorder of emotion rather than a disturbance of thought. It is a common and highly underdiagnosed and undertreated illness. Major depression, which affects approximately 20% of the population, is classified as either unipolar (characterized by a persistent unpleasant mood) or bipolar (characterized by alternating periods of depression and mania). Approximately 5% of the world's population has unipolar depression. The prevalence of unipolar depression among women is double that in men. The prevalence of bipolar disorder is approximately 1.5% in the population at large and is approximately equally distributed between men and women. Men more often have the manic phase in the initial episode, whereas women

more often have the depressed phase as the initial episode. Approximately 10% to 15% of adolescents who present with major depression develop bipolar disorder. The average age of onset of bipolar disorder is the mid- to late 20s, and for unipolar depression, the mid-30s; however, the age of onset of both disorders has been decreasing. In addition, the incidence of depression appears to be increasing. Prevalence of depression is higher in individuals from families with a history of mood disorders than in the population at large, indicating a genetic component to the etiology. Depression occurs less frequently in African Americans than in whites or Hispanics. Bipolar depression appears more frequently in the higher socioeconomic groups, whereas unipolar depression occurs more frequently in the lower socioeconomic groups.[19–22]

As with schizophrenia, genetic factors appear to play an important role in the development of mood disorders. Several studies have identified genetic loci that might contribute to the vulnerability to depression in families and individuals. However, the expression of affective disorders is not 100% in vulnerable families, which strongly suggests that environmental factors also play a critical role in the development of mood disorders.[9]

Manifestations

Depression is classified as a mood disorder and is characterized by the following: depressed mood, anhedonia (inability to experience pleasure), feelings of worthlessness or excessive guilt, decreased concentration, psychomotor agitation or retardation, insomnia or hypersomnia, decreased libido, change in weight or appetite, and thoughts of death or suicidal ideation. Depression can vary in intensity and often is recurrent. The earlier and more frequent the onset of symptoms, the more likely it is that the affected individual will require medications for symptom relief. Depression in the elderly often appears with an element of confusion and often is left untreated. A first episode of depression that occurs after 65 years of age can be a precursor to dementia and should precipitate both assessment and treatment of the depression, as well as a thorough evaluation for dementia. Early intervention often greatly retards the progression of dementia, maintaining the individual's independence and quality of life.

Unipolar Depression Unipolar depression has three subtypes distinguished by variable symptom patterns. The most common is melancholic depression, characterized by depression that is worse in the morning, insomnia with early morning awakening, anorexia with significant weight loss, psychomotor agitation and mental pain, loss of interest in activity, inability to respond to pleasurable stimuli, and a complete loss of capacity for joy. The symptoms of atypical depression are the opposite of melancholic depression; it is characterized by a depression that becomes worse as the day progresses, overeating, and hypersomnia (excessive sleep). The last type of unipolar depression is called *dysthymia* and is characterized by a persistent but mild depression that lasts for more than 2 years.[19–21]

Bipolar Depression Bipolar depression, or manic-depressive illness, also has multiple subtypes, all characterized by episodes of elation and irritability (mania) with or without episodes of depression, although the occurrence of mania without associated depression (unipolar mania) is rare.[21,23] When the person is experiencing mania, some of the common symptoms include decreased need for food and sleep, labile mood, irritability, racing thoughts, high distractibility, rapid and pressured speech, inflated self-esteem, and excessive involvement with pleasurable activities, some of which may be high risk. In its minor forms, the subjective experience of mania can be quite pleasurable to the individual, with a heightened sense of well-being and increased alertness.[24] The severity of manic symptoms runs the gamut from a condition called *cyclothymia*, in which mood fluctuates between mild elation and depression, to severe delusional mania.[23] Mania may begin abruptly within hours or days, or develop over a few weeks. Mixed states with features of both mania and depression present at the same time often are not well recognized. Bipolar episodes, left untreated, become more severe with age. Rapid cycling is said to occur when an individual has four or more shifts in mood from normal within a 1-year period. Women are more likely than men to be rapid cyclers.[25]

Kindling is a hypothesized phenomenon in which a stressor creates an electrophysiologic vulnerability to future stressful events by causing long-lasting changes in neuronal function. This may be the basis for the phenomenon of rapid cycling in bipolar depression. The more frequently a person has a shift in mood, cycling into either mania or depression, the easier it becomes to have another episode. There now is evidence that many psychiatric disorders, not just bipolar, are subject to this phenomenon. The better the control of the illness and the fewer cycles an individual has, the better his or her quality of life is likely to be.[26]

Diagnostic Criteria

The diagnostic criteria (DSM-IV classification) for a major depressive episode include the simultaneous presence of five or more of the aforementioned symptoms during a 2-week period, and these must represent a change from previous functioning.[19] Depression must be differentiated from grief reactions, medication side effects, and sequelae of medical illnesses. Bipolar depression is diagnosed on the basis of the pattern of occurrence of manic, hypomanic, and depressed episodes over time that are not due to medications or other therapies. The frequency, duration, and severity of the manic or depressive periods are unique to each individual.[19,21] Mania, particularly in its severe delusional forms, also needs to be differentiated from schizophrenia or drug-induced states.

Neurophysiology of Symptoms

In some cases of familial unipolar and bipolar depression, PET and MRI studies have demonstrated a 45% reduction in the volume of gray matter in the prefrontal cortex, with an associated decrease in activity in the region. Clinical studies have suggested that this area of the brain is important for mood states and has extensive connections with the limbic system. Physiologically, there is evidence of decreased functioning in the frontal and temporal lobes; although it is not known if this is a cause or an effect of depression, the activity returns to normal with the resolution of the symptoms.[22,27,28] The amygdala tends to have increased blood flow and oxygen consumption during depression.[22] Unlike those areas where function returns to normal with the resolution of depression, the amygdala continues to be excessively active for 12 to 24 months after the resolution of depression. It is hypothesized that relapse into depression is more likely to occur if medications are decreased or stopped before the amygdala returns to normal functioning. A number of neurotransmitters, serotonin and norepinephrine in particular, are implicated in depression.[19,21,29] The biogenic amine hypothesis suggests that decreased levels of these hormones in the synaptic cleft, due either to decreased presynaptic release or decreased postsynaptic sensitivity, is the underlying pathology in depression. The hypothesis is derived from the fact that drugs that depleted brain serotonin and norepinephrine caused depression, and drugs that increased brain levels of norepinephrine and serotonin decreased depression. It has become increasingly clear, however, that a simple decrease in the concentration of amines in neuronal synapses cannot entirely explain the complexities of depression. Neuromodulatory systems in the brain interact with each other in complex ways. For example, cholinergic and GABA-ergic pathways also may play a role in the development of depression because both of these pathways influence the activity of brain norepinephrine neurons.[19,21,29]

Disturbances in the function of the HPA axis also may play a critical role in depression. In the general population, cortisol levels usually are flat from late in the afternoon until a few hours before dawn, when they begin to rise. In persons with depression, cortisol levels spike erratically over the 24 hours of the day. The increased secretion of cortisol is the result of increased secretion of corticotropin-releasing hormone. Cortisol levels return to the normal pattern as depression resolves. In 40% of those diagnosed with depression, hypersecretion of cortisol is resistant to feedback inhibition by dexamethasone, which indicates a dysfunction of the HPA axis. However, so many factors affect cortisol levels that a skilled clinical interview is preferred to the test if the only reason for administering it is to confirm depression.[29]

Thyroid system dysfunction characterized by a decrease in triiodothyronine and thyroxine, a decrease in the release of thyroid-stimulating hormone, and an increase in thyrotropin-releasing hormone often is present in depression. If thyroid functioning is diminished, the individual is likely to have a less vigorous response to medical intervention.[20]

Circadian rhythms also are an area of serious research interest.[26] Alteration in the sleep-wake cycle is common in most mental illnesses and often is one of the prodromal signs of relapse. A specific type of depression known as *seasonal affective disorder* is triggered for persons in the winter by the shortening of daylight hours as fall commences, with symptoms of depression usually resolving in the spring when daylight hours again lengthen. Persons with depression often have what is called *dream pressure sleep.* Researchers have found that the normal sleep cycle is reversed in depression. The depressed individual falls into light and dream-state sleep early in the sleep cycle and reaches deep stage 4 sleep only late in the sleep cycle. This finding helps explain why many inpatients report they did not sleep all night and the staff reports that the patient was asleep all night. The sleep cycle reverts to normal after the resolution of the depression, but may not be completely normal for weeks to months. Decreasing or halting medications before the sleep disturbances resolve may lead to a relapse of depressive symptoms. Circadian rhythms are critical in symptom management for persons with bipolar depression. One of the fastest ways to precipitate a manic episode is for the individual to stay up all night. It is not unusual for a first manic episode to occur when someone "pulls an all-nighter" studying for final examinations. Persons with bipolar disorder should have a fairly rigid schedule for sleeping and awakening if cycling is to be minimized. Exercise is necessary, but the person with bipolar disorder should exercise before mid-afternoon to prevent the normal increase in metabolic rate from disrupting the sleep cycle.

Treatment

Effective treatments exist for unipolar and bipolar illnesses, including electroconvulsive therapy, antidepressant drugs, lithium, anticonvulsants, and psychotherapy.[19–21,30] Electroconvulsive therapy, a procedure that electrically stimulates a generalized seizure, is a highly effective treatment for depression, with 70% to 90% of clients showing a good response. The antidepressants most often used are MAOIs, which block the degradation of norepinephrine and serotonin; tricyclic compounds, which block the reuptake of norepinephrine and serotonin; and SSRIs, which block the reuptake of serotonin. The exact mechanism by which lithium works in bipolar depression is unknown. However, lithium blocks the enzymatic breakdown of inositol triphosphate (IP_3), increasing its intracellular concentration. IP_3 is an important regulator of intracellular calcium levels. Anticonvulsants (carbamazepine and valproate) also have proven to be efficacious in the treatment of bipolar depression, although the mechanism by which the drugs work is not completely understood. Psychotherapy is an important component of therapy for persons and families with major depressive disorder as well as with bipolar disorders. Individuals and families can learn how to deal with stressful life events and heal disrupted interpersonal relationships.

Many people who have bipolar disorder do not believe they need treatment, particularly during the manic phase of the illness, and tend to self-medicate with alcohol or recreational drugs. It is not unusual for people with bipolar depression to be diagnosed with substance abuse. When in the manic phase, they often feel exceptionally creative and talented. When helping people make the decision to enter treatment, it is important that they understand the treatment will not stop their creativity.

> In summary, depression is a disorder of emotion rather than of thought and is classified as unipolar, characterized by a persistent unpleasant mood, or bipolar, characterized by alternating periods of depression and mania. Depression is characterized by an inability to experience pleasure, feelings of worthlessness and excessive guilt, alterations in sleeping patterns and appetite, and thoughts of death or suicidal ideation. Mania is characterized by elation, irritability, high distractibility, and, often, engagement in high-risk pleasurable activities. As with schizophrenia, genetic factors appear to play an important role in the development of mood disorders. Neuroimaging techniques have revealed several anatomic and functional abnormalities in different regions of the brain. Abnormalities in neurotransmission also have been implicated in the development and maintenance of depression, including changes in concentration and activity of the neurotransmitters norepinephrine, serotonin, acetylcholine, and GABA. Treatment includes antidepressant drugs and psychotherapy.

Anxiety Disorders

After you have completed this section of the chapter, you should be able to meet the following objectives:

✦ Define the terms *panic disorder, generalized anxiety disorder, social phobia,* and *obsessive-compulsive disorder*
✦ Describe the epidemiology of panic disorder, generalized anxiety disorder, social phobia, and obsessive-compulsive disorder
✦ Describe the manifestations of panic disorder, generalized anxiety disorder, social phobia, and obsessive-compulsive disorder and the underlying neuropathophysiology of each
✦ Cite the diagnostic criteria for panic disorder, generalized anxiety disorder, social phobia, and obsessive-compulsive disorder according to the DSM-IV classification
✦ Describe the treatment for panic disorder, generalized anxiety disorder, social phobia, and obsessive-compulsive disorder

Anxiety disorders are extremely common, and the intensity of disability experienced by the person living with anxiety varies widely. Anxiety disorders affect approximately 15% of all individuals, women more often than men.

The common feature of anxiety disorders is increased fearfulness that sometimes is intense. The basic symptoms that are common to all anxiety disorders occur with the activation of the sympathetic cascade through the HPA axis. The core issue with anxiety disorders is that these symptoms occur without a precipitating potentially dangerous event. Anxiety disorders have a higher rate of occurrence among family members, but there is not yet any clearly delineated genetic process. According to the American Psychiatric Association DSM-IV anxiety is subdivided into five types, depending on clinical characteristics and response to pharmacologic agents. These five types include panic disorder, post-traumatic stress disorder (PTSD), generalized anxiety disorder, social phobia, and obsessive-compulsive disorder (OCD). See Chapter 9 for the discussion of PTSD.

PANIC DISORDER

Epidemiologic studies suggest that panic disorder has a lifetime prevalence of between 1.5% and 3%. First-degree relatives of persons with panic disorder have a 3- to 21-fold higher risk of developing panic disorder than unrelated persons. Panic disorder is characterized by neurologic symptoms (dizziness or lightheadedness, paresthesias, fainting), cardiac symptoms (tachycardia, chest pain, palpitations), respiratory symptoms (shortness of breath, feeling of smothering or choking), and psychological symptoms (feelings of impending doom, fear of dying, and a sense of unreality). The attacks, which are unexpected and not related to external events, usually last 15 to 30 minutes, but sometimes continue for an hour. Half of all clients with panic disorder also have a concomitant depression.[31]

Responses to medications suggest that multiple mechanisms and neurotransmitters are involved in initiating the panic attack. Persons experiencing panic attacks have been found to have somewhat lower levels of serotonin than do persons with no known mental illness, but the mechanism for that decrease is not known. The SSRIs are effective in the treatment of panic, but full response to medication can easily take 12 or more weeks. The tricyclic antidepressants also may be helpful, but their risk with overdose may limit their use in the treatment of panic in an effort to reduce suicides.[31,32]

Responses to yohimbine and clonidine indicate that the adrenergic system clearly is involved. Yohimbine, an α_2-adrenergic receptor blocker, precipitates panic attacks in persons who are susceptible to the attacks but not in others. This suggests that alterations in the adrenergic system may be part of the etiology of this disorder. The administration of clonidine, an α_2-adrenergic agonist, has been shown to block the panic-inducing effect of yohimbine. However, clonidine has not proved to be an efficacious treatment for panic disorder.[33]

γ-Aminobutyric acid is the third neurotransmitter system hypothesized to be involved in panic disorder. It has been suggested that persons experiencing panic disorder may have excess inverse agonists to GABA. The benzodiazepines, which act on GABA receptor sites, are effective in the treatment of panic. One of the risks is that of addiction among persons who may have a propensity for substance misuse. There has been some out-of-class use of the GABA-ergic anticonvulsants in the treatment of panic.[33]

Many individuals may require the use of more than one class of medication for the management of panic attacks. However, treatment is not fully effective unless psychotherapy focused on cognitive and behavioral changes is included as part of a comprehensive program. If inadequately treated, persons with panic disorder frequently develop phobias, particularly agoraphobia, which can be so debilitating that the person cannot leave his or her house.[31,33,34]

GENERALIZED ANXIETY DISORDER

In 1980, generalized anxiety disorder was first recognized as a separate entity from panic disorder in the DSM-III. Since then, the diagnostic criteria have been sharpened in an attempt to improve the ability of practitioners to discriminate the disorder. The central characteristic of generalized anxiety disorder is prolonged (>6 months), excessive worry that is not easily controlled by the person. The characteristics of the disorder include muscle tension, autonomic hyperactivity, and vigilance and scanning (exaggerated startle response, inability to concentrate). Drugs that are particularly effective in treating this disorder are the benzodiazepines (chlordiazepoxide, diazepam). These drugs increase the activity of the GABA$_A$ receptor, which increases the flow of chloride ions across the cell membrane, hyperpolarizing the membrane and thus inhibiting the firing of target cells.[19,33]

OBSESSIVE-COMPULSIVE DISORDER

Obsessive-compulsive disorder is characterized by obsessions (repeated thoughts) and compulsions (repeated acts) that are time consuming or distressing to the individual.[35,36] Usually, the person experiencing the symptoms recognizes that the rituals are unreasonable. For instance, the person may have to recheck the stove many times before she is able to leave for work or may have to repeatedly check the stairwells at work for debris to ensure that no one is injured. Between 2% and 3% of the world's population has OCD. This disorder is found with equal frequency among men and women, and there is a higher prevalence among family members. The average age of onset is approximately 20 years, although the disorder also may occur in children and, undiagnosed, may appear as behavior problems and angry outbursts that can seem impulsive and may be confused with attention deficit or hyperactivity disorders.[35,36]

There is no evidence of any neuroanatomic abnormalities in OCD, but there do seem to be consistent physiologic changes represented by increased activity in the anterior cingulate and the caudate. Some studies have suggested increased activity in the thalamus and the putamen, as well as a decrease in serotonin activity.[37] Treatment for OCD involves a combination of medication (SSRIs or certain tricyclic antidepressants) and psychotherapy. This disorder is particularly amenable to cognitive behavioral therapy. Studies indicate that there are physiologic changes in affected areas in response to this psychotherapeutic intervention.[35,36]

SOCIAL ANXIETY DISORDER

Social anxiety disorder is a generalized or specific, intense, irrational, and persistent fear of being scrutinized or negatively evaluated by others. Diagnostic criteria include the development of symptoms of anxiety when the person is exposed to the feared social situation, recognition by the person that the fear is irrational, avoidance by the person of the social situation, and interference of the anxiety or avoidance behavior with the person's normal routine. The fear must not be related to any physiologic effects of a substance and must be present for at least 6 months.[19,33,38]

Social phobia is a fairly common disorder with a lifetime prevalence of between 3% to 13%, with a slight tendency to occur more often in women than in men. Typically, the onset is between 11 and 19 years of age. The major adverse effects of social anxiety disorder are felt in employment and school, causing a loss of earning power and socioeconomic status. In addition, approximately one half of persons with social phobia also have a drug or alcohol problem. Several drugs have proved efficacious for the treatment of social phobia, including MAOIs, SSRIs, benzodiazepines, and β-adrenergic blockers. Social phobia also has been particularly responsive to behavioral and cognitive therapies.[19,33,38]

In summary, anxiety disorders include generalized anxiety, panic disorder, OCD, and social phobia. A common characteristic of the disorders is an intense fear that occurs in the absence of a precipitating dangerous event. The symptoms of anxiety disorders suggest an inappropriate and intense activation of the sympathetic nervous system. Panic disorder is characterized by neurologic, cardiac, respiratory, and psychological symptoms. The central characteristic of generalized anxiety disorder is excessive worry not easily controlled by the person and lasting more than 6 months. OCD is characterized by repetitive thoughts and acts. Social anxiety disorder is a generalized or specific, intense, irrational, and persistent fear of being scrutinized or negatively evaluated by others.

Related Web Sites

American Psychiatric Association   www.psych.org
American Psychiatric Nurses Association   www.apna.org
National Institute of Mental Health   www.nimh.nih.gov

References

1. Shorter E. (1997). *A history of psychiatry: From the era of the asylum to the age of Prozac.* New York: John Wiley & Sons.
2. Kandel E.R. (2000). Cellular mechanisms of learning and biological basis of individuality. In Kandel E.R., Schwartz J.H., Jessel T.M. (Eds.), *Principles of neural science* (4th ed., pp. 1247–1277). New York: McGraw-Hill.
3. Trimble M.R. (1996). *Biological psychiatry* (2nd ed., pp. 116–141, 325–378). West Sussex, England: John Wiley & Sons.
4. Callicott J.H., Weinberger D.R. (1999). Functional brain imaging: Future perspectives for clinical practice. In Weissman S., Sabshin M., Eist H. (Eds.), *Psychiatry in the new millennium* (pp. 119–135). Washington, DC: American Psychiatric Press.
5. Plomin R. (1996). Beyond nature vs. nurture. In Hall L.L. (Ed.), *Genetics and mental illness: Evolving issues for research and society* (pp. 29–50). New York: Plenum Press.
6. Hyman S.E. (1999). Looking to the future: The role of genetics and molecular biology in research on mental illness. In Weissman S., Sabshin M., Eist H. (Eds.), *Psychiatry in the new*

millennium (pp. 97–117). Washington, DC: American Psychiatric Press.
7. Taylor C.J.A., Macdonald A.M., Murray R.M. (1992). The genetics of psychiatric syndromes. In Weller M., Eysenck M. (Eds.), *The scientific basis of psychiatry* (2nd ed., pp. 270–300). Philadelphia: W.B. Saunders.
8. Gottesman I.I. (1996). Blind men and elephants: Genetic and other perspectives on schizophrenia. In Hall L.L. (Ed.), *Genetics and mental illness: Evolving issues for research and society* (pp. 51–77). New York: Plenum Press.
9. Tsuang M.T., Faraone S.V. (1996). The inheritance of mood disorders. In Hall L.L. (Ed.), *Genetics and mental illness: Evolving issues for research and society* (pp. 79–109). New York: Plenum Press.
10. Kandel E.R., Siegelbaum S.A. (2000). Overview of synaptic transmission. In Kandel E.R., Schwartz J.H., Jessel T.M. (Eds.), *Principles of neural science* (4th ed., pp. 175–185). New York: McGraw-Hill.
11. Kandel E.R. (2000). Neurotransmitters. In Kandel E.R., Schwartz J.H., Jessel T.M. (Eds.), *Principles of neural science* (4th ed., pp. 280–296). New York: McGraw-Hill.
12. Kandel E.R. (2000). Disorders of thought and volition: Schizophrenia. In Kandel E.R., Schwartz J.H., Jessel T.M. (Eds.), *Principles of neural science* (4th ed., pp. 1188–1207). New York: McGraw-Hill.
13. Marken P.A., Stanislav S.W. (1995). Schizophrenia. In Young L.L., Koda-Kimble M.A. (Eds.), *Applied therapeutics: The clinical use of drugs* (6th ed., pp. 75-1–75-23). Vancouver, WA: Applied Therapeutics.
14. Torrey E.F. (1988). *Surviving schizophrenia: A family manual.* New York: Harper & Row.
15. Turner T. (1997). ABC of mental health: Schizophrenia. *British Medical Journal* 315, 108–111.
16. Andreasen N.C. (1997). Linking mind and brain in the study of mental illnesses: A project for a scientific psychopathology. *Science* 275, 1585–1593.
17. Fortinash K.M. (2000). The schizophrenias. In Fortinash K.M., Holoday-Worret P.A. (Eds.). *Psychiatric mental health nursing* (2nd ed., pp. 294–328). St. Louis: Mosby.
18. Harrison P.J. (1999). The neuropathology of schizophrenia: A critical review of the data and their interpretation. *Brain* 122, 593–624.
19. Kandel E.R. (2000). Disorders of mood: Depression, mania, and anxiety disorders. In Kandel E.R., Schwartz J.H., Jessel T.M. (Eds.), *Principles of neural science* (4th ed., pp. 1209–1225). New York: McGraw-Hill.
20. Laird L.K., Benefield W.H. (1995). Mood disorders I: Major depressive disorders. In Young L.L., Koda-Kimble M.A. (Eds.), *Applied therapeutics: The clinical use of drugs* (6th ed., pp. 76-1–76-24). Vancouver, WA: Applied Therapeutics.
21. Love R.C., Grothe D.R. (1995). Mood disorders II: Bipolar affective disorders. In Young L.L., Koda-Kimble M.A. (Eds.), *Applied therapeutics: The clinical use of drugs* (6th ed., pp. 77-1–77-9). Vancouver, WA: Applied Therapeutics.
22. Doris A., Ebmeier K., Shajahan P. (1999). Depressive illness. *Lancet* 354, 1369–1375.
23. Manning J.S., Connor P.D., Sahai A. (1998). The bipolar spectrum: A review of current concepts and implications for the management of depression in primary care. *Archives of Family Medicine* 7 (1), 63–71.
24. Daly I. (1997). Mania. *Lancet* 349, 1157–1160.
25. Kilzieh N., Akiskal H.S. (1999). Rapid-cycling bipolar disorder: An overview of research and clinical experience. *Psychiatric Clinics of North America* 22, 585–607.
26. Haber J., Krainovich-Miller B., McMahon A., Price-Hoskins P. (1997). *Comprehensive psychiatric nursing* (5th ed., pp. 609–610). St. Louis: Mosby.

27. Soares J.C., Mann J.J. (1997). The anatomy of mood disorders: Review of structural neuroimaging studies. *Biological Psychiatry* 41, 86–106.

28. Videbech P. (2000). PET measurements of brain glucose metabolism and blood flow in major depressive disorder: A critical review. *Acta Psychiatrica Scandinavica* 101, 11–20.

29. McAllister-Williams R.H., Ferrier I.N., Young A.H. (1998). Mood and neuropsychological function in depression: The role of corticosteroids and serotonin. *Psychological Medicine* 28, 573–584.

30. Williams J.W., Mulrow C.D., Chiquette E., Noel P.H., Aguilar C., Cornell J. (2000). A systematic review of newer pharmacotherapies for depression in adults: Evidence report summary: Clinical guideline, part 2. *Annals of Internal Medicine* 132, 743–756.

31. Saeed S.A., Bruce T.J. (1998). Panic disorder: Effective treatment options. *American Family Physician* 57, 2412–2415, 2419–2420.

32. Roy-Byrne P.P, Cowley D.S. (1998). Search for pathophysiology of panic disorder. *Lancet* 352, 1646–1647.

33. Grimsley S.R. (1995). Anxiety disorders. In Young L.L., Koda-Kimble M.A. (Eds.), *Applied therapeutics: The clinical use of drugs* (6th ed., pp. 73-1–73-28). Vancouver, WA: Applied Therapeutics.

34. Gorman J.M., Kent J.M., Sullivan G.M., Coplan J.D. (2000). Neuroanatomical hypothesis of panic disorder, revised. *American Journal of Psychiatry* 157, 493–505.

35. Eddy M.F., Walbroehl G.S. (1998). Recognition and treatment of obsessive-compulsive disorder. *American Family Physician* 57, 1623–1628, 1632–1634.

36. Gedenk M., Nepps P. (1997). Obsessive-compulsive disorder: Diagnosis and treatment in the primary care setting [Medical Practice]. *Journal of the American Board of Family Practice* 10, 349–356.

37. Tibbo P., Warneke L. (1999). Obsessive-compulsive disorder in schizophrenia: Epidemiologic and biologic overlap. *Journal of Psychiatry and Neuroscience* 24, 15–24.

38. Bruce T.J., Saeed S.A. (1999). Social anxiety disorder: A common, underrecognized mental disorder. *American Family Physician* 60, 2311–2322.

Special Senses

Of all the ancient civilizations, it was the Greeks who led the way in understanding the body and its workings. One of the earliest Greek anatomists was Alcmaeon of Croton (c. 500 BC). Through his animal dissections, Alcmaeon came to recognize many structures and was the first to mention the eye in his writings. He described the optic nerve and decided that three things were necessary for vision—external light, the "fire" in the eye (he assumed there must be fire in the eye because a blow to the eye produces sparks, or stars), and the liquid in the eyeball.

The Greeks also developed early surgical procedures, among them techniques for the removal of cataracts. However, it was the Roman encyclopedist, Aulus Cornelius Celsus (1st century AD), whose most important surviving works are concerned with medicine, who provided a vivid description of the procedure:

The needle is to be sharp enough to penetrate, yet not too fine; and this to be inserted straight through . . . at a spot between the pupil of the eye and the angle adjacent to the temple, away from the middle of the cataract, in such a way that no vein is wounded. The needle, however, should not be inserted timidly. When the spot is reached, the needle is to be sloped against the colored area [lens] itself and rotated gently, guiding it little by little below the pupil; when the cataract has passed below the pupil, it is pressed upon more firmly in order that it may settle below.

Chapter 53

Control of Special Senses

Edward W. Carroll, Sheila M. Curtis,
and Robin L. Curtis

The Eye and Visual Function

After you have completed this section of the chapter, you should be able to meet the following objectives:

✦ Describe the structures and functions of the eyelids and lacrimal apparatus

✦ Name the layers of the eyeball and relate their structure to the overall function of the eye

✦ Compare the location and contents of the anterior and posterior chambers of the eye

✦ Discuss the function of the lens and distinguish between refraction and accommodation

✦ Explain the difference between myopia and hyperopia

✦ Characterize the structure of the retina, differentiating the three layers of neurons and the functions of rods and cones

✦ Trace a visual image from the time it reaches the retina to its perception in the visual and association cortices

The optic globe, or eyeball, is a remarkable, mobile, nearly spherical structure contained in a pyramid-shaped cavity of the skull called the *orbit* (Fig. 53-1). The eyeball consists of three layers: an outer supporting fibrous layer, the sclera; a vascular layer, the uveal tract; and a neural layer, the retina. Its interior is filled with transparent media, the aqueous and vitreous humors, which allow the penetration and transmission of light to photoreceptors in the retina. Exposed surfaces of the eyes are protected by the eyelids, which are mucous membrane-lined skin flaps that provide a means for shutting out most light. Tears bathe the anterior surface of the eye; they prevent friction between it and the lid, maintain hydration of the cornea, and protect the eye from irritation by foreign objects. The two eyes, with their associated extraocular muscles that permit directional rotation of the eyeball, provide different images of the same object. This results in binocular vision with depth perception.

ORBIT

The bony orbit of the skull houses and protects the eyeball. This protective shell is a pyramid-shaped cavity with walls formed by the union of seven cranial and facial bones: the frontal, maxillary, zygomatic, lacrimal, sphenoid, ethmoid,

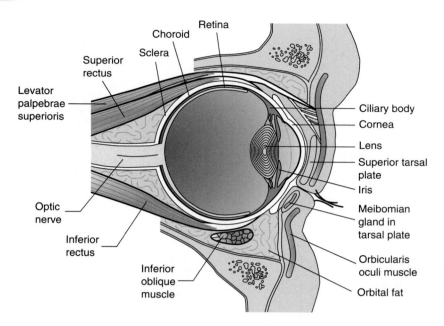

FIGURE 53-1 The eye and its appendages, lateral view. (Chaffee E.E., Lytle I.M. [1980]. *Basic physiology and anatomy* [4th ed.]. Philadelphia: J.B. Lippincott)

and palatine bones (Fig. 53-2). The superior surface of the maxillary bone forms the main floor of the orbit. Paired maxillary and lacrimal bones and the singular ethmoid bone form the medial wall of the orbit. Laterally, the orbit is triangular and is formed anteriorly by the zygomatic bone and posteriorly by the sphenoid bone, where it forms the thickest part of the orbit, particularly at the orbital margin, which is most likely to be exposed to trauma.

At the apex of the orbital pyramid, near the posterior medial part of the orbit, is an opening called the *optic foramen* through which pass the optic nerve, ophthalmic artery, and sympathetic nerves. A larger opening, the superior orbital fissure, permits passage of branches of the cranial nerves that provide motor innervation for the extrinsic and intrinsic eye muscles and sensory innervation to the orbit and its contents.

🔑 Vision

➤ Vision is a special sensory function that incorporates the visual receptor functions of the eyeball, the optic nerve, and visual pathways that carry and distribute sensory information from the optic globe to the central nervous system, and the primary and visual association cortices that translate the sensory signals into visual images.

➤ The eyeball is a hollow spherical structure that functions in the reception of the light rays that provide the stimuli for vision. The refractive surface of the cornea and accommodative properties of the lens serve to focus the light signals from near and far objects on the photoreceptors in the retina.

➤ Visual information is carried to the brain by axons of the retinal cells that form the optic nerve. The two optic nerves fuse in the optic chiasm, where axons of the nasal retina of each eye cross to the contralateral side and travel with axons of the ipsilateral temporal retina to form the fibers of the optic radiations that travel to the visual cortex.

➤ Binocular vision depends on the coordination of three pairs of extraocular nerves that provide for the conjugate eye movements, with optical axes of the two eyes maintained parallel to one another.

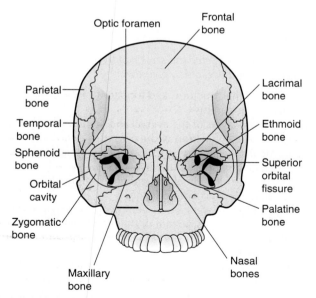

FIGURE 53-2 Anterior view of the skull shows the orbital cavity and optic foramen that form an opening for the optic nerve, blood vessels (*e.g.*, ophthalmic artery), and sympathetic nerves that supply the eye. (Chaffee E.E., Lytle I.M. [1980]. *Basic physiology and anatomy* [4th ed.]. Philadelphia: J.B. Lippincott)

Only the anterior one fifth of the orbit is occupied by the eyeball; the remainder is filled with muscles, nerves, the lacrimal gland, and adipose tissue that supports the normal position of the optic globe. A fascia known as *Tenon's capsule* surrounds the globe of the eye from the cornea to the posterior segment and separates the eye from the orbital fat.

EYELID

The upper and lower eyelids, the palpebrae, are modified folds of skin that protect the eyeball. The palpebral fissure is the oval opening between the upper and lower eyelids. At the corners of the eye, where the upper and lower lids meet, is an angle called the *canthus*; the lateral canthus is the outer, or temporal, angle, and the medial canthus is the inner, or nasal, angle. A line through the lateral and medial canthi defines the angle of the palpebral fissure and usually is horizontal. In children with Down syndrome (trisomy 21), this line has an upward and outward slant (see Chapter 7). A fold of skin, the epicanthic fold, covers the medial canthus and is characteristic of members of the Asian race and of persons with certain chromosomal abnormalities.

In each lid, a tarsus, or plate of dense connective tissue, gives the lid its shape (Fig. 53-3). Each tarsus contains modified sebaceous glands, called *meibomian glands*, the ducts of which open onto the eyelid margins. The sebaceous secretions of the meibomian glands enable airtight closure of the lids and prevent rapid evaporation of tears.

The lacrimal gland is the source of serous secretions called *tears*. This gland lies in the orbit, superior and lateral to the eyeball (Fig. 53-4). Approximately 12 small ducts connect the lacrimal gland to the superior conjunctival fornix. Tears, which comprise approximately 98% water, 1.5% sodium chloride, and the antibacterial enzyme lysozyme,

are essential to vision because of their lubricant and possibly antibacterial properties. Lubrication between the layers of the conjunctiva reduces friction between the eye and eyelids. Tears drain from the eye through a reddish elevation, the *lacrimal caruncle*, in the medial canthus into the nasolacrimal duct, which opens into the nasal cavity.

CONJUNCTIVA

The conjunctiva is a thin mucous membrane that lines the inner surface of both eyelids and covers the anterior surface of the optic globe to the limbus, or corneoscleral junction (Fig. 53-5). The portion of the conjunctiva that lines the eyelids is called the *palpebral conjunctiva*, and the part that covers the eyeball is called the *bulbar (ocular) conjunctiva*. When the eyes are closed, the conjunctiva lines the closed conjunctival sac. The conjunctiva is extremely sensitive to irritation and inflammation.

EYEBALL

Three distinct layers form the wall of the eyeball: the sclera or outer supporting layer, the choroid or middle vascular layer, and the retina, which is composed of the neuronal retinal layer and outer pigmented layer (see Fig. 53-5). The optic globe is separated into two cavities, an anterior, fluid-filled cavity and a posterior cavity, the vitreous body, which is filled with a gel-like material. The anterior cavity is further divided into an anterior and a posterior chamber by the lens and the ciliary body and its processes.

Sclera and Cornea
The outer layer of the eyeball consists of a tough, opaque, white, fibrous layer called the *sclera*. It is strong yet elastic, and maintains the shape of the globe. The sclera is continuous with the cornea anteriorly and with the cranial dural sheath that surrounds and protects the optic nerve posteriorly. This scleral sheath is continuous, but it is perforated posteriorly by many tiny holes called the *lamina cribrosa*. Approximately 1.5 million optic nerve fibers pass through these openings as they exit the retina.

At the anterior part of the eyeball, the sclera is continuous with and connects to the transparent cornea at the limbus. A major part of refraction (*i.e.*, bending) of light rays and focusing of vision occurs in the cornea. Three layers of tissue form the cornea: an extremely thin outer epithelial layer, which is continuous with the bulbar (ocular) conjunctiva; a middle layer called the *substantia propria* or *stroma*; and an inner endothelial layer, which lies next to the aqueous humor of the anterior chamber. The substantia propria is composed of regularly arranged collagen bundles embedded in a mucopolysaccharide matrix. This organization of the collagen fibers makes the substantia propria transparent and is necessary for light transmission. Hydration within a limited range is necessary to maintain the spacing of the collagen fibers and transparency.

Uveal Tract
The middle vascular layer, or uveal tract, of the eye includes the choroid, the ciliary body, and the iris. This tract is an

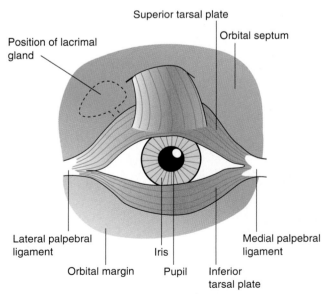

FIGURE 53-3 Anterior view of the right orbit shows the superficial structures. (Modified from Akesson A.J., Loeb J.A., Wilson-Pauwels, L. [1980]. *Thompson's core textbook of anatomy* [2nd ed.]. Philadelphia: J.B. Lippincott)

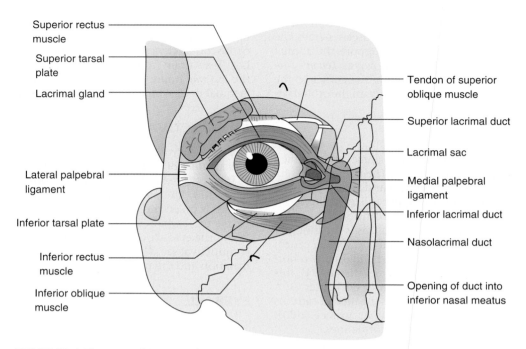

Superior rectus muscle

Superior tarsal plate

Lacrimal gland

Lateral palpebral ligament

Inferior tarsal plate

Inferior rectus muscle

Inferior oblique muscle

Tendon of superior oblique muscle

Superior lacrimal duct

Lacrimal sac

Medial palpebral ligament

Inferior lacrimal duct

Nasolacrimal duct

Opening of duct into inferior nasal meatus

FIGURE 53-4 The eye and its appendages: anterior view. (Chaffee E.E., Lytle I.M. [1980]. *Basic physiology and anatomy* [4th ed.]. Philadelphia: J.B. Lippincott)

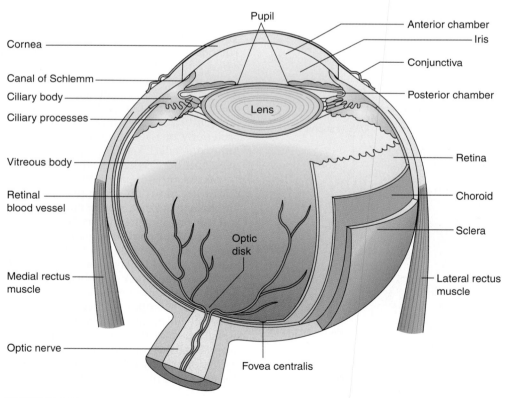

Pupil

Cornea

Canal of Schlemm

Ciliary body

Ciliary processes

Vitreous body

Retinal blood vessel

Medial rectus muscle

Optic nerve

Anterior chamber

Iris

Conjunctiva

Posterior chamber

Lens

Retina

Choroid

Sclera

Lateral rectus muscle

Optic disk

Fovea centralis

FIGURE 53-5 Transverse section of the eyeball. (Chaffee E.E., Lytle I.M. [1980]. *Basic physiology and anatomy* [4th ed.]. Philadelphia: J.B. Lippincott)

incomplete ball with gaps at the pupil and at the optic disk, where it is continuous with the arachnoid and pial layers surrounding the optic nerve. Melanocytes, which abound in the choroid, prevent the diffusion of light through the wall of the optic globe. Pigmentation in these cells absorbs light in the eyeball and light that penetrates the retina. This light-absorptive function prevents the scattering of light and is important for visual acuity, particularly with high background illumination levels. The choroid also is one of the most vascular tissues in the entire body.

The ciliary body is an anterior continuation of the choroid layer. It has both smooth muscle and secretory functions. Its smooth muscle function contributes to alteration in lens shape; its secretory function contributes to the production of aqueous humor.

Alterations in pupil diameter, and therefore in the amount of light entering the eye, are made by the muscular iris. Posteriorly, the surface of the iris is formed by a two-layer epithelium continuous with those layers covering the ciliary body. The anterior layer contains the dilator, or radial, muscles of the iris (Fig. 53-6). Just anterior to these muscles is the loose, highly vascular connective tissue stroma. Embedded in this layer are concentric rings of smooth muscle cells that comprise the sphincter muscle of the pupil. At its anterior surface, the iris forms a highly irregular anterior surface that contains many fibroblasts and melanocytes. Eye color differences result from the density of the pigment; pigment density decreases from dark brown eyes through shades of brown and gray to blue.

Several mutations affect the pigment of the uveal tract, including albinism. Albinism is a genetic (autosomal recessive trait) deficiency of tyrosinase, the enzyme needed for the synthesis of melanin by the melanocytes. Tyrosinase-negative albinism, also called *classic albinism*, is characterized by an absence of tyrosinase; affected persons have white hair, pink skin, and light blue eyes. In these persons, excessive light penetrates the unpigmented iris and choroid, and, to some extent, the anterior sclera. Their photoreceptors are flooded with excess light, and visual acuity is markedly reduced. Excess stimulation of the photoreceptors at normal or high illumination levels is experienced as painful photophobia.

Anterior and Posterior Chambers

The fluid-filled anterior cavity of the eye is divided by the iris into the anterior and posterior chambers, with the pupil forming the only passageway between the two chambers (see Fig. 53-5). The anterior chamber lies in front of the iris and the posterior chamber, the smaller of the two, is posterior to the iris and anterior to the lens. A gel-like vitreous humor fills the posterior cavity of the globe.

Aqueous humor, which fills the space between the cornea and lens, is secreted by the ciliary epithelium in the posterior chamber. This transparent humor flows slowly through the thin passageway between the lens and the iris and is reabsorbed by a specialized region at the iridocorneal angle. At the iridocorneal angle, the aqueous humor normally passes through a porous trabeculated region of the

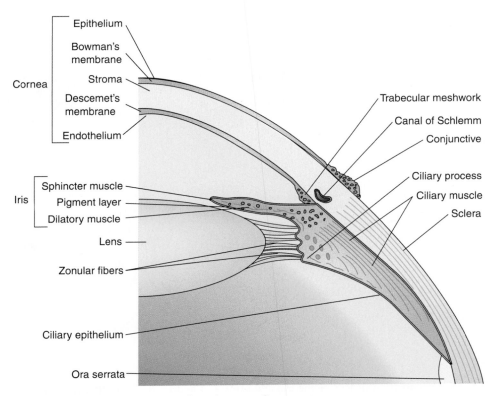

FIGURE 53-6 Anterior chamber angle and surrounding structures.

sclera (see Fig. 53-6) that permits entry into a circular venous ring called the *canal of Schlemm*. From the canal of Schlemm, the aqueous humor flows into the anterior ciliary veins.

LENS

The function of the eye is to transform light energy into nerve signals that can be transmitted to the cerebral cortex for interpretation. Optically, the eye is similar to a camera. It contains a lens system that inverts an image, an aperture (*i.e.*, the pupil) for controlling light exposure, and a retina that corresponds to the film and records the image (Fig. 53-7).

The lens is an avascular, transparent, biconvex body, the posterior side of which is more convex than the anterior side. A thin, highly elastic lens capsule is attached to the surrounding ciliary body by delicate suspensory radial ligaments called *zonules*, which hold the lens in place (see Fig. 53-6). In providing for a change in lens shape, the tough elastic sclera acts as a bow, and the zonule and the lens capsule act as the bow string. The suspensory ligaments and lens capsule normally are under tension, causing the lens to have a flattened shape for distant vision. Contraction of the muscle fibers of the ciliary body narrows the diameter of the ciliary body, relaxes the fibers of the suspensory ligaments, and allows the lens to relax to a more spherical or convex shape for near vision.

Refraction

When light passes from one medium to another, its velocity is decreased or increased, and the direction of light transmission is changed. This change in direction of light rays is called *refraction*. When light rays pass through the center of a lens, their direction is not changed; however, other rays passing peripherally through a lens are bent (Fig. 53-8). The refractive power of a lens usually is described as the distance (in meters) from its surface to the point at which the rays come into focus (*i.e.*, focal length). Usually, this is reported as the reciprocal of this distance (*i.e.*, diopters). For example, a lens that brings an object into focus at 0.5 m has a refractive power of 2 diopters (1.0/0.5 = 2.0). With a fixed-power lens, the closer an object is to the lens, the further behind the lens is its focus point. The closer the object, the stronger and more precise the focusing system must be.

In the eye, the major refraction of light begins at the convex corneal surface. Further refraction occurs as light moves from the posterior corneal surface to the aqueous humor, from the aqueous humor to the anterior lens surface, and from the posterior lens surface to the vitreous humor.

Disorders of Refraction. A perfectly shaped optic globe and cornea result in optimal visual acuity (*i.e.*, *emmetropia*), producing a sharp image in focus at all points on the retinal surface in the posterior part, or fundus, of the eye (see Fig. 53-8). Unfortunately, individual differences in formation and growth of the eyeball and cornea frequently result in inappropriate focal image formation. If the anterior-

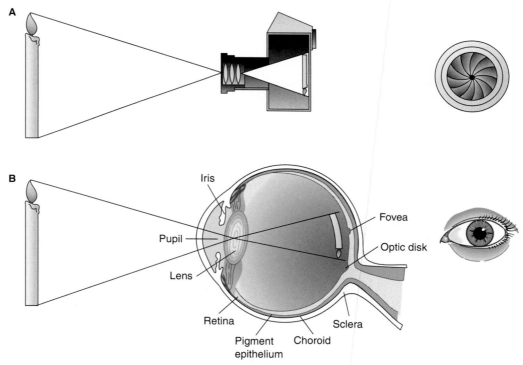

FIGURE 53-7 Comparison of lens of the eye and camera. (Kandel E.R., Schwartz J.H., Jessel T.M. [1991]. *Principles of neural science* [3rd ed.]. New York: Elsevier)

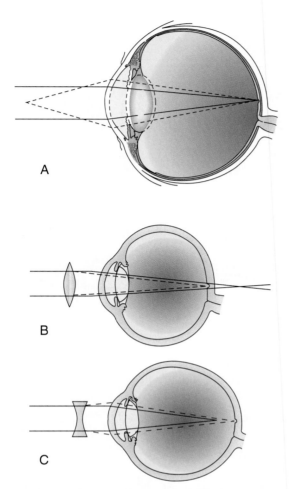

FIGURE 53-8 (**A**) Accommodation. The *solid lines* represent rays of light from a distant object, and the *dotted lines* represent rays from a near object. The lens is flatter for the former and more convex for the latter. In each case, the rays of light are brought to a focus on the retina. (**B**) Hyperopia corrected by a biconvex lens, shown by the *dotted lines*. (**C**) Myopia corrected by a biconcave lens, shown by the *dotted lines*. (Chaffee E.E., Lytle I.M. [1980]. *Basic physiology and anatomy* [4th ed.]. Philadelphia: J.B. Lippincott)

posterior dimension of the eyeball is too short, the image is focused posterior to (behind) the retina. This is called *hyperopia* or *farsightedness*. In such cases, the accommodative changes of the lens can bring distant images into focus, but near images become blurred. This type of defect is corrected by appropriate biconvex lenses. If the anterior-posterior dimension of the eyeball is too long, the focus point for an infinitely distant target is anterior to the retina. This condition is called *myopia* or *nearsightedness* (see Fig. 53-8). Persons with myopia can see close objects without problems because accommodative changes in their lens bring near objects into focus, but distant objects are blurred. Myopia can be corrected with an appropriate biconcave lens. Radial keratotomy, a form of refractive corneal surgery, can be performed to correct the defect. This surgical procedure involves the use of radial incisions to alter the corneal curvature.

Refractive defects of the corneal surface do not permit the formation of a sharp image. However, the accommodative reflex continues its unsuccessful attempts to alter the shape of the lens by ciliary muscle contraction to alter the lens shape. The discomfort or pain associated with continuous muscle contraction is experienced as eyestrain. Nonuniform curvature of the refractive medium (*e.g.*, horizontal vs. vertical plane) is called *astigmatism*. Astigmatism usually is the result of a defect in the cornea, but it can result from defects in the lens or the retina. Spherical aberration, another refractive error, involves a cornea with nonspherical surfaces. Lens correction is available for both of these refractive errors.

Accommodation

The focusing surface of the eye, the retina, is at a fixed distance from the lens; adjustability in the refractive power of the lens is needed to keep the image of close objects in focus on the retina. This ability to adjust the refractive power of the lens is called *accommodation*. Accommodation is the process by which a clear image is maintained as gaze is shifted from afar to a near object. The shape of the lens and the degree of pupillary opening must be under the control of a feedback system that makes these adjustments while evaluating image sharpness. All of this is accomplished by accommodation and pupillary reflexes under the control of the visual acuity centers in the primary visual and association cortices. These areas provide feedback control for modifying lens shape and therefore visual acuity.

Accommodation requires convergence of the eyes, pupillary constriction, and thickening of the lens through contraction of the ciliary muscle. Accommodation is controlled by the parasympathetic portion of the oculomotor cranial nerve (CN III). The cell bodies of this nerve are contained in the oculomotor nuclear complex in the midbrain, and its preganglionic axons synapse with postganglionic neurons of the ciliary ganglion in the orbit. Postganglionic axons enter the back of the eye and travel in the choroid layer to the ciliary muscle fibers. Visual function must be present to evaluate and adjust the clarity of the image. The functional integrity of the entire visual system, including the forebrain and midbrain circuitry, is necessary for accommodation. Accommodation does not occur in the totally blind, during sleep, or in the comatose person.

In near vision, pupillary constriction (*i.e.*, miosis) improves the clarity of the retinal image. This must be balanced against the resultant decrease in light intensity reaching the retina. During changes from near to far vision, pupillary dilation partially compensates for the reduced size of the retinal image by increasing the light entering the pupil. A third component of accommodation involves the reflex narrowing of the palpebral opening during near vision and widening during far vision.

Disorders of Accommodation. Paralysis of the ciliary muscle, with loss of accommodation, is called *cycloplegia*. Pharmacologic cycloplegia sometimes is necessary to aid ophthalmoscopic examination of the fundus of the eye, especially in small children who are unable to hold a steady fixation during the examination. Lens shape is totally controlled by the pretectal region and the parasympathetic pathways through the oculomotor nerve to the ciliary muscle. Accommodation is lost with destruction of this pathway.

The term *presbyopia* refers to changes in vision that occur because of aging. The lens consists of transparent fibers arranged in concentric layers, of which the external layers are the newest and softest. No loss of lens fibers occurs with aging; instead, additional fibers are added to the outermost portion of the lens. As the lens ages, it thickens, and its fibers become less elastic, so that the range of focus or accommodation is diminished to the point where reading glasses become necessary for near vision.

RETINA

Retinal Function and Organization

The function of the retina is to receive visual images, partially analyze them, and transmit this modified information to the brain. It is composed of two layers: the outer, melanin-containing layer and the inner neural layer. The light-sensitive neural retina covers the inner aspect of the eyeball. A non–light-sensitive portion of the retina, along with the retinal pigment epithelium, continues anteriorly to form the posterior surface of the iris. A wavy border called the *ora serrata* exists at the junction between the light-sensitive and the non–light-sensitive retinas. Separating the vascular portion of the choroid from the single layer of pigmented cells is a thin layer of elastic tissue, *Bruch's membrane*, which contains collagen fibrils in its superficial and deep portions. Cells of the pigmented layer receive their nourishment by diffusion from the choroid vessels. Tight junctions between the endothelial cells of the retinal blood vessels combine to form a blood-retina barrier.

The neural retina is composed of three layers of neurons: a posterior layer of photoreceptors, a middle layer of bipolar cells, and an inner layer of ganglion cells that communicate with the photoreceptors. A pattern of light on the retina falls on a massive array of photoreceptors. These photoreceptors synapse with bipolar and other interneurons before action potentials in ganglion cells relay the message to specific regions of the brain and the brain stem associated with vision. For rods, this microcircuitry involves the convergence of signals from many rods on a single ganglion cell. This arrangement maximizes spatial summation and the detection of stimulated (light vs. dark) receptors. The interneurons, composed of horizontal and amacrine cells, have cell bodies in the bipolar layer, and they play an important role in modulating retinal function. A superficial marginal layer contains the axons of the ganglion cells as they collect and leave the eye by way of the optic nerve (Fig. 53-9). These fibers lie beside the vitreous humor. Light must pass through the transparent inner layers of the sensory retina before it reaches the photoreceptors.

Photoreceptors

Two types of photoreceptors are present in the retina: rods, capable of black–white discrimination, and cones, capable of color discrimination. Both types of photoreceptors are thin, elongated, mitochondria-filled cells with a single, highly modified cilium (see Fig. 53-9). The cilium has a short base, or inner segment, and a highly modified outer segment. The plasma membrane of the outer segment is tightly folded to form membranous disks (rods) or conical

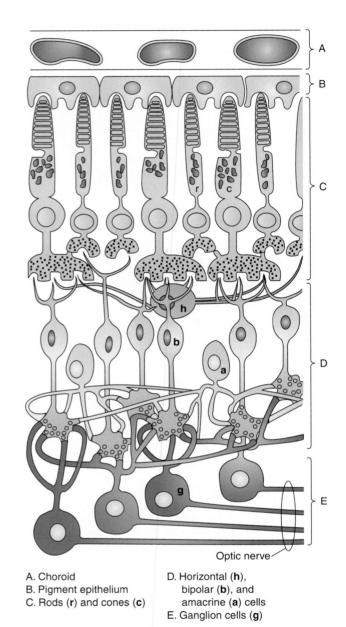

A. Choroid
B. Pigment epithelium
C. Rods (**r**) and cones (**c**)

D. Horizontal (**h**), bipolar (**b**), and amacrine (**a**) cells
E. Ganglion cells (**g**)

FIGURE 53-9 Organization of the human retina. The various layers are described in the text. (Modified from Dowling J.F., Boycott B.B. [1966]. Organization of the primate retina: Electron microscopy. *Proceedings of the Royal Society of London* 166, 80–111)

shapes (cones) containing visual pigment. These disks are continuously synthesized at the base of the outer segment and shed at the distal end. The discarded membranes are phagocytized by the retinal pigment cells. If this phagocytosis is disrupted, as in retinitis pigmentosa (see Chapter 54), the sensory retina degenerates.

Rods. Photoreception involves the transduction of light energy into an altered ionic membrane potential of the rod cell. Light passing through the eye penetrates the nearly transparent neural elements to produce decomposition of the photochemical substance (visual pigment) called *rhodopsin* in the outer segment of the rod. Light that is not trapped by a rhodopsin molecule is absorbed by the retinal pigment melanin or the more superficial choroid melanin. Rhodopsin consists of a protein called *opsin* and a vitamin A–derived pigment called *retinal*. During light stimulation, rhodopsin is broken down into its component parts, opsin and retinal; retinal subsequently is converted into vitamin A. The reconstitution of rhodopsin occurs during total darkness; vitamin A is transformed into retinal, and then opsin and retinal combine to form rhodopsin. Considerable stores of vitamin A are present in the retinal pigment cells and in the liver; therefore, a vitamin A deficiency must be present for weeks or months to affect the photoreceptive process. Reduced sensitivity to light, a symptom of vitamin A deficiency, initially affects night vision; however, this is quickly reversed by injection or ingestion of the vitamin.

Rod-based vision is particularly sensitive to detecting light, especially moving light stimuli, at the expense of clear pattern discrimination. Rod vision is particularly adapted for night and low-level illumination. Dark adaptation is the process by which rod sensitivity increases to the optimum level. This requires approximately 4 hours in total or near-total darkness and involves only rods or scotopic vision. During daylight or high-intensity bombardment, the concentration of vitamin A increases and the concentration of the photopigment retinal decreases. During dark adaptation, increased synthesis of retinal from vitamin A results in a higher concentration of rhodopsin available to capture light energy.

Cones and Color Sensitivity.   Cone receptors that are selectively sensitive to different wavelengths of light provide the basis for color vision. Three types of cones, or cone-color systems, respond to the blue, green, and red portions of the visible electromagnetic spectrum. This selectivity reflects the presence of one of three color-sensitive molecules to which the photochemical substance (visual pigment) is

bound. The decomposition and reconstitution processes of the cone visual pigments are believed to be similar to that of the rods. The color a person perceives depends on which set of cones or combination of sets of cones is stimulated in a given image.

Cones do not have the dark adaptation of rods. Consequently, the dark-adapted eye is a rod receptor eye with only black-gray-white experience (*scotopic* or *night vision*). The light-adapted eye (*photopic vision*) adds the capacity for color discrimination. Rhodopsin has its maximum sensitivity in the blue-green region of the electromagnetic spectrum. If red lenses are worn in daylight, the red cones (and green cones to some extent) are in use, whereas the rods and blue cones are essentially in the dark, and therefore dark adaptation proceeds. This method is used by military and night-duty airport control tower personnel to allow adaptation to take place before they go on duty in the dark.

Macula and Fovea.   An area approximately 1.5 mm in diameter near the center of the retina, called the *macula lutea* (*i.e.*, "yellow spot"), is especially adapted for acute and detailed vision. This area is composed entirely of cones. In the central portion of the macula, the *fovea centralis* (foveola), the blood vessels and innermost layers are displaced to one side instead of resting on top of the cones (Fig. 53-10). This allows light to pass unimpeded to the cones without passing through several layers of the retina. The density of cones drops off rapidly away from the fovea. Rods are not present in the fovea, but their numbers increase as the cones decrease in density toward the periphery of the retina. Many cones are connected one-to-one with ganglion cells. Retinal microcircuitry for cones emphasizes the detection of edges. This type of circuitry favors high acuity. A concentration of acuity-favoring cones at the fovea supports the use of this part of the retina for fine analysis of focused central vision.

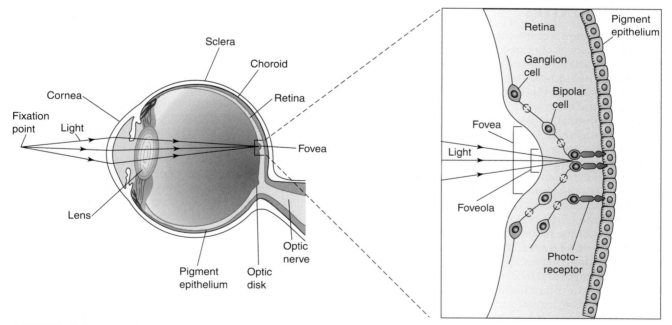

FIGURE 53-10 Location of fovea in the retina. (Kandel E.R., Schwartz J.H., Jessel T.M. [1991]. *Principles of neural science* [3rd ed.]. New York: Elsevier)

Color Blindness.   Color blindness is a misnomer for a condition in which persons appear to confuse or mismatch colors, or experience reduced acuity for color discrimination. Such persons often are unaware of their defect until they attempt to discriminate between red and green traffic lights or show difficulty matching colors. Most often the result of genetic factors, the deficit can result from the defective function of one or more of the three color-cone mechanisms. The deficiency usually is partial but can be complete. Rarely are two of the color mechanisms missing; when this occurs, usually red and green are missing. Persons with no color mechanisms are rare. For them, the world is experienced entirely as black, gray, and white.

The genetically color-blind person has never experienced the full range of normal color vision and is unaware of what he or she is missing. Color discrimination is necessary for everyday living, and color-blind persons, knowingly or unknowingly, make color discriminations based on other criteria, such as brightness or position. For example, the red light of a traffic signal is always the upper light, and the green is the lower light. Color-blind persons experience difficulties when brightness differences are small and discrimination must be based on hue and saturation qualities.

The genes responsible for color blindness affect receptor mechanisms rather than central acuity. The gene for the red and green mechanisms is sex linked (*i.e.*, on the X chromosomes), resulting in a much higher incidence among males of red, green, or red-green color blindness; however, the gene affecting the blue mechanism is autosomal. Acquired color defects are more complex but follow a general rule: disease of the more peripheral retina affects blue discrimination, and disease of the more central retina affects red and green discrimination because blue cones are not present in the central fovea.

NEURAL PATHWAYS AND CORTICAL CENTERS

Full visual function requires the normally developed brain-related functions of photoreception and the pupillary reflex. These functions depend on the integrity of all visual pathways, including retinal circuitry and the pathway from the optic nerve to the visual cortex and other visual regions of the brain and brain stem.

Visual information is carried to the brain by axons of the retinal ganglion cells, which form the optic nerve. Surrounded by pia mater, cerebrospinal fluid (CSF), arachnoid, and the dura mater, the optic nerve represents an outgrowth of the brain rather than a peripheral nerve. Exiting the optic globe and the orbit through the optic foramen, the optic nerve traverses the floor of the middle fossa to the optic chiasm at the base of the brain (Fig. 53-11). Axons from the nasal portion of the retina remain medial, and those from the temporal retina remain lateral in the optic nerve.

The two optic nerves meet and fuse at the optic chiasm, on the ventral and most rostral end of the brain stem, just in front of the infundibular stalk of the pituitary gland. In the optic chiasm, axons from the nasal retina of each eye cross to the opposite side and join with the axons of the temporal retina of the contralateral eye to form the optic

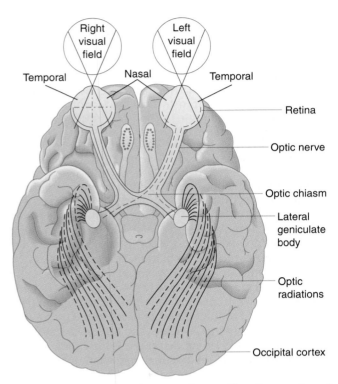

FIGURE 53-11 Diagram of optic pathways. Note the crossing of fibers from the medial half of each retina. (Chaffee E.E., Lytle I.M. [1980]. *Basic physiology and anatomy* [4th ed.]. Philadelphia: J.B. Lippincott)

tracts. One optic tract contains fibers from both eyes that transmit information from the same visual field.

Fibers of the optic tracts move laterally around the cerebral peduncles to synapse in the dorsal lateral geniculate nucleus (LGN) of the thalamus. Axons from these neurons in the LGN form the optic radiations to the primary visual cortex in the calcarine area of the occipital lobe. The LGN receives input from the visual cortex, the oculomotor centers in the brain stem, and the brain stem reticular formation; this input is thought to modify the pattern and strength of the retinal input.

The pattern of information transmission established in the optic tract is retained in the optic radiations. For example, the axons from the right visual field, represented by the nasal retina of the right eye and the temporal retina of the left eye, are united at the chiasm. They continue through the left optic tract and left optic radiation to the left visual cortex, where visual experience is first perceived. The left primary visual cortex receives two representations of the right visual field. Physical separation of information from the left and right visual fields is maintained in the visual cortex. Interaction between these disparate representations occurs and provides the basis for the sensation of depth in the near visual field.

Visual Cortex

The primary visual cortex (area 17 or V1) surrounds the calcarine fissure, which lies in the occipital lobe. It is at this level that visual sensation is first experienced (Fig. 53-12).

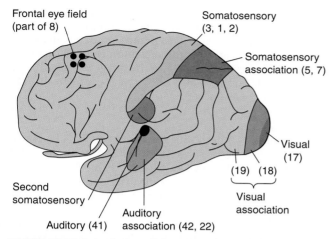

FIGURE 53-12 Lateral view of the cortex illustrating the location of the visual, visual association, auditory, and auditory association areas.

Immediately surrounding area 17 (V1) are the visual association cortices (areas 18 [V2, V3, V4] and 19 [V5]) and several other association cortices. These association cortices, with their thalamic nuclei, must be functional for added meaningfulness of visual perception. This higher-order aspect of the visual experience depends on previous learning.

Approximately 1 million retinal ganglion cell axons pass through the optic nerve and tract to reach the LGN in the thalamus; more than 100 million axons arising from geniculate neurons provide the input to the billions of neurons in the visual cortex. Here, the spatial representation of the visual field is retained in a distorted retinal map. The proportion of cells of the LGN and of the primary visual area devoted to analysis of the central visual field is greatly expanded compared with that of the peripheral retina. From 80% to 90% of the cellular mass and area of the primary visual cortex is concerned with central vision. This intense level of neural representation supports the high degree of visual acuity characteristic of central vision; it exists at the retina and all levels of the visual pathway.

Circuitry in the primary visual cortex and the visual association areas is extremely discrete with respect to the location of retinal stimulation. For example, specific neurons respond to the particular orientation of a moving edge, specific colors, or familiar shapes. This elaborate organization of the visual cortex, with its functionally separate and multiple representations of the same visual field, provides the major basis for visual sensation and perception. Because of this discrete circuitry, lesions of the visual cortex must be large to be detected clinically.

A flash of light delivered to the retina evokes potentials that can be measured and recorded by placing electrodes on the scalp over the occipital lobes. The waves of the evoked potentials, called pattern-reversed evoked potentials or visual evoked potentials, are useful for clinical evaluation of the functional integrity of successive levels of the visual pathway.

Pupillary Reflex

Changes in the size of the pupillary opening are mediated by the pupillary reflex, a functional component of the autonomic nervous system. The sphincter muscle that produces pupillary constriction is innervated by postganglionic parasympathetic neurons of the ciliary ganglion and other scattered ganglion cells between the scleral and choroid layers (Fig. 53-13). Part of the oculomotor (CN III) nucleus

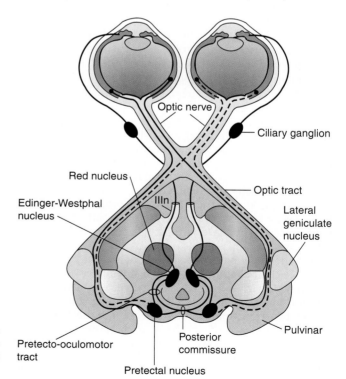

FIGURE 53-13 Diagram of the path of the pupillary light reflex. (Reproduced with permission from Walsh F.B., Hoyt W.F. [1969]. *Clinical neuro-ophthalmology* [3rd ed., vol. 1]. Baltimore: Williams & Wilkins)

is called the *Edinger-Westphal nucleus*. This autonomic nucleus, found in the midbrain, provides the preganglionic innervation for these parasympathetic axons. Innervation for the dilator muscle is derived from thoracic sympathetic preganglionic neurons that send axons along the sympathetic chain to innervate the postganglionic neurons in the superior cervical ganglion. Postganglionic neurons send axons along the internal carotid and ophthalmic arteries to the posterior surface of the optic globe. These axons travel between the scleral and choroid layers to reach the dilator muscles of the iris.

The pupillary reflex is controlled by a region in the midbrain called the *pretectum*. Pretectal areas on each side of the brain are connected, explaining the binocular aspect of the light reflex. These areas project axons to the Edinger-Westphal nuclei of the midbrain, which contain the parasympathetic preganglionic neurons that innervate the ciliary ganglion and control the sphincter muscle of the iris. Midbrain-level evaluation with feedback control provides an automatic brightness control mechanism. The functional importance of this reflex mechanism is its rapidity, compared with the slow light- and dark-adaptive retinal mechanism.

Visual Fields

The *visual field* refers to the area that is visible during fixation of vision in one direction. Because visual system deficits often are expressed as visual field deficits rather than as direct measures of neural function, the terminology for normal and abnormal visual characteristics usually is based on visual field orientation.

Most of the visual field is *binocular*, or seen by both eyes. This binocular field is subdivided into central and peripheral portions. Central portions of the retina provide high visual acuity and correspond to the field focused on the central fovea; the peripheral and surrounding portion provides the capacity to detect objects, particularly moving objects. Beyond the visual field shared by both eyes, the left lateral periphery of the visual field is seen exclusively by the left nasal retina, and the right peripheral field is seen by the right nasal retina.

As with a camera, the simple lens system of the eye inverts the image of the external world on each retina. In addition, the right and left sides of the visual field also are reversed. The right binocular visual field is seen by the left retinal halves of each eye: the nasal half of the right eye and the temporal half of the left eye.

Once the level of the retina is reached, the nervous system plays a consistent role. The upper half of the visual field is received by the lower half of the retinas of both eyes. The representations of this upper half of the field are carried in the lower half of each optic nerve: they synapse in the lower half of the LGN of each side of the brain. Neurons in this part of the LGN send their axons through the inferior half of the optic radiation, looping into the temporal lobe to terminate in the lower half of the primary visual cortex on each side of the brain. Because of the lateral separation of the two eyes, each eye contributes a different image of the world to the visual field. This is called *binocular disparity*. Disparity between the laterally displaced images seen by the two eyes provides a powerful source of three-dimensional depth perception for objects within a distance of 30 m. Beyond that distance, binocular disparity becomes insignificant: depth perception is based on other cues (*e.g.*, the superimposition of the image of near objects over that of far objects, and the faster movement of near objects than of far objects).

In summary, the optic globe, or eyeball, is a nearly spherical structure protected posteriorly by the bony structures of the orbit and anteriorly by the eyelids. A protective layer of tears constantly bathes the eye. A conjunctiva lines the inner surface of the eyelids and covers the optic globe to the junction of the cornea and sclera. The wall of the eye is made up of three layers: an outer fibrous coat that has a white, opaque region called the *sclera* and a transparent window known as the *cornea*; a highly pigmented middle vascular layer known as the *choroid*; and an inner neural layer, the retina. Interiorly, the eye is divided into a smaller, fluid-filled anterior cavity and a larger, vitreous-filled posterior segment. The anterior segment of the eye is divided into an anterior and posterior chamber, separated by the pupil and closely adjacent lens. Aqueous humor, secreted by the ciliary epithelium, flows through a thin passageway between the lens and iris; it then moves through a porous trabeculated region of the sclera into the canal of Schlemm and the venous system.

The function of the eye is similar to that of a camera. It contains a lens and an aperture for controlling light exposure (*i.e.*, pupil), and the retina corresponds to the film. The lens is a biconvex, avascular, colorless, and almost transparent structure suspended behind the iris. It is enclosed by a thin, homogeneous, highly elastic, carbohydrate-containing lens capsule held in place by suspensory ligaments called *zonules*. The shape of the lens is controlled by the ciliary muscle, which contracts and relaxes the zonule fibers, thus changing the tension on the lens capsule and altering the focus of the lens.

Refraction refers to the ability to focus an object on the retina. The refractive properties of the eye depend on the size and shape of the eyeball and the cornea and on the focusing ability of the lens. Errors in refraction occur when the visual image is not focused on the retina because of individual differences in the size or shape of the eyeball or cornea. In hyperopia, or farsightedness, the image falls behind the retina. In myopia, or nearsightedness, the image falls in front of the retina.

Accommodation is the process by which a clear image is maintained as the gaze is shifted from afar to a near object. It requires convergence of the eyes, pupillary constriction, and thickening of the lens through contraction of the ciliary muscle. Paralysis of the ciliary muscle with consequent loss of accommodation is called *cycloplegia*. Lens shape is totally controlled by the pretectal region, which sends parasympathetic fibers of the oculomotor nerve to the ciliary muscle. Accommodation is lost with the destruction of this pathway.

Presbyopia is a change in the lens that occurs because of aging such that the lens becomes thicker and less able to change shape and accommodate for near vision.

The retina covers the inner aspect of the posterior two thirds of the eyeball and is continuous with the optic nerve. It contains the photoreceptors for vision: the rods, for black and white discrimination, and the cones, for color vision. Visual information is carried to the brain by axons of the retinal ganglion cells forming the optic nerve. The two optic nerves meet and fuse in the optic chiasm. The axons of each nasal retina cross in the chiasm and join the uncrossed fibers from the temporal retina of the opposite eye in the optic tract. From the optic chiasm, crossed fibers of the nasal retina of one eye and the uncrossed temporal fibers of the eye pass to the LGN. After synapsing in the LGN, these fibers travel to the primary visual cortex, which lies in the calcarine fissure of the occipital lobe.

Eye Movements and Conjugate Gaze Reflex Mechanisms

After you have completed this section of the chapter, you should be able to meet the following objectives:

✦ Name the six extraocular muscles and relate their function to the movements of the optic globe during conjugate, vergent, and gaze movements of the eye
✦ Characterize conjugate gaze, slow pursuit, and saccadic and optokinetic eye movements
✦ Describe normal nystagmus eye movements

BINOCULAR COORDINATION OF EYE MOVEMENTS

For complete function of the eyes, it is necessary that the two eyes point toward the same fixation point and that the retinal and central nervous system (CNS) visual acuity

mechanisms function. Despite slight variations in the view of the external world for each eye (binocular disparity), it is important that these two images become fused (binocular fusion), which is a forebrain function. Binocular fusion is controlled by ocular reflex mechanisms that adjust the orientation of each eye to produce a single image. If these reflexes fail, diplopia or double vision occurs. To be effective, these reflexes must adjust eye movements for viewing objects at various distances. During distance vision, reflex mechanisms called *conjugate gaze* reflexes are required to maintain parallel orientation of the two eyes. In contrast to parallel or conjugate eye movements, at distances closer than approximately 30 feet, reflexes must alter eye orientation away from parallel if a common fixation point is to be obtained. These constitute a second category of reflexes, called *vergence reflexes*, that turn the eyes inward (convergence) as targeted objects approach the observer, or outward (divergence) when objects are receding.

The concept of "optical grasp" has been used to characterize the reflexes that enable the eyes to grasp and "hang onto" a visual target. Bilaterally linked or yoked rotation of the two eyes in response to visual, auditory, vestibular, or somesthetic stimuli depends on a basic repertoire of eye movement reflexes built into the circuitry of the CNS. These reflexes normally are operative at or within a few weeks of birth.

Conjugate and vergence movements are further subdivided into slow and very rapid, or saccadic, movements. Usually, the slow movements permit continuous fixation on a visual target during movements of the target or rotations of the head. The rapid or saccadic movements permit a resetting of the fixation point to a new location.

EXTRINSIC EYE MUSCLES AND THEIR INNERVATION

Binocular vision depends on three pairs of extraocular muscles—the medial and lateral recti, the superior and inferior recti, and the superior and inferior obliques (Fig. 53-14).

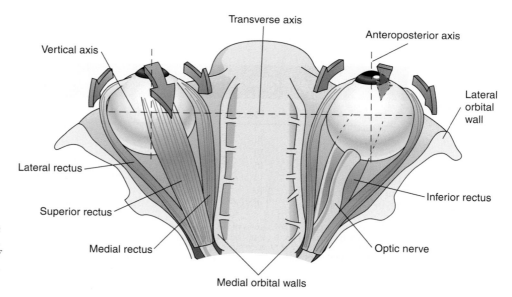

FIGURE 53-14 Extraocular eye muscles. (Williams & Warwick. [1975]. *Functional neuroanatomy of man* [p. 1126]. Philadelphia: W.B. Saunders)

Transverse axis
Vertical axis
Anteroposterior axis
Lateral orbital wall
Lateral rectus
Superior rectus
Medial rectus
Inferior rectus
Optic nerve
Medial orbital walls

Each of the three sets of muscles in each eye is reciprocally innervated so that one muscle relaxes when the other contracts. Reciprocal contraction of the medial and lateral recti moves the eye from side to side (adduction and abduction); the superior and inferior recti move the eye up and down (elevation and depression). The oblique muscles rotate (intorsion and extorsion) the eye around its optic axis. A seventh muscle, the levator palpebrae superioris, elevates the upper lid.

The extraocular muscles are innervated by three cranial nerves. The trochlear nerve (CN IV) innervates the superior oblique, the abducens nerve (CN VI) innervates the lateral rectus, and the oculomotor nerve (CN III) innervates the remaining four muscles. Motor units in the extraocular muscles are quite small, with one lower motoneuron (LMN) innervating 2 to 10 muscle fibers. This gives the CNS very delicate control of muscle-generated force through progressive recruitment of these very small units. Delicate control is necessary because a very small eye movement results in a very large shift in the location of a distant fixation point.

Table 53-1 describes the function and innervation of the extraocular muscles. The CN VI (abducens) nucleus, in the caudal pons, innervates the lateral rectus muscle, which rotates the ipsilateral (same side) eye laterally (abduction). The long pathway of CN VI along the floor of the cranial cavity from the pons to the orbit makes it vulnerable to damage from severe injury or fracture of the cranial base. Partial or complete damage to this nerve results in weakness or complete paralysis of the muscle. Medial gaze is normal, but the affected eye fails to rotate laterally with an attempted gaze toward the affected side, a condition called *medial strabismus*.

The CN IV (trochlear) nucleus, at the junction of the pons and midbrain, innervates the contralateral or opposite side superior oblique muscle, which rotates the top of the globe inward toward the nose, a movement called *intorsion*. In combination with other muscles, it also contributes strength to movement of the innervated eye downward and inward. The superior oblique muscle neurons cross over the roof of the midbrain, drop vertically through the roof of the cavernous sinus, and then enter the orbit. This short pathway rarely is damaged, and signs of dysfunction usually are the result of a small brain stem stroke affecting the CN IV nucleus or from damage to the midbrain-level vertical gaze networks.

The CN III (oculomotor) nucleus, which extends through a considerable part of the midbrain, contains clusters of LMNs for each of the five eye muscles it innervates: the ipsilateral superior rectus, inferior rectus, inferior oblique, and medial rectus. A fifth muscle, the levator palpebrae superioris, elevates the upper lid and is involved only in vertical gaze eye movements. As the eyes rotate upward, the upper lid is reflexively retracted, and in the downward gaze, the upper lid is lowered, restricting the exposure of the conjunctiva to air and reducing the effects of drying. The medial rectus, superior rectus, and inferior rectus rotate the eyes in the directions shown in Table 53-1. The inferior rectus is antagonistic to the superior rectus. Because of its plane of attachment to the globe, the inferior oblique rotates the eye in the frontal plane (*i.e.*, torsion), pulling the top of the eye laterally (*i.e.*, extorsion).

CONJUGATE EYE MOVEMENTS

The term *conjugate gaze* refers to the use of both eyes to look steadily in one direction. During conjugate eye movements, the optical axes of the two eyes are maintained parallel with

TABLE 53-1 ◆ Eye in Primary Position: Extrinsic Ocular Muscle Actions				
Muscle*	Innervation	Primary	Secondary	Tertiary
MR: medial rectus	III	Adduction		
LR: lateral rectus	VI	Abduction		
SR: superior rectus	III	Elevation	Intorsion	Adduction
IR: inferior rectus	III	Depression	Extorsion	Adduction
SO: superior oblique	IV	Intorsion	Depression	Abduction
IR: inferior oblique	III	Extorsion	Elevation	Abduction

*In the schema of the functional roles of the six extraocular muscles, the major directional force applied by each muscle is indicated on the top. These muscles are arranged in functionally opposing pairs per eye and in parallel opposing pairs for conjugate movements of the two eyes. The numbers associated with each muscle indicate the cranial nerve innervation: 3, oculomotor (III) cranial nerve; 4, trochlear (IV) cranial nerve; 6, abducens (VI) cranial nerve.

each other as the eyes rotate in their sockets. Although the conjugate reflexes are essential to efficient visual function during head movement or target movement, their circuitry is so deeply embedded in CNS function that they are present and can be elicited when the eyes are closed, during sleep, and in deep coma, and they function normally and accurately in congenitally blind persons.

Conjugate gaze movements include lateral gaze, vertical gaze, oblique gaze, and torsional gaze. Lateral gaze movements are in the horizontal plane and are controlled by lateral gaze centers. These gaze centers consist of interneurons in the abducens (CN VI) nucleus on the side of abduction (Fig. 53-15). Vertical gaze upward or downward is controlled by a vertical gaze center of interneurons in and near the oculomotor (CN III) nucleus. Oblique gaze involves a combination of lateral and vertical gaze controls. Torsional gaze movements involve ocular rotation around the optical axis of the eyes, and although they occur fre-

quently, they are more difficult to observe. The torsional gaze center involves interneurons in the bilaterally located trochlear (CN IV) nucleus on both sides. Each of these control centers maintains a moderate level of tonic activity (*i.e.,* low level of "spontaneous" action potentials) in each opposing pair of muscles. This maintains a neutral position of eye posture. More motor units are automatically recruited when an eye deviates from this neutral position. When released from a directional signal, the eyes automatically return to the neutral position.

Communication between the eye muscle nuclei of each side occurs primarily through the posterior commissure at the rostral end of the midbrain. Longitudinal communication among the three nuclei occurs along a fiber tract called the *medial longitudinal fasciculus* (MLF), which extends from the midbrain to the upper part of the spinal cord (see Fig. 53-15). Each pair of eye muscles is reciprocally innervated, by way of the MLF or other associated pathways, so that as one muscle contracts, the other relaxes. For example, the LMNs of CN VI produce lateral rotation (*i.e.,* abduction) of the left eye. Simultaneously, interneurons of the left CN VI, which communicate with the right CN III by way of the MLF, move the right eye medially (adduction). These MLF-linked communication paths are vulnerable to damage in the caudal midbrain and pons. Damage to the pontine MLF on one side results in a loss of this linkage such that lateral deviation in the ipsilateral eye no longer is linked to adduction on the contralateral side (*i.e.,* internuclear ophthalmoplegia). If the MLF is damaged bilaterally, the linkage is lost for lateral gaze in either direction.

Slow Conjugate Eye Movements

Slow conjugate gaze reflexes, which are integrated by the vestibular and visual systems, hold a steady visual fixation point on the fovea during brief head movements. The vestibular nuclei send controlling signals to the appropriate gaze centers, moving the eyes in the opposite direction to that of the head. These movements are at precisely the same rate as the head movement, thereby allowing the eyes to maintain a constant distant fixation point, whatever the direction of movement.

A specialized part of the conjugate gaze network, a nucleus in the floor of the fourth ventricle called the *nucleus prepositus hypoglossi*, converts the vestibular afferent signals into the appropriate velocity and range of gaze movements. This mechanism can adapt to alterations in vestibular input. Destruction of the vestibular nerve of one side results in a severe sensation of falling, reduced muscle tone, and nystagmus toward the damaged side. Adaptive recovery is rapid, with only minor signs remaining within a few weeks after damage. The adaptive mechanism involves vestibular afferent collaterals that project to the flocculus of the archicerebellum, which projects to the nucleus prepositus hypoglossi and to the vestibular nuclei. Destruction of this region of the cerebellar cortex prevents any further adaptive changes from occurring.

The vestibulo-ocular reflexes, although powerful, can be avoided or altered to some extent by learned forebrain mechanisms. For instance, spinning skaters and dancers learn to reduce the reflex by rotating their head in the di-

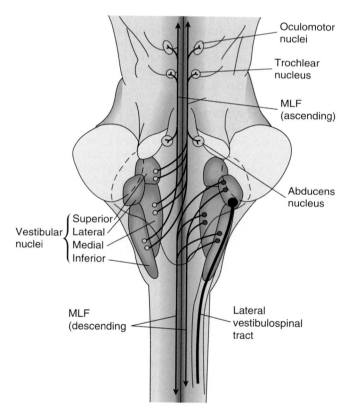

FIGURE 53-15 The ascending (*left*) and descending (*right*) vestibular pathways. Ipsilateral inhibitory and contralateral excitatory ascending projections from the vestibular nuclei course through the medial longitudinal fasciculus (MLF) and target motor neurons in the abducens, trochlear, and oculomotor nuclei. The ascending connections mediate the vestibulo-ocular reflex. Bilateral descending fibers in the MLF project primarily to motor neurons in the cervical spinal cord that innervate the dorsal neck muscles, forming the basis for the vestibulocochlear reflex. The lateral vestibulospinal tract arises from the lateral vestibular nuclei and descends ipsilaterally in the spinal cord, targeting primarily motor neurons that innervate axial extensor muscles that maintain posture. (Conn P.M. [1995]. *Neuroscience in medicine.* Philadelphia: J.B. Lippincott)

Figure labels: Oculomotor nuclei; Trochlear nucleus; MLF (ascending); Abducens nucleus; Vestibular nuclei — Superior, Lateral, Medial, Inferior; MLF (descending); Lateral vestibulospinal tract

rection opposite to the spin, reducing vestibular input and the conjugate movements. Fixing attention on a visual stimulus also can override the reflex.

The term *optokinetic* refers to eye movements that are driven by visual stimuli. The optokinetic slow gaze reflexes result in conjugate eye movements that follow a moving visual stimulus. These vestibulo-ocular reflexes hold the moving visual fixation point on the fovea while the head position remains stationary. They can be superseded by visual stimuli, if the stimulus has high contrast and high intensity. This reflex mechanism requires high-definition directional signals that move in consort as if the opposite were true (*i.e.*, as if the head were moving through a visual environment). Probably everyone has had the experience of moving through space, although the head is stationary, when a nearby bus or train moves in the opposite direction. If a rotating visual environment has less contrast, if the cortical visual system is functional, and if the person "attends" to a particular visual target in the moving visual field, optokinetic slow following of the target also occurs.

Conjugate following of a rotating visual environment can occur at a subcortical level or at a visual cortical level. Although the optokinetic conjugate eye movement reflexes provide a powerful experience of movement through space, they also operate in persons with damage to their visual cortex (*i.e.*, cortical blindness) but with functional subcortical visual reflex mechanisms. In this instance, visual perception of movement during the optokinetic conjugate movements does not occur.

Another class of slow conjugate gaze mechanisms are those involving smooth visual pursuit or tracking movements that maintain an object at a fixed point in the center of the visual fields of both eyes. The object may be moving and the eyes following it, or the object may be stationary and the head of the observer moving. In smooth pursuit, the visual cortical areas dominate and use the vestibular system's slow eye reflex systems through direct projections on the vestibular nuclei. The superior colliculus apparatus provides the specific directional motor control required to move the conjugate focal point to the moving target. The superior colliculus also operates through tectobulbar projection on the vestibular nuclei. Temporal and spatial smoothing adjustments are provided by visual cortical projections in the cerebellar vermis. Unlike the optokinetic reflexes, smooth visual pursuit reflexes depend on the perception of and attention to a clear, localized visual target. They do not occur with clouded vision or with cortical blindness. Testing for smooth pursuit requires the tester to move his or her finger or a small distinct target, such as a small flashlight, randomly in the plane of focus in front of the subject. While moving the target, the tester constantly observes whether the target-following conjugate gaze continuously (smoothly) follows the target location.

Fast Saccadic Eye Movements

Saccades are small, jerky movements that quickly move the eye from one point to another, allowing the entire visual field to be seen in a short time. When slow conjugate deviation reaches the limit to which the optic globes can rotate in the orbits, a reflex mechanism called *saccadic movement* occurs. This is an extremely rapid corrective conjugate rotation that functions in finding a new point at the edge of the visual field onto which fixation is shifted. Shifting or jumping from one point to another occurs at a rate of two to three jumps per second. During the saccade, a person does not experience the blur of the rapidly moving visual field. The mechanism by which visual experience is momentarily shut off is not understood. Saccades are a component of the vestibular, optokinetic, startle, and motor-driven scanning movements. Saccadic movements are automatic reflex movements that, in most situations, operate at the brain stem level.

Eye Tremor

An eye tremor refers to involuntary, rhythmic, oscillatory eye movements, occurring approximately 10 times per second. Because of this quivering motion, a constant movement of a stable optical image occurs over the retinal photoreceptors. Small-range optical tremors are a normal and useful independent function of each eye. Tremors occur because of the inequality in the number of motor units active at any moment that oppose the extraocular muscles. One function of the fine optic tremor is to constantly move a bright image onto a new bank of cones, permitting previously stimulated receptors quickly to recover from adaptation.

Optokinetic Nystagmus

The sequence of alternating slow ocular rotation and fast saccadic phase eye movements is called *optokinetic nystagmus*. This reflex occurs when a person fixates his or her vision on a uniformly moving visual stimulus pattern (*e.g.*, when a person is looking out of the side window of a railway car at objects in the seemingly moving scenery). Here, both eyes simultaneously follow the visual pattern as it moves in the opposite direction of that traveled by the train. When the object is no longer in view, a saccade returns the eyes to a new, more central fixation point. The same thing happens when a person tries to read the numbers on a measuring stick moved in front of him or her in a horizontal or vertical direction.

Optically induced nystagmus has been used to test visual acuity in infants and persons in whom conversation is ineffective. If the reflex can be induced by surrounding the infant with a set of rotating vertical black and white stripes, it suggests that the retinal and brain stem components are functional. The width of the stripes can then be systematically reduced until the reflex is lost, providing an objective, nonverbal method of testing the retinal level of visual acuity.

The Startle Reflex

Saccadic shifts of a gaze toward the source of a sudden, unexpected visual, auditory, tactile, or painful stimulus are a component of the startle pattern. This is functionally a visual grasping reflex, redirecting conjugate gaze in the direction of the startle stimulus. The startle saccade involves superior collicular domination of the conjugate gaze mechanism. Rapid head turning, turning of the body, and extension of the ipsilateral upper limb also occur. Learned shifting of conjugate gaze from one visual target to another involves the frontal eye fields under the domination of the motor, premotor, and prefrontal cortex. Visual input to the visual cortex and to the superior colliculus provides the required directional information. The frontal eye fields dominate the superior colliculus-saccadic gaze mechanism. Motor-driven shifts to a new visual target can occur only as saccades; therefore, blurs are not experienced.

Learned Motor Control of Saccadic Conjugate Eye Movements

Rapid, or saccadic, conjugate eye movements are not limited to vestibular, startle, or visual reflexes. A person learns to control the direction of visual fixation and to change from one fixation point to another during visual searching of the environment, as when reading a map or searching the woods for a singing bird. A specialized area of the lateral premotor cortex on the middle frontal gyrus, called the *frontal eye fields*, has direct control of saccadic eye movements (see Fig. 53-12). The frontal eye fields receive input from the visual cortex, the motion-sensitive parietal cortex (*i.e.*, parietal eye fields), the premotor cortex, and the lateral prefrontal cortex. Projections from the frontal eye fields are a part of the corticobulbar system, and they impinge on the directional motor fields of the superior colliculus and directly on the saccadic gaze centers. The frontal eye fields in each hemisphere control saccades toward the contralateral side and have subareas dedicated to the various directional dimensions of saccadic movement.

Frontal cortical control of saccadic eye movements becomes an integrated component of planned, learned motor patterns. A person learns to move her or his conjugate gaze smoothly from one fixation point to another fixation point. Instead the eyes always move between the fixation points in one saccade or a series of jerky saccades. This learned skill is an important but infrequently recognized aspect of the acquired motor skills necessary for daily survival. Motor control of saccadic eye movements supersedes vestibular system control, except during very rapidly accelerating head rotation.

VERGENCE EYE MOVEMENTS

Vergence (disconjugate) movements are those that move the eyes in opposite directions to keep the image of an object precisely positioned on the fovea of each eye. The vergence system is driven by retinal disparity (*i.e.*, differential placement of an object's image on each retina). A nearby target (<30 feet) moving in the same dimension as the optical axis elicits a reflex mechanism that provides redirection of the optical axes of each eye away from parallel (*i.e.*, in opposite directions) in the horizontal plane (*i.e.*, vergence gaze). This process permits a continued binocular focus on the near target. Convergence and divergence, which assist in maintaining a binocularly fixed image in near vision, have a major role in accurate depth perception. Perception of depth is a higher-order function of the cortical visual system and is based on one or more of several classes of stimuli, such as superimposition and relative movement. Retinal disparity, or differences in the retinal image of a visual target, is a major contributor to depth perception in near vision. Accurate depth perception is important for precise manipulation of tools or other objects with which humans are especially skilled.

> In summary, binocular vision depends on three pairs of extraocular muscles. These include the medial and lateral recti, which move the eye from side to side; the superior and inferior recti, which move the eye up and down; and the superior and inferior obliques, which rotate the eye around its optical axis. The extraocular muscles are innervated by three pairs of cranial nerves: (1) the trochlear nerve (CN IV), which innervates the superior oblique and turns the eye downward and laterally; (2) the abducens nerve (CN VI), which innervates the lateral rectus and moves the eye laterally; and (3) the oculomotor nerve (CN III), which innervates the medial rectus, which turns the eye medially, the superior rectus, which elevates the eye and rolls it upward, the inferior rectus, which depresses the eye and rolls it downward, and the inferior oblique, which elevates the eye and turns it laterally.
>
> For full visual function, it is necessary that the two eyes point toward the same fixation point and the two images become fused. Binocular fusion is controlled by ocular reflex mechanisms that adjust the orientation of each eye to produce a single image. The term *conjugate gaze* refers to the use of both eyes to look steadily in one direction. During conjugate eye movements, the optical axes of the two eyes are maintained parallel with each other as the eyes rotate upward, downward, or from side to side in their sockets. Saccadic eye movement consists of small jumping movements that represent rapid shifts in conjugate gaze orientation. The sequence of slow ocular rotation, a saccade, slow rotation, and so on is called *nystagmus*. Vergence movements (convergence and divergence) are necessary for maintaining the focus on a near image.

The Ear and Auditory and Vestibular Function

After you have completed this section of the chapter, you should be able to meet the following objectives:

✦ List the structures of the external, middle, and inner ear and cite their function
✦ Explain how the frequency and intensity of a tone are transformed into the experience of pitch at a particular level of sound
✦ Explain the function of the vestibular system with respect to postural reflexes and maintaining a stable visual field despite marked changes in head position

The ears are paired organs that are responsible for hearing and the maintenance of equilibrium and effective posture. Each ear consists of an external ear, a middle ear, and an inner ear. External and middle ear functions capture, transmit, and amplify sound. The inner ear contains the receptive organs that are selectively stimulated by sound waves (*i.e.*, hearing) or head position and motion (*i.e.*, vestibular function).

THE AUDITORY SYSTEM

Hearing is a specialized sense that provides the ability to perceive vibration of sound waves. Functions of the ear include receiving sound waves, distinguishing their frequency, translating this information into nerve impulses, and transmitting these impulses to the CNS. The auditory system can be divided into five parts: the external ear, the middle ear, the inner, auditory brain stem pathways, and the primary and auditory association cortices of the brain's temporal lobe.

The compression waves that produce sound have frequency and intensity. Frequency indicates the number of waves per unit time (reported in cycles per second [cps] or hertz [Hz]). Most persons cannot hear compression waves that have a frequency higher than 20,000 Hz. Waves of higher frequency are called *ultrasonic waves*, meaning that they are above the audible range. In the audible frequency range, the subjective experience correlated with sonic frequency is the pitch of a sound. Waves below

20 to 30 Hz are experienced as a rattle or drum beat rather than a tone. The human ear is most sensitive to waves in the frequency range of 1000 to 3000 Hz.

Wave intensity is represented by amplitude or units of sound pressure. By convention, the intensity (in power units, or ergs per square centimeter) of a sound is expressed as the ratio of intensities between the sound and a reference value. A 10-fold increase in sound pressure is called a bel, after Alexander Graham Bell. This representation often is too crude to be of use; the most often used unit is the decibel (dB), or 1/10 of a bel. In the normal sonic environment, approximately 1 dB of increased intensity (loudness) can be detected. The region of audible speech sounds falls between 42 and 70 dB.

External Ear

The external ear is called the *pinna*, or *auricle*. It is supported by elastic cartilage and shaped like a funnel. This funnel shape concentrates high-frequency sound entering from the lateral-forward direction into the external acoustic meatus, or ear canal (Fig. 53-16). This shape also helps to prevent front–back confusion of sound sources. The external ear canal extends from the auricle to the tympanic membrane, or eardrum. Its outer two thirds is supported by elastic cartilage, and its inner one third is supported by the temporal bone. It is "S" shaped and acts as a resonator, amplifying frequencies of approximately 3500 Hz. A thin layer of skin containing fine hairs, sebaceous glands, and ceruminous glands lines the ear canal. Ceruminous glands secrete cerumen, or earwax, which has certain antimicrobial properties and is thought to serve a protective function.

The anterior portion of the pinna and the external ear canal are innervated by branches of the mandibular division of the trigeminal nerve (CN V). Posterior portions of the ear, including the back of the external ear and the posterior wall of the ear canal, are innervated by auricular branches of the facial (CN VII), glossopharyngeal (CN IX), and vagus (CN X) nerves. Because of the vagal innervation, the insertion of a speculum or an otoscope into the external ear canal can stimulate coughing or vomiting reflexes, particularly in young children.

Middle Ear

The middle ear is a tiny cavity roughly the shape of a red blood cell set on edge. It occupies the petrous ("stony") portion of the temporal bone. Its lateral wall is formed by the tympanic membrane, and its medial wall is formed by the bone dividing the middle and inner ear. Posteriorly, the middle ear is connected with small air pockets in the temporal bone called *mastoid air spaces* or *cells*. In early life, these air spaces are filled with hematopoietic tissue. Replacement of hematopoietic tissue with air sacs begins during the third year of life and is completed at puberty. The eustachian tube, or auditory tube, connects the air-filled middle ear with the nasopharynx: it is lined with a mucous membrane that is continuous with the pharynx and mastoid air cells.

Three tiny bones, the auditory ossicles, are suspended from the roof of the middle ear cavity and connect the tympanic membrane with the oval window (see Fig. 53-17). They are connected by synovial joints and are covered with

Hearing

➤ Hearing is a special sensory function that incorporates the sound-transmitting properties of the external ear canal, the eardrum that separates the external and middle ear, the bony ossicles of the middle ear, the sensory receptors of the cochlea in the inner ear, the neural pathways of the vestibulocochlear or auditory nerve, and the primary auditory and auditory association cortices.

➤ The middle ear is an air-filled chamber that connects the external ear with the inner ear. It is separated from the external ear by the tympanic membrane, which transmits sound vibrations to the bony ossicles that amplify sound waves as they are transmitted to the fluid in the inner ear.

➤ The inner ear contains a fluid-filled membranous labyrinth with specialized sensory hair cells in the organ of Corti that function as the receptors for hearing.

➤ Afferent fibers from the hair cells in the organ of Corti travel through the vestibulocochlear nerve to the cochlear nucleus and then to central auditory pathways that merge with the auditory tracts that travel to the primary and associational cortices.

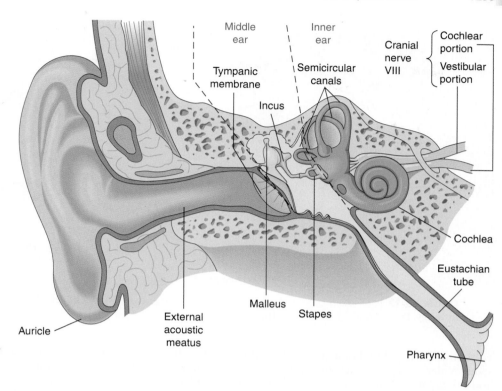

Middle
ear

Inner
ear

Tympanic
membrane

Semicircular
canals

Cranial
nerve
VIII

Cochlear
portion

Vestibular
portion

Incus

Cochlea

Eustachian
tube

Malleus

Stapes

External
acoustic
meatus

Auricle

Pharynx

FIGURE 53-16 External, middle, and internal subdivisions of the ear. (Modified from Chaffee E.E., Lytle I.M. [1980]. *Basic physiology and anatomy* [4th ed.]. Philadelphia: J.B. Lippincott)

the epithelial lining of the cavity. The *malleus* ("hammer") has its handle firmly fixed to the upper portion of the tympanic membrane. The head of the malleus articulates with the *incus* ("anvil"), which articulates with the *stapes* ("stirrup"), which is inserted and sealed into the oval window by an annular ligament. Arrangement of the ear ossicles is such that their lever movements transmit vibrations from the tympanic membrane to the oval window and from there to the fluid in the inner ear. Two tissue-covered openings in the medial wall, the oval and the round windows, provide for the transmission of sound waves between the air-filled middle ear and the fluid-filled inner ear. It is the piston-like action of the stapes footplate that sets up compression waves in the inner ear fluid.

Air and liquid offer different degrees of impedance (resistance) to the transmission of sound waves. The bones of the middle ear also serve as impedance-matching devices between the low impedance of the air and the high impedance of the cochlear fluid. This matching is accomplished by concentrating the pressure from the large area of the tympanic membrane (43 to 55 mm^2) to the small area of the oval window (approximately 3 mm^2); in addition, the air-transmitted sound waves are amplified into the force required to set up compression waves in the fluid of the inner ear. Amplification is accomplished by the ossicular lever system, which increases the pressures from the tympanic membrane to the oval window.

Two tiny skeletal muscles, the tensor tympani and the stapedius, insert into the ear ossicles. The tensor tympani, which is innervated by CN V, is positioned in the roof of the auditory tube and inserts on the handle of the malleus.

The functional role of this muscle is in dispute; however, the stapedius alters the movement of the stapes, reducing the displacement of fluid in the inner ear. The stapedial reflex, reflex contraction of this muscle by means of the facial nerve, provides a protective mechanism for the delicate inner ear structures when high-intensity sound occurs.

Inner Ear

The inner ear contains a labyrinth, or system of intercommunicating channels, and the receptors for hearing and position sense. An outer bony wall, the bony labyrinth, encloses a thin-walled, membranous duct system, the *membranous labyrinth* (Fig. 53-17). Two separate fluids are found in the inner ear. The *periotic fluid* or *perilymph* separates the bony labyrinth from the membranous labyrinth, and the *otic fluid* or *endolymph* fills the membranous labyrinth. Periotic fluid composition is similar to that of the CSF, and a tubular perilymphatic duct connects the periotic fluid with the CSF in the arachnoid space of the posterior fossa. Otic fluid has a potassium content that is similar to that of intracellular fluid. A small-diameter tubular extension, the endolymphatic sac, connects this system with the subdural space near the jugular foramen, providing an exit for the slowly circulating otic fluid.

The bony labyrinth occupies a volume with a diameter less than the size of a dime. It is divided into a series of perilymph-filled interconnected cavities: the cochlea, the semicircular ducts, the utricle, and the saccule. The membranous labyrinth floats in the bony labyrinth. Localized dilatations of the membranous labyrinth develop into three specialized sensory regions consisting of a columnar

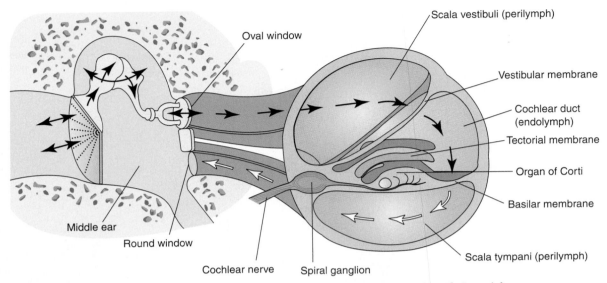

FIGURE 53-17 Path taken by sound waves reaching the inner ear. (Cormack D.H. [1993]. *Essential histology*. Philadelphia: J.B. Lippincott)

epithelium: the ciliated hair cells of the ampulla of each semicircular canal, the maculae of the utricle and sacculus, and the organ of Corti of the cochlear duct. The cochlea, which contains the auditory receptors, is enclosed in a bony tube shaped like a snail shell that winds around a central bone column called the *modiolus*. Receptors for head position sense are contained in the semicircular ducts, the utricle, and the saccule.

A membranous triangular cochlear duct stretches across the cochlea, separating it into two parallel tubes, each containing periotic fluid: the *scala vestibuli* and the *scala tympani* (Fig. 53-18). One side of the cochlear duct, the *basilar membrane*, stretches under tension laterally from the modiolus to an elastic spiral ligament. A second side, the *vestibular membrane (i.e.,* Reissner's membrane), is a delicate double layer of squamous epithelial cells. The third side

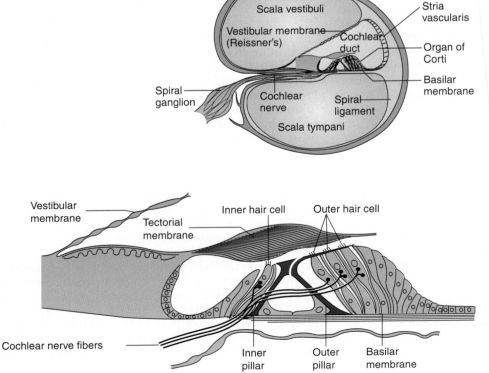

FIGURE 53-18 (**Top**) Portion of cochlea. Notice the relation of the cochlear duct to the scalae, vestibuli, and tympani. (**Bottom**) Spiral organ of Corti has been removed from the cochlear duct and greatly enlarged. (Modified from Chaffee E.E., Lytle I.M. [1980]. *Basic physiology and anatomy* [4th ed.]. Philadelphia: J.B. Lippincott)

consists of a well-vascularized epithelium, the *stria vascularis*, which is the source of otic fluid. The cochlear duct separates the scala vestibuli and the scala tympani from the base of the cochlea throughout its two and one-half spiral turns to its apex. An opening at the apex, called the *helicotrema*, permits fluid waves to move between the two scalae. Sound waves, delivered by the stapes footplate to the periotic fluid, travel throughout the fluid of the inner ear, including up the scala vestibuli, to the apex of the cochlea. These sound waves produce a fluid pressure wave leading to the compensatory displacements of the round window, thus compressing the air of the middle ear cavity and auditory canal.

The basilar membrane becomes progressively more massive from base to its distal apex and resonates to higher frequencies near the base and to lower frequencies toward the apex as the fluid pressure wave travels up the cochlear spiral. This "tuned" aspect of the basilar membrane results in increased amplitude of displacement at the resonant locations, responding to a particular sound frequency and greater firing of cochlear neurons innervating this region. This mechanism provides the major basis for the discrimination of sound frequency.

Perched on the basilar membrane and extending along its entire length is an elaborate arrangement of columnar epithelium called the *organ of Corti*. Continuous rows of hair cells separated into inner and outer rows can be found within the columnar arrangement. The cells have hairlike cilia that protrude through openings in an overlying supporting reticular membrane into the endolymph of the cochlear duct. A gelatinous mass, the tectorial membrane, extends from the medial side of the duct to enclose the cilia of the outer hair cells. The traveling compression waves moving from base to apex through the periotic fluid distort the organ of Corti, causing the hairs to bend against the less flexible tectorial membrane. Each inner hair cell is innervated by several nerve fibers, and the outer hair cells by many cochlear afferent neuron terminals.

Several theories exist concerning the transduction of mechanical sound into afferent nerve signals. These include the following mechanisms: (1) the vibrational effects of sound waves on the hair cells in the organ of Corti; and (2) the effects of the two ionically different fluids (*i.e.*, the periotic fluid and the otic fluid) on nerve impulse generation. It is generally agreed that the inner rows of hair cells, transducing different frequencies, are arranged sequentially, with those transducing the higher tones on the lower (basal) end of the cochlear duct, and those transducing lower tones near its apex (Fig. 53-19). Selective destruction of hair cells in a particular segment of the cochlea can lead to hearing loss of particular tones. The outer rows of hair cells appear to provide the signals on which the experience of loudness, a correlate of the sound's physical intensity, is based.

Neural Pathways

Afferent fibers from the organ of Corti have their cell bodies in the spiral ganglion in the central portion of the cochlea. Nerve fibers from the spiral ganglion (*i.e.*, vestibulocochlear or auditory nerve [CN VIII]) travel to the cochlear nuclei in the caudal pons. Many secondary nerve fibers from the

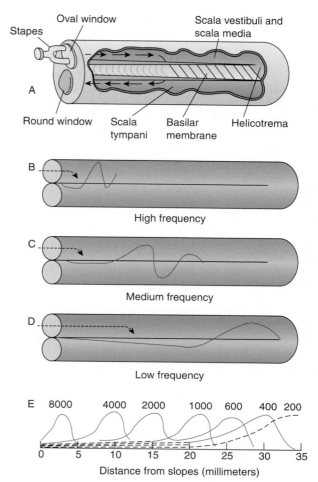

FIGURE 53-19 (**A**) Movement of fluid in the cochlea after forward thrust of the stapes. (**B,C,D**) "Traveling waves" along the basilar membrane for high-, medium-, and low-frequency sounds. (**E**) Amplitude pattern of vibration of the basilar membrane for a medium-frequency sound. Amplitude patterns for sounds of all frequencies between 200 and 8000 per second, showing the points of maximum amplitude (the resonance points) on the basilar membrane for the different frequencies. (Modified from Guyton A.C., Hall J.E. [1996]. *Textbook of medical physiology* [9th ed., pp. 665–666]. Philadelphia: W.B. Saunders)

cochlear nuclei pass to the opposite side of the pons. These secondary fibers may project to such cell groups as the trapezoid or the superior olivary nucleus, or rostrally toward the inferior colliculus of the midbrain. Ipsilateral projections and interconnections between the nuclei of the two sides occur throughout the central auditory system. Consequently, impulses from either ear are transmitted through the auditory pathways to both sides of the brain stem.

Many reflexes initiated by auditory stimuli involve the central auditory pathways in the brain stem. Very–high-intensity sound results in a protective stapedial reflex by which the movement of the middle ear ossicular chain is dampened, and this involves the trapezoid nuclei. Directional analysis of the sound based on comparison of the timing and intensity of the stimuli reaching the two ears initially occurs in the superior olivary nuclei. Sudden, intense sounds result in the auditory startle reflex in which the eyes, head, and body are suddenly turned toward the source, the ipsilateral shoulder is flexed, the elbow is extended, and body support is shifted to the contralateral leg. The heart rate rapidly increases, the skin blanches, the pupils dilate, and respiration stops momentarily. This startle response pattern involves the inferior colliculi, where the directional responses are organized. The trapezoid nuclei have extensive connections with the brain stem respiratory and cardiovascular centers, providing the linkage to the alarm aspects of the startle reflex.

From the inferior colliculus, the auditory pathway passes to the medial geniculate nucleus of the thalamus, where all the fibers synapse. Considerable evidence supports the capability of this level of organization to provide crude auditory experience, including crude tone and intensity discrimination and the directionality of a sound source. From the medial geniculate nucleus, the auditory tract spreads through the auditory radiation to the primary auditory cortex (area 41), located mainly in the superior temporal gyrus and insula (see Fig. 53-12). This area and its corresponding higher-order thalamic nucleus are required for high-acuity loudness discrimination and precise discrimination of pitch. The auditory association cortex (areas 42 and 22) borders the primary cortex on the superior temporal gyrus. This area and its associated higher-order thalamic nuclei are necessary for auditory gnosis, or the meaningfulness of sound, to occur. Experience and the precise analysis of momentary auditory information are integrated during this process.

THE VESTIBULAR SYSTEM

The vestibular receptive organs of the inner ear and their CNS connections contribute to the reflex activity necessary for effective posture and movement in a physical world governed by momentum and a gravitational field. The vestibular system senses motion and acceleration of the head. The vestibular system serves two general and related functions. It maintains and assists recovery of stable body and head position through control of postural reflexes, and it maintains a stable visual field despite marked changes in head position.

Peripheral Vestibular Structures

The peripheral apparatus of the vestibular system is contained in the bony labyrinth of the inner ear next to and continuous with the cochlea of the auditory system. The vestibular apparatus is divided into five prominent structures: three semicircular ducts, a utricle, and a saccule (Fig. 53-20). Receptors in these structures are differentiated into the angular acceleration-deceleration receptors of the semicircular ducts and the linear acceleration-deceleration and static gravitational receptors of the utricle and saccule. Both the utricle and saccule are widened membranous sacs in the bony vestibule. The utricle connects the ends of each semicircular duct, whereas the saccule communicates with the utricle through a small duct and with the cochlear duct of the auditory apparatus through the ductus reuniens.

Small patches of hair cells are located in the floor of the utricle (utricular macula), in the side wall of the saccule (sac-

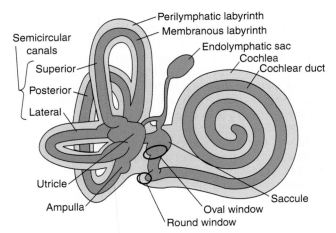

FIGURE 53-20 The labyrinth of the inner ear, showing the semicircular canals and the utricle and saccule, organs devoted to the sensation of rotary motion and static position. (Rhoades R.A., Tanner G.A. [1996]. *Medical physiology* [p. 83]. Boston: Little, Brown)

cular macula), at the base of each semicircular duct (cristae), and in the organ of Corti along the floor of the cochlear duct (Fig. 53-21). Each hair cell has several microvilli and one true cilium, called a *kinocilium*. At the apical end of each inner hair cell is a projecting bundle of rodlike structures called *stereocilia*. Ganglion cells, homologous with dorsal root ganglion cells, form three afferent ganglia: the superior vestibular ganglion, which innervates the hair cells of the utricular macula and the cristae of the superior and horizontal semicircular ducts; the inferior vestibular ganglion, which innervates the saccular macula and the cristae of the inferior semicircular duct; and the spiral, or acoustic, ganglion, which innervates the cochlear duct. The central axons of these ganglion cells become the superior and inferior vestibular nerves and the cochlear auditory nerve. They often are collectively called the *eighth cranial nerve*, and they enter the side of the nearby medullary-pontine junction of

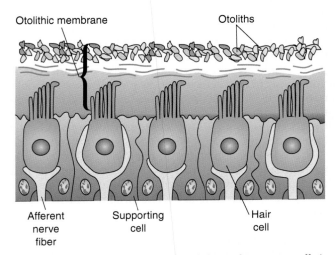

FIGURE 53-21 The relation of the otoliths to the sensory cells in the macula of the utricle and saccule. (Adapted from Selkurt F.D. [Ed.] [1982]. *Basic physiology for the health sciences* [2nd ed.]. Boston: Little, Brown)

the brain stem. Axons of the vestibular nerves terminate in the four vestibular nuclei (*i.e.*, superior, lateral, medial, and inferior vestibular nuclei).

Semicircular Ducts.   Three semicircular ducts, each subtending approximately two thirds of a circle, are arranged at right angles to one another, with the horizontal duct tilted approximately 12 degrees above the normal horizontal plane of the head (see Fig. 53-20). The horizontal ducts on the two sides of the head are in the same plane, whereas the superior (anterior) duct of one side is parallel with the inferior (posterior) duct on the other side, and the two function as a pair. Near its junction with the utricle, each semicircular duct has an enlargement, called the *ampulla*. Each ampulla contains a hair cell sensory surface raised into a crest, or crista, at right angles to the duct. The stereocilia of each hair cell extend into a flexible gelatinous mass, called the *cupula*, which essentially closes off fluid flow through the semicircular ducts.

When the head begins to rotate around the axis of a semicircular duct (*i.e.*, undergoes angular acceleration), the momentum of the otic fluid causes an increase in pressure on one side of the cupula. This is similar to the lagging behind of the water in a glass that is suddenly rotated, except that the otic fluid cannot flow past the cupula. Instead, the otic fluid applies a differential pressure to the two sides of the cupula, bending it and the stereocilia of the hair cells. All of the hair cells face in the same direction; when the stereocilia are bent toward the kinocilium, the frequency of action potentials in the primary afferent vestibular neuron leaving the ampulla is increased. Bending the hair cells in the other direction decreases the action potential frequency. Action potentials in the vestibular afferents are transmitted past the vestibular ganglia through the vestibular nerve (CN VIII) to the vestibular nuclei of the caudal pons.

Maximal stimulation of the afferents of a semicircular duct results when rotation of the head occurs exactly in the plane of the membranous duct. Because of the orientation of the semicircular ducts, angular accelerations of the head result in action potentials in at least one and usually more than one of the vestibular nerve branches to the three cristae. If the angular acceleration is reduced to a steady angular velocity, friction between the otic fluid and the duct wall gradually results in a reduction of pressure. Because of this pressure reduction, there is a loss of differential pressure on both sides of the cupula. This results in a form of sensory adaptation. On sudden reduction or cessation of head rotation, the momentum of the otic fluid applies pressure on the cupula from the opposite direction. The semicircular duct system provides a mechanism for signaling the direction and rate of accelerations and decelerations in head rotation to the CNS.

Utricle and Saccule.   The hair cell surface (*i.e.*, macula) of the utricle is oriented approximately in the horizontal plane. At right angles to the utricle, the macula of the saccule is oriented in the vertical plane. In both instances, the stereocilia of the hair cells extend into a gelatinous mass in the otic fluid. Myriad microscopic crystals of calcium carbonate and calcium phosphate, called *otoliths*, are embed-

ded in this gelatinous material, adding considerably to its total mass. The gelatinous mass with its otoliths is called the *otolithic membrane*. When the head is tilted, the gelatinous mass shifts its position because of the pull of the gravitational field, bending the stereocilia of the macular hair cells. Although each hair cell becomes hyperpolarized (less excitable) or hypopolarized (more excitable) depending on the direction in which the cilia are bending, the hair cells are oriented in all directions, making these sense organs sensitive to static or changing head position in relation to the gravitational field. Central connections from the maculae provide the mechanism by which head, body, and eye postural adjustments occur in response to tilting the head, maintaining a stable visual fixation point in the optic field and postural support of a stable head position. Projections to the forebrain provide the basis for sensations of head tilt away from the horizontal plane.

Besides this static tilt reception function, the utricle and saccule provide linear acceleration and deceleration reception. Differential movement between the head and the otolithic membranes provides the basis for compensatory reflex bracing of neck, trunk, and limbs. This happens when the head is accelerated linearly, such as the initial or terminal phase of an elevator ride or during automobile acceleration or deceleration. The utricle and saccule also provide the input data on which the air-righting reflexes are based. A cat dropped from an upside-down position lands on its feet and would do so even if blindfolded. Most vestibular reflexes, including air-righting, are functional at birth. If a neonate is supported in the prone position and the support is momentarily (and with great care) removed, the trunk and all four limbs are extended as falling begins. In the supine position, the trunk is flexed and the limbs are flexed as the fall progresses. However, the head-on-body vestibular reflexes of the infant are not sufficiently operational during the first 6 weeks or so after birth to maintain head posture. This is why the neonate's head must be supported when the neonate is lifted in the supine position.

Neural Pathways

The nerve fibers from the vestibular receptors travel in the vestibular portion of the vestibulocochlear nerve (CN VIII) to the superior, medial, lateral, and inferior vestibular nuclei at the junction of the medulla and pons (see Fig. 53-15). Primary vestibular afferent axons project to two areas of the cerebellar cortex: the midline, or vermis, and the flocculus. Vermal projections contribute to head, body, and limb coordination by providing constant information on head position relative to gravity and on linear or angular head velocity or acceleration. The floccular projection is part of the network that provides adaptability to the system, such as compensation for asymmetric function due to unilateral damage.

Neurons from the vestibular nuclei also project into the nearby reticular formation and provide powerful control for postural reflexes of the eyes, head, body, and limbs. Projections extend into the pons lateral gaze control center and to the vertical and torsional gaze control regions. These projections also extend to the trochlear cranial nerve nuclei, to the previously described MLF that extends from the midbrain to the upper part of the spinal cord, to the abducens and oculomotor nerve nuclei, and to cervical-level LMNs innervating the sternocleidomastoid and other neck muscles that control head turning and posture. The MLF projections primarily control horizontal or lateral turning and conjugate gaze. Extensive projections into and through the reticular formation follow the central tegmental fasciculus pathway that controls the vertical and rotatory (torsion) gaze reflexes.

The term *nystagmus* is used to describe the involuntary rhythmic and oscillatory eye movements that preserve eye fixation on stable objects in the visual field during angular and rotational movements of the head. These vestibular-controlled eye movements are initiated by impulses generated by the movement of the otic fluid in the semicircular ducts. This movement is transmitted to the vestibular nuclei and relayed through the MLF to the appropriate extraocular motor nuclei for controlling conjugate eye movement. As discussed in the section on extraocular eye movements, as the body and head begin rotation, the eyes move in a conjugate manner in exactly the opposite direction, maintaining the previous fixation point (Fig. 53-22). This is called the *slow phase of nystagmus.* If the rotation continues beyond the range of lateral eye movement, a quick (*i.e., rapid phase*

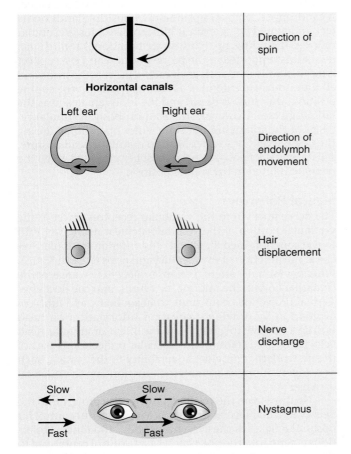

FIGURE 53-22 Effect of spinning a subject clockwise. (Sekurt F.E. [1982]. *Basic physiology for the health professions* [2nd ed., p. 140]. Boston: Little, Brown)

of nystagmus) conjugate eye correction (*i.e.,* saccadic return) occurs as if to obtain a new stable fixation point; afterward, the slow phase is reestablished. This nystagmus pattern continues as long as angular acceleration continues. When a steady rotational velocity is reached, compensatory nystagmus movements gradually wane as the disparity between the movement of endolymph and the semicircular duct wall is lost and the pressure on the two sides of the cupula is equalized. Clinically, the direction of nystagmus is named for the fast, or saccadic phase. The reflex circuitry is in precise control of motor units in the nuclei that innervate the extrinsic eye muscles by way of CNs III, IV, and VI. The precision of nystagmus movements is as great in persons whose eyes are closed and in the congenitally blind as in normal-sighted persons. If the eyes are not allowed to move, or if stimulation is strong, the head also moves in a nystagmus-like way because of vestibular control of the sternocleidomastoid muscles by CN XI.

Nystagmus can be classified according to the direction of eye movement: horizontal, vertical, rotary (torsional), or mixed. If head rotation is continued, friction between otic fluid and semicircular duct walls results in otic fluid rotating at the same velocity as the head, and nystagmus adapts to a stable eye posture. If rotation is suddenly stopped, vestibular nystagmus reappears in the direction precisely opposite to the angular accelerating nystagmus. This results because the inertia of the otic fluid is again bending ampullar hair cells of a now stationary ampulla. Because the observer does not have to rotate the subject, demonstration of postrotatory nystagmus often is used to evaluate the function of vestibular reflexes. Nystagmus always is abnormal if it occurs spontaneously or is sustained. Nystagmus eye movements can be tested by rotation or caloric stimulation (see Chapter 55).

Thalamic and Cortical Projections. Some neurons of the vestibular nuclei project their axons rostrally to the ventrolateral nuclei of the thalamus. Projections also go to the primary vestibular cortex near the somesthetic area of the parietal lobe. These thalamic and cortical projections provide the basis for the subjective experiences of position in space, rotation, and vertigo that accompany the onset or sudden cessation of head rotation. During such episodes, nystagmus is observed.

Postural Reflexes

Sudden changes in balance or orientation, such as falling to the right or left or backward or forward, result in powerful reflexes needed to maintain equilibrium and posture. The descending portion of the MLF, essentially a medial vestibulospinal tract, continues at least into thoracic cord levels and provides vestibular control of the muscle tone of axial muscles, including the dorsal back muscles. A rapidly conducting lateral vestibulospinal tract descends in or within the spinal cord to provide powerful vestibular control of the LMNs of the upper and lower limbs. As the head begins to tip (*i.e.,* rotate) on the neck or moves as part of general body tipping, the vestibular system activates the appropriate extensor muscles of the neck, trunk, and limbs, opposing the direction of the tilt. These powerful reflex adjustments in muscle tone assist in maintaining stable head and therefore body postural support during static posture and during passive or active movement.

All the vestibular nuclei receive input from the cerebellum and the vestibular nerve. The cerebellar connections of the vestibular system are necessary for adjustments of temporally smooth, coordinated movements to ongoing head movement, tilt, or angular acceleration. For instance, accurate grasping can occur during a fall, indicating cerebellar adjustments based on vestibular information during the performance of a smooth, accurate movement.

Vestibular reflexes are powerful, and considerable learning is required to inhibit or greatly modify them, as is necessary for acrobatic pilots, divers, and gymnasts. Dancers and skaters who engage in rapid spinning movements also learn to use or at least partially inhibit these reflexes.

Doll's-Head Eye Response

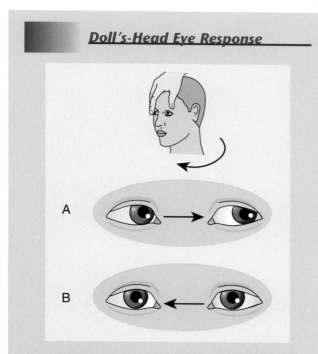

The *doll's-head eye response* demonstrates the always-present vestibular static reflexes without forebrain interference or suppression. Severe damage to the forebrain or to the brain stem rostral to the pons often results in loss of rostral control of these static vestibular reflexes. If the person's head is moved from side to side or up and down, the eyes will move in conjugate gaze to the opposite side (**A**), much like those of a doll with counterweighted eyes. If the doll's-head phenomenon is observed, brain stem function at the level of the pons is considered intact (in a comatose person). In the unconscious person without intact brain stem function and vestibular static reflexes, the eyes stay in midposition (fixed) or turn in the same direction (**B**) as the head is turned.

In summary, hearing is a specialized sense whose external stimulus is the vibration of sound waves. Our ears receive sound waves, distinguish their frequencies, translate this information into nerve impulses, and transmit them to the CNS. Anatomically, the auditory system consists of the outer ear, middle ear, and inner ear, the auditory pathways, and the auditory cortex. The middle ear is a tiny air-filled cavity in the temporal bone. A connection exists between the middle ear and the nasopharynx. This connection, called the *auditory tube*, allows equalization of pressure between the middle ear and the atmosphere. The inner ear contains the receptors for hearing.

The vestibular system plays an essential role in the equilibrium sense, which is closely integrated with the visual and proprioceptive (position) senses. Receptors for the vestibular system, in the semicircular ducts of the inner ear, respond to changes in linear and angular acceleration of the head. The vestibular nerve fibers travel in CN VIII to the vestibular nuclei at the junction of the medulla and pons; some fibers pass through the nuclei to the cerebellum. Cerebellar connections are necessary for temporally smooth, coordinated movements during ongoing head movements, tilt, and angular acceleration. The vestibular nuclei also connect with nuclei of the oculomotor (CN III), trochlear (CN IV), and abducens (CN VI) nerves. Vestibular control of conjugate eye movements preserves eye fixation on stable objects in the visual field during head movement. *Nystagmus* is a term used to describe vestibular-controlled eye movements that occur in response to angular and rotational movements of the head. Neurons of the vestibular nuclei also project to the thalamus, to the temporal cortex, and to the somesthetic area of the parietal cortex. The thalamic and cortical projections provide the basis for the subjective experiences of position in space and of rotation and vertigo.

Related Web Sites

Anatomy, Physiology and Pathology of the Human Eye
    members.aol.com/MonT714/tutorial/the_eye
History of Ophthalmology www.mrcophth.com/
    Historyofophthalmology
Ophthalmology Times http://www.findarticles.com/cf_1/
    m0VEY/10_25/62302869/print.jhtml
Retina International www.irpa.org

Bibliography

Brodal P. (1998). *The central nervous system: Structure and function* (2nd ed., pp. 245–295). New York: Oxford University Press.

Evans N.M. (1995). *Ophthalmology* (2nd ed.). New York: Oxford University Press.

Forrester J., Dick A., McMenamin P., Lee W. (1996). *The eye: Basic sciences in practice* (p. 208). Philadelphia: W.B. Saunders.

Goldberg M.E. (2000). The vestibular system. In Kandel E.R., Schwartz J.H., Jessel T.M. (Eds.), *Principles of neural science* (4th ed., pp. 801–815). New York: McGraw-Hill.

Goldberg M.E., Hudspeth A.J. (2000). Control of gaze. In Kandel E.R., Schwartz J.H., Jessel T.M. (Eds.), *Principles of neural science* (4th ed., pp. 782–800). New York: McGraw-Hill.

Guyton A.C., Hall J.E. (2000). *Textbook of medical physiology* (10th ed., pp. 566–612). Philadelphia: W.B. Saunders.

Marieb E.N. (2001). *Human anatomy and physiology* (5th ed., pp. 564–602). San Francisco: Addison Wesley Longman.

Martini F.H. (2001). *Fundamentals of anatomy and physiology* (5th ed., pp. 538–575). Upper Saddle River, NJ: Prentice Hall.

Oyster C.W. (1999). *The human eye: Structure and function.* Sunderland, MA: Sinauer Associates.

Pocock G., Richards C.D. (1999). *Human physiology: The basis of medicine* (pp. 118–143). Oxford: Oxford University Press.

Rind F.C., Simmons P.J. (1999). Seeing what is coming: Building collision-sensitive neurones. *Trends in Neuroscience 22,* 215–220.

Sanes D.H., Reh T.A., Harris W.A. (2000). *Development of the nervous system* (pp. 421–430). San Diego: Academic Press.

Sharpe L.T., Stockman A. (1999). Rod pathways: The importance of seeing nothing. *Trends in Neuroscience 22,* 497–504.

Spencer R.F. (1995). The oculomotor system. In Conn P.M. (Ed.), *Neuroscience in medicine* (pp. 249–260). Philadelphia: J.B. Lippincott.

Thibodeau G.A., Patton K.T. (1999). *Anatomy and physiology* (4th ed., pp. 454–473). St. Louis: Mosby.

Van De Graaff K.M., Fox S.I. (1999). *Concepts of human anatomy and physiology* (5th ed,. pp. 512–547). New York: McGraw-Hill.

Wong-Riley, M.T.T. (2000). *Neuroscience secrets* (pp. 69–140). Philadelphia: Hanley & Belfus.

Zigmond M.J., Bloom F.E., Landis S.C., Roberts J.L., Squire L.R. (1999). *Fundamental neuroscience* (pp. 791–849). San Diego: Academic Press.

Zolton B. (1996). *Vision, perception, and cognition* (3rd ed.). Thorofare, NJ: Slack.

Chapter 54

Alterations in Vision

Edward W. Carroll and Sheila M. Curtis

Almost 17.3 million persons in the United States have some degree of visual impairment; of these, 1.1 million are legally blind.[1] The prevalence of vision impairment increases with age. An estimated 26% of persons 75 years of age and older report visual impairment severe enough to interfere with recognizing a friend across the room or reading newspaper print even when wearing glasses.[1] At the other end of the age spectrum, an estimated 95,100 children younger than 18 years of age are severely visually impaired.[1]

Alterations in vision can result from disorders of the orbit and surrounding structures, intraocular pressure (glaucoma), lens (cataract), vitreous and retina, visual pathways and visual cortex, and extraocular muscles and eye movement. Visual impairment due to common types of eye disorders is illustrated in Figure 54-1.

Disorders of the Orbit and Surrounding Structures

After you have completed this section of the chapter, you should be able to meet the following objectives:

✦ Differentiate exophthalmos from proptosis
✦ Define *entropion* and *ectropion*
✦ Explain the differences between marginal blepharitis, a hordeolum, and a chalazion in terms of causes and manifestations
✦ State the causes and treatment of dry eye

Because the walls of the orbit are rigid, any space-occupying lesion results in protrusion of the eyeball, a condition called *exophthalmos*. Exophthalmos may be caused

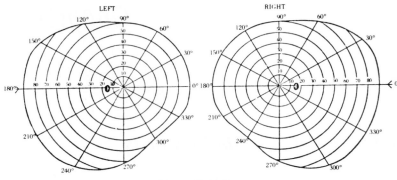

THE FIELD OF VISION (peripheral vision) with both eyes is 180° recorded on these charts.

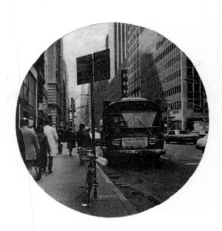

NORMAL VISION A person with normal or 20/20 vision sees this street scene.

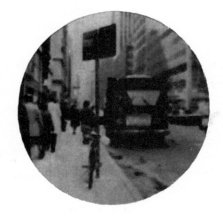

CATARACT Diminished acuity from an opacity of the lens. The field of vision is unaffected. There is no scotoma, but the person has an overall haziness of the view, particularly in glaring light conditions.

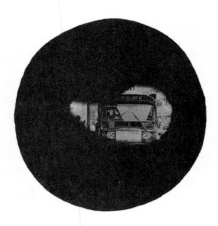

GLAUCOMA Advanced glaucoma involves loss of peripheral vision but the individual still retains most of his central vision.

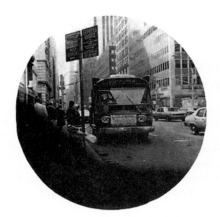

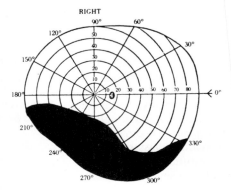

RETINAL DETACHMENT shown here in the active stage. There are many causes for detachment, but the hole or tear allows fluid to lift the retina from its normal position. This elevated retina causes a field or vision defect, seen as a dark shadow in the peripheral field. It may be above, or below as illustrated.

FIGURE 54-1 Photographs representing the eye diseases, done as if the camera were the right eye. The accompanying visual field chart showing the area of visual loss also represents the right eye. (Photo courtesy The Lighthouse, The New York Association for the Blind)

by swelling or trauma of orbital tissues, tumors of the orbit, or forward displacement of the eye because of endocrine disorders of pituitary or hypothalamic origin. It commonly is seen in persons with a form of hyperthyroidism called *Graves' disease* (see Chapter 40). When the eyelid also protrudes, the condition is known as *proptosis*. This condition causes a delay in lid closure (*i.e.*, lid lag) and, in severe cases, prevents the lids from closing completely, which results in constant exposure and subsequent drying of the cornea. Because the optic nerve has sufficient length in the orbit, protrusion greater than 5 mm is required before nerve damage occurs.

Enophthalmos, or deeply sunken eyes, may be an individual characteristic, but the condition also occurs with severe loss of orbital fat during malnutrition and starvation. Severe developmental defects during the first month of fetal life can result in the absence of one or both optic globes, called *anophthalmos*, and growth defects during the last 3 months of gestation can result in abnormally small eyes, called *microphthalmos*.

DISORDERS OF THE EYELIDS

The two striated muscles that provide movement of the eyelids are the levator palpebrae superioris and the orbicularis oculi, which is a circular ring of muscle that surrounds the eye (see Chapter 53). The levator palpebrae, which is innervated by the oculomotor cranial nerve (cranial nerve [CN] III), raises the upper lid. The orbicularis oculi, which is supplied by the facial nerve (CN VII), closes the lid. The palpebral portion of this muscle is used for gentle closure, and the orbital portion is used for forcible closure of the lids.

Eyelid Weakness

Drooping of the eyelid is called *ptosis*. It can result from weakness of the levator muscle that elevates the upper lid in conjunction with the unopposed action of the orbicularis oculi that forcefully closes the palpebral fissure. Weakness of the orbicularis oculi causes an open eyelid, but not ptosis. Neurologic causes of eyelid weakness include damage to the innervating cranial nerves or to the nerves' central nuclei in the midbrain and the caudal pons. Interruption of sympathetic innervation from the superior cervical ganglion to the smooth muscle in the upper eyelid can cause a mild form of ptosis, called *pseudoptosis*.

The facial nerve (CN VII) reaches the orbicularis oculi after exiting the skull under the parotid gland and traveling deep to the skin across the face. Trauma to the zygomatic and buccal branches of the facial nerve with resultant weakness of the orbicularis oculi muscle is relatively common. Weakness of the orbicularis oculi is tested by placement of the examiner's fingers on the muscular sphincter ring while the eye is open and then asking the person to close the eye. Bell's palsy, which involves paralysis of muscles on one side of the face due to a lesion of the facial nerve or its nucleus in the caudal pons, may result in eyelid weakness, hyperacusis (*i.e.*, acute sense of hearing or painful sensitivity to sound), and disorders of lacrimation and salivation from involvement of the lacrimal, submandibular, and sublingual glands.

Damage to the oculomotor nerve is much less common than damage to the facial nerve because the oculomotor nerve is protected by the skull throughout its path. However, ptosis resulting from CN III injury can occur in cases of midbrain stroke and basal skull fractures and from tumors located deep in the orbit or in the cavernous sinus.

Normally, the edges of the eyelids, or palpebrae, are in such a position that the palpebral conjunctiva that lines the eyelids is not exposed and the eyelashes do not rub against the cornea. Turning in of the lid is called *entropion*. It is usually caused by scarring of the palpebral conjunctiva or degeneration of the fascial attachments to the lower lid that occurs with aging. Turning inward of the eyelashes causes corneal irritation. *Ectropion* refers to eversion of the lower lid. The condition usually is bilateral and caused by relaxation of the orbicularis oculi muscle because of CN VII weakness or the aging process. Ectropion causes tearing and ocular irritation and may lead to inflammation of the cornea.

Entropion and ectropion can be treated surgically. Electrocautery penetration of the lid conjunctiva also can be used to treat mild forms of ectropion. Contraction of the scar tissue that follows tends to draw the lid up to its normal position.

Eyelid Inflammation

Blepharitis is a bilateral inflammation of the eyelid margins. Anterior blepharitis involves the eyelid skin, eyelashes, and associated glands. There are two main types of anterior blepharitis: seborrheic and staphylococcal. The seborrheic form usually is associated with seborrhea (*i.e.*, dandruff) of the scalp or brows. Staphylococcal blepharitis may be caused by *Staphylococcus aureus*, in which case it often is ulcerative, *Staphylococcus epidermidis*, or a coagulase-negative staphylococci.[2] The chief symptoms are irritation, burning, redness, and itching of the eyelid margins. Treatment includes careful cleaning with a wet applicator or clean washcloth to remove the scales. A nonirritating baby shampoo can be used. When the disorder is associated with a microbial infection, an antibiotic ointment is prescribed.

Posterior blepharitis is inflammation of the eyelids secondary to dysfunction of the meibomian glands. There may be bacterial infection, particularly with staphylococci. The lid margins are red and swollen. The meibomian glands and their orifices are inflamed, with dilation of the glands and abnormal secretions. The lid margins often are rolled inward to produce mild entropion, and the tears may be frothy and abnormally greasy from the meibomian secretions. Treatment of posterior blepharitis is determined by associated conjunctival and corneal changes. Long-term, low-dose systemic antibiotic therapy guided by results of bacterial cultures along with short-term topical steroids may be needed.

A hordeolum, or stye, is caused by infection of the sebaceous glands of the eyelid and can be internal or external. The main symptoms are pain, redness, and swelling. The treatment is similar to that for abscesses in other parts of the body. Heat in the form of warm compresses is applied, and antibiotic ointment may be used. Incision or expression of the infectious contents of the abscess may be necessary.

A chalazion is a granulomatous inflammation of a meibomian gland that may follow an internal hordeolum. It is characterized by a small, nontender nodule on the upper or lower lid. The conjunctiva in the area of the chalazion is red and elevated. If the chalazion is large enough, it may press on the eyeball and distort vision. Treatment consists of surgical excision.

DISORDERS OF THE LACRIMAL SYSTEM

Tears form a thin film that covers the cornea and conjunctival epithelium. The lacrimal system includes the major lacrimal gland, which produces the tears, the puncta and tear sac, which collect the tears, and the nasolacrimal duct, which empties the tears into the nasal cavity. The lacrimal gland lies in the orbit, superior and lateral to the eyeball (see Chapter 53, Fig. 53-4). Approximately 12 small ducts connect the lacrimal gland to the superior conjunctival fornix. Tears contain approximately 98% water, 1.5% sodium chloride, and small amounts of potassium, albumin, and glucose. The function of tears is to make a smooth optical surface by abolishing minute surface irregularities, to wet and protect the delicate surface of the cornea and conjunctiva, to flush and remove irritating substances and microorganisms, and to provide the cornea with necessary nutrient substances.[2] Tears also contain lysozymes and immunoglobulin A (IgA), IgG, and IgE, which synergistically act to protect against infection. Although IgA predominates, IgE concentrations are increased in some allergic conditions.[2]

Dry Eyes

The thin film of tears that covers the cornea is essential in preventing drying and damage of the outer layer of the cornea. The tear film is composed of three layers: the superficial lipid layer, derived from the meibomian glands and thought to retard evaporation; the aqueous layer, secreted by the lacrimal glands; and the mucinous layer, which overlies the cornea and epithelial cells.[2] Because the epithelial cell membranes are relatively hydrophobic and cannot be wetted by aqueous solutions alone, the mucinous layer plays an essential role in wetting these surfaces. Periodic blinking of the eyes is needed to maintain a continuous tear film over the ocular surface. Disruption of any of the tear film components or of the blinking action of the eyelids can lead to the interruption of the tear film and result in dry spots on the cornea.

Several conditions reduce the functioning of the lacrimal glands. With aging, the lacrimal glands tend to diminish their secretion, and as a result, many older persons awaken from a night's sleep with highly irritated eyes. Dry eyes also result from loss of reflex lacrimal gland secretion because of congenital defects, infection, irradiation, damage to the parasympathetic innervation of the gland, and medications such as antihistamines and drugs with an anticholinergic action. Wearing contact lenses tends to contribute to eye dryness through decreased blinking.

Sjögren's syndrome is a systemic disorder in which lymphocytes and plasma cells infiltrate the lacrimal and parotid glands. The disorder is associated with diminished salivary and lacrimal secretions, resulting in keratoconjunctivitis sicca (dry eye syndrome) and xerostomia (*i.e.*, dry mouth). The syndrome occurs mainly in women near menopause and often is associated with connective tissue disorders such as rheumatoid arthritis. Persons with dry eyes complain of a dry or gritty sensation in the eye, burning, itching, inability to produce tears, photosensitivity, redness, pain, and difficulty in moving the eyelids. Dry eyes and the absence of tears can cause keratinization of the cornea and conjunctival epithelium. In severe cases, corneal ulcerations can occur. Consequent corneal scarring can cause blindness.

The treatment of dry eyes includes frequent instillation of artificial tear solutions into the conjunctival sac. More prolonged duration of action can be obtained from topical preparations containing methylcellulose or polyvinyl alcohol. An ointment is useful for prolonged lubrication. In general, these artificial tear preparations are safe and without side effects. However, the preservatives necessary to maintain their sterility can be irritating to the cornea.[2,3]

Dacryocystitis

Dacryocystitis is an infection of the lacrimal sac. It occurs most often in infants or in persons older than 40 years of age. It usually is unilateral and most often occurs secondary to obstruction of the nasolacrimal duct. Often the cause of the obstruction is unknown, although there may be a history of severe trauma to the midface. The symptoms include tearing and discharge, pain, swelling, and tenderness. The treatment includes application of warm compresses and antibiotic therapy. In chronic forms of the disorder, surgical repair of the tear duct may be necessary.

In infants, dacryocystitis usually is caused by failure of the nasolacrimal ducts to open spontaneously before birth. When one of the ducts fails to open, a secondary dacryocystitis may develop. These infants usually are treated with gentle massage of the tear sac, instillation of antibiotic drops into the conjunctival sac, and, if that fails, probing of the tear duct.

In summary, the optic globe, or eyeball, is protected posteriorly by the bony structures of the orbit and anteriorly by the eyelids. It is continuously bathed by a protective film of tears. Protrusion of the eyes is called *exophthalmos*, and the condition of deeply sunken eyes is called *enophthalmos*.

The eyelids serve to protect the eye. Entropion, which refers to turning in the upper eyelid and eyelashes, is discomforting and causes corneal irritation. Ectropion, or eversion of the lower eyelid, causes tearing and the potential for corneal inflammation. Marginal blepharitis is the most common disorder of the eyelids. It commonly is caused by a staphylococcal infection or seborrhea (*i.e.*, dandruff). Ptosis refers to drooping of the upper lid, which is caused by injury to CN III. A milder form, pseudoptosis, can be caused by interruption of sympathetic innervation to portions of the principal elevator muscle of the upper eyelid (*i.e.*, levator palpebrae superioris).

The lacrimal system includes the major lacrimal gland, which produces the tears, the puncta and tear sac, which collect the tears, and the nasolacrimal duct, which empties the tears into the nasal cavity. Tears protect the cornea from drying and irritation. Impaired tear production or conditions that prevent blinking and the spread of tears produce drying of the eyes and predispose them to corneal irritation and injury. Dacryocystitis is an infection of the lacrimal sac.

Disorders of the Conjunctiva, Cornea, and Uveal Tract

After you have completed this section of the chapter, you should be able to meet the following objectives:

♦ Compare symptoms associated with red eye caused by conjunctivitis, corneal irritation, and acute glaucoma
♦ List at least four causes of red eye
♦ Describe the appearance of corneal edema
♦ Characterize the manifestations, treatment, and possible complications of bacterial, *Acanthamoeba*, and herpes keratitis

The outer wall of the eyeball (optic globe) is composed of the sclera, which is modified anteriorly to form the cornea, through which light rays enter the eye. The middle vascular layer, or uveal tract, of the eye includes the choroid, the ciliary body, and the iris. The choroid layer contains many of the blood vessels that nourish the structures of the eyeball. The choroid also contains many pigmented cells. These cells contain the pigment melanin, which absorbs stray light rays.

The conjunctiva is a thin layer of mucous membrane that lines the inner surface of the eyelid and covers the optic globe to the junction of the cornea and sclera.[2–4]

CONJUNCTIVITIS

Conjunctivitis, or inflammation of the conjunctiva (*i.e.*, red eye or pink eye), is one of the most common forms of eye disease. It varies from mild hyperemia with tearing (*i.e.*, hay fever conjunctivitis) to a severe necrotizing process (*i.e.*, membranous conjunctivitis). Conjunctivitis may result from bacterial or viral infection, allergens, chemical agents, physical irritants, or radiant energy. Infections may extend from areas adjacent to the conjunctiva or may be blood-borne, such as in measles or chickenpox. Newborns can contract conjunctivitis during the birth process.

The main symptoms of conjunctivitis are redness of the eye, which is most obvious peripherally; ocular discomfort or foreign body sensation; a gritty or burning sensation; and tearing. Severe pain suggests corneal rather than conjunctival disease. Itching is common in allergic conditions. A discharge, or exudate, may be present with all types of conjunctivitis and may cause transient blurring of vision. It usually is watery when the conjunctivitis is caused by al-

lergy, a foreign body, or viral infection and mucopurulent in the presence of bacterial or fungal infection. A characteristic of many forms of conjunctivitis is papillary hypertrophy. This occurs because the palpebral conjunctiva is bound to the tarsus by fine fibrils. As a result, inflammation that develops between the fibrils causes the conjunctiva to be elevated in mounds called *papillae*. When the papillae are small, the conjunctiva has a smooth, velvety appearance. A red papillary conjunctivitis suggests bacterial or chlamydial conjunctivitis. In allergic conjunctivitis, the papillae often become flat-topped, polygonal, and milky in color and have a cobblestone appearance.

The diagnosis of conjunctivitis is based on history, physical examination, and microscopic and culture studies to identify the cause. Because a red eye may be the sign of several eye conditions, it is important to differentiate between redness caused by conjunctivitis and that caused by more serious eye disorders, such as corneal lesions and acute glaucoma. In contrast to corneal lesions and acute glaucoma, conjunctivitis produces injection (*i.e.*, enlargement and redness) of the peripheral conjunctival blood vessels rather than those radiating around the corneal limbus, and it causes mild discomfort rather than moderate to severe discomfort associated with corneal lesions or the severe and deep pain associated with acute glaucoma. Conjunctivitis does not affect vision, nor does it cause pupillary dilation, as does acute glaucoma. It does not produce changes in the appearance of the cornea. The clarity of the cornea may be changed in corneal injury, depending on the cause, and is steamy or cloudy in acute glaucoma. Infectious forms of conjunctivitis often are bilateral and may involve other family members and close associates. Unilateral disease suggests sources of irritation such as foreign bodies or chemical irritation.

Infectious Conjunctivitis

Bacterial Conjunctivitis. Bacterial conjunctivitis may present as a hyperacute, acute, or chronic infection. Hyperacute conjunctivitis is a severe, sight-threatening ocular infection. The infection has an abrupt onset and is characterized by a copious amount of yellow-green drainage. The symptoms, which typically are progressive, include conjunctival redness and chemosis, lid swelling, and tender, swollen preaurical lymph nodes. The most common causes of hyperacute purulent conjunctivitis are *Neisseria gonorrhoeae* and *Neisseria meningitidis*, with *N. gonorrhoeae* being the most common.[3] Gonococcal ocular infections that are left untreated result in corneal ulceration with ultimate perforation, and sometimes permanent loss of vision.[3] Diagnostic methods include immediate Gram staining of ocular specimens and special cultures for *Neisseria* species. Treatment includes systemic antibiotics supplemented with ocular antibiotics. Because of the increasing prevalence of penicillin-resistant *N. gonorrhoeae*, antibiotic choice should be determined by current information regarding antibiotic sensitivity.

Acute conjunctivitis typically presents with burning, tearing, and mucopurulent or purulent discharge. Common agents of bacterial conjunctivitis are *Streptococcus pneu-*

moniae, S. aureus, and *Haemophilus influenzae.* The eyelids are sticky, and there may be excoriation of the lid margins. Treatment may include local application of antibiotics. The disorder usually is self-limited, lasting approximately 10 to 14 days if untreated. Scrupulous personal hygiene and prompt adequate treatment of infected persons and their contacts are effective.

Chronic bacterial conjunctivitis most commonly is caused by *Staphylococcus* species, although other bacteria may be involved. It often is associated with blepharitis and bacterial colonization of eyelid margins. The symptoms of chronic bacterial conjunctivitis vary and can include itching, burning, foreign body sensation, and morning eyelash crusting. There may be flaky debris and erythema along the lid margins, as well as eyelash loss and eye redness. Some people with chronic bacterial conjunctivitis also have recurrent styes and chalazia of the lid margins.[3] Treatment includes good eyelid hygiene and application of topical antibiotics.

Viral Conjunctivitis.   Etiologic agents of viral conjunctivitis include adenoviruses, herpesviruses, and enteroviruses. Adenovirus type 3 infection usually is associated with pharyngitis, fever, and malaise.[4,5] It causes generalized hyperemia, copious tearing, and minimal exudate. Children are affected more often than adults. Swimming pools contaminated because of inadequate chlorination are common sources of infection. Infections due to adenoviruses types 4 and 7 often are associated with acute respiratory disease. These viruses are rapidly disseminated when large groups mingle with infected individuals (*e.g.,* military recruits). Adenovirus type 8 epidemics are associated with inadequate sterilization of ophthalmic equipment. There is no specific treatment for this type of viral conjunctivitis; it usually lasts 7 to 14 days. Preventive measures include scrupulous personal hygiene and avoiding shared use of eyedroppers, eye makeup, goggles, and towels.

Herpes simplex virus conjunctivitis is characterized by unilateral infection, irritation, mucoid discharge, pain, and mild photophobia. Herpetic vesicles may develop on the eyelids and lid margins. Although the infection usually is caused by the type 1 herpesvirus, it also can be caused by the type 2 virus. It often is associated with herpes simplex virus keratitis, in which the cornea shows discrete epithelial lesions.

Treatment involves the use of systemic or local antiviral agents. Topical antiviral agents such as vidarabine, trifluridine, or idoxuridine usually provide prompt relief.[3] Local corticosteroid preparations increase the activity of the herpes simplex virus, apparently by enhancing the destructive effect of collagenase on the collagen of the cornea. The use of these medications should be avoided in those suspected of having herpes simplex conjunctivitis or keratitis.

Chlamydial Conjunctivitis.   Inclusion conjunctivitis usually is a benign suppurative conjunctivitis transmitted by the type of *Chlamydia trachomatis* (serotypes D through K) that causes venereal infections (see Chapter 52). It is spread by contaminated genital secretions and occurs in newborns

of mothers with *C. trachomatis* infections of the birth canal. It also can be contracted through swimming in unchlorinated pools. The incubation period varies from 5 to 12 days, and the disease may last for several months if untreated. The infection usually is treated with appropriate oral antibiotics.

A more serious form of infection is caused by a different strain of *C. trachomatis* (serotypes A through C). This form of chlamydial infection affects the conjunctiva and causes ulceration and scarring of the cornea. It is the leading cause of preventable blindness in the world. Although the agent is widespread, it is seen mostly in developing countries, particularly those of Africa, Asia, and the Middle East.[6] It is transmitted by direct human contact, contaminated objects (fomites), and flies.

Ophthalmia Neonatorum.   Ophthalmia neonatorum is a form of conjunctivitis that occurs in newborns younger than 1 month of age. It is usually contracted during or soon after vaginal delivery. There are many causes, including *N. gonorrhoeae, Pseudomonas,* and *C. trachomatis.*[7] Epidemiologically, these infections reflect those sexually transmitted diseases most common in a particular area. Once the most common form of conjunctivitis in the newborn, gonococcal ophthalmia neonatorum has an incidence of 0.3% of live births in the United States; *C. trachomatis* has an incidence of 8.2% of live births.[7] Drops of 0.5% erythromycin or 1% silver nitrate are applied immediately after birth to prevent gonococcal ophthalmia. Silver nitrate instillation may cause mild, self-limited conjunctivitis.

Signs of ophthalmia neonatorum include redness and swelling of the conjunctiva, swelling of the eyelids, and discharge, which may be purulent. The conjunctivitis caused by silver nitrate occurs within 6 to 12 hours of birth and clears within 24 to 48 hours.[7] The incubation period for *N. gonorrhoeae* is 2 to 5 days and for *C. trachomatis,* 5 to 14 days. Infection should be suspected when conjunctivitis develops 48 hours after birth.[7] Ophthalmia neonatorum is a potentially blinding condition, and it can cause serious and potentially systemic manifestations. It requires immediate diagnosis and treatment.

Allergic Conjunctivitis

Ocular allergy encompasses a spectrum of conjunctival conditions usually characterized by itching. The most common of these is seasonal allergic rhinoconjunctivitis, or hay fever. Seasonal allergic conjunctivitis is an IgE-mediated hypersensitivity reaction precipitated by small airborne allergens such as pollens. It typically causes bilateral tearing, itching, and redness of the eyes. The treatment of seasonal allergic rhinoconjunctivitis includes allergen avoidance, the use of cold compresses, oral antihistamines, and vasoconstrictor eye drops. Allergic conjunctivitis also has been successfully treated with topical mast cell stabilizers, histamine H_1 receptor antagonists, and topical nonsteroidal anti-inflammatory drugs. All three types of agents are well tolerated and have a rapid onset of action. In severe cases, a short course of topical corticosteroids is required to afford symptomatic relief.[4]

DISORDERS OF THE CORNEA

The cornea is avascular and obtains its nutrient and oxygen supply by diffusion from blood vessels of the adjacent sclera, from the aqueous humor at its deep surface, and from tears. The corneal epithelium is heavily innervated by sensory neurons (trigeminal nerve [CN V], ophthalmic division [CN V_1]). Epithelial damage causes discomfort that ranges from a foreign body sensation and burning of the eyes to severe, stabbing or knifelike, incapacitating pain. Reflex lacrimation is common. Disorders of the cornea include trauma and infections, abnormal corneal deposits, and arcus senilis.

Corneal Trauma

Trauma that causes abrasions of the cornea can be extremely painful, but if minor, the abrasions usually heal in a few days. The epithelial layer is capable of regeneration, and small defects heal without scarring. If the stroma is damaged, healing occurs more slowly, and the danger of infection is increased. Injuries to Bowman's membrane and the stromal layer heal with scar formation and permanent opacification. Opacities of the cornea impair the transmission of light. A minor scar can severely distort vision because it disturbs the refractive surface.

The integrity of the epithelium and the endothelium is necessary to maintain hydration of the cornea within a limited range. Damage to either structure leads to edema and loss of transparency. Among the causes of corneal edema are prolonged and uninterrupted wearing of hard contact lenses, which can deprive the epithelium of oxygen, disrupting its integrity. The edema disappears spontaneously when the cornea comes in contact with the atmosphere. Corneal edema also occurs when there is a sudden rise in intraocular pressure. If intraocular pressure rises rapidly above 50 mm Hg, as in acute glaucoma, subendothelial edema develops. With corneal edema, the cornea appears dull, uneven, and hazy. Visual acuity decreases, and iridescent vision (*i.e.*, rainbows around lights) occurs. Iridescent vision results from epithelial and subepithelial edema, which splits white light into its component parts, with blue in the center and red on the outside.

Keratitis

Keratitis refers to inflammation of the cornea. It can be caused by infections, hypersensitivity reactions, ischemia, defects in tearing, trauma, and interruption in sensory innervation, as occurs with local anesthesia. Scar tissue formation due to keratitis is the leading cause of blindness and impaired vision throughout the world. Most of this vision loss is preventable if the condition is diagnosed early and appropriate treatment is instituted.

Diagnosis of keratitis is based on history of trauma, medication use, and signs and symptoms associated with corneal irritation and disease. Because the cornea has many pain fibers, superficial or deep corneal abrasions cause discomfort, photophobia, and lacrimation. The discomfort may range from a foreign body sensation to severe pain. Defective vision results from the changes in transparency and curvature of the cornea that occur. Because of the discomfort involved, examination of the eye often is facilitated by instillation of a local anesthetic agent. Fluorescein staining can be used to outline an ulcerated area. The biomicroscope (slitlamp) is used for proper examination of the cornea. In cases of an infectious etiology, scrapings from the ulcer are obtained for staining and culture studies.

Keratitis can be divided into two types: ulcerative, in which parts of the epithelium, stroma, or both are destroyed, and nonulcerative, in which all the layers of the epithelium are affected by the inflammation, but the epithelium remains intact. Causes of ulcerative keratitis include infectious agents such as those causing conjunctivitis (*e.g.*, *Staphylococcus*, *S. pneumoniae*, *Chlamydia*), exposure trauma, and use of extended-wear contact lens. Bacterial keratitis tends to be aggressive and demands immediate care. Exposure trauma may result from deformities of the lid, paralysis of the lid muscles, or severe exophthalmos. Mooren's ulcer is a chronic, painful, indolent ulcer that occurs in the absence of infection. It usually is seen in older persons and may affect both eyes. Although the cause is unknown, an autoimmune origin is suspected.

Acanthamoeba is a free-living protozoan that thrives in contaminated water. *Acanthamoeba keratitis* is an increasingly serious and sight-threatening complication of wearing soft contact lens, particularly when homemade saline solutions are used for cleaning.[2] It also may occur in non–contact lens wearers after exposure to contaminated water or soil. It is characterized by pain that is disproportionate to the clinical manifestations, redness of the eye, and photophobia. The disorder commonly is misdiagnosed as herpes keratitis. Diagnosis is confirmed by scrapings and culture with specially prepared medium. In the early stages of infection, epithelial debridement may be beneficial. Treatment includes intensive use of topical antibiotics. However, the organism may encyst within the corneal stroma, making treatment more difficult. Keratoplasty may be necessary in advanced disease to arrest the progression of the infection.

Nonulcerative or interstitial keratitis is associated with a number of diseases, including syphilis, tuberculosis, and lupus erythematosus. It also may result from a viral infection entering through a small defect in the cornea. Treatment usually is symptomatic.

Herpes Simplex Keratitis

Herpes simplex virus keratitis is the most common cause of corneal ulceration in the United States. Most cases are caused by herpes simplex virus type 1 infections. However, in neonatal infections acquired during passage through the birth canal, approximately 80% are caused by herpes simplex virus type 2.[8] The disease can occur as a primary or recurrent infection. Primary infections cause follicular conjunctivitis and blepharitis, characterized by a rounded cobblestone pattern of avascular lesions. Epithelial keratitis may develop. After the initial primary infection, the virus may persist in a quiescent or latent state that remains in the trigeminal ganglion and possibly in the cornea without causing signs of infection. During childhood, mild primary herpes simplex virus infection may go unnoticed.[8]

Recurrent infection may be precipitated by various poorly understood, stress-related factors that reactivate the virus. Involvement usually is unilateral. The first symptoms are irritation, photophobia, and tearing. There may be some reduction in vision when the lesion affects the central part of the cornea. Because corneal anesthesia occurs early in the disease, the symptoms may be minimal, and the person may delay seeking medical care. There often is a history of fever blisters or other herpetic infection, but corneal lesions may be the only sign of recurrent herpes infection. Most typically, the corneal lesion involves the epithelium and has a typical branching pattern. These epithelial lesions heal without scarring. Topical antiviral agents such as trifluridine (Viroptic) drops, idoxuridine (IDU) drops, or vidarabine (Vira-A) ointment are used to promote healing. Corticosteroid drugs are contraindicated because they increase viral replication.

Lesions that involve the stromal layer of the cornea produce increasingly severe corneal opacities. They are thought to have an immune rather than an infectious cause. Stromal keratitis may be treated with topically applied corticosteroids to suppress the immune response. The most common cause of corneal blindness in the Western world is stromal scarring from herpes simplex keratitis.[8]

Abnormal Corneal Deposits

The cornea frequently is the site of deposition of abnormal metabolic products. In hypercalcemia, calcium salts can precipitate in the cornea, producing a cloudy band keratopathy. Cystine crystals are deposited in cystinosis, cholesterol esters in hypercholesterolemia, and a golden ring of copper (*i.e.*, Kayser-Fleischer ring) in hepatolenticular degeneration due to Wilson's disease. Pharmacologic agents, such as chloroquine, can result in crystal deposits in the cornea.

Arcus Senilis

Arcus senilis is an extremely common, bilateral, benign corneal degeneration that may occur at any age, but is more common in the elderly. It consists of a grayish-white infiltrate, approximately 2 mm wide, that occurs at the periphery of the cornea. It represents an extracellular lipid infiltration and commonly is associated with hyperlipidemia. Arcus senilis does not produce visual symptoms, and there is no treatment for the disorder.

Corneal Transplantation

Advances in ophthalmologic surgery permit corneal transplantation using a cadaver cornea. Unlike kidney or heart transplantation procedures, which are associated with considerable risk of rejection of the transplanted organ, the use of cadaver corneas entails minimal danger of rejection because this tissue is not exposed to the vascular and therefore the immunologic defense system. Instead, the success of this type of transplantation operation depends on the prevention of scar tissue formation, which would limit the transparency of the transplanted cornea.

UVEITIS

Inflammation of the entire uveal tract, which supports the lens and neural components of the eye, is called *uveitis*. It is one of several inflammatory disorders of ocular tissue with clinical features in common and an immunologically based cause.[8] One of the serious consequences of uveitis can be the involvement of the underlying retina. Parasitic invasion of the choroid can result in local atrophic changes that usually involve the retina; examples include toxoplasmosis and histoplasmosis. Sarcoid deposition in the form of small nodules results in irregularities of the underlying retinal surface.

> In summary, the conjunctiva lines the inner surface of the eyelids and covers the optic globe to the junction of the cornea and sclera. Conjunctivitis, also called *red eye* or *pink eye*, may result from bacterial or viral infection, allergens, chemical agents, physical agents, or radiant energy. It is important to differentiate between redness caused by conjunctivitis and that caused by more serious eye disorders, such as acute glaucoma or corneal lesions.
>
> Keratitis, or inflammation of the cornea, can be caused by infections, hypersensitivity reactions, ischemia, trauma, defects in tearing, or trauma. Trauma or disease that involves the stromal layer of the cornea heals with scar formation and permanent opacification. These opacities interfere with the transmission of light and may impair vision.
>
> The uveal tract is the middle vascular layer of the eye. It contains melanocytes that prevent diffusion of light through the wall of the optic globe. Inflammation of the uveal tract (uveitis) can affect visual acuity.

◼ Glaucoma

After you have completed this section of the chapter, you should be able to meet the following objectives:

✦ Describe the formation and outflow of aqueous humor from the eye and relate to the development of glaucoma
✦ Compare closed-angle and open-angle glaucoma
✦ Explain why glaucoma leads to blindness

Glaucoma includes a group of conditions that produce an elevation in intraocular pressure. If left untreated, the pressure may increase sufficiently to cause ischemia and degeneration of the optic nerve, leading to progressive blindness. Glaucoma is a major contributor to the incidence of more than 89,000 to 150,000 legally blind persons in the United States.[1,9] It is the second leading cause of irreversible blindness in the United States and the most common cause among African Americans. Although the latter have been reported to have an incidence four to six times that of whites, they are only twice as likely to receive appropriate health care.[1] The condition often is asymptomatic, and a significant loss of peripheral vision may occur before medical attention is sought, emphasizing the need for routine screening for early diagnosis and treatment of increased intraocular pressure in persons older than 40 years of age.

CONTROL OF INTRAOCULAR PRESSURE

The aqueous humor helps maintain intraocular pressure and serves a nutritive function, facilitating metabolism of the lens and posterior cornea. It contains a low protein concentration and a high concentration of ascorbic acid, glucose, and amino acids. It also mediates the exchange of respiratory gases.

The aqueous humor is produced by the ciliary epithelium in the posterior chamber and passes between the anterior surface of the lens and posterior surface of the iris, through the pupil and into the anterior chamber. It leaves through the iridocorneal angle between the iris and the sclera. Here it filters through the trabecular meshwork and enters the canal of Schlemm for return to the venous circulation (Fig. 54-2). The secretion of aqueous humor is an active process that continues regardless of the pressure exerted by the secreted fluid. The secretory activity of the ciliary epithelium requires the enzyme carbonic anhydrase.

The interior pressure of the eye must exceed atmospheric pressure to prevent the eyeball from collapsing. The hydrostatic pressure of the aqueous humor results from a balance of several factors, including the rate of secretion, resistance to flow through the narrow opening between the iris and the ciliary body at the entrance to the anterior chamber, and resistance to resorption at the trabeculated region of the sclera at the iridocorneal angle. Normally, the rate of aqueous production is equal to the rate of aqueous outflow, and the intraocular pressure is maintained within a normal range of 9 to 21 mm Hg. However, data suggest that the value is closer to 12 ± 1 mm Hg in young, healthy adults during daylight hours. The mean value increases by approximately 1 mm Hg per decade after 40 years of age.[10]

Intraocular pressure can be measured by means of a tonometer. Two common types of tonometry are used for measuring intraocular pressure: the contact applanation tonometer and the noncontact (air puff) tonometers.[2] The applanation method measures the amount of force that is required to flatten the central cornea. Applanation tonometry can be performed with a contact tonometer such as Goldmann's applanation tonometer, which is placed on the anesthetized eye. Applanation tonometry is the most accurate clinically applicable method to measure the intraocular pressure. With the noncontact air puff tonometer, a small puff of air is blown against the cornea. The air rebounding from the corneal surface hits a pressure-sensing membrane in the instrument. This method is not as accurate as applanation tonometry but does not require anesthetic drops because no instrument touches the eye. An additional method, impression tonometry, measures direct pressure on the eyeball and requires only a hand-held instrument—the Schiotz contact tonometer. It is less accurate than Goldmann's applanation tonometer but may be used when an irregular corneal surface precludes use of other devices.

TYPES OF GLAUCOMA

Abnormalities in the balance between aqueous production and outflow lead to increased intraocular pressure, a disease complex called *glaucoma*. Rarely is intraocular pressure increased by overproduction of aqueous humor; it usually results from interference with aqueous outflow from the anterior chamber. As intraocular pressure rises because of impaired outflow, the canal of Schlemm is compressed, causing a further reduction in aqueous outflow. Temporary or permanent impairment of vision results from pressure-induced degenerative changes in the retina and optic nerve and from corneal edema and opacification. Damage to optic nerve axons in the region of the optic nerve can be recognized on ophthalmoscopic examination. The normal optic disk has a centrally placed depression called the *optic cup*. With progressive atrophy of axons caused by increased intraocular pressure, pallor of the optic disk develops, and the size and depth of the optic cup increase. Because changes in the optic cup precede the visual field loss, regular ophthalmoscopic examination is important for detecting eye changes that occur with increased intraocular pressure. Stereoscopic viewing during slit-lamp examination improves the accuracy of evaluation.[11]

Advances in computer technology allow detection and quantification of visual changes due to glaucoma. These tests of vision include color vision analysis, blue-on-yellow visual field testing and testing of contrast sensitivity, dark adaptation, and other tests of retinal function. In the future, these tests are likely to be used in detecting visual field defects not currently detected by standard means.[9]

Glaucoma commonly is classified as closed-angle (*i.e.*, narrow-angle) or open-angle (*i.e.*, wide-angle) glaucoma, depending on the location of the compromised aqueous humor circulation and resorption. Glaucoma may occur as a congenital or an acquired condition, and it may manifest as a primary or a secondary disorder. Primary glaucoma occurs without evidence of preexisting ocular or systemic disease. Secondary glaucoma can result from inflammatory

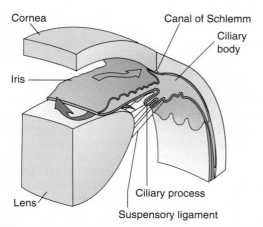

FIGURE 54-2 Enlarged view of the anterior portion of the eyeball. Arrows indicate the flow of aqueous humor. (Chaffee E.E., Lytle I.M. [1980]. *Basic physiology and anatomy* [4th ed.]. Philadelphia: J.B. Lippincott)

processes that affect the eye, from tumors, or from the blood cells of trauma-produced hemorrhage that obstruct the outflow of aqueous humor. Obstruction of the anterior chamber angle can accompany a number of pathologic processes, such as adhesions of the iris to the cornea or lens.

Closed-Angle Glaucoma

In closed-angle glaucoma, the anterior chamber is narrow and outflow becomes impaired when the iris thickens as the result of pupillary dilation (Fig. 54-3). As the iris thickens, it restricts the circulation between the base of the iris and the sclera, blocking the circulation between the posterior and anterior chambers and reducing or eliminating access to the angle where aqueous reabsorption occurs.[9] Approximately 5% to 10% of all cases of glaucoma fall into this category. Closed-angle glaucoma usually occurs as the result of an inherited anatomic defect that causes a shallow anterior chamber. This defect is exaggerated by the anterior displacement of the peripheral iris that occurs in older persons because of the increase in lens size that occurs with aging.

The depth of the anterior chamber can be evaluated by transillumination or by a technique called *gonioscopy*. Gonioscopy uses a special contact lens and mirrors or prisms so that the angle of the anterior chamber can be seen and measured. The transillumination method requires only a penlight. The light source is held at the temporal side of the eye and directed horizontally across the iris. In persons with a normal-sized anterior chamber, the light passes through the chamber to illuminate both halves of the iris. In persons with a narrow anterior chamber, only the half of the iris adjacent to the light source is illuminated (Fig. 54-4).

The symptoms of closed-angle glaucoma are related to sudden, intermittent increases in intraocular pressure. These occur after prolonged periods in the dark, emotional upset, and other conditions that cause extensive and prolonged dilation of the pupil. Administration of pharmacologic

agents such as atropine that cause pupillary dilation (mydriasis) also can precipitate an acute episode of increased intraocular pressure in persons with the potential for closed-angle glaucoma. Attacks of increased intraocular pressure are manifested by ocular pain and blurred or iridescent vision caused by corneal edema. The pupil may be enlarged and fixed. The symptoms often are spontaneously relieved by sleep and conditions that promote pupillary constriction. With repeated or prolonged attacks, the eye becomes reddened, and edema of the cornea may develop, giving the eye a hazy appearance. A unilateral, often excruciating, headache is common. Nausea and vomiting may occur, causing the headache to be confused with migraine.

Some persons with congenitally narrow anterior chambers never develop symptoms, and others develop symptoms only when they are elderly. Because of the dangers of vision loss, those with narrow anterior chambers should be warned about the significance of blurred vision, halos, and ocular pain. Sometimes, decreased visual acuity and an unreactive pupil may be the only clue to closed-angle glaucoma in the elderly.

The treatment of acute closed-angle glaucoma is primarily surgical. It involves creating an opening between the anterior and posterior chambers with laser or incisional iridectomy to allow aqueous humor to bypass the pupillary block. The anatomic abnormalities responsible for closed-angle glaucoma usually are bilateral, and prophylactic surgery often is performed on the other eye.

Primary Open-Angle Glaucoma

Primary open-angle glaucoma is the most common form of glaucoma. It tends to manifest after 35 years of age, with an incidence of 0.5% to 2% among persons 40 years of age and older.[8] The condition is characterized by an abnormal increase in intraocular pressure that occurs in the absence of obstruction at the iridocorneal angle, hence the name *open-angle glaucoma*. Instead, it usually occurs because of an abnormality of the trabecular meshwork that controls the flow of aqueous humor into the canal of Schlemm. Risk factors for this disorder include an age of 40 years and older, family history of the disorder, diabetes mellitus, and myopia. In some persons, the use of moderate amounts of topical corticosteroid medications can cause an increase in intraocular pressure. Sensitive persons also may sustain an increase in intraocular pressure with the use of systemic corticosteroid drugs.

Primary open-angle glaucoma usually is asymptomatic and chronic, causing progressive loss of visual field unless it is appropriately treated. Because the condition usually is asymptomatic, routine screening using applanation tonometry is the best means of detecting the disorder.

The elevation in intraocular pressure in persons with open-angle glaucoma usually is treated pharmacologically or, in cases where pharmacologic treatment fails, by increasing aqueous outflow through a surgically created pathway. Drugs used in the long-term management of glaucoma fall into five classes: β-adrenergic antagonists, prostaglandin analogues, adrenergic agonists, carbonic anhydrase inhibitors, and cholinergic agonists.[12] Most glaucoma drugs are applied topically. However, systemic side effects may occur.

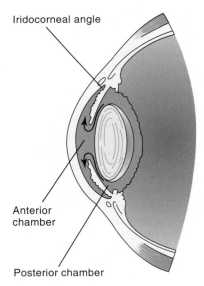

FIGURE 54-3 Narrow anterior chamber and iridocorneal angle in closed-angle (narrow-angle) glaucoma.

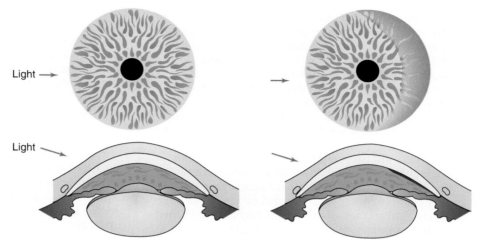

FIGURE 54-4 Transillumination of the iris. In the eye with a normal anterior chamber, the iris is evenly illuminated by light shining obliquely into the anterior chamber. In the eye with a narrow anterior chamber, the iris is unevenly illuminated and shadowed. (Bates B.B. [1995]. *A guide to physical examination and history taking* [6th ed.]. Philadelphia: J.B. Lippincott)

Topical β-adrenergic antagonists usually are the drugs of first choice for lowering intraocular pressure. The β-adrenergic antagonists are thought to lower intraocular pressure by decreasing aqueous humor production in the ciliary body. β-adrenergic antagonists decrease the production of aqueous humor by approximately one third.[12] Both nonselective (β$_1$ and β$_2$) and selective (β$_1$) β-blockers are available. The selection between a nonselective and selective β-adrenergic antagonist often is determined by the difference in their side effects. For example, the cardiac effects of β$_1$-adrenergic blockade include hypotension, decreased myocardial contractility, worsening of congestive failure, and bradycardia. These side effects might be contraindicated in someone with heart disease.

Prostaglandins are locally acting hormones, found in most tissues. At low concentrations, prostaglandin F$_{2α}$ increases uveoscleral outflow through the iris root and ciliary body, either by decreasing the extracellular matrix or by relaxing the ciliary musculature. A topical prostaglandin analog, Latanoprost (Xalatan), is the only drug of this class currently available in the United States.[12]

Adrenergic agonists cause an early decrease in production of aqueous humor by constricting the vessels supplying the ciliary body. Later, there is an increase in aqueous humor outflow mediated by α- and β-adrenergic stimulation. Nonselective adrenergic agents such as epinephrine stimulate both α and β receptors and tend to cause more systemic side effects such as tachycardia than nonselective drugs. Apraclonidine, an α$_2$ agonist, reduces intraocular pressure by decreasing aqueous humor formation. Dipivefrin is a prodrug that is converted to epinephrine in the eye and seldom causes side effects.

Carbonic anhydrase inhibitors reduce the secretion of aqueous humor by the ciliary epithelium. Until recently, these drugs (*i.e.*, methazolamide and acetazolamide) had to be taken orally, and systemic side effects were common. A topical carbonic anhydrase inhibitor, dorzolamide, acts locally, eliminating the side effects associated with the oral forms of the drug.

Acetylcholine is the postganglionic neuromediator for the parasympathetic system; it increases aqueous outflow through contraction of the ciliary muscle and pupillary constriction (miosis). Cholinergic drugs exert their effects by increasing the effects of acetylcholine. Acetylcholine is broken down by the enzyme acetylcholinesterase. The most commonly used miotic drug is pilocarpine, which functions as a direct cholinergic agonist. Echothiophate, another miotic agent, acts indirectly by inhibiting the breakdown of acetylcholine by acetylcholinesterase.

When a reduction in intraocular pressure cannot be maintained through pharmacologic methods, surgical treatment may become necessary. Until recently, the main surgical treatment for open-angle glaucoma was a filtering procedure in which an opening was created between the anterior chamber and the subconjunctival space. An argon or neodymium–aluminum-garnet (Nd:YAG) laser technique, in which multiple spots are applied 360 degrees around the trabecular meshwork, has been developed.[2] The microburns resulting from the laser treatment scar rather than penetrate the trabecular meshwork, a process that is thought to enlarge the outflow channels by increasing the tension exerted on the trabecular meshwork. Cryotherapy, diathermy, and high-frequency ultrasound may be used in some cases to destroy the ciliary epithelium and reduce aqueous humor production.

Congenital or Infantile Glaucoma

Congenital glaucoma is caused by a disorder in which the anterior chamber retains its fetal configuration, with aberrant trabecular meshwork extending to the root of the iris, or is covered by a membrane. An X-linked recessive mode of inheritance is common, producing a high incidence among males.[7] The earliest symptoms are excessive lacrimation and photophobia. Affected infants tend to be fussy, have poor eating habits, and rub their eyes frequently. Diffuse edema of the cornea usually occurs, giving the eye a grayish-white appearance. Chronic elevation of the intraocular pressure before the age of 3 years causes enlargement of the entire globe (*i.e.*, buphthalmos). Early surgical treatment is necessary to prevent blindness.

In summary, glaucoma is one of the leading causes of blindness in the United States. It is characterized by conditions that cause an increase in intraocular pressure and that, if untreated, can lead to atrophy of the optic disk and progressive blindness. The aqueous humor is formed by the ciliary epithelium in the posterior chamber and flows through the pupil to the angle formed by the cornea and the iris. Here, it filters through the trabecular meshwork and enters the canal of Schlemm for return to the venous circulation. Glaucoma results from overproduction or the impeded outflow of aqueous humor from the anterior chamber of the eye.

There are two major forms of glaucoma: closed-angle and open-angle. Closed-angle glaucoma is caused by a narrow anterior chamber and blockage of the outflow channels at the angle formed by the iris and the cornea. This occurs when the iris becomes thickened during pupillary dilation. Open-angle glaucoma is caused by microscopic obstruction of the trabecular meshwork. Open-angle glaucoma usually is asymptomatic, and considerable loss of the visual field often occurs before medical treatment is sought. Routine screening by applanation tonometry provides one of the best means for early detection of glaucoma before vision loss has occurred.

Cataracts

After you have completed this section of the chapter, you should be able to meet the following objectives:

✦ Describe the changes in eye structure that occur with cataract
✦ Cite risk factors associated with cataract
✦ Characterize the visual changes that occur with cataract
✦ Describe the treatment of persons with cataracts

A cataract is a lens opacity that interferes with the transmission of light to the retina. It has been estimated that 13 million persons in the United States 40 years of age or older are visually disabled because of cataracts.[1] Cataracts are the most common cause of age-related visual loss in the world; they are found in approximately 50% of those between 65 and 74 years of age and in 70% of those older than 75 years.[1] Cataract surgery is the most common surgical procedure covered by Medicare, with over 1 million procedures performed annually. Over 90% of persons undergoing cataract surgery experience visual improvement if there is no ocular comorbidity.[13]

CAUSES AND TYPES OF CATARACTS

The cause of cataract development is thought to be multifactorial, with different factors being associated with different types of opacities. The pathogenesis of cataracts is not completely understood. Several risk factors have been proposed, including the effects of aging, genetic influences, environmental and metabolic influences, drugs, and injury.[14] Metabolically induced cataracts are caused by disorders of carbohydrate metabolism (diabetes) or inborn errors of

metabolism. In a condition called *Lowe's syndrome*, abnormal synthesis of lens proteins leads to opacification.[15] Long-term exposure to sunlight (ultraviolet B radiation) and heavy smoking have been associated with increased risk of cataract formation.[14] In some cases, cataracts occur as a developmental defect (*i.e.*, congenital cataracts) or secondary to trauma or diseases.

Cataracts can result from a number of drugs. Dinitrophenol, a drug widely used for weight reduction during the 1930s, as well as triparanol, chlorpromazine, and the corticosteroid drugs have all been implicated as causative agents in cataract formation. Busulfan, a cancer treatment drug, has been clearly linked to cataract formation. Frequent examination of lens transparency should accompany the use of these and any other medications with potential cataract-forming effects.

Traumatic Cataract
Traumatic cataracts most often are caused by foreign body injury to the lens or blunt trauma to the eye. Foreign body injury that interrupts the lens capsule allows aqueous and vitreous humor to enter the lens and initiate cataract formation. Other causes of traumatic cataract are overexposure to heat (*e.g.*, glassblower's cataract) or to ionizing radiation. The radiation dose necessary to cause a cataract varies with the amount and type of energy; younger lenses are most vulnerable.

Congenital Cataract
A congenital cataract is one that is present at birth. Among the causes of congenital cataracts are genetic defects, toxic environmental agents, and viruses such as rubella. A maternal rubella infection during the first trimester can cause congenital cataract. Exposure of the embryo to ionizing radiation levels as low as 50 centigrays, such as occurs during a barium enema or fluoroscopy, also can induce congenital cataract. Cataracts and other developmental defects of the ocular apparatus depend on the total dose and the embryonic stage at the time of exposure. During the last trimester of fetal life, genetically or environmentally influenced malformation of the superficial lens fibers can occur. Most congenital cataracts are not progressive and are not dense enough to cause significant visual impairment. However, if the cataracts are bilateral and the opacity is significant, lens extraction should be done on one eye by the age of 2 months to permit the development of vision and prevent nystagmus. If the surgery is successful, the contralateral lens should be removed soon after.

Senile Cataract
Cataract is the most common cause of age-related vision loss in the world. With normal aging, the nucleus and the cortex of the lens enlarge as new fibers are formed in the cortical zones of the lens. In the nucleus, the old fibers become more compressed and dehydrated. Metabolic changes occur. Lens proteins become more insoluble, and concentrations of calcium, sodium, potassium, and phosphate increase. During the early stages of cataract formation, a yellow pigment and vacuoles accumulate in the lens fibers. The unfolding of protein molecules, cross-linking of sulfhydryl

groups, and conversion of soluble to insoluble proteins lead to the loss of lens transparency. The onset is gradual, and the only symptoms are increasingly blurred vision and visual distortion.

MANIFESTATIONS

The manifestations of cataract depend on the extent of opacity and whether the defect is bilateral or unilateral. With the exception of traumatic or congenital cataract, most cataracts are bilateral. Age-related cataracts, which are the most common type, are characterized by increasingly blurred vision and visual distortion (see Fig. 54-1). Vision for far and near objects decreases. Dilation of the pupil in dim light improves vision. With nuclear cataracts (those involving the lens nucleus), the refractive power of the anterior segment often increases to produce an acquired myopia. Persons with hyperopia may experience a "second sight" or improved reading acuity until increasing opacity reduces acuity. Central lens opacities may divide the visual axis and cause an optical defect in which two or more blurred images are seen. In addition to decreased visual acuity, cataracts tend to cause light entering the eye to be scattered, thereby producing glare or the abnormal presence of light in the visual field. On ophthalmoscopic examination, cataracts may appear as a gross opacity filling the pupillary aperture or as an opacity silhouetted against the red background of the fundus.

DIAGNOSIS AND TREATMENT

Diagnosis of cataract is based on the Snellen vision test and on the degree of visual impairment. A Snellen acuity of 20/50 is a common requirement for drivers of motor vehicles. Visual impairment is based on the person's assessment of visual function and disability due to glare. Other tests of potential vision (*e.g.,* the ability to see well after surgery), such as electrophysiologic testing in which the response to visual stimuli is measured electronically, may be done.

There is no effective medical treatment for cataract. Use of strong bifocals, magnification, appropriate lighting, and visual aids may be used as the cataract progresses. Surgery is the only treatment for correcting cataract-related vision loss. Surgery usually involves lens extraction and intraocular lens implantation. One of the greatest advances in cataract surgery has been the development of reliable lens implants. The use of extracapsular surgery, which leaves the posterior capsule of the lens intact, has further improved the outcomes of cataract surgery. The cataract lens usually is removed using phacoemulsification techniques. Phacoemulsification involves ultrasonic fragmentation of the lens into fine pieces, which then are aspirated from the eye. Opacification of the posterior capsule may develop in up to 50% of eyes with intraocular implants within 3 to 5 years.[13] Another advance in cataract surgery has been the use of an Nd:YAG laser to remove these capsular opacities. Surgery commonly is performed on an outpatient basis and with the use of local anesthesia.

The American Academy of Ophthalmology standard for when cataract surgery should be performed is when "best corrected" visual acuity is 20/50 or worse in the affected eye.[16] However, surgery still may be indicated when a person's best corrected acuity is 20/40 or better, if there is disabling glare or work-related disability or if the cataract threatens to cause other eye problems, such as secondary glaucoma or uveitis.

> In summary, a cataract is a lens opacity. It can occur as the result of congenital influences, metabolic disturbances, infection, injury, and aging. The most common type of cataract is the senile cataract that occurs with aging. The treatment for a totally opaque or mature cataract is surgical extraction. An intraocular lens implant may be inserted during the surgical procedure to replace the lens that has been removed; otherwise, thick convex lenses or contact lenses are used to compensate for the loss of lens function.

Disorders of the Vitreous and Retina

After you have completed this section of the chapter, you should be able to meet the following objectives:

◆ Relate the phagocytic function of the retinal pigment epithelium to the development of retinitis pigmentosa
◆ Cite the manifestations and long-term visual effects of papilledema and central artery and central venous occlusions
◆ Describe the pathogenesis of background and proliferative diabetic retinopathies and their mechanisms of visual impairment
◆ Explain how prematurity and oxygen administration interact in producing retinopathy of prematurity
◆ Discuss the cause of retinal detachment
◆ Explain the pathology and visual changes associated with macular degeneration

The posterior segment, which constitutes five sixths of the eyeball, contains the transparent vitreous humor and the neural retina. The innermost layer of the eyeball, the fundus, is visualized through the pupil with an ophthalmoscope.

DISORDERS OF THE VITREOUS

The vitreous humor (*i.e.,* vitreous body) is a colorless, amorphous biologic gel that fills the posterior cavity of the eye. It consists of approximately 99% water, some salts, glycoproteins, proteoglycans, and dispersed collagen fibrils. The vitreous is attached to the ciliary body and the peripheral retina in the region of the ora serrata and to the periphery of the optic disk.

Disease, aging, and injury can disturb the factors that maintain the water of the vitreous humor in suspension, causing liquefaction of the gel to occur. With the loss of gel structure, fine fibers, membranes, and cellular debris develop. When this occurs, floaters (images) often can be noticed as these substances move within the vitreous cavity during head movement. In disease, blood vessels may grow from the surface of the retina or optic disk onto the posterior surface of the vitreous, and blood may fill the vitreous cavity.

In a procedure called a *vitrectomy*, the removal and replacement of the vitreous with a balanced saline solution can restore sight in some persons with vitreous opacities resulting from hemorrhage or vitreoretinal membrane formations that cause legal blindness. In this procedure, a small probe with a cutting tip is used to remove the opaque vitreous and membranes. The procedure is difficult and requires complex instrumentation. It is of no value if the retina is not functional.

DISORDERS OF THE RETINA

The function of the retina is to receive visual images, partially analyze them, and transmit this modified information to the brain. Disorders of the retina and its function include derangements of the pigment epithelium (*e.g.*, retinitis pigmentosa); ischemic conditions caused by disorders of the retinal blood supply; disorders of the retinal vessels such as retinopathies that cause hemorrhage and the development of opacities; separation of the pigment and sensory layers of the retina (*i.e.*, retinal detachment); retinopathy of prematurity; and abnormalities of Bruch's membrane and choroid (*e.g.*, macular degeneration). Because the retina has no pain fibers, most diseases of the retina are painless and do not cause redness of the eye.

Retinitis Pigmentosa

Retinitis pigmentosa is a group of hereditary diseases that cause slow degenerative changes in the retinal receptors. There are several modes of inheritance, including dominant, recessive, sex-linked, and sporadic.[8] In the United States, the incidence for all types of retinitis pigmentosa is 1 case in 3500 persons; the incidence of the carrier state may be 1 in 80. Slow destruction of the rods occurs, progressing from the peripheral to the central regions of the retina. Based on research with animal models, one probable mechanism of the disorder is a defect in phagocytic mechanisms of the pigment cells that causes membrane debris to accumulate and destroy the photoreceptors. The destruction results in dark lines and areas in which the pigment of the retinal pigment layer is unmasked by receptor loss. Night blindness, the first symptom of the disorder, often begins in early youth, with gross visual handicap occurring in the middle or advanced years.

Disorders of Retinal Blood Supply

The blood supply for the retina is derived from two sources: the choriocapillaris of the choroid and the branches of the central retinal artery. The nutritional needs of the retina, including oxygen and the supply to the pigment cells and rods and cones, involve diffusion from blood vessels in the choroid. Because the choriocapillary layer provides the only blood supply for the fovea centralis (*i.e.*, foveola), de-

tachment of this part of the sensory retina from the pigment epithelium causes irreparable visual loss.

The bipolar, horizontal, amacrine, and ganglion cells, as well as the ganglion cell axons that gather at the optic disk, are supplied by branches of the retinal artery. The central artery of the retina is a branch of the ophthalmic artery. It enters the globe through the optic disk. Branches of this artery radiate over the entire retina, except for the central fovea, which is surrounded by, but is not crossed by, arterial branches. The retinal veins follow a distribution parallel to the arterial branches and carry venous blood to the central vein of the retina, which exits the back of the eye through the optic disk.

Funduscopic examination of the eye with an ophthalmoscope provides an opportunity to examine the retinal blood vessels and other aspects of the retina (Fig. 54-5). Because the retina is an embryonic outgrowth of the brain and the blood vessels are to a considerable extent representative of brain blood vessels, the ophthalmoscopic examination of the fundus of the eye permits the study and diagnosis of metabolic and vascular diseases of the brain and of pathologic processes that are specific to the retina.

The functioning of the retina, like that of other cellular portions of the central nervous system (CNS), depends on an oxygen supply from the vascular system. One of the earliest signs of decreased perfusion pressure in the head region is a graying-out or blackout of vision, which usually precedes loss of consciousness. This can occur during large increases in intrathoracic pressure, which interfere with the return of venous blood to the heart, as occurs with Valsalva's maneuver; with systemic hypotension; and during sudden postural movements under conditions of decreased vascular adaptability.

Ischemia of the retina occurs during general circulatory collapse. If a person survives cardiopulmonary arrest, for instance, permanently decreased visual acuity can occur as a result of edema and the ischemic death of retinal neurons.

Disorders of the Retinal Blood Supply

➤ The blood supply for the retina is derived from the central retinal artery, which supplies blood flow for the entire inside of the retina, and from vessels in the choroid, which supply the rods and cones.

➤ Central retinal occlusion interrupts blood flow to the inner retina and results in unilateral blindness.

➤ The retinopathies, which are disorders of the retinal vessels, interrupt blood flow to the visual receptors, leading to visual impairment.

➤ Retinal detachment separates the visual receptors from the choroid, which provides their major blood supply.

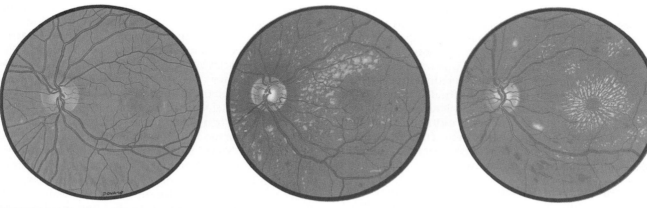

FIGURE 54-5 Fundus of the eye as seen in retinal examination with an ophthalmoscope: (**left**) normal fundus; (**middle**) diabetic retinopathy—combination of microaneurysms, deep hemorrhages, and hard exudates of background retinopathy; (**right**) hypertensive retinopathy with purulent exudates. Some exudates are scattered, while others radiate from the fovea to form a macular star. (Bates B. [1995]. *A guide to physical examination and history taking.* (pp. 208, 210). Philadelphia: J. B. Lippincott Company)

This is followed by primary optic nerve atrophy proportional to the extent of ganglionic cell death. The ophthalmic artery, the source of the central artery of the retina, takes its origin from the internal carotid artery. Intermittent retinal ischemia can accompany internal carotid or common carotid stenosis. In addition to ipsilateral intermittent blindness, contralateral hemiplegia or sensory deficits may accompany the episodes, depending on the competency of the circle of Willis in providing the brain with alternative arterial support. Treatment with anticoagulants or surgical endarterectomy may provide relief. Arteritis of the ophthalmic and central artery occurs more frequently in older persons and, if severe, it can result in occlusive disease and permanent visual deficits.

Papilledema. The central retinal artery enters the eye through the optic papilla in the center of the optic nerve. The central vein of the retina exits the eye along the same path. The entrance and exit of the central artery and vein of the retina through the tough scleral tissue at the optic papilla can be compromised by any condition causing persistent increased intracranial pressure. The most common of these conditions are cerebral tumors, subdural hematomas, hydrocephalus, and malignant hypertension.

The thin-walled, low-pressure veins are the first to collapse, with the consequent backup and slowing of arterial blood flow. Under these conditions, capillary permeability increases, and leakage of fluid results in edema of the optic papilla, called *papilledema*. The interior surface of the papilla normally is cup-shaped and can be evaluated through an ophthalmoscope. With papilledema, sometimes called *choked disk*, the optic cup is distorted by protrusion into the interior of the eye (Fig. 54-6). Because this sign does not occur until the intracranial pressure is significantly elevated, compression damage to the optic nerve fibers passing through the lamina cribrosa may have begun. As a warning sign, papilledema occurs quite late. Unresolved papilledema

results in the destruction of the optic nerve axons and blindness.

Central Retinal Artery Occlusion. Complete occlusion of the central artery of the retina results in sudden unilateral blindness (*i.e.*, anopsia). This is an uncommon disorder of older persons and most often is caused by embolism or atherosclerosis. Because the retina has a dual blood supply, the survival of retinal structures is possible if blood flow can be reestablished within approximately 90 minutes.[2] If blood flow is not restored, the infarcted retina swells and opacifies. Because the receptors of the central fovea are supplied with blood from the choroid, they survive (*i.e.*, macular sparing). A cherry-red spot, indicating a healthy fovea, is surrounded by the pale white, opacified retina. Although the nerve fibers

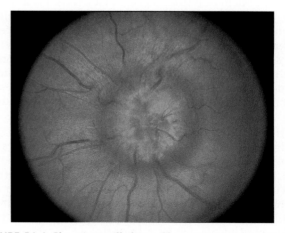

FIGURE 54-6 Chronic papilledema. The optic nerve head is congested and protrudes anteriorly toward the interior of the eye. It has blurred margins, and vessels within it are poorly seen. (Rubin E., Farber J.L. [1999]. *Pathology* [3rd ed., p. 1558]. Philadelphia: Lippincott-Raven)

of the optic disk are adequately supplied by the choroid, the disk becomes pale after death of the ganglion cells and their axonal processes (*i.e.*, optic nerve fibers), resulting in optic nerve atrophy.

Occlusions of branches of the central artery, called *branch arterial occlusions*, are essentially retinal strokes. These occur mainly as a result of emboli and local infarction in the neural retina. The opacification that follows often is slowly resolved, and retinal transparency is restored. Local blind spots or scotomas may occur after destruction of local elements of the retina. Loss of the axons of destroyed ganglion cells results in some optic nerve atrophy.

Central Retinal Vein Occlusion.   Occlusion of the central retinal vein results in venous dilation, stasis, and reduced flow through the retinal veins. It usually is monocular and causes rapid deterioration of visual acuity because of an accompanying increase in capillary wall fragility and a lack of arterial inflow. Superficial and deep hemorrhages may occur throughout the retina.

Among the causes of central retinal vein obstruction are hypertension, diabetes mellitus, and conditions such as sickle cell anemia that slow venous blood flow. The reduction in blood flow results in neovascularization with fibrovascular invasion of the space between the retina and the vitreous humor. In addition to obstructing normal visual function, the new vessels are fragile and prone to hemorrhage. Escaped blood may fill the space between the retina and vitreous, producing the appearance of a sudden veil over the visual field. The blood can find its way into the aqueous humor (*i.e.*, hemorrhagic glaucoma). Photocoagulation of the spreading new blood vessels with high-intensity light or laser beam is used to prevent blindness and eye pain. As the hemorrhage is resolved, degenerating blood products can produce contraction of the vitreous and formation of fibrous tissue within it, causing tears and detachment of the retina.

Much more common are local vein occlusions with regional and focal capillary microhemorrhages that produce the same but more restricted pathologic effects. These microhemorrhages result in the formation of rings of yellow exudate composed of lipid and lipoprotein blood breakdown products. Microhemorrhages deep in the neural retina are somewhat restricted by the vertical organization of the neural elements and result in dot hemorrhages. Microhemorrhages in the layer of ganglionic cell axon bundles result in the appearance of cotton-wool spots on the fundus.

Retinopathies

Disorders of the retinal vessels result in microaneurysms, neovascularization, hemorrhage, and formation of retinal opacities. Microaneurysms are outpouchings of the retinal vasculature. On ophthalmoscopic examination, they appear as minute, unchanging red dots associated with blood vessels. These microaneurysms tend to leak plasma, resulting in localized edema that gives the retina a hazy appearance. Microaneurysms can be identified with certainty using fluorescein angiography; the fluorescein dye is injected intravenously, and the retinal vessels subsequently are photographed using a special ophthalmoscope and fundus

camera. The microaneurysms may bleed, but areas of hemorrhage and edema tend to clear spontaneously. However, they reduce visual acuity if they encroach on the macula and cause degeneration before they are absorbed.

Neovascularization involves the formation of new blood vessels. They can develop from the choriocapillaris, extending between the pigment layer and the sensory layer, or from the retinal veins, extending between the sensory retina and the vitreous cavity and sometimes into the vitreous. These new blood vessels are fragile, leak protein, and tend to bleed. Neovascularization occurs in a number of conditions that impair retinal circulation, including stasis because of hyperviscosity of blood or decreased flow, vascular occlusion, sickle cell disease, sarcoidosis, diabetes mellitus, and retinopathy of prematurity. Research links the formation of new blood vessels with a vascular endothelial growth factor produced by the lining of blood vessels.[17] The cause of new blood vessel formation is uncertain. The vitreous humor is thought to contain a substance that normally inhibits neovascularization, and this factor apparently is suppressed under conditions in which the new blood vessels invade the vitreous cavity.

Hemorrhage can be preretinal, intraretinal, or subretinal. Preretinal hemorrhages occur between the retina and the vitreous. These hemorrhages tend to be large because the blood vessels are only loosely restricted; they may be associated with a subarachnoid or subdural hemorrhage and usually are regarded as a serious manifestation of the disorder. They usually reabsorb without complications unless they penetrate into the vitreous. Intraretinal hemorrhages occur because of abnormalities of the retinal vessels, diseases of the blood, increased pressure in the retinal vessels, or vitreous traction on the vessels. Systemic causes include diabetes mellitus, hypertension, and blood dyscrasias. Subretinal hemorrhages are those that develop between the choroid and pigment layer of the retina. A common cause of subretinal hemorrhage is neovascularization. Photocoagulation may be used to treat microaneurysms and neovascularization.

Light normally passes through the transparent inner portions of the sensory retina before reaching the photoreceptors. Opacities such as hemorrhages, exudate, cotton-wool patches, edema, and tissue proliferation can produce a localized loss of transparency observable with an ophthalmoscope. Exudates are opacities resulting from inflammatory processes. The development of exudates often results in the destruction of the underlying retinal pigment and choroid layer. Deposits are localized opacities consisting of lipid-laden macrophages or accumulated cellular debris. Cotton-wool patches are retinal opacities with hazy, irregular outlines. They occur in the nerve fiber layer and contain cell organelles. Cotton-wool patches are associated with retinal trauma, severe anemia, papilledema, and diabetic retinopathy.

Diabetic Retinopathy.   Diabetic retinopathy is the third leading cause of blindness for all ages in the United States. It ranks first as the cause of newly reported cases of blindness in persons between the ages of 20 and 74 years, and current estimates suggest it is responsible for 12,000 to 24,000 new cases of blindness in the United States each year.[18]

Diabetic retinopathy can be divided into two types: nonproliferative (*i.e.*, background) and proliferative. Background or nonproliferative retinopathy is confined to the retina. It involves thickening of the retinal capillary walls and microaneurysm formation (see Fig. 54-5). Ruptured capillaries cause small intraretinal hemorrhages, and microinfarcts may cause cotton-wool exudates. A sensation of glare (because of the scattering of light) is a common complaint. The most common cause of decreased vision in persons with background retinopathy is macular edema.[18,19] It represents fluid accumulation in the retina stemming from a breakdown in the blood-retina barrier.

Proliferative diabetic retinopathy represents a more severe retinal change than background retinopathy. It is characterized by formation of fragile blood vessels (*i.e.*, neovascularization) at the disk and elsewhere in the retina. These vessels grow in front of the retina along the posterior surface of the vitreous or into the vitreous. They threaten vision in two ways. First, because they are abnormal, they tend to bleed easily, leaking blood into the vitreous cavity and decreasing visual acuity. Second, the blood vessels attach firmly to the retinal surface and posterior surface of the vitreous, such that normal movement of the vitreous may exert a pull on the retina, causing retinal detachment and progressive blindness. Because early proliferative diabetic retinopathy is likely to be asymptomatic, it must be identified early, before bleeding occurs and obscures the view of the fundus or leads to fibrosis and retinal attachment.

The American Diabetes Association, American College of Physicians, and American Academy of Ophthalmology have developed screening guidelines for diabetic retinopathy.[19,20] These guidelines recommend that persons with type 1 diabetes be screened annually for retinopathy beginning 5 years after the onset of diabetes. In general, screening is not indicated before the start of puberty. Persons with type 2 diabetes should have an initial examination for retinopathy shortly after diagnosis. After the initial eye examination, every person with diabetes should have regular ocular follow-up visits, at least once each year and more frequently if warranted by the severity of the retinopathy. The ocular examination by the ophthalmologist should include acuity measurements, slit-lamp biomicroscopy, and direct and indirect ophthalmoscopy of the retina through fully dilated pupils. When indicated, color fundus photographs and fluorescein angiograms should be done. When planning pregnancy, women with preexisting diabetes should be counseled about the risk of developing retinopathy or progression of existing retinopathy. Women who become pregnant should have a comprehensive eye examination just before or soon after conception and at least every 3 months throughout pregnancy.

Preventing diabetic retinopathy from developing or progressing is considered the best approach to preserving vision. Growing evidence suggests that careful control of blood sugar levels in persons with diabetes mellitus may retard the onset and progression of retinopathy. The Diabetes Control and Complications Trial Research Group demonstrated that intensive management of persons with type 1 diabetes to maintain blood glucose levels at near-normal levels reduced the risk of retinopathy by 76% in persons with no retinopathy and slowed the progress by 54% in persons with early disease.[21] Both hypertension and hyperlipidemia are thought to increase the risk of diabetic retinopathy in persons with diabetes.[19]

Photocoagulation using an argon laser provides the major direct treatment modality for diabetic retinopathy.[19] Treatment strategies include laser photocoagulation applied directly to leaking microaneurysms and grid photocoagulation with a checkerboard pattern of laser burns applied to diffuse areas of leakage and thickening.[18] Because laser photocoagulation destroys the proliferating vessels and the ischemic retina, it reduces the stimulus for further neovascularization. However, photocoagulation of neovascularization near the disk is not recommended.[19] Laser phototherapy also decreases macular edema and increases the chance of visual improvement in persons with nonproliferative retinopathy.[22] Vitrectomy has proved effective in removing vitreous hemorrhage and severing vitreoretinal membranes that develop.

Hypertensive Retinopathy.   Long-standing systemic hypertension results in the compensatory thickening of arteriolar walls, which effectively reduces capillary perfusion pressure. Ordinarily, a retinal blood vessel is transparent and seen as a red line; in venules, the red cells resemble a string of boxcars. On ophthalmoscopy, arteries in persons with long-standing hypertension appear paler than veins because they have thicker walls. The thickened arterioles in chronic hypertension become opaque and have a copper-wiring appearance. Edema, microaneurysms, intraretinal hemorrhages, exudates, and cotton-wool spots all are observed[6] (see Fig. 54-5). Malignant hypertension involves swelling of the optic disk as a result of the local edema produced by escaped fluid. If the condition is permitted to progress long enough, serious visual deficits result.

Protective thickening of arteriolar walls cannot occur with sudden increases in blood pressure. Therefore, hemorrhage is likely to occur. Trauma to the optic globe or the head, sudden high blood pressure in eclampsia, and some types of renal disease characteristically are accompanied by edema of the retina and optic disk and by an increased likelihood of hemorrhage.

Atherosclerosis of Retinal Vessels.   In atherosclerosis, the lumen of the arterioles becomes narrowed. As a result, the retinal arteries become tortuous and narrowed. At sites where the arteries cross and compress veins, the red cell column of the vein appears distended. Exudate accumulates on arteriolar walls as "fluffy," white plaques (cotton wool patches). These patches are damaged axons that on cross-section resemble "crystalloid bodies." Deep and superficial hemorrhages are common. Atheromatous plaques of the central artery are associated with increased danger of stasis, thrombi of the central veins, and occlusion.

Retinopathy of Prematurity.   Retinopathy of prematurity is a potentially blinding abnormal proliferation of retinal blood vessels that is unique to the preterm infant. The condition previously was called *retrolental fibroplasia* because of the mass of scarred tissue that develops behind the lens in advanced cases. Improved survival rates of low–birth-weight premature infants have resulted in an increased incidence of retinopathy of prematurity.

The risk factors associated with retinopathy of prematurity are not fully known, but prematurity and low birth weight are major risk factors. Hyperoxia also is a major risk factor, as are other problems such as respiratory distress, apnea, infection, hypoxia, and acidosis. Generally the lower the birth weight, the greater the risk. The incidence of retinopathy of prematurity in infants weighing 500 to 750 g is almost 100%, with severe disease developing in approximately 30% of these infants; the incidence of retinopathy in those weighing 751 to 1000 g is almost 80%, with severe disease occurring in approximately 10% of the infants.[23]

The immature retina has two blood supplies, the choroidal and the inner retinal vessels. The choroidal blood vessels, which lie on the outside of the retina, develop early and are the sole supplier of nourishment for the immature retina. Vascularization of the inner retina begins during the 16th week of gestation as the retinal vessels grow and advance outward in a 360-degree circle from the optic nerve; they reach the ora serrata, the anterior serrated edge of the neural retina, at the nasal periphery by 32 weeks and reach the temporal periphery by approximately the 40th week of gestation.[7] Retinopathy of prematurity develops at the site of these newly forming retinal vessels. These vessels undergo abnormal proliferation, forming an abrupt, rather than a gradual, junction between the vascular and avascular retina. The newly formed vessels often are abnormal and weak and can grow into the vitreous body, where they may cause leakage of fluid or hemorrhage with resultant formation of scar tissue. As the scar tissue shrinks, it can exert traction on the retina, causing retinal detachment and permanent loss of vision[6] (Fig. 54-7).

Because of the risk of retinopathy in premature infants, it is recommended that all at-risk infants undergo regular ophthalmologic examinations.[7] Guidelines vary but usually include infants weighing less than 1500 g at birth and those born before 28 weeks of gestation. Infants weighing over 1500 g who have an unstable clinical course and are thought to be at high risk also should be examined.

Treatment consists of cryotherapy or laser surgery to the vascular portion of the retina. During cryotherapy, the trained ophthalmologist or ocular surgeon places the cryoprobe on the outside of the eye to produce transscleral freezing and destruction of the abnormal vessels. Because the incidence of myopia and astigmatism is greater among children treated with cryotherapy, infants requiring treatment should be closely followed by an ophthalmologist.

Retinal Detachment

Retinal detachment involves the separation of the sensory retina from the pigment epithelium (Fig. 54-8). It occurs when traction on the inner sensory layer or a tear in this layer allows fluid, usually vitreous, to accumulate between the two layers. Retinal detachment that results from breaks in the sensory layer of the retina is called *rhegmatogenous detachment* (*rhegma* in Greek, meaning "rent" or "hole"). The vitreous normally is adherent to the retina at the optic disk, macula, and periphery of the retina. When the vitreous shrinks, it separates from the retina at the posterior pole of the eye (posterior vitreous detachment), but at the periphery, the vitreous pulls on the attached retina, which can lead to tearing of the retina. Vitreous fluid can enter the tear and contribute to further separation of the retina from its overlying pigment layer.

Persons with high grades of myopia may have abnormalities in the peripheral retina that predispose to sudden detachment. Intraocular surgery such as cataract extraction may produce traction on the peripheral retina that causes eventual detachment months or even years after surgery.[18] Detachment may result from exudates that separate the two retinal layers. Exudative detachment may be caused by intraocular inflammation, intraocular tumors, or certain systemic diseases. Inflammatory processes include posterior scleritis, uveitis, or parasitic invasion. Retinal detachment also can follow trauma immediately or at some later time.

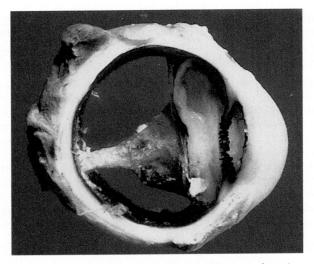

FIGURE 54-7 Retinopathy of prematurity. Horizontal section of an eye with advanced retinopathy of prematurity shows a totally detached retina adherent to a fibrovascular mass behind the lens. (Rubin E., Farber J.L. [1999]. *Pathology* [3rd ed., p. 1558]. Philadelphia: Lippincott-Raven)

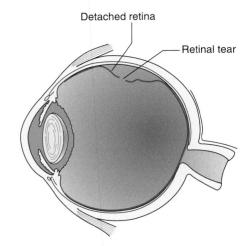

FIGURE 54-8 Detached retina.

Detachment of the neural retina from the retinal pigment layer separates the receptors from their major blood supply, the choroid. If retinal detachment continues for some time, permanent destruction and blindness of that part of the retina occur. The bipolar and ganglion cells survive because their blood supply, by way of the retinal arteries, remains intact. Without receptors, however, there is no visual function. The primary symptom of retinal detachment is loss of vision. Sometimes, flashing lights or sparks, followed by small floaters or spots in the field of vision, occur as the retina pulls away from the posterior pole of the eye. There is no pain. As detachment progresses, the person perceives a dark curtain progressing across the visual field (see Fig. 54-1). Because the process begins in the periphery and spreads circumferentially and posteriorly, initial visual disturbances may involve only one quadrant of the visual field. Large peripheral detachments may occur without involvement of the macula, so that visual acuity remains unaffected. The tendency, however, is for detachments to enlarge until all of the retina is detached.

Diagnosis is based on the ophthalmoscopic appearance of the retina. Treatment is aimed at closing retinal tears and reattaching the retina. Rhegmatogenous detachment usually requires surgical treatment. Scleral buckling or pneumatic retinopexy are the most commonly used surgical techniques. Scleral buckling is the primary surgical procedure performed to reattach the retina. The procedure requires careful location of the retinal break and treatment with diathermy, cryotherapy, or laser to produce chorioretinal adhesions that seal the retinal tears so that the vitreous can no longer leak into the subretinal space. With scleral buckling, a piece of silicone (*i.e.*, the buckle) is sutured and infolded into the sclera, physically indenting the sclera so it comes in contact with the separated pigment and retinal layers. Pneumatic retinopexy involves the intraocular injection of an expandable gas instead of a piece of silicone to form the indentation. An overall reattachment rate of 90% is reported, but the visual results depend on the preoperative status of the macula.[2] The most common cause of failure after surgical treatment for detached retina is the development of membranes on the retina. Intraocular instruments have been refined for microsurgical removal of membranes from the retinal surface and reattaching the retina.[18]

Macular Degeneration

Macular degeneration is characterized by destructive changes of the yellow-pigmented area surrounding the central fovea resulting from vascular disorders. Age-related macular degeneration is the most common cause of reduced vision in the United States. It is the leading cause of blindness among persons older than 75 years and of newly reported cases of blindness among those older than 65 years of age.[1] The cause of macular degeneration is unknown, although nutritional, hemodynamic, degenerative, and phototoxic factors are under investigation.

Macular degeneration is characterized by the loss of central vision, usually in both eyes. Age-related macular degeneration can be classified into early and late stages.[24] The early stage is associated with minimal visual impairment.

There are pigmentary abnormalities and pale yellow spots that may occur individually or in groups throughout the macula, called *drusen*. Only eyes with large drusen are at risk for late-stage age-related macular degeneration. Persons with late-stage disease often find it difficult to see at long distances (*e.g.*, in driving), do close work (*e.g.*, reading), see faces clearly, or distinguish colors. However, the person may not be severely incapacitated because the peripheral retinal function usually remains intact. With the help of low-vision aids, most persons with macular degeneration can continue their normal activities.

There are two types of age-related macular degeneration: an atrophic nonexudative or "dry" form and an exudative or "wet" form.[24] The atrophic form is characterized by a gradual, progressive bilateral vision loss from atrophy and degeneration of the rod and cone photoreceptors. It does not involve leakage of blood or serum; hence it is called *dry age-related macular degeneration*. The exudative form is characterized by the formation of a choroidal neovascular membrane that separates the pigmented epithelium from the neuroretina. These new blood vessels have weaker walls than normal and are prone to leakage: hence it is called *wet age-related macular degeneration*. The leakage of serous or hemorrhagic fluid into the subretinal space causes separation of the pigmented epithelium from the neurosensory retina. Over time, the subretinal hemorrhages organize to form scar tissue. When this happens, retinal tissue death and loss of all visual function in the corresponding macular area occurs. Between 80% and 85% of those with age-related macular degeneration have the atrophic form, but 80% to 85% of severe vision loss can be ascribed to the exudative form.[25]

Although there is no treatment for the dry form of macular degeneration, argon laser photocoagulation may be useful in treating the neovascularization that occurs with the wet form.[25,26] Another method that has been used to halt neovascularization is photodynamic therapy. It is a nonthermal process leading to localized production of reactive oxygen species that mediate cellular, vascular, and immunologic injury and destruction of new blood vessels.

Although rare, macular degeneration can occur as a hereditary condition in young persons and sometimes in adults. The genetic form of macular dystrophy, Stargardt's disease, becomes manifest in the middle of the first to second decade of life and is inherited as a classic recessive trait, requiring mutations in both alleles of a single disease-related gene.[27] The gene codes for an ABCR (ATP-binding cassette transporter—retina) transporter molecule located in the retina that functions in the transport of retinal lipids and peptides (see Chapter 53). It is thought that mutations in this gene allow degraded material to accumulate and interfere with retinal function.

Tests of Retinal Function

The diagnosis of retinal disease is based on history, tests of visual acuity, refraction, visual field tests, color vision tests, and often fluorescein angiography. Electroretinography can be used to measure the electrical activity of the retina in response to a flash of light. Recorded electroretinography represents the difference in electrical potential between an electrode placed in a corneal contact lens and one placed on the forehead. The test can be used to evaluate retinal function in persons with an opaque lens or vitreous body. The electro-oculogram records the electrical potentials between the front of the eye and the retina in the back of the eye. It is recorded from two electrodes, one placed above and the other lateral to the eye. The electro-oculogram measures eye movement and is used frequently in sleep studies.

> In summary, the retina covers the inner aspect of the posterior two thirds of the eyeball and is continuous with the optic nerve. It contains the neural receptors for vision, and it is here that light energy of different frequencies and intensities is converted to graded local potentials, which then are converted to action potentials and transmitted to visual centers in the brain. The photoreceptors normally shed portions of their outer segments. These segments are phagocytized by cells in the pigment epithelium. Failure of phagocytosis, as occurs in one form of retinitis pigmentosa, results in degeneration of the pigment layer and blindness.
>
> The retina receives its blood from two sources: the choriocapillaris, which supplies the pigment layer and the outer portion of the sensory retina adjacent to the choroid, and the branches of the retinal artery, which supply the inner half of the retina. The retinal blood vessels normally are apparent through the ophthalmoscope. Disorders of retinal vessels can result from a number of local and systemic disorders, including diabetes mellitus and hypertension. They cause vision loss through changes that result in hemorrhage, the production of opacities, and the separation of the pigment epithelium and sensory retina. Retinopathy of prematurity is a potentially blinding disorder of preterm infants who require oxygen therapy. The disorder involves the formation of new, fragile blood vessels that may cause leakage of fluid and hemorrhage with scar formation. Retinal detachment involves separation of the sensory receptors from their blood supply; it causes blindness unless reattachment is accomplished promptly.

Disorders of Neural Pathways and Cortical Centers

After you have completed this section of the chapter, you should be able to meet the following objectives:

✦ Characterize what is meant by a *visual field defect*
✦ Explain the use of perimetry in the diagnosis of a visual field defect
✦ Define the terms *hemianopia, quadrantanopia, heteronymous hemianopia,* and *homonymous hemianopia* and relate to disorders of the optic pathways
✦ Describe visual defects associated with disorders of the visual cortex and visual association areas
✦ Describe tests used in assessing the pupillary reflex and cite the possible causes of abnormal pupillary reflexes

Full visual function requires the normally developed brain-related functions of photoreception, visual sensation and perception, and the pupillary reflex. These functions depend on the integrity of all visual pathways, including the retinal circuitry and the pathway from the optic nerve.

VISUAL FIELD DEFECTS

Visual field defects result from damage to the visual pathways or the visual cortex. Perimetry or visual field testing, in which the visual field of each eye is measured and plotted in an arc, is used to identify defects and determine the location of lesions. The periphery of the opposite visual field is represented on the medial surface and in the depths of a deep medial calcarine sulcus of the occipital cortex (area 17). The central, high-acuity part of the visual half-field extends somewhat over the occipital pole. The visual association cortex surrounds the primary cortex on the superior, lateral, and inferior occipital lobe. This area is required for complex analysis and learned meaningfulness of visual stimuli.

All of us possess a hole, or scotoma, in our visual field, of which we are unaware. Because the optic disk, where the optic nerve fibers exit the retina, does not contain photoreceptors, the corresponding location in the visual field constitutes a blind spot. Local retinal damage caused by small vascular lesions (*i.e.*, retinal stroke) and other localized pathologies can produce additional blind spots. As with the normal blind spot, persons usually are not aware of the existence of scotomata in their visual fields unless they encounter problems seeing objects in certain restricted parts of the visual field.

Absences near or in the center of the bilateral visual field can be annoying and even disastrous. Although the hole is not recognized as such, the person finds that a part of a printed page appears or disappears, depending on where the fixation point is held. Most persons learn to position their eyes so as to use the remaining central foveal vision for high-acuity tasks. Defects in the peripheral visual field, including the monocular peripheral fields, are less annoying but potentially more dangerous. The person who is unaware of the defect, when walking or driving an automobile, does not see cars or bicyclists until their image reaches the functional visual field—sometimes too late to avert an accident. With careful education, a person can learn to shift the gaze constantly to obtain visual coverage of important parts of the visual field. If the damage is at the retinal or optic nerve level, only the monocular field of the damaged eye becomes a problem. A lesion affecting the central foveal vision of one eye can result in complaints of eye strain during reading and other close work, because only one eye really is being used. Localized damage to the optic tracts, lateral geniculate nucleus (LGN), optic radiation, or primary visual cortex affects corresponding parts of the visual fields of both eyes.

DISORDERS OF THE OPTIC PATHWAYS

The visual pathway extends from the front to the back of the head. It is much like a telephone line between distant points in that damage at any point along the pathway results in functional defects (Fig. 54-9). Among the disorders that can interrupt the visual pathway are vascular lesions, trauma, and tumors. For example, normal visual system function depends on vascular adequacy in the ophthalmic artery and its branches; the central artery of the retina; the anterior and middle cerebral arteries, which supply the intracranial optic nerve, chiasm, and optic tracts; and the posterior cerebral artery, which supplies the LGN, optic radiation, and visual cortex. The adequacy of posterior cerebral artery function depends on that of the vertebral and basilar arteries that supply the brain stem. Vascular insufficiency in any one of these arterial systems can seriously affect vision.

Examination of visual system function is of particular diagnostic use because lesions at various points along the pathway have characteristic symptoms that assist in the localization of pathologies. Visual field defects of each eye and of the two eyes together are useful in localizing lesions affecting the system. Blindness in one eye is called *anopia*. If half of the visual field for one eye is lost, the defect is called *hemianopia*; loss of a quarter field is called *quadrantanopia*. Enlarging pituitary tumors can produce longitudinal damage through the optic chiasm with loss of the medial fibers of the optic nerve representing both nasal retinas and both temporal visual half-fields. Loss of the temporal or peripheral visual fields on both sides results in a

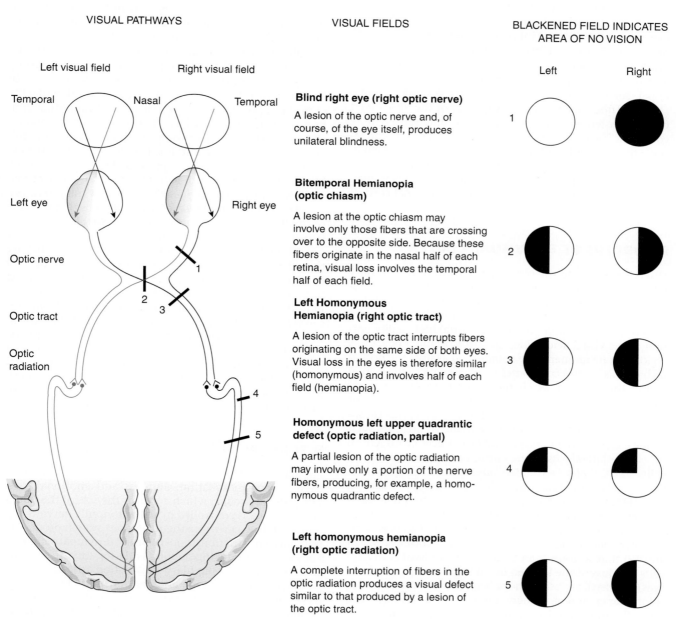

FIGURE 54-9 Visual field defects produced by selected lesions in the visual pathways. (Bates B.B. [1995]. *A guide to physical examination and history taking* [6th ed.]. Philadelphia: J.B. Lippincott)

narrow binocular field, commonly called *tunnel vision*. The loss of different half-fields in the two eyes is called a *heteronymous loss*, and the abnormality is called *heteronymous hemianopia*. Destruction of one or both lateral halves of the chiasm is common with multiple aneurysms of the circle of Willis. In this condition, the function of one or both temporal retinas is lost, and the nasal fields of one or both eyes are lost. The loss of the temporal fields (nasal retina) of both eyes is called *bitemporal heteronymous anopia*. With both eyes open, the person with bilateral defects still has the full binocular visual field.

Loss of the optic tract, LGN, full optic radiation, or complete visual cortex on one side results in loss of the corresponding visual half-fields in each eye. *Homonymous* means "the same" for both eyes. In left-side lesions, the right visual field is lost for each eye and is called *complete right homonymous hemianopia*. Partial injury to the left optic tract, LGN, or optic radiation can result in the loss of a quarter of the visual field in both eyes. This is called *homonymous quadrantanopia*, and depending on the lesion, it can involve the upper (superior) or lower (inferior) fields. Because the optic radiation fibers for the superior quarter of the visual field traverse the temporal lobe, superior quadrantanopia is more common. The LGN, optic radiation, and visual cortex all receive their major blood supply from the posterior cerebral artery; unilateral occlusion of this artery results in complete loss of the opposite field (*i.e.*, homonymous hemianopia). Bilateral occlusion of these arteries results in total cortical blindness.

DISORDERS OF THE VISUAL CORTEX

Discrete damage to the binocular portion of the primary visual cortex also can result in scotomata in the corresponding visual fields. If the visual loss is in the central high-acuity part of the field, severe loss of visual acuity and pattern discrimination occurs. The central high-acuity portion of the visual field is located at the occipital pole. This region can be momentarily compressed against the occipital bone (*i.e.*, contrecoup) after severe trauma to the frontal part of the cranium. Mechanical trauma to the cortex results in firing of neurons, experienced as flashes of light or "seeing stars." Destruction of the polar visual cortex causes severe loss of visual acuity and pattern discrimination. Such damage is permanent and cannot be corrected with lenses.

The bilateral loss of the entire primary visual cortex, called *cortical blindness*, eliminates all visual experience. Crude analysis of visual stimulation at reflex levels, such as eye-orienting and head-orienting responses to bright moving lights, pupillary reflexes, and blinking at sudden bright lights, may be retained even though vision has been lost. Extensive damage to the visual association cortex (areas 18 and 19) that surrounds an intact primary visual cortex results in a loss of the learned meaningfulness of visual images (*i.e.*, visual agnosia). The patient can see the patterns of color, shapes, and movement, but no longer can recognize formerly meaningful stimuli. Familiar objects can be described but not named or reacted to meaningfully. However, if other sensory modalities, such as hearing and touch,

can be applied, full recognition occurs. This disorder represents a problem of recognition rather than intellect.

TESTING OF VISUAL FIELDS

Crude testing of the binocular visual field and the visual field of each individual eye (*i.e.*, monocular vision) can be accomplished without specialized equipment. In the confrontation method, the examiner stands or sits 2 to 3 feet in front of the person to be tested and instructs the person to focus on an object such as a penlight with one eye closed. The object is moved from the center toward the periphery of the person's visual field and from the periphery toward the center, and the person is instructed to report the presence or absence of the object. By moving the object through the vertical, horizontal, and oblique aspects of the visual field, a crude estimate can be made of the visual field. If the test object is kept midway between the examiner and the person being tested, the examiner can close the corresponding eye and compare the person's monocular vision with his or her own. This test is based on the assumption that the examiner's peripheral field of vision is within normal limits. Large field defects can be estimated by the confrontation method, and it may be the only way for testing young children and uncooperative adults. Rapidly presenting the examiner's fingers toward the eyes and observing for a reflex blink to the threat sometimes is the only way to detect a visual field deficit in someone with decreased consciousness.

Accurate determination of the presence, size, and shape of smaller holes, or scotomata, in the visual field of a particular eye can be demonstrated by the ophthalmologist only through the use of perimetry. This is done by having the person look with one eye toward a central spot directly in front of the eye while the head is stabilized by a chin rest or bite board. A small dot of light or a colored object is moved back and forth in all areas of the visual field. The person reports whether the stimulus is visible and, if a colored stimulus is used, what the perceived color is. A hemispheric support is used to control and standardize the movement of the test object, and a plot of radial coordinates of the visual field is made. Perimetry provides a means of determining alterations from normal and, with repeated testing, a way of following the progress of the disease or treatment.

DISORDERS OF THE PUPILLARY REFLEX

Pupillary size normally varies with levels of ambient light, degree of accommodation, alertness, and emotional state. The pupillary reflex, which controls the size of the pupillary opening, is controlled by the autonomic nervous system, with the parasympathetic nervous system producing pupillary constriction (miosis) and the sympathetic nervous system producing pupillary dilation (mydriasis). The afferent stimuli for pupillary constriction arise in the ganglionic cells of the retina and are transmitted to the pretectal nuclei at the junction of the thalamus and the midbrain, and from there to preganglionic neurons in the oculomotor (CN III) nuclei (see Chapter 53, Fig. 53-13). The efferent pathway is through CN III to the ciliary ganglion in the orbit of the eye, and from there to the constrictor muscles in the iris. Dilation of the pupil is provided by sympathetic innervation under excitatory descending control from the hypothalamus. Innervation is derived from preganglionic neurons in the upper thoracic cord, which send axons along the sympathetic chain to synapse with postganglionic neurons in the superior ciliary ganglion. The postganglionic fibers travel along the surfaces of the carotid and smaller arteries to reach the eye.

The pupillary reflex can be tested by shining a penlight into one eye of the person being tested. To avoid a change in pupil size due to accommodation, the person is asked to stare into the distance. A rapid constriction of the pupil exposed to light should occur; this is called the *direct pupillary light reflex*. Because the reflex is normally bilateral, the contralateral pupil also should constrict, a reaction called the *consensual pupillary light reflex*. The circuitry of the light reflex is partially separated from the main visual pathway. This is illustrated by the fact that the pupillary reflex remains unaffected when lesions to the optic radiations or the visual cortex occur. The cortically blind person retains direct and consensual light reflexes.

The integrity of the dual autonomic control of pupillary diameter is vulnerable to trauma, tumor enlargement, or vascular disease. With diffuse damage to the forebrain involving the thalamus and hypothalamus, the pupils are typically small but respond to light. Damage to the CN III nucleus or nerve eliminates innervation of four of the six extraocular muscles and the levator muscle of the upper lid, and it results in permanent pupillary dilation in the affected eye. Lesions of the sympathetic pathways that control the iris dilator muscle can result in permanent pupillary constriction. Tumors of the orbit that compress structures behind the eye can eliminate all pupillary reflexes, usually before destroying the optic nerve.

Pupillary size is differentially affected by many pharmacologic agents. Bilateral pupillary constriction is characteristic of opiate usage. Pupillary dilation results when topical parasympathetic blocking agents such as atropine are applied and sympathetic pupillodilatory function is left unopposed. These medications are used by ophthalmologists to facilitate the examination of the transparent media and fundus of the eye. Miotic drugs such as pilocarpine have the opposite effect, facilitating aqueous humor circulation.

> In summary, visual information is carried to the brain by axons of the retinal ganglion cells that form the optic nerve. The two optic nerves meet and fuse in the optic chiasm. The axons of each nasal retina cross in the chiasm and join the uncrossed fibers of the temporal retina of the opposite eye in the optic tract. From the optic chiasm, the crossed fibers of the nasal retina of one eye and the uncrossed temporal fibers of the other eye pass to the LGN and then to the primary visual cortex, which is located in the calcarine fissure of the occipital lobe. Damage to the visual pathways or visual cortex leads to visual field defects that can be identified through visual field testing or perimetry and used to determine the lesion's location. Damage to the visual as-

sociation cortex can result in the phenomenon of seeing an object, but with loss of learned recognition (*i.e.*, visual agnosia).
>
> The pupillary reflex, which controls the size of the pupil, is controlled by the autonomic nervous system. The parasympathetic nervous system controls pupillary constriction, and the sympathetic nervous system controls pupillary dilation.

Disorders of Eye Movement

After you have completed this section of the chapter, you should be able to meet the following objectives:

✦ Explain the difference between paralytic and nonparalytic strabismus
✦ Define *amblyopia* and explain its pathogenesis
✦ Explain the need for early diagnosis and treatment of eye movement disorders in children

Normal vision depends on the coordinated action of the entire visual system and a number of central control systems. It is through these mechanisms that an object is simultaneously imaged on the fovea of both eyes and perceived as a single image. Strabismus and amblyopia are two disorders that affect this highly integrated system. Although strabismus may develop in later life, it is seen most commonly in children, among whom its incidence is approximately 2%.

STRABISMUS

Strabismus, or squint, refers to any abnormality of eye coordination or alignment that results in loss of binocular vision (Fig. 54-10). When images from the same spots in visual space do not fall on corresponding points of the two retinas, diplopia, or double vision, occurs.

In standard terminology, the disorders of eye movement are described according to the direction of movement. Esotropia refers to medial deviation, exotropia refers to lateral deviation, hypertropia refers to upward deviation, hypotropia refers to downward deviation, and cyclotropia refers to torsional deviation. The term *concomitance* refers to equal deviation in all directions of gaze. A nonconcomitant strabismus is one that varies with the direction of gaze. Strabismus may be divided into paralytic (nonconcomitant) forms, in which there is weakness or paralysis of one or more of the extraocular muscles, and nonparalytic (concomitant) forms, in which there is no primary muscle impairment. Strabismus is called *intermittent*, or *periodic*, when there are periods in which the eyes are parallel. It is monocular when the same eye always deviates and the fellow eye fixates. Figure 54-11 illustrates abnormalities in eye movement associated with esotropia and exotropia.

Strabismus affects approximately 4% of children younger than 6 years of age.[28] Because 30% to 50% of these children sustain permanent secondary loss of vision, or amblyopia, if the condition is left untreated, early diagnosis and treatment are essential.[29]

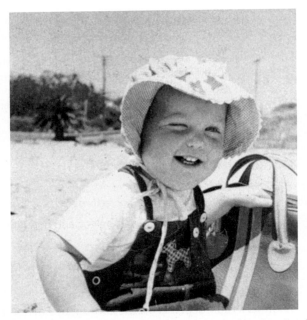

FIGURE 54-10 Photograph of a child with intermittent exotropia squinting in the sunlight. (Vaughn D.G., Asbury T., Riordon-Eva P. [1995]. *General ophthalmology* [p. 239]. Stamford, CT: Appleton & Lange)

Paralytic Strabismus

Paralytic strabismus results from paresis (*i.e.*, weakness) or plegia (*i.e.*, paralysis) of one or more of the extraocular muscles. When the normal eye fixates, the affected eye is in the position of primary deviation. In the case of esotropia, there is weakness of one of the lateral rectus muscles, usually the result of weakness of the abducens nerve (CN VI). When the affected eye fixates, the unaffected eye is in a position of secondary deviation. The secondary deviation of the unaffected eye is greater than the primary deviation of the affected eye. This is because the affected eye requires an excess of innervational impulse to maintain fixation; the excess impulses also are distributed to the unaffected eye, causing overaction of its muscles.[2]

Paralytic strabismus is uncommon in children but accounts for nearly all cases of adult strabismus; it can be caused by a number of conditions. Paralytic strabismus is seen most commonly in adults who have had cerebral vascular accidents and also may occur as the first sign of a tumor or inflammatory condition involving the CNS. One type of muscular dystrophy exerts its effects on the extraocular muscles. Initially, eye movements in all directions are weak, with later progression to bilateral optic immobility. Weakness of eye movement and lid elevation often is the first evidence of myasthenia gravis. The pathway of the oculomotor (CN III), trochlear (CN IV), and abducens

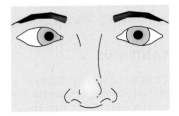

A   Primary position: right esotropia

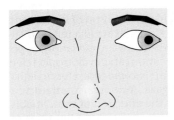

B   Left gaze: no deviation

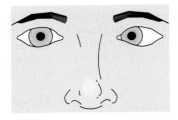

C   Right gaze: left esotropia

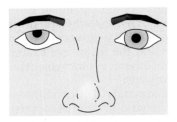

D   Right hypertropia

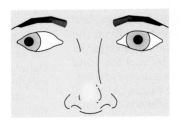

E   Right exotropia

FIGURE 54-11 Paralytic strabismus associated with paralysis of the right lateral rectus muscle: (**A**) primary position (looking straight ahead) of the eyes; (**B**) left gaze with no deviation; and (**C**) right gaze with left esotropia. (**D**) Primary position of the eyes with weakness of the right inferior rectus and right hypertropia; and (**E**) primary position of the eyes with weakness of the right medial rectus and right exotropia.

(CN VI) nerves through the cavernous sinus and the back of the orbit make them vulnerable to basal skull fracture and tumors of the cavernous sinus (*e.g.*, cavernous sinus syndrome) or orbit (*e.g.*, orbital syndrome).[30] In infants, paralytic strabismus can be caused by birth injuries affecting the extraocular muscles or the cranial nerves supplying these muscles. It also can result from congenital anomalies of the muscles. In general, paralytic strabismus in an adult with previously normal binocular vision causes diplopia. This does not occur in persons who have never developed binocular vision.

Nonparalytic Strabismus

In nonparalytic strabismus, there is no extraocular muscle weakness or paralysis, and the angle of deviation is always the same in all fields of gaze. With persistent deviation, secondary abnormalities may develop because of overaction or underaction of the muscles in some fields of gaze. Nonparalytic esotropia is the most common type of strabismus. The disorder may be accommodative, nonaccommodative, or a combination of the two. Accommodative strabismus is caused by disorders such as uncorrected hyperopia, in which the esotropia occurs with accommodation. The onset of this type of esotropia characteristically occurs between 18 months and 4 years of age because accommodation is not well developed until that time. The disorder most often is monocular but may be alternating. Approximately 50% of the cases of esotropia are accommodative. The causes of nonaccommodative strabismus are obscure. The disorder may be related to faulty muscle insertion, fascial abnormalities, or faulty innervation. There is evidence that idiopathic strabismus may have a genetic basis; siblings may have similar disorders.

Diagnosis and Treatment

All infants and children should be examined for visual alignment. Alignment of the visual axis occurs in the first 3 months of life. All infants should have consistent, synchronized eye movement by 5 to 6 months of age.[31] Infants who have reached this age and whose eyes are not aligned at all times during waking hours should be examined by a qualified practitioner.

Rapid assessment of extraocular muscle function is accomplished by three methods. First, in a somewhat darkened room and with the child staring straight ahead, a penlight is pointed at the midpoint between the two eyes, and a bright dot of reflected light can be seen on the cornea of each eye. With normal eye alignment, the reflected light should appear at the same spot on the cornea of each eye. Nonparallelism of the two eyes indicates muscle imbalance because of weakness or paralysis of the deviant eye. In a second method, the child is asked to follow the movement of a small object (*e.g.*, a pencil point, lighted penlight) as it is moved through the extremes of what are called the *six cardinal positions of gaze*. In extreme lateral gaze, normal subjects can show a few quick beats of a jerky or nystagmoid movement. Nystagmoid movement is abnormal if it is prolonged or present in any other eye posture. The third method, called the *cover-uncover test*, eliminates binocular fusion as a factor in maintaining parallelism between the eyes and is used to determine which eye is used for fixation. The child's attention is directed toward a fixed object such as a small picture or tongue blade. A light should not be used because it may not stimulate accommodation. If a mild weakness is present, the eye with blocked vision drifts into a resting position, the extent of which depends on the relative strength of the muscles. The eye should snap back when the card is removed. The test always is done for near and far fixation. Visual acuity is evaluated to obtain a comparison of the two eyes. A tumbling E chart (or similar test chart) can be used for young children.[32]

Treatment of strabismus is directed toward the development of normal visual acuity, correction of the deviation, and superimposition of the retinal images to provide binocular vision. Nonsurgical and surgical methods can be used. In children, early treatment is important; the ideal age to begin is 6 months. Nonsurgical treatment includes occlusive patching, pleoptics (*i.e.*, eye exercises), and prism glasses. Because prolonged occlusive patching leads to loss of useful vision in the covered eye, patching is alternated between the affected and unaffected eye. This improves the vision in the affected eye without sacrificing vision in the unaffected eye. Prism glasses compensate for an abnormal alignment of an optic globe. Occasionally, long-acting miotics in weak strengths (*e.g.*, echothiophate iodide solution [Phospholine Iodide] or pilocarpine [Pilocarpine HS]) are used to cause pharmacologic accommodation in place of or in combination with corrective lenses.[28] Surgical procedures may be used to strengthen or weaken a muscle by altering its length or attachment site.

AMBLYOPIA

Amblyopia describes a condition of diminished vision (uncorrectable by lenses) in which no detectable organic lesion of the eye is present.[33] This condition sometimes is referred to as *lazy eye*. Types of amblyopia include deprivation occlusion, strabismus, refractive, and organic amblyopia. It is caused by visual deprivation (*e.g.*, cataracts, severe ptosis) or abnormal binocular interactions (*e.g.*, strabismus, anisometropia) during visual immaturity. Normal development of the thalamic and cortical circuitry necessary for binocular visual perception requires simultaneous binocular use of each fovea during a critical period early in life (0 to 5 years). In infants with unilateral cataracts that are dense, central, and larger than 2 mm in diameter, this time is before 2 months of age.[2] In conditions causing abnormal binocular interactions, one image is suppressed to provide clearer vision. In esotropia, vision of the deviated eye is suppressed to prevent diplopia. A similar situation exists in anisometropia, in which the refractive indexes of the two eyes are different. Although the eyes are correctly aligned, they are unable to focus together, and the image of one eye is suppressed. In animal experiments, monocular deprivation results in reduced synaptic density in the LGN and the primary visual cortical areas that process input from the affected eye or eyes.[32]

The reversibility of amblyopia depends on the maturity of the visual system at the time of onset and the duration of the abnormal experience. If esotropia is involved, some persons alternate eyes and do not experience diplopia. With late adolescent or adult onset, this habit pattern must be unlearned after correction.

Peripheral vision is less affected than central foveal vision in amblyopia. Suppression becomes more evident with high illumination and high contrast. It is as if the affected eye did not possess central vision and the person learns to fixate with the nonfoveal retina. If bilateral congenital blindness or near blindness (*e.g.*, from cataracts) occurs and remains uncorrected during infancy and early childhood, the person remains without pattern vision and has only overall field brightness and color discrimination. This is essentially bilateral amblyopia.

The treatment of children with the potential for development of amblyopia must be instituted well before the age of 6 years to avoid the suppression phenomenon. Surgery for congenital cataracts and ptosis should be done early. Severe refractive errors should be corrected. In strabismus, alternately blocking vision in one eye and then the other forces the child to use both eyes for form discrimination. The duration of occlusion of vision in the good eye must be short (2 to 5 hours per day) and closely monitored, or deprivation amblyopia can develop in the good eye as well. Although amblyopia is not likely to occur after 8 or 9 years of age, some plasticity in central circuitry is evident even in adulthood.[34] For example, after refractive correction for long-standing astigmatism in adults, visual acuity improves slowly, requiring several months to reach normal levels.

In summary, disorders of eye movement include strabismus and amblyopia. Strabismus refers to abnormalities in the coordination of eye movements with loss of binocular eye alignment. This inability to focus a visual image on corresponding parts of the two retinas results in diplopia. Esotropia refers to medial deviation, exotropia refers to lateral deviation, hypertropia refers to upward deviation, hypotropia refers to downward deviation, and cyclotropia refers to torsional deviation. Paralytic strabismus is caused by weakness or paralysis of the extraocular muscles. Nonparalytic strabismus results from the inappropriate length or insertion of the extraocular muscles or from accommodation disorders. Amblyopia (*i.e.*, lazy eye) is a condition of diminished vision that cannot be corrected by lenses and in which no detectable organic lesion in the eye can be observed. It results from inadequately developed CNS circuitry because of visual deprivation (*e.g.*, cataracts) or abnormal binocular interactions (*e.g.*, strabismus, anisometropia) during the period of visual immaturity.

References

1. Leonard R. (1999). Statistics on visual impairment: A resource manual. Lighthouse International. [On-line]. Available: http://www.lighthouse.org.

2. Vaughan D.G., Ashbury T., Riordan-Eva P. (1999). *General ophthalmology* (15th ed., pp. 75, 84–90, 92–107, 119–140, 160, 188, 200–212, 216–233). Norwalk, CT: Appleton & Lange.

3. Morrow G.L., Abbott R.L. (1998). Conjunctivitis. *American Family Physician* 57(4), 735–746.

4. Hara J.H. (1996). The red eye: Diagnosis and treatment. *American Family Physician* 54, 2423–2430.

5. Riordan-Eva P., Vaughan D.G. (2001). Eye. In Tierney L.M., McPhee S.J., Papadakis M.A. (Eds.), *Current medical diagnosis and treatment* (40th ed., pp. 185–216). New York: Lange Medical Books/McGraw-Hill.

6. Klintworth G.K. (1999). The eye. In Rubin E., Farber J.L. (Eds.), *Pathology* (3rd ed., pp. 1537–1563). Philadelphia: Lippincott Williams & Wilkins.

7. Olitsky S.E., Nelson L. (2000). Disorders of the conjunctiva. In Behrman R.E., Kliegman R.M., Jenson H.B. (Eds.), *Nelson textbook of pediatrics* (16th ed., pp. 1911–1913, 1918, 1925–1926). Philadelphia: W.B. Saunders.

8. Evans N.M. (1995). *Ophthalmology* (2nd ed., pp. 43–44, 68–69, 113–116, 205). New York: Oxford University Press.

9. Rosenberg L.F. (1995). Glaucoma: Early detection and therapy for prevention of vision loss. *American Family Physician* 52, 2289–2298.

10. Martin X.D. (1992). Normal intraocular pressure in man. *Ophthalmologica* 205, 57–63.

11. Quigley H.A. (1993). Open-angle glaucoma. *New England Journal of Medicine* 328, 1097–1106.

12. Alward W.L.M. (1998). Medical management of glaucoma. *New England Journal of Medicine* 339, 1299–1307.

13. Quillen D.A. (1999). Common causes of vision loss in elderly patients. *American Family Physician* 60, 99–108.

14. Agency for Health Care Policy and Research, Cataract Management Guideline Panel. (1993). *Clinical practice guideline 4. Cataract in adults: Management of functional impairment*. AHCPR No. 93-0543. Bethesda, MD: U.S. Department of Health and Human Services.

15. Schmitt C., Hockwin O. (1990). The mechanisms of cataract formation. *Journal of Inherited Metabolic Disease* 13, 501–508.

16. Quality of Care Committee—Anterior Segment Panel. (1989). *Cataract in the otherwise healthy eye*. San Francisco: American Academy of Ophthalmology.

17. Albert D.M., Dryja T.P. (1999). The eye. In Cotran R.S., Kumar V., Collins T. (Eds.), *Robbins pathologic basis of disease* (6th ed., pp. 1359–1377). Philadelphia: W.B. Saunders.

18. D'Amico D.J. (1994). Diseases of the retina. *New England Journal of Medicine* 331, 95–106.

19. Ferris F.L., Davis M.D., Aiello L.M. (1999). Treatment of diabetic retinopathy. *New England Journal of Medicine* 341, 667–678.

20. Klein R. (1994). Eye care delivery for people with diabetes. *Diabetes Care* 17, 614–615.

21. Diabetes Control and Complications Trial Research Group. (1993). The effect of intensive treatment of diabetes on the development and progression of long-term complications in insulin-dependent diabetes mellitus. *New England Journal of Medicine* 329, 977–986.

22. Murphy R.P. (1995). Management of diabetic retinopathy. *American Family Physician* 51, 785–796.

23. Kretzer F.L., Hittner H.M. (1988). Retinopathy of prematurity: Clinical implications of retinal development. *Archives of Disease in Childhood* 63, 1151–1167.

24. Fine S.L., Berger J.W., MacGuire M., Ho A.C. (2000). Age-related macular degeneration. *New England Journal of Medicine* 342, 483–492.

25. Woods S. (1992). Macular degeneration. *Nursing Clinics of North America* 27, 755–761.
26. Macular Photocoagulation Study Group. (1991). Argon laser photocoagulation for neovascular maculopathy. *Archives of Ophthalmology* 109, 1109–1114.
27. Lewis R.A., Lupski J.R. (2000). Macular degeneration: The emerging genetics. *Hospital Practice* 35 (6), 41–58.
28. Mills M.D. (1999). The eye in childhood. *American Family Physician* 60, 907–918.
29. Lavrich J.B., Nelson L.B. (1993). Diagnosis and management of strabismus disorders. *Pediatric Clinics of North America* 40, 737–751.
30. Kline L.B., Bajandas F.J. (1996). *Neuro-ophthalmology review manual* (Chapters 4–7). Thorofare, NJ: Slack.
31. Broderick P. (1998). Pediatric vision screening for the family physician. *American Family Practitioner* 58(3), 691–704.
32. Scheiman M. (1997). *Understanding and managing vision defects* (pp. 26–27). Thorofare, NJ: Slack.
33. Rubein S.E., Nelson S.B. (1993). Amblyopia: Diagnosis and management. *Pediatric Clinics of North America* 40, 727–735.
34. Wong-Riley M.T.T., Carroll E.W. (1984). The effect of impulse blockage on cytochrome oxidative activity in the monkey visual system. *Nature* 307, 262–264.

Chapter 55

Alterations in Hearing and Vestibular Function

Susan A. Fontana

The ears are paired organs consisting of an external and middle ear, which function in capturing, transmitting, and amplifying sound, and an inner ear that contains the receptive organs that are stimulated by sound waves (*i.e.*, hearing) or head position and movement (*i.e.*, vestibular function). Otitis media, or inflammation of the middle ear, is a common disorder of childhood. Hearing loss is one of the most common disabilities experienced by persons in the United States, particularly among the elderly. Vertigo, a disorder of vestibular function, is also a common cause of disability among the elderly. This chapter is divided into two parts: the first focuses on disorders of the ear and auditory function and the second on disorders of the inner ear and vestibular function.

Alterations in Auditory Function

After you have completed this section of the chapter, you should be able to meet the following objectives:

✦ Describe two common disorders of the outer ear
✦ Relate the functions of the eustachian tube to the development of middle ear problems, including acute otitis media and otitis media with effusion

✦ Describe anatomic variations as well as risk factors that make infants and young children more prone to develop acute otitis media
✦ List three common symptoms of acute otitis media
✦ Describe the disease process associated with otosclerosis and relate it to the progressive conductive hearing loss that occurs
✦ Characterize tinnitus
✦ Differentiate between conductive, sensorineural, and mixed hearing loss and cite the more common causes of each
✦ Define the term *presbycusis* and describe factors that contribute to its development
✦ Describe methods used in the diagnosis and treatment of hearing loss

DISORDERS OF THE EXTERNAL EAR

The external ear is a funnel-shaped structure that conducts sound waves to the tympanic membrane. It consists of the pinna, the external acoustic meatus, and the lateral surface of the tympanic membrane (see Chapter 53, Fig. 53-16). The function of the external ear is disturbed when sound transmission is obstructed by impacted cerumen, inflammation (*i.e.*, otitis externa), or drainage from the external ear (otorrhea).

Impacted Cerumen

Cerumen, or earwax, is a protective secretion produced by the ceruminous glands of the skin that lines the ear canal. Although the ear normally is self-cleaning, the cerumen can accumulate and narrow the canal. Impaction is a common cause of reversible hearing loss.[1] Repeated unskilled attempts to remove the wax may pack it more deeply into the ear canal. Impacted cerumen usually produces no symptoms until the canal becomes completely occluded, at which point the person experiences a feeling of fullness, loss of hearing, tinnitus (*i.e.*, ringing in the ears), or coughing because of vagal stimulation.

In most cases, cerumen can be removed by gentle irrigation using a bulb syringe and warm tap water. Warm water is used to avoid inducing a feeling of disequilibrium due to the vestibular caloric response. The ear canal should be dried thoroughly after irrigation to avoid introducing an infection. Irrigation should be avoided in an only-hearing ear or one that is postsurgical, prone to infection, or suspect for perforation of the tympanic membrane. Alternatively, health care professionals may remove cerumen using an otoscope and a wire loop or blunt cerumen curette.

Cerumen that has become hardened or impacted can be softened by instillation of a few drops of a ceruminolytic agent available commercially (*e.g.*, dilute hydrogen peroxide solution) or by prescription. Typically, these agents are instilled in the affected ear one or two times daily for up to 4 days before irrigation. Ceruminolytic agents should not be used in ears that may have a perforated tympanic membrane.

Otitis Externa

Otitis externa is an inflammation of the external ear that can vary in severity from a mild eczematoid dermatitis to severe cellulitis. It can be caused by infectious agents, irritation (*e.g.*, wearing earphones), or allergic reactions. Predisposing factors include moisture in the ear canal after swimming (*i.e.*, swimmer's ear) or bathing and trauma resulting from scratching or attempts to clean the ear. Most infections are caused by gram-negative bacteria (*e.g.*, *Pseudomonas*, *Proteus*) or fungi that grow in the presence of excess moisture.[2] Otitis externa commonly occurs in the summer and is manifested by itching, redness, tenderness, and narrowing of the ear canal because of swelling. Inflammation of the pinna or canal makes movement of the ear painful. There may be watery or purulent drainage and intermittent hearing loss.

Treatment usually includes the use of ear drops containing an appropriate antimicrobial agent in combination with a corticosteroid to reduce inflammation. An antifungal agent may also be used. Protection of the ear from additional moisture and avoidance of trauma from scratching are important. Preventing recurrences is important, particularly in persons who swim frequently. Instillation of a dilute alcohol, acetic acid, or Burow's otic solution (available in over-the-counter ear drops) immediately after swimming usually is an effective prophylaxis.

Dermatoses (*i.e.*, seborrheic, contact, and atopic dermatitis) are common causes of inflammation of the external ear canal and can be precursors of acute inflammation caused by scratching and introduction of infectious organisms. They can be treated satisfactorily by instillation of an otic solution containing a corticosteroid.

Pruritus

Pruritus of the external ear and ear canal is a common problem. It is most commonly self-induced by overzealous cleaning with soap and water or use of cotton swabs to remove protective cerumen from the ear canal.

Treatment includes avoidance of scratching, irritation, and removal of cerumen. Corticosteroid ear drops may be used when inflammation is present. Severe pruritus also may be caused by allergy in persons with hay fever. Medications used for treatment of the allergy and corticosteroid ear drops usually are effective in relieving the pruritus.

DISORDERS OF THE MIDDLE EAR AND EUSTACHIAN TUBE

The middle ear consists of the tympanic membrane, or eardrum, which separates the outer ear from the middle ear; the *eustachian tube*, also called the *auditory tube*, which connects the middle ear with the nasopharynx; and the bony ossicles, which connect the tympanic membrane with the oval window (see Chapter 53, Fig. 53-16). It is located in an air-filled space in the petrous portion of the temporal bone. The tympanic membrane, which separates the external ear from the middle ear, has three layers: an outer layer of thin skin continuous with the lining of the external ear canal, a middle layer of tough collagenous fibers mixed with fibrocytes and some elastic fibers, and an inner epithelial layer continuous with the lining of the middle ear. It is attached in a manner that allows it to vibrate freely when audible sound waves enter the external auditory canal.

When viewed through an otoscope, the tympanic membrane appears as a shallow, almost circular cone pointing inward toward its apex, the umbo (Fig. 55-1). Light usually is reflected from the pars tensa at approximately the 4-o'clock position. Landmarks include the lightened stripe over the handle of the malleus; the umbo at the end of the handle; the pars tensa, which constitutes most of the drum; and the pars flaccida, the small area above the malleus attachment. The tympanic membrane is semitransparent, and a small, whitish cord, which traverses the middle ear from back to front, can be seen just under its upper edge. This is the *chorda tympani*, a branch of the intermedius component of the facial nerve (cranial nerve [CN] VII).

Eustachian Tube Dysfunction

The eustachian tube, which connects the nasopharynx with the middle ear, is located in a gap in the bone between the anterior and medial walls of the middle ear (Fig. 55-2). The middle ear is filled with the air that reaches it from the nasopharynx through the eustachian tube. The eustachian tube is lined with a mucous membrane that is continuous with the pharynx and the mastoid air cells. Infections from the nasopharynx can travel from the nasopharynx along the mucous membrane of the eustachian tube to the middle ear, causing acute otitis media. Toward the nasopharynx, the eustachian tube becomes lined by columnar epithelium with mucus-secreting cells. Hypertrophy of the mucus-

Disorders of the Middle Ear

➤ The middle ear is a small, air-filled compartment in the temporal bone. It is separated from the outer ear by the tympanic membrane; communication between the nasopharynx and the middle ear occurs through the eustachian tube; and tiny bony ossicles that span the middle ear transmit sound to the sensory receptors in the inner ear.

➤ Otitis media (OM) refers to inflammation of the middle ear, usually associated with an acute infection (acute OM) or an accumulation of fluid (OME). It commonly is associated with disorders of eustachian tube function.

➤ The function of the middle ear is to conduct sound waves from the external to the inner ear. Impaired conduction of sound waves and hearing loss occur when the tympanic membrane has been perforated; air in the middle ear has been replaced with fluid (OME); or the function of the bony ossicles has been impaired (otosclerosis).

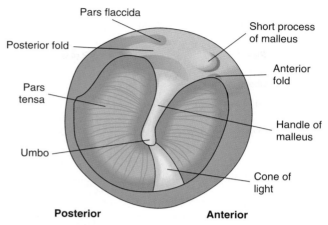

FIGURE 55-1 Right eardrum.

secreting cells is thought contribute to the mucoid secretions that develop during certain types of otitis media (OM).

The eustachian tube serves three basic functions: (1) ventilation of the middle ear, along with equalization of middle ear and ambient pressures; (2) protection of the middle ear from unwanted nasopharyngeal sound waves and secretions; and (3) drainage of middle ear secretions into the nasopharynx.[3] The nasopharyngeal entrance to the eustachian tube, which usually is closed, is opened by the action of the trigeminal (CN V)–innervated *tensor veli pala-*

tini muscles (Fig. 55-3). Opening of the eustachian tube, which normally occurs with swallowing and yawning reflexes, provides the mechanism for equalizing the pressure of the middle ear with that of the atmosphere. This equalization ensures that the pressures on both sides of the tympanic membrane are the same, so that sound transmission is not reduced and rupture does not result from sudden changes in external pressure, as occurs during plane travel.

Abnormalities in eustachian tube function are important factors in the pathogenesis of middle ear infections. There are two important types of eustachian tube dysfunction: abnormal patency and obstruction (see Fig. 55-3). The *abnormally patent tube* does not close or does not close completely. In infants and children with an abnormally patent tube, air and secretions often are pumped into the eustachian tube during crying and nose blowing.

Obstruction can be functional or mechanical. *Functional obstruction* results from the persistent collapse of the eustachian tube due to a lack of tubal stiffness or poor function of the tensor veli palatini muscle that controls the

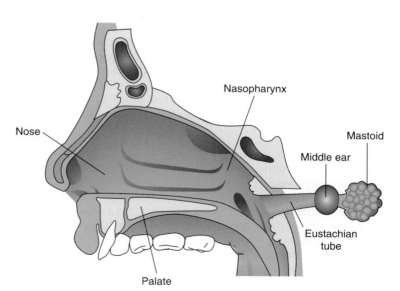

FIGURE 55-2 Nasopharynx–eustachian tube–mastoid air cell system. (Bluestone C.D. [1981]. Recent advances in pathogenesis, diagnosis, and management of otitis media. *Pediatric Clinics of North America* 28 [4], 36. Reproduced with permission)

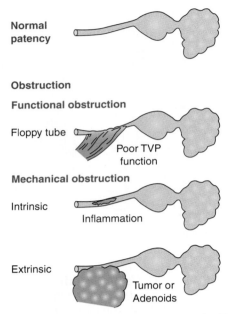

FIGURE 55-3 Pathophysiology of the eustachian tube. TVP, tensor veli palatini. (Bluestone C.D. [1981]. Recent advances in the pathogenesis, diagnosis, and management of otitis media. *Pediatric Clinics of North America* 28 [4], 737. Reproduced with permission)

opening of the eustachian tube. It is common in infants and young children because the amount and stiffness of the cartilage supporting the eustachian tube are less than in older children and adults. Changes in the craniofacial base also render the tensor muscle less efficient for opening the eustachian tube in this age group. In addition, craniofacial disorders, such as a cleft palate, alter the attachment of the tensor muscles, producing functional obstruction of the eustachian tube.

Mechanical obstruction results from internal obstruction or external compression of the eustachian tube. Ethnic differences in the structure of the palate may increase the likelihood of obstruction. The most common internal obstruction is caused by swelling and secretions resulting from allergy and viral respiratory infections. External compression by prominent or enlarged adenoidal tissue surrounding the opening of the eustachian tube may make drainage less effective. Tumors also may obstruct drainage. With obstruction, air in the middle ear is absorbed, causing a negative pressure and the transudation of serous capillary fluid into the middle ear.

Barotrauma

Barotrauma represents injury resulting from the inability to equalize the barometric stress on the middle ear imposed by air travel or, less commonly, by underwater diving. It occurs most often during air travel when there is a sudden change in atmospheric pressure. The pressure in the middle ear parallels atmospheric pressure; it decreases at high altitudes and increases at lower altitudes. The problem occurs during rapid airplane descent, when the negative pressure in the middle ear tends to cause the eustachian

tube to collapse. If air cannot pass back through the eustachian tube, hearing loss and discomfort develop.

This most often occurs in persons who travel while suffering from an upper respiratory tract infection. Autoinflation measures such as yawning, swallowing, and chewing gum facilitate opening of the eustachian tube, which equalizes air pressure in the middle ear. Intranasal (*e.g.*, phenylephrine HCl) or systemic decongestants may be used to prevent symptoms. Acute negative middle ear pressure that persists on the ground is treated with decongestants and attempts at autoinflation. More severe hearing loss or discomfort may require that the person consult an otolaryngologist. Myringotomy (*i.e.*, surgical incision in the tympanic membrane) provides immediate relief and may be used in cases of acute otalgia and hearing loss. Placement of ventilation tubes may be considered for persons with repeated episodes of barotrauma related to frequent air travel.

Otitis Media

Otitis media is an infection of the middle ear that is associated with a collection of fluid. Although OM may occur in any age group, it is the most common diagnosis made by health care providers who care for children. Almost all children have had at least one ear infection by 7 years of age, and one third have three or more episodes by 3 years of age.[4] Infants and young children are at highest risk for OM, with the peak occurrence between 6 and 13 months of age. The occurrence of the disease tends to decrease as a function of age, with a marked decline after 6 years of age.[5] The incidence is higher in boys, non–breast-fed infants, those who use pacifiers beyond infancy, children in large day care settings, children exposed to tobacco smoke, those with siblings or parents with a significant history of OM, those with allergic rhinitis, and children with congenital or acquired immune deficiencies (*e.g.*, acquired immunodeficiency syndrome).[4–6] The incidence of OM also is higher among children with craniofacial anomalies (*e.g.*, cleft palate, Down syndrome) and among Canadian and Alaskan Eskimos, and Native Americans.[7] It is more common during the winter months, reflecting the seasonal patterns of upper respiratory tract infections.

There are two reasons for the increased risk of OM in infants and young children: the eustachian tube is shorter, more horizontal, and wider in this age group than in older children and adults; and infection can spread more easily through the eustachian canal of infants who spend most of their day lying supine. Bottle-fed infants have a higher incidence of OM than breast-fed infants, probably because they are held in a more horizontal position during feeding, and swallowing while in the horizontal position facilitates the reflux of milk into the middle ear. Breast-feeding also provides for the transfer of protective maternal antibodies to the infant.

Otitis media may present as acute otitis media (AOM), recurrent OM, or OM with effusion (OME) or fluid in the middle ear. This effusion may be thin and watery (serous), thick and mucus-like (mucoid), or purulent (containing pus). The characteristics of the fluid vary depending on the type of OM.

Acute Otitis Media.   Acute OM is characterized by the presence of fluid in the middle ear in combination with signs and symptoms of an acute or systemic infection.[8] AOM can fail to resolve despite antibiotic treatment (persistent OM) or it may resolve and then recur (recurrent OM). It is estimated that AOM resolves spontaneously without treatment in approximately 60% of children.[9]

Most cases of AOM follow an upper respiratory tract infection that has been present for several days. The mucosal lining of the middle ear is continuous with the eustachian tube and nasopharynx, and most middle ear infections enter through the eustachian tube (see Fig. 55-2). AOM may be of either bacterial or viral origin. *Streptococcus pneumoniae*, *Haemophilus influenzae*, and *Moraxella catarrhalis* are the three major bacterial pathogens isolated from the middle ear in children with AOM.[8,10] There may be more than one type of bacteria present in some children. *S. pneumoniae* causes the largest proportion (40% to 50%) of cases generated by a single organism, and it is the least likely to resolve without treatment.[10] Emergence of a multiple–drug-resistant strain of *S. pneumoniae* (DRSP) has led to increased numbers of treatment failures. Children may be considered as at either high or low risk for DRSP. Children who are at high risk for DRSP include those younger than 2 years of age, those who attend day care, and those who have received antibiotics in the past 3 months.[4,8,11]

The role of viruses as etiologic agents in AOM is controversial. Viruses have been identified as a single pathogen in only a few middle ear aspirates obtained from children with AOM. Viruses may promote bacterial infection by impairing eustachian tube function and other host defenses.[9] The respiratory syncytial virus is the virus most frequently associated with AOM. Parainfluenza and influenza viruses are other common viral pathogens in AOM. As with bacterial infections, more than one type of respiratory virus may be present in the middle ear fluid of children with AOM.[12]

Manifestations.   Acute OM is characterized by otalgia (earache), fever (up to 104°F), and hearing loss. Children older than 3 years of age may have rhinorrhea or running nose, vomiting, and diarrhea. In contrast, younger children often have nonspecific signs and symptoms that manifest as ear tugging, irritability, nighttime awakening, and poor feeding. Ear pain usually increases as the effusion accumulates behind the tympanic membrane. Perforation of the tympanic membrane may occur acutely, allowing purulent material from the eustachian tube to drain into the external auditory canal. This may prevent spread of the infection into the temporal bone or intracranial cavity. Spontaneous perforation with discharge occurs most frequently in children of high-risk ethnic groups.

Diagnosis.   Diagnosis of AOM is made by associated signs and symptoms and otoscopic examination. In persons with AOM, a bulging yellow or red tympanic membrane with subsequent obliteration of the bony landmarks and cone of light is observed. Gentle movement of the pinna can help to differentiate OM from otitis externa. This maneuver does not produce pain in AOM but causes severe discomfort in otitis externa. Although diagnosis of AOM often can be made by otoscopic examination alone, pneumatic otos-

copy usually is performed to document middle ear effusion and immobility of the tympanic membrane.[13] The use of the pneumatic otoscope permits the introduction of air into the ear canal for the purpose of determining tympanic membrane flexibility. The movement of the tympanic membrane is decreased in some cases of AOM and absent in chronic middle ear infection.

The diagnosis of AOM can be confirmed using tympanometry or acoustic reflectometry. *Tympanometry* is helpful in detecting effusion in the middle ear or high negative middle ear pressure. A tympanogram is obtained by inserting a small probe into the external auditory canal; a tone of fixed characteristics is then presented through the probe, and the mobility of the tympanic membrane is measured electronically while the external canal pressure is artificially varied. The tympanogram provides a determination of the degree of negative pressure present in the middle ear. It detects disease when present but is less reliable when disease is absent. *Acoustic reflectometry* is used to reflect sound waves from the middle ear and provides information as to whether an effusion is absent or present. Increased reflected sound correlates with an increased likelihood of effusion. This technique is most useful in children older than 3 months, and its success depends on user technique.

Tympanocentesis may be done to relieve pain from an effusion or to obtain an organism for culture and sensitivity testing. The procedure involves the insertion of a needle through the inferior part of the tympanic membrane. Because of the cost, effort, and lack of availability, it is not routinely used in management of AOM.[13] In selected cases of refractory or recurrent middle ear disease, tympanocentesis can serve to improve diagnostic accuracy, guide treatment, and avoid unnecessary medical or surgical interventions. In instances where the tympanic membrane has perforated with resultant drainage into the external ear, a culture can be made and microbiologic studies done in selected cases to identify a microorganism.

Treatment.   The treatment of AOM includes the judicious use of antibiotic therapy in high-risk children, especially those younger than 2 years of age. The dramatic emergence of DRSP in the United States has led to increased treatment failures for AOM. Therefore, the Centers for Disease Control and Prevention report from the Drug-Resistant *S. pneumoniae* Therapeutic Working Group distinguishes among the antibiotic treatment options for initial AOM based on whether persons had received antibiotic treatment within the prior month, because recent antibiotic exposure increases the risk for infection with resistant pathogens.[10] According to this report, if there is no improvement in symptoms by day 3 of the initial antibiotic therapy, a switch to an antibiotic that targets resistant pathogens is recommended. Older children who have no fever or a low-grade fever do not require antibiotic treatment provided follow-up evaluation of symptoms occurs within 1 to 3 days. Regardless of whether antibiotic therapy is indicated, supportive therapy that includes analgesics, antipyretics, and local heat often is helpful. If the tympanic membrane is bulging and painful because of the accumulation of purulent drainage, a myringotomy may be done to relieve the pressure, thus reducing pain and hearing loss. In addition, this procedure prevents the ragged opening that can follow spontaneous rupture of the tympanic membrane.

Residual middle ear effusions are part of the continuum of AOM and persist regardless of whether antibiotics have been used. The effusion usually clears spontaneously within 1 to 3 months and does not require further treatment unless it persists beyond this period.

Recurrent Otitis Media. Recurrent OM is defined as three new AOM episodes within 6 months or four episodes in 1 year that occur with almost every upper respiratory tract infection. Reinforcement of environmental controls, such as avoidance of passive tobacco smoke, is important. Children with recurrent OM should be evaluated to rule out any anatomic variations (e.g., enlarged adenoids) and immunologic abnormalities. Children with immunoglobulin G subclass deficiencies (see Chapter 19) and poor responses to polysaccharide vaccines are more likely to develop recurrent OM.[5]

Traditionally, prophylactic antibiotics or antibiotics given at one-half the therapeutic dose may be given once daily for up to 6 months during winter and spring. Although children with recurrent OM respond well to such treatment, increasing concern regarding the emergence of bacterial resistance has emerged as a rationale for more judicious use of prophylactic antibiotics. Another approach to prevent recurrent OM is immunization with pneumococcal and influenza vaccines. Referral for placement of tympanostomy tubes is another alternative, particularly for children who have experienced five or more OM episodes within a 12-month period.

Otitis Media With Effusion. Otitis media with effusion is a condition in which the tympanic membrane is intact and there is an accumulation of fluid in the middle ear without signs or symptoms of infection. The type of effusion often is described as serous, nonsuppurative, or secretory, but these terms may not be correct in all cases. The duration of the effusion may range from less than 3 weeks to more than 3 months. The similarity between OME and AOM is that hearing loss may be present in both conditions. The major distinction is that signs and symptoms of infection are lacking in OME, although some children may complain of a feeling of ear fullness. Distinguishing between OME and AOM often is difficult because of the variability and overlap of symptoms, particularly in young children.

Diagnosis is based on otoscopic examination, which frequently reveals opacification of the tympanic membrane, making it difficult to visualize the effusion and, thus, characterize the type. If the tympanic membrane is translucent, a yellow or bluish fluid may be seen, as may an air–fluid level or bubbles, or both. Pneumatic otoscopy often reveals decreased mobility of the tympanic membrane, with a shape that is either retracted or convex. Alternatively, fullness or bulging may be noted.

Most cases of persistent middle ear effusion resolve spontaneously within a 3-week to 3-month period. The management options for this duration include observation only, antibiotic therapy, or combination antibiotic and corticosteroid therapy. Topical and systemic decongestants usually are of little value in clearing middle ear effusion.

Because there is concern over hearing loss and its effect on learning and speech, a hearing evaluation may be indicated and usually is done after 6 weeks.

If the effusion persists for 3 months or longer and is accompanied by hearing loss of 20 decibels (dB) or greater in children of normal development, tympanostomy tube placement may be indicated.[5] The tubes usually are placed under general anesthesia. The ears of children with tubes must be kept out of water. Spontaneous extrusion of tubes usually occurs after 5.5 to 7 months.[14] The adverse effects of tube placement include recurrent otorrhea; persistent perforation, scarring, and atrophy of the tympanic membrane; and cholesteatoma.

Complications. Since the advent of antimicrobial therapy, the intracranial suppurative complications of OM have been uncommon. However, extratemporal complications, including those affecting the middle ear, mastoid, and adjacent structures of the temporal bone, continue to occur.

Hearing loss, which is a common complication of OM, usually is conductive and temporary based on the duration of the effusion. Hearing loss that is associated with fluid collection usually resolves when the effusion clears. Permanent hearing loss may occur as the result of damage to the tympanic membrane or other middle ear structures. Cases of sensorineural hearing loss are rare. Persistent and episodic conductive hearing loss in children may impair their cognitive, linguistic, and emotional development. However, the degree and duration of hearing loss required to produce such effects are unknown.

Perforation of the tympanic membrane can occur spontaneously or result from surgical interventions. Temporary perforations are created for surgical treatment of AOM (myringotomy) or for tube placement. Usually the perforations heal spontaneously. Antimicrobial treatment for AOM with acute perforation is the same as for AOM without perforation.[5] When chronic drainage is present, cultures usually are performed and the antimicrobial regimen adjusted accordingly. Otic drops also may be instilled in the external ear to prevent or treat an external canal infection.[5] Healing of the tympanic membrane usually follows resolution of the middle ear infection.

Adhesive OM involves an abnormal healing reaction in an inflamed middle ear. It produces irreversible thickening of the mucous membranes and may cause impaired movement of the ossicles and possibly conductive hearing loss. Tympanosclerosis involves the formation of whitish plaques and nodular deposits on the submucosal surface of the tympanic membrane, with possible adherence of the ossicles and conductive hearing loss.

A *cholesteatoma* is a saclike mass containing silvery-white debris of keratin, which is shed by the squamous epithelial lining of the tympanic membrane. As the lining of the epithelium sheds and desquamates, the lesion expands and erodes the surrounding tissues. The lesion, which is associated with chronic middle ear infection, is insidiously progressive, and erosion may involve the temporal bone, causing intracranial complications. Treatment involves microsurgical techniques to remove the cholesteatomatous material.

The mastoid antrum and air cells constitute a portion of the temporal bone and may become inflamed as an extension of acute or chronic OM. The disorder causes necrosis of the mastoid process and destruction of the bony intercellular matrix, which are visible by radiologic examination. Mastoid tenderness and drainage of exudate through a perforated tympanic membrane can occur. Chronic mastoiditis can develop as the result of chronic middle ear infection. The usefulness of antibiotics for this condition is limited. Mastoid or middle ear surgery, along with other medical treatment, may be indicated. The incidence of mastoiditis has markedly decreased compared with the pre-antimicrobial era. It remains uncertain whether this decrease is due to antimicrobial treatment, changes in the natural history of OM, changes in organism virulence, or increased host resistance.[15]

Intracranial complications, although rare, can develop if the infection spreads through vascular channels, by direct extension, or through preformed pathways such as the round window. These complications are seen more often with chronic suppurative OM and mastoiditis. They include meningitis, focal encephalitis, brain abscess, lateral sinus thrombophlebitis or thrombosis, labyrinthitis, and facial nerve paralysis. Any child who develops persistent headache, tinnitus, stiff neck, or visual or other neurologic symptoms should be investigated for possible intracranial complications.

Otosclerosis

Otosclerosis refers to the formation of new spongy bone around the stapes and oval window, which results in progressive deafness.[16] In most cases, the condition is familial and follows an autosomal dominant pattern with variable penetrance. Otosclerosis may begin at any time in life but usually does not appear until after puberty, most frequently between the ages of 20 and 30 years. The disease process accelerates during pregnancy.

Otosclerosis begins with resorption of bone in one or more foci. During active bone resorption, the bone structure appears spongy and softer than normal (*i.e.*, osteospongiosis). The resorbed bone is replaced by an overgrowth of new, hard, sclerotic bone. The process is slowly progressive, involving more areas of the temporal bone, especially in front of and posterior to the stapes footplate. As it invades the footplate, the pathologic bone increasingly immobilizes the stapes, reducing the transmission of sound. Pressure of otosclerotic bone on inner ear structures or the vestibulocochlear nerve (CN VIII) may contribute to the development of tinnitus, sensorineural hearing loss, and vertigo.

The symptoms of otosclerosis involve an insidious hearing loss. Initially, the affected person is unable to hear a whisper or someone speaking at a distance. In the earliest stages, the bone conduction by which the person's own voice is heard remains relatively unaffected. At this point, the person's own voice sounds unusually loud, and the sound of chewing becomes intensified. Because of bone conduction, most of these persons can hear fairly well on the telephone, which provides an amplified signal. Many are able to hear better in a noisy environment, probably because the masking effect of background noise causes other persons to speak louder.

The treatment of otosclerosis can be medical or surgical. A carefully selected, well-fitting hearing aid may allow a person with conductive deafness to lead a normal life. Sodium fluoride has been used with some success in the medical treatment of osteospongiosis. Because much of the conductive hearing loss associated with otosclerosis is caused by stapedial fixation, surgical treatment involves stapedectomy with stapedial reconstruction using the patient's own stapes or a stapedial prosthesis. The argon laser may be used in the surgical procedure.

DISORDERS OF THE INNER EAR

The inner ear, which contains the receptors for hearing and vestibular function, is also called the *labyrinth* because of its complicated series of canals (see Chapter 53). Structurally, it consists of an outer bony labyrinth located in the temporal bone and an inner, fluid-filled membranous labyrinth.

Tinnitus

Tinnitus (from the Latin *tinniere*, meaning "to ring") is the perception of abnormal ear or head noises, not produced by an external stimulus.[17,18] Although it often is described as "ringing of the ears," it may also assume a hissing, roaring, buzzing, or humming sound. Tinnitus may be constant, intermittent, and unilateral or bilateral. It has been estimated that 35 million people in the United States have the disorder. Nearly 10 million of these are estimated to have severe or troubling tinnitus. The condition affects males and females equally, is most prevalent between 40 and 70 years of age, and occasionally affects children.[17]

Intermittent periods of mild, high-pitched tinnitus lasting for several minutes are common in normal-hearing persons. Impacted cerumen is a benign cause of tinnitus, which resolves after the ear wax is removed. Medications such as aspirin and stimulants such as nicotine and caffeine can cause transient tinnitus. Although tinnitus is subjective, for clinical purposes it is subdivided into objective and subjective tinnitus. *Objective tinnitus* refers to those rare cases in which the sound is detected or potentially detectable by another observer. Typical causes of objective tinnitus include vascular abnormalities or neuromuscular disorders. In some vascular disorders, for example, sounds generated by turbulent blood flow (*e.g.*, arterial bruits or venous hums) are conducted to the auditory system. Vascular disorders typically produce a pulsatile form of tinnitus. *Subjective tinnitus* refers to noise perception when there is no noise stimulation of the cochlea. The physiologic mechanism underlying subjective tinnitus is largely unknown. It seems likely that there are several mechanisms, including abnormal firing of auditory receptors, dysfunction of cochlear neurotransmitter function or ionic balance, and alterations in central processing of the signal.

Tinnitus is a symptom, and the diagnosis relies heavily on the person's description of the problem, including onset, frequency, description, and location of the tinnitus; perceived cause; and extent to which the person is bothered by the problem. A history of medication or stimulant use and dietary factors that may cause tinnitus should be obtained. Tinnitus often accompanies hearing disorders, and tests of auditory function usually are done. Causes of objective tinnitus, such serious vascular abnormalities, should be ruled out.

Treatment measures are designed to treat the symptoms rather than effect a cure. They include elimination of drugs or other substances such as caffeine, some cheeses, red wine, and foods containing monosodium glutamate that are suspected of causing tinnitus. The use of an externally produced sound (noise generators or tinnitus-masking devices) may be used to mask or inhibit the tinnitus. Medications, including antihistamines, anticonvulsant drugs, calcium channel blockers, benzodiazepines, and antidepressants, have been used for tinnitus alleviation, but most are not effective, and many produce undesirable side effects. For persistent tinnitus, psychological interventions may be needed to help the person deal with the stress and distraction associated with the condition. Tinnitus retraining therapy, which includes directive counseling and extended use of low-noise generators to facilitate auditory adaptation to the tinnitus, has met with considerable success. Surgical intervention (*i.e.*, cochlear nerve section, vascular decompression) is a last resort for persons in which all other interventions have failed and in whom the disorder is disabling.

Hearing Loss

Nearly 30 million Americans have hearing loss. It affects persons of all age groups. One of every 1000 infants born in the United States is completely deaf, and more than 3 million children have hearing loss.[19] Thirty percent to 40% of people older than 75 years of age have hearing loss.

The level of hearing is measured in decibels, where 0 dB is the threshold for perception of sound at a given frequency in persons with normal hearing.[20] A 10-fold increase in sound pressure level from 0 dB is measured as 20 dB. Hearing loss is qualified as mild, moderate, severe, or profound. "Hard of hearing" is defined as hearing loss greater than 20 to 25 dB in adults and greater than 15 dB in children. Profound deafness is defined as hearing loss greater than 100 dB[21] or 70 dB in children.[22] There are many causes of hearing loss or deafness. Most fit into the categories of conductive, sensorineural, or mixed deficiencies that involve a combination of conductive and sensorineural function deficiencies of the same ear.[20] Chart 55-1 summarizes common causes of hearing loss. Hearing loss may be genetic or nongenetic, sudden or progressive, unilateral or bilateral, partial or complete, reversible or irreversible. Age and suddenness of onset provide important clues as to the cause of hearing loss.

Conductive Hearing Loss. Conductive hearing loss occurs when auditory stimuli are not adequately transmitted through the auditory canal, tympanic membrane, middle ear, or ossicle chain to the inner ear. Temporary hearing loss can occur as the result of impacted cerumen in the outer ear or fluid in the middle ear. Foreign bodies, including pieces of cotton and insects, may impair hearing. More permanent causes of hearing loss are thickening or damage of the tympanic membrane or involvement of the bony structures (ossicles and oval window) of the middle ear due to otosclerosis or Paget's disease.

CHART 55-1

Common Causes of Conductive and Sensorineural Hearing Loss

Conductive Hearing Loss

- External ear conditions
  - Impacted ear wax or foreign body
  - Otitis externa
- Middle ear conditions
  - Trauma
  - Otitis media (acute and with effusion)
  - Otosclerosis
  - Tumors

Sensorineural Hearing Loss

- Trauma
  - Head injury
  - Noise
- Central nervous system infections (*e.g.*, meningitis)
- Degenerative conditions
  - Presbycusis
- Vascular
  - Atherosclerosis
  - Sudden deafness
- Ototoxic drugs (*e.g.*, aminoglycosides, salicylates, loop diuretics)
- Tumors
  - Vestibular schwannoma (acoustic neuroma)
  - Meningioma
  - Metastatic tumors
- Idiopathic
  - Ménière's disease

Mixed Conductive and Sensorineural Hearing Loss

- Middle ear conditions
  - Barotrauma
  - Cholesteatoma
  - Otosclerosis
- Temporal bone fractures

Hearing Loss

➤ Hearing loss represents impairment of the ability to detect and perceive sound.

➤ It can range from mild, affecting sounds of different tones and intensities, to moderate or profound.

➤ Hearing loss can be caused by conductive disorders, in which auditory stimuli are not transmitted through the structures of the outer and middle ears to the sensory receptors in the inner ear; by sensorineural disorders that affect the inner ear, auditory nerve, or auditory pathways; or by a combination of conductive and sensorineural disorders.

Sensorineural Hearing Loss. Sensorineural, or perceptive, hearing loss occurs with disorders that affect the inner ear, auditory nerve, or auditory pathways of the brain. With this type of deafness, sound waves are conducted to the inner ear, but abnormalities of the cochlear apparatus or auditory nerve decrease or distort the transfer of information to the brain. Tinnitus often accompanies cochlear nerve irritation. Abnormal function resulting from damage or malformation of the central auditory pathways and circuitry is included in this category.

Sensorineural hearing loss may have a genetic cause or may result from intrauterine infections such as maternal rubella, or developmental malformations of the inner ear. Genetic hearing loss may result from mutation in a single gene (monogenetic) or from a combination of mutations in different genes and environmental factors (multifactorial).[21] It has been estimated that 50% of profound deafness in children has a monogenetic basis.[21,23] The inheritance pattern for monogenetic hearing loss is autosomal recessive in approximately 75% of cases.[21] Hearing loss may begin before development of speech (prelingual) or after speech development (postlingual). Most prelingual forms are present at birth. Genetic forms of hearing loss also can be classified as being part of a syndrome in which other abnormalities are present, or as nonsyndromic, in which deafness is the only abnormality.

Sensorineural hearing loss also can result from trauma to the inner ear, tumors that encroach on the inner ear or sensory neurons, vascular disorders with hemorrhage, or thrombosis of vessels that supply the inner ear. Other causes of sensorineural deafness are infections and drugs. Sudden sensorineural hearing loss represents an abrupt loss of hearing that occurs instantaneously or on awakening. It most commonly is caused by viral infections, circulatory disorders, or rupture of the labyrinth membrane that can occur during tympanotomy.[24]

Environmentally induced deafness can occur through direct exposure to excessively intense sound, as in the workplace or at a concert. This is a particular problem in older adults who were working in noisy environments before the mid-1960s, when there were no laws mandating use of devices for protective hearing. This type of deafness was once called *boilermaker's deafness* because of the intense reverberating sound to which riveters were exposed when putting together boiler tanks. Sustained or repeated exposure to noise pollution at sound intensities greater than 100 to 120 dB can cause corresponding mechanical damage to the organ of Corti on the "tuned" basilar membrane. If damage is severe, permanent sensorineural deafness to the offending sound frequencies results. Wearing earplugs or ear protection is important under many industrial conditions and for musicians and music listeners exposed to high sound amplification. Noise pollution often is characterized by high-intensity sounds of a specific frequency that cause corresponding damage to the organ of Corti. Temporary threshold shift is a reversible hearing loss that occurs in individuals who attend loud concerts and hear ringing sounds after the event.

A number of infections can cause hearing loss. Deafness or some degree of hearing impairment is the most common serious complication of bacterial meningitis in infants and children, reportedly resulting in sensorineural hearing loss in 5% to 35% of persons who survive the infection.[23] The mechanism causing hearing impairment seems to be a suppurative labyrinthitis or neuritis resulting in the loss of hair cells and damage to the auditory nerve. Untreated suppurative OM also can extend into the inner ear and cause sensorineural hearing loss through the same mechanisms. Congenital and acquired syphilis can cause unilateral or bilateral sensorineural hearing loss. Hypothyroidism is a potential cause of sensorineural hearing loss in older persons.

Among the neoplasms that impair hearing are *acoustic neuromas*. Acoustic neuromas are benign Schwann cell tumors affecting CN VIII. These tumors usually are unilateral and cause hearing loss by compressing the cochlear nerve or interfering with blood supply to the nerve and cochlea. Other neoplasms that can affect hearing include meningiomas and metastatic brain tumors. The temporal bone is a common site of metastases. Breast cancer may metastasize to the middle ear and invade the cochlea.

Drugs that damage inner ear structures are labeled *ototoxic*. Vestibular symptoms of ototoxicity include lightheadedness, giddiness, and dizziness; if toxicity is severe, cochlear symptoms consisting of tinnitus or hearing loss occur. Hearing loss is sensorineural and may be bilateral or unilateral, transient or permanent. Several classes of drugs have been identified as having ototoxic potential, including the aminoglycoside antibiotics and some other basic antibiotics, antimalarial drugs, some chemotherapeutic drugs, loop diuretics, and salicylates. The symptoms of drug-induced hearing loss may be transient, as often is the case with salicylates and diuretics, or they may be permanent. The risk of ototoxicity depends on the total dose of the drug and its concentration in the bloodstream. It is increased in persons with impaired kidney functioning and in those previously or currently treated with another potentially ototoxic drug. Chart 55-2 lists drugs with the potential for producing ototoxicity.

Presbycusis. The term *presbycusis* is used to describe degenerative hearing loss that occurs with advancing age. Approximately 23% of persons between 65 and 75 years of age and 40% of the population older than 75 years of age are affected.[25] The degenerative changes that impair hearing may begin in the fifth decade of life and not be clinically apparent until later.[26] Onset may be associated with chronic noise exposure or vascular disorders.[26] The disorder involves loss of neuroepithelial (hair) cells, neurons, and the stria vascularis.[23] High-frequency sounds are affected more than low-frequency sounds, because high and low frequencies distort the base of the basilar membrane, but only low frequencies affect the distal (apical) region. Through the years, permanent mechanical damage to the organ of Corti is more likely to occur near the base of the cochlea, where the high sonic frequencies are discriminated. Men are affected earlier and experience a greater loss than women.

Diagnosis. Although approximately 10% of Americans have some degree of hearing loss, including one third of persons older than 65 years of age, hearing loss often is

CHART 55-2

*Drugs With Ototoxic Potential**

Aminoglycosides
  Amikacin
  Gentamicin
  Kanamycin
  Streptomycin
  Tobramycin
Other antibiotics
  Macrolides (erythromycin, azithromycin,
    clarithromycin)
  Vancomycin
Antimalarial drugs
  Chloroquine[†]
  Quinine[†]
Cancer drugs
  Cisplatin
Loop diuretics
  Ethacrynic acid
  Furosemide[†]
  Bumetide[†]
  Torsemide[†]
Salicylates[†]

* Not intended to be inclusive.
† Effects rarely are permanent.

underdiagnosed. Although visual impairments are readily accepted and vigorously treated, loss of hearing often is denied, minimized, or ignored. In a society that favors youth, glasses and contact lens are considered normal and even fashionable, whereas hearing aids often are regarded as a sign of "graceless aging."[20]

Diagnosis of hearing loss is aided by careful history of associated otologic factors such as otalgia, otorrhea, tinnitus, and self-described hearing difficulties; physical examination to detect the presence of conditions such as otorrhea, impacted cerumen, or injury to the tympanic membrane; and hearing tests. A history of occupational and noise exposure is important, as is the use of medications with ototoxic potential. Testing for hearing loss includes a number of methods, including a person's reported ability to hear an observer's voice, use of a tuning fork to test air and bone conduction, audioscopes, and auditory brain stem evoked responses (ABRs).

Tuning forks are used to differentiate conductive and sensorineural hearing loss. A 512-Hz or higher-frequency tuning fork is used because frequencies below this level elicit a tactile response. The Weber test evaluates conductive hearing loss by lateralization of sound. It is done by placing the lightly vibrating tuning fork on the forehead or vertex of the head. In persons with conductive losses, the sound is louder on the side with the hearing loss, but in persons with sensorineural loss, it radiates to the side with the better hearing. The Rinne test compares air and bone conduction. The test is done by alternately placing the tuning fork on the mastoid bone and in front of the ear canal. In conductive losses, bone conduction exceeds air conduction; in sensorineural losses, the opposite occurs.

Audioscopes can be used to assess a person's ability to hear pure tones at 1000 to 2000 Hz (usual speech frequencies). If a person cannot hear these tones, referral for a full audiogram should be done. The audiogram is an important method of analyzing a person's hearing, and is generally considered the gold standard for diagnosis of hearing loss. It is done by an audiologist and requires highly specialized sound production and control equipment. Pure tones of controlled intensity are delivered, usually to one ear at a time, and the minimum intensity needed for hearing to be experienced is plotted as a function of frequency.

The ABR is a noninvasive method that permits functional evaluation of certain defined parts of the central auditory pathways. Electroencephalographic (EEG) electrodes and high-gain amplifiers are required to produce a record of the electrical wave activity elicited during repeated acoustic stimulations of either or both ears. ABR recording involves subjecting the ear to loud clicks and using a computer to pick up nerve impulses as they are processed in the midbrain. With this method, certain of the early waves that come from discrete portions of the pons and midbrain auditory pathways can be correlated with specific sensorineural abnormalities. Imaging studies such as computed tomography scans and magnetic resonance imaging can be done to determine the site of a lesion and the extent of damage.[19]

Although hearing loss is a common problem in the elderly, many older persons are not appropriately assessed for hearing loss. When assessing an older person's ability to hear, it is important to ask both the person and the family about awareness of hearing loss. The ability to hear high-frequency sounds usually is lost first. Loss of high-frequency discrimination is characterized by difficulty in understanding words in noisy environments, in hearing a speaker in an adjacent room, or hearing a speaker whose back is turned. Hearing loss may be estimated by having the person report hearing of softly whispered, normally spoken, or shouted words. In the English language, vowels are low-frequency sounds, whereas consonants are of higher frequency. A ticking watch also may be used to test for the higher frequencies.

Because hearing impairment can have a major impact on the development of a child, early identification through screening programs is strongly advocated. The American Academy of Pediatricians endorses the goal of universal detection of hearing loss in infants before 3 months of age, with proper intervention no later than 6 months of age.[27] The currently recommended screening techniques are either the evoked otoacoustic emissions (EOAE) or the ABR. Both methodologies are noninvasive, relatively quick (<5 minutes), and easy to perform. The EOAE measures sound waves generated in the inner ear (cochlea) in response to clicks or tone bursts emitted and recorded by a minute microphone placed in the external ear canals of the infant. The ABR uses three electrodes pasted to the infant's scalp to measure the EEG waves generated by clicks. Many children become hearing impaired after the neonatal period and are not identified by neonatal screening programs. It often is not until children are in preschool or kindergarten that hearing screening takes place. Therefore, parents, caregivers, and health care providers should be alert to signs and symptoms of hearing impairment so that early interventions can be instituted.

Treatment. Untreated hearing loss can have many consequences. In infants and children, hearing loss can greatly affect language development and hearing-associated learning. Social isolation and depressive disorders are common in hearing-impaired elderly. Hearing-impaired people may avoid social situations where background noise makes conversation difficult to hear. Safety issues, both in and out of the home, may become significant. Treatment of hearing loss ranges from simple removal of impacted cerumen in the external auditory canal to surgical procedures such as those used to reconstruct the tympanic membrane. For other people, particularly the frail elderly, hearing aids remain an option. Cochlear implants also are an option for some people.

Hearing aids remain the mainstay of treatment for many persons with conductive and sensorineural hearing loss. With the advent of microcircuitry, hearing aids are now being designed with computer chips that allow multiple programs to be placed in a single hearing aid. The various programs allow the user to select a specific setting for different listening situations. The development of microcircuitry has also made it possible for hearing aids to be miniaturized to the point that, in many cases, they can be placed deep in the ear where they take advantage of the normal shape of the external ear and ear canal. Although modern hearing aids have improved greatly, they cannot replicate the hearing person's ability to hear both soft and loud noises. They also fail to consistently filter out distorted or background noise. Many persons who are fitted with hearing aids use them inconsistently, often because of social embarrassment, increase in background noise, or the sound of their own voice being transmitted through the hearing aid.[28] Other aids for the hearing impaired include alert and signal devices, assisted-listening devices from telephone companies, and dogs trained to respond to various sounds.

Most important, hearing impairment produces a loss of the important communicative function of auditory language, leading to social isolation. Although many assistance devices are available to persons with hearing loss, understanding on the part of family and friends is perhaps the most important.[20] The interpretation of speech involves both visual and auditory clues. It is important that people speaking to persons with hearing impairment face the person and articulate so that lip reading cues can be used. Adequate lighting is important. Distractions such as background noise can make communication difficult and should be avoided when possible.

Surgically implantable cochlear prostheses for the profoundly deaf have been developed. These prostheses are inserted into the scala tympani of the cochlea and work by providing direct stimulation to the auditory nerve, bypassing the stimulation that typically is provided by transducer cells but that is absent or nonfunctional in a deaf cochlea. For the implant to work, the auditory nerve must be functional. Early implants used a single electrode. Current implants use multielectrode placement, enhancing speech perception. Much of the progress in implant performance has been achieved through improvements in the speech processors that convert sound into electrical stimuli.

Advances in the development of the multichannel implant have improved performance such that cochlear implants have been established as an effective option for adults and children with profound hearing impairment. Most persons who are deafened after learning speech derive substantial benefit when cochlear implants are used in conjunction with lip reading; some are able to understand some speech without lip reading; and some are able to communicate by telephone. A National Institutes of Health Consensus Panel on Cochlear Implants in Adults and Children concluded that cochlear implantation improves the communication ability in most adults with severe to profound deafness and frequently leads to positive psychological and social benefits. The Consensus Panel recommended that children at least 2 years of age and adults with profound deafness should be considered as candidates for implantation.[29] The Panel also concluded that optimal educational and rehabilitation services are important for adults and critical for children to maximize the benefits available from the implant. One limitation is that the earliest age for implantation in children is no earlier than 2 years of age, which is beyond the critical period of auditory input for the acquisition of oral language.

DISORDERS OF THE CENTRAL AUDITORY PATHWAYS

The auditory pathways in the brain involve communication between the two sides of the brain at many levels. As a result, strokes, tumors, abscesses, and other focal abnormalities seldom produce more than a mild reduction in auditory acuity on the side opposite the lesion. For intelligibility of auditory language, lateral dominance becomes important. On the dominant side, usually the left side, the more medial and dorsal portion of the auditory association cortex is of crucial importance. This area is called *Wernicke's area*, and damage to it is associated with auditory receptive aphasia (and agnosia of speech). Persons with damage to this area of the brain can speak intelligibly and read normally but are unable to understand the meaning of major aspects of audible speech.

Irritative foci that affect the auditory radiation or the primary auditory cortex can produce roaring or clicking sounds, which appear to come from the auditory environment of the opposite side (*i.e.*, auditory hallucinations). Focal seizures that originate in or near the auditory cortex often are immediately preceded by the perception of ringing or other sounds preceded by a prodrome (*i.e.*, aura). Damage to the auditory association cortex, especially if bilateral, results in deficiencies of sound recognition and memory (*i.e.*, auditory agnosia). If the damage is in the dominant hemisphere, speech recognition can be affected (*i.e.*, sensory or receptive aphasia).

In summary, disorders of the auditory system include infections of the external and middle ear, otosclerosis, and conduction and sensorineural deafness. Otitis externa is an inflammatory process of the external ear. The middle ear is a tiny, air-filled cavity located in the temporal bone. The eustachian tube connects the middle ear to the nasopharynx and allows for equalization of pressure between the middle ear and the atmosphere. Infections can travel from the nasopharynx to the middle ear along the eustachian tube, causing OM or inflammation of the middle ear. The eustachian tube is shorter and more horizontal in infants and young children, and infections of the middle ear are a common problem in these age groups.

Otitis media is an infection of the middle ear that is associated with a collection of fluid. OM may present as AOM, recurrent OM, or OME. AOM usually follows an upper respiratory tract infection and is characterized by otalgia, fever, and hearing loss. The effusion that accompanies OM can persist for weeks or months, interfering with hearing and impairing speech development. Otosclerosis is a familial disorder of the otic capsule. It causes bone resorption followed by excessive replacement with sclerotic bone. The disorder eventually causes immobilization of the stapes and conduction deafness.

Deafness, or hearing loss, can develop as the result of a number of auditory disorders. It can be conductive, sensorineural, or mixed. Conduction deafness occurs when transmission of sound waves from the external to the inner ear is impaired. Sensorineural deafness can involve cochlear structures of the inner ear or the neural pathways that transmit auditory stimuli. Sensorineural hearing loss can result from genetic or congenital disorders, trauma, infections, vascular disorders, tumors, or ototoxic drugs. Treatment of hearing loss includes the use of hearing aids and, in some cases of profound deafness, implantation of a cochlear prosthesis.

Disorders of Vestibular Function

After you have completed this section of the chapter, you should be able to meet the following objectives:

✦ Relate the function of the vestibular system to nystagmus and vertigo

✦ Differentiate the structures of peripheral and central vestibular function

✦ Characterize the physiologic cause of motion sickness

✦ Compare the manifestations and pathologic processes associated with benign positional vertigo and Ménière's disease

✦ Differentiate the manifestations of peripheral and central vestibular disorders

The vestibular receptive organs, which are located in the inner ear, and their central nervous system (CNS) connections contribute to the reflex activity necessary for effective posture and movement. Because the vestibular apparatus is part of the inner ear and located in the head, it is head motion and acceleration that are sensed. The vestibular system serves two general and related functions.

It maintains and assists recovery of stable body and head position through control of postural reflexes, and it maintains a stable visual field despite marked changes in head position.

VESTIBULAR FUNCTION

The vestibular system plays an essential role in the equilibrium sense, which is closely integrated with the visual and proprioceptive (position) senses. The receptors for the vestibular system, which are located in the semicircular ducts of the inner ear, respond to changes in linear and angular acceleration of the head. The vestibular nerve fibers travel in the vestibulocochlear nerve (CN VIII) to the vestibular nuclei located at the junction of the medulla and pons. Some of the fibers pass through the nuclei to the cerebellum. The cerebellar connections are necessary for temporally smooth, coordinated movements during ongoing head movements, tilt, and angular acceleration. The vestibular nuclei also connect with the nuclei of the oculomotor (CN III), trochlear (CN IV), and abducens (CN VI) nerves. Vestibular control of conjugate eye movements serves to preserve eye fixation on stable objects in the visual field during head movement. Neurons of the vestibular nuclei also project to the thalamus, the temporal cortex, and the somesthetic area of the parietal cortex. The thalamic and cortical projections provide the basis for the subjective experiences of position in space and of rotation. The vestibular system also connects with a chemoreceptor trigger zone, which stimulates the vomiting center in the brain. This accounts for the nausea and vomiting that often is associated with vestibular disorders.

Disorders of vestibular function can be peripheral, involving the labyrinth, or central, involving the vestibular connections. Abnormal nystagmus, tinnitus, and hearing loss are other common manifestations of vestibular dysfunction, as are vertigo and autonomic manifestations such as perspiration, nausea, and vomiting.

NYSTAGMUS

The term *nystagmus* is used to describe the vestibulo-ocular reflexes that occur in response to ongoing head rotation (see Chapter 53). The vestibulo-ocular reflexes produce slow compensatory conjugate eye rotations that occur in the direction precisely opposite to ongoing head rotation and provide for continuous, ongoing reflex stabilization of the binocular fixation point.[30] This reflex can be demonstrated by holding a pencil vertically in front of the eyes and moving it from side to side through a 10-degree arc at a rate of approximately five times per second. At this rate of motion, the pencil appears blurred, because a different and more complex reflex, smooth pursuit, cannot compensate quickly enough. However, if the pencil is maintained in a stable position and the head is moved back and forth at the same rate, the image of the pencil is clearly defined. The eye movements are the same in both cases. The reason that the pencil image remains clear in the second situation is because the vestibulo-ocular reflexes keep the image of the pencil on the retinal fovea. The vestibulo-ocular reflexes are "hard

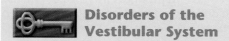

Disorders of the Vestibular System

➤ The receptors concerned with the sense of balance and position in space are located in fluid (endolymph)-filled semicircular canals of the vestibular system of the inner ear.

➤ The vestibular system has extensive interconnections with neural pathways controlling vision, hearing, and autonomic nervous system function. Disorders of the vestibular system are characterized by vertigo, nystagmus, tinnitus, nausea and vomiting, and autonomic nervous system manifestations.

➤ Disorders of vestibular function can result from repeated stimulation of the vestibular system such as during car, air, and boat travel (motion sickness); acute infection of the vestibular pathways (acute vestibular neuritis); dislodgment of otoliths that participate in the receptor function of the vestibular system (benign positional vertigo); or distention of the endolymphatic compartment of the inner ear (Ménière's disease).

wired" in the CNS and occur almost with the same precision with the eyes closed or in the congenitally blind. They can be modified, however, by visual control and by motor system intervention.

When compensatory vestibulo-ocular reflexes carry the conjugate eye rotations to their physical limit, a very rapid conjugate movement (*i.e.*, saccade) moves the eyes in the direction of head rotation to a new fixation point, followed by a slow vestibulo-ocular reflex as the head continues to rotate past the new fixation point. This pattern of slow–fast–slow movements is called *nystagmus*.

Spontaneous nystagmus that occurs without head movement or visual stimuli is always pathologic. It seems to appear more readily and more severely with fatigue and to some extent can be influenced by psychological factors. Nystagmus derived from the CNS, in contrast to peripheral end-organ or vestibulocochlear nerve sources, seldom is accompanied by vertigo. If present, the vertigo is of mild intensity.

VERTIGO

Disorders of vestibular function are characterized by a condition called *vertigo*, in which an illusion of motion occurs. The person is stationary and the environment is in motion (*i.e.*, objective vertigo), or the person is in motion and the environment is stationary (*i.e.*, subjective vertigo). Persons with vertigo frequently describe a sensation of spinning, "to-and-fro" motion, or falling.

Vertigo should be differentiated from light-headedness, faintness, unsteadiness, or syncope (loss of consciousness; Table 55-1).[31–33] Presyncope, which is characterized by a feeling of light-headedness or "blacking out," is commonly caused by postural hypotension (see Chapter 23) or a stenotic lesion in the cerebral circulation that limits blood flow. An inability to maintain normal gait may be described as dizziness despite the absence of objective vertigo. The unstable gait may be caused by disorders of sensory input (*e.g.*, proprioception), peripheral neuropathy, gait problems, or disorders other than vestibular function and usually are corrected by touching a stationary object such as the wall or a table.

Vertigo or dizziness can result from central or peripheral vestibular disorders. Approximately 85% of persons with vertigo have a peripheral vestibular disorder, whereas only 15% have a central disorder. Vertigo due to peripheral disorders tends to be severe in intensity and episodic or brief in duration. In contrast, vertigo due to central causes tends to be mild and constant and chronic in duration.

MOTION SICKNESS

Motion sickness is a form of normal physiologic vertigo. It is caused by repeated rhythmic stimulation of the vestibular system, such as is encountered in car, air, or boat travel. Vertigo, malaise, nausea, and vomiting are the principal symptoms. Autonomic signs, including lowered blood pressure,

TABLE 55-1 ✦ Differences in Pathology and Manifestations of Dizziness Associated With Benign Positional Vertigo, Presyncope, and Disequilibrium State

Type of Disorder	Pathology	Symptoms
Benign positional vertigo	Disorder of otoliths	Vertigo initiated by a change in head position, usually lasts less than a minute
Presyncope	Orthostatic hypotension	Light-headedness and feeling faint on assumption of standing position
Disequilibrium	Sensory (*e.g.*, vision, proprioception) deficits	Dizziness and unsteadiness when walking, especially when turning; relieved by additional proprioceptive stimulation such as touching wall or table

tachycardia, and excessive sweating, may occur. Hyperventilation, which commonly accompanies motion sickness, produces changes in blood volume and pooling of blood in the lower extremities, leading to postural hypotension and sometimes to syncope. Some persons experience a variant of motion sickness, complaining of sensing the rocking motion of the boat after returning to ground. This usually resolves after the vestibular system becomes accustomed to the stationary influence of being back on land.

Motion sickness can usually be suppressed by supplying visual signals that more closely match the motion signals being supplied to the vestibular system. For example, looking out the window and watching the environment move when experiencing motion sickness associated with car travel provides the vestibular system with the visual sensation of motion, but reading a book provides the vestibular system with the miscue that the environment is stable. Motion sickness usually decreases in severity with repeated exposure. Anti–motion sickness drugs also may be used to reduce or ameliorate the symptoms. These drugs work by suppressing the activity of the vestibular system.

DISORDERS OF PERIPHERAL VESTIBULAR FUNCTION

The peripheral vestibular system consists of a set of paired inner ear sensory organs, each sending messages to brain centers that interpret signals related to the body's position in space and control eye movement. Disorders of peripheral vestibular function occur when these signals are distorted, as in benign paroxysmal positional vertigo, or are unbalanced by unilateral involvement of one of the vestibular organs, as in Ménière's disease. The inner ear is vulnerable to injury caused by fracture of the petrous portion of the temporal bones; by infection of nearby structures, including the middle ear and meninges; and by blood-borne toxins and infections. Damage to the vestibular system can occur as an adverse effect of certain drugs or from allergic reactions to foods. The aminoglycosides (*e.g.*, streptomycin, gentamicin) have a specific toxic affinity for the vestibular portion of the inner ear. Alcohol can cause transient episodes of vertigo. The cause of peripheral vertigo remains unknown in approximately half of the cases.

Severe irritation or damage of the vestibular end-organs or nerves results in severe balance disorders reflected by instability of posture, dystaxia, and falling accompanied by vertigo. With irritation, falling is away from the affected side; with destruction, it is toward the affected side. Adaptation to asymmetric stimulation occurs within a few days, after which the signs and symptoms diminish and eventually are lost. After recovery, there usually is a slightly reduced acuity for tilt, and the person walks with a somewhat broadened base to improve postural stability. The neurologic basis for this adaptation to unilateral loss of vestibular input is not understood. After adaptation to the loss of vestibular input from one side, the loss of function of the opposite vestibular apparatus produces signs and symptoms identical to those resulting from unilateral rather than bilateral loss. Within weeks, adaptation is again sufficient for locomotion and even for driving a car. Such a person relies heavily on visual and proprioceptive input and has severe orientation difficulty in the dark, particularly when traversing uneven terrain.

Benign Paroxysmal Positional Vertigo

Benign paroxysmal positional vertigo (BPPV) is the most common cause of pathologic vertigo and usually develops after the fourth decade. It is characterized by brief periods of vertigo, usually lasting less than 1 minute, that are precipitated by a change in head position.[31,34] The most prominent symptom of BPPV is vertigo that occurs in bed when the person rolls into a lateral position. It also commonly occurs when the person is getting in and out of bed, bending over and straightening up, or extending the head to look up. It also can be triggered by amusement rides that feature turns and twists.

BPPV is thought to result from damage to the delicate sensory organs of the inner ear, the semicircular ducts, and otoliths (see Chapter 53, Fig. 53-21). In persons with BPPV, the calcium carbonate particles (otoliths) from the utricle become dislodged and become free-floating debris in the endolymph (otic fluid) of the posterior semicircular duct, which is the most dependent part of the inner ear.[34] Movement of the free-floating debris causes this portion of the vestibular system to become more sensitive, such that any movement of the head in the plane parallel to the posterior duct may cause vertigo and nystagmus. There usually is a several-second delay between head movement and onset of vertigo, representing the time it takes to generate the exaggerated endolymph activity. Symptoms usually subside with continued movement, probably because the movement causes the debris to be redistributed throughout the endolymph system and away from the posterior duct.

Diagnosis is based on tests that involve the use of a change in head position to elicit vertigo and nystagmus. BPPV often is successfully treated with drug therapy to control vertigo-induced nausea. Nondrug therapies using habituation exercises and canalith repositioning are successful in many people.[34] Canalith repositioning involves a series of maneuvers in which the head is moved to different positions in an effort to reposition the free-floating debris in the endolymph of the semicircular canals.

Acute Vestibular Neuronitis

Acute vestibular neuronitis is characterized by an acute onset (usually hours) of vertigo, nausea, and vomiting lasting several days and not associated with auditory or other neurologic manifestations. Most persons experience gradual improvement over 1 to 2 weeks, but some develop recurrent episodes.[35] A large percentage report an upper respiratory tract illness 1 to 2 weeks before onset of symptoms, suggesting a viral origin. The condition also can occur in persons with herpes zoster oticus. In some persons, attacks of acute vestibulopathy recur over months or years. There is no way to determine whether a person who experiences a first attack will have repeated attacks.

Ménière's Disease

Ménière's disease is a disorder of the inner ear due to distention of the endolymphatic compartment of the inner ear, causing a triad of hearing loss, vertigo, and tinnitus.[31,36–38] The primary lesion appears to be in the endolymphatic sac, which is thought to be responsible for endolymph filtration and excretion. A number of pathogenic mechanisms have been postulated, including an increased production of endolymph, decreased production of perilymph accompanied by a compensatory increase in volume of the endolymphatic sac, and decreased absorption of endolymph caused by malfunction of the endolymphatic sac or blockage of endolymphatic pathways.

Ménière's disease is characterized by fluctuating episodes of tinnitus, feelings of ear fullness, and violent rotary vertigo that often renders the person unable to sit or walk. There is a need to lie quietly with the head fixed in a comfortable position, avoiding all head movements that aggravate the vertigo. Symptoms referable to the autonomic nervous system, including pallor, sweating, nausea, and vomiting, usually are present. The more severe the attack, the more prominent are the autonomic manifestations. A fluctuating hearing loss occurs with a return to normal after the episode subsides. Initially the symptoms tend to be unilateral, resulting in rotary nystagmus caused by an imbalance in vestibular control of eye movements. Because initial involvement usually is unilateral and because the sense of hearing is bilateral, many persons with the disorder are not aware of the full extent of their hearing loss. However, as the disease progresses, the hearing loss stops fluctuating and progressively worsens, with both ears tending to be affected so that the prime disability becomes one of deafness.[37] The episodes of vertigo diminish and then disappear, although the person may be unsteady, especially in the dark.

The cause of Ménière's disease is unknown. A number of conditions, such as trauma, infection (*e.g.*, syphilis), and immunologic, endocrine (adrenal-pituitary insufficiency and hypothyroidism), and vascular disorders have been proposed as possible causes of Ménière's disease.[37,38] The most common form of the disease is an idiopathic form thought to be caused by a single viral injury to the fluid transport system of the inner ear. One area of investigation has been the relation between immune disorders and Ménière's disease.

Methods used in the diagnosis of Ménière's disease include audiograms, vestibular testing by electronystagmography, and petrous pyramid radiographs. The administration of hyperosmolar substances, such as glycerin and urea, often produces acute temporary hearing improvement in persons with Ménière's disease and sometimes is used as a diagnostic measure of endolymphatic hydrops. The diuretic furosemide also may be used for this purpose.

The management of Ménière's disease focuses on attempts to reduce the distention of the endolymphatic space, and can be medical or surgical. Pharmacologic management consists of suppressant drugs (*e.g.*, prochlorperazine, promethazine, diazepam), which act centrally to decrease the activity of the vestibular system. Diuretics are used to reduce endolymph fluid volume. Histamine analogs, which directly reduce inner ear fluid mainly by decreasing cochlear blood flow, are being studied.[36] A low-sodium diet is recommended in addition to these medications. The steroid hormone prednisone may be used to maintain satisfactory hearing and resolve dizziness. Gentamicin therapy has been used for ablation of the vestibular system.[37,39,40] Persons who are candidates for intratympanic gentamicin infusion include those who have frequent attacks of Ménière's disease, disease that involves one ear, good contralateral vestibular function, or normal or near-normal balance between episodes. This treatment is mainly effective in controlling vertigo and does not alter the underlying pathology.

Surgical methods include the creation of an endolymphatic shunt in which excess endolymph from the inner ear is diverted into the subarachnoid space or the mastoid (endolymphatic sac surgery), and vestibular nerve section. Advances in vestibular nerve section have facilitated the monitoring of CN VII and CN VIII potentials. These methods are used to prevent hearing damage. In unilateral cases, vestibular nerve section has a success rate of 90% to 95% in terms of providing complete relief of vertigo at 2 years after surgery.[37,38] The surgery, however, involves an intracranial procedure with possible postoperative morbidity.

DISORDERS OF CENTRAL VESTIBULAR FUNCTION

Abnormal nystagmus and vertigo can occur as a result of CNS lesions involving the cerebellum and lower brain stem. Central causes of vertigo include brain stem ischemia, tumors, and multiple sclerosis.[41] When brain stem ischemia is the cause of vertigo, it usually is associated with other brain stem signs such as diplopia, ataxia, dysarthria, or facial weakness. Compression of the vestibular nuclei by cerebellar tumors invading the fourth ventricle results in progressively severe signs and symptoms. In addition to abnormal nystagmus and vertigo, vomiting and a broad-based and dystaxic gait become progressively more evident. The central demyelinating effects of multiple sclerosis can present with vertigo up to 10% of the time, and up to one third of persons with multiple sclerosis experience vertigo and nystagmus some time in the course of the disease.[41]

Centrally derived nystagmus usually has equal excursion in both directions (*i.e.*, pendular). In contrast to peripherally generated nystagmus, CNS-derived nystagmus is relatively constant rather than episodic, can occur in any direction rather than being primarily in the horizontal or torsional (rotatory) dimensions, often changes direction through time, and cannot be suppressed by visual fixation. Repeated induction of nystagmus results in rapid diminution or "fatigue" of the reflex with peripheral abnormalities, but fatigue is not characteristic of central lesions. Abnormal nystagmus can make reading and other tasks that require precise eye positional control difficult.

DIAGNOSTIC TESTS OF VESTIBULAR FUNCTION

Diagnosis of vestibular disorders is based on a description of the symptoms, a history of trauma or exposure to agents that are destructive to vestibular structures, and physical examination. Tests of eye movements (*i.e.*, nystagmus) and muscle control of balance and equilibrium often are used. The tests of vestibular function focus on the horizontal semicircular reflex because it is the easiest reflex to stimulate rotationally and calorically and to record using electronystagmography.

Electronystagmography

Electronystagmography (ENG) is a precise and objective diagnostic method of evaluating nystagmus eye movements. Electrodes are placed lateral to the outer canthus of each eye and above and below each eye. A ground electrode is placed on the forehead. With ENG, the velocity, frequency, and amplitude of spontaneous or induced nystagmus and the changes in these measurements brought by a loss of fixation, with the eyes open or closed, can be quantified. The advantages of ENG are that it is easily administered, is noninvasive, does not interfere with vision, and does not require head restraint.[42]

Caloric Stimulation

Caloric testing involves elevating the head 30 degrees and irrigating each external auditory canal separately with 30 to 50 mL of ice water. The resulting changes in temperature, which are conducted through the petrous portion of the temporal bone, set up convection currents in the otic fluid that mimic the effects of angular acceleration. In an unconscious person with a functional brain stem and intact oculovestibular reflexes, the eyes exhibit a jerk nystagmus lasting 2 to 3 minutes, with the slow component toward the irrigated ear followed by rapid movement away from the ear. With impairment of brain stem function, the response becomes perverted and eventually disappears. An advantage of the caloric stimulation method is the ability to test the vestibular apparatus on one side at a time. The test is never done on a person who does not have an intact eardrum or who has blood or fluid collected behind the eardrum.

Rotational Tests

Rotational testing involves rotation using a rotatable chair or motor-driven platform. Unlike caloric testing, rotational testing depends only on the inner ear and is unrelated to conditions of the external ear or temporal bone. A major disadvantage of the method is that both ears are tested simultaneously.

Motor-driven platforms can be precisely controlled, and multiple graded stimuli can be delivered in a relatively short period. For rotational testing, the person is seated in a chair mounted on the motor-driven platform. Testing usually is performed in the dark without visual influence and with selected light stimuli. Eye movements are monitored using ENG. The Bárány chair, a rotatable chair that is much like a barber's chair, can be used for assessing postrotational vestibular reflexes. The person is strapped into the chair with the head positioned so that the plane of one pair of semicircular ducts is in the horizontal plane (*i.e.*, plane of rotation); each of the three primary planes of the ducts is tested in turn. The person is rotated until a steady rate of rotation is achieved. The chair is suddenly stopped, and the ensuing postrotational reflex nystagmus and the compensatory movements of the body and limbs are ob-

served. Vestibular reflexes are very powerful and extreme caution is needed when rotational tests are used to evaluate these reflexes.

Romberg Test

The Romberg test is used to demonstrate disorders of static vestibular function. The person being tested is requested to stand with feet together and arms extended forward so that the degree of sway and arm stability can be observed. The person then is asked to close his or her eyes. When visual clues are removed, postural stability is based on proprioceptive sensation from the joints, muscles, and tendons and from static vestibular reception. Deficiency in vestibular static input is indicated by greatly increased sway and a tendency for the arms to drift toward the side of deficiency.

If vestibular input is severely deficient, the subject falls toward the deficient side. Care must be taken because defects of proprioceptive projection to the forebrain also result in some arm drift and postural instability toward the deficient side. Only if two-point discrimination and vibratory sensation from the lower and upper limbs are bilaterally normal can the deficiency be attributed to the vestibular system.

TREATMENT OF VESTIBULAR DISORDERS

Pharmacologic Methods

Depending on the cause, vertigo may be treated pharmacologically. There are two types of drugs used in the treatment of vertigo.[43] First are the drugs used to suppress the illusion of motion. These include drugs such as antihistamines (*e.g.*, meclizine [Antivert], cyclizine [Marezine], dimenhydrinate [Dramamine], and promethazine [Phenergan]) and anticholinergic drugs (*e.g.*, scopolamine, atropine) that suppress the vestibular system. Although the antihistamines have long been used in treating vertigo, little is known about their mechanism of action. The second type includes drugs used to relieve the nausea and vomiting that commonly accompany the condition. Antidopaminergic drugs (*e.g.*, phenothiazines) and benzodiazepines commonly are used for this purpose.

Vestibular Rehabilitation

Vestibular rehabilitation, a relatively new treatment modality for peripheral vestibular disorders, has met with considerable success.[44–46] It commonly is done by physical therapists and uses a home exercise program that incorporates habituation exercises, balance retraining exercises, and a general conditioning program.[44] The habituation exercises take advantage of physiologic fatigue of the neurovegetative response to repetitive movement or positional stimulation and are done to decrease motion-provoked vertigo, lightheadedness, and unsteadiness. The exercises are selected to provoke the vestibular symptoms. The person moves quickly into the position that causes symptoms, holds the position until the symptoms subside (*i.e.*, fatigue of the neurovegetative response), relaxes, and then repeats the exercise for a prescribed number of times. The exercises usually are repeated twice daily. The habituation effect is characterized by decreased sensitivity and duration of symptoms. It may occur in as little as 2 weeks or take as long as 6 months.[46]

Balance-retraining exercises consist of activities directed toward improving individual components of balance that may be abnormal. General conditioning exercises, a vital part of the rehabilitation process, are individualized to the person's preferences and lifestyle. They should consist of motion-oriented activity that the person is interested in and should be done on a regular basis, usually four to five times per week.[46]

> In summary, nystagmus, an illusory sensation of motion of either oneself or one's surroundings (vertigo), tinnitus, and hearing loss are common manifestations of vestibular dysfunction, as are autonomic manifestations such as perspiration, nausea, and vomiting. Common disorders of the vestibular system include motion sickness, BPPV, and Ménière's disease.
>
> Benign paroxysmal positional vertigo is a condition believed to be caused by free-floating particles in the posterior semicircular canal. It presents as a sudden onset of dizziness or vertigo that is provoked by certain changes in head position. Ménière's disease, which is caused by an overaccumulation of endolymph, is characterized by severe, disabling episodes of tinnitus, feelings of ear fullness, and violent rotary vertigo. The diagnosis of vestibular disorders is based on a description of the symptoms, a history of trauma or exposure to agents destructive to vestibular structures, and tests of eye movements (*i.e.*, nystagmus) and muscle control of balance and equilibrium. Among the methods used in treatment of the vertigo that accompanies vestibular disorders are habituation exercises and antivertigo drugs. These drugs act by diminishing the excitability of neurons in the vestibular nucleus.

Related Web Sites

American Academy of Audiology   www.audiology.org
American Academy of Pediatrics—Screening Initiatives
   www.aap.org/policy
American Speech-Language-Hearing Association   www.asha.org
Centers for Disease Control and Prevention—Early Hearing
   Detection and Intervention Program   www.cdc.gov/nceh/
   cddh/ehdi.htm
Marion Downs National Center for Infant Hearing
   www.colorado.edu/slhs/mdnc
National Association of the Deaf   www.nad.org
National Institute on Deafness and Other Communication
   Disorders   www.nidcd.nih.gov

References

1. Grossan M. (2000). Safe, effective techniques for cerumen removal. *Geriatrics* 55, 83–86.
2. Jackler R.K., Kaplan M.J. (2001). Diseases of the ear. In Tierney L.M., McPhee S.J., Papadakis M.A. (Eds.), *Current medical diagnosis and treatment* (40th ed., pp. 217–231). New York: Lange Medical Books/McGraw-Hill.
3. Bluestone C.D., Klein J. (1995). *Otitis media in infants and children*. Philadelphia: W.B. Saunders.
4. Swanson J.A., Hoecker J.L. (1996). Otitis media in young children. *Mayo Clinic Proceedings* 71, 179–183.
5. Kenna M. (2000). The ear. In Behrman R.E., Kliegman R.M., Jenson H.B. (Eds.), *Nelson textbook of pediatrics* (16th ed., pp. 1951–1959). Philadelphia: W.B. Saunders.
6. Shapiro A.M., Bluestone C.D. (1995). Otitis media reassessed. *Postgraduate Medicine* 97 (5), 73–82.
7. Pichichero, M.E. (2000). Acute otitis media: Part II. Treatment in an era of increasing antibiotic resistance. *American Family Physician* 61, 2410–2415.
8. Berman S. (1995). Otitis media in children. *New England Journal of Medicine* 332, 1560–1565.
9. McCracken G.H. Jr. (1998). Treatment of acute otitis media in an era of increasing microbial resistance. *Pediatric Infectious Disease Journal* 17, 576–579.
10. Dowell S.F., Butler J.C., Giebink G.S., Jacobs M.R., Jernigan D., Musher D.M., et al. (1999). Acute otitis media: Management and surveillance in an era of pneumococcal resistance—a report from the Drug Resistant *Streptococcus pneumoniae* Therapeutic Working Group. *Pediatric Infectious Disease Journal* 18 (1), 1–9.
11. Tigges B.B. (2000). Acute otitis media and pneumococcal resistance: Making judicious management decisions. *Nurse Practitioner* 25 (1), 69–85.
12. Heikkinen T., Thint M., Chonmaitree T. (1999). Prevalence of various respiratory viruses in the middle ear during acute otitis media. *New England Journal of Medicine* 340, 260–264.
13. Pichichero M.E. (2000). Acute otitis media: Part I. Improving diagnostic accuracy. *American Family Physician* 61, 2051–2056.
14. Heald M.M., Matkin N.D., Merideth K.E. (1990). Pressure-equalization (PE) tubes in treatment of otitis media: National survey of otolaryngologists. *Otolaryngology–Head and Neck Surgery* 102, 334–338.
15. Culpepper L., Froom J. (1997). Routine antimicrobial treatment of acute otitis media: Is it necessary? *Journal of the American Medical Association* 278, 1643–1645.
16. Rubin E., Farber J.L. (1999). *Pathology* (3rd ed., pp. 1331–1332). Philadelphia: Lippincott Williams & Wilkins.
17. Fortune D.S. (1999). Tinnitus: Current evaluation and management. *Medical Clinics of North America* 83, 153–162.
18. Vesterager V. (1997). Fortnightly review: Tinnitus—investigation and management. *British Medical Journal* 314, 728–731.
19. Weissman J.L. (1996). Hearing loss. *Radiology* 199, 593–611.
20. Shohet J.A., Bent T. (1998). Hearing loss: The invisible disability. *Postgraduate Medicine* 104 (3), 81–83, 87–90.
21. Willems P.J. (2000). Genetic causes of hearing loss. *New England Journal of Medicine* 342, 1101–1109.
22. Kenna M. (2000). Hearing loss. In Behrman R.E., Kliegman R.M., Jenson H.B. (Eds.), *Nelson textbook of pediatrics* (16th ed., pp. 1940–1947). Philadelphia: W.B. Saunders.
23. Nadol J.G. (1993). Hearing loss. *New England Journal of Medicine* 329, 1092–1101.
24. Yamasoba T., Kikuchi S., O'uchi T., Higo R., Tokumaru A. (1993). Sudden sensorineural hearing loss associated with slow blood flow of the vertebrobasilar system. *Annals of Otorhinolaryngology* 102, 873–877.
25. Gates G.A. (Chairperson). (1989). Invitational Geriatric Otorhinolaryngology Workshop: Presbycusis. *Otolaryngology—Head and Neck Surgery* 100, 266–271.
26. Saeed S., Ramsden R. (1994). Hearing loss. *Practitioner* 238, 454–460.
27. Task Force on Newborn and Infant Hearing of the American Academy of Pediatrics. (1999). Newborn and infant hearing loss: Detection and intervention. *Pediatrics* 103, 527–530.

28. Committee on Disabilities of the Group for the Advancement of Psychiatry. (1997). Issues to consider in deaf and hard-of-hearing patients. *American Family Physician* 56 (8), 2057–2068.

29. NIH Consensus Development Panel on Cochlear Implants in Adults and Children. (1995). Cochlear implants in adults and children. *Journal of the American Medical Association* 274, 1955–1961.

30. Kandel E.R., Schwartz J.H., Jessel T.M. (2000). *Principles of neural science* (pp. 801–815). New York: McGraw-Hill.

31. Baloh, R.W. (1999). The dizzy patient: Presence of vertigo points to vestibular cause. *Postgraduate Medicine* 105 (5), 161–172.

32. Derebery J.M. (1999). The diagnosis and treatment of dizziness. *Medical Clinics of North America* 83, 163–176.

33. Ruckenstein M.J. (2001). The dizzy patient: How you can help. *Consultant* 41 (1), 29–33.

34. Furman J.M., Cass S.P. (1999). Benign paroxysmal positional vertigo. *New England Journal of Medicine* 341, 1590–1596.

35. Hotson J.R., Baloh R.W. (1998). Acute vestibular syndrome. *New England Journal of Medicine* 339, 680–685.

36. Dickins J.R.E., Graham S.S. (1990). Ménière's disease: 1983–1989. *American Journal of Otology* 11, 51–65.

37. Saeed S.R. (1998). Fortnightly review: Diagnosis and treatment of Ménière's disease. *British Medical Journal* 316, 368–372.

38. Hollis L., Bottrill I. (1999). Ménière's disease. *Hospital Medicine (London)* 60, 574–578.

39. Brooks C.B. (1996). The pharmacological treatment of Ménière's disease. *Clinical Otolaryngology* 21, 3–11.

40. Odkvist L.M., Bergenius J., Moller C. (1997). When and how to use gentamicin in the treatment of Ménière's disease. *Acta Oto-Laryngologica Supplement* 526, 54–57.

41. Derebery M.J. (1999). The diagnosis and treatment of dizziness. *Medical Clinics of North America* 83, 163–176.

42. Baloh R.W. (1989). Modern vestibular function testing. *Western Journal of Medicine* 150, 59–67.

43. Rascol O., Hain T.C., Brefel C., Benazet A.M., Horak F.G., Rycewiscz C., et al. (1995). Antivertigo drugs and drug-induced vertigo. *Drugs* 50, 777–789.

44. Horak F.B., Jones-Rycewicz C., Black F.W., et al. (1992). Effects of vestibular rehabilitation on dizziness and imbalance. *Otolaryngology—Head and Neck Surgery* 106, 175–180.

45. Smith-Whellock M., Shepard N.T., Telian S.A. (1991). Physical therapy program for vestibular rehabilitation. *American Journal of Otology* 12, 218–225.

46. Brandt T. (2000). Management of vestibular disorders. *Journal of Neurology* 247, 491–499.

Musculoskeletal Function

Some of the most significant investigations of the skeleton and muscles took place during the Renaissance—a time that celebrated the human body and lifted the knowledge of the body and its workings out of medieval murkiness.

The first comprehensive description of musculature was presented by Andreas Vesalius (1514–1564), a professor of anatomy and surgery at Padua. The product of his scrupulous dissections was the masterwork *De Humani Corporis Fabrica* (On the Structure of the Human Body), the second volume of which dealt with muscles and their structure. The work was beautifully illustrated with elegantly poised cadavers set against backgrounds of medieval Italy. Vesalius' effort successfully challenged many of the long-held pronouncements of Galen. The studies of artist Leonardo da Vinci (1452–1519) sought not to dispute or confirm previous teachings but to learn of the "divine form" so that it could be better rendered. A physician of the time wrote that "in order that he might be able to paint the various joints and muscles as they bend and extend according to the laws of nature, he [Leonardo] dissected in medical schools the corpses of criminals, indifferent to this inhuman and nauseating work." Although da Vinci was primarily a painter studying anatomy for the sake of art, there is little doubt that had his anatomic drawings been published during his lifetime or shortly after, science would have been advanced by years.

Structure and Function of the Skeletal System

Without the skeletal system, movement in the external environment would not be possible. The bones of the skeletal system serve as a framework for the attachment of muscles, tendons, and ligaments. The skeletal system protects and maintains soft tissues in their proper position, provides stability for the body, and maintains the body's shape. The bones act as a storage reservoir for calcium, and the central cavity of some bones contains the hematopoietic connective tissue in which blood cells are formed.

The skeletal system consists of the axial and appendicular skeleton. The axial skeleton, which is composed of the bones of the skull, thorax, and vertebral column, forms the axis of the body. The appendicular skeleton consists of the bones of the upper and lower extremities, including the shoulder and hip. For our purposes, the skeletal system is considered to include the bones and cartilage of the axial and appendicular skeleton, as well as the connective tissue structures (*i.e.*, ligaments and tendons) that connect the bones and join muscles to bone.

Characteristics of Skeletal Tissue

After you have completed this section of the chapter, you should be able to meet the following objectives:

✦ Cite the common components of cartilage and bone
✦ Compare the properties of the intercellular collagen and elastic fibers of skeletal tissue
✦ Cite the characteristics and name at least one location of elastic cartilage, hyaline cartilage, and fibrocartilage

✦ Name and characterize the function of the four types of bone cells
✦ State the function of parathyroid hormone, calcitonin, and vitamin D in terms of bone formation and metabolism
✦ State the location and function of the periosteum and the endosteum

Two types of connective tissue are found in the skeletal system: cartilage and bone. Each of these connective tissue types consists of living cells, nonliving intercellular protein fibers, and an amorphous (shapeless) ground substance. The tissue cells are responsible for secreting and maintaining the intercellular substances in which they are housed. These substances provide the structural characteristics of the tissue. For example, the intercellular matrix of bone is impregnated with calcium salts, providing the hardness that is characteristic of this tissue.

Two main types of intercellular fibers are found in skeletal tissue: collagenous and elastic. Collagen is an inelastic and insoluble fibrous protein. Because of its molecular configuration, collagen has great tensile strength; the breaking point of collagenous fibers found in human tendons is reached with a force of several hundred kilograms per square centimeter. Fresh collagen is colorless, and tissues that contain large numbers of collagenous fibers generally appear white. The collagen fibers in tendons and ligaments give these structures their white color. Elastin is the major component of elastic fibers that allows them to stretch several times their length and rapidly return to their original shape when the tension is released. Ligaments and structures that must undergo repeated stretching contain a high proportion of elastic fibers.

CARTILAGE

Cartilage is a firm but flexible type of connective tissue consisting of cells and intercellular fibers embedded in an amorphous, gel-like material. It has a smooth and resilient surface and a weight-bearing capacity exceeded only by that of bone.

Cartilage is essential for growth before and after birth. It is able to undergo rapid growth while maintaining a considerable degree of stiffness. In the embryo, most of the axial and appendicular skeleton is formed first as a cartilage model and is replaced by bone. In postnatal life, cartilage continues to play an essential role in the growth of long bones and persists as articular cartilage in the adult.

There are three types of cartilage: elastic cartilage, hyaline cartilage, and fibrocartilage. *Elastic cartilage* contains some elastin in its intercellular substance. It is found in areas, such as the ear, where some flexibility is important. Pure cartilage is called *hyaline cartilage* (from a Greek word meaning "glass") and is pearly white. It is the type of cartilage seen on the articulating ends of fresh soup bones found in the supermarket. *Fibrocartilage* has characteristics that are intermediate between dense connective tissue and hyaline cartilage. It is found in the intervertebral disks, in areas where tendons are connected to bone, and in the symphysis pubis.

The Skeletal System

➤ The skeletal system consists of the bones of the skull, thorax, and vertebral column, which form the axial skeleton, and the bones of the upper and lower extremities, which form the appendicular skeleton.

➤ Two types of connective tissue are found in the skeletal system: (1) cartilage, a semirigid and slightly flexible structure that plays an essential role in prenatal and childhood development of the skeleton and as a surface for the articulating ends of skeletal joints; and (2) bones, which provide for the firm structure of the skeleton and serve as a reservoir for calcium and phosphate storage.

➤ Both bone and cartilage are composed of living cells and a nonliving intercellular matrix that is secreted by the living cells.

➤ Bone matrix is maintained by three types of cells: osteoblasts, which synthesize and secrete the constituents of bone; osteoclasts, which resorb surplus bone and are required for bone remodeling; and the osteocytes, which make up the osteoid tissue of bone.

Hyaline cartilage is the most abundant type of cartilage. It forms much of the cartilage of the fetal skeleton. In the adult, hyaline cartilage forms the costal cartilages that join the ribs to the sternum and vertebrae, many of the cartilages of the respiratory tract, the articular cartilages, and the epiphyseal plates.

Cartilage cells, which are called *chondrocytes*, are located in lacunae. These lacunae are surrounded by an uncalcified, gel-like intercellular matrix of collagen fibers and ground substance. Cartilage is devoid of blood vessels and nerves. The free surfaces of most hyaline cartilage, with the exception of articular cartilage, is covered by a layer of fibrous connective tissue called the *perichondrium*.

It has been estimated that approximately 65% to 80% of the wet weight of cartilage is water held in its gel structure. Because cartilage has no blood vessels, this tissue fluid allows the diffusion of gases, nutrients, and wastes between the chondrocytes and blood vessels outside the cartilage. Diffusion cannot take place if the cartilage matrix becomes impregnated with calcium salts, and cartilage dies if it becomes calcified.

BONE

Bone is connective tissue in which the intercellular matrix has been impregnated with inorganic calcium salts so that it has great tensile and compressible strength but is light enough to be moved by coordinated muscle contractions. The intercellular matrix is composed of two types of substances—organic matter and inorganic salts. The organic matter, including bone cells, blood vessels, and nerves, constitutes approximately one third of the dry weight of bone; the inorganic salts make up the other two thirds.

The organic matter consists primarily of collagen fibers embedded in an amorphous ground substance. The inorganic matter consists of hydroxyapatite, an insoluble macrocrystalline structure of calcium phosphate salts, and small amounts of calcium carbonate and calcium fluoride. Bone may also take up lead and other heavy metals, thereby removing these toxic substances from the circulation. This can be viewed as a protective mechanism. The antibiotic tetracycline is readily bound to calcium deposited in newly formed bones and teeth. When tetracycline is given during pregnancy, it can be deposited in the teeth of the fetus, causing discoloration and deformity. Similar changes can occur if the drug is given for long periods to children younger than 6 years of age.

Types of Bone

There are two types of mature bones, cancellous and compact bone (Fig. 56-1). Both types are formed in layers and are therefore called *lamellar bone*. Cancellous (spongy) bone is found in the interior of bones and is composed of *trabeculae*, or *spicules*, of bone that form a latticelike pattern. These latticelike structures are lined with osteogenic cells and filled with red or yellow bone marrow. Cancellous bone is relatively light, but its structure is such that it has considerable tensile strength and weight-bearing properties. Compact (cortical) bone, which forms the outer shell of a bone, has a densely packed calcified intercellular matrix that makes it

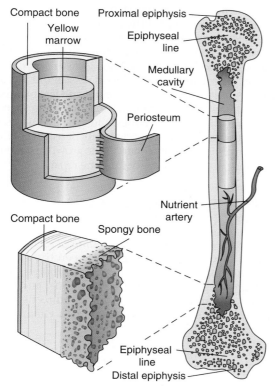

FIGURE 56-1 A long bone shown in longitudinal section. (Adapted with permission from Chaffee E.E., Lytle I.M. [1980]. *Basic physiology and anatomy* [4th ed.]. Philadelphia: J.B. Lippincott)

more rigid than cancellous bone. The relative quantity of compact and cancellous bone varies in different types of bones throughout the body and in different parts of the same bone, depending on the need for strength and lightness. Compact bone is the major component of tubular bones. It is also found along the lines of stress on long bones and forms an outer protective shell on other bones.

Bone Cells

Four types of bone cells participate in the formation and maintenance of bone tissue: osteogenic cells, osteoblasts, osteocytes, and osteoclasts (Table 56-1).

Osteogenic Cells. The undifferentiated osteogenic cells are found in the periosteum, endosteum, and epiphyseal plate of growing bone. These cells differentiate into osteoblasts and are active during normal growth; they may also be activated in adult life during healing of fractures and other injuries. Osteogenic cells also participate in the continual replacement of worn-out bone tissue.

Osteoblasts. The osteoblasts, or bone-building cells, are responsible for the formation of the bone matrix. Bone formation occurs in two stages: ossification and calcification. Ossification involves the formation of osteoid, or prebone. Calcification of bone involves the deposition of calcium salts in the osteoid tissue. The osteoblasts synthesize collagen and other proteins that make up osteoid tissue. They also participate in the calcification process of the osteoid tissue, probably by controlling the availability of calcium and phosphate. Osteoblasts secrete the enzyme *alkaline phosphatase*, which is thought to act locally in bone tissue to raise calcium and phosphate levels to the point at which precipitation occurs. The activity of the osteoblasts undoubtedly contributes to the rise in serum levels of alkaline phosphatase that follows bone injury and fractures.

Osteocytes. The osteocytes are mature bone cells that are actively involved in maintaining the bony matrix. Death of the osteocytes results in the resorption of this matrix. The osteocytes lie in a small lake filled with extracellular fluid, called a *lacuna*, and are surrounded by a calcified intercellular matrix. Extracellular fluid-filled passageways permeate the calcified matrix and connect with the lacunae of adjacent osteocytes. These passageways are called *canaliculi*. Because diffusion does not occur through the calcified matrix of bone, the canaliculi serve as communicating channels for the exchange of nutrients and metabolites between the osteocytes and the blood vessels on the surface of the bone layer.

The osteocytes, together with their intercellular matrix, are arranged in layers, or lamellae. In compact bone, 4 to 20 lamellae are arranged concentrically around a central haversian canal, which runs essentially parallel to the long axis of the bone. Each of these units is called a *haversian system*, or *osteon*. The haversian canals contain blood vessels

Type of Bone Cell	Function
TABLE 56-1 ✦ Function of Bone Cells	
Osteogenic cells	Undifferentiated cells that differentiate into osteoblasts. They are found in the periosteum, endosteum, and epiphyseal growth plate of growing bones.
Osteoblasts	Bone-building cells that synthesize and secrete the organic matrix of bone. Osteoblasts also participate in the calcification of the organic matrix.
Osteocytes	Mature bone cells that function in the maintenance of bone matrix. Osteocytes also play an active role in releasing calcium into the blood.
Osteoclasts	Bone cells responsible for the resorption of bone matrix and the release of calcium and phosphate from bone.

that carry nutrients and wastes to and from the canaliculi (Fig. 56-2). The blood vessels from the periosteum enter the bone through tiny openings called *Volkmann's canals* and connect with the haversian systems. Cancellous bone is also composed of lamellae, but its trabeculae usually are not penetrated by blood vessels. Instead, the bone cells of cancellous bone are nourished by diffusion from the endosteal surface through canaliculi, which interconnect their lacunae and extend to the bone surface.

Osteoclasts. Osteoclasts are bone cells that function in the resorption of bone, removing the mineral content and the organic matrix. Unlike the osteoblasts, which originate in osteogenic cells, the osteoclasts are formed by the fusion of blood-derived monocytes. Although the mechanism of osteoclast formation and activation remains elusive, it is known that parathyroid hormone (PTH) increases the number and resorptive function of the osteoclasts. Calcitonin is thought to reduce the number and resorptive function of the osteoclasts. The mechanism whereby osteoclasts exert their resorptive effect on bone is unclear. These cells may secrete an acid that removes calcium from the bone matrix, releasing the collagenic fibers for digestion by osteoclasts or mononuclear cells.

Periosteum and Endosteum

Bones are covered, except at their articular ends, by a membrane called the *periosteum* (see Fig. 56-1). The periosteum has an outer fibrous layer and an inner layer that contains the osteogenic cells needed for bone growth and development. The periosteum contains blood vessels and acts as an anchorage point for vessels as they enter and leave the bone. The endosteum is the membrane that lines the spaces of spongy bone, the marrow cavities, and the haversian canals of compact bone. It is composed mainly of osteogenic cells. These osteogenic cells contribute to the growth and remodeling of bone and are necessary for bone repair.

HORMONAL CONTROL OF BONE FORMATION AND METABOLISM

The process of bone formation and mineral metabolism is complex. It involves the interplay between the actions of PTH, calcitonin, and vitamin D. Other hormones, such as cortisol, growth hormone, thyroid hormone, and the sex hormones, also influence bone formation directly or indirectly. The actions of PTH, calcitonin, and vitamin D are summarized in Table 56-2.

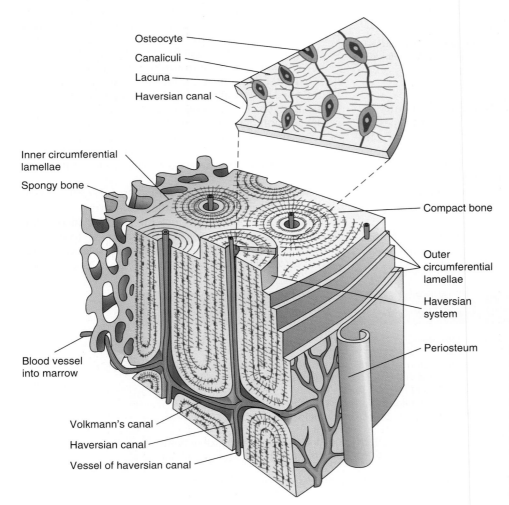

FIGURE 56-2 Haversian systems as seen in a wedge of compact bone tissue. The periosteum has been peeled back to show a blood vessel entering one of Volkmann's canals. (**Upper right**) Osteocytes lying within lacunae; canaliculi permit interstitial fluid to reach each lacuna. (Adapted with permission from Chaffee E.E., Lytle I.M. [1980]. *Basic physiology and anatomy* [4th ed.]. Philadelphia: J.B. Lippincott)

TABLE 56-2 ◆ Actions of Parathyroid Hormone, Calcitonin, and Vitamin D

Actions	Parathyroid Hormone	Calcitonin	Vitamin D
Intestinal absorption of calcium	Increases indirectly through increased activation of vitamin D	Probably not affected	Increases
Intestinal absorption of phosphate	Increases	Probably not affected	Increases
Renal excretion of calcium	Decreases	Increases	Probably increases, but less effect than PTH
Renal excretion of phosphate	Increases	Increases	Increases
Bone resorption	Increases	Decreases	$1,25\text{-}(OH)_2D_3$ increases
Bone formation	Decreases	Uncertain	$24,25\text{-}(OH)_2D_3$ increases (?)
Serum calcium levels	Produces a prompt increase	Decreases with pharmacologic doses	No effect
Serum phosphate levels	Prevents an increase	Decreases with pharmacologic doses	No effect

Parathyroid Hormone

PTH is one of the important regulators of calcium and phosphate levels in the blood. The hormone is secreted by the parathyroid glands. There are two pairs of parathyroid glands located on the dorsal surface of the thyroid gland.

PTH prevents serum calcium levels from falling below and serum phosphate levels from rising above normal physiologic concentrations. The secretion of PTH is regulated by negative feedback according to serum levels of ionized calcium (see Chapter 31). PTH, which is released from the parathyroid gland in response to a decrease in plasma calcium, restores the concentration of the calcium ion to just above the normal set point. This inhibits further secretion of the hormone. Other factors, such as serum phosphate and arterial blood pH, indirectly influence parathyroid secretion by altering the amount of calcium that is complexed to phosphate or bound to albumin.

PTH maintains serum calcium levels by initiation of calcium release from bone, by conservation of calcium by the kidney, by enhanced intestinal absorption of calcium through activation of vitamin D, and by reduction of serum phosphate levels (Fig. 56-3). PTH also increases the movement of calcium and phosphate from bone into the extracellular fluid. Calcium is immediately released from the canaliculi and bone cells; a more prolonged release of calcium and phosphate is mediated by increased osteoclast activity. In the kidney, PTH stimulates tubular reabsorption of calcium while reducing the reabsorption of phosphate. The latter effect ensures that increased release of phosphate from bone during mobilization of calcium does not produce an elevation in serum phosphate levels. This is important because an increase in calcium and phosphate levels could lead to crystallization in soft tissues. PTH increases intestinal absorption of calcium because of its ability to stimulate activation of vitamin D by the kidney.

Calcitonin

Whereas PTH increases blood calcium levels, the hormone calcitonin lowers blood calcium levels. Calcitonin, some-

times called *thyrocalcitonin*, is secreted by the parafollicular, or C, cells of the thyroid gland.

Calcitonin inhibits the release of calcium from bone into the extracellular fluid. It is thought to act by causing calcium to become sequestered in bone cells and by inhibiting osteoclast activity. Calcitonin also reduces the renal tubular reabsorption of calcium and phosphate; the decrease in serum calcium level that follows administration of pharmacologic doses of calcitonin may be related to this action.

The major stimulus for calcitonin synthesis and release is a rise in serum calcium. The role of calcitonin in overall mineral homeostasis is uncertain. There are no clearly

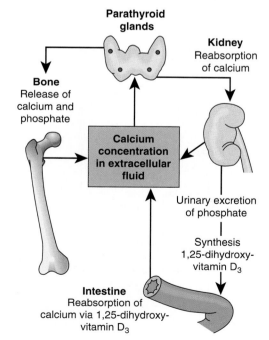

FIGURE 56-3 Regulation and actions of parathyroid hormone.

definable syndromes of calcitonin deficiency or excess, which suggests that calcitonin does not directly alter calcium metabolism. It has been suggested that the physiologic actions of calcitonin are related to the postprandial handling and processing of dietary calcium. This theory proposes that after meals, calcitonin maintains parathyroid secretion at a time when it normally would be reduced by calcium entering the blood from the digestive tract. Although excess or deficiency states associated with alterations in physiologic levels of calcitonin have not been observed, it has been shown that pharmacologic doses of the hormone reduce osteoclastic activity. Because of this action, calcitonin has proved effective in the treatment of Paget's disease (see Chapter 58). The hormone is also used to reduce serum calcium levels during hypercalcemic crises.

Salmon calcitonin, which differs from human calcitonin in 9 of 32 amino acids, is 100 times more potent than human calcitonin. The higher potency may be related to higher affinity for receptor sites and slower degradation by peripheral tissues. Calcitonin used clinically is often a synthetic preparation containing the amino acid sequence of salmon calcitonin.

Vitamin D

Vitamin D and its metabolites are not vitamins but steroid hormones. There are two forms of vitamin D: vitamin D_2 (ergocalciferol) and vitamin D_3 (cholecalciferol). The two forms differ by the presence of a double bond, but they have identical biologic activity. The term vitamin D is used to indicate both forms.

Vitamin D has little or no activity until it has been metabolized to compounds that mediate its activity. Figure 56-4 depicts sources of vitamin D and pathways for activation. The first step of the activation process occurs in the liver, where vitamin D is hydroxylated to form the metabolite 25-hydroxyvitamin D_3 [25-(OH)D_3]. From the liver, 25-

$(OH)D_3$ is transported to the kidneys, where it undergoes conversion to 1,25-dihydroxyvitamin D_3 [1,25-(OH)$_2D_3$] or 24,25-dihydroxyvitamin D_3 [24,25-(OH)$_2D_3$]. Other metabolites of vitamin D have been and still are being discovered.

There are two sources of vitamin D: intestinal absorption and skin production. Intestinal absorption occurs mainly in the jejunum and includes vitamin D_2 and vitamin D_3. The most important dietary sources of vitamin D are fish, liver, and irradiated milk. Because vitamin D is fat soluble, its absorption is mediated by bile salts and occurs by means of the lymphatic vessels. In the skin, ultraviolet radiation from sunlight spontaneously converts 7-dehydrocholesterol provitamin D_3 to vitamin D_3. A circulating vitamin D–binding protein provides a mechanism to remove vitamin D from the skin and make it available to the rest of the body.

With adequate exposure to sunlight, the amount of vitamin D that can be produced by the skin is usually sufficient to meet physiologic requirements. The importance of sunlight exposure is evidenced by population studies that report lower vitamin D levels in countries, such as England, that have less sunlight than the United States. Elderly persons who are housebound or institutionalized frequently have low vitamin D levels. The deficiency often goes undetected until there are problems such as pseudofractures or electrolyte imbalances. Seasonal variations in vitamin D levels probably reflect changes in sunlight exposure.

The most potent of the vitamin D metabolites is 1,25-$(OH)_2D_3$. This metabolite increases intestinal absorption of calcium and promotes the actions of PTH on resorption of calcium and phosphate from bone. Bone resorption by the osteoclasts is increased and bone formation by the osteoblasts is decreased; there is also an increase in acid phosphatase and a decrease in alkaline phosphatase. Intestinal absorption and bone resorption increase the amount of calcium and phosphorus available to the mineralizing surface of the bone. The role of 24,25-$(OH)_2D_3$ is less clear. There is evidence that 24,25-$(OH)_2D_3$, in conjunction with 1,25-$(OH)_2D_3$, may be involved in normal bone mineralization.

The regulation of vitamin D activity is influenced by several hormones. PTH and prolactin stimulate 1,25-$(OH)_2D_3$ production by the kidney. States of hyperparathyroidism are associated with increased levels of 1,25-$(OH)_2D_3$, and hypoparathyroidism leads to lowered levels of this metabolite. Prolactin may have an ancillary role in regulating vitamin D metabolism during pregnancy and lactation. Calcitonin inhibits 1,25-$(OH)_2D_3$ production by the kidney. In addition to hormonal influences, changes in the concentration of ions such as calcium, phosphate, hydrogen, and potassium exert an effect on 1,25-$(OH)_2D_3$ and 24,25-$(OH)_2D_3$ production. Under conditions of deprivation of phosphate and calcium, 1,25-$(OH)_2D_3$ levels are increased, whereas hyperphosphatemia and hypercalcemia decrease the levels of metabolite.

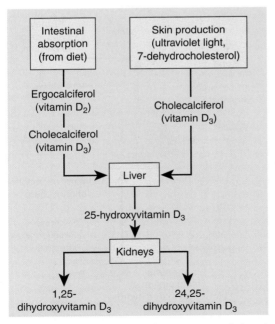

FIGURE 56-4 Sources and pathway for activation of vitamin D.

In summary, skeletal tissue is composed of two types of connective tissue: cartilage and bone. These skeletal structures are composed of similar tissue types; each has living cells and nonliving intercellular fibers and ground substance that is secreted by the cells. Cartilage is a firm, flexible type of skeletal tissue that is essential for growth before and after birth. There are three types of cartilage: elastic, hyaline, and fibrocartilage. Hyaline cartilage, which is the most abundant type, forms the costal cartilages that join the ribs to the sternum and vertebrae, many of the cartilages of the respiratory tract, and the articular cartilages.

The characteristics of the various skeletal tissue types are determined by the intercellular matrix. In bone, this matrix is impregnated with calcium salts to provide hardness and strength. There are four types of bone cells: osteocytes, or mature bone cells; osteoblasts, or bone-building cells; osteoclasts, which function in bone resorption; and osteogenic cells, which differentiate into osteoblasts. Densely packed compact bone forms the outer shell of a bone, and latticelike cancellous bone forms the interior. The periosteum, the membrane that covers bones, contains blood vessels and acts as an anchorage point for vessels as they enter and leave the bone. The endosteum is the membrane that lines the spaces of spongy bone, the marrow cavities, and the haversian canals of compact bone.

The process of bone formation and mineral metabolism involves the interplay among the actions of PTH, calcitonin, and vitamin D. PTH acts to maintain serum levels of ionized calcium; it increases the release of calcium and phosphate from bone, the conservation of calcium and elimination of phosphate by the kidney, and the intestinal reabsorption of calcium through vitamin D. Calcitonin inhibits the release of calcium from bone and increases renal elimination of calcium and phosphate, thereby serving to lower serum calcium levels. Vitamin D functions as a hormone in regulating body calcium. It increases absorption of calcium from the intestine and promotes the actions of PTH on bone.

▌ Skeletal Structures

After you have completed this section of the chapter, you should be able to meet the following objectives:

✦ Characterize the structure of bones based on their shape and list the structures of long bones
✦ State the characteristics of tendons and ligaments
✦ State the difference between synarthrodial and diarthrodial joints
✦ Describe the source of blood supply to a diarthrodial joint
✦ Explain why pain is often experienced in all the joints of an extremity when only a single joint is affected by a disease process
✦ Describe the structure and function of a bursa
✦ Explain the pathology associated with a torn meniscus of the knee

CLASSIFICATION OF BONES

Bones are classified by shape as long, short, flat, and irregular. Long bones are found in the upper and lower extremities. Short bones are irregularly shaped bones located in the

ankle and the wrist. Except for their surface, which is compact bone, these bones are spongy throughout. Flat bones are composed of a layer of spongy bone between two layers of compact bone. They are found in areas such as the skull and rib cage, where extensive protection of underlying structures is needed, or, as in the scapula, where a broad surface for muscle attachment must be provided. Irregular bones, because of their shapes, cannot be classified in any of the previous groups. This group includes bones such as the vertebrae and the bones of the jaw.

A typical long bone has a shaft, or *diaphysis*, and two ends, called *epiphyses*. Long bones usually are narrow in the midportion and broad at the ends so that the weight they bear can be distributed over a wider surface. The shaft of a long bone is formed mainly of compact bone roughly hollowed out to form a marrow-filled medullary canal. The ends of long bones are covered with articular cartilage that rests on a bony plate, the subchondral bone.

In growing bones, the part of the bone shaft that funnels out as it approaches the epiphysis is called the *metaphysis* (Fig. 56-5). It is composed of bony trabeculae that have cores of cartilage. In the child, the epiphysis is separated from the metaphysis by the cartilaginous growth plate. After puberty, the metaphysis and epiphysis merge, and the growth plate is obliterated.

Bone marrow occupies the medullary cavities of the long bones throughout the skeleton and the cavities of cancellous bone in the vertebrae, ribs, sternum, and flat bones of the pelvis. The cellular composition of the bone marrow varies with age and skeletal location. Red bone marrow contains developing red blood cells and is the site of blood cell formation. Yellow bone marrow is composed largely of

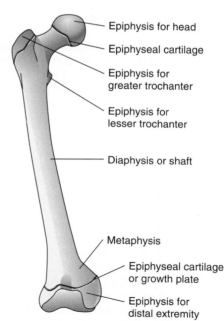

Epiphysis for head
Epiphyseal cartilage
Epiphysis for greater trochanter
Epiphysis for lesser trochanter
Diaphysis or shaft
Metaphysis
Epiphyseal cartilage or growth plate
Epiphysis for distal extremity

FIGURE 56-5 A femur, showing epiphyseal cartilages for the head, metaphysis, trochanters, and distal end of the bone. (Adapted with permission from Chaffee E.E., Lytle I.M. [1980]. *Basic physiology and anatomy* [4th ed.]. Philadelphia: J.B. Lippincott)

adipose cells. At birth, nearly all of the marrow is red and hematopoietically active. As the need for red blood cell production decreases during postnatal growth, red marrow is gradually replaced with yellow bone marrow in most of the bones. In the adult, red marrow persists in the vertebrae, ribs, sternum, and ilia.

TENDONS AND LIGAMENTS

In the skeletal system, tendons and ligaments are dense connective tissue structures that connect muscles and bones. Tendons connect muscles to bone, and ligaments connect the movable bones of joints. Tendons can appear as cordlike structures or as flattened sheets, called *aponeuroses*, such as in the abdominal muscles.

The dense connective tissue found in tendons and ligaments has a limited blood supply and is composed largely of intercellular bundles of collagen fibers arranged in the same direction and plane. This type of connective tissue provides great tensile strength and can withstand tremendous pull in the direction of fiber alignment. At the sites where tendons or ligaments are inserted into cartilage or bone, a gradual transition from pure dense connective tissue to bone or cartilage occurs. In cartilage, this transitional tissue is called *fibrocartilage*.

Tendons that may rub against bone or other friction-generating surfaces are enclosed in double-layered sheaths. An outer connective tissue tube is attached to the structures surrounding the tendon, and an inner sheath encloses the tendon and is attached to it. The space between the inner and outer sheath is filled with a fluid similar to synovial fluid.

JOINTS AND ARTICULATIONS

Articulations, or joints, are areas where two or more bones meet. The term *arthro* is the prefix used to designate a joint. For example, *arthrology* is the study of joints, and *arthroplasty* is the repair of a joint. There are two classes of joints, based on movement and the presence of a joint cavity: synarthroses and diarthroses.

Synarthroses

Synarthroses are joints that lack a joint cavity and move little or not at all. There are three types of synarthroses: synostoses, synchondroses, and syndesmoses. *Synostoses* are nonmovable joints in which the surfaces of the bones are joined by dense connective tissue or bone. The bones of the skull are joined by synostoses; they are joined by dense connective tissue in children and young adults and by bone in older persons. *Synchondroses* are joints in which bones are connected by hyaline cartilage and have limited motion. The ribs are attached to the sternum by this type of joint. *Syndesmoses* permit a certain amount of movement; they are separated by a fibrous disk and joined by interosseous ligaments. The symphysis pubis of the pelvis and the bodies of the vertebrae that are joined by intervertebral disks are examples of syndesmoses.

Skeletal Joints

➤ Joints, or articulations, are sites where two or more bones meet to hold the skeleton together and give it mobility.

➤ There are two types of joints: synarthroses, which are immovable joints, and diarthroses, which are freely movable joints.

➤ All limb joints are synovial diarthroidal joints, which are enclosed in a joint cavity containing synovial fluid.

➤ The articulating surfaces of synovial joints are covered with a layer of avascular cartilage that relies on oxygen and nutrients contained in the synovial fluid.

➤ Regeneration of articular cartilage of synovial joints is slow, and healing of injuries often is slow and unsatisfactory.

Diarthroses

Diarthrodial joints (*i.e.*, synovial joints) are freely movable joints. Most joints in the body are of this type. Although they are classified as freely movable, their movement ranges from almost none (*e.g.*, sacroiliac joint), to simple hinge movement (*e.g.*, interphalangeal joint), to movement in many planes (*e.g.*, shoulder or hip joint). The bony surfaces of these joints are covered with thin layers of articular cartilage, and the cartilaginous surfaces of these joints slide past each other during movement. As discussed in Chapter 59, diarthrodial joints are the joints most frequently affected by rheumatic disorders.

In a diarthrodial joint, the articulating ends of the bones are not connected directly but are indirectly linked by a strong fibrous capsule (*i.e.*, joint capsule) that surrounds the joint and is continuous with the periosteum (Fig. 56-6). This capsule supports the joint and helps to hold the bones in place. Additional support may be provided by ligaments that extend between the bones of the joint.

The joint capsule consists of two layers: an outer fibrous layer and an inner membrane, the synovium. The synovium surrounds the tendons that pass through the joints and the free margins of other intra-articular structures such as ligaments and menisci. The synovium forms folds that surround the margins of articulations but do not cover the weight-bearing articular cartilage. These folds permit stretching of the synovium so that movement can occur without tissue damage.

The synovium secretes a slippery fluid with the consistency of egg white called *synovial fluid*. This fluid acts as a lubricant and facilitates the movement of the articulating surfaces of the joint. Normal synovial fluid is clear or pale yellow, does not clot, and contains fewer than

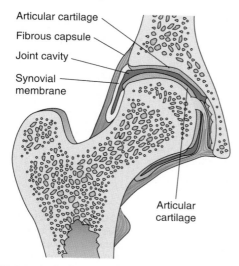

Articular cartilage
Fibrous capsule
Joint cavity
Synovial membrane

Articular cartilage

FIGURE 56-6 Diarthrodial joint, showing the articular cartilage, fibrous joint capsule, joint cavity, and synovial membrane. (Adapted with permission from Chaffee E.E., Lytle I.M. [1980]. *Basic physiology and anatomy* [4th ed.]. Philadelphia: J.B. Lippincott)

100 cells/mm³. The cells are predominantly mononuclear cells derived from the synovium. The composition of the synovial fluid is altered in many inflammatory and pathologic joint disorders. Aspiration and examination of the synovial fluid play an important role in the diagnosis of joint diseases.

The articular cartilage is an example of hyaline cartilage and is unique in that its free surface is not covered with perichondrium. It has only a peripheral rim of perichondrium, and calcification of the portion of cartilage abutting the bone may limit or preclude diffusion from blood vessels supplying the subchondral bone. Articular cartilage is apparently nourished by the diffusion of substances contained in the synovial fluid bathing the cartilage. Regeneration of most cartilage is slow; it is accomplished primarily by growth that requires the activity of perichondrium cells. In articular cartilage, which has no perichondrium, superficial injuries heal slowly.

Blood Supply and Innervation

The blood supply to a joint arises from blood vessels that enter the subchondral bone at or near the attachment of the joint capsule and form an arterial circle around the joint. The synovial membrane has a rich blood supply, and constituents of plasma diffuse rapidly between these vessels and the joint cavity. Because many of the capillaries are near the surface of the synovium, blood may escape into the synovial fluid after relatively minor injuries. Healing and repair of the synovial membrane usually are rapid and complete. This is important because synovial tissue is injured in many surgical procedures that involve the joint.

The nerve supply to joints is provided by the same nerve trunks that supply the muscles that move the joints. These nerve trunks also supply the skin over the joints. As a rule, each joint of an extremity is innervated by all the peripheral nerves that cross the articulation; this accounts for

the referral of pain from one joint to another. For example, hip pain may be perceived as pain in the knee.

The tendons and ligaments of the joint capsule are sensitive to position and movement, particularly stretching and twisting. These structures are supplied by the large sensory nerve fibers that form proprioceptor endings (see Chapter 47). The proprioceptors function reflexively to adjust the tension of the muscles that support the joint and are particularly important in maintaining muscular support for the joint. For example, when a weight is lifted, there is a proprioceptor-mediated reflex contraction and relaxation of appropriate muscle groups to support the joint and protect the joint capsule and other joint structures. Loss of proprioception and reflex control of muscular support leads to destructive changes in the joint.

The synovial membrane is innervated only by autonomic fibers that control blood flow. It is relatively free of pain fibers, as evidenced by the fact that surgical procedures on the joint are often done under local anesthesia. The joint capsule and the ligaments have pain receptors; these receptors are more easily stimulated by stretching and twisting than other joint structures. Pain arising from the capsule tends to be diffuse and poorly localized.

Bursae

In some diarthrotic joints, the synovial membrane forms closed sacs that are not part of the joint. These sacs, called *bursae*, contain synovial fluid. Their purpose is to prevent friction on a tendon. Bursae occur in areas where pressure is exerted because of close approximation of joint structures (Fig. 56-7). Such conditions occur when tendons are deflected over bone or where skin must move freely over bony tissue. Bursae may become injured or inflamed, causing discomfort, swelling, and limitation in movement of the involved area. A bunion is an inflamed bursa of the metatarsophalangeal joint of the great toe.

Intra-articular Menisci

Intra-articular menisci are fibrocartilage structures that develop from portions of the articular disk that occupied the space between articular cartilage surfaces during fetal development. Menisci may extend part way through the joint and have a free inner border, as at the lateral and medial articular surfaces of the knee, or they may extend through the joint, separating it into two separate cavities, as in the sternoclavicular joint. The menisci of the knee joint may be torn as the result of an injury (see Chapter 57).

> In summary, bones are classified on the basis of their shape as long, short, flat, or irregular. Long bones are found in the upper and lower extremities; short bones in the ankle and wrist; flat bones in the skull and rib cage; and irregular bones in the vertebrae and jaw. Tendons and ligaments are dense connective skeletal tissue that connect muscles and bones. Tendons connect muscles to bones, and ligaments connect the movable bones of joints.
>
> Articulations, or joints, are areas where two or more bones meet. Synarthroses are joints in which bones are

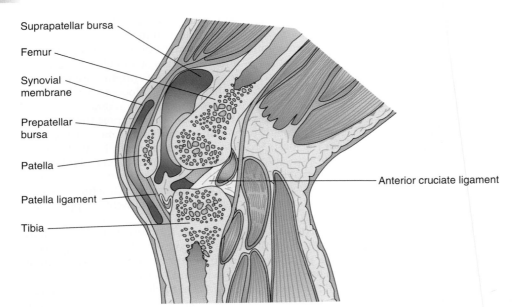

Suprapatellar bursa

Femur

Synovial membrane

Prepatellar bursa

Patella

Patella ligament

Tibia

Anterior cruciate ligament

FIGURE 56-7 Sagittal section of knee joint, showing prepatellar and suprapatellar bursae. (Adapted with permission from Chaffee E.E., Lytle I.M. [1980]. *Basic physiology and anatomy* [4th ed.]. Philadelphia: J.B. Lippincott)

joined together by fibrous tissue, cartilage, or bone; they lack a joint cavity and have little or no movement. Diarthrodial or synovial joints are freely movable. The surfaces of the articulating ends of bones in diarthrodial joints are covered with a thin layer of articular cartilage, and they are enclosed in a fibrous joint capsule. The joint capsule consists of two layers: an outer fibrous layer and an inner membrane, the synovium. The synovial fluid, which is secreted by the synovium into the joint capsule, acts as a lubricant and facilitates movement of the joint's articulating surfaces. Bursae, which are closed sacs containing synovial fluid, prevent friction in areas where tendons are deflected over bone or where skin must move freely over bony tissue.

Menisci are fibrocartilaginous structures that develop from portions of the articular disk that occupied the space between the articular cartilage during fetal development. The menisci may have a free inner border, or they may extend through the joint, separating it into two cavities. The menisci in the knee joint may be torn as a result of injury.

Bibliography

Cormack D.H. (1987). *Ham's histology* (9th ed., pp. 234–338). Philadelphia: J.B. Lippincott.

DeLuca H.F. (1988). The vitamin D story: A collaborative effort of basic science and clinical medicine. *FASEB Journal 2*, 236–242.

Guyton A.C., Hall J.E. (2000). *Textbook of medical physiology* (10th ed., pp. 899–912). Philadelphia: W.B. Saunders.

Junqueira L.C., Carneiro J., Kelly O. (1995). *Basic histology* (8th ed., pp. 124–151). Los Altos, CA: Lange Medical Publications.

Moore K.L., Dalley A.F. (1999). *Clinically oriented anatomy* (4th ed). Philadelphia: Lippincott Williams & Wilkins.

Rhoades R.A., Tanner G.A. (1996). *Medical physiology* (pp. 725–735). Boston: Little, Brown.

Chapter 57

Alterations in Skeletal Function: Trauma and Infection

Kathleen E. Gunta

The musculoskeletal system includes the bones, joints, and muscles of the body together with associated structures such as ligaments and tendons. This system, which constitutes more than 70% of the body, is subject to a large number of disorders. These disorders affect persons in all age groups and walks of life and cause pain, disability, and deformity. The discussion in this chapter focuses on the effects of trauma, infections, and ischemia on musculoskeletal structures such as bones, muscles, tendons, and ligaments.

Injury and Trauma of Musculoskeletal Structures

After you have completed this section of the chapter, you should be able to meet the following objectives:

✦ Describe the physical agents responsible for soft tissue trauma
✦ Name the three types of soft tissue injuries
✦ Compare muscle strains and ligamentous sprains
✦ Describe the healing process of soft tissue injuries
✦ Differentiate open from closed fractures
✦ List the signs and symptoms of a fracture
✦ Describe the fracture healing process

✦ Relate individual and local factors to the healing process in bone
✦ Explain the importance of immobilization for fracture healing
✦ Explain why muscle and joint function should be maintained during fracture healing
✦ Differentiate the early complications of fractures from later complications of fracture healing

Trauma, which commonly includes injury to musculoskeletal structures, is the third leading cause of death in the United States. Injuries cost the United States billions of dollars each year owing to the cost of medical care and lost production.

A broad spectrum of musculoskeletal injuries results from numerous physical forces, including blunt tissue trauma, disruption of tendons and ligaments, and fractures of bony structures. Many of the forces that cause injury to the musculoskeletal system are typical for a particular environmental setting, activity, or age group. Trauma resulting from high-speed motor accidents is ranked as the number one killer of adults younger than 45 years of age.[1] Motorcycle accidents are especially common in young men, with fractures of the distal tibia, midshaft femur, and radius occurring most often.

Trauma in children is usually the result of an accident. Childhood falls cause approximately 3 million emergency department visits each year,[2] and bicycle-related injuries, most of them involving the 5- to 14-year-old age group, account for another 50,000 visits.[1] More than 775,000 children younger than 15 years of age are treated each year in hospital emergency departments for sports injuries. Most of these injuries occur in unorganized football, basketball, and baseball sports activities.[2]

Falls are the most common cause of injury in people 65 years of age and older. Current statistics indicate that 30% of persons in this age group experience at least one fall each year.[3] Impaired vision and hearing, dizziness, and unsteadiness of gait contribute to falls in the older person. These falls often are compounded by osteoporosis, or bone atrophy, which makes fractures more likely. Fractures of the vertebrae, proximal humerus, and hip are particularly common in this age group.

ATHLETIC INJURIES

Athletic injuries are either acute injuries or overuse injuries. Acute injuries are caused by sudden trauma and include injuries to soft tissues (contusion, strains, and sprains) and to bone (fractures). Overuse represents a series of smaller injuries. They commonly occur in the elbow ("Little League elbow" or "tennis elbow") and in tissue where tendons attach to the bone, such as the heel, knee, and shoulder. Contact sports pose a greater threat for injury to the neck, spine, and growth plates in children and adolescents, who have not yet reached maturity. Injuries can be prevented by proper training, use of safety equipment, and competition according to skill and size rather than chronologic age.

SOFT TISSUE INJURIES

Most skeletal injuries are accompanied by soft tissue injuries. These injuries include contusions, hematomas, and lacerations. They are discussed here because of their association with musculoskeletal injuries.

A *contusion* is an injury to soft tissue that results from direct trauma and is usually caused by striking a body part against a hard object. With a contusion, the skin overlying the injury remains intact. Initially, the area becomes ecchymotic (*i.e.*, black and blue) because of local hemorrhage; later, the discoloration gradually changes to brown and then to yellow as the blood is reabsorbed. A large area of local hemorrhage is called a *hematoma*. Hematomas cause pain as blood accumulates and exerts pressure on nerve endings. The pain increases with movement or when pressure is applied to the area. The pain and swelling of a hematoma take longer to subside than that accompanying a contusion. A hematoma may become infected because of bacterial growth. Unlike a contusion, which does not drain, a hematoma may eventually split the skin because of increased pressures and produce drainage.

The treatment for a contusion and a hematoma consists of elevating the affected part and applying cold for the first 24 hours to reduce the bleeding into the area. A hematoma may need to be aspirated. After the first 24 hours,

heat or cold should be applied intermittently for 20 minutes at a time.

A *laceration* is an injury in which the skin is torn or its continuity is disrupted. The seriousness of a laceration depends on the size and depth of the wound and on whether there is contamination from the object that caused the injury. Puncture wounds from nails or rusted material may result in the growth of toxic bacteria, leading to gas gangrene or tetanus.

Lacerations are usually treated by wound closure, which is done after the area is sufficiently cleaned; the closed wound is covered with a sterile dressing. It is important to minimize contamination of the wound and to control bleeding. Contaminated wounds and open fractures are copiously irrigated and debrided, and the skin usually is left open to heal to prevent the development of an anaerobic infection or a sinus tract.

JOINT (MUSCULOTENDINOUS) INJURIES

Joints, or articulations, are sites where two or more bones meet. Joints (*i.e.*, diathrodial) are supported by tough bundles of collagenous fibers called *ligaments* that attach to the joint capsule and bind the articular ends of bones together, and by *tendons* that join muscles to the periosteum of the articulating bones. Joint injuries involve mechanical overloading or forcible twisting or stretching.

Strains and Sprains

Strains.   A *strain* is a stretching injury to a muscle or a musculotendinous unit caused by mechanical overloading. This type of injury may result from an unusual muscle contraction or an excessive forcible stretch. Although there usually is no external evidence of a specific injury, pain, stiffness, and swelling exist. The most common sites for muscle strains are the lower back and the cervical region of the spine. The elbow and the shoulder are also supported by musculotendinous units that are subject to strains. Foot strain is associated with the weight-bearing stresses of the

  Fracture Healing

- ➤ Fractures are caused by forces that disrupt the continuity of bone.

- ➤ Fracture healing depends on the extent of the injury, the ability to align the bone fragments, and immobilizing the fracture site so that healing can take place.

- ➤ Bone healing occurs by replacement of injured bone cells. It involves formation of a hematoma that provides the foundation for blood vessel and fibroblast infiltration, proliferation of bone repair cells (osteoblasts), callus formation, ossification of the callus, and remodeling of the fracture site.

feet; it may be caused by inadequate muscular and ligamentous support, overweight, or excessive exercise such as standing, walking, or running.

In the lumbar and cervical spine regions, muscle strains are more common than sprains. Mechanical low back pain is becoming increasingly common in the adolescent athlete. Overuse, especially hyperextension of the lumbar spine in such sports as track, wrestling, gymnastics, and diving, can tear the muscles, fascia, and ligaments. Careful diagnosis is necessary because chronic low back pain may indicate a stress fracture. Fractures near the top and bottom surface of the vertebrae can occur when the growing lumbar spine is overstressed, causing the disks to push into the bone. Early detection and treatment are important to prevent complications and disability. Treatment of back strains consists of bed rest, traction, application of heat, and massage. Cold should be used during the first 24 hours to reduce pain and swelling of the affected area. Exercises, correct posture, and good body mechanics help to reduce the risk of reinjury.

Sprains. A *sprain,* which involves the ligamentous structures surrounding the joint, resembles a strain, but the pain and swelling subside more slowly. It usually is caused by abnormal or excessive movement of the joint. With a sprain, the ligaments may be incompletely torn or, as in a severe sprain, completely torn or ruptured (Fig. 57-1). The signs of sprain are pain, rapid swelling, heat, disability, discoloration, and limitation of function. Any joint may be sprained, but the ankle joint is most commonly involved, especially in higher-risk sports such as basketball. Most ankle sprains occur in the lateral ankle when the foot is turned inward under a person, forcing the ankle into inversion beyond the structural limits. Other common sites of sprain are the knee (the collateral ligament and anterior cruciate ligament) and elbow (the ulnar side). As with a strain, the soft tissue injury that occurs with a sprain is not evident on the radiograph. Occasionally, however, a chip of bone is evident when the entire ligament, including part of its bony attachment, has been ruptured or torn from the bone.

Healing. Healing of the dense connective tissues in tendons and ligaments is similar to that of other soft tissues. If properly treated, injuries usually heal with the restoration of the original tensile strength. Repair is accomplished by fibroblasts from the inner tendon sheath or, if the tendon has no sheath, from the loose connective tissue that surrounds the tendon. Capillaries infiltrate the injured area during the initial healing process and supply the fibroblasts with the materials they need to produce large amounts of collagen. Formation of the long collagen bundles begins within 4 to 5 days, and although tensile strength increases steadily thereafter, it is not sufficient to permit strong tendon pulls for 4 to 5 weeks.[4] During the first 3 weeks, there is a danger that muscle contraction will pull the injured ends apart, causing the tendon to heal in the lengthened position. There is also a danger that adhesions will develop in areas where tendons pass through fibrous channels, such as in the distal palm of the hands, rendering the tendon useless.

Treatment. The treatment of muscle strains and ligamentous sprains is similar in several ways. For an injured extremity, elevation of the part followed by local application of cold may be sufficient. Compression, accomplished through the use of adhesive wraps or a removable splint, helps reduce swelling and provides support. A cast is applied for severe sprains, especially those severe enough to warrant surgical repair. Immobilization for a muscle strain is continued until the pain and swelling have subsided. In a sprain, the affected joint is immobilized for several weeks. Immobilization may be followed by graded active exercises. Early diagnosis, treatment, and rehabilitation are essential in preventing chronic ligamentous instability.

Dislocations

Dislocation of a joint is the loss of articulation of the bone ends in the joint capsule caused by displacement or separation of the bone end from its position in the joint. It usually follows a severe trauma that disrupts the holding ligaments. Dislocations are seen most often in the shoulder and acromioclavicular joints. A subluxation is a partial dislocation in which the bone ends in the joint are still in partial contact with each other.

Dislocations can be congenital, traumatic, or pathologic. Congenital dislocations occur in the hip and knee. Traumatic dislocations occur after falls, blows, or rotational injuries. For example, car accidents often cause dislocations of the hip and accompanying acetabular fractures because of the direction of impact. This is true of persons wearing seat belts and those who are unrestrained. In the shoulder and patella, dislocations may become recurrent, especially in athletes. They recur with the same motion but require less and less force each time.

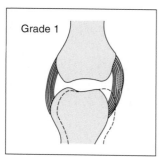
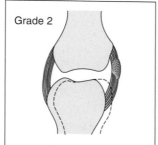
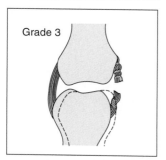
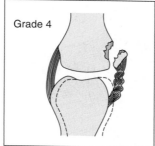

FIGURE 57-1 Degrees of sprain on the medial side of the right knee: grade 1, mild sprain of the medial collateral ligament; grade 2, moderate sprain with hematoma formation; grade 3, severe sprain with total disruption of the ligament; and grade 4, severe sprain with avulsion of the medial femoral condyle at the insertion of the medial collateral ligament. (Adapted from Spickler L.L. [1983]. Knee injuries of the athlete. *Orthopedic Nursing* 2 [5], 12–13)

Pathologic dislocation in the hip is a late complication of infection, rheumatoid arthritis, paralysis, and neuromuscular diseases. Dislocations of the phalangeal joints are not serious and are usually reduced by manipulation. Less common sites of dislocation, seen mainly in young adults, are the wrist and midtarsal region. They usually are the result of direct force, such as a fall on an outstretched hand.

Diagnosis of a dislocation is based on history, physical examination, and radiologic findings. The symptoms are pain, deformity, and limited movement. With recurrent dislocations, the person often experiences apprehension during tests of joint rotation, fearing that the joint will slip out of place.

The treatment depends on the site, mechanism of injury, and associated injuries such as fractures. Dislocations that do not reduce spontaneously usually require manipulation or surgical repair. Various surgical procedures also can be used to prevent redislocation of the patella, shoulder, or acromioclavicular joints. Immobilization is necessary for several weeks after reduction of a dislocation to allow healing of the joint structures. In dislocations affecting the knee, alternatives to surgery are isometric quadriceps-strengthening exercises and a temporary brace. Surgical procedures, such as joint replacement, may be necessary in certain pathologic dislocations.

Loose Bodies

Loose bodies are small pieces of bone or cartilage within a joint space. These can result from trauma to the joint or may occur when cartilage has worn away from the articular surface, causing a necrotic piece of bone to separate and become free floating. The symptoms are painful catching and locking of the joint. Loose bodies are commonly seen in the knee, elbow, hip, and ankle. The loose body repeatedly gets caught in the crevice of a joint, pinching the underlying healthy cartilage; unless the loose body is removed, it may cause osteoarthritis and restricted movement. The treatment consists of removal using operative arthroscopy.

Rotator Cuff and Shoulder Injuries

Rotator cuff injury occurs in one or more of the four muscles that lie deep in the shoulder, bridging the glenohumeral joint (Fig. 57-2). It can be caused by excessive use, a direct

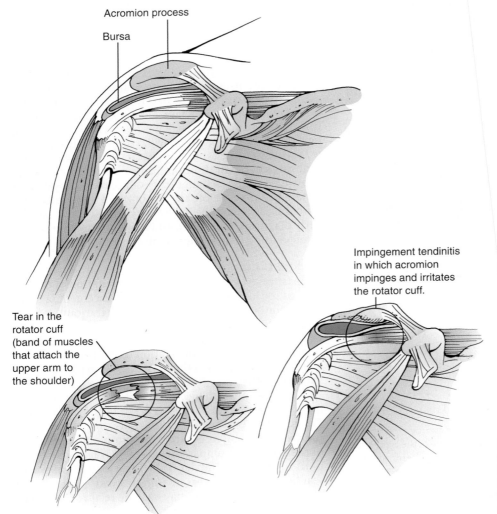

Acromion process

Bursa

Tear in the rotator cuff (band of muscles that attach the upper arm to the shoulder)

Impingement tendinitis in which acromion impinges and irritates the rotator cuff.

FIGURE 57-2 Muscles and tendons of the rotator cuff that hold the humerus into the shoulder socket (**top**). Tear in rotator cuff (**bottom left**) and impingement tendinitis (**bottom right**).

blow, or stretch injury, usually involving throwing or swinging, as with baseball pitchers or tennis players. Complete tears of the rotator cuff usually occur in young persons after severe trauma. Overuse syndrome has a slower onset and is seen in older persons with minor or no trauma. Rotator cuff tendinitis, also known as *shoulder impingement syndrome*, also is common, especially in swimmers. Severe tendinitis also can cause either a partial or complete rotator cuff tear.

Many physical examination maneuvers are used to define shoulder pathology. The history and mechanism of injury are important. In addition to standard radiographs, an arthrogram, computed tomography (CT) scan, or magnetic resonance imaging (MRI) scan may be obtained. Arthroscopic examination under anesthesia is done for diagnostic purposes and operative arthroscopy to repair severe tears. Conservative treatment with anti-inflammatory agents, corticosteroid injections, and physical therapy often is done. A period of rest is followed by a customized exercise and rehabilitation program to improve strength, flexibility, and endurance. The rotator cuff is not unlike other muscle groups of the body in that its risk of injury increases when it is required to perform a high-stress function in an unconditioned state.

Knee Injuries

The knee is a common site of injury, particularly sport-related injuries in which the knee is subjected to abnormal twisting and compression forces. These forces can result in injury to the menisci, patellar subluxation and dislocation, and chondromalacia. Knee injuries in young adulthood and both knee and hip injuries in middle age substantially increase the risk of osteoarthritis in the same joint later in life.[2]

Meniscus Injuries.

The menisci are C-shaped plates of fibrocartilage that are superimposed between the condyles of the femur and tibia. There are two menisci in each knee, a lateral and medial meniscus (Fig. 57-3). The menisci are thicker at their external margins and taper to thin, unattached edges at their interior margin. They are firmly attached at their ends to the intercondylar area of the tibia and they are supported by the coronary and transverse ligaments of the knee. The menisci play a major role in load bearing and shock absorption. They also help to stabilize the knee by deepening the tibial socket and maintaining the femur and tibia in proper position. In addition, the meniscus assists in joint lubrication and serves as source of nutrition for articular cartilage in the knee.

Any action of the knee that causes injury to the knee ligaments can also cause a meniscal tear.[5] Meniscus injury commonly occurs as the result of a rotational injury from a sudden or sharp pivot or a direct blow to the knee, as in hockey, basketball, or football. The final type and location of the meniscal tear is determined by the magnitude and direction of the force that acts on the knee and the position of the knee at the time of injury. Meniscus tears can be described by their appearance (*e.g.*, parrot-beak, bucket handle) or their location (*e.g.*, posterior horn, anterior horn). The injured knee is edematous and painful, especially with hyperflexion and hyperextension. A loose fragment may cause knee instability and locking.

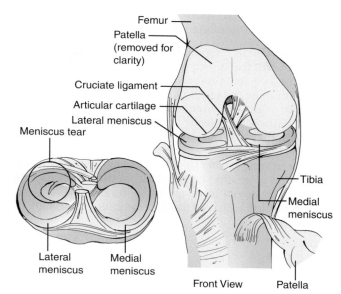

FIGURE 57-3 The knee showing the lateral and medial meniscus (with the patella removed for clarity). Insert (**lower left**) shows meniscus tear.

Diagnosis is made by examination and confirmed by methods such as arthroscopy and radiologic, CT scans, and radionuclide imaging. MRI has proven particularly useful in diagnosis of meniscal tears.[6] Initial treatment of meniscal injuries may be conservative. The knee may be placed in a removable knee immobilizer. Isometric quadriceps exercises may be prescribed. Activity usually is restricted until complete motion is recovered. Arthroscopic meniscectomy may be performed when there is recurrent or persistent locking, recurrent effusion, or disabling pain.

There is evidence that loss of meniscal function is associated with progressive degeneration of the knee.[5] Meniscal reconstruction procedures have been developed to preserve these functions before development of significant degenerative changes, thus preventing a total joint replacement later in life. Among the reconstruction methods used is replacement of the damaged meniscus with a meniscal transplant (fresh, frozen, or cryopreserved allografts).[6,7] Use of a synthetic collagen scaffold that allows fibrochondrocyte ingrowth is being investigated.[6]

Patellar Subluxation and Dislocations.

Recurrent subluxation and dislocation of the patella (*i.e.*, knee cap) are common injuries in young adults. They account for approximately 10% of all athletic injuries and are more common in women. Sports such as skiing or tennis may cause stress on the patella. These sports involve external rotation of the foot and lower leg with knee flexion, a position that exerts rotational stresses on the knee. Congenital knee variations are also a predisposing factor.

There is often a sensation of the patella "popping out" when the dislocation occurs. Other complaints include the knee giving out, swelling, crepitus, stiffness, and loss of range of motion.

Treatment can be difficult, but nonsurgical methods are used first. They include immobilization with the knee extended, bracing, administration of anti-inflammatory agents, and isometric quadriceps-strengthening exercises. Surgical intervention often is necessary.

Chondromalacia. Chondromalacia, or softening of the articular cartilage, is seen most commonly on the under-surface of the patella and occurs most frequently in young adults. It can be the result of recurrent subluxation of the patella or overuse in strenuous athletic activities. Persons with this disorder typically complain of pain, particularly when climbing stairs or sitting with the knees bent. Occasionally, the person experiences weakness of the knee.

The treatment consists of rest, isometric exercises, and application of ice after exercise. Part of the patella may be surgically removed in severe cases. In less severe cases, the soft portion is shaved using a saw inserted through an arthroscope.

FRACTURES

Fracture, or discontinuity of the bone, is the most common type of bone lesion. Normal bone can withstand considerable compression and shearing forces and, to a lesser extent, tension forces. A fracture occurs when more stress is placed on the bone than it is able to absorb. Grouped according to cause, fractures can be divided into three major categories: fractures caused by sudden injury, fatigue or stress fractures, and pathologic fractures. The most common fractures are those resulting from sudden injury. The force causing the fracture may be direct, such as a fall or blow, or indirect, such as a massive muscle contraction or trauma transmitted along the bone. For example, the head of the radius or clavicle can be fractured by the indirect forces that result from falling on an outstretched hand. A fatigue fracture results from repeated wear on a bone. Pain associated with overuse injuries of the lower extremities, especially posterior medial tibial pain, is one of the most common symptoms that physically active persons, such as runners, experience. Stress fractures in the tibia may be confused with "shin splints," a nonspecific term for pain in the lower leg from overuse in walking and running, because they frequently do not appear on x-ray films until 2 weeks after the onset of symptoms.

A pathologic fracture occurs in bones that already are weakened by disease or tumors. Fractures of this type may occur spontaneously with little or no stress. The underlying disease state can be local, as with infections, cysts, or tumors, or it can be generalized, as in osteoporosis, Paget's disease, or disseminated tumors.

Classification

Fractures usually are classified according to location, type, and direction or pattern of the fracture line (Fig. 57-4).

Location. A long bone is divided into three parts: proximal, midshaft, and distal (see Fig. 57-4). A fracture of the long bone is described in relation to its position in the bone. Other descriptions are used when the fracture affects the head or neck of a bone, involves a joint, or is near a prominence such as a condyle or malleolus.

Types. The type of fracture is determined by its communication with the external environment, the degree of break in continuity of the bone, and the character of the fracture

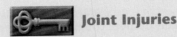

Joint Injuries

➤ Joints are the weakest part of the skeletal system and common sites for injury due to mechanical overloading or forcible twisting or stretching.

➤ Injury can include damage to the tendons, which connect muscle to bone; ligaments, which hold bones together; or the cartilage that covers the articular surface.

➤ Healing of the dense connective tissue involved in joint injuries requires time to restore the structures so that they are strong enough to withstand the forces imposed on the joint. Ligamentous injuries may require surgical intervention with approximation of many fibrous strands to facilitate healing.

➤ Injuries involving the articular cartilage may predispose to later joint disease.

pieces. A fracture can be classified as open or closed. When the bone fragments have broken through the skin, the fracture is called an *open* or *compound fracture.* Open fractures often are complicated by infection, osteomyelitis, delayed union, or nonunion. In a closed fracture, there is no communication with the outside skin.

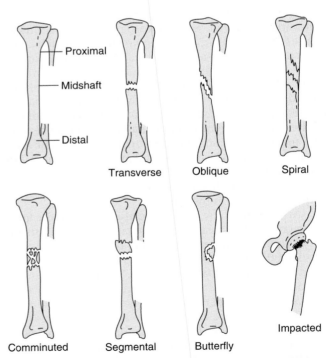

FIGURE 57-4 Classification of fractures. Fractures are classified according to location (proximal, midshaft, or distal), the direction of fracture line (transverse, oblique, spiral), and type (comminuted, segmental, butterfly, or impacted).

The degree of a fracture is described in terms of a partial or complete break in the continuity of bone. A *greenstick fracture*, which is seen in children, is an example of a partial break in bone continuity and resembles the kind seen when a young sapling is broken. This kind of break occurs because children's bones, especially until approximately 10 years of age, are more resilient than the bones of adults.

A fracture is also described by the character of the fracture pieces. A *comminuted fracture* has more than two pieces. A *compression fracture*, as occurs in the vertebral body, involves two bones that are crushed or squeezed together. A fracture is called *impacted* when the fracture fragments are wedged together. This type usually occurs in the humerus, often is less serious, and usually is treated without surgery.

Patterns.   The direction of the trauma or mechanism of injury produces a certain configuration or pattern of fracture. *Reduction* is the restoration of a fractured bone to its normal anatomic position. The pattern of a fracture indicates the nature of the trauma and provides information about the easiest method for reduction. *Transverse fractures* are caused by simple angulatory forces. A *spiral fracture* results from a twisting motion, or torque. A transverse fracture is not likely to become displaced or lose its position after it is reduced. On the other hand, spiral, oblique, and comminuted fractures often are unstable and may change position after reduction.

Manifestations

The signs and symptoms of a fracture include pain, tenderness at the site of bone disruption, swelling, loss of function, deformity of the affected part, and abnormal mobility. The deformity varies according to the type of force applied, the area of the bone involved, the type of fracture produced, and the strength and balance of the surrounding muscles.

In long bones, three types of deformities—angulation, shortening, and rotation—are seen. Severely angulated fracture fragments may be felt at the fracture site and often push up against the soft tissue to cause a tenting effect on the skin. Bending forces and unequal muscle pulls cause angulation. Shortening of the extremity occurs as the bone fragments slide and override each other because of the pull of the muscles on the long axis of the extremity (Fig. 57-5). Rotational deformity occurs when the fracture fragments rotate out of their normal longitudinal axis; this can result from rotational strain produced by the fracture or unequal pull by the muscles that are attached to the fracture fragments. A crepitus or grating sound may be heard as the bone fragments rub against each other. In the case of an open fracture, there is bleeding from the wound where the bone protrudes.

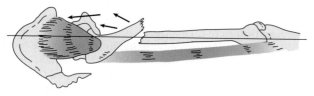

FIGURE 57-5 Displacement and overriding of fracture fragments of a long bone (femur) caused by severe muscle spasm.

Blood loss from a pelvic fracture or multiple long bone fractures can cause hypovolemic shock in a trauma victim.

Shortly after the fracture has occurred, nerve function at the fracture site may be temporarily lost. The area may become numb, and the surrounding muscles may become flaccid. This condition has been called *local shock*. During this period, which may last for a few minutes to half an hour, fractured bones may be reduced with little or no pain. After this brief period, pain sensation returns and, with it, muscle spasms and contractions of the surrounding muscles.

The early complications of fractures are associated with loss of skeletal continuity, injury from bone fragments, pressure from swelling and hemorrhage, involvement of nerve fibers, or development of fat emboli. The extent of early complications depends on the severity of the fracture and the area of the body that is involved. For example, bone fragments from a skull fracture may cause injury to brain tissue, or multiple rib fractures may lead to a flail chest and respiratory insufficiency. With flail chest, the chest wall on the fractured side becomes so unstable that it may move in the opposite direction as the person breathes (*i.e.*, in during inspiration and out during expiration).

Healing

Bone healing occurs in a manner similar to soft tissue healing. It is, however, a more complex process and takes longer. Although the exact mechanisms of bone healing are open to controversy, five stages of the healing process have been identified: (1) hematoma formation, (2) cellular proliferation, (3) callus formation, (4) ossification, and (5) remodeling (Fig. 57-6). The degree of response during each of these stages is in direct proportion to the extent of trauma.

Hematoma Formation.   Hematoma formation occurs during the first 48 to 72 hours after fracture. It develops as blood from torn vessels in the bone fragments and surrounding soft tissue leaks between and around the fragments of the fractured bone. Evidence suggests that the function of the hematoma is to be a source of signaling molecules that initiate the cellular events essential to fracture healing.[8] As the result of hematoma formation, clotting factors remain in the injured area to initiate the formation of a fibrin meshwork, which serves as a framework for the ingrowth of fibroblasts and new capillary buds. Granulation tissue, the result of fibroblasts and new capillaries, gradually invades and replaces the clot. When a large hematoma develops, healing is delayed because macrophages, platelets, oxygen, and nutrients for callus formation are prevented from entering the area.

Cellular Proliferation.   Three layers of bone structure are involved in the cellular proliferation that occurs during bone healing: the periosteum, or outer covering of the bone; the endosteum, or inner covering; and the medullary canal, which contains the bone marrow. During this process, the osteoblasts, or bone-forming cells, multiply and differentiate into a fibrocartilaginous callus. The fibrocartilaginous callus is softer and more flexible than callus. Cellular proliferation begins distal to the fracture, where there is a greater supply of blood. After a few days, a fibrocartilage "collar" becomes evident around the fracture site. The collar edges on

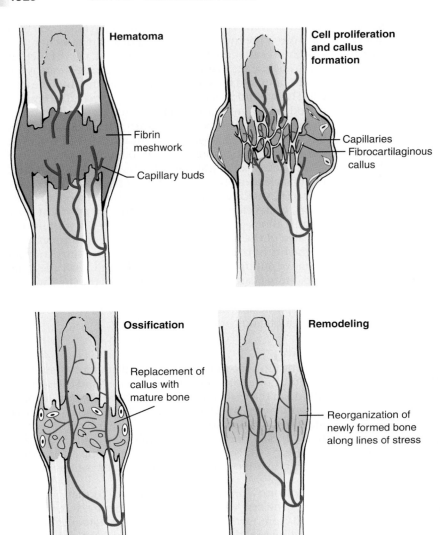

Hematoma

Fibrin meshwork

Capillary buds

Cell proliferation and callus formation

Capillaries
Fibrocartilaginous callus

Ossification

Replacement of callus with mature bone

Remodeling

Reorganization of newly formed bone along lines of stress

FIGURE 57-6 The stages of bone healing. The hematoma stage provides the fibrin mesh-work and capillary buds needed for subsequent cellular invasion. Cellular proliferation and callus formation represent the stages during which osteoblasts enter the area and form the fibrocartilaginous callus that joins the bone fragments. The ossification stage involves the mineralization of the fibrocartilaginous callus; and the remodeling stage, the reorganization of mineralized bone along the lines of mechanical stress.

either side of the fracture eventually unite to form a bridge, which connects the bone fragments.

Callus Formation. During the early stage of callus formation, the fracture becomes "sticky" as osteoblasts continue to move in and through the fibrin bridge to help keep it firm. Cartilage forms at the level of the fracture, where there is less circulation. In areas of the bone with muscle insertion, periosteal circulation is better, bringing in the nutrients necessary to bridge the callus. The bone calcifies as mineral salts are deposited. This stage usually occurs during the third to fourth week of fracture healing.

Ossification. Ossification involves the final laying down of bone. This is the stage at which the fracture has been bridged and the fracture fragments are firmly united. Mature bone replaces the callus, and the excess callus is gradually resorbed by the osteoclasts. The fracture site feels firm and immovable and appears united on the radiograph. At this point, it is safe to remove the cast.

Remodeling. Remodeling involves resorption of the excess bony callus that develops in the marrow space and encircles the external aspect of the fracture site. The remodeling process is directed by mechanical stress and direction of weight bearing. It continues according to Wolff's law—bone responds to mechanical stress by becoming thicker and stronger in relation to its function.

Healing Time. Healing time depends on the site of the fracture, the condition of the fracture fragments, hematoma formation, and other local and host factors. In general, fractures of long bones, displaced fractures, and fractures with less surface area heal slower. Function usually returns within 6 months after union is complete. However, return to complete function may take longer.

Factors that influence bone healing are specific to the person, the type of injury sustained, and local factors that disrupt healing (Chart 57-1). Individual factors that may delay bone healing are the patient's age; current medications; debilitating diseases, such as diabetes and rheumatoid

> ### CHART 57-1
>
> #### *Factors Affecting Fracture Healing*
>
> - Nature of the injury or the severity of the trauma, including fracture displacement, edema, and arterial occlusion with crushing injuries
> - Degree of bridge formation that develops during bone healing
> - Amount of bone loss (*e.g.*, it may be too great for the healing to bridge the gap)
> - Type of bone that is injured (*e.g.*, cancellous bone heals faster than cortical bone)
> - Degree of immobilization that is achieved (*e.g.*, movement disrupts the fibrin bridge and cartilage forms instead of bone)
> - Local infection, which retards or prevents healing
> - Local malignancy, which must be treated before healing can proceed
> - Bone necrosis, which prevents blood flow into the fracture site

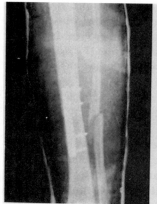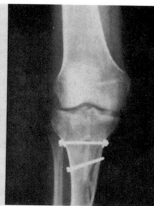

FIGURE 57-7 (Left) Internal fixation of the tibia with compression plate. **(Right)** Internal fixation of an intra-articular fracture of the upper tibia with a screw and bolt. (Adapted with permission from Farrell J. [1986]. *Illustrated guide to orthopaedic nursing* [3rd ed.]. Philadelphia: J.B. Lippincott)

arthritis; local stress around the fracture site; circulatory problems and coagulation disorders; and poor nutrition.

Diagnosis and Treatment

Diagnosis is the first step in the care of fractures and is based on history and physical manifestations. X-ray examination is used to confirm the diagnosis and direct the treatment. The ease of diagnosis varies with the location and severity of the fracture. In the trauma patient, the presence of other, more serious injuries may make diagnosis more difficult. A thorough history includes the mechanism, time, and place of the injury; first recognition of symptoms; and any treatment initiated. A complete history is important because a delay in seeking treatment or a period of weight bearing on a fracture may cause further injury or displacement of the fracture.

A *splint* is a device for immobilizing the movable fragments of a fracture. When a fracture is suspected, the injured part always should be splinted before it is moved. This is essential for preventing further injury. Further treatment depends on the general condition of the patient, the presence of associated injuries, the location of the fracture and its displacement, and whether the fracture is open or closed.

There are three objectives for treatment of fractures: reduction of the fracture, immobilization, and preservation and restoration of the function of the injured part.

Reduction. Reduction of a fracture is directed toward replacing the bone fragments to as near normal anatomic position as possible. This can be accomplished by closed manipulation or surgical (open) reduction. Closed manipulation uses methods such as manual pressure and traction. Fractures are held in reduction by external or internal fixation devices. Surgical reduction involves the use of various types of hardware to accomplish internal fixation of the fracture fragments (Fig. 57-7). Primary closure of crush injuries in the extremities is delayed until tissue viability is

determined. The wound is first debrided and immobilized with an external fixation device. Reconstruction is done later using cancellous bone grafts with microvascular composite tissue grafts, or by means of tissue regeneration with distraction devices.

Immobilization. Immobilization prevents movement of the injured parts and is the single most important element in obtaining union of the fracture fragments. Immobilization can be accomplished through the use of external devices, such as splints, casts, external fixation devices, or traction, or by means of internal fixation devices inserted during surgical reduction of the fracture.

Splints are made from many different materials. Metal splints or air splints may be used during transport to a health care facility as a temporary measure until the fracture has been reduced and another form of immobilization instituted. Plaster of Paris splints, which are molded to fit the extremity, work well. Splinting should be done if there is any suspicion of a fracture because motion of the fracture site can cause pain, bleeding, more soft tissue damage, and nerve or blood vessel compression. If the fracture has sharp fragments, movement can cause perforation of the skin and conversion of a closed fracture into an open one. When a splint is applied to an extremity, it should extend from the joint above the fracture site to the joint below it.

Casts, which are made of plaster or synthetic material such as fiberglass, are commonly used to immobilize fractures of the extremities. They often are applied with a joint in partial flexion to prevent rotation of the fracture fragments. Without this flexion, the extremity, which is essentially a cylinder, tends to rotate within the cylindrical structure of the cast. A brace may be used after a cast is removed or instead of a cast, as with a tibial stress fracture.

The application of a cast carries the risk of impaired circulation to the extremity because of blood vessel compression. A cast applied shortly after a fracture may not be large enough to accommodate the swelling that inevitably occurs in the hours that follow. After a cast is applied, the peripheral circulation must be observed carefully until this danger has passed. If the circulation becomes inadequate, the parts that are exposed at the distal end of the cast (*i.e.*, the toes with a leg cast and the fingers with an arm cast) usually become cold and cyanotic or pale. An increase in pain may occur initially, followed by paresthesia (*i.e.*, tingling or abnormal sensation) or anesthesia as the sensory neurons that supply the area are affected. There is a decrease in the amplitude or absence of the pulse in areas where the arteries can be palpated. Capillary refill time, which is assessed by applying pressure to the fingernail and observing the rate of blood return, is prolonged to longer than 3 seconds. This condition demands immediate measures, such as splitting the cast, to restore the circulation and prevent permanent damage to the extremity. A casted extremity always should be elevated above the level of the heart for the first 24 hours to minimize swelling.

With *external fixation devices*, pins or screws are inserted directly into the bone above and below the fracture site. They are secured to a metal frame and adjusted to align the fracture. This method of treatment is used primarily for open fractures, infections such as osteomyelitis and septic joints, unstable closed fractures, and limb lengthening.

Limb-lengthening devices are used for traumatic losses of bone and soft tissue. Limb-lengthening systems, such as the Ilizarov external fixator (Fig. 57-8), are used to lengthen or widen bones, correct angular or rotational defects, or immobilize fractures.[9] The apparatus is applied with a surgical technique called a *corticotomy*, which is a percutaneous

osteotomy that preserves the periosteal and endosteal tissues. A circular external apparatus is attached to bone by tensioned Kirschner wires. The corticotomy site is gradually distracted or pulled apart by approximately 1 mm/day until the desired length is achieved. The continuous distraction activates regeneration of bone, soft tissue, nerves, and blood vessels. New bone forms (*i.e.*, osteogenesis) in the distraction gap. This newly formed bone can fill posttraumatic defects or those formed after resection for osteomyelitis, consolidate nonunions, regenerate bone in limb lengthening, correct deformities, and eliminate the need for bone grafting. The apparatus is left on until the desired length is achieved and consolidation is complete.

Another method for achieving immobility and maintaining reduction is *traction*. Traction is a pulling force applied to an extremity or part of the body while a counterforce, or countertraction, pulls in the opposite direction. Countertraction usually is exerted by the body's weight on the bed. Traction is used to maintain alignment of the fracture fragments and reduce muscle spasm.

Effective traction prevents movement of the fracture site. Fractures caused by trauma are associated with muscle injury and spasm. These muscle contractions cause overriding and displacement of the bone fragments, particularly when the fractures affect long bones. The five goals of traction therapy are to correct and maintain the skeletal alignment of entire bones or joints; to reduce pressure on a joint surface; to correct, lessen, or prevent deformities such as contractures and dislocations; to decrease muscle spasm;

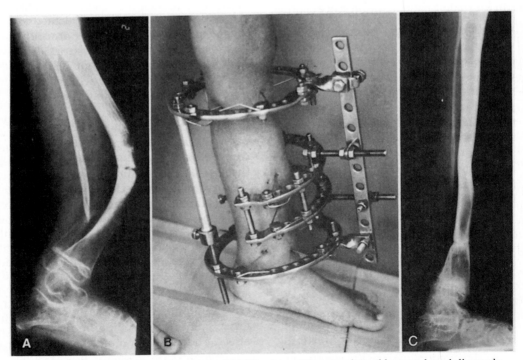

FIGURE 57-8 Ilizarov device used to treat a tibial fracture with anterolateral bow and medullary sclerosis: before (**A**), with Ilizarov device in place (**B**), and 3-year follow-up lateral roentgenograph (**C**). (Paley D., Catagni M., Argnani F. et al. [1992]. Treatment of congenital pseudoarthrosis of the tibia using Ilizarov technique. *Clinical Orthopaedics and Related Research, 280,* 84)

and to immobilize a part to promote healing. Traction may be used as a temporary measure before surgery or as a primary treatment method.

There are three types of traction: manual traction, skin traction, and skeletal traction. *Manual traction* consists of a steady, firm pull that is exerted by the hands. It is a temporary measure used to manipulate a fracture during closed reduction, for support of a neck injury during transport when a cervical spine fracture is suspected, or for reduction of a dislocated joint. *Skin traction* is a pulling force applied to the skin and soft tissue. It is accomplished by strips of adhesive, flannel, or foam secured to the injured part.

Skeletal traction is a pulling force applied directly to the bone. Pins, wires, or tongs are inserted through the skin and subcutaneous tissue into the bone distal to the fracture site. Skeletal traction provides an excellent pull and can be used for long periods with large amounts of weight. It is commonly used for fractures of the femur, the humerus, and the cervical spine (*e.g.*, Crutchfield tongs applied to the skull). Skeletal traction also is used in maintaining alignment of fractures that are casted and in certain types of reconstructive foot surgery. Pin tract infection is a complication of skeletal traction. Larger pins are associated with a greater risk of infection.

Preservation and Restoration of Function. During the period of immobilization required for fracture healing, the preservation and restoration of the function of muscles and joints are an ongoing process in the unaffected and affected extremities. Exercises designed to preserve function, maintain muscle strength, and reduce joint stiffness should be started early. Active range of motion, in which the person moves the extremity, is done on unaffected extremities, and isometric, or muscle-tensing, exercises are done on the affected extremities. In some instances, an electrical muscle stimulator is applied directly to the skin to stimulate isometric muscle contraction as a means of preventing disuse atrophy. After the fracture has healed, a program of physical therapy may be necessary. However, the most important factor in restoring function is the person's own active exercises.

Muscles tend to atrophy during immobilization because of lack of use. Joints stiffen as muscles and tendons contract and shorten. The degree of muscle atrophy and joint stiffness depends on several factors. In adults, the degree of atrophy and muscle stiffness is directly related to the length of immobilization, with longer periods of immobility resulting in greater stiffness. Children have a natural tendency to move on their own, and this movement maintains muscle and joint function. They usually have less atrophy and recover sooner after the source of immobilization has been removed. Associated soft tissue injury, infection, and pre-existing joint disease increase the risk of stiffness. Although limbs are immobilized in a functional position, casts are removed as soon as fracture healing has taken place so that joint stiffness does not occur.

Impaired Healing

Union of a fracture has occurred when the fracture is solid enough to withstand normal stresses and it is clinically and radiologically safe to remove the external fixation. In chil-

dren, fractures usually heal within 4 to 6 weeks; in adolescents, they heal within 6 to 8 weeks; and in adults, they heal within 10 to 18 weeks. The increased rate of healing among children compared with adults may be related to the increased cellularity and vascularity of the child's periosteum.[10] A number of factors can contribute to impaired bone healing, including the nature and extent of the injury, the health of the person with the fracture and his or her responses to injury, the adequacy of initial treatment, and pharmacologic factors. Chart 57-1 summarizes factors that influence fracture healing.

Malunion is healing with deformity, angulation, or rotation that is visible on x-ray films. Early, aggressive treatment, especially of the hand, can prevent malunion and result in earlier alignment and return of function. It is caused by inadequate reduction or alignment of the fracture.

Delayed union is the failure of a fracture to unite within the normal period (*e.g.*, 20 weeks for a fracture of the tibia or femur in an adult). Intra-articular fractures (those through a joint) may heal more slowly and may eventually produce arthritis. *Nonunion* is failure to produce union and cessation of the processes of bone repair. It is seen most often in the tibia, especially with open fractures or crushing injuries. It is characterized by mobility of the fracture site and pain on weight bearing. Muscle atrophy and loss of range of motion may occur. Nonunion usually is established 6 to 12 months after the time of the fracture. The complications of fracture healing are summarized in Table 57-1.

Treatment methods for impaired bone healing encompass surgical interventions, including bone grafts, bracing, external fixation, or electrical stimulation of the bone ends. The treatment for delayed union consists of determining and correcting the cause of the delay. Electrical stimulation is thought to stimulate the osteoblasts to lay down a network of bone. Three types of commercial bone growth stimulators are available: a noninvasive model, which is placed outside the cast; a semi-noninvasive model, in which pins are inserted around the fracture site; and a totally implantable type, in which a cathode coil is wound around the bone at the fracture site and operated by a battery pack implanted under the skin. The Ilizarov method of circular external fixation is used to treat nonunions, especially those that are infected.

COMPLICATIONS OF FRACTURES AND OTHER MUSCULOSKELETAL INJURIES

The complications of fractures and other orthopedic injuries are associated with loss of skeletal continuity, injury from bone fragments, pressure from swelling and hemorrhage (*e.g.*, fracture blisters, compartment syndrome), involvement of nerve fibers (*e.g.*, reflex sympathetic dystrophy and causalgia), or development of fat emboli.

Fracture Blisters

Fracture blisters are skin bullae and blisters representing areas of epidermal necrosis with separation of epidermis from the underlying dermis by edema fluid. They are seen with more severe, twisting types of injuries (*e.g.*, motor

TABLE 57-1 ✦ Complications of Fracture Healing

Complication	Manifestations	Contributing Factors
Delayed union	Failure of fracture to heal within predicted time as determined by x-ray	Large displaced fracture Inadequate immobilization Large hematoma Infection at fracture site Excessive loss of bone Inadequate circulation
Malunion	Deformity at fracture site Deformity or angulation on x-ray	Inadequate reduction Malalignment of fracture at time of immobilization
Nonunion	Failure of bone to heal before the process of bone repair stops Evidence on x-ray Motion at fracture site Pain on weight bearing	Inadequate reduction Mobility at fracture site Severe trauma Bone fragment separation Soft tissue between bone fragments Infection Extensive loss of bone Inadequate circulation Malignancy Bone necrosis Noncompliance with restrictions

vehicle accidents and falls from heights), but can also occur after excessive joint manipulation, dependent positioning, and heat application, or from peripheral vascular disease. They can be solitary, multiple, or massive depending on the extent of injury. Most fracture blisters occur in the ankle, elbow, foot, knee, or areas where there is little soft tissue between the bone and the skin. The development of fracture blisters reportedly is reduced by early surgical intervention in persons requiring operative repair.[11] This probably reflects the early operative release of the fracture hematoma, reapproximation of the disrupted soft tissues, ligation of bleeding vessels, and fixation of bleeding fracture surfaces. Prevention of fracture blisters is important because they pose an additional risk of infection.

Compartment Syndrome

Compartment syndrome is the result of increased pressure in a limited anatomic space that compromises circulation and threatens the viability and function of the nerves and muscles (see Chapter 22). It can be acute or chronic. Acute compartment syndrome can occur after a fracture or crushing injury when excessive swelling around the site of injury results in increased pressure (≥30 mm Hg) in a closed compartment. This increase in pressure occurs because fascia, which covers and separates muscles, is inelastic and unable to stretch and compensate for the extreme swelling. The most common sites are the four compartments of the lower leg (*i.e.*, deep posterior, superficial posterior, lateral, and anterior compartments) and the dorsal and volar compartments of the forearm.

The condition is characterized by pain that is out of proportion to original injury or physical findings.[12,13] Nerve compression may cause changes in sensation (*e.g.*, paresthesias such as burning or tingling or loss of sensation), dimin-ished reflexes, and eventually the loss of motor function. Symptoms usually begin within a few hours, but can be delayed up to 64 hours.[13] Compression of blood vessels may cause muscle ischemia and loss of function. Muscles and nerves may be permanently damaged if the pressure is not relieved. In contrast to the diminished or absent pulses that occur when ischemia is caused by a tight bandage or cast, the arterial pulses often are normal in compartment syndrome. Pallor and loss of the pulse, when they occur, are late findings.

Treatment of compartment syndrome is directed at reducing the compression of blood vessels and nerves. Constrictive dressings and casts are loosened. Intracompartmental pressure can be measured by means of a catheter or needle inserted into the compartment. A fasciotomy, or transection of the fascia that is restricting the muscle compartment, may be required when the pressure in the area rises above 30 mm Hg, which is roughly equal to the perfusion pressure in the capillary beds. Delay in diagnosis and treatment of compartment syndrome can lead to irreversible nerve and muscle damage.

Chronic compartment syndrome occurs most often in young adults after activity that involves repetitive strain on lower extremities, such as long-distance running or marching. Although the exact mechanism is unclear, exercise causes an increase in compartment size and intramuscular pressure that result in tissue ischemia and pain.[14] The compartment is stretched and becomes inflamed. The fascia is scarred, less elastic, and unable to compensate for further compartment volume. Pain is experienced during activity. Tissue pressure measurements usually are done. Conservative measures, such as shoe orthotics, stretching exercises, and activity modification are attempted. A fasciotomy is done for persistent symptoms.

Reflex Sympathetic Dystrophy and Causalgia

Reflex sympathetic dystrophy and causalgia represent soft tissue complications of musculoskeletal injuries that cause pain out of proportion to the injury and autonomic nervous system dysfunction manifested by hyperhidrosis (increased sweating) and vasomotor instability (either flushed and warm or cold and pale).[11] The disorder often produces long-term disability and chronic pain syndromes (see Chapter 48).

Pain, which is the prominent symptom of the disorder, is described as severe, aching, or burning. It usually increases in intensity with movement and with noxious and non-noxious stimuli. The pathophysiologic cause of the pain is unclear, but is thought to have a sympathetic nervous system component. Muscle wasting, thin and shiny skin, and abnormalities of the nails and bone can occur. Decreased muscle strength and disuse can lead to contractures and osteoporosis.

Treatment focuses on pain management and prevention of disability. Physical therapy interventions such as hot/cold baths and elevation of the limb are used to maximize range of motion and minimize pain. Medications include anti-inflammatory agents, vasodilators, and antidepressant medications. Sympathetic nerve blocks may be used.

Fat Embolism Syndrome

The fat embolism syndrome (FES) refers to a constellation of clinical manifestations resulting from the presence of fat droplets in the small blood vessels of the lung or other organs after a long-bone fracture or other major trauma. The main clinical features of fat embolism are respiratory failure, cerebral dysfunction, and skin petechiae.[11,15,16]

Clinically, the incidence of fat embolization is related to fractures of bones containing the most marrow (*i.e.*, long bones and the bones of the pelvis). An increase in intramedullary pressure in the femur is the most important pathogenic factor in the development of emboli. The use of conventional cement for fracture fixation of joint arthroplasty also increases the risk of FES.[17] Although fat embolization occurs with fractures or operative fixation of fractures, FES occurs only in a small percentage of cases, supporting the hypothesis that factors other than mechanical obstruction by fat globules may be necessary in the development of FES.

There are two theories about the mechanisms leading to the FES: mechanical and biochemical. The mechanical theory is that fat globules are released from the bone marrow or subcutaneous tissue at the fracture site into the venous system through torn veins and are lodged in the lungs, brain, or other organs.[11] Support for the mechanical theory resides with studies that have correlated the severity of pulmonary failure with the quantity of fat embolization.[18] The biochemical theory postulates that the fat emboli develop intravascularly secondary to an alteration in lipid stability caused by increased release of tissue lipases, catecholamines, glucagon, or other steroid hormones in response to the stress of injury.[11] The circulating free fatty acids affect the pneumocytes, producing abnormalities in gas exchange. The mechanical and biochemical theories are not mutually exclusive. Fat emboli also may be caused by exogenous sources of fat, such as blood transfusions, intravenous fat emulsions, or bone marrow transplantation.

Initial symptoms of FES begin to develop within a few hours to 3 to 4 days after injury and do not appear beyond 1 week after the injury. The first symptoms include a subtle change in behavior and signs of disorientation resulting from emboli in the cerebral circulation combined with respiratory depression. There may be complaints of substernal chest pain and dyspnea accompanied by tachycardia and a low-grade fever. Diaphoresis, pallor, and cyanosis become evident as respiratory function deteriorates. A petechial rash that does not blanch with pressure often occurs 2 to 3 days after the injury. This rash usually is found on the anterior chest, axillae, neck, and shoulders. It also may appear on the soft palate and conjunctiva. The rash is thought to be related to embolization of the skin capillaries or thrombocytopenia.

Three degrees of severity are seen: subclinical, overt clinical, and fulminating. Although the subclinical and overt clinical forms of FES respond well to treatment, the fulminating form often is fatal. There are three possible outcomes when fat emboli enter the pulmonary circulation: (1) small emboli can mold to vessel caliber, pass through the lung, and enter the systemic circulation, where they are trapped in the tissues or eliminated through the kidney; (2) the fat particles can be broken down by alveolar cells and eliminated through sputum; or (3) local lipolysis can occur with the release of free fatty acids.[19] Free fatty acids cause direct injury to the alveolar capillary membrane, which leads to hemorrhagic interstitial pneumonitis with disruption of surfactant production and development of the adult respiratory distress syndrome. The fat globules also become coated with platelets, causing thrombocytopenia. Serotonin released by the sequestered platelets causes bronchospasm and vasodilatation.

An important part of the treatment of fat emboli is early diagnosis. Arterial blood gases should be assayed immediately after recognition of clinical manifestations. Urinary fat bodies are so common after injury that they are of no diagnostic value. Treatment is directed toward correcting hypoxemia and maintaining adequate fluid balance. Mechanical ventilation may be required. Corticosteroid drugs are administered to decrease the inflammatory response of lung tissues, decrease the edema, stabilize the lipid membranes to reduce lipolysis, and combat the bronchospasm. Corticosteroids are also given prophylactically to high-risk persons. The only preventive approach to FES is early stabilization of the fracture.

In summary, many external physical agents can cause trauma to the musculoskeletal system. Particular factors, such as environments, activity, or age, can place a person at greater risk for injury. Some soft tissue injuries such as contusions, hematomas, and lacerations are relatively minor and easily treated. Muscle strains and ligamentous sprains are caused by mechanical overload on the connective tissue. They heal more slowly than the minor soft tissue injuries and require some degree of immobilization. Healing of soft tissue begins within 4 to 5 days of the injury and is primarily the function of fibroblasts, which produce collagen. Joint dislocation is caused by trauma to the supporting structures. Repeated trauma to the joint can cause articular softening (*i.e.*, chondromalacia) or the separation of small pieces of bone or cartilage, called *loose bodies*, in the joint.

Fractures occur when more stress is placed on a bone than the bone can absorb. The nature of the stress determines the type of fracture and the character of the resulting bone fragments. Healing of fractures is a complex process that takes place in five stages: hematoma formation, cellular proliferation, callus formation, ossification, and remodeling. For satisfactory healing to take place, the affected bone has to be reduced and immobilized. This is accomplished by a surgically implanted internal fixation device or devices such as splints, casts, or traction or external fixation apparatus. The complications associated with fractures can occur early when soft tissue, blood vessels, and nerves are damaged, or later when the healing process is interrupted. Local factors related to the healing environment and the person's general physical condition affect the healing process.

Bone Infections

After you have completed this section of the chapter, you should be able to meet the following objectives:

- ✦ Explain the implications of bone infection
- ✦ Describe the pathogenesis of osteomyelitis
- ✦ Differentiate among osteomyelitis due to spread from a contaminated wound, hematogenous osteomyelitis, and osteomyelitis due to vascular insufficiency in terms of etiologies, manifestations, and treatment
- ✦ Cite the characteristics of chronic osteomyelitis

Bone infections are difficult to treat and eradicate. Their effects can be devastating; they can cause pain, disability, and deformity. Chronic bone infections may drain for years because of a sinus tract. This occurs when a passageway develops from an abscess or cavity in the bone to an opening through the skin.

IATROGENIC BONE INFECTIONS

Iatrogenic bone infections are those inadvertently brought about by surgery or other treatment. These infections include complications of pin tract infection in skeletal traction, septic (infected) joints in joint replacement surgery, and wound infection after any surgery. Measures to prevent these infections include (1) preparation of the skin to reduce bacterial growth before surgery or insertion of traction devices or wires; (2) strict operating room protocols, including disinfection of the operative site and a wide surrounding field with draping to prevent egress of the patient's and operating room personnel's flora into the area, presence

Bone Infections

- ➤ Bone infections may be caused by a wide variety of microorganisms introduced during injury, during operative procedures, or from the bloodstream.

- ➤ Once localized in bone, the microorganisms proliferate, produce cell death, and spread within the bone shaft, inciting a chronic inflammatory response with further destruction of bone.

- ➤ Bone infections are difficult to treat and eradicate. Measures to prevent infection include careful cleaning and debridement of skeletal injuries and strict operating room protocols.

of laminar air flow systems, use of hoods for operating room personnel, and limiting the number of personnel in the room; (3) prophylactic use of antibiotics immediately before and for 24 hours after surgery and as a topical wound irrigation; and (4) maintenance of sterile technique after surgery when working with drainage tubes and dressing changes. Because of the danger of infection, orthopedic wounds are kept covered with a sterile dressing until they are closed.

OSTEOMYELITIS

Osteomyelitis represents an acute or chronic pyogenic infection of the bone. The term *osteo* refers to bone, and *myelo* refers to the marrow cavity, both of which are involved in this disease. Osteomyelitis can be caused by direct extension, or contamination of an open fracture or wound (contiguous invasion); seeding through the bloodstream (hematogenous spread); or from skin infections in persons with vascular insufficiency. In most cases, *Staphylococcus aureus* is the infecting organism.[20–22] *S. aureus* has two characteristics that favor its ability to produce osteomyelitis: (1) it is able to produce a collagen-binding adhesion molecule that allows it to adhere to the connective tissue elements of bone; and (2) it has the ability to be internalized and survive in osteoblasts, making the microorganism more resistant to antibiotic therapy.[22] The term *acute osteomyelitis* is used to describe a newly recognized bone infection. *Chronic osteomyelitis* refers to recurrence of a previously treated or untreated infection.

The pathogenesis of osteomyelitis includes the presence of the infecting agent, inflammation and the protective efforts of inflammatory cells, and bone destruction. The infective microorganisms present in osteomyelitis incite an inflammatory process with recruitment of phagocytic cells. In an attempt to contain the invading microorganisms, the phagocytes generate toxic oxygen radicals and release proteolytic enzymes that destroy surrounding tissues.[22] The purulent drainage that ensues spreads into blood vessels in the bone, raising intraosseous pressure, and impairing blood flow. The loss of blood flow leads to ischemic necrosis of bone. The blood supply to the bone may become obstructed by septic thrombi, in which case the ischemic bone becomes necrotic. As the process continues, the necrotic bone separates from the viable surrounding bone to form devascularized fragments, called *sequestra* (Fig. 57-9).

One of the characteristics of chronic osteomyelitis is the presence of necrotic bone and the absence of living osteocytes.

Infections Due to a Contiguous Area of Infection

The most common cause of osteomyelitis is the direct contamination of bone from an open wound. It may be the result of an open fracture, a gunshot wound, or a puncture wound. Inadequate irrigation or debridement, introduction of foreign material into the wound, and extensive tissue injury increase the bone's susceptibility to infection. If the infection is not sufficiently treated, the acute infection may become chronic. Osteomyelitis may also occur as a complication of surgery, such as in the sternum after open heart surgery or in extremities after bone allograft or total joint replacement.

Osteomyelitis after trauma or bone surgery usually is associated with persistent or recurrent fevers, increased pain at the operative or trauma site, and poor incisional healing, which often is accompanied by continued wound drainage and wound separation. Prosthetic joint infections present with joint pain, fever, and cutaneous drainage.

Diagnosis requires both confirming the infection and identifying the offending microorganism. The diagnosis of skeletal infection entails use of various imaging strategies, including conventional radiology, nuclear imaging studies, CT scans, and MRI. Bone biopsy may be used to identify the causative microorganisms.

Treatment includes the use of antibiotics and selective use of surgical interventions. Antibiotics should be administered prophylactically to persons undergoing bone surgery. For persons with osteomyelitis, early antibiotic treatment, before there is extensive destruction of bone, produces the best results. The choice of antibiotics and method of administration depend on the microorganisms causing the infection. In acute osteomyelitis that does not respond to antibiotic therapy, surgical decompression is used to release intramedullary pressure and remove drainage from the periosteal area.[22]

Hematogenous Osteomyelitis

Hematogenous osteomyelitis occurs as the result of localization of a bloodborne infection in the bone. It is seen most commonly in children younger than 10 years of age,[23] but is seen occasionally in the elderly.[22]

In children, it commonly begins in the metaphyseal region of long bones and usually is preceded by staphylococcal or streptococcal infections of the skin, sinuses, teeth, or middle ear. Thrombosis occurring as the result of local

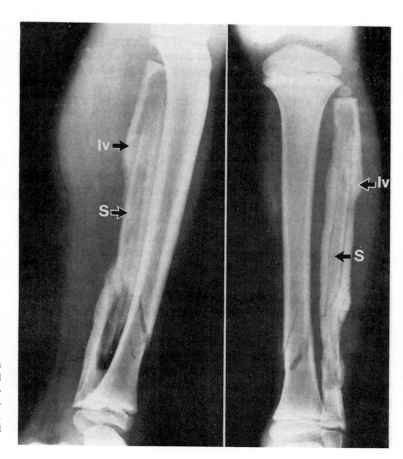

FIGURE 57-9 Hematogenous osteomyelitis of the fibula of 3 months' duration. The entire shaft has been deprived of its blood supply and has become a sequestrum (S) surrounded by new immature bone, involucrum (Iv). Pathologic fractures are present in the lower tibia and fibula. (Wilson F.C. [1980]. The musculoskeletal system. [2nd ed., p. 150]. Philadelphia: J.B. Lippincott)

trauma may predispose to localization of the infection consequent to bacteremia.[23]

In the adult, hematogenous osteomyelitis usually affects the axial skeleton and the irregular bones in the wrist and ankle. It is most common in debilitated patients and in those with a history of chronic skin infections, chronic urinary tract infections, and intravenous drug use and in those who are immunologically suppressed. Intravenous drug users are at risk for infections with *Streptococcus* and *Pseudomonas*.

The signs and symptoms of acute hematogenous osteomyelitis are those of bacteremia accompanied by symptoms referable to the site of the bone lesion. Bacteremia is characterized by chills, fever, and malaise. There often is pain on movement of the affected extremity, loss of movement, and local tenderness followed by redness and swelling. X-ray studies may appear normal initially, but they show evidence of periosteal elevation and increased osteoclastic activity after an abscess has formed. Changes are evident on a bone scan 10 to 14 days before any changes are seen on x-ray films.

Although the incidence of the acute form of osteomyelitis has declined, there is an apparent increase in the subacute form.[24] Subacute osteomyelitis has an insidious onset in which symptoms are typically present for 2 weeks or more before diagnosis. The infection usually begins in the metaphysis of the bone where the nutrient artery channels terminate and the blood flow is sluggish. Because of the bone's rigid structure, there is little room for swelling, and the purulent exudate that forms finds its way to the surface of the bone to form a subperiosteal abscess. There may be extensive ischemic necrosis of bone and formation of sequestra.

The treatment of acute osteomyelitis begins with identification of the causative organism through blood cultures, aspiration cultures, and Gram's stain.[25] Antibiotics are given first intravenously and then orally. The amount of time that the affected limb needs to be rested and pain control measures used are based on the person's symptoms. Debridement and surgical drainage also may be necessary.

Chronic Osteomyelitis

Chronic osteomyelitis has long been recognized as a disease. However, the incidence has decreased in the past century because of improvements in surgical techniques and antibiotic therapy. Chronic osteomyelitis includes all inflammatory processes of bone, excluding those in rheumatic diseases, that are caused by microorganisms. It may be the result of delayed or inadequate treatment of acute hematogenous osteomyelitis or osteomyelitis caused by direct contamination of bone. Acute osteomyelitis is considered to have become chronic when the infection persists beyond 6 to 8 weeks or when the acute process has been adequately treated and is expected to resolve but does not. Chronic osteomyelitis can persist for years; it may appear spontaneously, after a minor trauma, or when resistance is lowered.

The hallmark feature of chronic osteomyelitis is the presence of infected dead bone, a sequestrum, that has sep-

arated from the living bone. A sheath of new bone, called the *involucrum*, forms around the dead bone. Radiologic techniques such as x-ray films, bone scans, and sinograms are used to identify the infected site. Chronic osteomyelitis or infection around a total joint prosthesis can be difficult to diagnose because the classic signs of infection are not apparent and the blood leukocyte count may not be elevated. A subclinical infection may exist for years. Bone scans are used in conjunction with bone biopsy for a definitive diagnosis.[26]

The treatment of chronic bone infections begins with wound cultures to identify the microorganism and its sensitivity to antibiotic therapy. Although intravenous antibiotic therapy remains the primary treatment, antibiotic-laden beads implanted at the site are an effective measure, especially for open fractures. The goal in selecting antimicrobial treatment for osteomyelitis is to use the drug with the highest bactericidal activity and least toxicity and at the lowest cost.[25] High doses are needed for up to 6 weeks.

Initial antibiotic therapy is followed by surgery to remove foreign bodies (*e.g.*, metal plates, screws) or sequestra and by long-term antibiotic therapy. Immobilization of the affected part usually is necessary, with restriction of weight bearing on a lower extremity. External fixation devices are used. With this method, chronic refractory osteomyelitis frequently can be cured because the mass regeneration of new bone within the focus of infection serves as a highly vascularized bone graft.[27]

Osteomyelitis with Vascular Insufficiency

In persons with vascular insufficiency, osteomyelitis may develop from a skin lesion. It is seen most commonly associated with chronic or ischemic foot ulcers in persons with long-standing diabetes or other chronic vascular disorders. It is characterized by local cellulitis with inflammation and necrosis. Treatment depends on the oxygen tension of the involved tissues. Debridement and antibiotic therapy may benefit persons who have good oxygen tension in the infected site. Amputation is indicated when oxygen tension is inadequate.

TUBERCULOSIS OF THE BONE OR JOINT

Tuberculosis can spread from one part of the body, such as the lungs or the lymph nodes, to the bones and joints. When this happens, it is called *extrapulmonary* or *miliary tuberculosis*. It is caused by *Mycobacterium tuberculosis*. The disease is localized and progressively destructive but not as contagious as primary pulmonary tuberculosis. In approximately 50% of cases, it affects the vertebrae, but it also frequently is seen in the hip and knee.[28] Tuberculosis also can affect the joints and soft tissues. The disease is characterized by bone destruction and abscess formation. Local symptoms include pain, immobility, and muscle atrophy; joint swelling, mild fever, and leukocytosis also may occur. Diagnosis is confirmed by a positive culture. The most important part of the treatment is antituberculosis drug therapy. Conservative treatment is usually as effective as surgery, especially for earlier and milder cases.

Because of improved methods to prevent and treat tuberculosis, its incidence had diminished in recent decades. However, tuberculosis has reemerged as a health problem, affecting one third of the global population and 10 million people in the United States.[29] Tuberculosis has increased because of the spread of disease in communal settings (*e.g.*, jails, shelters, nursing homes), the human immunodeficiency virus epidemic, and the influx of immigrants who have come to the United States from countries where the disease is endemic.[30] Unfortunately, the diagnosis of tuberculosis in the bones and joints still may be missed, especially when the musculoskeletal infection is the sole presenting sign. CT scans and MRI can be used as aids for early diagnosis.

> In summary, bone infections occur because of the direct or indirect invasion of the skeletal circulation by microorganisms, most commonly *S. aureus*. Tuberculosis of the bone, which is characterized by bone destruction and abscess formation, is caused by spread of the infection from the lungs or lymph nodes. Osteomyelitis, or infection of the bone and marrow, can be an acute or chronic disease. Acute osteomyelitis is seen most often as a result of the direct contamination of bone by a foreign object. Chronic osteomyelitis is a long-term process that can recur spontaneously at any time throughout a person's life. The incidence of all types of bone infection has been dramatically reduced since the advent of antibiotic therapy. Iatrogenic infections are those inadvertently brought about by surgery or other treatments.

▉ Osteonecrosis

After you have completed this section of the chapter, you should be able to meet the following objectives:

✦ Define *osteonecrosis*
✦ Cite four major causes of osteonecrosis
✦ Characterize the blood supply of bone and relate it to the pathologic features of the condition
✦ Describe the methods used in diagnosis and treatment of the condition

Osteonecrosis, or death of a segment of bone, is a condition caused by the interruption of blood supply to the marrow, medullary bone, or cortex. It is a relatively common disorder and can occur in the medullary cavity of the metaphysis and the subchondral region of the epiphysis, especially in the proximal femur, distal femur, and proximal humerus. It is a common complicating disorder of Legg-Calvé-Perthes disease, sickle cell disease, steroid therapy, and hip surgery.[31,32] The rates of osteonecrosis among persons treated with corticosteroids range from 5% to 25%. More than 10% of 500,000 joint replacements performed annually in the United States are for treatment of osteonecrosis.[31]

Although bone necrosis results from ischemia, the mechanisms producing the ischemia are varied and include mechanical vascular interruption such as occurs with a fracture; thrombosis and embolism (*e.g.*, sickle cell disease, nitrogen bubbles caused by inadequate decompression during deep sea diving); vessel injury (*e.g.*, vasculitis, radiation therapy); and increased intraosseous pressure with vascular compression (*e.g.*, steroid-induced osteonecrosis). In many cases, the cause of the necrosis is uncertain. Other than fracture, the most common causes of bone necrosis are idiopathic (*i.e.*, those of unknown cause) and prior steroid therapy. Chart 57-2 lists disorders associated with osteonecrosis.

Bone has a rich blood supply that varies from site to site. The flow in the medullary portion of bone originates in nutrient vessels from an interconnecting plexus that supplies the marrow, trabecular bone, and endosteal half of the cortex. The outer cortex receives its blood supply from periosteal, muscular, metaphyseal, and epiphyseal vessels that surround the bone. Some bony sites, such as the head of the femur, have only limited collateral circulation so that interruption of the flow, such as with a hip fracture, can cause necrosis of a substantial portion of medullary and cortical bone and irreversible damage.

The pathologic features of bone necrosis are the same, regardless of cause. The site of the lesion is related to the vessels involved. There is necrosis of cancellous bone and marrow. The cortex usually is not involved because of collateral blood flow. In subchondral infarcts (*i.e.*, ischemia below the cartilage), a triangular or wedge-shaped segment of tissue that has the subchondral bone plate as its base and the center of the epiphysis as its apex undergo necrosis. When medullary infarcts occur in fatty marrow, death of bone results in calcium release and necrosis of fat cells with the formation of free fatty acids. Released calcium forms an insoluble "soap" with free fatty acids. Because bone lacks mechanisms for resolving the infarct, the lesions remain for life.

▉ CHART 57-2

Causes of Osteonecrosis

Mechanical disruption of blood vessels
    Fractures
    Legg-Calvé-Perthes disease
    Blount's disease
Thrombosis and embolism
    Sickle cell disease
    Nitrogen bubbles in decompression sickness
Vessel injury
    Vasculitis
    Connective tissue disease
        Systemic lupus erythematosus
        Rheumatoid arthritis
    Radiation therapy
    Gaucher's disease
Increased intraosseous pressure
    Steroid-induced osteonecrosis

One of the most frequent causes of osteonecrosis is that associated with administration of corticosteroids.[31,32] Despite numerous studies, the mechanism of steroid-induced osteonecrosis remains unclear. The condition may develop after the administration of very high, short-term doses; during long-term treatment; or even from intra-articular injection. Although the risk increases with the dose and duration of treatment, it is difficult to predict who will be affected. The interval between corticosteroid administration and onset of symptoms rarely is less than 6 months and may be more than 3 years. There is no satisfactory method for preventing progression of the disease.

The symptoms associated with osteonecrosis are varied and depend on the extent of infarction. Typically, subchondral infarcts cause chronic pain that is initially associated with activity but that gradually becomes more progressive until it is experienced at rest. Subchondral infarcts often collapse and predispose the patient to severe secondary osteoarthritis.

Diagnosis of osteonecrosis is based on history, physical findings, radiographic findings, and the results of special imaging studies, including CT scans and technetium-99m bone scans. MRI is particularly effective in the diagnosis of osteonecrosis. Plain radiographs are used to define and classify the course of the disease, particularly of the hip.

Treatment of osteonecrosis depends on the underlying pathology. In some cases, only short-term immobilization, nonsteroidal anti-inflammatory drugs, exercises, and limitation in weight bearing are used. Osteonecrosis of the hip is particularly difficult to treat. In persons with early disease, limitation of weight bearing through the use of crutches may allow the condition to stabilize. Although several surgical approaches have been used, the most definitive treatment of advanced osteonecrosis of the knee or hip is total joint replacement.

> In summary, osteonecrosis is a common condition that has long been recognized but is not fully understood. Death of bone is caused by disruption of the blood supply from intravascular or extravascular processes. Sites with poor collateral circulation, such as the femoral head, are most seriously affected. Causative factors include corticosteroids. Symptoms include pain that varies in severity, depending on the extent of infarction. Total joint replacement is the most frequently used treatment for advanced osteonecrosis.

References

1. Peters K.D., Kromchamek K., Murphy S.L. (1998). *Deaths: Final data for 1996*. National Vital Statistics Report (Vol. 47). Hyattsville, MD: National Center for Health Statistics.
2. American Academy of Orthopedic Surgeons. (1995). *Play it safe: A guide to safety for young athletes*. Des Plaines, IL: Author.
3. American Academy of Orthopedic Surgeons. (2000). *Don't let a fall be your last trip*. Rosemont, IL: Author.
4. Wright P.H., Brashear H.R. (1980). The local response to trauma. In Wilson F.C. (Ed.), *The musculoskeletal system: Basic processes and disorders* (2nd ed., p. 264). Philadelphia: J.B. Lippincott.
5. Muellner T., Nikolic A., Vecsei V. (1999). Recommendations for the diagnosis of traumatic meniscal injuries in athletes. *Sports Medicine* 27, 337–345.
6. Maitra R.S., Miller M.D., Johnson D.L. (1999). Meniscal reconstruction. Part I: Indications, techniques, and graft considerations. *American Journal of Orthopedics* 28 (4), 213–218.
7. Maitra R.S., Miller M.D., Johnson D.L. (1999). Meniscal reconstruction. Part II: Outcome, potential complications, and future directions. *American Journal of Orthopedics* 28 (5), 280–286.
8. Einhorn T.A. (1998). The cell and molecular biology of fracture healing. *Clinical Orthopaedics and Related Research* 355 (Suppl.), S7–S21.
9. Paley D., Catagni M., Argnani F., Prerot J., Bell D., Armstron P. (1992). Treatment of congenital pseudoarthrosis of the tibia using Ilizarov technique. *Clinical Orthopaedics and Related Research* 280, 81.
10. Hayda R.A., Brighton C.T., Esterhai J.L. (1998). Pathophysiology of delayed healing. *Clinical Orthopaedics and Related Research* 355 (Suppl.), S31–S36.
11. Hoover T.J., Siefert J.A. (2000). Soft tissue complications of orthopedic emergencies. *Emergency Medicine Clinics of North America* 18, 115–139.
12. Ross D. (1996). Chronic compartment syndrome. *Orthopedic Nursing* 15 (3), 23–27.
13. Swain R., Ross D. (1999). Lower extremity compartment syndrome. *Postgraduate Medicine* 105, 159–168.
14. Mohler L.R., Styf J.R., Pedowitz R., Hargens A.R., Gershuni D.H. (1997). Intramuscular deoxygenation during exercise in patients who have chronic anterior compartment syndrome of the leg. *Journal of Bone and Joint Surgery, American* 79 (6), 844–849.
15. Fabian T.C. (1993). Unraveling the fat embolism syndrome. *New England Journal of Medicine* 329, 961–963.
16. Richards R.R. (1997). Fat emboli syndrome. *Canadian Journal of Surgery* 40, 334–339.
17. Pitto R.P., Koessler M., Kuehle J.W. (1999). Comparison of fixation of the femoral component without cement and fixation with the use of a bone vacuum cementing technique for prevention of fat embolization during total hip arthroplasty. *Journal of Bone and Joint Surgery*. American 81, 831–843.
18. Pell A.C.H., Hughes D., Keating J., Christie J., Buscittil A., Sutherland G.R. (1993). Fulminating fat embolism syndrome caused by paradoxical embolism through patent foramen ovale. *New England Journal of Medicine* 329, 926–929.
19. Linquist B.G.P., Schoeman H.S., Dommisee G.F., et al. (1987). Fat embolism and the fat embolism syndrome. *Journal of Bone and Joint Surgery*. British 69, 128–131.
20. Rosenberg A. (1998). Bones, joints, and soft tissue tumors. In Cotran R.S., Kumar V., Collins T. (Eds.), *Robbins pathologic basis of disease* (6th ed., pp. 1231–1233). Philadelphia: W.B. Saunders.
21. Schiller A.L., Teitelbaum S.L. (1999). Bones and joints. In Rubin E., Farber J.L. (Eds.), *Pathology* (pp. 1359–1363). Philadelphia: Lippincott Williams & Wilkins.
22. Lew D.P., Waldvogel F.A. (1997). Osteomyelitis. *New England Journal of Medicine* 336, 999–1007.
23. Narashimhan N., Marks M. (1996). Osteomyelitis and septic arthritis. In Behrman R.F., Kliegman R.M., Arvin A.M. (Eds.), *Nelson textbook of pediatrics* (15th ed., pp. 724–728). Philadelphia: W.B. Saunders.
24. Jones N.S., Anderson D.J., Stiles P.J. (1987). Osteomyelitis in a general hospital. *Journal of Bone and Joint Surgery*. British 69, 779–783.

25. Mader J.T., Landon G.C., Calhoun J. (1993). Antimicrobial treatment of osteomyelitis. *Clinical Orthopaedics* 195, 87–95.

26. Haas D.W., McAndrew M.P. (1996). Bacterial osteomyelitis in adults: Evolving considerations in diagnosis and treatment. *American Journal of Medicine* 101, 550–561.

27. Green S.A. (1991). Osteomyelitis: The Ilizarov perspective. *Orthopedic Clinics of North America* 22, 515–521.

28. Childs S.G. (1996). Osteoarticular *Mycobacterium tuberculosis*. *Orthopedic Nursing* 15 (3), 28–33.

29. Silber J.S., Whitfield S.B., Anbari K., Vergillio J., Fitzgerald R.H., Jr. (2000). Insidious destruction of the hip by *Mycobacterium tuberculosis* and why early diagnosis is critical. *Journal of Arthroplasty* 15, 392–397.

30. Alland D., Kalkut G., Moss A., McAdam R.A., Hahn J.A., Bosworth W., et al. (1994). Transmission of tuberculosis in New York City: An analysis of DNA fingerprinting and epidemiologic methods. *New England Journal of Medicine* 330, 1710–1716.

31. Simkin P.S., Gardner G.C. (1994). Osteonecrosis: Pathogenesis and practicalities. *Hospital Practice* 29 (3), 73–84.

32. Mont M.A., Jones J.C., Einhorn T.A., Hungerford D.S., Reddi A.H. (1998) Osteonecrosis of the of the femoral head. *Clinical Orthopaedics and Related Research* 355 (Suppl.), S314–S335.

Chapter 58

Alterations in Skeletal Function: Congenital Disorders, Metabolic Bone Disease, and Neoplasms

Kathleen E. Gunta

During childhood, skeletal structures grow in length and diameter and sustain a large increase in bone mass. The term *modeling* refers to the formation of the macroscopic skeleton, which ceases at maturity, usually between 18 and 20 years of age. Bone remodeling replaces existing bone and occurs in children and adults. It involves resorption and formation of bone. With aging, bone resorption and formation are no longer perfectly coupled, and there is loss of bone.

Alterations in musculoskeletal structure and function may develop as a result of normal growth and developmental processes or as a result of impairment of skeletal development due to hereditary or congenital influences. Other skeletal disorders can occur later in life as a result of metabolic disorders or neoplastic growth.

Alterations in Skeletal Growth and Development

After you have completed this section of the chapter, you should be able to meet the following objectives:

♦ Describe the function of the epiphysis in skeletal growth
♦ Differentiate between toeing-in and toeing-out
♦ Describe common torsional deformities that occur in infants and small children, proposed mechanisms of development, diagnostic methods, and treatment
♦ Define genu varum and genu valgum
♦ List the problems that occur because of defective tissue synthesis in osteogenesis imperfecta
♦ Characterize the abnormalities associated with developmental dysplasia of the hip and methods of diagnosis
♦ Describe the treatment for a newborn with clubfoot
♦ Define the term *osteochondroses* and describe the pathology and symptomatology of Legg-Calvé-Perthes disease and Osgood-Schlatter disease
♦ Describe the pathology associated with a slipped capital femoral epiphysis and explain why early treatment is important
♦ Differentiate between infantile, idiopathic, and neuromuscular scoliosis
♦ Discuss the diagnosis and treatment of idiopathic scoliosis

BONE GROWTH AND REMODELING

Embryonic Development

The skeletal system develops from the mesoderm, the thin middle layer of embryonic tissue. Development of the vertebrae of the axial skeleton begins at approximately the fourth week in the embryo; during the ninth week, ossification begins with the appearance of ossification centers in the lower thoracic and upper lumbar vertebrae. The paddle-shaped limb buds of the lower extremities make their appearance late in the fourth week. The hand pads are developed by days 33 to 36, and the finger rays are evident on days 41 to 43 of embryonic development.[1]

Bone Growth in Childhood

During the first two decades of life, the skeleton undergoes general overall growth. The long bones of the skeleton, which grow at a relatively rapid rate, are provided with a specialized structure called the *epiphyseal growth plate*. As long bones grow in length, the deeper layers of cartilage cells in the growth plate multiply and enlarge, pushing the articular cartilage farther away from the metaphysis and diaphysis of the bone.[2] As this happens, the mature and enlarged cartilage cells at the metaphyseal end of the plate become metabolically inactive and are replaced by bone cells (Fig. 58-1). This process allows bone growth to proceed without changing the shape of the bone or causing disruption

of the articular cartilage. The cells in the growth plate stop dividing at puberty, at which time the epiphysis and metaphysis fuse.

Several factors can influence the growth of cells in the epiphyseal growth plate. Epiphyseal separation can occur in children as the result of trauma. The separation usually occurs in the zone of the mature enlarged cartilage cells, which is the weakest part of the growth plate. The blood vessels that nourish the epiphysis pass through the growth plate. These vessels are ruptured when the growth plate separates. This can cause cessation of growth and a shortened extremity.

The growth plate also is sensitive to nutritional and metabolic changes. Scurvy (*i.e.,* vitamin C deficiency) impairs the formation of the organic matrix of bone, causing slowing of growth at the epiphyseal plate and cessation of diaphyseal growth. In rickets (*i.e.,* vitamin D deficiency), calcification of the newly developed bone on the metaphyseal side of the growth plate is impaired. Thyroid and growth hormones are required for normal growth. Alterations in these and other hormones can affect growth (see Chapter 40).

Growth in the diameter of bones occurs as new bone is added to the outer surface of existing bone along with an accompanying resorption of bone on the endosteal or inner surface. Such oppositional growth allows for widening of the marrow cavity while preventing the cortex from becoming

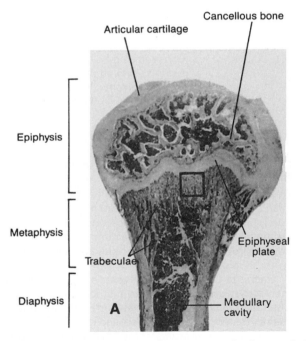
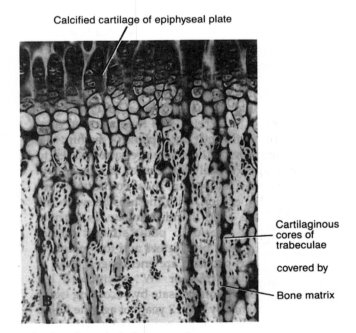

FIGURE 58-1 (**A**) Low-power photomicrograph of one end of a growing long bone (rat). Osteogenesis has spread from the epiphyseal center of ossification so that only the articular cartilage above and the epiphyseal disk below remain cartilaginous. On the diaphyseal side of the epiphyseal plate (disk), metaphyseal trabeculae extend down into the diaphysis. (**B**) Medium-power photomicrograph of the area indicated in **A**, showing trabeculae on the diaphyseal side of the epiphyseal plate (disk). These have cores of calcified cartilage on which bone has been deposited. The cartilaginous cores of the trabeculae were formerly partitions between columns of chondrocytes in the epiphyseal plate (disk). (Cormack D.H. [1987]. *Ham's histology* [9th ed.]. Philadelphia: J.B. Lippincott)

Developmental Skeletal Disorders

➤ Many disorders of early infancy are caused by intrauterine positions and resolve as the child grows.

➤ All infants and toddlers have lax ligaments that predispose to skeletal disorders caused by twisting or torsional forces.

➤ Bone growth in infants and children occurs at the epiphysis. Separation of the epiphyseal growth plate ruptures the blood vessels that nourish the epiphysis, causing cessation of growth and shortened extremity length.

➤ Nutritional and metabolic disorders impair the formation of the organic matrix of bone, causing slowing of growth at the epiphyseal plate.

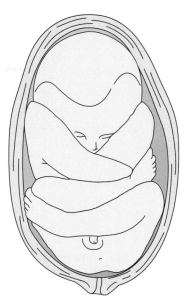

FIGURE 58-2 Position of fetus in utero, with tibial bowing and legs folded. (Dunne K.B., Clarren S.K. [1986]. The origin of prenatal and postnatal deformities. *Pediatric Clinics of North America* 33 [6], 1282)

too thick and heavy. In this way, the shape of the bone is maintained. As a bone grows in diameter, concentric rings are added to the bone surface, much as rings are added to a tree trunk; these rings form the lamellar structure of mature bone. Osteocytes, which develop from osteoblasts, become buried in the rings. Haversian channels form as periosteal vessels running along the long axis become surrounded by bone.

ALTERATIONS DURING NORMAL GROWTH PERIODS

Infants and children undergo changes in muscle tone and joint motion during growth and development. Toeing-in, toeing-out, bowlegs, and knock-knees occur frequently in infancy and childhood.[3] These changes usually cause few problems and are corrected during normal growth processes. The normal folded position of the fetus in utero causes physiologic flexion contractures of the hips and a froglike appearance of the lower extremities (Fig. 58-2). The hips are externally rotated, and the patellae point outward, whereas the feet appear to point forward because of the internal pulling force of the tibiae. During the first year of life, the lower extremities begin to straighten out in preparation for walking. Internal and external rotation become equal, and the hips extend. Flexion contractures of the shoulders, elbows, and knees also are commonly seen in newborns, but they should disappear by 4 to 6 months of age.[4] Musculoskeletal assessment of the newborn is important to identify abnormalities that require early intervention, facilitate treatment, establish baselines for future reference, and educate and counsel parents. There are many clinical deviations that are easily correctable in a newborn. Many others correct spontaneously as the child grows.

Torsional Deformities

All infants and toddlers have lax ligaments that become tighter with age and assumption of the weight-bearing posture. The hypermobility that accompanies joint laxity coupled with the torsional, or twisting, forces exerted on the limbs during growth are responsible for a number of variants seen in young children. Torsional forces caused by intrauterine positions or sleeping and sitting patterns twist the growing bones and can produce the deformities as a child grows and develops.

In infants, the femur normally is rotated to an anteverted position with the femoral head and neck rotated anteriorly with respect to the femoral condyles. Femoral anteversion (*i.e.*, medial rotation) decreases from an average 40 degrees at birth to approximately 15 degrees at maturity. The normal tibia is externally rotated approximately 5 degrees at birth and 15 degrees at maturity. Torsional abnormalities frequently demonstrate a familial tendency.

Toeing-in and Toeing-out.   The foot progression angle describes the angle between the axis of the foot and the line of progression. It is determined by watching the child walking and running. Figure 58-3 illustrates the position of the foot in toeing-in and toeing-out.

Toeing-in (*i.e.*, metatarsus adductus) is the most common congenital foot deformity, affecting boys and girls equally. It can be caused by torsion in the foot, lower leg, or entire leg. Toeing-in due to adduction of the forefoot (*i.e.*, congenital metatarsus adductus) usually is the result of the fetal position maintained in utero. It may occur in one foot or both feet. A supple deformity can be passively manipulated into a straight position and requires no treatment. Treatment consisting of serial long leg casting or a brace that pushes the metatarsals (not the hindfoot) into

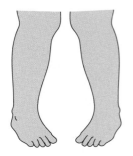
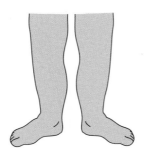

Toeing-in   Toeing-out

FIGURE 58-3 Position of feet in toeing-in and toeing-out.

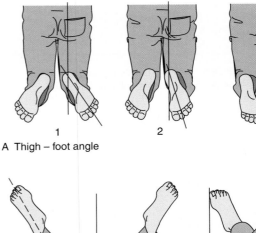

1   **2**   **3**

A Thigh – foot angle

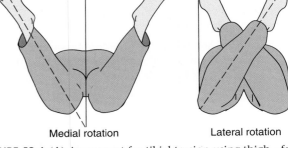

B   Medial rotation   Lateral rotation

FIGURE 58-4 (A) Assessment for tibial torsion using thigh—foot angle. When child is in the prone position with the knee flexed, with normal alignment there is slight external rotation (2); internal tibial torsion produces inward rotation (3), and external tibial torsion; outward rotation (1). **(B)** Hip rotation is measured with child prone and knees flexed at 90° angle. On outward rotation the leg produces internal (medial) hip and femoral rotation; on inward rotation the leg produces external hip and femoral rotation. (Adapted from Staheli L.T. [1986]. Torsional deformity. *Pediatric Clinics of North America* 33 [6], 1378, and Kliegman R.M., Neider M.I., Super D.M. [Eds.]. [1996]. *Practical strategies in pediatric diagnosis and therapy.* Philadelphia: W.B. Saunders.)

abduction usually is required in a fixed deformity (*i.e.,* one in which the forefoot cannot be passively manipulated into a straight position).

Toeing-out is a common problem in children and is caused by external femoral torsion. This occurs when the femur can be externally rotated to approximately 90 degrees but internally rotated only to a neutral position or slightly beyond. Because the femoral torsion persists when a child habitually sleeps in the prone position, an external tibial torsion also may develop. If external tibial torsion is present, the feet point lateral to the midline of the medial plane. External tibial torsion rarely causes toeing-out; it only intensifies the condition. Toeing-out usually corrects itself as the child becomes proficient in walking. Occasionally, a night splint is used. Toeing-in and toeing-out are less noticeable when the child is running or barefoot. Overcorrection of a supple foot deformity can cause flatfoot deformity, but a rigid deformity that is untreated can cause pain and improper fitting of footwear.

Tibial Torsion.   Tibial torsion is determined by measuring the thigh–foot angle, which is done with the ankle and knee positioned at 90 degrees (Fig. 58-4A). In this position, the foot normally rotates outward. *Internal tibial torsion (i.e.,* bowing of the tibia) is a rotation of the tibia that makes the feet appear to turn inward. It is the most common cause of toeing-in in children younger than 2 years of age. It is present at birth and may fail to correct itself if children sleep on their knees with the feet turned in or sit on in-turned feet. It is thought to be caused by genetic factors and intrauterine compression, such as an unstretched uterus during a first pregnancy or intrauterine crowding with twins or multiple fetuses. Tibial torsion improves naturally with growth, but this may take years.[5] The Denis Browne splint, a bar to which shoes are attached, may be used to put the feet into mild external rotation while the child is sleeping.

External tibial torsion, a much less common disorder, is associated with calcaneovalgus foot and is caused by a normal variation of intrauterine positioning or a neuromuscular disorder. It is characterized by an abnormally positive thigh–foot angle of 30 to 50 degrees. The condition corrects itself naturally, and treatment is observational. Significant improvement begins during the first year with the onset of

ambulation and usually is complete by 2 to 3 years of age.[4] The normal adult exhibits 20 degrees of tibial torsion.

Femoral Torsion.   *Femoral torsion* refers to abnormal variations in hip rotation. Hip rotation is measured at the pelvic level with the child in the prone position and the knees flexed at a 90-degree angle. In this position, the hip is in a neutral position. Rotating the lower leg outward produces internal or medial femoral rotation; rotating it inward produces external or lateral rotation (see Fig. 58-4B). During measurement of hip rotation, the legs are allowed to fall to full internal rotation by gravity alone; lateral rotation is measured by allowing the legs to fall inward and cross. Hip rotation in flexion and extension also can be measured with computed tomography (CT). By 1 year of age, there is normally approximately 45 degrees of internal and 45 degrees of external rotation.[4]

Internal femoral torsion, also called *femoral anteversion,* is a normal variant commonly seen during the first 6 years of life, especially in 3- and 4-year-old girls.[3] Characteristically, there is 80 to 90 degrees internal rotation of the hip in the prone position.[4] The condition is thought to be related to increased laxity of the anterior capsule of the hip such that it does not provide the stable pressure needed to correct the anteversion that is present at birth. Children are most comfortable sitting in the "W" position with their hips between their knees (Fig. 58-5). It is believed that this position allows the lower leg to act as a lever, producing torsional changes in the femur. When the child stands, the knees turn in and the feet appear to point straight ahead; when the child walks, knees and toes point in. Children with this problem are encouraged to sit cross-legged or in the so-called *tailor position*. If left untreated, the tibiae compensate by becoming externally rotated so that by 8 to 12 years of age the knees may turn in but the feet no longer do. This can result in patellofemoral malalignment with patellar subluxation or dislocation and pain. A derotational osteotomy may be done in severe cases or if there is functional disability.

External femoral torsion is an uncommon disorder. It usually is associated with slipped capital femoral epiphysis (discussed later). It is characterized by excessive external rotation of the hip. Idiopathic external femoral torsion usually is a bilateral disorder. When the disorder is unilateral, slipped capital femoral epiphysis should be excluded. External femoral torsion usually is benign and treatment is observational.

Genu Varum and Genu Valgum

Genu varum or *bowlegs* is an outward bowing of the knees greater than 1 inch when the medial malleoli of the ankles are touching (Fig. 58-6). Most infants and toddlers have some bowing of their legs up to age 2 years. If there is a large separation between the knees (>15 degrees) after 2 years of age, the child may require bracing. The child also should be evaluated for diseases such as rickets or tibia vara (*i.e.*, Blount's disease).

Genu valgum or *knock-knees* is a deformity in which there is decreased space between the knees (see Fig. 58-6). The medial malleoli in the ankles cannot be brought in contact with each other when the knees are touching. It is seen most fre-

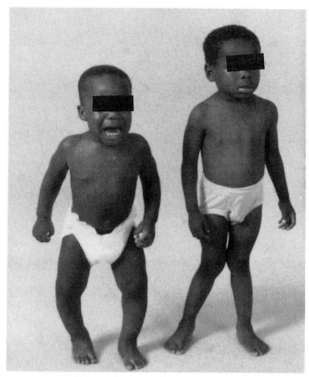

FIGURE 58-6 Normal genu varum (bowlegs) in a toddler *(left)* and genu valgum (knock-knees) in a toddler *(right),* which is often seen in children between 2 and 6 years of age. (From Weinstein S.L., Buckwalter J.A. [1994]. *Turek's orthopaedics* [5th ed.] Philadelphia: J.B. Lippincott.)

quently in children between the ages of 3 and 5 years and should resolve by 5 to 8 years of age.[4] The condition usually is the result of lax medial collateral ligaments of the knee and may be exacerbated by sitting in the "M" position. Genu valgum can be ignored up to age 7 years, unless it is more than 15 degrees, unilateral, or associated with short stature. It usually resolves spontaneously and rarely requires treatment. If genu varum or genu valgum persists and is uncorrected, osteoarthritis may develop in adulthood as a result of abnormal intra-articular stress. Genu varum can cause gait awkwardness and increased risk of sprains and fractures. Uncorrected genu valgum may cause subluxation and recurrent dislocation of the patella, with a predisposition to chondromalacia and joint pain and fatigue.

Idiopathic tibia vara, or *Blount's disease*, is a developmental deformity of the medial half of proximal tibial epiphysis that results in a progressive varus angulation below the knee (Fig. 58-7). It is the most common cause of pathologic genu varum and seen most often in black children, females, obese children, and early walkers.[6] Onset can occur early in infancy, or later, during adolescence. Adolescent Blount's disease occurs in the second decade of life, is seen in persons who are above the 95th percentile in height and weight, and is usually unilateral.[7] Long leg braces are used for treatment in early-onset disease. If progression occurs, or onset is late, surgery is done to correct the angulation and prevent further progression.

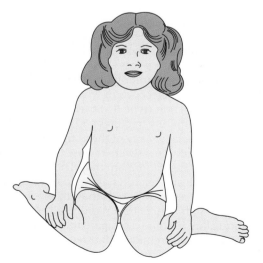

FIGURE 58-5 Typical sitting position of child with femoral anteversion. (Staheli L.T. [1986]. Torsional deformities. *Pediatric Clinics of North America 33* [6], 1382)

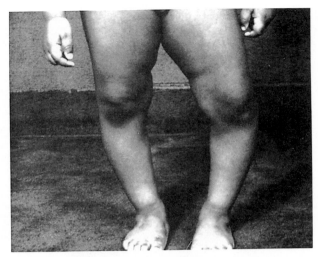

FIGURE 58-7 Rotational deformity of the proximal tibia, especially when unilateral, suggests tibia vera (Blount's disease). (From Weinstein S.L., Buckwalter J.A. [1994]. *Turek's orthopaedics* [5th ed.]. Philadelphia: J.B. Lippincott)

Flatfoot

Flatfoot (*i.e.,* pes planus) is a deformity characterized by the absence of the longitudinal arch of the foot. Infants normally have a wider and fatter foot than adults. The fat pads that normally are accentuated by pliable muscles create an illusion of fullness often mistaken for flatfeet. Until the longitudinal arch develops at 2 to 3 years of age, all children have flatfeet. The true criterion for flatfoot is that the head of the talus points medially and downward, so that the heel is everted and the forefoot must be inverted (toed-in) for the metatarsal heads to be planted equally on the ground. Weight bearing may cause pain in the longitudinal arch and up the leg.

There are two types of flatfeet—flexible and rigid. Most children with flexible (or supple) flatfeet have loose ligaments, allowing the feet to sag when they gain weight. In supple flatfeet, the arch disappears only with weight bearing. No special treatment is needed for flexible flatfeet, and it usually is recommended that children with the disorder wear regular shoes. The rigid flatfoot is fixed with no apparent arch in any position. It is seen in conjunction with congenitally tight heel cords, neuromuscular diseases such as cerebral palsy, or juvenile rheumatoid arthritis.

In the adult, treatment of flatfeet is conservative and aimed at relieving fatigue, pain, and tenderness. Supportive, well-fitting shoes with arch supports may be helpful and prevent ligaments from becoming overstretched. Women may complain of pain in the forefoot when wearing poorly fitting high heels. Surgery may be done in cases of severe and persistent symptoms.

HEREDITARY AND CONGENITAL DEFORMITIES

Congenital deformities are abnormalities that are present at birth. They range in severity from mild limb deformities, which are relatively common, to major limb malforma-

tions, which are relatively rare. There may be a simple webbing of the fingers or toes (syndactyly), the presence of an extra digit (*i.e.,* polydactyly), or the absence of a bone such as the phalanx, rib, or clavicle. Joint contractures and dislocations produce more severe deformity, as does the absence of entire bones, joints, or limbs. An epidemic of limb deformities occurred from 1957 to 1962 as a result of maternal ingestion of thalidomide. This drug was withdrawn from the market in 1961.

Congenital deformities are caused by many factors, some unknown. These factors include genetic influences, external agents that injure the fetus (*e.g.,* radiation, alcohol, drugs, viruses), and intrauterine environmental factors. Many of the organic bone matrix components have been identified only recently, and their interactions found to be more complex than originally thought. Diseases associated with abnormalities in bone matrix include those with deficient collagen synthesis and decreased bone mass. As discussed in Chapter 7, the fourth through the seventh week of gestation is the most vulnerable period for the development of limb deformities.

Osteogenesis Imperfecta

Osteogenesis imperfecta is a hereditary disease characterized by defective synthesis of type I collagen.[8] It is one of the most common hereditary bone diseases, with an occurrence rate of approximately 1 case in 10,000 births.[9] Although it usually is transmitted as an autosomal dominant trait, a distinct form of the disorder with multiple lethal defects is thought to be inherited as an autosomal recessive trait.[10] In some cases the defect is caused by a spontaneous mutation.

The clinical manifestations of osteogenesis imperfecta include a spectrum of disorders marked by extreme skeletal fragility. Four major subtypes have been identified[10] (Table 58-1). The disorder is characterized by thin and poorly developed bones that are prone to multiple fractures. These children have short limbs and a soft, thin cranium with bifrontal prominences that give a triangular appearance to the face. Other problems associated with defective connective tissue synthesis include short stature, thin skin, blue or gray sclera, abnormal tooth development, hypotonic muscles, loose-jointedness, scoliosis, and a tendency toward hernia formation. Hearing loss due to otosclerosis of the middle and inner ear is common in affected adults.

The most serious defects occur when the disorder is inherited as a recessive trait (type II). Severely affected fetuses have multiple intrauterine fractures and bowing and shortening of the extremities. Many of these infants are stillborn or die during infancy. Less severe disease occurs when the disorder is inherited as a dominant trait. The skeletal system is not so weakened, and fractures often do not appear until the child becomes active and starts to walk, or even later in childhood. These fractures heal rapidly, although with a poor-quality callus. In some cases, parents may be suspected of child abuse when the child is admitted to the health care facility with multiple fractures. There also is an increased incidence of complications such as hernias and congenital heart abnormalities.

There is no known medical treatment for correction of the defective collagen synthesis that is characteristic of

TABLE 58-1 ✦ Types of Osteogenesis Imperfecta

Type	Subtype	Inheritance	Major Features
I	Postnatal fractures, blue sclera	Autosomal dominant	Normal stature, skeletal fragility, hearing impairment, joint laxity, blue sclera
II	Perinatal, lethal	Autosomal recessive	Death in utero, or in days after birth
			Skeletal deformity with excessive fragility, multiple fractures, blue sclera
III	Progressive deformity	Autosomal dominant (75%) Autosomal recessive (25%)	Growth retardation, multiple fractures, progressive kyphoscoliosis, hearing impairment, blue sclera at birth
IV	Postnatal fractures, normal sclera	Autosomal dominant	Moderate skeletal fragility, short stature

(Developed from Cotran R.S., Kumar V., Collins T. [1999]. *Robbins pathologic basis of disease* [6th ed., p. 1222]. Philadelphia: W.B. Saunders)

osteogenesis imperfecta. Instead, treatment modalities focus on preventing and treating fractures. Precise alignment is necessary to prevent deformities. Nonunion is common, especially with repeated fractures at a progressively deforming site. Surgical intervention often is needed to correct deformities (*e.g.,* internal fixation of long bones may be done with an intramedullary rod that "grows" with the child), stabilize fractures, remove hardware devices after a nonunion, and, occasionally, amputate the site of a failed bone graft.

Developmental Dysplasia of the Hip

Developmental dysplasia of the hip, formerly known as *congenital dislocation of the hip,* is an abnormality in hip development that leads to a wide spectrum of hip problems in infants and children, including hips that are unstable, malformed, subluxated, or dislocated.[10–12] In less severe cases, the hip joint may be unstable, with excessive laxity of the joint capsule, or subluxated, so that the joint surfaces are separated and there is a partial dislocation (Fig. 58-8). With dislocated hips, the head of the femur is located outside of the acetabulum.

The results of newborn screening programs have shown that 1 of 100 infants have some evidence of hip instability; however, dislocation of the hip is seen in 1.5 of every 1000 live births.[12] The left hip is involved three times more frequently than the right hip because of the left occipital intrauterine positioning of most infants.[11] In white infants, developmental dysplasia of the hips occurs most frequently in first-born children and is six times more common in female than in male infants.[11] The cause of developmental dysplasia of the hip is multifactorial, with physiologic, mechanical, and postural factors playing a role. A positive family history and generalized laxity of the ligaments are related. The increased frequency in girls is thought to result from their susceptibility to maternal estrogens and other hormones associated with pelvic relaxation. Dislocation also may result from environmental factors such as fetal

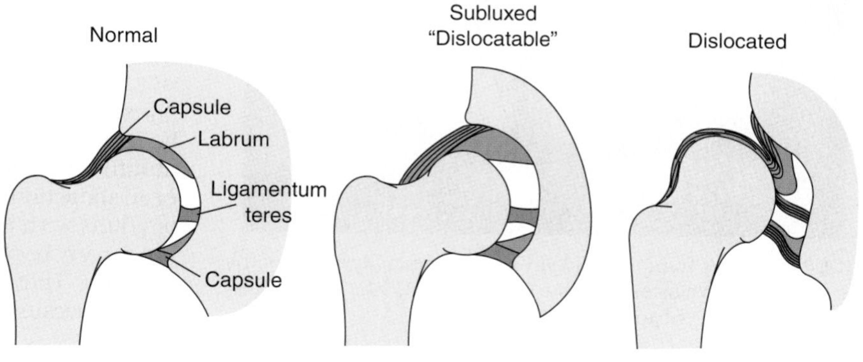

FIGURE 58-8 Normal and abnormal relationships of hip joint structure. (Adapted from Dunn P.M. [1969]. Congenital dislocation of the hip. *Proceedings of the Royal Society of Medicine* 62, 1035–1037)

position, a tight uterus that prevents fetal movement, and breech delivery.

Early diagnosis of a developmental dysplasia of the hip is important because treatment is easiest and most effective if begun during the first 6 months of life. Repeated dislocation causes damage to the femoral head and the acetabulum. Clinical examinations to detect dislocation of the hip should be done at birth and every several months during the first year of life. Several examination techniques are used to screen for a dislocatable hip. In infants, signs of dislocation include asymmetry of the hip or gluteal folds, shortening of the thigh so that one knee (on the affected side) is higher than the other, and limited abduction of the affected hip (Fig. 58-9). The asymmetry of gluteal folds is not definitive but indicates the need for further evaluation. The Galeazzi test is a measurement of the length of the femurs that is done by comparing the height at the knees while they are flexed at 90 degrees. A specific examination method involves an attempt manually to dislocate and reduce the abnormal hip while the infant is in the supine position with both knees flexed (*i.e.*, Barlow's maneuver). With gentle downward pressure being applied to the knees, the knee and thigh are manually abducted as an upward and medial pressure is applied to the proximal thigh (Fig. 58-10). In infants with the disorder, the initial downward pressure on the knee produces a dislocation of the hip, a positive Barlow's sign. This is followed by a palpable or audible click (*i.e.*, Ortolani's sign) as the hip is reduced and moves back into the acetabulum. In an older child, instability of the hip may produce a delay in standing or walking and eventually cause a characteristic waddling gait. When the thumbs are placed over the anterior iliac crest and the hands are placed over the lateral pelvis in examination, the levels of the thumbs are not even; the child is unable to elevate the opposite side of the pelvis (positive Trendelenburg's test). Diagnosis is confirmed by radiography. Ultrasound is used to diagnose newborns and infants from birth to 4 months of age.[11]

The treatment of a developmental dysplasia should be individualized and depends on whether the hip is subluxated or dislocated. Mild instability often resolves without

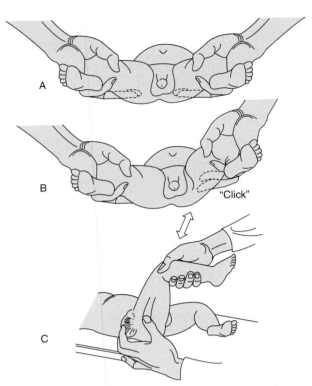

FIGURE 58-10 Examination for developmental dysplasia of the hip. (**A**) In the newborn, both hips can be equally flexed, abducted, and externally rotated without producing a "click." (**B**) A diagnosis of congenital dislocation of the hip may be confirmed by Ortolani's "click" test. The involved hip cannot be abducted as far as the opposite one, and there is a "click" as the hip reduces. (**C**) Telescoping of the femur to aid in the diagnosis of a congenitally dislocated hip. (Hoppenfeld S. [1976]. *Physical examination of the spine and extremities.* New York: Appleton-Century-Crofts)

treatment. The best results are obtained if the treatment is begun before changes in the hip structure (*e.g.,* 2 to 3 months) prevent it from being reduced by gentle manipulation or abduction devices. The Pavlik harness is used on newborns (up to 6 months) to maintain the femoral head in the acetabulum. The harness allows the child more mobility as the leg is slowly and gently brought into abduction. Infants with dislocated hips caused by anatomic changes and toddlers who may lack development of the acetabular socket require more aggressive treatment, such as open reduction and joint reconstruction. Treatment at any age includes reduction of the dislocation and immobilization of the legs in an abducted position. The most serious complication of any treatment is avascular necrosis of the femoral head as a result of the forced abduction. With children younger than 3 years of age, skin traction is used when reduction cannot be easily obtained. This treatment is followed by several months of immobilization in a hip spica cast, plaster splints, or an abduction splint such as an Ilfeld splint. Older children or adults with an unreduced dislocatable hip may require hip surgery because of damage to the articulating surface of the joint. These persons have considerable problems after surgery because of soft tissue contractures.

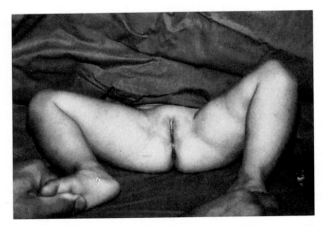

FIGURE 58-9 An 18-month-old girl has congenital dysplasia of the left hip. (From Weinstein S.L., Buckwalter J.A. [1994]. *Turek's orthopaedics* [5th ed.]. Philadelphia: J.B. Lippincott)

Congenital Clubfoot

Clubfoot, or talipes, is a congenital deformity of the foot that can affect one or both feet. Like congenital dislocation of the hip, its occurrence follows a multifactorial inheritance pattern. The condition has an incidence of 1 case per 1000 live births and occurs twice as often in males as in females.[13] Clubfoot is associated with chromosomal abnormalities and may be associated with other congenital syndromes that are transmitted by mendelian inheritance patterns (see Chapter 6). However, it is most commonly idiopathic and found in normal infants in whom no genetic or chromosomal abnormality or other extrinsic cause can be found.

In forefoot adduction, which accounts for approximately 95% of idiopathic cases, the foot is plantar flexed and inverted. This is the so-called *equinovarus type* in which the foot resembles a horse's hoof (Fig. 58-11). The other 5% of cases are of the calcaneovalgus type, or reverse clubfoot, in which the foot is dorsiflexed and everted. The reverse clubfoot can occur as an isolated condition or in association with multiple congenital defects. At birth, the feet of many infants assume one of these two positions, but they can be passively overcorrected or brought back into the opposite position. If the foot cannot be overcorrected, some type of correction may be necessary. Although the exact cause of clubfoot is unknown, three theories are generally accepted: an anomalous development occurs during the first trimester of pregnancy, the leg fails to rotate inward and move from the equinovarus position at approximately the third month, or the soft tissues in the foot do not mature and lengthen. Maternal smoking is associated with occurrence of clubfoot, and the risk increases enormously when combined with a family history.[14]

Clubfoot varies in severity from a mild deformity to one in which the foot is completely inverted. Treatment is begun as soon as the diagnosis is made. When treatment is initiated during the first few weeks of life, a nonoperative procedure is effective within a short period. Serial manipulations and casting are used to gently correct each component in the forefoot varus, the hindfoot varus, and the equinus. The treatment is continued until the foot is in a normal position with full correction evident clinically and on radiographic studies. Surgery may be required for severe deformities or when nonoperative treatment methods are unsuccessful. Approximately 30% to 50% of idiopathic deformities are corrected with casts; the others require surgery.[15] An external distractor such as the Ilizarov external fixator may be used to correct the deformity of a relapsed or neglected clubfoot.

JUVENILE OSTEOCHONDROSES

The term *juvenile osteochondroses* is used to describe a group of children's diseases in which one or more growth ossification centers undergoes a period of degeneration, necrosis, or inactivity that is followed by regeneration and usually deformity. The osteochondroses are separated into two groups according to their causes. The first group consists of the true osteonecrotic osteochondroses, so called because the diseases are caused by localized osteonecrosis of an apophyseal or epiphyseal center (*e.g.,* Legg-Calvé-Perthes disease, Freiberg's infraction, Panner's disease, Kienböck's disease). The second group of juvenile osteochondroses are caused by abnormalities in ossification of cartilaginous tissue resulting from a genetically determined normal variation or from trauma (*e.g.,* Osgood-Schlatter disease, Blount's disease, Sever disease, Scheuermann's disease). The discussion in this section focuses on Legg-Calvé-Perthes disease from the first group and Osgood-Schlatter disease from the second group.

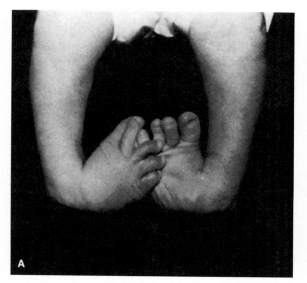
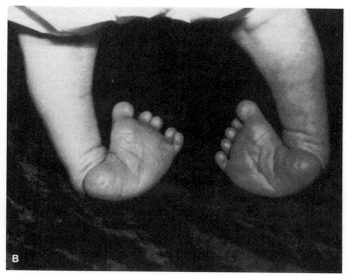

FIGURE 58-11 Severe clubfoot deformity. (**A**) The heel is in severe varus, and the forefoot is adducted and inverted. (**B**) The cavus deformity results from the slightly pronated position of the forefoot in relation to the hindfoot. (From Weinstein S.L., Buckwalter J.A. [1994]. *Turek's orthopaedics* [5th ed.]. Philadelphia: J.B. Lippincott.)

Legg-Calvé-Perthes Disease

Legg-Calvé-Perthes disease, or coxa plana, is an osteonecrotic disease of the proximal femoral (capital) epiphysis, which is the growth center for the head of the femur. It occurs in 1 of 1200 children, affecting primarily those between ages 2 and 13 years, with a peak incidence between 4 and 9 years.[16] It occurs primarily in boys and is much more common in whites than African Americans. Although no definite genetic pattern has been established, it occasionally affects more than one family member.

The cause of Legg-Calvé-Perthes disease is unknown. The disorder usually is insidious in onset and occurs in otherwise healthy children. It may, however, be associated with acute trauma. Affected children usually have a shorter stature. Undernutrition has been suggested as a causative factor. When girls are affected, they usually have a poorer prognosis than boys because they are skeletally more mature and have a shorter period for growth and remodeling than boys of the same age. Although both legs can be affected, in 85% of cases, only one leg is involved.[5]

The primary pathologic feature of Legg-Calvé-Perthes disease is an avascular necrosis of the bone and marrow involving the epiphyseal growth center in the femoral head. The disorder may be confined to part of the epiphysis, or it may involve the entire epiphysis. In severe cases, there is a disturbance in the growth pattern that leads to a broad, short femoral neck. The necrosis is followed by slow absorption of the dead bone over 2 to 3 years. Although the necrotic trabeculae eventually are replaced by healthy new bone, the epiphysis rarely regains its normal shape. The process occurs in four predictable stages.[16] The *first stage,* which lasts for 1 to 3 weeks, is the synovitis stage, which is characterized by synovial inflammation and increased joint fluid. The *second stage* is the aseptic or avascular stage, during which the ossification center becomes necrotic. This stage may last from several months to a year. Damage to the femoral head is determined by the degree of necrosis that occurs during this stage. The *third stage* is the regenerative or revascularization stage, during which resorption of the necrotic bone takes place. This stage usually lasts 1 to 3 years, during which the necrotic bone is gradually replaced by new immature bone cells and the contour of the bone is remodeled. The *fourth stage,* which is the healed or residual stage, involves the formation and replacement of immature bone cells by normal bone cells.

Legg-Calvé-Perthes disease has an insidious onset with a prolonged course. The main symptoms are pain in the groin, thigh, or knee and difficulty in walking. The child may have a painless limp with limited abduction and internal rotation and a flexion contracture of the affected hip. The age of onset is important because young children have a greater capability for remodeling of the femoral head and acetabulum, and thus less flattening of the femoral head occurs. Early diagnosis is important and is based on correlating physical symptoms with radiographic findings that are related to the stage of the disease.

The goal of treatment is to reduce deformity and preserve the integrity of the femoral head. Conservative and surgical interventions are used in the treatment of Legg-Calvé-Perthes disease. Children younger than 4 years of age with little or no involvement of the femoral head may require only periodic observation. In all other children, some intervention is needed to relieve the force of weight bearing, muscular tension, and subluxation of the femoral head. It is important to maintain the femur in a well-seated position in the concave acetabulum to prevent deformity. This is done by keeping the hip in abduction and mild internal rotation. Treatment involves abduction casts or braces to keep the legs separated in abduction with mild internal rotation. The Atlanta Scottish Rite brace, which does not extend below the knee, is the most widely used orthosis because it provides containment while allowing free knee motion and ambulation without crutches or external support[5,10] (Fig. 58-12). Surgery may be done to contain the femoral head in the acetabulum. This treatment usually is reserved for children older than 6 years of age who at the time of diagnosis have more serious involvement of the femoral head. The best surgical results are obtained when surgery is done early, before the epiphysis becomes necrotic.

Osgood-Schlatter Disease

Osgood-Schlatter disease involves microfractures in the area where the patellar tendon inserts into the tibial tubercle, which is an extension of the proximal tibial epiphysis.[4] This area is particularly vulnerable to injury caused by sudden or continued strain from the patellar tendon during periods of growth, particularly in athletic individuals. It occurs most frequently in boys between the ages of 11 and 15 years and in girls between 8 and 13 years.

The disorder is characterized by pain in the front of the knee that is associated with inflammation and thickening of the patellar tendon. The pain usually is associated with specific activities such as kneeling, running, bicycle rid-

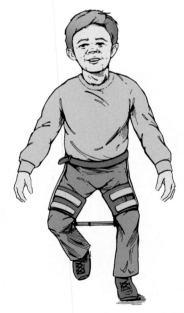

FIGURE 58-12 Scottish Rite brace for Legg-Calvé-Perthes disease produces containment for abduction and allows free knee motion. (Johnson K.B., Oski F.A. [1997]. *Oski's essential pediatrics.* Philadelphia: Lippincott-Raven)

ing, or stair climbing. There is swelling, tenderness, and increased prominence of the tibial tubercle. The symptoms usually are self-limiting. They may recur during growth periods, but usually resolve after closure of the tibial growth plate. In some cases, limitations on activity, tibial bands or braces to immobilize the knee, anti-inflammatory agents, and application of cold are necessary to relieve the pain. The objective of treatment is to release tension on the quadriceps to permit revascularization and reossification of the tibial tubercle. Complete resolution of symptoms through healing (physical close) of the tibia tubercle usually requires 12 to 24 months.[4] Occasionally, minor symptoms or an increased prominence of the tibial tubercle may continue into adulthood. In some cases, a high-riding patella can cause dislocation with chondromalacia of the patella and result in degenerative arthritis.

Slipped Capital Femoral Epiphysis

Normally, the proximal femoral epiphysis unites with the neck of the femur between 16 and 19 years of age. Before this time (10 to 14 years of age in girls and 10 to 16 years in boys), the femoral head may slip from its normal position directly at the head of the femur and become displaced medially and posteriorly.[16] The head is held in the acetabulum by the ligamentum teres, and the neck of the femur is pulled upward and outward. This produces an anterolateral and superior adduction with extension deformity. The condition occurs with an estimated frequency of between 1 in 100,000 to 1 in 800,000.[5] It is the most common disorder of the hip in adolescents.

The cause of slipped capital femoral epiphysis is obscure, but it may be related to the child's susceptibility to stress on the femoral neck as a result of genetics or abnormal structure. Boys are affected twice as often as girls, and in approximately one half of cases, the condition is bilateral. Affected children often are overweight with poorly developed secondary sex characteristics or, in some instances, are extremely tall and thin. In many cases, there is a history of rapid skeletal growth preceding displacement of the epiphysis. The condition also may be affected by nutritional deficiencies or endocrine disorders such a hypothyroidism, hypopituitarism, and hypogonadism. Rapid growth after administration of growth hormone has been associated with displacement of the epiphysis.

Children with the condition often complain of referred knee pain accompanied by difficulty in walking, fatigue, and stiffness. The diagnosis is confirmed by radiographic studies in which the degree of slipping is determined and graded according to severity. Early treatment is imperative to prevent lifelong crippling. Avoidance of weight bearing on the femur and bed rest are essential parts of the treatment. Traction or gentle manipulation under anesthesia is used to reduce the slip. Surgical insertion of pins to keep the femoral neck and head of the femur aligned is a common method of treatment for children with moderate or severe slips. Crutches are used for several months after surgical correction to prevent full weight bearing until the growth plate is sealed by the bony union.

Children with the disorder must be followed closely until the epiphyseal plate closes. Long-term prognosis depends on the amount of displacement that occurs. Complications include avascular necrosis, leg shortening, malunion, and problems with the internal fixation. Degenerative arthritis may develop, requiring joint replacement later in life.

SCOLIOSIS

Scoliosis is a lateral deviation of the spinal column that may or may not include rotation or deformity of the vertebrae. It has been estimated that more than 500,000 adults in the United States have scoliosis.[17] It is most commonly seen during adolescence and is eight times more common among girls than boys. Scoliosis can develop as the result of another disease condition, or it can occur without known cause. Idiopathic scoliosis accounts for 75% to 80% of cases of the disorder. The other 20% to 25% of cases result from more than 50 different causes, including poliomyelitis, congenital hemivertebrae, neurofibromatosis, and cerebral palsy. Although minor curves are relatively common (affecting approximately 2% of the population), it has been estimated that less than 0.1% of U.S. schoolchildren have severe idiopathic scoliosis. Earlier studies that indicated a more widespread problem probably were based on inclusion of children with serious systemic diseases such as poliomyelitis.

Types of Scoliosis

Scoliosis is classified as postural or structural. With postural scoliosis, there is a small curve that corrects with bending. It can be corrected with passive and active exercises. Structural scoliosis does not correct with bending. It is a fixed deformity classified according to the cause: congenital, neuromuscular, and idiopathic.

Congenital Scoliosis. Congenital scoliosis is caused by disturbances in vertebral development during the sixth to eighth week of embryologic development. There are structural anomalies in the vertebrae that can cause a severe curvature. The child may have other anomalies and neurologic complications if the spine is involved. Early diagnosis and treatment of progressive curves are essential for children with congenital scoliosis.

Neuromuscular Scoliosis. Neuromuscular scoliosis develops from neuropathic or myopathic diseases. Neuropathic scoliosis is seen with cerebral palsy, myelodysplasia, and poliomyelitis. There is often a long, "C"-shaped curve from the cervical to the sacral region. In children with cerebral palsy, severe deformity may make treatment difficult. Myopathic neuromuscular scoliosis develops with Duchenne's muscular dystrophy and usually is not severe.

Idiopathic Scoliosis. Idiopathic scoliosis is a structural spinal curvature for which no cause has been established. It seems likely that genetics is involved, and mother-daughter pairings are common. Growth and mechanical factors also seem to play a role.

Idiopathic scoliosis can be divided into three groups on the basis of age at onset: infantile (birth to 3 years), juvenile (4 to 10 years), and adolescent (11 years and older).[18] The infantile form is rare in the United States. It is seen primarily in the United Kingdom and Europe. It affects males more often than females and the curvature usually is convex and to the left rather than to the right, as in other forms of scoliosis. Although most forms of juvenile scoliosis regress spontaneously, some progress and are difficult to treat effectively. Juvenile idiopathic scoliosis is uncommon. However, in many children with the diagnosis of adolescent scoliosis, the onset may have occurred when they were juveniles but was not diagnosed until later. Adolescent scoliosis is the most common type, accounts for approximately 80% of cases, and is seen most commonly in girls. An increase in joint laxity, which causes excessive joint motion and is found commonly in girls, has been associated with development of idiopathic scoliosis. Delayed puberty and menarche are other risk factors for the development of scoliosis.[19]

Although the curve may be present in any area of the spine, the most common curve is a right thoracic curve, which produces a rib prominence on the convex side and hypokyphosis from rotation of the vertebral column around its long axis as the spine begins to curve. A spinal curvature of less than 10 degrees is considered a normal variant, not scoliosis.[17,20] Curves greater than 40 degrees usually are considered severe.

Manifestations

Scoliosis usually is first noticed because of the deformity it causes. A high shoulder, prominent hip, or projecting scapula may be noticed by a parent or in a school screening program. In girls, difficulty in hemming or fitting a dress may call attention to the deformity. Idiopathic scoliosis usually is a painless process, although pain may be present in severe cases, usually in the lumbar region. The pain may be caused by pressure on the ribs or on the crest of the ilium. There may be shortness of breath as a result of diminished chest expansion and gastrointestinal disturbances from crowding of the abdominal organs. Adults with less severe deformity may experience mild backache. If scoliosis is left untreated, the curve may progress to an extent that compromises cardiopulmonary function and creates a risk for neurologic complications.

Diagnosis and Treatment

Early diagnosis of scoliosis can be important in the prevention of severe spinal deformity. The cardinal signs of scoliosis are uneven shoulders or iliac crest, prominent scapula on the convex side of the curve, malalignment of spinous processes, asymmetry of the flanks, asymmetry of the thoracic cage, and rib hump or paraspinal muscle prominence when bending forward (Fig. 58-13). A complete physical examination is necessary for children with scoliosis because the defect may be indicative of other, underlying pathology.

School screening programs were instituted with the assumption that early detection and treatment of spinal curves would halt progression of the defect. The Scoliosis Research Society has recommended annual screening for all children between 10 and 14 years of age. The American Academy of Pediatrics has recommended screening during routine health supervision visits at the ages of 10, 12, 14, and

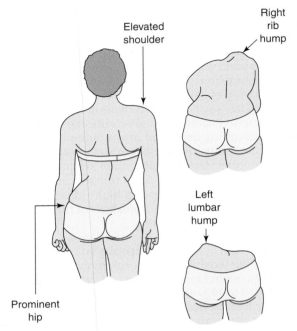

FIGURE 58-13 Scoliosis. Abnormalities to be determined at initial screening examination. (Gore D.R., Passhel R., Sepic S., Dalton A. [1981]. Scoliosis screening: Results of a community project. *Pediatrics* 67 [2]. Copyright 1981 by the American Academy of Pediatrics)

16 years. Scoliosis screening is required by law in 26 states.[21] The U.S. Preventative Task Force examined evidence regarding the effectiveness of routine screening for adolescent idiopathic scoliosis. After reviewing studies regarding the natural history of curve projection, accuracy of screening tests, effectiveness of treatment, potential adverse effects, costs, and burden of suffering, the Task Force issued a statement that "there is insufficient evidence to recommend for or against routine screening of asymptomatic adolescents for idiopathic scoliosis."[17] There is a great need for clinical research to demonstrate the effectiveness or ineffectiveness of routine screening. There are times when screening identifies many children as positive who really do not need treatment.[21]

Diagnosis of scoliosis is made by physical examination and confirmed by radiographs. A scoliometer should be used at the apex of the curvature to quantify a prominence; a scoliometer reading of greater than 10 degrees requires referral to a physician. The curve is measured by determining the amount of lateral deviation present on radiographs and is labeled "right" or "left" for the convex portion of the curve. Other radiographic procedures may be done, including CT, magnetic resonance imaging (MRI), and myelography.

The treatment of scoliosis depends on the severity of the deformity and the likelihood of progression. Larger curves are more likely to progress. Age of presentation also is important. Curves that are detected before menarche are more likely to progress than those detected after menarche. For persons with lesser degrees of curvature (10 to 20 degrees), the trend has been away from aggressive treatment and toward a "wait and see" approach, taking advantage of the more sophisticated diagnostic methods that now are available. Treatment is considered for physiologically immature patients with curves between 20 and 30 degrees. Curves between 30 and 40 degrees usually are considered for bracing, and those greater than 40 to 45 degrees are considered for surgery.

A brace may be used to control the progression of the curvature during growth and can provide some correction. A commonly used brace is the Milwaukee brace, which was developed by Blount and Schmitt in the 1940s (Fig. 58-14). This was the first brace to provide some degree of active correction. It involves a pelvic mold, various pads, and two metal upright supports around the throat. It is cumbersome, and compliance with wearing the brace has been shown to be poor. Studies across the United States found that fewer than 50% of patients consistently wore their braces. In an effort to improve compliance, a number of new bracing techniques were developed. They include underarm or thoracolumbosacral orthoses. These orthoses consist of easily concealed, prefabricated forms that are modified to suit the patient. Although probably less effective than the Milwaukee brace, they are more cosmetically acceptable. Another alternative is the Charleston brace, which provides more dramatic correction but is worn only at night. There is, however, indication that more time spent in a brace (*i.e.,* 23 hours per day for the Milwaukee Brace) halts progression of the curve more effectively.[22]

Surgical intervention with instrumentation and spinal fusion is done in severe cases—when the curvature has progressed to 40 degrees or more at the time of diagnosis or when curves of a lesser degree are compounded with imbalance or rotation of the vertebrae. Unlike bracing, which is intended to halt progression of the curvature, surgical intervention is used to decrease the curve. Instrumentation helps correct the curve and balance, and spinal fusion maintains the spine in the corrected position. Several methods of instrumentation (*i.e.,* rods that attach to the vertebral column) are used. Earlier methods included Harrington rod instrumentation and posterior spinal fusion, Dwyer (or Zielke) instrumentation and anterior spinal fusion, and segmental (Luque) spinal instrumentation and posterior spinal fusion. There are many newer systems using bilateral rods with wire hooks or screws that correct the spinal deformity and stabilize the spine. An anterior approach usually is used as the

first stage of a two-stage procedure. Combined anterior and posterior surgery is used for more severe curvatures. The newer systems provide better sagittal control and more stable fixation, which allow earlier mobility. Despite great advances in spinal surgery, no one method seems to be the best for all cases.

In summary, skeletal disorders can result from congenital or hereditary influences or from factors that occur during normal periods of skeletal growth and development. Newborn infants undergo normal changes in muscle tone and joint motion, causing torsional conditions of the femur or tibia. Many of these conditions are corrected as skeletal growth and development take place. Osteogenesis imperfecta is a rare autosomal hereditary disorder characterized by defective synthesis of connective tissue, including bone matrix. It results in poorly developed bones that fracture easily. Developmental dysplasia of the hip includes a range of structural abnormalities. Dislocated hips are always treated to prevent changes in the anatomic structure. Other childhood skeletal disorders, such as the osteochondroses, slipped capital femoral epiphysis, and scoliosis, are not corrected by the growth process. These disorders are progressive, can cause permanent disability, and require treatment. Disorders such as congenital dislocation of the hip and congenital clubfoot are present at birth. Both of these disorders are best treated during infancy. Regular examinations during the first year of life are recommended as a means of achieving early diagnosis of such disorders.

Metabolic Bone Disease

After you have completed this section of the chapter, you should be able to meet the following objectives:

✦ Name the three factors responsible for maintaining the equilibrium of bone tissue
✦ Cite the functions of osteoclasts and osteoblasts in bone remodeling and relate them to the actions of parathyroid hormone, vitamin D, and estrogen

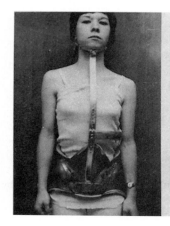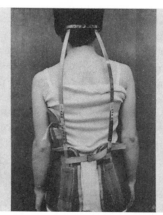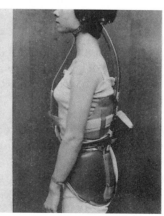

FIGURE 58-14 The Milwaukee brace as seen from front, back, and side. (Farrell J. [1986]. *Illustrated guide to orthopedic nursing* [3rd ed., p. 172]. Philadelphia: J.B. Lippincott)

- ✦ Describe risk factors that contribute to the development of osteoporosis and relate them to the prevention of the disorder
- ✦ Describe the primary features of osteoporotic bone
- ✦ Identify risk factors for the development of osteoporosis
- ✦ Define the female athlete triad
- ✦ Describe the action of estrogen, calcitonin, fluorides, and bisphosphonates in the treatment of osteoporosis
- ✦ Describe the pathogenesis and manifestations of osteomalacia and rickets
- ✦ Characterize the cause and manifestations of Paget's disease

Bone remodeling, or the process of bone resorption and formation, is continuous throughout life. There are two types of bone remodeling, structural and internal remodeling. Structural remodeling involves deposition of new bone on the outer aspect of the shaft at the same time that bone is resorbed from the inner aspect of the shaft. It occurs during growth and results in a bone having adult form and shape. Internal remodeling largely involves the replacement of trabecular bone and is continuous during adulthood.

In the adult, approximately 25% of trabecular bone is replaced each year, compared with 3% of compact bone.[23] In the adult skeleton, bone remodeling proceeds in cycles that involve resorption of old bone by osteoclasts and subsequent formation of new bone by osteoblasts (Fig. 58-15). After the bone formation has ceased, the bone is covered by a distinct type of terminally differentiated osteoblast.

The sequence of bone resorption and bone formation is activated by many stimuli, including the actions of parathyroid hormone and calcitonin. It begins with osteoclastic resorption of existing bone, during which the organic (protein matrix) and the inorganic (mineral) components are removed. The sequence proceeds to the formation of new bone by osteoblasts. In the adult, the length of one sequence (*i.e.,* bone resorption and formation) is approximately 4 months. Ideally, the replaced bone should equal the absorbed bone. If it does not, there is a net loss of bone. In the elderly, for example, bone resorption and formation no longer are perfectly coupled, and bone mass is lost.

The three major influences on the equilibrium of bone tissue are mechanical stress; calcium and phosphate levels in the extracellular fluid; and hormones and local growth factors and cytokines, which influence bone resorption and formation. Mechanical stress stimulates osteoblastic activ-

Metabolic Bone Disorders

- ➤ Metabolic bone disorders have their origin in the bone remodeling process that involves an orderly sequence of osteoclastic bone reabsorption, the formation of new bone by the osteoblasts, and mineralization of the newly formed osteoid tissue.

- ➤ Osteoporosis represents an increased loss of total bone mass due to an imbalance between bone absorption and bone formation, most often related to the aging process and decreased estrogen levels in postmenopausal women.

- ➤ Osteomalacia and rickets represent a softening of bone due to inadequate mineralization of the bone matrix caused by a deficiency of calcium or phosphate.

- ➤ Paget's disease is a disorder involving excessive bone destruction and repair, resulting in structural deformities of long bones, spine, pelvis, and cranium.

ity and formation of the organic matrix. It is important in preventing bone atrophy and in healing fractures. Bone serves as a storage site for extracellular calcium and phosphate ions. Consequently, alterations in the extracellular levels of these ions affect their deposition in bone (see Chapter 31). Vitamin C is required for proper collagen formation. A deficiency of vitamin C can result in a disease called *scurvy*. In the absence of vitamin C, the epiphyseal plates and bony shaft of growing bone are so thin and fragile that they are predisposed to fractures. In the adult, vitamin C deficiency affects bone maintenance rather than growth. Vitamin D is needed for intestinal absorption of calcium and phosphate. Blood levels of calcium and phosphate are regulated by parathyroid hormone and calcitonin. Parathyroid hormone promotes bone resorption, and calcitonin inhibits bone resorption.

Osteoclasts and osteoblasts are derived from progenitor cells in the bone marrow.[23] The osteoclasts originate from

| Quiescent bone surface covered by lining cells | Osteoclasts on the bone surface resorbing old bone | Osteoblasts filling the resorption cavity with osteoid | Osteoid becoming mineralized |

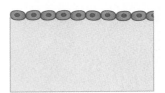 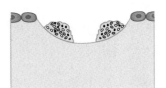 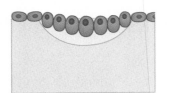 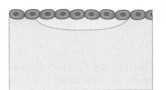

FIGURE 58-15 The process of bone resorption by the osteoclasts and subsequent bone formation by the osteoblasts.

hematopoietic precursors and osteoblasts from stromal (supporting) cells in the bone marrow. However, the development of osteoclasts from hematopoietic precursors cannot take place unless stromal-osteoblastic cells are present. The effects of systemic hormones and local influences on osteoclast development are mediated by stromal-osteoblastic cells. The differentiation and function of osteoclasts and osteoblasts are regulated by chemical messengers, including colony-stimulating factors and other cytokines (see Chapter 18). Interleukin-6, which is produced in response to systemic hormones such as parathyroid hormone and vitamin D, stimulates the early stages of osteoclast development. Interleukin-6 is thought to be involved in the abnormal bone resorption associated with Paget's disease. The inhibitory effects of estrogen on bone resorption are thought to be mediated through the inhibition of interleukin-6. With aging, the ability of the bone marrow to produce osteoblastic precursors is decreased.

OSTEOPENIA

Osteopenia is a condition that is common to all metabolic bone diseases. It is characterized by a reduction in bone mass greater than expected for age, race, or sex, and it occurs because of a decrease in bone formation, inadequate bone mineralization, or excessive bone deossification. *Osteopenia* is not a diagnosis but a term used to describe an apparent lack of bone seen on x-ray studies. The major causes of osteopenia are osteoporosis, osteomalacia, malignancies such as multiple myeloma, and endocrine disorders such as hyperparathyroidism and hyperthyroidism.

OSTEOPOROSIS

Osteoporosis refers to increased porosity of bone due to loss of bone mass. Although osteoporosis can occur as the result of an endocrine disorder or malignancy, it most often is associated with the aging process. After maximal bone mass is attained at 30 years of age, the rate of bone loss for both sexes is approximately 0.5% per year, and it increases to approximately 1% per year or more in menopausal women.[24] An estimated 25 million Americans are affected with osteoporosis, and more than 1.5 million sustain fractures related to osteoporosis each year. After menopause, a woman's lifetime risk of an osteoporosis fracture is 1 in 3.[25] Bone mass positively correlates with the amount of skin pigmentation; whites have the least bone mass, and African Americans have the most. Although osteoporosis is uncommon among African-American women, many cases are seen among postmenopausal women with brown and yellow skin.[26] One of the reasons for the increased risk in postmenopausal women of white or Asian descent may be that their original bone mass is less and that the losses associated with aging therefore affect them sooner. Osteoporosis is rare in children. When it does occur, it is related to such causes as the excess corticosteroid levels associated with Cushing's syndrome, colon disease, prolonged immobility, or osteogenesis imperfecta.

Premature osteoporosis is being seen in female athletes owing to an increased prevalence of eating disorders and amenorrhea.[27] The *female athlete triad* refers to a pattern of disordered eating that leads to amenorrhea and eventually osteoporosis. Poor nutrition, combined with intense training, can lead to an energy deficit that causes a lack of estrogen production by the ovary and secondary amenorrhea.[28] The lack of estrogen combined with the lack of calcium and vitamin D from dietary deficiencies results in a loss of bone density and increased risk of fractures.[28] There is a concern that athletes with low bone mineral density will be at increased risk for fractures during their competitive years. It is unclear if osteoporosis induced by amenorrhea is reversible. It most frequently affects women engaged in endurance sports such as running and swimming, in activities where appearance is important, such as figure skating, diving, and gymnastics, or sports with weight categories such as horse racing, martial arts, and rowing.[29]

The development of osteoporosis involves many factors, including hormone levels, physical fitness, and general nutrition. Postmenopausal women are particularly at risk. Estrogens are thought to act indirectly to suppress bone resorption, an action that is reduced after menopause. Persons with endocrine disorders such as hyperthyroidism, hyperparathyroidism, Cushing's syndrome, or diabetes mellitus also are at high risk for development of osteoporosis. Exercise may prevent osteoporosis by increasing peak bone mineral density during periods of growth.[30] Poor nutrition or an age-related decrease in intestinal absorption of calcium because of deficient activation of vitamin D may contribute to the development of osteoporosis, particularly in the elderly. The prolonged use of medications that increase calcium excretion, such as aluminum-containing antacids, corticosteroids, and anticonvulsants, also is associated with bone loss.[31] Excessive intake of diet soda that is high in phosphate also can deplete calcium stores. Fluoridated drinking water increases bone mineral density at the hip and spine, thus preventing hip fractures.[32] Other risk factors found to be associated with osteoporosis are a diet high in protein, cigarette smoking, alcohol ingestion, and a family history of osteoporosis. Persons with HIV infection or AIDS who are being treated with antiretroviral therapy may develop a lower bone density and signs of osteoporosis and osteopenia.[33]

Pathogenesis

The pathogenesis of osteoporosis is unclear, but most data suggest an imbalance between bone resorption and formation such that bone resorption exceeds bone formation. There appears to be a decrease in the number and activity of osteoblasts or bone-building cells and an increase in activity of osteoclasts or bone-resorbing cells.[34] Decreases in levels of sex hormones, which seem to act as intermediates to prevent bone loss in men and women, are somehow important in the pathogenesis of osteoporosis. During early menopause, there is osteoclast-mediated rapid bone loss. This is caused by increased remodeling activation and increased rate and depth of osteoclastic bone reabsorption. There are structural changes in the cancellous and cortical bone structure. In postmenopausal women, these changes can be reversed by estrogen therapy. Bone loss is slower after early menopause because of a decrease in remodeling by the osteoclasts. There is some evidence that osteoporosis is caused, at least in part, by abnormalities in local factors, such as prostaglandins, interleukins, and growth factors, that influence bone cell function.[26] Further study is needed, particularly because local factors cannot be measured directly but must be identified with in vitro organ culture methods and tissues from laboratory animals.

Osteoporotic changes occur in the diaphysis and metaphysis of bone. The diameter of the bone enlarges with age, causing the outer supporting cortex to become thinner. In severe osteoporosis, the bones begin to resemble the fragile structure of a fine porcelain vase. There is loss of trabeculae from cancellous bone and thinning of the cortex to such an extent that minimal stress causes fractures (Fig. 58-16). The changes that occur with osteoporosis have been explained by two distinct disease processes affecting women early and late in life.[26] Type I is caused by early postmenopausal estrogen deficiency and is manifested by loss of trabecular bone, with a predisposition to fractures of the vertebrae and distal radius. Type II (*i.e.,* senile osteoporosis) is caused by a calcium deficiency and is a slower process in which cortical and trabecular bone are lost. Hip fractures, which are seen later in life, result from the second type. The different pathogenic mechanisms and presentations make it difficult to generalize about osteoporosis.

Manifestations

The first clinical manifestations of osteoporosis are pain accompanied by skeletal fractures—a vertebral compression fracture or fractures of the hip, pelvis, humerus, or any other bone. Fractures usually represent an end stage of the disease. Fracture occurs with a force less than typically is needed, such as in a gymnast performing a common jump. Women who present with fractures are much more likely to sustain another fracture than are women of the same age without osteoporosis. Wedging and collapse of vertebrae causes a loss of height in the vertebral column and kyphosis, a condition commonly referred to as *dowager's hump.* Usually, there is no generalized bone tenderness. When pain occurs, it is related to fractures. Systemic symptoms such as weakness and weight loss suggest that the osteoporosis may be caused by underlying disease. Avascular necrosis of the hip and compression fractures are being seen as complications of antiretroviral therapy in persons with HIV infection or AIDS.

Diagnosis and Treatment

An important advance in diagnostic methods used for the identification of osteoporosis has been the use of bone density assessment. The clinical method of choice for bone density studies is dual-energy x-ray absorptiometry of the spine and hip. Simpler single- or dual-photon beams to assess density of the calcaneus (and the wrists, hips, or spine) also can be used. In the United States, the National Osteoporosis Foundation sets the diagnostic criterion at 2.0 standard deviations below peak value. According to these standards, most women would be candidates for treatment by 60 years of age.[26] Measurement of bone density has become increasingly common for early detection and fracture prevention. Excessive loss of height indicates some probability of low bone mass.[35] Measurement of serial heights in older adults is another simple way to screen for osteoporosis. A further advance in the diagnosis of osteoporosis is the refinement of risk factors, permitting better analysis of risk pertaining

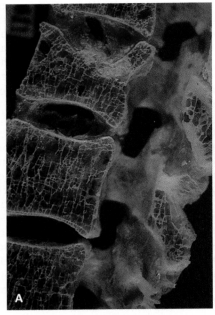
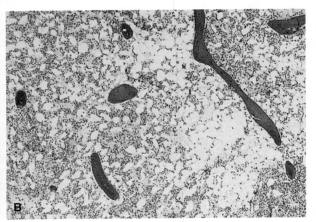

FIGURE 58-16 Osteoporosis. (**A**) A section of the vertebral column, in which the bone marrow has been washed out, demonstrates a loss of bone tissue and a compression fracture of a vertebral body *(top).* (**B**) A photomicrograph of a vertebral body shows very attenuated bony trabeculae. (Rubin E., Farber L.F., [1999]. *Pathophysiology* [3rd ed., p. 1367]. Philadelphia: Lippincott Williams & Wilkins)

to particular persons. Women older than 65 years of age who weigh less than 140 pounds at menopause or who have never used estrogens for more than 6 months should be screened for osteoporosis. The simple mnemonic ABONE (*A* = age, *B* = bulk, and *ONE* = never on estrogen) aids in remembering these criteria.[35]

Prevention and early detection of osteoporosis are essential to the prevention of the associated deformities and fractures. It is important to identify persons in high-risk groups so treatment can begin early. Postmenopausal women of small stature or lean body mass, those with sedentary lifestyles, those with poor calcium intake, and those with diseases that demineralize bone are at greatest risk. Other risk factors include an age of 80 years or greater, maternal history of hip fracture, caffeine intake exceeding two cups of coffee each day, previous hyperthyroidism, current anticonvulsant therapy, and current use of long-acting benzodiazepines. Risk factors for osteoporosis are listed in Chart 58-1.

Regular exercise and adequate calcium intake are important factors in preventing osteoporosis. Weight-bearing exercises such as walking, jogging, rowing, and weight lifting are important in the maintenance of bone mass. Studies have indicated that premenopausal women need more than 1000 mg and postmenopausal women need 1500 mg of calcium daily.[36,37] This means that adults should drink three to four glasses of milk daily or substitute other foods that are high in calcium. Because most older American women do not consume a sufficient quantity of dairy products to meet their calcium needs, calcium supplementation is recommended. Calcium tablets vary in content of elemental calcium. Calcium carbonate contains 40% elemental calcium but requires normal stomach acidity to be absorbed. Calcium citrate is 21% elemental calcium but can be absorbed in the absence of acidity.[35]

There still are conflicting data on recommendations for vitamin D supplementation. Deficient activation of vitamin D may be an important factor in the impaired intestinal absorption of calcium in the elderly. On the basis of this evidence, 1,25-dihydroxyvitamin D_3 is being studied as a treatment for osteoporosis. A daily intake of 400 to 800 IU of vitamin D is recommended because vitamin D optimizes calcium absorption and inhibits parathyroid secretion, which stimulates calcium resorption from bone.[35]

Estrogen therapy in postmenopausal women in the United States is relatively common and is becoming less controversial. It is the single most powerful intervention to reduce the incidence and progression of osteoporosis. If begun soon after menopause, estrogen prevents early-stage bone loss. Studies have indicated that the beneficial effects from administering estrogen to women continue into their eighth decade.[31] Although the incidence of endometrial cancer is increased by administration of estrogen, this risk is reduced by concurrent administration of progestin.[26] Whether estrogen increases the risk of breast cancer remains to be determined. However, most studies suggest little, if any, risk during the first 5 to 10 years of therapy.[26]

Active treatment of osteoporosis uses four types of agents: gonadal hormones (estrogen), calcitonin, fluorides, and bisphosphonates. Calcitonin can be used to decrease osteoclastic activity. It has some effect on bone pain, but until recently it was available only as an injectable drug. A nasal spray formulation now is available. Sodium fluoride's use has been studied, but its role remains questionable because of potential toxicity and inconsistent findings concerning its antifracture effects.[36] There is some indication that community water fluoridation may help prevent osteoporosis.

The bisphosphonates are analogs of endogenous inorganic pyrophosphate that the body cannot break down. In bone, they bind to hydroxyapatite and prevent bone resorption through the inhibition of osteoclast activity. Etidronate (Didronel), the prototypical first-generation agent, inhibits osteoblastic activity and bone formation. Second- and third-generation drugs, such as alendronate (Fosamax) and risedronate (Actonel), which inhibit bone resorption at rates 1000 times their effects on bone formation have largely replaced etidronate.[37] Long-term treatment with either alendronate or estrogen/progesterone has similar effects in reducing postmenopausal bone loss.[38] Further research is needed to determine if the increases in bone density seen with bisphosphonates can be maintained and if the bone deposits are of high quality.

Persons with osteoporosis have many special needs. In treating fractures, it is important to minimize immobility. Surgical intervention is done for stable fracture fixation

---

CHART 58-1

Risk Factors Associated With Osteoporosis

Personal Characteristics
Advanced age
Female
White (fair, thin skin)
Small bone structure
Postmenopausal
Family history

Lifestyle
Sedentary
Calcium deficiency (long-term)
High-protein diet
Excessive alcohol intake
Excessive caffeine intake
Smoking

Drug and Disease Related
Aluminum-containing antacids
Anticonvulsants
Heparin
Corticosteroids or Cushing's disease
Gastrectomy
Diabetes mellitus
Chronic obstructive lung disease
Malignancy
Hyperthyroidism
Hyperparathyroidism
Rheumatoid arthritis

that allows early restoration of mobility and function; for fractures of the lower extremities, this means early weight bearing. Walking and swimming are encouraged. Unsafe conditions that predispose persons to falls and fractures should be corrected or avoided.

OSTEOMALACIA AND RICKETS

In contrast to osteoporosis, which causes a loss of total bone mass and results in brittle bones, osteomalacia and rickets produce a softening of the bones and do not involve the loss of bone matrix. Approximately 60% of bone is mineral content, approximately 30% is organic matrix, and the remainder is living bone cells. The organic matrix and the inorganic mineral salts are needed for normal bone consistency. If the inorganic mineral salts are removed from fresh bone (by dilute nitric acid), the organic matrix that remains still resembles a bone, but it is so flexible that it can be tied in a knot. When a bone is placed over a hot flame, the organic material is destroyed, and the bone becomes brittle.

Osteomalacia

Osteomalacia is a generalized bone condition in which inadequate mineralization of bone results from a calcium or phosphate deficiency, or both. It is sometimes referred to as the adult form of rickets.

There are two main causes of osteomalacia: insufficient calcium absorption from the intestine because of a lack of calcium, or resistance to the action of vitamin D and phosphate deficiency due to increased renal losses or decreased intestinal absorption. Vitamin D is a fat-soluble vitamin that is absorbed intact through the intestine or produced in the skin with exposure to ultraviolet irradiation. Vitamin D that is absorbed from the intestine or synthesized in the skin is inactive. Vitamin D is activated in a two-step process that begins in the liver and is completed in the kidney. Vitamin D deficiency is caused most commonly by reduced vitamin D absorption as a result of biliary tract or intestinal diseases that impair fat and fat-soluble vitamin absorption. Lack of vitamin D in the diet is rare in the United States because many foods are fortified with the vitamin. Anticonvulsant medications, such as phenobarbital and phenytoin, induce hepatic hydroxylases that accelerate breakdown of the active forms of vitamin D.

A form of osteomalacia called *renal rickets* occurs in persons with chronic renal failure. It is caused by the inability of the kidney to activate vitamin D and excrete phosphate and is accompanied by hyperparathyroidism, increased bone turnover, and increased bone resorption. Another form of osteomalacia results from renal tubular defects that cause excessive phosphate losses. This form of osteomalacia is commonly referred to as *vitamin D–resistant rickets* and often is a familial disorder.[5] It is inherited as an X-linked dominant gene passed by mothers to one half of their children and by fathers to their daughters only. This form of osteomalacia affects boys more severely than girls. Long-standing primary hyperparathyroidism causes increased calcium resorption from bone and hypophosphatemia, which can lead to rickets in children and osteomalacia in adults. Another cause of phosphate deficiency is the

long-term use of antacids, such as aluminum hydroxide, that bind dietary forms of phosphate and prevent their absorption.

The incidence of osteomalacia is high among the elderly because of diets deficient in calcium and vitamin D and often is compounded by the intestinal malabsorption problems that accompany aging. Osteomalacia often is seen in cultures in which the diet is deficient in vitamin D, such as in northern China, Japan, and northern India. Women in these areas have a higher incidence of the disorder than men because of the combined effects of pregnancy, lactation, and more indoor confinement. Osteomalacia occasionally is seen in strict vegetarians, persons who have had a gastrectomy, and those on long-term anticonvulsant, tranquilizer, sedative, muscle relaxant, or diuretic drugs. There also is a greater incidence of osteomalacia in the colder regions of the world, particularly during the winter months, probably because of lessened exposure to sunlight.

The clinical manifestations of osteomalacia are bone pain, tenderness, and fractures as the disease progresses. In severe cases, muscle weakness often is an early sign. The cause of muscle weakness is unclear. The combined effects of gravity, muscle weakness, and bone softening contribute to the development of deformities. There may be a dorsal kyphosis in the spine, rib deformities, a heart-shaped pelvis, and marked bowing of the tibiae and femurs. Osteomalacia predisposes a person to pathologic fractures in the weakened areas, especially in the distal radius and proximal femur. In contrast to osteoporosis, it is not a significant cause of hip fractures. There may be delayed healing and poor retention of internal fixation devices. Osteomalacia usually is accompanied by a compensatory or secondary hyperparathyroidism stimulated by low serum calcium levels. Parathyroid hormone reduces renal absorption of phosphate and removes calcium from the bone. Serum calcium levels are only slightly reduced in osteomalacia.

Diagnostic measures are directed toward identifying osteomalacia and establishing its cause. Diagnostic methods include x-ray studies, laboratory workup, bone scan, and bone biopsy. X-ray findings typical of osteomalacia are the development of transverse lines or pseudofractures called *Looser's zones* or *milkman's fractures*.[5] These apparently are caused by stress fractures that are inadequately healed or by the mechanical inadequacy of penetrating nutrient vessels.[10] A bone biopsy may be done to confirm the diagnosis of osteomalacia in a person with nonspecific osteopenia who shows no improvement after treatment with exercise, vitamin D, and calcium.

The treatment of osteomalacia is directed at the underlying cause. If the problem is nutritional, restoring adequate amounts of calcium and vitamin D to the diet may be sufficient. The elderly with intestinal malabsorption also may benefit from vitamin D. The least expensive and most effective long-term treatment is a diet rich in vitamin D (*i.e.*, fish, dairy products, and margarine) along with careful exposure to the midday sun. Vitamin D is specific for adult osteomalacia and vitamin D–resistant rickets, but large doses usually are needed to overcome the resistance to its calcium-absorption action and to prevent renal loss of phosphate. The biologically active forms of vitamin D, 25-OH vitamin D (calciferol) or 1,25-$(OH)_2$ vitamin D (calcitriol), are available for use in the treatment of osteomalacia resistant to vitamin D (*i.e.*, osteomalacia resulting from chronic liver disease and kidney failure). If osteomalacia is caused by malabsorption, the treatment is directed toward correcting the primary disease. For example, adequate replacement of pancreatic enzymes is of paramount importance in pancreatic insufficiency. In renal tubular disorders, the treatment is directed at the altered renal physiology.

Rickets

Rickets is a disorder of vitamin D deficiency, inadequate calcium absorption, and impaired mineralization of bone in children. Children with rickets manifest inadequate mineralization not only of bone, but also of the cartilaginous matrix of the epiphyseal growth plate. Rickets occurs primarily in underdeveloped areas of the world and among immigrants to developed countries. The causes are inadequate exposure to sunlight (*e.g.*, children are often kept clothed and indoors) and prolonged breast-feeding without vitamin D supplementation.[39] Although the vitamin D content of human milk is low, the combination of breast milk and sunlight exposure usually provides sufficient vitamin D. Another cause of rickets is the use of commercial alternative milks (*e.g.*, soy or rice beverages) that are not fortified with vitamin D.[40] A dietary deficiency in calcium and phosphorous may also contribute to the development of rickets. A newly discovered genetic mutation also can cause vitamin D deficiency rickets, a condition that does not respond to simple vitamin supplementation. The mutation results in the absence of a critical enzyme in vitamin D metabolism.[41]

The pathology of rickets is the same as that of osteomalacia seen in adults. Because rickets affects children during periods of active growth, the structural changes seen in the bone are somewhat different. Bones become deformed; ossification at epiphyseal plates is delayed and disordered, resulting in widening of the epiphyseal cartilage plate. Any new bone that does grow is unmineralized.

The symptoms of rickets usually are noticed between 6 months and 3 years of age. The child usually has stunted growth, with a height sometimes far below the normal range. Weight often is not affected so that the children, many of whom present with a protruding abdomen (*i.e.*, rachitic potbelly), have been described as presenting a Buddha-like appearance when sitting. Early symptoms are lethargy and muscle weakness, which may be accompanied by convulsions or tetany related to hypocalcemia. Irritability is common. In severe cases, children lose their skin pigment, acquire flabby subcutaneous tissue, and have poorly developed musculature. The ends of long bones and ribs are enlarged. The thorax may be abnormally shaped, with prominent rib cartilage (*i.e.*, rachitic rosary). The legs exhibit bowlegged or knock-kneed deformities. The skull is enlarged and soft, and closure of the fontanels is delayed. Teeth are slow to develop, and the child may have difficulty standing.

Rickets is treated with a balanced diet sufficient in calcium, phosphorus, and vitamin D. Exposure to sunlight also is important, especially for premature infants and those on artificial milk feedings. Supplemental vitamin D in excess of normal requirements is given for several months.

Maintenance of good posture, positioning, and bracing in older children are used to prevent deformities. After the disease is controlled, deformities may have to be surgically corrected as the child grows.

PAGET'S DISEASE

Paget's disease (*i.e.*, osteitis deformans) is discussed separately because it is not a true metabolic disease. It is a progressive skeletal disorder that involves excessive bone destruction and repair and is characterized by increasing structural changes of the long bones, spine, pelvis, and cranium. The disease usually begins during mid-adulthood and becomes progressively more common thereafter.[10] In children, hyperostosis corticalis deformans juvenilis (a rare inherited disorder), hyperphosphatemia, and diseases that cause diaphyseal stenosis may mimic Paget's disease and sometimes are referred to as *juvenile Paget's disease.*

The cause of Paget's disease is unknown. It may be caused by a virus capable of inciting osteoclastic activity.[9,10] It has been suggested that the virus may induce secretion of interferon-6, which is a potent stimulator of osteoclastic recruitment and resorptive activity.[10] The disease usually begins insidiously and progresses slowly over many years. An initial osteolytic phase is followed by an osteoblastic sclerotic phase. During the initial osteolytic phase, abnormal osteoclasts proliferate. Bone resorption occurs so rapidly that new bone formation cannot keep up, and the bone is replaced by fibrous tissue. The two processes of destruction and rebuilding occur simultaneously. The bones increase in size and thickness because of accelerated bone resorption followed by abnormal regeneration. Irregular bone formation results in sclerotic and osteoblastic lesions. The result is a thick layer of coarse bone with a rough and pitted outer surface that has the appearance of pumice. Histologically, Paget's lesions show increased vascularity and bone marrow fibrosis with intense cellular activity. The bone has a somewhat mosaic-like pattern caused by areas of density outlined by heavy blue lines, called *cement lines.*

The disease varies in severity from a simple lesion to involvement of many bones. It may be present long before it is detected clinically. The clinical manifestations of Paget's disease depend on the specific area involved. Approximately 20% of persons with the disorder are totally asymptomatic, and the disease is discovered accidentally.[42] Involvement of the skull causes headaches, intermittent tinnitus, vertigo, and eventual hearing loss. In the spine, collapse of the anterior vertebrae causes kyphosis of the thoracic spine. The femur and tibia become bowed. Softening of the femoral neck can cause coxa vara (*i.e.*, reduced angle of the femoral neck). Coxa vara, in combination with softening of the sacral and iliac bones, causes a waddling gait. When the lesion affects only one bone, it may cause only mild pain and stiffness. Progressive deossification weakens and distorts the bone structure. The deossification process begins along the inner cortical surfaces and continues until the substance of the bone disappears. Pathologic fractures may occur, especially in the bones subjected to the greatest stress (*e.g.*, upper femur, lower spine, pelvic bones). These fractures often heal poorly, with excessive and poorly distributed callus.

Other manifestations of Paget's disease include nerve palsy syndromes from lesions in the upper extremities, mental deterioration, and cardiovascular disease. Cardiovascular disease is the most serious complication and is listed as the most common cause of death in those with advanced generalized Paget's disease. It is caused by vasodilation of the vessels in the skin and subcutaneous tissues overlying the affected bones. When one third to one half of the skeleton is affected, the increased blood flow may lead to high-output cardiac failure. Ventilatory capacity may be limited by rib and spine involvement.

Osteogenic sarcomas occur in 5% to 10% of persons with severe polyostotic disease.[10] One fifth of all osteogenic sarcomas in persons 50 years of age or older originate in people with Paget's disease.[43] The bones most often affected, in order of frequency, are the femur, pelvis, humerus, and tibia. There appears to be a close histopathogenic relationship between Paget's disease and the associated sarcoma.[43]

Diagnosis of Paget's disease is based on characteristic bone deformities and x-ray changes. Elevated levels of serum alkaline phosphatase and urinary hydroxyproline support the diagnosis, and continued surveillance of these levels may be used to monitor the effectiveness of treatment. Bone scans are used to detect the rapid bone turnover indicative of active disease and to monitor the response to treatment. The scan cannot identify bone activity resulting from malignant lesions. Bone biopsy may be done to differentiate the lesion from osteomyelitis or a primary or metastatic bone tumor.

The treatment of Paget's disease is based on the degree of pain and the extent of the disease. Pain can be reduced with nonsteroidal or other anti-inflammatory agents. Suppressive agents such as the hormone calcitonin, mithramycin, and bisphosphonates are used to manage pain and prevent further spread of the disease and neurologic defects. Calcitonin and etidronate, a bisphosphonate agent, inhibit osteoclast-mediated bone resorption. Nasal calcitonin is available as an alternative to parenterally administered forms, but must be taken in higher doses because less of the drug reaches the diseased bone. Bisphosphonates are the treatment of choice for Paget's disease. They act by binding directly to bone minerals, inhibiting bone loss by rapidly decreasing bone resorption, followed by a secondary slower decrease in the rate of bone formation. Treatment usually is continued for 3 to 4 months, although recent studies are evaluating shorter courses of treatment.[44] Mithramycin is a cytotoxic agent that causes osteoclasts to reduce their resorption of bone. Because this drug is toxic, it is reserved for resistant cases. Decreases in serum alkaline phosphatase and urinary hydroxyproline levels and radiologically evident improvement indicate a response to treatment. However, symptomatic improvement usually is considered the best measure of success.

In summary, in addition to its structural function, the skeleton is a homeostatic organ. Metabolic bone diseases such as osteoporosis, osteomalacia, rickets, and Paget's disease are the result of a disruption in the equilibrium of bone formation and resorption. Osteoporosis, which is the most common of the metabolic bone diseases, occurs when the rate of bone resorption is greater than that of bone formation. It is seen frequently in postmenopausal women and is the major cause of fractures in persons older than 45 years of age. Osteomalacia and rickets are caused by inadequate mineralization of bone matrix, primarily because of a deficiency of vitamin D. Paget's disease results from excessive osteoclastic activity and is characterized by the formation of poor-quality bone. The success rate of the various drugs and hormones that are used to treat metabolic bone diseases varies. Further research is needed to clarify the cause, pathology, and treatment of these diseases.

Neoplasms

After you have completed this section of the chapter, you should be able to meet the following objectives:

- ✦ Differentiate between the properties of benign and malignant bone tumors
- ✦ Name the three major symptoms of bone cancer
- ✦ Contrast osteogenic sarcoma and chondrosarcoma
- ✦ List the primary sites of tumors that frequently metastasize to the bone
- ✦ State the three primary goals for treatment of metastatic bone disease

Neoplasms in the skeletal system usually are referred to as *bone tumors*. Primary malignant tumors of the bone are uncommon, constituting approximately 1% of all adult cancers and 15% of pediatric malignancies.[43] Metastatic disease of the bone, however, is relatively common. Primary bone tumors may arise from any of the skeletal components, including osseous bone tissue, cartilage, and bone marrow. The discussion in this section focuses on primary benign and malignant bone tumors of osseous or cartilaginous origin and metastatic bone disease. Tumors of bone marrow origin (*i.e.,* leukemia and multiple myeloma) are discussed in Chapter 16.

Like other types of neoplasms, bone tumors may be benign or malignant. The benign types, such as osteochondromas and giant cell tumors, tend to grow rather slowly and usually do not destroy the supporting or surrounding tissue or spread to other parts of the body. Malignant tumors, such as osteosarcoma and Ewing's sarcoma, grow rapidly and can spread to other parts of the body through the bloodstream or lymphatics. Specific types of bone tumors affect different age groups. They are virtually unknown in infancy, rare in children younger than 10 years of age, and peak during the teenage years. Adolescents have the highest incidence, with a rate of 3 cases per 100,000.[43] The two major forms of bone cancer in children and young adults are osteosarcoma and Ewing's sarcoma. It is unusual for either condition to be seen after 20 years of age.[9] Chondrosarcoma is most common in those 40 years of age and older.[10] The classification of benign and malignant bone tumors is described in Table 58-2.

TABLE 58-2 ✦ Classification of Primary Bone Neoplasms

Tissue Type	Benign Neoplasm	Malignant Neoplasm
Bone	Osteoid osteoma Benign osteo- blastoma	Osteosarcoma Parosteal osteogenic sarcoma
Cartilage	Osteochondroma Chondroma Chrondroblastoma Chondromyxoid fibroma	Chondrosarcoma
Lipid	Lipoma	Liposarcoma
Fibrous and fibro- osseous tissue	Fibrous dysplasia	Fibrosarcoma Malignant fibrous histiocytoma
Miscellaneous	Giant cell tumor	Malignant giant cell Ewing's sarcoma
Bone marrow		Multiple myeloma Reticulum cell sarcoma

CHARACTERISTICS OF BONE TUMORS

There are three major symptoms of bone tumors: pain, presence of a mass, and impairment of function[45] (Chart 58-2). Pain is a feature common to almost all malignant tumors, but may or may not occur with benign tumors. For example, a benign bone cyst usually is asymptomatic until a fracture occurs. Pain that persists at night and is not relieved by rest suggests malignancy. A mass or hard lump may be the first sign of a bone tumor. A malignant tumor is suspected when a painful mass exists that is enlarging or eroding the cortex of the bone. The ease of discovery of a mass depends on the location of the tumor; a small lump

---

CHART 58-2

Symptoms of Bone Cancer

- Bone pain in an adult or child that comes on slowly but lasts for as long as a week, is constant or intermittent, and may be worse at night.
- Unexplained swelling or lump on the bones of the arms, legs, thighs, or other parts of the body that is firm and slightly tender and may be felt through the skin. It may interfere with normal movement and can cause the bone to break.

These symptoms are not sure signs of cancer. They also may be caused by other, less serious problems. Only a physician can tell for sure.

(Adapted from U.S. Department of Health and Human Services [1993]. *What you need to know about cancers of the bone.* NIH publication no. 93-1517. Bethesda, MD: U.S. Government Printing Office)

---

arising on the surface of the tibia is easy to detect, whereas a tumor that is deep in the medial portion of the thigh may grow to a considerable size before it is noticed. Benign and malignant tumors may cause the bone to erode to the point where it cannot withstand the strain of ordinary use. In such cases, even a small amount of bone stress or trauma precipitates a pathologic fracture. A tumor may produce pressure on a peripheral nerve, causing decreased sensation, numbness, a limp, or limitation of movement.

BENIGN NEOPLASMS

Benign bone tumors usually are limited to the confines of the bone, have well-demarcated edges, and are surrounded by a thin rim of sclerotic bone. The four most common types of benign bone tumors are osteoma, chondroma, osteochondroma, and giant cell tumor.

An *osteoma* is a small bony tumor found on the surface of a long bone, flat bone, or the skull. It usually is composed of hard, compact (ivory osteoma), or spongy (cancellous) bone. It may be excised or left alone.

A *chondroma* is a tumor composed of hyaline cartilage. It may arise on the surface of the bone (*i.e.,* ecchondroma) or within the medullary cavity (*i.e.,* endochondroma). These tumors may become large and are especially common in the hands and feet. A chondroma may persist for many years and then take on the attributes of a malignant chondrosarcoma. A chondroma usually is not treated unless it becomes unsightly or uncomfortable.

An *osteochondroma* is the most common form of benign tumor in the skeletal system, representing 50% of all benign bone tumors and approximately 15% of all primary skeletal lesions.[43] It grows only during periods of skeletal growth, originating in the epiphyseal cartilage plate and growing out of the bone like a mushroom. An osteochondroma is composed of cartilage and bone and usually occurs singly but may affect several bones in a condition called *multiple exostoses*. Malignant changes are rare, and excision of the tumor is done only when necessary.

A *giant cell tumor,* or *osteoclastoma,* is an aggressive tumor of multinucleated cells that often behaves like a

---

 Bone Neoplasms

➤ Neoplasms of the skeletal system can affect bone tissue, cartilage, or bone marrow.

➤ Benign tumors tend to grow slowly, do not spread to other parts of the body, and exert their effects through the space-occupying nature of the tumor and their ability to weaken bone structures.

➤ Malignant bone tumors are rare before 10 years of age, have their peak incidence in the teenage years, tend to grow rapidly, and have a high mortality rate.

malignant tumor, metastasizing through the bloodstream and recurring locally after excision. It occurs most often in young adults, predominantly females, and is found most commonly in the knee, wrist, or shoulder. The tumor begins in the metaphyseal region, grows into the epiphysis, and may extend into the joint surface. Pathologic fractures are common because the tumor destroys the bone substance. Clinically, pain may occur at the tumor site, with gradually increasing swelling. X-ray films show destruction of the bone with expansion of the cortex.

The treatment of giant cell tumors depends on their location. If the affected bone can be eliminated without loss of function, such as the clavicle or fibula, the entire bone or part of it may be removed. When the tumor is near a major joint, such as the knee or shoulder, a local excision is done. Irradiation may be used to prevent recurrence of the tumor.

MALIGNANT BONE TUMORS

In contrast to benign tumors, malignant tumors tend to be ill defined, lack sharp borders, and extend beyond the confines of the bone, showing that it has destroyed the cortex. Malignant bone tumors are rare before 10 years of age, have their peak incidence in the teenage years, and have a high mortality rate. There is much morbidity and trauma from the often-mutilating surgical excision.

The diagnosis of bone tumors includes radiologic staging and biopsy. Radiographs give the most general diagnostic information, such as malignant versus benign and primary versus metastatic status. The radiograph demonstrates the region of bone involvement, extent of destruction, and amount of reactive bone formed. Radioisotope scans are used to estimate the local intramedullary extent of the tumor and screen for other skeletal areas of involvement. CT scans further aid diagnosis and anatomic localization and can identify small pulmonary metastases not seen by conventional radiographs. MRI is the most accurate method of evaluating the intramedullary extent of bone tumor and can demarcate the soft structures in relation to neurovascular structures without the use of contrast media. It is best used in conjunction with a CT scan.[46] A biopsy also is done because the definitive treatment of most bone tumors is based on pathologic interpretation of the biopsy specimen. A bone biopsy is performed by means of a large needle or open surgical method. A biopsy is needed to stage the tumor.

The treatment of malignant bone tumors primarily involves surgical removal of the tumor, with amputation of the limb or wide resection of the tumor and surrounding tissue. Preoperative, intraoperative, or postoperative irradiation; chemotherapy; or chemotherapy plus irradiation are used. Radiation therapy is used as a definitive and adjuvant treatment to slow the progression of the cancer, decrease bone pain, and prevent pathologic fractures. A pathologic fracture spreads the tumor cells through formation of a hematoma. Because high-grade bone and soft tissue sarcomas produce clinically undetectable metastases called *micrometastases,* immunotherapy, irradiation, and chemotherapy often are used in combination as adjuvant therapy.

Chemotherapy is the most effective modality for controlling metastases. Extremely aggressive drug combinations have been developed, particularly for the pediatric and young adult age groups.

Many advances have been made in the limb salvage and reconstructive surgical procedures being used as alternatives to limb amputation. The tumor must have minimal soft tissue involvement and no involvement of major blood vessels. A prosthetic metal implant or allograft (*i.e.,* cadaveric bone transplant) is used to fill the bony defect resulting from surgery.

Osteosarcoma

Osteosarcoma represents 60% of all bone tumors occurring in children and adolescents. Osteosarcoma has a bimodal distribution, with 75% occurring in persons younger than 20 years of age. A second peak occurs in the elderly with predisposing factors such as Paget's disease, bone infarcts, or prior irradiation.[10] The male-to-female ratio increases to approximately 1.6 to 1 during late adolescence and adulthood. It is seen most commonly during periods of maximal growth. In younger persons, the primary tumor most often is located at the anatomic sites associated with maximum growth velocity—the distal femur, proximal tibia, and proximal humerus. Persons affected with osteosarcoma usually are tall and are found to have a high plasma level of somatomedin. Bone tumors in the elderly are more common in the humerus, pelvis, and proximal femur.

Osteosarcoma is a malignant tumor of mesenchymal cells, characterized by the direct formation of osteoid or immature bone by malignant osteoblasts. These cells synthesize thin, wispy, and purposeless fragments of bone. Osteogenic sarcomas are aggressive tumors that grow rapidly; they often are eccentrically placed in the bone and move from the metaphysis of the bone out to the periosteum, with subsequent spread to adjacent soft tissues.

The causes of osteosarcoma are unknown. The correlation of age and location of most of the tumors with the period of maximum growth suggests some relation to increased osteoblastic activity. Paget's disease, which is linked to osteosarcoma in adults, also is associated with increased osteoblastic activity. Irradiation from an internal source, such as the radioactive pharmaceutical technetium used in bone scans, or an external source, such as x-ray films, also has been associated with osteosarcoma.

The primary clinical feature of osteosarcoma is localized pain and swelling in the affected bone, usually of sudden onset. Patients and their families often associate the symptoms with recent trauma.[46] The skin overlying the tumor may be warm, shiny, and stretched, with prominent superficial veins. The range of motion of the adjacent joint may be restricted. Osteosarcoma usually begins as a firm white or reddish mass and later becomes softer with a viscous interior (Fig. 58-17). The tumor infrequently metastasizes to the lymph nodes because the cells are unable to grow in the node. Nodal metastases usually occur only in the late course of disseminated disease. Most often, the tumor cells exit the primary tumor through the venous end of the capillary, and early metastasis to the lung is common. Lung metastases, even if massive, usually are relatively asymptomatic. The

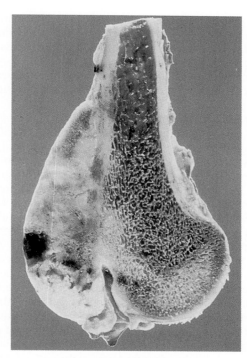

FIGURE 58-17 Juxtacortical osteosarcoma. The lower femur contains a malignant tumor arising from the periosteal surface of the bone and sparing the medullary cavity. (Rubin E., Farber L.F. [1999]. *Pathophysiology* [3rd ed., p. 1386]. Philadelphia: Lippincott Williams & Wilkins)

prognosis for a patient with osteosarcoma depends on the aggressiveness of the disease, radiologic features, presence or absence of pathologic fracture, size of the tumor, rapidity of tumor growth, and sex of the person.

The treatment for sarcomas is surgery in combination with multiagent chemotherapy used both before and after surgery.[46,47] Osteosarcomas are relatively resistant to radiation therapy. In the past, treatment usually entailed amputation above the level of the tumor. Limb salvage surgical procedures, using a metal prosthesis or cadaver allografts, are becoming a standard alternative. Studies have shown that limb salvage surgery has no adverse effects on the long-term survival of persons with osteosarcoma. The success of limb salvage appears to depend on the use of a wide surgical margin, improved radiographic imaging studies, multiagent chemotherapy, and more refined surgical reconstructive techniques. Advanced imaging techniques, including serum thallium scans, and the use of angiography assist the surgeon in determining the best type of treatment. Chemotherapy using various drug combinations is the most effective treatment for metastatic osteosarcoma.

Ewing's Sarcoma

Ewing's sarcoma is the third most common type of primary bone tumor, and it is highly malignant. It commonly occurs in males younger than 25 years of age, with the incidence highest among teenagers.[46] Ewing's tumor arises from immature bone marrow cells and causes bone destruction from within. It usually occurs in the shaft of long bones or

any portion of the pelvis and often metastasizes to bone marrow.

Manifestations of Ewing's tumor include pain, limitation of movement, and tenderness over the involved bone or soft tissue. It often is accompanied by systemic manifestations such as fever or weight loss, which may serve to confuse the diagnosis. There also may be a delay in diagnosis when the pain and swelling associated with the tumor are attributed to a sports injury. Pathologic fractures are common because of bone destruction.

Treatment methods incorporate a combination of multiagent chemotherapy, surgery, and radiation therapy. There is controversy about the potential superiority of surgical resection compared with radiation therapy.[46] Radiation therapy is associated with risk of radiation-induced second malignancies, especially osteosarcoma.

Chondrosarcoma

Chondrosarcoma, a malignant tumor of cartilage that can develop in the medullary cavity or peripherally, is the second most common form of malignant bone tumor. It occurs primarily in middle or later life and slightly more often in males. The tumor arises from points of muscle attachment to bone, particularly the knee, shoulder, hip, and pelvis. Chondrosarcomas can arise from underlying benign lesions such as osteochondroma, chrondroblastoma, or fibrous dysplasia.[10]

Chondrosarcomas are slow growing, metastasize late, and often are painless. They can remain hidden in an area such as the pelvis for a long time. This type of tumor, like many primary malignancies, tends to destroy bone and extend into the soft tissues beyond the confines of the bone of origin. Chondrosarcomas mainly affect the bones of the trunk, pelvis, or proximal femur and rarely develop in the distal portion of a bone. Irregular flecks and ringlets of calcification often are prominent radiographic findings. Early diagnosis is important because chondrosarcoma responds well to early radical surgical excision. It usually is resistant to radiation therapy and available chemotherapeutic agents. Not infrequently, these tumors transform into a highly malignant tumor, mesenchymal chondrosarcoma, which requires a more aggressive treatment, including combination chemotherapy.

METASTATIC BONE DISEASE

Skeletal metastases are the most common malignancy of osseous tissue. Approximately half of all people with cancer have bone metastasis at some point in their disease.[48] Metastatic lesions are seen most often in the spine, femur, pelvis, ribs, sternum, proximal humerus, and skull, and are less common in anatomic sites that are further removed from the trunk of the body. Tumors that frequently spread to the skeletal system are those of the breast, lung, prostate, kidney, and thyroid, although any cancer can ultimately involve the skeleton. More than 85% of bone metastases result from primary lesions in the breast, lung, or prostate.[49] The incidence of metastatic bone disease is highest in persons older than 40 years of age. There typically are several bony metastases, with or without metastatic spread to other organs. Solitary lesions are seen most commonly with cancers of the kidney and thyroid. Because of the effectiveness of current cancer treatment modalities, patients with cancer are living longer, and the incidence of clinically apparent skeletal involvement appears to be increasing in the long run. These skeletal metastases cause great pain, increase the risk of fractures, and increase the disability of the patient with cancer.

Metastasis to the bone frequently occurs without involving other organs because the blood flow in the veins of the skeletal system is sluggish. These are thin-walled, valveless veins, and there are many storage sites along the way. The pattern of metastasis often is related to the specific vascular pathway that is involved (*e.g.,* metastases to the shoulder girdle and pelvis occur when prostatic cancers invade the vertebral vein system). If metastasis is limited to the skeletal system, without other major organ involvement, a person can live for many years. Death usually is a consequence of metastasis to vital organs rather than a consequence of the primary tumor.

The major symptom of bone metastasis is pain with evidence of an impending pathologic fracture. It usually develops gradually, over weeks, and is more severe at night. Pain is caused by stretching of the periosteum of the involved bone or by nerve entrapment, as in the nerve roots of the spinal cord by the vertebral body. X-ray examinations are used along with CT or bone scans to detect, diagnose, and localize metastatic bone lesions. Approximately one third of persons with skeletal metastases have positive bone scans without radiologic findings. This is because 50% of the trabecular bone must be destroyed before a lesion is visible on plain radiographs.[50] Arteriography using radiopaque contrast media may be helpful in outlining the tumor margins. A bone biopsy usually is done when there is a question regarding the diagnosis or treatment. A closed-needle biopsy with CT localization is particularly useful with spine lesions. Serum levels of alkaline phosphatase and calcium often are elevated in persons with metastatic bone disease. Hypercalcemia occurs in 10% to 20% of persons with metastatic bone disease because of bone lysis.

The primary goals in treatment of metastatic bone disease are to prevent pathologic fractures and promote survival with maximum functioning, allowing the person to maintain as much mobility and pain control as possible. Treatment methods include chemotherapy, irradiation, and surgical stabilization. The discovery of new and more effective drugs along with the use of combination protocols has increased the effectiveness of chemotherapy in treating metastatic bone disease. Local irradiation can effect rapid pain relief within 1 to 2 weeks in more than 50% of patients.[49] Radiation therapy is primarily used as a palliative treatment to alleviate pain and prevent pathologic fractures. A prophylactic internal fixation may be done in a weight-bearing bone threatened by an expanding lesion. Bracing may be ordered for an unstable spine. It is difficult to find a comfortable fit when there is metastasis to the ribs or pelvis. Steroid drugs also may be helpful. The bisphosphonates inhibit osteoclastic activity and subsequent bone-induced osteolysis. Bisphosphonates are used in metastatic bone disease to relieve the symptoms, enable bone healing to occur, and delay complications.

Hypercalcemia occurs in 10% to 20% of persons with metastatic bone disease because of bone lysis.[49] Symptoms include dulling of consciousness, stupor, weakness, muscle flaccidity, and decreased neural excitability. A total serum calcium level greater than 12 mg/dL requires treatment with diuretics and intravenous sodium chloride (see Chapter 31).

Pathologic fractures occur in approximately 10% to 15% of persons with metastatic bone disease. The affected bone appears to be eaten away on x-ray images and, in severe cases, crumbles on impact, much like dried toast. Many pathologic fractures occur in the femur, humerus, and vertebrae. In the femur, fractures occur because the proximal aspect of the bone is under great mechanical stress. Lesions may be treated prophylactically with surgery and radiation therapy to prevent pathologic fractures. Flexible intramedullary rods may be used to stabilize long bones. After a pathologic fracture has occurred, bracing, intramedullary nailing of the femur, and spine stabilization may be done. Because adequate fixation often is difficult in diseased bone, cement (*i.e.,* methylmethacrylate) often is used with internal fixation devices to stabilize the bone. The selection of a treatment modality for prevention or treatment of pathologic fractures depends on the severity of the lesion, the degree of pain, and the life expectancy of the patient. The goal is to provide flexibility, mobility, and pain relief. Surgeons usually treat metastatic lesions aggressively so that patients can function as normally as possible, even if life expectancy is as short as 3 months.[49]

> In summary, bone tumors, like any other type of neoplasm, may be benign or malignant. Benign bone tumors grow slowly and usually do not destroy the surrounding tissues. Malignant tumors can be primary or metastatic. Primary bone tumors are rare, grow rapidly, metastasize to the lungs and other parts of the body through the bloodstream, and have a high mortality rate. Metastatic bone tumors usually are multiple, originating primarily from cancers of the breast, lung, and prostate. The incidence of metastatic bone disease probably is increasing because improved treatment methods enable persons with cancer to live longer. Advances in chemotherapy, radiation therapy, and surgical procedures have substantially increased the survival and cure rates for many types of bone cancers. A primary goal in metastatic bone disease is the prevention of pathologic fractures.

References

1. Moore K.L., Persaud T.V.N. (1998). *The developing human* (6th ed., pp. 90–106). Philadelphia: W.B. Saunders.
2. Cormack D.H. (1993). *Essential histology* (pp. 174–178). Philadelphia: J.B. Lippincott.
3. Bruce R.W. (1996). Torsional and angular deformities. *Pediatric Clinics of North America* 43, 867–881.
4. Thompson G.H., Scoles P.V. (2000). Bone and joint disorders. In Behrman R.E., Kliegman R.M., Jenson H.B. (Eds.), *Nelson textbook of pediatrics* (16th ed., pp. 2055–2112). Philadelphia: W.B. Saunders.

5. Johnson K.B., Oski F.S. (1997). *Oski's essential pediatrics* (pp. 149–169). Philadelphia: Lippincott-Raven.

6. Schoppee K. (1995). Blount disease. *Orthopedic Nursing* 14 (5), 31–34.

7. Pizzutillo P.D. (1994). The pediatric leg and knee. In Weinstein S.L., Buckwalter J.A. (Eds.), *Turek's orthopaedics: Principles and their application* (5th ed., pp. 573–584). Philadelphia: J.B. Lippincott.

8. National Institutes of Health. (1999). Osteoporosis and related bone diseases. Fast facts on osteogenesis imperfecta. [On-line]. Available: http://www.oif.org/tier2/fastfact.htm.

9. Schiller A.L., Teitelbaum S.L. (1999). Bones and joints. In Rubin E., Farber J.L. (Eds.), *Pathophysiology* (3rd ed., pp. 1352–1380). Philadelphia: Lippincott Williams & Wilkins.

10. Cotran R.S., Kumar V., Robbins S.L. (1999). *Robbins pathologic basis of disease* (6th ed., pp. 1221–1246). Philadelphia: W.B. Saunders.

11. American Academy of Pediatrics (2000). Clinical practice guideline: Early detection of developmental dysplasia of the hip. *Pediatrics* 105, 896–905.

12. Novacheck T.F. (1996). Developmental dysplasia of the hip. *Pediatrics* 43, 829–848.

13. Weinstein S.L. (1994). The pediatric foot. In Weinstein S.L., Buckwalter J.A. (Eds.), *Turek's orthopaedics: Principles and their application* (5th ed., pp. 615–653). Philadelphia: J.B. Lippincott.

14. Honein M., Paulozzi L.J., Moore C.A. (2000). Family history, maternal smoking, and clubfoot: An indication of a gene–environment interaction. *American Journal of Epidemiology* 152, 658–665.

15. Hoffinger S.A. (1996). Evaluation and management of pediatric foot deformities. *Pediatric Clinics of North America* 43, 1091–1101.

16. Koops S., Quanbeck D. (1996). Three common causes of childhood hip pain. *Pediatric Clinics of North America* 43, 1056–1065.

17. U.S. Preventative Services Task Force. (1993). Screening for adolescent idiopathic scoliosis. *Journal of the American Medical Association* 269, 2664–2672.

18. Weinstein S. (1994). The thoracolumbar spine. In Weinstein S.L., Buckwalter J.A. (Eds.), *Turek's orthopaedics: Principles and their application* (5th ed., pp. 447–483). Philadelphia: J.B. Lippincott.

19. Omey M.L., Micheli L.J., Gerbino P. G. (2000). Idiopathic scoliosis and spondylolysis in the female athlete: Tips for treatment. *Clinical Orthopaedics and Related Research* 372, 74–84.

20. Skaggs D.L., Bassett G.S. (1996). Adolescent idiopathic scoliosis: An update. *American Family Physician* 53, 2327–2334.

21. Yawn B.P., Yawn R.A., Hodge D., Kurland M., Shaughnessy W.J., Ilstrup D., Jacobsen S.J. (1999). A population-based study of school scoliosis screening. *JAMA* 282, 1427–1432.

22. Rowe D.E., Bernstein S.M., Riddick M.F., Adler F., Emens J.B., Gardner-Bonneau D. (1997). A meta-analysis of the efficacy of non-operative treatments for idiopathic scoliosis. *Journal of Bone and Joint Surgery*. American 79, 664–674.

23. Manolagas S.C., Jilka R.L. (1995). Bone marrow, cytokines, and bone remodeling. *New England Journal of Medicine* 332, 305–310.

24. Barzel U.S. (1996). Osteoporosis: Taking a fresh look. *Hospital Practice* 30 (5), 59–68.

25. Genant H.K., Guglielmi G., Jergus M. (Eds.). (1998). *Bone densitometry and osteoporosis*. Berlin: Springer-Verlag.

26. Riggs B.L., Melton L.J. (1992). The prevention and treatment of osteoporosis. *New England Journal of Medicine* 327, 620–627.

27. Dueck C.A., Matt K.S., Manore M.M., Skinner J.S. (1996). Treatment of athletic amenorrhea with a diet and training intervention program. *International Journal of Sport Nutrition* 6 (2), 24–40.

28. Otis C.L., Drinkwater B., Johnson M., Louck A., Wilmore J. (1997). American College of Sports Medicine position stand: The female athlete triad. *Medicine and Science in Sports and Exercise* 29 (5), i–ix.

29. Hobart J.A., Smucker D.R. (2000). The female athlete triad. *American Family Physician* 61, 3357–3367.

30. Karlsson M.K., Linden C., Karlsson C., Johnell O., Obrant K., Seeman E. (2000). Exercise during growth and bone mineral density and fractures in old age. *Lancet* 355, 460–470.

31. Gambert S.R., Schulz B.M., Hamdy B.C. (1995). Osteoporosis: Clinical features, prevention, and treatment. *Endocrinology and Metabolic Clinics of North America* 24, 317–371.

32. Phipps K.R., Orwoll E.S., Mason J., Cauley J.A. (2000). Fluoridated drinking water increases bone mineral density. *British Medical Journal* 321, 844–845, 860, 864.

33. Tebas P., Powerly W.G., Claxton S., Marin D., Tantisriwat W., Teitelbaum S.L., et al. (2000). Accelerated bone mineral loss in HIV-infected patients receiving potent antiretroviral therapy. *AIDS* 14 (4), F63–F67.

34. Hunt A.H. (1996). The relationship between height change and bone mineral density. *Orthopedic Nursing* 15 (3), 57–64.

35. Weinstein L., Ullery B. (2000). Age, weight, and estrogen use determine need for osteoporosis screen. *American Journal of Obstetrics and Gynecology* 183, 547–549.

36. Andrews W.C. (1998). What's new in preventing and treating osteoporosis. *Postgraduate Medicine* 104 (4), 89–97.

37. Bukata S.V., Rosier R.N. (2000). Diagnosis and treatment of osteoporosis. *Current Opinion in Orthopedics* 11, 336–340.

38. Ravn P., Bidstrup M., Wasnich R.D., Davis J.W., McClung M.R., Balske A., et al. (1999). Alendronate and estrogen-progestin in the long-term prevention of bone loss: Four-year results of the early postmenopausal intervention cohort study. A randomized, controlled trial. *Annals of Internal Medicine* 131 (2), 935–942.

39. Bishop M. (1999). Rickets today—Children still need milk and sunshine. *New England Journal of Medicine* 341, 602–604.

40. Centers for Disease Control. (2001). Severe malnutrition among young children—Georgia, January 1997–June 1999. *MMWR* 50 (12), 224–227.

41. Bouillon R. (1998). The many faces of rickets. *New England Journal of Medicine* 131, 935–942.

42. Hamdy R.C. (1990). Paget's disease of bone. *Hospital Practice* 25 (10), 33–41.

43. Rosen G., Forscher C.A., Mankin H.J., Selch M.T. (2000). Neoplasms of the bone and soft tissue. In Bast R. C., Kufe D.W., Pollock R.E., Weichselbaum R.R., Holland J.F., Frei E. (Eds.), *Cancer medicine* (pp. 1870–1902). Hamilton, Ontario: B.C. Decker.

44. Sadovsky R. (1997). Paget's disease of the bone: Bisphosphonate treatment. *American Family Physician* 55, 1400–1401.

45. U.S. Department of Health and Human Services. (1990). *What you need to know about cancers of the bone*. NIH publication no. 90-1571. Bethesda, MD: U.S. Government Printing Office.

46. Arndt C.S. (2000). Neoplasms of bone. In Behrman R.E., Kliegman R.M., Jenson H.B. (Eds.), *Nelson textbook of pediatrics* (16th ed., pp. 1558–1561). Philadelphia: W.B. Saunders.

47. Arndt C.A.S., Crist W.M. (1999). Common musculoskeletal tumors of childhood and adolescence. *New England Journal of Medicine* 431, 342–352.

48. American Cancer Society. (1999). Bone cancer. [On-line]. Available: http://www3.cancer.org.

49. O'Keefe R.J., Schwartz E.M., Boyce B.F. (2000). Bone metastasis: An update on bone resorption and therapeutic strategies. *Current Opinion in Orthopedics* 11, 353–359.

50. Rubens R.D., Coleman R.E. (1995). Bone metastases. In Abeloff M.D., Armitage J.O., Lichter A.S., Niederhuber J.E. (Eds.), *Clinical oncology* (pp. 643–666). New York: Churchill Livingstone.

Chapter 59

Alterations in Skeletal Function: Rheumatic Disorders

Debra Ann Bancroft and Janice Smith Pigg

*A*rthritis is a descriptive term applied to more than 100 rheumatic diseases, ranging from localized, self-limiting conditions to those that are systemic, autoimmune processes. Arthritis affects persons in all age groups and is the second leading cause of disability in the United States.[1,2] The common use of the term *arthritis* oversimplifies the nature of the varied disease processes, the difficulty in differentiating one form of arthritis or rheumatic disease from another, and the complexity of treatment of these usually chronic conditions. These diverse conditions share inflammation of the joint as a prominent or accompanying symptom. In the systemic rheumatic diseases—those affecting body systems in addition to the musculoskeletal system—the inflammation is primary, resulting from an immune response, probably autoimmune in origin. In rheumatic conditions limited to a single or few diarthrodial joints, the inflammation is secondary, resulting from the degenerative process and joint irregularities as the bone attempts to remodel itself.

The disabling effects of arthritis may be manifested in an individual's personal, social, and employment activities. To help persons with arthritis, health care providers must have a working knowledge of the specific disease and an understanding of the underlying pathologic processes. Basic education is fundamental in rectifying misconceptions.

Although arthritis cannot be cured, much can be done to control its progress. Fear of being crippled is a major concern that should be addressed so the disease can be perceived realistically. All aspects of treatment require that the person with arthritis accept responsibility for the health care program. Family members should be included in education programs; their support in integrating prescribed treatment regimens is important. Because many unproven remedies for arthritis are offered, patients need information on how to assess the validity of the available treatments. The Arthritis Foundation provides information and community services to persons with arthritis and their families.

This chapter focuses on systemic autoimmune rheumatic diseases, arthritis associated with spondylitis, osteoarthritis syndromes, metabolic diseases associated with arthritis, and rheumatic disease in children and the elderly. A review of normal joint structures is presented in Chapter 56.

Systemic Autoimmune Rheumatic Diseases

After you have completed this section of the chapter, you should be able to meet the following objectives:

- ✦ Describe the difficulty in defining the term *arthritis*
- ✦ Describe the pathologic changes that may be found in the joint of a person with rheumatoid arthritis
- ✦ List the extra-articular manifestations of rheumatoid arthritis
- ✦ Describe the immunologic process that occurs in systemic lupus erythematosus
- ✦ List four major organ systems that may be involved in systemic lupus erythematosus

Systemic autoimmune rheumatic diseases are a group of chronic disorders characterized by diffuse inflammatory vascular lesions and degenerative changes in connective tissue. These disorders share similar clinical features and may affect many of the same organs. Rheumatoid arthritis, systemic lupus erythematosus (SLE), polymyalgia rheumatica, temporal arteritis, and juvenile arthritis and dermatomyositis, which share an autoimmune systemic pathogenesis, are discussed in this chapter.

RHEUMATOID ARTHRITIS

Rheumatoid arthritis is a systemic inflammatory disease that affects 0.3% to 1.5% of the population, with women affected two to three times more frequently than men.[1] Although the disease occurs in all age groups, its prevalence increases with age. The peak incidence among women is between the ages of 40 and 60 years, with the onset at 30 to 50 years of age.

Etiology and Pathogenesis

Although the cause of rheumatoid arthritis remains somewhat mysterious, evidence points to the importance of immunologic events (see Chapters 18 and 19). Approximately 70% to 80% of those with the disease have a substance called the *rheumatoid factor*, which is an antibody that reacts with a fragment of immunoglobulin G (IgG), an autologous (self-produced) antibody, to form immune complexes.[3]

Why the body would begin to produce antibodies against its own IgG remains unclear. An infectious agent, such as a virus, may alter the immunoglobulin so that it is recognized as foreign. Another possibility is that genetic predisposition plays a role in the development of the response. Sixty percent of persons with rheumatoid arthritis

have the major histocompatibility complex (MHC) antigen, human leukocyte antigen (HLA) DR4.[1] HLA-DR4 may play a role in identifying susceptibility to rheumatoid arthritis and be related to the severity of the disease.

Rheumatoid factor has been found in the blood, synovial fluid, and synovial membrane of affected individuals. Much of the rheumatoid factor is produced by lymphocytes in the inflammatory infiltrate of the synovial tissue.[3] The role of the autoimmune process in joint destruction remains obscure. At the cellular level, polymorphonuclear leukocytes, macrophages, and lymphocytes are attracted to the area. The polymorphonuclear leukocytes and macrophages phagocytize the immune complexes and, in the process, release lysosomal enzymes capable of causing destructive changes in the joint cartilage (Fig. 59-1). The inflammatory response that follows attracts additional lymphocytes and plasma cells, setting into motion a chain of events that perpetuates the condition. As the inflammatory process advances, the synovial cells and the subsynovial tissue undergo reactive hyperplasia. Vasodilation and increased blood flow cause warmth and redness. Swelling results from the increased capillary permeability that accompanies the inflammatory process.

Characteristic of rheumatoid arthritis is the development of an extensive network of new blood vessels in the synovial membrane that contributes to the advancement of the rheumatoid synovitis. This destructive vascular granulation tissue, which is called *pannus*, extends from the synovium to involve the "bare area," a region of unprotected bone at the junction between cartilage and subchondral bone. Pannus is a feature of rheumatoid arthritis that differentiates it from other forms of inflammatory arthritis[4] (Fig. 59-2). The inflammatory cells found in the pannus have a destructive effect on the adjacent cartilage and bone. Eventually, pannus develops between the joint margins, leading to reduced joint motion and the possibility of eventual ankylosis. With progression of the disease, joint inflammation and the resulting structural changes can lead to joint instability, muscle atrophy from disuse, stretching of the ligaments, and involvement of the tendons and muscles. The effect of the pathologic changes on joint structure and function is related to the degree of disease activity, which can change at any time. Unfortunately, the destructive changes are irreversible.

Clinical Manifestations

Rheumatoid arthritis often is associated with extra-articular as well as articular manifestations. It usually has an insidious onset marked by systemic manifestations such as fatigue, anorexia, weight loss, and generalized aching and stiffness. The disease, which is characterized by exacerbations and remissions, may involve only a few joints for brief durations, or it may be relentlessly progressive and debilitating. Approximately 3% of those with the disease have a progressive, unremitting form that does not respond to aggressive therapy.[2]

Joint Manifestations. Joint involvement usually is symmetric and polyarticular. Any diarthrodial joint can be involved. The person may complain of joint pain and stiffness that lasts 30 minutes and frequently for several hours. The

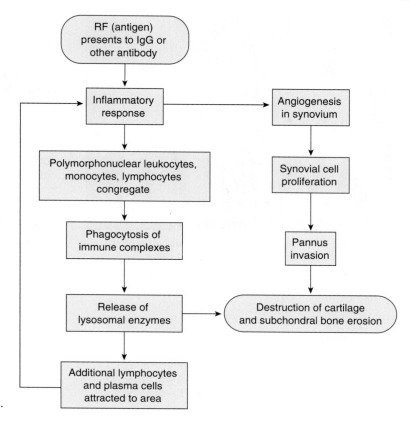

FIGURE 59-1 Disease process in rheumatoid arthritis.

limitation of joint motion that occurs early in the disease usually is because of pain; later, it is because of fibrosis. The most frequently affected joints initially are the fingers, hands, wrists, knees, and feet. Later, other diarthrodial joints may become involved. Spinal involvement usually is limited to the cervical region. In the hands, there usually is bilateral and symmetric involvement of the proximal interphalangeal (PIP) and metacarpophalangeal (MCP) joints in the early stages of rheumatoid arthritis; the distal interphalangeal (DIP) joints rarely are affected. The fingers often take on a spindle-shaped appearance because of inflammation of the PIP joints (Fig. 59-3).

Progressive joint destruction may lead to subluxation (*i.e.,* dislocation of the joint resulting in misalignment of the bone ends) and instability of the joint and in limitation of movement. Swelling and thickening of the synovium can result in stretching of the joint capsule and ligaments. When this occurs, muscle and tendon imbalances develop, and mechanical forces applied to the joints through daily activities produce joint deformities. In the MCP joints, the

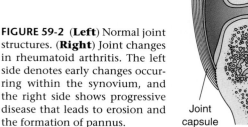

FIGURE 59-2 (Left) Normal joint structures. **(Right)** Joint changes in rheumatoid arthritis. The left side denotes early changes occurring within the synovium, and the right side shows progressive disease that leads to erosion and the formation of pannus.

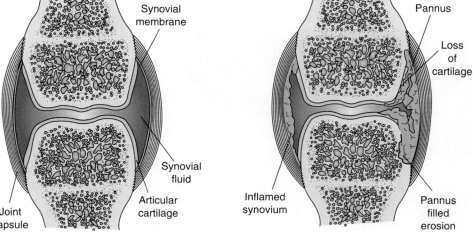

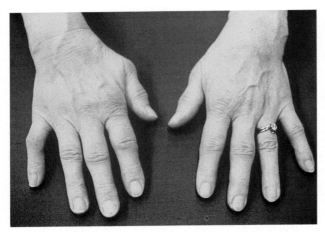

FIGURE 59-3 Inflammation of finger proximal interphalangeal joints in early stages of rheumatoid arthritis, giving the fingers a spindle-shaped appearance. (Reprinted from the ARHP Arthritis Teaching Slide Collection. Used with permission of the American College of Rheumatology.)

extensor tendons can slip to the ulnar side of the metacarpal head, causing ulnar deviation of the finger (Fig. 59-4). Subluxation of the MCP joints may develop when this deformity is present. Hyperextension of the PIP joint and partial flexion of the DIP joint is called a *swan neck deformity*. After this condition becomes fixed, severe loss of function occurs because the person can no longer make a fist. Flexion of the PIP joint with hyperextension of the DIP joint is called a *boutonnière deformity*.

The knee is one of the most commonly affected joints and is responsible for much of the disability associated with the disease.[1] Active synovitis may be apparent as visible swelling that obliterates the normal contour over the medial and lateral aspects of the patella. The *bulge sign*, which involves milking fluid from the lateral to the medial side of the patella, may be used to determine the presence of excess fluid when it is not visible. Joint contractures, instability, and genu valgus (knock-knee) deformity are other possible manifestations. Severe quadriceps atrophy can contribute to the disability. *Baker's cyst* may occur in the popliteal area behind the knee. This is caused by enlarge-

ment of the bursa and usually does not cause symptoms unless the cyst ruptures, in which case symptoms mimicking thrombophlebitis appear.

Disease activity can limit flexion and extension of the ankle, which can create difficulty in walking. Involvement of the metatarsophalangeal joints can cause subluxation, hallux valgus, and hammer toe deformities.

Neck discomfort is common. In rare cases, longstanding disease can lead to neurologic complications such as occipital headaches, muscle weakness, and numbness and tingling in the upper extremities. More severe but less common neurologic complications are dislocation of the first cervical vertebra and subluxation of the odontoid process of the second vertebra into the foramen magnum, which can lead to paralysis and is potentially fatal.

Extra-articular Manifestations.   Although characteristically a joint disease, rheumatoid arthritis can affect a number of other tissues. Extra-articular manifestations probably occur with a fair degree of frequency but usually are mild enough to cause few problems. They are most likely to occur in persons with rheumatoid factor.

Because rheumatoid arthritis is a systemic disease, it may be accompanied by complaints of fatigue, weakness, anorexia, weight loss, and low-grade fever when the disease is active. The erythrocyte sedimentation rate (ESR), which commonly is elevated during inflammatory processes, has been found to correlate with the amount of disease activity.[5] Anemia associated with a low serum iron level or low iron-binding capacity is common.[1] This anemia usually is resistant to iron therapy.

Rheumatoid nodules are granulomatous lesions that develop around small blood vessels. The nodules may be tender or nontender, movable or immovable, and small or large. Typically, they are found over pressure points such as the extensor surfaces of the ulna. The nodules may remain unless surgically removed, or they may resolve spontaneously.

Vasculitis is an uncommon manifestation of rheumatoid arthritis in persons with a long history of active arthritis and high titers of rheumatoid factor. It is possible that some persons have vasculitis that remains silent. Vasculitis is caused by the inflammatory process affecting the small and medium-sized arterioles (see Chapter 22). Manifesta-

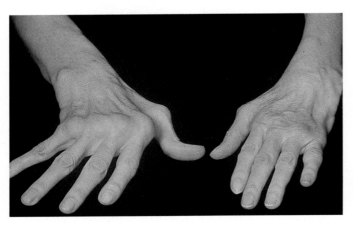

FIGURE 59-4 Subluxation of the metacarpophalangeal joints of the fingers in rheumatoid arthritis (swan neck deformity). (Reprinted from the ARHP Arthritis Teaching Slide Collection. Used with permission of the American College of Rheumatology.)

tions include ischemic areas in the nail fold and digital pulp that appear as brown spots. Ulcerations may occur in the lower extremities, particularly around the malleolar areas. In some cases, neuropathy may be the only symptom of vasculitis. The visceral organs, such as the heart, lungs, and gastrointestinal tract, also may be affected.

Other extra-articular manifestations include eye lesions such as episcleritis and scleritis, hematologic abnormalities, pulmonary disease, cardiac complications, infection, and Felty's syndrome (*i.e.*, leukopenia with or without splenomegaly).

Diagnosis and Treatment

The diagnosis of rheumatoid arthritis is based on findings of the history, physical examination, and laboratory tests. Information should be elicited regarding the duration of symptoms, systemic manifestations, stiffness, and family history. The criteria for rheumatoid arthritis developed by the American Rheumatism Association are useful in establishing the diagnosis (Chart 59-1). At least four of the criteria must be present to make a diagnosis of rheumatoid arthritis. Practitioners must realize that these criteria were developed for use in epidemiologic studies and are designed for classification purposes and not as diagnostic criteria, but they can be used as guidelines for diagnosing the illness in individual patients.

In the early stages, the disease often is difficult to diagnose. On physical examination, the affected joints show signs of inflammation, swelling, tenderness, and possibly warmth and reduced motion. The joints have a soft, spongy feeling because of the synovial thickening and inflammation. Body movements may be guarded to prevent pain. Changes in joint structure usually are not visible early in the disease.

CHART 59-1

Proposed 1987 Revised American Rheumatism Association Criteria for Rheumatoid Arthritis

Four or more of the following conditions must be present to establish a diagnosis of rheumatoid arthritis:
1. Morning stiffness for at least 1 hour and present for at least 6 weeks
2. Swelling of three or more joints for at least 6 weeks
3. Swelling of wrist, metacarpophalangeal, or proximal interphalangeal joints for 6 or more weeks
4. Symmetric joint swelling
5. Hand roentgenogram changes typical of rheumatoid arthritis that must include erosions or unequivocal bony decalcification
6. Rheumatoid nodules
7. Serum rheumatoid factor identified by a method that is positive in less than 5% of normal subjects

(From Arthritis Foundation. [1997]. *Primer on the rheumatic diseases* [11th ed.]. Atlanta: Author. Used with the permission of the Arthritis Foundation.)

Rheumatoid factor test results are not diagnostic for rheumatoid arthritis, but they can be of value in differentiating rheumatoid arthritis from other forms of arthritis. Between 1% and 5% of healthy persons have rheumatoid factor, and its presence seems to be more common with advancing age.[1] A person can have rheumatoid arthritis without having rheumatoid factor.[6] Radiologic findings also are not diagnostic in rheumatoid arthritis because joint erosions often are not seen on radiographic images in the early stages of the disorder. Synovial fluid analysis can be helpful in the diagnostic process. The synovial fluid has a cloudy appearance, the white blood cell count is elevated as a result of inflammation, and the complement components are decreased.

The treatment goals for a person with rheumatoid arthritis are to reduce pain, minimize stiffness and swelling, maintain mobility, and become an informed health care consumer. The treatment plan includes education about the disease and its treatment, rest, therapeutic exercises, and medications. Because of the chronicity of the disease and the need for continuous, long-term adherence to the prescribed treatment modalities, it is important that the treatment be integrated with the person's lifestyle.

Strategies to aid in symptom control also involve regulating activity by pacing, establishing priorities, and setting realistic goals. Support groups and group education experiences benefit some persons. The home and work environments should be assessed, and interventions should be incorporated as the situation warrants.

Both physical and emotional rest are important aspects of care. Physical rest reduces joint stress. Rest of specific joints is recommended to relieve pain. For example, sitting reduces the weight on an inflamed knee, and the use of light-weight splints reduces undue movement of the hand or wrist. Some persons find that discomfort increases with emotional stress; with emotional rest, muscles relax, and discomfort is reduced. Although rest is essential, therapeutic exercises also are important in maintaining joint motion and muscle strength. Range-of-motion exercises involve the active and passive movement of joints. Isometric (muscle-tensing) exercises may be used to strengthen muscles. These exercises frequently are taught by a physical therapist and performed daily at home. The difference between normal activity and therapeutic exercise should be emphasized. Aerobic exercise can be an important component of the treatment regimen of selected patients. Studies have shown that although persons with rheumatoid arthritis in general have low levels of physical fitness, they can benefit from individualized exercise programs without experiencing joint damage or flare-ups of the disease.[7]

Instruction in the safe use of heat and cold modalities to relieve discomfort and in the use of relaxation techniques also is important. Proper posture, positioning, body mechanics, and the use of supportive shoes can provide further comfort. There often is a need for information about the principles of joint protection and work simplification. Some persons need assistive devices to reduce pain and improve their ability to perform activities of daily living. The goals of pharmacologic therapy for rheumatoid

Management of Rheumatoid Arthritis

➤ Early diagnosis and treatment are necessary to improve long-term outcomes.

➤ Nonpharmacologic approaches include patient education, physical and occupational therapy, psychological support, and promotion of self-management strategies.

➤ Pharmacologic approaches include nonsteroidal anti-inflammatory drugs, traditional disease-modifying antirheumatic drugs, biologic agents, and corticosteroids.

arthritis are to reduce pain, decrease inflammation, maintain or restore joint function, and prevent bone and cartilage destruction. Medications used to achieve these goals are classified as those that provide relief of arthritis symptoms and those that have the potential for modifying the course of the disease.

The trend in management of rheumatoid arthritis is toward a more aggressive pharmacologic approach earlier in the disease. A window of opportunity for improved disease management occurs within 2 years of disease onset. Early treatment is based on the theory that T-cell–dependent pathways, which manifest early in the inflammatory process, are more responsive to treatment than later in the process, when disease progression may be controlled by activated fibroblasts and macrophages, and the disease may be more resistant to treatment.[5]

Nonsteroidal anti-inflammatory drugs (NSAIDs) usually are the first choice in the treatment of rheumatoid

CHART 59-2

Proposed Criteria for Clinical Remission in Rheumatoid Arthritis

Five or more of the following requirements must be fulfilled for at least 2 consecutive months:

1. Duration of morning stiffness not exceeding 15 minutes
2. No fatigue
3. No joint pain (by history)
4. No joint tenderness or pain on motion
5. No soft tissue swelling in joints or tendon sheaths
6. Erythrocyte sedimentation rate (Westergren method) less than 30 mm/hour for a female or 20 mm/hour for a male

(From Arthritis Foundation. [1997]. *Primer on rheumatic diseases* [11th ed.]. Atlanta: Author. Used with permission of the Arthritis Foundation.)

arthritis. The NSAIDs inhibit the production of prostaglandins, which have a damaging effect on joint structures. NSAIDs, including salicylates (*e.g.*, aspirin), provide analgesic and anti-inflammatory effects. Effectiveness, side effects, cost, and dosing schedules are considered when selecting an NSAID. There is a wide range of responses to the various NSAIDs, and the particular NSAID that works best for any one individual is not always predictable. The incidence of adverse reactions to the NSAIDs increases with age and long-term use; adverse reactions may include gastric irritation, kidney damage, changes in liver function, anemia, rashes, headaches, and confusion.

A new class of NSAIDs, the cyclooxygenase-2 (COX-2) inhibitors, has been developed with the goal of decreasing the gastrointestinal adverse effects seen with the traditional NSAIDs. COX-2 inhibitors have been shown to inhibit inflammatory processes, but do not inhibit the protective prostaglandin synthesis in the gastrointestinal tract.[8] The COX-2 agents (*e.g.*, celecoxib and rofecoxib) do not inhibit COX-1, which mediates the production of prostaglandins not only in the physiologic function of the gastrointestinal tract but in the maintenance of platelet aggregation and renal blood flow, thereby reducing the overall incidence of serious adverse events.[9]

Second-line drug therapy is initiated early in the disease if joint symptoms persist despite use of NSAIDs. Disease-modifying antirheumatic drugs (DMARDs) include gold salts, hydroxychloroquine, sulfasalazine, methotrexate, and azathioprine. Methotrexate has become the drug of choice because of its potency, and it is relatively fast acting (*i.e.*, improvement is seen in 1 month) compared with the slower-acting DMARDs, which can take 3 to 4 months to work. Methotrexate is thought to interfere with purine metabolism, leading to the release of adenosine, a potent anti-inflammatory compound. All of the DMARDs can be toxic and require close monitoring for adverse effects, especially those related to bone marrow suppression.[10]

Corticosteroid drugs may be used to reduce discomfort. To avoid long-term side effects, they are used only in specific situations for short-term therapy at a low dose level. They may be used for unremitting disease with extra-articular manifestations. Corticosteroids may interrupt the inflammatory and immune cascade at several levels, such as by interfering with inflammatory cell adhesion and migration, impairing prostaglandin synthesis, and inhibiting neutrophil superoxide production.[11] This medication does not modify the disease and is unable to prevent joint destruction. Intra-articular corticosteroid injections can provide rapid relief of acute or subacute inflammatory synovitis (after infection is excluded) in a few joints. They should not be repeated more than a few times each year.

Newer antirheumatic drugs include leflunamide, etanercept, and infliximab. Leflunamide (Arava) is a pyrimidine synthesis inhibitor that blocks the expansion of T cells. Its efficacy is equal to that of methotrexate.[12] Infliximab (Remicade) and etanercept (Enbrel) are biologic response–modifying agents that block tumor necrosis factor-α (TNF-α), one of the key proinflammatory cytokines in rheumatoid arthritis. Both of the anti–TNF-α agents have been shown to slow radiographic progression of rheumatoid arthritis.[13]

Another approach to rheumatoid arthritis treatment is combination therapy. This approach is still considered experimental, but it has been shown to be effective in early studies. Individual drugs with different mechanisms of action are given simultaneously to control the disease. A typical drug combination may include hydroxychloroquine, sulfasalazine plus methotrexate or cyclosporine, leflunamide, or etanercept plus methotrexate. These combinations are given in addition to an NSAID. Drugs then are tapered as symptoms subside and clinical remission is achieved.[14]

Apheresis is a newer approved treatment strategy for patients with severe rheumatoid arthritis and long-standing disease who have failed other DMARDs. A specific device, the Prosorba column, has been developed for the therapeutic removal of IgG and IgG-containing circulating immune complexes from plasma. The apheresis treatments are given weekly over 12 weeks, with approximately 30% of patients responding to the treatment.[15]

Surgery also may be a part of the treatment of rheumatoid arthritis. Synovectomy may be indicated to reduce pain and joint damage when synovitis does not respond to medical treatment. The most common soft tissue surgery is tenosynovectomy (*i.e.*, repair of damaged tendons) of the hand to release nerve entrapments. Total joint replacements (*i.e.*, arthroplasty) may be indicated to reduce pain and increase motion. Arthrodesis (*i.e.*, joint fusion) is indicated only in extreme cases when there is so much soft tissue damage and scarring or infection that a replacement is impossible.

Although the course of rheumatoid arthritis is unpredictable, increasingly effective treatments for the disease have been developed since the late 1990s. Patients with arthritis symptoms are being diagnosed and treated earlier, and criteria have been developed for remission in rheumatoid arthritis (Chart 59-2).

SYSTEMIC LUPUS ERYTHEMATOSUS

Systemic lupus erythematosus is a chronic inflammatory disease that can affect virtually any organ system, including the musculoskeletal system. It is a major rheumatic disease, with a prevalence of approximately 1 case per 2000 persons. Approximately 500,000 persons in the United States have this disease. There is a female predominance of 9 to 1, and this ratio is closer to 30 to 1 during the childbearing years. SLE is more common in African Americans, Hispanics, and Asians than whites, and the incidence in some families is higher than in others.[1]

Etiology and Pathogenesis
The cause of SLE is unknown. It is characterized by the formation of autoantibodies and immune complexes. Persons with SLE appear to have B-cell hyperreactivity and increased production of antibodies against self (*i.e.*, autoantibodies) and nonself antigens. These B cells are polyclonal, meaning that there are multiple B-cell clones, each producing a different type of antibody. Antibodies have been identified against an array of nuclear and cytoplasmic cell components. B-cell hyperreactivity could result from several mechanisms. In theory, excessive functioning of helper T cells or defective functioning of suppressor T cells could alter the B-cell response (see Chapter 18).

The development of autoantibodies can result from a combination of factors, including genetic, hormonal, immunologic, and environmental factors.[16] Genetic predisposition is evidenced by the occurrence of familial cases of SLE, especially among identical twins. The increased incidence among African Americans compared with whites also suggests genetic factors. As many as four genes may be involved in the expression of SLE in humans. Genes linked to the HLA-DR and HLA-DQ loci in the MHC class II molecules show strong support for a genetic link in the development of SLE.[17]

Studies also suggest that an imbalance in sex hormone levels may play a role in the development of the disease, especially because the disease is so prevalent among women. Androgens appear to protect and estrogens seem to favor the development of SLE. It has been suggested that an imbalance in sex hormone levels may lead to a heightened helper T-cell and weakened suppressor T-cell immune response that could lead to the development of autoantibodies.[1]

Possible environmental triggers include ultraviolet (UV) light, chemicals (*e.g.*, hydralazine, procainamide, hair dyes), some foods, and possibly infectious agents.[16] UV light, specifically UVB associated with exposure to the sun or unshielded fluorescent bulbs, may trigger exacerbations. Photosensitivity occurs in approximately one third of patients with SLE.

The pathologic process probably begins with the activation of polyclonal B cells, causing exaggerated production of autoantibodies. The autoantibodies combine with corresponding antigens to form immune complexes. These immune complexes are deposited in vascular and tissue surfaces, triggering an inflammatory response and ultimately causing local tissue injury. Some autoantibodies that have been identified in SLE are anti-nuclear antibodies (ANA), including anti-deoxyribonucleic acid (DNA). Other antibodies may be produced against various cells, including red blood cell surface antigens, platelets, coagulation factors, and other antibodies. Autoantibodies against red blood cells can lead to anemia and those against platelets to thrombocytopenia. Certain drugs may provoke a lupus-like disorder in susceptible persons, particularly in the elderly. The most common of these drugs are hydralazine and procainamide. Other drugs, such as quinidine, chlorpromazine, methyldopa, isoniazid, and phenytoin, also have been known to produce this syndrome. The disease usually recedes when the drug is discontinued.[16]

Clinical Manifestations
Systemic lupus erythematosus can manifest in a variety of ways. The disease has been called the *great imitator* because it has the capacity for affecting many different body systems, including the musculoskeletal system, the skin, the cardiovascular system, the lungs, the kidneys, the central nervous system (CNS), and the red blood cells and platelets. The onset may be acute or insidious, and the course of the disease is characterized by exacerbations and remissions. Rare cases result in death within weeks or months.

Arthralgias and arthritis are among the most commonly occurring early symptoms of SLE; approximately 90% of all persons with the disease complain of joint pain at some point during the course of their disease.[17] The polyarthritis of SLE initially can be confused with other forms of arthritis, especially rheumatoid arthritis, because of the symmetric arthropathy. However, on radiologic examination, articular destruction rarely is found. Ligaments, tendons, and the joint capsule may be involved, causing varied deformities in approximately 30% of persons with the disease. Flexion contractures, hyperextension of the interphalangeal joint, and subluxation of the carpometacarpal joint contribute to the deformity and subsequent loss of function in the hands. Other musculoskeletal manifestations of SLE include tenosynovitis, rupture of the intrapatellar and Achilles tendons, and avascular necrosis, frequently of the femoral head.

Skin manifestations can vary greatly and may be classified as acute, subacute, or chronic. The acute skin lesions include the classic malar or "butterfly" rash on the nose and cheeks (Fig. 59-5). This rash is seen in SLE but may be associated with other skin lesions, such as hives or livedo reticularis (*i.e.*, reticular cyanotic discoloration of the skin, often precipitated by cold) and fingertip lesions, such as periungual erythema, nail fold infarcts, and splinter hemorrhages. Hair loss is common. Mucous membrane lesions tend to occur during periods of exacerbation. Sun sensitivity may occur in SLE even after mild sun exposure.

Renal involvement occurs in approximately 50% of persons with SLE. Several forms of glomerulonephritis may occur, including mesangial, focal proliferative, diffuse proliferative, and membranous (see Chapter 33). Interstitial nephritis also may occur. Nephrotic syndrome causes proteinuria with resultant edema in the legs, abdomen, and around the eyes. Renal failure may or may not be preceded by the nephrotic syndrome. Kidney biopsy is the best determinant of renal damage and the extent of treatment needed.

Pulmonary involvement in SLE occurs in 40% to 50% of patients and is manifested primarily by pleural effusions or pleuritis. Less frequently occurring pulmonary problems include acute pneumonitis, pulmonary hemorrhage, chronic interstitial lung disease, and pulmonary embolism.

Pericarditis is the most common of the cardiac manifestation, occurring in up to 30% to 40% of persons with SLE and often accompanied by pleural effusions. Myocarditis affects as many as 25% of those with SLE. Congenital heart block can occur in infants of mothers with lupus who have a specific type of ANA (anti-Ro) in their serum. Secondary heart disease also is a problem in those with SLE. Hypertension may be associated with lupus nephritis and long-term corticosteroid use. Ischemic heart disease can occur in older patients with longer-duration SLE. Infective carditis is rare but can occur with valvular lesions.[17]

The CNS is involved in 30% to 75% of persons with SLE. The pathologic basis for the CNS symptoms is not entirely clear. It has been ascribed to an acute vasculitis that impedes blood flow, causing strokes or hemorrhage; an immune response involving anti-neuronal antibodies that attack nerve cells; or production of anti-phospholipid antibodies that damage blood vessels and cause blood clots in the brain. Seizures can occur and are more frequent when renal failure is present. Psychotic symptoms, including depression and unnatural euphoria, as well as decreased cognitive functioning, confusion, and altered levels of consciousness may develop. More research is being done on the role of psychological factors in triggering the onset of SLE.

Hematologic disorders may manifest as hemolytic anemia, leukopenia, lymphopenia, or thrombocytopenia. Lymphadenopathy also may occur in 50% of all patients with SLE.[17] Discoid SLE (*i.e.*, chronic cutaneous lupus) involves plaquelike lesions on the head, scalp, and neck. These lesions first appear as red, swollen patches of skin, and later there can be scarring, depigmentation, and plugging of hair follicles. Ninety percent of patients with discoid lupus have disease that involves only the skin.

Subacute cutaneous lupus erythematosus (SCLE) is a less severe form of lupus. The skin lesions in this condition may resemble psoriasis. These lesions are found in sun-exposed areas such as the face, chest, upper back, and arms. Patients with SCLE may have mild systemic problems, which usually are limited to joint and muscle pains. There is a low incidence of lupus nephritis among those with SCLE.

Diagnosis and Treatment

The diagnosis of SLE can be complicated and difficult. The American College of Rheumatology has defined 11 criteria to be considered in the diagnosis of the disease, but these are intended for use in clinical trials rather than for indi-

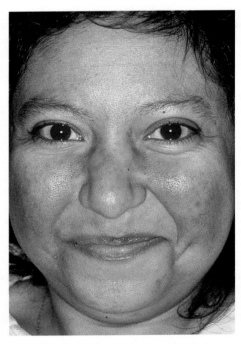

FIGURE 59-5 The butterfly (malar) rash of systemic lupus erythematosus. (Reprinted from the ARHP Arthritis Teaching Slide Collection. Used with permission of the American College of Rheumatology.)

Clinical Manifestations of Systemic Lupus Erythematosus

➤ SLE is known as the *great imitator*, with manifestations that resemble many other diseases.

- ➤ Constitutional—fevers, fatigue, anorexia, weight loss

- ➤ Musculoskeletal—arthritis, muscle weakness and atrophy, avascular necrosis

- ➤ Dermatologic—alopecia, photosensitivity, rash

- ➤ Cardiovascular—pericarditis, systolic murmurs, valvular complications

- ➤ Pulmonary—pleuritis, pneumonitis, pulmonary hypertension

- ➤ Renal—nephritis, glomerulonephritis

- ➤ Neuropsychiatric—cognitive dysfunction, depression, psychosis

vidual diagnosis.[18] Diagnosis is based on a complete history, physical examination, and analysis of blood work. No single test can diagnose SLE in all persons.

The most common laboratory test performed is the immunofluorescence test for ANA. Ninety-five percent of persons with untreated SLE have high ANA levels. The ANA test is not specific for lupus, and positive ANA results may be found in healthy persons or may be associated with other disorders. The anti-DNA antibody test is more specific for the diagnosis of SLE.[17] Other serum tests may reveal moderate to severe anemia, thrombocytopenia, and leukocytosis or leukopenia. Additional immunologic tests may be done to give support to the diagnosis or to differentiate SLE from other connective tissue diseases.

Treatment of SLE focuses on managing the acute and chronic symptoms of the disease. Communication and trust between health care providers and the person with SLE are the basis for long-term disease management. The person with SLE is the best source of information about the pattern of his or her disease activity. Teamwork can reduce the need for unnecessary hospitalization, testing, expense, and anxiety. The goals of treatment include preventing progressive loss of organ function, reducing the possibility of exacerbations, minimizing disability from the disease process, and preventing complications from medication therapy.[19] Treatment with medications may be as simple as a drug to reduce inflammation, such as an NSAID. NSAIDs can control fever, arthritis, and mild pleuritis. An antimalarial drug (*e.g.,* hydroxychloroquine) may be the next medication considered to treat cutaneous and musculoskeletal manifestations of SLE. Corticosteroids are used to treat more significant symptoms of SLE, such as renal and CNS disorders. High-dose corticosteroid treatment is used for acute symptoms, and the drug is tapered to the lowest ther-

apeutic dose as soon as possible to minimize the adverse effects. Immunosuppressive drugs are used in cases of severe disease. Cyclophosphamide, under closely monitored circumstances, has been found to be beneficial in the treatment of lupus nephritis.[20]

SYSTEMIC SCLEROSIS

Systemic sclerosis, often prefixed by the term *progressive*, is sometimes called *scleroderma*. The condition is systemic and may involve the lungs, esophagus, heart, duodenum, and kidneys. In this disorder, the skin is thickened through fibrosis, with an accompanying fixation to the subdermal structures, including the sheaths or fascia covering tendons and muscles. African Americans and women are more susceptible to this disease than white men. Clinical manifestations include muscular atrophy, pain, edema, calcification, and arthrodesis. Studies have indicated that if heart, lung, or kidney involvement is to become severe, it tends to do so early in disease and is a predictor of shortened survival; therefore, early detection and implementation of treatment are necessary. Patients who survive the first few years without developing severe organ involvement are less likely to develop life-threatening involvement later in their illness.[21] The cause of this rare disorder, although characterized by proliferative vascular changes, is not well understood.

A variant of systemic sclerosis is the CREST syndrome. This acronym represents the manifestations of calcinosis, Raynaud's phenomenon, esophageal dysmotility, sclerodactyly (localized scleroderma of the fingers), and telangiectasia.

POLYMYOSITIS AND DERMATOMYOSITIS

Polymyositis and dermatomyositis are chronic inflammatory myopathies. The pathogenesis is multifactorial and includes cellular and humoral immune mechanisms. Systemic manifestations are common, and cardiac and pulmonary complications often adversely affect the outcome. These conditions are characterized by symmetric proximal muscle weakness and occasional muscle pain and tenderness.

In summary, rheumatoid arthritis is a systemic inflammatory disorder that affects 0.3% to 1.5% of the population. Women are affected more frequently than men. This form of arthritis, the cause of which is unknown, has a chronic course and usually is characterized by remissions and exacerbations. Joint involvement is symmetric and begins with inflammatory changes in the synovial membrane. As joint inflammation progresses, structural changes can occur, leading to joint instability and eventual deformity. Systemic manifestations include weakness, anorexia, weight loss, and low-grade fever. Some extra-articular features include rheumatoid nodules and vasculitis. The treatment goals include reducing pain, stiffness, and swelling, maintaining mobility, and assisting the person to become an informed health care consumer.

Systemic lupus erythematosus is a chronic auto-immune disorder that affects multiple body systems. There is no known cause of SLE, but the disease may result from an immunoregulatory disturbance brought about by a combination of genetic, hormonal, and environmental factors. Some drugs have been shown to induce lupus, especially in the elderly. There is an exaggerated production of autoantibodies, which interact with antigens to produce an immune complex. These immune complexes produce an inflammatory response in affected tissues. Treatment focuses on preventing loss of organ function, controlling inflammation, and minimizing complications of medication therapy.

Systemic sclerosis, often prefixed by the term *progressive*, is sometimes called *scleroderma*. In this disorder, the skin is thickened through fibrosis with an accompanying fixation to the subdermal structures, including the sheaths or fascia covering tendons and muscles. Polymyositis and dermatomyositis are chronic inflammatory myopathies. The pathogenesis is multifactorial and includes cellular and humoral immune mechanisms.

Arthritis Associated With Spondylitis

After you have completed this section of the chapter, you should be able to meet the following objectives:

✦ Cite a definition of the seronegative spondyloarthropathies

✦ Cite the primary features of ankylosing spondylitis

✦ Describe how the site of inflammation differs in spondyloarthropathies from that in rheumatoid arthritis

✦ Contrast and compare ankylosing spondylitis, reactive arthritis, and psoriatic arthritis in terms of cause, pathogenesis, and clinical manifestations

The *spondyloarthropathies* are an interrelated group of multisystem inflammatory disorders that primarily affect the axial skeleton, particularly the spine. Inflammation develops at sites where ligament inserts into bone rather than in the synovium. Sacroiliitis is the pathologic hallmark. The person with spondyloarthropathy sometimes also has inflammation and involvement of the peripheral joints, in which case the signs and symptoms overlap with other inflammatory types of arthritis. However, the spondyloarthropathies differ from rheumatoid arthritis in that there is an absence of the rheumatoid factor; these disorders often are referred to as *seronegative spondyloarthropathies* (Table 59-1).

The seronegative spondyloarthropathies include ankylosing spondylitis, juvenile ankylosing spondylitis, reactive arthritis, enteropathic arthritis (*i.e.,* inflammatory bowel disease), and psoriatic arthritis. There is clinical evidence of overlap between the various seronegative spondyloarthropathies. In none of these disorders is the cause or pathogenesis well understood. There is a striking association with the HLA-B27 antigen, but the presence of the HLA-B27 antigen by itself is neither necessary nor sufficient for the development of any of the diseases.

ANKYLOSING SPONDYLITIS

Ankylosing spondylitis is a chronic, systemic inflammatory disease of the axial skeleton, including the sacroiliac joints, intervertebral disk spaces, and the apophyseal and costovertebral articulations. Bilateral sacroiliitis is a primary feature of the disease. Occasionally, large synovial joints (*i.e.,* hips, knees, and shoulders) may be involved. The small peripheral joints usually are not affected. The sites of ligament insertion into bone are eroded by inflammatory cells, with subsequent formation of woven bone. Ankylosing spondylitis may cause fibrosis, calcification, and ossification of joints, with progression to ankylosis. The joint becomes ankylosed when bone replaces ligament throughout its length.

The disease brings to mind an image of a person bent over looking at the floor and unable to straighten up. X-ray films show a rigid, bamboo-like spine. Fortunately, few persons develop a progressive disease pattern that leads to this outcome. The disease spectrum ranges from an asymptom-

TABLE 59-1 ✦ Comparison of the Spondyloarthropathies				
Characteristic	Ankylosing Spondylitis	Reiter's Syndrome	Psoriatic Arthritis	Inflammatory Bowel Disease
Age at onset	Young adult	Young to middle age	Any age	Any age
Type of onset	Gradual	Sudden	Variable	Gradual
Sacroiliitis	>95%	20%	20%	10%
Peripheral joint involvement	25%	90%	All (about 5% to 7% of those patients with psoriasis)	Occasional
HLA-B27 (in whites)	>90%	75%	<50%	<50%
Eye involvement	25% to 30%	Common	Occasional	Occasional

(Adapted from Arnett F.C., Khan M.A., Willikens R.F. [1989]. A new look at ankylosing spondylitis. *Patient Care* 23 [19], 82–101)

atic sacroiliitis to a progressive disease that can affect many body systems. The progressive disease pattern usually affects men.

Etiology and Pathogenesis

Ankylosing spondylitis is more common than once was believed, affecting approximately 2% to 8% of the HLA-B27–positive white population.[1] Epidemiologic findings indicate that genetic and environmental factors play a role in the pathogenesis of the disease. Clinical manifestations usually begin in late adolescence or early adulthood and are slightly more common in men than in women. The disease evolves more slowly and is less severe in women.

The pathogenesis of ankylosing spondylitis is not well understood. The presence of mononuclear cells in acutely involved tissue suggests an immune response. The HLA-B27 antigen remains one of the best-known examples of an association between a disease and a hereditary marker. Although approximately 90% of those with ankylosing spondylitis possess the HLA-B27 antigen and nearly 100% of those who also have uveitis or aortitis have the marker, the HLA-B27 antigen also is present in approximately 8% of the normal population. Several theories have been advanced to account for the association between the HLA-B27 antigen and ankylosing spondylitis. One possibility is that the gene that determines the HLA-B27 antigen may be linked to other genes that determine pathologic autoimmune phenomena or that lead to increased susceptibility to infections or environmental agents. A second theory postulates molecular mimicry; an autoimmune reaction to an antigenic determinant site in the host's tissues may occur as a consequence of an immunologic response to an identical or closely related antigen of a foreign agent, usually an infectious agent.

Clinical Manifestations

The person with ankylosing spondylitis typically complains of low back pain, which may be persistent or intermittent. The pain, which becomes worse when resting, particularly when lying in bed, initially may be blamed on muscle strain or spasm from physical activity. Lumbosacral pain also may be present, with discomfort in the buttocks and hip areas. Sometimes, pain can radiate to the thigh in a manner similar to that of sciatic pain. Prolonged stiffness is present in the morning and after periods of rest. Mild physical activity or a hot shower helps reduce pain and stiffness. Sleep patterns frequently are interrupted because of these manifestations. Walking or exercise may be needed to provide the comfort needed to return to sleep. Muscle spasm also may contribute to discomfort.

Loss of motion in the spinal column is characteristic of the disease. The severity and duration of disease activity influence the degree of mobility. Loss of lumbar lordosis occurs as the disease progresses, and this is followed by kyphosis of the thoracic spine and extension of the neck. A spine fused in the flexed position is the end result in severe ankylosing spondylitis. A kyphotic spine makes it difficult for the patient to look ahead and to maintain balance while walking. The heart and lungs are constricted in the chest cavity. Abnormal weight bearing can lead to degeneration and destruction of the hips, necessitating joint replacement procedures. Peripheral arthritis is more common in hips and shoulders. The incidence of hip joint involvement varies from 17% to 36% and potentially is more crippling than involvement in any other joint.[1] A lower age at onset and a presenting manifestation of hip joint involvement indicate a greater likelihood of progression to the need for total hip replacement. The most common extraskeletal involvement is acute anterior uveitis, which occurs in 25% to 30% of patients sometime in the course of their disease.[1] Systemic features of weight loss, fever, and fatigue may be apparent. Sometimes, the fatigue is a greater problem than pain or stiffness. Osteoporosis can occur, especially in the spine, which contributes to the risk of spinal fracture. Fusion of the costovertebral joints can lead to reduced lung volume.

The disease process varies considerably among individuals. Exacerbations and remissions are common; their unpredictability can create uncertainty in planning daily activities and in setting goals. Fortunately, most of those affected are able to lead productive lives. The prognosis for ankylosing spondylitis in general is good. The first decade of disease predicts the remainder. Severe disease usually occurs early and is marked by peripheral arthritis, especially of the hip. The mortality rate is low (6%), and significant disability occurs in fewer than 20% of persons with the disorder.

Diagnosis and Treatment

The early and precise diagnosis of ankylosing spondylitis is closely related to a favorable prognosis. Early recognition allows for implementation of a conservative and usually effective treatment program on a lifelong basis. The diagnosis of ankylosing spondylitis is based on history, physical examination, and x-ray examination. Several methods are available to assess mobility and detect sacroiliitis. These methods include pressure on the sacroiliac joints with the person in a forward-bending position to elicit pain and muscle spasm, measurement of the distance between the tips of fingers and the floor in a bent-over position with straight knees, and a modified Schöber's test in which contralateral flexion of the back is measured. Although these measures alone do not provide a diagnosis of ankylosing spondylitis or other spondyloarthropathies, they can provide useful measurements for monitoring the disease status. Chest expansion may be used as an indirect indicator of thoracic involvement, which usually occurs late in the disease course. Measurements are taken at the fourth intercostal space. Normally, the chest expands by 4 to 5 cm with inspiration. This measurement is more difficult to obtain in women and less specific in older persons with normally decreased expansion, in smokers, or in those with emphysema.

Laboratory findings frequently include an elevated ESR. The patient also may have a mild normocytic normochromic anemia. HLA typing is not diagnostic of the disease and should not be used as a routine screening procedure. Radiologic evaluations help differentiate sacroiliitis from other diseases. In early disease, x-ray images may be negative. Vertebrae normally are concave on the anterior border. In ankylosing spondylitis, the vertebrae take on a squared appearance (Fig. 59-6). Progressive spinal changes usually follow an ascending pattern up the spine.

Treatment is directed at controlling pain and maintaining mobility by suppressing inflammation. The patient should be instructed in proper posture and positioning. This includes sleeping in a supine position on a firm mattress and using one small pillow or no pillow. Sleeping in extension may reduce the possibility of flexion contractures. A bed board may be used to supply additional firmness. Therapeutic exercises are important to assist in maintaining motion in peripheral joints and in the spine. Muscle-strengthening exercises for extensor muscle groups also are prescribed. Heat applications or a shower or bath may be beneficial before exercise to improve ease of movement. These strategies also can be used in the morning or at bedtime to reduce stiffness and pain. Immobilizing joints is not recommended. Maintaining ideal weight reduces the stress on weight-bearing joints. Smoking should be discouraged because it can exacerbate respiratory problems. Swimming is an excellent general conditioning exercise that avoids joint stress and enhances muscle tone. Occupational counseling or job evaluation may be warranted because of postural abnormalities. NSAIDs are used to reduce inflammation, which helps to control pain and reduce muscle spasm. Phenylbutazone is highly effective, but its use should be limited to persons with severe disease in

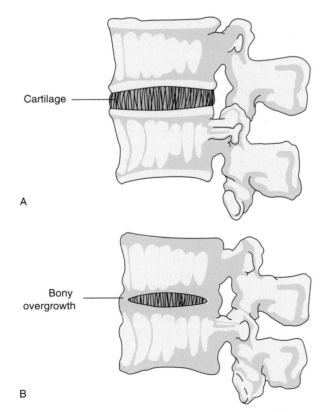

Cartilage

A

Bony overgrowth

B

FIGURE 59-6 The bony overgrowth (**B**) of the vertebra characteristic of ankylosing spondylitis is evident when compared with normal vertebra (**A**).

whom other agents have failed because of potential bone marrow suppression with long-term use. More recently, promising small-scale studies have been done suggesting anti–TNF-α agents are efficacious in the treatment of active ankylosing spondylitis.[22]

Most peripheral joint pain and limitations of motion occur in the hip. Total hip replacement surgery helps reduce pain and increase mobility. Anesthesia can be problematic for persons with cervical rigidity or reduced chest expansion. These factors must be weighed before surgery is considered.

REACTIVE ARTHRITIS

The reactive arthropathies may be defined as sterile inflammatory joint disorders that are distant in time and place from the initial inciting infective process. A reactive arthritis is a seronegative arthritis in which an infective trigger mechanism is suspected. The list of triggering agents is continuously increasing and may be divided into urogenic, enterogenic, and respiratory tract–associated, and the idiopathic arthritides. In some cases, the identity of the causative agent is unknown.

Rheumatic fever is a classic form of reactive arthritis. More recently recognized forms of reactive arthritis include those involving *Chlamydia pneumoniae* infection and hepatitis B vaccination. Reactive arthritis also has been observed in persons with acquired immunodeficiency syndrome (AIDS). Spondyloarthropathies such as Reiter's syndrome and psoriatic arthritis are more severe and frequent in human immunodeficiency virus (HIV)–infected patients than in the general population. It is thought the immune system response to HIV infection is selective and largely spares the natural killer cells, and these residual functioning components of the immune response may be critical in the pathogenesis of these conditions.[23,24] In contrast, rheumatoid arthritis and SLE dramatically improve as immunodeficiency develops. Reactive arthritis may result from the presence of a foreign substance in the joint tissue, as in silicone implants in the small joints of the hand or feet or after exposure to industrial gases and oils. However, there is no evidence of antigenicity of the causative substance. In the strictest sense, the definition of reactive arthritis includes a possibility of immunologic sensitization before arthritic development.[23] Having the HLA-B27 marker is not a prerequisite for development of reactive arthritis.

Similarities exist between reactive arthritis and bacterial arthritis. Several bacteria cause both diseases. When cultured bacteria are isolated from the synovial fluid, the diagnosis is bacterial arthritis. When they cannot be isolated, even though there has been a preceding infection, the diagnosis of reactive arthritis is made.

Reactive arthritis may follow a self-limited course; it may involve recurrent episodes of arthritis or, in a small number of cases, it may follow a continuous, unremitting course. The treatment is largely symptomatic. NSAIDs are used in treating the arthritic symptoms. Vigorous treatment of possible triggering infections is thought to prevent relapses of reactive arthritis, but in many cases, the triggering infection passes unnoticed or is mild, and the patient contacts a physician only with the onset of definite arthritis. Short antibiotic courses at this time are not effective.

Reiter's Syndrome

Reiter's syndrome is considered to be a clinical manifestation of reactive arthritis that may be accompanied by extra-articular symptoms such as uveitis, bowel inflammation, and carditis. Reiter's syndrome develops in a genetically susceptible host after an infection by bacteria, *Chlamydia trachomatis* in the genitourinary tract, or *Salmonella*, *Shigella*, *Yersinia*, or *Campylobacter* in the gastrointestinal tract.

The term *Reiter's syndrome* soon may be relegated to history as the pathogenesis becomes better understood. Alternative designations include SARA (sexually associated reactive arthritis) and the BASE syndrome (HLA-B27, arthritis, sacroiliitis, and extra-articular inflammation).[24] Reiter's syndrome was the first rheumatic disease to be recognized in association with HIV infection. Symptoms of arthritis may precede any overt signs of HIV disease. Treatment with agents such as methotrexate and azathioprine may further suppress the immune response and provoke a full expression of AIDS.

ENTEROPATHIC ARTHRITIS

Arthritis that is associated with an inflammatory bowel disease usually is considered an enteropathic arthritis because the intestinal disease is directly involved in the pathogenesis. Most cases of enteropathic arthritis are classified among the spondyloarthropathies. These include cases in which the arthritis is associated with inflammatory bowel disease (*i.e.*, ulcerative colitis and Crohn's disease), the reactive arthritides triggered by enterogenic bacteria, some of the undifferentiated spondyloarthropathies, Whipple's disease, and reactions after intestinal bypass surgery.[1] There is no direct relation between the activity of the bowel disease and the degree of arthritis activity.

PSORIATIC ARTHRITIS

Psoriatic arthritis is a seronegative inflammatory arthropathy. There seems to be a clinical similarity between reactive arthritis and psoriatic arthritis, suggesting a bacterial or other infectious trigger. Genetic susceptibility factors play an important role in expression of the psoriatic skin disease and the arthritis. The pathologic state of the synovium is similar to that in rheumatoid arthritis, with a few exceptions.

Although the arthritis can antedate detectable skin rash, the definitive diagnosis of psoriatic arthritis cannot be made without evidence of skin or nail changes typical of psoriasis. Psoriatic arthritis falls into five subgroups: oligoarticular, or asymmetric (48%); spondyloarthropathy (24%); polyarticular, or symmetric (18%); distal interphalangeal (8%); and mutilans (2%).[25] This heterogeneous clinical presentation suggests more than one disease is associated with psoriasis, or various clinical responses to a common cause. At least 20% of those with psoriatic arthritis have an elevated serum level of uric acid. The abnormally elevated serum uric acid level is caused by the rapid skin turnover of psoriasis, the breakdown of nucleic acid, and the metabolism to uric acid. This finding may lead to a misdiagnosis of gout. Psoriatic arthritis tends to be slowly progressive, but has a more favorable prognosis than rheumatoid arthritis.

Basic management is similar to the treatment of rheumatoid arthritis. Suppression of the skin disease may be important in helping control the arthritis. Often, affected joints are surprisingly functional and only minimally symptomatic.

> In summary, spondyloarthropathies affect the axial skeleton, particularly the spine. Inflammation develops at sites where ligaments insert into bone. They include ankylosing spondylitis, reactive arthritis, enteropathic arthritis, and psoriatic arthritis. Because they lack the rheumatoid factor, they are referred to as *seronegative spondyloarthropathies*. Ankylosing spondylitis is considered a prototype of this classification category. Bilateral sacroiliitis is the primary feature of ankylosing spondylitis. The disease spectrum ranges from asymptomatic sacroiliitis to a progressive disorder affecting many body systems. The cause remains unknown; however, a strong association between the HLA-B27 antigen and ankylosing spondylitis has been identified. Loss of motion in the spinal column is characteristic of the disease. Peripheral arthritis may occur in some persons. Other forms of spondyloarthritis include reactive arthritis, enteropathic arthritis, and psoriatic arthritis. Although there are overlapping features for each of the spondyloarthropathies, identifying etiologic differences and clinical manifestations is important for determining treatment.

◼ Osteoarthritis Syndrome

After you have completed this section of the chapter, you should be able to meet the following objectives:

✦ Compare rheumatoid arthritis and osteoarthritis in terms of joint involvement, level of inflammation, and local and systemic manifestations
✦ Describe the pathologic joint changes associated with osteoarthritis
✦ Characterize the treatment of osteoarthritis

Osteoarthritis, formerly called *degenerative joint disease*, is the most prevalent form of arthritis. It is second only to cardiovascular disease as the cause of chronic disability in adults.[26] Osteoarthritis is more of a disease process than a specific entity. The term encompasses a heterogeneous collection of syndromes. Clinical subsets include osteoarthritis of the hand, of the knee, of the hip, of the foot, and of the spine. It can lead to loss of mobility and chronic pain, often causing significant disability, especially when the involved joints are critical to carrying out daily activities. Fortunately, changes in the traditional conservative management of this underemphasized condition are occurring. Attitudes regarding the inevitability of the limitations imposed by this condition are changing on the part of health care providers and persons with the disease.

One third of all adults in the United States have radiographic evidence of osteoarthritis of the hand, foot, knee, or hip. Although the radiographic incidence of knee osteoarthritis increases with advancing age, the incidence of symptomatic osteoarthritis of the knee decreases.[27] The joint changes associated with osteoarthritis are progressive loss of articular cartilage and synovitis resulting from the inflammation caused by the attempts of the bone to remold itself, creating osteophytes or spurs. These changes are accompanied by joint pain, stiffness, limitation of motion, and possibly by joint instability and deformity. Although there may be periods of mild inflammation, it is not the severe, destructive type seen in the inflammatory forms of rheumatic diseases such as rheumatoid arthritis.

Osteoarthritis can occur as a primary idiopathic or a secondary disorder, although this distinction is not always clear. Idiopathic or primary variants of osteoarthritis occur as localized or generalized (*i.e.*, more than three joints) syndromes. Chart 59-3 lists examples of the post-traumatic disorders, anatomic and bony disorders, metabolic disorders, neuropathic arthritis, and hereditary disorders of collagen. Sex and age interact to influence the time of onset and, with race, the pattern of joint involvement. Men are affected more commonly at a younger age than women, but the rate of women affected exceeds that of men by middle age.

Hand osteoarthritis is more likely to affect white women, whereas knee osteoarthritis is more common in black women. The incidence of hip osteoarthritis is less among the Chinese than Europeans, perhaps representing the influence of other factors such as occupation, obesity, or heredity. Obesity is a risk factor for osteoarthritis of the knee in women and a contributory biomechanical factor in the pathogenesis of the disease. Weight loss reduces the risk of developing symptomatic osteoarthritis of the knee.[27] Excess fat may have a direct metabolic effect on cartilage beyond the effects of excess joint stress. Heredity influences the occurrence of hand osteoarthritis in the DIP joint. Bone mass may influence the risk of developing osteoarthritis. In theory, thinner subchondral bone mass may provide a greater shock-absorbing function than denser bone, allowing less direct trauma to the cartilage. Studies also implicate immunologic factors in the perpetuation and acceleration of osteoarthritic changes.[28]

PATHOGENESIS

Osteoarthritis is not a simple consequence of aging; it is an active metabolic disorder of the articular cartilage and subchondral bone (*i.e.*, bony plate that supports the articular cartilage) of diarthrodial joints (Fig. 59-7). Popularly known as *wear and tear* arthritis, the changes that occur in osteoarthritis are much more complex.

A balance between mechanical stress and the ability of the joint tissues to resist that stress exists in the diarthrodial joints. Osteoarthritis represents deterioration of

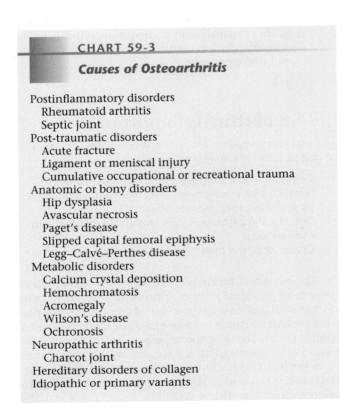

CHART 59-3

Causes of Osteoarthritis

Postinflammatory disorders
  Rheumatoid arthritis
  Septic joint
Post-traumatic disorders
  Acute fracture
  Ligament or meniscal injury
  Cumulative occupational or recreational trauma
Anatomic or bony disorders
  Hip dysplasia
  Avascular necrosis
  Paget's disease
  Slipped capital femoral epiphysis
  Legg–Calvé–Perthes disease
Metabolic disorders
  Calcium crystal deposition
  Hemochromatosis
  Acromegaly
  Wilson's disease
  Ochronosis
Neuropathic arthritis
  Charcot joint
Hereditary disorders of collagen
Idiopathic or primary variants

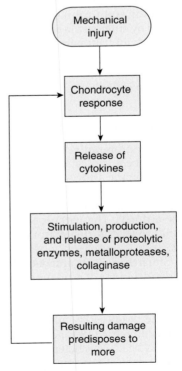

FIGURE 59-7 Disease process in osteoarthritis.

the articular cartilage caused by a physiologic imbalance between the stress applied to the joint tissues and the ability of the joint tissues to withstand the stress. Either the articular cartilage underlying bone is normal, but excessive loads applied to the joints cause the tissues to fail, or a physiologically reasonable load is applied to the joint, but the articular cartilage or bone is defective.

Articular cartilage plays two essential mechanical roles in joint physiology. First, the articular cartilage serves as a remarkably smooth weight-bearing surface. In combination with synovial fluid, the articular cartilage provides extremely low friction during movement of the joint. Second, the cartilage transmits the load down to the bone, dissipating the mechanical stress. The subchondral bone protects the overlying articular cartilage, providing it with a pliable bed and absorbing the energy of the force (Fig. 59-8).

Cartilage is a specialized type of connective tissue. As with other types of tissue, it consists of cells (*i.e.*, chondrocytes) nested in an extracellular matrix. In articular cartilage, the extracellular matrix is composed of water, proteoglycans, collagen, and ground substance. The proteoglycans, which are large macromolecules made up of disaccharides and amino acids, afford elasticity and stiffness, permitting articular cartilage to resist compression. The ground substance constitutes a highly hydrated, semisolid gel. Collagen molecules consist of polypeptide chains that form long fibrous strands. They provide form and tensile strength. The primary function of the collagen fibers is to provide a rigid scaffold to support the chondrocytes and ground substance of cartilage. The hydrated proteoglycan molecules, because of their macromolecular size and charge, are trapped in the collagen meshwork of the extracellular matrix. Because of the inextensibility of the collagen fibers, the proteoglycans are prevented from expanding to their maximum size. This confers a high osmotic pressure within the tissue.

Mechanical injury results in a chondrocyte response that leads to eventual degradation in the upper layers of cartilage. It is thought that injury leads to the release of cytokines such as interleukin-1. These chemical messengers stimulate production and release of extracellular proteolytic enzymes, metalloproteases, and collagenase. The resulting damage predisposes the chondrocytes to more injury. Inadequate repair mechanisms and imbalances between the proteases and their inhibitors may contribute further to disease progression (Fig. 59-9).

Under physiologic conditions of impact loading, the joint is protected with passive and active mechanisms. Passive mechanisms include microfractures and deformation of the subchondral bone. Deformation is essential for maximizing the contact area and for minimizing the stress (see Fig. 59-8). A progressive increase in the number of microfractures in subchondral bone may be detrimental to normal joint function because the remodeled trabeculae may be stiffer than normal and less effective as shock absorbers. Under such circumstances, the subchondral bone cannot deform normally with a load. The increased incongruity of joint surfaces that occurs normally with loading is diminished, and stress is concentrated at contact areas on the articular cartilage.

Under conditions of repeated movement, articular cartilage is highly resistant to wear. However, repetitive impact loading rapidly leads to joint failure, accounting for the high prevalence of osteoarthritis specific to vocational or avocational sites, such as the shoulders and elbows of baseball pitchers, ankles of ballet dancers, and knees of basketball players. Although this process is occurring in the cartilage, changes also are taking place in the underlying subchondral bone. The subchondral bone plate thickens and can become eburnated (*i.e.*, an ivory-like mass). Sclerosis, or formation of new bone and cysts, usually occurs in

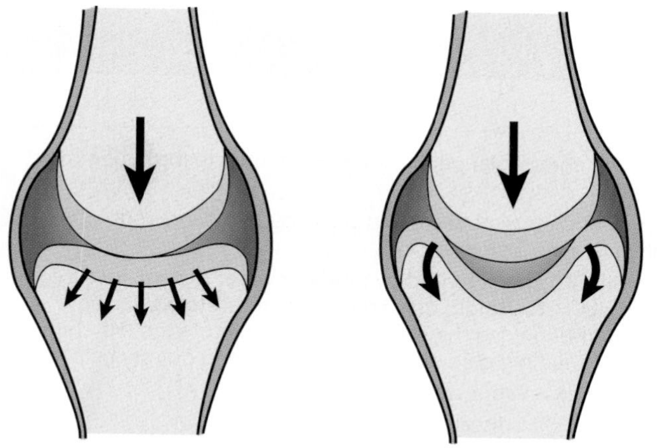

FIGURE 59-8 (**Left**) A joint normally undergoes deformation of the articular cartilage and the subchondral bone when carrying a load. This maximizes the contact area and spreads the force of the load. (**Right**) If the joint does not deform with a load, the stresses are concentrated and the joint breaks down. (Redrawn from Brandt K.D. & Radin E. [1987]. The physiology of articular stress: Osteoarthroses. *Hospital Practice* [January 15], 111)

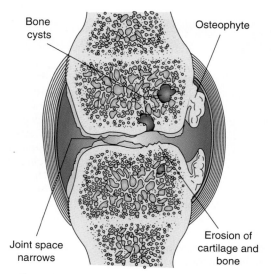

FIGURE 59-9 Joint changes in osteoarthritis. The left side denotes early changes and joint space narrowing with cartilage breakdown. The right side shows more severe disease progression with lost cartilage and osteophyte formation.

the juxta-articular bone (*i.e.*, bone near the joint). New bone that forms at the joint margins is called an *osteophyte*, or spur.

To understand further the pathology of osteoarthritis, the lubrication of the joint must be considered. Under high loads such as weight bearing, lubrication depends on a film of interstitial fluid squeezed out of the cartilage with compression of the opposing surfaces of the joint. The greater the load is, the better the lubrication. With depletion of proteoglycans from the cartilage matrix in osteoarthritis, the mechanisms that normally operate under high loads to produce a pressurized lubricating film may be impaired. Attempts to devise artificial lubricants have been unsuccessful because they impede the flow of interstitial fluid into and out of the cartilage surface.

Immobilization also can produce degenerative changes in articular cartilage. Cartilage degeneration due to immobility may result from loss of the pumping action of lubrication that occurs with joint movement. These changes are more marked and appear earlier in areas of contact but occur also in areas not subject to mechanical compression. By 3 weeks after remobilization, all biochemical, metabolic, and morphologic abnormalities in the cartilage that result from immobilization are reversed. Although cartilage atrophy is rapidly reversible with activity after a period of immobilization, impact exercise during the period of remobilization can prevent reversal of the atrophy. Slow, gradual remobilization may be important in preventing cartilage injury and has clinical implications with respect to instructions to patients concerning the recommended level of physical activity after removal of a cast. This balance between enough activity to lubricate and nourish cartilage and overloaded activity that further damages cartilage reasonably confuses patients who have difficulty in understanding whether they should use an affected joint or rest it.

Mild synovitis may occur in osteoarthritis. This inflammation represents a reactive process and is more likely to be seen in advanced disease. The synovitis may be related to the release of free cartilage proteoglycans from the deteriorating articular cartilage. Immunologic factors also may be involved. Calcium pyrophosphate and apatite crystals are common in osteoarthritic knee effusions.[1]

CLINICAL MANIFESTATIONS

The manifestations of osteoarthritis may occur suddenly or insidiously. Initially, pain may be described as aching and may be somewhat difficult to localize. It worsens with use or activity and is relieved by rest. In later stages of disease activity, night pain may be experienced during rest. Pain can occur at rest, several hours after the use of the involved joints. Crepitus and grinding may be evident when the joint is moved. As the disease advances, even minimal activity may cause pain because of the limited range of motion resulting from intra-articular and periarticular structural damage.

The most frequently affected joints are the hips, knees, lumbar and cervical vertebrae, proximal and distal joints of the hand, the first carpometacarpal joint, and the first metatarsophalangeal joints of the feet. Table 59-2 identifies the joints that commonly are affected by osteoarthritis and the common clinical features correlated with the disease activity of each particular joint. A single joint or several may be affected. Although a single weight-bearing joint may be involved initially, other joints often become affected because of the additional stress placed on them while trying to protect the original joint. It is not unusual for a person having a knee replacement to discover soon after the surgery is done that the second knee also needs to be replaced. Other clinical features are limitations of joint motion and joint instability. Joint enlargement usually results from new bone formation; the joint feels hard, in contrast to the soft, spongy feeling characteristic of the joint in rheumatoid

TABLE 59-2 ✦ **Clinical Features of Osteoarthritis**	
Joint	**Clinical Features**
Cervical spine	Localized stiffness; radicular or nonradicular pain; posterior osteophyte formation may cause vascular compression
Lumbar spine	Low back pain and stiffness; muscle spasm; decreased back motion; nerve root compression causing radicular pain; spinal stenosis
Hip	Most common in older male adults; characterized by insidious onset of pain, localized to groin region or inner aspect of the thigh; may be referred to buttocks, sciatic region, or knee; reduced hip motion; leg may be held in external rotation with hip flexed and adducted; limp or shuffling gait; difficulty getting in and out of chairs
First carpometacarpal joint	Tenderness at base of thumb; squared appearance to joint
Proximal interphalangeal joint—Bouchard's nodes	Same as for distal interphalangeal joint disease
Distal interphalangeal joint—Heberden's nodes	Occurs more frequently in women; usually involves multiple DIPs, lateral flexor deviation of joint, spur formation at joint margins, pain and discomfort after joint use
Knee	Localized discomfort with pain on motion; limitation of motion; crepitus; quadriceps atrophy due to lack of use; joint instability; genu varus or valgus; joint effusion
First metatarsophalangeal joint	Insidious onset; irregular joint contour; pain and swelling aggravated by tight shoes

arthritis. Sometimes, mild synovitis or increased synovial fluid can cause joint enlargement.

DIAGNOSIS AND TREATMENT

The diagnosis of osteoarthritis usually is determined by history and physical examination, x-ray studies, and laboratory findings that exclude other diseases. Although osteoarthritis often is contrasted with rheumatoid arthritis for diagnostic purposes, the differences are not always readily apparent. Other rheumatic diseases may be superimposed on osteoarthritis. Psychological factors, severity of joint disease, and educational level affect the expression of symptoms.[29]

Characteristic radiologic changes initially include medial joint space narrowing, followed by subchondral bony sclerosis, formation of spikes on the tibial eminence, and osteophytes. The results of laboratory studies usually are normal because the disorder is not a systemic disease. The ESR may be slightly elevated in generalized osteoarthritis or erosive inflammatory variations of the disease. If inflammation is present, there may be a slight increase in the blood cell count. The synovial fluid usually is normal.

Because there is no cure, the treatment of osteoarthritis is symptomatic and includes physical rehabilitative, pharmacologic, and surgical measures. Physical measures are aimed at improving the supporting structures of the joint and strengthening opposing muscle groups involved in cushioning weight-bearing forces. This includes a balance of rest and exercise, use of splints to protect and rest the joint, use of heat and cold to relieve pain and muscle spasm, and adjusting the activities of daily living. Weight reduction is helpful when the knee is involved. The involved joint should not be further abused, and steps should be taken to protect and rest it. This includes weight reduction (when weight-bearing surfaces are involved) and the use of a cane or walker if the hips and knees are involved. Muscle-strengthening exercises may help protect the joint and decrease pain.[29]

Oral medications are aimed at reducing inflammation or providing analgesia. The most popular medications used in the treatment of osteoarthritis are the NSAIDs, many of which are available without a prescription. Ongoing research may confirm that some NSAIDs impede the repair mechanisms in early cartilage lesions. There is growing concern about the side effects of NSAIDs, and the newer COX-2–inhibiting agents (see section on treatment of rheumatoid arthritis) also are indicated for the treatment of osteoarthritis. However, studies have shown that the pain of osteoarthritis may arise from causes other than an inflamed synovium. These causes include stretching of the joint capsule, ligaments, or nerve endings in the periosteum over osteophytes; nontrabecular microfractures; intraosseous hypertension; bursitis or tendinitis; or muscle spasm. In such cases, the pain may be relieved by an NSAID because of the analgesic action of the drug rather than an anti-inflammatory effect.[29] For many persons, acetaminophen in doses as high as 4000 mg/day may be as effective and less toxic than NSAIDs.

If the patient becomes more limited or the regimen is unsuccessful in adequately relieving symptoms, cortico-

Osteoarthritis

➤ Knee osteoarthritis affects approximately 11% of those 65 years of age and older.

➤ Losing weight, preventing injury, strengthening the muscles bridging joints, and modifying job tasks can help prevent knee and hip osteoarthritis.

➤ Addressing vitamin and postmenopausal hormone deficiencies may play a future role in osteoarthritis prevention.

steroid injections may be helpful, especially for those who have an effusion of the joint. Injections usually are limited to a total of four and not more than three within 1 year because their use is thought to accelerate joint destruction.

Viscosupplementation is a newer concept in treatment and is based on the hypothesis that joint lubrication is abnormal in osteoarthritis. Hyaluronate is injected into the joint weekly for 3 to 5 weeks. Controlled studies have shown this approach to be equally as efficacious as NSAIDs. Speculation that other agents may be chondroprotective has initiated other studies, but these results have not been confirmed in humans.

Surgery is considered when the person is having severe pain and joint function is severely reduced. Procedures include arthroscopic lavage and debridement, bunion resections, osteotomies to change alignment of the knee and hip joints, and decompression of the spinal roots in osteoarthritic vertebral stenosis. Total hip replacements have provided effective relief of symptoms and improved range of motion for many persons, as have total knee replacements, although the latter procedure has produced less consistent results. Joint replacement is available for the first carpometacarpal joint. Arthrodesis is used in advanced disease to reduce pain; however, this results in loss of motion.

Investigations are underway that use animal models of abrasion of the subchondral bone to permit vascular invasion to stimulate cartilage resorption and replacement with fibrocartilage and that place chondral grafts and progenitor cells under the periosteum.[30] Future management of osteoarthritis lies in the development of techniques to identify and monitor cartilage lesions at an earlier stage. Potential approaches include bone scanning, magnetic resonance imaging, and arthroscopy.

In summary, osteoarthritis, the most common form of arthritis, is a localized condition affecting primarily the weight-bearing joints. Risk factors for osteoarthritis progression include older age, osteoarthritis in multiple joints, neuropathy, and, for knees, obesity. The disorder is characterized by degeneration of the articular cartilage and subchondral bone. It has been suggested that the cellular events responsible for the development of osteoarthritis begin with some type of abnormal mechanical insult or stimulus, including hormones and growth factors, drugs, mechanical stresses, and the extracellular environment. Studies also implicate immunologic factors in the perpetuation and acceleration of the osteoarthritic change. As cartilage ages, biochemical events such as collagen fatigue and fracture occur with less stress. Attempts at repair by increased matrix synthesis and cellular proliferation maintain the integrity of the cartilage until failure of reparative processes allows the degenerative changes to progress. Joint enlargement usually results from new bone formation, which causes the joint to feel hard. Pain and stiffness are primary features of the disease. Inflammatory mediators (*e.g.*, prostaglandins) may increase the inflammatory and degenerative response.

Treatment is directed toward the relief of pain and maintenance of mobility while preserving the articular cartilage. Although there is no known cure for osteoarthritis, appropriate treatment can reduce pain, maintain or improve joint mobility, and limit functional disability.

Metabolic Diseases Associated With Rheumatic States

After you have completed this section of the chapter, you should be able to meet the following objectives:

✦ Relate the metabolism and elimination of uric acid to the pathogenesis of crystal-induced arthropathy

✦ State why asymptomatic hyperuricemia is a laboratory finding and not a disease

✦ Describe the clinical manifestations, diagnostic measures, and methods used in the treatment of gouty arthritis

Metabolic bone and joint disorders result from biochemical and metabolic disorders that affect the joints. Metabolic and endocrine diseases associated with joint symptoms include amyloidosis, osteogenesis imperfecta, diabetes mellitus, hyperparathyroidism, thyroid disease, AIDS, and hypermobility syndromes. The discussion in this chapter is limited to the crystal-induced arthropathy caused by monosodium urate deposition, or gout.

CRYSTAL-INDUCED ARTHROPATHIES

Crystal deposition in joints produces arthritis. In gout, monosodium urate or uric acid crystals are found in the joint cavity. Another condition in which calcium pyrophosphate dihydrate crystals are found in the joints sometimes is referred to as *pseudogout* or *chondrocalcinosis*. A brief discussion of pseudogout is found later in this chapter in the section on rheumatic diseases in the elderly.

GOUT

The manifestations of the heterogeneous group of diseases known as the *gout syndrome* include acute gouty arthritis with recurrent attacks of severe articular and periarticular inflammation; tophi or the accumulation of crystalline deposits in articular surfaces, bones, soft tissue, and cartilage; gouty nephropathy or renal impairment; and uric acid kidney stones. Primary gout is predominantly a disease of men, with a peak incidence in the fourth or sixth decade. Only 3% to 7% of cases occur in women, and most of these are in postmenopausal women.[6]

Uric Acid Metabolism and Elimination

Uric acid is a metabolite of the purines, adenine and guanine. Normally, approximately two thirds of the uric acid produced each day is excreted through the kidneys; the rest is eliminated through the gastrointestinal tract. Normal renal handling of uric acid involves three steps: filtration, reabsorption, and secretion. Uric acid is freely filtered in the glomerulus, completely reabsorbed in the proximal tubule, and secreted back into the tubular fluid by another mechanism in the distal end of the proximal tubule or distal tubule (see Chapter 30). The tubular secretion and postsecretory reabsorption determine the final concentration of uric acid in the urine.

Most persons with gout have reduced urate clearance. For them, the serum urate level becomes elevated so that a normal amount of urate can be excreted and urate homeostasis can be achieved. Most persons with increased production of urate have increased excretion of uric acid. However, with kidney damage, an increased amount of uric acid is eliminated by the gastrointestinal tract.

Small doses of uricosuric agents may preferentially reduce secretion and increase uric acid retention, but therapeutic doses block reabsorption and increase uric acid elimination. The salicylates reduce secretion and cause retention of uric acid when given at doses used for pain relief; very large doses are needed to block reabsorption and secretion. Consequently, aspirin and other salicylates are not recommended for use as an analgesic in persons with gout. Some of the diuretics, including the thiazides, which are weak acids, are secreted by the proximal tubular cells and also can interfere with the excretion of uric acid.

Etiology and Pathogenesis

Hyperuricemia reflects a metabolic derangement in extracellular fluids. Hyperuricemia is defined as a serum urate concentration greater than 7.0 mg/dL as measured by the specific uricase method.[31] Monosodium urate crystal deposition develops when hyperuricemia exists. Asymptomatic hyperuricemia is a laboratory finding and not a disease. Most persons with hyperuricemia do not develop gout. Hyperuricemia may occur because of overproduction of uric acid, underexcretion of uric acid, or a combination of the two. Primary and secondary forms of hyperuricemia exist. Primary forms result from genetic defects in purine metabolism. Secondary forms of hyperuricemia are related to certain disease conditions and medications.

An attack of gout occurs when monosodium urate crystals precipitate in the joint and initiate an inflammatory response. This may follow a sudden rise in the serum urate levels. The excess urate is not soluble and therefore precipitates. An attack also can occur with a sudden drop in the urate level. In either situation, crystals are released into the synovial fluid and an inflammatory response is initiated.

Phagocytosis of urate crystals by polymorphonuclear leukocytes occurs and leads to polymorphonuclear cell death with the release of lysosomal enzymes. As this process continues, the inflammation causes destruction of the cartilage and subchondral bone. Tophi are large, hard nodules that have irregular surfaces and contain crystalline deposits of monosodium urate that incite an inflammatory response. They are found most commonly in the synovium, olecranon bursa, Achilles tendon, subchondral bone, and extensor surface of the forearm and may be mistaken for rheumatoid nodules. Tophi usually do not appear until 10 years or more after the first gout attack. This stage of gout, called *chronic tophaceous gout*, is characterized by more frequent and prolonged attacks, which often are polyarticular.

Crystal deposition usually occurs in peripheral areas of the body, such as the great toe and the pinnae of the ear. Sodium urate is less soluble at temperatures below 37°C. The peripheral tissues are cooler than other parts of the body, and this may at least partially explain why gout occurs most frequently in peripheral joints.

Clinical Manifestations

The typical acute attack of gout is monoarticular and usually affects the first metatarsophalangeal joint. The tarsal joints, insteps, ankles, heels, knees, wrists, fingers, and elbows also may be initial sites of involvement. Acute gout often begins at night and may be precipitated by excessive exercise, certain medications, foods, alcohol, or dieting. The onset of pain typically is abrupt, and redness and swelling are observed. The attack may last for days or weeks. Pain may be severe enough to be aggravated even by the weight of a bed sheet covering the affected area.

In the early stages of gout after the initial attack has subsided, the person is asymptomatic, and joint abnormalities are not evident. This is referred to as *intercritical gout*. After the first attack, it may be months or years before another attack. As attacks recur with increased frequency, joint changes occur and become permanent.

Diagnosis and Treatment

Although hyperuricemia is the biochemical hallmark of gout, the presence of hyperuricemia cannot be equated with gout because many persons with this condition never develop gout. A definitive diagnosis of gout can be made only when monosodium urate crystals are in the synovial fluid or in tissue sections of tophaceous deposits. Synovial fluid analysis is useful in excluding other conditions, such as septic arthritis, pseudogout, and rheumatoid arthritis.[32] The next step is to determine if the disorder is related to overproduction or to underexcretion of uric acid. The uric

acid level is determined, and a 24-hour urine sample is collected. Ideally, the person should be on a purine-free diet during the time the urine specimen is being collected. Urate urine values above the normal range of 264 to 588 mg/day indicate an overproduction of uric acid.[33] The normal serum urate concentration is 5.0 to 5.7 mg/dL in men and 3.7 to 5.0 mg/dL in women.[1]

The objectives in the treatment of gout are the termination and prevention of the acute attacks of gouty arthritis and the correction of hyperuricemia, with consequent inhibition of further precipitation of sodium urate and absorption of urate crystal deposits already in the tissues. Management of acute gout is directed toward reducing joint inflammation. Hyperuricemia and related problems of tophi, joint destruction, and renal problems are treated after the acute inflammatory process has subsided. NSAIDs, particularly indomethacin and ibuprofen, are used for treating acute gouty arthritis. Alternative therapies include colchicine and intra-articular deposition of corticosteroids. Treatment with colchicine is used early in the acute stage. Although the drug usually is given orally, a more rapid response is obtained when colchicine is given intravenously. The nausea and diarrhea that may occur with large oral doses are avoided when the drug is given intravenously. The acute symptoms of gout usually subside within 48 hours after treatment with oral colchicine has been instituted and within 12 hours after intravenous administration of the drug.

The NSAIDs are effective during the acute stage when used at their maximum dosage and sometimes are preferred to colchicine because they have fewer toxic side effects. Phenylbutazone usually is effective but is used only on a short-term basis because long-term use can cause bone marrow suppression. The corticosteroid drugs are not recommended for treatment of gout unless all other medications have proved unsuccessful. Intra-articular injections of corticosteroid agents may be used when only one joint is involved and the person is unable to take colchicine or NSAIDs.

With the exception of phenylbutazone, the drugs used to treat acute gout have no effect on the serum urate level and are valueless in tophaceous gout and the control of hyperuricemia. After the acute attack has been relieved, the hyperuricemia is treated. One method is to reduce hyperuricemia through the use of allopurinol or a uricosuric agent (*i.e.,* probenecid or sulfinpyrazone, a phenylbutazone derivative). These compounds are not used in the treatment of acute gouty arthritis and, if given, tend only to exacerbate and prolong the inflammation. These uricosuric medications prevent the tubular reabsorption of urate. The serum urate concentrations are monitored to determine efficacy and dosage. These drugs usually are started in small doses and gradually increased over 7 to 10 days. Aspirin should not be used with these medications because it decreases the urinary excretion of uric acid. Allopurinol is the preferred antihyperuricemic therapy for patients with frequent attacks of gout, significant hyperuricemia (>9 to 11 mg/dL), significant hyperuricosuria (>800 to 1000 mg/day), tophi, uric acid urolithiasis, or urate nephropathy. Allopurinol inhibits xanthine oxidase, an enzyme needed for the conversion of hypoxanthine to xanthine and xanthine to uric acid. There is a slight possibility that xanthine kidney stones can develop if allopurinol is used for many years. It usually is reserved for the person who does not have an adequate response or is unable to tolerate other forms of treatment. Treatment of hyperuricemia is aimed at maintaining normal uric acid levels and is lifelong. Prophylactic colchicine or NSAIDs may be used between gout attacks. If the uric acid level is normal and the person has not had recurrent attacks of gout, these medications may be discontinued.[31]

Gout can be effectively controlled by medical management; often it is not because many persons with gout have a limited understanding of the disease and therefore a low compliance with treatment. Education about the disease and its management is fundamental to the treatment and management of gout. The sufferer should be made aware that the prognosis is very good and that the disease, although chronic, can be controlled in almost all cases. Some changes in lifestyle may be needed, such as maintenance of ideal weight, moderation in alcohol consumption, and avoiding purine-rich foods, such as liver, kidney, sardines, anchovies, and sweetbreads, particularly by patients with excessive tophaceous deposits. Adherence to the lifelong use of medications may be the only major lifestyle change necessary for many persons.

In summary, crystal-induced arthropathy is characterized by crystal deposition in the joint. However, hyperuricemia is a laboratory finding and not a disease. Gout is the prototype of this group. Acute attacks of arthritis occur with gout and are characterized by the presence of monosodium urate crystals in the joint. The disorder is accompanied by hyperuricemia, which results from overproduction of uric acid or from the reduced ability of the kidney to rid the body of excess uric acid. Management of acute gout is directed first toward the reduction of joint inflammation; then the hyperuricemia is treated. Hyperuricemia is treated with uricosuric agents, which prevent the tubular reabsorption of urate, or with medication that inhibits the production of uric acid. Although gout is chronic, it can be controlled with appropriate lifestyle changes by most patients.

Rheumatic Diseases in Children and the Elderly

After you have completed this section of the chapter, you should be able to meet the following objectives:

✦ List three types of juvenile rheumatoid arthritis and differentiate among their major characteristics
✦ Name one rheumatic disease that affects only the elderly population

RHEUMATIC DISEASES IN CHILDREN

Children can be affected with almost all of the rheumatic diseases. In addition to disease-specific differences, these conditions affect not only the child but the family. Growth and development require special attention. Adherence to the treatment program requires intervention with the child and parents. School issues also must be addressed.

Juvenile Rheumatoid Arthritis

Juvenile rheumatoid arthritis (JRA) is a chronic disease that affects approximately 60,000 to 200,000 children in the United States.[1] It is characterized by synovitis and can influence epiphyseal growth by stimulating growth of the affected side. Generalized stunted growth also may occur.

Systemic onset (*i.e.*, Still's disease) affects approximately 20% of children with JRA.[1] The symptoms of Still's disease include a daily intermittent high fever, which usually is accompanied by a rash, generalized lymphadenopathy, hepatosplenomegaly, leukocytosis, and anemia. Most of these children also have joint involvement by the disease. Systemic symptoms usually subside in 6 to 12 months. This form of JRA also can make an initial appearance in adulthood. Infections, heart disease, and adrenal insufficiency may cause death.

A second subgroup of JRA, pauciarticular arthritis, affects no more than four joints. This disease affects 55% to 75% of children with JRA. Pauciarticular arthritis affects two distinct groups. The first group generally consists of girls younger than 6 years of age with chronic uveitis. The results of ANA testing in this group usually are positive. The second group, characterized by late-onset arthritis, is made up mostly of boys. The HLA-B27 test results are positive in more than one half of this group. They are affected by sacroiliitis, and the arthritis usually occurs in the lower extremities.

The third subgroup of JRA, accounting for approximately 20% of the total, is polyarticular onset disease. It affects more than four joints during the first 6 months of the disease. This form of arthritis more closely resembles the adult form of the disease than the other two subgroups. Rheumatoid factor sometimes is present and may indicate a more active disease process. Systemic features include a low-grade fever, weight loss, malaise, anemia, stunted growth, slight organomegaly (*e.g.*, hepatosplenomegaly), and adenopathy.[1]

The prognosis for most children with rheumatoid arthritis is good. NSAIDs are the first-line drugs used in treating JRA. Salicylates have been replaced by agents such as naproxen, ibuprofen, and ketoprofen. The second-line agent is low-dose methotrexate or, less often, sulfasalazine. Gold salts, hydroxychloroquine, and D-penicillamine rarely are used.[34] Other aspects of treatment of children with JRA are similar to those used for the adult with rheumatoid arthritis. Children are encouraged to lead as normal a life as possible.

Systemic Lupus Erythematosus

The features of SLE in children are similar to those in adults. The incidence in children is 10 times lower, estimated to occur in 0.6 of 100,000 children. The occurrence in the sexes is almost equal until pubescence, after which it approaches the sex ratio seen in adults. The clinical manifestations of SLE in children reflect the extent and severity of systemic involvement. The best prognostic indicator in children is the extent of renal involvement, which is more common and more severe in children than in adults with SLE. Infectious complications are the most common cause of death (40%) in children with SLE.

Children with SLE may present with constitutional symptoms, including fever, malaise, anorexia, and weight loss. Symptoms of the integumentary, musculoskeletal, central nervous, cardiac, pulmonary, and hematopoietic systems are similar to those of adults. Endocrine abnormalities include Cushing's syndrome from long-term corticosteroid use and autoimmune thyroiditis. Adolescents often experience menstrual disturbances, which tend to resolve with disease remission.

Treatment of SLE in children is similar to that in adults. The use of NSAIDs, corticosteroids, antimalarials, and immunosuppressive agents depends on the symptoms. Corticosteroids may cause stunting of growth and necrosis of femoral heads and other joints. Immunization schedules should be maintained using attenuated rather than live vaccines. Rest periods should be balanced with exercise; children should be encouraged to maintain as normal a schedule as possible.[35] The diversity of the clinical manifestations of SLE in the young requires the establishment of a comprehensive program.

Juvenile Dermatomyositis

Juvenile dermatomyositis (JDMS) is an inflammatory myopathy primarily involving skin and muscle and associated with a characteristic rash. JDMS can affect children of all ages, with a mean age at onset of 8 years. There is an increased incidence among girls. The cause is unknown.

Symmetric proximal muscle weakness, elevated muscle enzymes, evidence of vasculitis, and electromyographic changes confirming an inflammatory myopathy are diagnostic for JDMS. Generalized vasculitis is not seen in the adult form of the disease. The rash may precede or follow the onset of proximal muscle weakness. Periorbital edema, erythema, and eyelid telangiectasia are common.

Calcifications can occur in 30% to 50% of children with JDMS and are by far the most debilitating symptom. The calcifications appear at pressure points or sites of previous trauma. JDMS is treated primarily with corticosteroids to reduce inflammation. Occasionally, immunosuppressives are used in cases of refractory disease.[1]

Juvenile Spondyloarthropathies

Ankylosing spondylitis, reactive arthritis, psoriatic arthritis, and spondyloarthropathies associated with ulcerative colitis and regional enteritis can affect children and adults. In children, spondyloarthritis manifests in peripheral joints first, mimicking pauciarticular JRA, with no evidence of sacroiliac or spine involvement for months to years after onset. The spondyloarthropathies are more common in boys and commonly occur in children who have a positive family history. HLA-B27 typing is helpful in diagnosing children because of the unusual presentation of the disease.

Management of the disease involves physical therapy, education, and attention to school and growth and development issues. Medication includes the use of salicylates or other NSAIDs such as tolmetin or indomethacin. More severe disease or symptoms may require systemic corticosteroids.[1]

RHEUMATIC DISEASES IN THE ELDERLY

Arthritis is the most common complaint of elderly persons. The pain, stiffness, and muscle weakness affect daily life, often threatening independence and quality of life. Symptoms of the rheumatic diseases also can have an indirect effect and even threaten the duration of life for the elderly. The weakness and gait disturbance that often accompany the rheumatic diseases can contribute to the likelihood of falls and fracture, causing suffering, increased health care costs, further loss of independence, and the potential for a decreased life span.

The elderly cope less well with mild to moderately severe disease that in younger persons is less likely to lead to serious disability for the same degree of impairment. Unfortunately, the elderly and often their health care providers think the problems associated with arthritis are an inevitable consequence of aging and fail to benefit from measures that can improve the quality of life.

Because arthritis is the leading cause of change in the functional status of older adults, a functional approach to the problems of the elderly is appropriate. Inactivity is a societal expectation of the elderly. What activity there is tends to be low impact (*e.g.*, leisurely walking), and deconditioning occurs.

Older patients often have multiple problems complicating diagnosis and management. The diagnosis of an elderly patient with a musculoskeletal problem must consider a wide variety of disorders that usually are regarded as outside the range of typical rheumatic disease. Among these are metastatic malignancy, multiple myeloma, musculoskeletal disorders accompanying endocrine or metabolic disorders, orthopedic conditions, and neurologic disease. The diagnosis may be missed if the assumption is that musculoskeletal problems in the older person are caused by osteoarthritis.

There is an increased incidence of false-positive test results for rheumatoid factor and ANA in the elderly population with or without rheumatic disease because older persons are better producers of autoantibodies than younger persons. There are differences in the manifestations, diagnosis, and treatment of some of the rheumatic diseases in the elderly. The usual presentation of these conditions was discussed earlier in this chapter. One form of rheumatic disease that has a predilection for the elderly is polymyalgia rheumatica.

Rheumatoid Arthritis

The prevalence of rheumatoid arthritis increases with advancing age, at least until 75 years of age.[36] Seropositive patients are more likely to have had an acute onset with systemic features and higher disease activity. Patients with seronegative, elderly-onset rheumatoid arthritis have a disease that usually follows a mild course. The close resemblance of the manifestations of seronegative rheumatoid arthritis in the elderly to those of polymyalgia rheumatica has led to speculation concerning the relation of these syndromes.[36] It may be that rheumatoid arthritis in the elderly is a broad disorder that includes a number of distinct subsets with characteristic manifestations, courses, and outcomes.

Systemic Lupus Erythematosus

Systemic lupus erythematosus is another condition with different manifestations in the elderly. The disease is accompanied less frequently by renal involvement. However, pleurisy, pericarditis, arthritis, and symptoms closely resembling polymyalgia rheumatica are more common than in younger patients. The characteristics of SLE in the elderly closely resemble those of drug-induced SLE, leading to speculation that the syndrome may result from one of the multiple drugs that are taken by many elderly patients.[37]

Osteoarthritis

Osteoarthritis is by far the most common form of arthritis among the elderly. It is the greatest cause of disability and limitation of activity in older populations. It has been suggested that osteoarthritis begins at a very young age, expressing itself in the elderly only after a long period of latency. Too often, it is accepted by the patient or expected by the physician. Osteoarthritis presents a major management problem, but there is much that can be done. Self-control by maintaining a positive attitude and sense of self-esteem is a frequent coping strategy.[38]

Crystal-Induced Arthropathies

The incidence of clinical gout increases with advancing age, in part because of the increased involvement of joints after years of continued hyperuricemia. High serum urate levels rarely occur in women before menopause; initial attacks of clinical gout occur around the age of 70 years, or 20 years after menopause.[31] Gouty attacks in elderly women may be precipitated by the use of diuretics.

The treatment of gout is more difficult in the elderly. Although colchicine may be effective in controlling the symptoms of chronic gout, it may cause diarrhea in some patients, limiting its effectiveness in maintenance therapy.

As part of the tissue-aging process, osteoarthritis develops with associated cartilage degeneration. Calcium pyrophosphate crystals are shed into the joint cavity. These crystals may produce a low-grade chronic inflammation—the chronic pseudogout syndrome. The accumulation of calcium pyrophosphate and related crystalline deposits in articular cartilage is common in the elderly. There are no medications that can remove the crystals from the joints. Although it may be asymptomatic, presence of the crystals may contribute to more rapid cartilage deterioration. This condition may coexist with severe osteoarthritis.

Polymyalgia Rheumatica

Of the forms of arthritis affecting the elderly, polymyalgia rheumatica is one of the more difficult to diagnose and one of the most important to identify. Elderly women are especially at risk. Polymyalgia rheumatica is a common syndrome of older patients, rarely occurring before age 50 and usually after age 60 years. The onset can be abrupt, with the patient going to bed feeling well and awakening with pain and stiffness in the neck, shoulders, and hips.

Diagnosis is based on the pain and stiffness persisting for at least 1 month and an elevated ESR. The diagnosis is confirmed when the symptoms respond dramatically to a small dose of prednisone, a corticosteroid. Biopsies have shown that the muscles are normal, despite the name, but that a nonspecific inflammation affecting the synovial tissue is present. It is possible that a number of patients are erroneously diagnosed as having rheumatoid arthritis or osteoarthritis. For patients with an elevated Westergren ESR (0.5 mm), the diagnosis usually is based on a 3-day trial of prednisone treatment.[39] Patients with polymyalgia rheumatica typically exhibit striking clinical improvement approximately the second day. Patients with rheumatoid arthritis also show improvement, although usually days later.

Treatment with NSAIDs provides relief for some patients, but most require continuing therapy with prednisone, with gradual reduction of the dose over the course of 1.5 to 2 years, using the patient's symptoms as the primary guide. Patients need close monitoring during the maintenance phase with prednisone. Because their symptoms are relieved, they often quit taking the prednisone and their symptoms recur, or doses are missed and the decreased dosage leads to an increase in symptoms. Unless careful assessment reveals the frequency of missed doses, the physician may be misled into increasing the dosage when it is not needed. Because of the side effects of the corticosteroids, the goal is to use the lowest dose of the drug necessary to control the symptoms. Weaning patients off low-dose prednisone therapy after this length of time can be a difficult and extended process. Health care providers must work closely with the elderly patient to make sure the correct dosage is taken as the amount is slowly decreased. Even a small error in dosage can set the tapering program back by weeks or months.

A certain percentage of patients with polymyalgia rheumatica also have giant cell arteritis (*i.e.*, temporal arteritis), frequently with involvement of the ophthalmic arteries. The two conditions are considered to represent different manifestations of the same disease. Giant cell arteritis, a form of systemic vasculitis, is a systemic inflammatory disease of large and medium-sized arteries (see Chapter 22). The inflammatory response seems to be a T-cell response to an antigen.

Clinical manifestations of giant cell arteritis usually begin insidiously and may exist for some time before being recognized[39] (Chart 59-4). It is potentially dangerous if missed or mistreated, especially if the temporal artery or other vessels supplying the eye are involved, in which case blindness can ensue quickly without treatment. The condition is responsive to appropriate therapy. For those patients at risk, adherence to the medication program is critical, with preservation of sight being the goal. Because this complication can occur so quickly and is relatively asymptomatic, it is vital that the patient understand the importance of taking the correct dose regularly as prescribed. Treatment consists of large doses of prednisone. The usual side effects occur, some of which (osteoporosis)

CHART 59-4

Signs and Symptoms of Giant Cell Arteritis

Constitutional symptoms
  Malaise
  Fatigue
  Fever (usually low grade)
  Weight loss
  Cough
  Sore throat
Polymyalgia rheumatica syndrome
  Limb girdle pain and stiffness
Manifestations related to vascular involvement
  New type of headache
  Scalp tenderness, especially over temporal area
  Visual loss
  Diplopia
  Aortic arch syndrome
Ischemic optic neuropathy
  Atrophy
Claudication of jaw or arm

or a COX-2 inhibitor to prevent ulcer formation, and the patient should be monitored for renal insufficiency.[40] Even such tasks as the frequent visits to the physician's office for the laboratory monitoring that is necessary with drugs such as methotrexate can be difficult or impossible for elderly patients who live in a cold climate during the winter. For the patient who no longer drives or does not want to, transportation can be a barrier. Elderly patients often hesitate to ask family or friends to take them to the doctor every week.

The elderly are more likely to conceal symptoms than to elaborate on them because they feel they are a part of the aging process or that "nothing can be done." One of the ways to enhance a person's ability to combat the symptoms of arthritis is by enforcing a greater sense of control. The elderly patient should be involved in the management and treatment program.

Joint arthroplasty is used for pain relief and increased function. Chronologic age is not a contraindication to surgical treatment of arthritis. In appropriately selected elderly candidates, survival and functional outcome after surgery are equivalent to those in younger age groups. The more sedentary activity level of the elderly makes them even better candidates for joint replacement, because they put less stress and demand on the new joint.

are more common than normally expected. This dosage is continued for 4 to 6 weeks and then decreased gradually.

Localized Musculoskeletal Disorders

The elderly also are prone to localized musculoskeletal syndromes. Years of wear frequently lead to a range of inflammatory disorders, including bursitis and tendinitis. These are known collectively as *impingement syndromes*. An example is a disorder in the shoulder where the rotator cuff rides against the acromion. Tennis elbow (only 5% of those with this problem actually play tennis), or humeral epicondylitis, also is seen frequently among the elderly. Other localized inflammatory conditions of the musculoskeletal system affecting the elderly are fibrositis or fibromyalgia and Dupuytren's contracture.

Management of Rheumatic Diseases in the Elderly

In addition to diagnosis-specific treatment, the elderly require special considerations. Management techniques that rely on modalities other than drugs are particularly important for the elderly. These include splints, walking aids, muscle-building exercise, and local heat. Muscle-strengthening and stretching exercises are particularly effective in the elderly person with age-related losses in muscle function and should be instituted early. Rest, the cornerstone of conservative therapy, is hazardous in the elderly, who can rapidly lose muscle strength.

The NSAIDs may be less well tolerated by the elderly, and their side effects are more likely to be serious. In addition to bleeding from the gastrointestinal tract and renal insufficiency, there may be cognitive dysfunction, manifested by forgetfulness, inability to concentrate, sleeplessness, paranoid ideation, and depression. Misoprostol should be considered in conjunction with treatment with NSAIDs

In summary, rheumatic diseases that affect children can be similar to the adult diseases, but there also are manifestations unique to the younger population. Children with chronic diseases also have to be approached with different priorities than adults. Managing rheumatic diseases in children requires a team approach to address issues of the family, school, growth and development, and coping strategies and requires a comprehensive disease management program.

Arthritis is the most common complaint of the elderly population. The pain, stiffness, and muscle weakness affect daily life, often threatening independence and quality of life. There is a difference in the manifestations, diagnosis, and treatment of some of the rheumatic diseases in the elderly compared with those in the younger population. Osteoarthritis is the most common form of arthritis among the elderly. The prevalence of rheumatoid arthritis and gout increases with advancing age. One form of rheumatic disease that has a predilection for the elderly is polymyalgia rheumatica. A certain percentage of patients with polymyalgia rheumatica also have giant cell arteritis, frequently with involvement of the ophthalmic arteries. If this condition is untreated, it carries a serious threat of blindness.

Related Web Links

American College of Rheumatology   www.rheumatology.org
Arthritis Foundation   www.arthritis.org
Lupus Foundation of America, Inc.   www.lupus.org/lupus
National Institutes of Arthritis and Musculoskeletal and Skin Diseases, National Institutes of Health   www.nih.gov/niams
Scleroderma Foundation   www.scleroderma.org
Sjögren's Syndrome Foundation, Inc.   www.sjogrens.com
Spondylitis Association of America   www.spondylitis.org

References

1. Klippel J.R. (Ed.). (1997). *Primer on the rheumatic diseases* (11th ed.). Atlanta: Arthritis Foundation.
2. Harris E.D. (2001). Clinical features of rheumatoid arthritis. In Ruddy S., Harris E.D., Sledge C.B. (Eds.), *Textbook of rheumatology* (6th ed., pp. 967–1000). Philadelphia: W.B. Saunders.
3. Green M., Marzo-Ortega H. McGonagle D., Wakefield R., Proudman S., Conaghan P., et al. (1999). Persistence of mild, early inflammatory arthritis: The importance of disease duration, rheumatoid factor, and the shared epitope. *Arthritis and Rheumatism* 42, 2184–2188.
4. Klippel J.H., Dieppe P.A. (1998). *Rheumatology* (2nd ed.). St. Louis: Mosby.
5. Irvine S., Munro R., Porter D. (1999). Early referral, diagnosis, and treatment of rheumatoid arthritis: Evidence for changing medical practice. *Annals of Rheumatic Disease* 58, 510–513.
6. Ramsburg K. (2000). Rheumatoid arthritis. *American Journal of Nursing* 100 (11), 40–43.
7. Iverson M.D., Fossel A.H., Daltroy L.H. (1999). Rheumatologist–patient communication about exercise and physical therapy in the management of rheumatoid arthritis. *Arthritis Care and Research* 12, 180–192.
8. Rodgers E. (1999). Treating pain with COX-2 inhibitors. *Nurse Practitioner* 24 (11), 95–102.
9. Simon K.S., Weaver A.L., Graham D.Y., Kivitz A., Lipsky P., Hubbard P., et al. (1999). Anti-inflammatory and upper gastrointestinal effects of celecoxib in rheumatoid arthritis. *Journal of the American Medical Association* 282, 1921–1928.
10. Halin J. (2000). Treatment of rheumatoid arthritis: Etanercept, a recent advance. *Journal of the American Academy of Nurse Practitioners* 12, 433–441.
11. Weaver A.L. (1999). The evolving therapy of rheumatoid arthritis. In *Today's challenges of rheumatoid arthritis patient management* [pp. 7–15]. University of Nebraska Medical Center CME proceedings. Omaha, NE: Impact Unlimited, Inc.
12. Smolen J.S., Kalden J.R., Scott D.L., Rozman B., Kvien T., Larsen A., et al. (1999). Efficacy and safety of leflunamide compared with placebo and sulfasalazine in active rheumatoid arthritis: A double-blind, randomized, multicenter trial. *Lancet* 353, 259–266.
13. Jones R. E., Moreland L.W. (1999). Tumor necrosis factor inhibitors for rheumatoid arthritis. *Bulletin on the Rheumatic Diseases* 48 (3).
14. Kremer J.M. (1999). Methotrexate and emerging therapies. *Clinical and Experimental Rheumatology* 17 (Suppl. 18), S43–S46.
15. Cypress Bioscience. (1999). *Prescribing information on Prosorbaprotein A immunoadsorption column*. San Diego, CA: Author.
16. Wallace D.J. (1999). Lupus for the non-rheumatologist. *Bulletin on the Rheumatic Diseases* 48 (9).
17. McCowan C.B. (1998). Systemic lupus erythematosus. *Journal of the American Academy of Nurse Practitioners* 10, 225–231.
18. Tan E.M., Cohen A.S., Fries J.C., Masi A., McShane D., Rothfield W., et al. (1982). The 1982 revised criteria for the classification of systemic lupus erythematosus. *Arthritis and Rheumatism* 25, 1271–1277.
19. Pigg J.S., Bancroft D.A. (2000). Management of patients with rheumatic diseases. In Smeltzer S.C., Bare B.C. (Eds.), *Brunner and Suddarth's textbook of medical-surgical nursing* (9th ed., pp. 1405–1433). Philadelphia: Lippincott Williams & Wilkins.
20. Ortman R.A., Klippel J.H. (2000). Update on cyclophosphamide for systemic lupus erythematosus. *Rheumatic Disease Clinics of North America* 26, 363–375.
21. Steen V.D., Medsger T.A. (2000). Severe organ involvement in systemic sclerosis with diffuse scleroderma. *Arthritis and Rheumatism* 43, 2437–2444.
22. Brandt J., Haibel H., Cornely D., Golder W., Gonzalez J., Reddig J., et al. (2000). Successful treatment of active ankylosing spondylitis with the anti-tumor necrosis factor α monoclonal antibody infliximab. *Arthritis and Rheumatism* 43, 1346–1352.
23. Schumacher H.R. (1998). Reactive arthritis. *Rheumatic Disease Clinics of North America* 24, 261–273.
24. Sigal L.H. (2001). Update on reactive arthritis. *Bulletin on the Rheumatic Diseases* 50 (4).
25. Smiley J.D. (1995). Psoriatic arthritis. *Bulletin on the Rheumatic Diseases* 44 (4).
26. Felson D.T. (1998). Preventing knee and hip osteoarthritis. *Bulletin on the Rheumatic Diseases* 47 (7).
27. Huang M., Chen C., Chen T., Weng M., Wang W., Wang Y. (2000). The effects of weight reduction on the rehabilitation of patients with knee osteoarthritis and obesity. *Arthritis Care and Research* 13, 398–405.
28. Leslie M. (1999). Hyaluronic acid treatment for osteoarthritis of the knee. *Nurse Practitioner* 24 (7), 38–48.
29. Puppione A.A. (1999). Management strategies for older adults with osteoarthritis: How to promote and maintain function. *Journal of the American Academy of Nurse Practitioners* 11, 167–171.
30. Dieppe P. (2000). The management of osteoarthritis in the third millennium. *Scandinavian Journal of Rheumatology* 29, 279–281.
31. Agudelo C.A., Wise K.M. (2000). Crystal-associated arthritis in the elderly. *Rheumatic Disease Clinics of North America* 26, 527–546.
32. Segal J.B., Albert D. (1999). Diagnosis of crystal-induced arthritis by synovial fluid examination for crystals: Lessons from an imperfect test. *Arthritis Care and Research* 12, 376–380.
33. Levinson D.J. (1989). Clinical gout and the pathogenesis of hyperuricemia. In McCarthy D.J. (Ed.), *Arthritis and allied conditions* (11th ed., pp. 1645–1677). Philadelphia: Lea & Febiger.
34. Lomater C., Gerloni V., Gattinara M., Mazzetti J., Cimaz R., Fantini F. (2000). Systemic onset juvenile idiopathic arthritis: A retrospective study of 80 consecutive patients followed for 10 years. *Journal of Rheumatology* 27, 491–496.
35. Klepper S. (1999). Effects of an 8 week physical conditioning program on disease signs and symptoms in children with chronic arthritis. *Arthritis Care and Research* 12, 52–60.
36. Yaziu Y., Paget S.A. (2000). Elderly-onset rheumatoid arthritis. *Rheumatic Disease Clinics of North America* 26, 517–526.
37. Kammer G.M., Misha N. (2000). Systemic lupus erythematosus in the elderly. *Rheumatic Disease Clinics of North America* 26, 475–492.
38. Rapp S.R., Rejeski W.J., Miller M.E. (2000). Physical function among older adults with knee pain: The role of coping skills. *Arthritis Care and Research* 13, 270–279.
39. Evans J.M., Hunder G.C. (2000). Polymyalgia rheumatica and giant cell arteritis. *Rheumatic Disease Clinics of North America* 26, 493–515.
40. American College of Rheumatology Ad Hoc Committee on Clinical Guidelines. (1996). Guidelines for monitoring drug therapy in rheumatoid arthritis. *Arthritis and Rheumatism* 30, 723–731.

Integumentary Function

Dermatoglyphics, or the study of the ridges on the skin of the fingertips and palms of the hand, has intrigued cultures throughout the ages. These ridges, which are unique to each individual, develop early in fetal life. In the days before written signatures, the fingerprint was often used as a personal seal on lands sales, loans, and other transactions. Some of the first evidence of the use of fingerprints comes from China, where the practice of imprinting fingers extends over centuries. In the 16th century, when the sale of children was common among the Chinese, whole palm and sole prints were often included on the deed of sale.

Although elements of symbolism, magic, and superstition abound with deciphering of palm creases and fingertip ridges in areas such as fortune-telling, scientific interest was delayed until the late 18th and early 19th centuries. In 1823, J.E. Purkinje (1787–1869) developed the first classification of patterns for fingertip ridges, providing the basis for the use of fingerprints as a means of personal identification. This was followed by an 1880 publication of Henry Faulds (1843–1930), who suggested that fingerprints left at the crime scene could serve as positive identification of offenders when apprehended.

Chapter 60

Control of Integumentary Function

Gladys Simandl

The skin is primarily an organ of protection. It is the largest organ of the body and forms the major barrier between the internal organs and the external environment. The skin accounts for roughly 16% of the body's weight. As the body's first line of defense, the skin is continuously subjected to potentially harmful environmental agents, including solid matter, liquids, gases, sunlight, and microorganisms. Although the skin may become bruised, lacerated, burned, or infected, it has remarkable properties that allow for a continuous cycle of healing, shedding, and cell regeneration.

In its protective role, the skin harbors a constant flora of microorganisms. Relatively harmless strains protect the skin surface from other, more virulent organisms. A thin layer of lipid film covers the skin and contains fatty acids that are bactericidal, protecting against the entry of harmful microorganisms. The skin also serves as an immunologic barrier. The Langerhans' cells detect foreign antigens, playing an important part in allergic skin conditions and skin graft rejections. As a chemical barrier, the skin controls substances entering or leaving the body.

The skin serves several other important functions, including temperature regulation, somatosensory function, and vitamin D synthesis. The skin is richly innervated with pain, temperature, and touch receptors. Skin receptors relay the numerous qualities of touch, such as pressure, sharpness, dullness, and pleasure, to the central nervous system for localization and fine discrimination.

As the outer covering of the body, the skin may demonstrate outwardly what occurs within the body. A number of systemic diseases are manifested by skin disorders (*e.g.*, rash associated with systemic lupus erythematosus and jaundice due to liver disease). In other words, although skin eruptions frequently represent primary diseases of the skin, they may also be a manifestation of systemic disease.

Structure of the Skin

After you have completed this chapter, you should be able to meet the following objectives:

- ✦ List and describe the functions of skin
- ✦ Describe the changes in a keratinocyte from its inception in the basal lamina to its arrival on the outer surface of the skin
- ✦ List the four specialized cells of the epidermis and describe what is known about their functions
- ✦ Describe the structure and function of the dermis and subcutaneous layers of skin
- ✦ Describe the following skin appendages and their functions: sebaceous gland, eccrine gland, apocrine gland, nails, and hair
- ✦ Characterize the skin in terms of sensory and immune functions

Because there are great variations in skin structure on different parts of the body, "normal skin" in any one area of the body is difficult to describe. Variations are found in the properties of the skin, such as the thickness of skin layers, the distribution of sweat glands, and the number and size of hair follicles. For example, the skin is thicker on the palms of the hands and soles of the feet (0.8 mm) than

Functions of the Skin

➤ The skin is the largest organ of the body.

➤ As an interface between the internal and external environments, the skin prevents body fluids from leaving the body, protects the body from potentially damaging environmental agents, and serves as an area for heat exchange; in addition, cells of the skin immune system provide protection against invading microorganisms.

➤ Receptors in the skin relay touch, pressure, temperature, and pain sensation to the central nervous system for localization and discrimination.

elsewhere on the body (0.07 to 0.12 mm). Hair follicles are densely distributed on the scalp, axillae, and genital areas, but they are sparse on the inner arms and abdomen. The apocrine sweat glands are confined to the axillae and the anogenital area.

Nevertheless, certain structural properties are common to all skin in all areas of the body. The skin is composed of two layers: the epidermis (outer layer) and the dermis (inner layer). The basal lamina (basement membrane) divides the two layers. The subcutaneous tissue, a layer of loose connective and fatty tissues, binds the dermis to the underlying tissues of the body (Fig. 60-1). Although the skin is described in the following pages as quite structured and layered, it is

Organization of Skin Structures

➤ The skin has two layers, an outer epidermis and an inner dermis, separated by a basement membrane.

➤ The epidermis, which is avascular, is composed of four to five layers of stratified squamous keratinized epithelial cells that are formed in the deepest layer of the epidermis and migrate to the skin surface to replace cells that are lost during normal skin shedding.

➤ The basement membrane is a thin adhesive layer that cements the epidermis to the dermis. This is the layer involved in blister formation.

➤ The dermis is a connective tissue layer that separates the epidermis from the underlying subcutaneous fat layer. It contains the blood vessels and nerve fibers that supply the epidermis.

never as static as this description implies. The skin is, in fact, a moving, dynamic organ.

EPIDERMIS

The functions of the skin depend on the properties of its outermost layer, the epidermis. The epidermis covers the body, and it is specialized in areas to form the various skin appendages: hair, nails, and glandular structures. The keratinocytes of the epidermis produce a fibrous protein called *keratin*, which is essential to the protective function of skin. In addition to the keratinocytes, the epidermis has three other types of cells that arise from its basal layer: melanocytes that produce a pigment called *melanin*, which is responsible for skin color, tanning, and protecting against ultraviolet radiation; Merkel's cells that provide sensory information; and Langerhans' cells that link the epidermis to the immune system. The epidermis contains openings for two types of glands: sweat glands, which produce watery secretions, and sebaceous glands, which produce an oily secretion called *sebum*.

Keratinocytes

The keratinocyte is the major cell of the epidermis. The epidermis is composed of stratified squamous keratinized epithelium, which, when viewed under the microscope, is seen to consist of five distinct layers, or strata, that represent a progressive differentiation or maturation of the keratinocytes: the stratum germinativum, or basal layer; the stratum spinosum; the stratum granulosum; the stratum lucidum; and the stratum corneum.

The deepest layer, the stratum germinativum or stratum basale, consists of a single layer of basal cells that are attached to the basal lamina. The basal cells, which are columnar, undergo mitosis to produce new keratinocytes that move toward the skin surface to replace cells lost during normal skin shedding. Unlike the other layers of the epidermis, the basal cells do not migrate toward the skin surface, but remain stationary in the stratum germinativum.

The next layer, the stratum spinosum, is formed as the progeny of the basal cell layer move outward toward the skin surface. The stratum spinosum is two to four layers thick, and its cells become differentiated as they migrate outward. The cells of this layer are commonly referred to as *prickle cells*, because they develop a spiny appearance as their cell borders interact.

The stratum granulosum is only a few cells thick; it consists of granular cells that are the most differentiated cells of the living skin. The cells in this layer are unique in that two opposing functions are occurring simultaneously: while some cells are losing cytoplasm and DNA structures, others continue to synthesize keratin.

The stratum lucidum, which lies just superficial to the stratum granulosum, is a thin, transparent layer mostly confined to the palms of the hands and soles of the feet. It consists of transitional cells that retain some of the functions of living skin cells from the layers below but otherwise resemble the cells of the stratum corneum.

The top or surface layer, the stratum corneum, consists of dead, keratinized cells. This layer contains the most cell

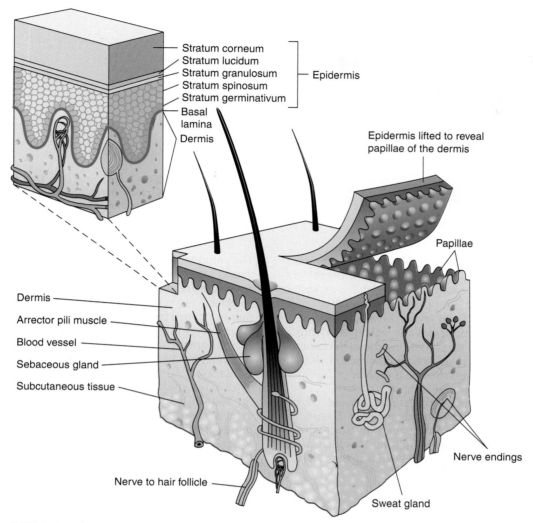

FIGURE 60-1 Three-dimensional view of the skin. (From Chaffee E.E., Lytel I.M. [1980]. *Basic physiology and anatomy.* Philadelphia: J.B. Lippincott)

layers and the largest cells of any zone of the epidermis. It ranges from 15 layers thick in areas such as the face to 25 layers or more on the arm. Specialized areas, such as the palms of the hands or soles of the feet, have 100 or more layers.

The keratinocyte that originates in the basal layer changes morphologically as it is pushed toward the outer layer of the epidermis. For example, in the basal layer, the keratinocyte is round. As it is pushed into the stratum spinosum, the keratinocyte becomes multisided. It becomes flatter in the granular layer and is flattened and elongated in the stratum corneum (Fig. 60-2). The migration time of a keratinocyte from the basal layer to the stratum corneum is 20 to 30 days. Keratinocytes also change cytoplasmic structure and composition as they are pushed outward. This transformation from viable cells to the dead cells of the stratum corneum is called *keratinization.*

The movement of the cells to the surface of the skin can best be described as random or nonsynchronized. Keratinocytes pass other keratinocytes, melanocytes, and Lan-

gerhans' cells as they migrate in a seemingly random fashion. However, the cells are connected with minute points of attachment called *desmosomes.* Desmosomes keep the cells from detaching and provide some structure to the skin while it is in perpetual motion. The basal layer provides the underlying structure and stability for the epidermis.

Melanocytes

Melanocytes are pigment-synthesizing cells that are located at or in the basal layer. They function to produce pigment granules called *melanin*, the black or brown substance that gives skin its color. The ability to synthesize melanin depends on the ability of the melanocytes to produce an enzyme called *tyrosinase*, which converts the amino acid tyrosine to a precursor of melanin. A genetic lack of this enzyme results in a clinical condition called *albinism*. Persons with this disorder lack pigmentation in the skin, hair, and iris of the eye. Tyrosinase is synthesized in the rough endoplasmic reticulum of the melanocytes and then routed to

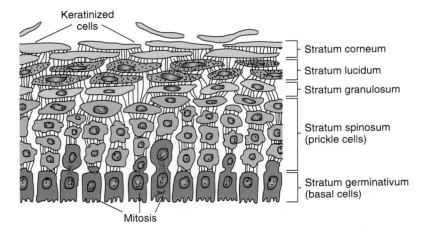

Keratinized cells

Stratum corneum

Stratum lucidum

Stratum granulosum

Stratum spinosum (prickle cells)

Stratum germinativum (basal cells)

Mitosis

FIGURE 60-2 Epidermal cells. The basal cells undergo mitosis, producing keratinocytes that change their size and shape as they move upward, replacing cells that are lost during normal cell shedding.

membranous vesicles in the Golgi complex called *melanosomes*. Melanin is subsequently synthesized in the melanosomes. Melanocytes have long, cytoplasm-filled extensions that extend between the keratinocytes. Although the melanocytes remain in the basal layer, the melanosomes are transferred to the keratinocytes through these dendritic processes. The dendrite tip containing the melanosome is engulfed by a nearby keratinocyte, and the melanin is transferred (Fig. 60-3). Each melanocyte is capable of supplying several keratinocytes with melanin.

Exposure to the sun's ultraviolet rays increases the production of melanin, causing tanning to occur. The primary function of melanin is to protect the skin from harmful ultraviolet sun rays, which are implicated in skin cancers. Melanin protects by absorbing and scattering the radiation.

The amount of melanin in the keratinocytes determines a person's skin color. Black-skinned and white-skinned people have the same amount of melanocytes. However, in the skin of blacks, more melanosomes are produced. The greater number of melanosomes produced and transferred to the keratinocyte is responsible for the darker pigmentation in African Americans; African Americans do not have more melanocytes than whites, but the production of pigment is increased. All people have relatively few or no melanocytes in the epidermis of the palms of the hands or soles of the feet. In light-skinned people, the number of melanocytes decreases with age; the skin becomes lighter and is more susceptible to skin cancer.

Merkel's Cells

Merkel's cells consist of free nerve endings attached to modified epidermal cells. Their origin remains unknown, and they are the least densely populated cells of the epidermis. Merkel's cells are found over the entire body, but are most plentiful on the skin of the fingers, toes, lips, oral cavity, and outermost sheath of hair follicles (*i.e.*, the touch areas). It is believed that Merkel's cells function as mechanoreceptors, or touch receptors. Other encapsulated sensory nerve endings (*e.g.*, pacinian corpuscles, Meissner's corpuscles, Ruffini's corpuscles, Krause's end bulbs) are present in the dermis.

Langerhans' Cells

Langerhans' cells are located in the suprabasal layers of the epidermis among the keratinocytes. They are few in number compared with the keratinocytes. They are derived from precursor cells originating in the bone marrow and continuously repopulate the epidermis. Like melanocytes, they have a dendritic shape and clear cytoplasm. *Birbeck's granules* that often resemble tennis racquets are their most distinguishing characteristic microscopically.

Langerhans' cells are the immunologic cells responsible for recognizing foreign antigens harmful to the body (Fig. 60-4). As such, Langerhans' cells play an important role in defending the body against foreign antigens. Langerhans' cells bind antigen to their surface, process it, and, bearing the processed antigen, migrate from the epidermis into lymphatic vessels and then into regional lymph nodes, where they become known as *dendritic cells*. During their migration

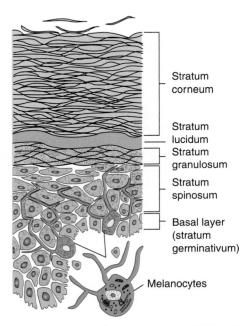

Stratum corneum

Stratum lucidum

Stratum granulosum

Stratum spinosum

Basal layer (stratum germinativum)

Melanocytes

FIGURE 60-3 Melanocytes. The melanocytes, which are located in the basal layer of the skin, produce melanin pigment granules that give skin its color. The melanocytes have threadlike cytoplasmic-filled extensions that are used in passing the pigment granules to the keratinocytes.

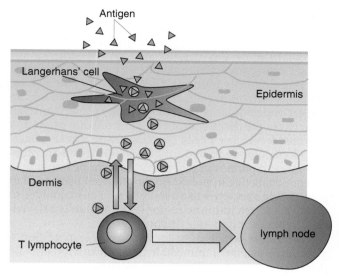

Antigen

Langerhans' cell

Epidermis

Dermis

T lymphocyte

lymph node

FIGURE 60-4 Langerhans' cells.

in the lymph channels, the Langerhans' cells become potent antigen-presenting cells (see Chapter 18). Langerhans' cells are innervated by sympathetic nerve fibers, which may explain why the skin's immune system is altered under stress. An example of this is the exacerbations of acne seen in persons under stress. Keratinocytes also are involved in the

immunologic functions of the skin. Langerhans' cells are antigen-presenting cells, and the keratinocytes produce a number of cytokines that stimulate maturation of skin-localizing T lymphocytes or T cells.

BASAL LAMINA

The basal lamina (basement membrane) is a layer of intercellular and extracellular matrices that serves as an interface between the dermis and the epidermis (Fig. 60-5). It provides for adhesion of the dermis to the epidermis and serves as a selective filter for molecules moving between the two layers. It is also a major site of immunoglobulin and complement deposition in skin disease. The basal lamina is involved in skin disorders that cause bullae or blister formation.

Hemidesmosomes, which resemble half-desmosomes, lie immediately at the basal plasma membrane and form the site or source of tonofilaments, which attach the dermis and epidermis. They also may relay signals between the intracellular keratin filament network and the extracellular basement membrane. The basal lamina consists of three distinct zones or layers—the lamina lucida, lamina densa, and lamina fibroreticularis—all of which contribute to the adhesion of the two skin layers. The *lamina lucida* is an electron-lucent layer where the adherence proteins are located. It consists of fine anchoring filaments and a cell adhesion glycoprotein, called *laminin*, that plays a role in organization of the macromolecules in the basement membrane zones and promotes

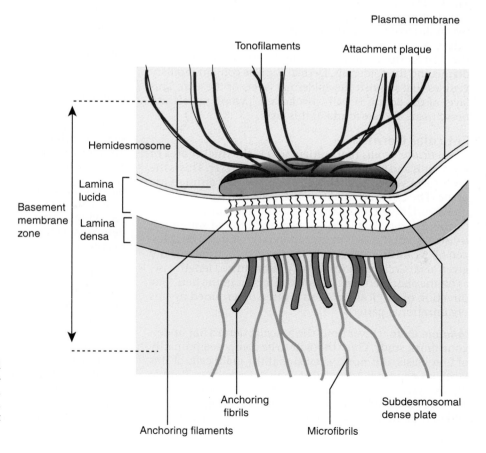

Plasma membrane

Tonofilaments

Attachment plaque

Hemidesmosome

Basement membrane zone

Lamina lucida

Lamina densa

Anchoring fibrils

Anchoring filaments

Microfibrils

Subdesmosomal dense plate

FIGURE 60-5 The dermal–epidermal interface and basement membrane layers. (Adapted from Rubin E., Farber J.L. [1999]. *Pathology* [3rd ed., p. 1244]. Philadelphia: Lippincott Williams & Wilkins)

attachment of cells to the extracellular matrix. The *lamina densa* contains an adhesive called *type IV collagen* as well as laminin. It is important in dermal-epidermal attachment. The *lamina fibroreticularis* contains many anchoring microfibrils. These are short, curved structures that insert into the lamina densa and the upper part of the dermis (superficial dermis), where they are known as *anchoring fibrils*. Type VII collagen, another adherent substance, has been found in the anchoring fibrils and plaques. Another component of the lamina fibroreticularis is elastic fiber bundles that extend to the dermis.

DERMIS

The dermis is the connective tissue layer that separates the epidermis from the subcutaneous fat layer. It supports the epidermis and serves as its primary source of nutrition. The two layers of the dermis, the papillary dermis and the reticular dermis, are composed of cells, fibers, ground substances, nerves, and blood vessels. The pilar (hair) structures and glandular structures are embedded in this layer and continue through the epidermis. In general, the black dermis is more compact than the white dermis, thereby lessening wrinkling in darker-skinned people.

Papillary Dermis

The *papillary dermis* (pars papillaris) is a thin, superficial layer that lies adjacent to the epidermis. It consists of collagen fibers and ground substance. This layer is densely covered with conical projections called *dermal papillae* (see Fig. 60-1). The basal cells of the epidermis project into the papillary dermis, forming *rete ridges*. Microscopically, the junction between the epidermis and the dermis appears like undulating ridges and valleys. It is believed that the dense structure of the dermal papillae serves to minimize the separation of the dermis and the epidermis. Dermal papillae contain capillary venules that nourish the epidermal layers of the skin. This layer of the dermis is well vascularized. Lymph vessels and nerve tissue also are found in this layer.

Reticular Dermis

The *reticular dermis* (pars reticularis) is the thicker area of the dermis and forms the bulk of the dermal layer. This is the layer from which the tough leather hides of animals are made. The reticular dermis is characterized by a complex meshwork of three-dimensional collagen bundles interconnected with large elastic fibers and ground substance, a viscid gel that is rich in mucopolysaccharides. The collagen fibers are oriented parallel to the body's surface in any given area. Collagen bundles may be organized lengthwise, as on the abdomen, or in round clusters, as in the heel. The direction of surgical incisions is often determined by this organizational pattern.

Immune Cells.   Over time, the reticular dermis has undergone much study. Once thought to be composed primarily of fibroblasts, it is now believed that the main cells of this layer are dendritic cells, called *dermal dendrocytes*. Dermal dendrocytes, having both phagocytic and dendritic properties, are believed to possess antigen-presenting functions and play an important part in the immunobiology of the dermis. In addition, it is possible that dermal dendrocytes may be able either to initiate or respond to immunologic occurrences in the epidermis. Dermal dendrocytes also are thought to be involved in processes such as wound healing, blood clotting, and inflammation.

Immune cells found in the dermis include macrophages, T cells, mast cells, and fibroblasts. Dermal macrophages and venular epithelial cells may present antigen to T cells in the dermis. Most of these T cells are previously activated or memory T cells. T-cell responses to macrophage- or endothelium-associated antigens in the dermis are probably more important in generating an immune response to antigen challenge in previously immunized persons than in initiating a response to a new antigen. The major type of T-cell–mediated immune response in the skin is delayed-type hypersensitivity (see Chapter 19).

Mast cells, which have a prominent role in immunoglobulin E–mediated immediate hypersensitivity, also are present in the dermis. These cells are strategically located at body interfaces such as the skin and mucous membranes and are thought to interact with antigens that come in contact with the skin.

Blood Vessels.   The arterial vessels that nourish the skin form two plexuses (*i.e.*, collection of blood vessels), one located between the dermis and the subcutaneous tissue and the other between the papillary and reticular layers of the dermis. The pink color of skin in white persons results primarily from blood seen in the vessels of this plexus. Capillary flow that arises from vessels in this plexus also extends up and nourishes the overlaying epidermis by diffusion. Blood leaves the skin by way of small veins that accompany the subcutaneous arteries. The lymphatic system of the skin, which aids in combating certain skin infections, also is limited to the dermis.

The skin is richly supplied with arteriovenous anastomoses in which blood flows directly between an artery and a vein, bypassing the capillary circulation. These anastomoses are important in terms of temperature regulation. They can open up, letting blood flow through the skin vessels when there is a need to dissipate body heat, and close off, conserving body heat if the environmental temperature is cold.

Innervation.   The innervation of the skin is complex. The skin, with its accessory structures, serves as an organ for receiving sensory information from the environment. The dermis is well supplied with sensory neurons as well as nerves that supply the blood vessels, sweat glands, and arrector pili muscles.

The receptors for touch, pressure, heat, cold, and pain are widely distributed in the dermis (see Chapter 48). The papillary layer of the dermis is supplied with free nerve endings that serve as nociceptors (*i.e.*, pain receptors) and thermoreceptors. The dermis also contains encapsulated pressure-sensitive receptors that detect pressure and touch. The largest of these are the *pacinian corpuscles*, which are widely distributed in the dermis and subcutaneous tissue. The afferent nerve endings of the pacinian corpuscle are surrounded by concentric layers of modified Schwann cells such that they resemble an onion when sectioned. Flat, encapsulated nerve endings found on the palmar surfaces of the fingers and hands and planter surfaces of the feet are called *Meissner's corpuscles*. These are highly sensitive mechanoreceptors for touch. The deep dermis is supplied with small, spindle-shaped mechanoreceptors called *Ruffini's corpuscles*. They register tension in the supporting collagen fibers. A few regions of the skin are supplied by *Krause's end bulbs*, nerve endings contained in an ill-defined capsule. Although their function is uncertain, they are thought to function as mechanoreceptors.

Because of the variations in function among the different types of nerve endings, it is generally agreed that sensory modalities are not associated with a particular type of receptor. For example, the sensations of pain, touch, and pressure probably result from multiple stimuli. The final sensation may be the result of central summation in the central nervous system, which mediates patterned responses.

Most of the skin's blood vessels are under sympathetic nervous system control. The sweat glands are innervated by cholinergic fibers but controlled by the sympathetic nervous system. Likewise, the sympathetic nervous system controls the arrector pili (pilomotor) muscles that cause elevation of hairs on the skin. Contraction of these muscles tends to cause the skin to dimple, producing "goose bumps."

SUBCUTANEOUS TISSUE

The subcutaneous tissue layer consists primarily of fat and connective tissues that lend support to the vascular and neural structures supplying the outer layers of the skin. There is controversy about whether the subcutaneous tissue should be considered an actual layer of the skin. Because the eccrine glands and deep hair follicles extend to this layer and several skin diseases involve the subcutaneous tissue, the subcutaneous tissue may be considered part of the skin.

SKIN APPENDAGES

The skin houses a variety of appendages, including hair, nails, and sebaceous and sweat glands. The distribution and functions of the appendages vary.

Sweat Glands

There are two types of sweat glands: eccrine and apocrine. *Eccrine sweat glands* are simple tubular structures that originate in the dermis and open directly to the skin surface. They are numerous (several million), vary in density, and are located over the entire body surface. Their purpose is to transport sweat to the outer skin surface to regulate body temperature. *Apocrine sweat glands* are less numerous than eccrine sweat glands. They are larger and located deep in the dermal layer. They open through a hair follicle, even though a hair may not be present, and are found primarily in the axillae and groin. The major difference between these glands and the eccrine glands is that apocrine glands secrete an oily substance. In animals, apocrine secretions give rise to distinctive odors that enable animals to recognize the presence of others. In humans, apocrine secretions are sterile until mixed with the bacteria on the skin surface; then they produce what is commonly known as body odor.

Sebaceous Glands

The sebaceous glands are located over the entire skin surface except for the palms, soles, and sides of the feet. They are part of the *pilosebaceous unit*. They secrete a mixture of lipids, including triglycerides, cholesterol, and wax. This mixture is called *sebum*; it lubricates hair and skin. Sebum is not the same as the surface lipid film. Sebum prevents undue evaporation of moisture from the stratum corneum during cold weather and helps to conserve body heat. Sebum production is under the control of genetic and hormonal influences. Sebaceous glands are relatively small and inactive until an individual approaches adolescence. The glands then enlarge, stimulated by the rise in sex hormones. Gland size directly influences the amount of sebum produced, and the level of androgens influences gland size. The sebaceous glands are the structures that become inflamed in acne (see Chapter 61).

Hair

Hair is a structure that originates from hair follicles in the dermis. Most hair follicles are associated with sebaceous glands, and these structures combine to form the pilosebaceous unit. The entire hair structure consists of the hair follicle, sebaceous gland, hair muscle (arrector pili), and, in some instances, the apocrine gland (Fig. 60-6). Hair is a

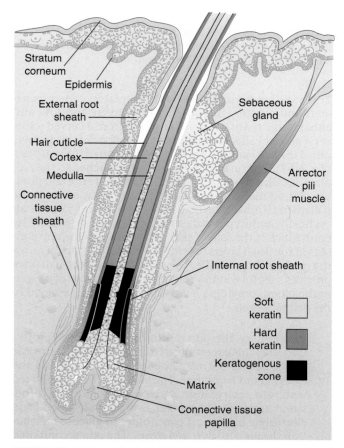

FIGURE 60-6 Parts of a hair follicle. (From LeBond C.P. [1951]. *Annals of the New York Academy of Sciences* 53, 464.)

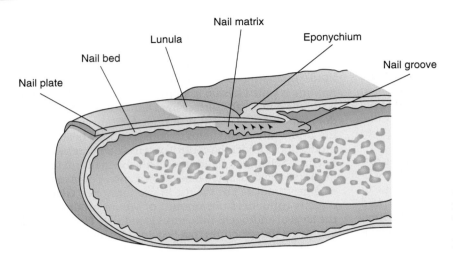

FIGURE 60-7 Parts of a fingernail. *Arrowheads* indicate the direction of displacement of nail cells in the germinal region of the nail plate. (From: Cormack D.H. [1993]. *Essential histology.* Philadelphia: J.B. Lippincott)

keratinized structure that is pushed upward from the hair follicle. Growth of the hair is centered in the bulb (*i.e.*, base) of the hair follicle, and the hair undergoes changes as it is pushed outward. Hair has been found to go through cyclic phases identified as anagen (the growth phase), catagen (the atrophy phase), and telogen (the resting phase). A vascular network at the site of the follicular bulb nourishes and maintains the hair follicle. Melanocytes are found in the bulb and are responsible for the color of the hair. The arrector pili muscle, located under the sebaceous gland, provides a thermoregulation function by contracting to cause "goose bumps," thereby reducing the skin surface area that is available for the dissipation of body heat.

Nails

The nails are hardened keratinized plates, called *fingernails* and *toenails*, that protect the fingers and toes and enhance dexterity. The nails grow out from a curved transverse groove called the *nail groove*. The floor of this groove, called the *nail matrix*, is the germinal region of the nail plate (Fig. 60-7). The underlying epidermis, attached to the nail plate, is called the *nail bed*. Like hair, nails are the end product of dead matrix cells that are pushed outward from the nail matrix. Unlike hair, nails grow continuously rather than cyclically, unless permanently damaged or diseased. The epithelium of the fold of skin that surrounds the nail consists of the usual layers of skin. The stratum corneum forms the *eponychium* or cuticle. The nearly transparent nail plate provides a useful window for viewing the amount of oxygen in the blood, providing a view of the color of the blood in the dermal vessels.

In summary, the skin is primarily an organ of protection. It is the largest organ of the body and forms the major barrier between the internal organs and the external environment. The skin is richly innervated with pain, temperature, and touch receptors; it synthesizes vitamin D and plays an essential role in fluid and electrolyte balance. It contributes to glucose metabolism through its glycogen stores. The skin is composed of two layers, the epidermis and the dermis, separated by a basal lamina. A layer of subcutaneous tissue binds the dermis to the underlying organs and tissues of the body. The epidermis, the outermost layer of the skin, contains five layers, or strata. The major cells of the epidermis are the keratinocytes, melanocytes, Langerhans' cells, and Merkel's cells. The stratum germinativum, or basal layer, is the source of the cells in all five layers of the epidermis. The keratinocytes, which are the major cells of the epidermis, are transformed from viable keratinocytes to dead keratin as they move from the innermost layer of the epidermis (*i.e.*, stratum germinativum) to the outermost layer (*i.e.*, stratum corneum). The melanocytes are pigment-synthesizing cells that give skin its color. The dermis provides the epidermis with support and nutrition and is the source of blood vessels, nerves, and skin appendages (*i.e.*, hair follicles, sebaceous glands, nails, and sweat glands). Sensory receptors for touch, pressure, heat, cold, and pain are widely distributed in the dermis. The skin serves as a first line of defense against microorganisms and other harmful agents. The epidermis contains Langerhans' cells, which process foreign antigens for presentation to T cells, and the dermis contains macrophages, T cells, mast cells, and fibroblasts.

Related Web Sites

American Academy of Dermatology www.aad.org
University of California, Irvine Libraries www.lib.uci.edu

Bibliography

Eady R.A.J., Leigh I.H., Pope F.M. (1998). Anatomy and organization of human skin. In Champion R.H., Burton J.L., Burns D.A., Breathnach S.M. (Eds.), *Textbook of dermatology* (6th ed., pp. 37–111). Oxford: Blackwell Science.

Harrist T.J., Schapiro B., Quinn T.R., Clark W.H. (1999). The skin. In Rubin E., Farber J.L. (Eds.), *Pathology* (3rd ed., pp. 1237–1246). Philadelphia: Lippincott Williams & Wilkins.

Headington J.T. (1993). Dermal dendrocytes. In Nickoloff B.J. (Ed.), *Dermal immune system* (pp. 8–23). Ann Arbor: CRC Press.

Wysocki A.B. (2000). Skin anatomy, physiology, and pathophysiology. *Nursing Clinics of North America* 34, 777–798.

Chapter 61

Alterations in Skin Function and Integrity

Gladys Simandl

The skin is a unique organ in that numerous signs of disease or injury are immediately observable on the skin. Skin serves as an interface between the body's internal and external environments. Therefore, skin disorders represent the culmination of environmental forces and the internal functioning of the body. Sunlight, insects and other arthropods, infectious agents, chemicals, and physical agents all play a role in the pathogenesis of skin disorders. The skin also relays signs of other organ dysfunction.

The skin also has an elusive quality of reflecting emotional states, regardless of disease. It is through the skin that warmth and human affection are given and received. The skin conveys a sense of health, beauty, integrity, and emotion. Human beings emphasize the body and, in particular,

the skin to the degree that even slight imperfections may evoke a wide variety of responses. With the wealth of scientific research and knowledge about the skin, it is increasingly important that people's emotional and psychological responses to their skin conditions be considered.

Manifestations of Skin Disorders

After you have completed this section of the chapter, you should be able to meet the following objectives:

✦ Describe the following skin rashes and lesions: macule, patch, papule, plaque, nodule, tumor, wheal, vesicle, bulla, and pustule

◆ Describe the characteristics and causes of blisters, calluses, and corns

◆ Cite two physiologic explanations for pruritus

◆ Identify the major cause of dry skin

◆ Compare the actions of emollients, humectants, and occlusive moisturizing agents

◆ State common variations found in black skin

No two skin disorders look exactly alike, nor are they necessarily caused by the same agents. The appearance of many skin disorders is influenced by the discomfort, such as itching, a disorder produces or by self-treatment of a disorder. Skin color also may influence the appearance. Nevertheless, most skin disorders have some unique characteristics. Recognition of these characteristics contributes to accurate diagnosis and treatment. This section of the chapter covers lesions and rashes, dry skin, pruritus, skin disorders due to mechanical forces, and variations in black skin.

LESIONS AND RASHES

Rashes are temporary eruptions of the skin, such as those associated with childhood diseases, heat, diaper irritation, or drug-induced reactions. The term *lesion* refers to a traumatic or pathologic loss of normal tissue continuity, structure, or function. The components of a rash sometimes are referred to as *lesions*. Rashes and lesions may range in size from a fraction of a millimeter (*e.g.*, the pinpoint spots of petechiae) to many centimeters (*e.g.*, decubitus ulcer, or pressure sore). They may be blanched (white), erythematous (reddened),

Skin Lesions

➤ Skin disorders may present as a primary skin disease or as evidence of disease of other organ systems.

➤ Skin disorders are characterized by lesions and rashes that vary in size, color, and change in skin structure and integrity.

➤ The skin is amply supplied with pain and itch receptors that cause varying degrees of pain, pruritus, and discomfort in persons with skin lesions.

➤ There are normal differences in terms of skin color, texture, and other properties among persons of different ages and ethnic groups that need to be considered when evaluating skin disorders.

➤ Because the skin is the part of the body that others see and touch, skin disorders can have a great impact on emotional and psychological well-being.

hemorrhagic or purpuric (containing blood), or pigmented. Repeated rubbing and scratching can lead to lichenification (thickened and roughened skin characterized by prominent skin markings due to repeated scratching or rubbing) or excoriation (lesion caused by breakage of the epidermis, producing a raw linear area). Skin lesions may occur as primary lesions arising in previously normal skin, or they may develop as secondary lesions resulting from other disease conditions. Figure 61-1 illustrates various types of skin lesions.

A *blister* is a vesicle or fluid-filled papule. Blisters of mechanical origin form from the friction caused by repeated rubbing on a single area of the skin. Friction blisters most commonly occur on the palmar and plantar surfaces of the hands and feet where the skin is thick enough to form a bleb. Blisters also develop from first-degree and second-degree partial-thickness burns. Histologically, there is degeneration of epidermal cells and a disruption of intercellular junctions that causes the layers of the skin to separate. As a result, fluid accumulates, and a noticeable bleb forms on the skin surface. Blisters are best protected by adding layers of padding (*e.g.*, adhesive bandages and gauze) to prevent further blister formation. Breaking the skin of a blister to remove the fluid is inadvisable because of the risk of secondary infections.

A *callus* is a hyperkeratotic plaque of skin due to chronic pressure or friction. It represents a hyperplasia of the dead keratinized cells that make up the cornified or horny layer of the skin. Increased cohesion between cells results in hyperkeratosis and decreased skin shedding. A callus may be filed down but is likely to recur if pressure continues in the localized area.

Corns are small, well-circumscribed, conical keratinous thickenings of the skin. They usually appear on the toes from rubbing or ill-fitting shoes. The actual corn may be either hard with a central horny core or soft, as commonly seen between the toes. They may appear on the hands as an occupational hazard. Corns on the feet often are painful, whereas corns on the hands may be asymptomatic. Corns may be abraded or surgically removed, but they recur if the causative agent is not removed.

PRURITUS

Pruritus, or the sensation of itch, is a symptom common to many skin disorders. Generalized itching in the absence of a primary skin disease may be symptomatic of other organ disorders, such as chronic renal disease, diabetes, or biliary disease. Warmth, touch, and vibration also can act locally to trigger the itch phenomenon.

Itch is mediated by cutaneous receptors. Both itch and pain sensation, which are thought to be closely related, are carried by small unmyelinated afferent C fibers found in the dermis of the skin, mucous membranes, and cornea (see Chapter 48). The C fibers enter the dorsal horn of the spinal cord, synapse, cross the midline to the opposite side of the cord, and ascend in the spinothalamic tract to the thalamus. From there, the impulse travels to the sensory cortex. A variety of mediators stimulate the C fiber endings and induce itching. Substances such as histamine, bradykinin,

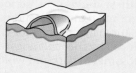

Circumscribed, flat, nonpalpable changes in skin color	Palpable elevated solid masses	Circumscribed superficial elevations of the skin formed by free fluid in a cavity within the skin layers

Macule—Small, up to 1 cm. Example: freckle, petechia
Patch—Larger than 1 cm. Example: vitiligo

Papule—Up to 0.5 cm. Example: elevated nevus
Plaque—A flat, elevated surface larger than 0.5 cm, often formed by the coalescence of papules
Nodule—0.5 cm to 1–2 cm; often deeper and firmer than a papule
Tumor—Larger than 1–2 cm
Wheal—A somewhat irregular, relatively transient, superficial area of localized skin edema. Example: mosquito bite, hive

Vesicle—Up to 0.5 cm; filled with serous fluid. Example: herpes simplex
Bulla—Greater than 0.5 cm; filled with serous fluid. Example: 2nd-degree burn
Pustule—Filled with pus. Examples: acne, impetigo

FIGURE 61-1 Primary lesions may arise from previously normal skin. Authorities vary somewhat in their definitions of skin lesions by size. Dimensions given should be considered approximate. (Bates B.B. [1995]. *A guide to physical examination and history taking* [6th ed.]. Philadelphia: J.B. Lippincott)

substance P, and bile salts act locally to stimulate the itch receptors. Prostaglandins are modulators of the itch response, lowering the threshold for other mediators. One type of itch, sometimes referred to as *central itch*, is perceived as occurring on the skin, but originates in the central nervous system (CNS).[1] For example, the pain reliever morphine promotes itch by acting on central opioid receptors in the CNS.

Scratching, the well-known response to itch, is a neurologic reflex that to varying degrees can be controlled by the individual. Although scratching may temporarily relieve itch, many types of itch are not easily localized and are not relieved by scratching. In many people, excoriations and thickened papular areas develop at the site of repeated scratching or rubbing.

Because excoriated skin is more susceptible to infectious processes, measures to determine the source of itch and to prevent scratching are important. Most treatment measures for pruritus are palliative, largely because it is poorly understood. Measures such as using the entire hand to rub over large areas and keeping the fingernails trimmed often can relieve itch and prevent skin damage.[2] Because vasodilation tends to increase itching, cold applications may provide relief. Cool showers before bed, light sleepwear, and cool home temperatures also may be helpful. Self-limited or seasonal cases of pruritus may respond to such treatment measures as moisturizing lotions, bath oils, and the use of humidifiers. Application of topical corticosteroids may be helpful in some cases, such as itch related to allergy-mediated urticaria. Systemic antihistamines and corticosteroids may be indicated for persons with severe pruritus.

Opioid antagonists may be used for pruritus caused by opioid medications such as morphine.

DRY SKIN

Dry skin, also called *xerosis*, may be a natural occurrence, as in the drying of skin associated with aging, or it may be symptomatic of underlying skin or systemic disorders. Most cases of dry skin are caused by dehydration of the stratum corneum. A decrease in the secretion of moisture from the sweat glands and oil from the sebaceous glands may contribute to dry skin in older persons. Any number of symptoms may accompany dry skin, such as pruritus or discomfort.

Treatment should be directed toward alleviating dry skin with moisturizing agents that maintain skin hydration. Moisturizing agents can be emollients, humectants, or occlusives. *Emollients* are fatty acid–containing lotions that replenish the oils on the skin surface, but usually do not leave a residue on the skin. Emollients have a short duration of action and need to be applied frequently. *Humectants* are the additives in lotions, such as urea, that draw out water from the deeper skin layers and hold it on the skin surface. *Occlusives* are thick creams that contain petroleum or some other moisture-proof material. They prevent water loss from the skin. Occlusives are the most effective agents for relieving skin dryness, but because of their greasiness and lack of cosmetic appeal, some persons do not wish to use them. Use of room humidifiers and keeping the room temperature as low as possible to prevent water loss from the skin also may be helpful.

VARIATIONS IN BLACK SKIN

Some skin disorders common to African Americans are not commonly found in European Americans. Similarly, some skin disorders, such as skin cancers, affect light-skinned persons more commonly than dark-skinned persons. Because of these differences, serious skin disorders may be overlooked, and normal variations in darker skin may be mistaken for anomalies. Skin color is determined by the melanin produced by the melanocytes. Although the number of melanosomes in dark and white skin are the same, black skin produces more melanin and produces it faster than does white skin. Because of their skin color, blacks are better protected against skin cancer and the premature wrinkling and aging of the skin that occurs with sun exposure.

Some conditions common in people with black skin are too much or too little color. Areas of the skin may darken after injury, such as a cut or scrape, or after disease conditions such as acne.[3] These darkened areas may take many months or years to fade. Dry or "ashy" skin also can be a problem for people with black skin. It often is uncomfortable, and it also is easily noticed because it gives the skin an ashen, or grayish, appearance. Although using a moisturizer may help relieve the discomfort, it may cause a worsening of acne in predisposed persons.

Normal variations in skin structure and skin tones often make evaluation of dark skin difficult (Table 61-1). The darker pigmentation can make skin pallor, cyanosis,

and erythema more difficult to observe. Therefore, verbal histories must be relied on to assess skin changes. The verbal history should include clients' descriptions of their normal skin tone. Changes in skin color, in particular hypopigmentation and hyperpigmentation, often accompany ethnic skin disorders and are very important signs to observe for when diagnosing skin conditions. The appearances of skin disorders common to dark skin are listed in Table 61-2.

In summary, skin lesions and rashes are the most common manifestations of skin disorders. Rashes are temporary skin eruptions. Lesions result from traumatic or pathologic loss of the normal continuity, structure, or function of the skin. Lesions may be vascular in origin; they may occur as primary lesions in previously normal skin; or they may develop as secondary lesions resulting from primary lesions. Blisters, calluses, and corns result from rubbing, pressure, and frictional forces applied to the skin. Pruritus and dry skin are symptoms common to many skin disorders. Scratching because of pruritus can lead to excoriation, infection, and other complications. Normal variations in black skin often make evaluation difficult and result in some disorders being overlooked. Changes in color, especially hypopigmentation or hyperpigmentation, often accompany the skin disorders of dark-skinned people.

TABLE 61-1 ✦ Common Normal Variations in Dark Skin

Variation	Appearance
Futcher (Voigt's) line	Demarcation between darkly pigmented and lightly pigmented skin in upper arm; follows spinal nerve distribution; common in black and Japanese populations
Midline hypopigmentation	Line or band of hypopigmentation over the sternum, dark or faint, lessens with age; common in Latin American and black populations
Nail pigmentation	Linear dark bands down nails or diffuse nail pigmentation, brown, blue or blue-black
Oral pigmentation	Blue to blue-gray pigmentation of oral mucosa; gingivae also affected
Palmar changes	Hyperpigmented creases, small hyperkeratotic papules, and tiny pits in creases
Plantar changes	Hyperpigmented macules, can be multiple with patchy distribution, irregular borders, and variance in color

(Developed from information in Rosen T., Martin S. [1981]. *Atlas of black dermatology.* Boston: Little, Brown)

Skin Damage Due to Ultraviolet Radiation

After you have completed this section of the chapter, you should be able to meet the following objectives:

✦ Describe the three types of ultraviolet radiation and relate them to sunburn, aging skin changes, and the development of skin cancer
✦ Describe the manifestations and treatment of sunburn
✦ List three drugs that produce photosensitivity
✦ State the properties of an effective sunscreen

The skin is the protective shield against harmful ultraviolet rays from the sun. The increased production of melanin as a result of exposure to ultraviolet radiation is believed to be the body's protective response. Skin cancers and other skin disorders such as early wrinkling and aging of the skin have been attributed to the damaging effects of sunlight.

ULTRAVIOLET RAYS

The earth's sunlight is measured in wavelengths ranging from approximately 290 nm in the ultraviolet region up to approximately 2500 nm in the infrared region. Ultraviolet radiation accounts for roughly 5% of solar radiation, but the amount of radiation human beings are exposed to has increased because of artificial sources, such as tanning salons and occupational exposure.

TABLE 61-2 ✦ **Appearance of Common Disorders of Black Skin**

Disorder	Appearance
Hot-comb alopecia	Well-defined patches of scalp alopecia on crown; extends down; decreased number of follicular orifices, hair loss irreversible; due to use of hot comb with petroleum, more common with Afro hairstyles
Infantile acropustulosis	Crops of vesicopustules for 7 to 10 days, followed by a 2- to 3-week remission before recurrence; pruritus; affects palms and soles of feet in children 2 to 10 months of age; resolves by 3 years of age
Keloids	Firm, smooth, shiny, hairless, elevated scars, sometimes hyperpigmented; often with symptomatic pruritus, tenderness, or pain; extremely common even with simple wounds on ears, neck, jaw, cheeks, upper chest, shoulders, and back
Mongolian spot	Very common; ill-defined light blue to slate-gray macule in lumbosacral area; usually disappears but may persist through adulthood
Atopic dermatitis	Follicular lesion development that progresses to a lichenification stage; hyperpigmented lichenifications are interspersed with excoriated pink patches; common in blacks
Pityriasis rosea	Lesions are salmon-pink, dull red, or dark brown; profuse, fine scales, not commonly seen in white skin; postinflammatory pigmentary changes are more common in blacks
Psoriasis	Does not commonly occur in blacks; distribution is similar, but the plaques are bright red, violet, or blue-black; pigment changes may persist after treatment
Tinea versicolor	Common in blacks, increased incidence in tropical climates; hypopigmented or extremely hyperpigmented patches, gray to dark brown; occurs more often on the face in blacks than in whites
Lichen planus	Papules are deep purple from pigmentary leakage; oral lesions are uncommon; hypertrophic lesions are more common in blacks than in whites

(Developed from information in Rosen T., Martin S. [1981]. *Atlas of black dermatology.* Boston: Little, Brown)

Ultraviolet radiation is divided into three types: UVC, UVB, and UVA. UVC rays are short (100 to 289 nm) and do not pass through the earth's atmosphere. However, they can be produced artificially and are damaging to the eyes. UVB rays are 290 to 320 nm. These are the rays that are primarily responsible for nearly all the skin effects of sunlight. They are more commonly referred to as *sunburn rays*. UVA rays are 321 to 400 nm. These rays, which can pass through window glass, are more commonly referred to as *suntanning rays*. In general, it takes approximately 1000 times more UVA to match the untoward effects of UVB. Nonetheless, UVA contributes to many skin alterations. Artificial sources of UVA, such as tanning salons, may produce the same effects as UVB.[4,5]

The wavelength of sunlight is determined by the ozone layer in the atmosphere. Ozone absorbs wavelengths shorter than 320 nm; the shortest wavelength of sunlight reaching the earth is approximately 290 nm. The diminishing ozone layer is believed to be a critical factor in increased ultraviolet light exposure and the concomitant increased incidence over the past several decades of cancerous skin lesions.[4] Smoke and fog may play a part in reducing the intensity of ultraviolet radiation.

With ultraviolet radiation exposure, skin cells release vasoactive and injurious chemicals, resulting in vasodilation and sunburn. Melanin in the stratum corneum absorbs ultraviolet radiation. The skin responds to ultraviolet radiation exposure with an increase in melanin content as a means of preventing destruction of the lower skin layers. Components of the immune system in the skin, especially Langerhans' cells, are also involved. The number of immune cells is decreased and cell activity is lessened by ultraviolet radiation exposure.[6] It is thought that the immune cells are important in removing sun-damaged cells with malignant potential.[7]

Ultraviolet Radiation Exposure

➤ The ultraviolet rays of sunlight have the potential for directly damaging skin cells, accelerating the effect of aging on skin, and producing changes that predispose to development of skin cancer.

➤ Protection from the sun's harmful rays should include avoidance of sun exposure, use of protective clothing, and use of sunscreens.

SUNBURN

Sunburn is caused by excessive exposure of the epidermal and dermal layers of the skin to ultraviolet radiation, resulting in an erythematous inflammatory reaction. Sunburn ranges from mild to severe. A mild sunburn consists of various degrees of skin redness. Inflammation, vesicle eruption, weakness, chills, fever, malaise, and pain accompany more severe forms of sunburn. Scaling and peeling follow any overexposure to sunlight. Black skin also burns and may appear grayish or gray-black.

Severe sunburns are treated with wet Burow's solution soaks and topical creams and lotions to limit inflammation and pain.[8] Extensive second- and third-degree burns may require hospitalization and specialized burn care techniques, as described under Burns.

DRUG-INDUCED PHOTOSENSITIVITY

Some drugs are classified as photosensitive drugs because they produce an exaggerated response to ultraviolet light when the drug is taken in combination with sun exposure. Examples include some of the anti-infective agents (sulfonamides, tetracyclines, nalidixic acid), antihistamines (cyproheptadine, diphenhydramine), antineoplastic agents (fluorouracil, methotrexate, procarbazine), antipsychotic agents (phenothiazines, haloperidol), diuretics (thiazides, acetazolamide, amiloride), hypoglycemic agents (sulfonylureas), and nonsteroidal anti-inflammatory drugs (phenylbutazone, ketoprofen, naproxen).[9]

Drug-induced photosensitivity, such as UVA photosensitivity induced by the psoralens, may be used in treating skin conditions, such as psoriasis, that respond well to ultraviolet radiation exposure. Because an increased incidence of cancerous lesions has been reported in people who have been treated with these agents, their use requires caution and careful surveillance.

SUNSCREENS AND OTHER PROTECTIVE MEASURES

The ultraviolet rays of sunlight or other sources can be either completely or partially blocked from the skin surface by sunscreens. The U.S. Food and Drug Administration (FDA) requires a sun protection factor (SPF) rating on all commercial suntan preparations based on their ability to obstruct ultraviolet radiation absorption. The ratings usually are on a scale of 1 to 30; higher ratings block more sunlight.[10] Products with a higher SPF screen out more UVB rays, which are responsible for acute sun damage.

There are two primary types of sunscreens available on the market—chemical (soluble) agents and physical (insoluble) agents.[10] Chemical agents protect the skin from absorbing sunlight and physical agents work by reflecting sunlight. Although most sunscreen agents contain para-aminobenzoic acid (PABA), a chemical blocking agent that protects against UVB, some do not contain PABA. People who are sensitive to benzocaine, procaine, sulfonamides, or thiazide diuretics should use sunscreens that do not contain PABA. Broad-spectrum suntan lotions protect against UVA. These products contain a benzophenone such as oxybenzone, dioxybenzone, or avobenzone. Newer agents such as micronized titanium dioxide and microfine zinc act by reflecting as well as absorbing sunlight. They protect against most of the ultraviolet spectrum. Sunless suntan creams, such as dihydroxyacetone, produce a tan without exposure to the sun.

Sunscreens are available as lotions, creams, oils, gels, and sprays. They also are incorporated into cosmetics and lip balms. Sunscreens should be used diligently and according to the person's tendency to burn rather than tan. It is recommended that they be applied 30 minutes before sun exposure and reapplied every 2 hours. Water-resistant preparations maintain sunburn protection after being in the water for up to 40 minutes. Early morning and late afternoon sun exposures are less harmful because the ultraviolet rays are longer. Because many skin cancers are correlated with childhood sunburns, children younger than 18 years of age should use sunscreens that have a blocking agent with an SPF of at least 15. However, sunscreens may encourage a false sense of security. Prolonged sun exposure as a result of using sunscreens may still increase the chance of getting skin cancers, particularly melanoma.[10]

Other protective measures include knowledge about sunlight and how to protect the skin. Shade does not necessarily protect persons from the sun's rays because ultraviolet rays are reflected from many surfaces. Sand is a good reflector of sunlight. A person can become sunburned even while sitting under an umbrella on a sandy beach. Water absorbs ultraviolet radiation rather than reflecting it. However, ultraviolet radiation penetrates the upper few inches of clear water. This, combined with the scattered reflection of water, can increase the exposure to ultraviolet radiation. Shielding the skin with clothing and hats or head coverings helps decrease ultraviolet radiation exposure.

> In summary, there has been an alarming increase in skin cancers since the early 1980s, and repeated exposure to the ultraviolet rays of the sun has been implicated as its principal cause. Solar and artificial sources of radiation contribute to the amount of radiation to which human beings are exposed. Sunburn, which is caused by excessive exposure to ultraviolet radiation, is an erythematous inflammatory reaction, ranging from mild to severe. Photosensitive drugs can also produce an exaggerated response to ultraviolet light when they are taken in combination with sun exposure. Sunscreens are protective agents that work by either reflecting sunlight or preventing its absorption.

▌ Primary Disorders of the Skin

After you have completed this section of the chapter, you should be able to meet the following objectives:

- ✦ Describe common pigmentary disorders of the skin
- ✦ Identify the major treatment methods for vitiligo, albinism, and melasma
- ✦ Relate the behavior of fungi to the production of superficial skin lesions associated with tinea or ringworm
- ✦ State the cause and describe the appearance of impetigo and ecthyma
- ✦ Compare the viral causes, manifestations, and treatments of verrucae, herpes simplex, and herpes zoster lesions
- ✦ Compare acne vulgaris, acne conglobata, and rosacea in terms of appearance and location of lesions
- ✦ Describe the pathogenesis of acne vulgaris and relate it to measures used in treating the disorder
- ✦ Differentiate allergic and contact dermatitis and atopic and nummular eczema

◆ Describe the differences and similarities between erythema multiforme minor, Stevens-Johnson syndrome, and toxic epidermal necrolysis

◆ Define the term *papulosquamous* and use the term to describe the lesions associated with psoriasis, pityriasis rosea, and lichen planus

◆ Relate the life cycle of *Sarcoptes scabiei* to the skin lesions seen in scabies

◆ Use knowledge of the life cycles of *Pediculus humanus corporis* and *Pediculus humanus capitis* to explain the lesions associated with body and head lice

◆ Explain the mechanism whereby ticks transmit disease to humans, and name the organisms and state the major manifestations of Rocky Mountain spotted fever and Lyme disease

Primary skin disorders are those originating in the skin. They include pigmentary skin disorders, infectious processes, acne and rosacea, papulosquamous dermatoses, allergic disorders and drug reactions, and arthropod infestations. Although most of these disorders are not life threatening, they can affect the quality of life.

Primary Skin Disorders

➤ Primary skin disorders originate in the skin and are those that result from changes in pigmentation; fungal, bacterial, and viral infections; hypersensitivity and allergic reactions; and arthropod infestations.

➤ Pigmentary skin disorders involve increased, decreased, or absent melanocyte function.

➤ Infectious skin disorders are caused by organisms that invade the skin, incite inflammatory responses, and otherwise cause rashes and lesions that disrupt the skin surface.

➤ Acne involves occlusion of the pilosebaceous unit with noninflammatory and inflammatory lesions resulting from occlusion, inflammation due to the irritating effects of sebum, and infection caused by the *P. acnes* organism.

➤ Allergic and hypersensitivity responses are caused by antigen-antibody responses resulting from sensitization to topical or systemic antigens.

➤ The papulosquamous dermatoses constitute a group of disorders characterized by scaling papules and plaques that result from uncontrolled keratinocyte proliferation.

➤ Arthropod skin infestations are caused by bugs, ticks, and parasites that attach to and invade skin structures. They are transmitted from person to person, from animals to humans, or from inanimate objects to humans.

PIGMENTARY SKIN DISORDERS

Pigmentary skin disorders involve the melanocytes. In some cases, there is an absence of melanin production, as in vitiligo or albinism. In other cases, there is an increase in melanin or some other pigment, as in mongolian spots or melasma. In either case, the emotional impact can be devastating. Because pigmentary changes can result in social ostracism, it is important to treat the emotional and social components of these skin disorders as well.

Vitiligo

Vitiligo is a pigmentary problem of concern to darkly pigmented persons of all races. It also affects whites, but not as often; and the effects usually are not as socially problematic. The classic sign of vitiligo is the sudden appearance of white patches on the skin. The lesion is a depigmented macule with definite smooth borders on the face, axillae, neck, or extremities (Fig. 61-2). The patches vary in size from small macules to ones involving large skin surfaces. The large macular type is more common. Depigmented areas appear white, pale colored, or sometimes grayish-blue. Histologically, the depigmented areas may contain no melanocytes or amounts of melanocytes that are greatly altered or decreased; in some cases the melanocytes no longer produce melanin. These areas burn easily in sunlight, and they enlarge over time. Vitiligo often is asymptomatic, although pruritus may occur.

Vitiligo appears at any age, but the peak incidence is in the second and third decades. Women have a higher incidence. It has been on the rise in India, Pakistan, and East Asian countries. Although the cause is unknown, autoimmune factors have been implicated because it often accompanies other autoimmune diseases, such as diabetes mellitus and pernicious anemia. Vitiligo also may be a cutaneous expression of a systemic disorder, especially thyroid disease. Although there is a familial tendency, vitiligo may be precipitated by emotional stress or physical trauma, such as sunburn.

Although there are many treatment regimens for vitiligo, none is curative. Self-tanning lotions, skin stains, and cosmetics are used for camouflage. Self-tanning compounds

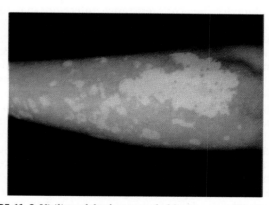

FIGURE 61-2 Vitiligo of the forearm of a black person. (Neutrogena Skin Care Institute.) (Sauer G.C., Hall J.C. [1996]. *Manual of skin diseases* [7th ed.]. Philadelphia: Lippincott-Raven)

contain a chemical called *dihydroxyacetone* that does not need melanocytes to color the skin.[11] Topical corticosteroids have been used, and the combination of psoralen and UVA (PUVA) treatment has been somewhat successful in people with large areas of skin involvement. If extensive skin surfaces are involved, the treatment may be reversed and the pigmented areas bleached to match the remainder of the skin color.

Albinism

Albinism is a congenital disorder in which there is a normal number of melanocytes, but they lack tyrosinase, the enzyme needed for synthesis of melanin. Although there are over 10 different types of albinism, the most common type is recessively inherited oculocutaneous albinism. It affects the skin, hair, and eyes. Individuals have pale or pink skin, white or yellow hair, and light-colored or sometimes pink eyes. Persons with albinism have ocular problems, such as extreme sensitivity to light, refractive errors, and nystagmus. There is no cure for albinism. Treatment efforts for people with albinism are aimed at reducing their risk for cancer through protection from solar radiation and screening for malignant skin changes.

Melasma

Melasma is a disorder characterized by darkened macules on the face. It is common in all skin types, but most prominent in brown-skinned people from Asia, India, and South America. It occurs in men but is more common in women, particularly during pregnancy or while using oral contraceptives. It may or may not resolve after giving birth or discontinuing hormonal birth control. Melasma is exacerbated by sun exposure. Treatment measures are palliative, mostly consisting of limiting exposure to the sun and using sunscreens. Bleaching agents, tretinoin cream, and azelaic acid have been useful in treating severe cases.

INFECTIOUS PROCESSES

The skin is subject to invasion by a number of microorganisms, including fungi, bacteria, and viruses. Normally, the skin flora, sebum, immune responses, and other protective mechanisms guard the skin against infection. Depending on the virulence of the infecting agent and the competence of the host's resistance, infections may result.

Superficial Fungal Infections

Fungi are free-living, saprophytic, plantlike organisms, certain strains of which are considered part of the normal skin flora (see Chapter 17). Fungal or mycotic infections of the skin are traditionally classified as superficial or deep. The superficial mycoses, more commonly known as *tinea* or *ringworm*, invade only the superficial keratinized tissue (skin, hair, and nails). Deep fungal infections involve the epidermis, dermis, and subcutis. Infections that typically are superficial may exhibit deep involvement in immunosuppressed individuals.

Most of the superficial mycoses (or *dermatophytoses*) are caused by the dermatophytes, a group of closely related fungi classified into three genera: *Microsporum* (*M. audouinii, M. canis, M. gypseum*), *Epidermophyton* (*E. floccosum*), and *Trichophyton* (*T. schoenleinii, T. violaceum, T. tonsurans*).[12] Another way of classifying the dermatophytes is according to their ecologic origin—human, animal, or soil. Anthropophilic species (*M. audouinii, M. tonsurans, T. violaceum*) are parasitic on humans and are spread by other infected humans. Zoophilic species (*M. canis* and *T. mentagrophytes*) cause parasitic infections in animals, some of which can be spread to human beings. Geophilic species originate in the soil, but may infect animals, which in turn serve to infect human beings.

The fungi that cause superficial mycoses live on the dead keratinized cells of the epidermis. They emit an enzyme that enables them to digest keratin, which results in superficial skin scaling, nail disintegration, or hair breakage, depending on the location of the infection. An exception to this is the invading fungus of tinea versicolor, which does not produce a keratolytic enzyme. Deeper reactions involving vesicles, erythema, and infiltration are thought to be caused by the inflammation that results from exotoxins liberated by the fungus. Fungi also are capable of producing an allergic or immune response. Superficial fungal infections affect various parts of the body, with the lesions varying according to site and fungal species. Tinea can affect the body (tinea corporis), face and neck (tinea faciei), scalp (tinea capitis), hands (tinea manus), feet (tinea pedis), or nails (tinea unguium).

Diagnosis of superficial fungal infections is primarily done by microscopic examination of skin scrapings for fungal spores, the reproducing bodies of fungi. Potassium hydroxide (KOH) preparations are used to prepare slides of skin scrapings. KOH disintegrates human tissue and leaves behind the threadlike filaments, called *hyphae*, that grow from the fungal spores. Cultures also may be done using a dermatophyte test medium or a microculture slide that produces color changes and allows for direct microscopic identification. The Wood's light (ultraviolet light) is another method that can assist with the diagnosis of tinea. Some types of fungi (*e.g., M. canis* and *M. audouinii*) fluoresce a yellow-green color when the light is directed onto the affected area.[13]

Superficial fungal infections may be treated with topical or systemic antifungal agents. Treatment usually follows diagnosis confirmed by KOH preparation or culture, particularly if a systemic agent is to be used. Topical agents, both prescription and over-the-counter preparations, are commonly used in the treatment of tinea infections; however, outcome success often is limited because of the lengthy duration of treatment, poor compliance, and high rates of relapse at specific body sites.

The oral systemic antifungal agents include griseofulvin, the azoles, and the allylamines. Griseofulvin is a fungicidal agent derived from a species of *Penicillium* that is used only in the treatment of dermatophytoses. It acts by binding to the keratin of newly forming skin, protecting the skin from new infection. Because its action is to prevent new infection, it must be administered for 2 to 6 weeks to allow for skin replacement. The azoles are a group of synthetic antifungal drugs that act by inhibiting the fungal enzymes needed for the synthesis of ergosterol, which is an essential part of fungal cell membranes. The azoles are classified as either imidazoles or triazoles. The imidazoles consist of ketoconazole, miconazole, and clotrimazole. The latter two drugs are used only in topical therapy. The triazoles include itraconazole and fluconazole, both of which are used for the systemic treatment of fungal infections. Terbinafine, a synthetic allylamine, acts by interrupting ergosterol synthesis, causing the accumulation of a metabolite that is toxic to the fungus. In contrast to griseofulvin, the synthetic agents are fungicidal (*i.e.*, kill the fungus) and therefore are more effective over shorter treatment periods.[13] Some of the oral agents can produce serious side effects, such as hepatic toxicity, or interact adversely with other medications being taken. A number of the synthetic fungicides (*e.g.*, ketoconazole, miconazole, clotrimazole, and terbinafine) are available as topical preparations and produce less severe side effects. Topical corticosteroids may be used in conjunction with antifungal agents to relieve itching and erythema secondary to inflammation.

Tinea of the Body or Face. *Tinea corporis* (ringworm of the body) can be caused by any of the fungi, but it usually is caused by *M. canis* or *M. audouinii;* less frequently, it is caused by *T. rubrum* or *T. mentagrophytes*. Although tinea corporis affects all ages, children seem most prone to infection. Transmission is most commonly from kittens, puppies, and other children who have infections.

The lesions vary, depending on the fungal agent. The most common types of lesions are oval or circular patches on exposed skin surfaces and the trunk, back, or buttocks (Fig. 61-3). Less common are foot and groin infections. The lesion begins as a red papule and enlarges, often with a central clearing. Patches have raised red borders consisting of vesicles, papules, or pustules. The borders are sharply defined, but lesions may coalesce. Pruritus, a mild burning sensation, and erythema frequently accompany the skin lesion.

Tinea faciale, or ringworm of the face, is an infection caused by *T. mentagrophytes* or *T. rubrum*. Tinea faciale may mimic the annular, erythematous, scaling, pruritic lesions characteristic of tinea corporis. It also may appear as flat erythematous patches. In either case, misdiagnosis is not uncommon.

Topical antifungal agents usually are effective in treating tinea corporis and tinea faciale. Oral antifungal agents may be used in resistant cases.

Tinea of the Scalp. There are two common types of *tinea capitis* (ringworm of the scalp): primary (noninflammatory) and secondary (inflammatory). Depending on the invading fungus, the lesions of the noninflammatory type can vary from grayish, round, hairless patches to balding spots or black dots on the head. The lesions vary in size and are most commonly seen on the back of the head (Fig. 61-4). Mild erythema, crust, or scale may be present. The individual usually is asymptomatic, although pruritus may exist. In the United States, 90% of the cases of noninflammatory tinea capitis are caused by *T. tonsurans,* which does not fluoresce green with a Wood's lamp.[14] Children between 3 and 14 years of age are primarily affected, although there are increasing numbers of adults being diagnosed. The lesser incidence among adults has been partially attributed to the higher content of fatty acids in the sebum after puberty.

The inflammatory type of tinea capitis is caused by virulent strains of *T. mentagrophytes, T. verrucosum,* and *M. gypseum*. The onset is rapid, and lesions usually are localized to one area. The initial lesion consists of a pustular, scaly, round patch with broken hairs. A secondary bacterial infection is common and may lead to a painful, circumscribed, boggy, and indurated lesion called a *kerion*. The highest incidence is among children and farmers who work with infected animals.

The treatment for both forms of tinea capitis is oral griseofulvin or synthetic antifungals. Topical ointments or shampoos are sometimes indicated in addition to oral medications. Because of the lower fatty acid content in sebum of young children, several of the topical antifungal agents are prepared with fatty acid bases. These antifungal agents have

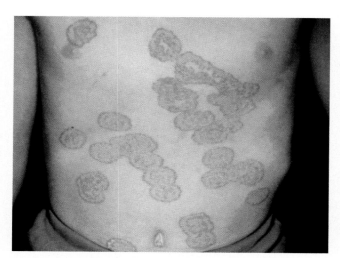

FIGURE 61-3 Tinea of the body caused by *Microsporum canis*. (Sauer G.C., Hall J.C. [1996]. *Manual of skin diseases* [7th ed.]. Philadelphia: Lippincott-Raven)

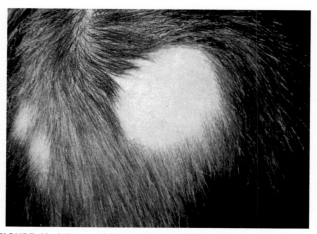

FIGURE 61-4 Tinea of the scalp caused by *Microsporum audouinii*. (Sauer G.C., Hall J.C. [1996]. *Manual of skin diseases* [7th ed.]. Philadelphia: Lippincott-Raven)

revolutionized treatment, replacing the old remedies in which children often were subjected to head shavings and the use of harsh shampoos and salves. Wet packs, medicated shampoos, and antibiotics may be prescribed for secondary infections that occur.

Tinea of the Foot and Hand. *Tinea pedis* (athlete's foot, or ringworm of the feet) is a common dermatosis primarily affecting the spaces between the toes, the soles of the feet, or the sides of the feet (Fig. 61-5). It is caused by *T. mentagrophytes* and *T. rubrum*. The lesions vary from a mildly scaling lesion to a painful, exudative, erosive, inflamed lesion with fissuring. Lesions often are accompanied by pruritus, pain, and foul odor. Some persons are prone to chronic tinea pedis. Mild forms are more common during dry environmental conditions. Exacerbations of the mild form occur as a result of hot weather, sweating, and exercise or when the feet are exposed to moisture, occlusive shoes, and communal swimming. Tinea pedis may occur alone or in combination with bacterial infections of the foot or other fungal skin infections such as tinea corporis or tinea cruris.

Tinea manus (ringworm of the hands) usually is a secondary infection with tinea pedis as the primary infection. In contrast to other skin disorders such as contact dermatitis and psoriasis, which affect both hands, tinea manus usually occurs only on one hand. The characteristic lesion is a blister on the palm or finger surrounded by erythema (Fig. 61-6). Chronic lesions are scaly and dry. Cracking and fissuring may occur. The lesions may spread to the plantar surfaces of the hand. If chronic, tinea manus may lead to tinea of the fingernails.

Simple forms of tinea pedis and tinea manus are treated with topical applications of antifungals. Complex cases are treated with oral griseofulvin, ketoconazole, or terbinafine.[15] Other treatment and preventive measures include careful cleaning and drying of affected areas. Persons with tinea pedis should wear clean and dry socks, changing them at least once daily. When bathed, the feet should be dried after other parts of the body to prevent spread of the infection.

Tinea of the Nail. *Tinea unguium* is a dermatophyte infection of the nails. It is a subset of *onychomycosis,* which

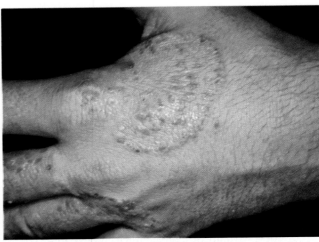

FIGURE 61-6 Tinea of the dorsum of the hand caused by *Trichophyton mentagrophytes.* (Duke Laboratories, Inc.) (Sauer G.C., Hall J.C. [1996]. *Manual of skin diseases* [7th ed.]. Philadelphia: Lippincott-Raven)

includes dermatophyte, nondermatophyte, and candidal infections of the nails. Toenails are involved more commonly than fingernails. Toenail infection is common in persons prone to chronic infections of tinea pedis. Often, the infection in the toenails becomes a ready source for future infections of the foot. It may begin from a crushing injury to a toenail or from the spread of tinea pedis.

Distal and lateral subungual onychomycosis, the most common form of tinea unguium, usually is caused by *T. rubrum* or *T. mentagrophytes*. The infection often begins at the tip of the nail, where the fungus digests the nail keratin. Initially, the nail appears opaque, white, or silvery (Fig. 61-7). The nail then turns yellow or brown. The condition often remains unchanged for years. During this time it may involve only one or two nails and may produce little

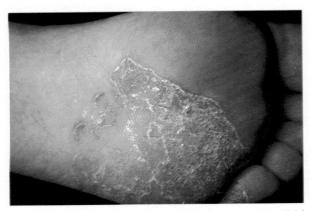

FIGURE 61-5 Chronic tinea of sole of the foot caused by *Trichophyton rubrum.* (Schering Corp.) (Sauer G.C., Hall J.C. [1996]. *Manual of skin diseases* [7th ed.]. Philadelphia: Lippincott-Raven)

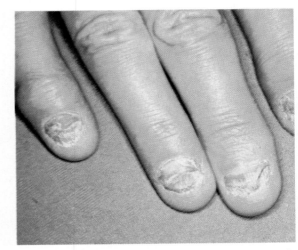

FIGURE 61-7 Tinea of the fingernail caused by *Trichophyton rubrum.* (Duke Laboratories, Inc.) (Sauer G.C., Hall J.C. [1996]. *Manual of skin diseases* [7th ed.]. Philadelphia: Lippincott-Raven)

or no discomfort. Gradually, the nail thickens and cracks as the infection spreads and includes the nail plate. Permanent discoloration and distortion result as the nail plate separates from the nail bed. Less common forms of tinea unguium are superficial white onychomycosis, in which areas of the nails become powdery white and erode, and proximal subungual onychomycosis (PSO), in which there is rapid invasion of the nail, leaving it white with no additional thickening of the nail. Although it is one of the less common forms of tinea unguium, PSO has increased among people with acquired immunodeficiency syndrome (AIDS).

Treatment of tinea unguium usually requires oral antifungal therapy.[16,17] Fingernail infections are more easily treated, in part because the fingernails are more easily exposed to air. Itraconazole, terbinafine, and, to a lesser extent, griseofulvin have been effective in treating fingernail infections. Itraconazole and terbinafine usually are used for toenail infections. Fluconazole also may be used, particularly if *Candida* is involved. Itraconazole is administered in pulses (intermittent weeks of therapy), whereas terbinafine or fluconazole is administered for 12 to 15 weeks. All of the oral agents require careful monitoring for side effects. A new nail may require 3 to 12 months to grow out; thus, people being treated with these antifungal agents need to be reminded that the resolution of the infection requires 4 to 6 months for fingernails and longer for toenails. Some authorities recommend removal of the infected toenails, with or without antifungal therapy. Many cases of tinea unguium would be prevented if the primary infection of tinea pedis were diagnosed and treated promptly.

Tinea Versicolor. Tinea versicolor is a fungal infection involving the upper chest, the back, and sometimes the arms. The causative agent is a yeast called *Malassezia furfur*. The infection occurs primarily in young adults in tropical and temperate regions, but cases have been reported in the northern states. The characteristic lesion is a yellow, pink, or brown sheet of scaling skin. The name *versicolor* is derived from the multicolored variations of the lesion. The patches are depigmented and do not tan when exposed to ultraviolet light. The skin has an overall appearance of being "dirty." These cosmetic defects often bring the patient to the health care provider in the summer months. It is believed that the fungus filters the ultraviolet light, preventing tanning. In darker-skinned persons, the depigmented areas are more apparent.

Selenium sulfide, found in several shampoo preparations, has been an effective fungistatic treatment measure. Miconazole or ketoconazole creams or shampoos, because of their fungicidal properties, have become the drugs of choice. The infection may recur after drug therapy. Boiling or steam-pressing clothes may help prevent recurrence.

Tinea Incognito. Tinea incognito is a form of dermatophyte infection that developed with the widespread use of topical corticosteroids. It often is seen in cases where tinea infections are misdiagnosed as eczema and treated with corticosteroids. Because the corticosteroids suppress the inflammation, scaling and erythema may not be present. There also has been an increased incidence of tinea in-

cognito in persons with AIDS. Persons with the disorder often present with thickened plaques with lichenification, papules, pustules, and nodules. Telangiectases, atrophy, and striae may be present. Tinea incognito is seen most often on the groin, the hand, or the dorsal aspect of the hand.

Treatment measures include discontinuing topical corticosteroids while using low-dose oral corticosteroids to prevent the flare-up associated with discontinuing potent topical steroids. Topical or oral antifungal agents may be used, depending on the severity of the infection. Persons who must remain on potent topical corticosteroids are difficult to treat.

Dermatophytid Reaction. A secondary skin eruption may occur in persons allergic to the fungus responsible for the dermatophytes. This dermatophytid or allergic reaction may occur during an acute episode of a fungal infection. The most common reaction occurs on the hands in response to tinea pedis. The lesions are vesicles with erythema extending over the palms and fingers of the hand and sometimes to other areas. Less commonly, a more generalized reaction occurs in which papules or vesicles erupt on the trunk or extremities. These eruptions may resemble tinea corporis. Lesions may become excoriated and infected with bacteria. Treatment is directed at the primary site of infection. The intradermal reaction resolves in most cases without intervention if the primary site is cleared.

Candidal Infections. Candidiasis (moniliasis) is a fungal infection caused by *Candida albicans*. This yeastlike fungus is a normal inhabitant of the gastrointestinal tract, mouth, and vagina (see Chapter 46). The skin problems result from the release of irritating toxins on the skin surface. Some persons are predisposed to candidal infections by conditions such as diabetes mellitus, antibiotic therapy, pregnancy, use of birth control pills, poor nutrition, and immunosuppressive diseases. Oral candidiasis may be the first sign of infection with human immunodeficiency virus (HIV).

C. albicans thrives in warm, moist intertriginous areas of the body. The rash is red with well-defined borders. Patches erode the epidermis, and there is scaling. Mild to severe itching and burning often accompany the infection. Severe forms of infection may involve pustules or vesiculopustules. In addition to microscopy, a candidal infection often can be differentiated from a tinea infection by the presence of satellite lesions. These satellite lesions are maculopapular and are found outside the clearly demarcated borders of the candidal infection. Satellite lesions often are diagnostic of diaper rash complicated by *Candida*. The appearance of candidal infections varies according to the site (Table 61-3).

Diagnosis usually is based on microscopic examination of skin or mucous membrane scrapings placed in KOH solution. Treatment measures vary according to the location. Preventive measures such as wearing rubber gloves are encouraged for persons with infections of the hands. Intertriginous areas often are separated with clean cotton cloth and allowed to air dry as a means of decreasing the macerating effects of heat and moisture. Depending on the site of infection and extent of involvement, topical and oral antifungal agents are used in treatment.

TABLE 61-3 ✦ Candidal Infections: Locations and Appearance of Lesions

Location	Appearance
Breasts, groin, axillae, anus, umbilicus, toe or fingerwebs	Red lesions with well-defined borders and presence of satellite lesions; lesions may be dry or moist
Vagina	Red, oozing lesions with sharply defined borders and inflamed vagina; cervix may be covered with moist, white plaque; cheesy, foul-smelling discharge; presence of pruritus and burning
Glans penis (balanitis)	Red lesions with sharply defined borders; penis may be covered with white plaque; presence of pruritus and burning
Mouth (thrush)	Creamy white flakes on a red, inflamed mucous membrane; papillae on tongue may be enlarged
Nails	Red, painful swelling around nail bed; common in persons who often have their hands in water

Bacterial Infections

Bacteria are considered normal flora of the skin. Most bacteria are not pathogenic, but when pathogenic bacteria invade the skin, superficial or systemic infections may develop. Bacterial skin infections are commonly classified as primary or secondary infections. Primary infections are superficial skin infections such as impetigo or ecthyma. Secondary infections consist of deeper cutaneous infections such as infected ulcers. Diagnosis usually is based on cultures taken from the infected site. Treatment measures include antibiotic therapy and measures to promote comfort and prevent the spread of infection.

Impetigo. Impetigo is a common superficial bacterial infection caused by *staphylococci* or *group A β-hemolytic streptococci* (GABHS), or both. Impetigo is common among infants and young children, although older children and adults occasionally contract the disease. Its occurrence is highest during the warm summer months or in warm, moist climates. It is highly communicable in the younger population. Impetigo initially appears as a small vesicle or pustule or as a large bulla on the face or elsewhere on the body. As the primary lesion ruptures, it leaves a denuded area that discharges a honey-colored serous liquid that hardens on the skin surface and dries as a honey-colored crust with a "stuck-on" appearance (Fig. 61-8). New vesicles erupt within hours. Pruritus often accompanies the lesions, and the skin excoriations that result from scratching multiply the infection sites. A possible complication of untreated GABHS impetigo is poststreptococcal glomerulonephritis (see Chapter 33). Topical mupirocin (Bactroban), which has few side effects, may be effective for limited disease. If the area is large or if there is concern about complications, systemic antibiotics are used.

Ecthyma is an ulcerative form of impetigo, usually secondary to minor trauma. It is caused by GABHS, *Staphylococcus aureus*, or *Pseudomonas*. It frequently occurs on the

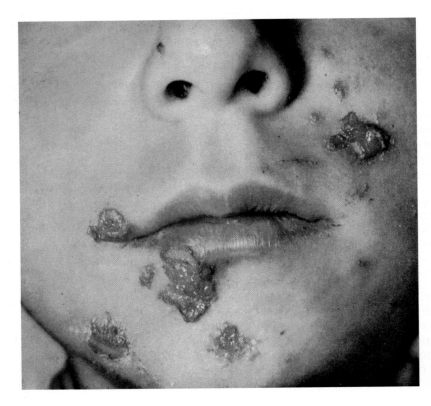

FIGURE 61-8 Impetigo of the face. (Abner Kurten, *Folia Dermatologica*. No. 2. Geigy Pharmaceuticals.) (Sauer G.C., Hall J.C. [1996]. *Manual of skin diseases* [7th ed.]. Philadelphia: Lippincott-Raven)

buttocks and thighs of children (Fig. 61-9). The lesions are similar to those of impetigo. A vesicle or pustule ruptures, leaving a skin erosion or ulcer that weeps and dries to a crusted patch, often resulting in scar formation. With extensive ecthyma, there is a low-grade fever and extension of the infection to other organs. Treatment usually involves the use of systemic antibiotics.

A less common form of *S. aureus* infection, called *Ritter's disease*, manifests with a diffuse, scarlet fever–like rash, followed by skin separation and sloughing (Fig. 61-10). It also is called *staphylococcal scalded-skin syndrome* because the skin looks scalded. Ritter's disease affects children younger than 5 years of age, but immunosuppressed adults also are at risk. The disorder is considered a deeper skin infection because the superficial layers of the epidermis are separated and shed. The onset of the rash may be preceded by malaise, fever, irritability, and extreme tenderness over the skin. The conjunctiva often is inflamed with a purulent drainage. The manifestations of the disorder are caused by the hematologic spread of toxins from another foci of infection such as the nasopharynx or a superficial skin abrasion. Although the fluid in the unbroken bullae is sterile, cultures usually are obtained from suspected sites of local infection and from the blood. Systemic antibiotics, either oral or parenteral, are used to treat the disorder. Healing usually occurs in 10 to 14 days without scarring.

Viral Infections

Viruses are intracellular pathogens that rely on live cells of the host for reproduction. They have no organized cell structure but consist of a DNA or RNA core surrounded by a protein coat. The viruses seen in skin lesion disorders tend to be DNA-containing viruses. Viruses invade the keratinocyte, begin to reproduce, and cause cellular proliferation or cellular death. The rapid increase in viral skin diseases has been attributed to the use of corticosteroid drugs, which have immunosuppressive qualities, and the use of antibiotics, which alter the bacterial flora of the skin. As the number of bacterial infections has decreased, there has been a proportional rise in viral skin diseases.

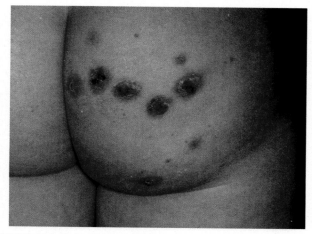

FIGURE 61-9 Ecthyma on the buttocks of a 13-year-old boy. (Glaxo-Wellcome Co.) (Sauer G.C., Hall J.C. [1996]. *Manual of skin diseases* [7th ed.]. Philadelphia: Lippincott-Raven)

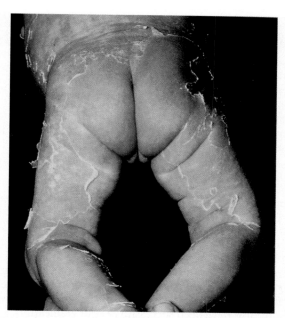

FIGURE 61-10 Staphylococcal scalded-skin syndrome. (Fitzpatrick T.B., Johnson R.A., Polono M.K., Suurmond D., Wolff K. [1992]. *Color atlas and synopsis of clinical dermatology* [2nd ed., p. 297]. New York: McGraw-Hill)

Verrucae. Verrucae, or warts, are common, benign papillomas caused by DNA-containing human papillomaviruses (HPV). Although warts vary in appearance depending on their location, they all have a similar histologic appearance (Table 61-4). The wart is not a mass of uniform tumor cells, but is like other skin diseases in that it is an exaggeration of the normal skin structure. There is an irregular thickening of the stratum spinosum and greatly increased thickening of the stratum corneum.

There are more than 50 types of HPVs found on the skin and mucous membranes of humans that cause several different kinds of warts, including skin warts and genital warts.[18] Many are genital warts that are sexually transmitted; some types of HPV may increase the risk of cervical cancer (see Chapter 45). The remainder account for warts that commonly appear on the hands and feet (Fig. 61-11). The nongenital warts, caused by HPV types 1, 2, 3, and 4, usually are not precancerous. They are known as common warts, flat warts, and plantar warts. HPV transmission usually occurs through breaks in skin integrity. For example, plantar warts, which occur on the soles of the feet, frequently are transmitted to the abraded, softened heels of children in swimming areas. Common hand warts can be transmitted by biting the cuticles surrounding the nail. Shaving may cause transmission of warts on the beard area.

Treatment usually is directed at inducing a "wart-free" period without producing scarring. Warts resolve spontaneously when immunity to the virus develops. The immune response may be delayed for years. Removal is usually done by applying a keratolytic agent, such as salicylic acid gel solution or plaster that breaks down the wart tissue, or by freezing with liquid nitrogen. Podophyllum resin, a cytotoxic agent that prevents growth of wart tissue, may be used

TABLE 61-4 ✦ Types and Characteristics of Verrucae (Warts)		
Type	Location	Appearance
Verruca vulgaris (common warts)	Anywhere on the skin, usually on the hands	Ragged dome shape with growth above the skin surface
Verruca filiformis	Eyelids, face, neck	Long, fingerlike projections
Verruca plana (flat wart)	Forehead, dorsum of hand	Small, flat tumors; may be barely visible
Verruca plantaris (plantar wart)	Sole of foot	Flat to slightly raised growth extending deep into skin; painful; bleeding occurs with superficial trimming; coalesced plantar warts are referred to as mosaic warts
Condyloma acuminata	Mucous membrane of the penis, female genitalia, perianal areas, and rectum	Large, moist projections with rough surfaces; usually pink or purple

in treating anogenital warts. It should not be used during pregnancy because of possible cytotoxic effects on the fetus. Various types of laser surgery, electrosurgery, and antiviral therapy also have been successful in wart eradication.

Herpes Simplex. Herpes simplex virus (HSV) infections of the skin and mucous membrane (*i.e.,* cold sore or fever blister) are common. Two types of herpesviruses infect humans: type 1 and type 2. HSV-1 usually is confined to the oropharynx, and the organism is spread by respiratory droplets or by direct contact with infected saliva. Genital herpes usually is caused by HSV-2 (see Chapter 46), although HSV-1 also can cause genital herpes. HSV-1 may be transmitted to other parts of the body through the occupational hazards that exist in athletics and some professions, such as dentistry and medicine.

Infection with HSV-1 may present as a primary or recurrent infection. Primary HSV-1 infections usually are asymptomatic. Symptomatic disease occurs most frequently in young children (1 to 5 years of age). Symptoms include fever, sore throat, painful vesicles, and ulcers of the tongue, palate, gingiva, buccal mucosa, and lips. Primary infection results in the production of antibodies to the virus so that recurrent infections are more localized and less severe.

After an initial infection, the herpesvirus persists in the trigeminal and other dorsal root ganglia in the latent state. It is likely that many adults were exposed to HSV-1 during childhood and therefore have antibodies to the virus.

The recurrent lesions of HSV-1 usually begin with a burning or tingling sensation. Vesicles and erythema follow and progress to pustules, ulcers, and crusts before healing (Fig. 61-12). The lesion is most common on the lips, face, and mouth. Pain is common, and healing takes place within 10 to 14 days. Precipitating factors may be stress, sunlight exposure, menses, or injury. Individuals who are immunocompromised may have severe attacks.

There is no cure for oropharyngeal herpes simplex; most treatment measures are palliative. Penciclovir cream, a topical antiviral agent, applied at the first symptom may be used to reduce the duration of an attack. Application of over-the-counter topical preparations containing antihistamines, antipruritics, and anesthetic agents along with aspirin or acetaminophen may be used to relieve pain. Oral acyclovir, an antiviral drug that inhibits herpesvirus replication, may be used prophylactically to prevent recurrences. The antiviral drugs valacyclovir and famciclovir also may be used for prophylaxis. Sunscreen preparations

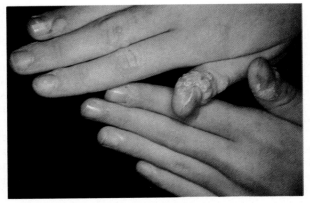

FIGURE 61-11 Common and periungual warts. (Reed & Carnrick Pharmaceuticals.) (Sauer G.C., Hall J.C. [1996]. *Manual of skin diseases* [7th ed.]. Philadelphia: Lippincott-Raven)

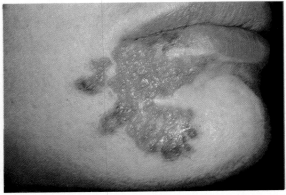

FIGURE 61-12 Recurrent herpes simplex of the face. (Dermik Laboratories, Inc.) (Sauer G.C., Hall J.C. [1996]. *Manual of skin diseases* [7th ed.]. Philadelphia: Lippincott-Raven)

applied to the lips can prevent sun-induced herpes simplex. Efforts to develop vaccines that would prevent herpesvirus infections are in process. They may be the best hope for control of the disease.[19]

Herpes Zoster.   Herpes zoster (shingles) is an acute, localized vesicular eruption distributed over a dermatomal segment of the skin. It is caused by the same herpesvirus, varicella-zoster, that causes chickenpox. It is believed to be the result of reactivation of a latent varicella-zoster virus that was dormant in the sensory dorsal root ganglia since a childhood infection. During an episode of herpes zoster, the reactivated virus travels from the ganglia to the skin of the corresponding dermatome. Although herpes zoster is not as contagious as chickenpox, the reactivated virus can be transmitted to nonimmune contacts.

The incidence of herpes zoster increases with age; it occurs 8 to 10 times more frequently in persons older than 60 years of age than in younger persons.[20] The normal age-related decrease in cell-mediated immunity is thought to account for the increased viral activation in this age group.[21] Other persons at increased risk because of impaired cell-mediated immunity are those with conditions such as HIV infection and certain malignancies, chronic corticosteroid users, and those undergoing cancer chemotherapy and radiation therapy.

The lesions of herpes zoster typically are preceded by a prodrome consisting of a burning pain, tingling sensation, extreme sensitivity of the skin to touch, and pruritus along the affected dermatome (Chapter 48). This may be present for 1 to 3 days or longer before the appearance of the rash. During this time, the pain may be mistaken for a number of other conditions such as heart disease, pleurisy, various musculoskeletal disorders, or gastrointestinal disorders.

The rash appears as an eruption of vesicles with erythematous bases that are restricted to skin areas supplied by sensory neurons of a single or associated group of dorsal root ganglia (Figs. 61-13 and 61-14). In immunosuppressed persons, the lesions may extend beyond the dermatome.

Eruptions usually are unilateral in the thoracic region, trunk, or face. New crops of vesicles erupt for 3 to 5 days along the nerve pathway. The vesicles dry, form crusts, and eventually fall off. The lesions usually clear in 2 to 3 weeks.

Serious complications can accompany eruptions. Eye involvement can result in permanent blindness and occurs in a large percentage of cases involving the ophthalmic division of the trigeminal nerve (see Chapter 54). Pain can persist for several months after the rash disappears. Postherpetic neuralgia, which is pain that persists longer than 1 to 3 months after the resolution of the rash, is an important complication of herpes zoster.[21] It is seen most commonly in persons who are 50 years of age or older and reportedly affects more than 40% of persons older than age 60 years.[20] Affected persons complain of a sharp, burning type pain that often occurs in response to non-noxious stimuli. Even the slightest pressure of clothing and bed sheets may elicit pain. It usually is a self-limited condition that persists for months, with symptoms abating over time. Less than 5% of persons continue to have pain at 1 year.[21]

The treatment of choice for herpes zoster is the administration of an antiviral agent. Acyclovir, the prototype antiviral drug, may be given orally or intravenously. Other antiviral agents, specifically valacyclovir and famciclovir, appear to be at least as effective as acyclovir. The treatment is most effective when started within 72 hours of rash development.[22] When given in the acute vesicular stage, the antiviral drugs have been shown to decrease the amount of lesion development and pain.[22] Narcotic analgesics, tricyclic antidepressants or anticonvulsant drugs, and nerve blocks may be used for management of herpetic pain. Oral corticosteroids sometimes are used to reduce the inflammation that may be contributing to the pain. Local treatment measures include Burow's solution compresses, aqueous alcohol lotions, calamine lotion, and starch shake lotions. Local application of capsaicin cream or lidocaine patches may be used in selected cases. There is current interest in the use of the varicella-zoster (chickenpox) vaccine for preventing or modifying the course of herpes zoster in the elderly.[23,24]

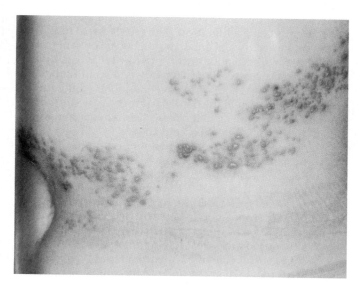

FIGURE 61-13 Herpes zoster in a common presentation, with involvement of a single dermatome. (Habif T.P. [1996]. *Clinical dermatology* [3rd ed., p. 351]. St Louis: CV Mosby)

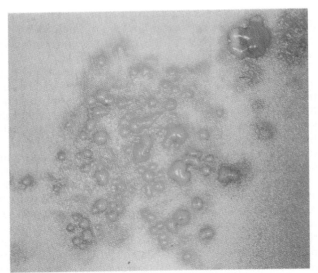

FIGURE 61-14 Herpes zoster is characterized by various sizes of vesicles. Vesicles of herpes simplex are uniform in size. (Habif T.P. [1996]. *Clinical dermatology* [3rd ed., p. 353]. St Louis: CV Mosby)

ACNE AND ROSACEA

Acne is a disorder of the pilosebaceous unit (hair follicle and sebaceous gland). The hair follicle is a tubular invagination of the epidermis in which hair is produced (see Chapter 60, Fig. 60-6). The sebaceous glands empty into the hair follicle, and the pilosebaceous unit opens to the skin surface by means of a widely dilated opening called a *pore*. The sebaceous glands produce a complex lipid mixture called *sebum*, from the Latin word meaning *tallow* or *grease*. Sebum consists of a mixture of free fatty acids, triglycerides, diglycerides, monoglycerides, sterol esters, wax esters, and squalene. Sebum production occurs through what is called a *holocrine process*, in which the sebaceous gland cells that produce the sebum are completely broken down and their lipid contents are emptied through the sebaceous duct into the hair follicle. The amount of sebum produced depends on two factors: the size of the sebaceous gland and the rate of sebaceous cell proliferation. The sebaceous glands are largest on the face, scalp, and scrotum, but are present in all areas of the skin except for the soles of the feet and palms of the hands. Sebaceous cell proliferation and sebum production are uniquely responsive to direct hormonal stimulation by androgens. In men, testicular androgens are the main stimulus for sebaceous activity; in women, adrenal and ovarian androgens maintain sebaceous activity.

Acne lesions consist of comedones (whiteheads and blackheads), papules, pustules, nodules, and, in severe cases, cysts. *Blackheads* are plugs of material that accumulate in sebaceous glands that open to the skin surface. The color of blackheads results from melanin that has moved into the sebaceous glands from adjoining epidermal cells. *Whiteheads* are pale, slightly elevated papules with no visible orifice. Papules are raised areas less than 5 mm in diameter. *Pustules* have a central core of purulent material. *Nodules* are larger than 5 mm in diameter and may become suppurative

or hemorrhagic. Suppurative nodules often are referred to as *cysts* because of their resemblance to inflamed epidermal cysts. Acne lesions are divided into noninflammatory and inflammatory lesions. Noninflammatory acne consists primarily of comedones. Inflammatory acne consists of papules, pustules, nodules, and cysts. The inflammatory lesions are believed to develop from the escape of sebum into the dermis and the irritating effects of the fatty acids contained in the sebum.

Two types of acne occur during different stages of the life cycle: acne vulgaris, which is the most common form among adolescents and young adults, and acne conglobata, which develops later in life. Other types of acne occur in association with various etiologic agents and influences.

Acne Vulgaris

The prevalence of acne vulgaris during adolescence is approximately 100% because almost all teenagers experience at least a few comedones. The difference is in the severity of the condition, rather than incidence.[25] In women, acne may begin earlier and persist until 30 years of age; however, the overall incidence and severity are greater in men. There is a genetic predisposition to acquiring acne, and stress is thought to play an important part in the longer prevalence of the condition among women. The exact link between stress and acne is unknown, but it is believed that stress increases androgen production.[25]

Acne vulgaris lesions form primarily on the face and neck and, to a lesser extent, on the back, chest, and shoulders (Fig. 61-15). The lesions may consist of comedones (whiteheads and blackheads) or inflammatory lesions (pustules, nodules, and cysts). The cause of acne vulgaris remains unknown. Several factors are believed to contribute to acne, including (1) the influence of androgens on sebaceous cell activity, (2) increased proliferation of the keratinizing epidermal cells that form the sebaceous cells, (3) increased sebum production in relation to the severity of the disease, (4) decreased amounts of linoleic acid in the sebum, and (5) the presence of *Propionibacterium acnes*.[25,26] These factors probably are interrelated. Increased androgen production results in increased sebaceous cell activity, with a resultant plugging of the pilosebaceous ducts. The excessive sebum provides a medium for the growth of *P. acnes*. The *P. acnes* organism contains lipases that break down the free fatty acids that produce the acne inflammation.

Over the years, several factors such as poor hygiene, acne as an infectious process, diets high in fatty content, and certain foods (*e.g.*, chocolate) have been studied empirically and rejected as causal or contributing factors in the development of acne. Although general hygienic measures are important, obsessive scrubbing can traumatize the skin and worsen the condition.[27,28] Instead, it is recommended that the affected areas be washed gently and patted dry. Water-based, rather than oil-based, cosmetics and moisturizers should be used. Mechanical trauma, such as squeezing, rubbing, or picking comedones, should be avoided. Even resting the chin, forehead, or cheek on a hand can exacerbate the condition. Hats, sweatbands, and shirt collars can also traumatize the skin and contribute to a worsening of acne. Although rigid dietary restrictions have not been shown to

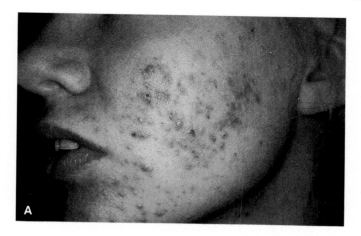

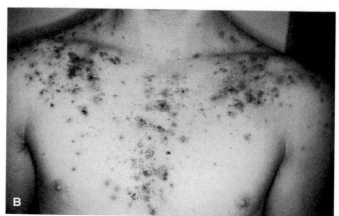

FIGURE 61-15 (**A**) Acne of the face and (**B**) acne of the chest. (Hall J.C. [1999]. *Sauer's manual of skin diseases* [8th ed., p. 118]. Philadelphia: Lippincott Williams & Wilkins)

be beneficial in acne management, a balanced diet is recommended. Women should be informed that acne often becomes worse during the week before menses.

The treatment of acne focuses on clearing up existing lesions, preventing new lesions from forming, and limiting scar formation. Management includes education regarding the causes of acne and protective skin care measures. Topical or systemic treatment may be used, depending on the extent of involvement and the type of lesion (comedonal or inflammatory) present. Long-term treatment usually is required. Significant improvement may not be apparent for 3 to 6 weeks after initiation of treatment, and maximum effects may not be apparent for months. An important treatment measure is sensitivity to the client's emotional needs.

Milder forms of acne usually respond to topical application of acne creams, ointments, or lotions. The treatment measures for moderate to severe acne are directed at correcting the defect in epidermal cell proliferation, decreasing sebaceous gland activity, reducing the *P. acnes* population, and limiting the inflammatory process. Often, a combination of comedolytic and antibacterial agents is used.

A number of topical comedolytic and antibacterial agents are available for the treatment of acne. The type of vehicle (cream, gel, or lotion) may be an important consideration in selection of an agent.[29] Persons with drier skin may benefit from creams, whereas persons with oily skin

may have better results using a gel or lotion. Many acne creams and lotions containing keratolytic agents such as sulfur, salicylic acid, phenol, and resorcinol are available as over-the-counter preparations. These agents act chemically to break down keratin, loosen comedones, and exert a peeling effect on the skin. With the advent of more effective products, these preparations are used less frequently than in the past.

Benzoyl peroxide is a topical agent that has both antibacterial and comedolytic properties. It is the topical agent most effective in reducing the *P. acnes* population. Bacterial proteins are oxidized by the oxygen free radicals released from the metabolism of benzoyl peroxide on the skin. Because of its mechanism of action, bacterial resistance does not develop to benzoyl peroxide. The irritant effect of the drug also causes vasodilation and increased blood flow, which may hasten resolution of the inflammatory lesions. Azelaic acid (Azelex), derived from wheat, rye, and barley, has actions similar to benzoyl peroxide. It decreases the proliferation of keratocytes and has antibacterial actions against *P. acnes*. Azelaic cream is moisturizing and causes only minimal skin irritation.

Tretinoin (Retin-A), an acid derivative of vitamin A, is a topical agent. Its action in acne has been attributed to decreased cohesiveness of epidermal cells and increased epidermal cell turnover. This is thought to result in increased extrusion of open comedones and transformation of closed comedones into open ones. All tretinoin formulations are irritating to the skin, an effect that is increased with sun exposure. Because of the known teratogenic effect of oral vitamin A products, there is concern over the use of tretinoin during pregnancy. A new delivery system of tretinoin (Retin-A Micro) is now available. It works by entrapping the drug in microspheres that move into the follicle and serve as reservoirs for drug release. Newer retinoid drugs such as adapalene and tazarotene have actions similar to tretinoin. Adapalene appears to be as effective as tretinoin, but is less irritating to the skin.[29,30]

Topically applied antibiotics also are effective in treating mild to moderate acne. Topical tetracycline, erythromycin, and clindamycin are used most commonly. They do not affect existing lesions but prevent future lesions by decreasing the amount of *P. acnes* on the skin, thereby reducing subsequent inflammation formed from the presence of sebaceous fatty acid metabolites. Treatment failure can result from development of antibiotic resistance. Combination drugs, such as Benzamycin (benzoyl peroxide and erythromycin), also have been effective.

Oral low-dose tetracycline has been used effectively for many years. Tetracycline has no effect on sebum production, but it decreases bacterial growth and the amount of free fatty acids produced. Tetracycline requires a sufficient treatment period to establish effective blood levels. Side effects are minimal, which is why the drug has remained so useful. However, it does have teratogenic effects on skeletal and tooth development and should not be given to pregnant or lactating women, or children. Erythromycin also is effective in acne treatment. Of the antimicrobial drugs, dapsone has been effective in severe cases of cystic acne. However, side effects are many. The drug should be used with caution and close monitoring.

Isotretinoin (Accutane), an orally administered synthetic retinoid or acid form of vitamin A, has revolutionized the treatment of recalcitrant cases of acne and cystic acnes. In carefully planned doses, oral isotretinoin has cleared major cases of acne and initiated long-term remissions of the disease. It is administered for 3- to 4-month treatment periods. Although the exact mode of action is unknown, it decreases sebaceous gland activity, prevents new comedones from forming, reduces the *P. acnes* count through sebum reduction, and has an anti-inflammatory effect. Because of its many side effects, it is used only in persons with severe acne. Side effects include dryness of the mouth and other mucous membranes, conjunctivitis, and musculoskeletal system abnormalities. Because the drug also can produce elevated serum lipid levels, abnormal liver enzyme test results, and hematologic disorders, careful clinical and laboratory monitoring is necessary. Isotretinoin also is a teratogen that causes brain, heart, and ear malformations. Women taking isotretinoin are strongly advised not to become pregnant.

Estrogens reduce the size and secretion of the sebaceous gland, but because of the high dosages required, they are contraindicated in men. In women, birth control pills that combine estrogen with a progestin that has low androgenic activity usually are used.[27,28] Corticosteroid therapy is limited primarily to severe, resistant cases. The therapy results in remarkable healing, but acne usually returns after the therapy has been terminated.

Other treatment measures for acne include surgery, ultraviolet irradiation, cryotherapy, and intralesional glucocorticosteroid injection. Acne surgery involves the aspiration of comedones with small-bore needles or devices designed to extract comedonal contents. Scarring is a common sequela if surgery is done improperly. The use of ultraviolet irradiation, which involves exposure to hot or cold quartz lights for specified periods, remains controversial. It continues to be used in treatment of some forms of acne. Cryotherapy (*i.e.*, freezing with carbon dioxide slushes, liquid nitrogen, dry ice, or acetone) has been effective in promoting healing of lesions by removing the outer layers of skin. Intralesional injection of corticosteroids using a syringe or needleless injector is limited to severe nodulocystic forms of acne. It has been effective in promoting cyst healing, but usually has to be repeated frequently.

Acne Conglobata

Acne conglobata occurs later in life and is a chronic form of acne. Comedones, papules, pustules, nodules, abscesses, cysts, and scars occur on the back, buttocks, and chest. Lesions occur to a lesser extent on the abdomen, shoulders, neck, face, upper arms, and thighs. The comedones have multiple openings. Their discharge is odoriferous, serous, and purulent or mucoid. Healing leaves deep keloidal lesions. Affected persons have anemia with increased white blood cell counts, sedimentation rates, and neutrophil counts. The treatment is difficult and stringent. It often includes debridement, systemic corticosteroid therapy, oral retinoids, and systemic antibiotics.

Other Forms of Acne

There are several forms of acne with various etiologic agents and influences. The symptoms vary depending on the source or age of onset. Treatment measures for these acnes depend on the precipitating agent and the extent of the lesions. Many of the previously discussed treatment measures have been used with various degrees of success.

Acne fulminans is manifested by a sudden eruption of large, inflamed lesions on the back and chest that ulcerate, heal, and scar. The lesions are extremely painful, and the person often walks in a bent-over position. Teenage boys, often with a mild form of acne, are most affected by this type. *Steatocystoma multiplex* consists of an eruption of many cystic lesions of various sizes on the trunk of men and women of young adult age. *Neonatal acne* occurs on newborn infants, mostly males. Typically, it is found on the nose and cheeks; it usually clears without treatment. *Drug acnes* occur as an untoward reaction to certain pharmacologic agents, most commonly steroids, iodides (in cough mixtures), and bromides (in sedatives). Acne that results from exposure to occupational compounds or chemicals is called *occupational acne*. Many of the precipitating agents are the same as those that cause allergic responses; cutting oils are the most offensive.

Acne cosmetica is believed to be caused by women's use of cosmetic, cleaning, and self-adornment products. The exact causes are unknown because of the variety of cosmetic agents used by women. Even after cosmetic use has been discontinued, this acne usually persists and is difficult to heal. *Acne detergicans* is believed to be caused by compulsive washing of the face with soaps, whereas *acne mechanica* develops from repeated trauma to the skin. A common form of acne mechanica is seen on football players from the rubbing of their helmets. *Pomade acne* follows the hairline and is most commonly seen on African-American men. *Acne excoriée des jeunes filles* is a mild form of acne seen in adolescent girls. The lesions spread from scratching and picking behavior that is believed to be of emotional origin.

Rosacea

Rosacea, formerly called *acne rosacea*, is a chronic inflammatory process that occurs in middle-aged and older adults. It is easily confused with acne and may coexist with it. In the early stage of development, there are repeated episodes of blushing, eventually becoming a permanent dark red erythema on the nose and cheeks that sometimes extends to the forehead and chin (Fig. 61-16). This stage often occurs before 20 years of age. As the person ages, the erythema persists, and telangiectasia with or without acneiform components (*e.g.*, comedones, pustules, nodules) develops. After years of affliction, acne rosacea may develop into an irregular bullous hyperplasia (thickening) of the nose, known as *rhinophyma*. The sebaceous follicles and openings enlarge, and the skin color changes to a purple-red. The cause remains unknown. It often is accompanied by gastrointestinal symptoms, yet there is little support for *Helicobacter pylori* as a possible causal factor.[31] More common in fair-skinned persons, it has been called "the curse of the Celts." An early characteristic and diagnostic sign is seen in persons who "flush and blush." It is more common in women; rhinophyma is more common in men.

Alcoholic intake has been rejected as a causative agent. However, persons with rosacea are heat sensitive. They are instructed to avoid vascular stimulating agents such as heat, cold, sunlight, hot liquids, highly seasoned foods, and alcohol. Treatment measures are similar to those used for acne vulgaris. Topical metronidazole and azelaic acid have been effective. Rhinophyma can be treated surgically.

ECZEMATOUS DERMATOSES

Eczema is an inflammatory response of the skin to multiple exogenous and endogenous agents. It is characterized by epidermal edema with separation of epidermal cells. Eczematous dermatoses may be related to hypersensitivity reactions and include irritant contact dermatitis, allergy contact dermatitis, atopic eczema, and nummular eczema.

Contact Dermatitis

Contact dermatitis is a common inflammation of the skin. There are two types of contact dermatitis: irritant and allergic contact dermatitis. Irritant contact dermatitis is caused by chemicals (soaps, detergents, organic solvents) that irritate the skin. Allergic contact dermatitis is a cell-mediated, type IV hypersensitivity response brought about by sensitization to an allergen. More than 2000 allergens have been identified as capable of producing an inflammatory skin response. Crude forms of many naturally occurring substances are in general less allergenic than alloys and synthetic products. Additives such as dyes and perfumes account for the major sources of known allergens. Some of the common topical agents causing allergic rashes are antimicrobial agents (especially neomycin), antihistamines, local anesthetic agents (benzocaine), preservatives (*e.g.*, parabens), and adhesive tape. Additional examples are poison ivy and metal alloys found in jewelry. Of recent concern is the increased incidence of contact dermatitis from the heavy use of synthetic latex products, specifically latex gloves and condoms used to prevent communicable diseases.

The lesions of allergic contact dermatitis range from a mild erythema with edema to vesicles or large bullae (Fig. 61-17). Secondary lesions from bacterial infection may occur. Lesions can occur almost anywhere on the body. The

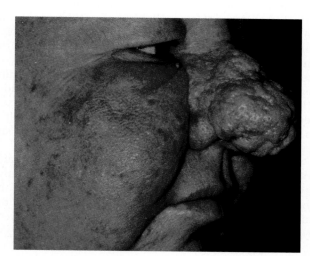

FIGURE 61-16 Chronic rosacea with rhinophyma. (Hoechst Marion Roussel Pharmaceuticals, Inc.) (Sauer G.C., Hall J.C. [1996]. *Manual of skin diseases* [7th ed.]. Philadelphia: Lippincott-Raven)

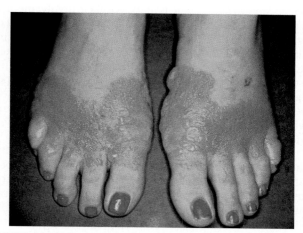

FIGURE 61-17 Contact dermatitis from shoe material. (Glaxo-Wellcome Co.) (Sauer G.C., Hall J.C. [1996]. *Manual of skin diseases* [7th ed.]. Philadelphia: Lippincott-Raven)

typical poison ivy lesion consists of vesicles or bullae in a linear pattern. The vesicles and bullae break and weep, leaving an excoriated area. Irritant contact dermatitis occurs in persons who are in contact with a sufficient amount of the irritant to cause a reaction. It can occur from mechanical means such as rubbing (*e.g.*, wool, fiberglass), chemical irritants (*e.g.*, household cleaning products), or environmental irritants (*e.g.*, plants, urine). An example is the skin burn that may occur from contact with cement products. Irritant contact dermatitis ranges from acute to chronic cases. Skin reactions range from mild erythema and scaling to acute necrotic burns.

With allergic contact dermatitis and irritant contact dermatitis, the location of the lesions is of great benefit in diagnosing the causative agent. Patch testing, in which a small amount of the suspected antigen is applied to the skin, is used to identify the allergens.

Treatment measures for both types of contact dermatitis are aimed at removing the source of the irritant or allergen. This may mean that the person needs to modify his or her behavior or even change employment to avoid contact with the irritant or allergen. Minor cases are treated by washing the affected areas to remove further contamination by the irritant or allergen, applying antipruritic creams or lotions, and bandaging the exposed areas. Topical corticosteroids may be helpful in these cases. Systemic treatment regimens differ according to the type of irritant or allergen and the severity of the reaction. More extreme cases are treated with wet dressings, systemic corticosteroids, and oral antihistamines.

Atopic Eczema and Nummular Eczema

Atopic eczema (atopic dermatitis) is a common skin disorder that occurs in two clinical forms, infantile and adult.[32,33] It is associated with a type I hypersensitivity reaction (see Chapter 19). There usually is a family history of asthma, hay fever, or atopic dermatitis. The infantile form is characterized by vesicle formation, oozing, and crusting with excoriations. It usually begins in the cheeks and may progress to involve the scalp, arms, trunk, and legs (Fig. 61-18). The skin of the cheeks may be paler, with extra creases under the eyes, called *Dennie-Morgan folds.* There is marked follicle involvement in persons with black skin. Lesions may be hypopigmented or hyperpigmented or both on a black-skinned person. The infantile form usually becomes milder as the child ages, often disappearing by the age of 15 years. Adolescents and adults usually have dry, leathery, and hyperpigmented or hypopigmented lesions located in the antecubital and popliteal areas. These may spread to the neck, hands, feet, eyelids, and behind the ears. Itching may be severe with both forms. Secondary infections are common.

Treatment of atopic eczema is designed to target the underlying abnormalities such as dryness, pruritus, superinfection, and inflammation. It involves allergen control, basic skin care, and medications. Avoiding exposure to environmental irritants and foods that cause exacerbation of the symptoms is recommended. Because dry skin and pruritus often exacerbate the condition, hydration of the skin is essential to treating atopic dermitis. Once-daily bathing for 5 to 10 minutes with warm (not hot) water is recommended.

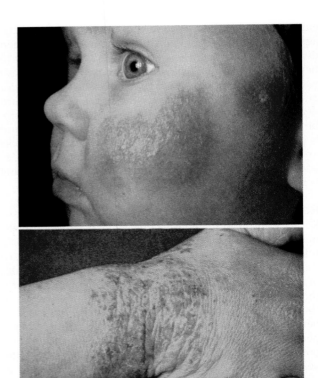

FIGURE 61-18 Atopic eczema on an infant's face and wrist. (Dome Chemicals.) (Sauer G.C., Hall J.C. [1996]. *Manual of skin diseases* [7th ed.]. Philadelphia: Lippincott-Raven)

Soap should be avoided if possible. A moisturizer should be applied immediately after bathing (and before the skin is completely dry). Ointments are superior to creams and lotions, but they are greasy and therefore poorly tolerated.[33] Mild or healing lesions may be treated with lotions containing a mild antipruritic agent. Acute weeping lesions are treated with soothing lotions, soaks, or wet dressings. Soaks in sodium bicarbonate or colloidal oatmeal (Aveeno) can be used to treat pruritus. Pruritus that is refractory to moisturizers and conservative measures can be treated with antihistamines or tricyclic antidepressants. Topical corticosteroids provide an effective form of treatment, but can cause local and systemic side effects. Because of their side effects, systemic corticosteroids usually are reserved for severe cases. Avoiding temperature changes and stress helps to minimize abnormal and cutaneous vascular and sweat responses.

The lesions of nummular eczema (discoid eczema) are coin-shaped (nummular) papulovesicular patches mainly involving the arms and legs (Fig. 61-19). Lichenification and secondary bacterial infections are common. It is not unusual for the initial lesions seemingly to heal, followed by a secondary outbreak of mirror-image lesions on the opposite side of the body. Most nummular eczema is chronic, with weeks to years between exacerbations. Exacerbations are more frequent in the cold winter months. The exact cause of nummular eczema is unknown. There usually is a

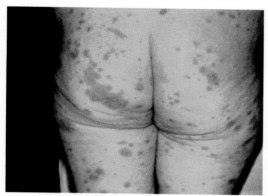

FIGURE 61-19 Nummular eczema of the buttocks. (Johnson & Johnson.) (Sauer G.C., Hall J.C. [1996]. *Manual of skin diseases* [7th ed.]. Philadelphia: Lippincott-Raven)

history of asthma, hay fever, or atopic dermatitis. Ingestion of iodides and bromides usually aggravates the condition. Treatment is palliative. Frequent bathing, foods rich in iodides and bromides, and stress should be reduced, whereas the environmental humidity should be increased. Topical corticosteroids, coal tar preparations, and ultraviolet light treatments are prescribed as necessary.

URTICARIA

Urticaria, or hives, is characterized by edematous plaques, called *wheals*, that are accompanied by intense itching. Wheals typically appear as raised pink or red areas surrounded by a paler halo. They blanch with pressure and vary in size from a few millimeters to centimeters. Thicker lesions that result from massive transudation of fluid into the dermis or subcutaneous tissue are referred to as *angioedema*. Although angioedema lesions can occur on any skin surface, they typically involve the larynx, causing hoarseness or sore throat, or mucosal surface of the gastrointestinal tract, causing abdominal pain.

Histamine is the most common mediator of urticaria. Histamine causes hyperpermeability of the microvessels of the skin and surrounding tissue, allowing fluid to leak into the tissues, causing edema and wheal formation.[34,35] Histamine is contained in the granules of mast cells. A variety of immunologic, nonimmunologic, physical, and chemical stimuli can cause mast cell degranulation with release of histamine into the surrounding tissues and circulation.

Urticaria can be acute or chronic. Daily or almost daily episodes of urticaria persisting for longer than 6 weeks are considered to be chronic. The most common causes of acute urticaria are foods or drinks, medications, or exposure to pollens or chemicals. Food is the most common cause of acute urticaria in children. Although nonsteroidal anti-inflammatory drugs, including aspirin, do not normally cause urticaria, they may exacerbate preexisting disease.

Chronic urticaria affects primarily adults and is twice as common in women as in men. Usually its cause cannot be determined despite extensive laboratory tests. Some forms of chronic urticaria are associated with histamine-releasing autoantibodies. In rare cases, urticaria is a manifestation of underlying disease, such as certain cancers, collagen diseases, and hepatitis. There is an association between chronic urticaria and autoimmune thyroid disease (*e.g.*, Hashimoto's thyroiditis, Graves' disease, toxic multinodular thyroiditis). A hereditary deficiency of a C1 (complement 1) inhibitor also can cause urticaria and angioedema.

Physical urticarias constitute another form of chronic urticaria.[35] Physical urticarias are intermittent, usually last less than 2 hours, are produced by appropriate stimuli, have distinctive appearances and locations, and are seen most frequently in young adults. Dermographism, or skin writing, is one form of physical urticaria in which wheals appear in response to simple rubbing of the skin (Fig. 61-20). The wheals follow the pattern of the scratch or rubbing, appearing within 10 minutes, and dissolving completely within 20 minutes. Other types of physical urticaria are cholinergic (*i.e.*, exercise-induced), cold, delayed pressure, solar (*i.e.*, sunlight), aquagenic (*i.e.*, water), vibratory, and external (localized heat-induced). Table 61-5 summarizes the features of common types of physical urticaria. Appropriate challenge tests (*e.g.*, application of an ice cube to the skin to initiate development of cold urticaria) are used to differentiate physical urticaria from chronic urticaria due to other causes.

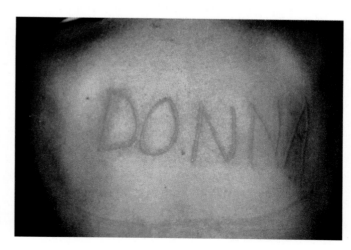

FIGURE 61-20 Dermographism on a patient's back. (Dermik Laboratories, Inc.) (Sauer G.C., Hall J.C. [1996]. *Manual of skin diseases* [7th ed.]. Philadelphia: Lippincott-Raven)

TABLE 61-5 ✦ Clinical Features of Physical Urticaria

Type	Clinical Features
Dermographism	Itchy linear wheals with surrounding bright red flair; last no longer than 15 to 30 minutes
Cholinergic urticaria	Small wheals with surrounding bright red flare and intense pruritus that develop in response to a rise in core temperature, as with exercise, external heat, emotion, or eating spicy foods; last no longer than 1 to 2 hours
Cold urticaria	Itchy, pale or red swelling at site of contact with cold surfaces, air, or water; lasts no longer than 30 to 60 minutes
Pressure urticaria	Large, painful, or itchy swelling at site of pressure (*e.g.,* waist, palms, hands); appears 1 to 4 hours after pressure application and lasts 24 hours or more
Solar urticaria	Itchy, pale or red swelling at site of exposure to ultraviolet light

Most types of urticaria are treated with antihistamines: drugs that block histamine type 1 (H_1) and, less frequently, H_1 in combination with histamine type 2 (H_2). They control urticaria by inhibiting vasodilation and escape of fluid into the surrounding tissues. Second-generation antihistamines are equally effective without the side effects, such as drowsiness.[36] Severe urticaria and angioedema are treated with epinephrine. Oral corticosteroids may be used in the treatment of refractory urticaria. Tricyclic antidepressant drugs, particularly those with antihistamine actions, also may be used. Starch or colloid-type (*e.g.,* Aveeno) baths may be used as comfort measures. Nontraditional measures, such as acupuncture, have been used successfully in practice, but not studied empirically.[37]

DRUG-INDUCED SKIN ERUPTIONS

Without exception, any drug can cause a localized or generalized skin eruption. Topical drugs usually are responsible for a localized contact dermatitis type of rash, whereas systemic drugs cause generalized skin lesions. Most drug eruptions are morbilliform (*i.e.,* measles-like) or exanthematous. They usually disappear in a few days. Some progress to more severe skin eruptions, necessitating prompt medical attention. Drug-induced skin reactions mimic almost all other skin lesions described in this chapter.

The diagnosis of a drug sensitivity depends almost entirely on accurate reporting by the person because the lesions from drug sensitization vary greatly. Treatment of mild cases is aimed at eliminating the offending drug while treating the symptoms. Severe drug eruptions often require systemic corticosteroid therapy and antihistamines.

Three types of bullous skin manifestations that result from drug reactions end in epidermal skin detachment: erythema multiforme minor, Stevens-Johnson syndrome (erythema multiforme major), and toxic epidermal necrolysis. The latter two are rare occurrences, but they can be life threatening. Both usually are caused by sensitivity to such drugs as sulfonamides and anticonvulsants. Although erythema multiforme minor may be drug induced, it more

frequently occurs after infections, especially with herpes simplex. It is self-limiting, with a small amount of skin detachment at the lesion sites.

The lesions of erythema multiforme minor and Stevens-Johnson syndrome are similar. The primary lesion of both is a round, erythematous papule, resembling an insect bite. Within hours to days, these lesions change into several different patterns. The individual lesions may enlarge and coalesce, producing small plaques, or they may change to concentric zones of color appearing as "target" or "iris" lesions (Fig. 61-21). The outermost rings of the target lesions usually are erythematous; the central portion usually is opaque white, yellow, or gray (dusky). In the center, small blisters on the dusky purpuric macules may form, giving them their characteristic target-like appearance. Although there is wide distribution of lesions over the body surface

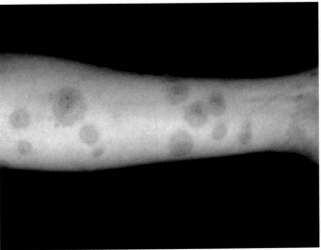

FIGURE 61-21 Erythema-multiforme–like eruption on the patient's arm. Notice the dusky, target-like appearance. (Dermik Laboratories, Inc.) (Sauer G.C., Hall J.C. [1996]. *Manual of skin diseases* [7th ed.]. Philadelphia: Lippincott-Raven)

area, there is a propensity for them to occur on the face and trunk. With Stevens-Johnson syndrome, there is more skin detachment.

Toxic epidermal necrolysis is the most serious and life-threatening drug reaction. The person experiences a prodromal period of malaise, low-grade fever, and sore throat. Within a few days, widespread erythema and large, flaccid bullae appear, followed by the loss of the epidermis. This leaves a denuded and painful dermis. The skin surrounding large denuded areas may have the typical target-like lesions seen with Stevens-Johnson syndrome. The skin separates easily from the dermis with lateral pressure; this is called *Nikolsky's sign*. The epithelium of mucosal surfaces, especially the mouth and eyes, may be involved.

These three types of bullous skin eruptions are seemingly quite similar. The diagnostic boundary for erythema multiforme minor is that it usually occurs after herpes simplex infection and is self-limiting. Precise diagnostic boundaries between Stevens-Johnson syndrome and toxic epidermal necrolysis have not been established. However, it is generally agreed that cases involving less than 10% of the body surface area are called *Stevens-Johnson syndrome*, and detachment of more than 30% of the epidermis is labeled *toxic epidermal necrolysis*.[38,39] The mortality rate for Stevens-Johnson syndrome is less than 5%, and that for toxic epidermal necrolysis is 30% or greater.[39]

The skin detachment of these drug reactions is different from the desquamation (*i.e.*, peeling) discussed with other skin disorders. For example, with scarlet fever there is peeling of the stratum corneum, the dead keratinized layer. In the bullous disorders discussed here, there is full-thickness detachment (*i.e.*, peeling of the entire epidermis down to the dermis). This leaves the person vulnerable to multiple problems, such as loss of body fluid and thermal control, nutritional deficits, and electrolyte imbalance.

Treatment of erythema multiforme minor and less severe cases of Stevens-Johnson syndrome includes relief of symptoms using compresses, antipruritic drugs, and topical anesthetics. Corticosteroid therapy may be indicated in moderate cases, although its use is controversial. For severe cases of Stevens-Johnson syndrome or toxic epidermal necrolysis, hospitalization is required for fluid replacement, antibiotics, respiratory care, analgesics, and moist dressings. When large areas of skin are detached, the care is similar to that of thermal burn patients.

PAPULOSQUAMOUS DERMATOSES

Papulosquamous dermatoses are a group of skin disorders characterized by scaling papules and plaques. Among the major papulosquamous diseases are psoriasis, pityriasis rosea, and lichen planus, which are discussed in this section of the chapter.

Psoriasis

Psoriasis is a common papulosquamous disease characterized by circumscribed red, thickened plaques with an overlying silvery-white scale. Psoriasis occurs worldwide, although the incidence is lower in warmer, sunnier climates. In the United States, it affects 2.6% or 6 million Ameri-

cans.[40] The average age of onset is in the third decade; its prevalence increases with age. Approximately one third of patients have a genetic history, indicating a hereditary factor. Childhood onset of the disease is more strongly associated with a family history than psoriasis occurring in adults older than 30 years of age.[41] The disease, which can persist throughout life and exacerbate at unpredictable times, is classified as a chronic ailment. A few cases, however, have been known to clear and not recur. There appears to be an association between psoriasis and arthritis. Psoriatic arthritis occurs in 5% to 7% of persons with psoriasis (see Chapter 59).

The primary cause of psoriasis is uncertain. The unintended, yet dramatic, clearing of severe, disabling psoriasis with cyclosporine provided strong evidence that psoriasis may be an autoimmune disease: a T-lymphocyte–mediated dermal immune response to an unidentified antigen.[42–44] It is thought that activated T lymphocytes (mainly CD4 helper cells) produce chemical messengers called *cytokines*, which stimulate keratinocyte proliferation. Accompanying inflammatory changes are caused by infiltration of neutrophils and monocytes (see Chapter 18). Skin trauma (*i.e.*, prepsoriasis) is a common precipitating factor in people predisposed to the disease. The reaction of the skin to an original trauma of any type is called the *Köebner reaction*. Stress, infections, trauma, xerosis, and use of medications such as angiotensin-converting enzyme inhibitors, β-adrenergic blocking drugs, lithium, and the antimalarial agent hydroxychloroquine (Plaquenil) may precipitate or exacerbate the condition.

Histologically, psoriasis is characterized by increased epidermal cell turnover with marked epidermal thickening, a process called *hyperkeratosis*. The migration time of the keratinocyte from the basal cell layer of the stratum corneum decreases from the normal 14 days to approximately 4 to 7 days. The granular layer (stratum granulosum) of the epidermis is thinned or absent, and neutrophils are found in the stratum corneum. There also is an accompanying thinning of the epidermal cell layer that overlies the tips of the dermal papillae (suprapapillary plate), and the blood vessels within dermal papillae become tortuous and dilated. These capillary beds show permanent damage even when the disease is in remission or has resolved. The close proximity of the vessels in the dermal papillae to the hyperkeratotic scale accounts for multiple, minute bleeding points that are seen when the scale is lifted.[18]

There are several variants or types of psoriasis, including plaque-type psoriasis, guttate psoriasis, pustular psoriasis (localized and generalized), and erythrodermic psoriasis.[43] Plaque-type psoriasis (*psoriasis vulgaris*), which is the most common type, is a chronic stationary form of psoriasis. The lesions may occur anywhere on the skin, but most often involve the elbows, knees, and scalp (Fig. 61-22). The primary lesions are papules that vary in shape. The papules form thick red plaques with a silvery scale. In darker-skinned persons, the plaques may appear purple. There may be excoriation, thickening, or oozing from the lesions. A differential diagnostic finding is that the plaques bleed from minute points when removed, which is known as *Auspitz sign*. *Guttate psoriasis*, which occurs in children and young

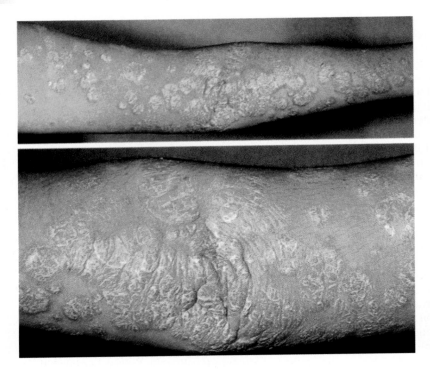

FIGURE 61-22 Psoriasis on the elbows of a 17-year-old girl. (Roche Laboratories.) (Sauer G.C., Hall J.C. [1996]. *Manual of skin diseases* [7th ed.]. Philadelphia: Lippincott-Raven)

adults, is characterized by teardrop-shaped, pink to salmon, scaly lesions. Its lesions are usually limited to the upper trunk and extremities. This form of psoriasis usually is brought on by a streptococcal infection. Sometimes guttate psoriasis resolves after several weeks, or it may progress to psoriasis vulgaris. *Pustular psoriasis* is characterized by papules or plaques studded with pustules. Localized pustular psoriasis usually is limited to the palms of the hands and soles of the feet. Generalized pustular psoriasis is characterized by a more general involvement and may be associated with systemic symptoms such as fever, malaise, and diarrhea. The person may or may not have had preexisting psoriasis. *Erythrodermic psoriasis* is a rare form of psoriasis affecting all body surfaces, including the hands, feet, nails, trunk, and extremities. It is characterized by a process in which the lesions scale and become confluent, leaving much of the body surface a bright red, with continuous skin shedding. It often is accompanied by severe itching and pain. Severe complications may develop related to loss of body fluids, proteins, and electrolytes and disturbances in temperature regulation.

Treatment. There is no cure for psoriasis. The goal of treatment is to suppress the signs and symptoms of the disease: hyperkeratosis, epidermal inflammation, and abnormal keratinocyte differentiation. Treatment depends on the severity of the disease, as well as the person's age, sex, treatment history, and level of treatment compliance. Treatment measures are divided into topical and systemic approaches. Usually, topical agents are used first in any treatment regimen and when less than 20% of the body surface is involved.[42,45] Combination therapies that are tailored to the needs of the client are most effective. Also, rotating the various therapies may decrease the side effects of any one therapy.

Topical agents include emollients, keratolytic agents, coal tar products, anthralin, corticosteroids, and calcipotriene. Emollients hydrate and soften the psoriatic plaques. Petroleum-based products are more effective than water-based ones, but they are less acceptable cosmetically to persons with psoriasis. Keratolytic agents are peeling agents. Salicylic acid is the most widely used. It softens and removes plaques. It has been used alone or in conjunction with other topical agents. Coal tar, the byproduct of the processing of coke and gas from coal, is one of the oldest yet more effective forms of treatment. The skin is covered with a film of coal tar for up to several weeks. The exact mechanism of action of the tar products is unknown, but side effects of the treatment are few. Newer preparations of coal tar lotions and shampoos are more aesthetically pleasing, but the odor remains a problem.

Anthralin, a synthesized product of Goa powder from Brazilian araroba tree bark, has remained a topical treatment of choice. It has been effective in resolving lesions in approximately 2 weeks. A disadvantage to anthralin is that it stains the uninvolved skin and clothes brown or purple. A treatment variation, called the *Ingram method*, involves coal tar applications and UVB radiation, followed by anthralin paste application.

Topical corticosteroids are widely used and relatively effective. They are generally more acceptable because they do not stain and are easy to use. Topical corticosteroids are available as low-, medium-, and high-potency preparations. Treatment usually is started with a medium-potency agent. Low-potency drugs usually are used on the face and areas of the body, such as the groin and axillary areas, where the skin tends to be thinner. High-potency preparations are reserved for treatment of thick chronic plaques that do not respond to less potent preparations. Although the corticosteroids are rapidly effective in the treatment of psoriasis, they are associated with flare-ups after discontinuation and they have many potential side effects. Their effectiveness is increased when used under occlusive dressings, but there is an increase in side effects. *Calcipotriene*, a topical vitamin D derivative, has been effective for the treatment of psoriasis. It inhibits epidermal cell proliferation and enhances cell differentiation. *Tazarotene*, a synthetic retinoid, also has been effective. It is classified as a pregnancy category X drug and its use should be avoided in women of childbearing age.

Systemic treatments include phototherapy, photochemotherapy, methotrexate, retinoids, corticosteroids, and cyclosporine. The positive effects of sunlight have long been established. Climatotherapy (warm climate and saltwater baths for 4 to 6 weeks) and heliotherapy (sunbathing in a suitable climate) have been effective treatment measures for those who can afford to travel. Phototherapy with UVB is a widely used treatment. Newly developed UVB equipment emitting only a narrow band of light useful for treating psoriasis is expected to improve phototherapy.[46]

Photochemotherapy involves using a light-activated form of the drug methoxsalen. Methoxsalen, a psoralen, exerts its actions when exposed to UVA radiation in 320- to 400-nm wavelengths. The combination treatment regimen of psoralen and UVA is known by the acronym PUVA. Methoxsalen is given orally before UVA exposure. Activated by the UVA energy, methoxsalen inhibits DNA synthesis, thereby preventing cell mitosis and decreasing the hyperkeratosis that occurs with psoriasis. Although viewed as one of the safest therapies since its introduction in the mid-1970s, PUVA increases the risk for squamous cell carcinoma, and it may increase the risk for development of melanoma.

Retinoids are derivatives of vitamin A. Etretinate has been effective, whereas isotretinoin (used for treatment of acne) is less effective in treating psoriasis. Etretinate suppresses inflammation and DNA synthesis in the epidermis. The drug also is used as short-term adjunctive therapy in combination with PUVA and UVB treatment.

Systemic corticosteroids have been effective in treating severe or pustular psoriasis. However, they cause severe side effects, including Cushing's syndrome. Intralesional injection of triamcinolone has proven effective in resistant lesions.

Methotrexate, which is used for cancer treatment, is an antimetabolite that inhibits DNA synthesis and prevents cell mitosis. Oral methotrexate has been effective in treating psoriasis when other approaches have failed. The drug has many side effects, including nausea, malaise, leukopenia, thrombocytopenia, and liver function abnormalities. Cyclosporine is a potent immunosuppressive drug used to prevent rejection of organ transplants. It suppresses inflammation and the proliferation of T cells in persons with psoriasis. Its use is limited to severe psoriasis because of serious toxic and side effects, including nephrotoxicity, hypertension, and increased risk of cancers. Intralesional cyclosporine also has been effective. Psoriasis treatment centers have successfully treated clients with recalcitrant cases of psoriasis. These centers have equipment, professionals, and therapists to assist clients in gaining control over the disease process and restoring normality to their lives.

Pityriasis Rosea

Pityriasis rosea is a rash that primarily affects young adults. The origin of the rash is unknown, but it is believed to be caused by an infective agent. Numerous viruses have been investigated, thus far with no conclusive evidence. The incidence is highest in winter. Cases occur in clusters and among persons who are in close contact with each other, indicating an infectious spread. However, there are no data to support communicability. It may be an immune response to any number of agents.

The characteristic lesion is an oval macule or papule with surrounding erythema (Fig. 61-23). The lesion spreads with central clearing, much like tinea corporis. This initial lesion is a solitary lesion called the *herald patch* and is usually on the trunk or neck. As the lesion enlarges and begins to fade away (2 to 10 days), successive crops of lesions appear on the trunk and neck. The lesions on the back have a characteristic "Christmas tree" pattern. The extremities, face, and scalp may be involved. Mild to severe pruritus may occur.

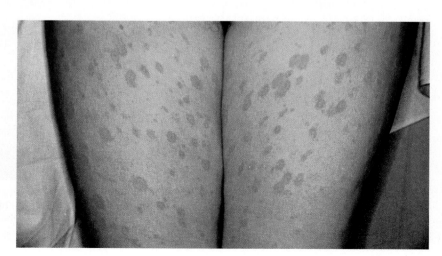

FIGURE 61-23 Pityriasis rosea of the thighs. (Syntex Laboratories.) (Sauer G.C., Hall J.C. [1996]. *Manual of skin diseases* [7th ed.]. Philadelphia: Lippincott-Raven)

The disease is self-limited and usually disappears within 6 to 8 weeks. Treatment measures are palliative and include topical steroids, antihistamines, and colloid baths. Systemic corticosteroids may be indicated in severe cases.

Lichen Planus

The term *lichen* is of Greek origin and means "tree moss." The term is applied to skin disorders characterized by small (2 to 10 mm), flat-topped papules with irregular, angulated borders (Fig. 61-24). Lichen planus is a relatively common chronic, pruritic disease. It involves inflammation and papular eruption of the skin and mucous membranes. There are variations in the pattern of lesions (*e.g.*, annular, linear) and differences in the sites (*e.g.*, mucous membranes, genitalia, nails, scalp). The characteristic lesion is a purple, polygonal papule covered with a shiny, white, lacelike pattern. The lesions appear on the wrist, ankles, and trunk of the body. Most persons who have skin lesions also have oral lesions, appearing as milky white lacework on the buccal mucosa or tongue.

The etiology of lichen planus is unknown. There is increasing evidence of a cell-mediated response involving the epidermal-dermal junction with damage to the basal cell layer. Although the cause of most cases of lichen planus is unknown, some are linked to medication use or hepatitis C virus infection. The most common offending agents include gold, antimalarial agents, thiazide diuretics, beta blockers, nonsteroidal anti-inflammatory agents, quinidine, and angiotensin-converting enzyme inhibitors.[47]

Diagnosis is based on the clinical appearance of the lesions and the histopathologic findings from a punch biopsy. For most persons, lichen planus is a self-limited disease. Treatment measures include discontinuation of all medications, followed by treatment with topical corticosteroids and occlusive dressings. Occlusion may be used to enhance the effect of topical medications. Antipruritic agents are helpful in reducing itch. Systemic corticosteroids may be indicated in severe cases. Intralesional corticosteroid injections also may be used. Acetretin, an orally administered retinoid agent, also may be effective. Because retinoids are teratogenic, this drug should be avoided in women of childbearing age.

Lichen Simplex Chronicus

Lichen simplex chronicus is a localized lichenoid dermatitis. The term *lichen simplex* denotes that there was no known predisposing skin disorder in the affected person. It is characterized by the occurrence of itchy, reddened, thickened, and scaly patches of dry skin (Fig. 61-25). Persons with the condition may have a single or, less frequently, multiple lesions. The lesions are seen most commonly at the nape of the neck, wrist, ankles, or anal area. The condition usually begins as a small pruritic patch, which culminates in a repetitive cycle of itching and scratching that develops into a chronic dermatosis. Because of the chronic itching and scratching, excoriations and lichenification with thickening of the skin develops, often giving the appearance of tree bark. Treatment consists of measures to decrease

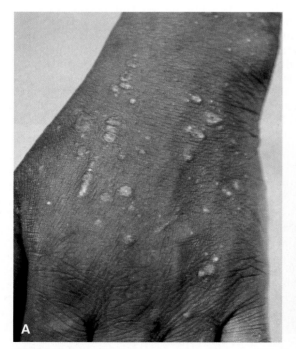
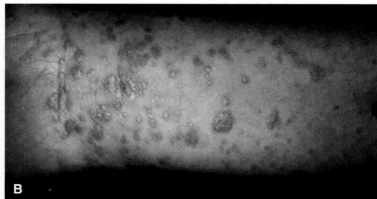

FIGURE 61-24 (**A**) Lichen planus of the dorsum of the hand and wrist. Notice the violacenous color of the papules and the linear Köebner's phenomenon. (**B**) Lichen planus. (E.R. Squibb, Johnson & Johnson.) (Sauer G.C., Hall J.C. [1996]. *Manual of skin diseases* [7th ed.]. Philadelphia: Lippincott-Raven)

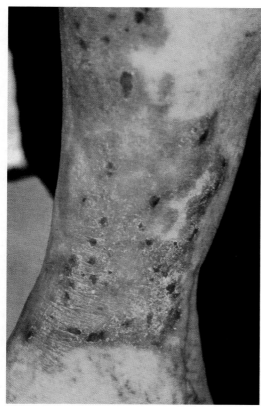

FIGURE 61-25 Localized lichen simplex chronicus of the leg. (Duke Laboratories, Inc.) (Sauer G.C., Hall J.C. [1996]. *Manual of skin diseases* [7th ed.]. Philadelphia: Lippincott-Raven)

scratching of the area. A moderate-potency corticosteroid is often prescribed to decrease the itching and subsequent inflammatory process.

ARTHROPOD INFESTATIONS

The skin is susceptible to a variety of disorders as a result of an invasion or infestation by bugs, ticks, or parasites. The type of rash or sometimes singular lesion depends on the causative agent.

Scabies

Scabies is caused by a mite, *Sarcoptes scabiei*, that burrows into the epidermis. After a female mite is impregnated, she burrows into the skin and lays two to three eggs each day for 4 or 5 weeks. The eggs hatch after 3 to 4 days, and the larvae migrate to the skin surface. At this point, they burrow into the skin only for food or protection. The larvae molt and become nymphs; they molt once more to become adults. After the new adult females are impregnated, the cycle is repeated.

The characteristic lesion is a small burrow, approximately 2 mm long, that may be red to reddish brown. Small vesicles may cover the burrows. The areas most commonly affected are the interdigital web of the finger, flexor surface of the wrist, inner surface of the elbow, axilla, female nipple, penis, belt line, and gluteal crease. Pruritus is common and may result from the burrows, the fecal material of the mite, or both. Excoriations may develop from scratching. Secondary bacterial infections and severe skin lesions may occur if the condition is untreated.

Scabies is transmitted by person-to-person contact, including sexual contact. It also is transmitted by contact with mite-infested sheets in hospitals and nursing homes because the mite can live up to 2 days on sheets or clothing. Scabies affects all people in all socioeconomic classes, although African Americans seem more resistant. Usually more prevalent in times of war and famine, scabies reached pandemic proportions in the 1970s, perhaps as a result of poverty, sexual promiscuity, and worldwide travel. Outbreaks continue to occur, but they are mostly sporadic and localized to nursing homes and families.

Diagnosis is done by skin scrapings. A positive diagnosis relies on the presence of mites, ova, or feces. The treatment is simple and curative. After bathing, permethrin, malathion, or other effective mite-killing agents are applied over the entire skin surface for 12 hours. Repeated applications may be recommended in certain cases, but one treatment usually is sufficient. Care must be taken to ensure that close contacts are treated. Clothes and towels are disinfected with hot water and detergent or they can be isolated for 4 weeks. If symptoms persist after treatment, the patient should be advised not to retreat the condition without consulting a health care provider. A red-brown nodule, thought to be an allergic response from the mite parts left on the skin, may form after treatment.

Pediculosis

Pediculosis is the term for infestation with lice (genus *Pediculus*). Lice are gray, gray-brown, or red-brown, oval, wingless insects that live off the blood of humans and animals. Lice are host specific; lice that live on animals do not transfer to humans, and vice versa. Lice also are host dependent; they cannot live apart from the host beyond a few hours. As with scabies, the incidence of pediculosis increased in the 1970s to pandemic levels, probably because of increases in poverty, sexual activity, and worldwide travel.

Three types of lice affect humans: *Pediculus humanus corporis* (body lice), *Phthirus pubis* (pubic lice), and *Pediculus humanus capitis* (head lice). Although these three types differ biologically, they have similar life cycles. The life cycle of a louse consists of an unhatched egg or "nit," three molt stages, an adult reproductive stage, and death. Before adulthood, lice live off the host and are incapable of reproduction. After fertilization, the egg is laid by the female louse along a hair shaft. These nits appear pearl gray to brown. Depending on the site, a female louse can lay between 150 and 300 nits in her life. The life span of a feeding louse is 30 to 50 days. Lice are equipped with stylets that pierce the skin. Their saliva contains an anticoagulant that prevents host blood from clotting while the louse is feeding. A louse takes up to 1 mL of blood during a feeding.

Pediculosis Corporis. Pediculosis corporis is infestation with *P. humanus corporis,* or body lice. The lice are transferred chiefly through contact with an infested person, clothing, or bedding. The lice live in clothes fibers, coming out only to feed. Unlike the pubic louse and the head louse, the body louse can survive 10 to 14 days without the host.

The typical lesion is a macule at the site of the bite. Papules and wheals may develop. The infestation is pruritic and evokes scratching that brings about a characteristic linear excoriation. Eczematous patches are found frequently. Secondary lesions may become scaly and hyperpigmented and leave scars. Areas typically affected are the shoulders, trunk, and buttocks. The presence of nits in the seams of clothes confirms a diagnosis of body lice.

Treatment measures consist of eradicating the louse and nits on the body and on clothing. Dry-cleaning clothes, washing them in hot water, or steam pressing are recommended methods. Special attention is given to the seams. Merely storing clothing in plastic bags for 2 weeks also rids clothes of lice. Many health care providers prefer not to treat the body unless nits are in evidence on hair shafts. If treatment is indicated, shampoos or topical preparations containing malathion or other pediculicides are recommended. Care must be taken to ensure that close contacts are treated.

Pediculosis Pubis.

Pediculosis pubis, the infestation known as crabs or pubic lice, is a nuisance disease that is uncomfortable and embarrassing. The disease is spread by intimate contact with someone harboring *P. pubis*. Lice and nits are located in the pubic area of men and women. Occasionally, they may be found in sites of secondary sex characteristics, such as the beard in men or the axilla in both sexes. Symptoms include intense itching and irritation of the skin. Diagnosis is made on the basis of symptoms and microscopic examination. The treatment is the same as for head lice.

Pediculosis Capitis.

Pediculosis capitis, or infestation with head lice, primarily affects white-skinned persons; it is relatively unknown in darker-skinned persons. The incidence is higher among girls, although hair length has not been indicated as a contributing factor. Infestations of head lice usually are confined to the nape of the neck and behind the ears. Less frequently, head lice are found on the beard, pubic areas, eyebrows, and body hairs. Although head lice can be transmitted by sharing combs and hats, they usually are spread from hair shaft to hair shaft through close personal contact.[48] A positive diagnosis depends on the presence of firmly attached nits or live adult lice on hair shafts. Pruritus and scratching of the head are the primary indicators that head lice may be present. The scalp may appear red and excoriated from scratching. In severe cases, the hair becomes matted together in a crusty, foul-smelling "cap." An occasional morbilliform rash, which may be misdiagnosed as rubella, may occur with lymphadenopathy.

Head lice are treated with permethrin or malathion shampoos or rinses. Retreatment may be needed to eliminate the hatching nits. Dead nits may be removed with a fine-toothed comb or over-the-counter nit removal hair rinses. Over the years, permethrin- and malathion-resistant lice have evolved.[49] There has been a resurgence of older

remedies, such as removing all nits using a nit comb or asphyxiation with olive oil or petroleum products left on the hair from 24 hours to several months. Rotating therapies also may be helpful.

Ticks

Ticks are insects that live in woods and underbrush. They attach to human and animal hosts and burrow into the epidermis, where they feed on blood. The tick bite is not problematic; the dangers stem from the infectious bacteria or viruses that they carry to human hosts. There are many tickborne illnesses, including Central European encephalitis, Q fever, and relapsing fever. Common tickborne diseases in the United States include Rocky Mountain spotted fever and Lyme disease.

Rocky Mountain Spotted Fever.

Rocky Mountain spotted fever (RMSF) is the most severe tickborne infection in the United States. It is caused by the tick that carries *Rickettsia rickettsii*. RMSF used to be limited to the Rocky Mountain states, but it now occurs throughout the United States from April to September. The initial tick bite appears as a papule or macule, with or without a central punctum. The tick burrows in and enlarges as it feeds. The tick must be attached to the human host for 4 to 6 hours before the rickettsiae are activated by the blood. The rickettsiae, found in the tick feces and body parts, enter the bloodstream and multiply in the body tissues. The incubation period is 2 to 14 days.

RMSF presents with fever, headache, muscle aches, nausea, and vomiting. The characteristic rash is macular or maculopapular that starts on the wrist or ankle then spreads to the rest of the body. Except in mild cases, the rash becomes hemorrhagic and is accompanied by generalized edema, conjunctivitis, petechial lesions, photophobia, lethargy, confusion, and cranial nerve deficits. Death may result if the disease is not promptly diagnosed and treated.

Treatment requires hospitalization and antibiotic therapy. The most important measure is to prevent tick bites by using insect repellents while engaged in activities in the woods. After a tick has attached itself, it is important to remove all the body parts to limit the possibility of infection.[50] It is important not to handle the tick with bare hands because infectious material may enter through breaks in the skin.

Lyme Disease.

Lyme disease, which was named after the town in Connecticut where the disease was discovered, is the most common tickborne disease in the United States. It characterized by a distinctive skin lesion called *erythema chronicum migrans* (ECM). The ECM is a red macule or papule that expands in an annular fashion with a central clearing at the bite site. The average time from the bite to the appearance of the ECM ranges from 1 day to 28 days.

The disease is caused by the spirochete *Borrelia burgdorferi* and is transmitted to humans by the bite of a small tick. Transmission of the disease occurs only if the tick has fed for several hours on the host. Incidence rates are highest in three geographic areas in the United States: coastal northeastern states (*i.e.*, Massachusetts to Maryland), midwestern states (*i.e.*, Minnesota and Wisconsin), and western states (*i.e.*, California, Utah, Nevada, Oregon, and Washington).

The manifestations of Lyme disease occur in three stages that may overlap. In the first or acute stage, there is the appearance of the ECM, often accompanied by flulike symptoms such as malaise, fatigue, fever, headache, and lymphadenopathy. In the second or intermediate stage, which occurs weeks to months later, there may be arthralgia and arthritis, neurologic manifestations, cardiac disease, in addition to the recurrence of the ECM. The third or chronic stage begins months to years later with chronic skin, nervous system, and joint involvement. Occasionally, chronic neurologic problems develop.

Preventive measures include using tick repellents, wearing clothing that covers the body, regularly checking for ticks, and promptly removing all attached ticks. A recombinant vaccine (LYMErix) using a highly conserved region of *B. burgdorferi* has been approved by the FDA.

The diagnosis of Lyme disease is based on both clinical manifestations and laboratory findings. Laboratory confirmation requires identification of specific antibodies to *B. burgdorferi* in the serum. Treatment involves the use of antibiotic therapy. Tetracycline is effective against the spirochete, and penicillin is moderately so. Antibiotics such as doxycycline, amoxicillin, cefuroxime axetil, erythromycin, and ceftriaxone can be used. The antibiotic that is chosen, the method of administration (oral versus parenteral), and the duration of treatment usually are determined by the stage of the disease and extent of the manifestations. Corticosteroids and other anti-inflammatory drugs may be used to provide relief from musculoskeletal manifestations.

> In summary, primary disorders of the skin include pigmentary skin disorders, infectious processes, inflammatory conditions, immune disorders, allergic reactions, and arthropod infestations. Pigmentary skin disorders include vitiligo, albinism, and melasma. Although the causes of the disorders vary, all involve changes in the amount of melanin produced by the melanocytes. These disorders appear in people of every skin type; however, the manifestations of the disorders vary among light-skinned and dark-skinned persons. Superficial fungal infections are called *dermatophytoses* and are commonly known as *tinea* or *ringworm*. Impetigo, which is caused by staphylococci or β-hemolytic streptococci, is the most common superficial bacterial infection. Viruses are responsible for verrucae (warts), herpes simplex type 1 lesions (cold sores or fever blisters), and herpes zoster (shingles). Noninfectious inflammatory skin conditions such as acne, lichen planus, psoriasis, and pityriasis rosea are of unknown origin. They usually are localized to the skin and are rarely associated with specific internal disease. Allergic skin responses involve the body's immune system and are caused by hypersensitivity reactions to allergens, environmental agents, drugs, and other substances. The skin is sensitive to invasion or infestation by bugs or parasites. Although tick bites in themselves are not problematic, the dangers stem from the infectious organisms that they carry to their human hosts.

Nevi and Skin Cancers

After you have completed this section of the chapter, you should be able to meet the following objectives:

✦ Describe the origin of nevi and state their relationship to skin cancers

✦ Compare the appearance and outcome of basal cell carcinoma, squamous cell carcinoma, and malignant melanoma

NEVI

Nevi, or moles, are common congenital or acquired tumors of the skin that are benign. Almost all adults have nevi, some in greater numbers than others. Nevi can be pigmented or nonpigmented, flat or elevated, and hairy or nonhairy.

Nevocellular nevi are pigmented skin lesions resulting from proliferation of melanocytes in the epidermis or dermis. Nevocellular nevi are tan to deep brown, uniformly pigmented, small papules with well-defined and rounded borders. They are formed initially by melanocytes with their long dendritic extensions that are normally interspersed among the basal keratinocytes (see Chapter 60, Fig. 60-3).[18] These melanocytes are transformed into round or oval melanin-containing cells that grow in nests or clusters along the dermal-epidermal junction. Because of their location, these lesions are called *junctional nevi* (Fig. 61-26). Eventually, most junctional nevi grow into the surrounding dermis as nests or cords of cells. *Compound nevi* contain epidermal and dermal components. In older lesions, the epidermal nests may disappear entirely, leaving a *dermal nevi*. Compound and dermal nevi usually are more elevated than junctional nevi.

Another form of nevi, the *dysplastic nevi*, are important because of their capacity to transform to malignant melanomas. Although the association between nevocellular nevi and malignant melanoma was made over 175 years

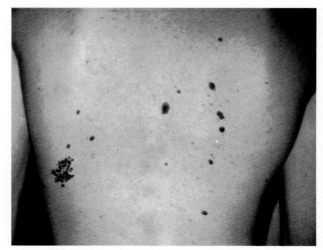

FIGURE 61-26 Junctional nevi of the back of a 16-year-old patient. (Owen Laboratories, Inc.) (Sauer G.C., Hall J.C. [1996]. *Manual of skin diseases* [7th ed.]. Philadelphia: Lippincott-Raven)

ago, it was not until 1978 that the role of dysplastic nevi as a precursor of malignant melanoma was described in detail. Dysplastic nevi are larger than other nevi (often >5 mm in diameter). Their appearance is one of a flat, slightly raised plaque with a pebbly surface, or a target-like lesion with a darker, raised center and irregular border. They vary in shade from brown and red to flesh tones and have irregular borders. A person may have hundreds of these lesions. Unlike other moles or nevi, they occur on both sun-exposed and covered areas of the body. Dysplastic nevi have been documented in multiple members of families prone to development of malignant melanoma.[18]

Because of the possibility of malignant transformation, any mole that undergoes a change warrants immediate medical attention. The changes to observe and report are changes in size, thickness, or color, and itching or bleeding.

SKIN CANCER

There has been an alarming increase in skin cancers over the past several decades. Since the 1970s, the incidence rate of malignant melanoma, the most serious form of skin cancer, has increased significantly on an average of 4% per year, from 5.7 per 100,000 in 1973 to 13.8 per 100,000 in 1996.[51] There are approximately 47,700 new cases and 9600 deaths each year from melanoma. There also are approximately 1.3 million cases each year of highly curable basal cell and squamous cell cancers.

The rising incidence of skin cancer may be attributed primarily to increased sun exposure associated with societal and lifestyle shifts in the United States. The thinning of the ozone layer in the earth's stratosphere is thought to be an important factor in this incidence rate. Society's emphasis on suntanning also is implicated. Persons have more leisure time and spend increasing amounts of time in the sun with uncovered skin.

Although the factors linking sun exposure to skin cancer are incompletely understood, both total cumulative exposure and altered patterns of exposure (in the case of melanoma) are strongly implicated. Basal cell and squamous cell carcinomas are associated with total cumulative exposure to ultraviolet radiation, whereas melanomas are associated with intense intermittent exposure. Thus, basal

 Skin Cancers

➤ An increase in skin cancers over the past several decades has been attributed to increased sun exposure.

➤ There are three major types of skin cancers: malignant melanomas, which are a rapidly progressive and metastatic form of skin cancer, and the basal cell carcinomas and squamous cell carcinomas, which are highly curable.

cell and squamous cell carcinomas occur more commonly on maximally sun-exposed parts of the body, such as the face and back of the hands and forearms. In contrast, melanomas occur most commonly in areas of the body that are exposed to the sun intermittently, such as the back in men and the lower legs in women. It is more common in persons with indoor occupations whose exposure to sun is limited to weekends and vacations.

Malignant Melanoma

Malignant melanoma is a malignant tumor of the melanocytes. It is a rapidly progressing, metastatic form of cancer. As previously mentioned, there has been a dramatic increase in the incidence of malignant melanoma over the past several decades. The increased incidence of melanoma is thought to be related to sun exposure. The risk is greatest in fair-skinned people, particularly those with blond or red hair who sunburn and freckle easily. Fortunately, the increased risk of melanoma has been associated with a concomitant increase in the 5-year survival rate, from approximately 40% in the 1940s to 90% at present.[52] Public health screening measures, early diagnosis, increased knowledge of precursor lesions, and greater public knowledge of the disease may account for earlier intervention.

Severe, blistering sunburns in early childhood and intermittent intense sun exposures (trips to sunny climates) contribute to increased susceptibility to melanoma in young and middle-aged adults. Roughly 90% of malignant melanomas in whites occur on sun-exposed skin. However, in African Americans and Asians, roughly 67% occur on non–sun-exposed areas, such as mucous membranes and subungual, palmar, and plantar surfaces.[53] Although sun exposure remains a significant risk factor for melanoma, other potential risk factors have been identified, including atypical mole/dysplastic nevus syndrome, immunosuppression, prior PUVA therapy, and exposure to ultraviolet light at tanning salons. Using statistical analysis, it has been determined that six risk factors independently influence the risk for development of malignant melanoma: family history of malignant melanoma, presence of blond or red hair, presence of marked freckling on the upper back, history of three or more blistering sunburns before 20 years of age, history of 3 or more years of an outdoor job as a teenager, and presence of actinic keratosis. Persons with two of these risk factors had a 3.5-fold increased risk of malignant melanoma and those with three or more risk factors had a 20-fold increased risk.[52]

Malignant melanomas differ in size and shape. Usually, they are slightly raised and black or brown. Borders are irregular and surfaces are uneven. Most seem to arise from preexisting nevi or new molelike growths (Fig. 61-27). There may be surrounding erythema, inflammation, and tenderness. Periodically, melanomas ulcerate and bleed. Dark melanomas are often mottled with shades of red, blue, and white. These three colors represent three concurrent processes: melanoma growth (blue), inflammation and the body's attempt to localize and destroy the tumor (red), and scar tissue formation (white). Malignant melanomas can appear anywhere on the body. Although they frequently are found on sun-exposed areas, sun exposure

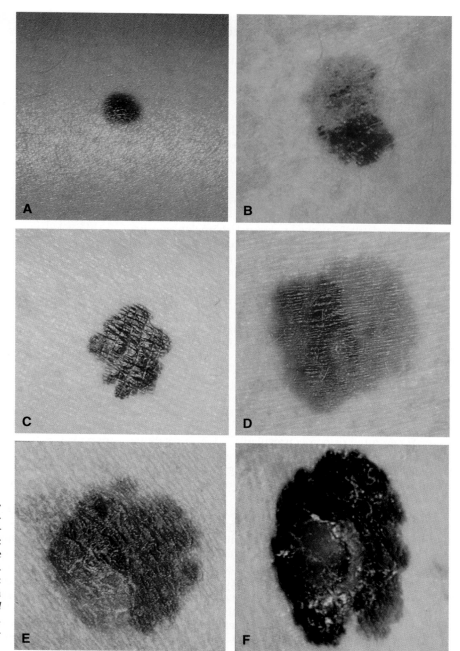

FIGURE 61-27 (**A**) Normal mole with even, round contour and sharply defined borders. (**B**) Changes in appearance of a mole: *asymmetry.* (**C**) Changes in appearance of a mole: *border irregularity.* (**D**) Changes in appearance of a mole: *color and uneven pigmentation.* (**E**) Changes in the appearance of a mole: *diameter greater than 6 mm.* (**F**) Changes in the surface of a mole: *scaliness, oozing, and bleeding.* (American Cancer Society. [1995]. *What you should know about melanoma.* Dallas: American Cancer Society)

alone does not account for their development. In men, they are found frequently on the trunk, head, neck, and arms; in women, they also are found on the legs.

Four types of melanomas have been identified: superficial spreading, nodular, lentigo maligna, and acral lentiginous.[54] *Superficial spreading melanoma* is characterized by a raised-edged nevus with lateral growth. It has a disorderly appearance in color and outline. This lesion tends to have biphasic growth, horizontally and vertically. It typically ulcerates and bleeds with growth. This type of lesion accounts for 70% of all melanomas and is most prevalent in persons who sunburn easily and have intermittent sun ex-

posure. *Nodular melanomas,* which account for 15% to 30% of melanomas, are raised, dome-shaped lesions that can occur anywhere on the body. They are commonly a uniform blue-black color and tend to look like blood blisters. Nodular melanomas tend to rapidly invade the dermis from the start with no apparent horizontal growth phase. *Lentigo maligna* melanomas, which account for 4% to 10% of all melanomas, are slow-growing, flat nevi that occur primarily on sun-exposed areas of elderly persons. Untreated lentigo maligna tends to exhibit horizontal and radial growth for many years before it invades the dermis to become lentigo maligna melanoma. *Acral lentiginous melanoma,* which accounts for 2 to 8% of melanomas, occurs primarily on the palms of the hands, soles of the feet, nail beds, and mucous membranes. It has the appearance of lentigo maligna. Unlike other types of melanomas, it has a similar incidence in all ethnic groups.

The prognosis for malignant melanoma varies. It depends on factors such as tumor thickness (measured in millimeters), anatomic site, type of lesion, and levels of invasion (degree of penetration in the anatomic layers of the skin). Tumor thickness is an important factor in determining prognosis in persons with malignant melanoma. Eight-year survival rates after definitive therapy for primary melanoma related to tumor thickness in millimeters are as follows: less than 0.76 mm, 93%; 0.76 to 1.69 mm, 86%; 1.7 to 3.6 mm, 60%; more than 3.60 mm, 33%.[55]

Because virtually all the known risks of melanoma are related to susceptibility and magnitude of ultraviolet light exposure, protection from the sun's rays plays a critical role in the prevention of malignant melanoma. Protection includes using a combination regimen of protective clothing, avoidance of midday sun, and regular use of broad-spectrum sunscreen with a high SPF.

Early detection is critical with malignant melanoma. Regular self-examination of the total skin surface in front of a mirror under good lighting provides a method for early detection. It requires that a person undress completely and examine all areas of the body using a full mirror, handheld mirror, and handheld hair dryer (to examine the scalp). An *ABCD* rule has been developed to aid in early diagnosis and timely treatment of malignant melanoma.[52] The acronym stands for *a*symmetry, *b*order irregularity, *c*olor variegation, and *d*iameter greater than 0.6 cm (pencil eraser size). People should be taught to watch for these changes in existing nevi or the development of new nevi, as well as other alterations such as bleeding or itching.

Diagnosis of melanoma is based on biopsy findings from a suspect lesion. Treatment is usually surgical excision, the extent of which is determined by the thickness of the lesion, invasion of the deeper skin layers, and spread to regional lymph nodes. Deep and wide excisions, with possible use of skin grafts, are used. Current cancer treatment, such as immunotherapy and chemotherapy, is indicated when the disease becomes systemic. Interferon alfa-2b is approved by the FDA for treatment of melanoma.[52] An area of active research in melanoma therapy involves vaccine development.

Basal Cell Carcinoma

Basal cell carcinoma is the most common skin cancer in white-skinned people (Fig. 61-28). It is less common among darker-skinned people. Like other skin cancers, basal cell carcinoma has increased in incidence over the past several decades. Fair-skinned persons with a history of significant long-term sun exposure are more susceptible. Black- and brown-skinned persons are affected occasionally.

Basal cell carcinoma usually is a nonmetastasizing tumor that extends wide and deep if left untreated. These tumors are most frequently seen on the head and neck. They also occur less frequently on other skin surfaces that were not exposed to the sun. However, basal cell carcinoma usu-

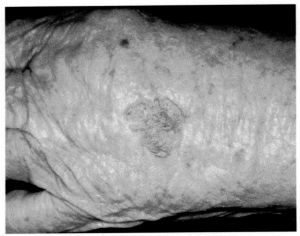

FIGURE 61-28 Basal cell carcinoma and wrinkling of the hand. (Syntex Laboratories.) (Sauer G.C., Hall J.C. [1996]. *Manual of skin diseases* [7th ed.]. Philadelphia: Lippincott-Raven)

ally occurs in persons who were exposed to great amounts of sunlight. The incidence is twice as high among men as women and greatest in the 55- to 75-year-old age group.[56]

Although there are several histologic types of basal cell carcinoma, nodular ulcerative and superficial basal cell carcinomas are the most frequently occurring types. *Nodular ulcerative basal cell carcinoma* is the most common type. It is a nodulocystic structure that begins as a small, flesh-colored or pink, smooth, translucent nodule that enlarges over time. Telangiectatic vessels frequently are seen beneath the surface. Over the years, a central depression forms that progresses to an ulcer surrounded by the original shiny, waxy border. Basal cell carcinoma in darker-skinned persons usually is darkly pigmented and frequently misdiagnosed as other skin diseases, including melanoma.

The second most common form is *superficial basal cell carcinoma*, which is seen most often on the chest or back. It begins as a flat, nonpalpable, erythematous plaque. The red, scaly areas slowly enlarge, with nodular borders and telangiectatic bases. This type of skin cancer is difficult to diagnose because it mimics other dermatologic problems.

All suspected basal cell carcinomas are biopsied for diagnosis. The treatment depends on the site and extent of the lesion. The most important treatment goal is complete elimination of the lesion. Also important is the maintenance of function and optimal cosmetic effect. Curettage with electrodesiccation, surgical excision, irradiation, and chemosurgery are effective in removing all cancerous cells. Patients should be checked at regular intervals for recurrences.

Squamous Cell Carcinoma

Squamous cell carcinomas are malignant tumors of the outer epidermis. The increase in the incidence of squamous cell carcinomas is consistent with increased ultraviolet radiation exposure. It is the most frequent skin cancer in blacks.[57] Metastasis is more common with squamous cell carcinoma than with basal cell carcinoma. There are two types of squamous cell carcinoma: intraepidermal and invasive. *Intraepidermal squamous cell carcinoma* remains confined to the epidermis for a long time. However, at some unpredictable time, it may penetrate the basement membrane to the dermis and metastasize to the regional lymph nodes. It then converts to *invasive squamous cell carcinoma.* The invasive type can develop from intraepidermal carcinoma or from a premalignant lesion (*e.g.*, actinic keratoses). It may be slow growing or fast growing with metastasis.

Squamous cell carcinoma is a red-scaling, keratotic, slightly elevated lesion with an irregular border, usually with a shallow chronic ulcer (Fig. 61-29). Later lesions grow outward, show large ulcerations, and have persistent crusts and raised, erythematous borders. The lesions occur on sun-exposed areas of the skin, particularly the nose, forehead, helixes of the ears, lower lip, and back of the hands. In blacks, the lesions may appear as hyperpigmented nodules and occur more frequently on non–sun-exposed areas.

The mechanisms of squamous cell carcinoma development are unclear. Sunlight is implicated as a causative factor. Most squamous cell cancers occur in sun-exposed areas of the skin, and persons who spend much time outdoors, have lighter skin, and live in lower latitudes are more af-

fected. Other suspected causes include exposure to arsenic (*i.e.*, Bowen's disease), gamma radiation, tars, and oils.

Treatment measures are aimed at the removal of all cancerous tissue using methods such as electrosurgery, excision surgery, chemosurgery, or radiation therapy. After treatment, the person is observed for the remainder of his or her life for signs of recurrence. The recurrence rate is roughly 50%, with a 70% metastatic rate.[58]

> In summary, nevi are moles that usually are benign. Because they may undergo cancerous transformation, any mole that undergoes a change warrants immediate medical attention. There has been an alarming increase in skin cancers over the past few decades. Repeated exposure to the ultraviolet rays of the sun has been implicated as the principal cause of skin cancer. Neoplasms of the skin include malignant melanoma, basal cell carcinoma, and squamous cell carcinoma. Malignant melanoma is a malignant tumor of the melanocytes. It is a rapidly progressing, metastatic form of cancer. Clinically, malignant melanoma of the skin usually is asymptomatic. The most important clinical sign is the change in size, shape, and color of pigmented skin lesion, such as a mole. As the result of increased public awareness, most melanomas can be cured surgically. Squamous cell carcinoma and basal cell carcinoma are of epidermal origin. Basal cell carcinomas are the most common form of skin cancer among whites. They are slow-growing tumors that rarely metastasize. Squamous cell carcinoma is most common in blacks and the elderly. The two types of squamous cell carcinoma are intraepidermal and invasive. Intraepidermal squamous cell carcinoma remains confined to the epidermis for a long time. Invasive squamous cell carcinoma can develop from intraepidermal carcinoma or from premalignant lesions such as actinic keratoses.

Burns

After you have completed this section of the chapter, you should be able to meet the following objectives:

- Compare the tissue involvement for first-degree, second-degree partial-thickness, second-degree full-thickness, and third-degree burns
- State how the Rule of Nines is used in determining the body surface area involved in a burn
- Cite the determinants for grading burn severity using the American Burn Association classification of burns
- Describe the systemic complications of burns
- Describe major considerations in treatment of burn injury

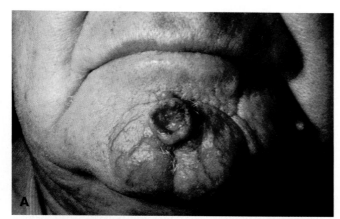

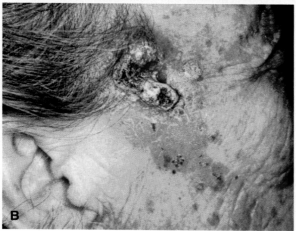

FIGURE 61-29 (**A**) Squamous cell carcinoma of the chin. (**B**) Squamous cell carcinoma and keratosis of aged skin. (Syntex Laboratories, Westwood Pharmaceuticals.) (Sauer G.C., Hall J.C. [1996]. *Manual of skin diseases* [7th ed.]. Philadelphia: Lippincott-Raven)

Most burns occur accidentally in the home or workplace. Patients with severe burns are surviving at higher rates than they did previously. The number of deaths has decreased proportionately since the 1970s. Approximately 60,000 to 80,000 persons with burns are admitted to the hospital annually.[59] Of those admitted, 5500 die.[60] The remainder of those with serious burns require extensive medical burn treatment, which has improved greatly over the years.

Inhalation injury remains the major problem contributing to mortality from burns. Sepsis and pneumonia are other important factors contributing to mortality. Burns are caused by a number of sources. Flame burns occur because of exposure to direct fire. Scald burns result from hot liquids spilled or poured on the skin surface. In a child, a scald burn may be indicative of child abuse. Chemical burns occur from industrial agents used in occupational sites. Electrical burns occur from contact with live electrical wires in fields or in the home. Electrical burns are usually more extensive because of internal tissue injury and the entrance and exit wounds. Lightning, electromagnetic radiation, and ionizing radiation also can cause skin burns.

CLASSIFICATION

The four classifications for the depth of burn injuries are first-degree, second-degree partial-thickness, second-degree full-thickness, and third-degree burns. The depth of a burn is largely influenced by the length of time exposed to the heat source and the temperature of the heating agent.

First-degree burns (superficial partial-thickness burns) involve only the outer layers of the epidermis. They are red or pink, dry, and painful. There usually is no blister formation. A mild sunburn is an example. The skin maintains its ability to function as a water vapor and bacterial barrier and heals in 3 to 10 days. First-degree burns usually require only palliative treatment, such as pain relief measures and adequate fluid intake. Extensive first-degree burns on infants, the elderly, and persons who receive radiation therapy for cancer may need more care.

Second-degree partial-thickness burns involve the epidermis and various degrees of the dermis. They are painful, moist, red, and blistered. Underneath the blisters is weeping, bright pink or red skin that is sensitive to temperature changes, air exposure, and touch. The blisters prevent the loss of body water and superficial dermal cells. Excluding excision of large burn areas, it is important to maintain intact blisters after injury because they serve as a good bandage and may promote wound healing.[61] These burns heal in approximately 1 to 2 weeks.

Second-degree full-thickness burns involve the entire epidermis and dermis. Structures that originate in the subcutaneous layer, such as hair follicles and sweat glands, remain intact. These burns can be very painful because the pain sensors remain intact. Tactile sensors may be absent or greatly diminished in the areas of deepest destruction. These burns appear as mottled pink, red, or waxy white areas with blisters and edema. The blisters resemble flat, dry tissue paper, rather than the bullous blisters seen with superficial partial-thickness injury. After healing, in approximately 1 month, these burns maintain their softness and elasticity, but there may be the loss of some sensation. Scar formation is usual. These burns heal with supportive medical care aimed at preventing further tissue damage, providing adequate hydration, and ensuring that the granular bed is adequate to support reepithelialization.

Third-degree full-thickness burns extend into the subcutaneous tissue and may involve muscle and bone. Thrombosed vessels can be seen under the burned skin, indicating that the underlying vasculature is involved. Third-degree burns vary in color from waxy white or yellow to tan, brown, deep red, or black. These burns are hard, dry, and leathery. Edema is extensive in the burn area and surrounding tissues. There is no pain because the nerve sensors have been destroyed. However, there is no such thing as a "pure" third-degree burn. Third-degree burns are almost always surrounded by second-degree burns, which are surrounded by an area of first-degree burns. The injury sometimes has an almost target-like appearance because of the various degrees of burn. Full-thickness burns wider than 1.5 inches usually require skin grafts because all the regenerative (i.e., dermal) elements have been destroyed. Smaller injuries usually heal from the margins inward toward the center, the dermal elements regenerating from the healthier margins. However, regeneration may take many weeks and leave a permanent scar, even in smaller burns.

In addition to the depth of the wound, the extent of the burn also is important. Extent is measured by estimating the amount of total body surface area (TBSA) involved. Several tools exist for estimating the TBSA. For example, the *Rule of Nines* counts anatomic body parts as multiples of 9% (the head is 9%, each arm 9%, each leg 18%, anterior trunk 18%, posterior trunk 18%), with the perineum 1%.[61] The Lund and Browder chart includes a body diagram table that estimates the TBSA by age and anatomic part.[62] Children are more accurately assessed using this method because it takes into account the difference in relative size of body parts.

The estimates of TBSA are then converted to the American Burn Association Classification of Extent of Injury (Table 61-6). Together, the depth and the extent of the burn indicate the severity of the burn and the need for treatment. Other factors, such as age, location, other injuries, and preexisting conditions, are taken into consideration for a full assessment of burn injury. These factors can increase the severity of the burn assessment and the length of treatment.

 Burns

➤ Burns represent heat-induced injuries of the skin and subcutaneous tissues.

➤ The extent and depth of injury, the effect on physiologic functioning, and the degree and mechanism of healing are determined by the length of time exposed to the heat source, the temperature of the heating agent, and the amount of surface area that is involved.

➤ Burns affecting the epidermis heal by regeneration, whereas burns involving the deeper dermal and subcutaneous tissues heal by scar tissue replacement.

TABLE 61-6 ✦ American Burn Association Grading of Burn Severity

Burn Type	Minor	Moderate	Major
Partial thickness	<15% TBSA, adult <10% TBSA, child	15–25% TBSA, adult 10–20% TBSA, child	>25% TBSA, adult >20% TBSA, child
Full thickness	<2% TBSA, adult	2–10% TBSA, adult	≥10% TBSA, adult

TBSA, total body surface area.
(American Burn Association [1976]. *American Burn Association Committee on Specific Optimal Criteria for Hospital Resources for Care of Patients with Burn Injury.* San Antonio: American Burn Association)

For example, a first-degree burn is reclassified as a more severe burn if other factors exist, such as burns to the hands, face, and feet; inhalation injury; electrical burns; other trauma; or existence of psychosocial problems. Genital burns almost always require hospitalization because edema may cause difficulty voiding and the location complicates maintenance of a bacteria-free environment.

SYSTEMIC COMPLICATIONS

Burn victims often are confronted with hemodynamic instability, impaired respiratory function, hypermetabolic response, major organ dysfunction, and sepsis. The magnitude of the response is proportional to the extent of injury, usually reaching a plateau when approximately 60% of the body is burned. The treatment challenge is for immediate resuscitation efforts and for more long-term maintenance of physiologic function. Pain and emotional problems are additional problems faced by persons with burns.

Hemodynamic Instability

Hemodynamic instability begins almost immediately with injury to capillaries in the burned area and surrounding tissue. Because of a loss of vascular volume, major burn victims often present in the emergency room in a form of hypovolemic shock (Chapter 26) known as *burn shock*. The patient has a decrease in cardiac output, increased peripheral vascular resistance, and impaired perfusion of vital organs. Burn shock is proportional to the extent and depth of injury. Fluid is lost from the vascular, interstitial, and cellular compartments. Sodium is lost from the vascular and interstitial fluid compartments, and potassium is lost from the intracellular compartment.

The major hemodynamic derangement results from a rapid shift of plasma from the vascular system into the interstitial fluid compartment, resulting in edema. The loss of plasma fluid and proteins decreases vascular colloidal osmotic pressure and results in additional edema formation in both burned and nonburned areas. Because plasma fluid rather than whole blood is lost from the vascular compartment, there is an increase in hematocrit and a concentration of other blood components. Consequently, damaged red cells in the capillaries may sludge, leading to thrombosis and further impairment of blood flow to vital organs. Because of the increased concentration of coagulation factors,

burn victims are at increased risk for development of disseminated intravascular coagulation (see Chapter 14). In persons with hemodynamic instability, adequate fluid resuscitation is essential to survival. The amounts of fluid needed are great. The type and amount of fluid are calculated according to the extent of the burn and the age and weight of the person, balanced with the increased fluid expended through burn sites. In persons receiving adequate fluid resuscitation, cardiac output usually returns to normal in approximately 24 hours.

Respiratory Dysfunction

Smoke inhalation and postburn lung dysfunction are frequent problems in burn victims. Victims often are trapped in a burning structure and inhale significant amounts of smoke, carbon monoxide, and other toxic fumes. Water-soluble gases, such as ammonia, sulfur dioxide, and chlorine, that are found in smoke from burning plastics and rubber react with mucous membranes to form strong acids and alkalis that induce ulceration of the mucous membrane, bronchospasm, and edema. Lipid-soluble gases, such as nitrous oxide and hydrogen chloride, are transported to the lower airways, where they produce damage. These substances damage cell membranes and impair the function of the mucociliary blanket. There also may be thermal injury to the respiratory passages.

Symptoms of inhalation injury include hoarseness, drooling, an inability to handle secretions, rales and rhonchi, strider, hacking cough, and labored and shallow breathing. Serial blood gases show a fall in PO_2. Signs of mucosal injury and airway obstruction often are delayed for 24 to 48 hours after a burn. It is necessary continually to monitor the patient for early signs of respiratory distress. Humidified oxygen is administered to prevent drying and sloughing of the mucosa. Intubation and ventilatory support may be needed. Other pulmonary conditions, such as pneumonia, pulmonary embolism, or pneumothorax, may occur secondarily to the burn.

Hypermetabolic Response

The stress of burn injury increases metabolic and nutritional requirements. Secretion of stress hormones such as catecholamines and cortisol is increased in an effort to maintain homeostasis. Heat production is increased in an effort to balance heat losses from the burned area. Hypermetabolism, characterized by increased oxygen consumption, increased glucose use, and protein and fat wasting, is a characteristic response to burn trauma and infection. The metabolic rate of persons with burns covering 40% of TBSA often is twice the normal rate.[63] The hypermetabolic state peaks at approximately 7 to 17 days after the burn, and tissue breakdown diminishes as the wounds heal.

Persons with 40% TBSA burns have been shown to lose 25% of their preadmission weight by 3 weeks after the injury. Nutritional support is essential to recovery from burn injury. Enteral and parenteral hyperalimentation is used to deliver sufficient nutrients to prevent tissue breakdown and postburn weight loss.

Organ Dysfunction

Burn shock results in impaired perfusion of vital organs. The patient may have impaired function of the kidneys, the gastrointestinal tract, and the nervous system. Although the initial insult often is one of hypovolemic shock and impaired organ perfusion, sepsis may contribute to impaired organ function after the initial resuscitation period.

Renal insufficiency can occur in burn patients as a result of the hypovolemic state, damage to the kidneys at the time of the burn, or from drugs that are administered. Immediately after the burn, a person goes into a short period of relative anuria, followed by a phase of hypermetabolism characterized by increased urine output and nitrogen loss. The effects of burn injury on the gastrointestinal tract include gastric dilation and decreased peristalsis. These effects are compounded by immobility and narcotic analgesics. Burn victims are observed carefully for vomiting and fecal impaction. Acute ulceration of the stomach and duodenum (called *Curling's ulcer*) is a relatively common complication in burn victims and is thought to be the result of stress and gastric ischemia. Enteral feeding tubes are inserted almost immediately. Tube feeding is intended to mitigate ulcer formation, maintain the integrity of the intestinal mucosa, and provide sufficient calories and protein for the hypermetabolic state. Burn patients are encouraged to begin eating as soon as possible to maintain gastrointestinal integrity.

Neurologic changes can occur from periods of hypoxia. Neurologic damage may result from head injuries, drug or alcohol abuse, carbon monoxide poisoning, fluid volume deficits, and hypovolemia. With an electrical burn, the brain or spine can be directly injured. The responses to physiologic damage may include confusion, memory loss, insomnia, lethargy, and combativeness.

Musculoskeletal effects include fractures that occur at the time of the accident, deep burns extending to the muscles and bone, hypertrophic scarring, and contractures. The hypermetabolic state increases tissue catabolism and severe protein and fat wasting.

Sepsis and Immune Function

A significant complication of the acute phase of burn injury is sepsis. It may arise from the burn wound, pneumonia, urinary tract infection, infection elsewhere in the body, or the use of invasive procedures or monitoring devices. Immunologically, the skin is the body's first line of defense. When the skin is no longer intact, the body is open to bacterial infection. Destruction of the skin also prevents the delivery of cellular components of the immune system to the site of injury. There also is loss of normal protective skin flora and a shift to colonization by more pathogenic flora.

Suppression of the immune system after burn trauma contributes to the development of sepsis. B-cell and T-cell immunity are involved. The cause of immunosuppression is unclear, but undoubtedly multiple factors are involved. It has been suggested that immunosuppression factors are produced by tissues away from the site of injury (*e.g.*, liver, gastrointestinal tract, endocrine system) and by the burned tissue itself. The capillary leak that occurs in the immediate postburn period removes immune cells and immunoglobulins from the circulation. Stress also contributes to immunosuppression through the hypothalamic-pituitary-adrenal axis (see Chapter 9). Persons with prior immunodeficiency, those with chronic debilitating conditions, and known alcoholics are particularly at risk. The very young and the elderly also are at risk for immunosuppression.

Pain

Burn injuries are extremely painful, and pain management must be a major priority in the care of these patients. The degree of pain in the resuscitative and acute phases of care is influenced by the depth and extent of the burn injury. During this stage, pain medications usually are given intravenously because of injury to the skin and because of impaired blood flow to the subcutaneous and intramuscular tissues.

Emotional Trauma

Burns are emotionally devastating because of the impact of disfigurement, pain, and lengthy recovery. These are persons who at one moment were well and extensively burned the next. Burn patients are faced with enormous physiologic, psychological, and social challenges. Any number of human responses are expected and normal for the person experiencing a major burn. Patients may exhibit responses such as anger, denial, and refusal to cooperate. The patient and family usually need psychological support in addition to all the physiologic forms of life support.

TREATMENT

Regardless of the type of burn, the first step in any burn situation is preventing the causal agent from producing further tissue damage. Copious amounts of water over the burned area are extremely helpful. Immediate submersion is more important than removal of clothing, which may delay cooling the involved areas. Cold (ice) applications are not recommended because ice can further limit blood flow to an area, turning a partial-thickness into a full-thickness burn. Depending on the depth and extent of the burn, medical treatment is necessary. Emergency care consists of resuscitation and stabilization with intravenous fluids while maintaining cardiac and respiratory function. Once hospitalized, the treatment regimen includes fluid replacement, maintenance of nutritional demands, antibiotic therapy, maintenance of cardiac and respiratory functions, pain alleviation, and emotional support.

After hemodynamic stability and pulmonary stability have been established, treatment is directed toward initial care of the wound. The wound is cleaned, debrided, and covered with a topical antimicrobial agent. Because of alterations in immune function, protective isolation measures may be instituted.

The sloughed tissue, or *eschar*, produced by the burn is excised as soon as possible. This decreases the chance of infection and allows the skin to regenerate faster.[64] Antimicrobial agents, such as silver sulfadiazine, mafenide acetate, or silver nitrate, are applied to burned areas, which are dressed with various gauzes. Systemic antibiotics seldom are useful at the burn sites because of the loss of the functional components of the skin. The dressings are changed according to the specific practice of the health care provider.

Burns that encircle the entire surface of the body or a body part (*e.g.*, arms, legs, torso) act like tourniquets and can cause major tissue damage to the muscles, tendons, and vasculature under the area of the leathery eschar skin. These burns are called *circumferential burns*. The eschar is incised longitudinally (escharotomy), and sometimes a fasciotomy (surgical incision through the fascia of the muscle) is performed. The timing of these incisions is important. Incision is done after the patient's circulatory condition stabilizes to some degree, thereby limiting some of the massive fluid loss. However, the incisions must occur before the eschar formation can cause hypoxia and necrosis of the tissues and organs under it. This is extremely important when torso burns occur because the pressure placed on a chest can result in inability to breathe and decreased blood return to the heart.

Skin grafts are surgically implanted as soon as possible, often at the same time the burns are debrided, to promote new skin growth, limit fluid loss, and act as a dressing. Skin grafts can be permanent or temporary and split-thickness or full-thickness. Permanent skin grafts are used over newly excised tissue. Temporary skin grafts are used to cover a burned area until the tissue underneath it has healed.

A *split-thickness skin graft* is one that includes the epidermis and part of the dermis. The thickness of these grafts depends on the donor site and the needs of the burn patient. A split-thickness skin graft can be sent through a skin mesher that cuts tiny slits into the skin, allowing it to expand up to nine times its size. These grafts are used frequently because they can cover large surface areas and there is less autorejection. *Full-thickness skin grafts* include the entire thickness of the dermal layer. They are used primarily for reconstructive surgery or for deep, small areas. The donor site of a full-thickness skin graft requires a split-thickness skin graft to help it heal.

Various sources of skin grafts exist: *autograft* (skin obtained from the person's own body), *homograft* (skin obtained from another human being, alive or recently dead), and *heterograft* (skin obtained from another species, such as pigs). The best choice is autografting when there is enough uninterrupted skin on the person's body. A two-layered (dermal and epidermal) synthetic skin graft, called *Alpligraf*, is now available and approved by the FDA.[65]

REHABILITATION

Treatment measures include positioning, splinting, and physical therapy to prevent contractures and maintain muscle tone. Because the normal body response to disuse is flexion, the contractures that occur with a burn are disfiguring and cause loss of limb or appendage use. Once the wounds have healed sufficiently, elastic pressure garments, sometimes for the full body, often are used to prevent hypertrophic scarring.

Psychological and emotional resources also are provided to burn patients and their families. Rehabilitation can take long periods, considering the numerous hospitalizations, skin grafting procedures, and plastic surgeries. Burn centers across the country specialize in total care for patients and have many of the additional supportive services needed for burn patients.

> In summary, burns cause damage to skin structures, ranging from first-degree burns, which damage the epidermis, to third-degree full-thickness burns, which extend into the subcutaneous tissue and may involve muscle and bone. The extent of injury is determined by the thickness of the burn and the total body surface area involved. In addition to skin involvement, burn injury can cause hemodynamic instability with hypovolemic shock, inhalation injury with respiratory involvement, a hypermetabolic state, organ dysfunction, immune suppression and sepsis, pain, and emotional trauma. Treatment methods vary with the severity of injury and include immediate resuscitation and maintenance of physiologic function, wound cleaning and debridement, application of antimicrobial agents and dressings, and skin grafting. Efforts are directed toward preventing or limiting disfigurement and disability.

Age-Related Skin Manifestations

After you have completed this section of the chapter, you should be able to meet the following objectives:

+ Differentiate a strawberry hemangioma from a port-wine stain hemangioma in terms of appearance and outcome
+ Describe the distinguishing features of rashes associated with the common infectious childhood diseases: roseola infantum, rubeola, rubella, chickenpox, and scarlet fever
+ Characterize the physiologic changes of aging skin
+ Describe the appearance of skin tags, keratoses, lentigines, and vascular lesions that are commonly seen in the elderly

Many skin problems occur more commonly in certain age groups. Because of aging changes, infants, children, and elderly persons tend to have different skin problems.

SKIN MANIFESTATIONS OF INFANCY AND CHILDHOOD

Skin Disorders of Infancy

Infancy connotes the image of perfect, unblemished skin. For the most part, this is true. However, several congenital skin lesions, such as mongolian spots, hemangiomas, and nevi, are associated with the early neonatal period.

Vascular and Pigmented Birthmarks. Pigmented and vascular lesions comprise most birthmarks.[66] Pigmented birthmarks represent abnormal migration or proliferation of melanocytes. Mongolian spots are caused by selective pigmentation. They usually occur on the buttocks or sacral area and are seen commonly in Asians and blacks. Nevi or moles are small, tan to brown, uniformly pigmented solid macules. *Nevocellular nevi* are formed initially from aggregates of melanocytes and keratinocytes along the dermal-epidermal border. *Congenital melanocytic nevi* are collections of melanocytes that are present at birth or develop within the first year of life. They present as macular, papular, or plaquelike pigmented lesions of various shades of brown, with a black or blue focus. The texture of the lesions varies and they may be with or without hair. They usually are found on the hands, shoulders, buttocks, entire arm, or trunk of the body. Some involve large areas of the body in garment-like fashion. They usually grow proportionately with the child. Congenital melanocytic nevi are clinically significant because of their association with malignant melanoma.

Vascular birthmarks are cutaneous anomalies of angiogenesis and vascular development.[66] Two types of vascular birthmarks commonly are seen in infants and small children: bright red, raised strawberry hemangiomas and flat, reddish-purple port-wine stains.

The strawberry hemangiomas begin as small, red lesions that are noticed shortly after birth. Hemangiomas are benign vascular tumors produced by proliferation of the endothelial cells. They are seen in approximately 5% to 10% of 1-year-old children.[67] Female infants are three times as likely as male infants to have hemangiomas, and there is an increased incidence in premature infants. Approximately 35% of these lesions are present at birth, and the remainder develop within a few weeks after birth. Hemangiomas typically undergo an early period of a proliferation during which they enlarge, followed by a period of slow involution where the growth is reversed, and finally complete resolution. Most strawberry hemangiomas disappear before 5 to 7 years of age without leaving an appreciable scar. Hemangiomas can occur anywhere in the body. Hemangiomas of the airway can be life threatening. Ulceration, the most frequent complication, can be painful and carries the risk of infection, hemorrhage, and scarring.[67]

Port-wine stains are pink or red patches that can occur anywhere on the body and are very noticeable (Fig. 61-30). They represent slow-growing capillary malformations that grow proportionately with the child and persist throughout life. Port-wine stains usually are confined to the skin, but may be associated with vascular malformations of the eye or leptomeninges over the cortex, leading to cognitive disorders, seizures, and other neurologic deficits. Cover-up cosmetics are used in an attempt to conceal their disfiguring effects. Laser surgery has been used effectively in the treatment of port-wine stains.

Diaper Rash. Because of its newness, infant skin is sensitive to irritation, injury, and extremes of temperature. The contents of soiled diapers, if not changed frequently, can lead to contact dermatitis and bacterial infections. Prolonged exposure to a warm, humid environment can lead to prickly heat, and too-frequent bathing can cause dryness that leads to skin problems. Baby lotions are helpful in maintaining skin moisture, whereas baby powder acts as a drying agent. Both are useful aids when used selectively and according to the nature of the skin problem (*i.e.,* excessive moisture or dryness). Unnecessary bathing should be avoided, and clothing appropriate to the environment should be worn.

The appearance of diaper rash ranges from simple (*i.e.,* widely distributed macules on the buttocks and anogenital areas) to severe (*i.e.,* beefy, red, excoriated skin surfaces in the diaper area). It results from a combination of ammonia and other breakdown products of urine. The treatment in-

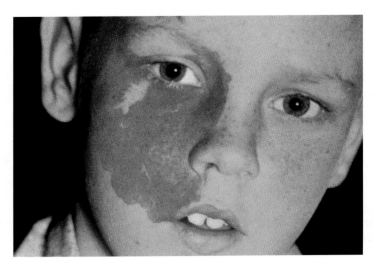

FIGURE 61-30 Port-wine stain on the face of a boy. (Ortho Dermatology Corp.) (Sauer G.C., Hall J.C. [1996]. *Manual of skin diseases* [7th ed.]. Philadelphia: Lippincott-Raven)

cludes measures to minimize or prevent skin wetness. It includes frequent diaper changes with careful cleaning of the irritated area to remove the waste products. This is particularly important in hot weather. Exposing the irritated area to air is helpful.

There is controversy regarding the effects of cloth versus disposable diapers in preventing diaper rash. In the early days of disposable diapers, infants who wore cloth diapers without plastic pants had fewer diaper rashes than those who wore disposable diapers.[68] It has been suggested that this may not be true with the newer disposable diapers that have absorbent gelling material.[65] These superabsorbent diapers have the smallest increase in skin wetness compared with conventional disposable diapers and cloth diapers. When cloth diapers are used, they should be washed in gentle detergent and thoroughly rinsed to remove all traces of waste products. Plastic pants should be discouraged. For intractable, severe cases, the child should be seen by a health care provider for treatment of any secondary infections. Secondary candidal (*i.e.*, yeast) infections are common (Fig. 61-31).

Prickly Heat. Prickly heat (heat rash) results from constant maceration of the skin because of prolonged exposure to a warm, humid environment. Maceration leads to midepidermal obstruction and rupture of the sweat glands. Although commonly seen during infancy, prickly heat may occur at any age. The treatment includes removing excessive clothing, cooling the skin with warm water baths, drying the skin with powders, and avoiding hot, humid environments.

Cradle Cap. Cradle cap is a greasy crust or scale formation on the scalp. It usually is attributed to infrequent and inadequate washing of the scalp. Cradle cap is treated by mild shampooing and gentle combing to remove the scales. Sometimes oil can be left on the head for minutes to several hours, softening the scales before scrubbing. Other emulsifying ointments or creams may be helpful in difficult cases. The scalp may need to be rubbed firmly to remove the buildup of keratinized cells.

Skin Manifestations of Common Infectious Diseases

Infectious childhood diseases that produce rashes include roseola infantum, rubella, rubeola, varicella, and scarlet fever. Although these diseases are seen less frequently because of successful immunization programs and the use of antibiotics, they still occur.

Roseola Infantum. Roseola infantum (*i.e.*, exanthema subitum) is a contagious viral disease of infants and young children, most frequently between 6 and 18 months of age. It is caused by human herpesvirus-6 and produces a characteristic maculopapular rash covering the trunk and spreading to the appendages. The rash is preceded by an abrupt onset of high fever (≤105°F), inflamed tympanic membranes, and coldlike symptoms usually lasting 3 to 4 days. These symptoms improve at approximately the same time the rash appears. Unlike rubella, no cervical or postauricular lymph node adenopathy occurs. Roseola infantum frequently is mistaken for rubella. Rubella usually can be excluded by the age of the child and the absence of lymph node adenopathy. In general, rubella does not develop in children younger than 6 to 9 months of age because they retain some maternal antibodies. Blood antibody titers may be taken to determine the actual diagnosis. In most cases, there are no long-term effects from this disease.

Rubella. Rubella (*i.e.*, 3-day measles or German measles) is a childhood disease caused by the rubella virus (a togavirus). It is characterized by a diffuse, punctate, macular rash that begins on the trunk and spreads to the arms and legs (Fig. 61-32). Mild febrile states occur; usually the fever is less than 100°F. Postauricular, suboccipital, and cervical lymph node adenopathy is common. Coldlike symptoms usually accompany the disease in the form of cough, congestion, and coryza.

Rubella usually has no long-lasting sequelae; however, the transmission of the disease to pregnant women early in their gestation periods may result in congenital rubella

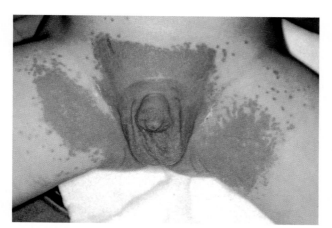

FIGURE 61-31 *Candida* intertrigo after a course of oral antibiotics in a 1-year-old child. (Owen Laboratories, Inc.) (Sauer G.C., Hall J.C. [1996]. *Manual of skin diseases* [7th ed.]. Philadelphia: Lippincott-Raven)

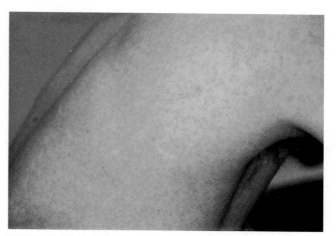

FIGURE 61-32 Rubella (*i.e.*, German or 3-day measles) rash of the trunk. (Fitzpatrick T.B., Johnson R.A., Polono M.K., Suurmond D., Wolff K. [1992]. *Color atlas and synopsis of clinical dermatology* [2nd ed., p. 289]. New York: McGraw-Hill)

syndrome. Among the clinical signs of congenital rubella syndrome are cataracts, microcephaly, mental retardation, deafness, patent ductus arteriosus, glaucoma, purpura, and bone defects. Most states have laws requiring immunization to prevent transmission of rubella. Immunization is accomplished by live-virus injection. A single injection after 12 to 15 months of age has produced a 98% immunity response in immunized children and is considered adequate in the prevention of rubella.[63] Many states require a second preschool or later dose of rubella vaccine to increase immunity. Cases of rubella in nonimmunized children are rare when the level of immunization in the general population remains high.

Rubeola.   Rubeola (measles, hard measles, 7-day measles) is an acute, highly communicable viral disease caused by morbillivirus. The characteristic rash is macular and blotchy; sometimes the macules become confluent (Fig. 61-33). The rubeola rash usually begins on the face and spreads to the appendages. There are several accompanying symptoms: a fever of 100°F or greater, Koplik's spots (i.e., small, irregular red spots with a bluish-white speck in the center) on the buccal mucosa, and mild to severe photosensitivity. The patient commonly has coldlike symptoms, general malaise, and myalgia. In severe cases, the macules may hemorrhage into the skin tissue or onto the outer body surface. This form is called *hemorrhagic measles.* The course of measles is more severe in infants, adults, and malnourished children. There may be severe complications, including otitis media, pneumonia, and encephalitis. Antibody titers are determined for a conclusive diagnosis of rubeola.

Measles is a disease preventable by vaccine, and immunization is required by law in the United States. Immunization is accomplished by the injection of a live-virus vaccine.

A single injection at 12 to 15 months of age is sufficient to produce initial immunity.[63] A second injection should be given on entry to elementary school, although it can be given in middle school. Measles outbreaks occur among nonimmunized and underimmunized children.

Varicella.   Varicella (chickenpox) is a common communicable childhood disease. It is caused by the varicella-zoster virus, which also is the agent in herpes zoster (shingles). The characteristic skin lesion occurs in three stages: macule, vesicle, and granular scab. The macular stage is characterized by development within hours of macules over the trunk of the body, spreading to the limbs, buccal mucosa, scalp, axillae, upper respiratory tract, and conjunctiva (Fig. 61-34). During the second stage, the macules form vesicles with depressed centers. The vesicles break open and a scab forms during the third stage. Crops of lesions occur successively, so that all three forms of the lesion usually are visible by the third day of the illness.

Mild to extreme pruritus accompanies the lesions, which can lead to scratching and subsequent development of secondary bacterial infections. Chickenpox also is accompanied by coldlike symptoms, including cough, coryza (i.e., nasal discharge), and sometimes photosensitivity. Mild febrile states usually occur, typically beginning 24 hours before lesion outbreak. Side effects, such as pneumonia, septic complications, and encephalitis, are rare.

Varicella in adults may be more severe, with a prolonged recovery rate and greater chances for development of varicella pneumonitis or encephalitis. Immunocompromised persons may experience a chronic, painful type.

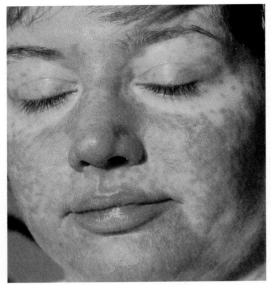

FIGURE 61-33 Rubeola rash on the face of a young woman. (Fitzpatrick T.B., Johnson R.A., Polono M.K., Suurmond D., Wolff K. [1992]. *Color atlas and synopsis of clinical dermatology* [2nd ed., p. 291]. New York: McGraw-Hill)

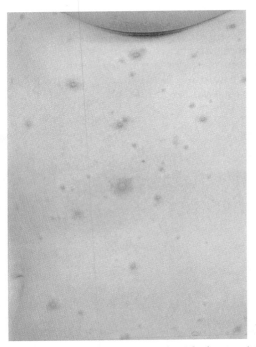

FIGURE 61-34 Varicella (*i.e.,* chickenpox), with characteristic erythematous papules and vesicles. (Fitzpatrick T.B., Johnson R.A., Polono M.K., Suurmond D., Wolff K. [1992]. *Color atlas and synopsis of clinical dermatology* [2nd ed., p. 289]. New York: McGraw-Hill)

Live attenuated varicella vaccine has been demonstrated to be highly effective in the prevention of chickenpox in healthy children (85% to 95%).[63] The vaccine is available in the United States and required by law in several states.

Scarlet Fever. Scarlet fever (scarlatina) is a systemic reaction to the toxins produced by group A β-hemolytic streptococci. The circulating toxin is responsible for the rash and systemic symptoms. Scarlet fever frequently is associated with streptococcal sore throat (strep throat). Scarlet fever was a feared disease in the 19th and early 20th centuries, when it was more virulent and before the advent of penicillin. It is characterized by a pink punctate skin rash on the neck, chest, axillae, groin, and thighs. When palpated, the rash feels like fine sandpaper. The patient has flushing of the face with circumoral pallor. Other symptoms include high fever, nausea, vomiting, strawberry tongue (white-coated tongue through which enlarged and red lingual papillae project), raspberry tongue (bright red), and skin desquamation. Complications of scarlet fever include otitis media, peritonsillar abscess, rheumatic fever, and acute glomerulonephritis.

SKIN MANIFESTATIONS AND DISORDERS IN THE ELDERLY

Elderly persons experience a variety of age-related skin disorders and exacerbations of earlier skin problems. Aging skin is believed to involve a complex process of actinic (solar) damage, normal aging, and hormonal influences.[69] Actinic changes primarily involve increased occurrence of lesions on sun-exposed surfaces of the body.

Normal Age-Related Changes

Normal aging consists of changes that occur on areas of the body that have not been exposed to the sun. They include thinning of the dermis and the epidermis, diminution in subcutaneous tissue, a decrease in and thickening of blood vessels, and a decrease in the number of melanocytes, Langerhans' cells, and Merkel's cells. The keratinocytes shrink, but the number of dead keratinized cells at the surface increases. This results in less padding and thinner skin, with color and elasticity changes. The skin also loses its resistance to environmental and mechanical trauma. Tissue repair takes longer.

With aging, there is also less hair and nail growth, and there is permanent hair pigment loss. Hormonally, there is less sebaceous gland activity, although the glands in the facial skin may increase in size. Hair growth reduction also may be hormonally influenced. Although the reason is poorly understood, the skin in most elderly persons older than 70 years of age becomes dry, rough, scaly, and itchy. When there is no underlying pathology, it is called *senile pruritus*. Itching and dryness become worse during the winter, when the need for home heating lowers the humidity.

The aging of skin, however, is not just a manifestation of age itself. Most skin changes associated with the elderly are the result of cumulative actinic or environmental damage. For example, the wrinkled, leathery look of aged skin, as well as odd scars and ecchymotic spots, are due to solar elastotic degenerative change.[69]

Skin Lesions Common Among the Elderly

The most common skin lesions in the elderly are skin tags, keratoses, lentigines, and vascular lesions. Most are actinic manifestations; they occur as a result of exposure to sun and weather over the years.

Skin Tags. Skin tags are soft, brown or flesh-colored papules. They occur on any skin surface, but most frequently the neck, axilla, and intertriginous areas. They range in size from a pinhead to the size of a pea. Skin tags have the normal texture of the skin. They are benign and can be removed with scissors or electrodesiccation for cosmetic purposes.

Keratoses. A *keratosis* is a horny growth or an abnormal growth of the keratinocytes. A *seborrheic keratosis* (i.e., seborrheic wart) is a benign, sharply circumscribed, wartlike lesion that has a stuck-on appearance (Fig. 61-35). They vary in size up to several centimeters. They are usually round or oval, tan, brown, or black lesions. Less pigmented ones may appear yellow or pink. Keratoses can be found on the face or trunk, as a solitary lesion or sometimes by the hundreds. Seborrheic keratoses are benign, but they must be watched for changes in color, texture, or size, which may indicate malignant transformation to a melanoma.

Actinic keratoses are the most common premalignant skin lesions that develop on sun-exposed areas. The lesions usually are less than 1 cm in diameter and appear as dry, brown scaly areas, often with a reddish tinge. Actinic keratoses often are multiple and more easily felt than seen (Fig. 61-36). They often are indistinguishable from squamous cell carcinoma without biopsy. A hyperkeratotic form also exists that is more prominent and palpable. Often, there is a weathered appearance of the surrounding skin. Slight changes, such as enlargement or ulceration, may indicate malignant transformation. Most actinic keratoses

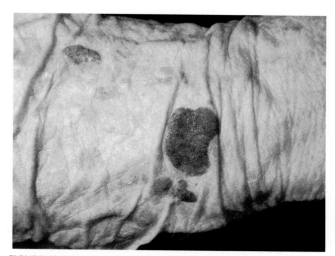

FIGURE 61-35 Large seborrheic keratoses on the hand of an 84-year-old woman. (Sauer G.C., Hall J.C. [1996]. *Manual of skin diseases* [7th ed.]. Philadelphia: Lippincott-Raven)

are treated with 5-fluorouracil cream, which erodes the lesions. Roughly 20% of actinic keratoses convert to squamous cell carcinomas.

Lentigines.   A *lentigo* is a well-bordered brown to black macule, usually less than 1 cm in diameter. *Solar lentigines* are tan to brown, benign spots on sun-exposed areas (Fig. 61-37). They are commonly referred to as liver spots. Creams and lotions containing hydroquinone (*e.g.,* Eldoquin, Solaquin) may be used temporarily to bleach the spots. These agents inhibit the synthesis of new pigment without destroying existing pigment. Higher concentrations are available by prescription. Successful treatment depends on avoiding sun exposure and consistent use of sunscreens. Liquid nitrogen applications have been successful in eradicating senile lentigines.

Lentigo maligna (*i.e.,* Hutchinson's freckle) is a slowly progressive (≤20 years) preneoplastic disorder of melanocytes. It occurs on sun-exposed areas, particularly the face. The lesion is a pigmented macule with a well-defined border and grows to 5 cm or sometimes larger. As it grows over the years, it may become slightly raised and wartlike. If untreated, a true malignant melanoma often develops. Surgery, curettage, and cryotherapy have been effective at removing the lentigines. Careful monitoring for conversion to melanoma is important.

Vascular Lesions.   Vascular lesions are vascular tumors with chronically dilated blood vessels. The small blood vessels lie in the middle to upper dermis. *Senile angiomas* (cherry angiomas) are smooth, cherry-red or purple, dome-shaped papules. They usually are found on the trunk. *Telangiectases* are single dilated blood vessels, capillaries, or terminal arteries that appear on areas exposed to sun or harsh weather, such as the cheeks and the nose. The lesions can become large and disfiguring. Pulsed dye lasers have been effective in removing them. *Venous lakes* are small, dark blue, slightly raised papules that have a lakelike appearance. They occur on exposed body parts, particularly

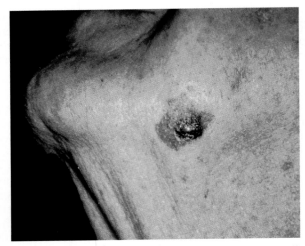

FIGURE 61-37 Malignant melanoma in lentigo, on jaw area. (Syntex Laboratories.) (Sauer G.C., Hall J.C. [1996]. *Manual of skin diseases* [7th ed.]. Philadelphia: Lippincott-Raven)

the backs of the hands, ears, and lips. They are smooth and compressible. Venous lakes can be removed by electrosurgery, laser therapy, or surgical excision if a person desires.

> In summary, some skin problems occur in specific age groups. Common in infants are diaper rash, prickly heat, and cradle cap. Infectious childhood diseases that are characterized by rashes include roseola infantum, rubella, rubeola, varicella, and scarlet fever. Vaccines are available to protect against rubella, rubeola, and varicella. Changes in skin that occur with aging involve a complex process of actinic damage, normal aging, and hormonal influences. With aging, there is thinning of the dermis and the epidermis, diminution in subcutaneous tissue, lessening and thickening of blood vessels, and a slowing of hair and nail growth. Dry skin is common among the elderly, becoming worse during the winter months. Among the skin lesions seen in the elderly are skin tags, keratoses, lentigines, and vascular skin lesions.

Related Web Sites

American Cancer Society Cancer Resource Center   www3. cancer.org/cancerinfo
CancerNet melanoma information (National Cancer Institute site)   cancernet.nci.nih.gov/cancer_types/melanoma. shtml
American Academy of Dermatology (excellent source of information on skin diseases)   www.aad.org
National Skin Centre (Singapore) Information of Common Skin Diseases   www.nsc.gov.sg/commskin/skin.html
Dermanet (information on skin anatomy, diseases, links to other sites with information on skin diseases)   www. dermatology1.org.uk
DermNet (New Zealand Dermatological Society; useful information on skin diseases)   www.dermnet.org.nz

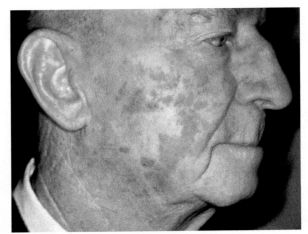

FIGURE 61-36 Multiple actinic keratoses of the face of an 80-year-old man. (Dermik Laboratories, Inc.) (Sauer G.C., Hall J.C. [1996]. *Manual of skin diseases* [7th ed.]. Philadelphia: Lippincott-Raven)

References

1. Greaves M.H. (1998). In Champion R.H., Burton J.L., Burns D.A., Breathnach S.M. (Eds.), *Textbook of dermatology* (6th ed., p. 617–618). Oxford: Blackwell Science.
2. Greco P.J., Ende J. (1992). An office-based approach to the patient with pruritus. *Hospital Practice* 27 (5A), 121–128.
3. American Academy of Dermatology. (1987). Black skin. [On-line]. Available: http://www.aad.org/pamphlets/black.html.
4. Diffey B.L. (1992). Human exposure to ultraviolet violet radiation. In Marks R., Plewig G. (Eds.), *The environmental threat to the skin* (pp. 3–9). London: Martin Dunitz.
5. Armstrong R.B. (1992). Photobiology of ultraviolet radiation. In Abel E.A. (Ed.), *Photochemotherapy in dermatology* (pp. 17–31). New York: Igaku-Shoin.
6. Jeevan A., Kripke M.L. (1995). Ozone depletion and the immune system. *Lancet* 342, 1159–1160.
7. Gilchrest B.A., Eller M.S., Geller A.C., Yaar M. (1999). The pathogenesis of melanoma induced by ultraviolet radiation. *New England Journal of Medicine* 340, 1341–1348.
8. Hall J.C. (1999). *Sauer's manual of skin diseases* (8th ed., p. 295). Philadelphia: Lippincott Williams & Wilkins.
9. Drug Facts and Comparisons Staff. (2000). *Drug facts and comparisons 2000* (54th ed., p. 1714). St. Louis: Facts and Comparisons.
10. Epstein J., Kaplan L., Levine N. (2000). The value of sunscreens. *Patient Care* 34 (11), 103–107.
11. American Academy of Dermatology. (1994). Vitiligo. [On-line]. Available: http://www.aad.org/pamphlets/vitiligo.html.
12. Brooks G.F., Butel J.S., Ornston L.N. (1995). *Medical microbiology* (20th ed., pp. 531–536). Norwalk, CT: Appleton & Lange.
13. Noble S.L., Forbes R.C. (1998). Diagnosis and management of common tinea infections. *American Family Physician* 58, 177.
14. Evans E.G.V., Dodman B., Williamson D.M., Brown G.J., Bowen R.G. (1993). Comparison of terbinafine and clotrimazole in treating tinea pedis. *British Medical Journal* 307, 645–647.
15. Nesbitt L.T. (2000). Treatment of tinea capitis. *International Journal of Dermatology* 39, 261–262.
16. Epstein E. (1998). How often does oral treatment of toenail onychomycosis produce a disease-free nail? An analysis of published data. *Archives of Dermatology* 134, 1551–1554.
17. Gupta A.K. (1999). The new oral antifungal agents for onychomycosis of the toenails. *Journal of the European Academy of Dermatology and Venereology* 13, 1–13.
18. Cotran R.S., Kumar V., Collins T. (1999). *Robbins pathologic basis of disease* (6th ed., pp. 1174–1177, 1198, 1199, 1208, 1209). Philadelphia: W.B. Saunders.
19. Stanberry L.R., Cunningham A.L., Mindel A., Scott L.L., Spruance S.L., Aoki F.Y., Lacey C.J. (2000). Prospects for control of herpes simplex virus disease through immunization. *Clinical Infectious Diseases* 30, 549–566.
20. Gilden D.H., Kleinschmidt-DeMasters B.K., LaGuardia J.J., Cohrs R.J. (2000). Neurologic complications of reactivation of varicella-zoster virus. *New England Journal of Medicine* 342, 635–645.
21. Stankus S.J., Dlugopolski M., Packer D. (2000). Management of herpes zoster (shingles) and postherpetic neuralgia. *American Family Physician* 61, 2437–2444, 2447–2448.
22. Tyring S.K. (1996). Early treatment of herpes zoster. *Hospital Practice* 31, 137–144.

23. Landow K. (2000). Acute and chronic herpes zoster. An ancient scourge yields to timely therapy. *Postgraduate Medicine* 107 (7), 107–118.
24. Levin M.J., Barber D., Goldblatt E., Jones M., LaFleur B., Chan C., Stinson D., Zerbe G.O., Hayward A.R. (1998). Use of a live attenuated varicella vaccine to boost varicella-specific immune responses in seropositive people 55 years of age and older: Duration of booster effect. *Journal of Infectious Diseases* 178, 109–112.
25. Plewig G., Klingman A.M. (1993). *Acne and rosacea* (2nd ed., pp. 3, 341). New York: Springer-Verlag.
26. Usantine R.P., Quan M.A., Strick R. (1998). Acne vulgaris: A treatment update. *Hospital Practice* 33 (2), 111–127.
27. Krowchuk D.P. (2000). Managing acne in adolescents. *Pediatric Clinics of North America* 47, 841–857.
28. Leyden J.J. (1997). Therapy for acne vulgaris. *New England Journal of Medicine* 336, 1156–1163.
29. Russell J.J. (2000). Topical therapy for acne. *American Family Physician* 61, 357–366.
30. Weiss J.S. (1997). Current options for the topical treatment of acne vulgaris. *Pediatric Dermatology* 14, 480–488.
31. Bamford J.T., Tilden R.L., Blankush J.L., Gangeness D.E. (1999). Effect of treatment of *Helicobacter pylori* infection on rosacea. *Archives of Dermatology* 135, 659–663.
32. Correale C.E., Walker C., Craig T.J. (1999). Atopic dermatitis: A review of diagnosis and treatment. *American Family Physician* 60, 1191–1210.
33. Kristal L., Klein P.A. (2000). Atopic dermatitis in infants and children. *Pediatric Clinics of North America* 47, 877–894.
34. Scott C.B., Moloney M.F. (1996). Physical urticaria. *Nurse Practitioner* 21 (11), 42–59.
35. Greaves M.W. (1995). Chronic urticaria. *New England Journal of Medicine* 332, 1767–1772.
36. Monroe E.W. (1997). Loratadine in the treatment of urticaria. *Clinical Therapeutics* 19, 3232–3242.
37. Chen C.J. (1998). Acupuncture treatment of urticaria. *Archives of Dermatology* 134, 1397–1398.
38. Bastuji-Garin S., Rzany B., Stern R.S., Shear N.H., Naldi L., Roujeau J.C. (1993). Clinical classification of cases of toxic epidermal necrolysis, Stevens-Johnson syndrome, and erythema multiforme. *Archives of Dermatology* 129, 92–96.
39. Roujeau J.C., Stern R.S. (1994). Severe adverse cutaneous reactions to drugs. *New England Journal of Medicine* 331, 1272–1284.
40. Koo J.Y. (1999). Current consensus and update on psoriasis therapy: A perspective from the U.S. *Journal of Dermatology* 26, 723–733.
41. Camisa C. (1994). *Psoriasis* (pp. 3, 30, 31, 55). Boston: Blackwell.
42. Phillips T.J. (1996). Current treatment options in psoriasis. *Hospital Practice* 31, 155–166.
43. Pardasani A.G., Feldman S.R., Clark A.R. (2000). Treatment of psoriasis: An algorithm based approach for primary care physicians. *American Family Physician* 61, 725–733, 736.
44. Camisa C. (1998). *Handbook of psoriasis* (p. 51). Malden, MA: Blackwell Science.
45. Federman D.G., Froelich C.W., Kirsner R.S. (1999). Topical psoriasis therapy. *American Family Physician* 59 (4), 957–964.
46. D'Epiro N. (1999). Psoriasis: New clues to causation, new ways to treat. *Patient Care for the Nurse Practitioner* 24, 42–50.
47. Katta R. (2000). Lichen planus. *American Family Physician* 61, 3319–3324, 3327–3328.
48. Stephens M.B. (2000). Controlling head lice. *Primary Care for Nurse Practitioners* (Sept. 15), 99–107.
49. Pollack R.J., Kiszewski A., Armstrong P., Hahn C., Wolfe N., Rahman H.A., Laserson K., Telford S.R., Spielman A. (1999).

Differential permethrin susceptibility of head lice sampled in the United States and Borneo. *Archives of Pediatrics and Adolescent Medicine* 153, 969–973.

50. Habif T.P. (1996). *Clinical dermatology* (3rd ed., p. 474). St. Louis: Mosby.

51. American Cancer Society. (2000) Skin Cancer Statistics. [Online]. Available: http://www.cancer.org.

52. Rigel D.S., Carucci J.A. (2000). Malignant melanoma: Prevention, early detection, and treatment in the 21st century. *CA: A Cancer Journal for Clinicians* 50, 215–236.

53. Halder R.M., Bridgeman-Shah S. (1995). Skin cancer in African Americans. *Cancer* 75, 667–673.

54. Jerant A.F., Johnson J.T., Sheridan C.M., Caffrey T.J. (2000). Early detection and treatment of cancer. *American Family Physician* 62, 357–368, 375–376, 381–382.

55. Rubin E., Farber J.L. (Eds.). (1999). *Pathology* (3rd ed., pp. 1288–1294). Philadelphia: Lippincott Williams & Wilkins.

56. Preston D.S., Stern R.S. (1992). Nonmelanoma cancers of the skin. *New England Journal of Medicine* 327, 1649–1662.

57. Johnson B.L., Moy R.L., White G.M. (1998). *Ethnic skin: Medical and surgical nursing* (p. 9). St. Louis: Mosby.

58. Frankel D.H. (1992). Squamous cell carcinoma of the skin. *Hospital Practice* 27, 99–106.

59. Nguyen T.T., Gilpin D.A., Meyer N.A., Herndon D.N. (1996). Current treatment of severely burned patients. *Annals of Surgery* 223, 14–25.

60. Brigham P.A., McLoughlin E. (1996). Burn incidence and medical care use in the United States: Estimates, trends, and data sources. *Journal of Burn Care Rehabilitation* 17, 95–107.

61. Wilson Y., Goberdhan N., Dawson R.A., Smith J., Freelander E., MacNeil S. (1994). Investigation of the presence and role of calmodulin and other mitogens in human burn blister fluid. *Journal of Burn Care and Rehabilitation* 61, 303–314.

62. Hudak C.M., Gallo B.M. (1997). *Critical care nursing* (7th ed., pp. 978–1011). Philadelphia: Lippincott-Raven.

63. Behrman R.E., Kliegman R.M, Jensen H.B. (2000). *Nelson textbook of pediatrics* (16th ed., pp. 291, 870–872, 892–894). Philadelphia: W.B Saunders.

64. Caldwell F.T., Wallace B.H., Cone J.B. (1996). Sequential excision and grafting of the burn injuries of 6107 patients treated between 1967 and 1986: End results and the determinants of death. *Journal of Burn Care and Rehabilitation* 17, 137–146.

65. Parenteau N. (1999). Skin: The first tissue-engineered products. *Scientific American* 280 (4), 83–84.

66. Dohil M.A., Baugh W.P., Eichenfield L.F. (2000). Vascular and pigmented birthmarks. *Pediatric Clinics of North America* 47, 783–810.

67. Drolet B.A., Esterly N.B., Frieden I.J. (1999). Hemangiomas in children. *New England Journal of Medicine* 341, 173–181.

68. Kazaks E.L., Lane A.T. (2000). Diaper dermatitis. *Pediatric Clinics of North America* 47, 909–918.

69. Bolognia J.L. (1995). Aging skin. *American Journal of Medicine* 98, 99S–103S.

Lab Values

Prefixes Denoting Decimal Factors

Prefix	Symbol	Factor
mega	M	10^6
kilo	k	10^3
hecto	h	10^2
deci	d	10^{-1}
centi	c	10^{-2}
milli	m	10^{-3}
micro	μ	10^{-6}
nano	n	10^{-9}
pico	p	10^{-12}
femto	f	10^{-15}

Hematology

Test	Conventional Units	SI Units
Erythrocyte count (RBC count)	M. $4.2–5.4 \times 10^6/\mu L$	M. $4.2–5.4 \times 10^{12}/L$
	F. $3.6–5.0 \times 10^6/\mu L$	F. $3.6–5.0 \times 10^{12}/L$
Hematocrit (Hct)	M. 40–50%	M. 0.40–0.50
	F. 37–47%	F. 0.37–0.47
Hemoglobin (Hb)	M. 14.0–16.5 g/dL	M. 140–165 g/L
	F. 12.0–15.0 g/dL	F. 120–150 g/L
Mean corpuscular hemoglobin (MHC)	27–34 pg/cell	0.40–0.53 fmol/cell
Mean corpuscular hemoglobin concentration (MCHC)	31–35 g/dL	310–350 g/L
Mean corpuscular volume (MCV)	80–100 fL	
Reticulocyte count	1.0–1.5% total RBC	
Leukocyte count (WBC count)	$4.4–11.3 \times 10^3/\mu L$	$4.4–11.3 \times 10^9/L$
Basophils	0–2%	
Eosinophils	0–3%	
Lymphocytes	24–40%	
Monocytes	4–9%	
Neutrophils (segmented [Segs])	47–63%	
Neutrophils (bands)	0–4%	

Blood Chemistry*

Test	Conventional Units	SI Units
Alanine aminotransferase (ALT, SGPT)	0–35 U/L	0–0.58 µkat/L
Alkaline phosphatase	41–133 U/L	0.7–2.2 µkat/L
Ammonia	18–16 µg/dL	11–35 µmol/L
Amylase	20–110 U/L[†]	0.33–1.83 µkat/L[†]
Aspartase amino transferase (AST, SGOT)	0–35 U/L[†]	0–0.58 µkat/L[†]
Bicarbonate	24–31 mEq/L	24–31 mmol/L
Bilirubin (total)	0.1–1.2 mg/dL	2–21 µmol/L
Direct	0.1–0.4 mg/dL	<7 µmol/L
Indirect	0.1–0.7 mg/dL	<12 µmol/L
Blood urea nitrogen (BUN)	8–20 mg/dL	2.9–7.1 mmol/L
Calcium	8.5–10.5 mg/dL	2.1–2.6 mmol/L
Carbon dioxide	24–29 mEq/L	24–29 mmol/L
Chloride	98–106 mEq/L	98–106 mmol/L
Creatine kinase (CK, CPK)	32–267 U/L[†]	0.53–4.45 µkat/L[†]
Creatine kinase (MB)	<16 IU/L[†] or 4% of total CK	<0.27 µkat/L[†]
Creatinine (serum)	0.6–1.2 mg/dL[‡]	50–100 µmol/L[‡]
Gamma-glutamyl-transpeptidase (GGT)	9–85 U/L[†]	0.15–1.42 µkat/L[†]
Glucose (blood)	60–115 mg/dL	3.3–6.3 mmol/L
Glycosylated hemoglobin (HbA$_{1c}$)	3.9–6.9%	
Lactate dehydrogenase (LDH)	88–230 U/L[†]	1.46–3.82 µkat/L[†]
Lipids		
Cholesterol	<200 mg/dL (desirable)	<5.2 mmol/L
Triglycerides	<165 mg/dL	<1.65 g/L
Lipase	0–160 U/L[†]	0.266 µkat/L[†]
Magnesium	1.84–3.0 mg/dL	0.99–1.23 mmol/L
Osmolality	275–295 mOsm/kg H$_2$O	275–295 mmol/kg H$_2$O
Phosphorus (inorganic)	2.5–4.5 mg/dL	0.77–1.45 mmol/L
Potassium	3.5–5.0 mEq/L	3.5–5.0 mmol/L
Prostate specific antigen (PSA)	0–4 ng/mL	0–4 µg/L
Protein total	6.0–8.6 g/dL	60–86 g/L
Albumin	3.8–5.6 g/dL	38–56 g/L
Globulin	2.3–3.5 g/dL	23–35 g/L
A/G ratio	1.0–2.2	1.0–2.2
Thyroid Tests		
Thyroxine (T$_4$) total	5.0–11.0 µg/dL	64–142 nmol/L
Thyroxine, free (FT$_4$)	9–24 pmol/L[†]	
Triiodothyronine (T$_3$) total	95–190 ng/dL	1.5–2.9 nmol/L
Thyroid stimulating hormone (TSH)	0.4–6.0 µU/mL	0.4–6.0 mU/L
Thyroglobin	3–42 ng/mL	3–42 µg/L
Sodium	135–145 mEq/L	135–145 mmol/L
Uric acid	M. 2.4–7.4 mg/dL	M. 140–440 µmol/L
	F. 1.4–5.8 mg/dL	F. 80–350 µmol/L

U, units.
* Values may vary with laboratory. The values supplied by the laboratory performing the test should always be used since the ranges may be method specific.
† Laboratory and/or method specific
‡ Varies with age and muscle mass
(Values obtained from Tierney LM., McPhee S.J., Papadakis M.A. [1997]. *Current medical diagnosis and treatment* [36th ed.]. Stamford, CT: Appleton & Lange, pp. 1495–1501; Fischbach F. [1995]. *Quick reference to common diagnostic and laboratory tests*. Philadelphia: Lippincott-Raven, and other sources.)

Glossary

Abduction The act of abducting (moving or spreading away from a position near the midline of the body or the axial line of a limb) or the state of being abducted.

Abrasion The wearing or scraping away of a substance or structure, such as the skin, through an unusual or abnormal mechanical process.

Abscess A collection of pus that is restricted to a specific area in tissues, organs, or confined spaces.

Accommodation The adjustment of the lens (eye) to variations in distance.

Acromion The lateral extension of the spine of the scapula, forming the highest point of the shoulder. (Noun: acromial)

Acuity The clearness or sharpness of perception, especially of vision.

Adaptation The adjustment of an organism to its environment, physical or psychological, through changes and responses to stress of any kind.

Adduction The act of adducting (moving or drawing toward a position near the midline of the body or the axial line of a limb) or the state of being adducted.

Adhesin The molecular components of the bacterial cell wall that are involved in adhesion processes.

Adrenergic Activated by or characteristic of the sympathetic nervous system or its neurotransmitters (i.e., epinephrine and norepinephrine).

Aerobic Growing, living, or occurring only in the presence of air or oxygen.

Afferent Bearing or conducting inward or toward a center, as an afferent neuron.

Agglutination The clumping together of particles, microorganisms, or blood cells in response to an antigen-antibody reaction.

Agonist A muscle whose action is opposed by another muscle (antagonist) with which it is paired; or a drug or other chemical substance that has affinity for or stimulates a predictable physiologic function.

Akinesia An abnormal state in which there is an absence or poverty of movement.

Allele One of two or more different forms of a gene that can occupy a particular locus on a chromosome.

Alveolus A small saclike structure, as in the alveolus of the lung.

Amine An organic compound containing nitrogen.

Amblyopia A condition of vision impairment without a detectable organic lesion of the eye.

Amorphous Without a definite form; shapeless.

Ampulla A saclike dilatation of a duct, canal, or any other tubular structure.

Anabolism A constructive metabolic process characterized by the conversion of simple substances into larger, complex molecules.

Anaerobic Growing, living, or occurring only in the absence of air or oxygen.

Analog A part, organ, or chemical having the same function or appearance but differing in respect to a certain component, such as origin or development.

Anaplasia A change in the structure of cells and in their orientation to each other that is characterized by a loss of cell differentiation, as in cancerous cell growth.

Anastomosis The connection or joining between two vessels; or an opening created by surgical, traumatic, or pathologic means.

Androgen Any substance, such as a male sex hormone, that increases male characteristics.

Anergy A state of absent or diminished reaction to an antigen or group of antigens.

Aneuploidy A variation in the number of chromosomes within a cell involving one or more missing chromosomes rather than entire sets.

Aneurysm An outpouching or dilation in the wall of a blood vessel or the heart.

Ankylosis Stiffness or fixation of separate bones of a joint, resulting from disease, injury, or surgical procedure. (Verb: ankylose)

Anorexia Lack or loss of appetite for food. (Adjective: anorexic)

Anoxia An abnormal condition characterized by the total lack of oxygen.

Antagonist A muscle whose action directly opposes that of another muscle (agonist) with which it is paired; or a drug or other chemical substance that can diminish or nullify the action of a neuromediator or body function.

Anterior Pertaining to a surface or part that is situated near or toward the front.

Antigen A substance that generates an immune response by causing the formation of an antibody or reacting with antibodies or T cell receptors.

Apex The uppermost point, the narrowed or pointed end, or the highest point of a structure, such as an organ.

Aphagia A condition characterized by the refusal or the loss of ability to swallow.

Aplasia The absence of an organ or tissue due to a developmental failure.

Apnea The absence of spontaneous respiration.

Apoptosis A mechanism of programmed cell death, marked by shrinkage of the cell, condensation of chromatin, formation of cytoplasmic blebs, and fragmentation of the cell into membrane-bound bodies eliminated by phagocytosis.

Apraxia Loss of the ability to carry out familiar, purposeful acts or to manipulate objects in the absence of paralysis or other motor or sensory impairment.

Articulation The place of connection or junction between two or more bones of a skeletal joint.

Ascites An abnormal accumulation of serous fluid in the peritoneal cavity.

Asepsis The condition of being free or freed from pathogenic microorganisms.

Astereognosis A neurologic disorder characterized by an inability to identify objects by touch.

Asterixis A motor disturbance characterized by a hand-flapping tremor, which results when the prolonged contraction of groups of muscles lapses intermittently.

Ataxia An abnormal condition characterized by an inability to coordinate voluntary muscular movement.

Athetosis A neuromuscular condition characterized by the continuous occurrence of slow, sinuous, writhing movements that are performed involuntarily. (Adjective: athetoid)

Atopy Genetic predisposition toward the development of a hypersensitivity or an allergic reaction to common environmental allergens.

Atresia The absence or closure of a normal body orifice or tubular organ, such as the esophagus.

Atrophy A wasting or diminution of size, often accompanied by a decrease in function, of a cell, tissue, or organ.

Autocrine A mode of hormone action in which a chemical messenger acts on the same cell that secretes it.

Autosome Any chromosome other than a sex chromosome.

Axillary Of or pertaining to the axilla, or armpit.

Bacteremia The presence of bacteria in the blood.

Bactericide An agent that destroys bacteria. (Adjective: bactericidal)

Bacteriostat An agent that inhibits bacterial growth. (Adjective: bacteriostatic)

Ballismus An abnormal condition charcterized by violent flailing motions of the arms and, occasionally, the head, resulting from injury to or destruction of the subthalamic nucleus or its fiber connections.

Baroreceptor A type of sensory nerve ending such as those found in the aorta and the carotid sinus that is stimulated by changes in pressure.

Basal Pertaining to, situated at, or forming the base; or the fundamental or the basic.

Benign Not malignant; or of the character that does not threaten health or life.

Bipolar neuron A nerve cell that has a process at each end—an afferent process and an efferent process.

Bolus A rounded mass of food ready to swallow or such a mass passing through the gastrointestinal tract; or a concentrated mass of medicinal material or other pharmaceutic preparation injected all at once intravenously for diagnostic purposes.

Borborygmus The rumbling, gurgling, or tinkling noise produced by the propulsion of gas through the intestine.

Bruit A sound or murmur heard while auscultating an organ or blood vessel, especially an abnormal one.

Buccal Pertaining to or directed toward the inside of the cheek.

Buffer A substance or group of substances that prevents change in the concentration of another chemical substance.

Bulla A thin-walled blister of the skin or mucous membranes greater than 5 mm in diameter containing serous or seropurulent fluid.

Bursa A fluid-filled sac or saclike cavity situated in places in the tissues at which friction would otherwise develop, such as between certain tendons and the bones beneath them.

Cachexia A condtion of general ill health and malnutrition, marked by weakness and emaciation.

Calculus A stony mass formed within body tissues, usually composed of mineral salts.

Capsid The protein shell that envelops and protects the nucleic acid of a virus.

Carcinogen Any substance or agent that causes the development or increases the incidence of cancer.

Carpal Of or pertaining to the carpus, or wrist.

Caseation A form of tissue necrosis in which the tissue is changed into a dry, amorphous mass resembling crumbly cheese.

Catabolism A metabolic process through which living organisms break down complex substances to simple compounds, liberating energy for use in work, energy storage, or heat production.

Catalyst A substance that increases the velocity of a chemical reaction without being consumed by the process.

Catecholamines Any one of a group of biogenic amines having a sympathomimetic action and composed of a catechol molecule and the aliphatic portion of an amine.

Caudal Signifying an inferior position, toward the distal end of the spine.

Cellulitis An acute, diffuse, spreading, edematous inflammation of the deep subcutaneous tissues and sometimes muscle, characterized most commonly by an area of heat, redness, pain, and swelling, and occasionally by fever, malaise, chills, and headache.

Cephalic Of or pertaining to the head, or to the head end of the body.

Cerumen The waxlike secretion produced by vestigial apocrine sweat glands in the external ear canal.

Cheilosis A noninflammatory disorder of the lips and mouth characterized by chapping and fissuring.

Chelate A chemical compound composed of a central metal ion and an organic molecule with multiple bonds, arranged in ring formation, used especially in treatment of metal poisoning.

Chemoreceptor A sensory nerve cell activated by chemical stimuli, as a chemoreceptor in the carotid that is sensitive to changes in the oxygen content in the bloodstream and reflexly increases or decreases respiration and blood pressure.

Chemotaxis A response involving cell orientation or cell movement that is either toward (positive chemotaxis) or away from (negative chemotaxis) a chemical stimulus.

Chondrocyte Any one of the mature polymorphic cells that form the cartilage of the body.

Chromatid One of the paired threadlike chromosome filaments, joined at the centromere, that make up a metaphase chromosome.

Chromosome Any one of the structures in the nucleus of a cell containing a linear thread of DNA, which functions in the transmission of genetic information.

Chyme The creamy, viscous, semifluid material produced during digestion of a meal that is expelled by the stomach into the duodenum.

Cilia The eyelid or its outer edge; or the small hairs growing on the edges of the eyelids. (Singular: cilium)

Circadian Being, having, pertaining to, or occurring in a period or cycle of approximately 24 hours.

Circumduction The active or passive circular movement of a limb or of the eye.

Cisterna An enclosed space, such as a cavity, that serves as a reservoir for lymph or other body fluids.

Clone One or a group of genetically identical cells or organisms derived from a single parent.

Coagulation The process of transforming a liquid into a semisolid mass, especially of blood clot formation.

Coarctation A condition of stricture or contraction of the walls of a vessel.

Cofactor A substance that must unite with another substance in order to function.

Colic Sharp, intermittent abdominal pain localized in a hollow or tubular organ, resulting from torsion, obstruction, or smooth muscle spasm. (Adjective: colicky)

Collagen The protein substance of the white, glistening, inelastic fibers of the skin, tendons, bone, cartilage, and all other connective tissue.

Collateral Secondary or accessory rather than direct or immediate; or a small branch, as of a blood vessel or nerve.

Complement Any one of the complex, enzymatic serum proteins that are involved in physiologic reactions, including antigen-antibody reaction and anaphylaxis.

Confluent Flowing or coming together; not discrete.

Congenital Present at, and usually before, birth.

Conjugate To pair and fuse in conjugation; or a form of sexual reproduction seen in unicellular organisms in which genetic material is exchanged during the temporary fusion of two cells.

Contiguous In contact or nearly so in an unbroken sequence along a boundary or at a point.

Contralateral Affecting, pertaining to, or originating in the opposite side of a point or reference.

Contusion An injury of a part without a break in the skin, characterized by swelling, discoloration, and pain.

Convolution An elevation or tortuous winding, such as one of the irregular ridges on the surface of the brain, formed by a structure being infolded upon itself.

Corpuscle Any small mass, cell, or body, such as a red or white blood cell.

Costal Pertaining to a rib or ribs.

Crepitus A sound or sensation that resembles a crackling or grating noise.

Cutaneous Pertaining to the skin.

Cyanosis A bluish discoloration, especially of the skin and mucous membranes, caused by an excess of deoxygenated hemoglobin in the blood.

Cytokine Any of a class of polypeptide immunoregulatory substances that are secreted by cells, usually of the immune system, that affect other cells.

Cytology The study of cells, including their origin, structure, function, and pathology.

Decibel A unit for expressing the relative power intensity of electric or acoustic signal power that is equal to one tenth of a bel.

Decomposition The separation of a compound substance into simpler chemical forms by whatever process.

Defecation The evacuation of feces from the digestive tract through the rectum.

Deformation The process of adapting in form or shape; also the product of such alteration.

Degeneration The deterioration of a normal cell, tissue, or organ to a less functionally active form. (Adjective: degenerative)

Deglutition The act or process of swallowing.

Degradation The reduction of a chemical compound to a compound less complex, usually by splitting off one or more groups.

Dehydration The condition that results from excessive loss of water from the body tissues.

Delirium An acute, reversible organic mental syndrome characterized by confusion, disorientation, restlessness, incoherence, fear, and often illusions.

Dendrite One of the branching processes that extends and transmits impulses toward a cell body of a neuron. (Adjective: dendritic)

Depolarization The reduction of a cell membrane potential to a less negative value than that of the potential outside the cell.

Dermatome The area of the skin supplied with afferent nerve fibers of a single dorsal root of a spinal nerve.

Desmosome A small, circular, dense area within the intercellular bridge that forms the site of adhesion between intermediate filaments and cell membranes.

Desquamation A normal process in which the cornified layer of the epidermis is shed in fine scales or sheets.

Dialysis The process of separating colloids and crystalline substances in solution, which involves the two distinct physical processes of diffusion and ultrafiltration; or a medical procedure for the removal of urea and other elements from the blood or lymph.

Diapedesis The outward passage of red or white blood corpuscles through the intact walls of the vessels.

Diaphoresis Perspiration, especially the profuse perspiration associated with an elevated body temperature, physical exertion, exposure to heat, and mental or emotional stress.

Diarthrosis A specialized articulation that permits, to some extent, free joint movement. (Adjective: diarthrodial)

Diastole The dilatation of the heart; or the period of dilatation, which is the interval between the second and the first heart sound and is the time during which blood enters the relaxed chambers of the heart from the systemic circulation and the lungs.

Differentiation The act or process in development in which unspecialized cells or tissues acquire more specialized characteristics, including those of physical form, physiologic function, and chemical properties.

Diffusion The process of becoming widely spread, as in the spontaneous movement of molecules or other particles in solution from an area of higher concentration to an area of lower concentration, resulting in an even distribution of the particles in the fluid.

Diopter A unit of measurement of the refractive power of lenses equal to the reciprocal of the focal length in meters.

Diploid Pertaining to an individual, organism, strain, or cell that has two full sets of homologous chromosomes.

Disseminate To scatter or distribute over a considerable area.

Distal Away from or being the farthest from a point of reference.

Diurnal Of, relating to, or occurring in the daytime.

Diverticulum A pouch or sac of variable size occurring naturally or through herniation of the muscular wall of a tubular organ.

Dorsum The back or posterior. (Adjective: dorsal)

Dysgenesis Defective or abnormal development of an organ or part, typically occurring during embryonic development. (Also called dysgenesia.)

Dyslexia A disturbance in the ability to read, spell, and write words.

Dyspepsia The impairment of the power or function of digestion, especially epigastric discomfort following eating.

Dysphagia A difficulty in swallowing.

Dysphonia Any impairment of the voice that is experienced as a difficulty in speaking.

Dysplasia The alteration in size, shape, and organization of adult cell types.

Ecchymosis A small hemorrhagic spot, larger than a petechia, in the skin or mucous membrane caused by the extravasation of blood into the subcutaneous tissues.

Ectoderm The outermost of the three primary germ layers of the embryo, and from which the epidermis and epidermal tissues, such as nails, hair, and glands of the skin, develop.

Ectopic Relating to or characterized by an object or organ being situated in an unusual place, away from its normal location.

Edema The presence of an abnormal accumulation of fluid in interstitial spaces of tissues. (Adjective: edematous)

Efferent Conveyed or directed away from a center.

Effusion The escape of fluid from blood vessels into a part or tissue, as an exudation or a transudation.

Embolus A mass of clotted blood or other formed elements, such as bubbles of air, calcium fragments, or a bit of tissue or tumor, that circulates in the bloodstream until it becomes lodged in a vessel, obstructing the circulation. (Plural: emboli)

Empyema An accumulation of pus in a cavity of the body, especially the pleural space.

Emulsify To disperse one liquid throughout the body of another liquid, making a colloidal suspension, or emulsion.

Endocytosis The uptake or incorporation of substances into a cell by invagination of its plasma membrane, as in the processes of phagocytosis and pinocytosis.

Endoderm The innermost of the three primary germ layers of the embryo, and from which epithelium arises.

Endogenous Growing within the body; or developing or originating from within the body or produced from internal causes.

Endoscopy The visualization of any cavity of the body with an endoscope.

Enteropathic Relating to any disease of the intestinal tract.

Enzyme A protein molecule produced by living cells that catalyzes chemical reactions of other organic substances without itself being destroyed or altered.

Epiphysis The expanded articular end of a long bone (head) that is separated from the shaft of the bone by the epiphyseal plate until the bone stops growing, the plate is obliterated, and the shaft and the head become united.

Epithelium The covering of the internal and the external surfaces of the body, including the lining of vessels and other small cavities.

Erectile Capable of being erected or raised to an erect position.

Erythema The redness or inflammation of the skin or mucous membranes produced by the congestion of superficial capillaries. (Adjective: erythematous)

Etiology The study or theory of all factors that may be involved in the development of a disease, including susceptibility of an individual, the nature of the disease agent, and the way in which an individual's body is invaded by the agent; or the cause of a disease.

Euploid Pertaining to an individual, organism, strain, or cell with a balanced set or sets of chromosomes, in any number, that is an exact multiple of the normal, basic haploid number characteristic of the species; or such an individual, organism, strain, or cell.

Evisceration The removal of the viscera from the abdominal cavity, or disembowelment; or the extrusion of an internal organ through a wound or surgical incision.

Exacerbation An increase in the severity of a disease as marked by greater intensity in any of its signs and symptoms.

Exfoliation Peeling and sloughing off of tissue cells in scales or layers. (Adjective: exfoliative)

Exocytosis The discharge of cell particles, which are packaged in membrane-bound vesicles, by fusion of the vesicular membrane with the plasma membrane and subsequent release of the particles to the exterior of the cell.

Exogenous Developed or originating outside the body, as a disease caused by a bacterial or viral agent foreign to the body.

Exophthalmos A marked or abnormal protusion of the eyeball.

Extension A movement that allows the two elements of any jointed part to be drawn apart, increasing the angle between them, as extending the leg increases the angle between the femur and the tibia.

Extrapyramidal Pertaining to motor systems supplied by fibers outside the corticospinal or pyramidal tracts.

Extravasation A discharge or escape, usually of blood, serum, or lymph, from a vessel into the tissues.

Extubation The process of withdrawing a previously inserted tube from an orifice or cavity of the body.

Exudate Fluid, cells, or other substances that have been slowly exuded or have escaped from blood vessels and have been deposited in tissues or on tissue surfaces.

Fascia A sheet or band of fibrous connective tissue that may be separated from other specifically organized structures, as the tendons, the aponeuroses, and the ligaments.

Febrile Pertaining to or characterized by an elevated body temperature, or fever.

Fibrillation A small, local, involuntary contraction of muscle, resulting from spontaneous activation of a single muscle fiber or of an isolated bundle of nerve fibers.

Fibrin A stringy, insoluble protein formed by the action of thrombin on fibrinogen during the clotting process.

Fibrosis The formation of fibrous connective tissue, as in the repair or replacement of parenchymatous elements.

Filtration The process of passing a liquid through or as if through a filter, which is accomplished by gravity, pressure, or vacuum.

Fimbria Any structure that forms a fringe, border, or edge or the processes that resemble such a structure.

Fissure A cleft or a groove, normal or otherwise, on the surface of an organ or a bony structure.

Fistula An abnormal passage or communication from an internal organ to the body surface or between two internal organs.

Flaccid Weak, soft, and lax; lacking normal muscle tone.

Flatus Air or gas in the intestinal tract that is expelled through the anus. (Adjective: flatulent)

Flexion A movement that allows the two elements of any jointed part to be brought together, decreasing the angle between them, as bending the elbow.

Flora The microorganisms, such as bacteria and fungi, both normally occurring and pathological, found in or on an organ.

Focal Relating to, having, or occupying a focus.

Follicle A sac or pouchlike depression or cavity.

Fontanel A membrane-covered opening in bones or between bones, such as the soft spot covered by tough membranes between the bones of an infant's incompletely ossified skull.

Foramen A natural opening or aperture in a membranous structure or bone.

Fossa A hollow or depressed area, especially on the surface of the end of a bone.

Fovea A small pit or depression in the surface of a structure or an organ.

Fundus The base or bottom of an organ or the portion farthest from the mouth of an organ.

Ganglion One of the nerve cell bodies, chiefly collected in groups outside the central nervous system. (Plural: ganglia)

Genotype The entire genetic constitution of an individual, as determined by the particular combination and location of the genes on the chromosomes; or the alleles present at one or more sites on homologous chromosomes.

Glia The neuroglia, or supporting structure of nervous tissue.

Globulin One of a broad group of proteins classified by solubility, electrophoretic mobility, and size.

Gluconeogenesis The formation of glucose from any of the substances of glycolysis other than carbohydrates.

Glycolysis A series of enzymatically catalyzed reactions, occurring within cells, by which glucose is converted to adenosine triphosphate (ATP) and pyruvic acid during aerobic metabolism.

Gonad A gamete-producing gland, as an ovary or a testis.

Gradient The rate of increase or decrease of a measurable phenomenon expressed as a function of a second; or the visual representation of such a change.

Granuloma A small mass of nodular granulation tissue resulting from chronic inflammation, injury, or infection. (Adjective: granulomatous)

Hapten A small, nonproteinaceous substance that is not antigenic by itself but that can act as an antigen when combined with a larger molecule.

Haustrum A structure resembling a recess or sacculation. (Plural: haustra)

Hematoma A localized collection of extravasated blood trapped in an organ, space, or tissue, resulting from a break in the wall of a blood vessel.

Hematopoiesis The normal formation and development of blood cells.

Hemianopia Defective vision or blindness in half of the visual field of one or both eyes.

Heterozygous Having two different alleles at corresponding loci on homologous chromosomes.

Heterogeneous Consisting of or composed of dissimilar elements or parts; or not having a uniform quality throughout. (Noun: heterogeneity)

Histology The branch of anatomy that deals with the minute (microscopic) structure, composition, and function of cells and tissue. (Adjective: histologic)

Homolog Any organ or part corresponding in function, position, origin, and structure to another organ or part, as the flippers of a seal that correspond to human hands. (Adjective: homologous)

Homozygous Having two identical alleles at corresponding loci on homologous chromosomes.

Humoral Relating to elements dissolved in the blood or body fluids.

Hydrolysis The chemical alteration or decomposition of a compound into fragments by the addition of water.

Hyperemia An excess or engorgement of blood in a part of the body.

Hyperesthesia An unusual or pathologic increase in sensitivity of a part, especially the skin, or of a particular sense.

Hyperplasia An abnormal multiplication or increase in the number of normal cells of a body part.

Hypertonic A solution having a greater concentration of solute than another solution with which it is compared, hence exerting more osmotic pressure than that solution.

Hypertrophy The enlargement or overgrowth of an organ that is due to an increase in the size of its cells rather than the number of its cells.

Hypesthesia An abnormal decrease of sensation in response to stimulation of the sensory nerves. (Also called hypoesthesia.)

Hypotonic A solution having a lesser concentration of solute than another solution with which it is compared, hence exerting less osmotic pressure than that solution.

Hypoxia An inadequate supply of oxygen to tissue that is below physiologic levels despite adequate perfusion of the tissue by blood.

Iatrogenic Induced inadvertently through the activity of a physician or by medical treatment or diagnostic procedures.

Idiopathic Arising spontaneously or from an unknown cause.

Idiosyncrasy A physical or behavioral characteristic or manner that is unique to an individual or to a group. (Adjective: idiosyncratic)

Incidence The rate at which a certain event occurs (e.g., the number of new cases of a specific disease during a particular period of time in a population at risk).

Inclusion The act of enclosing or the condition of being enclosed; or anything that is enclosed.

Infarction Necrosis or death of tissues due to local ischemia resulting from obstruction of blood flow.

In situ In the natural or normal place; or something, such as cancer, that is confined to its place of origin and has not invaded neighboring tissues.

Interferon Any one of a group of small glycoproteins (cytokines) produced in response to viral infection and which inhibit viral replication.

Interleukin Any of several multifunctional cytokines produced by a variety of lymphoid and nonlymphoid cells, including immune cells, that stimulate or otherwise affect the function of lympopoietic and other cells and systems in the body.

Interstitial Relating to or situated between parts or in the interspaces of a tissue.

Intramural Situated or occurring within the wall of an organ.

Intrinsic Pertaining exclusively to a part or situated entirely within an organ or tissue.

In vitro A biologic reaction occurring in an artificial environment, such as a test tube.

In vivo A biologic reaction occurring within the living body.

Involution The act or instance of enfolding, entangling, or turning inward.

Ionize To separate or change into ions.

Ipsilateral Situated on, pertaining to, or affecting the same side of the body.

Ischemia Decreased blood supply to a body organ or part, usually due to functional constriction or actual obstruction of a blood vessel.

Juxtaarticular Situated near a joint or in the region of a joint.

Juxtaglomerular Near to or adjoining a glomerulus of the kidney.

Karyotype The total chromosomal characteristics of a cell; or the micrograph of chromosomes arranged in pairs in descending order of size.

Keratin A fibrous, sulfur-containing protein that is the primary component of the epidermis, hair, and horny tissues. (Adjective: keratinous)

Keratosis Any skin condition in which there is overgrowth and thickening of the cornified epithelium.

Ketosis A condition characterized by the abnormal accumulation of ketones (organic compounds with a carboxyl group attached to two carbon atoms) in the body tissues and fluid.

Kinesthesia The sense of movement, weight, tension, and position of body parts mediated by input from joint and muscle receptors and hair cells. (Adjective: kinesthetic)

Kyphosis An abnormal condition of the vertebral column, characterized by increased convexity in the curvature of the thoracic spine as viewed from the side.

Lacuna A small pit or cavity within a structure, especially bony tissue; or a defect or gap, as in the field of vision.

Lateral A position farther from the median plane or midline of the body or a structure; or situated on, coming from, or directed towards the side.

Lesion Any wound, injury, or pathologic change in body tissue.

Lethargy The lowered level of consciousness characterized by listlessness, drowsiness, and apathy; or a state of indifference.

Ligament One of many predominantly white, shiny, flexible bands of fibrous tissue that binds joints together and connects bones or cartilages.

Ligand A group, ion, or molecule that binds to the central atom or molecule in a chemical complex.

Lipid Any of the group of fats and fatlike substances characterized by being insoluble in water and soluble in nonpolar organic solvents, such as chloroform and ether.

Lipoprotein Any one of the conjugated proteins that is a complex of protein and lipid.

Lobule A small lobe.

Lordosis The anterior concavity in the curvature of the lumbar and cervical spine as observed from the side.

Lumen A cavity or the channel within a tube or tubular organ of the body.

Luteal Of or pertaining to or having the properties of the corpus luteum.

Lysis Destruction or dissolution of a cell or molecule through the action of a specific agent.

Maceration Softening of tissue by soaking, especially in acidic solutions.

Macroscopic Large enough to be visible with the unaided eye or without the microscope.

Macula A small, flat blemish, thickening, or discoloration that is flush with the skin surface. (Adjective: macular)

Malaise A vague feeling of bodily fatigue and discomfort.

Manometry The measurement of tension or pressure of a liquid or gas using a device called a manometer.

Marasmus A condition of extreme protein-calorie malnutrition that is characterized by growth retardation and progressive wasting of subcutaneous tissue and muscle and occurs chiefly during the first year of life.

Matrix The intracellular substance of a tissue or the basic substance from which a specific organ or kind of tissue develops.

Meatus An opening or passage through any body part.

Medial Pertaining to the middle; or situated or oriented toward the midline of the body.

Mediastinum The mass of tissues and organs in the middle of the thorax, separating the pleural sacs containing the two lungs.

Meiosis The division of a sex cell as it matures, so that each daughter nucleus receives one half of the number of chromosomes characteristic of the somatic cells of the species.

Mesoderm The middle layer of the three primary germ layers of the developing embryo, lying between the ectoderm and the endoderm.

Metabolism The sum of all the physical and chemical processes by which living organisms are produced and maintained, and also the transformation by which energy is provided for vital processes and activities.

Metaplasia Change in type of adult cells in a tissue to a form that is not normal for that tissue.

Metastasis The transfer of disease (e.g., cancer) from one organ or part to another not directly connected with it. (Adjective: metastatic)

Miosis Contraction of the pupil of the eye.

Mitosis A type of indirect cell division that occurs in somatic cells and results in the formation of two daughter nuclei containing the identical complements of the number of chromosomes characteristic of the somatic cells of the species.

Molecule The smallest mass of matter that exhibits the properties of an element or compound.

Morbidity A diseased condition or state; the relative incidence of a disease or of all diseases in a population.

Morphology The study of the physical form and structure of an organism; or the form and structure of a particular organism. (Adjective: morphologic)

Mosaicism In genetics, the presence in an individual or in an organism of cell cultures having two or more cell lines that differ in genetic constitution but are derived from a single zygote.

Mutagen Any chemical or physical agent that induces a genetic mutation (an unusual change in form, quality, or some other characteristic) or increases the mutation rate by causing changes in DNA.

Mydriasis Physiologic dilatation of the pupil of the eye.

Myoclonus A spasm of a portion of a muscle, an entire muscle, or a group of muscles.

Myoglobin The oxygen-transporting pigment of muscle consisting of one heme molecule containing one iron molecule attached to a single globin chain.

Myopathy Any disease or abnormal condition of skeletal muscle, usually characterized by muscle weakness, wasting, and histologic changes within muscle tissue.

Myotome The muscle plate or portion of an embryonic somite that develops into a voluntary muscle; or a group of muscles innervated by a single spinal segment.

Necrosis Localized tissue death that occurs in groups of cells or part of a structure or an organ in response to disease or injury.

Neutropenia An abnormal decrease in the number of neutrophilic leukocytes in the blood.

Nidus The point where a morbid process originates, develops, or is located.

Nociception The reception of painful stimuli from the physical or mechanical injury to body tissues by nociceptors (receptors usually found in either the skin or the walls of the viscera).

Nosocomial Pertaining to or originating in a hospital, such as a nosocomial infection; an infection acquired during hospitalization.

Nystagmus Involuntary, rapid, rhythmic movements of the eyeball.

Oncogene A gene that is capable of causing the initial and continuing conversion of normal cells into cancer cells.

Oocyte A primordial or incompletely developed ovum.

Oogenesis The process of the growth and maturation of the female gametes, or ova.

Organelle Any one of the various membrane-bound particles of distinctive morphology and function present within most cells, as the mitochondria, the Golgi complex, and the lysosomes.

Orthopnea An abnormal condition in which a person must be in an upright position in order to breathe deeply or comfortably.

Osmolality The concentration of osmotically active particles in solution expressed in osmols or milliosmols per kilogram of solvent.

Osmolarity The concentration of osmotically active particles in solution expressed in osmols or milliosmols per liter of solution.

Osmosis The movement or passage of a pure solvent, such as water, through a semipermeable membrane from a solution that has a lower solute concentration to one that has a higher solute concentration.

Osteophyte A bony project or outgrowth.

Palpable Perceptible by touch.

Papilla A small nipple-shaped projection, elevation, or structure, as the conoid papillae of the tongue.

Papule A small circumscribed, solid elevation of the skin less than one centimeter in diameter. (Adjective: papular)

Paracrine A mode of hormone action in which a chemical messenger that is synthesized and released from a cell acts on nearby cells of a different type and affects their function.

Paralysis An abnormal condition characterized by the impairment or loss of motor function or the loss of sensation, or both, due to a lesion of the neural or muscular mechanism.

Paraneoplastic Relating to alterations produced in tissue remote from a tumor or its metastases.

Parenchyma The basic tissue or elements of an organ as distinguished from supporting or connective tissue or elements. (Adjective: parenchymal)

Paresis Slight or partial paralysis.

Paresthesia Any abnormal touch sensation, which can be experienced as numbness, tingling, or a "pins and needles" feeling, often in the absence of external stimuli.

Parietal Pertaining to the outer wall of a cavity or organ; or pertaining to the parietal bone of the skull or the parietal lobe of the brain.

Parous Having borne one or more viable offspring.

Pathogen Any microorganism capable of producing disease.

Pedigree A systematic presentation, such as in a table, chart, or list, of an individual's ancestors that is used in human genetics in the analysis of inheritance.

Peptide Any of a class of molecular chain compounds composed of two or more amino acids joined by peptide bonds.

Perfusion The process or act of pouring over or through, especially the passage of a fluid through a specific organ or an area of the body.

Peripheral Pertaining to the outside, surface, or surrounding area of an organ or other structure; or located away from a center or central structure.

Permeable A condition of being pervious, or permitting passage, so that fluids and certain other substances can pass through, as a permeable membrane.

Pervasive Pertaining to something that becomes diffused throughout every part.

Petechia A tiny, perfectly round purplish red spot that appears on the skin as a result of minute intradermal or submucous hemorrhage. (Plural: petechiae)

Phagocytosis The process by which certain cells engulf and consume foreign material and cell debris.

Phalanx Any one of the bones composing the fingers of each hand and the toes of each foot.

Phenotype The complete physical, biochemical, and physiologic makeup of an individual, as determined by the interaction of both genetic makeup and environmental factors.

Pheresis A procedure in which blood is withdrawn from a donor, a portion (plasma, leukocytes, etc.) are separated and retained, and the remainder is reperfused into the donor. It includes plasmapheresis and leukopheresis.

Pili Hair; or in microbiology, the minute filamentous appendages of certain bacteria. (Singular: pilus)

Plexus A network of intersecting nerves, blood vessels, or lymphatic vessels.

Polygene Any of a group of nonallelic genes that interact to influence the same character in the same way so that the effect is cumulative, usually of a quantitative nature, as size, weight, or skin pigmentation. (Adjective: polygenic)

Polymorph One of several, or many, forms of an organism or cell. (Adjective: polymorphic)

Polyp A small, tumor-like growth that protrudes from a mucous membrane surface.

Presbyopia A visual condition (farsightedness) that commonly develops with advancing years or old age in which the lens loses elasticity causing defective accommodation and inability to focus sharply for near vision.

Prevalence The number of new and old cases of a disease that are present in a population at a given time or occurrences of an event during a particular period of time .

Prodrome An early symptom indicating the onset of a condition or disease. (Adjective: prodromal)

Prolapse The falling down, sinking, or sliding of an organ from its normal position or location in the body.

Proliferation The reproduction or multiplication of similar forms, especially cells.

Pronation Assumption of a position in which the ventral, or front, surface of the body or part of the body faces downward. (Adjective: prone)

Propagation The act or action of reproduction.

Proprioception The reception of stimuli originating from within the body regarding body position and muscular activity by proprioceptors (sensory nerve endings found in muscles, tendons, joints, and the vestibular apparatus).

Prosthesis An artificial replacement for a missing body part; or a device designed and applied to improve function, such as a hearing aid.

Protagonist An agent, such as a substance or drug, that causes or supports the action of a neuromediator or body function; or a muscle that by its contraction causes a particular movement.

Proteoglycans Any one of a group of polysaccharide-protein conjugates occurring primarily in the matrix of connective tissue and cartilage.

Protooncogene A normal cellular gene that with alteration, such as by mutation, becomes an active oncogene.

Proximal Closer to a point of reference, usually the trunk of the body, than other parts of the body.

Pruritus The symptom of itching, an uncomfortable sensation leading to the urge to rub or scratch the skin to obtain relief. (Adjective: pruritic)

Purpura A small hemorrhage, up to about 1 cm in diameter, in the skin, mucous membrane, or serosal surface; or any of several bleeding disorders characterized by the presence of purpuric lesions.

Purulent Producing or containing pus.

Quiescent Quiet, causing no disturbance, activity, or symptoms.

Reflux An abnormal backward or return flow of a fluid, such as stomach contents, blood, or urine.

Regurgitation A flow of material that is in the opposite direction from normal, as in the return of swallowed food

into the mouth or the backward flow of blood through a defective heart valve.

Remission The partial or complete disappearance of the symptoms of a chronic or malignant disease; or the period of time during which the abatement of symptoms occurs.

Resorption The loss of substance or bone by physiologic or pathologic means, for example, the loss of dentin and cementum of a tooth.

Retrograde Moving backward or against the usual direction of flow; reverting to an earlier state or worse condition (degenerating); catabolic.

Retroversion A condition in which an entire organ is tipped backward or in a posterior direction, usually without flexion or other distortion.

Rostral Pertaining to or resembling a beak.

Sacroiliitis Inflammation in the sacroiliac joint.

Sclerosis A condition characterized by induration or hardening of tissue resulting from any of several causes, including inflammation, diseases of the interstitial substance, and increased formation of connective tissues.

Semipermeable Partially but not wholly permeable, especially a membrane that permits the passage of some (usually small) molecules but not of other (usually larger) particles.

Senescence The process or condition of aging or growing old.

Sepsis The presence in the blood or other tissues of pathogenic microorganisms or their toxins; or the condition resulting from the spread of microorganisms or their products. (Adjective: septic)

Serous Relating to or resembling serum; or containing or producing serum, such as a serous gland.

Shunt To divert or bypass bodily fluid from one channel, path, or part to another; a passage or anastomosis between two natural channels, especially between blood vessels, established by surgery or occurring as an abnormality.

Soma The body of an organism as distinguished from the mind; all of an organism, excluding germ cells; the body of a cell.

Spasticity The condition characterized by spasms or other uncontrolled contractions of the skeletal muscles. (Adjective: spastic)

Spatial Relating to, having the character of, or occupying space.

Sphincter A ringlike band of muscle fibers that constricts a passage or closes a natural orifice of the body.

Stenosis An abnormal condition characterized by the narrowing or stricture of a duct or canal.

Stria A streak or a linear scarlike lesion that often results from rapidly developing tension in the skin; or a narrow band-like structure, especially the longitudinal collections of nerve fibers in the brain.

Stricture An abnormal temporary or permanent narrowing of the lumen of a duct, canal, or other passage, as the esophagus, because of inflammation, external pressure, or scarring.

Stroma The supporting tissue or the matrix of an organ as distinguished from its functional element, or parenchyma.

Stupor A lowered level of consciousness characterized by lethargy and unresponsiveness in which a person seems unaware of his or her surroundings.

Subchondral Beneath a cartilage.

Subcutaneous Beneath the skin.

Sulcus A shallow groove, depression, or furrow on the surface of an organ, as a sulcus on the surface of the brain, separating the gyri.

Supination Assuming the position of lying horizontally on the back, or with the face upward. (Adjective: supine)

Suppuration The formation of pus, or purulent matter.

Symbiosis Mode of living characterized by close association between organisms of different species, usually in a mutually beneficial relationship.

Sympathomimetic An agent or substance that produces stimulating effects on organs and structures similar to those produced by the sympathetic nervous system.

Syncope A brief lapse of consciousness due to generalized cerebral ischemia.

Syncytium A multinucleate mass of protoplasm produced by the merging of a group of cells.

Syndrome A complex of signs and symptoms that occur together to present a clinical picture of a disease or inherited abnormality.

Synergist An organ, agent, or substance that aids or cooperates with another organ, agent, or substance.

Synthesis An integration or combination of various parts or elements to create a unified whole.

Systemic Pertaining to the whole body rather than to a localized area or regional portion of the body.

Systole The contraction, or period of contraction, of the heart that drives the blood onward into the aorta and pulmonary arteries.

Tamponade Stoppage of the flow of blood to an organ or a part of the body by pathologic compression, such as the compression of the heart by an accumulation of pericardial fluid.

Tetratogen Any agent or factor that induces or increases the incidence of developmental abnormalities in the fetus.

Thrombus A stationary mass of clotted blood or other formed elements that remains attached to its place of origin along the wall of a blood vessel, frequently obstructing the circulation. (Plural: thrombi)

Tinnitus A tinkling, buzzing, or ringing noise heard in one or both ears.

Tophus A chalky deposit containing sodium urate that most often develops in periarticular fibrous tissue, typically in individuals with gout. (Plural: tophi)

Torsion The act or process of twisting in either a positive (clockwise) or negative (counterclockwise) direction.

Trabecula A supporting or anchoring stand of connective tissue, such as the delicate fibrous threads connecting the inner surface of the arachnoid to the pia mater.

Transmural Situated or occurring through the wall of an organ.

Transudate A fluid substance passed through a membrane or extruded from the blood.

Tremor Involuntary quivering or trembling movements caused by the alternating contraction and relaxation of opposing groups of skeletal muscles.

Trigone A triangular-shaped area.

Ubiquitous The condition or state of existing or being everywhere at the same time.

Ulcer A circumscribed excavation of the surface of an organ or tissue, which results from necrosis that accompanies some inflammatory, infectious, or malignant processes. (Adjective: ulcerative)

Urticaria A pruritic skin eruption of the upper dermis, usually transient, characterized by wheals (hives) of various shapes and sizes.

Uveitis An inflammation of all or part of the uveal tract of the eye.

Ventral Pertaining to a position toward the belly of the body; or situated or oriented toward the front or anterior of the body.

Vertigo An illusory sensation that the environment or one's own body is revolving.

Vesicle A small bladder or sac, as a small, thin-walled, raised skin lesion, containing liquid.

Visceral Pertaining to the viscera, or internal organs of the body.

Viscosity Pertaining to the physical property of fluids, caused by the adhesion of adjacent molecules, that determines the internal resistance to shear forces.

Zoonosis A disease of animals that may be transmitted to humans from its primary animal host under natural conditions.

Index

Page numbers followed by *f* indicate figures; those followed by *t* indicate tables; and those followed by *c* indicate charts.

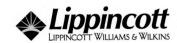

PREFIXES

a-, an- without, lack of
apnea (without breath)
anemia (lack of blood)

ab- separation, away from
abductor (leading away from)
aberrant (away from the usual course)

ad- to, toward, near to
adductor (leading toward)
adrenal (near the kidney)

ana- up, again, excessive
anapnea (to breathe again)
anasarca (severe edema)

ante- before, in front of
antecubital (in front of the elbow)
antenatal (occurring before birth)

anti- against, counter
anticoagulant (opposing coagulation)
antisepsis (against infection)

ap-, apo- separation, derivation from
apocrine (type of glandular secretion
that contains cast-off parts of the
secretory cell)

aut-, auto- self
autoimmune (immunity to self)
autologous (pertaining to self graft or
blood transfusion)

bi- two, twice, double
biarticulate (pertaining to two joints)
bifurcation (two branches)

brady- slow
bradyesthesia (slowness or dullness of
perception)

cata- down, under, lower, negative, against
catabolism (breaking down)
catalepsy (diminished movement)

circum- around, about
circumflex (winding around)
circumference (surrounding)

contra- against, counter
contraindicated (not indicated)
contralateral (opposite side)

de- away from, down from, remove
dehydrate (remove water)
deaminate (remove an amino group)

dia- through, apart, across, completely
diapedesis (ooze through)
diagnosis (complete knowledge)

dis- apart, reversal, separation
discrete (made up of separated parts)
disruptive (bursting apart)

dys- difficulty, faulty, painful
dysmenorrhea (painful menstruation)
dyspnea (difficulty breathing)

e-, ex- out from, out of
enucleate (remove from)
exostosis (outgrowth of bone)

ec- out from
eccentric (away from center)
ectopic (out of place)

ecto- outside, situated on
ectoderm (outer skin)
ectoretina (outer layer of retina)

em-, en- in, on
empyema (pus in)
encephalon (in the brain)

endo- within, inside
endocardium (within heart)
endometrium (within uterus)

epi- upon, after, in addition
epidermis (on skin)
epidural (upon dura)

eu- well, easily, good
eupnea (easy or normal respiration)
euthyroid (normal thyroid function)

exo- outside
exocolitis (inflammation of outer
coat of colon)
exogenous (originating outside)

extra- outside of, beyond
extracellular (outside cell)
extrapleural (outside pleura)

hemi- half
hemialgia (pain affecting only one
side of the body)
hemilingual (affecting one side of the
tongue)

hyper- extreme, above, beyond
hyperemia (excessive blood)
hypertrophy (overgrowth)

hypo- under, below
hypotension (low blood pressure)
hypothyroidism (underfunction of
thyroid)

im-, in- in, into, on
immersion (act of dipping in)
injection (act of forcing fluid into)

im-, in- not
immature (not mature)
inability (not able)

infra- beneath
infraclavicular (below the clavicle)
infraorbital (below the eye)

inter- among, between
intercostal (between the ribs)
intervene (come between)

intra- within, inside
intraocular (within the eye)
intraventricular (within the ventricles)

intro- into, within
introversion (turning inward)
introduce (lead into)

iso- equal, same
isotonia (equal tone, tension, or
activity)
isotypical (of the same type)

juxta- near, close by
juxtaglomerular (near an adjoining
glomerulus in the kidney)
juxtaspinal (near the spinal column)

macro- large, long, excess
macrocephaly (excessive head size)
macrodystrophia (overgrowth of a part)

mal- bad, abnormal
maldevelopment (abnormal growth or
development)
malfunction (to function imperfectly
or badly)

mega- large, enlarged, abnormally
large size
megaprosopous (having a large face)
megasoma (great size and stature)

meso- middle, intermediate, moderate
mesoderm (middle germ layer of
embryo)
mesocephalic (pertaining to a skull
with an average breadth–length
index)

meta- beyond, after, accompanying
metacarpal (beyond the wrist)
metamorphosis (change of form)

micro- small size or amount
microbe (a minute living organism)
microtiter (a titer of minute
quantity)

neo- new, young, recent
neoformation (a new growth)
neonate (newborn)

oligo- few, scanty, less than normal
oligogenic (produced by a few genes)
oligospermia (abnormally low number of spermatozoa in the semen)

para- beside, beyond
paracardiac (beside the heart)
paraurethral (near the urethra)

per- through
perforate (bore through)
permeate (pass through)

peri- around
peribronchia (around the bronchus)
periosteum (around bone)

poly- many, much
polyphagia (excessive eating)
polytrauma (occurrence of multiple
injuries)

post- after, behind in time or place
postoperative (after operation)
postpartum (after childbirth)

pre-, pro- in front of, before in time or
place
premaxillary (in front of the maxilla)
prognosis (foreknowledge)

pseud-, pseudo- false, spurious
pseudocartilaginous (made up of a
substance resembling cartilage)
pseudopregnancy (false pregnancy)

retro- backward, located behind
retrocervical (located behind cervix)
retrograde (going backward)

semi- half, partly
semiflexion (a limb midway between
flexion and extension)
semimembranous (composed in part
of membrane)